Brief TOC

Overview of CDC Hand Hygiene Guidelines

The Centers for Disease Control and Prevention have developed recommendations for hand hygiene in health care settings. Hand hygiene is a term that applies to handwashing, use of an antiseptic hand rub, or surgical hand antisepsis. Evidence suggests that hand antisepsis, the cleansing of hands with an antiseptic hand rub is more effective in reducing nosocomial infections than plain handwashing.

Follow These Guidelines in the Care of *All Patients*.

- Continue to wash hands with either plain soap or an antimicrobial soap and water (see Skill 7-1, page 175) whenever the hands are visibly soiled.
- Use an alcohol-based hand rub to routinely decontaminate the hands in the following clinical situations (NOTE: If alcohol-based hand rubs are not available, the alternative is handwashing.):
  - Before and after patient contact.
  - Before donning sterile gloves when inserting central intravascular catheters.
  - Before performing nonsurgical invasive procedures (e.g., urinary catheter insertion, nasotracheal suctioning).
  - After contact with body fluids or excretions, mucous membranes, nonintact skin, and wound dressings.
  - If moving from a contaminated body site (rectal area or mouth) to a clean body site (surgical wound, urinary meatus) during patient care.
  - After contact with inanimate objects (including medical equipment) in the immediate vicinity of the patient.
  - After removing gloves.
- Before eating and after using a restroom, wash hands with a nonantimicrobial or an antimicrobial soap and water.
- Antimicrobial-impregnated wipes (i.e., towelettes) are not a substitute for using an alcohol-based hand rub or antimicrobial soap.
- If exposure to *Bacillus anthracis* is suspected or proven, wash hands with a nonantimicrobial or an antimicrobial soap and water. The physical action of washing and rinsing hands is recommended because alcohols, chlorhexidine, iodophors, and other antiseptic agents have poor activity against spores.

Method for decontaminating hands

When using an alcohol-based hand rub, apply product to palm of one hand and rub hands together, covering all surfaces of hands and fingers, until hands are dry. Follow the manufacturer's recommendations regarding the volume of product to use.

Follow These Guidelines for Surgical Hand Antisepsis.

- Surgical hand antisepsis reduces the resident microbial count on the hands to a minimum. See Skill 37-1, page 968, for the surgical hand scrub procedure.
- The CDC recommends using an antimicrobial soap, and to scrub hands and forearms for the length of time recommended by the manufacturer, usually 2 to 6 minutes. The Association of Operating Room Nurses recommends 3 to 5 minutes. Refer to agency policy for time required.
- When using an alcohol-based surgical hand-scrub product with persistent activity, follow the manufacturer's instructions. Before applying the alcohol solution, prewash hands and forearms with a nonantimicrobial soap and dry hands and forearms completely. After application of the alcohol-based product as recommended, allow hands and forearms to dry thoroughly before donning sterile gloves.

General Recommendations for Hand Hygiene.

- Use hand lotions or creams to minimize the occurrence of irritant contact dermatitis associated with hand antisepsis or handwashing.
- Do not wear artificial fingernails or extenders when having direct contact with patients at high risk (e.g., those in intensive-care units or operating rooms).
- Keep natural nails tips less than ¼ inch long.
- Wear gloves when contact with blood or other potentially infectious materials, mucous membranes, and nonintact skin could occur.
- Remove gloves after caring for a patient. Do not wear the same pair of gloves for the care of more than one patient.
- Change gloves during patient care if moving from a contaminated body site to a clean body site.

(Modified from Centers for Disease Control and Prevention: Guidelines for Hand Hygiene in Health Care Settings, 2002. Available at http://www.cdc.gov/handhygiene; Centers for Disease Control and Prevention: *Guidelines for isolation precautions: preventing transmission of infectious agents in health care settings*, 2007. Available at http://www.cdc.gov/ncidod/dhqp/pdt/isolation2007.pdf.)

Clinical Nursing Skills & Techniques

Clinical Nursing Skills & Techniques

7th *Edition*

Anne Griffin Perry, RN, EdD, FAAN
Associate Dean and Professor
School of Nursing
Southern Illinois University–Edwardsville
Edwardsville, Illinois

Patricia A. Potter, RN, MSN, PhD, FAAN
Research Scientist
Siteman Cancer Center at Barnes-Jewish Hospital and
Washington University School of Medicine
St. Louis, Missouri

Section Editor
Wendy Ostendorf, RN, MS, EdD
Associate Professor of Nursing
Neumann College
Aston, Pennsylvania

With over 1200 illustrations

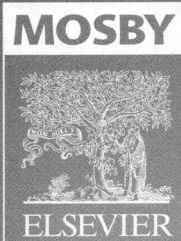

MOSBY

ELSEVIER

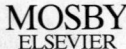
MOSBY
ELSEVIER

11830 Westline Industrial Drive
St. Louis, Missouri 63146

Clinical Nursing Skills & Techniques

ISBN: 978-0-323-05289-4

NOTICE

Previous editions copyrighted 2006, 2004, 2002, 1998, 1994, 1990, 1986

NCLEX, NCLEX-RN, and NCLEX-PN are federally registered trademarks and service marks of the National Council of State Boards of Nursing, Inc.

ISBN 978-0-323-05289-4

Executive Editor: Susan Epstein
Managing Editor: Jean Sims Fornango
Publishing Services Manager: Anne Altepeter
Senior Project Manager: Beth Hayes
Design Direction: Paula Catalano

Printed in the United States of America

Last digit is the print number: 9 8 7 6 5 4

*This book is dedicated to the many professional colleagues
I am proud to be associated with at Barnes-Jewish Hospital.
They practice at a level of excellence few achieve.*

Patricia A. Potter

*As always, this book is dedicated to my children. To be their mother
brings more joy, honor, and sense of pride than I could ever
imagine. They and their loved ones are truly my shining stars. As
they grow, things change, and I now dedicate this book to:*

*My daughter, Rebecca Lacey Perry Bryan, and her husband, Robert
Donald Bryan, and their two daughters Cora Elizabeth Bryan and
Amalie Mary Bryan, and my son: Horace Mitchell "Mitch" Perry.*

Anne G. Perry

Contributors

Jeanette S. Adams, PhD, ACNS-BC, CRNI
Faculty
University of Miami School of Nursing and Health Studies
Coral Gables, Florida

Sylvia K. Baird, BSN, MM
Manager, Nursing Quality
Spectrum Health
Grand Rapids, Michigan

Barbara A. Caton, RN, MSN
Assistant Professor
Missouri State University–West Plains
West Plains, Missouri

Aurelie Chinn, BN, MSN
Academic Nursing Skills Specialist and Simulation Coordinator/
    Instructor
Cabrillo College
Aptos, California

Janice C. Colwell, RN, MS, CWOCN, FAAN
Clinical Nursing Specialist
University of Chicago Medical Center
Chicago, Illinois

Kelly Jo Cone, RN, BSN, MS, PhD, CNE
Associate Professor–Graduate Program
Saint Francis College of Nursing
Peoria, Illinois

Ruth Curchoe, RN, MSN, CIC
Director, Infection Prevention and Control
Unity Health Systems
Rochester, New York

Wanda Cleveland Dubuisson, PhD, RN
Associate Professor and Director MSN Program
Joseph and Nancy Fail School of Nursing
William Carey University
Hattiesburg, Mississippi

Jane Fellows, RN, MSN, CWOCN
Ostomy Clinical Nurse Specialist
Duke University Health System
Durham, North Carolina

Susan Jane Fetzer, RN, BA, BSN, MSN, MBA, PhD
Associate Professor
College of Health and Human Services
University of New Hampshire
Durham, New Hampshire

Cathy Flasar, MSN, APRN, BC, FNP
Assistant Professor of Nursing
Barnes-Jewish College
St. Louis, Missouri

Amy Hall, RN, BSN, MS, PhD
Chair, Department of Nursing and Health Sciences
University of Evansville
Evansville, Indiana

Lori Klingman, MSN, RN
Advisor and Faculty
Ohio Valley School of Nursing
McKees Rocks, Pennsylvania

Nancy Laplante, PhD, RN
Assistant Professor
Neumann College
Aston, Pennsylvania

Nelda K. Martin, RN, ANP-BC, CCNS
Critical Care Clinical Nurse Specialist/Adult Nurse Practitioner
Barnes-Jewish Hospital Heart Services
St. Louis, Missouri

Lynne M. Murphy, RN, MSN
Nutrition Support Clinical Specialist
Private Practice/Consultant
Annandale, Virginia

Elaine K. Neel, RN, MSN
Nursing Instructor
Graham Hospital School of Nursing
Canton, Illinois

Mary Jane Ruhland, MSN, RN, BC
Performance Improvement Engineer
Progress West HealthCare Center
O'Fallon, Missouri

Jackie Raybuck Saleeby, PhD, RN, MSN
Associate Professor
Maryville University
Town and Country, Missouri

Julie S. Snyder, MSN, RN-BC
Adjunct Faculty
Old Dominion University, School of Nursing
Norfolk, Virginia

Kelly Schwartz, BSN, RN
Practice Consultant
Center for Practice Excellence
Barnes-Jewish Hospital
St. Louis, Missouri

Patricia A. Stockert, RN, BSN, MS, PhD
Associate Dean Undergraduate Program
Saint Francis Medical Center College of Nursing
Peoria, Illinois

Lynne Tier, RN, MSN, LNC
Associate Professor of Nursing
Learning Center Coordinator
Florida Hospital College of Health Science
Orlando, Florida

Nancy Tomaselli, RN, MSN, CS, CRPM, CWOCN
President and CEO
Premier Health Solutions, LLC
Cherry Hills, New York

Terry L Wood, PhD, RN
Lecturer
Southern Illinois University–Edwardsville
Edwardsville, Illinois

Rita Wunderlich, MSN, PhD
Director Baccalaureate Nursing Program
Assistant Professor
Saint Louis University School of Nursing
St. Louis, Missouri

Rhonda Yancey, BSN, RN
Practice Consultant
Center for Practice Excellence
Barnes-Jewish Hospital
St. Louis, Missouri

Valerie Yancey, PhD, RN, HNC, CHPN
Associate Professor
School of Nursing
Southern Illinois University–Edwardsville
Edwardsville, Illinois

Reviewers

Janet T. Adams, MSN, RT, RN
Nursing Instructor
Southeast Missouri State University
Cape Girardeau, Missouri

Joni Adams, RN, BSN, MSN
Assistant Professor
Ivy Tech Community College of Indiana
Evansville, Indiana

Colleen Andreoni, MSN, APRN, BC-NP
Instructor
Niehoff School of Nursing
Loyola University–Chicago
Chicago, Illinois

Ronda Bales, MN, RN
Adjunct Assistant Professor
Montana State University–Bozeman College of Nursing
Billings, Montana

Martha Baker, PhD, RN, APRN-BC
Director BSN Program
Professor of Nursing
St. John's College of Nursing–Southwest Baptist College
Springfield, Missouri

Doris Bartlett, BSN, MSN
Assistant Professor
Bethel College
Mishawaka, Indiana

Jennifer Beck, MSN, RN
Associate Professor; Chair, Undergraduate Studies
Our Lady of the Lake College
Baton Rouge, Louisiana

Brenda Becker, BSN, MA, RN
Nursing Faculty
North Hennepin Community College
Brooklyn Park, Minnesota

Karen Benjamin, RN, MSN
Assistant Professor
University of Wyoming
Fay W. Whitney School of Nursing
Laramie, Wyoming

Janet E. Bitzan, RN, PhD
Clinical Associate Professor
University of Wisconsin–Milwaukee
Milwaukee, Wisconsin

Phyllis Bonham, PhD, RN, MSN, CWOCN
Associate Professor, Director of Wound Care Education Program
College of Nursing, Medical University of South Carolina
Charleston, South Carolina

Patricia Buchsel, RN, MSN, FAAN
Clinical Instructor
Seattle University College of Nursing
Seattle, Washington

Barbara Caton, MSN, BSN
Assistant Professor of Nursing
Southwest Missouri State University–West Plains
West Plaines, Missouri

Aurelie Chinn, RN, MSN
Academic Nursing Skills and Simulation Specialist/Instructor
Cabrillo College
Monterey, California

Lissa Clark, MSN, RN, CNE
Instructor
Adult Health and Illness Department
College of Nursing
University of Nebraska Medical Center
Omaha, Nebraska

Kim Clevenger, MSN, RN, BC
Assistant Professor of Nursing
Morehead State University
Morehead, Kentucky

Patricia Conley, RN, BSN, MSN
Staff Nurse
Research Medical Center of Kansas City
Progressive Cardio-Pulmonary Care Unit
Kansas City, Missouri

Suzanne Costello, RN, MSN
Professional Nurse Educator
Jameson Hospital School of Nursing
New Castle, Pennsylvania

Neva Crogan, PhD, APRN, BC, GNP, FNGNA
Associate Professor
The University of Arizona College of Nursing
Tucson, Arizona

Barbara Derwinski-Robinson, MSN, RNC
Associate Professor
Montana State University–Billings Campus
Billings, Montana

Julie Potter-Dunlop, MN, RN
Assistant Professor
University of Hawaii–Maui
Kahului, Maui, Hawaii

Patricia Duckworth, MSN, APRN
Assistant Professor
University of Hawaii–Maui Community College
Kahului, Hawaii

Kathleen Ellstrom, RN, PhD, APRN, BC
Pulmonary Clinical Nurse Specialist
VA Loma Linda Healthcare System
Loma Linda, California

Susan Erue, RN, BSN, MS, PhD
Professor and Chair, Division of Nursing
Iowa Wesleyan College
Mount Pleasant, Iowa

Debbie Fischer, RN, MSN, CCRN
Adjunct Clinical Professor
University of Delaware School of Nursing
Newark, Delaware

Linda Kay Fluharty, RNC, MSN
Associate Professor
Ivy Tech Community College of Indiana
Indianapolis, Indiana

Cira Fraser, PhD, APRN, BC, MSCN
Associate Professor and Graduate Faculty
Marjorie K. Unterberg School of Nursing and Health Studies
Monmouth University
West Long Branch, New Jersey

Carole Gabriele, RN, BSN, MA, CNOR
Director
Bridgeport Hospital School of Nursing
Bridgeport, Connecticut

Teresa J. Getha-Eby, MSN, RN,C
Instructor
Education and Research Facilitator at Deaconess Hospital
Good Samaritan College of Nursing and Health Science
Cincinnati, Ohio

Margaret Gigstad, MS, RN, CSN
Clinical Assistant Professor
University of Arizona–College of Nursing
Tucson, Arizona

Margaret Gingrich, RN, MSN
Professor of Nursing
Harrisburg Area Community College
Harrisburg, Pennsylvania

Laurie Glover, MN, APRN, FNP, BC
Adjunct Assistant Professor
College of Nursing
Montana State University
Great Falls, Montana

Kathy Ham, RN, EdD
Assistant Professor
Southeast Missouri State University
Cape Girardeau, Missouri

John Harper, MSN, RN-BC
QM&I Reviewer; Clinical Educator
Taylor Hospital
Ridley Park, Pennsylvania

Melissa Henry, BSN, FNP, PhD
Assistant Professor
University of Northern Colorado
Greeley, Colorado

Janice Hoffman, RN, PhD
Instructor
Johns Hopkins School of Nursing
Clinical Nurse
Neurosciences Critical Care Unit
Johns Hopkins Hospital
Baltimore, Maryland

Patricia Hutchison, MSN, RN, CDE
Education Coordinator
Grove City Medical Center
Grove City, Pennsylvania

Helena Jermalovic, MSN, RN
Assistant Professor
University of Alaska–Anchorage
Anchorage, Alaska

Karen Johnson, RN, MSN, FNP-C
Nursing Instructor
Pittsburg State University
Pittsburg, Kansas

Stephanie Johnson, MSN, RN, BC, CNE
Assistant Professor of Nursing
Morehead State University
Morehead, Kentucky

Susan Kamath, MN, RN
Hospital Laboratory Coordinator/Professor of Nursing
Colin Count Community College
McKinney, Texas

Fran Kamp, RN, MSN
Nursing Faculty
Georgia Baptist College of Nursing of Mercer University
Atlanta, Georgia

Susan Porterfield, PhD, ARNP-C, MSN, BSN, MSHRMD, BA
Assistant Professor
Florida State University
Tallahassee, Florida

Theresa Schwindenhammer, RN, MSN
Assistant Professor of Nursing
Methodist College of Nursing
Peoria, Illinois

Corinne Settecase-Wu, MA, RN
Director of Experimental Learning
New York University–College of Nursing
New York, New York

Janet Somlyay, MSN, CNS, CPNP-AC/PC, CNE
Assistant Lecturer
Fay W. Whitney School of Nursing
University of Wyoming
Laramie, Wyoming

Marsha Ray, MSN, RN
Assistant Professor
Weber State University
Logan, Utah

Cherie R. Rebar, MSN, MBA, RN, FNP
Chair, Associate Degree Nursing Program
Assistant Professor
Kettering College of Medical Arts
Kettering, Ohio

Anita Reed, MSN, RN
Clinical Nursing Instructor/Faculty
Saint Joseph's College
Rensselaer, Indiana

Jill Reed, APRN, MSN
Instructor
University of Nebraska Medical Center College of Nursing–
Kearney Division
Kearney, Nebraska

Doreen Rogers, MSN, RN, CCRN
Instructor
St. Elizabeth College of Nursing
Utica, New York

Julie Ryhal, MEd, BSN, LCCE
Education Coordinator
Grove City Medical Center
Grove City, Pennsylvania

Maura Schlairet, RN, MSN, EdD
Assistant Professor
Valdosta State University College of Nursing
Valdosta, Georgia

Angela Stone Schmidt, MSNc, RNP, RN
Assistant Professor of Nursing
College of Nursing and Health Professions
Arkansas State University
Jonesboro, Arkansas

Debra L. Servello, RNP, MSN
Assistant Professor of Nursing
Rhode Island College
Providence, Rhode Island

Gale Sewell, RN, MSN, CNE
Assistant Professor of Nursing
Indiana Wesleyan University
Marion, Indiana

Ann Sprengel, EdD, RN
Professor
Department of Nursing
Southeast Missouri State University
Cape Girardeau, Missouri

Scott C. Thigpen RN, MSN, CCRN, CEN
Assistant Professor of Nursing
South Georgia College
Douglas, Georgia

Donna Thompson, MSN, CRNP, CCCN
Assistant Professor
Neumann College
Aston, Pennsylvania

Della F. Wagner, RN, MSN
Clinical Instructor
University of Texas Health Science Center–San Antonio
San Antonio, Texas

Michelle Lynne Williams, MSN, RN
Assistant Professor
Coordinator of Adult Health I
Austin Peay State University School of Nursing
Clarksville, Tennessee

Kathleen Williamson, BSN, MSN, PhD, RN
Assistant Professor of Nursing
Florida State University
Tallahassee, Florida

Janet Willis, MS, BSN
Senior Professor
Harrisburg Area Community College
Harrisburg, Pennsylvania

Paige Wimberley, RN, APN, CNE
Assistant Professor of Nursing
Arkansas State University
Jonesboro, Arkansas

Toni Wortham, RN, BSN, MSN
Professor of Nursing
Madisonville Community College
Madisonville, Kentucky

Jean Yockey, MSN, FNP, CNE
Assistant Professor
University of South Dakota
Vermillion, South Dakota

Clinical Reviewers

Liz Allibonne, PGCTLP, BSc, RGN
Nurse Teacher
Royal Brompton and Harefield NHS Trust
London, United Kingdom

Pam Bellefeuille, MN, APRN, BC, CNS, CEN
Associate Clinical Professor
University of California–San Francisco
San Francisco, California

Laura M. Criddle, MS, RN, CEN, CCNS
Clinical Nursing Specialist
Premier Jets/Lifeguard Air Ambulance

Ruth M. Curchoe, RN, MSN, CIC
Director, Infection Prevention and Control
Unity Health System
Rochester, New York

Lynn M. Czaplewski, MS, RN, CRNI, OCN
Clinical Assistant Professor
Columbia College of Nursing
Milwaukee, Wisconsin

Stephanie Gilbertson-White
Clinical Nurse Specialist for Pain Management
University of California San Francisco Medical Center
San Francisco, California

Elisabeth Harvey, RN, MSN, CWOCN
Memorial Medical Center
Modesto, California

Gina L. Heard, BSN
Nurse Coordinator for Nutrition Support
Barnes-Jewish Hospital
St. Louis, Missouri

Judith A. Jennrich, RN, PhD
Associate Professor of Nursing
Niehoff School of Nursing, Loyola University
Chicago, Illinois

Elizabeth Lemiska, BSN, RN, CWOCN
Wound, Ostomy, Continence Nurse Specialist
Middlesex Hospital
Middletown, Connecticut

Kathleen Murphy-Ende, RN, PhD, AOCNP
Nurse Practitioner
University of Wisconsin Hospitals and Clinics
Madison, Wisconsin

Kathleen A. Stevens, PhD, RN, CRRN
Quality Improvement Manager, Nursing and Allied Health
Rehabilitation Institute of Chicago
Chicago, Illinois

Marion F. Winkler, MS, RD, LDN, CNSD
Senior Clinical Teaching Associate of Surgery and Surgical
    Nutrition Specialist
Brown University Medical School and Rhode Island Hospital
Providence, Rhode Island

Cynthia Ann Worley, BSN, RN, CWOCN
Wound, Ostomy, Continence Nurse
The University of Texas M.D. Anderson Cancer Center
Houston, Texas

Contributors to Previous Editions

We would like to acknowledge the following people who contributed to previous editions of *Clinical Nursing Skills & Techniques*.

Jeannette Adams, PhD, MSN, APRN, CRNI
Nursing Consultant
Coconut Grove, Florida

Della Aridge, RN, MSN
Clinical Nurse Specialist
Abdominal Organ Transplant Service
Saint Louis University Health Sciences Center
St. Louis, Missouri

Elizabeth A. Ayello, PhD, MS, BSN, RN, CS, CWOCN
Clinical Assistant Professor
New York University, Division of Nursing
New York, New York

Margaret Benz, RN, MSN, CSANP
Adjunct Assistant Professor
Saint Louis University
St. Louis, Missouri

Barbara J. Berger, MSN, RN
Clinical Nurse Specialist for Nursing Practice and Nursing Informatics
Southwest General Health Center Partnering With University Hospitals Health Systems
Middleburg Heights, Ohio

Lyndal Guenther Brand, RN, BSN, MSN
Instructor, Missouri Baptist Medical Center
School of Nursing
St. Louis, Missouri

Peggy Breckinridge, RN, BSN, MSN, FNP
Associate Professor of Nursing
College of Health Sciences
Roanoke, Virginia

Victoria M. Brown, RN, BSN, MSN, PhD
Associate Professor, School of Nursing
Georgia College and State University
Milledgeville, Georgia

Gina Bufe, RN, BSN, MSN(R), PhD, CS
Psychiatric Clinical Nurse Specialist
Private Practice
Hyannis, Massachusetts

Gale Carli, MSN, MHed, BSN, RN
Assistant Professor
Ohlone College
Fremont, California

Ellen Carson, PhD
Associate Professor
Pittsburg State University
Pittsburg, Kansas

Maureen Carty, MSN, OCN
Oncology Clinical Nurse Specialist
Genesis Medical Center
Davenport, Iowa

Mary F. Clarke, MA, RN
Informatics Nurse Specialist
Genesis Medical Center
Davenport, Iowa

Janice C. Colwell, RN, MS, CWOCN
Clinical Nurse Specialist
University of Chicago Hospitals
Chicago, Illinois

Dorothy McDonnell Cooke, RN, PhD
Associate Professor of Nursing
Saint Louis University Health Sciences Center
St. Louis, Missouri

Eileen Costantinou, RN, BSN, MSN
Professional Practice Consultant
Barnes-Jewish Hospital
St. Louis, Missouri

Sheila A. Cunningham, RN, BSN, MSN
Assistant Professor of Nursing
Neumann College
Aston, Pennsylvania

Rick Daniels, RN, BSN, MSN, PhD
Associate Professor of Nursing
Oregon Health Sciences University at Southern
Ashland, Oregon

Carolyn Ruppel d'Avis, RN, BSN, MSN
Director, Baccalaureate Program/Adjunct Assistant Professor
The Catholic University of America
Washington, DC

Mardell Davis, RN, MSN, CETN
School of Nursing
University of Alabama
Birmingham, Alabama

Patricia A. Dettenmeier, RN, BSN, MSN(R), CCRN
Assistant Clinical Professor, School of Nursing
Instructor in Medicine, School of Medicine
Saint Louis University
St. Louis, Missouri

Wanda Cleveland Dubuisson, BSN, MN
Assistant Professor
University of Southern Mississippi, College of Nursing
Hattiesburg, Mississippi

Sharon J. Edwards, RN, MSN, PhD
Assistant Professor
College of Nursing
University of South Florida
Tampa, Florida

Martha E. Elkin, RN, MSN
Lactation Counselor
Stephens Memorial Hospital
Norway, Maine

Deborah Oldenburg Erickson, RN, BSN, MSN
Instructor, School of Nursing
Methodist Medical Center of Illinois
Peoria, Illinois

Debra Farrell, BSN, CNOR
Operating Room Staff Nurse
Saint Anthony's Medical Center
St. Louis, Missouri

Linda Fasciani, RN, BSN, MSN
Assistant Professor of Nursing
County College of Morris
Randolph, New Jersey

Susan Jane Fetzer, RN, BA, BSN, MSN, MBA, PhD
Associate Professor
University of New Hampshire
Durham, New Hampshire

Marlene S. Foreman, BSN, MN, RNCS
Associate Professor of Nursing
Louisiana State University at Eunice
Eunice, Louisiana

Carol P. Fray, RN, MA
Associate Professor, Adult Health Nursing
College of Nursing
University of North Carolina at Charlotte
Charlotte, North Carolina

Leah W. Frederick, RN, MS, CIC
Consultant
Infection Control Consultants
Scottsdale, Arizona

Paula Goldberg, RN, MS, MSN
Oncology Clinical Coordinator
Barnes Hospital
St. Louis, Missouri

Thelma Halberstadt, EdD, MS, BS, RN
Professor
Northern Essex Community College
Lawrence, Massachusetts

Amy Hall, PhD, MS, BSN, RN
Assistant Professor
Saint Francis Medical Center, College of Nursing
Peoria, Illinois

Linda C. Haynes, PhD, RN
Associate Professor
University of Northern Colorado
Greeley, Colorado

Diane Hildwein, RN, BC, MA
Director of Nursing Clinical Education
St. Luke's Hospital
Chesterfield, Missouri

Maureen B. Huhmann, MS, RD
Clinical Instructor and Clinical Dietician
University of Medicine and Dentistry of New Jersey
Newark, New Jersey

Nancy C. Jackson, RN, BSN, MSN, CCRN
Pulmonary Clinical Nurse Specialist
St. Mary's Health Center
St. Louis, Missouri

Ruth L. Jilka, RD, CDE
Diabetes Educator
Barnes Hospital
St. Louis, Missouri

Teresa M. Johnson, RN, MSN, CCRN
Clinical Nurse Specialist
The Medical Center of Central Georgia
Macon, Georgia

Judith Ann Kilpatrick, RN, DNSC
Assistant Professor
Widener University School of Nursing
Chester, Pennsylvania

Carl Kirton, RN, BSN, MA, CCRN, ACRN, ANP
Clinical Assistant, Professor of Nursing
New York University
New York, New York

Marilee Kuhrik, RN, MSN, PhD
Associate Professor
Colorado Mountain College
Glenwood Springs, Colorado

Nancy S. Kuhrik, RN, MSN, PhD
Associate Professor
Colorado Mountain College
Glenwood Springs, Colorado

Diane M. Kyle, RN, BSN, MS
Doctoral Candidate
Supervisor of Clinical Services/Clinical Nurse Specialist
East Hartford Visiting Nurse Association, Inc.
East Hartford, Connecticut

Louise K. Leitao, RN(c), BSN, MA
Director of Clinical Services
East Hartford Visiting Nurses Association, Inc.
East Hartford, Connecticut

Gail B. Lewis, RN, MSN
Associate Professor
Barnes College
St. Louis, Missouri

Ruth Ludwick, PhD, MSN, BSN, RNC, CNS
Associate Professor
Kent State University
Kent, Ohio

Mary Kay Macheca, MSN(R), RN, CS, ANP, CDE
Certified Adult Nurse Practitioner and Certified Diabetes Educator
The Bortz Diabetes Control Center
Richmond Heights, Missouri

Jill Feldman Malen, RN, MS, NS, ANP
Clinical Nurse Specialist
Barnes-Jewish Hospital at Washington University Medical Center
St. Louis, Missouri

Mary K. Mantese, RN, MSN
Director of Patient Care Services/Chief Nurse Executive
Barnes-Jewish West County Hospital
St. Louis, Missouri

Elizabeth Mantych, RN, MSN
Faculty
University of Missouri at St. Louis School of Nursing
St. Louis, Missouri

Tina Marrelli, MSN, MA, RN
Professor and Director
Transculutral Nursing Institute and MSN Program
Kean University
Union, New Jersey

Nelda K. Martin, APRN, BC, CCNS, ANP
Critical Care Clinical Nurse Specialist and Adult Nurse Practitioner
Barnes-Jewish Hospital at Washington University Medical Center
St. Louis, Missouri

Mary Mercer, RN, MSN
Coordinator, Cardiac Rehabilitation
St. John's Mercy Medical Center
Creve Coeur, Missouri

Rita Mertig, MS, BSN, RNC, CNS
Professor
John Tyler Community College
Richmond, Virginia

Norma Metheny, PhD, MSN, BSN, FAAN
Professor and Dorothy A. Votsmier Chair in Nursing
Saint Louis University School of Nursing
St. Louis, Missouri

Mary Dee Miller, RN, BSN, MS, CIC
Nurse Epidemiologist
Mercy Hamilton/Fairfield Hospitals
Hamilton, Ohio

Sharon M. J. Muhs, MSN, RN
Registered Nurse
Saint Luke's Hospital
Chesterfield, Missouri

Kathleen Mulryan, RN, BSN, MSN
Professor of Nursing
LaGuardia Community College
Long Island City, New York

Elaine K. Neel, RN, BSN, MSN
Nursing Instructor
Graham Hospital School of Nursing
Canton, Illinois

Meghan G. Noble, PhD, RN
Staff Nurse
MICU, Strong Memorial Hospital
University of Rochester Medical Center
Rochester, New York

Marsha Evans Orr, RN, BS, MS, CS
Zone Clinical Manager
Apria Healthcare
Phoenix, Arizona

Dula F. Pacquiao, EdD, RN, CTN
Professor and Director
Transcultural Nursing Institute and MSN Program
Kean University
Union, New Jersey

Sharon Phelps, RN, BSN, MS
Nursing Practice Consultant
Barnes-Jewish Hospital
St. Louis, Missouri

Catherine A. Robinson, BA, RN
Clinical Nurse Manager
Barnes-Jewish Hospital

Judith Roos, RN, MSN
Associate Professor
Jewish Hospital College of Nursing and Allied Health
St. Louis, Missouri

Jane Ruhland, RN, MSN, BSN
Education Coordinator
Barnes-Jewish St. Peters Hospital
St. Peters, Missouri

Jan Rumfelt, RNC, MSN, EdD
Associate Professor, School of Nursing
Southern Illinois University–Edwardsville
Edwardsville, Illinois

Jacqueline Raybuck Saleeby, PhD, RN, CS
Associate Professor
Jewish Hospital College of Nursing and Allied Health
St. Louis, Missouri

Linette M. Sarti, RN, BSN, CNOR
Operating Room Charge Nurse
Bayfront Medical Center
St. Petersburg, Florida

Kelly M. Schwartz, RN, BSN
Professional Practice Consultant
Barnes-Jewish Hospital
St. Louis, Missouri

April Sieh, RN, BSN, MSN
Assistant Professor
Delta College
University Center, Michigan

Marlene Smith, RN, BSN, MEd
Staff Development Specialist
St. Louis Regional Medical Center
St. Louis, Missouri

Julie Snyder, MSN, RNC
Faculty
Louise Obici School of Nursing
Suffolk, Virginia

Laura Sofield, MSN, APRN, BC
Director of Clinical Practice
Meridian Institute for Aging, Senior Health Center
Manchester, New Jersey

Sharon Souter, MSN, BSN
Director of Nursing Program
New Mexico State University at Carlsbad
Carlsbad, New Mexico

Martha A. Spies, RN, MSN
Assistant Professor
Deaconess College of Nursing
St. Louis, Missouri

Patricia A. Stockert, RN, BSN, MS, PhD
Associate Dean of Undergradute Program
Saint Francis Medical Center College of Nursing
Peoria, Illinois

Sandra Ann Szekely, RN, BSN
Director, Clinical and Infusion Services
Comfort Care of Michigan
Troy, Michigan

Nancy Tomaselli, RN, MSN, CS, CRNP, CWOCN, CLNC
President and CEO
Premier Health Solutions, LLC
Cherry Hills, New York

Riva Touger-Decker, PhD, RD, FADA
Associate Professor and Program Director
Graduate Programs in Clinical Nutrition,
Department of Primary Care, SHRP
Division of Nutrition, Department of Diagnostic Sciences
New Jersey Dental School
Newark, New Jersey

Joan Domigan Wentz, MSN, RN
Assistant Professor
Barnes-Jewish College of Nursing and Allied Health
St. Louis, Missouri

Terry L. Wood, PhD, RN
Assistant Professor
Barnes-Jewish College of Nursing and Allied Health
St. Louis, Missouri

Anne Falsone Vaughan, MSN, BSN, CCRN
Clinical Instructor
Bellarmine College, Lansing School of Nursing
Louisville, Kentucky

Cynthia Vishy, RN, BSN
Manager, Clinical Education
St. Louis Children's Hospital
St. Louis, Missouri

Pamela Becker Weilitz, MSN(R), RN, CS, ANP
Adult Nurse Practitioner
South City Health, LLC
St. Louis, Missouri

Laurel Wiersema, RN, MSN
Surgical Clinical Nurse Specialist
Barnes Hospital
St. Louis, Missouri

Rita Wunderlich, PhD(C), MSN(R), CCRN
Doctoral Candidate, Saint Louis University
Instructor
Clinical Nurse
Saint Louis University Hospital
St. Louis, Missouri

Rhonda Yancey, BSN, RN
Consultant, Professional Practice
Barnes-Jewish Hospital
St. Louis, Missouri

Preface to the Student

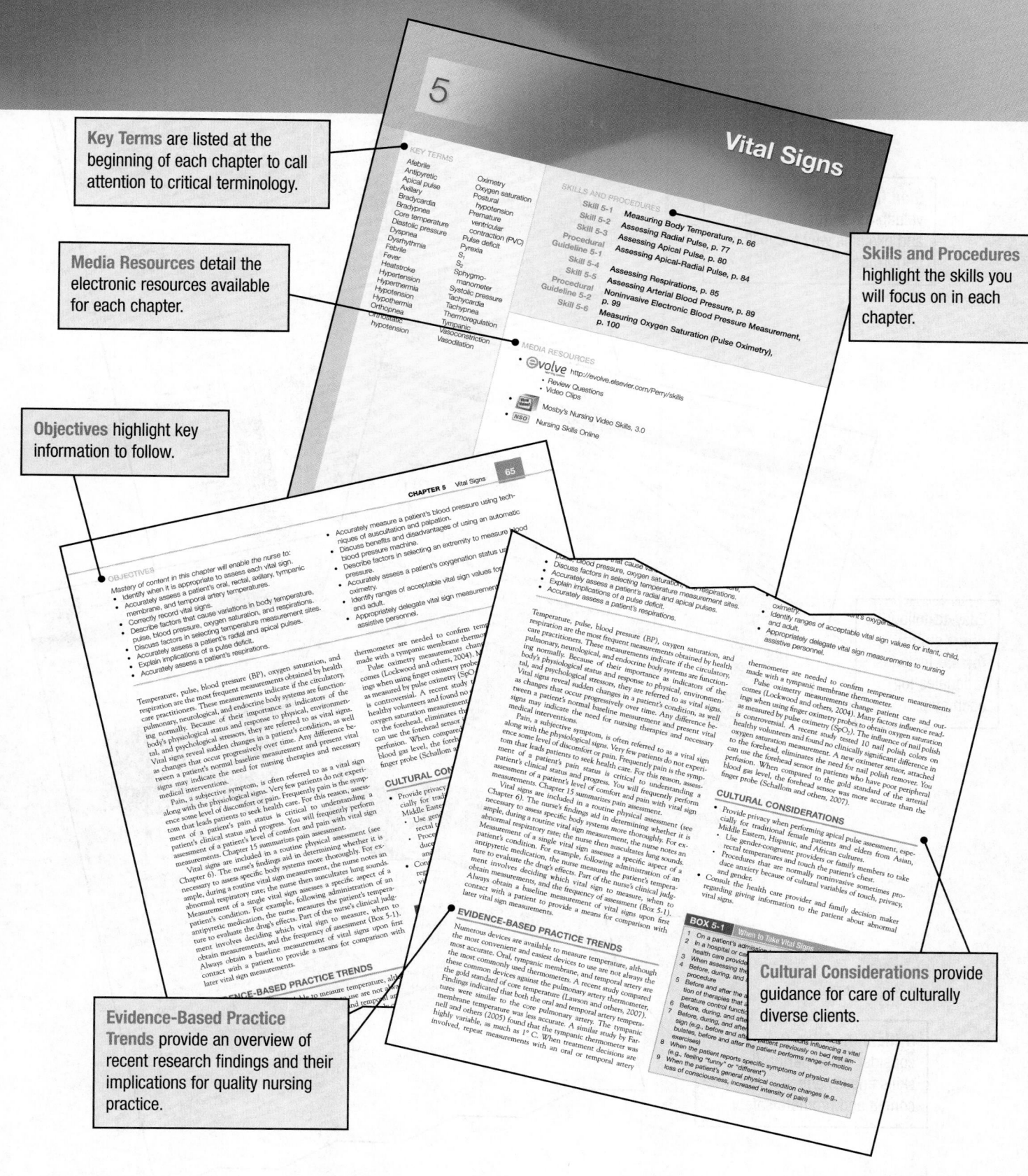

Key Terms are listed at the beginning of each chapter to call attention to critical terminology.

Media Resources detail the electronic resources available for each chapter.

Objectives highlight key information to follow.

Evidence-Based Practice Trends provide an overview of recent research findings and their implications for quality nursing practice.

Skills and Procedures highlight the skills you will focus on in each chapter.

Cultural Considerations provide guidance for care of culturally diverse clients.

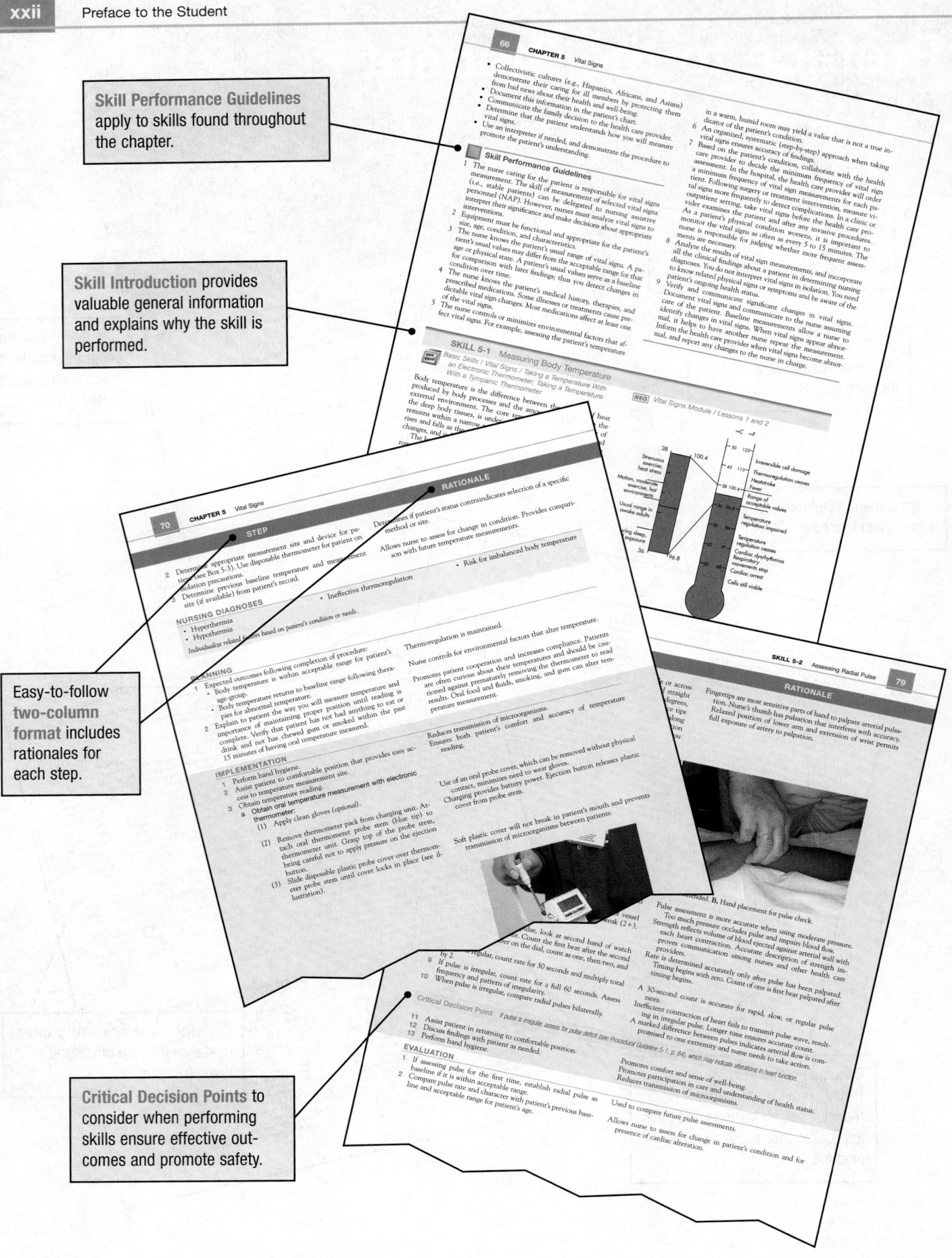

Skill Performance Guidelines apply to skills found throughout the chapter.

Skill Introduction provides valuable general information and explains why the skill is performed.

Easy-to-follow **two-column format** includes rationales for each step.

Critical Decision Points to consider when performing skills ensure effective outcomes and promote safety.

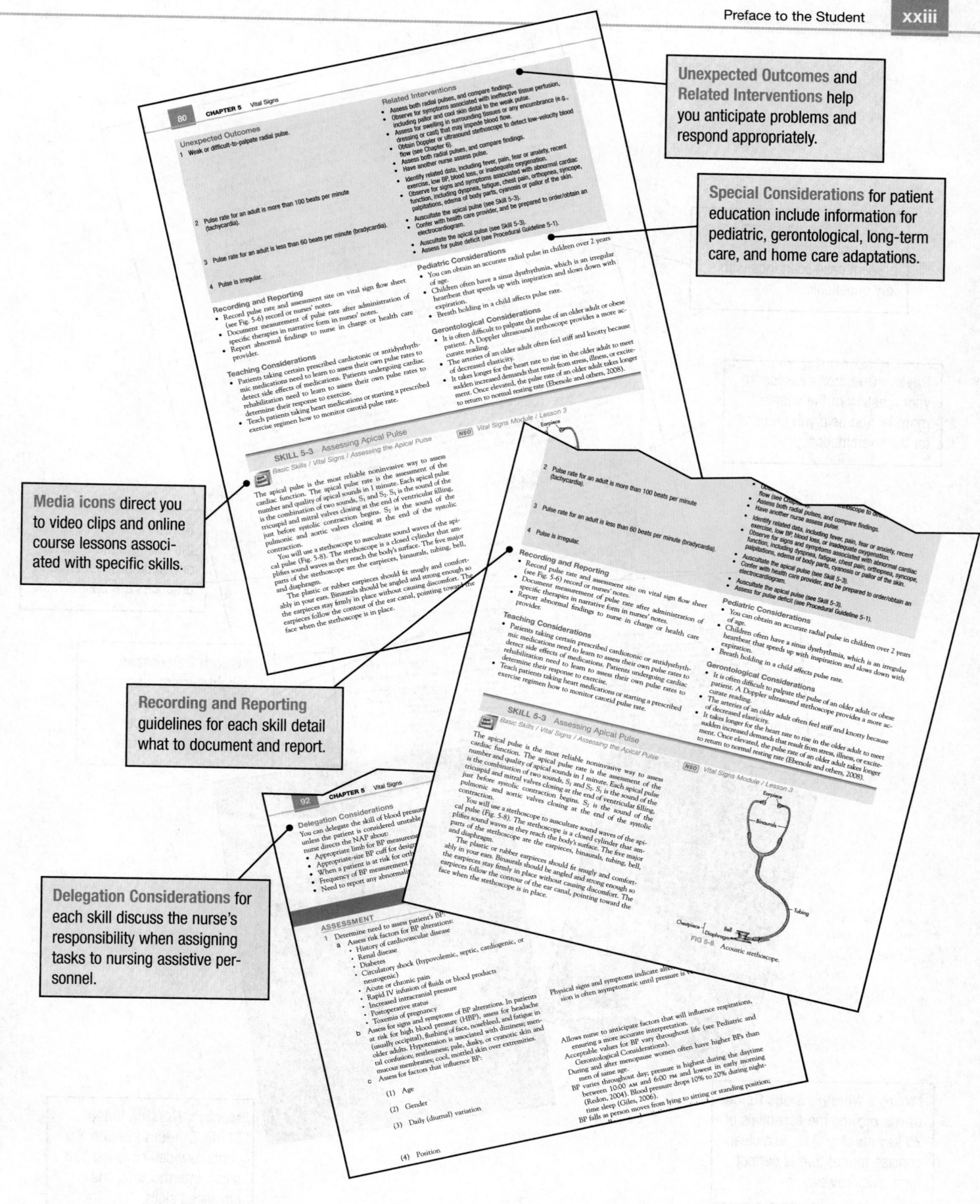

Unexpected Outcomes and **Related Interventions** help you anticipate problems and respond appropriately.

Special Considerations for patient education include information for pediatric, gerontological, long-term care, and home care adaptations.

Media icons direct you to video clips and online course lessons associated with specific skills.

Recording and Reporting guidelines for each skill detail what to document and report.

Delegation Considerations for each skill discuss the nurse's responsibility when assigning tasks to nursing assistive personnel.

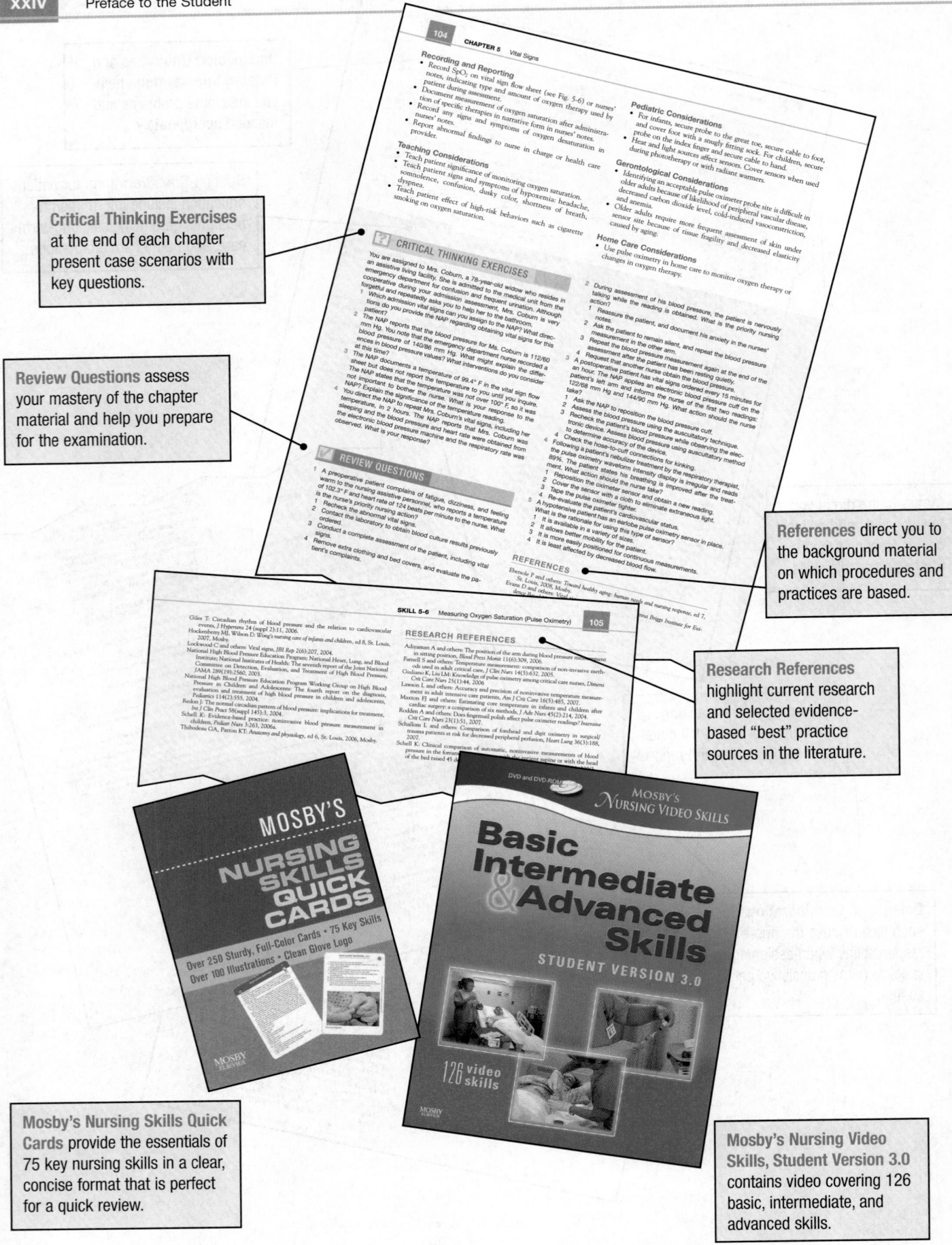

Critical Thinking Exercises at the end of each chapter present case scenarios with key questions.

Review Questions assess your mastery of the chapter material and help you prepare for the examination.

References direct you to the background material on which procedures and practices are based.

Research References highlight current research and selected evidence-based "best" practice sources in the literature.

Mosby's Nursing Skills Quick Cards provide the essentials of 75 key nursing skills in a clear, concise format that is perfect for a quick review.

Mosby's Nursing Video Skills, Student Version 3.0 contains video covering 126 basic, intermediate, and advanced skills.

Preface to the Instructor

Nursing education is incorporating an increasing amount of technology for patient care, adding the demand of technology literacy to the many demands already facing nursing students today. However, the need to develop fundamental knowledge and the critical thinking skills to apply that knowledge to individual patient needs continues to be far more important to the overall quality of care a nurse is able to deliver. This seventh edition of *Clinical Nursing Skills & Techniques* continues our tradition of teaching students both the how and the why of nursing care. Because successful performance is based on understanding, students are presented with both the evidence-based practice trends and the rationales for techniques. Students are reminded to consider many factors influencing patients, including age and cultural background. Analysis and critical thinking are promoted by completely new end-of-chapter exercises focused on clinical practice and NCLEX®-style review with additional review questions available on the companion Evolve site.

As always, *Clinical Nursing Skills & Techniques* provides your students with a comprehensive resource that will serve them well for many years to come.

Classic Features

- **Over 200 basic, intermediate, and advanced nursing skills and procedures** are presented.
- **Five-step nursing process** format provides a consistent presentation that helps students apply the process while learning each skill.
- **Skills and Procedures List, Objectives,** and **Key Terms** open each chapter.
- **Over 1200 full-color photos and drawings** help students master the material covered.
- **Skill Performance Guidelines** appear early in each chapter to focus student attention on the key principles of each skill.
- **Evidence-Based Practice Trends** in each chapter present students with the newest scientific evidence for the procedures and protocols presented. Recent research findings are discussed and their implications for patient care explored.
- **Rationales** are given for steps within skills so students learn the *why*, as well as the *how* for each skill. When relevant, rationales include citations from the current literature.
- **Critical Decision Points** alert students to key steps that affect patient safety and help them modify care as needed to meet individual patient needs.
- **Recording and Reporting** sections follow the evaluation discussion and alert students to what information should be documented in each situation.
- **Delegation Considerations** discuss the nurse's responsibility when delegating to nursing assistive personnel and highlight which tasks are appropriate for delegation and which are not.
- **Unexpected Outcomes** and **Related Interventions** remind students to be alert for potential problems and help them determine appropriate nursing interventions.
- **Teaching Considerations** remind students to incorporate teaching into their skills performance and highlight those points most important to convey to patients.

- **Home Care Considerations** teach students how to adapt skills for the home setting.
- **Glossary** includes all key terms.

New Features

- **Over 200 new photos** illustrate procedures and equipment.
- **Expanded panel of clinical specialists** reviewed 18 key chapters for accuracy and currency.
- **Content was streamlined** and the flow of information improved by the application of readability analysis techniques.
- More basic skills are presented in the streamlined **Procedural Guidelines** format.
- *Nursing Skills Online* icon integrates media content with chapter content to assist students in using the material in a complementary manner.
- *Mosby's Nursing Video Skills 3.0* icon integrates media content with chapter content to assist students in using the material in a complementary manner.
- New Coverage
  - *New* **Chapter on Using Evidence in Nursing Practice** familiarizes students with the steps of evidence-based practice, including how to develop a PICO question, how to locate the best evidence, how to critique evidence, and how to apply and evaluate use of evidence in nursing practice.
  - **Assessing Head and Neck**
  - **Assessing Genitals and Rectum**
  - **Breast Self-Examination**
  - **Genital Self-Examination**
  - **Special Tuberculosis Precautions**
  - **Use of Peak Flow Meter**
  - **Pacemaker Management**
  - **Use of Smart IV Pumps**
  - **Managing Triple Mix Parenteral Nutrition**
  - **Wound Assessment**
  - **Teaching Self-Catheterization**
- **Completely new end-of-chapter review questions** for every chapter.

Ancillaries

For Instructors

- **Evolve Instructor Resources (978-0-323-05479-9), including:**
  - ExamView test bank expanded to 1500 questions.
  - Instructor's Resource Manual with Educational Strategies, Clinical Activities, Independent Learning Activities, Media Integrator, Answers to End-of-Chapter Exercises, and Cross-Curriculum Guides.
  - Checklists (PDF format).
  - Answer key to additional review questions on Student Evolve Resources.
  - Answer Key to Review Questions included in *Mosby's Nursing Video Skills 3.0*.

- *Mosby's Nursing Video Skills* 3.0 DVDs available for use in the lab or classroom. Discs for computer (networkable) or DVD player included in each. Basic Skills (978-0-323-05294-8), Intermediate Skills (978-0-323-05295-5), Advanced Skills (978-0-323-05293-1), or packaged together (978-0-323-05601-4).

For Students

- *Skills Performance Checklists* (available separately [978-0-323-05485-0] or packaged with the text [978-0-323-05651-9]).
- Evolve Learning Resources with Video Clips, additional Review Questions, an Audio Glossary, and Checklists PDF files (*free with text*).
- *Nursing Skills Online* for *Clinical Nursing Skills & Techniques*, 7th edition (available separately [978-0-323-05481-2] or packaged with text [978-0-323-05480-5]).

- *Mosby's Nursing Video Skills* 3.0: *Basic, Intermediate, & Advanced, Student Version* DVD (978-0-323-05292-4).
- *Mosby's Nursing Skills Quick Cards* (illustrated flash cards) for 75 key skills (978-0-323-04615-2).
- Evolve Mobile download of Video Clips and Checklists PDFs available for iPod or MP3 players.

Acknowledgments

Special thanks are extended to everyone at Christiana Health Care System, for hosting our photo shoot in their Christiana Hospital in Newark, Delaware. Director of Nursing Resources, Ruth Morse, RN, MSN, CEN, was instrumental in helping us coordinate the many new photos taken during that visit.

Contents

Clinical Nursing Skills & Techniques

Using Evidence in Nursing Practice

MEDIA RESOURCES

- **evolve** *learning system* http://evolve.elsevier.com/Perry/skills

  - Review Questions

Mastery of content in this chapter will enable the nurse to:
- Define the key terms listed.
- Discuss the benefits of evidence-based practice.
- Describe the six steps of evidence-based practice.
- Develop a PICO question.

- Explain the levels of evidence in the literature.
- Discuss elements to review when critiquing the scientific literature.
- Discuss ways to apply evidence in practice.

Cathy works on a medical oncology floor, a unit where patients undergo extensive chemotherapy and radiation for leukemia, lymphoma, and other serious forms of cancer. The age of patients ranges from young to very old adults. Because of their chemotherapy, many patients experience drops in their platelet counts and clotting factors, increasing their risk for bleeding. Cathy recently cared for a 42-year-old woman, who fell while trying to get to the bathroom and hit her head against the bed frame, resulting in a serious intracranial bleed. Cathy discusses the situation with two nurse colleagues and asks, "How can we reduce the number of falls and injuries in our patients on the oncology unit?" The nurse specialist for the unit tells Cathy, "I heard about an approach to fall prevention on one of the surgical floors; it involves hourly rounding. Let's ask this question, 'Will the incidence of and injuries related to falls decline following use of hourly rounding compared with our current fall prevention protocol?'" Feeling frustrated that their existing fall prevention protocol was not effective in reducing falls, the group agreed that the question was the right one to search in the literature.

The nurse specialist conducted a literature search on the basis of the question and identified four articles pertaining to risk factors for falls and outcomes from hourly rounding. During their unit practice committee meeting, Cathy and her colleagues reviewed the articles carefully and chose three that offered good evidence for a way to implement hourly rounding and identify risk for and prevent falls. The staff noted that one of the articles recommended hourly rounding during daytime hours and rounding every 2 hours during evening and night hours. Another article summarized fall risks for patients in an acute care hospital and highlighted factors such as medications (e.g., antihistamines, sedatives, analgesics, and antiemetics), weakness, altered mental status, history of falls, and toileting needs to include in a nursing assessment.

Based on their experience and a review of their unit fall index reports, the staff knew that patients on the oncology unit commonly experienced falls during all hours of the day. The unit practice committee recommended incorporating a new hourly rounds program along with focused nursing assessments for key fall risk factors. Registered nurses (RNs) would begin to round on patients on all even hours and conduct focused assessments of fall risk factors such as weakness, pain, or the need to go to the bathroom. Nurses would carefully monitor patients receiving antihistamines before blood transfusions. Nursing assistive personnel (NAP) would round on odd hours and do follow-up observations to be sure patients had toileting needs met, were comfortable, and had no further needs. Each hour the nursing staff would inform patients that someone from the nursing team would return in an hour for another check. The unit practice committee planned a staff orientation and set a date for the start of the hourly rounding protocol.

Three months after implementing the rounding protocol, the medical oncology unit was cautiously optimistic. Their average fall index dropped from 5.1 to 3.7, and the injury rate also dropped. Another benefit was the decline in patients' use of call lights, which was attributed to patients knowing their nurses would visit frequently. All nursing staff on the unit were enthused by the change and agreed that hourly rounding needed to be a routine part of their unit culture. The staff was also able to see that the protocol improved patient outcomes and gave them more time to coordinate care because there were fewer distractions from patient calls. Six months after starting the new protocol, the fall index continued to remain low. An added outcome was a significant increase in patient satisfaction. Cathy submitted their protocol for an abstract in the hospital's Nursing Research Day. Cathy's abstract, "Using Evidence to Prevent Falls" was well accepted by her peers and became a standard for other nursing units in the hospital.

This clinical case study highlights the value in finding current and relevant information to make informed changes in the way you care for patients. The evidence from research studies and the opinions of oncology nurse experts provided a basis for Cathy and her colleagues to make evidence-based changes to their fall prevention protocol. The use of evidence in practice enables clinicians like Cathy to provide the highest quality of care to their patients and families. So, how does a nurse routinely use evidence in practice? It takes a new philosophy of thinking. Evidence-based practice (EBP) requires nurses to always think about their practice, raise good clinical questions, search for the evidence that pertains to their questions, apply relevant evidence in practice changes, and evaluate the outcomes.

A CASE FOR EVIDENCE

Evidence-based practice is a guide for making accurate, timely, and appropriate clinical decisions. In this textbook, you will learn that use of evidence in nursing procedures or skills provides scientific guidelines for how to perform skills more effectively and to improve patient outcomes. It is very important to translate best evidence into best practices at the patient's bedside. For example, using a sliding board to transfer a patient from bed to stretcher instead of lifting, and using the research-based Braden scale to routinely assess a patient's risk for skin breakdown are examples of using evidence at the bedside. Evidence-based practice is a problem-solving approach to clinical practice that integrates the conscientious use of best evidence along with a clinician's expertise and patient preferences and values in making decisions about patient care (Melnyk and Fineout-Overholt, 2005; Sackett and others, 2000).

As a professional nurse, you need to stay informed and be aware of the most current evidence. Typically, new students will diligently read their textbooks and the assigned scientific articles. A good textbook incorporates current evidence into the practice guidelines and nursing skills it describes. However, a textbook relies on the scientific literature; thus portions of a book often become outdated by the time it is published. Articles from nursing and the health care literature are available on almost any topic involving nursing practice. New research is reported every day. Although the scientific basis of nursing practice has grown, some practices are still not "research based" (based on findings from well-designed research studies), because findings are inconclusive or because researchers have not yet studied the practices (Titler and others, 2001). For example, in the past nurses applied antibiotic ointment to intravenous (IV) sites, assuming this would reduce the incidence of infection at the site. However, research showed that topical antibiotics offer no benefit, and thus the current standard of care is to simply apply a sterile transparent or gauze dressing to an intravenous site (Infusion Nurses Society [INS], 2006). The challenge is to obtain the very best, most current information at the right time, when you need it for patient care.

The best evidence comes from well-designed, systematically conducted research studies, found in scientific journals. Unfortunately, much of that evidence does not reach the bedside. Many health care settings do not have a process to help staff adopt new evidence in practice. Nurses in practice settings, unlike educational settings, do not have easy access to databases for scientific literature. Instead, nurses often care for patients on the basis of tradition or convenience. Because there are obstacles to research-based practice in clinical settings, it is important for administrators to provide a supportive environment and adequate facilitation of change (Rycroft-Malone and others, 2004).

There are sources of evidence that do not originate from research. This includes quality improvement and risk management data; infection control data, retrospective or concurrent chart reviews; and clinicians' expertise. Although non–research-based evidence is often very valuable, it is important that you learn to not rely on it alone. Research-based evidence is more likely to be timely and relevant. When you face a clinical problem, always seek the best source of evidence that helps you find the best solution in caring for patients.

Even when you use the best evidence available, application and outcomes will differ based on your patients' values, preferences, concerns, and/or expectations (Oncology Nursing Society [ONS], 2005). As a nurse, you will develop critical thinking skills to determine whether evidence is relevant and appropriate to your patients and to a clinical situation. For example, a single research article suggests that therapeutic massage administered 60 minutes after an analgesic will enhance pain relief. However, if you care for a patient from a culture in which touch is a taboo, the use of massage is inappropriate. Using your clinical expertise and considering patients' cultures, values, and preferences ensure that you will apply the evidence available in practice both ethically and appropriately. Evidence-based practice requires good nursing judgment; it is not finding research evidence and blindly applying it.

STEPS OF EVIDENCE-BASED PRACTICE

Evidence-based practice is a systematic approach to rational decision making that facilitates achievement of best practices (Newhouse and others, 2005). Using a step-by-step approach ensures that you will obtain the strongest available evidence to apply in patient care. There are six steps of EBP (Melnyk and Fineout-Overholt, 2005):

1 Ask a clinical question.
2 Collect the most-relevant and best evidence.
3 Critically appraise the evidence you gather.
4 Apply or integrate evidence along with your clinical expertise, patient preferences, and values in making a practice decision or change.
5 Evaluate the practice decision or change.
6 Communicate your results.

Ask the Clinical Question

Always think about your practice when caring for patients. Question what does not make sense to you, and question what you think needs clarification. As demonstrated in the previous case study, think about a problem or area of interest that is time consuming, costly, or not logical (Callister and others, 2005). Often The Joint Commission standards (e.g., the annual patient safety goals) offer questions to pose about your patients. If you keep a clinical journal, your entries are a rich source for clinical questions. Titler and others (2001) suggest using problem- and knowledge-focused triggers to ask clinical questions. A problem-focused trigger is one you face while caring for a patient or a trend you see on a nursing unit. For example, a problem-focused trigger might arise while caring for an unconscious patient: "What is the best antiinfective solution to use when giving oral care to this patient?" Examples of problem-focused trends include the increase in number of pressure ulcers or incidence of urinary tract infections on a nursing unit. Such trends should lead you to ask, "How do I reduce pressure ulcers on my unit?" or "What is the best way to prevent urinary tract infections in catheterized patients?"

A knowledge-focused trigger is a question regarding new information about a topic. For example, "What is the current evidence to reduce phlebitis in peripheral intravenous catheters?" Important sources of this type of information are standards and practice guidelines available from national agencies such as the Agency for Healthcare Research and Quality (AHRQ), the Infusion Nurses Society (INS), and the American Association of Critical Care Nurses (AACN).

When you ask a question and search the scientific literature, you do not want to read 100 articles in order to find the handful that are most helpful. You want to be able to read the best 4 to 6 articles that specifically address your practice question.

Melnyk and Fineout-Overholt (2005) suggest using a PICO format to state your question. Box 1-1 summarizes the four elements of a PICO question. The more focused a question you ask, the easier it is to search for evidence in the scientific literature. Examples of well-designed PICO questions follow: *In abdominal surgery patients (P), is epidural analgesia (I) compared with patient-controlled analgesia (C) more effective in reducing pain severity (O)? Is an adult patient's (P) blood pressure more accurate (O) while measuring with the patient's legs crossed (I) versus the patient's feet flat on the floor (C)?* A well-designed PICO question does not have to include all four elements, nor does it have to follow the PICO sequence. However, the goal is to ask a question that contains as many of the PICO elements as possible in a logically framed question. Inappropriately formed questions (e.g., What is the best way to reduce pressure ulcers? What is the best way to measure blood pressure?) lead to many irrelevant articles in a literature search, making it difficult to find the best evidence.

A clearly stated PICO question identifies knowledge gaps within a clinical situation. When you form well thought-out questions, the type of evidence you lack for clinical practice becomes

---

BOX 1-1 Developing a PICO Question

P = Patient population of interest
Identify your patients by age, gender, ethnicity, disease, or health problem

I = Intervention of interest
What is the intervention you think is worthwhile to use in practice (e.g., a treatment, diagnostic test, prognostic factor)?

C = Comparison of interest
What is the usual standard of care or current intervention you use now in practice?

O = Outcome
What result do you wish to achieve or observe as a result of an intervention (e.g., change in patient's behavior, physical finding, change in patient's perception)?

more clear. Examples of different knowledge gaps include the following (ONS, 2005):

- *Diagnosis:* Questions about the selection and interpretation of diagnostic tests. *Example:* Does the use of a disposable oral thermometer compared with an electronic oral thermometer measure body temperature accurately in a patient with an endotracheal tube?
- *Prognosis:* Questions about a patient's likely clinical outcome. *Example:* Is there a difference in the incidence of deep vein thrombosis in surgical patients wearing sequential compression stockings compared to those who perform range-of-motion (ROM) exercises?
- *Therapy:* Questions about the selection of the most beneficial treatments. *Example:* What bowel regimen is most effective in relieving constipation caused by the administration of opioid therapy in patients with chronic pain?
- *Prevention:* Questions about screening and prevention methods to reduce the risk of disease. *Example:* Does performance of a prostate specific antigen (PSA) test in an older adult who is asymptomatic of prostate disease decrease his risk for mortality from prostate cancer?
- *Education:* Questions about best teaching strategies for colleagues, patients, or family members. *Example:* Is the use of visual aids compared with low-literacy teaching booklets more effective to educate low-literacy adults about therapeutic diets?
- *Meaning:* Questions that seek understanding of a phenomenon. *Example:* How do patients with cervical cancer perceive their quality of life?

Remember, do not be satisfied with clinical routines. Always question and use critical thinking to consider better ways to provide patient care.

Collect the Best Evidence

Once you have a clear and concise PICO question, you are ready to search for evidence. Evidence exists in a variety of sources: agency policy and procedure manuals, quality improvement data, existing clinical practice guidelines, or computerized bibliographical databases. Do not hesitate to ask for help to find appropriate evidence. Your faculty is a key resource. When you are assigned to a health care setting, consider using experts such as advanced practice nurses, staff educators, risk managers, and infection control nurses.

When searching the scientific literature for evidence, seek the assistance of a medical librarian when possible. A medical librarian knows the relevant databases (Box 1-2). A database is an electronic library of published scientific studies, including peer-reviewed research. A peer-reviewed article is one that has been evaluated by a panel of experts familiar with the article's topic or subject matter. The librarian helps translate the elements of your PICO question into the language or key words that will yield the best evidence search. For example, in the PICO question "Does the use of computerized home instruction compared with a group class improve surgical patients' knowledge of postoperative activities?," the key words are *surgical patient, computerized instruction, group class, knowledge,* and *postoperative activities.* When conducting a search, it is necessary to enter and manipulate the different key words until you get the combination that gives you the articles you want to read about your question. When you enter a key word to search a database, be prepared for some confusion with the evidence you obtain. The vocabulary within published articles is often vague. The word you select sometimes has one meaning to one author and a very different meaning to another. A medical librarian helps you learn how to choose alternative words or terms that identify your PICO question

BOX 1-2	Searchable Scientific Literature Databases and Sources
CINAHL	Cumulative Index of Nursing and Allied Health Literature. Includes studies in nursing, allied health, and biomedicine.
	http://www.cinahl.com
MEDLINE	Includes studies in medicine, nursing, dentistry, psychiatry, veterinary medicine, and allied health.
	http://www.ncbi.nim.nih.gov
EMBASE	Biomedical and pharmaceutical studies.
	http://www.embase.com
PsycINFO	Psychology and related health care disciplines.
	http://www.apa.org/psycinfo
Cochrane Database of Systematic Reviews	Full text of regularly updated systematic reviews prepared by the Cochrane Collaboration. Includes completed reviews and protocols.
	http://www.cochrane.org/reviews
National Guidelines Clearinghouse	Repository for structured abstracts (summaries) about clinical guidelines and their development. Also includes condensed version of guideline for viewing.
	http://www.guideline.gov
PubMed	Health science library at the National Library of Medicine. Offers free access to journal articles.
	http://www.nlm.nih.gov
On-Line Journal of Knowledge Synthesis for Nursing	Electronic journal containing articles that provide a synthesis of research and an annotated bibliography for selected references.
	http://nursingsociety.org/publications/journals

and to obtain relevant evidence. In Fig. 1-1 we demonstrate the difference in the results of literature searches on two different questions. Question A is more general and not in a PICO format. Question B is a focused question using a PICO format. Note the difference in the number of articles in the last step of the search. Which group of articles would you prefer to review?

MEDLINE, CINAHL, and PubMed are among the most comprehensive databases and represent the scientific knowledge base of health care (Melnyk and Fineout-Overholt, 2005). Among the many databases, some are available through vendors at a cost, some are free of charge, and some offer both options. Nursing students and nurses who work in academic medical centers usually have access to an institutional subscription through a vendor. One of the more common vendors is OVID, which offers several different databases. There are also databases available free on the Internet, such as PubMed and the Cochrane Library. The Cochrane Database of Systematic Reviews is a valuable source of synthesized evidence (i.e., preappraised evidence). The Cochrane database includes the full text of regularly updated systematic reviews and protocols for reviews currently happening. The National Guidelines Clearinghouse (NGC) is a database supported by the Agency for Healthcare Research and Quality (AHRQ). It contains clinical guidelines, systematically developed statements about a plan of care for a specific set of clinical circumstances involving a specific

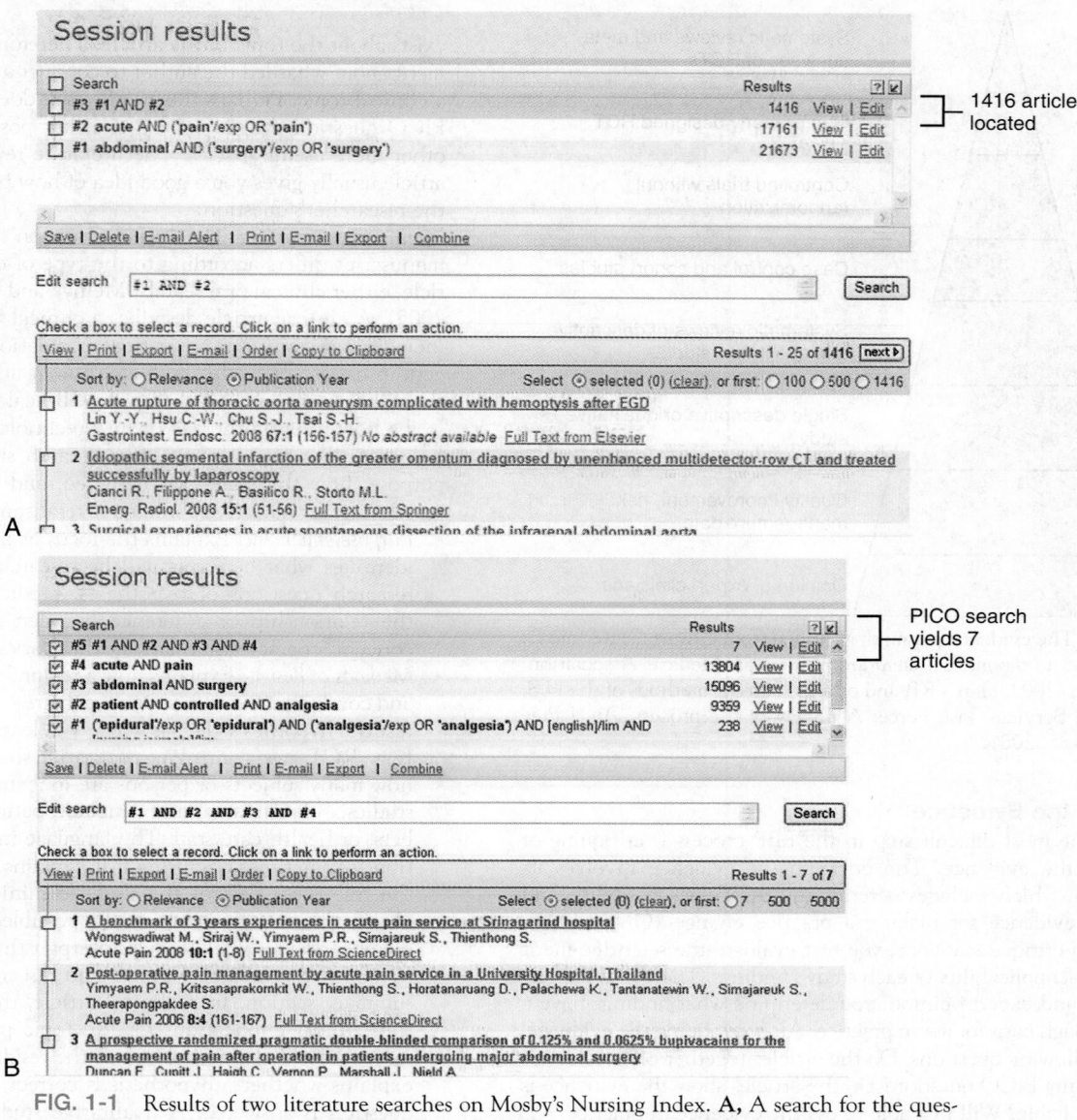

FIG. 1-1   Results of two literature searches on Mosby's Nursing Index. **A,** A search for the question "What type of pain control reduces pain in patients who have had abdominal surgery?" **B,** A search for the PICO question "Does the use of epidural analgesia reduce pain severity compared with patient-controlled analgesia in patients who have had abdominal surgery?"

patient population. The NGC is a valuable source when you want to develop a plan of care for a patient.

The pyramid in Fig. 1-2 represents a hierarchy of available evidence. At this point in your nursing career, you are probably not an expert on all aspects of the types of studies conducted. But you can learn enough about the types of studies to help you know which ones have the best scientific evidence. Table 1-1, p. 7, describes types of studies in the evidence hierarchy, beginning with the study at the top of the hierarchy, a systematic review.

If your PICO question leads you to a systematic review, celebrate! A systematic review is the perfect answer to a PICO question. Basically a researcher has asked the same PICO question you have asked and then examined all of the well-designed randomized controlled trials (RCTs) that ask the same question. A systematic review explains if the evidence that you are searching for exists and whether there is good cause to change practice. In the Cochrane Library, all entries include information on systematic reviews.

Individual RCTs are the gold standard for research (Titler and others, 2001). An RCT establishes cause and effect and is excellent for testing therapies. Historically there have been few RCTs conducted in nursing. The nature of nursing causes researchers to ask questions that are not always answered best by an RCT. Nurses care for patients' responses to disease or health problems. For example, we assist patients with problems such as knowledge deficits, symptom management, and coping with psychological distress. An RCT cannot easily be designed to learn how patients experience health problems. Often descriptive studies or qualitative approaches are more helpful. What is most important is to have the research question match the appropriate research method.

The use of clinical experts is at the bottom of the evidence pyramid, but do not consider clinical experts a poor source of evidence. Expert clinicians frequently use evidence as they build their own practice, and they are rich sources of information for clinical problems.

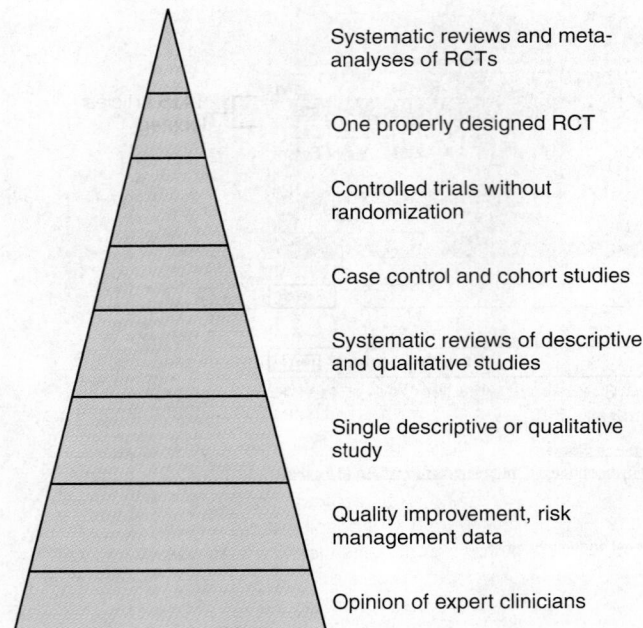

FIG 1-2   The evidence pyramid. Modified from Guyatt G, Rennie D: *User's guides to the medical literature.* American Medical Association: AMA Press, 2002. Harris RP, and others: Current methods of the U.S. Preventive Services Task Force: A review of the process. *Am J Prev Med* 20:21-35, 2001.

Critique the Evidence

Perhaps the most difficult step in the EBP process is critiquing or analyzing the evidence. The critiquing of evidence involves its evaluation, which includes determining the value, feasibility, and utility of evidence for making a practice change (ONS, 2005). When you critique evidence, you first evaluate the scientific merit and clinical applicability of each study's findings. Then with a group of studies and expert opinion, you determine what findings have a strong enough basis for use in practice. After critiquing the evidence, ask the following questions: Do the articles together offer evidence to answer my PICO question? Do the articles show the evidence is true and reliable? Will I be able to use the evidence in practice?

It takes time to acquire the skills to critique evidence like an expert. When you read an article from the literature, do not let the statistics or technical wording cause you to put the article down and walk away. Know the elements of an article, and use a careful approach when reviewing each one. Evidence-based articles include the following elements:

- *Abstract:* A brief summary of the article that quickly tells you if the article is research or clinically based. An abstract summarizes the purpose of the study or clinical topic, the major themes or findings, and the implications for nursing practice.
- *Introduction:* Contains information about the article's purpose and the importance of the topic for the audience who reads the article. It usually contains brief supporting evidence as to why the topic is important from the author's point of view.

Together, the abstract and introduction help determine if you want to continue to read the entire article. You will know if the topic of the article is similar to your PICO question or related closely enough to provide you useful information. Continue to read the next elements of the article:

- *Literature review or background:* A good author offers a detailed background of the level of scientific or clinical information that

exists about the topic of the article. Therefore it offers an argument about what led the author to conduct a study or report on a clinical topic. Perhaps the article itself does not address your PICO question the way you desire, but possibly leads you to other more useful articles. The literature review of a research article usually gives you a good idea of how past research led to the researcher's question.

- *Manuscript narrative:* The "middle section" or narrative of a manuscript differs according to the type of evidence-based article, either clinical or research (Melnyk and Fineout-Overholt, 2005). A clinical article describes a clinical topic, which often includes a description of a patient population, the nature of a certain disease or health problem, how it affects patients, and the appropriate nursing therapies. Clinical articles often describe how to use a therapy or new technology. A research article describes the conduct of a research study, including its purpose, how the study was designed, and the results. A research article's narrative contains several standard subsections:
  - *Purpose statement:* Explains the focus or intent of a study. It identifies what concepts will be researched. This includes research questions or hypotheses, predictions made about the relationship or difference between study variables (a concept, characteristic, or trait that varies within subjects).
  - *Methods or design:* Explains how a research study is organized and conducted in order to answer the research question or to test the hypothesis. This is where you learn the type of study (e.g., RCT, case control, or qualitative study). You also learn how many subjects or persons are in a study. In health care studies, subjects sometimes include patients, family members, or health care staff. The language in the methods section is sometimes confusing if it explains details about how the researcher designs the study to minimize bias so as to obtain the most accurate results possible. Use your faculty member as a resource to help interpret this section.
  - *Results or conclusions:* Clinical and research articles have a summary section. In a clinical article, the author explains the clinical implications for the topic presented. In a research article, the author details the results of the study and explains whether a hypothesis is correct or how a research question is answered. A qualitative study presents a thorough summary of the descriptive themes and ideas that arise from the researcher's analysis of data. A quantitative study includes a statistical analysis. It is important to become familiar with common statistical terms, especially in clinical trials, to know if a tested intervention had a significant effect or if the effect size was large enough to adopt in practice. When reading the statistical analysis, ask these questions: Does the researcher describe the results? Were the results significant? What was the size of the effect of the intervention? What was the sample size? A good author will discuss any limitations to a study in the results section. The information on limitations helps you to decide if you want to use the evidence with your patients.
  - *Clinical implications:* A research article includes a section that explains if the findings from the study have clinical implications. The researcher explains how to apply findings in a practice setting for the type of subjects studied.

After you critique each article for your PICO question, synthesize or combine the findings from all of the articles to determine the state of the evidence. Use critical thinking to consider the scientific rigor or accurateness of the evidence and how well

TABLE 1-1	Types of Studies in the Evidence Hierarchy	
Study Type	**Description**	**Example**
Systematic review or meta-analysis	A panel of experts reviews the evidence from randomized controlled trials about a specific clinical question and summarizes the state of the science. In a meta-analysis, there is the addition of a statistical analysis that combines data from all studies.	Nine studies examined the use of continuous epidural analgesia (CEA) compared with intravenous opioid patient-controlled analgesia (PCA) in relieving postoperative abdominal pain. The review revealed that CEA is superior in relieving pain for up to 72 hours (Werawatganon and Charuluxanum, 2004).
Randomized controlled trial	A researcher tests an intervention against the usual standard of care. Participants are randomly assigned to either a control group (receives standard care) or a treatment group (receives the experimental intervention), with both measured on the same outcomes to see if there is a difference.	Researchers randomly assigned 107 critical care patients to receive intermittent nasogastric feedings (treatment group) or continuous feedings (control group). Patients in the intermittent feeding group had a higher total intake at day 7, earlier extubation, and a lower risk of aspiration pneumonia (Chen and others, 2006).
Case control study	Researchers study one group of subjects with a certain condition (e.g., obesity) at the same time as another group of subjects who do not have the condition to determine if there is an association between the condition and predictor variables (e.g., exercise pattern, family history, history of depression).	Researchers from Singapore compared 61 patients with known ocular keratitis with 188 population-based and 178 hospitalized patients to determine what contact lens cleaning methods contributed to keratitis. The use of a specific contact lens cleaning solution was found to increase the risk for keratitis (Saw and others, 2007).
Descriptive study	Study that describes the concepts under study. It sometimes examines the prevalence, magnitude, and/or characteristics of a concept.	Researchers explored nurses' and health care providers' perceptions of infection control practices in relation to management of infectious disease (Watkins and others, 2006).
Qualitative study	Studies examine individuals' experiences with health problems or life experiences and the contexts in which the experiences occur.	Researchers asked 392 nurses to discuss a care episode from their practice. Cases describing patients with cancer involved nurses' use of powerful emotive language. The influence of patients' cancer experience affects nurses personally and professionally (Kendall, 2007).
Quality improvement data, risk management information	Data collected within a health care agency offers important trending information about clinical conditions and problems. Staff in the agency review the data periodically to identify problem areas and to then seek solutions.	Article reviews use of quality improvement (QI) process in a nursing home setting where staff adopted best practices for pressure ulcer care for residents (Berlowitz and Frantz, 2007).
Clinical experts	Accessing clinical experts on a nursing unit is an excellent way to learn about current evidence. Clinical experts often write clinical articles on topics that require application of evidence in the literature.	Clinical article describes an evidence-based practice project, in which a team of nurses applied evidence from the literature to change their hospital's approach to intravenous (IV) site care and IV catheter stabilization (Winfield and others, 2007).

it answers your area of interest. Scientific rigor is the extent to which a study's findings are valid, reliable, and relevant to your patient population of interest. Consider the evidence in light of your patients' concerns and preferences. Your review of articles offers a snapshot conclusion based on combined evidence about one focused topical area. As a clinician, judge whether to use the evidence for a particular patient or group of patients who usually have complex medical histories and patterns of responses (Melnyk and Fineout-Overholt, 2005). Ethically it is important to consider evidence that will benefit patients and do no harm. Decide if the evidence is relevant, easily applicable in your setting of practice, and has the potential for improving patient outcomes.

Apply the Evidence
Once you decide that the evidence is strong and applicable to your patients and clinical situation, incorporate the recommended evidence into practice. One way you may choose to use evidence is by applying the evidence in your care for a patient. For example, perhaps you find evidence for a new noninvasive pain therapy (e.g., music therapy). Use the article reference as the rationale for the intervention in your written care plan. Then try the intervention with a patient who is receptive to the therapy.

Another option, particularly if you are working with a group of other nurses or health care providers, is to apply evidence in the form of new teaching tools, clinical practice guidelines, policies and procedures, and new assessment or documentation tools. Typically members of a nursing staff will define a clinical problem. After reviewing and critiquing the literature, the staff integrates the available evidence into a process that all health care providers can use. For example, it is common for hospitals to routinely review the evidence as part of their annual nursing policy and procedure review process. As in the case of this textbook, current evidence provides the foundation for routine nursing procedures.

When you propose to change a procedure or policy on the basis of evidence, be sure to consider and review if your place of work is able to adopt the change. For example, evidence shows that toothbrushes are more effective than foam applicators in cleaning teeth and gums (Pearson and Hutton, 2002). Is your organization willing to purchase the toothbrushes? What planning is necessary to familiarize staff to any new hygiene guidelines? Any time you change a nursing procedure or adopt a new protocol, you will need to prepare all staff and communicate the change to your organization.

As a nursing student integrating evidence, your focus will begin with searching for and applying the best evidence to improve the care you directly provide your patients. The evidence available within nursing gives you an almost unlimited access to innovative and effective nursing interventions. Using an evidence-based practice approach will improve your skills and knowledge as a nurse and improve your patients' outcomes.

Evaluate the Practice Decision or Change

After applying evidence in your practice, your next step is to evaluate the effect. You do this by measuring outcomes; outcome measurement will tell you how an intervention worked. How effective was the clinical decision for your patient or practice setting? Sometimes your evaluation is as simple as determining if the expected outcomes you set for an intervention are met. For example, after the use of a new transparent IV dressing, does the IV dislodge or does the patient develop the complication of phlebitis? When using a new approach to preoperative teaching, does the patient learn what to expect after surgery?

When an evidence-based practice change occurs on a larger scale, an evaluation is more formal. For example, after reviewing evidence about factors contributing to pressure ulcers, a nursing unit adopts a new skin care protocol. To evaluate the protocol, the nurses track the incidence of pressure ulcers over a course of time (e.g., 6 months to a year). In addition, the nurses collect data to describe both the patients who develop ulcers and those who do not. This comparative information is valuable in determining the effects of the protocol and whether modifications are necessary.

Communicating a Practice Change

After applying evidence, it is important to communicate the change in practice as well as the results to nursing and other health care colleagues. This is true if the results are successful or unsuccessful. There are many ways to communicate the outcomes of evidence-based practice: talking with a colleague, sharing results in staff meetings, presenting in workshops or seminars, submitting an abstract for a poster presentation, and publishing an article. As a professional, you are responsible for communicating important information about nursing practice. Sharing evidence and the effects of any practice change motivates others and gets them excited about practice improvements. When you have successfully adopted an evidenced-based practice way of thinking, it becomes very natural to talk about available evidence and to continue seeking solutions for problems in patient care.

IMPACT OF EVIDENCE-BASED PRACTICE ON NURSING

Numerous factors within the health care environment have created the initiatives for evidence-based practice. Patient safety and medical errors, the economics of health care, and variability in how disease conditions are treated are just some of the factors that have led government and private groups to support evidence-based practice. The use of evidence-based practice has the potential to improve the quality of care nurses provide, patient outcomes, and clinicians' satisfaction with their practice.

This chapter provides a brief introduction to evidence-based practice. Of all of the initiatives introduced in health care, evidence-based practice may be the most important. With the rapid, ongoing expansion of research knowledge in health care, it is essential to remain accountable by applying evidence in patient care. When evidence exists on ways to improve patient outcomes, it becomes important for that evidence to reach the bedside. Your patients expect nursing professionals to be informed and to use the safest and most appropriate interventions. Use of evidence enhances nursing, improving patients' perceptions of excellent nursing care.

? CRITICAL THINKING EXERCISES

Maria Gonzalez is a 45-year-old Hispanic woman who is admitted to the hospital with ulcerative colitis, which she has had for 2 years. The disease is an inflammation and ulceration of the colon. As a result, Maria has a recurrence of bloody diarrhea, abdominal cramping, and a fever. During her hospital stay Maria received intravenous fluids, corticosteroids, and antiinfective drugs. Jeanne is the nurse assigned to coordinate Maria's discharge home. Jeanne is concerned about Maria's diet at home and wonders how it might affect her disease, particularly the frequency of diarrhea. Jeanne learns that Maria eats a diet with sources of high carbohydrates. In consultation with the dietitian Jeanne asks if a low-carbohydrate diet might be best for Maria. The dietitian suggests they do a literature search to see what the most current evidence suggests.

1 Given this clinical case study, write the PICO question that is the basis of Jeanne's inquiry.
2 The librarian helps Jeanne conduct a literature search. Among the articles located in the search is a systematic review. Explain why a systematic review is the best source of evidence.
3 One of the articles found by the librarian describes a study in which a researcher studied 45 patients with ulcerative colitis and 52 patients with normal intestinal function to determine if there is an association between frequency of diarrhea and ingestion of high protein intake. What type of study did this researcher conduct?

4 If Jeanne decides to educate Maria about changing her diet, what should she consider before applying the evidence that would be unique to Maria?

✓ REVIEW QUESTIONS

1 Which statement best explains the goal of evidence-based practice?
  1 Changes made in patient care are from suggestions in the literature.
  2 It is based solely on current trends seen on the nursing unit.
  3 It answers clinical questions by using appropriate, researched resources.
  4 It makes changes in patient care after conferring with the patients' health care providers.
2 There are many steps of evidence-based practice. Select all that apply.
  1 Ask a clinical question.
  2 Obtain permission from the health care providers.
  3 Communicate the findings.
  4 Collect the most-relevant evidence.
  5 Publish results of the project immediately.
  6 Make certain the changes fit within the patients' culture.

3 A question focusing on the best solution to use to clean infected incisions would be what type of trigger?
1 Problem-focused
2 Knowledge-focused
3 Peer-focused
4 PICO-focused

4 Which question contains the primary components of a PICO question?
1 Are oral steroids or inhaled steroidal medications better for female adults with adult-onset asthma?
2 What steroid preparations are best for male teenagers with activity-induced asthma who play sports?
3 How can school-age asthmatic children be best controlled using steroidal preparations?
4 Do pulse oximetry readings or peak flows provide better monitoring of the effectiveness of inhaled steroids in asthmatic children between the ages of 7 and 9?

5 Which activity would require the most critical thinking?
1 Determining whether data are relevant for the situation
2 Counting the number of related articles to support the new interventions
3 Assessing patients to determine if they meet the study criteria
4 Designing the table that will be used to report the data

REFERENCES

Berlowitz DR, Frantz RN: Implementing best practices in pressure ulcer care, the role of continuous quality improvement, *J Am Med Dir Assoc* 8(suppl 3):S37, 2007.
Callister LC and others: Inquiry in baccalaureate nursing education: fostering evidence-based practice, *J Nurs Educ* 44(2):59, 2005.
Guyatt G, Rennie D: *User's guides to the medical literature,* 2002, AMA Press (online).
Harris RP and others: Current methods of the U.S. Preventive Services Task Force: a review of the process, *Am J Prev Med* 20:21, 2001.
Infusion Nurses Society: Infusion nursing standards of practice, *J Intraven Nurs* 29(suppl 1):S1, 2006.
Melnyk BM, Fineout-Overholt E: *Evidence-based practice in nursing and healthcare: a guide to best practice,* Philadelphia, 2005, Lippincott Williams & Wilkins.
Newhouse R and others: Evidence-based practice: a practical approach to implementation, *J Nurs Adm* 35(1):35, 2005.
Oncology Nursing Society: *Evidence based practice resource area,* http://www.onsop-content.ons.org/toolkits/evidence/Definitions/index.shtml, accessed November 2005.
Sackett DL and others: *Evidence-based medicine: how to practice and teach EBM,* London, 2000, Churchill Livingstone.

RESEARCH REFERENCES

Chen YC and others: The effect of intermittent nasogastric feeding on preventing aspiration pneumonia in ventilated critically ill patients, *J Nurs Res* 14(3):167, 2006.
Kendall S: Witnessing tragedy: nurses' perceptions of caring for patients with cancer, *Int J Nurs Pract* 13(2):111, 2007.
Pearson LS, Hutton JL: A controlled trial to compare the ability of foam swabs and toothbrushes to remove dental plaque, *J Adv Nurs* 39(5):480, 2002.
Rycroft-Malone J and others: An exploration of the factors that influence the implementation of evidence into practice, *J Clin Nurs* 13:313, 2004.
Saw SM and others: Risk factors for contact lens related fusarium keratitis: a case control study in Singapore, *Arch Ophthalmol* 125(5):611, 2007.
Titler MG and others: The Iowa Model of Evidence-Based Practice to Promote Quality Care, *Crit Care Nurs Clin North Am* 13(4):497, 2001.
Watkins RE and others: Perceptions of infection control practices among health professionals, *Contemp Nurse* 22(1):109, 2006.
Werawatganon T, Charuluxanum S: Patient controlled intravenous opioid analgesia versus continuous epidural analgesia for pain after intra-abdominal surgery, *The Cochrane Database Rev* 2005:1.
Winfield C and others: Evidence: the first word in safe I.V. practice, *Am Nurse Today* 2(5):31, 2007.

2

Admitting, Transfer, and Discharge

MEDIA RESOURCES

- evolve *learning system* http://evolve.elsevier.com/Perry/skills
  - Review Questions

OBJECTIVES

Mastery of content in this chapter will enable the nurse to:
- Describe the nurse's role in maintaining continuity of care through a patient's admission, transfer, and discharge from an acute care facility.
- Explain the purpose and importance of advance directives.
- Identify the ongoing needs of patients in the process of discharge planning.
- Explain the role of a patient's family in the admission, transfer, or discharge process.

Patients receive health care services in multiple settings from numerous caregivers. It is important for patient care to be integrated across a variety of settings, services, health care practitioners, and care levels to make a continuum of care. The Joint Commission (2007) defines the continuum of care as matching an individual's ongoing needs with the appropriate level and type of medical, psychological, health, or social care or services within an organization or across multiple organizations. This continuum flows from preadmission to the admission process, throughout the acute care hospitalization as the discharge plan is developed, and posthospitalization upon discharge to home or to another health care setting. All disciplines work collaboratively in assisting a patient's transition from one level of care or service to another.

The nurse plays a key role in coordinating resources for a patient's care from admission to discharge to the next level of care. The nurse identifies patients' ongoing health care needs; anticipates physical, psychological, and social deficits that have implications for resuming normal activities; involves family and significant others in a plan of care; provides health education; and assists in making health care resources available to patients. To separate the processes of admission and discharge is a critical error; the two are simultaneous and continuous. Discharge planning begins at the time of admission. Patients and families need to be involved in the planning and decision making. They also need to understand the implications of any health problems and the responsibilities for continued care either in the home or next level of care setting.

EVIDENCE-BASED PRACTICE TRENDS

Evidence shows that good communication is a key part of admitting, transferring, and discharging patients. During the admission interview, be concise and specific in documenting information. Poor communication and incomplete information during transfer and discharge often lead to patient care problems, including life-threatening inaccuracies or delays in diagnosis or treatment and inadequate monitoring or follow-up treatment. When doing discharge teaching, use a combination of verbal and written information. The combined teaching methods provide patients standardized care information, which shows improved patient knowledge and satisfaction (Johnson and others, 2007). The use of computer-generated summaries and giving patients copies of pertinent discharge information are effective communication strategies to improve patient care after discharge (Kripalani and others, 2007).

The Joint Commission identified the 2008 National Patient Safety Goals to promote specific improvements in patient safety. Goal 8 is "Accurately and completely reconcile medications across the continuum of care." Medication reconciliation compares a patient's home medication list with the medication orders at admission, transfer, or discharge to avoid medication errors such as omissions, duplications, dosing errors, or drug interactions (Schwartz and Wyskiel, 2006; The Joint Commission [TJC], 2006). Completing and documenting an accurate medication history from a patient is the important first step in the medication reconciliation process (Kramer and others, 2007). In the older adult population, the increased number of home medications contributes to an increase in the medication discrepancy rate upon admission. Often the list does not contain strength or frequency of the medication, which leads to medication errors (Lessard and others, 2006). The use of the medication reconciliation process has decreased medication errors and improved cost savings by decreasing adverse drug events (Schwartz and Wyskiel, 2006). Research shows that patients at discharge who had electronically reconciled medication lists had a better understanding of medication administration instructions and potential adverse effects of the discharge medications (Kramer and others, 2007).

A patient's perception of readiness for discharge is related to postdischarge coping and improved outcomes (Weiss and others, 2007). High-quality discharge teaching improves a patient's readiness for discharge. A positive perception of readiness helps a patient to successfully manage care and continue recovery at home without placing a burden on the family. A patient's perception of lack of readiness for discharge places an increased burden on the family for support rather than the medical system (Weiss and Piacentine, 2006). Two factors associated with decreased readiness for discharge are living alone and poor care coordination before discharge (Weiss and others, 2007). The Readiness for Hospital Discharge Scale is one reliable and valid measure of a patient's readiness for discharge (Weiss and Piacentine, 2006). Readiness for discharge assessment needs to be part of the discharge process (Weiss and others, 2007). A discharge-planning checklist provides another approach to help a patient and family consider practical aspects to being discharged home (Grimmer and others, 2006).

CULTURAL CONSIDERATIONS

When admitting, transferring, or discharging patients from diverse cultures and religions, it is important to understand their cultural and religious practices. Assess use of cultural healers and other healing modalities to determine the impact the use of these have on a patient's decisions related to medical care (Giger and Davidhizar, 2004). A patient's cultural practices include family decision making. For example, in the Mexican or Gypsy cultures the adult male leader is the decision maker. Develop trust by working with the established family and social hierarchy, recognizing those in authority and allowing them to participate in making decisions about the patient's care.

For patients who are Orthodox Jews, schedule the admission, transfer, or discharge so the patients can begin observance of the Sabbath (sundown on Friday to sundown on Saturday) undisturbed. Orthodox Jews follow the beliefs of their religion closely (Giger and Davidhizar, 2004). Have kosher meals and snacks available (e.g., fruits and vegetables, meats that have the blood drained or cooked out, and no snacks or meals in which meats and dairy are eaten together).

Be aware of a cultural group's beliefs related to the use of eye contact and touch as you admit or discharge a patient. For example, in the American Indian, Vietnamese, and Chinese American cultures, eye contact is considered disrespectful and rude. Avoid or limit eye contact with these groups while you are taking a history or doing an assessment. Chinese Americans and Orthodox Jews find excessive touching offensive. Limit the amount of touching done during the admission assessment (Giger and Davidhizar, 2004).

 Skill Performance Guidelines

1 Screen all patients on admission to a health care setting for possible discharge needs.

2 Include the patient, family, and relevant health care professionals early in planning for all moves through the health care system.
3 Consider a patient's past experiences in health care settings.
4 Consider a patient's cultural, socioeconomic, and educational background when discharge planning.
5 Coordinate the health care providers who contribute to a patient's care needs to develop a plan of care for discharge.
6 Assist other health care personnel in assessing appropriate resources needed as patients move through the health care system.

SKILL 2-1   Admitting Patients

A patient enters the health care system in a variety of ways (e.g., hospital, clinic, or physician's office). There are common types of procedures for admitting patients to these settings (Box 2-1). However, a patient's condition determines the extent of the admitting procedure. For example, a patient entering through the emergency department (ED) is often not in a condition to undergo the same registration process that takes place in a hospital admitting office. Family members usually provide pertinent information for the hospital's records while the staff is caring for the patient. In contrast, an older adult patient with self-care limitations undergoes extensive screening before being accepted as a nursing home resident.

Admitting officers, secretaries, and technicians are the personnel involved with the preliminary admission procedures, such as interviewing patients and reviewing information about insurance, demographic data, and agency procedures. Technicians usually collect routine specimens and perform screening procedures such as electrocardiograms (ECGs). The nurse performs the admitting assessment.

ROLE OF THE ADMITTING CLERK OR SECRETARY

The admitting clerk or secretary initiates and maintains a courteous and professional relationship with patients while providing for patients' safety, legal rights, and privacy. A private interview area gives patients and families a place to reveal important identifying information, including a patient's full legal name, age, birth date, address, next of kin, physician, religious preference, occupation, and type of insurance. If a patient does not speak English or has a severe hearing impairment, the clerk has access to an interpreter to assist during the admission procedure.

At this time, the clerk secures an identification (ID) band legibly stating the patient's full legal name, hospital or agency number, physician, and birth date to the patient's wrist. Health care providers use the ID band to identify a patient when performing therapies or procedures. If a patient is unconscious, identification is often not made until family members arrive. A patient who has been a victim of crime is safer with an anonymous name under an agency's "blackout" or "do not publish" procedure.

A patient's legal rights are met by instructing the patient or legal guardian to read the general consent form for treatment. During admission, all patients receive information regarding their rights related to health care services. In 1999 the Centers for Medicare and Medicaid Services (CMS) introduced a Patients' Rights Condition of Participation that all hospitals are required to meet to receive Medicare and Medicaid reimbursement. This new condition required each patient to be notified of his or her rights (Box 2-2). Other regulatory agencies, such as The Joint Commission, also require institutions to provide for specific patient rights (Box 2-3). Each institution has policies and procedures describing a patient's rights and the role of the nurse in ensuring those rights.

The Patient Self-Determination Act, effective December 1, 1991, requires all Medicare- and Medicaid-recipient hospitals to provide patients with information about their right to accept or reject medical treatment. At the time of registration, patients receive information about advance directives and are referred to appropriate resources if they want to discuss advance directives or receive help in completing an advance directive document (Box 2-4).

The patient must be provided with information about the Health Insurance Portability and Accountability Act (HIPAA). HIPAA is a federal law to protect the privacy of patient health information, referred to as PHI or protected health information. Three key concepts of HIPAA are (1) institutions are required to inform patients of the privacy rights they have and how the institution will handle their PHI; (2) the institution and the health care providers are to use or disclose a patient's PHI only for the purposes of treatment or payment or for health care operations; and (3) health care providers disclose only the minimum amount of PHI necessary, on a need-to-know basis, to accomplish the purpose of the use (U.S. Department of Health ad Human Services [USDHHS], 2003).

The HIPAA privacy regulations also give patients the right to access their records, request amendments to the PHI contained in their records, request restriction of certain uses or disclosures of their PHI, request that they be sent information at an alternative address or telephone number, and request an accounting of PHI disclosures. Know your institution-specific policies and procedures related to HIPAA.

BOX 2-1   Common Procedures for Admission to a Health Care Agency

- Placement of patient in appropriate receiving area
- Explanation of patient's rights and elements of advance directives
- Orientation to the health care agency's policies and procedures
- Assessment of patient's health care problems and needs
- Preliminary testing and screening (specific for each agency and patient's condition)
- Development of an individualized plan of care
- Determination of patient's payment source for health care

BOX 2-2 | Patients' Rights Provided for by CMS

Code of Federal Regulations Title 42, Chapter IV Part 482 Sec. 482.13 Condition of Participation: Patients' Rights.

Standard 1: Notice of Rights
- A hospital must protect and promote each patient's rights.
- A hospital must inform each patient whenever possible, or when appropriate, the patient's representative, of the patient's rights, in advance of furnishing or discontinuing patient care.
- The hospital must have a process for prompt resolution of patient grievances and must inform each patient whom to contact to file a grievance.

Standard 2: Exercise of Rights
- The patient has the right to participate in the development and implementation of his or her plan of care.
- The patient or his or her representative has the right to make informed decisions regarding his or her care.
- The patient's rights include being informed of his or her health status, being involved in care planning and treatment, and being able to request or refuse treatment. This right must not be construed as a mechanism to demand the provision of treatment or services deemed medically unnecessary or inappropriate.
- The patient has the right to formulate advance directives and to have hospital staff and practitioners who provide care in the hospital comply with these directives.
- The patient has the right to have a family member or representative of his or her choice and his or her own physician notified promptly of his or her admission to the hospital.

Standard 3: Privacy and Safety
- The patient has the right to personal privacy.
- The patient has the right to receive care in a safe setting.
- The patient has the right to be free from all forms of abuse or harassment.

Standard 4: Confidentiality of Patient Record
- The patient has the right to the confidentiality of his or her clinical records.
- The patient has the right to access information contained in his or her clinical records within a reasonable time frame.

Standard 5: Restraint or Seclusion
- The patient has the right to be free from physical or mental abuse and corporal punishment.
- The patient has the right to be free from restraints or seclusion of any form that are not medically necessary or are used as a means of coercion, discipline, convenience, or retaliation by staff. A restraint is any manual method or physical or mechanical device, material, or equipment attached or adjacent to the patient's body that he or she cannot easily remove that restricts freedom of movement or normal access to one's body. A drug used as a restraint is a medication used to control behavior or to restrict the patient's freedom of movement and is not a standard treatment for the patient's medical or psychiatric condition. Seclusion is the involuntary confinement of a patient alone in a room or area from which the patient is physically prevented from leaving.
  - A restraint or seclusion can only be used if needed to improve the patient's well-being and less restrictive interventions have been determined to be ineffective.
  - The use of a restraint or seclusion must be selected only when other less restrictive measures have been found to be ineffective to protect the patient or others from harm; and in accordance with the order of a physician or other licensed independent practitioner.
  - This order must never be written as a standing or on an as needed basis (i.e. prn); and be followed by consultation with the patient's treating physician, as soon as possible, if the restraint or seclusion is not ordered by the patient's treating physician or health care provider.
  - The use of a restraint or seclusion must be:
    In accordance with a written modification to the patient's plan of care
    Implemented in the least restrictive manner possible
    In accordance with safe and appropriate restraining techniques
    Ended at the earliest possible time
- The condition of the restrained or secluded patient must be continually assessed, monitored, and reevaluated.
- All staff who have direct patient contact must have ongoing education and training in the proper and safe use of restraints and seclusion.

Modified from Centers for Medicare and Medicaid Services: Medicare and Medicaid programs, hospital conditions of participation: patients' rights; final rule, *Federal Register* 71(236):71378, 2006.

BOX 2-3 | The Joint Commission Patients' Rights Standards

- The hospital respects the rights of patients.
- Patients receive information about their rights.
- Patients are involved in decisions about care, treatment, and services provided.
- Informed consent is obtained.
- Consent is obtained for recording or filming made for purposes other than the identification, diagnosis, or treatment of the patients.
- Patients receive adequate information about the person(s) responsible for the delivery of their care, treatment, and services.
- Patients have the right to refuse care, treatment, and services in accordance with law and regulation.
- The hospital addresses the wishes of the patient relating to end-of-life care decisions.

- Patients and, when appropriate, their families are informed about the outcomes of care, treatment, and services, including unanticipated outcomes.
- The hospital addresses the resolution of complaints from patients and their families.
- The hospital respects the needs of patients for confidentiality, privacy, and security.
- Patients have a right to an environment that preserves dignity and contributes to a positive self-image.
- Patients have the right to be free from mental, physical, sexual, and verbal abuse, neglect, and exploitation.
- Patients have the right to pain management.
- Patients have a right to access protective and advocacy services.
- The hospital protects research subjects and respects their rights during research, investigation, and clinical trials involving human subjects.

From The Joint Commission: *Comprehensive accreditation manual for hospitals: the official handbook*, Chicago, 2007, The Joint Commission.

- An advance directive is a document that gives a patient's directions about future medical care or designates another person(s) to make medical decisions if the individual loses decision-making capacity.
- An advance directive conveys the patient's choice in continuing medical care when the patient is unable to speak or make decisions.
- Advance directives may include a living will, power of attorney for health care, or a notarized handwritten document.

- A copy of the document should be available in the patient's medical record. If not available, the substance of the advance directive should be documented in the medical record, and a family member should be asked to bring the advance directive to the hospital.
- The attending physician or health care provider is notified of the patient's advance directive.
- Witnesses for an advance directive document should not be medical personnel, nor should they be related to the patient or heirs to the patient's estate. A social worker often fulfills this requirement.

ROLE OF THE NURSE

Nurses assist in assigning patients to rooms, complete a thorough nursing assessment, review any advance directives, ensure that necessary diagnostic testing is completed, and provide for continuity of care when a patient is admitted (Fig. 2-1). Admitting personnel consult with nursing staff to ensure that a patient's room assignment is based on the patient's condition, health care needs, developmental level, activity level, expected length of stay, and personal preferences. For example, the best room for an older patient who is acutely ill, at risk for falls, and receiving multiple treatments is a room close to the nurses' station. The nurse identifies any known allergies and, if any exist, places an allergy band on the patient and properly documents the known allergies in the medical record.

When a patient is admitted through the ED, the nurse notifies the nursing division and reports on the patient's admission information, including the patient's name, admitting physician, chief complaint, any treatments or testing completed and the outcome, diagnosis, and pertinent information related to the patient's condition (e.g., initial vital signs, allergies, level of consciousness, and intravenous [IV] fluid infusing). An escort takes the patient and family members to the nursing division and introduces them to the nurse assuming the patient's care. The ED nurse shares pertinent observations about the patient's behavior (e.g., anxiety or fear or level of knowledge regarding need for health care) with the nursing staff to foster continuity of care and assist the patient and family in coping with a new environment and procedures.

Patients admitted on the morning of a surgical procedure or treatment are "same day" admissions. The nurse provides basic instructions about the purpose of the surgery or treatment, preparatory procedures, and postsurgical or posttreatment care. Admission and consent forms, diagnostic tests, patient teaching, and instructions are usually completed before the actual day of surgery. A variety of resources such as classes, videotapes, information booklets, and calls to home are used for patient teaching.

The nurse is active in coordinating the initial admission process for all patients. A patient's condition influences the extent and type of admission activities. Always note the patient's level of fatigue and comfort. For example, when a critically ill patient reaches a hospital's nursing division, the patient undergoes extensive examination and treatment procedures immediately. Little time is available for the nurse to orient the patient and family to the division or learn of the patient's fears or concerns. When a patient enters a hospital for elective treatment, the nurse has more time to prepare the patient psychologically for hospitalization.

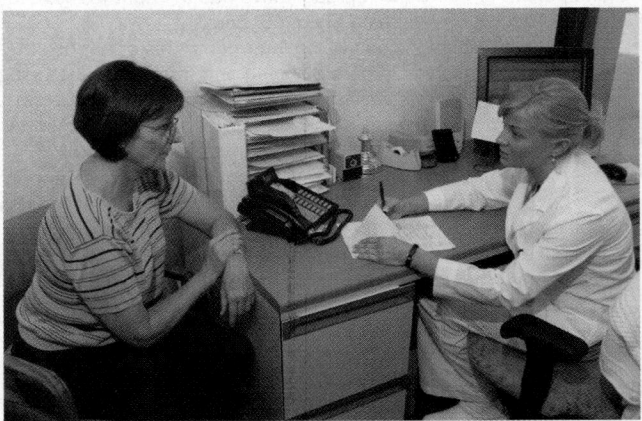

FIG 2-1 The nurse gathers important information from the patient.

Early psychological preparation when the patient is still at home prepares patients for hospitalization.

Delegation Considerations

The nursing assessment conducted during admission to a health care facility cannot be delegated to nursing assistive personnel (NAP). You cannot delegate admission obtaining vital signs because they provide a baseline for all further comparisons. The nurse directs the NAP to:

- Prepare the patient's room with necessary equipment needed before admission
- Gather and secure the patient's personal care items
- Escort and orient the patient and family to the nursing unit
- Collect ordered specimens

Equipment

- ☐ Hospital gown
- ☐ Bedpan and urinal
- ☐ Washbasin, bath towel, and washcloth
- ☐ Toiletry items (e.g., soap, toothpaste, hand lotion; *optional* in some hospitals)
- ☐ Facial tissues
- ☐ Water pitcher and drinking cup
- ☐ Kidney or emesis basin
- ☐ Disposable thermometer (see agency policy)
- ☐ Sphygmomanometer
- ☐ Stethoscope
- ☐ Pulse oximeter (*optional*)
- ☐ Documentation forms (see agency policy)

STEP	RATIONALE

ROOM PREPARATION

1 Perform hand hygiene, and prepare room equipment and furniture. Prepare bed by adjusting it to the lowest horizontal position if patient is ambulatory. Place bed in high position if patient is arriving by stretcher. Turn down top sheet and spread. Arrange room furniture for easy access to bed. Adjust lights, temperature, and ventilation.

Promotes patient's comfort by preventing delays during care. Proper position of bed lessens likelihood of patient falls and of back injuries to staff assisting patient into bed.

2 Be sure equipment is in working order. Then assemble any special equipment (e.g., suction, oxygen supplies, or IV pole) in patient's room.

Prevents delays in delivering immediate treatment and provides for smooth transition between caregivers.

ASSESSMENT

1 Greet patient and family cordially by name. Introduce yourself by name and job title; explain your responsibilities in patient's care. (Primary nurse is usually assigned at this time.)

Providing personalized care reduces anxiety about admission, clarifies staff roles, and expedites patient requests (Wu and Coyer, 2007).

2 If patient does not speak English or has a severe hearing impairment, arrange for a translation service so that you are able to conduct a nursing assessment.

Translation services are preferable to using family members to ensure correct translation of medical terminology.

3 Assess patient's general appearance, noting signs or symptoms of physical distress.

Provides baseline assessment.

Critical Decision Point *If patient is having acute physical problems, postpone routine admission procedures until you meet patient's immediate needs. Complete a focused assessment at this point.*

4 Escort patient and family to assigned room. Introduce them to roommate if semiprivate room is assigned at this time.

Orientation begins with introduction to roommate.

5 Assess patient's and family's psychological status by noting nonverbal behaviors and verbal responses to greetings and explanations.

Anxiety influences how well patient adapts to a health care environment and retains instruction.

6 Assess vital signs (see Chapter 5) and height and weight (see Chapter 6).

Provides baseline measurement to compare future findings. Determines alterations from normal range.

7 Assess for fall risk using scale with grading criteria as per agency policy. Consider patient's risk factors (e.g., neurological disorders, history of previous falls, urinary urgency or incontinence, use of sedatives, antihypertensives, and analgesics, history of unsteady gait, use of assistive devices, history of orthostatic hypotension, memory deficits).

Provides data to determine patient's risk for injury and whether patient needs to be placed on fall precautions.

8 Have family or friends leave room unless patient wishes to have them assist with changing into a hospital gown or pajamas. Close door and curtains. Help patient undress, and assist patient into comfortable position.

Provides for privacy and prepares patient for examination.

9 Obtain nursing history as soon as possible after patient's arrival to nursing division. Apply standards of nursing care adopted by hospital (e.g., functional health patterns). Data include:

Each patient is to have an admission assessment prepared by a registered nurse (RN) (TJC, 2007). Each institution sets a time frame for completion of admission assessment (maximum time 24 hours).

a Patient's perception of illness and health care needs

Establishes a baseline of patient's clinical status.

b Past medical history

c Presenting signs and symptoms and reason for hospitalization

Identifies signs and symptoms in case the patient's condition deteriorate.

d Completion of a review of health status based on standards such as elimination, nutrition and metabolism, activity and exercise, self-concept, values and beliefs, cultural factors, social support, and cognitive function

A comprehensive health history provides a holistic view of patient's health problems and response to those problems.

e Risk factors for illness

Allows nurse to institute preventive care measures and to educate patient about health promotion behaviors.

f History of allergies, including type of substance and a description of the reaction that patient has previously experienced.

Patients often have sensitivity to a drug or substance rather than a true allergy; this needs to be clarified. Specify all allergens to prevent accidental exposure.

STEP	RATIONALE

g Detailed medication history, including prescribed, over-the-counter (OTC), and alternative therapies such as herbs and hormones	Helps to assess potential for drug interactions and often explains patient's presenting signs and symptoms.
h Patient's knowledge of health problems and expectations of care	Enables the nurse to recognize and meet patient expectations when possible.
10 Conduct physical assessment of appropriate body systems (see Chapter 6). If not obtained in admitting, instruct patient to provide a urine specimen. Inform patient if collecting blood specimens or performing tests.	Provides objective data for identifying health problems. When unannounced procedures are performed, patients become anxious. Preparation of patient relieves anxiety.
11 Check physician's orders for treatment measures that need to be initiated immediately.	Delay causes deterioration of patient's condition.
12 Orient patient to nursing division.	
a Introduce staff members who enter room. Always introduce patient by last name unless patient indicates otherwise.	Helps patient to recognize caregivers. Shows respect for patient.
b Tell patient and family the name of nurse manager in charge of the division, and explain that person's role in solving problems.	Provides means for patient to communicate problems.
c Explain visiting hours and their purpose.	Provides knowledge and increases willingness to observe visiting hours policy, which ensures patient will receive adequate rest.
d Discuss smoking policy, and identify smoking areas for patient and family.	A hospitalwide smoking policy that prohibits the use of smoking materials throughout the hospital is required. In some cases, an exception is made for a patient by a physician prescription (TJC, 2007).
e Demonstrate use of equipment (e.g., bed, over-bed table, lighting).	Patient's safety depends on patient understanding correct use of equipment.
f Show patient how to use nurse call light, and position it in a convenient place. Have patient demonstrate use of light.	Ensures patient knows how to call for assistance.
g Escort patient to bathroom (if able to ambulate).	Patient's safety depends in part on understanding how to use toilet facilities.

h Explain hours for mealtime and nourishments to patient and family.	Family often wishes to visit during evening to assist with meals.
i Describe services available (e.g., chaplain, beauty shop, activity therapy).	Offers patient options for making decisions.

NURSING DIAGNOSES

- Anxiety
- Deficient knowledge regarding hospital procedures and planned therapies
- Fear
- Ineffective coping, individual or family
- Ineffective role performance
- Powerlessness
- Risk for injury

Individualize related factors based on patient's condition or needs.

PLANNING

1 Expected outcomes following completion of procedure:	
• Patient is able to explain purpose and schedule of planned treatments and procedures.	Understanding treatment plan gives patient a better sense of control and reduces anxiety about the unknown.
• Patient demonstrates how to call for nurse when assistance is needed.	Falls commonly occur when patients attempt to get out of bed without assistance.
• Patient is able to ambulate (if condition permits) in room free of obstacles and safely and efficiently use equipment in the room.	Equipment used in care of patient frequently poses hazards; assists in reducing some anxiety.
• Patient verbalizes understanding of smoking policy, visiting hours, mealtimes, and services available.	Knowledge of hospital policies assists patient in adapting to the health care environment.

STEP	RATIONALE

IMPLEMENTATION

1 Complete patient medication reconciliation by checking home medication list for duplication, omission, or potential drug interactions with newly ordered medications. Update medication list based on physician orders for treatment.

Medication reconciliation upon admission helps to make sure that patient is taking the correct medications and helps to avoid medication errors (TJC, 2006).

2 Inform patient about procedures or treatments scheduled for the next shift or day (e.g., visits by physician or dietitian). These vary based on nature of patient's condition.

Patient has right to be informed of any scheduled procedures or treatments. Being able to anticipate planned therapies minimizes anxiety.

3 Complete learning needs assessment for patient and family.

Identifies patient's and family's educational needs and learning preferences.

4 Give patient and family chance to ask questions about procedures or therapies. (If patient is unresponsive or unable to understand, review with family.)

Provides opportunity to clarify expectations and misconceptions.

5 Collect valuables patient chooses to keep at facility. Complete clothing and valuables listing sheet (see agency policy). Have patient or family member sign it. Place valuables in agency safe, or send home with family.

Accounts for placement of valuables and prevents loss.

6 Ensure patient and family have time together alone, if desired.

Admission is often stressful and fatiguing. Allows time for decision making.

7 Be sure call light is within easy reach and bed is in low position. (Check agency policy regarding use of side rails.)

Provides for patient's safety. Side rails enhance patient's ability to position in bed, but are considered a restraint if the side rail obstructs patient's ability to get out of bed when desired (TJC, 2007).

8 Perform hand hygiene.

Reduces spread of microorganisms.

EVALUATION

1 Have patient explain hospital policies, tests, and procedures through discussion and questions.

Patient demonstrates learning and understanding through patient feedback.

2 Have patient demonstrate use of call light.

Return demonstration confirms learning.

3 Monitor patient's ability to ambulate independently.

Provides data to judge patient's safety in ambulating without injury.

4 Check patient's room setup regularly.

Determines if care area is free of obstacles.

Unexpected Outcomes

1 Patient denies understanding hospital policies or knowing purpose or schedule for tests and procedures.

2 Patient becomes restless, expresses concerns, or displays tension in body movements.

3 Patient falls or is injured.

Related Interventions

- Schedule a follow-up session with patient.
- Keep information focused and specific to patient's situation. Include family if helpful.
- Give patient time to discuss fears and concerns.
- Show caring and compassion so that patient becomes willing to communicate openly.
- Attend to patient's immediate physical needs, inform physician of the injury or fall, reassess the patient's environment, alter care plan as needed, ensure that the environment is free of safety hazards, and complete incident report (see Chapter 13).

Recording and Reporting

- Record history and assessment findings on appropriate forms.
- If patient has an advance directive, place copy in the medical record. In the absence of the actual advance directive, document the substance of the directive in the medical record (TJC, 2007).
- Notify physician of patient's arrival; report any unusual findings. Secure admission orders if not previously provided.
- Begin to develop nursing plan of care. Confer with patient and family as needed.

- Teaching occurs throughout the admission process. Provide information regarding physical assessment findings, nature of patient's illness, planned diagnostic procedures, medications needed for treatment, and hospital routines. Do not begin a formal teaching plan until you have completed the assessment and developed a care plan.
- In an emergency situation or if patient is unable to perform aspects of his or her care, instruct family members in the rationale for any procedures and routines to be used in patient's care.

Teaching Considerations

- Explain to patient that a different nurse provides care on each shift. Explain time frame for how assignments are made.

Pediatric Considerations

- Hospitalization is a major crisis for children who feel stress from separation, loss of control, bodily injury, and pain. Separation anxiety is most common from middle infancy throughout the toddler years, especially ages 16 to 30 months. The child experiences protest, despair, and detachment. Preschoolers are better able to tolerate brief periods of separation, but their protest behaviors are more subtle than those in younger children (e.g., refusal to eat, difficulty sleeping, withdrawing from others). School-age children are able to cope with separation but have an increased need for parental security and guidance (Hockenberry and Wilson, 2007). Explain the institution's rooming-in and visiting policies. Allow and encourage parental involvement in the child's care. Allow parents to assist with routine care activities (e.g., bathing, eating) and when possible to remain with the child during procedures.

- Incorporate the child's usual routines such as favorite food, bedtime practices, and toileting into the plan of care. Encourage parent to bring the child a favorite toy, blanket, or other items to make child feel more comfortable in the unfamiliar setting.

Gerontological Considerations

- Hospitalized older adults with functional disabilities often rapidly regress into a helpless state during hospitalization. Interventions that retain functional status include daily orientation cues for patient, allowing the patient to be independent as tolerated, and reassurance regarding probability of transient delirium. Get patient up and out of room at least daily, and use physical therapy (PT) and occupational therapy (OT) daily. Keep the environment pleasant and comfortable, and personalize the environment (Ebersole and others, 2004).
- Patients who typically fall in the hospital are those who have been recently admitted and are unfamiliar with surroundings, have several pathological conditions, take medications with sedative or tranquilizing effects, or have had multiple recent transfers. In addition, visual changes that occur with aging often lead to falls in hospitalized older adult patients (Ebersole and others, 2004).

SKILL 2-2 Transferring Patients

Patients transfer to new patient care units and new agencies to receive different forms and levels of therapy and services and to have essential care continued closer to home. When patients transfer, you need to ensure continuity of nursing care. The aim is to continue health care so as to avoid therapeutic interruptions that may hinder progress toward recovery. Collaborate early with physicians and members of the other health care disciplines to ensure efficient patient transfer with good patient outcomes. Open collaboration and effective communication help to ensure quality patient care is realized.

When transferring a patient from one division to another within an agency, it is usually easy to complete the process without interrupting care activities. Policies and procedures are usually similar throughout the institution. The nurse first provides a telephone report to the receiving nurse. This allows the receiving nurse to prepare for the patient (e.g., preparing the room and securing necessary equipment). As clinically appropriate, the nurse or a technician accompanies the patient during transport, providing the receiving nurse with the patient's medical record, introducing the patient to the receiving nurse, and providing an updated report including any changes in clinical status or plan of care.

In the ED, when a patient is transferred from one institution to another, the nurse completes the transfer in compliance with the Emergency Medical Treatment and Labor Act (EMTALA) (CMS, 2003). EMTALA is a federal law intended to protect patients from being transferred against their wishes and thus defines how an appropriate facility-to-facility transfer is accomplished. An appropriate transfer includes:

- Informing the patient of the risks and benefits of the transfer
- Obtaining the patient's written consent for transfer

- Having the transferring hospital provide medical treatment within its capacity
- Having available space and qualified personnel for treatment of the patient at the receiving institution and agreement to accept transfer of the patient and to provide treatment
- Making copies of all relevant medical records, including a transfer form, sent by the transferring institution to the receiving facility
- Transporting the patient using qualified personnel and transportation equipment (e.g., ambulance with advanced cardiac life support [ACLS] versus basic life support [BLS])

Although this law primarily affects the ED, know the institution's EMTALA policies and transfer policies for inpatient transfers. Many institutions follow the same policies for all patient transfers.

Delegation Considerations

The assessment and decision making conducted during transfers cannot be delegated to NAP. The nurse directs the NAP to:

- Assist the patient with dressing
- Gather and secure the patient's personal belongings and any equipment that goes with the patient
- Escort the patient to the nursing unit or transport area

Equipment

- ☐ Transfer forms
- ☐ Copies of medical records, radiology films, laboratory test results, etc. (as appropriate)
- ☐ Special equipment as needed: wheelchair or stretcher, emesis basin, bedpan and urinal, oxygen tank and tubing, IV pole, cardiac monitor, and emergency medications

---

STEP	RATIONALE

ASSESSMENT

1 Obtain transfer order from sending physician. Order includes name of receiving agency (when applicable), receiving physician's name, and statement of patient's stability for transfer.

Physician is legally responsible for releasing patient from medical care and arranging for receiving physician. Patient has legal right to refuse transfer against medical advice.

STEP	RATIONALE
2 In collaboration with the physician and members of other health care disciplines, assess reason for patient's transfer (e.g., change in condition, services available at agency, patient or family preferences regarding patient's location).	Patient needs to have access to agency with best resources to meet health care needs. Physician determines patient's physical stability for transfer.
3 Explain purpose of transfer thoroughly, and provide time to discuss patient's and family's feelings about the change in care setting. As necessary, obtain patient's written consent to transfer. If patient is unable to consent, patient's family provides this consent.	Patients need to be informed of transfer plans in a timely manner (TJC, 2007). Patient requires adequate psychological preparation. In the event of a clinical emergency in which patient and patient's family are unable to consent, this consent is waived and patient is transferred to a higher level of care based on the clinical judgment of the physician requesting the transfer.
4 Assess patient's current physical condition, and determine method for transport. When transferring to new agency, assess method of transport to transferring vehicle (e.g., wheelchair or stretcher) (consult agency policy).	Patient's condition often changes quickly and influences stability for transfer and type of support needed during transport.

Critical Decision Point   *Determine if patient's status and safety require life support equipment. Staff assisting with transfer needs training in life support measures. When transporting to new agency, a vehicle equipped with life support equipment is necessary.*

STEP	RATIONALE
5 Assess if patient requires pain relief or other medications for symptom management.	Ensures patient's comfort during transfer
6 Ensure that staff have notified patient's family or significant others of transfer as desired by patient.	Provides adequate communication with family or significant others to assist with patient's emotional and psychological adjustment to the transfer (TJC, 2007).

NURSING DIAGNOSES

- Anxiety
- Deficient knowledge regarding transfer procedure
- Fear
- Pain, acute and chronic
- Powerlessness
- Risk for relocation stress syndrome

Individualize related factors based on patient's condition or needs.

PLANNING

1 Expected outcomes following completion of procedure:	
• Patient's vital signs and physiological status remain the same following transfer.	Treatments are planned so as not to interrupt physical support of patient during transfer.
• Patient incurs no injury during transport procedures.	Safety measures are successful in transferring patient from wheelchair or stretcher to transport vehicle.
• Patient or family explains purpose of transfer and procedure for transport.	Understanding provides patient with sense of control.
• Receiving nursing staff acquires and confirms written plan of care.	Ensures continuity of care.
2 Arrange for patient's transport to an agency by chosen vehicle (sometimes you will require support from social worker).	Transfer needs to occur without delays so that patient has access to all needed resources at all times.
3 When transfer is to a new agency, contact the agency and arrange for bed in appropriate setting. Confirm willingness of agency to accept patient (usually social worker or discharge coordinator will complete).	Prevents delays when patient arrives at destination. Receiving hospital ensures that there is available space and qualified personnel to treat patients. Hospital also agrees in advance to transfer.

IMPLEMENTATION

1 Make sure documentation in patient's record is complete. Individualize nursing care measures based on patient need.	Accurate information is necessary for receiving agency to assume patient's care.
2 Complete nursing care transfer form according to agency policy. (When transfer is to a different nursing unit, entire medical record accompanies patient.)	Form provides summary of patient's pertinent nursing care needs to ensure continuity of care and prevents unnecessary duplication of services.
3 Complete medication reconciliation per institution policy. Check the patient's current orders against the most recent medication administration record and the original home medication list. Communicate updated medication list to next provider of care.	Ensures that patient receives correct medications at new facility and decreases medication errors (TJC, 2006).

STEP	RATIONALE
4 Gather patient's personal care items, clothing, and valuables. Check the entire room and all storage areas. Secure in suitcase or container.	Prevents loss of articles during transfer.
5 Anticipate problems patient frequently develops just before or during transfer. Perform necessary nursing therapies such as suctioning or changing a dressing.	Ensures patient's comfort and safety during transport.
6 Assist in transferring patient to stretcher or wheelchair using safe patient handling techniques (see Chapters 9 and 10).	It is easier to move patient transported to outside agency by stretcher into transport vehicle.
7 Perform and document final assessment of patient's physical stability.	Minimizes risk of patient developing complications during transfer.

Critical Decision Point *Priority assessment includes vital signs, clear airway, patency of intravenous lines and accuracy of infusion rate, and patient's level of consciousness.*

STEP	RATIONALE
8 When transfer occurs to an outside agency, accompany patient to transport vehicle.	Ensures medically qualified personnel are in attendance until patient leaves agency/unit.
9 Call receiving agency/unit and notify of impending transfer and patient's status (check agency policy).	Notification of nurse in charge or nurse assuming care of patient ensures better continuity of care at time of patient's arrival.

EVALUATION

1 During the final assessment compare data with the previous findings.	Determines if patient's condition is changing.
2 Inspect patient's alignment and positioning on stretcher/wheelchair.	Proper alignment and positioning reduces risk of an injury occurring during transport.
3 Confirm patient understands transfer and procedures through discussion and questions.	Feedback helps to ensure learning.
4 Determine if receiving agency/nurse has questions about patient's care.	Provides for clear communication and continuity of care.

Unexpected Outcomes	Related Interventions
1 Patient's physical status deteriorates during preparation.	• Call physician immediately. • Initiate necessary interventions to stabilize patient's condition.
2 Patient sustains injury during transfer to wheelchair or stretcher.	• Stabilize patient and call physician. • Complete incident (occurrence) report (see Chapter 4).
3 Patient is confused or uncertain about transfer.	• Provide clarification or additional explanation.
4 Receiving staff misinterprets directions for patient's care.	• Sending agency has nurse or physician call to confirm that there are no questions regarding patient's care.

Recording and Reporting

- Nurse sending patient documents patient's status, including vital signs and other assessment findings, nursing plan of care, date and time of transfer, and method of transport.
- Nurse receiving patient documents patient's arrival at agency by recording date and time of arrival, reason for transfer, method of transport, patient's condition, and care provided at time of arrival.

Teaching Considerations

- A transfer frequently creates anxiety for patient and family members. Carefully repeat instructions regarding transfer at a time when patient and family are better able to understand your explanation. In this situation, be sure to have patient restate any critical information.

Pediatric Considerations

- Children need their parents' comfort and security; thus make sure parents are well informed. Involve older children in any discussion regarding transfers. Allow a parent to accompany the child in the transfer.

Gerontological Considerations

- When transferring an older adult patient to a new facility, relocation is stressful. Ensure that significant support persons are still accessible and that patient is thoroughly oriented to new surroundings. Also make sure that patient is able to take important memorabilia and has opportunity to make decisions about care.

Long-Term Care Considerations

- It is important that patients receive the level of services appropriate to their physical and mental health needs. Participation of social worker or discharge planner in transfer process ensures that transfer to a long-term care facility is appropriate.
- Upon patient's arrival at long-term care agency, complete Resident Assessment Instrument (RAI). The RAI consists of the minimum data set (MDS), resident assessment protocols, and utilization guidelines specified in state operations guidelines (Meiner and Lueckenotte, 2006).

BOX 2-5	Federal Requirements for Discharge Planning Process

- Hospitals must identify at an early stage of hospitalization patients who are likely to suffer adverse health consequences on discharge if there is no planning.
- The hospital must provide a discharge planning evaluation.
- A registered nurse, social worker, or other qualified person must develop or supervise development of the evaluation.
- Discharge planning must include an evaluation of the likelihood of the patient needing posthospital services and of the availability of the services.
- Discharge planning must include an evaluation of the likelihood of a patient's capacity for self-care.
- On request of the patient's physician or health care provider, the

- hospital must arrange for development and implementation of the patient's discharge plan.
- The evaluation must be completed on a timely basis so that appropriate arrangements for posthospital care are made before discharge and to avoid unnecessary delays in discharge.
- The discharge planning evaluation must be in the patient's medical record, and the results must be discussed with the patient and/or significant others.
- The patient and family members must be counseled to prepare them for posthospital care.
- The discharge plan must be reassessed on an ongoing basis to ensure that the plan is responsive to the patient's discharge needs.

Modified from Centers for Medicare and Medicaid Services: Chapter IV: Centers for Medicare and Medicaid Services, Department of Health and Human Services, Part 482.43, Condition of participation: discharge planning, http://www.access.gpo.gov/nara.cfr.waisdx_04/42cfr482_04.html, accessed on August 1, 2007.

SKILL 2-3   Discharging Patients

Discharge planning facilitates the transition of a patient from a health care agency to the most independent level of care, whether that is home or another agency. The overall goal of discharge planning is to provide the most appropriate level and quality of care throughout all stages of a patient's illness. The discharge planning process is comprehensive and multidisciplinary, including all caregivers who are involved in the care of the patient. Every hospitalized patient requires discharge planning. The trend toward a shortened length of stay in the acute care setting makes discharge planning increasingly difficult, but all the more essential (Wells and others, 2002). Federal regulations identify the elements of a comprehensive discharge planning model (Box 2-5).

Development of a plan with outcomes mutually accepted by the patient and caregivers and ongoing communication about its progress are essential (Cleary and others, 2003). The discharge process occurs in three phases: acute, transitional, and continuing care (Fig. 2-2). In the acute phase, medical attention dominates discharge planning efforts. During the transitional phase, the need for acute care is still present, but its urgency declines and patients begin to address and plan for their future health care needs. In the continuing care phase, patients are able to participate in planning and implementing continuing care activities needed after discharge.

The greatest challenge in effective discharge planning is communication. You minimize the communication problem when an organization has a discharge coordinator or case manager responsible for discharge planning (Zander, 2002). Staff in these roles are responsible for thoroughly assessing a patient's health care needs at

discharge, identifying available and needed resources, and linking the patient and family to the proper resources. Staff are also responsible for coordinating services (as appropriate), and following up on the patient's progress after discharge.

Discharge from an agency is stressful for a patient and family. Before a patient is discharged, the patient and family need to know how to manage care in the home and what to expect in regard to any continuing physical problems. Without the necessary equipment and professional resources, a patient risks loss of rehabilitation gains made before discharge. Failure to understand restrictions or implications of health problems often causes a patient to develop complications. Poor discharge planning ignores a patient's needs within the home and increases the chance of the patient needing to reenter the health care system prematurely.

Delegation Considerations

The assessment, care planning, and instruction included in discharging patients cannot be delegated to NAP. The nurse directs the NAP to:
- Gather and secure the patient's personal items and any supplies that accompany the patient
- Transport the patient to the discharge transport vehicle

Equipment
- ❑ Wheelchair or stretcher
- ❑ Discharge documentation forms (see agency policy)
- ❑ Patient instruction sheets
- ❑ Plastic bag for personal belongings

STEP	RATIONALE

ASSESSMENT

1 From time of admission, assess patient's discharge needs using nursing history, discussions with patient, and care plan; focus on ongoing assessments of patient's physical health, functional status, psychosocial support system, financial resources, health values, cultural and ethnic background, level of education, and barriers to care.

Planning for discharge begins at admission and continues throughout patient's stay in agency. Discharge planning interventions focus on assisting patients in achieving maximal functioning.

2 Assess patient's and family's need for health teaching related to how to perform home therapies, use of home medical equipment, restrictions resulting from health alterations, and possible complications.

Improves understanding of health care needs and ability to achieve self-care at home. Inclusion of family member in teaching sessions provides patient with available resource.

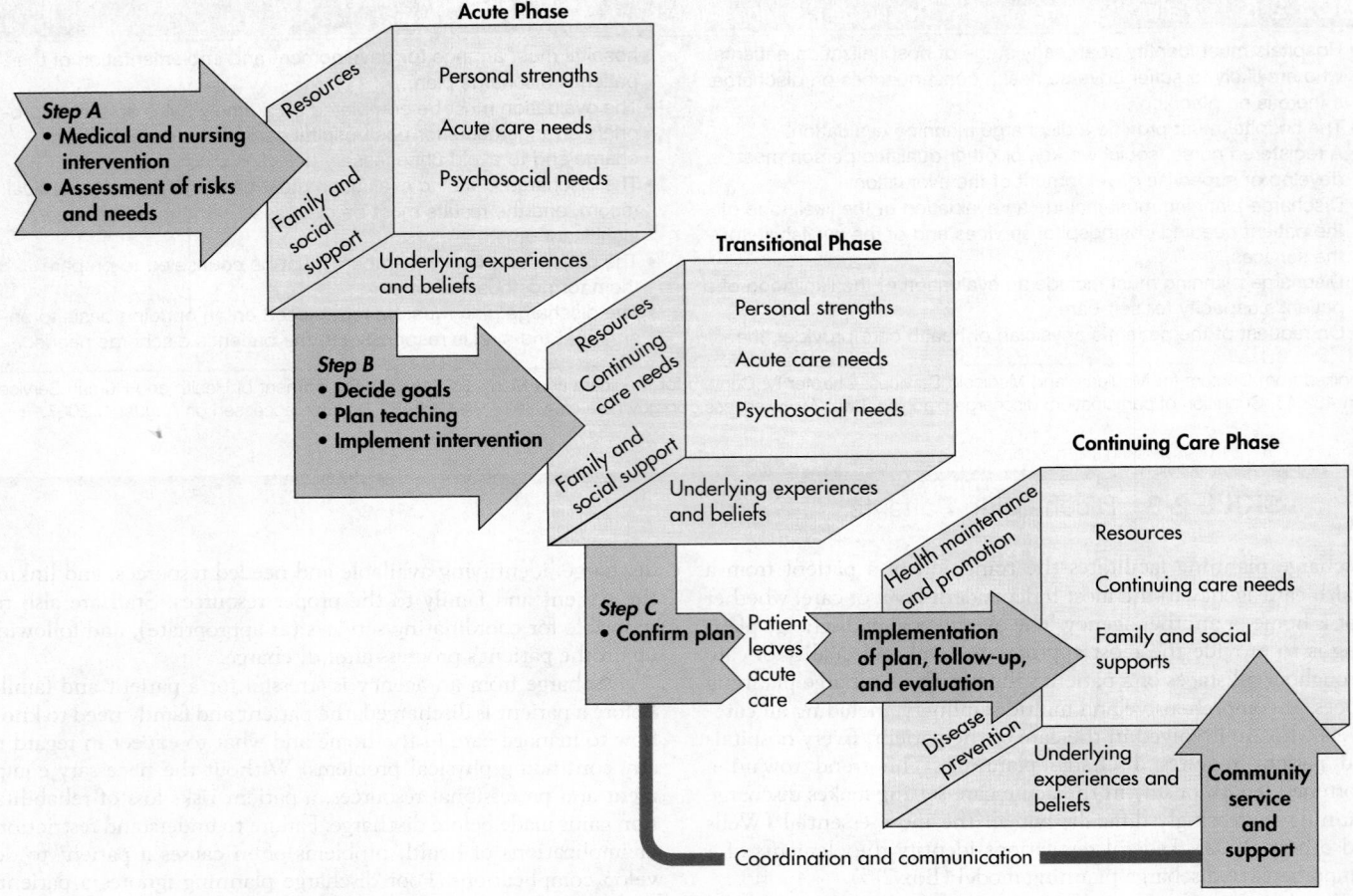

FIG 2-2   Phases of discharge planning process. (Redrawn from Rorden JW, Taft E: *Discharge planning guide for nurses*, Philadelphia, 1990, WB Saunders.)

STEP	RATIONALE
3 Assess for barriers to learning.	Determines timing and approach to instruction. Different types of educational materials are effective with different individual learning styles. If printed material is to be used, be sure material at proper reading level is available.
4 Assess for environmental factors within home that interfere with self-care (e.g., size of rooms, doorway clearances, steps, bathroom facilities). (A home care nurse is usually available on referral to assist with assessment.)	Environmental factors within patient's home pose safety risks or problems for self-care. For example, throw rugs are a fall hazard for a patient discharged with crutches or a walker (see Chapter 41).
5 Collaborate with physician and multidisciplinary staff (e.g., physical therapy) in assessing need for referral for skilled home care services or extended care facility.	Patients eligible for home care must be confined to home as result of illness, are under physician's care, and require skilled nursing care on an intermittent basis.
6 Assess patient's and family's perceptions of continued health care needs outside the hospital. Include an assessment of family caregivers' perceived ability to provide care to patient, including ability to adjust to demands of patient care, impact of care demands on their lives (e.g., reducing noise levels in home, preparing special diets), and potential ongoing nature of patient's needs.	Patients and family members often disagree on health care needs of patient after discharge. Identifying these discrepancies early helps in more accurately developing the discharge plan. Family caregiving is frequently a highly stressful experience. Family members who are not properly prepared for their role as caregivers are frequently overwhelmed by patient's needs, which can lead to neglect or unnecessary hospital readmissions.

Critical Decision Point   *It is often necessary to talk with patient and family separately to learn about true concerns or doubts.*

7 Assess patient's acceptance of health problems and related restrictions.	Affects willingness to follow therapies and restrictions.

STEP	**RATIONALE**
8 Consult other health care team members (e.g., dietitian, social worker) about anticipated needs after discharge. Make appropriate referrals in a timely manner.	Members of all health care disciplines collaborate to determine patient's needs and functional abilities.

NURSING DIAGNOSES

- Anxiety
- Caregiver role strain
- Deficient knowledge regarding home care restrictions
- Impaired home maintenance
- Ineffective therapeutic regimen management
- Interrupted family processes
- Relocation stress syndrome
- Self-care deficit: feeding, toileting, dressing/grooming, bathing/hygiene

Individualize related factors based on patient's condition or needs.

PLANNING

1 Expected outcomes following completion of procedure:	
• Patient or family caregiver explains how health care is to continue in home (or other facility), what treatments or medications patient needs, and when to seek medical attention for problems.	Increases likelihood of care not being interrupted in home (or other facility).
• Patient is able to demonstrate self-care activities (or family member is able to administer care measures).	Feedback ensures learning.
• Remove obstacles to patient's mobility and hazards to ambulation in home setting.	Patient is often physically weakened or has physical changes resulting from illness that predispose to injury.

IMPLEMENTATION

1 Preparation before day of discharge:	
a Suggest ways to change physical arrangement of home to meet patient's needs (see Chapter 41).	Maintains patient's level of independence and ability to retain function within safe environment.
b Provide patient and family with information about community health care resources (e.g., medical equipment companies, Meals on Wheels, adult day care). Referrals are usually made while patient is in hospital.	Community resources offer services patient or family cannot provide (Smith and Liles, 2007).
c Conduct teaching sessions with patient and family as soon as possible during hospitalization (e.g., signs and symptoms of complications, information regarding medications, use of medical equipment, follow-up care, diet, exercise, restrictions imposed by illness or surgery). Review and give the patient discharge materials such as pamphlets, books, or multimedia resources. Refer patient to resources on the Internet.	Gives patient opportunities to practice new skills, ask questions, and obtain necessary feedback to ensure learning. A combination of written and verbal information is effective in improving patient satisfaction and knowledge (Johnson and others, 2007).
d Communicate patient's and family's response to teaching and proposed discharge plan to other health care team members.	Facilitates development of individualized discharge plan.
2 Procedure on day of discharge:	
a Let patient and family ask questions or discuss issues related to home care. A final opportunity to demonstrate learned skills is helpful.	Allows for final clarification of information previously discussed. Helps relieve anxiety.
b Check physician's discharge orders for prescriptions, change in treatments, or need for special medical equipment. (Make sure orders are written as early as possible.) Make arrangements for delivery and setup of equipment before the patient arrives home (e.g., hospital bed, oxygen, feeding pump).	Only a physician is able to authorize a discharge. Early check of orders permits nurse to attend to any last-minute treatments or procedures well before discharge.
c Determine whether patient or family has arranged for transportation.	Patient's condition at discharge determines method of transport.
d Provide privacy and assistance as patient dresses and packs all personal belongings. Check all closets and drawers for belongings. Obtain copy of valuables list signed by patient, and have security or appropriate administrator deliver valuables to patient.	Prevents loss of personal items. Patient's signature verifies receipt of items and relieves nursing department of liability for losses.

STEP	RATIONALE
e Complete medication reconciliation per institution policy. Check discharge medication orders against the medication administration record and home medication list. Provide patient with prescriptions or pharmacy-dispensed medications ordered by physician. Offer a final review of information needed to facilitate safe medication self-administration.	Medication reconciliation decreases risk of medication errors and ensures that patient is receiving correct medication at home (TJC, 2006). Review of drug information provides feedback to determine patient's success in learning about medications.
f Provide information on follow-up appointments to the physician's office. Provide phone number of unit.	Provides patient with contact for questions that arise after discharge. Ensures continuity of care to prevent rehospitalization.
g Contact agency's business office to determine whether patient needs to finalize arrangements for payment of bill. Arrange for patient or family to visit business office.	Source of concern for many patients is whether agency has accepted insurance or other payment forms.
h Acquire utility cart to move patient's belongings. Obtain wheelchair for patient. Transport patients leaving by ambulance on ambulance stretchers.	Provides for safe transport.
i Assist patient to wheelchair or stretcher using safe patient handling and transfer techniques (see Chapter 9). Escort patient to entrance of agency where source of transportation is waiting (see agency policy) (see illustrations). Lock wheelchair wheels. Assist patient in transferring into transport vehicle. Help place personal belongings in vehicle.	Prevents injury to nurse and patient. Agency policy requires escort to ensure patient's safe exit. Agency's liability ends once patient is safely in vehicle.
j Return to division. Notify admitting or appropriate department of time of discharge. Notify housekeeping of need to clean patient's room.	Allows agency to prepare for admission of next patient.

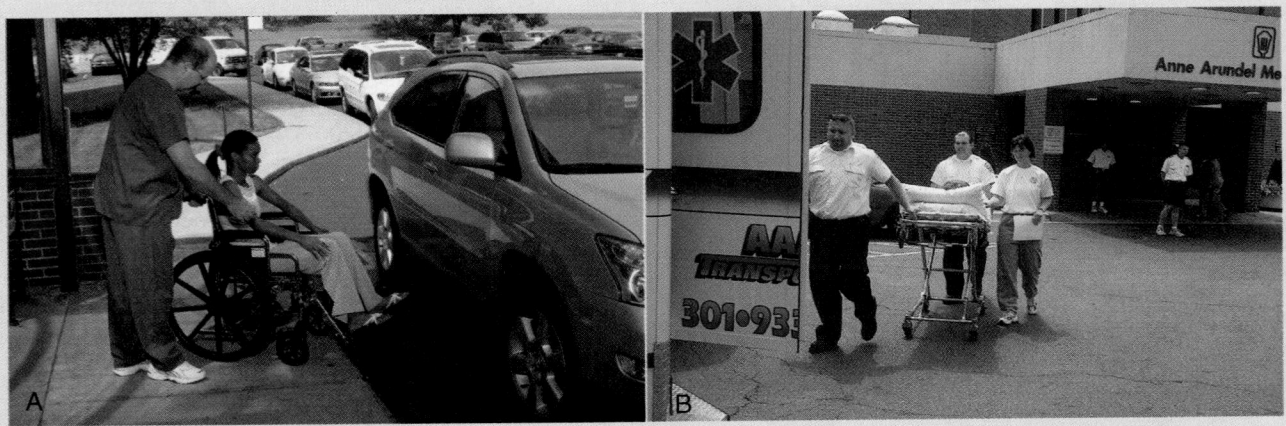

STEP 2i **A,** Nurse escorts the patient to the transport vehicle at the time of discharge via a wheelchair. **B,** Many patients are discharged via stretcher.

EVALUATION

1 Ask patient or family member to describe nature of illness, treatment regimens, and physical signs or symptoms to be reported to a physician.	Measures patient's or family's learning.
2 Have patient or family member perform any treatments that will continue in the home.	Return demonstrations allow nurse to evaluate level of learning.
3 Home care nurse inspects home, identifies obstacles that pose risks for patient, and recommends revisions.	Provides continuity of care.

Unexpected Outcomes	Related Interventions
1 Patient or family is unable to explain self-care measures.	• Provide immediate clarification, or offer additional instruction.
2 Patient or family demonstrates treatment measures incorrectly.	• Plan additional time to demonstrate treatment measures to patient and family.
	• Ask patient to explain what aspect of procedure is difficult to perform and why.
	• If patient or family continues to be unable to correctly demonstrate treatment measures, request referral for home care of public health services.

Unexpected Outcomes

3 Environmental risks are still present in home.

4 Patient or family resists discharge plans and refuses assimilation of new roles needed for home care.

5 Patient refuses continued treatment and requests to leave the hospital before planned discharge.

Related Interventions

- Family or patient often discounts risk or does not have resources to make needed changes.
- Home care nurse attempts to problem solve and seek appropriate solution.
- Contact additional resources (e.g., social work, home care, pastoral care) to assist patient and family with home care needs.
- Talk with patient to determine reason for request to leave the hospital. Attempt to resolve the pressing issue for the patient; involve family and social worker as appropriate.
- Notify physician to talk with patient and explain the risks of leaving the hospital with unresolved health care needs and the benefits of continued treatment.
- Inform patient that his or her health insurance provider may not pay for hospitalization due to leaving against medical advice (AMA).
- Request that patient sign discharge AMA form documenting that he or she understands the risk involved in leaving.
- Complete incident report, and document thoroughly all communications/action taken in attempt to have patient continue treatment (see Chapter 4).

Recording and Reporting

- Complete documentation of patient's discharge on discharge summary form (Box 2-6). Give patient a signed copy of form.
- Document unresolved problems and description of arrangements made for resolution in nurses' notes.
- Document patient's vital signs and status of health problems at time of discharge in nurses' notes.

Teaching Considerations

- Assess patient's fatigue and pain levels before beginning any instruction. Keep focused on the important teaching topics to cover.

Pediatric Considerations

- Once family members have learned how to perform any necessary caregiver skills, have them assume care before child returns home. Many hospitals incorporate a trial period requiring family to manage care before child's discharge home (Hockenberry and Wilson, 2007).

Gerontological Considerations

- Older persons have been found to be interested in more information about community resources and how to access information once discharged (Smith and Liles, 2007).

- Older adults and their families often overestimate their ability to manage care after discharge. They also disagree about what postdischarge care includes. Make referrals to home care as needed to address needs associated with functional decline and to help prevent readmission to the hospital.
- Older adults frequently need assistance with bathing and household activities. Assess bathroom for safety issues. Make referral to community agencies that provide assistance to older adults with bathing and other household chores (McKeown, 2007).

Home Care Considerations

- Assess availability and skill of primary caregiver (e.g., spouse or neighbor): assess time availability, ability and willingness to give care, emotional and physical stamina, and knowledge of caregiving. Assess additional resources, including friends or neighbors who are available to help.
- Refer patients who meet the eligibility criteria to home care agencies for assistance.
- Inform patient or family member and patient's physician as to decision to accept or not accept patient for admission to home care agency.

BOX 2-6	Elements of a Written Discharge Summary Form

- Mode of discharge: ambulatory, wheelchair, stretcher
- Instructions for self-care activities: activity, diet, medications, special treatments such as wound care, self-catheterization, tracheostomy care
- Reconciled list of discharge medications with dose, frequency, route, reasons for change in medication or for newly prescribed medications
- Signs and symptoms of complications or drug reactions to be observant for

- Signs and symptoms that are to be normally expected by the patient
- Correct settings for any equipment required
- Planned follow-up appointment at physician's office, clinic
- Name and contact information of physician and/or nursing unit
- Explanation of pertinent emergency procedures
- Patient's signature, showing understanding of instructions

Modified from Kripalani S and others: Deficits in communication and information transfer between hospital-based and primary care physicians: implications for patient safety and continuity of care, *JAMA* 297(8):831, 2007.

CRITICAL THINKING EXERCISES

Mrs. Hampton, a 68-year-old retired school teacher, is transferring from intensive care to your nursing unit following a cerebrovascular accident (CVA). She entered the ED 2 days ago with slurred speech and weakness of the right arm and leg. She has a history of primary hypertension, coronary artery disease, and type 2 diabetes. Her condition is stabilized. The intensive care nurse calls you to give report on Mrs. Hampton. The nurse notes the admitting diagnosis, vital signs, pain level, and transferring physician orders.

1 What other information would you like to have about Mrs. Hampton?

2 The nurse arrives with Mrs. Hampton in a wheelchair; she is accompanied by her husband. What interventions would you select to reduce Mr. and Mrs. Hampton's anxiety related to the transfer out of the intensive care unit?

3 Mr. Hampton states his wife has an advance directive. What is the role of the nurse in understanding a patient's advance directive?

4 Mr. Hampton tells you that his wife is going home in a few days because she is doing so well. She will be going home using a walker. He says that he hopes he will be able to take care of her once she is at home. How do you respond to Mr. Hampton? What interventions do you need to take before Mrs. Hampton's discharge?

REVIEW QUESTIONS

1 In which steps of the admission process can the admission clerk participate? Select all that apply.
1 Explain information about a patient's rights to health care services.
2 Attach an identification band after verifying the information is correct.
3 Review the details of a patient's advance directive for clarity.
4 Explain how HIPAA is enforced in the institution.
5 Print a patient's allergies on the allergy band before attaching it to the patient.
6 Help a patient know what is included in the basic admission process.

2 Who is responsible for developing a patient's discharge plan?
1 The primary nurse
2 The medical social worker
3 The nurse caring for the patient the longest
4 The patient's health care team

3 Which statement best explains why it is essential to assess and document the clinical status of a patient immediately before transfer or discharge?
1 Increased reimbursement to the hospital that occur because of additional diagnosis codes.
2 Potential changes in a patient's clinical needs that require nursing interventions to provide for patient safety during transport.
3 Hospital documentation requirements could prevent transfer of a patient unless the information is current.
4 The necessary information needs to be reflective of a discharge plan for visiting accrediting agencies.

4 A toddler, 20 months old, is hospitalized for the first time. Which strategy is most effective to make the child feel more comfortable?
1 Have the parents visit only sporadically so the toddler does not get upset.
2 Have the child bring a favorite blanket for comfort.
3 Ask the parents what time the toddler usually goes to bed.
4 Find out the toddler's favorite foods and beverages.

5 An alert patient is admitted to the hospital for an elective surgical procedure. He does not want to stay in his room and is constantly going into the rooms of other patients, bothering them. Which approach is most appropriate to deal with the situation?
1 Obtain a physician's order to sedate the patient.
2. Apply a jacket restraint until the physician can evaluate him.
3 Begin the discharge summary form.
4 Spend some time talking with the patient to obtain some insight about his behavior.

REFERENCES

Centers for Medicare and Medicaid Services: 42 CFR Parts 413, 482, and 489 Medicare Program, Clarifying policies related to the responsibilities of Medicare-participating hospitals in treating individuals with emergency medical conditions: final rule, *Federal Register* 68(174):53222, 2003.

Centers for Medicare and Medicaid Services: 42 CFR 482.13 (b)(2) Medicare and Medicaid programs, hospital condition of participation: patients' rights, final rule, *Federal Register* 71(236):71378, 2006.

Centers for Medicare and Medicaid Services: *Chapter IV: Medicare and Medicaid Services, Department of Health and Human Services Centers, Part 482.43, Condition of participation, discharge planning,* http://www.access.gpo.gov/nara.cfr.waisdx_04/42cfr482_04.html, accessed August 1, 2007.

Ebersole P and others: *Toward healthy aging: human nature and nursing response,* ed 6, St. Louis, 2004, Mosby.

Giger JN, Davidhizar RE: *Transcultural nursing: assessment and intervention,* ed 4, St. Louis, 2004, Mosby.

Hockenberry MJ, Wilson D: *Wong's nursing care of infants and children,* ed 8, St. Louis, 2007, Mosby.

Meiner SE, Lueckenotte AG: *Gerontologic nursing,* ed 3, St. Louis, 2006, Mosby.

Schwartz M, Wyskiel R: Medication reconciliation: developing and implementing a program, *Crit Care Nurs Clin North Am* 18:503, 2006.

The Joint Commission: Using medication reconciliation to prevent errors, *Sentinel Event Alert* Jan 23(35):1, 2006.

The Joint Commission: *Comprehensive accreditation manual for hospitals: the official handbook,* Chicago, 2007, The Joint Commission.

U.S. Department of Health and Human Services: *Summary of the HIPAA privacy rule,* Washington, DC, 2003, Office for Civil Rights.

Wu DF, Coyer F: Reconsidering the transfer of patient from the intensive care unit to the ward: a case study approach, *Nurs Health Sci* 9:48, 2007.

Zander K: Nursing case management in the 21st century: intervening where margin meets mission, *Nurs Adm Q* 26(5):58, 2002.

RESEARCH REFERENCES

Cleary M and others: Consumer feedback on nursing care and discharge planning, *J Adv Nurs* 42(3):269, 2003.

Grimmer K and others: Incorporating patient and career concerns in discharge plans: the development of a practical patient-centered checklist, *Internet J Allied Health Sci Pract* 4(1):1, 2006.

Johnson A and others: Written and verbal information versus verbal information only for patients discharged from acute hospital settings to home, *Cochrane Database Syst Rev* 3: no page, 2007.

Kramer JS and others: Implementation of an electronic system for medication reconciliation, *Am J Health Syst Pharm* 64:404, 2007.

Kripalani S and others: Deficits in communication and information transfer between hospital-based and primary care physicians: implications for patient safety and continuity of care, *JAMA* 297(8):831, 2007.

Lessard S and others: Medication discrepancies affecting senior patient at hospital admission, *Am J Health Syst Pharm* 63:740, 2006.

McKeown F: The experiences of older people on discharge from hospital following assessment by the public health nurse, *J Clin Nurs* 16:469, 2007.

Smith J, Liles C: Information needs before hospital discharge of myocardial infarction patients: a comparative, descriptive study, *J Clin Nurs* 16:662, 2007.

Weiss ME, Piacentine LB: Psychometric properties of the Readiness for Hospital Discharge Scale, *J Nurs Meas* 14(3):163, 2006.

Weiss ME and others: Perceived readiness for hospital discharge in adult medical-surgical patients, *Clin Nurs Spec* 21(1):31, 2007.

Wells DL and others: Evaluation of an integrated model of discharge planning: achieving quality discharges in an efficient and ethical way, *Can J Nurs Res* 34(3):103, 2002.

Communication

SKILLS AND PROCEDURES

KEY TERMS

Active listening

Cadence

Clarifying

Comforting

De-escalation

Empathy

Interviewing

Orientation phase

Paraphrasing

Reflecting

Restating

Summarizing

Termination phase

Therapeutic silence

Working phase

MEDIA RESOURCES

- **evolve** *learning system* http://evolve.elsevier.com/Perry/skills
  - Video Clips
  - Review Questions

OBJECTIVES

Mastery of content in this chapter will enable the nurse to:
- Identify guidelines to use in therapeutic communication.
- Explain the communication process.
- Identify the purposes of therapeutic communication, communication in various phases of the nurse-patient relationship, and special issues related to communication.
- Develop skills for therapeutic communication in various phases of the nurse-patient relationship.
- Develop therapeutic communication skills for communicating with anxious, angry and depressed patients.

It is critical that nurses have effective and adaptable communication skills (Gruber and Hartman, 2007). A nurse's responsibility to effectively communicate extends beyond the patient to include family members/significant others and members of the health care team. This chapter does not intend to give a complete introduction to the complicated process of communication. Rather, the purpose of this chapter is to provide a framework for you to develop therapeutic skills that are essential to the communication process.

Communication is an interaction between two or more persons that involves the exchange of information between a sender and a receiver (Fig. 3-1). It is an essential component of the human experience, involving the expression of emotions, ideas, and thoughts through verbal (words or written language) and nonverbal (behaviors) exchanges. Therapeutic communication is an application of the process of communication to promote the well-being of a patient.

Verbal communication includes both spoken and written words. The sender of verbal communication needs to be aware of the tone, volume, and cadence (pace or rate) of voice to send an accurate message. In addition, the sender of verbal communication needs to be aware of cultural differences between sender and receiver, such as the use of dialect or slang. Other issues the sender must consider with written communication include barriers such as cognitive and visual impairments of the receiver. In addition, consider the developmental perspectives of the receiver because these influence the method of communication used.

Nonverbal communication describes all behaviors that convey messages without the use of words. This type of communication includes body movement, physical appearance, personal space, and touch. As a nurse, be aware of body language, which includes posture, body position, gestures, eye contact, facial expression, and movement (Fig. 3-2). For clarity, make sure nonverbal communication is consistent with the spoken word. When assessing a patient's needs, assess the nonverbal messages received from the patient and validate them. For example, if you observe a patient wringing her hands and sighing often, ask, "You seem anxious today. Is there anything on your mind?" You avoid problems in language behavior through the consistent use of clear, mutually understood verbal terminology and nonverbal gestures. Be aware of any cultural norms or values (e.g., eye contact) that patients may have to avoid misinterpretation of nonverbal cues (see Skill 3-1).

Therapeutic communication is essential to excellent nursing practice. Nurses use communication skills in caring for patients by providing information and comfort, promoting understanding, clarifying misinformation, assisting in developing plans of care, and facilitating wellness through patient teaching. The nurse-patient relationship promotes a connection, which is an essential component of the healing process.

EVIDENCE-BASED PRACTICE TRENDS

Effective therapeutic communication with patients across the life span is essential for successful nursing practice. Research identifies the following health outcomes as a result of effective therapeutic communication: emotional health, symptom resolution, functional and psychological status, satisfaction with care, and pain control (O'Gara and Fairhurst, 2004). Nurse researchers and clinicians have developed creative modes of communicating with patients. For example, when interacting with patients with severe communication impairments, nurses use alternative modes of communication. These include use of additional communicative devices, including picture books, communication software, and electronic communication methods (e.g., fax, short message service with mobile phones, and telephone typewriters). Recent data indicate that deaf persons are expanding their social network with hearing people through the use of the above-mentioned devices (Power and others, 2007). In addition, research has improved communication with patients with aphasia. Conversation analysis is a methodology that considers the behaviors of the conversing partner. Conversation analysis is a procedure to analyze recorded, naturally occurring talk produced in everyday human interaction, such as pausing during speaking. This is a useful tool in engaging in meaningful dialogue with patients with aphasia (Beeke and others, 2007). The use of computer-mediated communication is another example of how electronic communication increases the so-

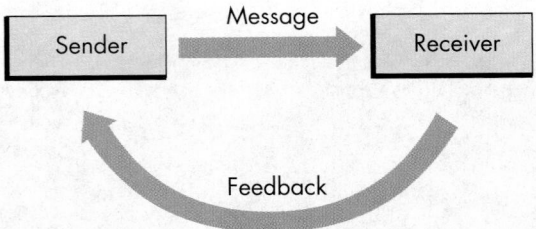

FIG 3-1   Communication is a two-way process.

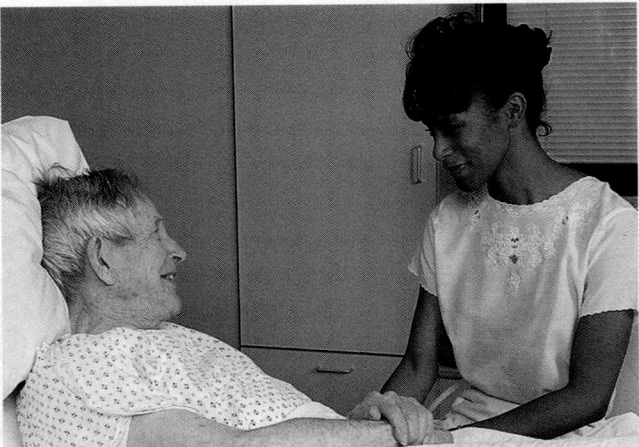

FIG 3-2   An open, relaxed posture conveys interest.

ciability of patients. This method of communication, the use of computers and the Internet, provides a forum for social communication for those who are socially anxious and shy. Computer-mediated communication aids people who are stigmatized in forming relationships with others using a traditional face-to-face interaction (Sheeks and Birchmeier, 2007).

Managing patients with behavioral and/or cognitive impairments requires communication skills to assess and redirect patients and to modify any negative behaviors. Research shows that specific behavior management strategies learned during formal staff training are effective in reducing agitation and improving interactions with behaviorally disturbed patients who reside in nursing homes (see Skills 3-2 and 3-3) (Burgio and others, 2002). In addition, nurses who participated in video training programs on the use of effective communication skills reported having increased knowledge and competence when interacting with patients who have communication difficulties. When patients are aggressive and violent, it is critical that nurses use therapeutic communication techniques to de-escalate them. Data show that promoting a therapeutic nurse-patient relationship is necessary in order to manage aggressive behaviors effectively. In addition, it is crucial to consider the perspectives of both the staff and the patients, because patients have reported perceived environmental conditions and poor communication to be a significant precursor to aggressive behavior (Duxbury and Whittington, 2005).

Nurses often use elder-speak, using a slower rate of speech, exaggerated intonation, greater repetition, and simpler vocabulary and grammar than normal adult speech, when caring for older adults. However, many older patients perceive this type of communication as patronizing and believe this implies incompetence, stereotyping older adults. A study was conducted with nurses who work with older adults. The nurses participated in an educational program that provided a framework for communication using alternative strategies other than elder-speak. The study results yield interesting findings, namely, nurses need to first be self-aware and recognize their use of elder-speak before modifying communication practices, with the ultimate goal of enhancing interpersonal skills with patients (Williams and others, 2004). Nurses should use affirming talk, balancing care for and control of a patient, thereby recognizing that the patient is competent and independent.

Physiological factors such as pain hinder communication between nurses and patients. Often, inadequate communication about pain or pain management occurs between patients and health care providers. Some research examined nurses' responses to pain communication from patients using clinical vignettes; the results indicate that nurses use relatively few of the recommended pain management strategies to respond to pain problems. Nurses did not incorporate other pain measures, reassess pain following an intervention, or discuss the strategy of altering dose/level of pain medication with members of the health care team (McDonald and others, 2007).

COMMUNICATING WITH CULTURALLY DIVERSE PATIENTS

Nurses face challenges when communicating with culturally and linguistically diverse patients. Effective communication between culturally diverse patients and nurses is essential to improving health outcomes (Flaskerud, 2007). Research shows that providing both general and disease-specific information to patients in a cul-

turally sensitive manner improves chronic illness self-management. Conversely, a language barrier prevents the delivery of timely health care, thereby worsening existing health problems and causing new health issues (Dysart-Gale, 2007).

The following factors are essential to effectively care for culturally and linguistically diverse patients: (1) use of appropriate linguistic services (e.g., interpreter or bilingual health care workers) and/or other communication strategies, (2) a display of empathy and respect, (3) use of accurate health history taking for diagnostic and treatment purposes and health teaching, and (4) use of patient-centered communication behaviors, including participatory decision making (Schouten and Meeuwesen, 2006). It is also helpful to speak plainly; avoid mimicking a patient's accent or dialect. Understand that members of certain cultures use cultural phrases or slang common to their culture and this is not an indication they do not understand English.

When nurses communicate with patients of diverse cultures, an interpreter is sometimes necessary. When using an interpreter, address the patient and family directly; do not direct questions or comments to the interpreter. Take care to determine if the patient understood. Speak slowly in normal tones, and avoid overly technical jargon or terms unique to a culture (Box 3-1). Adopting a flexible, respectful attitude that also communicates interest in the patient bridges any communication barriers that exist because of cultural differences between patient and caregiver. When interacting with a community, culturally competent communication strategies use the language and the dialect of the community and use communication vehicles (e.g., preferred media outlets and familiar distribution sites) that are significant to the community served (Flaskerud, 2007). A study of the care of Somali women reveals that the use of same-gender clinicians and interpreters to assist in their care was helpful to these women in their preventive health care (Carroll and others, 2007).

Not all cultures express anxiety, anger, and depression in the same way as in Western culture. Sometimes these present as somatic complaints because some cultures view illness as holistic and combine physical, psychological, and spiritual symptoms together (Park and others, 2002). For example, a patient speaks of lack of sleep and appetite but denies the sensation of anxiety. East Asian cultures, Cambodians, and Laotians often describe communicating with dead ancestors as a coping mechanism for anxiety, and this is normal within their culture (Yick and Gupta, 2002). In addition, some patients internalize anger and express it in somatic complaints of heat, indigestion, or tachycardia.

BOX 3-1	Special Approaches to Patients Who Speak Different Languages

- Use a caring tone of voice and facial expressions to help alleviate patients' fears and anxieties.
- Speak slowly and distinctly, but not loudly.
- Use gestures, pictures, and playacting to help the patient understand.
- Repeat the message in different ways if necessary.
- Be alert to and use words the patient seems to understand.
- Keep messages simple.
- Avoid jargon.
- Use an appropriate language dictionary.

From Giger J, Davidhizar R: *Transcultural nursing: assessment and interventions,* ed 5, St. Louis, 2007, Mosby.

Skill Performance Guidelines

1 Listen to what and how a patient communicates, including content and verbal and nonverbal messages. Some patients express themselves clearly without difficulty. Often, however, indirect and nonverbal cues communicate a patient's needs.

2 Nonverbal communication involves transmission of messages without the use of words. Personal appearance, tone of voice, facial expression, posture, gait, gestures, and touch are ways to convey nonverbal messages.

3 Know your own attitudes toward the patient or situation. Being unaware of personal feelings leads to negative consequences in communication. You need to be aware of your personal feelings in order to control how you communicate issues.

4 Control external factors in both the environmental setting (temperature of room, privacy issues) and the psychological setting (emotional state of the nurse and patient) that influence or hinder communication. When you are talking with a patient about the patient's personal concerns, privacy is important. When teaching, try to have a family member/significant other present with whom to reinforce the content of the instruction. If a patient is experiencing subjective distress in the form of pain or anxiety, take measures to minimize these subjective experiences. Controlling noise level and interruptions is also important.

5 Establish and understand the purpose of interaction. This is an essential quality of effective communication. Without this quality, communication is casual and superficial.

6 Guide the interaction depending on the patient's condition and response. Patient needs remain the focus of the interaction. For example, you establish that the purpose of the interaction is patient teaching; however, the patient just learned about the death of a loved one and expresses the need to talk about the death. You would assist the patient with grieving first, remaining flexible and creative in the interaction.

SKILL 3-1   Establishing the Nurse-Patient Relationship

A therapeutic nurse-patient relationship is the foundation of nursing care and involves using patient-centered therapeutic communication skills. Communication is essential in nursing, because the job requires ongoing involvement with patients and their families in a variety of health care settings (Barrere, 2007). The primary goal of therapeutic communication for the nurse is to promote wellness and personal growth in patients. Therapeutic communication empowers patients to make decisions but differs from social communication in that it is patient centered and goal directed with limited disclosure from the professional. Social communication involves equal opportunity for personal disclosure, and both participants seek to have personal needs met (Keltner and others, 2006). Nurses do not share intimate details of their personal lives with patients. However, nurses use personal self-disclosure cautiously and only in selected situations. Personal self-disclosure by the nurse is useful for the following goals: (1) to educate the patient, (2) to build the therapeutic alliance with the patient, and (3) to encourage the patient's independence (Fortinash and Holoday-Worret, 2007). For example, you share selected personal thoughts and life experiences with a patient to show that you understand what the patient is experiencing.

Skills essential to therapeutic communication include active listening, broad openings, humor, sharing perceptions, clarifying, focusing, informing, paraphrasing, reflecting, restating, summarizing, suggesting, use of therapeutic silence, and use of open-ended statements/questions. Most of these skills are defined with case illustrations identifying therapeutic and nontherapeutic examples of their use (Box 3-2). Paraphrasing involves restating a patient's original message by transforming the message into the nurse's own words without losing the meaning. You achieve empathy in communication through the use of all the aforementioned skills. Empathy is being sensitive and understanding of a patient's feelings and communicating this understanding to the patient. It differs from sympathy in that sympathy is nonobjective and noncritical.

Barriers to therapeutic communication include giving an opinion, offering false reassurance, being defensive, showing approval or disapproval, stereotyping, and asking "why?" The use of "why" questions causes increased defensiveness in a patient and hinders communication. The therapeutic nurse-patient relationship is goal directed, with the patient moving toward productive modes of interpersonal functioning. Three overlapping phases characterize the nurse-patient relationship: orientation, working, and termination. The orientation phase involves learning about the patient and any initial concerns and needs. In the orientation phase, you clarify your role and that of other health care providers, establish rapport with the patient, collect information, establish goals, and clarify misunderstandings. When the orientation phase is successful and the patient is ready, work toward effective goal attainment begins with the working phase of the nurse-patient relationship. The termination phase consists of evaluation and summary of progress toward prescribed goals. Prepare for termination generally at the beginning of the relationship. The nurse must communicate effectively with patients throughout all three phases of the nurse-patient relationship.

Delegation Considerations

Therapeutic communication is a goal of all patient interactions, delegated or not. The skill of establishing therapeutic communication can be delegated to nursing assistive personnel (NAP) following appropriate instruction. The nurse directs the NAP about:

- The proper way to interact verbally and nonverbally with select patients.
- Environmental considerations, such as privacy and confidentiality.
- Special considerations pertaining to communication with patients who are cognitively or sensorially impaired older children, anxious, and potentially violent.

BOX 3-2 Therapeutic Communication Techniques

Technique: Listening

Definition: An active process of receiving information and examining one's reaction to messages received

Example: Consider the cultural practice of your patient, maintain appropriate eye contact, and be receptive to nonverbal communications.

Therapeutic Value: Nonverbally communicates nurse's interest and acceptance to patient

Nontherapeutic Threat: Failure to listen, interrupting patient

Technique: Broad Openings

Definition: Encouraging patient to select topics for discussion

Example: "What are you thinking about?"

Therapeutic Value: Indicates acceptance by nurse and value of patient's initiative

Nontherapeutic Threat: Domination of interaction by nurse; rejecting responses

Technique: Restating

Definition: Repeating main thought patient has expressed

Example: "You say that your mother left you when you were 5 years old."

Therapeutic Value: Indicates nurse is listening and validates, reinforces, or calls attention to something important that has been said

Nontherapeutic Threat: Lack of validation of nurse's interpretation of message; being judgmental; reassuring; defending

Technique: Clarification

Definition: Attempting to improve the nurses' understanding of words, vague ideas, or unclear thoughts of the patient or asking the patient to explain what he or she means

Example: "I'm not sure what you mean. Could you tell me again?"

Therapeutic Value: Helps to clarify patient's feelings, ideas, and perceptions and to provide an explicit correlation between them and the patient's actions

Nontherapeutic Threat: Failure to probe; assumed understanding

Technique: Reflection

Definition: Directing back to patient ideas, feelings, questions, or content

Example: "You're feeling tense and anxious, and it's related to a conversation you had with your sister last night?"

Therapeutic Value: Validates nurse's understanding of what patient is saying and signifies empathy, interest, and respect for patient

Nontherapeutic Threat: Stereotyping patient's responses, inappropriate timing of reflections; inappropriate depth of feeling of reflections; inappropriate to the cultural experience and educational level of the patient

Technique: Humor

Definition: Discharging of energy through comic enjoyment of the imperfect

Example: "This gives a whole new meaning to 'Just relax.'"

Therapeutic Value: Can promote insight by making conscious repressed material, resolving paradoxes, tempering aggression, and revealing new options and is a socially acceptable form of sublimation

Nontherapeutic Threat: Indiscriminate use; belittling patient; screen to avoid therapeutic intimacy

Technique: Informing

Definition: Demonstrating skills or giving information

Example: "I think it would be helpful for you to know more about how your medication works."

Therapeutic Value: Helpful in patient education about relevant aspects of patient's well-being and self-care

Nontherapeutic Threat: Giving advice

Technique: Focusing

Definition: Asking questions or making statements that help patients expand on a topic of importance

Example: "I think it would be helpful if we talk more about your relationship with your father."

Therapeutic Value: Allows patient to discuss central issues related to problem and keeps communication process goal directed

Nontherapeutic Threat: Allowing abstractions and generalizations; changing topics

Technique: Sharing Perceptions

Definition: Asking patient to verify nurse's understanding of what patient is thinking or feeling

Example: "You're smiling, but I sense that you are really very angry with me."

Therapeutic Value: Conveys nurse's understanding to patient and has potential for clearing up confusing communication

Nontherapeutic Threat: Challenging patient; accepting literal responses; reassuring; testing; defending

Technique: Theme Identification

Definition: Clarifying underlying issues or problems experienced by patient that emerge repeatedly during nurse-patient relationship

Example: "I've noticed that in all the relationships that you have described, you've been hurt or rejected by the man. Do you think this is an underlying issue?"

Therapeutic Value: Allows nurse to best promote patient's exploration and understanding of important problems

Nontherapeutic Threat: Giving advice; reassuring; disapproving

Technique: Silence

Definition: Using silence or nonverbal communication for a therapeutic reason

Example: Sitting with patient and nonverbally communicating interest and involvement

Therapeutic Value: Allows patient time to think and gain insights, slows the pace of the interaction, and encourages patient to initiate conversation, while conveying nurse's support, understanding, and acceptance

Nontherapeutic Threat: Questioning patient: asking for "why" responses; failure to break a nontherapeutic silence

Technique: Suggesting

Definition: Presenting of alternative ideas for patient's consideration relative to problem solving

Example: "Have you thought about responding to your boss in a different way when he raises that issue with you? For example, you could ask him whether a specific problem has occurred."

Therapeutic Value: Increases patient's perceived options or choices

Nontherapeutic Threat: Giving advice, inappropriate timing; being judgmental

Modified from Keltner N and others: *Psychiatric nursing,* ed 5, St. Louis, 2006, Mosby.

STEP	RATIONALE

ASSESSMENT

1 The first contact a nurse has with a patient occurs during the orientation phase. Address patient by name, and introduce self and role on health care team ("Hello, my name is Sally, and I am the registered nurse assigned to take care of you today . . ."). Use clear, specific communication (verbal and nonverbal) to provide information and clarify concerns.

Congruent verbal and nonverbal communication expresses warmth and respect and helps to establish rapport. Clear, specific communication decreases confusion and anxiety (Dyche, 2007).

2 Assess the following behaviors: patient's needs, coping strategies, defenses, and adaptation styles.

Recurrent themes in patient's response help to identify problem areas related to health status (e.g., avoidance of questions, request for information, expression of a loss).

3 Determine patient's need to communicate (e.g., patient who constantly uses call light, patient who is crying, patient who does not understand an illness, patient who has just been admitted).

Patients in need of support, comfort, knowledge, or encouragement will benefit from meaningful communication.

4 Assess reason patient needs health care.

Nature of illness affects patient's coping ability and effectiveness in communicating needs and concerns.

5 Assess factors about self and patient that normally influence communication: perceptions, values, and beliefs; emotions; sociocultural background; severity of illness; knowledge; age; verbal ability; roles and relationships; environmental setting; physical comfort or discomfort (see illustration).

Communication is a dynamic process influenced by interpersonal and intrapersonal processes. By assessing factors that influence communication, you can more accurately assess patients' experiences of patients (Verklan, 2007).

6 Assess personal barriers to communication with patient (e.g., bias toward patient's condition, anxiety from inexperience).

Barriers prevent you from conveying empathy and caring and obtaining relevant assessment information.

7 Assess patient's language and ability to speak. Does patient have difficulty finding words or associating ideas with accurate word symbols? Does patient have difficulty with expression of language and/or reception of messages? What is patient's primary language?

Determines need for special communication techniques (e.g., picture boards; aids, such as an interpreter) (see illustration).

8 Assess patient's literacy level. Determine if patient skips over uncommon or hard words, does patient avoid asking questions or have difficulty discussing concepts about illness? *Option:* To assess health literacy in detail use a standardized instrument such as the, Rapid Estimate of Adult Literacy in Medicine (REALM).

Health literacy has a direct effect on health outcomes. Assessing patient's level of health literacy will allow you to design more effective communication and teaching approaches.

9 Assess patient's ability to hear. Be sure hearing aid is functional if worn. Be sure patient hears and understands words.

Patients with hearing deficits require techniques to enhance hearing reception (e.g., speaking in normal tone, speaking so patient can see face).

10 Observe patient's pattern of communication and verbal or nonverbal behavior (e.g., gestures, tone of voice, eye contact).

Patient's patterns of communication determine type of and manner of communication you will use.

11 Assess resources available in selecting communication methods:

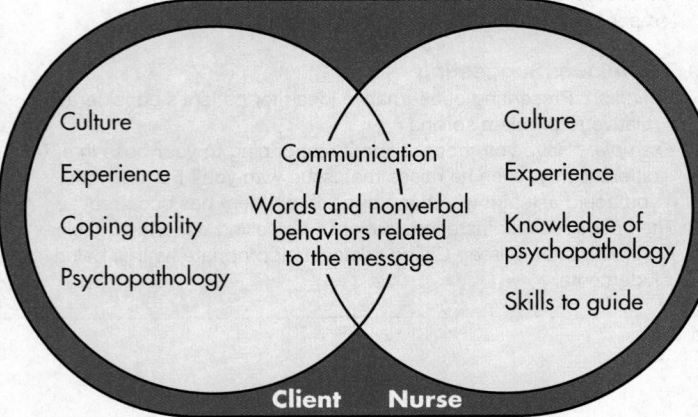

STEP 5   Essential and influencing variables of the therapeutic communication environment. *(Modified from Keltner N and others: Psychiatric nursing, ed 5, St. Louis, 2006, Mosby.)*

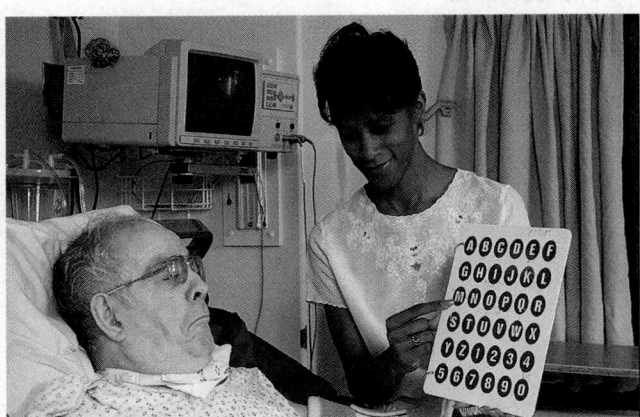

STEP 7   Tracheostomy interferes with speech.

STEP	RATIONALE
a Review information available through chart, care plan, and past experience.	Relying totally on information from patient restricts the quality of interaction. Additional resources provide insight into best methods of communicating.
b Consult with family, physician, and other health care team members concerning patient's condition, problems, and impressions.	Collaboration with other health care team members facilitates nurse's response to patient based on integration of knowledge.
12 Before initiating the working phase of nurse-patient relationship, assess patient's readiness to work toward goal attainment.	Patient's goals are identified and agreed upon by effective communication skills such as restating and clarifying.
13 Consider when patient is due to be discharged or transferred from health care agency.	Allows nurse to anticipate the amount of time available to work with patient and when termination of relationship is to occur.

NURSING DIAGNOSES

- Anxiety
- Deficient knowledge
- Fear
- Impaired social interaction
- Impaired verbal communication
- Ineffective coping
- Noncompliance
- Readiness for enhanced decision making

Individualize related factors based on patient's condition or needs.

PLANNING

1 Expected outcomes following completion of procedure: • Patient expresses ideas, fears, and concerns clearly and openly with relief of anxiety.	Once patients are able to talk directly about emotions, the focus is on coping more effectively with them (Keltner and others, 2006).
• Patient goals are identified and achieved.	Interaction remains patient focused.
• Patient verbalizes understanding of information communicated by nurse.	This provides a means to build trust and develop a knowledge base for patient to make decisions.
2 Prepare for communication during orientation phase: provide a warm and accepting environment, establish trust, formulate individualized patient goals, consider time allocation, formulate initial questions, and mentally prepare to keep one's mind clear of other concerns or distractions.	Preparation is part of planned process that facilitates communication and interaction. Planning for orientation phase assists in identifying actual or potential problems, current health status, and experience. Without preparation, a risk exists of casual non–goal-oriented communication.
3 Prepare patient and environment physically: provide a quiet environment, maintain privacy, reduce distractions or interruptions, and take care of patient's physical needs (e.g., comfort or hygiene) before beginning discussion.	Taking care of basic needs promotes an environment for interaction and decreases patient distractions and interruptions.
4 Prepare for communication during working phase. Identify strategies to develop a realistic plan to meet identified health goals of patients.	Preparation promotes goal attainment and avoids risk of misinterpretation.
5 Prepare for communication during termination phase by identifying methods of summarizing and synthesizing information pertinent for aftercare.	Effective communication by summarizing and synthesizing information reinforces behavior change.

IMPLEMENTATION

1 Establishing the nurse-patient relationship during the orientation phase:	
a Create a climate of warmth and acceptance. Be aware of nonverbal cues that are both sent and received. Provide comfort and support to patient.	This facilitates open exchange without fear or anxiety.
b Use appropriate nonverbal behaviors (e.g., good eye contact, open relaxed position, sitting eye level with patient [see Fig 3-2]).	This facilitates communication by providing a nonverbal message that you are interested in what patient has to say.
c Observe patient's nonverbal behaviors, including body language. If patient's verbal behaviors do not match nonverbal behaviors, seek clarification.	Congruence between patient's verbal and nonverbal behaviors ensures you receive the correct message.
d Explain purpose of interaction when information is to be shared.	Information and explanation can decrease anxiety about the unknown.
e Use active listening.	Conveys interest in the patient's needs, concerns, and problems; conveys empathy.

STEP	RATIONALE
f Identify patient's expectations in seeking health care.	This conveys a level of interest in patient's needs.
g Interview the patient about the health status, lifestyle, support systems, patterns of health and illness, and strengths and limitations.	Facilitates a positive nurse-patient relationship and facilitates the development of trust, putting the patient at ease.
h Encourage patient to ask for clarification at any time during the communication.	This gives patient a sense of control and keeps channels of communication open.
i Use therapeutic communication techniques when interacting with patient (refer to Box 3-2, p. 31).	Techniques establish a greater understanding of messages sent and received.
2 Setting mutual goals during the working phase:	
a Use therapeutic communication skills such as restating, reflecting, and paraphrasing to identify and clarify strategies for attainment of mutually agreed-upon goals.	Effective communication ensures clear understanding on part of patient and improves ability of patient to participate in care (Ammentorp and other, 2007).
b Discuss and prioritize problem areas.	A patient, nonjudgmental, supportive approach minimizes patient anxiety.
c Provide information to patient, and help patient express needs and feelings.	Patient is able to respond to help, develop workable solutions based on goals, and fully participate in a realistic plan for his or her well-being.
d Use questions carefully and appropriately. Ask one question at a time, and allow sufficient time to answer. Use direct questions. Use open-ended statements as much as possible, such as "Tell me about how you are feeling today."	Assists patient in expressing self and allows nurse to obtain thorough information about patient's needs and concerns.

Critical Decision Point *Avoid asking questions about information that may not have yet been disclosed to the patient (e.g., human immunodeficiency virus [HIV] status). Avoid asking "why" questions; this causes increased defensiveness in the patient and will prevent communication.*

STEP	RATIONALE
e Avoid communication barriers as discussed earlier in this chapter.	Communication breakdown occurs when a message is not received, is distorted, or is not understood.
3 Communicating with the patient during the termination phase:	
a Use effective communication skills to discuss discharge/termination issues and to guide discussion related to specific patient changes in thoughts and behaviors.	Communication skills reinforce behaviors/skills learned during working phase of relationship.
b Summarize with patient what you discussed during interaction, including goal achievement.	Signals close of interaction and allows nurse and patient to depart with same idea. Provides a sense of closure and mutual understanding.

EVALUATION

1 Observe patient's verbal and nonverbal responses to your communication, noting patient's willingness to share information and concerns during orientation phase.	Both verbal and nonverbal feedback reveal patient's interest and willingness to communicate and reflect patient's ability to form a therapeutic relationship with nurse.
2 Note your response to patient and patient's response to you. Reflect on effectiveness of therapeutic techniques used in establishing rapport with patient.	Sensitivity to one's own ability in using therapeutic communication skills helps improve ability to adjust techniques when necessary.
3 During working phase, evaluate patient's ability to work toward identified goals. Elicit feedback (verbal and nonverbal) to determine success of goal attainment. Evaluate patient's health status in relation to identified goals. Reevaluate and identify barriers if patient goals are not met.	Feedback is an essential step in evaluating new behaviors. Modifications are necessary if goals cannot be met.
4 During termination phase, use communication skills such as summarizing and restating. Reinforce patient's strengths, outline issues still requiring work, and develop an action plan.	Evaluates patient progress in terms of attainment of mutually agreed-upon goals.

Unexpected Outcomes	Related Interventions
1 Patient verbally and nonverbally expresses feelings of anxiety, fear, anger, confusion, distrust, and helplessness. Patient is often responding to internal and external factors and cues.	• Reassess patient's level of anxiety, fear, and distrust. • Repeat message to patient at a later time. • Use a caring tone of voice and facial expression to help calm fears of patient who speaks a different language.
2 Feedback between nurse and patient reveals a lack of understanding. Barriers to communication exist.	• Assess for barriers to communication.

Unexpected Outcomes

3 Nurse's own personal issues interfere with establishment of a therapeutic nurse-patient relationship.

4 Nonverbal cues (e.g., poor eye contact, facial expressions, gestures) indicate ineffective communication.

5 Patient possibly speaks a different language.

6 Nurse is unable to acquire information about patient's ideas, fears, and concerns. Communication techniques do not promote patient's willingness to communicate openly. Trust is not established. Goals are not identified and therefore cannot be achieved.

Related Interventions

- Make appropriate adjustments to communication style.
- Use special approaches (gesture, pictures, play acting) for patients who speak a different language (Carroll and others, 2007).
- Consider cultural norms associated with eye contact, use of touch, personal space, and nonverbal behaviors.
- Repeat message in different ways if necessary.
- Avoid using medical terms that patient does not understand.
- Be alert to words patient seems to understand, and use them frequently. Consider use of interpreter.
- Use alternative communication techniques to promote patient's willingness to communicate openly.
- Offer another professional for patient to talk with to obtain necessary information.

Recording and Reporting

- Record in nurses' notes communication pertinent to patient's health, response to illness or therapies, and responses that demonstrate understanding or lack of understanding (include verbal and nonverbal cues).
- Report any relevant information obtained through patient's verbal and nonverbal behaviors to members of health care team.

Teaching Considerations

- Use gestures, pictures, and playacting to help patient understand. Be alert to literacy status; determine if patient is able to access health information adequately. Be alert to words patient seems to understand, and use them frequently.
- Individualize patient teaching to meet needs of patient. Always conduct teaching toward meeting patient's learning needs with consideration for patient's preferred methods for learning.

Pediatric Considerations

- Communicating with children requires an understanding of feelings and thought process from the child's perspective (Hockenberry and Wilson, 2007).
- Use vocabulary that is familiar to child, based on child's level of understanding (age and development appropriate). Try to be on the same eye level as the patient.

- Understand the child's cognitive, developmental, and functional level to select most appropriate communication techniques. Some age-appropriate communication techniques include storytelling and drawing (Hockenberry and Wilson, 2007).

Gerontological Considerations

- Be aware of any cognitive or sensory impairment. Assess each patient individually, and avoid stereotyping older adults who have cognitive or sensory impairments.
- It is important to understand the value of good communication skills and importance of history and personality within older adult population in terms of providing both human and therapeutic responses. Regression to earlier defenses is normal and adaptive with this population, particularly when facing illness.
- Make sure older patient with visual impairments uses assistive devices such as eyeglasses and large-print reading material to aid in communication.

Home Care Considerations

- Identify primary caregiver for patient, and adapt techniques to assess level of understanding regarding patient's condition.
- Incorporate communication into patient's daily activities (e.g., bathing and dressing).

SKILL 3-2 Communicating With an Anxious Patient

Patients in the health care setting sometimes experience anxiety for a variety of reasons. A newly diagnosed illness, separation from loved ones, threat associated with diagnostic tests or surgical procedures, and expectations of life changes are just a few factors that cause anxiety. How successfully a patient copes with anxiety depends in part on previous experiences, the presence of other stressors, the significance of the event causing anxiety, and the availability of supportive resources. You can be a support to the patient. You help to decrease anxiety through effective communication. Communication methods reviewed in this skill will assist you in helping an anxious patient clarify factors causing anxiety and to cope more effectively. There are four stages of anxiety with corresponding behavioral manifestations: mild, moderate, severe, and panic (Box 3-3).

BOX 3-3 | Behavioral Manifestations of Anxiety: Stages of Anxiety

Mild Anxiety
- Increased auditory and visual perception
- Increased awareness of relationships
- Increased alertness
- Able to problem solve

Moderate Anxiety
- Selective inattention
- Decreased perceptual field
- Focus only on relevant information
- Muscle tension; diaphoresis

Severe Anxiety
- Focus on fragmented details
- Headache, nausea, dizziness
- Unable to see connections between details
- Poor recall

Panic State of Anxiety
- Does not notice surroundings
- Feeling of terror
- Unable to cope with any problem

Delegation Considerations

Communication with an anxious patient is best managed by a professional nurse. However, therapeutic communication is important in all patient interactions. The nurse directs the nursing assistive personnel (NAP) about:

- The proper way to interact verbally and nonverbally with specific patients.
- The reason for a patient's anxiety.
- The necessary skills for communicating with an anxious patient.

STEP	RATIONALE

ASSESSMENT

1 Provide brief, simple introduction; introduce yourself, and explain purpose of interaction.	Anxiety limits amount of information patient can understand.
2 Assess for physical, behavioral, and verbal cues that indicate patient is anxious, such as dry mouth, sweaty palms, tone of voice, frequent use of call light, difficulty concentrating, wringing of hands, and statements such as "I am scared."	Anxiety interferes with usual manner of communication and thus interferes with patient's care and treatment. Extreme anxiety interferes with comprehension, attention, and problem-solving abilities.
3 Assess for possible factors causing patient anxiety (e.g., hospitalization, unknown diagnosis, fatigue).	Understanding the source of anxiety will assist in patient support and communication.
4 Assess factors influencing communication with patient (e.g., environment, timing, presence of others, values, experiences, need for personal space because of heightened anxiety).	Helps in identifying effective communication strategies.
5 Discuss with family members the possible causes of patient's anxiety.	Gathering information about patient from a family perspective is useful because family may provide new information or understanding of situation (Keltner and others, 2006).

NURSING DIAGNOSES

- Anxiety
- Decisional conflict
- Defensive coping
- Deficient knowledge
- Fear
- Impaired social interaction
- Impaired verbal communication
- Ineffective coping

Individualize related factors based on patient's condition or needs.

PLANNING

1 Expected outcomes following completion of procedure:	
• Patient will sense less anxiety during interactions with nurse.	Gives patient resource to cope with stressor(s).
• Patient is able to discuss area of concern.	Communication techniques ease anxiety and allow patient to focus on problem.

Critical Decision Point *First acknowledge and take care of anxious patient's physical and emotional discomfort, but avoid dwelling on physical complaints. Focus on understanding patient, providing feedback and assisting in problem solving, and providing atmosphere of warmth and acceptance.*

2 Prepare for communication by considering the following: patient goals, time allocation, and resources.	Effective communication allows patient to establish rapport, to achieve a sense of calm, and to begin to analyze source of anxiety.
3 Recognize personal level of anxiety and consciously try to remain calm (breathe slowly and deeply). Be aware of nonverbal cues that indicate own anxiety (e.g., body language, posture, cadence of speech).	Nurse's own anxiety will increase patient's anxiety.
4 Prepare physical environment: provide a quiet, calm area, allowing ample personal space.	Decreasing stimuli has a calming effect. Invasion of personal space increases anxiety.

IMPLEMENTATION

1 Use appropriate nonverbal behaviors and active listening skills, such as staying with patient at bedside and having a relaxed posture.	Nonverbal messages to patient express interest and help to alleviate anxiety.
2 Use appropriate verbal techniques that are clear and concise to respond to anxious patient. Use brief statements that acknowledge current feeling state and provide direction to patient, such as "It seems to me that you are anxious" or "I notice that you seem anxious, would you like to go rest in your room?"	Appropriate techniques and statements provide reassurance and prevent further escalation of anxiety.

STEP	RATIONALE
3 Help patient acquire alternative coping strategies, such as progressive relaxation, slow deep-breathing exercises, and visual imagery (see Chapter 15). 4 Provide necessary comfort measures.	Coping mechanisms provide foundation for effective communication so that patient can explore causes of anxiety and steps to alleviate anxious feelings. Pain heightens patient's anxiety.

EVALUATION

1 Observe for continuing presence of physical signs and symptoms or behaviors reflecting anxiety.	Observation determines extent to which planned interaction relieved patient's anxiety.
2 Have patient discuss ways to cope with anxiety in the future and make decisions about own care.	This measures patient's ability to assume more health-promoting behavior.
3 Evaluate patient's ability to discuss factors causing anxiety.	This measures patient's ability to attend or focus on area of concern.

Unexpected Outcomes

1 Physical signs and symptoms of anxiety continue. Nurse's interaction has increased patient's anxiety, or source of anxiety is not resolved.

2 Patient displays difficulty in decision making. Patient avoids nurse's efforts at focusing discussion or is unable to discuss real concerns. Anxiety continues to prevent problem solving.

3 Anxiety continues to escalate.

Related Interventions

- Use refocusing or distraction skills, such as relaxation or guided imagery (Fortinash and Holoday-Worret, 2007).
- Be clear and direct when communicating with patient to avoid misunderstanding.
- Touch, when used appropriately, helps control feelings of panic.
- Continue to use previous steps.
- Be very direct and clear when making requests. If patient needs to deal with stimulus causing anxiety, reintroduce when patient is less anxious.
- Touch, while therapeutic, requires individualized assessment of patient's anxiety level and need for personal space, and some patients perceive this as threatening. When used appropriately, reassurance through human touch helps control feelings of panic.
- As a last resort, administer an antianxiety medication (per orders).

Recording and Reporting

- Record in nurses' notes cause of patient's anxiety and any exhibited signs and symptoms of behaviors.
- Report methods used to relieve anxiety and patient's response to ensure continuity of care between nurses

Teaching Considerations

- Teaching patient to identify possible sources of anxiety, such as illness, hospitalization, knowledge deficits, or other known stressors, gives patient knowledge of anxiety and increases patient's sense of control.
- Remember that patients and their family members who are under stress often require repeated explanations.

Pediatric Considerations

- Children often demonstrate anxiety through physical and behavioral signs but are unable to express anxiety verbally. Some children express anxiety through restless behavior, physical complaints, or behavioral regression. It is important to note any changes in child's behavior that occur during illness or hospitalization (Hockenberry and Wilson, 2007).

Gerontological Considerations

- Anxiety is one of the most common symptoms seen in older adults. Patients often become ritualistic and intent on performing activities a certain way. Anxiety develops as a result of a specific event or a general pattern of change (e.g., decline in health) (Meiner and Lueckenotte, 2006).

- Anxiety is sometimes present in long-term care settings, such as residential care facilities and assisted living facilities. Manage anxiety based on patient's presenting behaviors with consideration of any cognitive/physical impairments.
- Psychosocial factors such as anxiety and confusion, lack of mobility, and spatial organization of long-term care institution are factors that decrease social contacts, thus hindering communication with peers and health care providers. This leads to further feelings of isolation, boredom, and increased anxiety.
- Older adults who are socially isolated have multiple medical problems and are more likely to have anxious and/or depressive symptoms. In addition, they are less likely to seek care for these symptoms.

Home Care Considerations

- Anxiety occurs in home care settings. Manage anxiety based on patient's presenting behaviors with a consideration of any cognitive/physical impairments.
- Anticipation of a home care visit increases a patient's anxiety and leads to exacerbation of symptoms. Therefore some patients avoid home care visits (Fortinash and Holoday-Worret, 2007).

SKILL 3-3 Communicating With an Angry Patient Through De-escalation

Anger is the common underlying factor associated with potential for violence. Patients become angry for a variety of reasons. The anger is often directly related to a patient's experience with illness, or it is associated with problems that existed before the patient entered the health care setting. In the health care setting, you will have frequent contact with a patient and thus often become the target of the patient's anger. It is important for you to understand that in many cases a patient's ability to express anger is important to recovery. For example, when a patient has experienced a significant loss, anger becomes a means to help cope with grief. Some patients express anger toward the nurse, but the anger often hides a specific problem or concern. For example, a patient diagnosed as having cancer voices displeasure with the nurse's care instead of expressing a fear of dying.

It is very stressful dealing with an angry patient. Anger often represents rejection or disapproval of the nurse's care. Your efforts at satisfying an angry patient's needs can result in a failure to meet the priorities of other patients. Allow patients to express anger openly, and do not feel threatened by their words. However, do not allow a patient's anger to threaten or compromise care. Skills for communicating with an angry patient or a potentially violent patient allow you to assist the patient in dealing with anger constructively and in refocusing emotional energy toward effective problem solving. De-escalation skills are useful techniques that you can use to manage a potentially violent patient; these skills range from using nonthreatening verbal and nonverbal messages to safely disengaging and controlling the aggressor physically (Fortinash and Holoday-Worret, 2007).

Delegation Considerations

De-escalation is a skill that cannot be delegated to NAP. The nurse directs the NAP by:

- Informing them about the proper way to interact verbally and nonverbally with the patient.
- Explaining their role as the nurse uses de-escalation techniques.
- Reviewing approaches that have been successful and unsuccessful.

STEP	RATIONALE

ASSESSMENT

1. Observe for behaviors that indicate the patient is angry (e.g., pacing, clenched fist, loud voice, throwing objects) and/or expressions that indicate anger (e.g., repeat questioning of nurse, not following requests, aggressive outbursts, threats).

    Anger is a normal expression of frustration or response to feeling threatened. However, its expression often interferes with or blocks communication and interactions.

2. Assess factors that influence communication of angry patient, such as refusal to comply with treatment goals, use of sarcasm or hostile behavior, having a low frustration level, or being emotionally immature.

    Allows nurse to accurately assess situation or the experiences of patient that block or facilitate communication (Duxbury and Whittington, 2005).

3. Consider resources (e.g., health care team or family) available to assist in communicating with potentially violent patient.

    Assists in clarifying cause and intervention required to deal with patient's anger.

Critical Decision Point *With some violent behaviors (e.g., physical aggression) you may not be able to de-escalate the situation. When this potential exists, know whom to call for assistance (e.g., trained psychology technicians, security staff).*

NURSING DIAGNOSES

- Anxiety
- Defensive coping
- Fear

- Impaired social interaction
- Impaired verbal communication
- Ineffective coping

- Risk for other-directed violence
- Risk for self-directed violence

Individualize related factors based on patient's condition or needs.

PLANNING

1. Expected outcomes following completion of procedure:
   - Patient no longer exhibits verbal and nonverbal expressions of anger.

    De-escalation techniques successfully allow patient to express anger in a constructive way.

2. Prepare for interaction with an angry patient:
   a. Pause to collect own thoughts, feelings, and reactions.

    Awareness and control of your own reaction and responses will facilitate more constructive interaction.

   b. Determine what patient is saying.
   c. Attempt a calm, firm, assertive approach. Try to talk in comfortable, reassuring voice.

3. Prepare the environment to de-escalate a potentially violent patient:

    Potentially violent patient needs to be in an environment with decreased stimuli and to have protection from injury to self or against others.

STEP	RATIONALE
a Encourage other people, particularly those who provoke anger, to leave room or area.	Encourages patient's expression of anger rather than provokes it.
b Maintain adequate distance.	Avoids pressuring patient; helps to prevent injury if anger becomes out of control.
c Maintain open exit. Position self closest to the door to facilitate escape from a potentially violent situation. Do not block exit so patient feels escape is unattainable; this may cause a violent outburst.	Prevents feeling of being trapped for both nurse and patient.
d Make sure gestures are slow and deliberate rather than sudden and abrupt.	Less chance of misinterpretation of message and less threatening.
e When anger begins to disturb others, close door. This is particularly important if patient is becoming agitated.	Agitation and anxiety can spread to others. Some hospital rooms are equipped with security windows or cameras to allow for observation of patient.

Critical Decision Point *Some patients are disruptive to each other, especially those who are hyperactive, intrusive, threatening, or exhibiting bizarre behaviors. For these patients, first try least-restrictive measures before using more-restrictive measures, such as seclusion.*

STEP	RATIONALE
f Reduce disturbing factors in room (e.g., noise, drafts, inadequate lighting).	Reduces irritants that may heighten anger.
g Take care of patient's physical and emotional needs and discomforts (e.g., offer analgesic for pain).	Physical and emotional needs are often factors in patient's anger; sometimes patient is not aware of these needs.

IMPLEMENTATION

1 Responding to a potentially violent patient:	
a Maintain nonthreatening verbal and nonverbal communication skills when interacting with angry or potentially violent patient.	A relaxed atmosphere will prevent further escalation. Creates climate of acceptance for patient.
b Use therapeutic silence, and allow the patient to vent feelings.	Often de-escalates anger. Anger expends emotional and physical energy; patient runs out of momentum and energy to maintain anger at high level.
c Answer questions as appropriate; if patient asks power struggle type of question (challenging or confrontational type), redirect and set limits by giving clear, concise expectations. Inform patient of potential consequences without sounding threatening, and follow through with consequences if patient does not change behaviors.	Setting limits on power-struggle questions provides structure and helps diffuse anger.
d If patient is making verbal threats to harm others, remain calm yet professional and continue to set limits on inappropriate behavior.	Angry patient loses ability to process information rationally and therefore may impulsively express anger through intimidation.

Critical Decision Point *If strong likelihood of imminent harm to other is present upon discharge, notify proper authorities (e.g., nurse manager).*

e Maintain personal space and safety with patient who is making verbal threats of violence directed at others. Maintain nonthreatening position and nonverbal behavior, including body language, position, and cadence.	Avoiding sudden movements and loud tones prevents giving the appearance of an attack.

Critical Decision Point *A potentially violent patient can be impulsive and explosive, and therefore you need to keep personal safety skills in mind. In this case, avoid touch.*

f If patient appears to be calm and anger is defused, explore alternatives to situation or feelings of anger.	Processing with patient will possibly prevent future explosive outbursts and teach patient effective ways of dealing with anger.

EVALUATION

1 Observe for continuing behaviors of verbal expressions of anger.	Indicates success of communication efforts.
2 Note patient's ability to answer questions and problem solve.	Determines whether anger has lessened so that patient is able to focus on alternative coping skills.

Unexpected Outcomes

1 Patient continues to demonstrate behaviors or verbal expression of anger or violence. Nurse is unable to assist patient in relieving source of anger or in expressing anger openly without violent acts.

Related Interventions

- Reassess factors contributing to anger. Also remove or alter factors contributing to anger.
- Take charge with calm, firm directions. Give as-needed (prn) medications as ordered for agitation/escalating behaviors.
- Direct patient to a quiet area for a "time out."
- Make sure fellow staff is available to assist if necessary.

Recording and Reporting

- Record in nurses' notes cause of patient's anger (if determined) and behaviors patient exhibits.
- Record and report technique used to de-escalate and patient's response.

Teaching Considerations

- Patients experiencing emotionally charged situations do not always comprehend instruction. Focus on understanding patient, providing feedback and assisting in problem solving, and providing an atmosphere of safety, warmth, and acceptance.
- Teaching patient to identify possible factors that contribute to angry outbursts, such as inadequate coping skills, low frustration levels, illness, hospitalization, knowledge deficits, or other known stressors, may give patient a sense of control.
- Once anger has been de-escalated, teach patient new adaptive methods of coping with anger.

Pediatric Considerations

- Set limits for inappropriate behaviors exhibited by child, such as a time out. Apply such limits immediately because children tend to have less internal control over their own behaviors (Hockenberry and Wilson, 2007).

Gerontological Considerations

- Patients who have cognitive impairments often exhibit tantrumlike behaviors in response to real or perceived frustration. Use distraction techniques to remove cognitively impaired older adult patient from disturbing stimuli, or redirect patient to activity that is pleasurable (Meiner and Lueckenotte, 2006).

Home Care Considerations

- Personal safety for nurse against potentially violent patient or family member extends to all health care settings, including patient's home. You may be in potentially dangerous situation while giving care to patient at home because you may be giving care to patient without support from other staff members.
- Be aware of physical surroundings of home, including possible exits.
- If de-escalation does not occur and you feel your safety is threatened, call for assistance or remove yourself from situation.

SKILL 3-4   Communicating With a Depressed Patient

Depression is a feeling state that is more than just sadness. It is a common psychiatric condition that affects a person's ability to function in day-to-day activities. There are many symptoms of depression, the most common being apathy, feelings of sadness, fatigue, guilt, poor concentration, sleep disturbances, and suicidal thoughts. Depression results in both subjective and objective behaviors (Box 3-4). Subjective behaviors include report of feelings of sadness, tearfulness, report of no energy, and increase in physical complaints. Some patients report feeling anxious when depressed. Objective signs include decrease in performance of activities of daily living (ADLs), and decreased time spent in social activities (altered social interaction).

Many patients in acute care settings suffering from either acute or chronic health conditions have symptoms of depression. Some patients have been formally diagnosed and treated with medications and/or psychotherapy, and yet others may not have been diagnosed and therefore have not been treated. Use the nursing process to develop nursing interventions, expected outcomes, and evaluation of those outcomes for patients with depression. The intervention strategies emphasize use of therapeutic communication techniques.

Delegation Considerations

Communication with a depressed patient is best managed by a professional nurse. However, communicating effectively with a depressed patient is a skill that can be delegated to NAP. The nurse directs the NAP by:

- Informing them of the proper way to interact verbally and nonverbally with the specific patient.
- Explaining the possible causes and signs and symptoms of the patient's depression.
- Reviewing the skills necessary for communicating with a depressed patient.

BOX 3-4   Symptoms of Depression

Common Symptoms	Other Symptoms
• Apathy	• Fatigue
• Sadness	• Thoughts of death
• Sleep disturbances	• Decreased libido
• Hopelessness	• Ruminations of inadequacy
• Helplessness	• Psychomotor agitation
• Worthlessness	• Verbal berating of self
• Guilt	• Spontaneous crying
• Anger	• Dependency, passiveness

From Keltner N and others: *Psychiatric nursing,* ed 5, St. Louis, 2006, Mosby.

STEP	RATIONALE

ASSESSMENT

1 Assess for physical, behavioral, and verbal cues that indicate patient is depressed, such as feelings of sadness, tearfulness, difficulty concentrating, increase in reports of physical complaints, and statements such as "I am sad/depressed."

Depression interferes with usual manner of communication and thus interferes with patient's care and treatment. If depression is severe, it will interfere with comprehension, attention, and problem-solving abilities.

2 Assess for possible factors causing patient's depression (e.g., acute or chronic illness, personal vulnerability, past history).

Patient's depressive state is sometimes unknown to nurse. Understanding the possible cause of depression assists in patient support and communication.

3 Assess factors influencing communication with patient (e.g., environment, timing, presence of others, values, experiences, poor concentration).

Understanding factors that influence communication helps nurse identify effective communication strategies.

4 You may need to discuss possible causes of patient's depression with family members, including past history of the illness.

Gathering information about patient from a family perspective is useful because family provides new information or understanding of situation (Keltner and others, 2006).

NURSING DIAGNOSES

- Decisional conflict
- Hopelessness
- Impaired social interaction
- Impaired verbal communication
- Ineffective coping
- Ineffective role performance
- Risk for self-directed violence
- Spiritual distress

Individualize related factors based on patient's condition or needs.

PLANNING

1 Expected outcomes following completion of procedure:
- Patient's depression is reduced.

Patient is given resources to cope with feelings of depression.

2 Prepare for communication by considering patient goals, time allocation, and resources.

Effective communication allows patient to establish rapport, to achieve a sense of calm, and to begin to analyze source(s) of depression.

3 Be aware of your own nonverbal cues that affect communication with depressed patient (e.g., body language, posture, cadence of speech). Remain nonjudgmental.

Nurse's personal feelings regarding depression may negatively affect interaction with patient.

4 Prepare environment physically by providing a quiet, calm area, allowing ample personal space.

Decreasing stimuli has a calming effect. Invasion of personal space increases anxiety, thereby preventing communication with the depressed patient.

Critical Decision Point   *First acknowledge and take care of depressed patient's physical and emotional discomfort, but avoid dwelling on physical complaints. Focus on understanding patient, providing feedback and assisting in problem solving, and providing atmosphere of warmth and acceptance.*

IMPLEMENTATION

1 Provide brief, simple introduction; introduce yourself, and explain purpose of interaction.

Symptoms associated with depression limit amount of information patient can understand.

2 Accept patient as he or she is and focus on positive aspects of patient. Provide positive feedback.

Depressed patients often have low self-esteem, and this approach helps to focus on their strengths.

3 Be honest and empathic.

Facilitates the development of trust.

4 Use appropriate nonverbal behaviors and active listening skills, such as staying with patient at bedside.

Nonverbal messages to patient express your interest and help to alleviate depressive symptoms.

5 Use appropriate verbal techniques that are clear and concise to respond to depressed patient. Use observational statements that both acknowledge current feeling state and provide direction to patient.

Appropriate techniques and statements provide reassurance to depressed patient. Expresses empathy.

6 Use open-ended questions, such as "Tell me about how you are feeling" or "You seem sad, tell me about your sadness."

Encourages the patient to continue talking, facilitating an in-depth discussion of symptoms.

7 Reward small decisions and independent actions. When necessary, make decisions that patients are not ready to make. Present situations that require no decision making.

Depressed patients are often overly dependent and indecisive.

8 Respond to anger therapeutically; avoid becoming defensive or angry, and encourage verbal expression of anger.

Some depressed patients are angry; understand that anger is a symptom of their depression. Verbal expression often reduces tension.

9 Provide necessary comfort measures.

Depressed patients often have multiple somatic complaints; address and adequately treat the physical complaints (e.g., pain, nause

STEP	RATIONALE
10 Spend time with patient who is withdrawn.	Communicates the patient's worth.
11 Ask patient about suicidal ideation and presence of a plan.	Depressed patients are at increased risk for suicide. Other risk factors include general medical conditions, hopelessness, male gender, and increased age. The more developed the plan, the greater the risk of suicide (Keltner and Wilson, 2006).

EVALUATION

1 Observe for continuing presence of physical signs and symptoms or behaviors reflecting depression.	Observation determines extent to which planned interaction relieved patient's depressive symptoms.
2 Have patient discuss ways to cope with depression in the future and make decisions about own care.	This measures patient's ability to assume more health-promoting behavior.
3 Evaluate patient's ability to discuss factors causing depression.	Measures patient's ability to attend or focus on area of concern.

Unexpected Outcomes	Related Interventions
1 Depressive behaviors continue. Nurse's interaction has been ineffective at relieving depressive symptoms.	• Continue to use therapeutic communication skills when interacting with depressed patient. • Refer patient to mental health professional for consultation regarding use of pharmacological agents and/or formal psychotherapy to treat depression.
2 Patient reports suicidal ideation with/without plan.	• Refer patient to mental health professional for evaluation and possible admission to an inpatient psychiatric treatment facility.

Recording and Reporting

• Record in nurses' notes both objective and subjective behaviors (associated with depression) patient is displaying and objective behaviors (associated with depression) observed by the nurse.
• Report methods used to improve these behaviors and patient's response to ensure continuity of care between nurses.

Teaching Considerations

• Teaching patient to identify possible sources of depression, such as acute/chronic illness, personal vulnerability, ineffective coping, or other known stressors, gives patient knowledge of depression and increases patient's sense of control over feelings of depression.
• Make teaching modifications with a consideration of impaired concentration and memory related to patient's depressed status (e.g., present a small amount of material at a time).

Pediatric Considerations

• Children often demonstrate symptoms of depression that differ from those of adults. They manifest depression through physical (increased somatic complaints) and behavioral signs (poor school performance, social isolation) and are often unable to express depression verbally. Some children express depression through restless behavior or behavioral regression. It is important to note any changes in child's behavior that occur during illness or hospitalization (Hockenberry and Wilson, 2007).

Gerontological Considerations

• Depression among older adults is a major health concern. It is important to differentiate between depression and any underlying medical illness in this population because the symptoms sometimes overlap. In addition, suicide risk is increased in older adults (Keltner and others, 2006).

Home Care Considerations

• Depression is often present in home care settings. Manage depression based on patient's presenting behaviors with a consideration of any cognitive/physical impairments.

? CRITICAL THINKING EXERCISES

You are assigned to care for Mrs. Garcia, an 82-year-old woman who was admitted to the hospital 5 days ago after falling at her son's home. She recently moved from Mexico to the United States, following the death of her husband. She has only one child, a son, whom she moved in with following her move to the United States. She had emergency surgery to repair a fractured right hip. During shift report on a medical-surgical unit, the nurse tells you that Mrs. Garcia is a problematic patient. She is agitated and never seems satisfied with anything. In addition, her grasp of the English language is poor. None of the nursing staff speaks Spanish. When you approach her to perform an initial assessment, she is babbling incoherently in Spanish and seems disoriented. She appears disheveled, and her lunch tray is untouched. She is wincing and grimacing. You ask the patient if she is complaining of pain, but you get a response that you cannot understand. After repeating the question, "Are you in pain? Please rate your pain on a scale from 0 to 10," the patient yells at you in Spanish and throws the water pitcher across the room.

1 What steps are necessary to effectively communicate with this linguistically diverse patient?
2 What should you do first to prepare to respond to Mrs. Garcia? Explain your choice(s).
3 Describe two ways to alter the environment so as to deescalate Mrs. Garcia's anger. Explain your rationale.
4 The interpreter learns what Mrs. Garcia is concerned about, being unable to move about. How do you approach answering the question?

✓ REVIEW QUESTIONS

1 Which approach reflects an obstacle to nurse-patient communication?
   1 Discussing fears about a patient with members of the health care team
   2 Obtaining information about a critically ill patient from his or her family
   3 Admitting a mistake to a patient's family
   4 Avoiding issues that are uncomfortable for a patient

2 The nurse is caring for a postoperative patient who is still having pain despite analgesia administration. Which statement by the nurse best reflects therapeutic communication?
   1 "I think your doctor needs to know that you are still in pain."
   2 "What do you want me to do about your pain problem?"
   3 "When it comes to pain, your doctor tends to undermedicate his patients."
   4 "Your pain will be a lot better in the morning."

3 A patient recovering from a bilateral mastectomy for breast cancer tearfully tells the nurse she is feeling depressed and worthless as a woman. Which communication phrase is inappropriate?
   1 "Many women have body image concerns after undergoing this surgery."
   2 "Tell me more about how you feel."
   3 "Why do you feel depressed and worthless?"
   4 "How long have you been feeling this way?"

4 Which approach would be best when initially working with an anxious patient?
   1 Tell the patient that everything he or she says will be kept private.
   2 Ask the patient what he or she believes is causing his or her anxiety.
   3 Watch the patient's behavior for the amount of anxiety being exhibited.
   4 Explain what the patient can expect in terms he or she can understand.

5 A nurse is working with a potentially threatening patient. Which nursing intervention is most appropriate?
   1 Speaking clearly and slightly louder so the patient does not need the nurse to repeat what was said
   2 Positioning himself or herself near the exit of the room to prevent being blocked by the patient
   3 Bringing in other team members so the patient knows there are others to help him or her gain control
   4 Asking the patient what comfort measures he or she uses when he or she becomes out of control

REFERENCES

Barrere C: Discourse analysis of nurse-patient communication in a hospital setting: implications for staff development, *J Nurses Staff Dev* 23(3):114, 2007.

Dyche L: Interpersonal skill in medicine: the essential partner of verbal communication, *J Gen Intern Med* 22(7):1035, 2007.

Fortinash K, Holoday-Worret P: *Psychiatric mental health nursing,* ed 4, St. Louis, 2007, Mosby.

Giger J, Davidhizar R: *Transcultural nursing: assessment and interventions,* ed 5, St. Louis, 2007, Mosby.

Gruber M, Hartman R: Don't overlook "communication competence," *Nurs Manage* 38(3):12, 2007.

Hockenberry MJ and Wilson D: *Wong's nursing care of infants and children,* ed 8, St. Louis, 2007, Mosby.

Keltner N and others: *Psychiatric nursing,* ed 5, St. Louis, 2006, Mosby.

Meiner S, Lueckenotte A: *Gerontologic nursing,* ed 3, St. Louis, 2006, Mosby.

O'Gara P, Fairhurst W: Therapeutic communication. I. General approaches that enhance the quality of the consultation, *Accid Emerg Nurs* 12(3):166, 2004.

Verklan M: Johari window: a model for communicating to each other, *J Perinat Neonatal Nurs* 21(2):173, 2007.

RESEARCH REFERENCES

Ammentorp J and others: The effect of training in communication skills on medical doctors' and nurses' self-efficacy: a randomized controlled trial, *Patient Educ Couns* 66(3):270, 2007.

Beeke S and others: Using conversation analysis to assess and treat people with aphasia, *Semin Speech Lang* 28(2):136, 2007.

Burgio LD and others: Teaching and maintaining behavior management skills in the nursing home, *Gerontologist* 42(4):487, 2002.

Carroll J and others: Caring for Somali women: implications for clinician-patient communication, *Patient Educ Couns* 66(3):337, 2007.

Duxbury J, Whittington R: Causes and management of patient aggression and violence: staff and patient perspectives, *J Adv Nurs* 50(5):469, 2005.

Dysart-Gale D: Clinicians and medical interpreters: negotiating culturally appropriate care for patients with limited English ability, *Fam Community Health* 30(3):237, 2007.

Flaskerud J: Cultural competence: what else is necessary? *Issues Ment Health Nurs* 28(2): 219, 2007.

Kovach CR and others: Use of the assessment of discomfort in dementia protocol, *Appl Nurs Res* 14(4):193, 2001.

McDonald D and others: Nurses' response to pain communication from patients: a post-experimental study, *Int J Nurs Stud* 44(1):29, 2007.

Park Y-J and others: The conceptual structure of Hwa-Byuun in middle-aged Korean women, *Health Care Women Int* 23:389, 2002.

Power M and others: Deaf people communicating via SMS, TTY, relay service, fax, and computers in Australia, *J Deaf Stud Deaf Ed* 12(1):80, 2007.

Schouten B, Meeuwesen L: Cultural differences in medical communication: a review of the literature, *Patient Educ Couns* 64(1-3):21, 2006.

Sheeks M, Birchmeier Z: Shyness, sociability, and the use of computer-mediated communication in relationship development, *Cyberpsychol Behav* 10(1):64, 2007.

Williams K and others: Enhancing communication with older adults: overcoming elderspeak, *J Gerontol Nurs* 30(10):17, 2004.

Yick AG, Gupta R: Chinese cultural dimensions of death, dying, and bereavement: focus group findings, *J Cult Divers* 9(2):32, 2002.

4

Reporting and Recording

MEDIA RESOURCES

- **evolve** *learning system*   http://evolve.elsevier.com/Perry/skills

Mastery of content in this chapter will enable the nurse to:
- List guidelines for effective communication and reporting.
- Describe measures to maintain confidentiality of patient information.
- Identify the purpose of the patient record.
- Describe elements of a change-of-shift report.
- Complete an incident report accurately.
- Write a nurse's progress note using SOAP, SOAPIE, PIE, focus, and SBAR charting formats.

- Describe information found in a patient care profile and nursing Kardex.
- Accurately complete a nursing flow sheet.
- Explain guidelines used in documentation of home care and long-term care.
- Describe the role of critical pathways in multidisciplinary documentation.
- Discuss the role of computerization in documentation.

Nursing documentation continues to be an essential and important component of health care delivery. Documentation is anything written or printed in a patient record. A Joint Commission evaluation found that more than 70% of sentinel events in accredited health care organizations were caused by communication problems, concluding that effective communication among caregivers is critical to patient safety (The Joint Commission [TJC], 2007b). Nursing documentation ensures continuity of care, provides legal evidence, and evaluates patient outcomes (Cheevakasemsook and others, 2006). One of the challenges you face is documenting quality patient care within the constraints imposed by regulations, limited resources, and finances. Your documentation provides a detailed account of the plan of care and documentation of assessment and treatment. Effective documentation ensures continuity of care, maintains standards, and reduces errors (Durkin, 2006; McGeehan, 2007). The quality of documentation depends on your ability to communicate effectively in both the written and spoken word. Furthermore, technology now offers new tools to improve documentation and improve patient care (Brandeis and others, 2007). You are held accountable for the accuracy of documentation that is in the patient record, and this information is confidential and needs to be protected.

Accreditation agencies such as The Joint Commission specify guidelines for documentation and require health care facilities to monitor and evaluate patient outcomes and appropriateness of care. This evaluation process occurs through an audit of information that is documented in patient records. The Joint Commission provides requirements for documentation in standards (TJC, 2008).

CONFIDENTIALITY

All members of the health care team are legally and ethically obligated to keep patient information confidential. Do not discuss a patient's examinations, observations, conversations, or treatments with other patients or staff not involved in the patient's care, unless permission is granted by the patient. Sometimes patients request copies of their records, and they have a right to read their records. One exemption to information access involves patients with mental illness. These patients can be denied access from their general right of access where such access would be "likely to cause serious harm to the physical or mental health or condition of the data, subject, or any other person" (Dolan, 2004). Agencies have specific policies for controlling the manner in which records are shared; usually agencies require patients to provide written permission for the release of medical information.

The Health Insurance Portability and Accountability Act (HIPAA) protects patients' private health information (U.S. Department of Health and Human Services [USDHSS], 2003). This governs all areas of health information management, which in-

cludes, for example, reimbursement, coding, security, and patient records. Previously the rule required written consent for disclosure of all patient information. Under new regulations, to eliminate barriers that delay access to care, providers are only to notify patients of their privacy policy and make a reasonable effort to get written acknowledgment of this notification. As a result of this act, patients have more control over their personal health care information and who has access to this information (USDHHS, 2003).

When you are a student in a clinical setting, confidentiality and compliance with HIPAA legislation are part of professional practice. You review the medical record only for information needed to provide safe, efficient care. For example, when you are assigned to provide complete care for a patient, you need to review the current medical record and plan of care. However, do not share information with other classmates or access the medical records of other patients on the specific clinical area. To further maintain confidentiality and protect patient privacy, do not have patient identifiers on written materials used in your student clinical practice. These identifiers may include room number, date of birth, medical record number, or other identifiable demographic information.

STANDARDS

Current Joint Commission standards require that all patients who are admitted to a health care institution have an assessment of physical, psychosocial, environmental, self-care, patient education, and discharge planning needs (TJC, 2008). The Joint Commission standards require documentation to be within the context of the nursing process, including evidence of patient and family teaching and discharge planning. Institutional standards or policies often state the frequency of assessment, so it is essential to know the standards of your health care organization.

The documentation of care and patient information is vital for ensuring patient safety in health care organizations. Electronic records and information create complexities in information management. The goal of information management is to support decision making and improve patient outcomes, improve health care documentation, ensure patient safety, and improve performance in patient care, treatment and services, governance, management; and support processes (TJC, 2007b).

MULTIDISCIPLINARY COMMUNICATION WITHIN THE HEALTH CARE TEAM

Patient care requires effective communication among the members of the health care team. Records and reports communicate specific information about a patient's health status and the interventions that all health care team members contribute toward improving

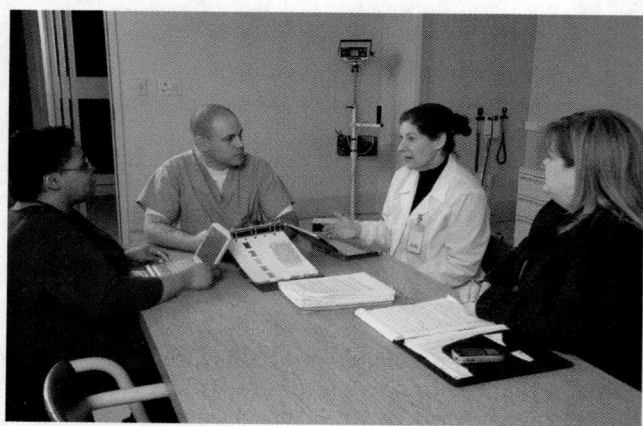

FIG 4-1 Communication among members of the health care team.

the patient's health. Multidisciplinary communication and documentation are necessary to provide more efficient health care and improve patient outcomes (Ballard, 2006).

A patient's record or chart is a confidential, permanent legal document containing information relevant to a patient's health care. Information about the patient's health care is recorded after each patient contact. The record is a continuing account of the patient's health status and needs, treatments delivered, results of diagnostic tests, and the patient's response to therapy.

Reports are oral, written, or audiotaped exchanges of information between caregivers (Fig. 4-1). Patient information may be received or reported verbally, by fax, or via paging system. Reports include information about a patient's clinical status, observations made about the patient's behavior, data pertaining to diagnostic tests, and directions for changes in therapy. Common reports given by nurses include change-of-shift (handoff) reports (see Procedural Guideline 4-1), telephone reports, transfer reports, and incident reports (see Procedural Guideline 4-3, p. 61). In addition, a physician or health care provider sometimes calls a nursing unit to receive a verbal report on critical test results, a patient's condition, and progress.

You also communicate information through discussions or conferences among health care team members. For example, a discharge planning conference often involves members of all disciplines (e.g., nursing, medicine, social work, physical therapy, and dietary), who meet to discuss a patient's progress toward established discharge goals. You need to document this information in a patient's permanent record so that all caregivers benefit from the information and plan the patient's care accordingly.

GUIDELINES FOR QUALITY DOCUMENTATION AND REPORTING

Quality documentation and reporting enhance efficient, safe, individualized patient care, and you achieve this through the use of standard guidelines. Accurate documentation is one of the best defenses of legal claims associated with nursing care (McGeehan, 2007; Sullivan, 2004). Five common issues in malpractice caused by inadequate or incorrect documentation include (1) failure to document the correct time of events, (2) failing to record verbal orders or failing to have them signed, (3) charting actions in advance to save time, (4) documenting incorrect data, and (5) failing to give a report, or giving an incomplete report, to an oncoming shift (Table 4-1).

To limit liability, nursing documentation must clearly indicate that the nurse provided individualized, goal-directed nursing care to a patient based on the nursing assessment. The recorded information in a patient's record must describe exactly what happened to the patient. This is best achieved when you chart immediately after you provide care (Sullivan, 2004). Include all assessment findings, care plans, interventions, patient responses to interventions, and consultations/referrals in the medical record. Quality documentation and reporting have six characteristics: they are factual, accurate, complete, current, organized, and confidential.

Factual

A record or report contains descriptive, objective information about what you see, hear, feel, and smell. An objective description is the result of direct observation and measurement such as "respiratory rate 20 and unlabored." Avoid terms such as *appears*, *seems*, or *apparently*, which are often subject to interpretation. For example, the description "the patient seems to be in pain" does not accurately communicate the facts to another caregiver. The phrase *seems* is not supported by any objective facts. Objective documentation needs to include your observations of patient behavior. For example, objective signs of pain include increased pulse rate, increased respiration, diaphoresis, or guarding of a body part.

The only subjective data included in a record are what the patient actually verbalizes. Write subjective information with quotation marks, using the patient's exact words whenever possible. For example, you record "Patients states, 'My stomach hurts.'" You will also include complementary objective findings so the database is descriptive.

Accurate

The use of exact measurements in documentation establishes accuracy. For example, charting that an abdominal wound is "5 cm in length without redness, edema, or drainage" is more descriptive than "large wound healing well." It is essential to avoid unnecessary words and irrelevant details. For example, the fact that a patient is watching TV is only necessary when this activity is significant to the patient's status and plan of care.

The Joint Commission requires health care organizations to standardize abbreviations, symbols, acronyms, and dose designations and establish a list of abbreviations that should never be used (TJC, 2007b). Use abbreviations carefully to avoid misinterpretation, and minimize errors by spelling out confusing abbreviations. It is essential to know the institution's abbreviation list, and use only the accepted abbreviations, symbols, and measures (e.g., metric), so that all documentation is accurate and in compliance with standards. For example, the abbreviation for *every day (qd)* **is no longer used** (see Chapter 20). If a treatment or medication is needed daily, the written order or care plan should write out the word *"daily"* or *"every day."* The abbreviation *qd (every day)* can be misinterpreted to mean O.D. *(right eye)*.

Correct spelling demonstrates a level of competency and attention to detail. Many terms are easy to misinterpret because they sound similar: for example, dysphagia or dysphasia and dram or gram. Some spelling errors result in serious treatment errors; for example, the names of certain medications such as digitoxin and digoxin or morphine and Numorphan are similar and you need to transcribe them carefully to ensure that the patient receives the correct medication.

The Joint Commission standards (2008) require that "all entries in medical records be dated and a method is established to identify the authors of entries." Therefore each entry in a patient's

TABLE 4-1 Legal Guidelines for Recording

Guidelines	Rationale	Correct Action
Do not erase, apply correction fluid, or scratch out errors made while recording.	Charting becomes illegible: it appears as if you were attempting to hide information or deface record.	Draw single line through error, write word *error* above it, and sign your name or initials. Then record note correctly. Check agency policy.
Do not write retaliatory or critical comments about patient or care by other health care professionals.	Statements can be used as evidence for non-professional behavior or poor quality of care.	Enter only objective descriptions of patient's behavior; use quotations for patient's comments.
Need to add additional patient information.	New information is acquired.	If additional information is to be added to an existing entry, write the date and time of the new entry on the next available space, and mark it as an addendum (date and time of prior note) (Sullivan, 2004).
	Forgot to chart during a shift.	Write the current date and time in the next available space, and mark it as a late entry (date and time/shift missed) (Sullivan, 2004).
Correct all errors promptly.	Errors in recording can lead to errors in treatment.	Avoid rushing to complete charting; be sure information is accurate.
Record all facts.	Record must be accurate and reliable.	Be certain entry is factual; do not speculate or guess.
Do not leave blank spaces in nurses' notes.	Another person can add incorrect information in space.	Chart consecutively, line by line; if space is left, draw line horizontally through it, and sign your name at end.
Record all entries legibly and in black ink.	Illegible entries can be misinterpreted, causing errors and lawsuits; ink cannot be erased; black ink is more legible when records are photocopied or transferred to microfilm.	Never erase entries or use correction fluid, and never use pencil.
If order is questioned, record that you sought clarification.	If you perform an order known to be incorrect, you are just as liable for prosecution as the physician or health care provider is.	Do not record "physician made error." Instead, chart that "Dr. Smith was called to clarify order for analgesic."
Chart only for yourself.	You are accountable for information you enter into chart.	Never chart for someone else. **Exception:** If caregiver has left unit for day and calls with information that needs to be documented, include the name of the source of information in the entry, and include that the information was provided via telephone.
Avoid using generalized, empty phrases such as "status unchanged" or "had good day."	Specific information about patient's condition or case can be accidentally deleted if information is too generalized.	Use complete, concise descriptions of care.
Begin each entry with time, and end with your signature and title.	This guideline ensures that correct sequence of events is recorded; signature documents who is accountable for care delivered.	Do not wait until end of shift to record important changes that occurred several hours earlier; be sure to sign each entry.
For computer documentation, keep your password to yourself.	Maintains security and confidentiality.	Once logged on to the computer, do not leave the computer screen unattended.

record ends with the caregiver's full name or initials and status. Sometimes you will document interventions performed by another caregiver. For example, "Patient ambulated by Sue Smith, NA." As a nursing student, you need to enter full name, student nurse abbreviation (e.g., SN, NS), and educational institution, such as "David Jones, SN [student nurse], CMTC (Central Maine Technical College)."

Records need to reflect accountability during the time frame of the entry, which you accomplish best when you chart your own observations and actions. The signature holds that nurse accountable for information recorded. If information was inadvertently omitted from the record, it is acceptable for nurses to ask colleagues to chart information after they leave work. The entry needs to clearly show what was done and by whom (e.g., "At 11 AM Sam Turner, RN, called and reported that at 8 AM Demerol 100 mg IM

was administered to patient for abdominal pain"). The nurse recording the information then signs this entry.

Complete

The information within a recorded entry or a report must be complete, containing appropriate and essential information. Criteria for thorough communication exist for certain health problems or nursing activities (Table 4-2). Make written entries in a patient's medical record, describing nursing care that you administer and the patient's response. For example:

1915 Patient verbalizes sharp, throbbing pain localized along lateral side of right ankle, beginning approximately 15 minutes ago after twisting his foot on the stairs. Patient rates pain as 7 on a scale of 0 to 10. Pain increased to an 8 with movement, relieved to a 6 with

TABLE 4-2 Examples of Criteria for Reporting and Recording

Topic	Criteria to Report or Record
Assessment	
Subjective data	Description of episode/event in patient's words in quotation marks Clarify onset, location, description of condition (severity; duration; frequency; precipitating, aggravating, and relieving factors)
Patient behavior (e.g., anxiety, confusion, hostility)	Onset, behaviors exhibited, precipitating factors
Objective data (e.g., rash, tenderness, breath sounds)	Onset, location, description of condition (severity; duration; frequency; precipitating, aggravating, and relieving factors)
Nursing Interventions and Evaluation	
Treatments (e.g., enema, bath, dressing change)	Time administered, equipment used (if appropriate), patient's response (objective and subjective changes) compared to previous treatment; for example, rated pain 2 on a scale of 0-10 during dressing change or "patient reported no abdominal cramping during enema"
Medication administration	Immediately after administration document: time medication given, dose, route, any preliminary assessment (e.g., pain level, vital signs), patient response or effect of medication; for example, "1200 Pain reported at 7 (scale 0-10). Tylenol 500 mg given PO 1230: Patient reports pain level 2 (scale 0-10) at 1330" or "Pruritus and hives developed over lower abdomen 1 hour after penicillin was given."
Patient teaching	Information presented, method of instruction (e.g., discussion, demonstration, videotape, booklet), patient response, including questions and evidence of understanding such as return demonstration or change in behavior
Discharge planning	Measurable patient goals or expected outcomes, progress toward goals, need for referrals

elevation. Pedal pulses equal bilaterally. Right ankle circumference 1 cm larger than left. Ice applied. Percocet 2 tabs by mouth given for pain.

1945 Patient states pain somewhat relieved following application of ice and rates pain as 6 on a scale of 0 to 10. Physician notified for new analgesic order. Lee Turno, RN.

You include routine activities such as vital signs, daily hygiene, and ambulation on graphic records and flow sheets. Changes in functional ability or status require more detailed documentation. For example, your patient was unable to move from the bed to the chair without shortness of breath and now is no longer short of breath during this transfer. This change warrants additional documentation.

Current

Effective documentation includes making timely entries in a patient's record, which avoids omissions and delay in patient care (TJC, 2008). To increase accuracy and decrease unnecessary duplication, many health care agencies use records kept near a patient's bedside, which facilitate immediate documentation of care activities. Document the following activities or findings at the time of occurrence:

- Vital signs
- Pain assessment
- Administration of medications and treatments
- Preparation for diagnostic tests or surgery
- Change in patient's status and who was notified
- Treatment for a sudden change in patient's status
- Patient response to intervention
- Admission, transfer, discharge, or death of a patient

Many health care agencies use military time, a 24-hour system that avoids misinterpretation of AM and PM times. The military clock ends with midnight at 2400 and begins 1 minute after mid-

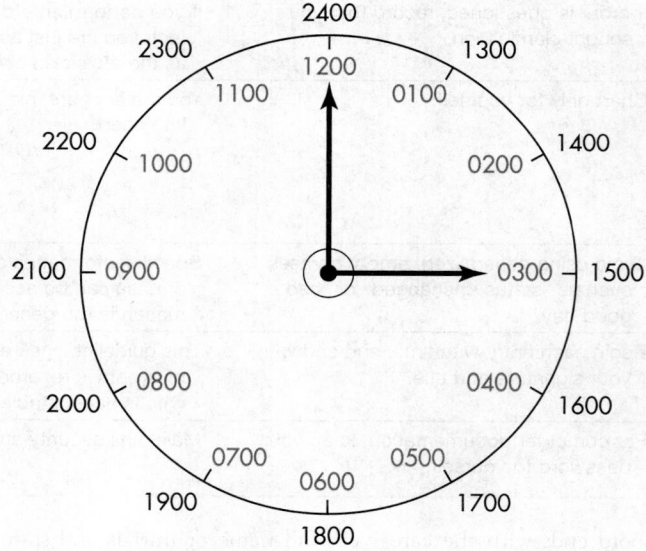

FIG 4-2 Military time clock. Instead of two 12-hour cycles, the military clock is one 24-hour time cycle (e.g., 3 PM is 1500 military time).

night at 0001. For example, 1:00 PM is 1300 military time; 10:22 AM is 1022 military time. Fig. 4-2 compares military and civilian times.

Organized

You need to present written communication in logical order beginning with assessments, the nursing interventions, and finally patient responses. Communication is also more effective when it is clear, concise, and brief. Entries are more organized and clear if you make a list of what to include before beginning to write in the permanent legal record.

COMMON RECORD-KEEPING FORMS

The patient chart or record provides evidence of a patient's health status. The chart includes a variety of forms to facilitate quick and comprehensive documentation. Use of these forms helps avoid duplication of information within the record.

Admission Nursing History Forms

A comprehensive nursing history form provides baseline assessment data and is completed when a patient is admitted to a nursing care unit. You will use the admission data later to compare it to any changes in the patient's condition. The form guides the admitting nurse through a complete assessment to identify relevant nursing diagnoses or problems for the patient's care plan. Each institution designs these forms based on the standards of practice and philosophy of nursing care.

Flow Sheets and Graphic Records

Flow sheets and graphic records permit concise documentation of nursing information and patient data over time. Records include documentation of routine observations or repeated specific measurements for a patient such as vital signs (see Chapter 6), intake and output hygiene, medication administration (see Chapter 20), and pain assessment. Flow sheets use a system for entry of information (Fig. 4-3). When documenting a significant change that appears on a flow sheet, you describe the change in the progress notes, including the patient's response to nursing interventions. For example, if a patient's blood pressure becomes dangerously low, record in the progress notes the blood pressure; relevant assessment, such as pallor, dizziness; and any interventions to raise the blood pressure. Also, include an evaluation of the interventions, such as repeated blood pressures and relief of dizziness. Flow sheets provide a quick, easy reference for the health care team members in assessing a patient's status.

Patient Education Record

Patient teaching and education are essential nursing interventions. Many health care organizations have an education record that identifies a patient's knowledge base about his or her diagnosis, treatment, and medications. The goal of patient and family education is to promote health behavior and self-care by involving the patient and/or family in decisions, which improves health outcomes. Standards for patient education include assessment of needs, functional abilities, learning styles, and readiness to learn. You base patient education needs on the assessment and usually include safe and effective use of medications, nutrition and dietary modifications, safe use of medical equipment, pain control, rehabilitative methods to promote and improve functional abilities, and self-care activities (TJC, 2008).

Patient Care Summary or Kardex

Many health care organizations now have computerized systems that provide concise, summarative information in the form of a patient care summary. This summary prints out for each patient during each shift. Data are automatically updated as new orders and nursing decisions enter the system.

In some health care settings, a Kardex ("flip-over" file) kept at the nurses' station provides information for daily patient care needs. It has two parts: an activity and treatment section and a nursing care plan section. The updated information in the Kardex eliminates the need for repeated referral to the chart for routine information throughout the day. The Kardex does not always become part of the permanent record. Information commonly found on the patient care summary or Kardex includes the following:

- Basic demographic data (e.g., age, religion)
- Primary medical diagnosis
- Current physician's or health care provider's orders (e.g., diet, activity, dressing changes)
- A nursing care plan
- Nursing orders or nursing interventions (e.g., intake and output, comfort measures, teaching)
- Scheduled tests and procedures
- Safety precautions used in the patient's care
- Factors related to activities of daily living
- Nearest relative/guardian or person to contact in an emergency
- Emergency code status
- Allergies

Acuity Records

Health care organizations use a patient acuity system as a method of determining the intensity of nursing care required for a group of patients. Acuity measurements for patients on a unit serve as a guide for determining staffing needs. An acuity recording system determines the hours of nursing care and number of staff required for a nursing unit.

Typically, nurses enter acuity data into a computerized documentation system in the morning. The administrative staff collects the acuity data electronically and uses it to make appropriate staffing decisions. Acuity levels allow the nursing staff to compare patients with one another. For example, an acuity system might rate bathing patients from 1 to 5 (1 is totally dependent, 5 is independent), whereas a patient returning from surgery who requires frequent monitoring and extensive care has an acuity level of 1. On the same continuum, another patient awaiting discharge after a successful recovery from surgery has an acuity level of 5. Accurate acuity ratings justify the number and qualifications of staff needed to safely care for patients on a particular unit.

Standardized Care Plans

Some health care organization use standardized care plans for more efficient documentation. The plans, based on the institution's standards of nursing practice, are preprinted, established guidelines used to care for patients with similar health problems. After completing a nursing assessment, place an appropriate standardized care plan in the patient chart. You individualize standardized care plans for each patient. Most standardized care plans allow for the addition of patient-specific outcomes and target dates for achievement of these outcomes.

One advantage of standardized care plans is the establishment of evidence-based standards of care. By using standardized plans, nurses learn to recognize the accepted requirements of care for patients. The standardized care plans also improve continuity of care among professional nurses. The Joint Commission supports the use of standardized care plans and no longer requires a written care plan for each patient.

One disadvantage of standardized care plans is an increased risk that the unique, individualized therapies needed by patients will go unrecognized. Standardized care plans do not replace your professional judgment and decision making. In addition, care plans need updating on a regular basis to ensure that content is current and appropriate. The trend among many health care organizations is to computerize care plans. These systems provide daily computer-generated care plans, which incorporate several nursing diagnoses

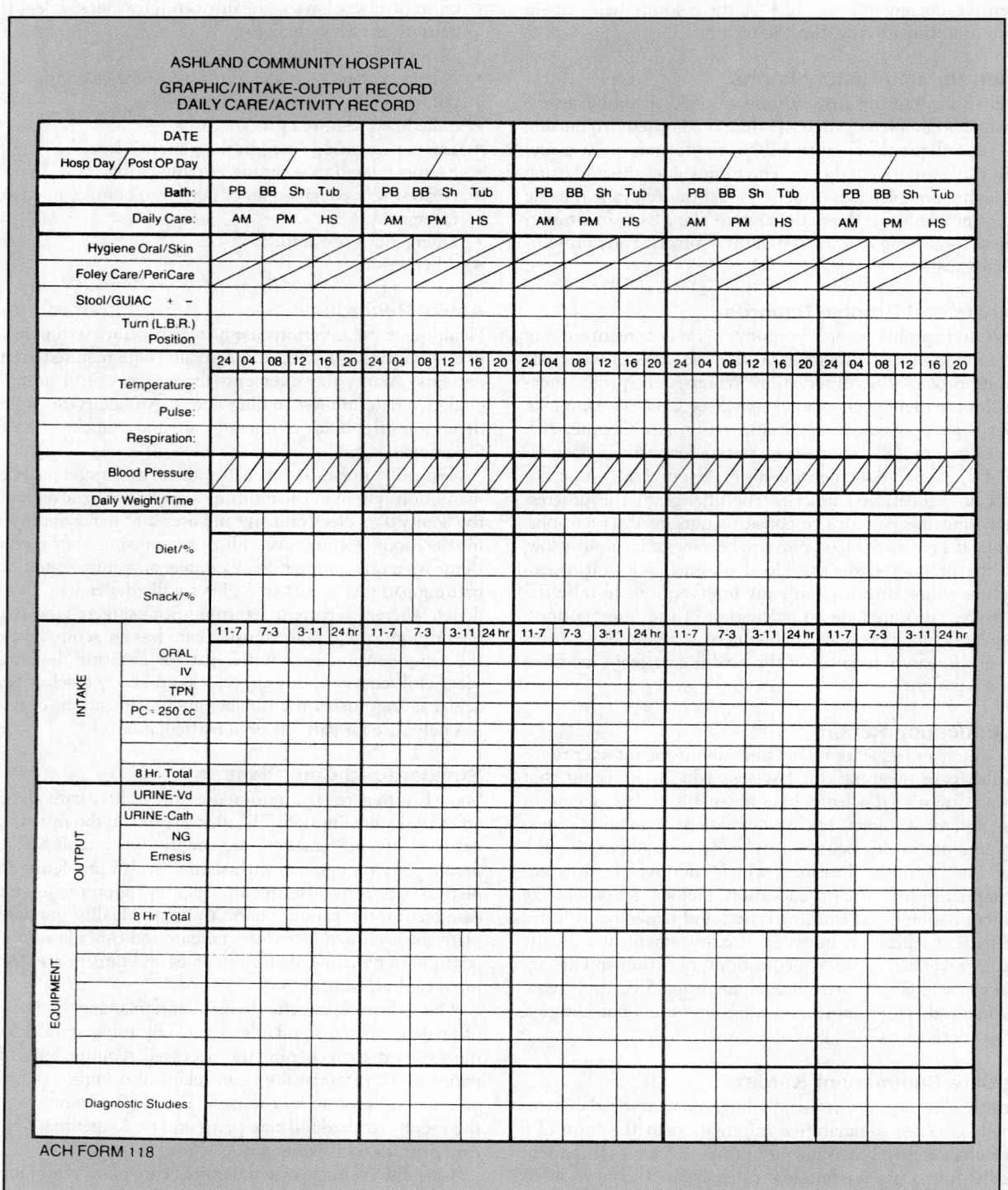

FIG 4-3   Graphic and intake-output record. (*Courtesy Ashland Community Hospital, Ashland, Ore.*)

or problems in a single care plan. These systems enhance nursing knowledge and improve descriptions of patient problems and care strategies (Lee, 2006).

Discharge Summary Forms

Discharge planning is a comprehensive process with emphasis placed on preparing a patient for discharge from a health care organization. Discharge planning, case management, and utilization review are complementary processes in patient care (Birmingham, 2007). A prospective payment system based on diagnosis-related groups (DRGs) encourages health care organizations to be more efficient and discharge a patient as soon as possible. Early hospital discharge improves the hospital's chances of full reimbursement. It is important to ensure that a patient's discharge results in desirable outcomes. You enhance discharge planning when you are responsive to changes in a patient's condition and involve the patient and family in the planning process (Chapman, 2007). The discharge summary includes essential information for the patient, family, and health care organization (Box 4-1).

Discharge planning begins at admission and becomes a more prominent part of care as a patient gets closer to discharge. There needs to be evidence of the involvement of the patient and family members in the discharge planning process so that the patient and family have the necessary information and resources to return home (Chapman, 2007). The Joint Commission (2007a) has standards for patient and family education necessary for effective discharge planning. When a patient is discharged from a health care organization, the members of the health care team prepare a discharge summary. A discharge summary provides important information relating to the patient's ongoing health problems and need for health care after discharge. Discharge planning achieves specific outcomes that include identifying patients with ongoing health needs, collaborating with other health care professions to determine level of care, matching patients with appropriate referrals and resources, and streamlining the transition to the next level of care (Birmingham, 2007; Foust, 2007; Walker and others, 2007). Include in the discharge summary the reason for hospitalization, significant findings, current status of the patient, and the teaching plan that is given to the patient or family, home care, rehabilitation, or long-term care agency (TJC, 2008). Discharge summary forms make the summary concise and instructive. Discharge summary forms emphasize previous learning by the patient and family and care that needs to continue in any restorative care setting.

BOX 4-1	Discharge Summary Information

- Use clear, concise descriptions in patient's own language.
- Provide step-by-step description of how to perform a procedure (e.g., home medication administration). Reinforce explanation with printed instructions.
- Identify precautions to follow when performing self-care or administering medications.
- Review any restrictions that may relate to activities of daily living (e.g., bathing, ambulating, driving).
- Review signs and symptoms of complications to report to the health care provider.
- List names and phone numbers of health care providers and community resources for the patient to contact.
- Identify any unresolved problem, including plans for follow-up and continuous treatment.
- List actual time of discharge, mode of transportation, and who accompanied the patient.

CHARTING SYSTEMS

There are a variety of documentation forms and systems for recording patient information and progress. The documentation system selected by nursing reflects the philosophy of the health care organization. The same documentation system is used throughout a specific agency, but there are several acceptable methods for recording health care data.

Narrative Documentation

Narrative documentation is the traditional method for recording nursing care and activities. In many settings, other methods such as focus charting have begun to replace narrative charting. Narrative charting uses a storylike format to document specific information about a patient's conditions and nursing care, usually presented in chronological order. Narrative charting is useful in emergency situations when the time and order of events is important. Organize a narrative in a clear, concise way, for example, by using the nursing process to order the data. The major disadvantage of narrative charting is that information is found throughout the chart, which can lead to incomplete or inadequate communication among the health care team.

Problem-Oriented Medical Records

The problem-oriented medical record (POMR) is a structured method of documentation that emphasizes a patient's problems. This method is organized using the nursing process, which facilitates communication about patient needs. Data are organized by problem or diagnosis. Ideally, all members of the health care team contribute to the list of identified patient problems. This approach assists in coordinating an individualized plan of care with the following sections: database, problem list, care plan, and progress notes.

Patient Database

A patient's database contains all available assessment information pertaining to the patient. This section is the foundation for identifying patient problems and planning care. The database remains active and current for each patient and is revised as new data become available.

Problem List

The problem list develops after a patient's assessment data are analyzed. The problem list includes the patient's physiological, psychological, sociocultural, spiritual, developmental, and environmental needs. Identify and list priority problems in chronological order to serve as an organizing guide for the patient's care. Add new problems as they are identified during the ongoing nursing assessment. When a problem is resolved, you record the date and draw a line through the problem and its number.

Nursing Care Plan

All disciplines involved in a patient's care contribute to the development of a plan of care for a specific problem. For example, in the case of a patient having a nutritional deficit, a nurse will recommend feeding approaches and a registered dietitian will recommend types of diet supplements. Care plan standards require that a plan of care be developed for all patients on admission to a health care organization (TJC, 2008). Generally these plans of care include nursing diagnoses, expected outcomes, and interventions.

Progress Notes

Health care team members use progress notes to monitor and record the progress of a patient's problem (Box 4-2). Narrative notes, flow sheets, and discharge summaries are formats used to document patient progress (see Procedural Guideline 4-2, p. 59).

BOX 4-2 Formats for Recording Progress Notes

Narrative Note

Describes patient data in a narrative paragraph.

Example:

Patient states, "I am dreading this surgery because last time I had a terrible reaction to the anesthesia and had such terrible pain when they made me get out of bed." Noted muscle tension and loud, agitated voice. Notified anesthesiologist, Dr. M, of patient's prior experience. Discussed alternatives for anesthesia and pain-control options. Stressed importance of activity for circulation/healing. Encouraged to keep nurses informed of pain level/need for medication and that pain may be present, but manageable.

SOAP (Acronym for Subjective Data, Objective Data, Assessment, and Plan)

Usually based on a numbered list of problems or nursing diagnoses.

Example:

S (Subjective data) (the patient's statements regarding the problem): Patient states, "I am dreading this surgery because last time I had a terrible reaction to the anesthesia and had such terrible pain when they made me get out of bed."

O (Objective data) (observations that support or are related to subjective data): Noted muscle tension and loud, agitated voice.

A (Assessment/Analysis) (conclusions reached based on data): Fear related to pain/anesthesia.

P (Plan) (the plan for dealing with the situation): Notified anesthesiologist, Dr. M, of patient's prior experience. Discussed alternatives for anesthesia/pain control options. Stressed importance of activity for circulation/healing. Encouraged to keep nurses informed of pain level/need for medication and that pain may be present, but manageable.

PIE (Acronym for Problem, Intervention, and Evaluation)

Problem-oriented system in which progress notes are written based on a list of identified problems, and detailed data may be entered by any member of the health care team.

Example:

P (Problem): Patient states, "I am dreading this surgery because last time I had a terrible reaction to the anesthesia and had such terrible pain when they made me get out of bed." Noted muscle tension and loud, agitated voice.

I (Intervention): Notified anesthesiologist, Dr. M, of patient's prior experience. Discussed alternatives for anesthesia and pain-control options. Stressed importance of activity for circulation/healing. Encouraged to keep nurses informed of pain level/need for medication and that pain may be present, but manageable.

E (Evaluation): Patient stated she was "very relieved." Stated she would tell the nurses about pain.

Focus or DAR Charting

A way to organize progress notes to make them more clear and organized.

Example:

D (Data): Patient states, "I am dreading this surgery because last time I had a terrible reaction to the anesthesia and had such terrible pain when they made me get out of bed." Noted muscle tension and loud, agitated voice.

A (Nursing Action): Notified anesthesiologist, Dr. M, of patient's prior experience. Discussed alternatives for anesthesia and pain-control options. Stressed importance of activity for circulation/healing. Encouraged to keep nurses informed of pain level/need for medication and that pain may be present, but manageable.

R (Patient Response): Patient stated she was "very relieved." Stated understanding of the importance of informing the nurses about pain.

NOTE: Some agencies add P (Plan) and refer to this as DARP charting.

Example:

P (Plan): Assess pain level at least every 4 hours postoperatively. Provide nonpharmacological pain management techniques, and administer medication as needed.

SBAR (Acronym for Situation, Background, Assessment, and Recommendation)

SBAR is a system of structured communication used to share information about a patient condition.

Example:

S (Situation): Patient verbalized preoperative fears. Nurse noted muscle tension and loud, agitated voice.

B (Background): Patient fearful of surgery because of past experiences with anesthesia and pain.

A (Actions taken): Notified anesthesiologist, Dr. M, of patient's prior experience. Discussed alternatives for anesthesia and pain-control options. Stressed importance of activity for circulation/healing. Encouraged to keep nurses informed of pain level/need for medication and that pain may be present, but manageable.

R (Recommendation): Assess pain level at least every 4 hours postoperatively. Provide nonpharmacological pain management techniques, and administer medication as needed.

SOAP Documentation. You can use structured notes to document patient progress in the SOAP format. SOAP is a mnemonic for the following:

S: Subjective data (patient statements about the problem)

O: Objective data (data that are measured and observed or related to subjective data)

A: Assessment/Analysis (conclusions based on the subjective and objective data)

P: Plan (what the caregiver plans to do)

Some institutions add an *I* and *E* (i.e., SOAPIE). The *I* stands for *intervention*, and the *E* represents *evaluation*. The logic for SOAP(IE) notes is similar to that of the nursing process: Collect data about a patient's problems, draw conclusions, and develop a plan of care. Number each SOAP note, and title it according to the problem on the list.

PIE Documentation. The PIE note format of documentation is similar to SOAP charting in its problem-oriented nature. How-

ever, it differs from the SOAP method in that PIE charting has a nursing origin, whereas SOAP originated from a medical model. PIE is a mnemonic for the following:

P: Problem or nursing diagnosis for the patient

I: Interventions or actions taken

E: Evaluation of the outcomes of nursing interventions

The PIE format simplifies documentation by combining the care plan and progress note into one record. The PIE format differs from SOAP because there is no assessment data in the narrative note. Assessment data is included in documentation on each shift's flow sheets. You will number or label the PIE notes according to a patient's problems. Resolved problems are dropped from daily documentation after your review. Continuing problems are documented daily.

Focus Charting. Another narrative format is focus charting or DAR (data, action, response). One distinction of focus charting is it places less importance on patient problems and focuses on patient concerns such as a sign or symptom, condition, a nursing diagnosis, a behavior, a significant event, or a change in condition. Each documentation includes data (both subjective and objective), actions or nursing interventions, and patient response (e.g., evaluation of effectiveness). Nurses need to broaden their thinking to include any patient concerns, not just problem areas, and to apply critical thinking. Focus charting saves time because it is easy for caregivers to understand and is adaptable to most health care settings, and it enables all caregivers to track a patient's condition and progress.

SBAR Documentation. Structured communication provides a model for data about a patient's condition. You apply this method to both written and verbal communication. SBAR is a mnemonic for the following:

S: Situation (state what is happening at the present time)
B: Background (explain the circumstances leading up to the situation)
A: Assessment (what do you think the problem is?)
R: Recommendation (what would you do to correct the problem?)

SBAR is a technique that provides a framework for communication between members of the health care team about a patient's condition. SBAR is a concrete mechanism used for framing conversation, especially critical ones, requiring a nurse's immediate attention and action. It allows for an easy and focused way to set expectations for what the team will communicate. SBAR promotes the provision of safe, efficient, timely, and patient-centered communication (Haig and others, 2006).

Source Records

In a source record a patient's chart is organized so that each discipline (e.g., nursing, medicine, social work, and respiratory therapy) has a separate section in which to record data. The advantage of a source record is that it is easy for caregivers to locate the proper section of the record in which to make entries.

A disadvantage of the source record is that information about a specific problem may be distributed throughout the record. For example, the nurse describes the character of a patient's fractured femur pain and use of repositioning and narcotic analgesia in the nurses' notes. The physician or health care provider notes in a separate section of the record the patient's bone healing and the plan for casting or surgery. The results of x-ray examinations that show bone healing are in the radiology results section of the record. The method makes it difficult to find chronological information about patient care or how the team is coordinating care to meet all of the patient's needs.

Charting by Exception

Charting by exception (CBE) is a system of documentation that aims to eliminate redundancy, makes documentation of routine care more concise, emphasizes abnormal findings, and identifies trends in clinical care. Documentation is more effective, nurses spend less time charting, data is easy to retrieve, and communication is improved (Guido, 2006). CBE is a shorthand method for documenting based on clearly defined standards of practice and predetermined criteria for nursing assessments and interventions. This system involves completing a flow sheet that incorporates standard assessment and intervention criteria by placing a check mark in the appropriate standard box on the flow sheet to indicate normal findings and routine interventions. You write a narrative nurse's note *only* when there is an exception to the established standard or abnormal data are present. Assessments are standard-ized on forms so that all health care providers evaluate and document findings consistently (Fig. 4-4).

The presumption with CBE is that the nurse did assess the patient and all standards are met unless otherwise documented. Changes in a patient's condition require thorough and precise descriptions of what happened, actions taken, and patient response to treatment. Legal risks in using CBE include difficulty in proving safe care if nurses are not disciplined in documenting exceptions. To avoid miscommunication or misinterpretation when using CBE, writing "N/A" on flow sheets when an item does not apply avoids leaving areas blank (Sullivan, 2004).

Case Management Plan and Critical Pathways

Case management is a delivery of care model that coordinates and links health care services to patients and families while streamlining costs and maintaining quality (Dadich, 2007). Collaboration and communication are promoted in a multidisciplinary approach using critical or collaborative pathways for a specific disease or condition that is summarized into a standardized care plan. Case management plans incorporate standardized documents that include short care plans for the problem, key interventions, and expected outcomes for patients with a specific disease or condition (Fig. 4-5). These pathways provide the ideal sequence and timing of interventions for all members of the health care team. Use of critical pathways minimizes care delays, maximizes resource utilization, improves quality care, and monitors and documents patient progress (Coffey and others, 2005). The goal of a critical pathway is to improve the quality of care, reduce risks, increase patient satisfaction, and improve outcomes (DeBleser and others, 2006).

Case management programs use a multidisciplinary plan of care summarized into critical pathways. The critical pathways are multidisciplinary care plans that include key interventions and expected outcomes within an established time frame (see Fig. 4-5). Critical pathways are evidence based, and the assessment/monitoring, interventions, and expected outcomes are based on research and/or clinical evidence within the literature.

Critical pathways state the goals and important elements of care based on best practice and patient expectations by documenting, monitoring, and evaluating variances and providing resources and outcomes. Variances are unexpected occurrences, unmet goals, and interventions not specified within the critical pathway time frame and reflect a positive or negative change. A positive variance occurs when a patient progresses more rapidly than the case management plan expected (e.g., use of a Foley catheter is discontinued a day early). A negative variance occurs when the activities on the critical pathway do not happen as predicted or outcomes are unmet (e.g., oxygen therapy is necessary for a new-onset breathing problem). Your responsibility is to document the variance and include causative factors, actions taken, patient response, and outcomes. Over time the reoccurrence of similar variances will lead the health care team to revise a critical pathway, particularly if it affects quality of care or length of stay.

STANDARDIZED LANGUAGE

Standardized language is recognized as the means by which nurses communicate consistent information to describe a clinical situation to reduce complexity, improve completion time, and increase staff satisfaction in care planning (Thomas, 2006). Nursing care is more effective and appropriate to patient needs when nurses use the same language to identify patient problems and plan patient outcomes. There are several classification systems that provide

Working Copy

BARNES-JEWISH HOSPITAL

Nursing Shift Assessment C-6

Requested by: CAROL

789651458 X

Collins, Phil

S.S.

Dr.

Unit: Bed:

Search Interval   From: 05-Dec-2009 at 07:00
To: 06-Dec-2009 at 14:51

Patient Assessment

		Monday 12/06 07:00
N/S	**NEUROSENSORY STANDARD** Alert and awake. If asleep awakens to name. Verbal appropriate, clear, and understandable. Swallows without coughing. Oriented to time, place, person and situation. Behavior is appropriate to situation. Moves all extremities well, ambulates with steady gait.	Within Normal Limits
RESP	**RESPIRATORY STANDARD** Respirations are even and unlabored. Nailbeds and mucous membranes are pink. Patent airway. Lung sounds clear to auscultation. No cough noted	Within Normal Limits
CARD	**CARDIOVASCULAR STANDARD** Regular palpable pulses. Skin pallor within patient's norm. Skin warm and dry. No edema.	Within Normal Limits
SKIN	**SKIN INTEGRITY STANDARD** Skin and mucous membranes intact without notable lesions or impaired integrity. Mucous membranes moist and pink. Braden Score greater than 17.	* Exception as noted below
	Braden Risk Assessment	Mobility: Slightly Limited (3) Sensory: Slightly Limited (3) Moisture: Occasionally Moist (3) Activity: Walks Occasionally (3) Nutrition: Adequate (3) Friction/Shear: Potential Problem (2) Total Score 17
	Casts, Splints, Braces Type: Fiberglass Cast Site: Right Lower Leg	Maintains correct anatomical position No pressure areas noted Distal extremity pink warm to touch Palpable distal pulse Capillary Refill <3 seconds Sensation normal Able to move distal phalanges.
	VASCULAR ACCESS STANDARD IV SITE: Site free of redness, swelling, pain, bleeding, drainage, IV patent, dressing occlusive and intact.	
NUTR	**NUTRITION STANDARD** Tolerating prescribed diet without nausea and vomiting. Eating at least 75% of each meal without difficulty. Feeds self.	Within normal limits
	Diet Type	Regular
GI	**GASTROINTESTINAL STANDARD** Abdomen soft. Bowel sounds active all 4 quadrants. No pain with palpation. Having bowel movements within patient's normal pattern, consistency, and color.	Within Normal Limits
GU	**GENITOURINARY STANDARD** Continent of urine. Urine clear and yellow to amber color.	Within Normal Limits
PSYCH	**PSYCHOSOCIAL STANDARD** Accepts situation and facial expressions are appropriate. family support available and patient receives visitors. Able to communicate without assistance.	Within Normal Limits
EDU	Health Status Teaching	
	Tests/Procedures/Therapies	
	Medication Teaching	
	Nutrition Teaching	
	Medical Equipment Teaching	
HMGT	Equipment	
Charted By		cl

Signatures:
cl   C. Logan, RN

Printed: 06-Dec-2009 at 14:51

FIG 4-4   Charting by exception—assessment form. When standards in far left column are not met, a detailed note explaining findings must be entered. (*Courtesy Barnes-Jewish Hospital, BJC Health System, St. Louis, Mo.*)

Norman Regional Hospital CareMap®
Community Acquired Pneumonia

Page 1

Check (✓) Precautions

☐ Falls ☐ Skin ☐ DNR

Admitting Physician: Primary Care Physician: Consulting Physician(s):   Expected LOS   M&R LOS

Allergy/Reaction   Secondary Diagnosis

Prob	Patient Problem	Expected Outcome (Responsible Discipline)	Outcome	Date	Signature
#1 ★	Infection	Blood cultures obtained prior to start of antibiotics? (RN)	☐ YES ☐ NO		
#2	Activity Tolerance	Patient is at or above baseline activity (endurance) level? (RN)	☐ YES ☐ NO		
#3	Knowledge Deficit	Patient able to verbalize understanding of pneumonia signs and symptoms? (RN)	☐ YES ☐ NO		
#4 ★	Timeliness of Antibiotic Administration	First dose of antibiotic administered within 2 hours of order? (RN, RPh)	☐ YES ☐ NO		
#5 ★	Discharge Preparation	Patient switched from IV to oral antibiotic within 48hrs after delivery of 1st dose? (RN, RPh)	☐ YES ☐ NO		

★ = Key Exception
<u> </u> = Documentation Required

Copyright© 2000 Norman Regional Hospital

Authors: **Rosalie Lavon, M.D., Jerry Leu, M.D., John McCarter, M.D., Tom Merrill, M.D., Bruce Naylor, M.D., J. Kin Pirtle, M.D., Joe Riddle, M.D., Christian Sieck, M.D., Jackie Evans, Linda Fielder, Vicki Johnson, Wanda Maddox, Yvette Morrison, Wanda Morrow, Joyce Nolen, Barbara Poe, Michelle Rausch, Darin Smith, Brenda Wilson**

Date: 7/00   Form# CMAP 114   Revised:

Statement of Intent:
The CareMap® serves as an optional guideline for patient care and is subject to alteration based on the individual needs of the patient.
(CareMap® used with permission of the Center for Case Management.)

Patient Sticker

FIG 4-5   Example of a critical pathway for pneumonia. *(From Norman Regional Hospital CareMap, Community Acquired Pneumonia. Copyright 2000, Norman Regional Hospital. Used with permission of Normal Regional Hospital, Norman, Okla.)*

Norman Regional Hospital CareMap®
Community Acquired Pneumonia CareMap® Summary

		Day #1 (ER/Floor) Date _____	Day #2 Date _____
PATIENT STICKER	**Time Admitted:** _____		
	Assessments/Monitoring	VS qshift (and Temp q4h if T>99.5) Nursing Assessment qshift Weight I&O Pain Assessment	VS qshift (and Temp q4h if T>99.5) Nursing Assessment qshift I&O Pain Assessment
	Consults	Respiratory Therapy Assess need for Social Work Consult	
	Procedures/Tests	CBC with diff, Basic Metabolic Panel, UA, Sputum gram stain + C&S Stat (induce if necessary), Blood cultures x2 (15 minutes apart), CXR (PA & Lateral)	CBC with diff
	Treatments	Oxygen Therapy per protocol C&DB q2hr Suction prn Albuterol AN treatments/MDI per RT/RN if ordered Incentive Spirometry q2hr WA @ bedside if ordered	Continue oxygen therapy per protocol, evaluate for discontinuation of O2 RT to convert to MDI pm Incentive Spirometry q2hr WA @ bedside if ordered
	Medications/IV	Initial Antibiotic STAT (to be administered within one hour of order) IV Fluids	Cont Abx-consider oral switch Evaluate and change to HL or DC IV if applicable
	Nutrition	Diet as tolerated Encourage oral fluids if appropriate	Diet as tolerated Encourage oral fluids if appropriate Goal: 3-4 glasses H2O if not fluid restricted
	Activity/Safety	Activity as tolerated (Encourage up in chair for meals) Fall prevention program initiated if appropriate	Activity as tolerated (Encourage up in chair for meals) Goal: Ambulate 25-50ft x 2
	Patient/Family Education	Assess knowledge level concerning disease process and medication Teach use of MDI if applicable	Reasses patient's ability to use MDI Reinforce med education, activity and follow-up
	Discharge Planning	RN/SW initiates discharge planning	Interview patient/family re: discharge planning
	Psychosocial/Emotional/ Spiritual	Explain procedures Encourage verbalization of feelings	Notify Chaplain to visit if requested
	CMAP # 114		

Page 2

Additional Daily Treatments/Other

Isolation Precautions

Special Procedures/Surgeries:

Additional Daily Lab:
Order for CareMap entered into computer: initial (RN/US) _____

Other Pertinent Information:

Family Spokesperson:

Emergency Phone #: _____

FIG 4-5, cont'd

standardized language. NANDA International (NANDA-I) (2007) develops standardized nursing diagnoses to describe patients' responses to health problems. The Nursing Interventions Classification (NIC) provides a label name, a definition, and a list of activities that a nurse performs to complete the intervention (Dochterman and Bulechek, 2004). Use of this standardized language in documentation may prove useful to communicate patient care needs more clearly.

Another standard form of language being used throughout health care is patient outcomes. The Nursing Outcomes Classification (NOC) provides an outcome label, a definition, and a list of interventions that will possibly result in the outcome (Moorhead and others, 2004). The use of outcomes is essential when evaluating the achievement of patient care goals and the appropriateness of patient interventions.

Outcome statements require a target date for completion and evaluation of a patient's progress toward achievement at specific intervals. Evaluation of progress determines if the patient's problem or diagnosis is resolved or if you need to revise or extend the plan. You individualize each outcome for the particular patient using specific measurement criteria. Such a process promotes continuity of care across the continuum of a patient's care and centers on the patient's and family's ability to restore, maintain, or improve the patient's health. The implementation of NANDA-I, NIC, and NOC nursing diagnoses, interventions, and outcomes can lead to higher quality of nursing diagnosis documentation, etiology-specific nursing interventions, and nursing-specific patient outcomes (Muller-Staub and others, 2007).

CULTURAL CONSIDERATIONS

Culturally focused nursing care is essential with the changing demographics of the United States. The Joint Commission (2006) developed standards to ensure that health care providers collect data on a patient's race, ethnicity, and spoken and written language in health records, integrate it into the management information system, and update this periodically. One step in providing this care is via the nursing care plan, which is integrated into the care of patients in most health care organizations. It is available in a variety of formats, including standardized care plans, concept maps, or critical pathways via computer or patient record. The intent is that this plan of care guides the health care team in targeting the needs and resources for any patient with diversity. The ultimate goal is to promote respect and provide quality patient care for every individual, including those with unique diversities. Compliance with government guidelines is evidenced within the clinical documentation system that integrates care plans and nursing documentation. The care plan provides a prompt for referral to the multidisciplinary team to organize care and prioritize resources for these patients. The computerized care plan can focus on the unique qualities, opportunities, and challenges of working with diverse populations (Walsh, 2004).

HOME CARE DOCUMENTATION

Home care continues to grow with shorter hospitalizations and increasing numbers of older adults requiring home care services. Medicare has specific guidelines for establishing eligibility for home care reimbursement (Struk, 2007). Skilled home nursing care is divided into four categories: observation and assessment, teaching and training, skilled treatments and procedures, and management and evaluation of a care plan (Carusa and others, 2004). When you provide care in the home, documentation has different

implications than in other areas of nursing. One primary difference is that the patient and family rather than the nurse witness the majority of care. In addition, documentation systems need to provide the entire health care team with the necessary information to work together effectively (Box 4-3). The documentation is both the quality control and the justification for reimbursement from Medicare, Medicaid, or private insurance companies (Carusa and others, 2004). It is important to consistently document all your services for reimbursement (e.g., direct skilled care, patient instructions, skilled observation, and evaluation visits) (TJC, 2007b).

Duplication of documentation is necessary, or agency policies state what forms you need to leave at the office versus what forms you need to take into the home. Computerized patient records are evolving as a method of addressing these different needs. With the use of electronic information systems and mobile computing technology, it is possible for records to be available in multiple locations, which allows greater access to the multidisciplinary needs that are present in home care (Brandeis and others, 2007; Doran and others, 2007).

LONG-TERM HEALTH CARE DOCUMENTATION

Increasing numbers of older adults and disabled people in the United States require care in long-term health care facilities. Nursing personnel face documentation challenges much different from those in the acute care setting. Documentation is essential to communicate among the health care providers, demonstrate appropriateness and quality of care, and evaluate effectiveness of treatments and interventions (McCloskey, 2006). Changes in the Medicare program determine the standards and policies for reimbursement and documentation in long-term care. The federally mandated Long Term Care Facility Resident Assessment Instrument provides standardized protocols for assessment and care planning and promotes quality improvement within and among facilities (Taunton and others, 2004). Records are reviewed for reimbursement, and there are expectations that standards and requirements have been met (Durkin, 2006).

Each resident in long-term care is assessed using the Long Term Care Facility Resident Assessment Instrument mandated by the Omnibus Budget Reconciliation Act of 1989 (OBRA) and updated in 1998 (Health Care Financing Administration [HCFA], 1998). A registered nurse is responsible for coordinating the plan of care. Documentation supports the assessment and planning process for patients using a multidisciplinary approach. Communication among health care providers, including nurses, social workers,

---

BOX 4-3 Home Care Forms for Documentation

The usual forms used to document home care include the following:
- Patient assessment
- Referral source information/intake form
- Discipline-specific care plans
- Physician's plan of treatment
- Medication sheet
- Clinical progress notes
- Miscellaneous (conference notes, verbal order forms, telephone calls)
- Discharge summary
- Reports to third-party payers

Modified from Iyer PW, Camp NH: *Nursing documentation: a nursing process approach*, ed 4, St. Louis, 2005, Mosby.

recreational therapists, and dietitians, is essential in regulation of the documentation process. The fiscal support for long-term care residents depends on the justification of nursing care as demonstrated in sound documentation of the services rendered. The overall goal is a system of clinical documentation that identifies potential or actual problems and provides improved actions for each problem that result in improved care for residents and increased reimbursement for that care (Bott and others, 2007).

DOCUMENTATION

Comprehensive computer systems in health care delivery have unlimited potential for improving the accuracy, efficiency, and quality of documentation. Researchers estimate that only a small percentage of health care facilities have some type of electronic record (Ashish and others, 2007; Blumenthal and Glaser, 2007). However, the traditional paper medical record is no longer meeting the needs of today's health care industry. A paper record is episode-oriented, with a separate record for each patient visit to a health care agency (Hebda, 2005). Key information, such as client allergies, current medications, and treatment complications may be lost from one episode of care (e.g., hospitalization or clinic visit) to the next, risking a patient's safety. The electronic health record (EHR) is a longitudinal electronic record of client health information generated by one or more encounters in a care delivery setting (Health Information and Management Systems Society, 2007). The EHR provides access to a patient's health record information at the time and place that clinicians need it.

Although an EHR is the wave of the future, many agencies have computerized medical record systems. Computerized documentation has features that potentially can improve documentation accuracy, timeliness and completeness of data entry, and communication among health care disciplines (Smith and others, 2005). In addition, computerized documentation systems are designed to reduce errors and provide standardized care plans or treatment protocols. Such a system relies on many data collection components; including flow sheets, medication records, and clinical care summaries. Software programs allow quick access to assessment data, and information automatically transfers to different reports. New technology allows for the use of pen-based or voice recognition programs.

The transition to computerized documentation presents both opportunities and challenges to nurses and nurse managers (Fig. 4-6). The Security Rule of HIPAA provides standards for the protection of electronic health information (DeVore and others, 2007; Gallagher, 2004). The successful implementation of a computerized documentation system requires preparation, involvement, and commitment of the entire nursing staff. Awareness of legal risks and confidentiality issues are important challenges in the transition from paper to computerized systems. Numerous nursing and medical professional organizations have developed guidelines and strategies for safe computer charting:

1 Do not share personal password or computer signature with other caregivers.
2 Avoid leaving the computer terminal unattended when logged on.
3 Follow the agency protocol for correcting errors.
4 Never create, change, or delete records unless your agency provides you with this authority.

5 Software systems have a system for backup files. If you inadvertently delete part of the permanent record, follow agency policy. It is necessary to type an explanation into the computer file with the date, time, and your initials and submit an explanation in writing to your manager.
6 Avoid leaving information about a patient displayed on a monitor when others are able to see it. Keep a log that accounts for every copy of a computerized file that you have generated from the system.
7 Follow the agency's confidentiality procedures for documenting sensitive material, such as diagnosis of human immunodeficiency virus (HIV) infection.
8 Protect printouts from computerized records. Shredding of printouts and the logging in of the number of copies generated by each caregiver minimizes duplicate records and protects the confidentiality of patient information.

EVIDENCE-BASED PRACTICE TRENDS

Computer-based health care records, informatics, and implementation of the electronic patient record all have major implications for the practice of nursing and the documentation of nursing care. Computer-based documentation systems are integral to improving and documenting quality nursing care (Mahler and others, 2007). This type of system maintains a continual record of care planned and/or provided to a patient by nurses and other members of the health care team and shows improvement in meeting selected agency's documentation standards (Currell and Urquhart, 2005). Studies show that the inclusion of the nursing process within the computerized record and in the care plan positively influences acceptance of the new system (Ammenwerth and Shaw, 2005; Lee, 2006). There are important criteria for the successful implementation of computer-based nursing documentation systems, including a high level of acceptance, careful preparation of standardized care plans, and organizational preparation and inclusion of future users in the development process (Lee, 2006; Nelson, 2007). Positive attitude toward technology is a major factor in acceptance of computerized documentation systems (Dillon and others, 2005). Getting nurses to the design table is often the key to success in implementing computerized systems.

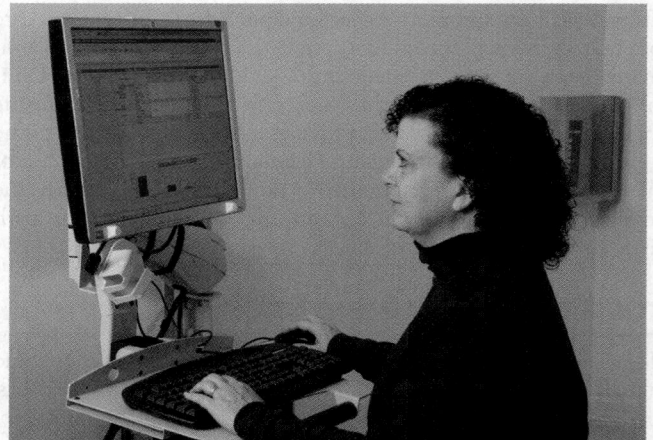

FIG 4-6   Computerized documentation provides many benefits.

PROCEDURAL GUIDELINE 4-1   Giving a Change-of-Shift (Handoff) Report

In addition to written documentation, the primary nurse provides a change-of-shift report to another caregiver assuming responsibility for patient care. The purpose of the report is to provide continuity of care for the patient. Recently, The Joint Commission (2008) *2009 National Patient Safety Goals* for health care organizations standardize an approach to "hand off" communication that includes opportunities to ask and respond to questions. Nurses give a change-of-shift report face-to-face, by audiotape recording, via telephone conversation, through a written report, in a computer format, or during "walking-planning" rounds at each patient's bedside. It is important to have some type of guidelines for reporting to avoid repetitive, irrelevant, and speculative communication (Benson and others, 2007; Wilson, 2007). It is essential to schedule an opportunity for oncoming nurses to ask questions for clarification after listening to the report. Regardless of the form of the change-of-shift report, you must maintain confidentiality.

Delegation Considerations
The skill of giving a change-of-shift report cannot be delegated to nursing assistive personnel (NAP). The nurse directs the NAP about:
- Licensed practical nurses (LPNs) may report on patients they care for directly.
- What to report to the nurse (e.g., increased pain, changes in vital signs), so the nurse can reassess, validate, and report any changes in the change-of-shift report.

Equipment
- ❏ Worksheets, nursing Kardex or patient care profile, nursing care plan, critical pathway, or multidisciplinary treatment plan
- ❏ Tape recorder (according to agency policy)

Procedural Steps
1 Develop an organized format for delivering report that provides a description of patient needs and problems.
2 Gather information from worksheets, NAP report, or other relevant documents.

> **Critical Decision Point**   *Report only relevant information to next shift to ensure staff's timely responsiveness.*

3 Prioritize information based on patient's needs and problems.
4 For each patient include:
  a *Background information*: Patient's name, gender, age, current primary reason for hospitalization, and brief history. Also include any known allergies, emergency code status (i.e., do not resuscitate [DNR]), and special needs as related to any physical challenges (e.g., blind, hearing deficit, amputee).
  b *Assessment data*: Provide objective observations and measurements made by the nurse during the shift. Describe patient's condition, and emphasize any recent changes. Include any relevant information reported by patient, family, or health care team members, such as laboratory data and diagnostic test results.
  c *Nursing diagnoses*: If appropriate, state the nursing diagnoses appropriate for patient. (Some agencies do not include nursing diagnoses in report.)
  d *Interventions, outcomes, and evaluation*: (steps can be combined in a report)
    (1) Describe therapies or treatments administered during shift and expected outcomes (e.g., medication changes, use of oxygen, referral visits). Specify how you implemented interventions uniquely for this patient. Report on evaluation by explaining patient's response and whether outcomes are met. Do not explain basic steps of procedure.
    (2) Describe instructions or education given in the teaching plan and patient's/family's ability to demonstrate learning.
  e *Family information*: Report on family visitation or involvement, specifically as it influenced patient. Explain if you included family members in care procedures or instruction.
  f *Discharge plan*: Review patient's progress toward discharge during each change-of-shift report. Discuss education progress, communication with referral agencies, and family preparation for discharge. This plan also identifies roles and responsibilities of the multidisciplinary team and their follow-up visits.
  g *Current priorities*: Clearly explain the priorities to which oncoming nurse must attend.
    (1) Report significant clinical changes.
    (2) Report on immediate treatment planned for any new admission.
    (3) Explain status of activities for patients preparing for procedures and treatments.
    (4) Describe current physical status of patients returning from diagnostic or operative procedures.
5 Ask the staff from oncoming shift if they have any questions regarding information provided.
6 If using a tape recorder, periodically evaluate for clarity, organization, rate of speaking, and volume level.

PROCEDURAL GUIDELINE 4-2   Documenting Nurses' Progress Notes

There are a variety of forms and formats to communicate information about a patient's health status and care. Accurate documentation reflects the quality of care and provides evidence of each health care team member's accountability in giving care. The purpose of a patient's record is to provide information for communication, education, assessment, research, financial billing, auditing, and legal documentation (Table 4-3).

Because the nursing process directs a nurse's approach to patient care, documentation needs to reflect this process. Nurses record assessment data, changes in a patient's condition, nursing interventions, and an evaluation of the patient's progress toward established outcomes. Prompt documentation of this data increases accuracy and promotes effective communication to all members of the health care team.

Continued

PROCEDURAL GUIDELINE 4-2 Documenting Nurses' Progress Notes—cont'd

Progress notes provide a format for documenting a patient's health status and progress. You can use a variety of formats when writing notes, including SOAP, SOAPIE, PIE, DAR, and SBAR. All caregivers need to be able to read the progress note and have a clear picture of the problem, level of care required, and results of interventions. The nurse caring for the patient is responsible for writing and signing each progress note, which includes your full name and title.

Delegation Considerations

The skill of writing a progress note cannot be delegated to NAP. The nurse directs the NAP about:

- What repetitive care activities to document on flow sheets (e.g., vital signs, intake and output [I&O], routine care).
- What to report to the nurse (e.g., increased pain, changes in vital signs), so the nurse can reassess, validate, and document any changes in the progress note.

Equipment

- ❑ Worksheets, nursing Kardex or patient care profile, nursing care plan, critical pathway, or multidisciplinary treatment plan
- ❑ Black pen

Procedural Steps

1 Review all necessary assessments and nursing interventions required by patient. Evaluate patient's response and status of each diagnosis.

2 Identify the forms you need to maintain and where they are located.

   a Forms at bedside or on chart holder just outside door may include graphic chart for vital signs, intake and output record, checklist or flow sheet for routine care or a critical pathway, medication administration record, and nurses' progress notes.

   b Additional nursing forms are sometimes included: intravenous (IV) flow sheets; diabetic record; pain management flow sheet; admission, transfer, and discharge forms; and teaching forms. Follow guidelines for charting (see Table 4-1) to ensure quality documentation.

3 After each patient contact, identify information that needs to be documented. Consider:

   a Abnormal findings

   b Changes in status

   c New problems identified

4 Document in a timely fashion without leaving open spaces between notes, and include date and time.

5 Using agency format, document the following:

   a Pertinent, factual, objective data

   b Selected subjective data that validates or clarifies

   c Nursing actions taken

   d Patient responses to actions taken

   e Additional plans needing to be implemented

   f To whom information has been reported, including name and status

6 Sign progress note with full name or first initial and last name and status according to agency policy. Do not leave any open space between this note and the previously written note. Students are usually required to indicate their level of education and school affiliation.

TABLE 4-3	Purposes of Records
Purpose	**Description**
Communication	The record is a means for health care team members to communicate the patient's *needs* (e.g., individual therapies, patient education, discharge planning) and the patient's *progress* (e.g., response to therapies). Anyone reading the record should have a clear understanding of the plan of care.
Education	The record contains a variety of information, including medical and nursing diagnoses, signs and symptoms of disease, successful and unsuccessful therapies, diagnostic findings, and patient behaviors. Students of nursing, medicine, and other health-related disciplines use records as educational resources.
Assessment	Records provide data that nurses use to identify and support nursing diagnoses and plan proper interventions for care. Information from records adds to the nurse's own observations and assessment. Information in medical progress notes allows the nurse to anticipate the status of the patient and to conduct an assessment that augments, validates, or confirms physician or health care provider findings.
Research	Statistical data relating to the frequency of clinical disorders, complications, use of specific medical and nursing therapies, recovery from illness, and death can be gathered from patient records. Records describe characteristics of the patient populations in a health care agency.
Financial billing	The medical record is a document that shows the extent to which hospitals should be reimbursed for services. For the facility to obtain full reimbursement, the record needs to show that all physicians' or health care providers' orders were completed adequately and correctly, and it must reflect results of those orders.
Auditing and monitoring	A regular review of information in patient records gives a basis for evaluation of the quality and appropriateness of care provided in an institution. The Joint Commission requires health care organizations to establish quality assessment and improvement programs to conduct objective, ongoing reviews of patient care. Review of records will reveal information about the processes and outcomes of care.
Legal documentation	A medical record must be accurate because it is a legal document. In case of a lawsuit, the medical record, not the nursing care, is on trial. Nursing care may have been excellent; however, care not documented is care not done as far as a court of law is concerned.

PROCEDURAL GUIDELINE 4-3   Incident Reporting

An incident is any event not consistent with the routine operation of a health care unit or routine care of a patient. Examples include patient falls, needle-stick injuries, medication errors, or a visitor becoming ill. Completion of an incident report occurs when there is actual or potential patient injury and is not part of the patient record. Document in the patient's record an objective description of what you observed and follow-up actions taken without reference to the incident report. Reporting of incidents helps in the identification of high-risk trends in nursing care or daily unit operations that warrant correction. You complete the report even if an injury does not occur or is not apparent. The information from incident reports helps nursing staff find solutions to prevent repeated incidents. The reports are an important part of a unit's quality improvement program (Table 4-4).

Incident reports are not a part of the permanent medical record but are an important source of risk management data for identifying and addressing the causes of errors in health care organizations (Burkoski, 2007).

Delegation Considerations

The skill of incident reporting cannot be delegated to NAP. The nurse directs the NAP to:

- Report to the nurse any event such as a fall, incorrect treatment, or adverse reaction.
- Report to the nurse any pertinent information about the incident so an incident report can be completed.

Equipment

- ❏ Incident report form
- ❏ Black pen

Procedural Steps

1 Use critical thinking skills to systematically and carefully determine what was involved in the incident. Either report the incident as witnessed, or determine from NAP what specifically occurred. Record the exact sequence of events involved in incident, including time and type of incident; injury to patient, nurse, or other staff; and observation of factors that possibly may have contributed to the incident (e.g., wet floor discovered in area of patient fall).

Critical Decision Point   *Prepare an incident report on any questionable event. Do not avoid incident reporting because you believe that punitive actions will occur if incident reports are filed.*

2 Assess extent of any injury to patient or others, including patient's subjective report and objective physical examination findings.
3 If incident involves an injury, take steps to restore individual's safety, such as stabilizing patient's position after a fall and assessing for further injuries.
4 When patient sustains an injury, call health care provider immediately.
5 When visitor or staff member sustains an injury, refer to emergency department or appropriate treatment setting.
6 Complete incident report form.

Critical Decision Point   *Document on incident report form as quickly as possible. The closer to the event, the more accurate the recording. (NOTE: This also necessitates that staff readily know where incident forms are kept and which forms to use for patients, visitors, and staff).*

   a Record time of incident, and describe exactly what occurred or was observed, using objective findings and observations (see Table 4-4). Use language that does not allow for subjective interpretation. Do not include personal opinions or feelings. Document the victim's interpretation of incident by using quotes.
   b Objectively describe patient's or staff member's condition when incident was discovered or observed.
   c Describe measures taken by any caregivers at time of incident.
   d Send completed report to designated department.
7 When patient is involved, document events of incident in patient's chart.
   a Do not duplicate all information from incident report.
   b Do not record that incident report was completed.
   c Only enter objective description of what happened.
   d Record any assessment and intervention activities initiated as a result of incident.
8 If patient was injured, implement any ordered therapies and begin routine assessment of body systems influenced by injury.

TABLE 4-4	Examples of Incident Report Entries	
Correct Entry		**Incorrect Entry**
6 PM Patient found on floor at foot of bed; able to respond to name when called. 2-cm abrasion noted across left forehead. Vital signs stable. Dr. Smith notified and arrived on floor at 6:15 PM. Placed patient on fall-prevention protocol.		Patient found on floor at foot of bed, probably fell on way to bathroom. Small abrasion over left forehead. Dr. Smith notified. Patient instructed to use call light when needing to go to bathroom.
Administered morphine sulfate 10 mg Sub-Q in right vastus lateralis at 4 PM for complaints of incisional pain; 6 mg ordered. Monitored vital signs q 15 minutes; called Dr. Jones; vital signs remain stable.		Administered 10 mg morphine sulfate at 4 PM without checking order before administering. 6 mg morphine sulfate ordered.
Needle stick to right index finger; caused minimal bleeding. Notified employee health department.		Needle stick to right index finger, likely due to needle left in bed linen after blood drawing. Notified employee health.

CRITICAL THINKING EXERCISES

You and the nursing assistive personnel (NAP) are caring for a 55-year-old woman with type 2 diabetes who is scheduled for an appendectomy that evening. Elements of her care include monitoring vital signs every 2 hours, pain assessment, preoperative preparation, and glucose monitoring every 4 hours.

1 Noting the four elements of care listed above, list those elements for which documentation may be delegated to NAP.

2 As you correctly noted, preoperative preparation cannot be delegated. Because the NAP will be providing other aspects of care, what information do you need to include in a report to the NAP about pain assessment, glucose monitoring, and preoperative preparation?

3 When you assess the patient's pain, it is important that you record your findings. Select the method of recording used in your agency, and do a sample recording of the pain assessment.

4 The NAP walks the patient to the bathroom and reports to you that the patient stated she "feels dizzy and sweaty" after walking. List your actions in order of priority.

5 The NAP notifies you that the patient did not understand the preoperative teaching that has been completed. What are your actions in order of priority?

REVIEW QUESTIONS

1 Recorded or reported information must be recorded in a timely manner and correctly. The nurse should question which guideline for documentation of information?
   1 Data are recorded immediately after care or treatment.
   2 Record information provided by another nurse.
   3 Begin each new entry with the time.
   4 Draw a single line through an error entry.

2 Military time is frequently used to document care. If oral hygiene was performed at 4:00 PM, what time would it be if documented according to military time?
   1 0400
   2 1400
   3 1600
   4 2400

3 There are multiple types of charting. Which components would be found in focus charting?
   1 Data-Action-Response
   2 Problem-Intervention-Evaluation
   3 Subjective-Objective-Assessment-Plan
   4 Subjective-Evaluation-Assessment-Plan-Implementation-Evaluation

4 There are four purposes for charting by exception. Three of these purposes are to eliminate redundancy, to ensure concise documentation for routine care, and to emphasize abnormal findings. Which statement best explains the fourth purpose?
   1 To identify a change in a patient's condition
   2 To identify a change in a patient's medical orders
   3 To identify trends in clinical care
   4 To identify trends in resource utilization

5 Change-of-shift report is an important component of care. What is the major outcome of an effective exchange of information during this process?
   1 It ensures notification of new physician orders.
   2 It helps to identify any new trends in care.
   3 The patient receives continuity of care based on his or her needs.
   4 The patient's risk status will be stabilized.

REFERENCES

Ammenworth E, Shaw N: Bad health informatics can kill: is evaluation the answer? *Methods Inf Med* 44(1):2, 2005.

Ashish K and others: How common are electronic health records in the United States? A summary of evidence, *Health Affairs* 25(6):496, 2007.

Benson E and others: Improving nursing shift-to-shift report, *J Nurs Care Qual* 22(1):80, 2007.

Birmingham J: Case management: two regulations with coexisting functions, *Prof Case Manag* 12(1):16, 2007.

Blumenthal D, Glaser J: Information technology comes to medicine, *Health Policy Rep* 356(24):2527, 2007.

Bott M and others: Care planning efficiency for nursing facilities, *Nurs Econ* 25(2):85, 2007.

Brandeis G and others: Electronic health record implementation in community homes, *J Am Med Dir Assoc* 8(1):31, 2007.

Burkoski V: Identifying risk: the limitations of incident reporting, *Can Nurse* 103(3):13, 2007.

Carusa JT and others: Making sense of Medicare: a Medicare house call, *Am J Nurs* 104(7):71, 2004.

Chapman L: Discharge planning: a family affair, *Nursing* 37(5):12, 2007.

Coffey R and others: An introduction to critical paths, *Qual Manage Health Care* 14(1):45, 2005.

Dadich KA: Care delivery strategies. In Yoder-Wise PS, editor: *Leading and managing in nursing*, ed 4, St. Louis, 2007, Mosby.

DeBleser L and others: Defining pathways, *J Nurs Manag* 14(7):553, 2006.

DeVore D and others: Preparing for electronic charting, *Nursing Homes: Long Term Care Management* 56(1):29, 2007.

Dochterman J, Bulechek GM: *Nursing Interventions Classification (NIC)*, ed 4, St. Louis, 2004, Mosby.

Dolan B: Medical records: disclosing confidential clinical information, *Psychiatr Bull* 28:53, 2004.

Doran D and others: Evidence in the palm of your hand: development of an outcomes-focused knowledge translation intervention, *Worldviews Evid Based Nurs* 4(2):69, 2007.

Durkin N: Using record review as a quality improvement process, *Home Healthc Nurse* 24(8): 492, 2006.

Gallagher P: Maintain privacy with electronic charting, *Nurs Manage* 35(2):16, 2004.

Guido G: *Legal and ethical issues in nursing*, ed 4, Upper Saddle River, NJ, 2006, Prentice Hall.

Haig K and others: SBAR: a shared mental model for improving communication between clinicians, *J Qual Patient Safety* 32(3):168, 2006.

Health Care Financing Administration: *Long term care facility resident assessment instrument (RAI) user's manual*, Washington, DC, 1998, Health Care Financing Administration.

Healthcare Information and Management Systems society: The electronic health record, http://himss.org/ASP/topics_her.asp, accessed July 21, 2007.

Hebda T and others: *Handbook of informatics for nurses and health care professionals*, ed 3, Upper Saddle River, NJ, 2005, Pearson Prentice Hall.

Iyer PW, Camp NH: *Nursing documentation: a nursing process approach*, ed 4, St. Louis, 2005, Mosby.

McCloskey R: Documentation: challenges and recommendations specific to long-term care, *Can Nurs Home* 17(3):4, 2006.

McGeehan R: Best practice in record keeping, *Nurs Stand* 21(17):51, 2007.

Moody L and others: Electronic health records documentation in nursing, *Comput Nurs* 23(3):334, 2004.

Moorhead S and others: *Nursing outcomes classification (NOC)*, ed 3, St. Louis, 2004, Mosby.

NANDA International: *Nursing diagnoses: definitions and classification 2007-2008*, Philadelphia, 2007, NANDA International.

National Institutes of Health: *Standards for privacy of individually identifiable health information*: the privacy rule—final modification, http://www.cms.hhs.gov/hipaa.

Nelson R: Electronic health records: useful tools or high-tech headache? *Am J Nurs* 107(3):26, 2007.

Smith K and others: Evaluating the impact of computerized clinical documentation, *Comput Nurs* 23(3):132, 2005.

Struk C: The focus on quality: an overview of quality initiatives, *Comput Inform Nurs* 25(4):241, 2007.

Sullivan GH: Legally speaking, does your charting measure up? *RN* 67(3):61, 2004.

Taunton R and others: Care planning for nursing home residents: incorporating the minimum data set requirements into practice, *J Gerontol Nurs* 30(12):40, 2004.

The Joint Commission: *Office of minority health national culturally and linguistically appropriate services (CLAS) standards*, http://www.jointcommission.org, Oakbrook Terrace, Ill, 2006, The Commission, accessed July 2007.

The Joint Commission: *Setting the standard: The Joint Commission and healthcare safety and quality*, http://www.jointcommission.org/PatientSafety, Oakbrook Terrace, Ill, 2007a, The Commission, accessed July 2007.

The Joint Commission: *2008 National patient safety goals hospital program*, http://www.jointcommission.org, Oakbrook Terrace, Ill, 2007b, The Commission, accessed July 2007.

The Joint Commission: *Comprehensive accreditation manual for hospitals* (CAMH), Oakbrook Terrace, Ill, 2008, The Commission.

US Department of Health and Human Services: Standards for privacy of individuals, Health Insurance Portability and Accountability Act of 1996, 64 *Federal Register* 60053 (1999), Identifiable health information, August 2003, http://www.os.dhhs.gov/ocr/hipaa/finalreg.htm.

Walker C and others: Hospital discharge of older adults: how nurse can ease the transition, *Am J Nurs* 107(6):60, 2007.

Walsh S: Formulation of a plan of care for culturally diverse patients, *Int J Nurs Terminol Classif* 15(1):17, 2004.

Wilson MJ: A template for safe and concise handovers, *Medsurg Nurs* 16(3):201, 2007.

RESEARCH REFERENCES

Ballard E: Exploration of nurses' information environment, *Nurse Res* 13(4):50, 2006.

Dillon T and others: Nursing attitudes and images of electronic patient record systems, *Comput Inform Nurs* 23:3, 2005.

Cheevakasemsook A and others: The study of nursing documentation complexities, *Int J Nurs Pract* 12(6):366, 2006.

Foust J: Discharge planning as part of daily nursing practice, *Appl Nurs Res* 20(2):72, 2007.

Lee T: Nurses' perceptions of their documentation experiences in a computerized-nursing care planning system, *J Clin Nurs* 15(110):1376, 2006.

Mahler C and others: Effects of a computer-based nursing documentation system on the quality of nursing documentation, *J Med Syst* 31(4):274, 2007.

Muller-Staub M and others: Improved quality of nursing documentation: results of nursing diagnoses, interventions, and outcomes implementation study, *Int J Nurs Terminol Classif* 18(1):5, 2007.

Thomas C: The benefits of standardized nursing languages in complex adaptive systems such as hospitals, *J Nurs Adm* 36(9):426, 2006.

Vital Signs

KEY TERMS

Afebrile
Antipyretic
Apical pulse
Axillary
Bradycardia
Bradypnea
Core temperature
Diastolic pressure
Dyspnea
Dysrhythmia
Febrile
Fever
Heatstroke
Hypertension
Hyperthermia
Hypotension
Hypothermia
Orthopnea
Orthostatic
  hypotension

Oximetry
Oxygen saturation
Postural
  hypotension
Premature
  ventricular
  contraction (PVC)
Pulse deficit
Pyrexia
S_1
S_2
Sphygmo-
  manometer
Systolic pressure
Tachycardia
Tachypnea
Thermoregulation
Tympanic
Vasoconstriction
Vasodilation

SKILLS AND PROCEDURES

MEDIA RESOURCES

- **evolve** http://evolve.elsevier.com/Perry/skills
  - Review Questions
  - Video Clips

- Mosby's Nursing Video Skills, 3.0

- NSO Nursing Skills Online

OBJECTIVES

Mastery of content in this chapter will enable the nurse to:

- Identify when it is appropriate to assess each vital sign.
- Accurately assess a patient's oral, rectal, axillary, tympanic membrane, and temporal artery temperatures.
- Correctly record vital signs.
- Describe factors that cause variations in body temperature, pulse, blood pressure, oxygen saturation, and respirations.
- Discuss factors in selecting temperature measurement sites.
- Accurately assess a patient's radial and apical pulses.
- Explain implications of a pulse deficit.
- Accurately assess a patient's respirations.
- Accurately measure a patient's blood pressure using techniques of auscultation and palpation.
- Discuss benefits and disadvantages of using an automatic blood pressure machine.
- Describe factors in selecting an extremity to measure blood pressure.
- Accurately assess a patient's oxygenation status using pulse oximetry.
- Identify ranges of acceptable vital sign values for infant, child, and adult.
- Appropriately delegate vital sign measurements to nursing assistive personnel.

Temperature, pulse, blood pressure (BP), oxygen saturation, and respiration are the most frequent measurements obtained by health care practitioners. These measurements indicate if the circulatory, pulmonary, neurological, and endocrine body systems are functioning normally. Because of their importance as indicators of the body's physiological status and response to physical, environmental, and psychological stressors, they are referred to as vital signs. Vital signs reveal sudden changes in a patient's condition, as well as changes that occur progressively over time. Any difference between a patient's normal baseline measurement and present vital signs may indicate the need for nursing therapies and necessary medical interventions.

Pain, a subjective symptom, is often referred to as a vital sign along with the physiological signs. Very few patients do not experience some level of discomfort or pain. Frequently pain is the symptom that leads patients to seek health care. For this reason, assessment of a patient's pain status is critical to understanding a patient's clinical status and progress. You will frequently perform assessment of a patient's level of comfort and pain with vital sign measurements. Chapter 15 summarizes pain assessment.

Vital signs are included in a routine physical assessment (see Chapter 6). The nurse's findings aid in determining whether it is necessary to assess specific body systems more thoroughly. For example, during a routine vital sign measurement, the nurse notes an abnormal respiratory rate; the nurse then auscultates lung sounds. Measurement of a single vital sign assesses a specific aspect of a patient's condition. For example, following administration of an antipyretic medication, the nurse measures the patient's temperature to evaluate the drug's effects. Part of the nurse's clinical judgment involves deciding which vital sign to measure, when to obtain measurements, and the frequency of assessment (Box 5-1). Always obtain a baseline measurement of vital signs upon first contact with a patient to provide a means for comparison with later vital sign measurements.

EVIDENCE-BASED PRACTICE TRENDS

Numerous devices are available to measure temperature, although the most convenient and easiest devices to use are not always the most accurate. Oral, tympanic membrane, and temporal artery are the most commonly used thermometers. A recent study compared these common devices against the pulmonary artery thermometer, the gold standard of core temperature (Lawson and others, 2007). Findings indicated that both the oral and temporal artery temperatures were similar to the core pulmonary artery. The tympanic membrane temperature was less accurate. A similar study by Farnell and others (2005) found that the tympanic thermometer was highly variable, as much as 1° C. When treatment decisions are involved, repeat measurements with an oral or temporal artery thermometer are needed to confirm temperature measurements made with a tympanic membrane thermometer.

Pulse oximetry measurements change patient care and outcomes (Lockwood and others, 2004). Many factors influence readings when using finger oximetry probes to obtain oxygen saturation as measured by pulse oximetry (SpO_2). The influence of nail polish is controversial. A recent study tested 10 nail polish colors on healthy volunteers and found no clinically significant difference in oxygen saturation measurement. A new oximeter sensor, attached to the forehead, eliminates the need for nail polish remover. You can use the forehead sensor in patients who have poor peripheral perfusion. When compared to the gold standard of the arterial blood gas level, the forehead sensor was more accurate than the finger probe (Schallom and others, 2007).

CULTURAL CONSIDERATIONS

- Provide privacy when performing apical pulse assessment, especially for traditional female patients and elders from Asian, Middle Eastern, Hispanic, and African cultures.
  - Use gender-congruent providers or family members to take rectal temperatures and touch the patient's chest.
  - Procedures that are normally noninvasive sometimes produce anxiety because of cultural variables of touch, privacy, and gender.
- Consult the health care provider and family decision maker regarding giving information to the patient about abnormal vital signs.

BOX 5-1	When to Take Vital Signs

1. On a patient's admission to a health care facility
2. In a hospital or care facility on a routine schedule according to a health care provider's order or institution's standards of practice
3. When assessing the patient during home care visits
4. Before, during, and after a surgical or invasive diagnostic procedure
5. Before and after the administration of medications or application of therapies that affect cardiovascular, respiratory, or temperature control functions
6. Before, during, and after a transfusion of blood products
7. Before, during, and after nursing interventions influencing a vital sign (e.g., before and after a patient previously on bed rest ambulates, before and after the patient performs range-of-motion exercises)
8. When the patient reports specific symptoms of physical distress (e.g., feeling "funny" or "different")
9. When the patient's general physical condition changes (e.g., loss of consciousness, increased intensity of pain)

- Collectivistic cultures (e.g., Hispanics, Africans, and Asians) demonstrate their caring for ill members by protecting them from bad news about their health and well-being.
- Document this information in the patient's chart.
- Communicate the family decision to the health care provider.
- Determine that the patient understands how you will measure vital signs.
- Use an interpreter if needed, and demonstrate the procedure to promote the patient's understanding.

Skill Performance Guidelines

1 The nurse caring for the patient is responsible for vital signs measurement. The skill of measurement of selected vital signs (i.e., stable patients) can be delegated to nursing assistive personnel (NAP). However, nurses must analyze vital signs to interpret their significance and make decisions about appropriate interventions.

2 Equipment must be functional and appropriate for the patient's size, age, condition, and characteristics.

3 The nurse knows the patient's usual range of vital signs. A patient's usual values may differ from the acceptable range for that age or physical state. A patient's usual values serve as a baseline for comparison with later findings; thus you detect changes in condition over time.

4 The nurse knows the patient's medical history, therapies, and prescribed medications. Some illnesses or treatments cause predictable vital sign changes. Most medications affect at least one of the vital signs.

5 The nurse controls or minimizes environmental factors that affect vital signs. For example, assessing the patient's temperature

in a warm, humid room may yield a value that is not a true indicator of the patient's condition.

6 An organized, systematic (step-by-step) approach when taking vital signs ensures accuracy of findings.

7 Based on the patient's condition, collaborate with the health care provider to decide the minimum frequency of vital sign assessment. In the hospital, the health care provider will order a minimum frequency of vital sign measurements for each patient. Following surgery or treatment intervention, measure vital signs more frequently to detect complications. In a clinic or outpatient setting, take vital signs before the health care provider examines the patient and after any invasive procedures. As a patient's physical condition worsens, it is important to monitor the vital signs as often as every 5 to 15 minutes. The nurse is responsible for judging whether more frequent assessments are necessary.

8 Analyze the results of vital sign measurements, and incorporate all the clinical findings about a patient in determining nursing diagnoses. You do not interpret vital signs in isolation. You need to know related physical signs or symptoms and be aware of the patient's ongoing health status.

9 Verify and communicate significant changes in vital signs. Document vital signs and communicate to the nurse assuming care of the patient. Baseline measurements allow a nurse to identify changes in vital signs. When vital signs appear abnormal, it helps to have another nurse repeat the measurement. Inform the health care provider when vital signs become abnormal, and report any changes to the nurse in charge.

SKILL 5-1   Measuring Body Temperature

 Basic Skills / Vital Signs / Taking a Temperature With an Electronic Thermometer; Taking a Temperature With a Tympanic Thermometer

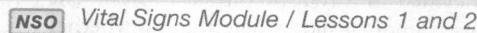 **NSO** *Vital Signs Module / Lessons 1 and 2*

Body temperature is the difference between the amount of heat produced by body processes and the amount of heat lost to the external environment. The core temperature, or temperature of the deep body tissues, is under control of the hypothalamus and remains within a narrow range. Skin or body surface temperature rises and falls as the temperature of the surrounding environment changes, and it fluctuates dramatically.

The body tissues and cells function best within a relatively narrow temperature range, from 36° to 38° C (96.8° to 100.4° F), but no single temperature is normal for all people. For healthy young adults the average oral temperature is 37° C (98.6° F). In clinical practice, nurses learn the temperature range of individual patients. No single temperature is normal for all people. An acceptable temperature range for adults depends on age, gender, range of physical activity, hydration status, and state of health (Fig. 5-1).

Many factors affect body temperature. Physiological and behavioral control mechanisms act to maintain a constant core temperature. For example, the mechanism of peripheral vasodilation increases blood flow to the skin, which increases the amount of heat radiated to the environment. Control mechanisms have failed when heat produced by the body is not equal to heat lost to the environment. For example, patients without sweat gland function are unable to tolerate warm temperatures because they cannot adequately cool themselves. Fever occurs when heat loss mechanisms are unable to keep pace with excess heat production, resulting in

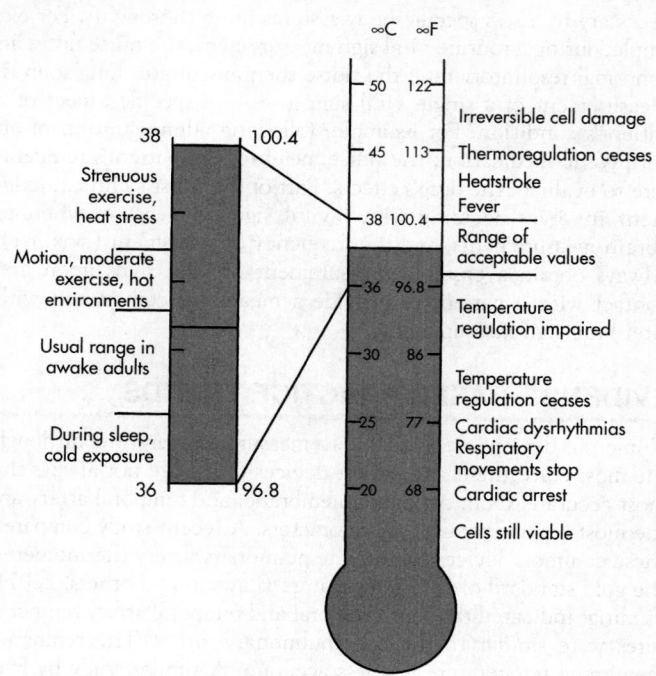

FIG 5-1   Ranges of normal temperature values and physiological consequences of abnormal body temperature. (*Modified from Thibodeau GA, Patton KT: Anatomy and physiology, ed 6, St. Louis, 2006, Mosby.*)

an abnormal rise in body temperature. When an individual has a febrile condition, pyrexia, initiate temperature-control measures such as controlling environmental temperatures, removing external coverings, and administering ordered antipyretics to achieve better temperature control.

The purpose of measuring body temperature is to obtain a representative average temperature of core body tissues. Average usual temperature varies depending on the measurement site used. Research findings from numerous studies are contradictory; however, it is generally accepted that rectal temperatures are usually 0.5° C (0.9° F) higher than oral temperatures. Axillary and tympanic temperatures are usually 0.5° C (0.9° F) lower than oral temperatures. Sites reflecting core temperature are more reliable indicators of body temperature than sites reflecting surface temperatures (Box 5-2).

To ensure accurate temperature readings you need to measure each site correctly. Use the same site when repeated measurements are necessary or when comparing temperature measurements over time. Each site has advantages and disadvantages (Box 5-3). You need to determine the safest and most accurate site for the patient.

Two types of thermometers are commonly available to measure body temperature: electronic and disposable. A third type, mercury-in-glass thermometer, was once the standard device found in the clinical setting. However, most municipalities have prohibited the sale or use of mercury-containing medical devices because of the potential hazards. However, mercury-in-glass thermometers are sometimes found in patients' homes.

The electronic thermometer consists of a rechargeable, battery-powered display unit, a thin wire cord, and a temperature-processing probe covered by a disposable probe cover (Fig. 5-2). Separate probes are available for oral (blue tip probe) and rectal (red tip probe) use. You can also use the oral probe for axillary temperature measurement. Electronic thermometers provide two modes of operation: a 4-second predictive temperature and a 3-minute standard temperature. In day-to-day clinical situations, the 4-second predictive is most common.

Two other types of electronic thermometers are available. The tympanic membrane thermometer consists of an otoscope-like speculum with an infrared sensor tip that detects heat radiated from the tympanic membrane of the ear (Fig. 5-3). Within seconds after the thermometer is placed in the auditory canal and the scan button is pressed, a sound signals when the peak temperature has been measured and a reading appears on the display unit. The temporal artery thermometer measures blood flow through the superficial temporal artery. You sweep a handheld scanner with an infrared sensor across the forehead and just behind the ear (Fig. 5-4). After scanning is complete, a reading appears on the display unit.

Single-use or reusable chemical dot thermometers are thin strips of plastic with a temperature sensor at one end. The sensor consists of a matrix of chemically impregnated dots that change color at different temperatures, usually within 60 seconds. In the Celsius version, there are 50 dots, each representing temperature increments of 0.1° C over a range of 35.5° to 40.4° C. The Fahrenheit version has 45 dots with increments of 0.2° F and a range of 96.0° to 104.8° F. Most chemical dot thermometers are for single use (Fig. 5-5). In one brand that is reusable for a single patient, the chemical dots return to the original color within a few seconds. The chemical dot thermometers are most commonly used for oral temperatures. You can also use them for axillary or rectal measurements, the latter covered by a plastic sheath, with a placement time of 3 minutes. Chemical dot thermometers are useful for screening temperatures or when caring for a patient on protective isolation. Use electronic thermometers to confirm measurements made with chemical dot thermometers when treatment decisions are indicated.

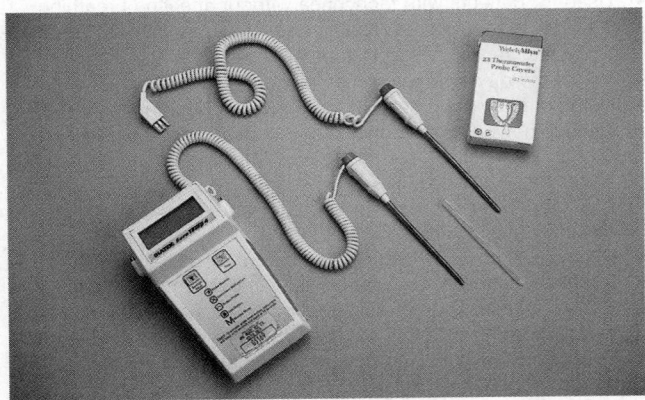

FIG 5-2   Electronic thermometer with disposable plastic sheath.

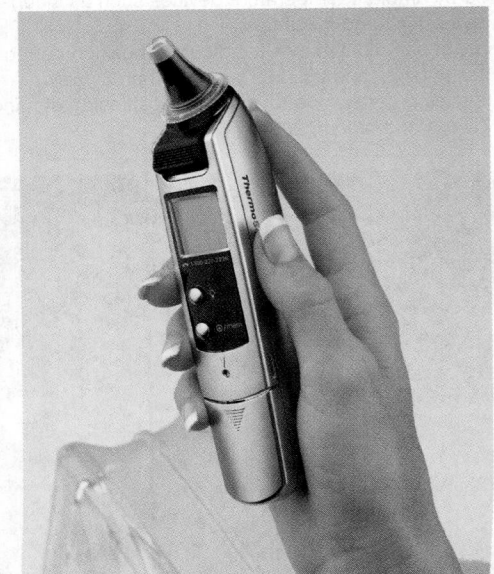

FIG 5-3   Tympanic membrane thermometer. (*Photo courtesy Welch Allyn.*)

BOX 5-2	Core and Surface Temperature Measurement Sites

Core Site	Surface Site
• Rectum	• Skin
• Tympanic membrane	• Oral cavity
• Temporal artery	• Axilla
• Esophagus	
• Pulmonary artery	
• Urinary bladder	

BOX 5-3 | Advantages and Limitations of Select Temperature Measurement Sites

Oral

Advantages

- Easily accessible—requires no position change
- Comfortable for patient
- Provides accurate surface temperature reading
- Reflects rapid change in core temperature
- Shown to be reliable route to measure temperature in intubated patients

Limitations

- Causes delay in measurement if patient recently ingested hot/cold fluids or foods or smoked.
- Should not be used with patients who have had oral surgery, trauma, history of epilepsy, or shaking chills
- Should not be used with infants, small children, or confused, unconscious, or uncooperative patients
- Risk for body fluid exposure

Tympanic Membrane Sensor

Advantages

- Easily accessible site
- Minimal patient repositioning required; can be obtained without disturbing, waking, or repositioning the patient
- Used for patients with tachypnea without affecting breathing
- Provides accurate core reading because eardrum close to hypothalamus; sensitive to core temperature changes
- Very rapid measurement (2 to 5 seconds)
- Unaffected by oral intake of food or fluids or smoking
- Used in newborns to reduce infant handling and heat loss

Limitations

- More variability of measurement than with other core temperature devices (Lawson and others, 2007)
- Requires removal of hearing aids before measurement
- Requires disposable sensor cover with only one size available
- Otitis media and cerumen impaction can distort readings (Lockwood and others, 2004)
- Should not be used with patients who have had surgery of the ear or tympanic membrane
- Does not accurately measure core temperature changes during and after exercise
- Cannot obtain continuous measurement
- Affected by ambient temperature devices such as incubators, radiant warmers, and facial fans
- Anatomy of ear canal makes it difficult to position correctly in neonates, infants, and children younger than 3 years
- Inaccuracies reported due to incorrect positioning of handheld unit (Maxton and others, 2004)

Rectal

Advantages

- Argued to be more reliable when oral temperature cannot be obtained

Limitations

- Lags behind core temperature during rapid temperature changes (Maxton and others, 2004)
- Not for patients with diarrhea, patients who have had rectal surgery, rectal disorders, bleeding
- Requires positioning and is often source of patient embarrassment and anxiety
- Risk for body fluid exposure
- Requires lubrication
- Not for routine vital signs in newborns
- Impacted stool influences readings (Maxton and others, 2004)

Axilla

Advantages

- Safe and inexpensive
- Used with newborns and unconscious patients

Limitations

- Long measurement time
- Requires continuous positioning by nurse
- Measurement lags behind core temperature during rapid temperature changes
- Not recommended for detecting fever in infants and young children
- Requires exposure of thorax, which can result in temperature loss, especially in newborns
- Affected by exposure to the environment, including time to place thermometer (Maxton and others, 2004)
- Underestimates core temperature (Lawson and others, 2007)

Skin

Advantages

- Inexpensive
- Provides continuous reading
- Safe and noninvasive
- Used for neonates

Limitations

- Measurement lags behind other sites during temperature changes, especially during hyperthermia
- Diaphoresis or sweat can impair adhesion
- Affected by environmental temperature
- Cannot be used for patients with allergy to adhesive

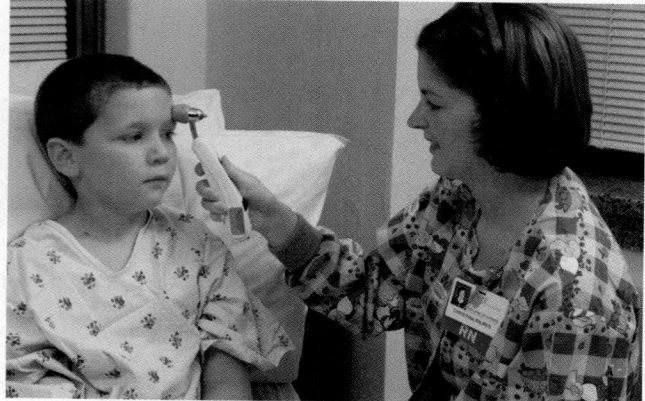

FIG 5-4 A temporal artery thermometer measures blood flow through the superficial temporal artery.

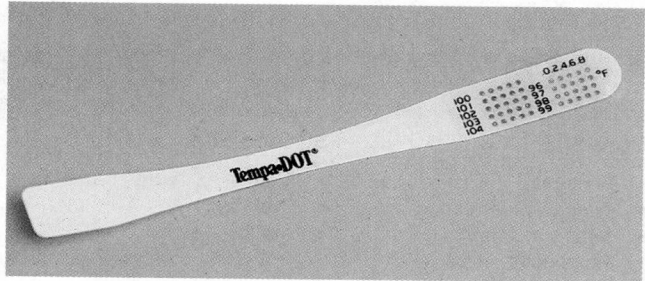

FIG 5-5 Disposable, single-use thermometer.

Delegation Considerations

You can delegate the skill of temperature measurement to nursing assistive personnel (NAP). The nurse directs the NAP to:

- Select appropriate route and device to measure temperature.
- Take appropriate precautions for patients who have difficulty positioning properly for rectal temperature measurement.
- Consider specific patient-related factors that falsely raise or lower temperature.
- Obtain temperature measurement for the patient with ordered frequency.
- Be aware of the usual values for the patient.
- Report any abnormalities to the nurse.

Equipment

- ☐ Appropriate thermometer
- ☐ Soft tissue or wipe
- ☐ Alcohol swab
- ☐ Water-soluble lubricant (for rectal measurements only)
- ☐ Pen, pencil, vital sign flow sheet or record form
- ☐ Clean gloves, plastic thermometer sleeve, disposable probe or sensor cover

STEP	RATIONALE

ASSESSMENT

1 Determine need to measure patient's body temperature:

a Note patient's risks for temperature alterations:
- Expected or diagnosed infection
- Open wounds or burns
- White blood cell count below 5000/mm^3 or above 12,000/mm^3
- Immunosuppressive drug therapy
- Injury to hypothalamus
- Exposure to temperature extremes
- Blood product infusion
- Hypothermia or hyperthermia therapy
- Postoperative status

Certain conditions place patients at risk for temperature alterations and require more frequent temperature measurement and nursing assessment.

b Assess for signs and symptoms that accompany temperature alteration:
- *Hyperthermia:* Decreased skin turgor, dry mucous membranes; tachycardia; hypotension; decreased venous filling; concentrated urine
- *Heatstroke:* Hot, dry skin; tachycardia; hypotension; excessive thirst; muscle cramps; visual disturbances; confusion or delirium
- *Hypothermia:* Pale skin; skin cool or cold to touch; bradycardia and dysrhythmias; uncontrollable shivering; reduced level of consciousness; shallow respirations

Physical signs and symptoms alert nurse to alteration in body temperature.

c Assess for factors that normally influence temperature:

Allows nurse to accurately assess for presence and significance of temperature alteration.

(1) Age

Older adults have a narrower range of temperature than younger adults.

Critical Decision Point *No single temperature is normal for all people. A temperature within an acceptable range in an adult may reflect a fever in an older adult. Undeveloped temperature control mechanisms in infants and children cause temperature to rise and fall rapidly.*

(2) Exercise

Muscle activity raises heat production.

(3) Hormones

Women have wider temperature fluctuations than men because of menstrual cycle hormonal changes; body temperature varies during menopause.

(4) Stress

Stress elevates temperature.

(5) Environmental temperature

Infants and older adults are more sensitive to environmental temperature changes.

(6) Medications

Some drugs impair or promote sweating, vasoconstriction, vasodilation, or interfere with the ability of the hypothalamus to regulate temperature.

(7) Daily fluctuations

Body temperature normally changes 0.5° to 1° C (0.9 to 1.8° F) during a 24-hour period. Temperature is lowest during early morning. Most patients have maximum temperature elevation between 5 PM and 7 PM; temperature falls gradually during night.

STEP	RATIONALE
2 Determine appropriate measurement site and device for patient (see Box 5-3). Use disposable thermometer for patient on isolation precautions.	Determines if patient's status contraindicates selection of a specific method or site.
3 Determine previous baseline temperature and measurement site (if available) from patient's record.	Allows nurse to assess for change in condition. Provides comparison with future temperature measurements.

NURSING DIAGNOSES

- Hyperthermia
- Hypothermia
- Ineffective thermoregulation
- Risk for imbalanced body temperature

Individualize related factors based on patient's condition or needs.

PLANNING

1 Expected outcomes following completion of procedure: • Body temperature is within acceptable range for patient's age-group.	Thermoregulation is maintained.
• Body temperature returns to baseline range following therapies for abnormal temperature.	Nurse controls for environmental factors that alter temperature.
2 Explain to patient the way you will measure temperature and importance of maintaining proper position until reading is complete. Verify that patient has not had anything to eat or drink and not has chewed gum or smoked within the past 15 minutes of having oral temperature measured.	Promotes patient cooperation and increases compliance. Patients are often curious about their temperatures and should be cautioned against prematurely removing the thermometer to read results. Oral food and fluids, smoking, and gum can alter temperature measurement.

IMPLEMENTATION

1 Perform hand hygiene.	Reduces transmission of microorganisms.
2 Assist patient to comfortable position that provides easy access to temperature measurement site.	Ensures both patient's comfort and accuracy of temperature reading.
3 Obtain temperature reading.	
a Obtain oral temperature measurement with electronic thermometer:	
(1) Apply clean gloves (*optional*).	Use of an oral probe cover, which can be removed without physical contact, minimizes need to wear gloves.
(2) Remove thermometer pack from charging unit. Attach oral thermometer probe stem (blue tip) to thermometer unit. Grasp top of the probe stem, being careful not to apply pressure on the ejection button.	Charging provides battery power. Ejection button releases plastic cover from probe stem.
(3) Slide disposable plastic probe cover over thermometer probe stem until cover locks in place (see illustration).	Soft plastic cover will not break in patient's mouth and prevents transmission of microorganisms between patients.

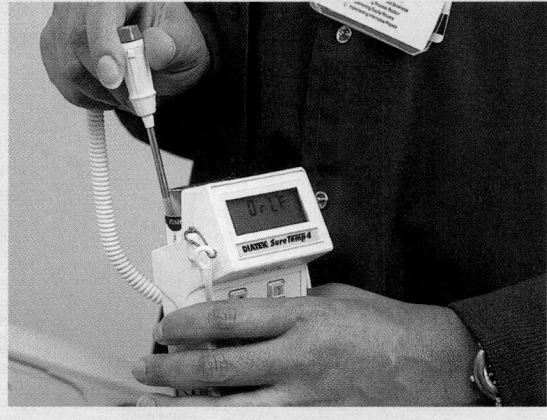

STEP 3a(3) Nurse inserts electronic thermometer probe stem into probe cover. Cover snaps in place.

STEP	RATIONALE

(4)   Ask patient to open mouth; then gently place thermometer probe under tongue in posterior sublingual pocket lateral to center of lower jaw (see illustration).

Heat from superficial blood vessels in sublingual pocket produces temperature reading. With electronic thermometer, temperatures in right and left posterior sublingual pocket are significantly higher than in area under front of tongue.

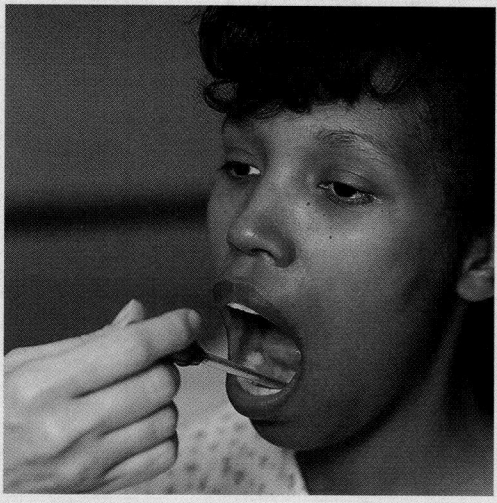

STEP 3a(4)   Probe under tongue in posterior sublingual pocket.

(5)   Ask patient to hold thermometer probe with lips closed.

Maintains proper position of thermometer during recording.

(6)   Leave thermometer probe in place until audible signal indicates completion and patient's temperature appears on digital display; remove thermometer probe from under patient's tongue.

Probe must stay in place until signal occurs to ensure accurate reading.

(7)   Push ejection button on thermometer probe stem to discard plastic probe cover into an appropriate receptacle.

Reduces transmission of microorganisms.

(8)   Return thermometer probe stem to storage holder of thermometer unit.

Protects probe stem from damage. Returning thermometer probe stem automatically causes digital reading to disappear.

(9)   If wearing gloves, remove and dispose in appropriate receptacle.

Reduces transmission of microorganisms.

(10)   Perform hand hygiene.

Reduces transmission of microorganisms.

(11)   Return thermometer to charger.

Maintains battery charge of thermometer unit.

b   Obtain rectal temperature measurement with electronic thermometer:

(1)   Draw curtain around bed and/or close room door. Assist patient to side-lying Sims' position with upper leg flexed. Move aside bed linen to expose only anal area. Keep patient's upper body and lower extremities covered with sheet or blanket.

Maintains patient's privacy, minimizes embarrassment, and promotes comfort.

(2)   Apply clean gloves.

Maintains standard precautions when exposed to items soiled with body fluid.

(3)   Remove thermometer pack from charging unit. Attach rectal thermometer probe stem (red tip) to thermometer unit. Grasp top of probe stem, being careful not to apply pressure on the ejection button.

Ejection button releases plastic cover from probe stem.

(4)   Slide disposable plastic probe cover over thermometer probe stem until cover locks in place.

Soft plastic probe cover prevents transmission of microorganisms between patients.

(5)   Squeeze liberal portion of lubricant on tissue. Dip thermometer's blunt end into lubricant, covering 2.5 to 3.5 cm (1 to 1½ inches) for adult.

Lubrication minimizes trauma to rectal mucosa during insertion. Tissue avoids contamination of remaining lubricant in the container.

STEP	RATIONALE

(6) With nondominant hand, separate patient's buttocks to expose anus. Ask patient to breathe slowly and relax.

Fully exposes anus for thermometer insertion. Relaxes anal sphincter for easier thermometer insertion.

(7) Gently insert thermometer into anus in direction of umbilicus 3.5 cm (1½ inches) for adult. Do not force thermometer.

Ensures adequate exposure against blood vessels in rectal wall.

(8) If you feel resistance during insertion, withdraw immediately. Never force thermometer.

Prevents trauma to mucosa.

Critical Decision Point   *If you cannot adequately insert thermometer into rectum or resistance is felt during insertion, remove thermometer and consider alternative method for obtaining temperature.*

(9) Once thermometer probe is positioned, hold it in place until audible signal indicates completion and patient's temperature appears on digital display; remove thermometer probe from anus (see illustration).

Probe must stay in place until signal occurs to ensure accurate reading.

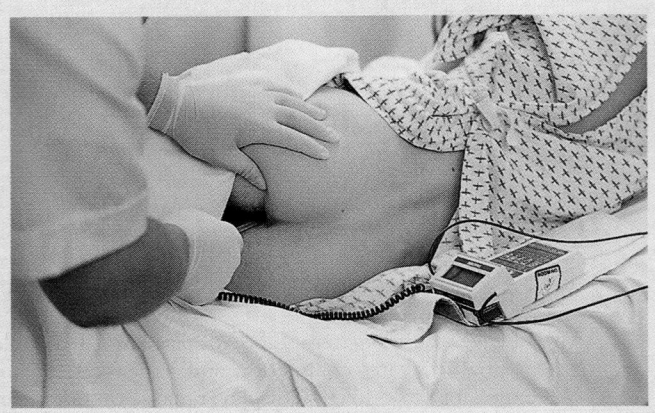

STEP 3b(9)   Probe removed smoothly from anus.

(10) Push ejection button on thermometer stem to discard plastic probe cover into an appropriate receptacle. Wipe probe stem with alcohol swab, paying particular attention to ridges where probe stem connects to probe.

Reduces transmission of microorganisms.

(11) Return thermometer stem to storage position of recording unit.

Protects probe stem from damage. Returning thermometer stem automatically causes digital reading to disappear.

(12) Wipe patient's anal area with soft tissue to remove lubricant or feces, and discard tissue. Assist patient in assuming a comfortable position.

Provides for comfort and hygiene.

(13) Remove and dispose of gloves in appropriate receptacle. Perform hand hygiene.

Reduces transmission of microorganisms.

(14) Return thermometer to charger.

Maintains battery charge of thermometer unit.

c Obtain axillary temperature measurement with electronic thermometer:

(1) Draw curtain around bed and/or close room door. Assist patient to supine or sitting position. Move clothing or gown away from shoulder and arm.

Maintains patient's privacy, minimizes embarrassment, and promotes comfort. Exposes axilla for correct thermometer probe placement.

(2) Remove thermometer pack from charging unit. Attach oral thermometer probe stem (blue tip) to thermometer unit. Grasp top of thermometer probe stem, being careful not to apply pressure on the ejection button.

Charging provides battery power. Ejection button releases plastic cover from probe stem.

STEP	RATIONALE
(3) Slide disposable plastic probe cover over thermometer stem until cover locks in place.	Soft plastic probe cover prevents transmission of microorganisms between patients.
(4) Raise patient's arm away from torso. Inspect for skin lesions and excessive perspiration; if needed, dry axilla. Insert thermometer probe into center of axilla, lower arm over probe, and place arm across patient's chest.	Maintains proper position of thermometer against blood vessels in axilla.

Critical Decision Point   *Do not use axilla if skin lesions are present because local temperature is sometimes altered and area may be painful to touch.*

STEP	RATIONALE
(5) Once thermometer probe is positioned, hold it in place until audible signal indicates completion and patient's temperature appears on digital display; remove thermometer probe from axilla.	Thermometer probe must stay in place until signal occurs to ensure accurate reading.
(6) Push ejection button on thermometer stem to discard plastic probe cover into appropriate receptacle.	Reduces transmission of microorganisms.
(7) Return thermometer stem to storage position of recording unit.	Returning thermometer stem to storage position automatically causes digital reading to disappear. Protects stem from damage.
(8) Assist patient in assuming a comfortable position, replacing linen or gown.	Restores comfort and sense of well-being.
(9) Perform hand hygiene.	Reduces transmission of microorganisms.
(10) Return thermometer to charger.	Maintains battery charge of thermometer unit.
d Obtain tympanic membrane temperature with infrared thermometer:	
(1) Assist patient in assuming comfortable position with head turned toward side, away from nurse. If patient has been lying on one side, use upper ear. If you are right-handed, obtain temperature from patient's right ear. If you are left-handed, obtain temperature from patient's left ear.	Ensures comfort and facilitates exposure of auditory canal for accurate temperature measurement. Heat trapped in ear facing down will cause false high temperature reading The less acute the angle of approach, the better the probe seal.
(2) Note if there is an obvious presence of cerumen (earwax) in the patient's ear canal.	Cerumen impedes the lens cover of speculum. Switch to other ear, or select alternative measurement site.
(3) Remove thermometer handheld unit from charging base, being careful not to apply pressure to the ejection button.	Charging base provides battery power. Removal of handheld unit from base prepares it to measure temperature. Ejection button releases plastic probe cover from thermometer tip.
(4) Slide disposable speculum cover over the otoscope-like lens tip until it locks in place. Be careful not to touch lens cover.	Soft plastic probe cover prevents transmission of microorganisms between patients. Lens cover should not have dust, fingerprints, or cerumen obstructing optical pathway.
(5) Insert speculum into ear canal following manufacturer's instructions for tympanic probe positioning:	Correct positioning of probe with respect to ear canal allows maximum exposure of tympanic membrane.
(a) Pull ear pinna backward, up, and out for an adult. For children less than 3 years of age, pull pinna down and back, point covered probe toward midpoint between eyebrow and sideburns (see illustration).	The ear tug straightens the external auditory canal, allowing maximum exposure of tympanic membrane. Some manufacturers recommend movement of speculum tip in a figure-eight pattern that allows sensor to detect maximum tympanic membrane heat radiation. Gentle pressure seals ear canal from ambient air temperature, which alters readings as much as 2.8° C or 5° F.

STEP	RATIONALE

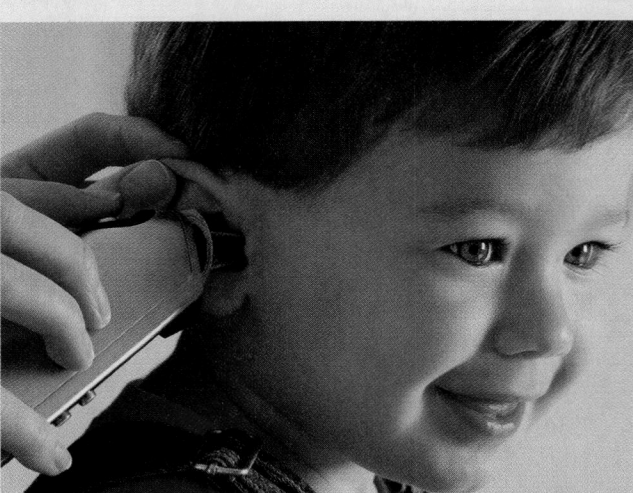

STEP 3d(5)(a)   Tympanic membrane thermometer with probe cover placed in child's ear. *(Photo courtesy Welch Allyn.)*

    (b)   Move thermometer in a figure-eight pattern.
    (c)   Fit speculum tip snug in canal, pointing toward the nose.

   (6)   Once positioned, press scan button on handheld unit. Leave speculum in place until audible signal indicates completion and patient's temperature appears on digital display.

Pressing scan button causes detection of infrared energy. The speculum tip must stay in place until signal occurs to ensure accurate reading.

   (7)   Carefully remove speculum from auditory meatus. Push ejection button on handheld unit to discard speculum cover into appropriate receptacle.

Reduces transmission of microorganisms. Automatically causes digital reading to disappear.

   (8)   If temperature is abnormal or second reading is necessary, replace probe cover, and wait 2 to 3 minutes before repeating in same ear or repeat measurement in other ear. Consider an alternative site or instrument.

Lens cover must be free of cerumen to maintain optical path. Time allows ear canal to regain usual temperature.

   (9)   Return handheld unit to thermometer base.
  (10) Assist patient in assuming a comfortable position.
  (11) Perform hand hygiene.
 4 Inform patient of temperature reading, and record measurement.

Protects sensor tip from damage.
Restores comfort and sense of well-being.
Reduces transmission of microorganisms.
Promotes participation in care and understanding of health status.

EVALUATION

1 If you are assessing temperature for the first time, establish temperature as baseline if it is within acceptable range.

Used to compare future temperature measurements.

2 Compare temperature reading with patient's previous baseline and acceptable temperature range for patient's age-group.

Body temperature fluctuates within narrow range; comparison reveals presence of abnormality. Improper placement or movement of thermometer can cause inaccuracies. Second measurement confirms initial findings of abnormal body temperature.

3 If patient has fever, take temperature approximately 30 minutes after administering antipyretics, and every 4 hours until temperature stabilizes.

Will determine if temperature begins to fall in response to therapy.

Unexpected Outcomes

1 Temperature is 1° C or more above usual range.

2 Temperature is 1° C or more below usual range.

3 No temperature obtained.

Related Interventions

- Initiate measures to lower body temperature:
  - Cool room environment.
  - Reduce external covering on patient's body to promote heat loss, but do not induce shivering.
  - Keep clothing and bed linen dry.
  - Apply hypothermia blanket as ordered (see Chapter 40).
  - Limit physical activity and sources of emotional stress.
  - Administer antipyretics as ordered.
  - Increase fluid intake to at least 3 L daily (unless contraindicated).
  - Initiate measures to stimulate appetite, and provide nutrients to meet increased energy needs.
  - Prevent or control spread of infection.
  - Provide wound care (see Chapter 38).
  - Perform pulmonary hygiene (see Chapter 24).
  - Promote adequate urinary elimination (see Chapter 33).

- Initiate measures to raise body temperature:
  - Apply warm blankets, and unless contraindicated offer warm liquids.
  - Apply hyperthermia blankets if ordered (see Chapter 40).
  - Remove wet clothing or linen.

- Reassess correct placement of temperature probe or sensor.
- Choose alternative temperature measurement site.
- Obtain alternative temperature measurement device.

Recording and Reporting

- Record temperature and route on vital sign flow sheet (Fig. 5-6, p. 76) or record form.
- Document measurement of temperature after administration of specific therapies in narrative form in nurses' notes.
- Report abnormal findings to nurse in charge or health care provider.

Teaching Considerations

- Identify patient's ability to initiate preventive health measures and recognize alteration in body temperature. Educate patients and family members about measures to prevent body temperature alterations.
- Educate patients about risk factors for hypothermia and frostbite: fatigue; malnutrition; hypoxemia; cold, wet clothing; alcohol intoxication.
- Educate patients about risk factors for heatstroke: strenuous exercise in hot, humid weather; tight-fitting clothing in hot environments; exercising in poorly ventilated areas; sudden exposures to hot climates; poor fluid intake before, during, and after exercise.
- Educate patients regarding the importance of taking and continuing antibiotics as directed until course of treatment for infection is completed.

Pediatric Considerations

- Infants and young children may lose more heat to the environment because of their increased body surface area/volume ratios. Neonates and infants less than 6 months old may suffer from cold stress that goes undetected and places greater oxygen demands on the infant in an attempt to regulate the infant's temperature.
- Critically ill children sometimes have cool skin but a high core temperature because of poor perfusion to the skin.
- Use axillary temperatures for screening purposes only, not to detect fevers in infants and young children. Use lower axilla to record temperature in side-lying infants.

- Children may assume prone position for rectal temperature measurement.
- With children who cry or become restless, it is best to take temperature as the last vital sign.

Gerontological Considerations

- The temperature of older adults is at the lower end of the acceptable temperature range: 36° C (96.8° F).
- Temperatures considered within normal range often reflect a fever in an older adult.
- Adults without teeth or older adults with poor muscle control may be unable to close their mouth tightly enough to obtain accurate oral temperature readings.
- Older adults are very sensitive to environmental temperature changes because their thermoregulatory systems are not as efficient (Ebersole and others, 2008).
- With aging, cerumen tends to be drier and cilia become stiff, contributing to buildup of cerumen impaction, which interferes with accurate tympanic temperature measurement.
- A decrease in sweat gland reactivity in the older adult results in a higher threshold for sweating at high temperatures, which can lead to hyperthermia.
- With aging, a loss of subcutaneous fat reduces the insulating capacity of the skin.
- Older adults are at high risk for hypothermia because of diminished sensation to cold, abnormal vasoconstrictor responses, and impaired shivering.

Home Care Considerations

- Assess temperature and ventilation of patient's environment to determine existence of any environmental conditions that influence patient's temperature.
- In the home, some patients continue to use mercury-in-glass thermometers. Assess safe storage of mercury-in-glass thermometers to protect from breakage and mercury spills. Educate patient and caregiver on proper use of the thermometer, mercury hazards, and proper disposal of any mercury-containing devices. Suggest alternative temperature measurement devices for home use.

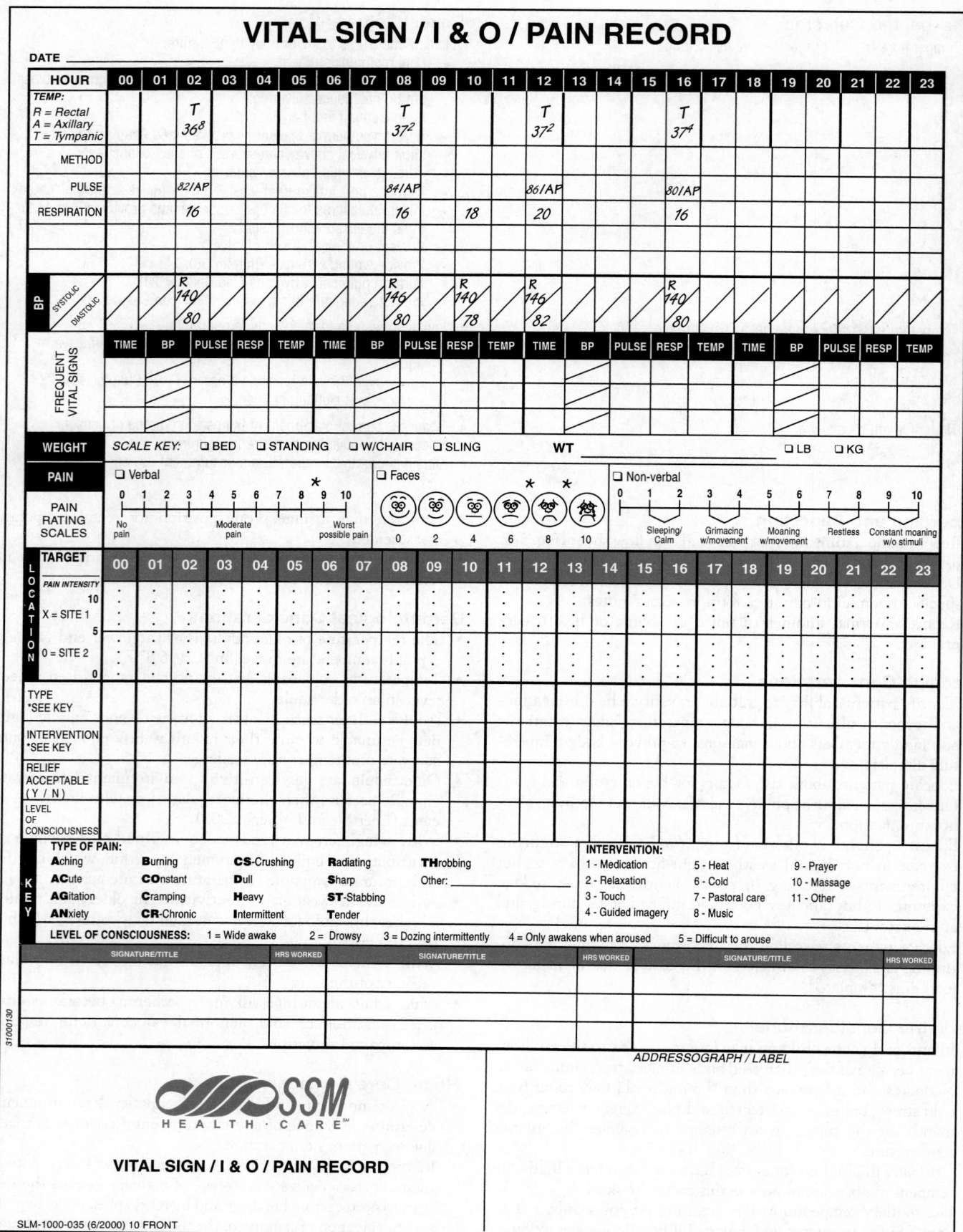

FIG 5-6   Temperature, pulse, and respiration recording on vital sign flow sheet. (*Form courtesy SSM Health Care, St. Mary's Health Center, St. Louis, Mo. [*Pain Rating Scale from McCaffery M, Pasero C: Pain clinical manual, ed 2, St. Louis, 1999, Mosby; **Wong-Baker FACES Pain Rating Scale from Hockenberry MJ and Wilson D: Wong's nursing care of infants and children, ed 8, St. Louis, 2007, Mosby.]*)

SKILL 5-2   Assessing Radial Pulse

Basic Skills / Vital Signs / Assessing Radial Pulse   NSO   *Vital Signs Module / Lesson 3*

The ejection of blood from the heart distends the walls of the aorta. Because of the force of the blood exiting the heart, aortic distention creates a pulse wave that travels rapidly toward the extremities. When the pulse wave reaches a peripheral artery, you can feel it by palpating the artery lightly against underlying bone or muscle. The pulse is the palpable bounding of the blood flow. The number of pulsing sensations occurring in 1 minute is the pulse rate.

Assessing the patient's peripheral pulse sites offers valuable data for determining the integrity of the cardiovascular system. An abnormally slow, rapid, or irregular pulse indicates the heart's inability to deliver adequate blood to the body; a pulse deficit may be present (see Procedural Guideline 5-1, p. 84). The strength or amplitude of a pulse reflects the volume of blood ejected against the arterial wall with each heart contraction. If the volume decreases, the pulse often becomes weak and difficult to palpate. In contrast, a full bounding pulse is an indication of increased volume.

The integrity of peripheral pulses indicates the status of blood perfusion to the area distributed by the pulse (Table 5-1). For example, assessment of the right femoral pulse determines whether blood flow to the right leg is adequate. If a peripheral pulse distal to an injured or treated area of an extremity feels weak on palpation, the volume of blood reaching tissues below the affected area may be inadequate and surgical intervention may be necessary.

You can assess any artery for pulse rate, but the radial and carotid arteries are commonly used because they are easy to palpate (Fig. 5-7). When a patient's condition suddenly worsens, the carotid site is recommended for quickly finding a pulse. Assessment of other peripheral pulse sites, such as the brachial or femoral artery, is unnecessary when routinely obtaining vital signs. Other peripheral pulses are assessed when a complete physical (see Chapter 6) is conducted or when the radial artery is not available for assessment because of surgery, trauma, or impaired blood flow.

Delegation Considerations

The skill of radial pulse measurement can be delegated to NAP unless the patient is considered unstable or the nurse is evaluating a response to a treatment or medication. The nurse directs the NAP to:

- Consider specific factors related to the patient history, usual values, or risk for abnormally slow, rapid, or irregular pulse.
- Obtain appropriate pulse measurement frequency and position for the patient.
- Report any abnormalities to the nurse.

Equipment

- ❑ Wristwatch with second hand or digital display
- ❑ Pen, pencil, vital sign flow sheet or record form

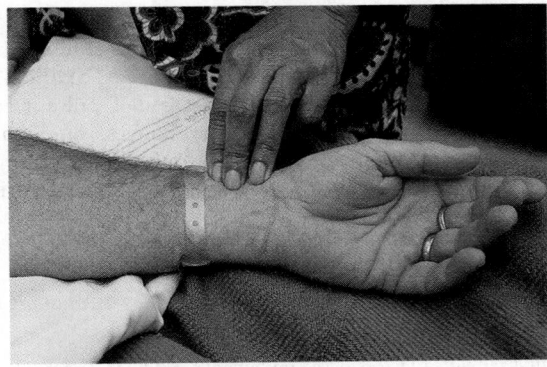

FIG 5-7   Palpating the right radial pulse. (*From Sorrentino S, Gorek B: Basic skills for nursing assistants in long-term care, St. Louis, 2005, Mosby.*)

TABLE 5-1	Pulse Sites	
Site	**Location**	**Rationale for Selection**
Temporal	Over temporal bone of the head, above and lateral to the eye	Easily accessible site to assess pulse in children
Carotid	Along medial edge of sternocleidomastoid muscle in the neck	Easily accessible site to assess character of peripheral pulse; used during physiological shock or cardiac arrest when other sites are not palpable
Apical	Fourth to fifth intercostal space at left midclavicular line	Site used to auscultate apical pulse
Brachial	Groove between biceps and triceps muscles at the antecubital fossa	Site used to auscultate upper extremity blood pressure; assess status of circulation to lower arm
Radial	Radial or thumb side of forearm at the wrist	Common site to assess character of peripheral pulse; assesses status of circulation to hand
Ulnar	Ulnar side of forearm at the wrist	Site used to assess status of circulation to ulnar side of hand; used to perform Allen's test
Femoral	Below the inguinal ligament, midway between symphysis pubis and anterior superior iliac spine	Site used to assess character of pulse during physiological shock or cardiac arrest when other pulses are not palpable; assess status of circulation to the leg
Popliteal	Behind the knee in popliteal fossa	Site used to auscultate lower extremity blood pressure; assess status of circulation to the lower leg
Posterior tibial	Inner side of each ankle, below medial malleolus	Site used to assess status of circulation to the foot
Dorsalis pedis	Along top of foot between extension tendons of great and first toe	Site used to assess status of circulation to the foot

STEP	RATIONALE

ASSESSMENT

1 Determine need to assess radial pulse:

   a Assess for any risk factors for pulse alterations:
   - A history of heart disease
   - Cardiac dysrhythmia
   - Onset of sudden chest pain or acute pain from any site
   - Invasive cardiovascular diagnostic tests
   - Surgery
   - Sudden infusion of large volume of intravenous (IV) fluid
   - Internal or external hemorrhage
   - Administration of medications that alter cardiac function

   Certain conditions place patients at risk for pulse alterations. A history of peripheral vascular disease often alters pulse rate and quality.

   b Assess for signs and symptoms of altered cardiac function such as presence of dyspnea, fatigue, chest pain, orthopnea, syncope, palpitations (person's unpleasant awareness of heartbeat), edema of dependent body parts, cyanosis or pallor of skin (see Chapter 6).

   Physical signs and symptoms often indicate alteration in cardiac function, which affects radial pulse rate and rhythm.

   c Assess for signs and symptoms of peripheral vascular disease such as pale, cool extremities; thin, shiny skin with decreased hair growth; thickened nails (see Skill 6-4).

   Physical signs and symptoms indicate alteration in local arterial blood flow.

   d Assess for factors that influence radial pulse rate and rhythm: age, exercise, position changes, fluid balance, medications, temperature, sympathetic stimulation.

   Allows nurse to anticipate factors that will alter pulse, ensuring accurate interpretation.

2 Determine patient's previous baseline pulse rate (if available) from patient's record.

   Allows nurse to assess for change in condition. Provides comparison with future pulse measurements.

NURSING DIAGNOSES

- Activity intolerance
- Decreased cardiac output
- Deficient fluid volume
- Ineffective tissue perfusion

Individualize related factors based on patient's condition and needs.

PLANNING

1 Expected outcomes following completion of procedure:
   - Radial pulse is palpable, within usual range for patient's age.
   - Rhythm is regular.
   - Radial pulse is strong, firm, and elastic.

   Usual range for adults is 60 to 100 beats per minute.
   Cardiac status is stable.
   Radial artery is patent.

2 Explain to patient that you will assess radial pulse rate (HR). Encourage patient to relax as much as possible. If patient has been active, wait 5 to 10 minutes before assessing pulse. If patient has been smoking, wait 15 minutes before assessing pulse.

   Anxiety, activity, or smoking elevates heart rate. Assessing radial pulse rate at rest allows for objective comparison of values.

IMPLEMENTATION

1 Perform hand hygiene.

   Reduces transmission of microorganisms.

2 If necessary, draw curtain around bed and/or close door.

   Maintains privacy and minimizes embarrassment.

3 Assist patient with assuming a supine or sitting position.

   Provides easy access to pulse sites.

STEP	RATIONALE
4 If supine, place patient's forearm straight alongside or across lower chest or upper abdomen with wrist extended straight (see illustration A). If sitting, bend patient's elbow 90 degrees, and support lower arm on chair or on nurse's arm. Place tips of first two or middle three fingers of hand over groove along radial or thumb side of patient's inner wrist (see illustration B). Slightly extend or flex wrist with palm down until you note strongest pulse.	Fingertips are most sensitive parts of hand to palpate arterial pulsation. Nurse's thumb has pulsation that interferes with accuracy. Relaxed position of lower arm and extension of wrist permits full exposure of artery to palpation.

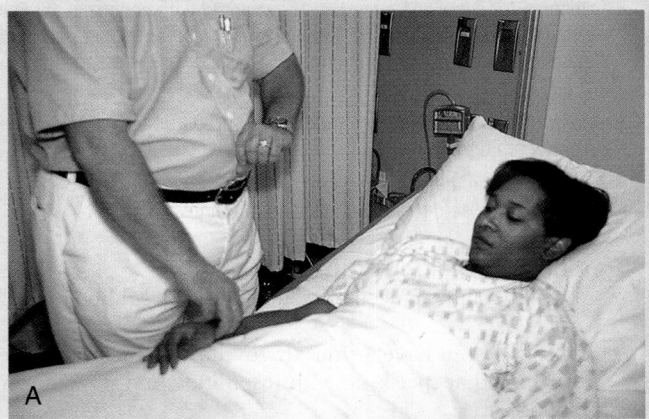 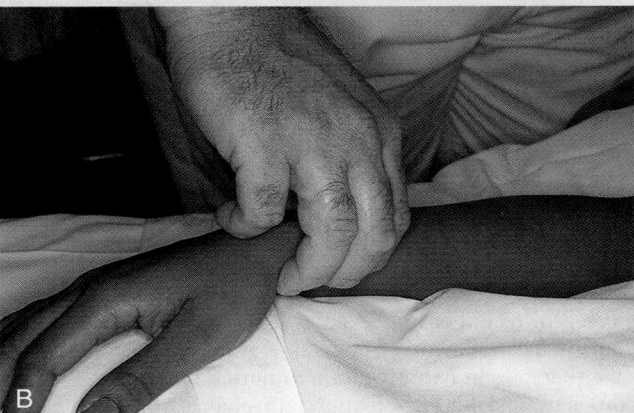

STEP 4 **A,** Pulse check with patient's forearm at side with wrist extended. **B,** Hand placement for pulse check.

STEP	RATIONALE
5 Lightly compress against radius, obliterate pulse initially, and then relax pressure so pulse becomes easily palpable.	Pulse assessment is more accurate when using moderate pressure. Too much pressure occludes pulse and impairs blood flow.
6 Determine strength of pulse. Note whether thrust of vessel against fingertips is bounding (4+), strong (3+), weak (2+), thready (1+), or absent (0).	Strength reflects volume of blood ejected against arterial wall with each heart contraction. Accurate description of strength improves communication among nurses and other health care providers.
7 After feeling a regular pulse, look at second hand of watch and begin to count rate. Count the first beat after the second hand hits the number on the dial, count as one, then two, and so on.	Rate is determined accurately only after pulse has been palpated. Timing begins with zero. Count of one is first beat palpated after timing begins.
8 If pulse is regular, count rate for 30 seconds and multiply total by 2.	A 30-second count is accurate for rapid, slow, or regular pulse rates.
9 If pulse is irregular, count rate for a full 60 seconds. Assess frequency and pattern of irregularity.	Inefficient contraction of heart fails to transmit pulse wave, resulting in irregular pulse. Longer time ensures accurate count.
10 When pulse is irregular, compare radial pulses bilaterally.	A marked difference between pulses indicates arterial flow is compromised to one extremity and nurse needs to take action.

Critical Decision Point *If pulse is irregular, assess for pulse deficit (see Procedural Guideline 5-1, p. 84), which may indicate alterations in heart function.*

STEP	RATIONALE
11 Assist patient in returning to comfortable position.	Promotes comfort and sense of well-being.
12 Discuss findings with patient as needed.	Promotes participation in care and understanding of health status.
13 Perform hand hygiene.	Reduces transmission of microorganisms.

EVALUATION

1 If assessing pulse for the first time, establish radial pulse as baseline if it is within acceptable range.	Used to compare future pulse assessments.
2 Compare pulse rate and character with patient's previous baseline and acceptable range for patient's age.	Allows nurse to assess for change in patient's condition and for presence of cardiac alteration.

Unexpected Outcomes

1   Weak or difficult-to-palpate radial pulse.

Related Interventions

- Assess both radial pulses, and compare findings.
- Observe for symptoms associated with ineffective tissue perfusion, including pallor and cool skin distal to the weak pulse.
- Assess for swelling in surrounding tissues or any encumbrance (e.g., dressing or cast) that may impede blood flow.
- Obtain Doppler or ultrasound stethoscope to detect low-velocity blood flow (see Chapter 6).
- Assess both radial pulses, and compare findings.
- Have another nurse assess pulse.

2   Pulse rate for an adult is more than 100 beats per minute (tachycardia).

- Identify related data, including fever, pain, fear or anxiety, recent exercise, low BP, blood loss, or inadequate oxygenation.
- Observe for signs and symptoms associated with abnormal cardiac function, including dyspnea, fatigue, chest pain, orthopnea, syncope, palpitations, edema of body parts, cyanosis or pallor of the skin.

3   Pulse rate for an adult is less than 60 beats per minute (bradycardia).

- Auscultate the apical pulse (see Skill 5-3).
- Confer with health care provider, and be prepared to order/obtain an electrocardiogram.

4   Pulse is irregular.

- Auscultate the apical pulse (see Skill 5-3).
- Assess for pulse deficit (see Procedural Guideline 5-1).

Recording and Reporting

- Record pulse rate and assessment site on vital sign flow sheet (see Fig. 5-6) record or nurses' notes.
- Document measurement of pulse rate after administration of specific therapies in narrative form in nurses' notes.
- Report abnormal findings to nurse in charge or health care provider.

Teaching Considerations

- Patients taking certain prescribed cardiotonic or antidysrhythmic medications need to learn to assess their own pulse rates to detect side effects of medications. Patients undergoing cardiac rehabilitation need to learn to assess their own pulse rates to determine their response to exercise.
- Teach patients taking heart medications or starting a prescribed exercise regimen how to monitor carotid pulse rate.

Pediatric Considerations

- You can obtain an accurate radial pulse in children over 2 years of age.
- Children often have a sinus dysrhythmia, which is an irregular heartbeat that speeds up with inspiration and slows down with expiration.
- Breath holding in a child affects pulse rate.

Gerontological Considerations

- It is often difficult to palpate the pulse of an older adult or obese patient. A Doppler ultrasound stethoscope provides a more accurate reading.
- The arteries of an older adult often feel stiff and knotty because of decreased elasticity.
- It takes longer for the heart rate to rise in the older adult to meet sudden increased demands that result from stress, illness, or excitement. Once elevated, the pulse rate of an older adult takes longer to return to normal resting rate (Ebersole and others, 2008).

SKILL 5-3   Assessing Apical Pulse

 Basic Skills / Vital Signs / Assessing the Apical Pulse   NSO *Vital Signs Module / Lesson 3*

The apical pulse is the most reliable noninvasive way to assess cardiac function. The apical pulse rate is the assessment of the number and quality of apical sounds in 1 minute. Each apical pulse is the combination of two sounds, S_1 and S_2. S_1 is the sound of the tricuspid and mitral valves closing at the end of ventricular filling, just before systolic contraction begins. S_2 is the sound of the pulmonic and aortic valves closing at the end of the systolic contraction.

You will use a stethoscope to auscultate sound waves of the apical pulse (Fig. 5-8). The stethoscope is a closed cylinder that amplifies sound waves as they reach the body's surface. The five major parts of the stethoscope are the earpieces, binaurals, tubing, bell, and diaphragm.

The plastic or rubber earpieces should fit snugly and comfortably in your ears. Binaurals should be angled and strong enough so the earpieces stay firmly in place without causing discomfort. The earpieces follow the contour of the ear canal, pointing toward the face when the stethoscope is in place.

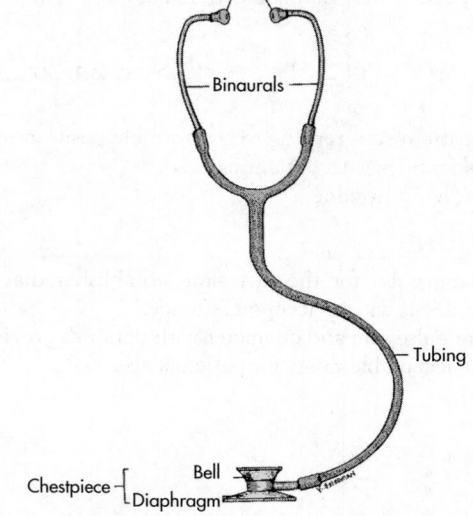

FIG 5-8   Acoustic stethoscope.

The polyvinyl tubing should be flexible and 30 to 45 cm (12 to 18 inches) in length; longer tubing decreases sound transmission. The tubing should be thick walled and moderately rigid to eliminate transmission of environmental noise and to prevent kinking. Stethoscopes can have one or two tubes.

The chestpiece consists of a bell and diaphragm that you rotate into position depending on which part you choose to use. To test, lightly tap to determine which side is functioning. Some stethoscopes have one chestpiece that combines features of the bell and diaphragm. When you apply light pressure, the chestpiece is a bell, whereas exerting more pressure converts the bell into a diaphragm.

The diaphragm is a circular flat-surfaced portion of the chestpiece covered with a plastic disk. It transmits high-pitched sounds created by high-velocity movement of air and blood. Position the diaphragm to make a tight seal against the patient's skin. Exert enough pressure to complete the seal, leaving a temporary red ring on the patient's skin after you remove the diaphragm.

The bell is the cone-shaped portion of the chestpiece usually surrounded by a rubber ring to avoid chilling the patient during placement. It transmits low-pitched sounds created by the low-velocity movement of blood. Hold the bell lightly against the skin for sound amplification.

Delegation Considerations

Often you measure the apical pulse when you suspect an irregularity in the radial pulse or when a patient's condition requires a more accurate assessment. In this situation, pulse assessment cannot be delegated to NAP. When measurement of apical pulse is a routine practice, you can delegate it to NAP. The nurse directs the NAP about:

- Specific factors related to the patient history, usual values, or risk for abnormally slow, rapid, or irregular pulse.
- Frequency of assessment needed
- Need to report any abnormalities in rate or rhythm to the nurse.

Equipment

- ❑ Stethoscope
- ❑ Wristwatch with second hand or digital display
- ❑ Pen, pencil, vital sign flow sheet or record form
- ❑ Alcohol swab

STEP	RATIONALE

ASSESSMENT

1 Determine need to assess apical pulse:
  a Assess for any risk factors for apical pulse alteration: Certain conditions place patients at risk for pulse alterations.
    • Heart disease
    • Cardiac dysrhythmias
    • Onset of sudden chest pain or acute pain from any site
    • Invasive cardiovascular diagnostic tests
    • Surgery
    • Sudden infusion of large volume of IV fluid
    • Internal or external hemorrhage
    • Administration of medications that alter heart function

  b Assess for signs and symptoms of altered cardiac function such as dyspnea, fatigue, chest pain, orthopnea, syncope, palpitations, edema of dependent body parts, cyanosis or pallor of skin (see Chapter 6).   Physical signs and symptoms indicate alteration in cardiac output or stroke volume.

  c Assess for factors that normally influence apical pulse rate and rhythm: Allows nurse to anticipate factors that will alter apical pulse, ensuring an accurate interpretation.
    (1) Age   Infant's heart rate at birth ranges from 100 to 160 beats per minute at rest; by age 2, pulse rate slows to 90 to 140 beats per minute; by adolescence, rate varies between 60 and 100 beats per minute and remains so throughout adulthood.
    (2) Exercise   Physical activity increases HR; a well-conditioned patient may have a slower-than-usual resting HR that returns more quickly to resting rate after exercise.
    (3) Position changes   Heart rate increases temporarily when changing from lying to sitting or standing position.
    (4) Medications   Antidysrhythmics, sympathomimetics, and cardiotonics affect rate and rhythm of pulse; large doses of narcotic analgesics can slow HR; general anesthetics slow HR; central nervous system stimulants such as caffeine can increase HR.
    (5) Temperature   Fever or exposure to warm environments increases HR; HR declines with hypothermia.
    (6) Sympathetic stimulation   Emotional stress, anxiety, or fear results in stimulation of the sympathetic nervous system, which increases HR.

2 Determine previous baseline apical rate (if available) from patient's record.   Allows nurse to assess for change in condition.

3 Determine any report of latex allergy. If patient has latex allergy, ensure that stethoscope is latex free.

STEP	RATIONALE

NURSING DIAGNOSES

- Activity intolerance
- Decreased cardiac output
- Ineffective tissue perfusion

Individualize related factors based on patient's condition or needs.

PLANNING

1 Expected outcomes following completion of procedure:
   - Apical heart rate is within acceptable range.
   - Rhythm is regular.
2 Explain to patient that you will assess apical pulse rate. Encourage patient to relax, and ask patient not to speak. If patient has been active, wait 5 to 10 minutes before assessing pulse. If patient has been smoking, wait 15 minutes before assessing pulse.

Adults average 60 to 100 beats per minute.
Cardiovascular status is stable.
Anxiety, activity, and smoking elevate heart rate. Patient's voice interferes with nurse's ability to hear sound when measuring apical pulse. Assessing apical pulse rate at rest allows for objective comparison of values.

IMPLEMENTATION

1 Perform hand hygiene.
2 If necessary, draw curtain around bed and/or close door.
3 Assist patient to supine or sitting position. Move aside bed linen and gown to expose sternum and left side of chest.
4 Locate anatomical landmarks to identify the point of maximal impulse (PMI), also called the apical impulse (see Chapter 6). Heart is located behind and to left of sternum with base at top and apex at bottom. Find Angle of Louis just below suprasternal notch between sternal body and manubrium; it feels like a bony prominence (see illustration A). Slip fingers down each side of angle to find second intercostal space (ICS) (illustration B). Carefully move fingers down left side of sternum to fifth ICS and laterally to the left midclavicular line (MCL) (illustration C). A light tap felt within an area 1 to 2 cm (½ to 1 inch) of the PMI is reflected from the apex of the heart (illustration D).

Reduces transmission of microorganisms.
Maintains privacy and minimizes embarrassment.
Exposes portion of chest wall for selection of auscultatory site.

Use of anatomical landmarks allows correct placement of stethoscope over apex of heart. This position enhances ability to hear heart sounds clearly. If unable to palpate the PMI, reposition patient on left side. In the presence of serious heart disease, you may locate the PMI to the left of the MCL or at the sixth ICS.

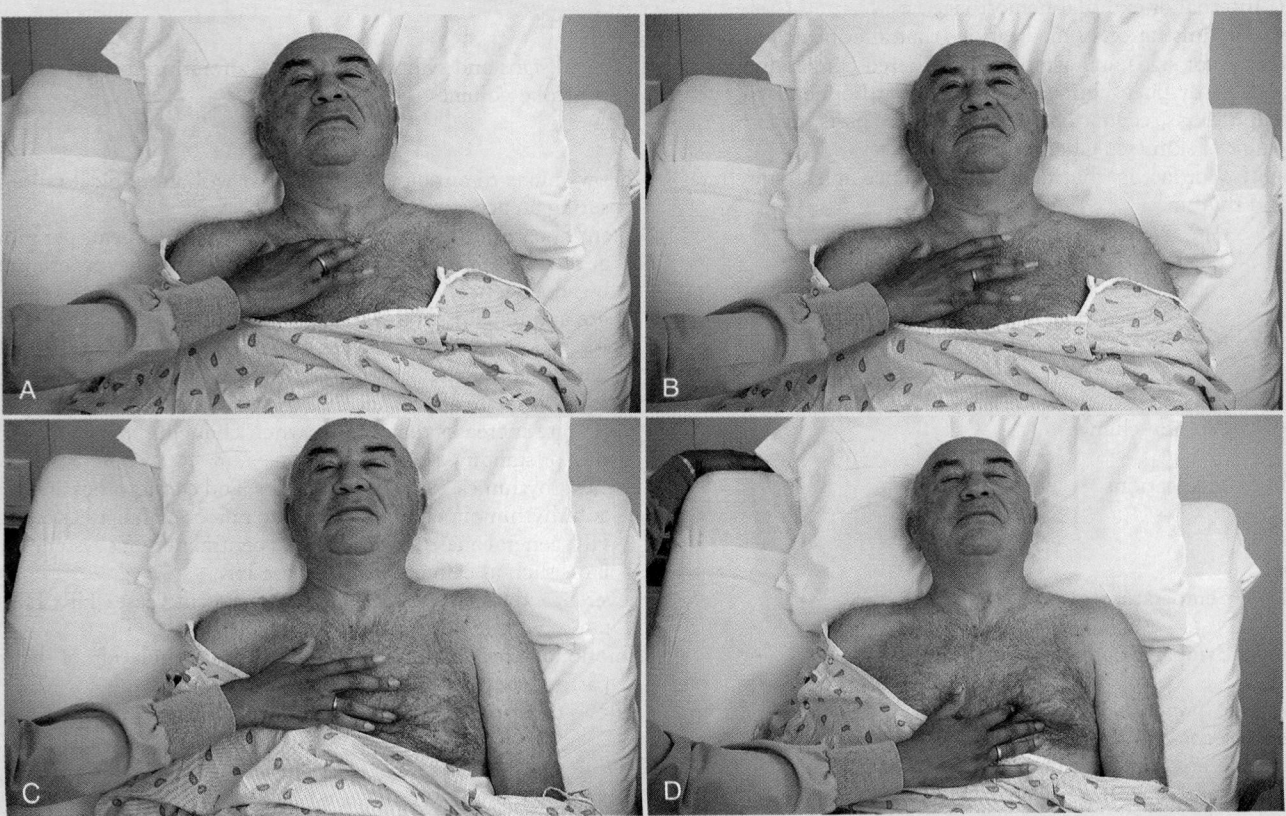

STEP 4   A, Nurse locates sternal notch. **B,** Nurse locates second intercostal space. **C,** Nurse locates fifth intercostal space. **D,** Nurse locates point of maximal impulse at intercostal space at the midclavicular line.

STEP	RATIONALE
5 Place diaphragm of stethoscope in palm of hand for 5 to 10 seconds.	Warming of metal or plastic diaphragm prevents patient from being startled and promotes comfort.
6 Place diaphragm of stethoscope over PMI at the fifth ICS, at the left MCL, and auscultate for normal S_1 and S_2 heart sounds (heard as "lub-dub") (see illustrations).	Allow stethoscope tubing to extend straight without kinks that would distort sound transmission. Normal sounds S_1 and S_2 are high pitched and best heard with the diaphragm.

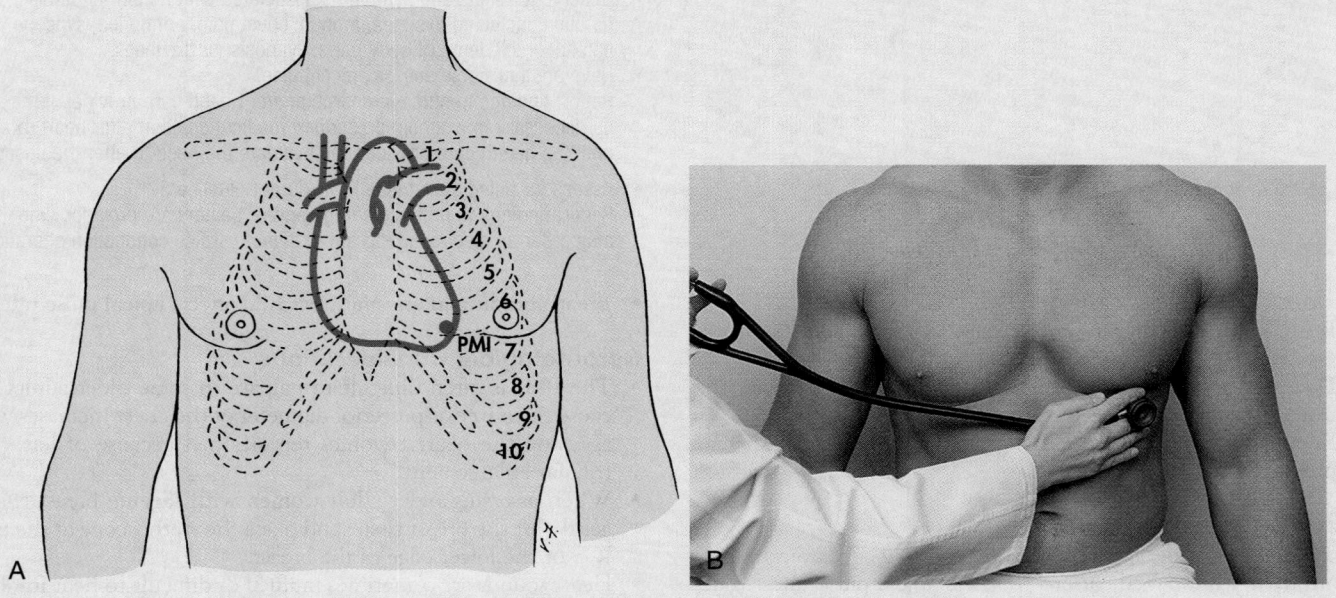

STEP 6   A, Location of point of maximal impulse (PMI) in adult. **B,** Stethoscope over PMI.

STEP	RATIONALE
7 When you hear S_1 and S_2 with regularity, use second hand of watch and begin to count rate: when sweep hand hits number on dial, start counting with zero, then one, two, and so on.	Apical rate is determined accurately only after you are able to auscultate sounds clearly. Timing begins with zero. Count of one is first sound auscultated after timing begins.
8 If apical rate is regular, count for 30 seconds and multiply by 2.	You can assess regular apical rate within 30 seconds.
9 If heart rate is irregular, or patient is receiving cardiovascular medication, count for a full 1 minute (60 seconds).	Irregular rate is more accurately assessed when measured over longer interval (Evans and others, 2004).
10 Note regularity of any dysrhythmia (S_1 and S_2 occurring early or late after previous sequence of sounds; e.g., every third or every fourth beat is skipped).	Regular occurrence of dysrhythmia within 1 minute indicates inefficient contraction of heart and potential alteration in cardiac output.
11 Replace patient's gown and bed linen; assist patient in returning to comfortable position.	Restores comfort and promotes sense of well-being.

Critical Decision Point   *If apical rate is abnormal or irregular, repeat measurement or have another nurse conduct measurement. Original measurement may be incorrect. Second measurement confirms initial findings of abnormal HR.*

STEP	RATIONALE
12 Discuss findings with patient as needed.	Promotes participation in care and understanding of health status.
13 Perform hand hygiene.	Reduces transmission of microorganisms.
14 Clean earpieces and diaphragm of stethoscope with alcohol swab routinely after each use.	Stethoscopes are frequently contaminated with microorganisms. Regular disinfection can control nosocomial infections.

EVALUATION

1 If assessing pulse for the first time, establish apical rate as baseline if it is within an acceptable range.	Used to compare future pulse assessments.
2 Compare apical rate and character with patient's previous baseline and acceptable range of heart rate for patient's age.	Allows nurse to assess for change in patient's condition and for presence of cardiac alteration.

Unexpected Outcomes

1 Apical pulse is greater than 100 beats per minute (tachycardia).

2 Apical pulse is less than 60 beats per minute (bradycardia).

3 Apical rhythm is irregular.

Related Interventions

- Identify related data, including fever, pain, fear or anxiety, recent exercise, low BP, blood loss, or inadequate oxygenation.
- Observe for signs and symptoms associated with abnormal cardiac function, including dyspnea, fatigue, chest pain, orthopnea, syncope, palpitations, edema of body parts, cyanosis, or dizziness.
- Assess for factors that decrease heart rate, such as digoxin and antiarrhythmic drugs.
- Observe for signs and symptoms associated with abnormal cardiac function, including dyspnea, fatigue, chest pain, orthopnea, syncope, palpitations, edema of body parts, cyanosis, or dizziness.
- Have another nurse assess apical pulse.
- Report findings to nurse in charge and/or health care provider. It may be necessary to withhold prescribed medications that alter heart rate until the health care provider can evaluate the need to alter the dosage.
- Assess for pulse deficit (see Procedural Guideline 5-1).
- Report findings to nurse in charge and/or health care provider, who may order an electrocardiogram to detect cardiac conduction alteration.

Recording and Reporting

- Record apical pulse rate and rhythm on vital sign flow sheet (see Fig. 5-6) or nurses' notes.
- Document measurement of apical pulse rate after administration of specific therapies in nurses' notes.
- Report abnormal findings to nurse in charge or health care provider.

Teaching Considerations

- Teach caregivers of patients taking prescribed cardiotonic or antidysrhythmic medications to assess apical pulse rates to detect side effects of medications.

Pediatric Considerations

- Point of maximal impulse of an infant is usually located at the third to fourth ICS near the left sternal border.
- In infants and children younger than 2 years, an apical pulse is more reliable and you should count it for 1 full minute because of possible irregularities in rhythm.

- Breath holding in an infant or child affects apical pulse rate.

Gerontological Considerations

- The PMI is often difficult to palpate in some older adults because the anterior-posterior diameter of the chest increases with age, and the heart becomes repositioned because of left ventricular enlargement.
- When assessing older adult women with sagging breast tissue, gently lift the breast tissue and place the stethoscope at the fifth ICS or the lower edge of the breast.
- Heart sounds are sometimes muffled or difficult to hear in older adults because of an increase in air space in the lungs.
- The older adult has a decreased heart rate at rest (Ebersole and others, 2008).

Home Care Considerations

- Assess home environment to determine which room affords a quiet environment for auscultation of apical rate.

PROCEDURAL GUIDELINE 5-1 Assessing Apical-Radial Pulse

Basic Skills / Vital Signs / Assessing the Apical-Radial Pulse

An inefficient contraction of the heart that fails to transmit a pulse wave to the peripheral pulse site creates a pulse deficit. Pulse deficits are frequently associated with dysrhythmias and warn of potential decreased cardiac function. To assess for a pulse deficit, the nurse and a colleague assess a peripheral pulse rate and the apical pulse rate simultaneously and compare the measurements. The difference between the rates is the pulse deficit.

Delegation Considerations

The skill of radial pulse palpation can be delegated to NAP while the nurse assesses the apical pulse. However, the nurse is responsible for determining the presence of a pulse deficit and follow-up assessments.

Equipment

- ❑ Stethoscope
- ❑ Watch with second hand or digital display
- ❑ Pen, pencil, and vital sign flow sheet or record form
- ❑ Alcohol swab

Procedural Steps

1 Determine need to assess for pulse deficit. Irregular heart rate and signs and symptoms such as dyspnea, fatigue, chest pain, and palpitations may indicate abnormal cardiac function.
2 Perform hand hygiene.
3 Draw curtain around bed and/or close door.
4 Assist patient to supine or sitting position. Move aside bed linen and gown to expose sternum and left side of chest.
5 Locate apical and radial pulse sites. If two nurses are available, one nurse auscultates the apical pulse (see Skill 5-3) and one nurse palpates the radial pulse (see Skill 5-2).
6 The nurse measuring the radial pulse and holding the watch states "start" to ensure that the pulse rate is measured simultaneously.
7 Both nurses count the pulse rate for 60 seconds simultaneously. The count ends when the nurse taking the radial pulse states "stop." Sixty seconds is required when a discrepancy between the pulse sites is expected or when the rhythm is irregular.

PROCEDURAL GUIDELINE 5-1   Assessing Apical-Radial Pulse—cont'd

8 Subtract the radial rate from the apical rate to obtain the pulse deficit. The pulse deficit reflects the number of ineffective cardiac contractions in 1 minute.

9 If a pulse deficit is noted, assess for other signs and symptoms of decreased cardiac output (see Chapter 6).

10 Discuss findings with patient as needed.

11 Perform hand hygiene; clean earpieces and diaphragm of stethoscope with alcohol swab routinely after each use.

12 Record the apical pulse, the radial pulse, and the pulse deficit in the nurses' notes. Inform the nurse in charge or health care provider of the presence of a pulse deficit.

SKILL 5-4   Assessing Respirations

 Basic Skills / Vital Signs / Assessing Respirations

The mechanism of respiration exchanges oxygen (O_2) and carbon dioxide (CO_2) between cells of the body and the atmosphere. Three processes are involved in respiration: ventilation, mechanical movement of gases into and out of the lungs; diffusion, movement of oxygen and carbon dioxide between the alveoli and the red blood cells; and perfusion, distribution of red blood cells to and from the pulmonary capillaries. You assess ventilation by observing the rate, depth, and rhythm of respiratory movements. Accurate assessment of respiration depends on recognizing normal thoracic and abdominal movements. Normal breathing is both active and passive. On inspiration the diaphragm contracts, causing abdominal organs to move downward and forward, thereby increasing the vertical size of the chest cavity. At the same time, the ribs lift upward and outward and the sternum lifts outward to aid the transverse expansion of the lungs. On expiration the diaphragm relaxes upward, the ribs and sternum return to their relaxed position, and the abdominal organs return to their original position (Fig. 5-9). During quiet breathing, the chest wall gently rises and falls. The body uses more energy during inspiration than during expiration. Expiration is an active process only during exercise, voluntary hyperventilation, and certain disease states.

Delegation Considerations

The skill of respiration measurement can be delegated to NAP unless the patient is considered unstable (i.e., complaints of dyspnea). The nurse directs the NAP to:

NSO *Vital Signs Module / Lesson 4*

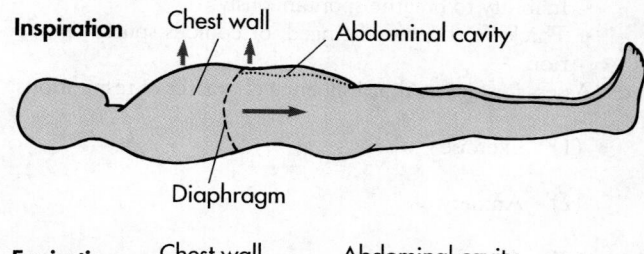

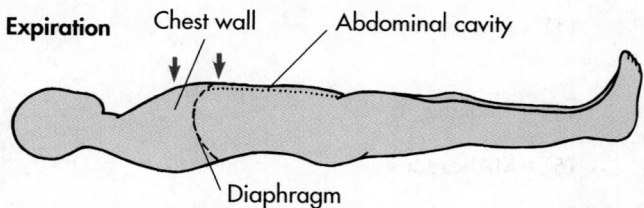

FIG 5-9 Diaphragmatic and chest wall movement during inspiration and expiration.

- Consider specific factors related to patient history or risk for increased or decreased respiratory rate or irregular respirations.
- Report any abnormalities in respiratory rate or rhythm to the nurse.

Equipment

☐ Wristwatch with second hand or digital display
☐ Pen, pencil, and vital sign flow sheet or record form

STEP	RATIONALE

ASSESSMENT

1 Determine need to assess patient's respirations:

  a Assess for risk factors of respiratory alterations:
- Fever
- Pain and anxiety
- Diseases of chest wall or muscles
- Constrictive chest or abdominal dressings
- Presence of abdominal incisions
- Gastric distention
- Chronic pulm onary disease (emphysema, bronchitis, asthma)
- Traumatic injury to chest wall with or without collapse of underlying lung tissue
- Presence of a chest tube
- Respiratory infection (pneumonia, acute bronchitis)
- Pulmonary edema and emboli
- Head injury with damage to brain stem
- Anemia

Certain conditions place patient at risk for ventilatory alterations detected by changes in respiratory rate, depth, and rhythm.

STEP	RATIONALE

b Assess for signs and symptoms of respiratory alterations, such as the following:
- Bluish or cyanotic appearance of nail beds, lips, mucous membranes, and skin
- Restlessness, irritability, confusion, reduced level of consciousness
- Pain during inspiration
- Labored or difficult breathing
- Orthopnea
- Use of accessory muscles
- Adventitious breath sounds (see Chapter 6)
- Inability to breathe spontaneously
- Thick, frothy, blood-tinged, or copious sputum production

Physical signs and symptoms indicate alterations in respiratory status.

c Assess for factors that influence character of respirations:

Allows nurse to anticipate factors that will influence respirations, ensuring a more accurate interpretation.

(1) Exercise

Respirations increase in rate and depth to meet the need for additional oxygen and rid the body of carbon dioxide.

(2) Anxiety

Anxiety causes increase in respiration rate and depth due to sympathetic nervous system stimulation.

(3) Acute pain

Pain alters rate and rhythm of respirations; breathing becomes shallow. Patient inhibits or splints chest wall movement when pain is in area of chest or abdomen.

(4) Smoking

Chronic smoking changes pulmonary airways, resulting in an increased respiratory rate at rest when not smoking.

(5) Medications

Narcotic analgesics, general anesthetics, and sedative hypnotics depress rate and depth; amphetamines and cocaine increase rate and depth, bronchodilators cause dilation of airways that ultimately slows respiratory rate.

(6) Body position

Standing or sitting erect promotes full ventilatory movement and lung expansion; stooped or slumped posture impairs ventilatory movement; lying flat prevents full chest expansion.

(7) Neurological injury

Damage to the brain stem impairs the respiratory center and inhibits rate and rhythm.

(8) Hemoglobin function

Decreased hemoglobin levels lower the amount of oxygen carried in the blood, which results in increased respiratory rate to increase oxygen delivery. An increase in altitude lowers the amount of saturated hemoglobin, which increases respiratory rate and depth.

2 Assess pertinent laboratory values:

a *Arterial blood gases (ABGs):* Normal ranges (values vary slightly among institutions):
- pH, 7.35 to 7.45
- $PaCO_2$, 35 to 45 mm Hg
- PaO_2, 80 to 100 mm Hg
- SaO_2, 95% to 100%

Arterial blood gas values measure arterial blood pH, partial pressure of oxygen and carbon dioxide, and arterial oxygen saturation, which reflect patient's oxygenation status.

b *Pulse oximetry (SpO2):* Normal SpO_2, 90% to 100%; 85% to 89% is acceptable for certain chronic disease conditions; less than 85% is abnormal (see Skill 5-6).

SpO_2 less than 85% is often accompanied by changes in respiratory rate, depth, and rhythm.

c *Complete blood count (CBC):* Normal CBC for adults (values vary within institutions):
- Hemoglobin: 14 to 18 g/100 mL, males; 12 to 16 g/100 mL, females
- Hematocrit: 40% to 54%, males; 38% to 47%, females
- Red blood cell count: 4.7 to 6.1 million/mm^3, males; 4.2 to 5.4 million/mm^3, females

Complete blood count measures red blood cell count, volume of red blood cells, and concentration of hemoglobin, which reflects patient's capacity to carry oxygen.

3 Determine previous baseline respiratory rate (if available) from patient's record.

Allows nurse to assess for change in condition. Provides comparison with future respiratory measurements.

STEP	RATIONALE

NURSING DIAGNOSES

- Activity intolerance
- Ineffective airway clearance
- Ineffective breathing pattern
- Impaired gas exchange
- Impaired spontaneous ventilation

Individualize related factors based on patient's condition or needs.

PLANNING

1 Expected outcomes following completion of procedure:
  - Respiratory rate is within acceptable range.
  - Respirations are regular and of normal depth.

  Adults average 12 to 20 respirations per minute.
  Respiratory status is stable.

2 If patient has been active, wait 5 to 10 minutes before assessing respirations.

  Exercise increases respiratory rate and depth. Assessing respirations while patient is at rest allows for objective comparison of values.

3 Assess respirations after pulse measurement in adult.

  Inconspicuous assessment of respirations immediately after pulse assessment prevents patient from consciously or unintentionally altering rate and depth of breathing.

4 Be sure patient is in comfortable position, preferably sitting or lying with the head of the bed elevated 45 to 60 degrees.

  Sitting erect promotes full ventilatory movement. Position of discomfort will cause patient to breathe more rapidly.

Critical Decision Point *Assess patients with difficulty breathing (dyspnea), such as those with heart failure, abdominal ascites, or in late stages of pregnancy, in the position of greatest comfort. Repositioning may increase the work of breathing, which will increase respiratory rate.*

IMPLEMENTATION

1 Draw curtain around bed and/or close door. Perform hand hygiene.

  Maintains privacy. Prevents transmission of microorganisms.

2 Be sure patient's chest is visible. If necessary, move bed linen or gown.

  Ensures clear view of chest wall and abdominal movements.

3 Place patient's arm in relaxed position across the abdomen or lower chest, or place nurse's hand directly over patient's upper abdomen (see illustration).

  A similar position used during pulse assessment allows respiratory rate assessment to be inconspicuous. Patient's or nurse's hand rises and falls during respiratory cycle.

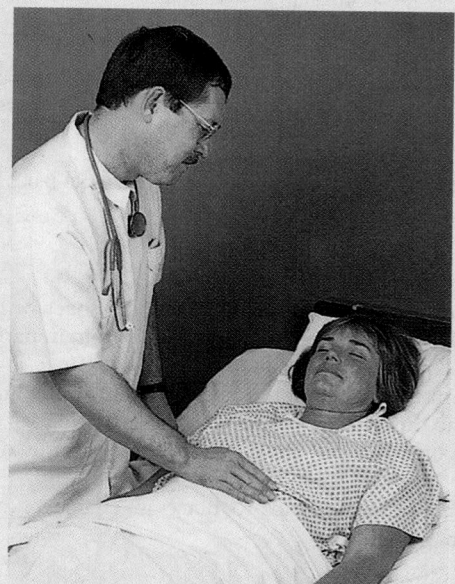

STEP 3   Nurse's hand over patient's abdomen to check respiration.

4 Observe complete respiratory cycle (one inspiration and one expiration).

  Rate is accurately determined only after nurse has viewed respiratory cycle.

5 After observing cycle, look at watch's second hand and begin to count rate: when sweep hand hits number on dial, begin time frame, counting one with first full respiratory cycle.

  Timing begins with count of one. Respirations occur more slowly than pulse; thus, timing does not begin with zero.

STEP	RATIONALE
6 If rhythm is regular, count number of respirations in 30 seconds and multiply by 2. If rhythm is irregular, less than 12, or greater than 20, count for 1 full minute.	Respiratory rate is equivalent to number of respirations per minute. Suspected irregularities require assessment for at least 1 minute (Box 5-4).
7 Note depth of respirations by observing degree of chest wall movement while counting rate. Also, assess depth by palpating chest wall excursion or auscultating the posterior thorax after you have counted rate (see Chapter 6). Describe depth as shallow, normal, or deep.	Character of ventilatory movement reveals specific disease states restricting the volume of air from moving into and out of the lungs.
8 Note rhythm of ventilatory cycle. Normal breathing is regular and uninterrupted. Do not confuse sighing with abnormal rhythm.	Character of ventilations reveals specific types of alterations. Periodically people unconsciously take single deep breaths or sighs to expand small airways prone to collapse.

Critical Decision Point   *Any irregular respiratory pattern or periods of apnea (cessation of respiration for several seconds) are symptoms of underlying disease in the adult and you need to report this to the health care provider or nurse in charge. Further assessment and immediate intervention is often necessary.*

9 Replace bed linen and patient's gown.	Restores comfort and promotes sense of well-being.
10 Perform hand hygiene.	Reduces transmission of microorganisms.
11 Discuss findings with patient as needed.	Promotes participation in care and understanding of health status.

EVALUATION

1 If assessing respirations for the first time, establish rate, rhythm, and depth as baseline if within acceptable range.	Used to compare future respiratory assessment.
2 Compare respirations with patient's previous baseline and usual rate, rhythm, and depth.	Allows nurse to assess for changes in patient's condition and for presence of respiratory alterations.
3 Correlate respiratory rate, depth, and rhythm with data obtained from pulse oximetry and arterial blood gas measurements if available.	Evaluation of ventilation, perfusion, and diffusion are interrelated.

Unexpected Outcomes

1 Respiratory rate is below 12 breaths per minute (bradypnea) or above 20 breaths per minute (tachypnea). Breathing pattern is sometimes irregular (see Box 5-4). Depth of respirations increased or decreased. Patient complains of feeling short of breath.

2 Patient demonstrates Kussmaul's, Cheyne-Stokes, or Biot's respirations (see Box 5-4).

Related Interventions

- Assess for related factors, including obstructed airway, abnormal breath sounds, productive cough, restlessness, anxiety, and confusion (see Chapter 6).
- Assist patient to supported sitting position (semi- or high-Fowler's) unless contraindicated.
- Provide oxygen as ordered (see Chapter 23).
- Assess for environmental factors that influence patient's respiratory rate, such as secondhand smoke, poor ventilation, or gas fumes.
- Notify health care provider or nurse in charge if alteration continues.
- Notify health care provider for additional evaluation and possible medical intervention.

Recording and Reporting

- Record respiratory rate on vital sign flow sheet or record (see Fig. 5-6). Record abnormal depth and rhythm in narrative form in nurses' notes.
- Document measurement of respiratory rate after administration of specific therapies in narrative form in the nurses' notes.
- Indicate type and amount of oxygen therapy, if used, in nurses' notes.
- Report abnormal findings to nurse in charge or health care provider.

Teaching Considerations

- Patients who demonstrate decreased ventilation often benefit from learning deep breathing and coughing exercises (see Chapter 23).
- Instruct family caregiver to contact home care nurse or health care provider if unusual fluctuations in respiratory rate occur.

Pediatric Considerations

- Assess respiratory rates before other vital signs or assessments, if you are able to view movement of chest wall or abdomen. This will allow assessment of rate and rhythm before the child becomes anxious due to stranger anxiety or fear of other assessment procedures.
- Average respiratory rate (breaths per minute) for newborns is 30 to 60; infant (6 months to 1 year) is 30 to 50; toddler (2 years) is 25 to 32; and child from 3 to 12 years is 20 to 30.
- Children up to age 7 breathe abdominally so respirations are observed by abdominal movement.
- An irregular respiratory rate and short apneic spells are normal for newborns.
- Nurses can simply observe infant or young child while chest and abdomen are exposed.
- A young child may breathe slowly for a few seconds and then suddenly breathe more rapidly.
- Use cardiorespiratory monitors for infants or newborns that are at risk for respiratory compromise or sustained apnea.

Gerontological Considerations

- Aging causes ossification of costal cartilage and downward slant of ribs, resulting in a more rigid rib cage, which reduces chest wall expansion. Kyphosis and scoliosis, frequent in older adults, may also restrict chest expansion.
- Depth of respirations tends to decrease with aging.
- The change in lung function with aging results in respiratory rates generally higher in older adults with a range of 16 to 25 breaths per minute.

- Some older adults depend more on accessory abdominal muscles during respiration than weakened thoracic muscles.

Home Care Considerations

- Assess for environmental factors in the home that influence patient's respiratory rate, such as secondhand smoke, poor ventilation, or gas fumes.

BOX 5-4	Alterations in Breathing Pattern
Alteration	**Description**
Bradypnea	Rate of breathing is regular but abnormally slow (fewer than 12 breaths per minute).
Tachypnea	Rate of breathing is regular but abnormally rapid (more than 20 breaths per minute).
Hyperpnea	Respirations are increased in depth; occurs normally during exercise.
Hyperventilation	Rate and depth of respirations increase. Hypocarbia, an abnormally low level of carbon dioxide in the blood, may occur.
Hypoventilation	Respiratory rate is abnormally low; depth of ventilation may be depressed. Hypercarbia, an abnormally elevated level of carbon dioxide in the blood, may occur.
Apnea	Respirations cease for several seconds. Persistent cessation results in respiratory arrest.
Cheyne-Stokes respiration	Respiratory rate and depth are irregular, characterized by alternating periods of apnea and hyperventilation. Respiratory cycle begins with slow, shallow breaths that gradually increase to abnormal rate and depth. The pattern reverses, breathing slows and becomes shallow, climaxing in apnea before respiration resumes.
Kussmaul's respiration	Respirations are abnormally deep, regular, and increased in rate. Common in diabetic ketoacidosis.
Biot's respiration	Respirations are abnormally shallow for two to three breaths followed by irregular period of apnea.

SKILL 5-5 Assessing Arterial Blood Pressure

 Basic Skills / Vital Signs / Obtaining Blood Pressure by the One-Step Method and Obtaining Blood Pressure by the Two-Step Method

NSO *Vital Signs Module / Lesson 5*

Blood pressure (BP) is the force exerted by blood against the vessel walls. During a normal cardiac cycle, BP reaches a peak, followed by a trough, or low point, in the cycle. The peak pressure occurs when the heart's ventricular contraction, or systole, forces blood under high pressure into the aorta. When the ventricles relax, the blood remaining in the arteries exerts a minimum or diastolic pressure. Diastolic pressure is the minimal pressure exerted against the arterial wall at all times.

The standard unit for measuring BP is millimeters of mercury (mm Hg). The measurement indicates the height to which the BP can sustain the column of mercury. The most common technique of measuring BP is auscultation using a sphygmomanometer and stethoscope. As the sphygmomanometer cuff is deflated, the five different sounds heard over an artery are called Korotkoff phases. The sound in each phase has unique characteristics (Fig. 5-10). Blood pressure is recorded with the systolic reading (first Korotkoff sound) before the diastolic (beginning of the fifth Korotkoff sound). The difference between systolic pressure and diastolic pressure is the pulse pressure. For a BP of 120/80, the pulse pressure is 40.

HYPERTENSION

Hypertension is a major factor underlying death from heart attack and stroke in the United States and Canada. The Joint National Committee on Prevention, Detection, Evaluation, and Treatment of High Blood Pressure (National High Blood Pressure Education Program [NHBPEP], 2003) has set criteria for determining categories of hypertension (Table 5-2). Prehypertension is a designation for patients at high risk for developing hypertension. In these patients, early intervention by adoption of healthy lifestyles reduces

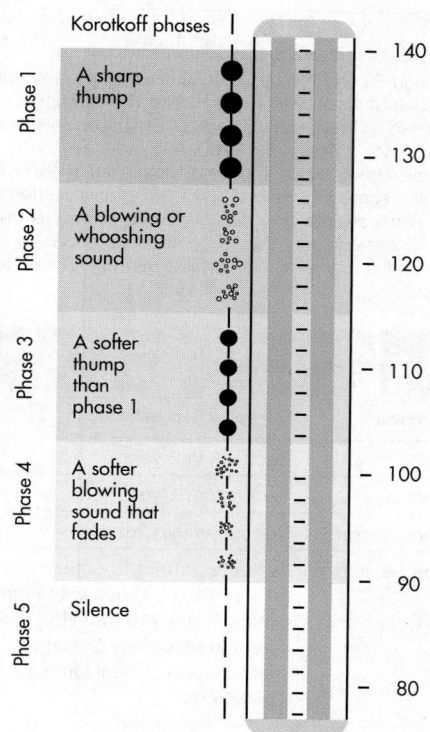

FIG 5-10 The sounds auscultated during blood pressure measurement can be differentiated into five Korotkoff phases. In this example, the blood pressure is 140/90 mm Hg.

the risk or prevents hypertension. Hypertension is defined as systolic blood pressure (SBP) of 140 mm Hg or greater, diastolic blood pressure (DBP) of 90 mm Hg or greater or taking antihypertensive medication (NHBPEP, 2003). The diagnosis of hypertension in adults requires the average of two or more readings taken at each of two or more visits after an initial screening.

One BP recording revealing a high SBP or DBP does not qualify as a diagnosis of hypertension. However, if you assess a high reading (e.g., 150/90 mm Hg), encourage the patient to return for another checkup within 2 months (Table 5-3).

HYPOTENSION

Hypotension occurs when the SBP falls to 90 mm Hg or below. Although some adults normally have a low BP, for the majority of people low BP is an abnormal finding associated with illness (e.g., hemorrhage or myocardial infarction). Orthostatic hypotension, also referred to as postural hypotension, occurs when a normotensive person develops symptoms (e.g., light-headedness or dizziness) and low BP when rising to an upright position. In severe cases, loss of consciousness may occur. Normally, when a healthy individual changes from a lying to sitting or standing position, the peripheral blood vessels in the legs constrict, the heart rate and contractility increase, and BP remains adequate to perfuse the heart and brain.

Orthostatic changes in vital signs are good indicators of blood volume depletion. Some medications cause orthostatic hypotension if misused, especially in young patients and older adults.

BLOOD PRESSURE EQUIPMENT

You measure arterial blood pressure either directly (invasively) or indirectly (noninvasively). The direct method requires electronic monitoring equipment and the insertion of a thin catheter into an artery. The risks of invasive BP monitoring require use in an intensive care setting.

The more common noninvasive method requires use of the sphygmomanometer and stethoscope. A sphygmomanometer includes a pressure manometer, an occlusive cloth or disposable vinyl cuff that encloses an inflatable rubber bladder, and a pressure bulb with a release valve that inflates the bladder (Fig. 5-11). There are two types of manometers: aneroid and mercury. The aneroid manometer has a glass-enclosed circular gauge containing a needle that registers millimeter calibrations. Metal parts in the aneroid manometer are subject to temperature expansion and contraction and must be recalibrated at least every 6 months to verify their accuracy. Before using the aneroid manometer, make sure the needle is pointing to zero.

Mercury manometers, once the gold standard, are less common because they contain mercury, a hazardous substance. Many states have prohibited the sale or use of mercury-containing devices. However, some facilities or nursing units still have mercury manometers. Pressure created by inflation of the compression cuff moves the column of mercury up the tube against the force of gravity. Millimeter calibrations mark the height of the mercury column. To ensure accurate readings, the mercury column should fall freely when you release pressure and it should always be at zero when the cuff is deflated. Mercury manometers are wall mounted or portable. You obtain accurate readings by looking at the height or meniscus level of the mercury at eye level. Looking up or down at the mercury results in distorted readings.

The release valves of both mercury and aneroid sphygmomanometers must be clean and freely movable in either direction. The valve, when closed, holds the pressure constant. A sticky valve makes pressure cuff deflation hard to regulate.

TABLE 5-2	Classification of Blood Pressure for Adults Age 18 Years and Older*		
Category	**Systolic (mm Hg)**		**Diastolic (mm Hg)**
Normal	<120	and	<80
Prehypertension	120-139	or	80-89
Stage 1	140-159	or	90-99
Stage 2	≥160	or	≥100

From National High Blood Pressure Education Program; National Heart, Lung, and Blood Institute; National Institutes of Health: The seventh report of the Joint National Committee on Prevention, Detection, Evaluation and Treatment of High Blood Pressure, *JAMA* 289(19):2560, 2003.

*Based on the average of two or more readings taken at each of two or more visits after an initial screening. Patient is not taking antihypertensive drugs and not acutely ill. When systolic and diastolic blood pressures fall into different categories, the higher category should be selected to classify the individual's blood pressure status. For example, 160/92 mm Hg should be classified as stage 2 hypertension.

TABLE 5-3	Recommendations for Blood Pressure Follow-up
Initial Blood Pressure	**Follow-up Recommended***
Normal	Recheck in 2 years.
Prehypertension	Recheck in 1 year.†
Stage 1 hypertension	Confirm within 2 months.†
Stage 2 hypertension	Evaluate or refer to source of care within 1 month. For those with higher pressure (e.g., >180/110 mm Hg), evaluate and treat immediately or within 1 week, depending on clinical situation and complications.

*Modify the scheduling of follow-up according to reliable information about past blood pressure measurements, other cardiovascular risk factors, or target organ damage.
†Provide advice about lifestyle modifications.

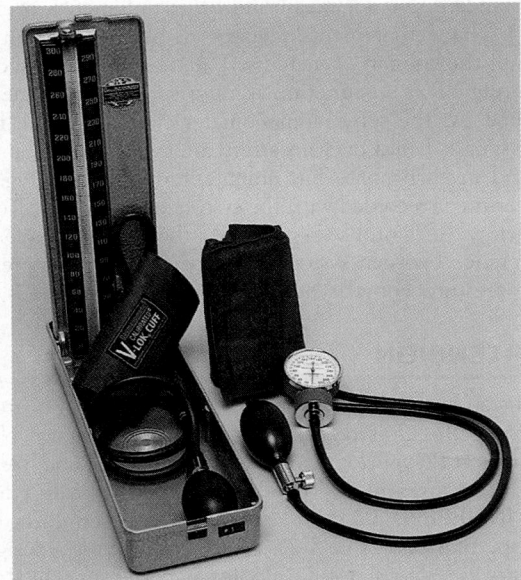

FIG 5-11   Mercury and aneroid sphygmomanometers.

Cloth or disposable vinyl compression cuffs contain an inflatable bladder and come in several different sizes. The size selected is proportional to the circumference of the limb you are assessing (Fig. 5-12). Ideally the width of the cuff should be 40% of the circumference (or 20% wider than the diameter) of the midpoint of the limb on which the cuff is to be used. The bladder enclosed within the cuff should encircle at least 80% of the upper arm (NHBPEP, 2003). Many adults require a large adult cuff. A regular-size cuff holds a bladder in the width of 12 to 13 cm (4.8 to 5.2 inches) and the length of 22 to 23 cm (8.5 to 9 inches). An improperly fitting cuff produces inaccurate BP measurements (Box 5-5).

Electronic or automatic blood pressure machines consist of an electronic sensor positioned inside a blood pressure cuff attached to an electronic processor (see Procedural Guideline 5-2). Electronic devices have their limitations but are useful when frequent measurements are necessary (Box 5-6).

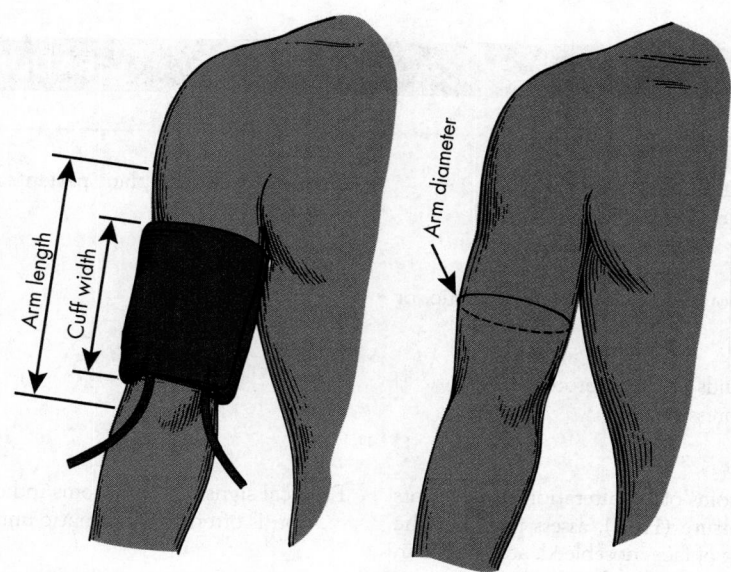

FIG 5-12 Guidelines for proper blood pressure cuff size. Cuff width equals 20% more than upper arm diameter, or 40% of circumference and two thirds of upper arm length.

BOX 5-5	Common Mistakes in Blood Pressure Assessment

Error	Effect
Bladder or cuff too wide	False low reading
Bladder or cuff too narrow or too short	False high reading
Cuff wrapped too loosely or unevenly	False high reading
Deflating cuff too slowly	False high diastolic reading
Deflating cuff too quickly	False low systolic and false high diastolic reading
Arm below heart level	False high reading
Arm above heart level	False low reading
Arm not supported	False high reading
Stethoscope that fits poorly or impairment of the examiner's hearing, causing sounds to be muffled	False low systolic and false high diastolic reading
Stethoscope applied too firmly against antecubital fossa	False low diastolic reading
Inflating too slowly	False high diastolic reading
Repeating assessments too quickly	False high diastolic reading
Inaccurate inflation level	False low systolic reading
Multiple examiners using different Korotkoff sounds for diastolic readings	False high systolic and false low diastolic reading

BOX 5-6	Advantages and Limitations of Electronic Blood Pressure Machines

Advantages
- Ease of use
- Efficient when frequent repeated measurements are indicated
- Stethoscope not required.
- Allows blood pressure to be recorded more frequently, as often as every 15 seconds with accuracy

Limitations
- Expensive
- Requires source of electricity
- Requires space to position machine

- Sensitive to outside motion interference and cannot be used in patients with seizures, tremors, or shivers or patients unable to cooperate
- Not accurate for hypotensive patients or in conditions with reduced blood flow (e.g., hypothermia)
- Accuracy standards for electronic blood pressure machine manufacturers are voluntary
- Vulnerable to error in clinical circumstances, including irregular heart rates, obese extremity

Delegation Considerations

You can delegate the skill of blood pressure measurement to NAP unless the patient is considered unstable (i.e., hypotensive). The nurse directs the NAP about:

- Appropriate limb for BP measurement.
- Appropriate-size BP cuff for designated extremity.
- When a patient is at risk for orthostatic hypotension.
- Frequency of BP measurement for specific patient.
- Need to report any abnormalities to the nurse.

Equipment

- ☐ Aneriod sphygmomanometer
- ☐ Cloth or disposable vinyl pressure cuff of appropriate size for patient's extremity
- ☐ Stethoscope
- ☐ Alcohol swab
- ☐ Pen, pencil, vital sign flow sheet or record form

STEP	RATIONALE

ASSESSMENT

1 Determine need to assess patient's BP:

a Assess risk factors for BP alterations:

- History of cardiovascular disease
- Renal disease
- Diabetes
- Circulatory shock (hypovolemic, septic, cardiogenic, or neurogenic)
- Acute or chronic pain
- Rapid IV infusion of fluids or blood products
- Increased intracranial pressure
- Postoperative status
- Toxemia of pregnancy

Certain conditions place patients at risk for BP alteration.

b Assess for signs and symptoms of BP alterations. In patients at risk for high blood pressure (HBP), assess for headache (usually occipital), flushing of face, nosebleed, and fatigue in older adults. Hypotension is associated with dizziness; mental confusion; restlessness; pale, dusky, or cyanotic skin and mucous membranes; cool, mottled skin over extremities.

Physical signs and symptoms indicate alterations in BP. Hypertension is often asymptomatic until pressure is very high.

c Assess for factors that influence BP:

Allows nurse to anticipate factors that will influence respirations, ensuring a more accurate interpretation.

(1) Age

Acceptable values for BP vary throughout life (see Pediatric and Gerontological Considerations).

(2) Gender

During and after menopause women often have higher BPs than men of same age.

(3) Daily (diurnal) variation

BP varies throughout day; pressure is highest during the daytime between 10:00 AM and 6:00 PM and lowest in early morning (Redon, 2004). Blood pressure drops 10% to 20% during night-time sleep (Giles, 2006).

(4) Position

BP falls as person moves from lying to sitting or standing position; normally, postural variations are minimal.

(5) Exercise

Increases in oxygen demand by the body for activity increase BP.

(6) Weight

Obesity is an independent predictor of hypertension.

(7) Sympathetic stimulation

Pain, anxiety, or fear stimulates the sympathetic nervous system, causing BP to rise. Anxiety raises BP as much as 30 mm Hg.

(8) Medications

Antihypertensives, diuretics, beta-adrenergic blockers, vasodilators, calcium channel blockers, angiotensin-converting enzyme (ACE) inhibitors, angiotensin receptor blockers (ARBs), and antidysrhythmics lower BP; opioids and general anesthetics also cause a drop in BP.

(9) Smoking

Smoking results in vasoconstriction, a narrowing of blood vessels. BP rises acutely and returns to baseline in about 15 minutes after stopping smoking (NHBPEP, 2003).

(10) Ethnicity

Incidence of hypertension is higher in African Americans than in European Americans. African Americans tend to develop more severe hypertension at an earlier age and have twice the risk for the complications of hypertension (i.e., stroke and heart attack). Hypertension-related deaths are also higher among African Americans.

STEP	RATIONALE
2 Determine best site for BP assessment. Avoid applying cuff to extremity when intravenous fluids are infusing, an arteriovenous shunt or fistula is present, or breast or axillary surgery has been performed on that side. Also, avoid applying the cuff to extremity that has been traumatized, diseased, or requires a cast or bulky bandage. Use the lower extremities when the brachial arteries are inaccessible.	Inappropriate site selection may result in poor amplification of sounds, causing inaccurate readings. Application of pressure from inflated bladder temporarily impairs blood flow and can further compromise circulation in extremity that already has impaired blood flow.
3 Determine previous baseline BP and site (if available) from patient's record. Determine any report of latex allergy.	Allows nurse to assess for change in condition. Provides comparison with future BP measurements. If patient has latex allergy, verify that stethoscope and BP cuff are latex free.

NURSING DIAGNOSES

- Decreased cardiac output
- Deficient fluid volume
- Deficient knowledge regarding medication adherence for BP control
- Excess fluid volume
- Ineffective tissue perfusion

Individualize related factors based on patient's condition or needs.

PLANNING

1 Expected outcome following completion of procedure: • Blood pressure is within acceptable range for patient's age.	Cardiovascular status is stable.
2 Explain to patient that you will assess BP. Have patient rest at least 5 minutes before measuring lying or sitting BP and rest 1 minute before measuring standing (NHBPEP, 2003). Ask patient not to speak while you are measuring BP (NHBPEP, 2003).	Reduces anxiety that falsely elevates readings. Exercise causes false elevations in BP. Talking to a patient during BP assessment increases readings 10% to 40%.
3 Be sure patient has not exercised, ingested caffeine, or smoked for 30 minutes before assessment of BP (NHBPEP, 2003).	Caffeine or nicotine causes false elevations in BP. Smoking increases BP immediately and lasts up to 15 minutes. The effects of coffee or caffeine increase BP up to 3 hours.
4 Have patient assume sitting or lying position. Be sure room is warm, quiet, and relaxing.	Maintains patient's comfort during measurement. The patient's perceptions that the physical or interpersonal environment is stressful affect the BP measurement.
5 Select appropriate cuff size (see Fig. 5-12).	Use of improper-size cuff causes false low or false high reading (see Box 5-5).
6 Perform hand hygiene.	Reduces transmission of microorganisms.

IMPLEMENTATION

1 Assess BP by auscultation: upper extremities a With patient sitting or lying, position patient's forearm, supported if needed at heart level, with palm turned up (see illustration). If sitting, instruct patient to keep feet flat on floor without legs crossed. If supine, patient should not have legs crossed.	If arm is extended and not supported, patient will perform isometric exercise that can increase diastolic pressure (Adiyaman and others, 2006). Placement of arm above the level of the heart causes false low reading. Even in the supported position, a diastolic pressure effort up to 3 to 4 mm Hg can occur for each 5-cm change in heart level. Leg crossing can falsely increase systolic and diastolic BP.

STEP	RATIONALE

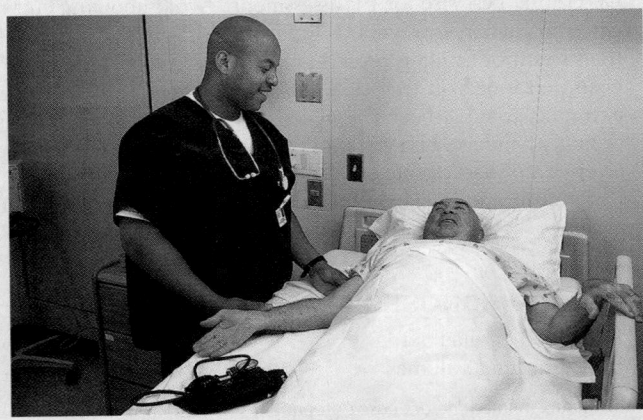

STEP 1a   Patient's forearm supported on bed.

b   Expose upper arm fully by removing constricting clothing.

c   Palpate brachial artery (see illustration A). Position cuff 2.5 cm (1 inch) above site of brachial pulsation (antecubital space). Apply compression cuff above artery by centering arrows marked on cuff over artery (see illustration B). If there are not any center arrows on cuff, estimate the center of the bladder and place this center over artery. With cuff fully deflated, wrap cuff evenly and snugly around upper arm (see illustration C).

Ensures proper cuff application. Do not place BP cuff over clothing.

Inflating bladder directly over brachial artery ensures that you apply proper pressure during inflation. Loose-fitting cuff causes false high readings.

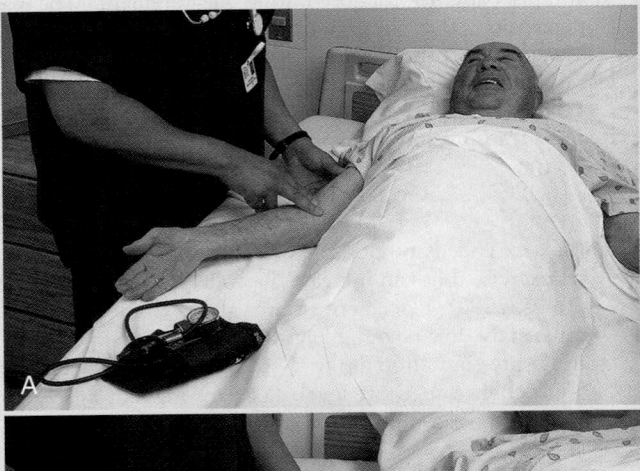

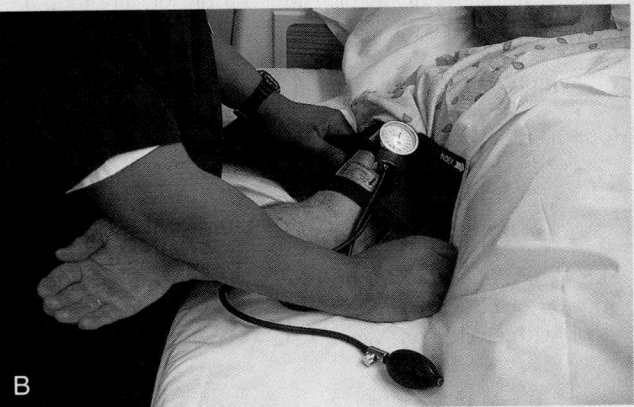

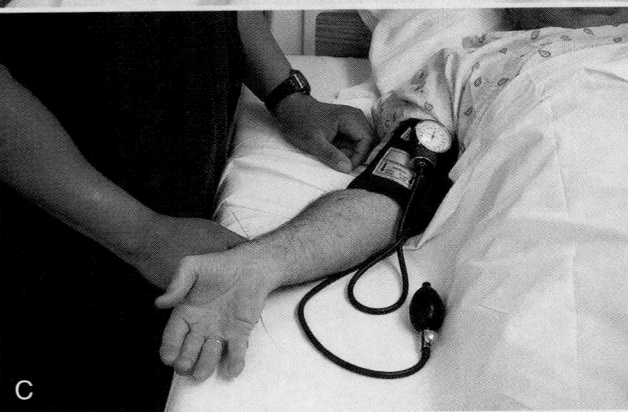

STEP 1c   A, Nurse palpating patient's brachial artery. B, Center bladder of cuff above artery.
C, Blood pressure cuff wrapped around upper arm.

STEP	RATIONALE

d   Position manometer vertically at eye level. Observer should be no farther than 1 meter (approximately 1 yard) away.

Looking up or down at the scale can result in distorted readings.

e   Measure BP.

(1)   Two-step method

(a)   Relocate brachial pulse. Palpate the artery distal to the cuff with fingertips of nondominant hand while inflating cuff rapidly to a pressure 30 mm Hg above point at which pulse disappears. Slowly deflate cuff, and note point when pulse reappears. Deflate cuff fully and wait 30 seconds.

Estimating prevents false low readings. Determine maximal inflation point for accurate reading by palpation. If unable to palpate artery because of weakened pulse, use an ultrasonic stethoscope (see Chapter 6). Completely deflating cuff prevents venous congestion and false high readings.

(b)   Place stethoscope earpieces in ears, and be sure sounds are clear, not muffled.

Each earpiece follows angle of ear canal to facilitate hearing.

(c)   Relocate brachial artery, and place the bell or diaphragm chestpiece of stethoscope over it. Do not allow chestpiece to touch cuff or clothing (see illustration).

Proper stethoscope placement ensures best sound reception. Stethoscope improperly positioned causes muffled sounds that often result in false low systolic and false high diastolic readings. The bell provides better sound reproduction, whereas the diaphragm is easier to secure with fingers and covers a larger area.

(d)   Close valve of pressure bulb clockwise until tight. Quickly inflate cuff to 30 mm Hg above patient's estimated systolic pressure (see illustration).

Tightening of valve prevents air leak during inflation.
Rapid inflation ensures accurate measurement of systolic pressure.

(e)   Slowly release pressure bulb valve, and allow manometer needle to fall at rate of 2 to 3 mm Hg/second.

Too rapid or slow a decline causes inaccurate readings.

(f)   Note point on manometer when you hear first clear sound. The sound will slowly increase in intensity.

First Korotkoff sound reflects systolic BP.

(g)   Continue to deflate cuff gradually, noting point at which sound disappears in adults. Note pressure to nearest 2 mm Hg. Listen for 20 to 30 mm Hg after the last sound, and then allow remaining air to escape quickly.

Beginning of the fifth Korotkoff sound is an indication of diastolic pressure in adults (NHBPEP, 2003). Fourth Korotkoff sound involves distinct muffling of sounds and is an indication of diastolic pressure in children.

(2)   One-step method

(a)   Place stethoscope earpieces in ears, and be sure sounds are clear, not muffled.

Earpieces should follow angle of ear canal to facilitate hearing.

(b)   Relocate brachial artery, and place bell or diaphragm chestpiece of stethoscope over it. Do not allow chestpiece to touch cuff or clothing.

Proper stethoscope placement ensures optimal sound reception. Stethoscope improperly positioned causes muffled sounds that often result in false low systolic and false high diastolic readings. The bell provides better sound reproduction, whereas the diaphragm is easier to secure with fingers and covers a larger area.

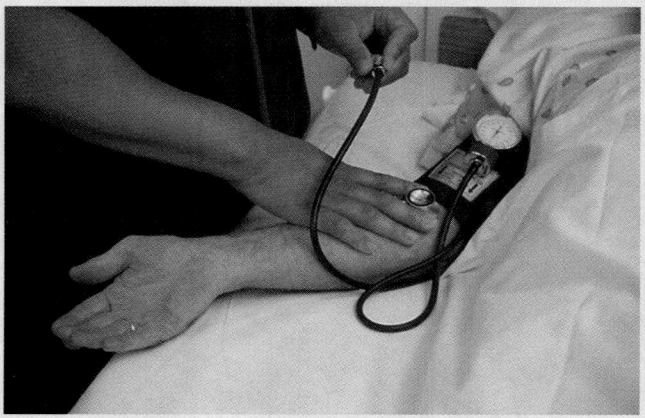

STEP 1e(1)(c)   Stethoscope over brachial artery to measure blood pressure.

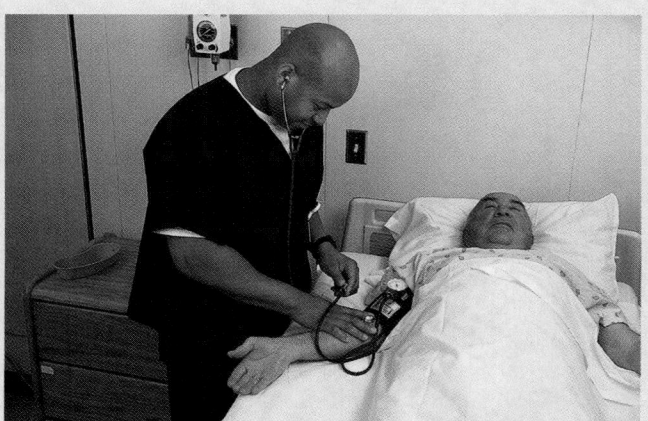

STEP 1e(1)(d)   Inflating blood pressure cuff.

STEP	RATIONALE

(c) Close valve of pressure bulb clockwise until tight. Quickly inflate cuff to 30 mm Hg above patient's usual systolic pressure.

Tightening of valve prevents air leak during inflation. Inflation above systolic level ensures accurate measurement of systolic pressure.

(d) Slowly release pressure bulb valve and allow manometer needle to fall at rate of 2 to 3 mm Hg/second. Note point on manometer when you hear first clear sound. The sound will slowly increase in intensity.

Too rapid or slow a decline in mercury level causes inaccurate readings. The first Korotkoff sound reflects systolic pressure.

(e) Continue to deflate cuff gradually, noting point at which sound disappears in adults. Note pressure to nearest 2 mm Hg. Listen for 10 to 20 mm Hg after the last sound, and then allow remaining air to escape quickly.

Beginning of the fifth Korotkoff sound is an indication of diastolic pressure in adults (NHBPEP, 2003). Fourth Korotkoff sound involves distinct muffling of sounds and is an indication of diastolic pressure in children.

f The Joint National Committee (NHBPEP, 2003) recommends the average of two sets of BP measurements, 2 minutes apart. Use the second set of BP measurements as the patient's baseline.

Two sets of BP measurements help to prevent false positive readings based on a patient's sympathetic response (alert reaction). Averaging minimizes the effect of anxiety, which often causes a first reading to be higher than subsequent measures (NHBPEP, 2003).

g Remove cuff from patient's arm unless you need to repeat measurement.

Continuous cuff inflation causes arterial occlusion, resulting in numbness and tingling of patient's arm.

h If this is first assessment of patient, repeat procedure on other arm.

Comparison of BP in both arms detects circulatory problems. (Normal difference of 5 to 10 mm Hg exists between arms.)

i Assist patient in returning to comfortable position, and cover upper arm if previously clothed.

Restores comfort and provides sense of well-being.

j Discuss findings with patient as needed.

Promotes participation in care and understanding of health status. Makes patient accountable for follow-up assessment.

k Perform hand hygiene. Clean earpieces and diaphragm of stethoscope with alcohol swab as needed (*optional*).

Reduces transmission of microorganisms.
Controls transmission of microorganisms when nurses share stethoscope

2 Assess BP by auscultation: lower extremities

a Assist patient to prone position. If patient is unable to assume position, assist patient to supine position with knee slightly flexed.

Prone position provides best access to popliteal artery.

b Move aside bed linen and any constrictive clothing from leg.

Ensures proper cuff positioning.

c Locate popliteal artery behind knee.

Artery palpation site lies just below patient's thigh, behind knee, just lateral to the midline in popliteal space.

d Apply large leg cuff 2.5 cm (1 inch) above popliteal artery around posterior aspect of middle thigh. Center arrows marked on cuff over artery (see illustration).

Proper cuff size is necessary for accurate reading. Cuff must be wide and long enough to allow for larger girth of the thigh. Narrow cuff causes false high readings.

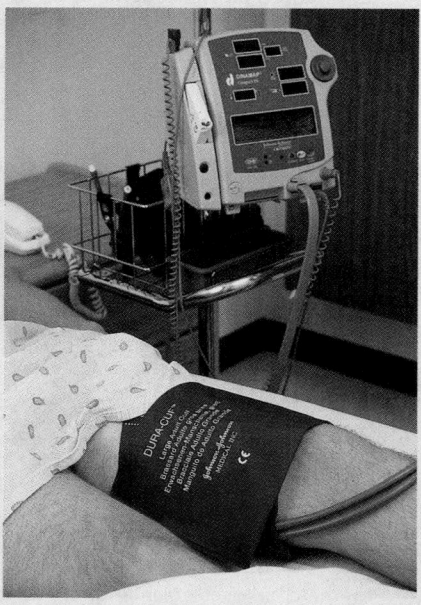

STEP 2d Blood pressure cuff applied around thigh.

STEP	RATIONALE
e Position manometer vertically at eye level. You should be no farther than 1 meter (approximately 1 yard) away.	Looking up or down at the scale can result in distorted readings.
f Using the popliteal artery, follow Step 1e(2)(a) through 1e(2)(e) of one-step method for auscultation of upper extremity.	
g If this is first assessment of patient, repeat procedure on other leg.	Comparison of BP in both legs detects circulatory problems.
h Assist patient in returning to comfortable position, and cover leg if previously clothed.	Restores comfort and promotes sense of well-being.
i Discuss findings with patient as needed.	Promotes participation in care and understanding of health status. Makes patient accountable for follow-up assessment. Systolic BP in the legs is usually higher by 10 to 40 mm Hg than in the brachial artery, but diastolic BP is the same.
j Perform hand hygiene. Clean earpieces and diaphragm of stethoscope with alcohol swab as needed.	Reduces transmission of microorganisms.
3 Assess systolic BP by palpation	
a Follow Steps 1a through 1d of auscultation method for upper extremity or Steps 2a through 2e of auscultation method for lower extremity.	
b Locate and then continually palpate brachial, radial, or popliteal artery with fingertips of one hand. Inflate cuff to a pressure 30 mm Hg above point at which you can no longer palpate pulse.	Ensures accurate detection of true systolic pressure once pressure valve is released.

Critical Decision Point   *If unable to palpate artery because of weakened pulse, use a Doppler ultrasonic stethoscope (see Fig. 5-13).*

STEP	RATIONALE
c Slowly release valve and deflate cuff, allowing manometer needle to fall at rate of 2 mm Hg/second. Note point on manometer when pulse is again palpable.	Too rapid or slow a decline results in inaccurate readings. Palpation helps identify the systolic pressure only.
d Deflate cuff rapidly and completely. Remove cuff from patient's extremity unless you need to repeat measurement.	Continuous cuff inflation causes arterial occlusion, resulting in numbness and tingling of extremity.
e Assist patient in returning to comfortable position, and cover extremity if previously clothed.	Restores comfort and promotes sense of well-being.
f Discuss findings with patient as needed.	Promotes participation in care and understanding of health status.
g Perform hand hygiene.	Reduces transmission of microorganisms.

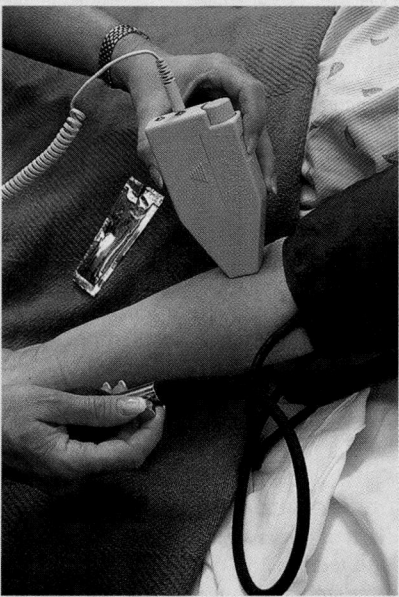

FIG 5-13 Doppler ultrasonic stethoscope over brachial artery to measure blood pressure.

STEP	RATIONALE

EVALUATION

1 If assessing BP for the first time, establish BP as baseline if it is within acceptable range.

Used to compare future BP measurements.

2 Compare BP reading with patient's previous baseline and usual BP for patient's age.

Allows nurse to assess for change in condition. Provides comparison with future BP measurements.

Unexpected Outcomes	Related Interventions
1 Blood pressure is above acceptable range.	• Repeat measurement in other extremity, and compare findings. • Verify correct selection and placement of BP cuff. • Have another nurse repeat measurement in 1 to 2 minutes. • Observe for related symptoms that are not apparent unless BP is extremely high, including headache, facial flushing, nosebleed, and fatigue in older patient. • Report BP to nurse in change or health care provider to initiate appropriate evaluation and treatment. • Administer antihypertensive medications as ordered.
2 Blood pressure is not sufficient for adequate perfusion and oxygenation of tissues.	• Compare BP value to baseline. • Position patient in a supine position to enhance circulation, and restrict activity that decreases BP further. • Repeat BP measurement with sphygmomanometer. Electronic BP devices are less accurate in low flow conditions. • Assess for signs and symptoms associated with hypotension including tachycardia, weak, thready pulse, weakness, dizziness, confusion, and cool, pale, dusky, or cyanotic skin. • Assess for factors that contribute to a low BP, including hemorrhage, dilation of blood vessels resulting from hyperthermia, anesthesia, or medication side effects. • Report BP to nurse in charge or health care provider to initiate appropriate evaluation and treatment. • Increase rate of IV infusion, or administer vasoconstricting drugs if ordered.
3 Unable to obtain BP reading.	• Determine that no immediate crisis is present by obtaining pulse and respiratory rate. • Assess for signs and symptoms of decreased cardiac output; if present, notify nurse in charge or health care provider immediately. • Use alternative sites or procedures to obtain BP: auscultate BP in lower extremity; use a Doppler ultrasonic instrument (see Chapter 6); palpate systolic BP.
4 Patient experiences orthostatic hypotension.	• Maintain patient safety. • Return patient to safe position in bed or chair. • Restrict activity that may drop BP further.
5 A difference of more than 20 mm Hg systolic or diastolic between BP measurements on upper extremities.	• Report abnormal findings to nurse in charge or health care provider.

Recording and Reporting

• Record BP and site assessed on vital sign flow sheet (see Fig. 5-6) or nurses' notes.
• Document measurement of BP after administration of specific therapies in narrative form in nurses' notes.
• Record any signs or symptoms of BP alterations in narrative form in nurses' notes.
• Report abnormal findings to nurse in charge or health care provider.

Teaching Considerations

• Educate patient about risks for hypertension. Persons with family history of hypertension, premature heart disease, lipidemia, or renal disease are at significant risk. Obesity, cigarette smoking, heavy alcohol consumption, high blood cholesterol and triglyceride levels, and continued exposure to stress from psychosocial and environmental conditions are factors linked to hypertension (NHBPEP, 2003).
• Primary prevention of hypertension includes lifestyle modifications (e.g., lose weight, exercise daily, reduce sodium and saturated fat intake, and maintain adequate intake of dietary potassium and calcium). Cigarette smoking is a powerful risk factor, so encourage patients to avoid tobacco in any form (NHBPEP, 2003).
• Instruct primary caregiver to take BP at same time each day and after patient has had a brief rest. Take BP sitting or lying down; use same position and arm each time you take pressure.
• Instruct primary caregiver that if the pressure is difficult to hear, it is probably due to one of the following reasons: the cuff is too loose, not big enough, or too narrow; the stethoscope is not over arterial pulse; cuff deflated too quickly or too slowly; or cuff not pumped high enough for systolic readings.

Pediatric Considerations

- BP measurement is not a routine part of assessment in children younger than 3 years (Schell, 2006a).
- The right arm is preferred for BP measurement in children (National High Blood Pressure Education Program Working Group, 2004). Thigh BP is least preferred and most uncomfortable for children (Schell, 2006a).
- BP measurement can frighten children. Prepare child for squeezing feeling of inflated BP cuff by comparing sensation to elastic band on finger or a tight hug on the arm.
- Obtain BP in child before performing anxiety-producing tests or procedures (Schell, 2006a).
- When a child reaches adolescence, BP varies by body size. Assess the level of a child or adolescent with respect to body size and age. Heavier and taller children have a higher BP than smaller children of the same age. During adolescence, BP continues to vary according to body size. Normal range for 10- to 17-year-olds at the 90th percentile is 124 to 136/77 to 84 mm Hg for boys and 124 to 127/63 to 74 mm Hg for girls (Hockenberry and others, 2007).
- Korotkoff sounds are difficult to hear in children because of low frequency and amplitude. A pediatric stethoscope bell is often helpful.

Gerontological Considerations

- Older adults, especially frail older adults, have lost upper arm mass, requiring special attention to selection of BP cuff size.
- Skin of older adults is more fragile and susceptible to cuff pressure when BP measurements are frequent. More frequent assessment of skin under cuff or rotation of BP sites is recommended.
- Older adults have an increase in systolic pressure related to decreased vessel elasticity.
- Older adults often experience a fall in BP after eating.
- Instruct older adults to change position slowly and wait after each change to avoid postural hypotension and prevent injuries.

Home Care Considerations

- Assess home noise level to determine the room that will provide the quietest environment for assessing BP.
- Instruct patient in the importance of an appropriate-size blood pressure cuff for home use.
- Assess family's financial ability to afford a sphygmomanometer for performing BP evaluations on a regular basis. Recommend electronic devices or aneroid sphygmomanometers that have proven to be accurate according to standard testing as well as appropriate-size cuffs. Finger blood pressure monitors are inaccurate (NHBPEP, 2003).

PROCEDURAL GUIDELINE 5-2   Noninvasive Electronic Blood Pressure Measurement

 Basic Skills / Vital Signs / Obtaining Blood Pressure by the One-Step Method or Obtaining Blood Pressure by the Two-Step Method

NSO *Vital Signs Module, Lesson 5*

Many different styles of electronic blood pressure (BP) machines are available to determine BP automatically (Fig. 5-14). Electronic BP machines rely on an electronic sensor to detect the vibrations caused by the rush of blood through an artery. Although electronic BP machines are fast and free the care provider for other activities, the nurse must consider the advantages and limitations of electronic BP machines (see Box 5-6). The devices are used when frequent assessment is required, such as in critically ill or potentially unstable patients, during or after invasive procedures, or when therapies require frequent monitoring.

Delegation Considerations

The use of an electronic BP machine can be delegated to NAP unless the patient is considered unstable (i.e., hypotensive). The nurse directs the NAP about:

- Appropriate limb for blood pressure measurement.

- Appropriate-size BP cuff for designated extremity.
- Any specific factors that might influence patient's BP.
- Frequency of BP measurement for specific patient.
- Need to inform nurse of any abnormalities.

Equipment

- ❑ Electronic BP machine
- ❑ Source of electricity
- ❑ BP cuff of appropriate size, as recommended by manufacturer
- ❑ Pen, pencil, and vital sign flow sheet or record form

Procedural Steps

1 Determine the appropriateness of using electronic BP measurement. Patients with irregular heart rate, peripheral vascular disease, seizures, tremors, and shivering are not candidates for this device.

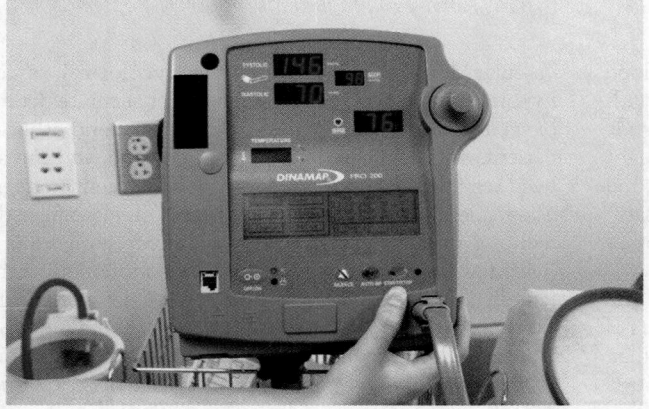
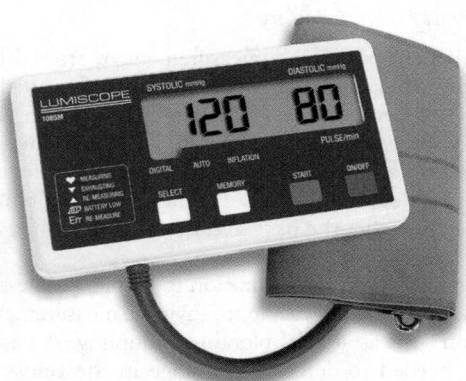

FIG 5-14   Variety of noninvasive electronic blood pressure machines. (*Photo courtesy the Lumiscope Company.*)

Continued

PROCEDURAL GUIDELINE 5-2 Noninvasive Electronic Blood Pressure Measurement—cont'd

2 Determine best site for cuff placement (see Skill 5-5, Assessment Step 2).

3 Assist patient to comfortable position, either lying or sitting. Plug in and place device near patient, ensuring that connector hose, between cuff and machine, will reach.

4 Locate on/off switch, and turn on machine to enable device to self-test computer systems.

5 Select appropriate cuff size for patient extremity (see Fig. 5-12) and appropriate cuff for machine. Electronic BP cuff and machine must be matched by manufacturer and are not interchangeable.

6 Expose extremity by removing constricting clothing to ensure proper cuff application. Do not place BP cuff over clothing.

7 Prepare BP cuff by manually squeezing all the air out of the cuff and connecting cuff to connector hose.

8 Wrap flattened cuff snugly around extremity, verifying that only one finger can fit between cuff and patient's skin. Make sure the "artery" arrow marked on the outside of the cuff is placed correctly (see illustration).

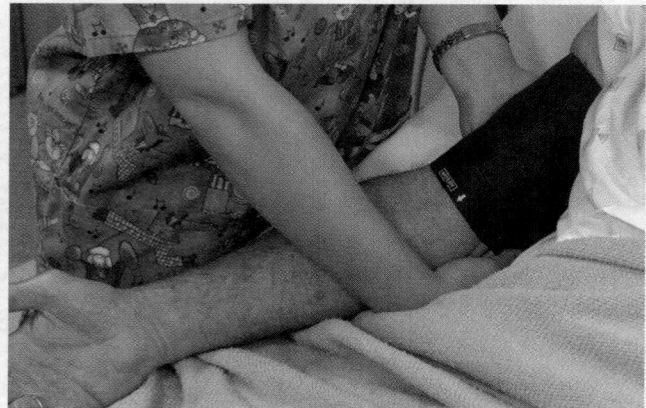

STEP 8 Aligning blood pressure cuff arrow with brachial artery.

9 Verify that connector hose between cuff and machine is not kinked. Kinking prevents proper inflation and deflation of cuff.

10 Following manufacturer's directions, set the frequency control for automatic or manual, then press the start button. The first BP measurement will pump the cuff to a peak pressure of about 180 mm Hg. After this pressure is reached, the machine begins a deflation sequence that determines the BP. The first reading determines the peak pressure inflation for additional measurements.

11 When deflation is complete, digital display will provide most recent values and flash time in minutes that has elapsed since the measurement occurred.

Critical Decision Point *If unable to obtain BP with electronic device, verify machine connections (e.g., plugged into working electrical outlet, hose-cuff connections tight, machine on, correct cuff). Repeat electronic BP; if unable to obtain, use auscultatory technique (see Skill 5-5).*

12 Set frequency of BP measurements, upper and lower alarm limits for systolic, diastolic, and mean BP readings. Intervals between BP measurements can be set from 1 to 90 minutes. The nurse determines frequency and alarm limits based on patient's acceptable range of BP, nursing judgment, and health care provider order.

13 Obtain additional readings at any time by pressing the start button. Pressing the cancel button immediately deflates the cuff.

14 If frequent BP measurements are required, the cuff may be left in place. Remove cuff at least every 2 hours to assess underlying skin integrity and if possible, alternate BP sites. Patients with abnormal bleeding tendencies are at risk for microvascular rupture from repeated inflations. When the patient no longer requires frequent BP monitoring, remove and clean BP cuff according to facility policy to reduce transmission of microorganisms.

15 Discuss findings with patient. Perform hand hygiene.

16 Compare electronic BP readings with auscultatory BP measurements to verify the accuracy of electronic BP device.

17 Record BP and site assessed on vital sign flow sheet (see Fig. 5-6) or nurses' notes; record any signs or symptoms of BP alterations in narrative form in nurses' notes; report abnormal findings to nurse in charge or health care provider.

SKILL 5-6 Measuring Oxygen Saturation (Pulse Oximetry)

 Basic Skills / Vital Signs / Measuring Oxygen Saturation With Pulse Oximetry

NSO *Airway Management Module / Lesson 2*

Pulse oximetry is the noninvasive measurement of arterial blood oxygen saturation—the percent to which hemoglobin is filled with oxygen. A pulse oximeter is a probe with a light-emitting diode (LED) connected by cable to an oximeter. The LED emits light wavelengths that are absorbed differently by the oxygenated and deoxygenated hemoglobin molecules. The more hemoglobin saturated by oxygen, the higher the oxygen saturation. Normally SpO_2 is greater than 90%.

The measurement of oxygen saturation is simple, painless, and has few of the risks associated with more invasive measurements of oxygen saturation such as arterial blood gas sampling. A vascular, pulsatile area is needed to detect the change in the transmitted light when making measurements with a digit or earlobe probe. Conditions that decrease arterial blood flow, such as peripheral

vascular disease, hypothermia, pharmacological vasoconstrictors, hypotension, or peripheral edema, affect accurate determination of oxygen saturation in these areas (Schallom and others, 2007). For patients with decreased peripheral perfusion, you can apply a forehead reflectance sensor. Factors that affect light transmission, such as outside light sources or patient motion, also affect the measurement of oxygen saturation. Avoid direct sunlight or fluorescent lighting when using an oximeter. Carbon monoxide in the blood, jaundice, and intravascular dyes can influence the light reflected from hemoglobin molecules.

In adults you can apply reusable and disposable oximeter probes to the earlobe, finger, toe, bridge of the nose, or forehead (Box 5-7). Pulse oximetry is indicated in patients who have an unstable oxygen status or are at risk for impaired gas exchange.

Delegation Considerations

The skill of oxygen saturation measurement can be delegated to NAP. The nurse directs the NAP about:

- Specific factors related to patient that can falsely lower oxygen saturation.
- Appropriate sensor site and probe to select.
- Obtaining frequency of oxygen saturation measurements for specific patient.
- Notifying nurse immediately of any reading lower than SpO_2 of 90%.

- Refrain from using pulse oximetry as an assessment of heart rate because oximeter will not detect an irregular pulse.

Equipment

- ❏ Oximeter
- ❏ Oximeter probe appropriate for patient and recommended by oximeter manufacturer
- ❏ Acetone or nail polish remover if needed
- ❏ Pen, pencil, vital sign flow sheet or record form

BOX 5-7	Characteristics of Pulse Oximeter Sensor Probes and Sites

Reusable Probe
Digit Probe
- Easy to apply, conforms to various sizes.

Earlobe Probe
- Clip-on smaller and lighter though more positional than digit probe.
- Yields strong correlation with oxygen saturation.
- Research suggests greater accuracy at lower saturations.
- Good when uncontrollable or rhythmic movements (e.g., hand tremors), exercise are present.
- Vascular bed least affected by decreased blood flow.

Forehead Sensor
- Research suggests greater accuracy during decreased perfusion (Schallom and others, 2007).

- Reliable for patients on vasoactive medications (Schallom and others, 2007).
- Detects desaturation quicker than other sites.
- Does not require a pulsatile vascular bed.
- Good when uncontrollable or rhythmic movements (e.g., hand tremors) are present.
- Requires headband to secure sensor.

Disposable Sensor Pad
- Can be applied to a variety of sites: earlobe of adult, nose bridge, palm or sole of infant.
- Less restrictive for continuous oxygen saturation monitoring.
- Expensive.
- Contains latex.
- Skin under adhesive may become moist and harbor pathogens.
- Available in variety of sizes; pad can be matched to infant weight.

STEP	RATIONALE

ASSESSMENT

1. Determine need to measure patient's oxygen saturation:
   a. Assess risk factors for decreased oxygen saturation:
      - Acute or chronic compromised respiratory function
      - Recovery from general anesthesia or conscious sedation
      - Traumatic injury to chest wall with or without collapse of underlying lung tissue
      - Ventilator dependence
      - Changes in supplemental oxygen therapy
      - Activity intolerance

   Certain conditions place patients at risk for decreased oxygen saturation.

   b. Assess for signs and symptoms of alterations in oxygen saturation:
      - Altered respiratory rate, depth, or rhythm
      - Adventitious breath sounds (see Chapter 6)
      - Cyanotic appearance of nail beds, lips, mucous membranes, and skin
      - Restlessness, irritability, confusion
      - Reduced level of consciousness
      - Labored or difficulty breathing

   Physical signs and symptoms indicate abnormal oxygen saturation.

2. Assess for factors that influence measurement of SpO_2, such as oxygen therapy, respiratory therapy such as postural drainage and percussion, hemoglobin level, hypotension, temperature, and medications such as bronchodilators.

   Allows nurse to anticipate factors that influence oxygen saturation, thus ensuring accurate interpretation. Peripheral vasoconstriction related to hypothermia can interfere with SpO_2 determination.

3. Review patient's medical record for health care provider's order, or consult agency's procedure manual for standard of care for measurement of SpO_2.

   Medical order is sometimes required to assess oxygen saturation with pulse oximetry.

4. Determine previous baseline SpO_2 (if available) from patient's record.

   Baseline information provides basis for comparison and assists in assessment of status and evaluation of interventions.

5. Determine most appropriate patient-specific site (e.g., finger, earlobe, bridge of nose, forehead) for sensor probe placement by measuring capillary refill (see Chapter 6). If capillary refill is less than 3 seconds, select alternative site.

   Changes in SpO_2 are reflected in the circulation of finger capillary bed within 30 seconds and the capillary bed of earlobe within 5 to 10 seconds.

STEP	RATIONALE

a   Site must have adequate local circulation and be free of moisture.

b   A finger free of polish or acrylic nail is preferred.

c   If patient has tremors or is likely to move, use earlobe or forehead.

d   If patient is obese, clip-on probe may not fit properly; obtain a disposable (tape-on) probe.

Finger and earlobe sensor requires pulsating vascular bed to identify hemoglobin molecules that absorb emitted light. Forehead sensor detects saturation in low perfusion conditions.

Moisture impedes ability of sensor to detect oxygen saturation levels.

Research on the influence of nail polish is contradictory. Brown and blue nail polish can falsely lower SpO_2, but it is not clinically significant (Rodden and others, 2007).

Detection of motion by the sensor probe creates false waves, or motion artifact, and is the most common cause of inaccurate readings (Giuliano and Liu, 2006).

NURSING DIAGNOSES

- Activity intolerance
- Ineffective airway clearance
- Ineffective breathing pattern
- Impaired gas exchange
- Impaired spontaneous ventilation
- Dysfunctional ventilatory weaning response

Individualize related factors based on patient's condition or needs.

PLANNING

1   Expected outcomes following completion of procedure:
   - Patient's SpO_2 remains between 90% and 100%.
   - Patient's oxygenation therapies are adjusted without requiring invasive assessment measures.

2   Obtain appropriate equipment and place at bedside.

3   Explain purpose of procedure to patient and how you will measure oxygen saturation.

Indicates adequate oxygenation.

Oximetry provides accurate SpO_2 measurement.

Mixing probes from different manufacturers can result in burn injury to patient. If patient has a latex sensitivity or latex allergy, avoid adhesive sensor that contains latex.

Promotes patient cooperation and increases compliance.

IMPLEMENTATION

1   Perform hand hygiene.

2   Position patient comfortably. Instruct patient to breathe normally. If finger is the monitoring site, support lower arm.

3   If using the finger, remove fingernail polish from digit with acetone or polish remover.

4   Attach sensor to monitoring site (see illustration). Instruct patient that clip-on probe will feel like a clothespin on the finger but will not hurt.

Reduces transmission of microorganisms.

Prevents large fluctuations in minute ventilation and possible changes in SpO_2. Ensures probe positioning and decreases motion artifact that interferes with SpO_2 determination.

Opaque coatings decrease light transmission; nail polish containing blue pigment absorbs light emissions and alters measurement of saturation.

Select sensor site based on peripheral circulation and extremity temperature. Peripheral vasoconstriction alters SpO_2. Pressure of sensor's spring tension on a finger or earlobe is sometimes uncomfortable.

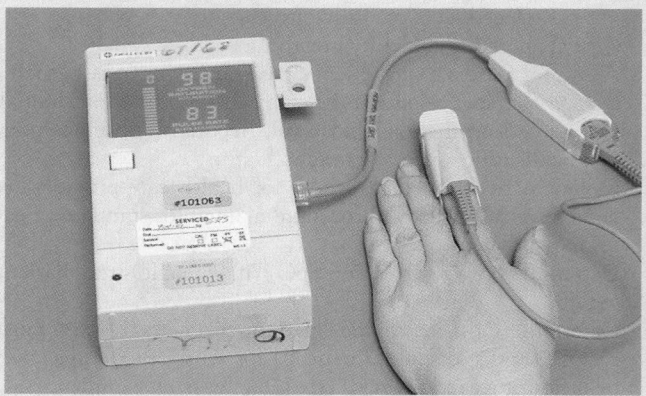

STEP 4   Oximeter sensor attached to finger.

STEP	RATIONALE

Critical Decision Point   *Do not attach probe to finger, ear, or bridge of nose if area is edematous or skin integrity is compromised. Do not use earlobe and bridge of the nose sensors for infants and toddlers because of skin fragility. Do not attach sensor to fingers that are hypothermic. Select ear or bridge of nose if adult patient has a history of peripheral vascular disease. Do not use disposable adhesive sensors if patient has a latex allergy. Do not place sensor on same extremity as electronic BP cuff because blood flow to finger will be temporarily interrupted when cuff inflates and cause inaccurate reading that can trigger alarms.*

5 Once sensor is in place, turn on oximeter by activating power. Observe pulse waveform/intensity display and audible beep. Correlate oximeter pulse rate with patient's radial pulse.	Pulse waveform/intensity display enables detection of valid pulse or presence of interfering signal. Pitch of audible beep is proportional to SpO_2 value. Double checking pulse rate ensures oximeter accuracy.

Critical Decision Point   *If you have measured oximeter pulse rate, patient's radial pulse, and apical pulse at the same time and they are different, reevaluate oximeter probe placement and reassess pulse rates.*

6 Leave sensor in place until oximeter readout reaches constant value and pulse display reaches full strength during each cardiac cycle. Inform patient that oximeter alarm will sound if sensor falls off or if patient moves sensor. Read SpO_2 on digital display.	Reading usually takes 10 to 30 seconds, depending on site selected.
7 If you plan to monitor oxygen saturation continuously, verify SpO_2 alarm limits preset by the manufacturer at a low of 85% and a high of 100%. Determine limits for SpO_2 and pulse rate as indicated by patient's condition. Verify that alarms are on. Assess skin integrity under sensor probe every 2 hours; relocate sensor at least every 4 hours and more frequently if skin integrity is altered or tissue perfusion compromised.	Alarms must be set at appropriate limits and volumes to avoid frightening patients and visitors. Spring tension of sensor or sensitivity to disposable sensor adhesive causes skin irritation and leads to disruption of skin integrity.
8 If you plan on intermittent or spot-checking SpO_2, remove probe, and turn oximeter power off. Store sensor in appropriate location.	Batteries will die if oximeter is left on. Sensors are expensive and vulnerable to damage.
9 Discuss findings with patient as needed and record findings.	Promotes participation in care and understanding of health status.
10 Assist patient in returning to comfortable position.	Restores comfort and promotes sense of well-being.
11 Perform hand hygiene.	Reduces transmission of microorganisms.

EVALUATION

1 If assessing oxygen saturation for the first time, establish SpO_2 as baseline if it is within acceptable range.	Used to compare future assessments of oxygen saturation.
2 Compare SpO_2 with patient's previous baseline and acceptable SpO_2. Note use of oxygen therapy.	Allows nurse to assess for change in patient's condition and presence of respiratory alteration.
3 During continuous monitoring, assess skin integrity underneath probe at least every 2 hours, based on patient's peripheral circulation.	Prevents tissue ischemia.

Unexpected Outcomes	Related Interventions
1 SpO_2 is less than 90%.	• Verify that oximeter probe is intact and that outside light is not influencing probe. Reposition probe if needed. • Assess for signs and symptoms of decreased oxygenation, including anxiety, restlessness, tachycardia, and cyanosis. • Verify that supplemental oxygen is delivered as ordered and is functioning properly. • Minimize factors that decrease SpO_2, such as lung secretions, increased activity, and hyperthermia. • Implement measures to reduce energy consumption. • Assist patient to a position that maximizes ventilatory effort; for example, place an obese patient in a high-Fowler's position.
2 Pulse waveform/intensity display is dampened or irregular.	• Locate different peripheral vascular bed, and reposition pulse oximeter probe. • Use another sensor if available. • Protect sensor from room light by covering sensor site with opaque covering or washcloth.
3 Pulse rate indicated on oximeter is less than radial or apical pulse rate.	• Reposition sensor probe to an alternative site with increased blood flow. • Assess apical and radial pulse along with other signs and symptoms indicating compromised cardiac status or decreased peripheral blood flow.

Recording and Reporting

- Record SpO_2 on vital sign flow sheet (see Fig. 5-6) or nurses' notes, indicating type and amount of oxygen therapy used by patient during assessment.
- Document measurement of oxygen saturation after administration of specific therapies in narrative form in nurses' notes.
- Record any signs and symptoms of oxygen desaturation in nurses' notes.
- Report abnormal findings to nurse in charge or health care provider.

Teaching Considerations

- Teach patient significance of monitoring oxygen saturation.
- Teach patient signs and symptoms of hypoxemia: headache, somnolence, confusion, dusky color, shortness of breath, dyspnea.
- Teach patient effect of high-risk behaviors such as cigarette smoking on oxygen saturation.

Pediatric Considerations

- For infants, secure probe to the great toe, secure cable to foot, and cover foot with a snugly fitting sock. For children, secure probe on the index finger and secure cable to hand.
- Heat and light sources affect sensors. Cover sensors when used during phototherapy or with radiant warmers.

Gerontological Considerations

- Identifying an acceptable pulse oximeter probe site is difficult in older adults because of likelihood of peripheral vascular disease, decreased carbon dioxide level, cold-induced vasoconstriction, and anemia.
- Older adults require more frequent assessment of skin under sensor site because of tissue fragility and decreased elasticity caused by aging.

Home Care Considerations

- Use pulse oximetry in home care to monitor oxygen therapy or changes in oxygen therapy.

? CRITICAL THINKING EXERCISES

You are assigned to Mrs. Coburn, a 78-year-old widow who resides in an assistive living facility. She is admitted to the medical unit from the emergency department for confusion and frequent urination. Although cooperative during your admission assessment, Mrs. Coburn is very forgetful and repeatedly asks you to help her to the bathroom.

1 Which admission vital signs can you assign to the NAP? What directions do you provide the NAP regarding obtaining vital signs for this patient?

2 The NAP reports that the blood pressure for Ms. Coburn is 112/60 mm Hg. You note that the emergency department nurse recorded a blood pressure of 140/86 mm Hg. What might explain the differences in blood pressure values? What interventions do you consider at this time?

3 The NAP documents a temperature of 99.4° F in the vital sign flow sheet but does not report the temperature to you until you inquire. The NAP states that the temperature was not over 100° F, so it was not important to bother the nurse. What is your response to the NAP? Explain the significance of the temperature reading.

4 You direct the NAP to repeat Mrs. Coburn's vital signs, including her temperature, in 2 hours. The NAP reports that Mrs. Coburn was sleeping and the blood pressure and heart rate were obtained from the electronic blood pressure machine and the respiratory rate was observed. What is your response?

✓ REVIEW QUESTIONS

1 A preoperative patient complains of fatigue, dizziness, and feeling warm to the nursing assistive personnel, who reports a temperature of 102.3° F and heart rate of 124 beats per minute to the nurse. What is the nurse's priority nursing action?
   1 Recheck the abnormal vital signs.
   2 Contact the laboratory to obtain blood culture results previously ordered.
   3 Conduct a complete assessment of the patient, including vital signs.
   4 Remove extra clothing and bed covers, and evaluate the patient's complaints.

2 During assessment of his blood pressure, the patient is nervously talking while the reading is obtained. What is the priority nursing action?
   1 Reassure the patient, and document his anxiety in the nurses' notes.
   2 Ask the patient to remain silent, and repeat the blood pressure measurement in the other arm.
   3 Repeat the blood pressure measurement again at the end of the assessment after the patient has been resting quietly.
   4 Request that another nurse obtain the blood pressure.

3 A postoperative patient has vital signs ordered every 15 minutes for an hour. The NAP applies an electronic blood pressure cuff on the patient's left arm and informs the nurse of the first two readings: 122/68 mm Hg and 144/90 mm Hg. What action should the nurse take?
   1 Ask the NAP to reposition the blood pressure cuff.
   2 Assess the blood pressure using the auscultatory technique.
   3 Recheck the patient's blood pressure while observing the electronic device. Assess blood pressure using auscultatory method to determine accuracy of the device.
   4 Check the hose-to-cuff connections for kinking.

4 Following a patient's nebulizer treatment by the respiratory therapist, the pulse oximetry waveform intensity display is irregular and reads 89%. The patient states his breathing is improved after the treatment. What action should the nurse take?
   1 Reposition the oximeter sensor and obtain a new reading.
   2 Cover the sensor with a cloth to eliminate extraneous light.
   3 Tape the pulse oximeter tighter.
   4 Re-evaluate the patient's cardiovascular status.

5 A hypotensive patient has an earlobe pulse oximetry sensor in place. What is the rationale for using this type of sensor?
   1 It is available in a variety of sizes.
   2 It allows better mobility for the patient.
   3 It is more easily positioned for continuous measurements.
   4 It is least affected by decreased blood flow.

REFERENCES

Ebersole P and others: *Toward healthy aging: human needs and nursing response*, ed 7, St. Louis, 2008, Mosby.

Evans D and others: Vital signs: a systematic review, *Joanna Briggs Institute for Evidence Based Nursing and Midwifery*, p.1, 2004

Giles T: Circadian rhythm of blood pressure and the relation to cardiovascular events, *J Hypertens* 24 (suppl 2):11, 2006.

Hockenberry MJ, Wilson D: *Wong's nursing care of infants and children,* ed 8, St. Louis, 2007, Mosby.

Lockwood C and others: Vital signs, *JBI Rep* 2(6):207, 2004.

National High Blood Pressure Education Program; National Heart, Lung, and Blood Institute; National Institutes of Health: The seventh report of the Joint National Committee on Detection, Evaluation, and Treatment of High Blood Pressure, *JAMA* 289(19):2560, 2003.

National High Blood Pressure Education Program Working Group on High Blood Pressure in Children and Adolescents: The fourth report on the diagnosis, evaluation and treatment of high blood pressure in children and adolescents, *Pediatrics* 114(2):555, 2004.

Redon J: The normal circadian pattern of blood pressure: implications for treatment, *Int J Clin Pract* 58(suppl 145):3, 2004.

Schell K: Evidence-based practice: noninvasive blood pressure measurement in children, *Pediatr Nurs* 3:263, 2006a.

Thibodeau GA, Patton KT: *Anatomy and physiology,* ed 6, St. Louis, 2006, Mosby.

RESEARCH REFERENCES

Adiyaman A and others: The position of the arm during blood pressure measurement in sitting position, *Blood Press Monit* 11(6):309, 2006.

Farnell S and others: Temperature measurement: comparison of non-invasive methods used in adult critical care, *J Clin Nurs* 14(5):632, 2005.

Giuliano K, Liu LM: Knowledge of pulse oximetry among critical care nurses, *Dimens Crit Care Nurs* 25(1):44, 2006

Lawson L and others: Accuracy and precision of noninvasive temperature measurement in adult intensive care patients, *Am J Crit Care* 16(5):485, 2007.

Maxton FJ and others: Estimating core temperature in infants and children after cardiac surgery: a comparison of six methods, *J Adv Nurs* 45(2):214, 2004.

Rodden A and others: Does fingernail polish affect pulse oximeter readings? *Intensive Crit Care Nurs* 23(1):51, 2007.

Schallom L and others: Comparison of forehead and digit oximetry in surgical/trauma patients at risk for decreased peripheral perfusion, *Heart Lung* 36(3):188, 2007.

Schell K: Clinical comparison of automatic, noninvasive measurements of blood pressure in the forearm and upper arm with the patient supine or with the head of the bed raised 45 degrees: a follow-up study, *Am J Crit Care* 15(2):16, 2006b.

Health Assessment

MEDIA RESOURCES

- evolve learning system http://evolve.elsevier.com/Perry/skills

  - Review Questions
  - Video Clip

- View Video! Mosby's Nursing Video Skills, 3.0

OBJECTIVES

Mastery of content in this chapter will enable the nurse to:
- Discuss the purposes of physical assessment.
- Describe the techniques used with each assessment skill.
- Describe proper positioning for a patient during each phase of the examination.
- Describe how to conduct a physical examination on patients from diverse cultures.
- List techniques to promote a patient's physical and psychological comfort during an examination.
- Make environmental preparations before an assessment.
- Identify data to collect from the nursing history before an examination.
- Discuss normal physical findings for patients across the life span.
- Discuss ways to incorporate health promotion and health teaching into an assessment.
- Identify self-screening assessments commonly performed by patients.
- Use physical assessment techniques and skills during routine nursing care.
- Document assessment findings on appropriate forms.
- Communicate abnormal findings to appropriate personnel.

Nurses perform systematic physical assessments on a regular basis in nearly every health care setting. In acute care settings you perform a brief physical assessment at the beginning of each shift to identify changes in the patient's status for comparison with the previous assessment. This routine physical assessment takes 10 to 15 minutes and reveals information that supplements the patient's database. In nursing homes and home care settings you perform similar assessments weekly or monthly and more frequently when a change in health status occurs.

Nurses perform a more comprehensive assessment when a patient is admitted to a health care agency. This assessment involves a detailed review of a patient's condition, and includes a nursing history and a behavioral and physical examination. The health history involves an interview with a patient to gather subjective data about any presenting conditions. A physical assessment is a head-to-toe review of each body system that offers objective information about the patient. The patient's condition and response affect the extent of the examination. After gathering data, the nurse groups significant findings into patterns of data that reveal actual or at risk nursing diagnoses (Table 6-1). Each abnormal finding directs the nurse to gather additional data. Initial assessment and examination provide a baseline for a patient's functional abilities and serve as a comparison for future assessment findings. In addition, the information is useful in selecting the best nursing measures to manage the patient's health problems.

Nurses are often the first to detect changes in patients' conditions. For this reason the ability to think critically and interpret patient behaviors and physiological changes is essential. The skills of physical assessment are powerful tools with which to detect subtle as well as obvious changes in a patient's health. During the physical assessment is an ideal time to offer patient teaching and encourage promotion of health practices, such as breast (Box 6-1) and genital (Box 6-2, p. 109) self-examination. The American Cancer Society (ACS) (2008b) recommends guidelines for early detections.

ASSESSMENT TECHNIQUES

Inspection, palpation, percussion, auscultation, and olfaction are the five basic assessment techniques. Each skill enables the nurse to collect a broad range of physical data about patients. Nurses need experience to recognize normal variations among patients, as well as ranges of normal for individual patients. Remember, cultural diversity is one factor that influences both normal variations and potential alterations that you find during the assessment. It is important to take the time needed to carefully assess each body part. Hurrying will cause you to overlook significant signs and make incorrect conclusions about a patient's condition.

Inspection is the visual examination of body parts or areas. An experienced nurse learns to make multiple observations, almost simultaneously, while becoming very perceptive of abnormalities. The secret is to always pay attention to the patient. Watch all movements, and look carefully at the body part you are inspecting. It is important to recognize normal physical characteristics of patients of all ages before trying to distinguish abnormal findings.

Inspection requires good lighting and full exposure of body parts. Inspect each area for size, shape, color, symmetry, position, and the presence of abnormalities. If possible, inspect each area compared with the same area on the opposite side of the body. When necessary, use additional light, such as a penlight, to inspect body cavities such as the mouth and throat. *Do not hurry. Pay attention to detail.* Verify and clarify all abnormalities with subjective

TABLE 6-1	Development of Individualized Nursing Diagnoses		
Assessment Method	**Findings**	**Patterns**	**Nursing Diagnosis**
Inspection of skin	Skin along sacral area is intact. There is a 3-cm area of redness around coccyx; skin blanches on palpation. No skin lesions are observed.	There is pressure area around coccyx.	Risk for impaired skin integrity
Palpation of skin	Skin is moist from diaphoresis. There is tenderness to palpation at sacral area. Skin turgor is elastic.	Skin moisture promotes maceration.	
Historical data	Patient suffered fractured left leg. Patient is immobilized due to left leg traction.	Continued pressure is exerted over sacrum.	

patient data. In other words, ask the patient for further information about each abnormality or change.

Palpation uses the sense of touch. Through palpation the hands make delicate and sensitive measurements of specific physical signs. Palpation detects resistance, resilience, roughness, texture, temperature, and mobility. You normally use palpation with or after visual inspection. You use different parts of the hand to detect specific characteristics. For example, the dorsum (back) of the hand is sensitive to temperature variations. The pads of the fingertips detect subtle changes in texture, shape, size, consistency, and pulsation of body parts. The palm of the hand is especially sensitive to vibration. The nurse measures position, consistency, and turgor by lightly grasping the body part with the fingertips.

BOX 6-1   Breast Self-Examination

BSE should be done once a month so that you become familiar with the usual appearance and feel of your breast. Familiarity makes is easier to notice any changes in the breast from one month to another. Early discovery of a change from what is "normal" is the main idea behind BSE.

For women who menstruate, the best time to do BSE is 2 or 3 days after a period ends, when the breasts are least likely to be tender or swollen. For women who no longer menstruate, pick a day, such as the first day of the month, to remind yourself to do BSE.

Procedure

1   Stand before a mirror. Inspect both breasts for anything unusual, such as any discharge from the nipples, puckering, dimpling, or scaling of the skin.
2   Watching closely in the mirror, clasp hands behind your head and press head forward. Note how the chest muscles tighten.
3   Next, press hands firmly on hips and bow slightly toward the mirror as you pull your shoulders and elbows forward.

The next part of the examination may be done in the shower. Gliding fingers over soapy skin makes it easier to appreciate the texture underneath.

4   Raise your left arm. Use three or four fingers of your right hand to explore your left breast firmly, carefully, and thoroughly. Beginning at the outer edge, press the flat part of your fingers in small circles, moving the circles slowly around the breast. Gradually work toward the nipple. Be sure to cover the entire breast. Pay special attention to the area between the breast and the armpit itself. Feel for any unusual lump or mass under the skin.
5   Gently squeeze the nipple and look for discharge. Repeat the exam on your right breast.
6   Lie flat on your back, right arm over your head, and a pillow or folded towel under your left shoulder. This position flattens the breast and makes it easier to examine. Use the same circular motion described earlier. Repeat on your left breast.
Call your physician if you find a lump or other abnormality.

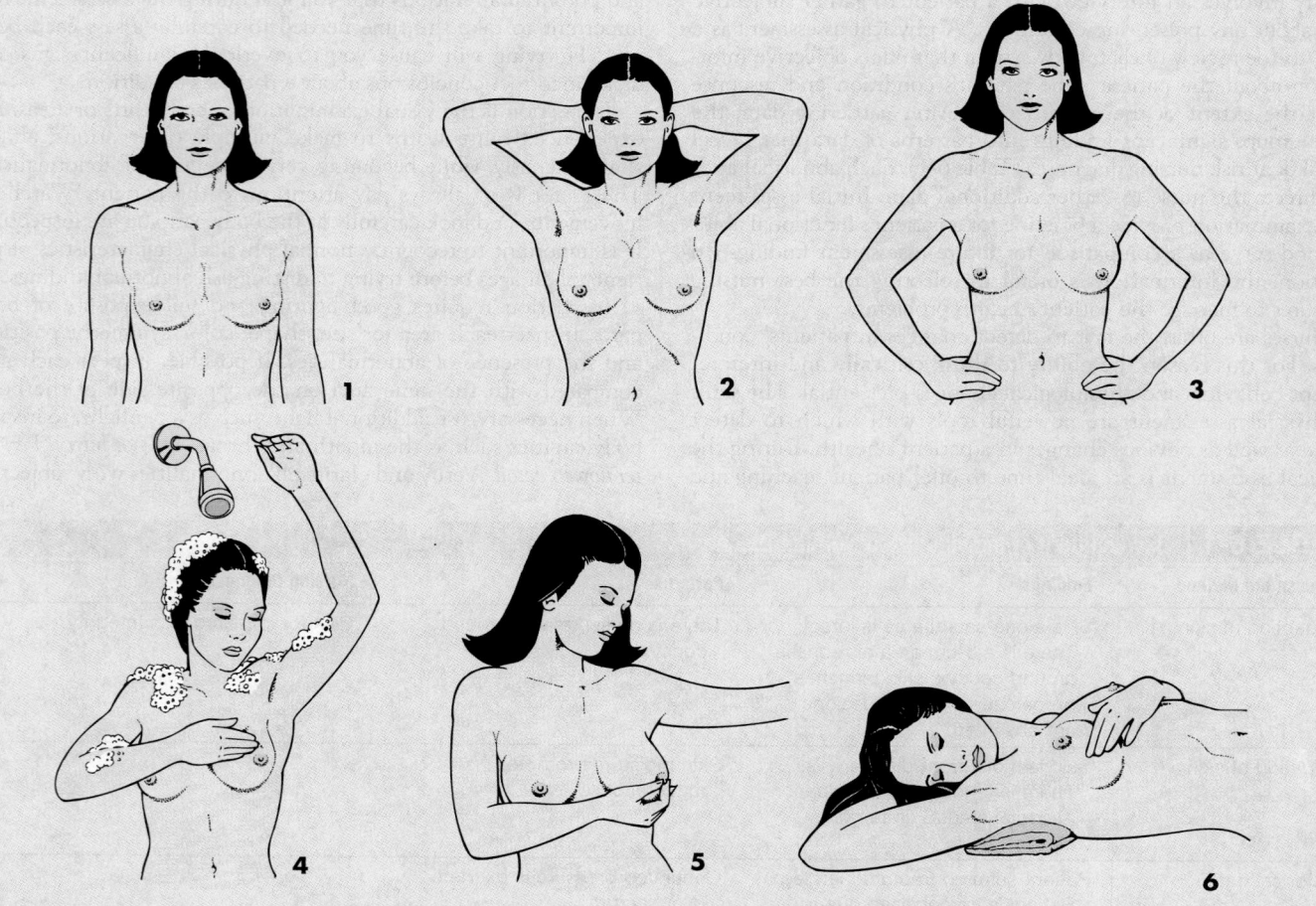

From Seidel HM and others: *Mosby's guide to physical examination*, ed 6, St. Louis, 2006, Mosby.
BSE, Breast self-examination.

Assist the patient in relaxing and positioning comfortably because muscle tension during palpation impairs the ability to palpate correctly. Asking the patient to take slow, deep breaths enhances muscle relaxation. Palpate tender areas last. Ask the patient to point out areas that are more sensitive, and note any nonverbal signs of discomfort. Palpation is either light or deep, and you control it by the amount of pressure you apply with the fingers or hand. Light palpation precedes deep palpation. Consider the patient's condition, the area being palpated, and the reason for using palpation. For example, when a patient is admitted to the emergency department following an automobile accident, consider the factors surrounding the patient's injury and inspect the chest wall carefully before performing any palpation around the area of the ribs.

For light palpation, apply pressure slowly, gently, and deliberately, depressing about 1 cm (½ inch) (Fig. 6-1, A). Check tender areas further, using light intermittent pressure. After light palpation, use deeper palpation to examine the condition of organs (Fig. 6-1, B). Depress the area you are examining by approximately 2 cm (1 inch). Caution is the rule. Bimanual palpation involves one hand placed over the other while applying pressure. The upper hand exerts downward pressure as the other hand feels the subtle characteristics of underlying organs and masses. Seek the assistance of a qualified instructor before attempting deep palpation.

Percussion involves tapping the body with the fingertips to evaluate the size, borders, and consistency of body organs and to

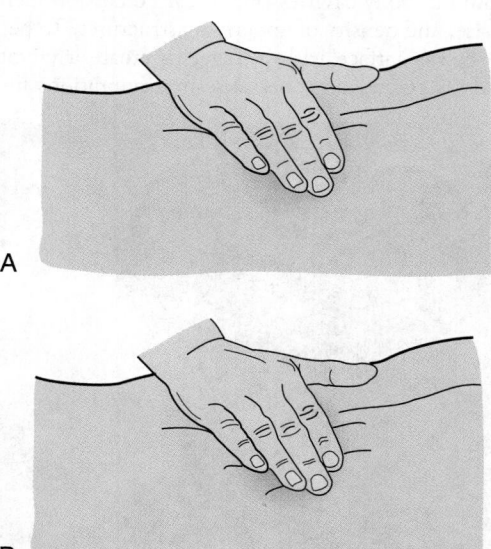

Fig. 6-1   A, During light palpation, gentle pressure against underlying skin and tissues can be used to detect areas of irregularity and tenderness. **B,** During deep palpation, depress tissue to assess condition of underlying organs.

| **BOX 6-2** | Genital Self-Examination |

All men 15 years and older should perform this examination monthly. Perform the examination after a warm bath or shower when the scrotal sac is relaxed. Call your physician if you find a lump or any other abnormality.

Penile Examination
1   Stand naked in front of a mirror and hold the penis in your hand and examine the head. Pull back the foreskin if uncircumcised.
2   Inspect and palpate the entire head of the penis in a clockwise motion, looking carefully for any bumps, sores, or blisters.
3   Look for any bumpy warts.
4   Look at the opening at the end of the penis for discharge.
5   Look along the entire shaft of the penis for the same signs.
6   Separate pubic hair at the base of the penis and carefully examine the skin underneath.

Testicular Examination
1   Look for swelling or lumps in the skin of the scrotum while looking in the mirror.
2   Use both hands, placing the index and middle fingers under the testicles and the thumb on top.
3   Gently roll the testicle, feeling for lumps, thickening, or a change in consistency (hardening).
4   Find the epididymis (a cordlike structure on the top and back of the testicle; it is not a lump).
5   Feel for small, pea-sized lumps on the front and side of the testicle. The lumps are usually painless and are abnormal.

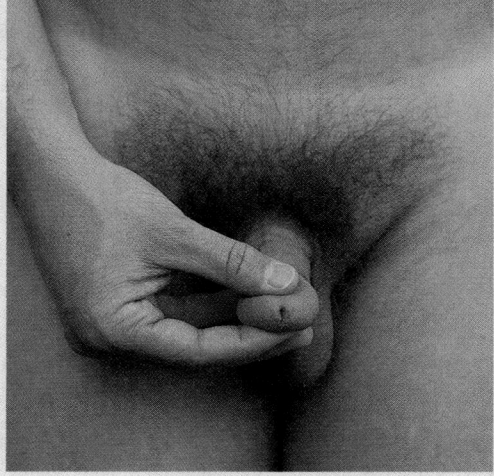

STEP 1

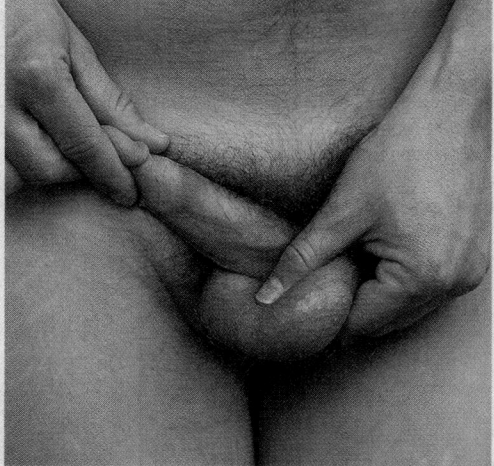

STEP 2

From Seidel HM and others: *Mosby's guide to physical examination*, ed 6, St. Louis, 2006, Mosby.

discover fluid in body cavities (Fig. 6-2). Percussion identifies the location, size, and density of underlying structures. To percuss, you strike the body's surface with a finger to create a vibration. You hear sounds as percussion tones arise from vibrations in body tis-

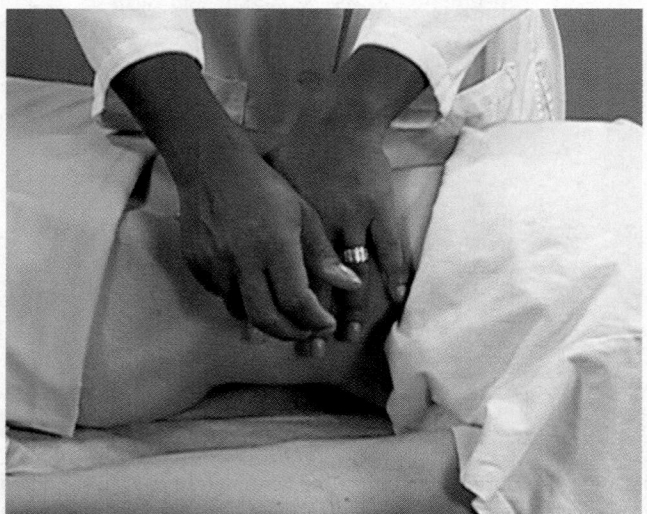

Fig. 6-2 Indirect percussion of the abdomen. (*From Seidel HM and others:* Mosby's guide to physical examination, *ed 6, St. Louis, 2006, Mosby.*)

sues (Seidel and others, 2006). The character of sound depends on the density of underlying tissues. Advanced practice nurses (APNs) typically use this technique because it requires practice and skill

There are two methods of percussion: direct and indirect. The direct method involves striking the body surface directly with one or two fingers. Perform the indirect technique by placing the middle finger of your nondominant hand firmly against the body surface. With palm and fingers remaining off the skin, the tip of the middle finger of the dominant hand strikes the base of the distal joint of the finger. Use a quick, sharp stroke, keeping the forearm stationary. Relax the wrist to deliver the proper blow. Once the finger has struck, the wrist snaps back. If the blow is not sharp, if the hand is held loosely, or if the palm rests on the body surface, the sound is softened and you will not detect the presence of underlying structures. A light, quick blow produces the clearest sounds. Table 6-2 describes the five different percussion sounds.

Auscultation is listening with a stethoscope to sounds produced by the body. To auscultate correctly, listen in a quiet environment for both the presence of sound and its characteristics. To be successful in auscultation, you must first recognize normal sounds from each body structure, including the passage of blood through an artery, heart sounds, and movement of air through the lungs. These sounds vary according to the location. Likewise, nurses become familiar with areas that normally do not emit sounds. It is important for you to listen to many normal sounds in order to recognize abnormal sounds when they arise.

TABLE 6-2	Sounds Produced by Percussion				
Sound	**Intensity**	**Pitch**	**Duration**	**Quality**	**Common Location**
Tympany	Loud	High	Moderate	Drumlike	Enclosed, air-containing space; gastric air bubble, puffed-out cheek
Resonance	Moderate to loud	Low	Long	Hollow	Normal lung
Hyperresonance	Very loud	Very low	Longer than resonance	Booming	Emphysematous lung
Dullness	Soft to moderate	High	Moderate	Thudlike	Liver, spleen, gallbladder
Flatness	Soft	High	Short	Flat	Muscle

BOX 6-3	Using a Stethoscope

1 Place earpieces in both ears with tips of earpieces turned toward the face. *Lightly* blow into the diaphragm. Again place earpieces in your ears, this time with ends turned toward the back of the head. *Lightly* blow into the stethoscope's diaphragm. You will find that you hear clearer sounds with the earpiece turned toward the face. After you have learned the right fit for the loudest sound, wear the stethoscope the same way each time.

2 Put the stethoscope on, and *lightly* blow into the diaphragm. If sound is barely audible, *lightly* blow into the bell. Sound is carried through only one part of the chest piece at a time. If the sound is greatly amplified through the diaphragm, the diaphragm is in position for use. If sound is barely audible through the diaphragm, the bell is in position for use.

3 Place the diaphragm over the anterior part of your chest. Ask a friend to speak in a normal conversational tone. Environmental noise seriously detracts from hearing the noise created by body organs. When using a stethoscope, the patient and the examiner need to remain quiet.

4 Put the stethoscope on, and gently tap the tubing. It is often difficult to avoid stretching or moving the stethoscope's tubing. Position yourself so that the tubing hangs free. Moving or touching the tubing creates extraneous sounds.

5 Care of the stethoscope: Remove earpieces regularly, and clean or remove cerumen (earwax). Keep the bell and diaphragm free of dust, lint, and body oils. Keep the tubing away from nurse's body oils. Avoid draping the stethoscope around the neck next to the skin. To clean, wipe the entire stethoscope (diaphragm, tubing, etc.) with alcohol or soapy water. Be sure to dry all parts thoroughly. Follow the manufacturer's recommendations.

6 Infection control: Harmful bacteria, even antibiotic-resistant microorganisms, can be transferred from patient to patient when using portable equipment such as stethoscopes (Truscott, 2005). Follow institution infection control guidelines, especially contact precautions to decrease this risk. The stethoscope (diaphragm/bell) is cleansed with a disinfectant before reuse on another patient. Using a disinfectant such as isopropyl alcohol (with or without chlorhexidine), benzalkonium, and sodium hypochlorite is effective in reducing the number of bacterial colonies. Earpieces of stethoscopes are sources of transferable bacteria as well when you inadvertently touch your ears and then care for the patient. Potential pathogens could contaminate earpieces. Using hand hygiene, before and after patient contact, decreases the risk of transmitting microorganisms from your ear to your patient.

To auscultate, you need good hearing acuity, a good stethoscope, and knowledge of how to use the stethoscope properly (Box 6-3). Nurses with hearing disorders may purchase stethoscopes with greater sound amplification and may need to ask colleagues to verify some findings through auscultation. It is essential to place the stethoscope directly on the patient's skin because clothing obscures and changes sound.

Through auscultation the nurse notes the following characteristics of sound:

Frequency: Number of sound wave cycles generated per second by a vibrating object. The higher the frequency, the higher the pitch of a sound and vice versa.

Loudness: Amplitude of a sound wave. Auscultated sounds are described as loud or soft.

Quality: Sounds of similar frequency and loudness from different sources. Terms such as blowing or gurgling describe quality of sound.

Duration: Length of time that sound vibrations last. Duration of sound is short, medium, or long. Layers of soft tissue dampen the duration of sounds from deep internal organs.

A nurse cannot be successful at auscultation without knowing how to use a stethoscope properly. Chapter 5 describes the parts of the acoustic stethoscope and use of the bell and diaphragm.

Olfaction uses the sense of smell to detect abnormalities that go unrecognized by any other means. Some alterations in body function and certain bacteria create characteristic odors (Table 6-3).

PREPARATION FOR ASSESSMENT

The process of assessment begins the moment you see the patient and continues with each care encounter. Always be aware of the patient's health history and the reason for seeking care. Also be alert for any changes or problems that have developed since the last assessment.

Preparation of the environment, equipment, and patient promotes a smooth assessment. To promote patient comfort and efficiency it is essential to provide privacy for the patient (e.g., a separate room; curtains or dividers to enclose the patient's bed; or in the home, use a bedroom). A comfortable environment includes a warm, comfortable temperature; a loose-fitting gown or pajamas for the patient; adequate direct lighting; control of outside noises; and precautions to prevent interruptions by visitors or other health care personnel. If possible, place the bed or examination table at waist level so that you can assess the patient easily.

Preparing the Patient

Prepare the patient both physically and psychologically for an accurate assessment. A tense, anxious patient may have difficulty understanding, following directions, or cooperating with your instructions. To prepare the patient:

1 Make patient comfortable by allowing the opportunity to empty the bowel or bladder (a good time to collect needed specimens).

2 Provide privacy.

3 Minimize patient's anxiety and fear by conveying an open, receptive, and professional approach. Using simple terms, thoroughly explain what you will do, what the patient should expect to feel, and how the patient can cooperate. Even if the patient appears unresponsive, it is still essential to explain your actions.

4 Provide access to body parts while draping areas that are not being examined.

5 Reduce distractions. Turn down volume or turn off radio/television.

6 Eliminate drafts, control room temperature, and provide warm blankets.

7 Help the patient assume positions during the assessment so that body parts are accessible and the patient stays comfortable (Table 6-4). A patient's ability to assume positions will depend on physical strength and limitations. Some positions are uncomfortable or embarrassing; keep a patient in position no longer than is necessary.

8 Pace assessment according to the patient's physical and emotional tolerance.

TABLE 6-3	Assessment of Characteristic Odors	
Odor	**Site or Source**	**Potential Causes**
Alcohol	Oral cavity	Ingestion of alcohol; diabetes
Ammonia	Urine	Urinary tract infection, renal failure
Body odor	Skin, particularly in areas where body parts rub together (e.g., under arms, breasts, perineal area)	Poor hygiene, excess perspiration (hyperhidrosis), foul-smelling perspiration (bromhidrosis)
	Wound site	Wound abscess
	Vomitus	Abdominal irritation, contaminated food
Feces	Vomitus/oral cavity (fecal odor)	Bowel obstruction
	Rectal area	Fecal incontinence
Foul-smelling stools in infant	Stool	Malabsorption syndrome
Halitosis	Oral cavity	Poor dental and oral hygiene, gum disease
Sweet, fruity ketones	Oral cavity	Diabetic acidosis
Stale urine	Skin	Uremic acidosis
Sweet, heavy, thick odor	Draining wound	*Pseudomonas* (bacterial) infection
Musty odor	Casted body part	Infection inside cast
Fetid, sweet odor	Tracheostomy or mucus secretions	Infection of bronchial tree (*Pseudomonas* bacteria)

TABLE 6-4 | Positions for Physical Assessment

Position	Areas Assessed	Rationale	Limitations
Sitting	Head and neck, back, posterior thorax and lungs, anterior thorax and lungs, breasts, axillae, heart, vital signs, and upper extremities	Sitting upright provides full expansion of lungs and provides better visualization of symmetry of upper body parts.	Physically weakened or developmentally disabled patient is sometimes unable to sit. Use supine position with head of bed elevated instead.
Supine	Head and neck, anterior thorax and lungs, breasts, axillae, heart, abdomen, extremities, pulses	This is most normally relaxed position. It provides easy access to pulse sites.	If patient becomes short of breath easily, raise head of bed.
Dorsal recumbent	Head and neck, anterior thorax and lungs, breasts, axillae, heart, abdomen	Position is for abdominal assessment because it promotes relaxation of abdominal muscles.	Patients with painful disorders are more comfortable with knees flexed.
Lithotomy	Female genitalia and genital tract	This position provides maximal exposure of genitalia and facilitates insertion of vaginal speculum.	Lithotomy position is embarrassing and uncomfortable, so examiner minimizes time that patient spends in it. Keep patient well draped. Patients with arthritis or other joint deformities may be unable to tolerate the position.
Sims'	Rectum and vagina	Flexion of hip and knee improves exposure of rectal and genitourinary areas.	Joint deformities hinder patient's ability to bend hip and knee.
Prone	Musculoskeletal system	This position is for assessing extension of hip joint, skin, and buttocks.	Patients with respiratory difficulties do not tolerate this position well.
Lateral recumbent	Heart	This position aids in detecting murmurs.	Patients with respiratory difficulties do not tolerate this position well.
Knee-chest	Rectum	This position provides maximal exposure of rectal area.	This position is embarrassing and uncomfortable. Patients with arthritis or other joint deformities may be unable to assume position.

9 Use a relaxed voice tone and facial expressions to put patient at ease.

10 Encourage the patient to ask questions and report discomfort felt during the examination.

11 Have a third person of the patient's gender in the room during assessment of genitalia. This prevents the patient from accusing the nurse of behaving in an unethical manner.

12 At conclusion of the assessment, ask the patient if there are any concerns or questions.

PHYSICAL ASSESSMENT OF VARIOUS AGE-GROUPS

Children and Adolescents

1 Routine assessments of children focus on health promotion and illness prevention (Hockenberry and Wilson, 2007). Focus on growth and development, vision and hearing screening, dental examination, and behavioral assessment.

2 It is helpful to gain a child's trust before doing any type of an examination. Talk and play with the child first. It also helps to perform parts of the examination that you can do visually before actually touching the child.

3 Children will feel safer during an examination if it is initiated from the periphery and then moves to the central. For example, examine the extremities before moving to the chest.

4 Children who are chronically ill, disabled, in foster care, or adopted from a foreign country may require additional assessment because of their unique health risks.

5 When obtaining histories of infants and children, gather all or part of the information from parents or guardians.

6 Parents may think they are being tested or judged by the examiner. Offer support during examination, and do not pass judgment.

7 Call children by their preferred name, and address parents as "Mr. and Mrs. Brown" rather than by first names.

8 Open-ended questions often allow parents to share more information and to describe more of the child's problems.

9 Older children and adolescents tend to respond best when treated as adults and individuals and often can provide details about their health history and severity of symptoms.

10 The adolescent has a right to confidentiality. After talking with parents about historical information, arrange to be alone with the adolescent to speak further privately and to perform the examination. It is recommended to use a chaperone.

Older Adults

1 Do not assume that aging is always accompanied by illness or disability. Older adults are able to adapt to change and maintain functional independence (Meiner and Lueckenotte, 2006).

2 Allow extra time, and be patient, relaxed, and unhurried with older adults.

3 Provide adequate space for an examination, particularly if the patient uses a mobility aid.

4 Plan the history and examination, taking into account the older adult's energy level, physical limitations, pace, and adaptability. More than one session is sometimes necessary to complete the assessment (Meiner and Lueckenotte, 2006).

5 Measure performance under the most favorable conditions. Take advantage of natural opportunities for assessment (e.g., during bathing, grooming, mealtime) (Meiner and Lueckenotte, 2006).

6 Sequence an examination to keep position changes to a minimum. Be efficient throughout the examination to limit patient movement.

7 Be sure an examination of an older adult includes review of mental status.

CULTURAL CONSIDERATIONS

Respect cultural differences when completing an examination. It is important to remember that cultural differences influence a patient's behaviors. Consider the patient's health beliefs, use of alternative therapies, nutritional habits, relationships with family, and comfort with your physical closeness during the history and examination.

- Learn to use open-ended questions to assess sociocultural and religious values that influence health/illness beliefs and practices.
- Communicate respect through proper use of distance, attention, eye contact, tone, and loudness of voice.
- Use a professional interpreter familiar with the patient's culture and language.

- Allow time for responses.
- Observe language and communication patterns of patients.
- Work with the established family hierarchy as identified by the patient.
- Develop knowledge of words that are offensive to the culture. For example, some Southeast Asian groups do not use words such as vagina, penis, and breasts because they find them offensive.
- Assess meaning of symptoms to the patient and family.
- Write down patient's own words to describe these meanings.
- Obtain prior knowledge of health risks common to the cultural group.
- Certain diseases are prevalent in some groups. For example, malaria is prevalent among Africans and Asians and parasitic worms are prevalent among migrants from the Third World.
- Integrate knowledge of cultural differences in growth and development, physical characteristics, and norms in interpreting assessment data.
- Biological/racial characteristics influence physical traits such as skin and mucosal color, hair texture/color, and height and weight.
- Recognize Mongolian spots common among infants and children of color as physiological differences in skin pigmentation rather than ecchymosis (bruising).
- Develop awareness of healing modalities used by some cultures, especially Asians, which may leave the skin discolored or scratched, such as cupping, coining, and pinching.
  - These treatments are for expelling bad wind and restoring balance in cold conditions.
  - In cupping, the skin appears reddened initially because of the application of heated cups, which changes to ecchymotic or discolored circular spots after a few days. The skin returns to normal color after a week.
  - In coining, heated oil is rubbed on the skin, and the edge of a coin is scratched against the skin, leaving superficial scratch marks on the chest and back.
  - After rubbing the skin with warm oil, it is pinched symmetrically and appears reddened after the treatment (Seidel and others, 2006).
- It is not unusual for patients from ethnocultural groups to ask for a family member to be present during the examination to interpret for them or provide moral support.
- Accommodate patient's request for presence of family member.
- Carefully weigh questions you ask in the presence of the family member because patients from collectivistic groups often provide only safe answers in the presence of family members.
- Use gender-congruent providers to perform the physical assessment.
- Ask permission before you touch the patient (Box 6-4).
- Drape the patient thoroughly, and use the bedside screen or curtains.

EVIDENCE-BASED PRACTICE TRENDS

Health Promotion: A Balanced Approach to Sun Exposure

Melanoma caused approximately 10,850 deaths in 2007; other skin cancer–related deaths were estimated to reach 2,740 (ACS, 2008a). There are several risk factors for melanoma: major factors are positive family history of melanoma, a prior melanoma, and multiple or unusual moles (nevi). Other factors include fair complexion/skin that is sensitive to the sun; excessive exposure to the sun (especially before age 18), and the use of tanning beds/booths. Research has indicated that skin can-

BOX 6-4 Cultural Awareness of Touch During Physical Examination

Physical contact with a patient can convey a variety of meanings, depending on the patient's cultural background. Consider these guidelines, but remember that each patient is an individual and may respond differently.

Hispanics
- Highly tactile
- Very modest (men and women)
- May ask for health care provider of same gender
- Women may refuse to be examined by male health care provider

Asians/Pacific Islanders
- Avoid touching (patting head is strictly taboo)
- Touching during an argument equals loss of control (shame)

- Public display of affection toward members of same gender is permissible (but not toward members of opposite gender)

African Americans
- May not like to be touched without permission
- May exercise level of distrust or caution initially with care provider

American Indians
- Shake hands lightly
- May not like to be touched without permission
- Nonverbal communication is important

Data from Meiner SE, Lueckenotte A: *Gerontologic nursing*, ed 3, St. Louis, 2006, Mosby; Seidel HM and others: *Mosby's guide to physical examination*, ed 6, St. Louis, 2006, Mosby.

cer, when detected early and treated properly, is highly curable. Overall survival rates for melanoma at the 5-year mark are 92% with 99% for localized melanoma; when it is grouped in regional and distant stages, the survival rates dramatically decrease (ACS, 2008a). Therefore early intervention is of utmost importance.

The results from research studies have made it a nursing responsibility to promote self-screening for all patients and their family members. Instruct your patients to conduct a complete monthly self-examination of the skin and scalp, noting nevi, blemishes, and birthmarks. They can perform the examination after a bath or shower, including a head-to-toe check. Use a well-lit room and mirrors to examine all skin surfaces. If necessary, have the patient ask a family member/significant other to aid in the investigation. The ACS (2008b) outlines the warning signs of skin cancer using the ABCD mnemonic: *A* is for Asymmetry—look for uneven shape; *B* is for Border irregularity—look for edges that are blurred, notched, or ragged; *C* is for Color—pigmentation is not uniform; blue, black, brown variegated, tan, or areas of unusual colors such as pink, white, gray, or red; and *D* is for Diameter—greater than the size of a typical pencil eraser. Also, teach your patients to contact their health care provider if a skin lesion or nevi starts to bleed or ooze or feels different (swollen, hard, lumpy, itchy, or tender to the touch). Especially instruct older adults, who tend to have delayed wound healing. Inform your patients of ways to prevent skin cancer by avoiding overexposure to the sun:
- Wear sunglasses
- Wear wide-brimmed hats that shade the ears, neck, and face; wear long sleeves and long pants.
- Apply broad-spectrum sunscreens with SPF of 15 or greater to protect against ultraviolet B (UVB) and ultraviolet A (UVA) rays approximately 30 minutes to 1 hour before going into the sun and after swimming, perspiring, or bathing.
- Avoid tanning under the direct sun at midday (10 AM to 4 PM).
- Do not use indoor sunlamps or tanning beds because these are sources of UV radiation.

Also, inform patients who are on mediations that make the skin more sensitive to the sun (e.g., oral contraceptives, antibiotics, antiinflammatories, immunosuppressives, antihypertensives) to take extra precautions when spending time in the sun. Inform patients to protect their children from the sun. Severe sunburns in childhood greatly increase melanoma risk later in life (ACS, 2008b). These interventions will provide the patient with self-screening measures to detect, prevent, and seek early treatment for

skin cancer. More information is available at the American Cancer Society website at http://www.cancer.org.

Data from American Cancer Society: *Cancer facts and figures 2008*, Atlanta, 2008a, The Society; and American Cancer Society: *Cancer prevention and early detection facts and figures 2008*, Atlanta, 2008b, The Society.

Skill Performance Guidelines

1 Prioritize the assessment based on a patient's presenting signs and symptoms or health care needs. For example, for a patient who develops sudden shortness of breath, first assess the lungs and thorax. If a patient is acutely ill, you may choose to assess only the involved body systems. Use judgment to ensure that an examination is relevant and inclusive.

2 Organize the examination. Compare both sides of the body for symmetry. If a patient becomes fatigued, offer rest periods. Perform painful procedures near the end of the examination.

3 Use a head-to-toe approach following the sequence of inspection, palpation, percussion, and auscultation (except during the abdominal assessment). This sequence facilitates an effective assessment.

4 Encourage the patient to actively participate. Patients usually know about their physical condition. Often the patient can let you know when certain findings are normal or when actual changes have occurred.

5 Always identify the patient using established agency policy.

6 Follow standard precautions for infection control. During an assessment, you may have contact with body fluids and discharge. Always wear clean gloves when there are breaks in the skin, lesions, or wounds, or when having contact with mucous membranes. In some circumstances you will need to wear a gown.

7 Consider the possibility of latex allergy. The incidence of serious allergic reaction to latex has increased dramatically (Seidel and others, 2006).

8 Record quick notes to facilitate accurate documentation.

9 Use assessment skills during each patient contact, including activities such as bathing, administration of medications, or other therapies or while conversing with a patient.

10 Integrate health promotion and education into physical assessment activities. There are "teachable moments" when you can share findings and educate patients about health promotion.

11 Record a summary of the assessment using appropriate medical terminology and in the sequence that you gather the findings. Use commonly accepted medical abbreviations to keep notes concise.

SKILL 6-1   General Survey

The general survey begins a review of the patient's primary health problems, and it includes assessment of the patient's vital signs, height and weight, general behavior, and appearance. The survey provides information about characteristics of an illness, a patient's hygiene, skin condition and body image, emotional state, recent changes in weight, and developmental status. The survey reveals important information about the patient's behavior that influences how you will communicate instructions to the patient and continue the assessment.

Delegation Considerations

The general survey cannot be delegated to nursing assistive personnel (NAP). The nurse directs the NAP to:

- Measure the patient's height and weight.
- Obtain vital signs (not the initial set, but subsequent measurements if patient is stable).
- Monitor oral intake and urinary output.
- Report a patient's subjective signs and symptoms to the nurse.

Equipment
- ❑ Stethoscope
- ❑ Sphygmomanometer and cuff
- ❑ Thermometer
- ❑ Digital watch or wristwatch with second hand
- ❑ Tape measure
- ❑ Clean gloves

STEP	RATIONALE

ASSESSMENT

1 Note if patient has had any acute distress: difficulty breathing, pain, anxiety. If such signs are present, reschedule general survey.

Signs establish priorities regarding what part of the examination to conduct first.

Critical Decision Point   *Findings may change the direction of the examination. Any patient in acute distress will require an immediate assessment of the body system(s) affected.*

2 Review graphic sheet for temperature, pulse, respirations, and blood pressure, and consider factors or conditions that will alter reading of vital signs (see Chapter 5).

Provides baseline and historical data regarding patient's vital signs.

3 Determine patient's primary language. If you identify a need for an interpreter, it is best to obtain services of a professional interpreter rather than a family member. Have the interpreter translate verbatim if possible.

Facilitates the presence of an interpreter familiar with medical terminology. If possible, have interpreter of the same gender and one who is older.

4 Reconfirm (after reviewing history) primary reason patient has sought health care.

Keeps assessment focused on patient to ensure that patient's expectations are addressed.

5 Identify patient's normal height and weight. If a sudden gain or loss in weight has occurred, determine amount of weight change and period of time in which it occurred. Assess if patient has recently been dieting or following an exercise program. Use growth chart for children age 18 and under.

Generally, weight of 10% to 20% above standard indicates excess body fat (Moore, 2005); however, fluid retention is one factor that must be ruled out. A person's weight can fluctuate daily because of fluid loss or retention (1 L of water weighs 1 kg, or 2.2 lb).

6 Review patient's past fluid intake and output (I&O) records.

Fluid and electrolyte balance maintains health and function in all body systems. Intake includes all liquids taken orally, by feeding tube, and parenterally. Liquid output includes urine, diarrhea stool, fistulas, vomitus, drainage from gastric suction, and drainage from postsurgical tubes, such as chest tubes or Jackson-Pratt drains.

7 Identify patient's general perceptions about personal health.

Assessment of patient's general appearance coupled with patient's own perceptions may reveal specific problem areas.

8 Assess for evidence of latex allergy, which includes contact dermatitis or systemic reactions. Ask if patient has risk factors such as food allergies (papaya, avocado, banana, peach, kiwi, tomato); high latex exposure (housekeepers, food handlers, health care worker); or must avoid products containing latex (rubber bands, adhesive tape, certain paints or carpets).

These are risk factors for latex allergy. Gloves will be worn during certain aspects of the assessment. Repeated exposure to latex may result in more serious reactions, including asthma, itching, and anaphylaxis (Seidel and others, 2006).

NURSING DIAGNOSES

- Anxiety
- Bathing/hygiene self-care deficit
- Deficient fluid volume or excess fluid volume
- Fear

- Imbalanced nutrition: less than body requirements or more than body requirements
- Impaired bed mobility
- Impaired physical mobility

- Impaired skin integrity
- Ineffective breathing pattern
- Ineffective peripheral tissue perfusion
- Pain (acute, chronic)

Individualize related factors based on patient's condition or needs.

STEP	RATIONALE

PLANNING

1 Expected outcomes following completion of procedure:
  • Patient demonstrates alert, cooperative behavior without evidence of physical or emotional distress during assessment.
  • Patient provides appropriate subjective data related to physical condition.

Nurse uses calm and confident approach during assessment. Patient has no abnormal findings.

Patient able to cooperate with assessment.

2 *Prepare patient:* Tell the patient you will be doing a routine process to check for areas of concern. Ask patient to tell you if any area you examine hurts when touched.

Understanding promotes patient's cooperation. Pain is an important finding during assessment.

IMPLEMENTATION

1 Throughout assessment note patient's verbal and nonverbal behaviors. Determine the level of consciousness and orientation by observing and talking to patient (Box 6-5, p. 120).

Behaviors may reflect specific physical abnormalities. Dementia and level of consciousness influence ability to cooperate.

2 Obtain temperature, pulse, respirations, and blood pressure unless taken within last 3 hours or if you notice a serious change (e.g., change in level of consciousness or difficulty breathing) (see Chapter 5). Inform patient of vital signs.

Vital signs provide important information regarding physiological changes in relation to oxygenation and circulation.

3 Observe the following aspects of appearance: gender, race, and age. Note the patient's physical features.

Gender influences type of examination performed and manner in which you make assessments. Different physical characteristics and predisposition to illnesses are related to gender and race.

4 If uncertain whether patient understands a question, rephrase or ask a similar question.

Inappropriate response from a patient may be caused by language or deterioration of mental status, preoccupation with illness, or decreased hearing acuity.

5 If a patient's responses are inappropriate, ask short, to-the-point questions regarding information the patient should know, for example: "Tell me your name." "What is the name of this place?" "Tell me where you live." "What day is this?" "What month is this?" or "What season of the year is this?"

Measures patient's orientation to person, place, and time. Note this in documentation as "Oriented × 3." If disoriented in any way, include subjective and/or objective data rather than just documenting "disoriented."

6 If patient is unable to respond to questions of orientation, offer simple commands, for example, "Squeeze my fingers" or "Move your toes."

Levels of consciousness exist along a continuum including full responsiveness, inability to consciously initiate meaningful behaviors, and unresponsiveness to stimuli.

7 Assess affect and mood: note if verbal expressions match nonverbal behavior and if appropriate to situation.

Reflects patient's mental status, consciousness, feelings, and emotional status.

8 Observe patient interaction with spouse or partner, older adult child, or caregiver. Be alert for indications of fear, hesitancy to report health status, or willingness to let caregiver control assessment interview. Does partner or caregiver have a history of violence, alcoholism, or drug abuse? Is the person unemployed, ill, or frustrated with caring for patient? Note if patient has any obvious physical injuries.

Suspect abuse in patients who have suffered obvious physical injury or neglect, show signs of malnutrition, or have ecchymoses (bruises) on the extremities or trunk. Some partners or caregivers have history of abusive or addictive behaviors.

Critical Decision Point *Be discreet in how you conduct the interview. Ask direct questions about abuse in private. It is often necessary to delay assessment to a later time, when the partner or caregiver is not present. Asking a partner or caregiver to leave during an assessment creates an awkward situation. Patients are more likely to reveal any problems when the suspected abuser is absent from the room (Kovach, 2004).*

9 Observe for signs of abuse:
  a *For a child:* Blood on underclothing, pain in genital area, difficulty sitting or walking, pain while urinating, vaginal or penile discharge pain, itching or unusual color in genital area. Physical injury inconsistent with parent's or caregiver's account of how injury occurred.

Suggestive of child physical abuse (Anbarghalami and others, 2007; Dougherty, 2006).

  b *For a female patient:* Injury or trauma inconsistent with reported cause, obvious injuries to head, face, neck, breasts, abdomen, and genitalia (black eyes, abrasions, bruises/welts, broken nose, lacerations, broken teeth, strangulation marks, burns, human bites, orbital fractures, fractured skull).

Indicates domestic abuse (Kovach, 2004). These signs also apply to male patient being abused by female partner.

STEP	RATIONALE

c *For an older adult:* Injury or trauma inconsistent with reported cause, injuries in unusual locations (such as neck or genitalia), pattern injuries (left when an object with which a person is struck leaves an imprint), parallel injuries (such as bilateral ecchymosis on the upper arms suggesting the patient was held and shaken), burns (shaped like a cigarette, iron, rope, or immersion with a clear line of demarcation), fractures, poor hygiene, and poor nutrition.

Indicates elder abuse/neglect (Geroff and Olshaker, 2006; Muehlbauer and Crane, 2006). Prolonged interval between injury and time patient sought medical care is also indicative of older adult abuse or neglect.

Critical Decision Point *A pattern of findings indicating abuse usually mandates a report to a social service center (refer to state guidelines). Obtain immediate consultation with physician, social worker, and other support staff to facilitate placement in a safer environment.*

10 Assess posture and position, noting alignment of shoulders and hips while patient stands and/or sits. Observe whether the patient has a slumped, erect, or bent posture (see illustration).

Reveals musculoskeletal problem, mood, or presence of pain.

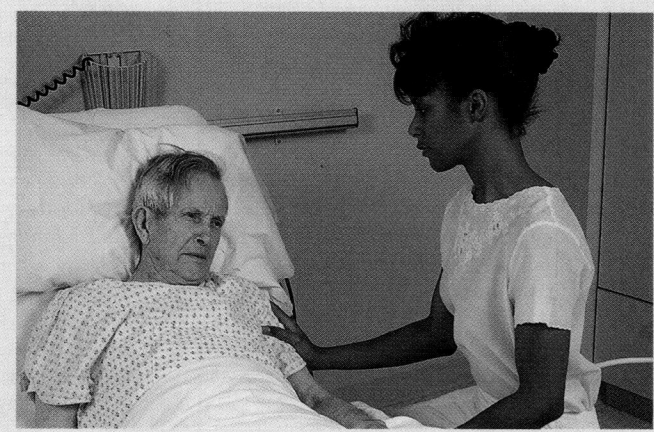

STEP 10 Observe patient's position and posture.

a Assess body movements. Are they purposeful? Are there tremors of the extremities? Are any body parts immobile? Are movements coordinated or uncoordinated?

11 Assess speech. Is it understandable and moderately paced? Is there an association with the person's thoughts?

Alterations reflect neurological impairment, injury or impairment of mouth, improperly fitting dentures, differences in dialect or language, and some mental illnesses.

12 Observe hygiene and grooming for presence or absence of makeup, type of clothes (hospital or personal), and cleanliness.

Grooming reflects activity level before examination, resources available to purchase grooming supplies, patient's mood, and self-care practices. May also reflect culture, lifestyle, economic status, and personal preferences.

a Observe the color, distribution, quantity, thickness, texture, and lubrication of hair.

Changes in hair distribution reflect hormonal changes, changes from aging, poor nutrition, or use of certain hair care products.

b Inspect the condition of nails (hands and feet).

Changes indicate inadequate nutrition or grooming practices, nervous habits, or systemic diseases.

c Assess the presence or absence of body odor.

Body odor may result from physical exercise, deficient hygiene, or physical or mental abnormalities. Inadequate oral hygiene or unhealthy teeth cause bad breath.

13 Inspect exposed areas of the skin, and ask if patient has noted any changes in the skin, including:
a Pruritus, oozing, bleeding

Incidence of melanoma, an aggressive form of skin cancer, has increased significantly. It is more than 10 times higher in whites than in African Americans (ACS, 2008a). The cancer can spread to other parts of the body quickly. Early detection and prompt treatment are critical (Box 6-6, p. 121).

STEP	RATIONALE

    b Change in the appearance of a mole (nevus), bump, or nodule; a change in sensation; itchiness, tenderness, or pain

    c Petechiae (pinpoint-size red or purple spots on the skin caused by small hemorrhages in the skin layers)

Petechiae indicate serious blood clotting disorder, drug reaction, or liver disease.

14 Inspect skin surfaces, comparing color of symmetrical body parts. Scan the entire body, noting areas unexposed to sun. Look for any patches or areas of skin color variation.

Changes in color are indicative of pathological alterations (Table 6-5, p. 121).

Critical Decision Point   *Be alert for basal cell carcinomas, such as an open sore that does not heal, shiny nodule, a pink or reddish growth, or scarlike area. These are often seen in sun-exposed areas and frequently occur in sun-damaged skin.*

15 Carefully inspect color of face, oral mucosa, lips, conjunctiva, sclera, and nail beds.

Abnormalities are easier to identify in areas of body where melanin production is lowest.

Critical Decision Point   *When assessing the skin of a patient with bandages, cast, restraints, or other restrictive devices, note areas of pallor and decreased temperature, which indicates impaired circulation. Immediate release of pressure from the restrictive device is often necessary.*

16 Use ungloved fingertips to palpate skin surfaces to feel moisture of intact skin.

Moisture is directly related to degree of hydration and condition of outer lipid layer of the skin surface. Older adults are prone to xerosis, which is evident as dry, scaly skin (Meiner and Lueckenotte, 2006).

    a Stroke skin surfaces lightly with fingertips to detect texture of skin's surface. Note whether skin is smooth or rough, thick or thin, tight or supple and if localized areas of hardness or lesions are present.

Localized texture changes result from trauma, surgical wounds, or lesions.

    b Palpate any areas that appear irregular in texture.

Allows detection of localized areas of hardness and/or tenderness within subcutaneous skin layers.

Critical Decision Point   *If patient receives routine injections (e.g., insulin, heparin), localized areas of hardness are usually over injection sites. Develop a plan to rotate injection sites systematically. Site rotation prevents local skin changes from repeated injections (Monahan and others, 2007; Roberts, 2007).*

17 While wearing clean gloves, inspect character of any secretions; note color, odor, amount, and consistency (e.g., thin and watery, thick and oily). Remove gloves.

Character of secretions from skin lesions helps to indicate type of lesion, presence of infection, or wound healing.

18 Using dorsum (back) of hand, palpate for temperature of skin surfaces. (If wearing a glove, remove temporarily.) Compare symmetrical body parts. Compare upper and lower body parts. Note distinct temperature differences. Note localized areas of warmth.

The skin of a stage I pressure ulcer is warm and erythematous (redness). Environmental temperature and anxiety affect skin temperature. Skin temperature reflects increase or decrease in blood flow. Skin on dorsum of hand is thin, which allows detection of subtle temperature changes.

STEP	RATIONALE

19 Assess skin turgor by grasping fold of skin on the sternum or forearm with the fingertips. Release skinfold, and note ease and speed with which skin returns to place (see illustration).

With reduced turgor, skin remains suspended or "tented" for a few seconds before slowly returning to place. This indicates decreased elasticity and possible dehydration (Elkin and others, 2007). Altered turgor increases the patient's risk for pressure ulcers, and it is essential to provide preventive measures.

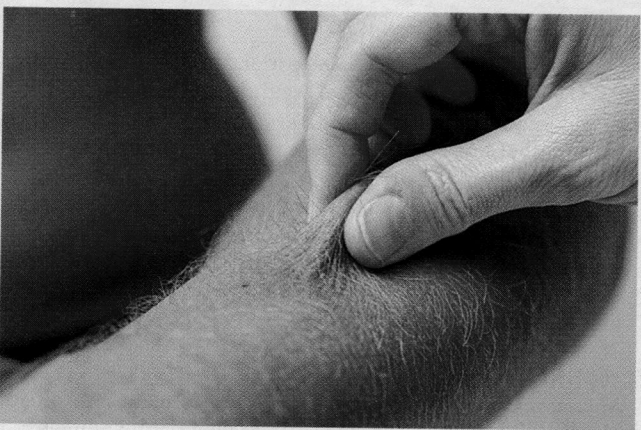

STEP 19   Checking skin turgor.

20 Assess condition of skin for pressure areas, paying particular attention to regions of pressure (e.g., sacrum, greater trochanter, heels, occipital area, clavicles). If you notice areas of redness, place fingertip over area and apply gentle pressure, then release.

Normal reactive hyperemia (redness) is the visible effect of localized vasodilation, body's normal response to lack of blood flow to underlying tissue. Affected area of skin will blanch with fingertip pressure.

Critical Decision Point *With evidence of normal reactive hyperemia, reposition the patient and develop a turning schedule if patient is dependent (see Chapter 18).*

21 When you detect a lesion, use adequate lighting to inspect its color, location, texture, size, shape, and type (Box 6-7, p. 122). Note also grouping (e.g., clustered, linear) and distribution (localized or generalized).

You identify certain skin lesions by a characteristic pattern of features.

  a Gently palpate any lesion to determine mobility, contour (flat, raised, or depressed), and consistency (soft or hard). If lesion is moist or draining, apply clean gloves before palpation.

Gentle palpation prevents accidental rupture of underlying cysts. Gloves reduce transmission of microorganisms.

  b Note if patient reports tenderness during palpation.

Tenderness indicates possible inflammation or pressure on body part.

  c Measure size of lesion (height, width, and depth) with centimeter ruler.

Provides for baseline to assess changes in lesion over time.

EVALUATION

1 Observe throughout the assessment for evidence of physical or emotional distress.

Interaction during assessment reveals emotional problems. Maneuvers used during physical examination reveal presence of physical problems.

2 Compare assessment findings with previous observations.

Determines if change has occurred.

3 Ask the patient if there is information about physical condition that you have not discussed.

Some patients feel they are bothering you by asking questions unless the opportunity for questions is provided.

Unexpected Outcomes

1 Patient demonstrates acute distress (e.g., respiratory distress, acute pain, severe anxiety).

2 Patient has abnormal skin condition (dry texture, reduced turgor, lesions).

3 Patient is unwilling or unable to provide adequate information relating to identified concerns.

Related Interventions

- Respond immediately to identified need (repositioning, oxygen, or medication as appropriate).
- Obtain vital signs.
- Notify health care provider.

- Identify contributing factors, and prevent continued irritation or damage as appropriate (see Chapter 18).

- Seek information from family members if present.
- Review patient's record for baseline data.

Recording and Reporting

- Record patient's vital signs on vital sign flow sheet.
- Record description of alterations in patient's general appearance.
- Describe patient's behaviors using objective terminology. Include patient's self-report of signs and symptoms.
- Report abnormalities and acute symptoms to nurse in charge or health care provider.

Teaching Considerations

- During general survey, inform patient about normal range of vital signs for age and physical condition and normal weight for height and body frame.
- Explain that it is best to weigh self in the morning after voiding and before eating or drinking.
- If patient is on established diet, discuss any problems patient has in diet preparation or food selection. The best form of weight reduction is to achieve gradual weight loss by increasing exercise and decreasing caloric intake. Refer to clinical dietitian for specific information.

Pediatric Considerations

- Measurement of physical growth is a key element in evaluation of a child's health status. These physical growth parameters include height, length, weight, skinfold thickness, and arm and head circumference (Hockenberry and Wilson, 2007). Use growth charts specific to child's age and condition.
- Weigh infants nude. Weigh children in light underclothes or gown.
- A child's interactions with parents provide valuable information regarding the child's behavior.

Gerontological Considerations

- An older adult's presenting signs and symptoms are sometimes deceiving. An older adult has a diminished physiological reserve that sometimes masks the usual, or "classic," signs and symptoms of a disease. In older adults signs and symptoms are often blunted or atypical (Meiner and Lueckenotte, 2006).

- Nutritional problems are frequently noted in older adults. Skipping meals is a common practice. The amount of nutrition becomes questionable. The following factors pose risks for malnutrition in older adults: fixed income, lack of socialization/loneliness, abuse of alcohol and other central nervous system depressants, confusion, memory loss, forgetfulness, inability to feed self, reduced strength and mobility, decreased vision, and vulnerability to advertising and food fads (Moore, 2005).
- Common skin changes with aging include dryness, wrinkling, reduced elasticity, and "liver spots" in areas exposed to sun. Common lesions include seborrheic keratosis (pigmented macular-papular lesion that are warty, scaly, or greasy); cherry angioma (bright, ruby-red or purplish papular lesion); skin tags (soft pinkish-tan to light-brown pedunculated lesions); and senile lentigines (gray-brown irregular macular lesions on sun-exposed areas) (Meiner and Lueckenotte, 2006).
- Inspection of the feet is critically important in the presence of impaired circulation, impaired vision, and diabetes. Common podiatric conditions include ulceration, fungal infection, corns, calluses, bunions, plantar warts, and hammer toe (Meiner and Lueckenotte, 2006).

Home Care Considerations

- In the home the focus of an examination is often on the patient's ability to perform basic self-care tasks. Be sure that the home assessment builds on all health concerns identified in other settings.

Long-Term Care Considerations

- The Minimum Data Set (MDS) is a tool that includes a comprehensive assessment of residents in the long-term care setting. It provides an ongoing comprehensive assessment of each resident, emphasizing functional ability and both a physical and a psychosocial profile. Only a registered nurse (RN) can function as the assessment coordinator (Meiner and Lueckenotte, 2006). All members of the health team make contributions.

BOX 6-5	Possible Symptoms of Dementia

Learning and Retaining New Information
- Trouble remembering recent conversations, events, and appointments
- Frequently misplaces objects

Language
- Increasing difficulty with expressing self
- Difficulty following conversations

Handling Complex Tasks
- Difficulty following a complex train of thought
- Difficulty performing tasks that require many steps

Behavior
- Appears more passive and less responsive
- More irritable and suspicious than usual
- Misinterprets visual and auditory stimuli

Reasoning Ability
- Unable to develop plan to address problems at work or home
- Displays uncharacteristic disregard for rules of social conduct

Spatial Ability and Orientation
- Difficulty driving
- Difficulty in organizing objects around the house
- Difficulty finding way around familiar places

BOX 6-6 | Malignant Melanoma Mnemonics

The ABCD Rule of Melanoma (ACS, 2007)

Here is a simple way to remember the characteristics that should alert you to the possibility of malignant melanoma.

A *Asymmetry* of lesion
B *Borders:* irregular
C *Color:* blue/black or variegated, pigmentation is not uniform, variations/multiple colors—tan, brown, black; areas of pink, white, gray, blue, or red
D *Diameter* greater than 6 mm

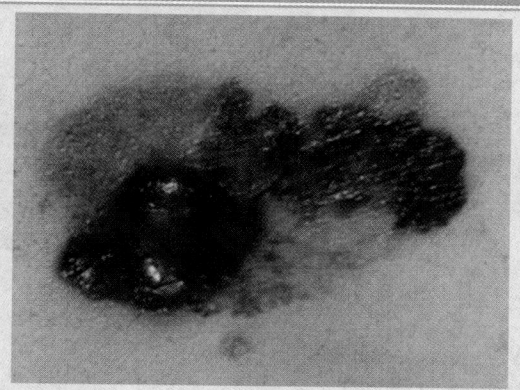

Malignant melanoma. *(From Zitelli B, Davis H: Atlas of pediatric physical diagnosis, ed 5, St. Louis, 2007, Mosby.)*

TABLE 6-5 | Skin Color Variations

Color	Condition	Causes	Assessment Locations
Bluish (cyanosis)	Increased amount of deoxygenated hemoglobin (associated with hypoxia)	Heart or lung disease, cold environment	Nail beds, lips, base of tongue, skin (severe cases)
Pallor (decrease in color)	Reduced amount of oxyhemoglobin Reduced visibility of oxyhemoglobin resulting from decreased blood flow	Anemia Shock	Face, conjunctivae, nail beds, palms of hands Skin, nail beds, conjunctivae, lips
Loss of pigmentation	Vitiligo	Congenital or autoimmune condition causing lack of pigment	Patchy areas on skin over face, hands, arms
Yellow-orange (jaundice)	Increased deposit of bilirubin in tissues	Liver disease, destruction of red blood cells	Sclera, mucous membranes, skin
Red (erythema)	Increased visibility of oxyhemoglobin caused by dilation or increased blood flow	Fever, direct trauma, blushing, alcohol intake	Face, area of trauma, sacrum, shoulders, other common sites for pressure ulcers
Tan-brown	Increased amount of melanin	Suntan, pregnancy	Areas exposed to sun: face, arms; areolae, nipples

BOX 6-7 Types of Primary Skin Lesions

Macule: Flat, nonpalpable change in skin color, smaller than 1.0 cm (e.g., freckle, petechia)

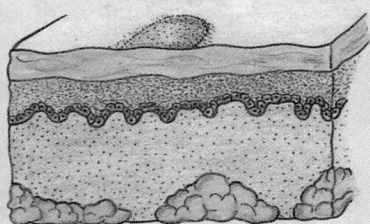

Vesicle: Circumscribed elevation of skin filled with serous fluid, smaller than 0.5 cm (e.g., herpes simplex, chickenpox)

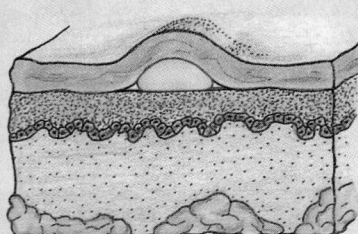

Papule: Palpable, circumscribed, solid elevation in skin, smaller than 0.5 cm (e.g., elevated nevus)

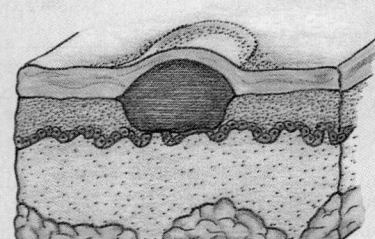

Pustule: Circumscribed elevation of skin similar to vesicle but filled with pus, varies in size (e.g., acne, staphylococcal infection)

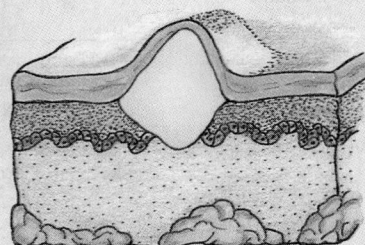

Nodule: Elevated solid mass, deeper and firmer than papule, 0.5 to 2.0 cm (e.g., wart)

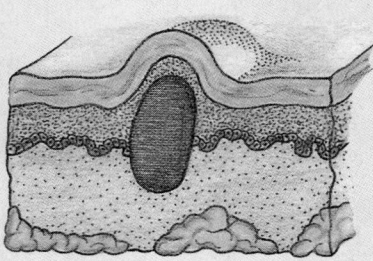

Ulcer: Deep loss of skin surface that may extend to dermis and frequently bleeds and scars, varies in size (e.g., venous stasis ulcer)

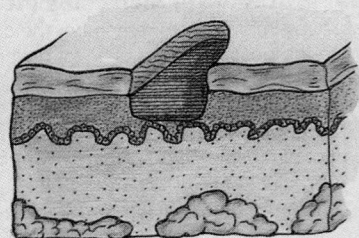

Tumor: Solid mass that may extend deep through subcutaneous tissue, larger than 1.0 to 2.0 cm (e.g., epithelioma)

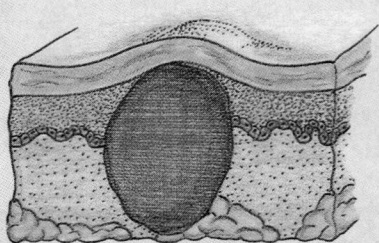

Atrophy: Thinning of skin with loss of normal skin furrow with skin appearing shiny and translucent, varies in size (e.g., arterial insufficiency)

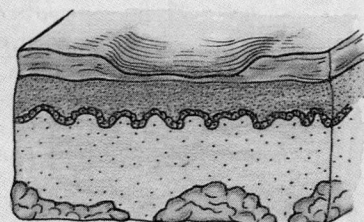

Wheal: Irregularly shaped, elevated area or superficial localized edema, varies in size (e.g., hive, mosquito bite)

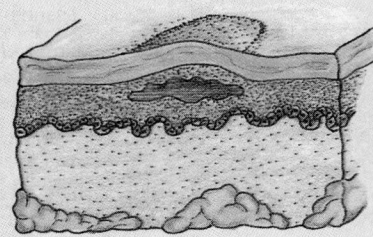

SKILL 6-2 Assessing the Head and Neck

Examination of the head and neck includes assessment of the head, eyes, ears, nose, mouth, and sinuses. Assessment of the head and neck uses inspection, palpation, and auscultation, with inspection and palpation often used simultaneously.

Delegation Considerations

The skills of assessing the head and neck cannot be delegated to NAP. The nurse directs the NAP to:

- Observe for nasal discharge and nasal bleeding.

- Report any findings found during routine care (e.g., oral care, bathing) to the nurse for further assessment.

Equipment

- ❏ Stethoscope
- ❏ Clean gloves
- ❏ Tongue blade
- ❏ Pen light

STEP	RATIONALE
ASSESSMENT	
1 Assess for history of headache, dizziness, pain, or stiffness.	Headaches and dizziness are signs of stress, a symptom of another underlying problem such as high blood pressure, or a result of injury.
2 Determine if the patient has a history of eye disease, diabetes, or hypertension.	Common conditions predispose patients to visual alterations requiring physician referral.
3 Ask if the patient has experienced blurred vision, flashing lights, or reduced visual field.	These common symptoms indicate visual problems.
4 Ask if the patient has experienced ear pain, itching, discharge, vertigo, tinnitus (ringing of the ears), or change in hearing.	These signs and symptoms indicate infection or hearing loss.
5 Review patient's occupational history.	Patient's occupation creates a risk of injury, potential for eye fatigue, or prolonged noise exposure.
6 Ask if the patient has a history of allergies, nasal discharge, epistaxis (nosebleeds), or postnasal drip.	History is useful in determining source of nasal and sinus drainage.
7 Determine if the patient smokes or chews tobacco.	Tobacco users have greater risk for mouth and throat cancer (ACS, 2008a).

NURSING DIAGNOSES

- Deficient knowledge
- Disturbed sensory perception
- Health-seeking behavior
- Impaired oral mucous membranes
- Ineffective health maintenance

Individualize related factors based on patient's condition or needs.

PLANNING	
1 Patient exhibits good visual acuity, normal hearing, moist and intact oral mucosa, and head and neck without masses or lesions. Expected outcomes following completion of procedure:	No abnormalities identified.
• Patient recognizes warning signs and symptoms of eye, ear, sinus, and mouth disease.	Awareness of risks and safety precautions improves compliance with healthful behaviors.
• Patient takes appropriate safety precautions for occupational injury related to the head and neck.	
2 Prepare patient. Tell patient you will be completing a routine examination of the head and neck to check for areas of concerns.	Understanding promotes patient's cooperation.

IMPLEMENTATION	
1 Position patient sitting upright if possible.	Provides for a more thorough examination of the head and neck structures.
2 Inspect the head.	
a Note head position and facial features.	Head tilting to one side indicates hearing or visual loss.
b Note the patient's facial features for symmetry.	Neurological disorders such as paralysis sometimes affect the symmetry of the face.
3 Assess the eyes:	
a Inspect position of eyes, color, condition of conjunctiva, and movement.	Asymmetrical positioning or eye movement reflects trauma or tumor growths. Differences in color are sometimes congenital; changes in color of conjunctiva may be due to local infection or symptomatic of another abnormality (e.g., pale conjunctiva is associated with anemia).

STEP	RATIONALE

b Assess patient's near vision (ability to read newspaper or magazines) and far vision (follow movement, ability to read the clock, television, or signs at a distance).

If patient has visual acuity or visual field loss, make adjustments to support self-care measures (e.g., feeding, bathing and hygiene, dressing) and teaching.

c Inspect pupils for size, shape, and equality (see illustration).

Normal pupils are round, regular, and equal in size and shape.

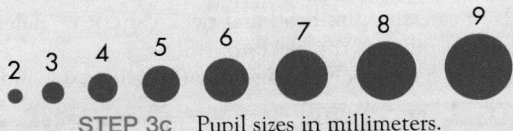

STEP 3c   Pupil sizes in millimeters.

d Test pupillary reflexes. To test reaction to light, dim room lights. If you cannot dim lights, cup hand over eye to temporarily shield the light. As patient looks straight ahead, move penlight from side of patient's face and direct light on pupil. Observe pupillary response of both eyes, noting briskness and equality of reflex (see illustrations).

Darkened room normally ensures brisk response of pupils to light. Pupil that is illuminated constricts. Pupil in other eye should constrict equally (consensual light reflex).

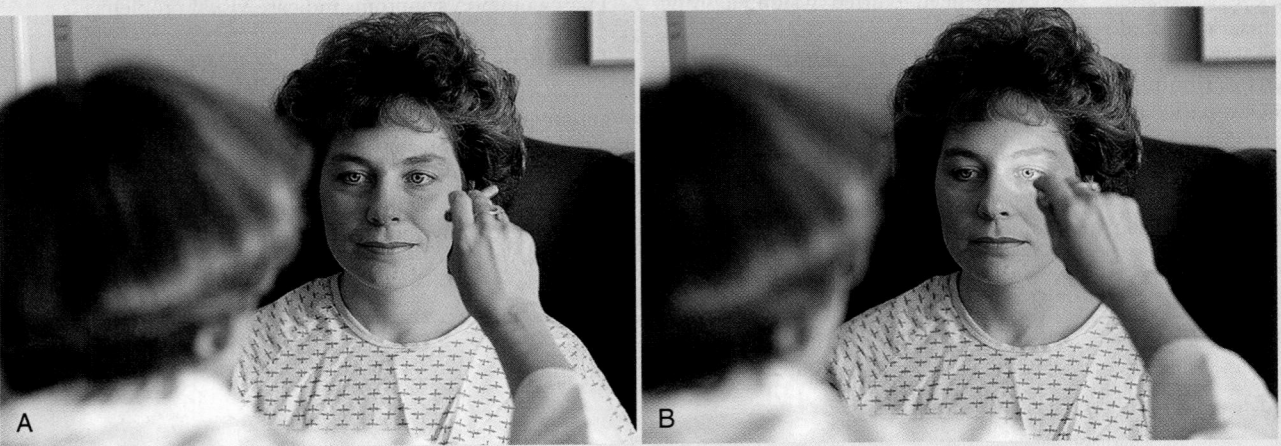

STEP 3d   **A,** Holding penlight to side of patient's face. **B,** Illumination of pupil causes pupillary constriction.

4 Assess hearing. Note the patient's response to questions and the presence/use of a hearing aid. If hearing loss is suspected, test by asking patient to repeat random words spoken by the nurse. Use one- or two-syllable words. Repeat, gradually increasing voice intensity until patient correctly repeats the words.

Seidel and others (2006) report that patients normally hear words or numbers clearly when whispered, responding correctly at least 50% of the time. For patient with obvious hearing impairment, speak clearly and concisely, stand so that patient can see your face, stand toward patient's good ear, speak in low pitch, and avoid yelling.

Critical Decision Point   *If hearing deficit is present, have a qualified nurse inspect patient's ears because impaired hearing may be due to impacted cerumen, external otitis, or swelling in ear canal due to allergic reactions to materials in hearing aids.*

5 Inspect nose externally for shape, skin color, alignment, drainage, and presence of deformity or inflammation. Note color of mucosa and any lesions, discharge, swelling, or presence of bleeding. If drainage appears infectious, consult with health care provider about obtaining a specimen.

Character of discharge and inflammation indicate allergy or infection. Perforation and erosion of the septum and puffiness and/or increased vascularity of the mucosa indicate habitual use of drugs.

6 In patients with a nasogastric, nasointestinal, or nasotracheal tube, inspect nares for excoriation or inflammation. Stabilize tube as needed.

Swallowing or coughing causes movement of tubes against nares, and pressure against tissues and mucosa can result in tissue erosion.

7 Assess the sinuses by palpation over frontal and maxillary areas.

Infection, allergy, or drug use sometimes causes tenderness.

8 Assess the mouth:

a Use a tongue blade to lightly depress the tongue, and inspect the oral cavity with a penlight. Inspect oral mucosa, tongue, teeth, and gums for hydration, discoloration, and obvious lesions (see illustration).

STEP	RATIONALE

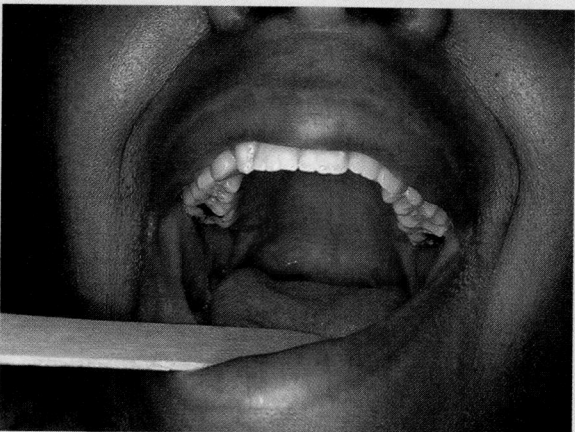

STEP 8a   Inspect mouth.

b Determine if patient wears dentures or retainers and if they are comfortable. Remove dentures to properly visualize and palpate gums.

Ill-fitting dentures and retainers chronically irritate mucosa and gums and put patient at risk for mouth cancer.

9 Inspect and palpate the neck. Ask the patient if there is a history of neck pain or difficulty with movement of the neck.

This determines that all neck structures are present, including neck muscles, lymph nodes of the head and neck, thyroid gland, and trachea. Indicates muscle strain, head injury, local nerve injury, or swollen lymph nodes.

a Neck muscles: Inspect neck for bilateral symmetry of muscles. Ask patient to flex and hyperextend neck and turn head side to side.

Detects muscle weakness, strain, and range of motion (ROM).

b Lymph nodes:

(1) With patient's chin raised and head tilted slightly, inspect area where lymph nodes are distributed and compare both sides (see illustration).

Lymph nodes are sometimes enlarged from infection or from various diseases such as cancer.

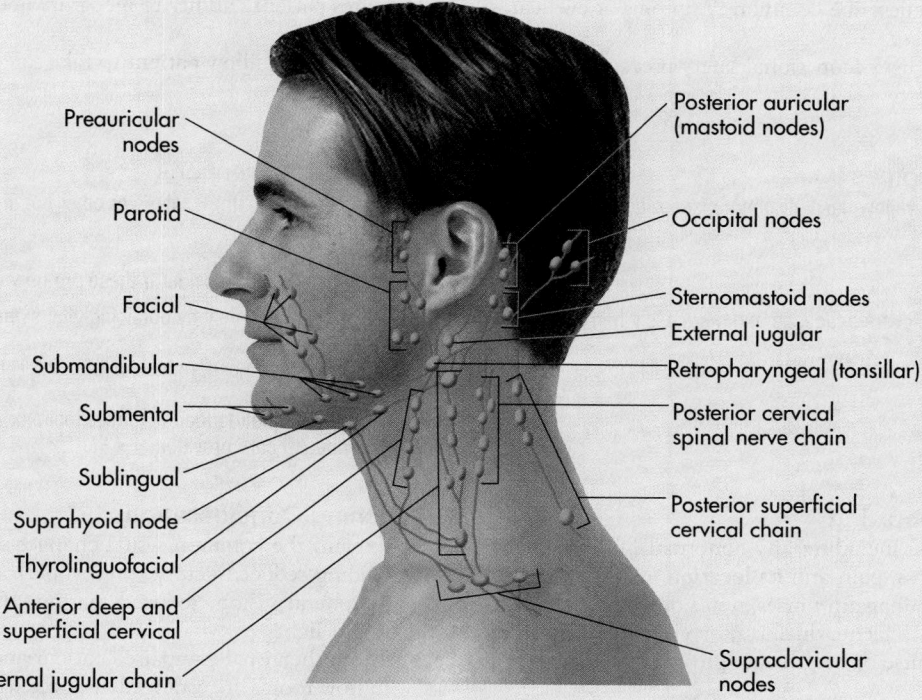

Preauricular nodes

Parotid

Facial

Submandibular

Submental

Sublingual

Suprahyoid node

Thyrolinguofacial

Anterior deep and superficial cervical

Internal jugular chain

Posterior auricular (mastoid nodes)

Occipital nodes

Sternomastoid nodes

External jugular

Retropharyngeal (tonsillar)

Posterior cervical spinal nerve chain

Posterior superficial cervical chain

Supraclavicular nodes

STEP 9b(1)   Palpable lymph nodes of head and neck. (*From Seidel HM and others:* Mosby's guide to physical examination, *ed 6, St. Louis, 2006, Mosby.*)

STEP	RATIONALE

(2) To examine lymph nodes, have patient relax with neck flexed slightly forward. To palpate, face or stand to the side of patient and use pads of middle three fingers of hand. Palpate gently in a rotary motion for superficial lymph nodes (see illustration).

This position relaxes tissues and muscles.

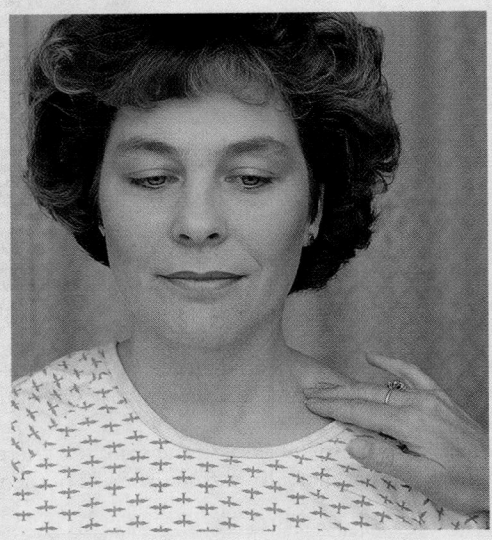

STEP 9b(2)   Palpation of cervical lymph nodes. (*From Elkin M and others:* Nursing interventions and clinical skills, *ed 4, St. Louis, 2007, Mosby.*)

(3) Note if lymph nodes are large, fixed, inflamed, or tender.

Large, fixed, inflamed, or tender lymph nodes indicate local infection, systemic disease, or neoplasm.

EVALUATION

1 Compare assessment findings with previous observations.
2 Ask the patient to describe common symptoms of eye, ear, sinus, or mouth disease.
3 Ask the patient to list occupational safety precautions.

Identifies changes in patient's condition.
Measures patient's ability to recognize abnormalities.

Knowledge will allow patient to take safety precautions.

Unexpected Outcomes

1 Patient demonstrates yellow nasal discharge, sneezing, and complaint of sinus pain.

2 Patient complains of severe headache and dizziness when standing.

Related Interventions

- Reposition into semi-Fowler's or other comfortable position to relieve sinus pain.
- Monitor temperature for fever.
- Notify health care provider if these are new findings.

- Respond immediately by obtaining vital signs, especially blood pressure.
- Return patient to bed in position of comfort to minimize dizziness and relieve headache.
- Identify contributing factors (stress, pain, or elevated blood pressure).
- Notify health care provider.

Recording and Reporting

- Record all findings, including any abnormal findings such as hearing or visual loss, pain and its location, current infection, and character of drainage in nurses' notes or flow sheet.
- Report increased headache, dizziness, or visual changes immediately to charge nurse or health care provider.

Teaching Considerations

- Explain the common visual changes associated with aging, including reduced acuity (presbyopia), loss of or a reduction in peripheral vision, reduced tearing, and sensitivity to glare or bright lights.
- Teach the visually impaired patient and family that adjustments in how rooms are arranged at home will aid in safe ambulation. Self-help aids are available to assist patient with functioning independently with daily activities.

Pediatric Considerations
- Some infants resist eye examination by closing eyes. Holding them in an upright position over their caregivers' shoulders causes eyes to open (Ball and Bindler, 2006).
- Any problem with ocular alignment or visual impairment requires immediate referral to a pediatrician or pediatric ophthalmologist (Engel, 2006).
- Headaches in children are usually caused by loss of sleep, poor nutrition, eye fatigue, and allergies. Children as young as 3 years of age can develop severe migraine headaches, but the symptoms are vague and difficult to diagnose.

Gerontological Considerations
- Older adults commonly have loss of peripheral vision caused by changes in the lens.
- Instruct patients older than age 65 to have regular hearing checks.
- Measurement of visual acuity helps determine level of assistance patient requires with daily living activities and ability of patient to safely ambulate and function independently within home.

SKILL 6-3 Assessing the Thorax and Lungs

Assessment of respiratory function is one of the most critical assessments because alterations can quickly become life threatening. Routine physical assessment is essential because changes in respiration can occur quickly as a result of a variety of factors, including immobility, infection, and fluid overload. Physical assessment includes auscultation, which assesses the movement of air through the tracheobronchial tree. Recognizing the sounds created by normal airflow allows you to detect sounds caused by obstruction of the airways. Assessment also includes inspection, palpation, and percussion.

Auscultation of the lungs requires familiarity with the anatomical landmarks of the chest wall (Fig. 6-3). During the assessment keep a mental image of the location of the lung lobes (Fig. 6-4) and the position of each rib. To locate the position of each rib anteriorly, locate the angle of Louis at the manubriosternal junction, where the second rib articulates with the sternum. Count the ribs and intercostal spaces from this point.

Examination of the lungs and thorax is most effective when the patient is undressed to the waist. Begin with the patient sitting for assessment of the posterior and lateral chest; the patient may sit or lie down for examination of the anterior chest. A female patient may keep a gown draped loosely over her chest while you examine the posterior chest. Good lighting is essential. You will need to assess the patient's ability to tolerate position changes and level of distress. Often a patient confined to bed rest or a patient with chest pain has limited lung expansion.

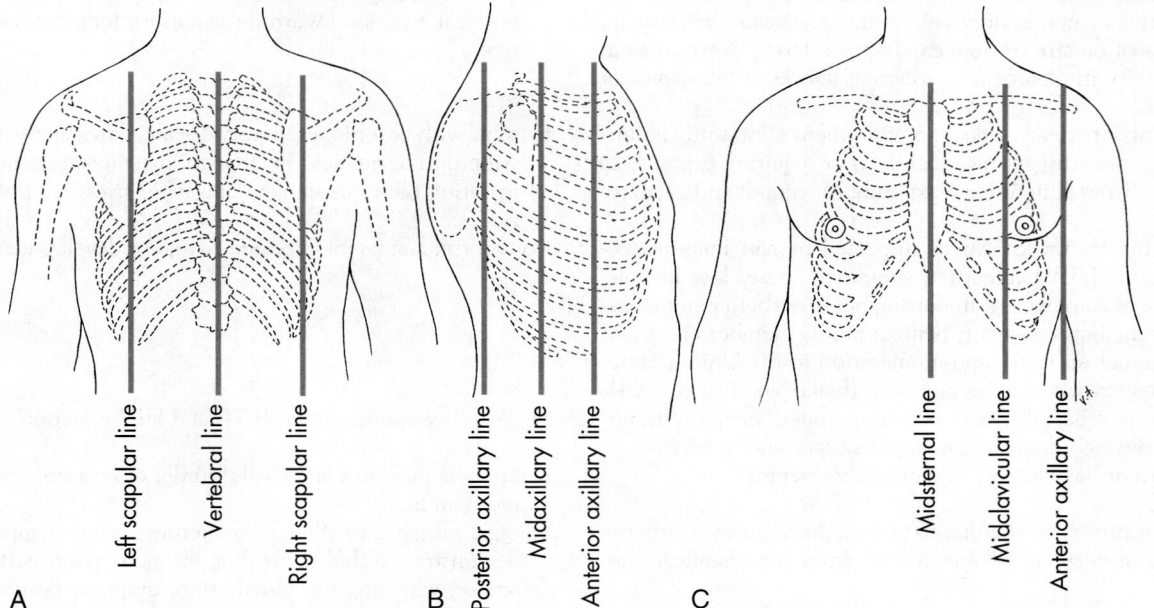

Fig. 6-3 Anatomical landmarks of chest wall. **A,** Posterior view. **B,** Lateral view. **C,** Anterior view.

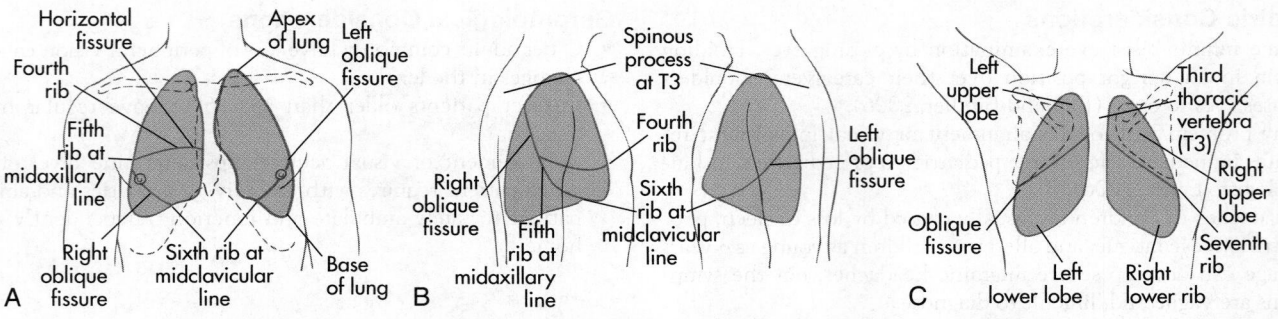

Fig. 6-4 Position of lung lobes in relation to anatomical landmarks. **A,** Anterior. **B,** Lateral. **C,** Posterior.

Delegation Considerations

The skill of assessing the lungs and thorax cannot be delegated to NAP. The nurse directs the NAP to:

- Measure the patient's respirations after determining stability.
- Report respiratory distress, difficulty breathing, and changes in rate and depth.

- Keep head of bed elevated for a patient who has respiratory difficulties.

EQUIPMENT

☐ Stethoscope
☐ Clean gloves

STEP	RATIONALE

ASSESSMENT

1 Assess history of tobacco or marijuana use, including type of tobacco, duration, and amount in pack-years. (Pack-years equal number of years smoking times the number of packs per day.) If patient has quit, determine the length of time since smoking stopped.

Smoking is a major cause of lung cancer, cerebrovascular disease, heart disease, and chronic lung disease (emphysema and chronic bronchitis). Smoking accounts for 29% of all lung cancer deaths in the United States (ACS, 2008a).

2 Ask if patient experiences any of the following: *persistent cough* (productive or nonproductive), *sputum production,* chest pain, shortness of breath, orthopnea, dyspnea during exertion or at rest, activity intolerance, or *recurrent attacks of pneumonia or bronchitis.*

Symptoms of respiratory alterations help nurse localize objective physical findings. (Warning signals for lung cancer are in italic type.)

3 Determine if patient works in environment containing pollutants (e.g., asbestos, arsenic, coal dust) or requiring exposure to radiation. Does patient have exposure to secondhand cigarette smoke?

Patients with chronic respiratory disease, particularly asthma, have symptoms aggravated by change in temperature and humidity, irritating fumes or smoke, emotional stress, and physical exertion.

4 Review history for known or suspected human immunodeficiency virus (HIV) infection, substance abuse, low income, residence or employment in nursing home or shelter, homelessness, recent imprisonment, being a family member of patient with tuberculosis (TB), and immigration to the United States from a country where TB is prevalent (Frakes and Evans, 2004).

Known risk factors for exposure to and/or development of TB.

5 Ask if patient has history of persistent cough, hemoptysis, unexplained weight loss, fatigue, night sweats, and/or fever.

Signs and symptoms for both TB and HIV infection.

6 Does patient have history of chronic hoarseness?

Hoarseness indicates laryngeal disorder or abuse of cocaine or opioids (sniffing).

7 Assess for history of allergies to pollen, dust, or other airborne irritants, as well as to any foods, drugs, or chemical substances.

Allergic response to allergens sometimes causes symptoms patient demonstrates: choking feeling, bronchospasm with respiratory stridor, wheezing on auscultation, dyspnea, cyanosis, and diaphoresis.

8 Review family history for cancer, TB, allergies, or chronic obstructive pulmonary disease (COPD).

Familial history places patient at risk for lung disease.

NURSING DIAGNOSES

- Fatigue
- Impaired gas exchange

- Ineffective airway clearance
- Ineffective breathing pattern

- Pain (acute, chronic)
- Risk for infection

Individualize related factors based on patient's condition or needs.

STEP	RATIONALE

PLANNING

1 Expected outcomes following completion of procedure:
   - Respirations are passive, diaphragmatic or costal, and regular (12 to 20/min in adult) with symmetrical expansion.
   - Breath sounds are clear to auscultation and equal bilaterally.
   - Patient is able to describe factors that predispose to lung disease.
   - Patient assumes appropriate posture for best ventilation.

Characteristics of normal respirations.

Air flows without interference or obstruction. Corresponding side to side should sound the same.

Awareness of risks can improve patient compliance with healthful behavior.

Patient can learn about benefits of good posture as examination maneuvers are performed.

IMPLEMENTATION

1 Position and prepare patient for examination:
   a Position patient sitting upright. For bedridden patient, elevate head of bed 45 to 90 degrees. If unable to tolerate sitting, supine position and side-lying positions are used.

   b Remove gown or drape first from posterior chest, keeping legs covered. As examination progresses, remove gown from area being examined.

   c Explain all steps of procedure, encouraging patient to relax and breathe normally through the mouth.

2 Inspect posterior thorax:
   a If possible, stand behind patient to inspect thorax for shape, deformities, position of the spine, slope of the ribs, retraction of intercostal spaces during inspiration, and bulging of intercostal spaces during expiration.

Promotes full lung expansion during examination. Patients with chronic respiratory disease will likely need to sit up throughout the examination because of shortness of breath. Assistance of another caregiver may be required to position unresponsive patients.

Avoids unnecessary exposure and provides full visibility of thorax. Allows direct placement of diaphragm or bell on the patient's skin, which enhances clarity of sounds.

Anxiety alters respiratory function. Breathing through the mouth decreases extraneous sounds from air passing through the nose.

Allows for identification of any factors that impair chest expansion and any symptoms of respiratory distress. In a child, shape of chest is almost circular, with anteroposterior diameter in 1:1 ratio. In the adult the anteroposterior (AP) diameter is less than the lateral diameter. Chronic lung disease causes the ribs to be more horizontal and increases the AP diameter. This causes a "barrel chest." Patients with breathing problems assume postures that improve ventilation.

Critical Decision Point *When a patient holds the chest wall during breathing this indicates localized chest pain. Assess the nature of pain, including onset, severity, precipitating factors, quality, region, and radiation.*

---

   b Determine the rate and rhythm of breathing (see Chapter 5). Have patient relaxed.
   c Systematically palpate posterior chest wall, costal spaces, and intercostal spaces, noting any masses, pulsations, unusual movement, or areas of localized tenderness (see illustration). If you detect a suspicious mass or swollen area, palpate for size, shape, and typical qualities of lesion (see Skill 6-1). Do not palpate painful areas deeply.

This is a good time to count respirations, with patient unaware of inspection. Awareness could alter respirations.

Palpation assesses further characteristics and confirms or supplements findings from inspection. Localized swelling or tenderness indicates trauma to ribs or underlying cartilage. A fractured rib fragment could be displaced.

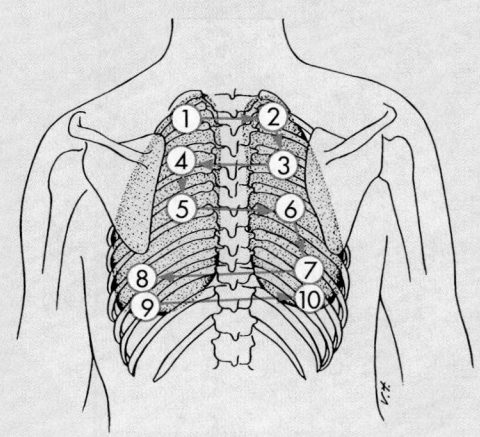

STEP 2c Pattern for assessment of posterior thorax.

STEP	RATIONALE

d Standing behind patient, place thumbs along the spinal processes at the tenth rib, with the palms lightly contacting the posterolateral surfaces (see illustration A). Keep your thumbs about 5 cm (2 inches) apart, with the thumbs pointing toward the spine and the fingers pointing laterally. Press hands toward patient's spine to form small skinfold between thumbs. After exhalation, patient takes deep breath. Note movement of thumbs (see illustration B), and note symmetry of chest wall movement. Normally symmetrical separation of the thumbs occurs during chest excursion 3 to 5 cm (1½ to 2 inches).

Palpation of chest excursion assesses depth of patient's breathing. This technique is good measure to evaluate patient's ability to perform deep-breathing exercises (see Chapter 36). Limited movement on one side indicates that patient is voluntarily splinting during ventilation because of pain. Avoid allowing the hands to slide over the skin, which gives a false measure of excursion.

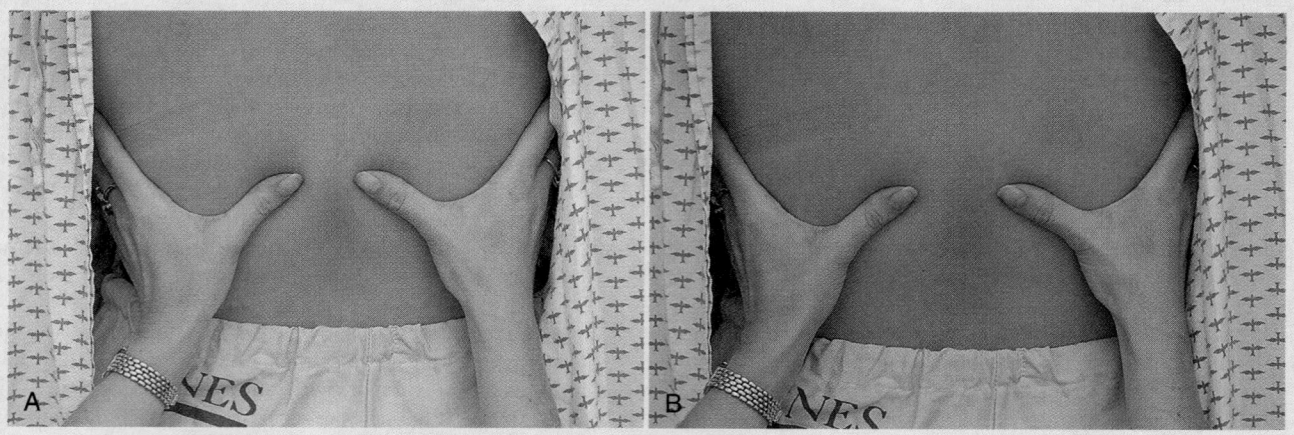

STEP 2d   **A,** Position of hands for palpation of posterior thorax excursion. **B,** As patient inhales, movement of chest excursion separates nurse's thumbs.

e Auscultate breath sounds. Have patient take slow, deep breaths with the mouth slightly open. For adult, place diaphragm of stethoscope firmly on chest wall over intercostal spaces (see illustration). Listen to entire inspiration and expiration at each stethoscope position. (See pattern in Step 2c.) Systematically compare breath sounds over right and left sides. If sounds are faint, ask patient to breathe a little deeper temporarily.

Assesses movement of air through tracheobronchial tree (Table 6-6, p. 133). Recognition of normal airflow sounds allows detection of sounds caused by mucus or airway obstruction. Characterize sounds by length of inspiratory and expiratory phases.

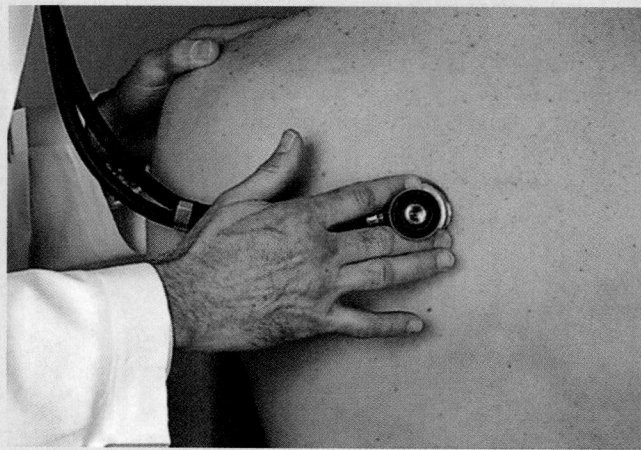

STEP 2e   Use of diaphragm of stethoscope to auscultate breath sounds. *(From Seidel HM and others:* Mosby's guide to physical examination, *ed 6, St. Louis, 2006, Mosby.)*

STEP	RATIONALE

f If you auscultate adventitious sounds, have patient cough and listen again to determine if sound has cleared with coughing (Table 6-7, p. 133).

Coughing may clear adventitious sounds. Rhonchi often are eliminated or altered by coughing. Crackles and wheezes are not.

3 Inspect lateral thorax:

a Instruct patient to raise arms, and inspect chest wall for same characteristics as reviewed for posterior chest.

Improves access to lateral thoracic structures.

b Extend palpation and auscultation of posterior thorax to lateral sides of chest, except for excursion measurement (see illustration).

Allows for location of abnormalities in lateral lung fields.

4 Inspect anterior thorax:

a Inspect accessory muscles of breathing: sternocleidomastoid, trapezius, and abdominal muscles, noting effort to breathe.

Extent to which accessory muscles are used reveals degree of effort to breathe. Generally these muscles are not used for breathing.

b Inspect width or spread of angle made by costal margins and tip of sternum. Angle is usually larger than 90 degrees between margins.

Indicates congenital, acquired, or traumatic alterations that influence patient's chest expansion.

c Observe the patient's breathing pattern, observing symmetry and degree of chest wall and abdominal movement. Respiratory rate and rhythm are more often assessed on the anterior chest wall.

Assesses patient's effort to breathe; symmetrical, passive movement indicates no respiratory distress.

d Palpate anterior thoracic muscles and ribs for lumps, masses, tenderness, or unusual movement following pattern across and down (see illustration).

Localized swelling or tenderness indicates trauma to underlying ribs or cartilage.

e Palpate anterior chest excursion. Place hands over each lateral rib cage, with thumbs approximately 5 cm (2 inches) apart and angled along each costal margin. As patient inhales deeply, thumbs should symmetrically move apart 3 to 5 cm (1½ to 2 inches), with each side expanding equally.

Assesses depth of patient's breathing and ability to perform deep-breathing exercises. Certain abnormalities are evident if expansion is not symmetrical.

f With patient sitting, auscultate anterior thorax. Begin above clavicles; move across and then down as during palpation.

Using a systematic pattern of assessment comparing sides helps to identify abnormal sounds.

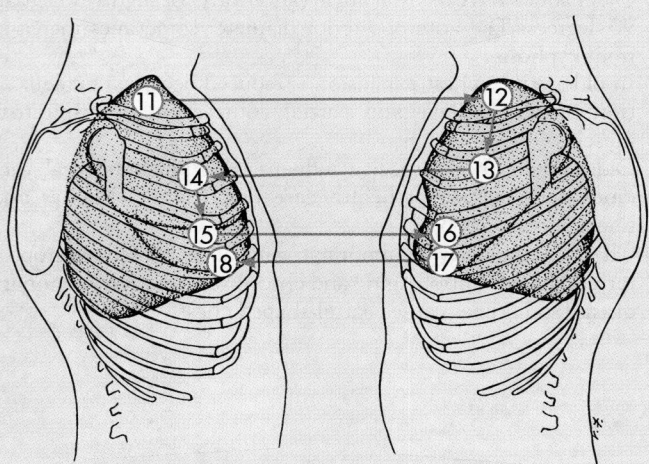

STEP 3b Pattern for assessment of lateral thorax.

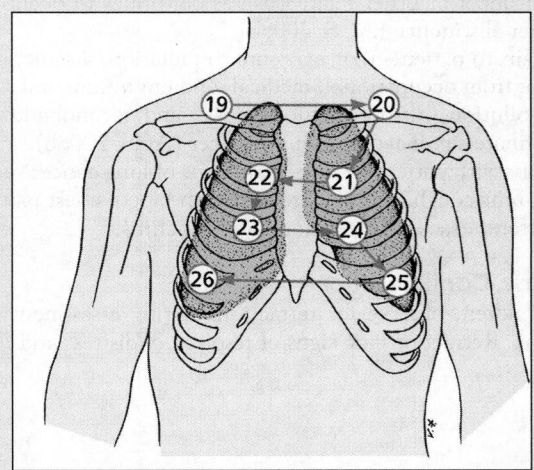

STEP 4d Pattern for assessment of anterior chest.

EVALUATION

1 Compare findings with normal assessment characteristics for thorax and lungs.

Determines presence of abnormalities.

2 Have patient identify factors leading to lung disease.

Demonstrates learning.

Unexpected Outcomes	Related Interventions
1 Patient has productive cough, and mucus is purulent.	• Obtain a specimen. • Auscultate lungs for adventitious sounds.
2 You observe posturing, with patient leaning over table or splinting side of chest with hand. Indicates breathing difficulties (chronic lung disease and pain, respectively).	• Assist patient into a position to improve lung expansion (e.g., high-Fowler's position).
3 Respirations are rapid or slow and irregular (see Chapter 5), and bulging of intercostal spaces is present.	• Position patient. • Auscultate lungs for adventitious sounds. • Notify health care provider.
4 Chest excursion is reduced. Depth of breathing is reduced by pain, postural deformity, or fatigue.	• Reposition patient. • Administer analgesic if appropriate.
5 Percussion note is dull or flat over lung tissue. Dullness occurs over the scapula, ribs, sternum, or spine. Dullness over lung tissue may be created by consolidation or a lung mass.	• Have patient cough and deep breathe. • Notify health care provider. • Obtain chest x-ray examination if ordered.
6 Abnormal breath sounds (adventitious sounds) are auscultated over one or both lungs.	• Have patient cough to determine if clear. • Notify health care provider.
7 Patient is unfamiliar with risks for lung disease.	• Education is necessary.
8 Patient does not assume preferred posture for optimal ventilation.	• This is difficult to change quickly; may require exercise and further discussion.

Recording and Reporting

• Record observations and findings in nurses' notes or assessment flow sheet.
• Record respiratory rate and character on vital signs flow sheet.
• Report abnormalities to nurse in charge or health care provider.

Teaching Considerations

• Educate patients about risks of cigarette smoking. Cigarette smoking alone causes approximately 29% of all cancer deaths. Individuals who stop smoking live longer than those who continue to smoke. The probability of these individuals dying from lung cancer or other related causes continues to decline with further abstinence (ACS, 2008b).
• Explain to patients that exposure to radiation, arsenic, and asbestos from occupational, medical, and environmental sources, air pollution, history of tuberculosis, and secondhand smoke contribute significantly to lung cancer (ACS, 2008b).
• Discuss with patients the warning signs of lung cancer such as a persistent cough, sputum streaked with blood, chest pains, and recurrent attacks of pneumonia or bronchitis.

Pediatric Considerations

• In children, observe for retractions during assessment of the thorax. Retractions are signs of respiratory distress and involve the intercostal suprasternal, or supraclavicular muscles (Hockenberry and Wilson, 2007).
• Children younger than age 7 exhibit noticeable abdominal or diaphragmatic movement. Older children and adults exhibit more costal or thoracic movement. Use bell to auscultate breath sounds in children. Breath sounds are louder in children because of their thin chest walls.
• Head bobbing and nasal flaring in infants are signs of significant respiratory distress (Hockenberry and Wilson, 2007).

Gerontological Considerations

• Older adults have a costal angle (anteriorly) of slightly less than 90 degrees. The anteroposterior diameter sometimes increases from kyphosis.
• In older adults chest expansion is reduced because of calcification of rib cartilage and partial contraction of inspiratory muscles.
• Older adults should receive influenza and pneumococcal vaccines upon advice of health care practitioner (Meiner and Lueckenotte, 2006).
• Chest contour may be abnormal, with an increased anteroposterior diameter ratio. Aging and chronic obstructive pulmonary disease sometimes causes barrel-shaped chest.

TABLE 6-6	Normal Breath Sounds		
Type	**Description**	**Location**	**Origin**
Bronchial	Loud and high-pitched with hollow quality. Expiration lasts longer than inspiration (3:2 ratio).	Best heard over trachea	Created by air moving through trachea close to chest wall
Bronchovesicular	Medium-pitched and blowing sounds of medium intensity. Inspiratory phase is equal to expiratory phase.	Best heard posteriorly between scapulae and anteriorly over bronchioles lateral to sternum at first and second intercostal spaces	Created by air moving through large airways
Vesicular	Soft, breezy, and low-pitched sounds. Inspiratory phase is 3 times longer than expiratory phase.	Best heard over lung's periphery (except over scapula)	Created by air moving through smaller airways

TABLE 6-7	Adventitious Breath Sounds		
Sound	**Site Auscultated**	**Cause**	**Character**
Crackles (also called rales)	Are most common in dependent lobes: right and left lung bases	Random, sudden reinflation of groups of alveoli; also related to increase in fluid in small airways	Fine, short, interrupted crackling sounds heard during end of inspiration, expiration, or both. May or may not change with coughing; sound like crushing cellophane. Medium crackles are lower, more moist sounds heard during middle of inspiration; not cleared with coughing. Coarse crackles are loud bubbly sounds heard during inspiration; not cleared with coughing
Rhonchi (sonorous wheeze)	Are primarily heard over trachea and bronchi; if loud enough, can be heard over most lung fields	Muscular spasm, fluid, or mucus in larger airways, causing turbulence	Loud, low-pitched, continuous sounds heard more during expiration; sometimes cleared by coughing. Sounds like blowing air through fluid with a straw
Wheezes (sibilant wheeze)	Heard over all lung fields	High-velocity airflow through severely narrowed or obstructed bronchus	High-pitched, musical sounds like a squeak heard continuously during inspiration or expiration; usually louder on expiration. Do not clear with coughing
Pleural friction rub	Heard over anterior lateral lung field (if patient is sitting upright)	Inflamed pleura, parietal pleura rubbing against visceral pleura	Has grating quality heard best during inspiration; does not clear with coughing; heard loudest over lower lateral anterior surface

Data from Seidel HM and others: *Mosby's guide to physical examination,* ed 6, St. Louis, 2006, Mosby.

SKILL 6-4   Cardiovascular Assessment

A patient who presents with signs or symptoms of heart (cardiac) problems, such as chest pain, may be suffering a life-threatening condition requiring immediate attention. In this situation, you act quickly and perform the portions of the examination that are absolutely necessary. When a patient's condition is stable, a more thorough assessment can reveal baseline heart function and any risks for heart disease. Patients tend to seek information about heart disease because it remains a leading cause of death in the United States. The heart, neck vessels, and peripheral circulation are assessed together because the systems work in unison.

You assess the integrity of the peripheral vascular system by noting the adequacy of blood flow to the extremities and by measuring arterial pulses and inspecting the condition of the skin and nails. Inadequate tissue perfusion results in an inadequate delivery of oxygen and nutrients to cells, a condition called ischemia. This is caused by constriction of vessels or by occlusion (blockage) from clot formation. The effects of ischemia depend on the duration of the problem and the metabolic needs of the tissues. Ischemia results in pain. If lack of oxygen to tissues is unrelieved, tissue necrosis (death) occurs. An embolus is a blood clot that breaks loose and travels through the circulation. If the clot obstructs circulation to the lungs or the brain, it can be life threatening.

You begin assessment of the heart after examining the lungs because the patient is already in a suitable position with the chest exposed. Assessment then proceeds to the neck vessels and ends with evaluating peripheral circulation. The skills of inspection, palpation, auscultation, and percussion are used during the examination.

Delegation Considerations

A cardiovascular assessment cannot be delegated to NAP. The nurse directs the NAP to:

- Count apical pulse and peripheral pulses if patient is stable.
- Recognize skin and color changes of affected extremities and report any changes to the nurse.

Equipment

- ❑ Stethoscope
- ❑ Doppler stethoscope (optional)
- ❑ Conducting gel (if a Doppler is used)

STEP	RATIONALE
ASSESSMENT	
1 Assess patient for history of smoking, alcohol intake, caffeine intake (coffee, tea, soft drinks, energy drinks, and chocolate), use of "recreational" drugs, exercise habits, and dietary patterns and intake.	These contribute to risk factors for cardiovascular disease. In addition, caffeine and alcohol cause tachycardia.
2 Determine if patient is taking medications for cardiovascular function (e.g., antidysrhythmics, antihypertensives, antianginals) and if patient knows their purpose, dosage, and side effects.	Allows nurse to assess patient's compliance with and understanding of drug therapies. Patient cannot take medications for cardiovascular function intermittently.
3 Ask if patient has experienced dyspnea, chest pain or discomfort, palpitations, excess fatigue, cough, leg pain or cramps, edema of the feet, cyanosis, fainting, and orthopnea. Ask if symptoms occur at rest or during exercise.	These are the cardinal symptoms of heart disease. Cardiovascular function is sometimes adequate during rest but not during exercise.
4 If patient reports chest pain, determine onset (sudden or gradual), precipitating factors, quality, region, severity, and if it radiates. Anginal pain is usually a deep pressure or ache that is substernal and diffuse, radiating to one or both arms, neck, or jaw.	Symptoms reveal acute coronary syndrome or coronary artery disease (CAD).
5 Assess family history for heart disease, diabetes, high cholesterol and/or lipid levels, hypertension, stroke, or rheumatic heart disease.	Family history of these conditions increases risk for heart and vascular disease.
6 Ask patient about a history of heart trouble (e.g., heart failure, congenital heart disease, coronary artery disease, dysrhythmias, murmurs), heart surgery, or vascular disease (hypertension, phlebitis, varicose veins).	Knowledge reveals patient's level of understanding of condition. A preexisting condition influences examination techniques used by nurse and expected findings.
7 Determine if patient experiences leg cramps, numbness or tingling in extremities, sensation of cold hands or feet, pain in legs, or swelling or cyanosis of feet, ankles, or hand.	These signs and symptoms indicate vascular disease.
8 If patient experiences leg pain or cramping in lower extremities, ask if walking or standing for long periods or sleep aggravates or relieves it.	Relationship of symptoms to exercise will clarify whether problem is vascular or musculoskeletal. Pain caused by vascular condition tends to increase with activity. Musculoskeletal pain is not usually relieved when exercise ends.
9 Ask women if they wear tight-fitting garters or hosiery and sit or lie in bed with legs crossed.	Tight hosiery around lower extremities and crossing legs can impair venous return.

STEP	RATIONALE

NURSING DIAGNOSES

- Activity intolerance
- Decreased cardiac output
- Deficient knowledge regarding risks for heart disease
- Ineffective peripheral tissue perfusion
- Pain (acute, chronic)
- Risk for peripheral neurovascular dysfunction

Individualize related factors based on patient's condition or needs.

PLANNING

1 Expected outcomes following completion of procedure:

- Heart rate is 60 to 100 beats per minute (adolescent through adult) and without extra sounds or murmurs.   Indicates normal rhythm and rate, normal sinus rhythm (NSR).
- Point of maximal impulse (PMI) is palpable at fifth intercostal space at left midclavicular line in children older than age 7 years and in adults. PMI is at fourth intercostals space at left midclavicular line in children younger than age 7 years (Hockenberry and Wilson, 2007).   Indicates normal heart position.
- Patient describes changes in own behavior that may improve cardiovascular function.   Information may improve patient's health care habits.
- Patient describes schedule, dosage, purpose, and benefits of medications being taken for cardiovascular function.   Information related to health benefits may improve compliance with therapy.
- Blood pressure is within normal limits for patient (see Chapter 5).   Normal cardiovascular function.
- Carotid pulse is localized, strong, elastic, and equal bilaterally. No change occurs during inspiration or expiration and without carotid bruit.   Vessel is patent.
- Jugular veins distend when patient lies supine and flatten when patient is in sitting position.   Venous pressure is normal.
- Peripheral pulses equal and strong (2+), extremities are warm and pink, with capillary refill less than 2 seconds. There is no dependent edema.   Peripheral circulation is intact.

IMPLEMENTATION

1 Assist patient in being as relaxed and comfortable as possible.   An anxious or uncomfortable patient can have mild tachycardia that may alter findings.

2 Have patient assume semi-Fowler's or supine position.   Provides adequate visibility and access to left thorax and mediastinum. Patient with heart disease often experiences shortness of breath while lying flat.

3 Explain procedure. Avoid facial gestures reflecting concern.   Some patients with previously normal cardiac history become anxious if nurse shows concern.

4 Be sure that room is quiet.   Subtle, low-pitched heart sounds are difficult to hear.

5 Assess the heart:

   a Form a mental image of the exact location of the heart (see illustration). The base of the heart is the upper portion, and the apex is the bottom tip. The surface of the right ventricle constitutes most of the heart's anterior surface.   Visualization improves ability to assess findings accurately and determines possible source of abnormalities.

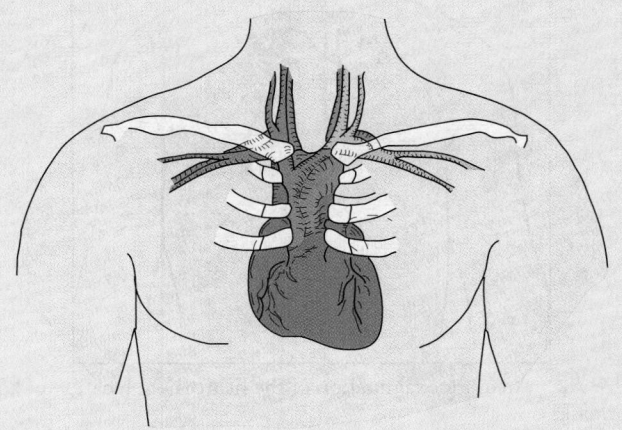

STEP 5a Anatomical position of the heart.

STEP	RATIONALE
b Find the angle of Louis at the manubriosternal junction, a visible and palpable angulation where the second rib articulates with the sternum. Slip fingers down each side of angle to feel adjacent ribs. The intercostal spaces are just below each rib.	Anatomical point used to locate intercostal spaces to assess corresponding heart sounds.
c Find the following anatomical landmarks (see illustration): (1) The aortic area is at the second intercostal space, right of the patient's sternum (1). (2) The pulmonic area is at the second intercostal space, left of the patient's sternum (2). (3) To find the second pulmonic area, move down left side of sternum to the third intercostal space (3), also referred to as Erb's point. (4) The tricuspid area (4) is located at the fourth left intercostal space along the sternum. (5) To find the mitral area, move fingers laterally to patient's left to locate fifth intercostal space at left midclavicular line (5). (6) The epigastric area (6) is at the inferior tip of the sternum.	Familiarity with landmarks allows nurse to describe findings more clearly and ultimately improves assessment.
d Stand to the patient's right to inspect and palpate the precordium with the patient supine. Note any visible pulsations and more exaggerated lifts at the anatomical landmarks. Closely inspect the area of the apex. Palpate for pulsations (using the proximal halves of the four fingers together and then alternating with ball of hand) at all anatomical landmarks.	Reveals size and symmetry of the heart. The apical impulse is normally visible at the midclavicular line in the fifth intercostal space. The apical impulse (PMI) becomes visible only when the patient sits up, bringing the heart closer to the anterior wall. It is difficult to see in obese patients. Normally you cannot feel any pulsations or vibrations in the second, third, or fourth intercostal spaces.
e Locate the PMI by palpating with fingertips along fifth intercostal space in midclavicular line (see illustration). Note a light, brief pulsation in an area 1 to 2 cm (½ to 1 inch) in diameter at the apex.	In the presence of serious heart disease, the PMI will be located to the left of the midclavicular line related to enlarged left ventricle. In chronic lung disease the PMI is often to the right of the midclavicular line as a result of right ventricular enlargement.

Critical Decision Point   *Presence of a palpable thrill is not normal and indicates a disruption of blood flow caused by a defect in closure of a heart valve or atrial septal defect. Report to health care provider.*

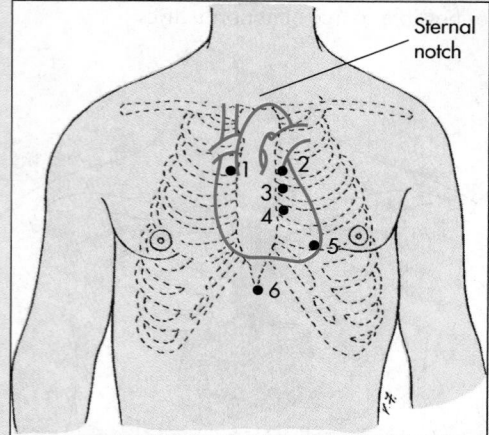

STEP 5c   Areas for examination of the heart (note location of bony landmarks).

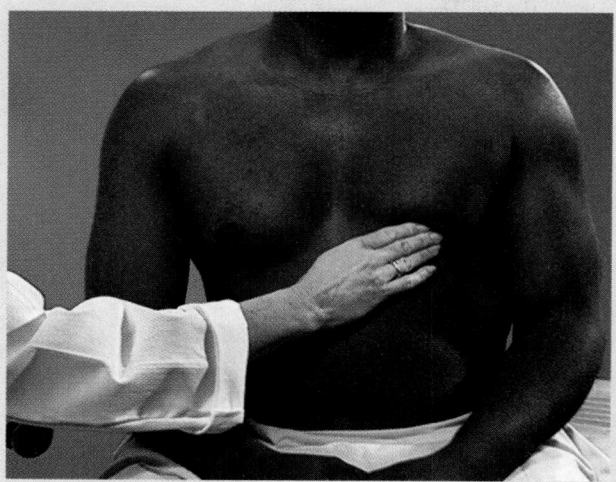

STEP 5e   Palpation of PMI. (*From Seidel HM and others: Mosby's guide to physical examination, ed 6, St. Louis, 2006, Mosby.*)

STEP	RATIONALE

Critical Decision Point   *A stronger than expected impulse is a heave or lift, which indicates increased cardiac output or left ventricular hypertrophy.*

f If palpating PMI is difficult, turn patient onto left side.

g Inspect the epigastric area and palpate the abdominal aorta. Note a localized strong beat.

h Auscultate heart sounds. Begin by having patient sit up and lean slightly forward; then have patient lie supine, and end the examination with patient in a left lateral recumbent position (see illustrations). In a female patient it is often necessary to lift the left breast to hear heart sounds more effectively.

Maneuver moves the heart closer to the chest wall.

Rules out reduced blood flow or diffuse pulse, which indicates a number of abnormalities.

Different positions help to clarify type of sounds heard. Sitting position is best to hear high-pitched murmurs (if present). Supine is a common position to hear all sounds. Left lateral recumbent is the best position to hear low-pitched sounds.

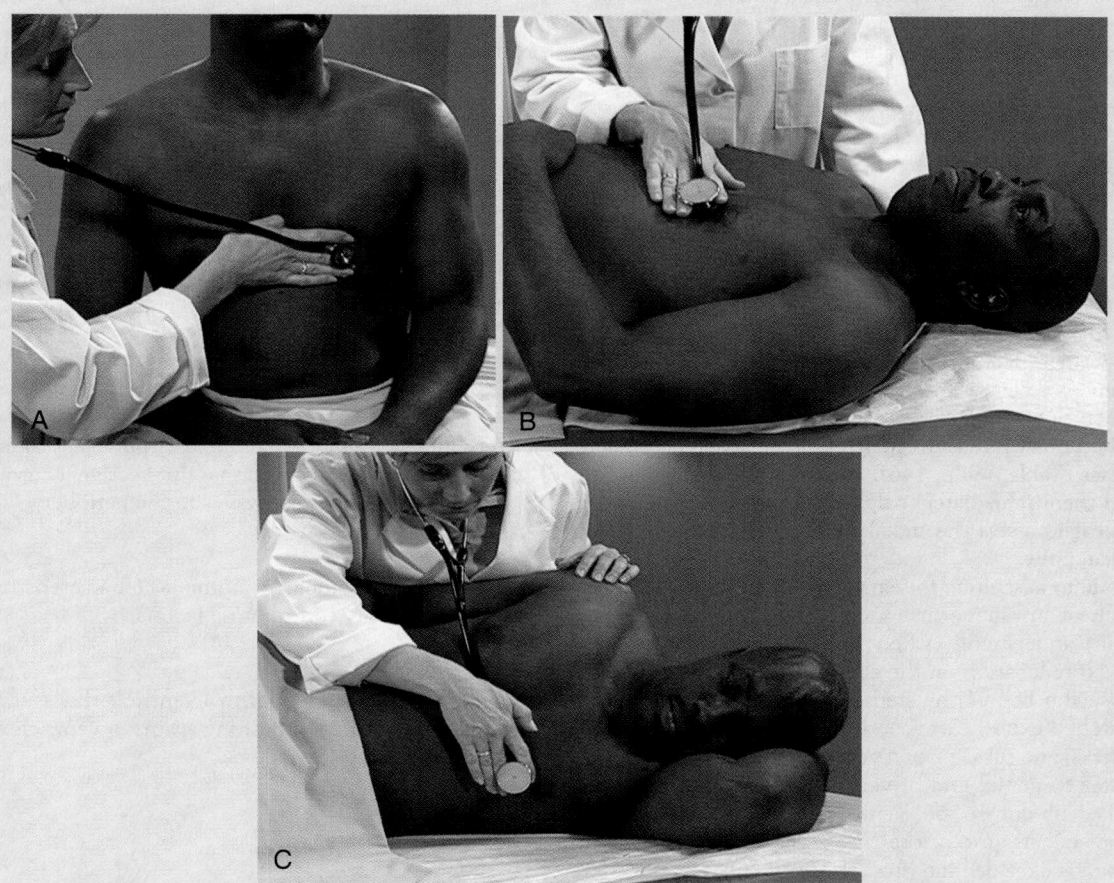

STEP 5h Patient positions for auscultation of heart sounds. **A,** Sitting. **B,** Supine. **C,** Left lateral. (*From Seidel HM and others:* Mosby's guide to physical examination, *ed 6, St. Louis, 2006, Mosby.*)

STEP	RATIONALE

(1) While auscultating sounds at each anatomical landmark, ask patient not to speak but to breathe comfortably. Begin with the diaphragm of the stethoscope; then alternate with the bell. Use very light pressure for the bell. Inch the stethoscope along; avoid jumping from one area to another. Do not try to hear all heart sounds at once.

Auscultation requires the examiner to isolate each heart sound at all auscultation sites.

(2) Begin at the apex or PMI; then move systematically to the tricuspid area, second pulmonic area, and pulmonic and aortic areas. (NOTE: Some examiners use reverse sequence.) Listen for the S_1 at each site. It sounds like "lub." You hear S_1 best at the apex, and it is simultaneous with the carotid pulse.

At normal slow rates S_1 is high pitched and dull in quality and sounds like a "lub." This sound precedes the systolic phase of heart contraction.

(3) Listen for S_2 at each site. It precedes the diastolic phase and sounds like "dub." You hear this best at the aortic area. Heart sounds will vary by pitch, loudness, and duration, depending on the auscultatory site (Table 6-8, p. 146).

Normal sounds S_1 and S_2 are high pitched and best heard with the diaphragm.

(4) After you hear both sounds clearly as "lub-dub," count each combination of S_1 and S_2 as one heartbeat. Count the number of beats for 1 minute.

Determines apical pulse rate.

(5) Assess heart rhythm by noting the time between S_1 and S_2 (systole) and then the time between S_2 and the next S_1 (diastole). Listen to the full cycle at each auscultation area. Note regular intervals between each sequence of beats. There should be a distinct pause between S_1 and S_2.

Failure of heart to beat at regular intervals is a dysrhythmia, which interferes with heart's ability to pump effectively.

(6) When heart rate is irregular, compare apical and radial pulses (Table 6-9, p. 146). Auscultate the apical pulse, and then immediately palpate the radial pulse. Have a colleague assess the radial pulse while you assess the apical pulse.

Determines if a pulse deficit (radial pulse is slower than apical) exists. Deficit indicates that ineffective contractions of the heart fail to send pulse waves to the periphery.

i Continue to auscultate for extra heart sounds at each site. If you hear any abnormal sounds, note pitch, loudness, duration, and timing (when in relation to the cardiac cycle). Note location on the chest wall.

Abnormal sounds include murmurs. Characteristics of murmurs help to identify contributing factors.

(1) Use the bell of the stethoscope, and listen for low-pitched extra heart sounds such as S_3 and S_4 gallops, clicks, and rubs. S_3, or a ventricular gallop, occurs just after S_2 at the end of ventricular diastole. It sounds like "lub-dub-ee" or "Ken-tuc-ky." S_4, or an atrial gallop, occurs just before S_1 or ventricular systole. It sounds like "dee-lub-dub" or "Ten-nes-see."

Premature rushes of blood into a ventricle that is stiff or dilated or an atrial contraction pushing against a ventricle that is not accepting blood cause gallops.

(2) Listen for clicks as short, high-pitched extra sounds.

Abnormalities such as mitral valve prolapse or prosthetic valves cause clicks.

(3) With patient leaning forward or lying on the left side, listen for friction rubs as squeaky or rubbing sounds. Instruct patient to hold breath as you continue to listen.

Rubs result from lungs or inflamed visceral and parietal layers of the pericardium of the heart rubbing against one another. If the sound is present only while the patient is breathing, the origin of the rub is pulmonary rather than cardiac.

j Auscultate for heart murmurs over each of the auscultation sites.

Murmurs are sustained swishing or blowing sounds heard at the beginning, middle, or end of systole or diastole. Increased blood flow through a normal valve, forward flow through a stenotic valve or into a dilated vessel or chamber, or backward flow through a valve that fails to close causes murmurs.

STEP	RATIONALE

k When you detect a murmur, listen carefully to note where you can hear the murmur best. Note the intensity of the murmur.

Intensity is related to rate of blood flow through the heart or the amount of blood regurgitated. A thrill is a continuous palpable sensation like the purring of a cat. A thrust is the upward lift felt when palpating the chest wall.

l Note if the murmur is low, medium, or high in pitch, using the bell for low-pitched sounds.

Pitch depends on velocity of blood flow through the valves.

6 Assess neck vessels:

a Assess carotid arteries: Have patient remain in sitting position.

Allows easier mobility of neck to expose artery for inspection and palpation.

b Inspect neck on both sides for obvious pulsations of artery. Ask patient to turn head slightly away from artery being examined. Sometimes you can see a pulse wave. Carotids are the only sites to assess quality of pulse wave (see illustration). Experience is required to evaluate wave in relation to events of cardiac cycle.

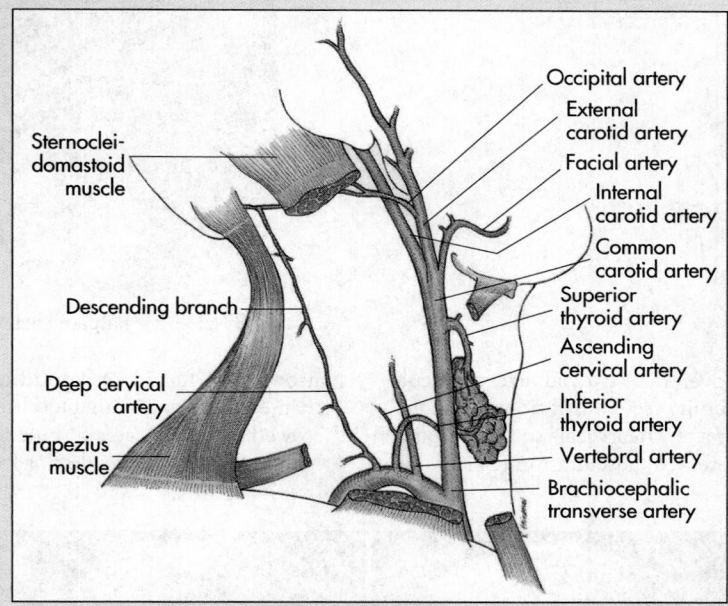

STEP 6b Anatomical position of carotid artery.

c   Palpate each carotid artery separately with index and middle fingers around medial edge of sternocleidomastoid muscle. Ask patient to raise chin slightly, keeping the head straight (see illustration). Note rate and rhythm, strength, and elasticity of artery. Also note if pulse changes as patient inspires and expires.

If both arteries were occluded simultaneously, patient could lose consciousness from reduced circulation to the brain. Turning the head improves access to artery. A change indicates a sinus dysrhythmia.

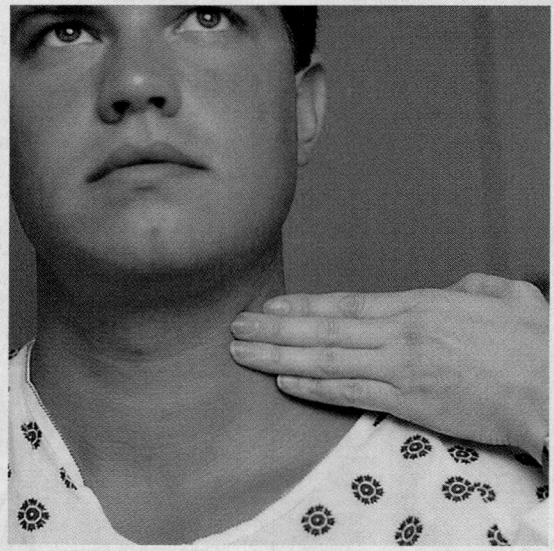

STEP 6c   Palpate each carotid artery separately.

d   Place bell of stethoscope over each carotid artery, auscultating for blowing sound (bruit) (see illustrations). Ask the patient to hold a breath for a few heartbeats so that respiratory sounds will not interfere with auscultation (Seidel and others, 2006).

Narrowing of lumen of carotid artery by arteriosclerotic plaques causes disturbance in blood flow. Blood passing through narrowed section creates turbulence and emits blowing or swishing sound. Normally you do not hear a bruit.

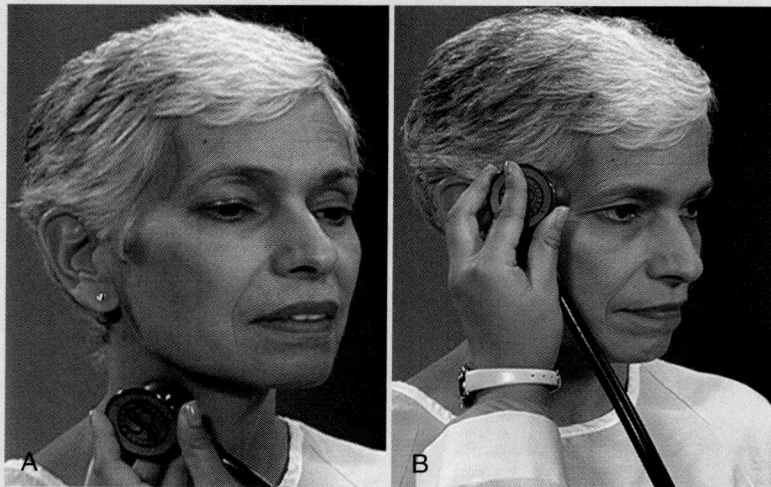

STEP 6d   Auscultation for carotid artery bruit. (*From Seidel HM and others:* Mosby's guide to physical examination, *ed 6, St. Louis, 2006, Mosby.*)

Critical Decision Point   *Do not vigorously palpate or massage the carotid artery. Stimulation of carotid sinus causes a reflex drop in heart rate and blood pressure.*

STEP	RATIONALE

e To assess jugular venous pressure have patient assume a supine position. Then raise the head of the bed 45 degrees. Avoiding neck hyperextension or flexion. Locate the highest point along the internal jugular vein where a pulsation can be seen (tangential lighting helps). Locate the sternal angle with a centimeter ruler, and measure the vertical distance between the sternal angle and the meniscus of the internal jugular vein (see illustration).

Normal veins are flat when patient is sitting, and pulsations become evident as you lower patient's head. A height of pulsation greater than 2.5 cm indicates fluid overload or right-sided heart failure.

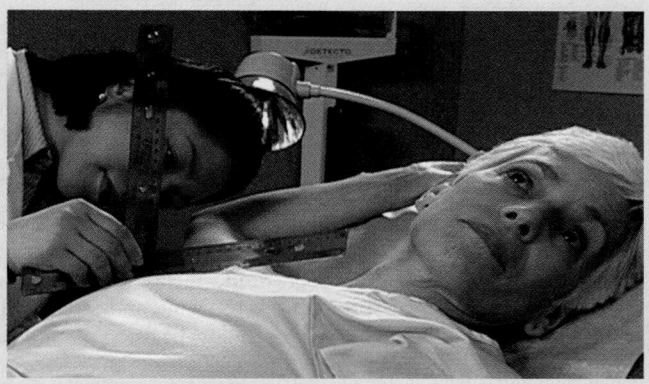

STEP 6e   Position for assessment of jugular vein distention. *(From Seidel HM and others:* Mosby's guide to physical examination, *ed 6, St. Louis, 2006, Mosby.)*

7 Peripheral vascular assessment:

a Inspect lower extremities for changes in color and condition of the skin (Table 6-10, p. 146). Note skin and nail texture, hair distribution, venous patterns, edema, and scars or ulcers. Compare skin color lying and standing.

Changes reflect impaired peripheral circulation.

b Palpate edematous areas, noting mobility, consistency, and tenderness.

Assists in determining extent of edema.

c Assess for pitting edema by pressing area firmly with the thumb for 5 seconds, then releasing. Depth of indentation determines severity (see illustration).
2 mm: 1 + edema
4 mm: 2 + edema
6 mm: 3 + edema
8 mm: 4 + edema
Use a tape measure to measure the circumference of the extremity.

Unilateral edema of affected leg is the most common physical finding of deep vein thrombosis (DVT), although half of all patients with DVT may present with no obvious signs (Bartley, 2006).
Edema results from fluid in tissues. Inadequate venous return causes edema in the sacrum if patient is confined to bed or in the feet and ankles if sitting.

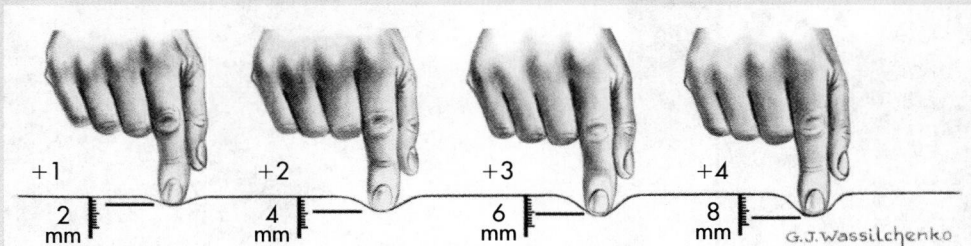

STEP 7c   Pitting edema. *(From Seidel HM and others:* Mosby's guide to physical examination, *ed 6, St. Louis, 2006, Mosby.)*

STEP	RATIONALE
d Check capillary refill by grasping patient's fingernail or toenail and noting color of nail bed. Next, apply gentle, firm pressure to the nail bed. Release quickly, watching for color change. Circulation is restored and normally returns to pink color in less than 2 seconds.	Capillary refill is measured in seconds; less than 2 seconds is brisk, whereas greater than 4 seconds is sluggish. Cold environmental temperature, with vasoconstriction, and vascular disease can delay refill. Local pressure from a cast or bandage also slows refill.
e Ask if the patient experiences pain or tenderness, and then palpate for heat, firmness, or localized swelling of the calf muscle, which are signs of phlebitis or DVT.	Patients who have been immobilized for several days and those who have bone or joint disease, lengthy surgery, surgical correction of joint or bone, heart failure, shock, varicose veins, or pain are at risk for impaired tissue perfusion (Bartley, 2006; Glover, 2005). Some patients have DVT and only complain of calf pain (Bartley, 2005).

Critical Decision Point   *Homans' sign is no longer considered a reliable indicator for the presence or absence of DVT (Bartley, 2005, 2006; Glover, 2005) and should not be considered a reliable test. Trauma to the vein or muscle, reduced mobility, and increased blood clotting are reliable risk factors. If calf is swollen, tender, or red, notify patient's health care provider for further assessment and evaluation. If there is a strong suspicion of DVT, testing for Homans' sign is contraindicated. If a clot is present, it may become dislodged from its original site during this test. This could result in a pulmonary embolism.*

f Starting at the most distal part of each extremity, palpate each peripheral artery for equality, comparing side to side; elasticity of vessel wall: depress and release artery, noting ease with which it springs back to shape and strength of pulse (force of blood against arterial wall) using the following rating scale (Seidel and others, 2006):	Comparison of both arteries allows nurse to determine any localized obstruction or disturbance in blood flow. Pulses are normally symmetrical side to side. If you notice asymmetry, look for other factors related to impaired circulation.
0 No pulse palpable	
1+ Diminished, pulse barely palpable, weak and thready, and easy to obliterate	
2+ Normal pulse, easy to palpate	
3+ Full, easy to palpate, and not easy to obliterate	
4+ Strong, bounding against fingertips, and cannot be obliterated	
g Palpate radial pulse by lightly placing tips of first and second fingers in groove formed along radial side of forearm, lateral to flexor tendon of wrist (see illustration).	Pulse is relatively superficial and should not require deep palpation.
h Palpate ulnar pulse by placing fingertips along ulnar side of forearm (see illustration).	Palpated when arterial insufficiency to hand is expected or when nurse assesses effects that radial occlusion (e.g., during arterial blood gas sampling) might have on circulation to hand (see Chapter 44).

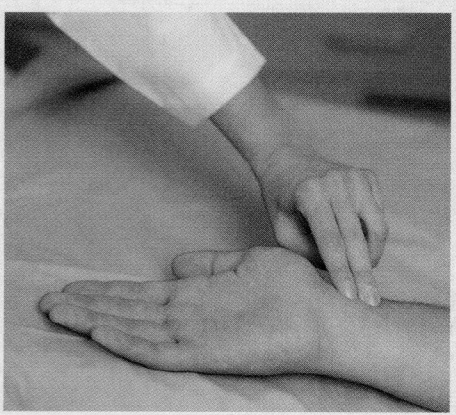

STEP 7g   Palpation of radial pulse.

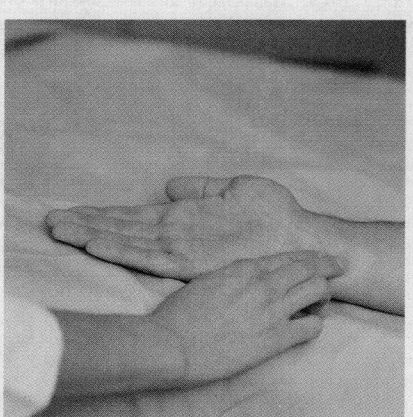

STEP 7h   Palpation of ulnar pulse.

STEP	RATIONALE

i   Palpate brachial pulse by locating groove between biceps and triceps muscles above elbow at antecubital fossa (see illustration). Place tips of first two fingers in muscle groove.

Artery runs along medial side of extended arm, requiring moderate palpation.

j   Have patient lie supine with feet relaxed, and palpate dorsalis pedis pulse. Gently place fingertips between great and first toe; slowly move fingers along groove between extensor tendons of great and first toe until pulse is palpable (see illustration).

Artery lies superficially and does not require deep palpation. Pulse is sometimes congenitally absent.

k   If pulses are difficult to palpate, or are not palpable, use a Doppler instrument over the pulse site:
   (1)   Apply conducting gel to the patient's skin over the pulse site or onto transducer tip of probe.
   (2)   Turn Doppler on. Gently apply ultrasound probe to the skin, changing Doppler angle until pulsation is audible. Adjust volume as needed (see illustration). Wipe off gel from patient and Doppler.

Doppler amplifies sounds, allowing you to hear low-velocity blood flow through peripheral arteries.

l   Palpate posterior tibial pulse by having patient relax and slightly extend feet. Place fingertips behind and below medial malleolus (ankle bone) (see illustration).

Artery is easily palpable with foot relaxed.

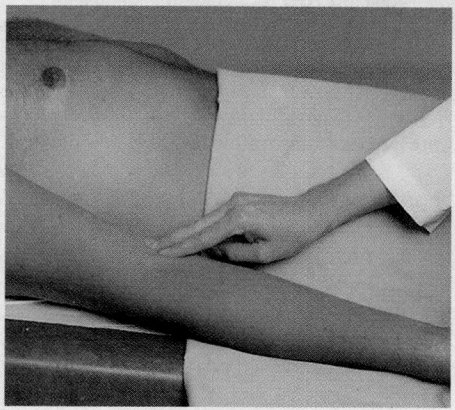

STEP 7i   Palpation of brachial pulse.

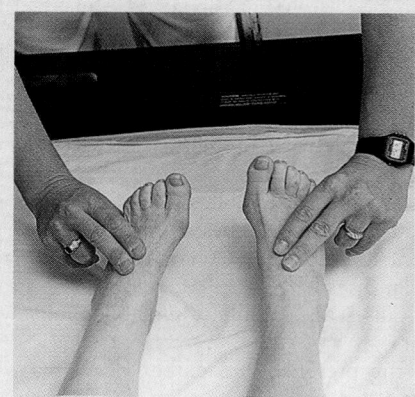

STEP 7j   Palpation of dorsalis pedis pulses.

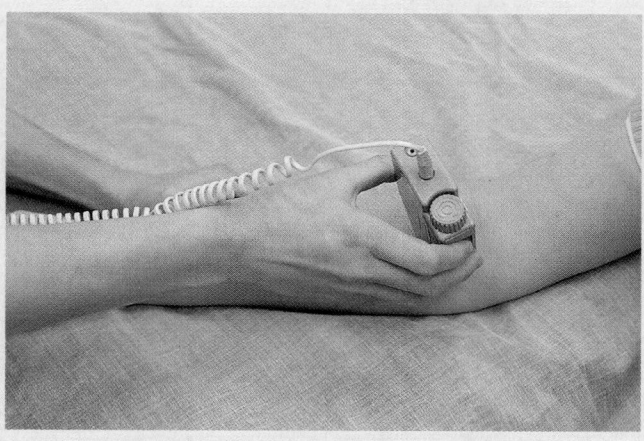

STEP 7k(2)   Use of Doppler for brachial pulse.

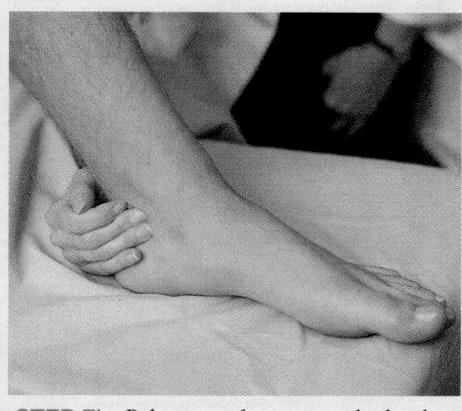

STEP 7l   Palpation of posterior tibial pulse.

STEP	RATIONALE

m   Palpate popliteal pulse by having patient slightly flex knee with foot resting on table or bed. Instruct patient to keep leg muscles relaxed. Palpate deeply into popliteal fossa with fingers of both hands placed just lateral to midline. Patient may also lie prone to achieve exposure of artery (see illustration).

Flexion of knee and muscle relaxation improve accessibility of artery. Popliteal pulse is one of the more difficult pulses to palpate.

n   With patient supine, wearing clean gloves, palpate femoral pulse by placing first two fingers over inguinal area below inguinal ligament, midway between pubic symphysis and anterosuperior iliac spine (see illustration).

Supine position prevents flexion in groin area, which interferes with artery access.

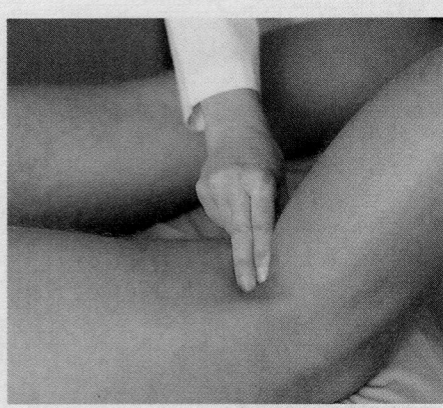

STEP 7m   Palpation of popliteal pulse with patient prone.

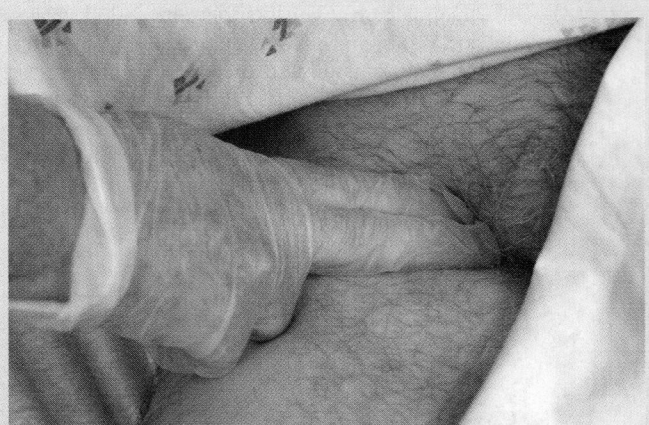

STEP 7n   Palpation of femoral pulse.

EVALUATION

1   Compare findings with normal assessment characteristics of heart and vascular system.

Determines presence of abnormalities.

2   If heart sounds are not audible, or if pulses are not palpable, ask another nurse to confirm assessment.

Validates abnormal assessment findings.

3   Ask patient to describe behaviors that increase risk for heart and vascular disease.

Demonstrates learning.

4   Compare pulses and capillary refill bilaterally with previous assessment.

Demonstrates change from baseline measures.

5   Compare the presence and extent of edema with previous assessment.

Identifies increased or decreased edema.

Unexpected Outcomes

1. Abnormal findings that are new to the assessment data require you to notify the health care provider. These include:
   - Pulsations, vibrations, or both are palpable. These are result of valvular problem, murmur, or both.
   - Point of maximal impulse is to the left of midclavicular line, which is the result of cardiomegaly.
   - Extra heart sounds S_3 or S_4 are auscultated. Extra sounds indicate atrial or ventricular gallop.
   - Murmur is auscultated. Impaired blood flow through heart indicates need for immediate medical attention. Some murmurs are benign.
   - Jugular venous pressure is elevated. This is a sign of right-sided heart failure or fluid overload.

2. Heart rate is irregular, with rate less than 60 beats per minute or more than 100 beats per minute.

3. Pulse deficit is noted. There is risk for inadequate cardiac output.

4. Patient is unable to explain risks for heart or vascular disease.

5. Previously palpable dorsalis pedis pulses are diminished or absent, indicating circulatory compromise.

6. Patient's lower extremities have pale, cool, thin, and shiny skin, with reduced hair growth and thickened nails, indicating chronic arterial insufficiency.

Related Interventions

- Notify health care provider.
- Prepare to order ECG.

- Check blood pressure. If low, dysrhythmia is possibly contributing to inadequate cardiac output.
- Observe for sensations or reports of dizziness or feeling "faint."
- Notify health care provider.
- Prepare to order ECG.
- Obtain vital signs.
- Notify health care provider.
- Additional education is needed.
- Notify health care provider.
- Elevate extremity.
- Instruct patient in proper foot care.
- Refer to podiatrist for nail trimming.
- Inspect feet for signs of impaired skin integrity.

Recording and Reporting

- Record all findings for heart and vascular assessment in nurses' notes or flow sheet.
- Record any instruction provided to patient and patient's response.
- Report immediately to health care provider any irregularities in heart function and indications of impaired arterial blood flow.
- Patients with dysrhythmias or pulse deficits often require an electrocardiogram or Holter monitor per physician's order.
- Report changes in peripheral circulation evidenced by edema or diminished or absent pulses or capillary refill, which indicates circulatory compromise that can result in permanent nerve damage or tissue death if untreated.

Teaching Considerations

- Explain risk factors for heart disease: high dietary intake of saturated fat or cholesterol, lack of regular aerobic exercise, smoking, excess weight, stressful lifestyle, hypertension, and family history of heart disease.
- Refer patient (if appropriate) to resources available for controlling or reducing risks (e.g., nutritional counseling, exercise class, and stress reduction programs).
- Explain that research shows clinical benefit from reducing dietary intake of cholesterol and saturated fats. Tell patient that about 70% to 75% of saturated fatty acids come from meats, poultry, fish, and dairy products. The American Heart Association recommends a diet that includes an intake of total fat less than 35% of calories, saturated fatty acids less than 10% of calories, and cholesterol less than 300 mg/100 mL (Moore, 2005).
- Encourage patient to have regular measurement of total blood cholesterol levels and triglycerides. Desirable levels are less than 200 mg/100 mL. You need more than one cholesterol measurement to assess the blood cholesterol level accurately. Low-density lipoprotein (LDL) cholesterol is the major compo-

nent of atherosclerotic plaques. Separate measurement of LDL cholesterol is wise in a patient with high total blood cholesterol levels. In an individual with no other risk factors, an LDL cholesterol level of 160 mg/100 mL or higher is high risk (Moore, 2005).

- Encourage patient to discuss with health care provider about the need for periodic C-reactive protein (CRP) testing. CRP levels assess a patient's cardiovascular disease risk.
- Advise patient to quit smoking because this lowers the risk for coronary heart disease and coronary vascular disease (ACS, 2007). Nicotine in cigarette smoke causes vasoconstriction.
- Patients who are at risk benefit from taking a daily low dose of aspirin. Consult health care provider before starting therapy.

Pediatric Considerations

- Perform cardiac assessment on infant or toddler while quiet, before more uncomfortable procedures.
- Capillary refill in infants is usually less than 1 second.
- It is not uncommon for children to have third heart sounds (S_3). Sinus arrhythmia occurs normally in many infants and children (Hockenberry and Wilson, 2007).
- Children have louder, higher-pitched heart sounds because of their thin chest walls.

Gerontological Considerations

- PMI is sometimes difficult to find in an older adult because anteroposterior diameter of the chest deepens.
- Accidental massage of the carotid sinus during palpation of the carotid artery is a particular problem for older adults, causing a sudden drop in heart rate from vagal nerve stimulation (Meiner and Lueckenotte, 2006).
- Older adults with hypertension benefit from regular monitoring of blood pressure (daily, weekly, or monthly). Home monitoring kits are available. Teach patient how to use them correctly.

TABLE 6-8 | Heart Sounds According to Auscultatory Area

	Aortic	Pulmonic	Second Pulmonic	Mitral	Tricuspid
Pitch	$S_1 < S_2$	$S_1 < S_2$	$S_1 < S_2$	$S_1 < S_2$	$S_1 < S_2$
Loudness	$S_1 < S_2$	$S_1 < S_2$	$S_1 < S_2$*	$S_1 > S_2$†	$S_1 > S_2$
Duration and others	$S_1 > S_2$	$S_1 > S_2$	$S_1 > S_2$	$S_1 > S_2$	$S_1 > S_2$

Modified from Seidel HM and others: *Mosby's guide to physical examination,* ed 6, St. Louis, 2006, Mosby.
*S_1 is relatively louder in second pulmonic area than in aortic area.
†S_1 may be louder in mitral area than in tricuspid area.

TABLE 6-9 | Common Types of Dysrhythmias

Type	Definition	Cause
Atrial fibrillation	Rapid, random contractions of atria cause irregular ventricular beats at 120-150 beats per minute.	Atria discharge very rapidly, with some impulses not reaching ventricles. This condition occurs in rheumatic heart disease and mitral stenosis. It causes reduced cardiac output.
Sinus arrhythmia	Pulse rate changes during respiration, increasing at peak of inspiration and decreasing during expiration.	Blood is momentarily trapped in lungs during inspiration, causing a fall in heart's stroke volume.
Sinus bradycardia	Pulse rhythm is regular, but rate is slower than normal at 40-60 beats/min.	Sinoatrial node fires less frequently. This is common in well-conditioned athletes and with use of antidysrhythmic medications.
Sinus tachycardia	Pulse rhythm is regular, but rate is accelerated to more than 100 beats/min.	Exercise, emotional stress, and caffeine or alcohol ingestion are common factors that cause increased firing of sinoatrial node.
Premature ventricular contraction	Premature beat occurs before regularly expected heart contraction.	Ventricle contracts prematurely because of electrical impulse bypassing normal conduction pathway. It may occur so early that it is difficult to detect as second beat. It may be followed by a pause.

TABLE 6-10 | Signs of Venous and Arterial Insufficiency

Assessment Criterion	Venous	Arterial
Pain	Aching, increases in evening and with dependent position	Burning, throbbing, cramping, increases with exercise
Paresthesia	None	Numbness, tingling, decreased sensation
Temperature	Normal to touch	Cool to touch
Color	Normal or cyanotic	Pale; worsened by elevation of the extremity; dusky red when extremity is lowered
Capillary refill	Not applicable	>2 seconds
Pulse	Present	Decreased or absent
Skin changes	Brown pigmentation around ankles	Thin, shiny skin; decreased hair growth; thickened nails
Ulcerations	Shallow ulcers around ankles (chronic venous stasis); edema apparent	Deep, well defined at site of trauma or tips of toes

Abdominal assessment is complex because of the multiple organs located within and near the abdominal cavity. This area of the body is associated with many health complaints, and many people are embarrassed by bowel or bladder dysfunction, reproductive problems, or urinary elimination problems. Abdominal pain is one of the most common symptoms patients report when seeking medical care. Abdominal pain could be caused by alterations in organs such as the stomach, gallbladder, or intestines; or the pain may be the result of spinal or muscular injury. An accurate assessment requires matching the patient's history with a careful assessment of the location of physical symptoms (Table 6-11).

To perform an effective assessment you need a detailed knowledge of the underlying structures involved, including the lower pelvis, kidneys, rectum, genitalia, liver, gallbladder, stomach, spleen, intestines, and reproductive organs (Fig. 6-5). An abdominal assessment is routine after abdominal surgery and for any patient who has undergone invasive diagnostic tests of the gastrointestinal tract (see Chapter 44). You complete an external genitalia

TABLE 6-11	Common Causes of Abdominal Pain	
Conduction	**Physical Alteration**	**Physical Signs and Symptoms**
Appendicitis	Obstruction of the appendix associated with inflammation, perforation, and peritonitis. Patient often lies on back or side with knees flexed to decrease pain.	Sharp pain directly over the irritated peritoneum 2-12 hours after onset. Often pain localizes at McBurney's point in the right lower quadrant between the anterior iliac crest and the umbilicus. Associated with rebound tenderness. Accompanied often by anorexia, nausea, and vomiting. Patient often lies on back or side with knees flexed to decrease pain.
Cholecystitis	Obstruction of the cystic duct causing inflammation or distention of the gallbladder.	*Murphy's sign:* Apply gentle pressure below the right subcostal arch and below the liver margin. Sharp pain and inspiratory arrest occur when the patient takes a deep breath (Seidel and others, 2006).
Constipation	Symptom of infrequent bowel movements. Disruption in normal bowel pattern, defecation may occur with opioid use or inadequate fiber and fluid intake.	Generalized discomfort accompanied by distention and palpation of a hard mass in the left lower quadrant. Nausea and vomiting may begin after several days.
Crohn's disease	A chronic inflammatory lesion of the ileum. Cause is unknown.	Steady colicky pain in the right lower quadrant or may be diffuse, with cramping, tenderness, flatulence, nausea, fever, and diarrhea. Often associated with bloody stools, weight loss, weakness, and fatigue. A tender mass of thickened intestine may be palpated in right lower quadrant.
Gastroenteritis	Inflammation of the stomach and intestinal tract.	Generalized abdominal discomfort accompanied by anorexia, nausea, vomiting, diarrhea, abdominal cramping.
Intestinal (bowel) obstruction	Blockage of the lumen of the intestine.	Colicky pain, nausea, vomiting, constipation, and abdominal distention. Bowel sounds are hyperactive with a rushing sound (early obstruction) or absence of bowel sounds (late obstruction).
Pancreatitis	Inflammation of the pancreas associated with alcoholism and gallbladder disease.	Steady severe epigastric pain close to the umbilicus radiates to the back. Associated with abdominal rigidity and vomiting. Pain is unrelieved by vomiting, worsens by lying supine. Decreased or absent bowel sounds.
Paralytic ileus	Obstruction of the small bowel that occurs after abdominal surgery, from abdominal radiation, or use of anticholinergic medications.	Generalized severe abdominal distention, nausea, and vomiting. Decreased/absent bowel sounds.
Peptic ulcers (gastric and duodenal)	Damage of gastrointestinal (GI) mucosa at any area of the GI tract. Caused by bacterial infection *(Helicobacter pylori)* or nonsteroidal antiinflammatory drugs (NSAIDs). Thought to be unrelated to stress. Aggravated by smoking and excessive alcohol use.	*Gastric ulcer:* Dull epigastric pain, localized midline. Early satiety; not usually relieved by food or antacids. *Duodenal ulcer:* Pain is episodic in nature, lasting 30 minutes to 2 hours. Pain is located midline epigastric region, may radiate around costal border to back; described as aching, burning, or gnawing. Typically occurs 1-3 hours after meals and at night (12 midnight to 3 AM). Often relieved by food/antacid. *Both (dyspepsia syndrome):* Complaints of fullness, epigastric discomfort, vague feeling of nausea, abdominal distention, and bloating; anorexia; weight loss (Monahan and others, 2007).

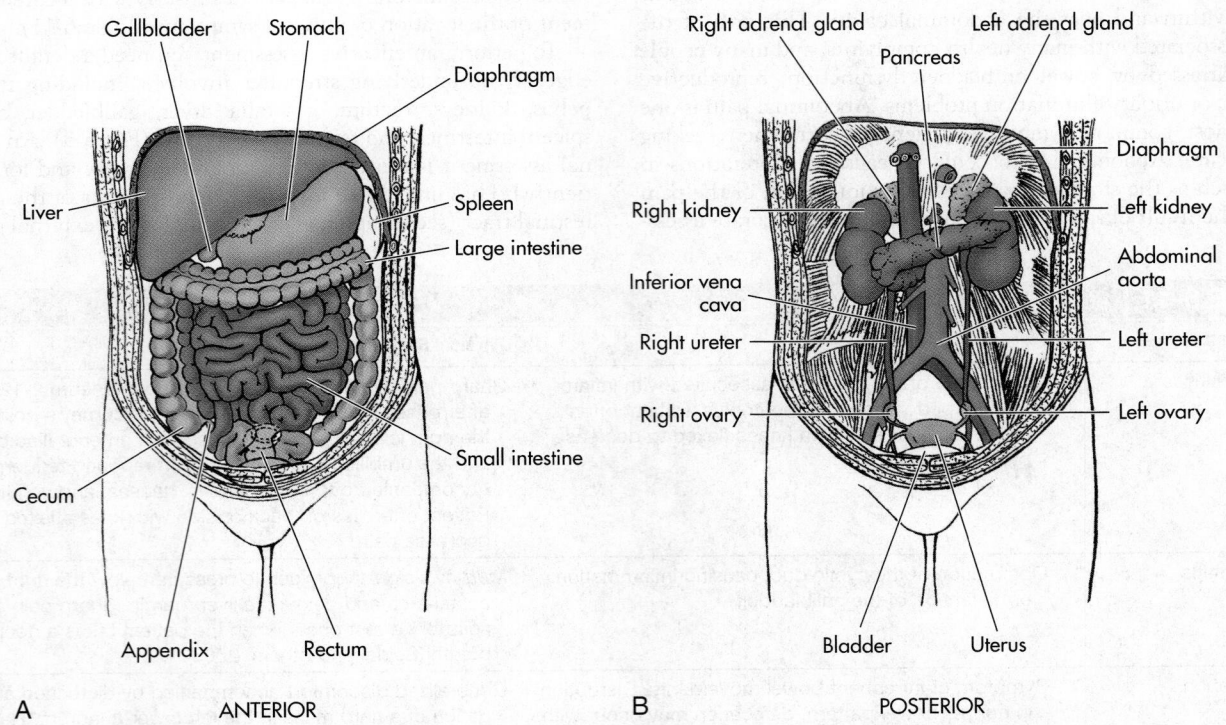

Fig. 6-5 Location of organs in the abdomen. **A,** Anterior. **B,** Posterior. (*Modified from* Mosby's *expert 10 minute physical examinations, ed 2, St. Louis, 2005, Mosby.*)

examination while performing routine hygiene measures or preparing to insert a urinary catheter. An examination of female and male external genitalia is part of preventive health screenings. You examine adolescents and young adults because of the growing incidence of sexually transmitted infections (STIs). The average age of menarche among young girls has declined, and the majority of male and female teenagers are sexually active by age 19 (Hockenberry and Wilson, 2007). You can easily combine rectal and anal assessments with this examination because the patient assumes a lithotomy or dorsal recumbent position.

The order of an abdominal assessment differs from that of other assessments. You begin with inspection and follow with auscultation. It is important to auscultate before palpation and percussion because these maneuvers alter the frequency and character of bowel sounds.

Delegation Considerations

The skill of assessing the abdomen, genitalia, rectum, and anus cannot be delegated to NAP. The nurse directs the NAP to:

- Report development of patient's abdominal pain and changes in the patient's bowel habits or dietary intake to the nurse.
- Report changes in patient's genitourinary function.

Equipment

- ❑ Stethoscope
- ❑ Tape measure
- ❑ Examination light
- ❑ Marking pen
- ❑ Clean gloves
- ❑ Drapes

STEP	RATIONALE

ASSESSMENT

1   General patient survey:
    a   If patient has abdominal or low back pain, assess the character of pain in detail (location, onset, frequency, precipitating factors, aggravating factors, type of pain, severity, course).

Pattern of characteristics of pain helps determine its source.

STEP	**RATIONALE**
b Carefully observe patient's movement and position, such as lying still with knees drawn up, moving restlessly to find a comfortable position, or lying on one side or sitting with knees drawn up to chest.	Positions assumed by patient reveal nature and source of pain. Movement aggravates the pain of peritonitis, patients will lie still. The supine position worsens acute pancreatitis pain; a flexed knee, curved-back position brings relief (Monahan and others, 2007). Patient with appendicitis lies on side or back with knees flexed in an attempt to decrease muscle strain on the abdominal wall (Monahan and others, 2007).
c Assess patient's normal bowel habits: frequency of stools; character of stools; recent changes in character of stools; measures used to promote elimination, such as laxatives, enemas, dietary intake; and eating and drinking habits.	Data compared with physical findings help identify cause and nature of elimination problems.
d Determine if patient has had abdominal surgery, trauma, diagnostic tests of the gastrointestinal (GI) tract, previous illness or surgery involving urinary or reproductive organs, including STIs.	Surgical or traumatic alterations of abdominal organs cause changes in expected areas (e.g., position of underlying organs). Diagnostic tests change character of stool.
e Assess if patient has had recent weight changes or intolerance to diet (nausea, vomiting, cramping, especially in last 24 hours).	Data possibly indicate alterations in upper GI tract (e.g., stomach or gallbladder) or lower colon.
f Assess for difficulty in swallowing, belching, flatulence, bloody emesis (hematemesis), black or tarry stools (melena), heartburn, diarrhea, or constipation.	Indicative of GI alterations.
g Determine if patient takes antiinflammatory medications (e.g., aspirin, steroids, and nonsteroidal antiinflammatory drugs [NSAIDs]), or antibiotics.	These pharmacological agents cause GI upset or bleeding.
h Inquire about family history of cancer, kidney disease, alcoholism, hypertension, or heart disease.	Data reveals risk for significant abdominal alterations. Chronic alcohol ingestion causes GI and liver problems.
i Review patient's history for health care occupation, hemodialysis, intravenous drug use, household or sexual contact with hepatitis B virus (HBV) carrier, sexually active heterosexual person (more than one sex partner in previous 6 months), sexually active homosexual or bisexual man, international traveler in area of high HBV prevalence.	Risk factors for HBV exposure. Abdominal findings for hepatitis include jaundice, hepatomegaly, anorexia, abdominal and gastric discomfort, tea-colored urine, and clay-colored stools (Seidel and others, 2006).
2 Assessment of female patients:	
a Determine if patient has signs and symptoms of vaginal discharge, painful or swollen perianal tissues, or genital lesions.	These signs and symptoms indicate presence of an STI or other pathological condition.
b Determine if patient has symptoms or history of genitourinary problems, including burning during urination (dysuria), frequency, urgency, nocturia, hematuria, or incontinence.	Urinary problems are associated with gynecological disorders, including STIs.
c Ask if patient has had signs of bleeding outside of normal menstrual period or after menopause or has had unusual vaginal discharge.	These are warning signs for cervical and endometrial cancer or vaginal infection.
d Determine if patient has received human papillomavirus (HPV) vaccine.	HPV vaccine is recommended for females to prevent cervical cancer (ACS, 2008b).
e Determine if patient has history of HPV (condyloma acuminatum, herpes simplex, or cervical dysplasia); has multiple sex partners; smokes cigarettes; has had multiple pregnancies.	These are risk factors for cervical cancer (ACS, 2008b). Vaccines are available for HPV for females 9 to 26 years of age.
f Determine if patient is older than 40, obese, and has history of ovarian dysfunction, breast or endometrial cancer, irradiation of pelvic organs, or endometriosis; has family history of ovarian, breast, or colon cancer; has history of infertility or nulliparity; or use of estrogen (alone) hormone replacement therapy.	These are risk factors for ovarian cancer (ACS, 2008a).

STEP	RATIONALE
g Determine if patient is postmenopausal, obese, or infertile; had early menarche; had late menopause; has history of hypertension, diabetes, gallbladder disease, or polycystic ovary disease; has family history of endometrial, breast, or colon cancer; or has a history of estrogen-related exposure (estrogen replacement therapy, tamoxifen use).	These are risk factors for endometrial cancer (ACS, 2008a).

3 Assessment of male patients:

STEP	RATIONALE
a Review normal urinary elimination pattern, including frequency of voiding; history of nocturia; character and volume of urine; daily fluid intake; symptoms of burning, urgency, and frequency; difficulty starting stream; and hematuria.	Urinary problems are directly associated with genitourinary problems because of anatomical structure of men's reproductive and urinary systems.
b Ask if patient has noted penile pain or swelling, genital lesions, or urethral discharge.	These signs and symptoms indicate STI.
c Determine if patient has noticed heaviness or painless enlargement of testis or irregular lumps. If patient reports an enlargement in inguinal area, assess if it is intermittent or constant, associated with straining or lifting, and painful and whether coughing, lifting, or straining at stool causes pain.	Theses signs and symptoms are early warning signs for testicular cancer. Signs and symptoms reflect potential inguinal hernia
d Ask if he has experienced weak or interrupted urine flow, inability to urinate, difficulty in starting or stopping urine flow, polyuria, nocturia, hematuria, or dysuria. Does patient have continuing pain in lower back, pelvis, or upper thighs?	These are warning signs of prostatic cancer (ACS, 2008a). Symptoms also suggest infection or prostate enlargement.

4 Assessment of all patients:

STEP	RATIONALE
a Determine whether patient has experienced bleeding from rectum, black or tarry stools (melena), rectal pain, or change in bowel habits (constipation or diarrhea).	These are warning signs of colorectal cancer (ACS, 2008a) or other GI alterations.
b Determine whether patient has personal or strong family history of colorectal cancer, polyps, or chronic inflammatory bowel disease. Ask if patient is over age 40.	These are risk factors for colorectal cancer (ACS, 2008a).
c Inquire about dietary habits, including high fat intake, diet high in processed or red meats, or deficient fiber content (inadequate fruits and vegetables).	Bowel cancer is often linked to dietary intake of fat or insufficient fiber intake (ACS, 2008b).
d Determine if patient is obese, physically inactive, smokes, or consumes alcohol.	Risk factors for colorectal cancer.
e Assess medication history for use of laxatives or cathartic medications.	Repeated use causes diarrhea and eventual loss of intestinal muscle tone.
f Assess for use of codeine or iron preparations.	Codeine causes constipation. Iron turns feces black and tarry.

NURSING DIAGNOSES

- Constipation
- Deficient knowledge
- Diarrhea
- Health-seeking behavior
- Imbalanced nutrition: less than body requirements
- Imbalanced nutrition: more than body requirements
- Ineffective health maintenance
- Pain (acute, chronic)

Individualize related factors based on patient's condition or needs.

PLANNING

1 Expected outcomes following completion of procedure:

• Abdomen is soft and symmetrical, with smooth and even contour. No mass, distention, or tenderness is palpable. There are no forceful visible pulsations.	Normal findings.
• Bowel sounds are active and audible in all four quadrants.	Indicates normal peristaltic activity.
• No costovertebral angle (CVA) tenderness is present.	No inflammation of kidney.
• Patient denies discomfort or worsening of existing discomfort following examination.	Proper examination procedures have been implemented.
• Patient is able to list warning signs of colorectal cancer; female patient: cervical, endometrial, and ovarian cancer; male patient: testicular and prostate cancer.	Demonstrates learning.

STEP	RATIONALE

IMPLEMENTATION

1 Prepare patient for abdominal assessment:

   a Ask if patient needs to empty bladder or defecate.

      Palpation of full bladder causes discomfort and feeling of urgency and makes it difficult for patient to relax.

   b Keep upper chest and legs draped.

      Maintains patient's comfort during examination, promoting relaxation.

   c Be sure that room is warm.

      Promotes patient's comfort.

   d Have patient lie supine or in a dorsal recumbent position with arms down at sides and knees slightly bent. Place a small pillow under patient's knees.

      Placing the arms under the head or keeping knees fully extended causes the abdominal muscles to tighten. Tightening of muscles prevents adequate palpation.

   e Expose area from just above the xiphoid process down to the symphysis pubis.

      Provides full visualization of abdomen.

Critical Decision Point   *Observe respirations as patient changes position. If abdomen is distended, lying flat will result in increased respiratory difficulty due to pressure on the diaphragm (Mosby's expert 10 minute physical examinations, 2005).*

   f Maintain conversation during assessment except during auscultation. Explain steps calmly and slowly.

      Patient's ability to relax during assessment improves accuracy of findings. Talking will prevent clear detection of bowel sounds.

   g Ask patient to point to tender areas.

      Assess painful areas last. Manipulation of body part increases patient's pain and anxiety and makes remainder of assessment difficult to complete.

2 Abdominal assessment:

   a Identify landmarks that divide abdominal region into quadrants. Boundary is from the tip of xiphoid process to symphysis pubis with line crossing and intersecting the umbilicus, dividing abdomen into four equal sections (see illustration).

      Location of findings by common reference point helps successive examiners to confirm findings and locate abnormalities.

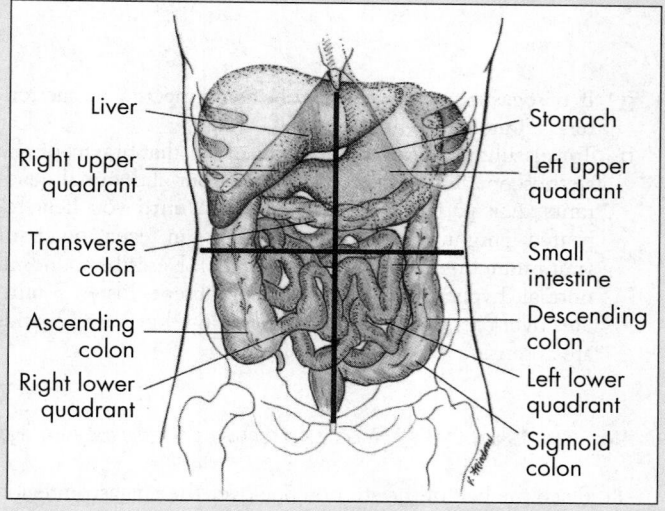

STEP 2a   Division of abdomen into quadrants.

   b Inspect skin of abdomen's surface for color, scars, venous patterns, rashes, lesions, silvery white striae (stretch marks), and artificial openings. Observe lesions for characteristics described in Skill 6-1.

      Scars reveal evidence that patient has had past trauma or surgery. Striae indicate stretching of tissue from growth, obesity, pregnancy, ascites, or edema. Venous patterns reflect liver disease (portal hypertension). Artificial openings indicate bowel or urinary diversion (see Chapter 35).

   c If you notice bruising, ask if patient self-administers injections (e.g., heparin or insulin).

      Frequent injections cause bruising and hardening of underlying tissues. Bruising also indicates physical abuse, accidental injury, or bleeding disorders.

   d Inspect the contour, symmetry, and surface motion of the abdomen. Note any masses, bulging, or distention. (Flat abdomen forms a horizontal plane from xiphoid process to symphysis pubis. Round abdomen protrudes in convex sphere from horizontal plane. Concave abdomen sinks into muscular wall. All are normal.)

      Changes in symmetry or contour reveal underlying masses, fluid collection, or gaseous distention. An everted umbilicus (protruding outward) indicates distention. A hernia also causes the umbilicus to protrude upward.

STEP	RATIONALE

e If abdomen appears distended, note if distention is generalized. Look at the flanks on each side.

Distention may be caused by the nine F's (fat, flatus, feces, fluids, fibroid, full bladder, false pregnancy, fatal tumor, and fetus) (Seidel and others, 2006). If gas causes distention, flanks do not bulge. If fluid causes distention, flanks bulge. Tumor causes a more unilateral bulging or distention. Pregnancy causes symmetrical bulge in lower abdomen.

f If you suspect distention, measure size of abdominal girth by placing tape measure around abdomen at level of umbilicus (see illustration). Use the marking pen to indicate where you applied tape measure.

Consecutive measurements will show any increase or decrease in abdominal distention. Make subsequent measurements at same level of umbilicus to provide objective means to evaluate changes. Use a water-based pen to make a mark on abdomen for subsequent measurements.

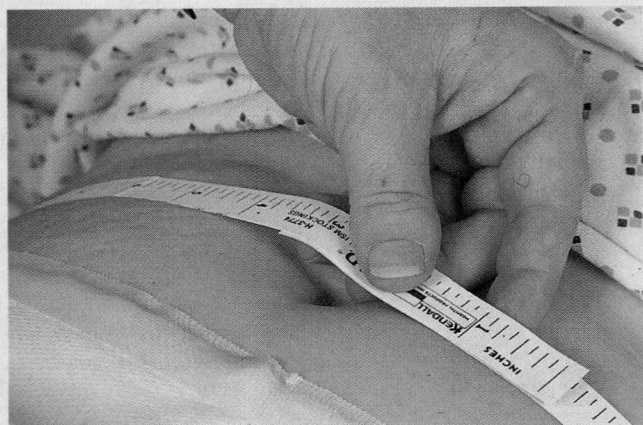

STEP 2f   Measuring abdominal girth at the level of the umbilicus.

g If nasogastric or intestinal tube is connected to suction, turn off momentarily.

Sound of suction machine obscures bowel sounds.

h To auscultate bowel sounds, place the diaphragm of the stethoscope lightly over each of the four abdominal quadrants. Ask patient not to talk. Listen until you hear repeated gurgling or bubbling sounds in each quadrant (minimum of once in 5 to 20 seconds). Describe sounds as normal, hyperactive, hypoactive, or absent. Listen 5 minutes over each quadrant before deciding that bowel sounds are absent.

Normal bowel sounds occur irregularly every 5 to 15 seconds. Absence of sounds indicates cessation of gastric motility. Hyperactive bowel sounds not related to hunger or a recent meal indicate diarrhea or early intestinal obstruction. Hypoactive or absent bowel sounds indicate paralytic ileus or peritonitis (Monahan and others, 2007; *Mosby's expert 10-minute physical examinations*, 2005). It is common for bowel sounds to be hypoactive postoperatively for 24 hours or more, especially following abdominal surgery.

Critical Decision Point   *Nausea and vomiting, increasing distention, and inability to pass flatus sometimes accompany severe paralytic ileus.*

i Place the bell of the stethoscope over the epigastric region of the abdomen and each quadrant. Auscultate for vascular (whooshing) sounds.

Determines presence of turbulent blood flow (bruit) through thoracic or abdominal aorta.

Critical Decision Point   *If you auscultate aortic bruit, which indicates the presence of an aneurysm, stop assessment and notify physician immediately. Percussion or palpation over abdominal bruit could cause rupture of an already weakened vessel wall in the presence of an abdominal aneurysm.*

j With patient supine, gently percuss each of four abdominal quadrants systematically. Note areas of tympany and dullness.

Reveals presence of air or fluid in stomach and intestines. Normal percussion is tympanic because of swallowed air in GI tract. Presence of fluid or underlying masses is revealed by dull percussion.

k To determine if fluid or air is causing distention, percuss for a fluid wave:

If you do feel a fluid wave, air is causing the distention. Presence of a fluid wave indicates ascites, found in cirrhosis, peritonitis, metastatic carcinoma, ovarian carcinoma, and pancreatitis. Jaundice, pruritus, dependent edema, and enlarged superficial abdominal veins often accompany ascites from liver congestion (Monahan and others, 2007).

STEP	RATIONALE

(1) Ask another person to assist by pressing gently and firmly at midline of abdomen (see illustration).

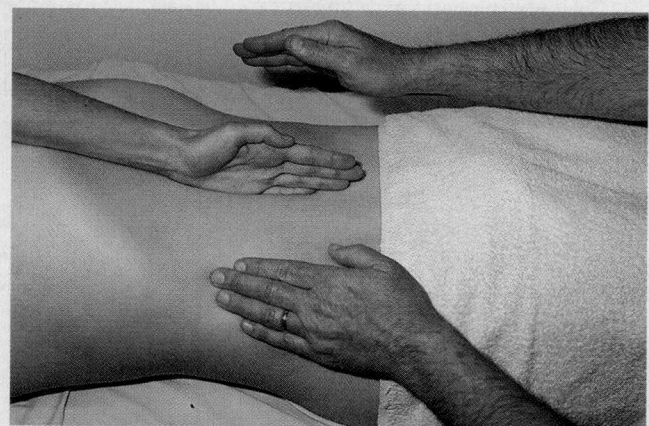

STEP 2k(1)   Testing for fluid wave. (*From Seidel HM and others: Mosby's guide to physical examination, ed 6, St. Louis, 2006, Mosby.*)

(2) Place your fingertips along both sides of the lower abdomen in the lumbar region. Thrust quickly into the patient's side with your dominant hand, keeping the nondominant hand in place.

(3) Palpate for a fluid wave with the nondominant hand.

l Ask patient if abdomen feels unusually tight, and determine if this is a recent development.

Continued sensation of fullness helps to detect distention. A feeling of fullness after a heavy meal causes only temporary distention. Tightness is not felt with obesity.

m With patient sitting, gently but firmly percuss over each costovertebral angle along scapular lines (see illustration A). Use ulnar surface of fist indirectly by placing nondominant hand flat against costovertebral angle and percussing with dominant hand or percuss directly against patient's skin (see illustration B). Note if patient experiences pain.

Determines presence of kidney inflammation.

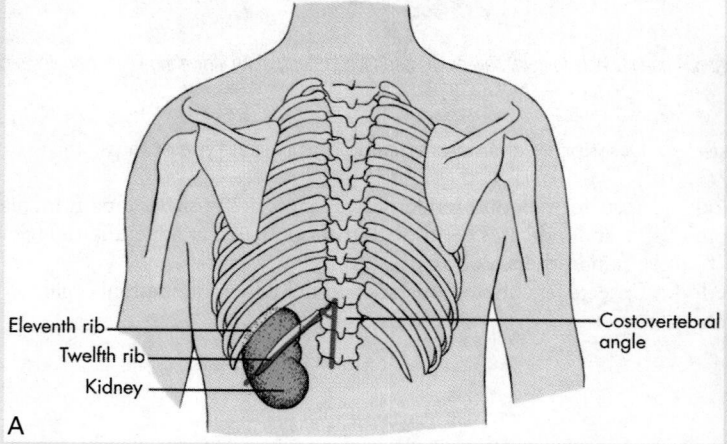

Eleventh rib
Twelfth rib
Kidney
Costovertebral angle

A

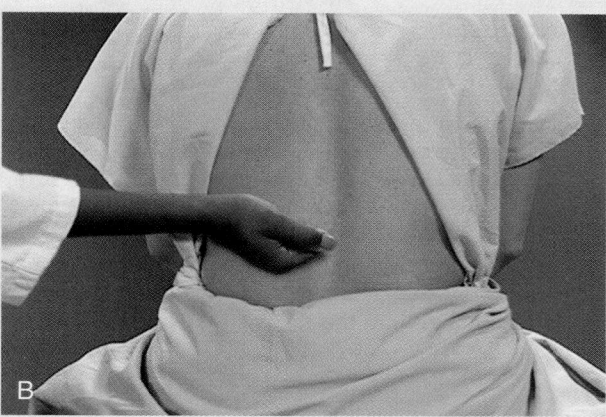

B

STEP 2m   **A,** Position of kidney in relation to costovertebral angle. **B,** Direct percussion of the kidney for costovertebral angle (CVA) tenderness. (*From Seidel HM and others:* Mosby's guide to physical examination, *ed 6, St. Louis, 2006, Mosby.*)

STEP	RATIONALE

n Lightly palpate over each abdominal quadrant, laying the palm of the hand with fingers extended and approximated lightly on the abdomen. Keep the palm and forearm horizontal. The pads of the fingertips depress the skin approximately 1 cm (½ inch) in a gentle dipping motion (see illustration). Palpate painful areas last.

Detects areas of localized tenderness, degree of tenderness, and presence and character of underlying masses. Palpation of sensitive area causes guarding (voluntary tightening of underlying abdominal muscles).

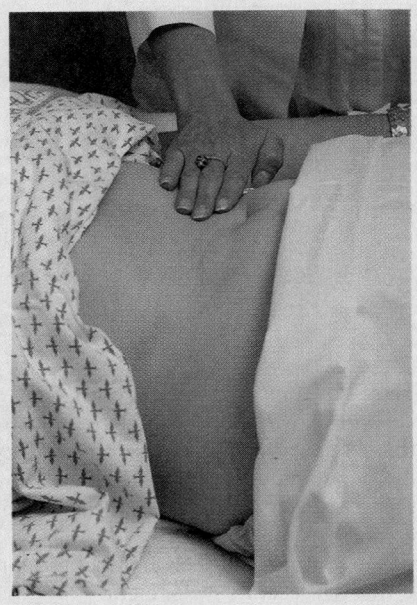

STEP 2n Light palpation of the abdomen.

  (1) Note muscular resistance, distention, tenderness, and superficial masses or organs while observing patient's face for signs of discomfort.

  (2) Note if abdomen is firm or soft to touch.

o Just below umbilicus and above symphysis pubis, palpate for a smooth, rounded mass. While applying light pressure, ask if patient has sensation of need to void.

Patient's verbal and nonverbal cues indicate discomfort from tenderness. Firm abdomen indicates active obstruction with fluid or gas building up.

Soft abdomen is normal or reveals that obstruction is resolving.

Detects presence of dome of distended bladder.

Critical Decision Point *Routinely check for distended bladder if patient has been unable to void, patient has been incontinent, or an indwelling Foley catheter is not draining well.*

p If masses are palpated, note size, location, shape, consistency, tenderness, mobility, and texture.

q When tenderness is present, press one hand slowly and deeply into the involved area and then let go quickly. Note if pain is aggravated.

r Perform deep palpation. Make sure the patient is relaxed. Depress the palm and fingers approximately 2.5 to 7.5 cm (1 to 3 inches) into the abdomen (see illustration).

Descriptive characteristics help to reveal type of mass.

Tests for rebound tenderness. Results are positive if pain increases and indicates peritoneal irritation (such as appendicitis) (Seidel and others, 2006).

Detects less obvious masses and delineates abdominal organs.

STEP	RATIONALE

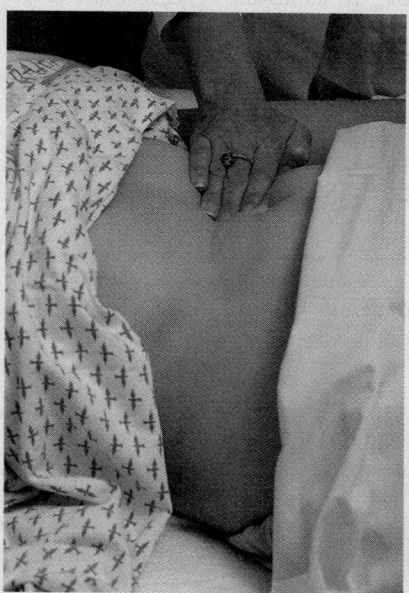

STEP 2r   Deep palpation of the abdomen.

3   Female genitalia examination:
  a   Implement Steps 1a through 1d.
  b   Expose only perineal area.
  c   Apply clean gloves. Inspect surface characteristics of perineum, then retract labia majora; observe for inflammation, edema, lesions, or lacerations. Note if there is any vaginal discharge. Presence of discharge may indicate need for a culture.

Skin of perineum is smooth, clean, and slightly darker than other skin. Mucous membranes are dark pink and moist. Labia majora are symmetrical, may be dry or moist. Normally there is no vaginal discharge.

4   Male genitalia examination:
  a   Have patient void.
  b   Be sure room is warm.
  c   Have patient lie supine with chest, abdomen, and lower legs draped OR have stand during examination.
  d   Apply clean gloves. Observe genitalia for lice, rashes, excoriations, or lesions.

Size of scrotum varies with temperature change.
Position and exposure of body maintains privacy.

Normally the skin is clear without lesions or parasites.

  e   Inspect and palpate penile surfaces:
    (1)   Inspect the corona, prepuce (foreskin), glans, urethral meatus, and shaft. Retract the foreskin in uncircumcised males. Observe for discharge, lesions, edema, and inflammation.

Glans looks smooth and pink along all surfaces. Urethral meatus is slitlike and normally positioned at tip of the glans. The foreskin usually retracts easily; a bit of white cheesy discharge sometimes collects here. The area between the foreskin and glans is a common site for venereal lesions.

  f   Inspect and palpate the scrotum:
    (1)   Inspect size, color, shape, and symmetry; also gently palpate for lesions and edema.

The left testicle is normally lower than the right. Scrotal skin is usually loose, surface is coarse, and skin color is more deeply pigmented than body skin.

  g   Palpate testes:
    (1)   Note size, shape, and consistency of tissue.

Testes are normally ovoid and approximately 2 by 4 cm in size, feel smooth and rubbery, and are free from nodules. Most common symptom of testicular cancer is an irregular, nontender fixed mass.

    (2)   Determine if patient experiences tenderness with palpation.

Testes are normally sensitive, but not tender.

5   Rectal assessment:
  a   Female patient remains in dorsal recumbent position or assumes a side-lying (Sims') position.

These positions allow for optimum visualization.

STEP	RATIONALE
b Male patient stands and bends forward with hips flexed and upper body resting across examination table; examine non-ambulatory patient in Sims' position.	
c View the perianal and sacrococcygeal areas by gently retracting the buttocks using your nondominant hand.	Perianal skin is smooth, more pigmented, and coarser than skin covering the buttocks.
d Inspect anal tissue for skin characteristics, lesions, external hemorrhoids (dilated veins that appear as reddened skin protrusion), ulcers, inflammation, rashes, and excoriation.	Anal tissues are moist and hairless; the voluntary sphincter holds the anus closed.

EVALUATION

1 Compare assessment findings with previous assessment characteristics to identify changes.	Determines presence of abnormalities.
2 Ask patient to describe signs and symptoms of colorectal cancer.	Demonstrates learning.

Unexpected Outcomes	Related Interventions
1 Abdomen is asymmetrical, with palpable mass, and dull to percussion.	• Report to health care provider because findings indicate enlarged liver, spleen, or tumor.
2 Abdomen protrudes symmetrically, with skin taut; patient complains of tightness and/or bowel sounds are absent. Gastrointestinal motility has ceased. Patient is vomiting.	• Keep patient on nothing by mouth (NPO) status, and encourage ambulation. • Notify health care provider; findings indicate an obstruction. • Gastric decompression following insertion of nasogastric tube sometimes becomes necessary.
3 Hyperactive bowel sounds are evident with gastrointestinal motility. Commonly they result from anxiety, diarrhea, overuse of laxatives, inflammation of the bowel, or reaction of the intestines to certain foods.	• Patient may need to be NPO. • Contact health care provider if patient needs antidiarrheal medication.
4 Rebound abdominal tenderness is found.	• Avoid palpating area. • Notify health care provider if this is a new finding. • Place patient on NPO status.
5 Bladder is palpable over symphysis pubis. Bladder is distended.	• Facilitate voiding by placing patient in sitting position or encouraging patient to bear down (if not contraindicated). • If unable to void, urinary catheterization is necessary.
6 Internal organs (liver, spleen) are enlarged.	• Do not continue to palpate area. • Notify health care provider. • Place patient on NPO status. • Enlargement is due to cancerous involvement, hepatitis, or cirrhosis.
7 Abdominal girth is increased, accompanied by a fluid wave. Fluid has built up within peritoneal cavity.	• Notify health care provider. • Place patient on NPO status.
8 Patient is unable to describe signs and symptoms of colorectal cancer.	• Additional education is necessary.

Recording and Reporting

- Record results of assessment in nurses' notes or flow sheet.
- Record patient's ability to void and defecate, including description of output.
- Record content of any patient instruction.
- Report serious abnormalities, such as absent bowel sounds, presence of a mass, or acute pain, to nurse in charge and health care provider.

Teaching Considerations

- Explain that factors such as diet, regular exercise, limited use of over-the-counter drugs causing constipation, establishment of regular elimination schedule, and adequate fluid intake promote normal bowel elimination.
- Explain activities or positions to avoid if patient has acute pain.
- If patient is a health care worker or has contact with blood or body fluids of affected persons, encourage patient to receive series of three hepatitis B vaccine doses.

- Discuss the guidelines of the ACS (2008b) for early detection of colorectal cancer for both men and women. The ACS (2008b) recommends the following examination schedules beginning at age 50:
  - Tests that detect polyps and cancer; one of the following: (1) flexible sigmoidoscopy (every 5 years), (2) colonoscopy (every 10 years), (3) double-contrast barium enema (every 5 years), (4) computed tomographic colonoscopy (every 5 years).
  - Test that primarily detect cancer: (1) guaiac-based fecal occult blood test (g fobt), or fecal immunochemical test (FIT) with high sensitivity for cancer (every year), (2) stool DNA (interval unclear).
- Discuss warning signs of colorectal cancer, including long-term progressive weight loss, change in bowel habits, and blood in stools.
- Discuss dietary planning and healthy lifestyle choice to maintain or improve colon health.

- Warn patient against problems caused by overuse of laxatives, cathartic medications, codeine, or enemas.

Female Health Teaching Considerations
- Instruct patient about purpose and recommended frequency of Papanicolaou (Pap) smears and gynecological examinations.
- Explain warning signs of STIs: pain or burning on urination, pain during sex, pain in pelvic area, bleeding between menstruation, itchy rash around vagina, and abnormal vaginal discharge.
- Teach measures to prevent STIs (e.g., male partner's use of condoms, restricting number of sexual partners, avoiding sex with persons who have several other partners, perineal hygiene measures).
- Reinforce the importance of performing perineal hygiene (as appropriate).

Male Health Teaching Considerations
- Explain warning signs of STIs: pain on urination and during sex, abnormal penile discharge, swollen lymph nodes, or rash or ulcer on skin or genitalia. Teach measures to prevent STIs: use of condoms, avoiding sex with infected partner, avoiding sex with persons who have multiple partners, and using regular perineal hygiene. Tell patients with an STI to inform their sexual partners of the need to have an examination. Instruct patient to seek treatment as soon as possible if partner becomes infected with an STI.
- Instruct patient in how to perform genital self-examination (see Box 6-2).

Pediatric Considerations
- Most common palpable abdominal mass in child is feces, usually palpated in right lower quadrant (Hockenberry and Wilson, 2007).

- Have a child stand erect and then lie supine during inspection of abdominal surface. Normal abdomen of infants and young children is cylindrical in erect position and flat in supine position. School-age children may have a rounded abdomen until 13 years of age when standing.
- In infants and children skin is usually taut and without wrinkles or creases.
- Infants and children (until the age of 7 years) are abdominal breathers.
- Some children perceive superficial palpation as tickling. Drawing attention to their laughter only causes it to increase. Have the children help by placing their hand on top of yours, or have them place their hand on their abdomen with their fingers separated and then palpate between their fingers.

Gerontological Considerations
- Older adult often lacks abdominal tone; underlying organs are more easily palpable (Reuben and others, 2005).
- Some older adults have increased fat deposits over the abdomen.
- A weakened intestinal musculature and decreased peristalsis affect the large intestine.
- Constipation along with nausea, flatulence, and heartburn are common.
- Stress to older adults importance of adequate fluid intake, regular exercise, and a diet with at least four servings daily of fresh fruit and vegetables and high-fiber foods to promote normal defecation.

SKILL 6-6   Musculoskeletal and Neurological Assessment

The nurse uses the skills of inspection and palpation during the musculoskeletal and neurological assessments. Initial assessment involves a general inspection of gait, posture, and body position. A more thorough assessment of major bone, joint, and muscle groups and the nervous system is indicated in the presence of abnormalities or as required by patient's condition. You can perform much of the assessment while examining the other body systems. For example, while assessing head and neck structures assess neck range of motion (ROM) and examine select cranial nerves. Integrate these assessments into routine activities of care, for example, while bathing or positioning a patient. Assessment of these systems is important when a patient reports pain, loss of sensation, or impairment of joint and/or muscle function.

Prolonged illness or immobility results in muscle weakness and atrophy. Some hospitalized patients experience neurovascular dysfunction as a result of high or low blood pressure or constriction of the extremities with dressings or a cast.

Delegation Considerations
The skill of assessing musculoskeletal and neurological function cannot be delegated to NAP. However, the nurse directs the NAP to:

- Recognize patients' problems with gait and ROM.
- Report any problems noted in ROM or muscle strength.
- Take precautions during ROM exercises to avoid forcing a joint beyond the patient's current ROM.
- Be informed of patients at risk for falls.
- Assist patients with muscular weakness with transfer and ambulation.

Equipment
- ❑ Cotton balls or cotton-tipped applicators
- ❑ Penlight
- ❑ Opposite tip of cotton swab or tongue blade broken in half
- ❑ Tape measure
- ❑ Tongue blade
- ❑ Tuning fork
- ❑ Reflex hammer

STEP	RATIONALE

ASSESSMENT

1 Review patient history for use of alcohol and/or caffeine; cigarette smoking; constant dieting; calcium intake less than 500 mg daily; thin and light body frame; females who have never been pregnant (nulliparous status); estrogen deficiency; menopause before age 45; postmenopausal status; family history of osteoporosis; white, Asian, American Indian, or northern European ancestry; advanced age; sedentary lifestyle; chronic diseases (Cushing's, hyperthyroidism and hypothyroidism, malabsorption/malnutrition disorders, neoplasms); long-term use of corticosteroids, methotrexate, phenytoin, heparin, and aluminum-containing antacids; lack of weight-bearing exercise; lack of exposure to sunlight (Holcomb, 2005, 2006).

These are risk factors for osteoporosis.

2 Determine if patient has been screened for osteoporosis.

Women age 65 and older need routine screening for osteoporosis (Holcomb, 2006; North American Menopause Society, 2006). Men are equally at risk for development of osteoporosis.

3 Ask patient to describe history of bone, muscle, or joint function (e.g., recent fall, trauma, lifting heavy objects, bone or joint disease with sudden or gradual onset) and location of alteration.

History assists in assessing nature of musculoskeletal problem. Osteoporosis-related fractures occur in half of all postmenopausal women; of those, 25% will have vertebral deformities, and 15% will suffer from hip fractures (U.S. Preventive Services Task Force, 2003).

4 Assess nature and extent of patient's musculoskeletal pain: location, duration, severity, predisposing and aggravating factors, relieving factors, and type of pain. If patient reports pain or cramping in the lower extremities, ask if it is relieved or aggravated by walking. Assess the distance walked and characteristics of pain before, during, and after activity.

Pain frequently accompanies alterations in bone, joints, or muscle. This has implications not only for comfort, but also ability to perform activities of daily living. Pain caused by certain vascular conditions tends to increase with activity.

5 Determine how alteration influences ability to perform activities of daily living (e.g., bathing, feeding, dressing, toileting, ambulating) and social functions (e.g., household chores, work, recreation, sexual activities).

The extent to which patient is able to perform self-care will determine the level of nursing care. Type and degree of restriction in continuing social activities influence topics for patient education and ability of nurse to identify alternative ways to maintain function.

6 Assess for a decrease in height in women older than 50 by subtracting current height from recall of maximum adult height.

Measurement is useful screening tool to predict osteoporosis. A loss of height is frequently the first clinical sign of osteoporosis.

7 Determine patient use of analgesics, alcohol, sedatives, hypnotics, antipsychotics, antidepressants, nervous system stimulants, or recreational drugs.

These medications alter level of consciousness or cause behavioral changes. Abuse sometimes causes tremors, ataxia, and changes in peripheral nerve function.

8 Determine if patient has recent history of seizures/convulsions: clarify sequence of events (aura, fall to ground, motor activity, loss of consciousness); character of any symptoms; and relationship of seizure to time of day, fatigue, or emotional stress.

Seizure activity often originates from central nervous system alteration. Characteristics of seizure help determine its origin.

9 Screen patient for headache, tremors, dizziness, vertigo, numbness or tingling of body part, visual changes, weakness, pain, or changes in speech.

These symptoms frequently originate from alterations in central nervous system or peripheral nervous system function. Identification of specific patterns aids in diagnosis of pathological condition.

10 Discuss with patient's family recent changes in patient's behavior (e.g., increased irritability, mood swings, memory loss, change in energy level).

Behavioral changes sometimes result from intracranial pathological states.

11 Assess patient for history of change in vision, hearing, smell, taste, or touch.

Major sensory nerves originate from brain stem. These symptoms help to localize nature of problem.

12 If a patient displays sudden acute confusion (delirium), review history for drug toxicity (anticholinergics, digoxin, antihistamines, antipsychotics, benzodiazepines, opioid analgesics, sedative/hypnotics, steroids), serious infections, metabolic disturbances (such as diabetes mellitus), heart failure, and severe anemia.

Delirium is one of the most common mental disorders in older persons but also occurs in children (Gray-Vickery, 2005).

STEP	RATIONALE

13   Review past history for head or spinal cord injury, meningitis, congenital anomalies, neurological disease, or psychiatric counseling.

Factors cause neurological symptoms or behavioral changes to develop, focusing assessment on possible cause.

NURSING DIAGNOSES

- Activity intolerance
- Disturbed body image
- Impaired physical mobility
- Impaired walking
- Ineffective peripheral tissue perfusion

- Pain (acute, chronic)
- Risk for injury
- Risk for peripheral neurovascular dysfunction

- Risk for trauma
- Self-care deficit (bathing/hygiene, dressing/grooming, feeding, or toileting)

Individualize related factors based on patient's condition or needs.

PLANNING

1   Expected outcomes following completion of procedure:

- Patient demonstrates erect posture, strong grasp, steady gait, with arms swinging freely at side.

  Indicates normal alignment, gait, and neuromuscular muscle strength.

- There is bilateral symmetry of extremities in length, circumference, alignment, position, and skinfolds (Seidel and others, 2006).

- Full active ROM is present in all joints with good muscle tone and absence of contractures, spasticity, or muscular weakness.

  Indicates normal ROM of joints.

- Patient is alert and oriented to person, place, and time. Behavior and appearance appropriate for condition/situation.

  Indicates normal cerebral function.

- Patient demonstrates the following: pupils equal, reactive, respond to light and accommodation (PERRLA), direct and consensual; external ocular muscles (EOMs) intact; facial sensation intact; symmetrical facial expressions; soft palate and uvula midline and rise upon phonation; gag reflex intact; speech clear without hoarseness; no difficulty swallowing.

  Indicates normal functioning of cranial nerves (CNs) III, IV, VI, V, VII, IX, and X.

- Patient distinguishes between sharp and dull sensations and light touch on symmetrical areas of extremities. Able to distinguish vibratory sensations on symmetrical distal joints of toes and fingers. Position sense intact to lower extremities.

  Indicates normal function of sensory nerves.

- Gait coordinated, steady with appropriate stance and swing phases. Romberg test negative.

  Indicates normal cerebellar and motor system functioning.

IMPLEMENTATION

1   Prepare patient:

   a   Integrate musculoskeletal and neurological assessments during other portions of physical assessment or during nursing care.

   Conserves patient's energy and allows observation of patient performing activities more naturally.

   b   Plan time for short rest periods during assessment.

   Movement of body parts and various maneuvers fatigue patient. It is especially important to consider rest periods with older adult and very ill patients.

2   Musculoskeletal assessment:

   a   Observe ability to use arms and hands for grasping objects (see illustration).

   Assesses coordination and muscle strength.

   b   Assess muscle strength of upper extremities by applying gradual increase in pressure to muscle group.

   Upper and lower extremity on patient's dominant side is normally stronger than that on nondominant side. Pain, rather than weakness, causes reduced muscle strength; however, long-term pain can lead to muscle weakening.

   c   To assess hand grasp strength, have patient grasp fingers of both of your hands and squeeze them as hard as possible. To avoid discomfort, you may cross index and middle fingers (see illustration).

   It is common for the patient's dominant hand to be slightly stronger than the nondominant hand. By crossing hands, patient's right hand grasps your right hand.

STEP	RATIONALE

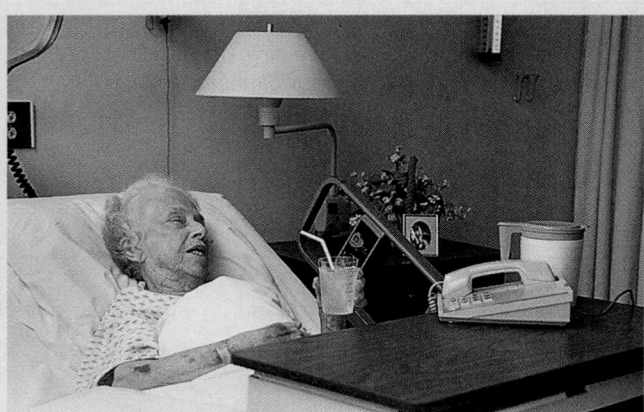

STEP 2a   Observe use of arms and hands.

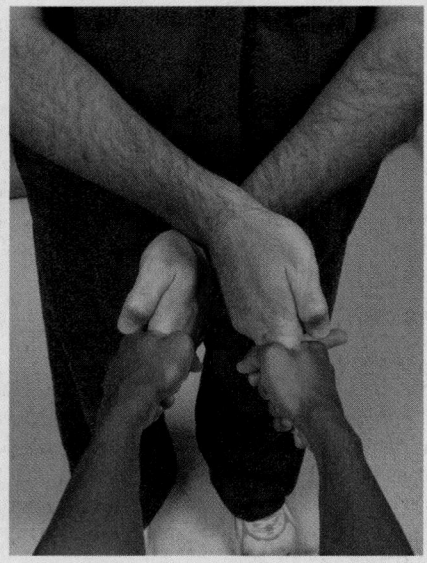

STEP 2c   Assessing strength of hand grasps, comparing sides.

d   Place hand on lower arm or leg, and have patient move major joint (e.g., elbow, knee) against resistance. For example, instruct patient to push hand against yours. Have patient maintain pressure until told to stop. Compare symmetrical muscle groups. Note weakness, and compare right with left.

Compares strength of symmetrical muscle groups. Rate muscle strength on scale of 0 to 5: Grade as follows:
0—No voluntary contraction
1—Slight contractility, no movement
2—Full range of motion, passive
3—Full range of motion, active
4—Full range of motion against gravity, some resistance
5—Full range of motion against gravity, full resistance
Indicates degree of atrophy.

e   If you identify muscle weakness, measure muscle size with tape measure placed around body of muscle. Compare with same muscle on opposite side of body.

f   Observe body alignment for sitting, supine, prone, or standing positions. Muscles and joints should be exposed and free to move to allow for accurate measurement.

Each joint or muscle group requires different position for measurement.

g   Inspect gait as patient walks and stands. Observe for foot dragging, shuffling or limping, balance, presence of obvious deformity in lower extremities, and position of the trunk in relation to the legs.

Gait is more natural if patient is unaware of nurse's observation. Assesses for a neuromusculoskeletal disorder.

h   Stand behind patient, and observe postural alignment (position of hips relative to shoulders). Look sideways at cervical, thoracic, and lumbar curves (see illustrations).

Abnormal curves of posture include lordosis (swayback, increased lumbar curvature), kyphosis (hunchback, exaggerated posterior curvature of thoracic spine), and scoliosis (lateral spinal curvature). Postural changes indicate muscular, bone, or joint deformity; pain; or muscular fatigue. Head should be held erect.

STEP	RATIONALE

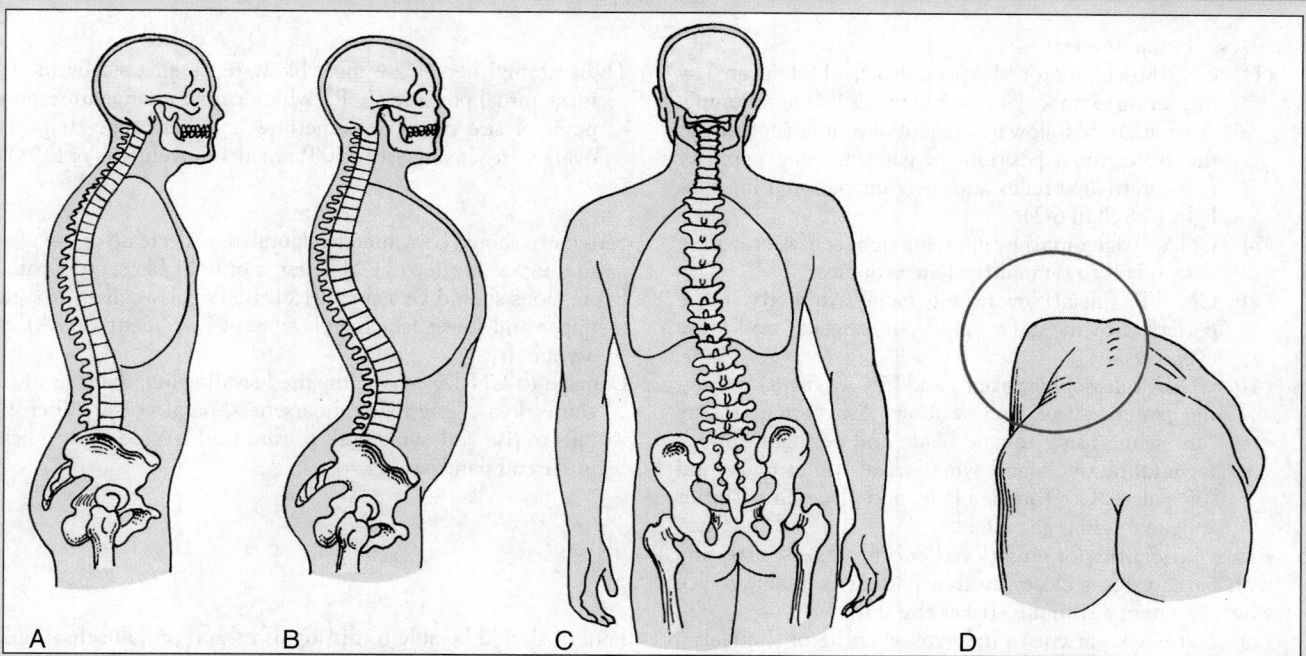

STEP 2h Spinal deformities. **A,** Kyphosis. **B,** Lordosis. **C,** Scoliosis. **D,** Scoliosis with patient bending forward.

i Make a general observation of the extremities. Look at overall size, gross deformity, bony enlargement, alignment, and symmetry.

General review helps to pinpoint areas requiring in-depth assessment.

j Gently palpate bones, joints, and surrounding tissues where patient reports pain. Note any heat, tenderness, edema, or resistance to pressure.

Reveals changes resulting from trauma or chronic disease. Do not attempt to move joint when fracture is suspected or when joint is apparently "frozen" by lack of movement over a long period of time.

k Ask patient to put major joint through its full ROM (Table 6-12, p. 165). Observe equality of motion in same body parts:

Assessment of patient's normal ROM provides baseline for assessing later changes after surgery or inactivity. Patients with deformities, reduced mobility, joint fixation, or weakness often require passive motion assessment.

(1) Active motion (patient needs no support or assistance and is able to move joint independently): Instruct patient in moving each joint through its normal range. Sometimes it is necessary to demonstrate movements and ask patient to mimic your movements.

Identifies muscle strength and detects limited range of motion.

(2) Passive motion (joint has full ROM but patient does not have the strength to move it independently): Have patient relax and move the same joints passively until the end of the range is felt. Support extremity at joint. Do not force the joint if there is pain or muscle spasm.

Determines ability to perform joint motion in the presence of muscle weakness. Forcing joint will cause injury and pain.

l Palpate joint for swelling, stiffness, tenderness, and heat; note any redness.

Indicates acute or chronic inflammation. Range of motion causes pain or injury.

m Assess muscle tone in major muscle groups. Normal tone causes mild, even resistance to movement through entire ROM.

If muscle has increased tone (hypertonicity), any sudden movement of joint is met with considerable resistance. Hypotonic muscle moves without resistance. Muscle feels flabby.

3 Neurological assessment

a Assess level of consciousness and orientation by asking patient to identify name, location, day of week, and year; note behavior and appearance.

A fully conscious patient responds to questions spontaneously. As consciousness declines, may show irritability, shortened attention span, or an unwillingness to cooperate. As consciousness deteriorates, patient becomes disoriented to name, time, and place. Behavior and appearance reveal information about the patient's mental status.

STEP	RATIONALE

b Assess cranial nerves:

(1) CN III (oculomotor), IV (trochlear), VI (abducens) by measuring extraocular movement (EOM) functioning. Ask patient to follow movement of your finger through the six cardinal positions of gaze; measure pupillary reaction to light reflex and accommodation using penlight (see Skill 6-2).

These cranial nerves are most likely to be affected by increasing intracranial pressure (ICP), which causes change in response of pupil or size of pupil; sometimes pupils change shape (more oval) or react sluggishly. ICP impairs movements of EOMs.

(2) CN V (trigeminal) by applying light sensation with a cotton ball to symmetrical areas of face.

Sensations should be symmetrical; unilateral decrease or loss of sensation is possibly due to CN V lesion or in higher sensory pathways.

(3) CN VII (facial) by noting facial symmetry. Have patient frown, smile, puff out cheeks, and raise eyebrows.

Expressions should be symmetrical; Bell's palsy causes drooping of upper and lower face; cerebrovascular accident (CVA) causes asymmetry.

(4) CN IX (glossopharyngeal) and CN X (vagus) by having patient speak and swallow. Ask patient to say "ah" while using tongue blade and penlight. Check for midline uvula and symmetrical rise of uvula and soft palate. Use tongue blade, and place on posterior tongue to elicit gag reflex.

Damage to CN IX causes impaired swallowing; damage to CN X causes loss of gag reflex, hoarseness, nasal voice. When palate fails to rise and uvula pulls toward normal side, this indicates a unilateral paralysis.

c Assess extremities for sensation. Perform all sensory testing with patient's eyes closed so that patient is unable to see when or where a stimulus strikes the skin.

(1) *Pain:* Ask patient to indicate when he or she feels a sharp or dull sensation as you alternately apply sharp and blunt ends of tongue blade to skin surface. Apply in symmetrical areas of extremities.

Patient should be able to distinguish sharp or dull sensations. Impaired sensations indicate disorders of the spinal cord or of peripheral nerve roots.

(2) *Light touch:* Apply light wisp of cotton to different points along skin's surface in symmetrical areas of extremities.

Patient should be able to distinguish when touched.

(3) *Vibration:* Apply stem of vibrating tuning fork to distal joints of toes and fingers. Have patient voice when and where vibration is felt and when sensation stops.

Loss of vibratory sensation occurs with peripheral neuropathy.

(4) *Position:* Grasp finger or toe, holding it by its sides with your thumb and index finger. Alternate moving finger or toe up and down. Ask patient to state when finger is up or down. Repeat with toes.

Patient should be able to distinguish movements of a few millimeters. Decreased/absent position sense may occur in spinal anesthesia, paralysis, or other neurological disorders.

d Assess motor and cerebellar function:

(1) *Gait:* Have patient walk across the room, turn, and come back. Similarly, note use of assistive devices.

Neurological and musculoskeletal disorders impair gait and balance.

(2) *Romberg's test:* Have patient stand with feet together, arm at sides, both with eyes open and eyes closed (for 20 to 30 seconds). Protect patient's safety by standing at side; observe for swaying.

Romberg test should be negative; slight swaying is considered normal.

e Assess deep tendon reflexes (DTRs):

(1) In patients with back pain or surgery, CVA, or spinal cord compression, it is appropriate to assess DTRs (Seidel and others, 2006). In most settings this is not part of the routine physical assessment.

Muscle spasticity and hyperactive reflexes may result from disorders such as stroke and paralysis. Diminished DTR and muscle weakness may suggest lower motor neuron disorders such as amyotrophic lateral sclerosis (ALS) or Guillain-Barré syndrome.

(2) For each reflex tested, compare sides and assign a grade on the following scale:

Grade indicates extent of neuron dysfunction.

Clonus is described as repeated spasms of muscular contraction and relaxation.

0　No response

1+　Sluggish or diminished response

2+　Normal, active or expected response

3+　More brisk than expected; slightly hyperactive

4+　Very brisk; hyperactive, with clonus.

STEP	RATIONALE
(3) *Knee reflex:* Palpate the patellar tendon just below the patella. Tap the pointed end of the reflex hammer briskly on the tendon.	Knee reflex is the most common DTR assessment performed. The normal response is knee extension (see illustration).
(4) *Plantar response (Babinski's reflex):* Using the handle end of the reflex hammer, stroke the lateral aspect of the sole, from the heel to the ball of the foot.	The toes should flex inward and downward (see illustration).
(5) After stroking the soles of the feet, if Babinski's reflex is present, the great toe will dorsiflex, accompanied by fanning of the other toes.	Indicates CNS dysfunction. Dorsiflexion of the great toe and fanning of the others is normal in a child younger than age 2 (Hockenberry and Wilson, 2007).

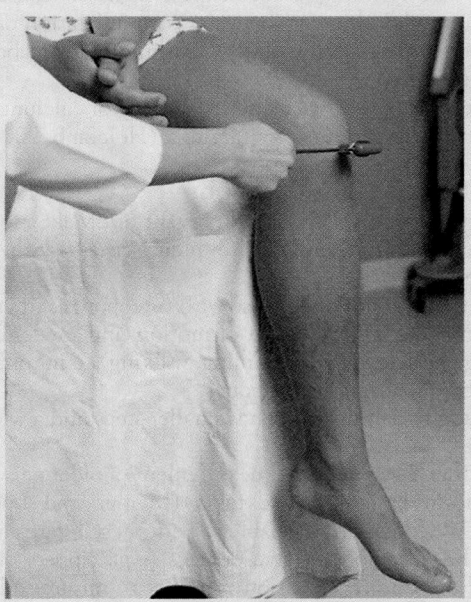

STEP 3e(3)   Position for testing patellar tendon reflexes. Lower leg will normally extend.

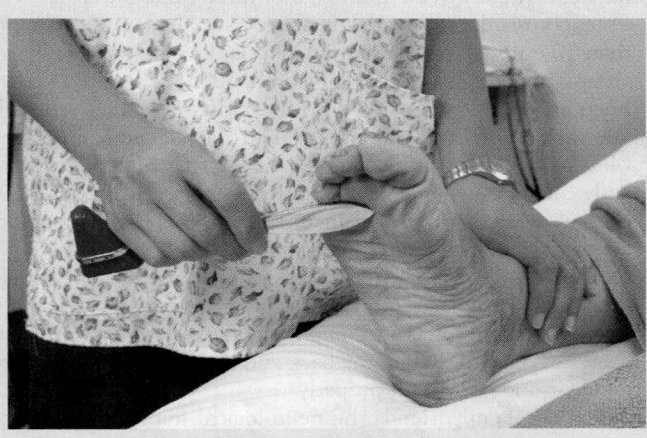

STEP 3e(4)   Toes should flex inward and downward.

EVALUATION

1 Compare muscle strength and ROM with previous physical assessment.	Determines presence of abnormalities.
2 Compare neurological status with previous physical assessment.	Determines presence of abnormalities.
3 Evaluate level of patient's discomfort following procedure using appropriate pain scale.	Determines if manipulation of musculoskeletal structures intensifies patient's discomfort.

Unexpected Outcomes	Related Interventions
1 Joints are prominent, swollen, and tender with nodules or overgrowth of bone in distal joints, indicating signs of arthritis.	• Instruct patient in proper ROM. • Determine patient's knowledge regarding use of antiinflammatory medications and nonphamacological measures (see Chapter 15).
2 Reduced ROM in one or more major joints: shoulder, elbow, wrist, fingers, knee, hip.	• Assess further for pain during movement, with joint unstable, stiff, painful, or swollen or with obvious deformity. • Notify health care provider. • Reduce mobility in extremity until cause of abnormal joint motion is determined.
3 Patient demonstrates weakness in one or more major muscle groups, or gait demonstrates unsteady balance with shuffling or stumbling of feet.	• Place patient on fall precautions. • Provide patient safety when ambulating (see Chapter 10). • Notify health care provider.
4 Patient has changes in mental status and pupillary response or other neurological deficits.	• Notify physician immediately. • Continue to assess patient's vital signs and level of consciousness closely. • Place on fall precautions.

Recording and Reporting

- Record posture, gait, muscle strength, and ROM in nurses' notes or appropriate assessment flow sheet.
- Record level of consciousness, orientation, pupillary response, sensation, and reflex responses in nurses' notes or appropriate assessment flow sheet.
- Report to nurse in charge or health care provider acute pain or sudden muscle weakness, change in level of consciousness, or change in size or pupillary reaction, which is indicative of condition requiring immediate treatment.

Teaching Considerations

- Instruct patient about correct postural alignment. Consult with physical therapist to provide patient with exercises for improving posture.
- Exercise regularly to strengthen muscles and bones.
- To reduce bone demineralization, instruct older adult patient in a proper weight-bearing exercise program (e.g., walking, low-impact aerobics) to be followed 3 or more times a week.
- Osteoporosis does not just affect older women; it affects more than 10 million American women and men and strikes all age-groups, including children (Holcomb, 2005).
- Encourage intake of calcium to meet the recommended daily allowance. Increased vitamin D will aid calcium absorption (400 to 800 international units daily). Recommendation for daily calcium supplements for adults over age 25: 1000 to 1500 mg/day. Instruct patient to take no more than 500 mg of calcium supplements at one time (Holcomb, 2006).
- Explain to patients with low back pain that they can benefit from modification of worker risk factors (e.g., lifting heavy weights, use of protective equipment), regular aerobic exercise, exercises that strengthen the back and increase trunk flexibility, and learning how to lift properly.
- Explain to family/friends the neurological implications of any behavioral or mental impairment the patient demonstrates.
- Explain measures to ensure safety (e.g., use of ambulation aids or safety bars in bathrooms or stairways) for patients with sensory or motor impairments.

Pediatric Considerations

- Examine infants carefully for musculoskeletal anomalies resulting from genetic or fetal insults. An examination includes review of posture, generalized movement, symmetry and skin creases of the extremities, muscle strength, and hip alignment.
- Normally the back of a newborn is rounded or C-shaped from the thoracic and pelvic curves.
- Scoliosis, lateral curvature of the spine, is an important childhood problem, especially in females, usually identified before puberty. (For closer examination, have child stand erect, wearing only underclothes. Observe from behind, looking for asymmetry of shoulders and hips. Then observe from the back as the child bends forward.) Uneven dress hems or trouser hems or uneven fit of clothing at the waist is an indication of scoliosis.
- Watching a child during play reveals information about musculoskeletal function.
- Children age 9 to 19 years need 1300 mg of calcium daily with 400 international units of vitamin D (Holcomb, 2006).

Gerontological Considerations

- Instruct older adults about fall prevention. Make modifications in the home environment to reduce the risk of falls (see Chapter 42).
- Instruct older adults and those with osteoporosis in proper body mechanics, as well as range-of-motion and moderate weight-bearing exercises (e.g., swimming, walking) to minimize trauma and subsequent fracture of bones.
- Older adult's gait normally has smaller steps and a wider base of support.
- Functional assessment is a measurement of older person's ability to perform basic self-care tasks (Meiner and Lueckenotte, 2006). When patient is unable to perform self-care easily, determine the need for assistive devices (e.g., zippers on clothing instead of buttons, elevation of chairs to minimize bending of knees and hips).
- Instruct older adult patient to pace activities to compensate for loss in muscle strength.
- Older adults tend to assume a stooped, forward-bent posture, with hips and knees somewhat flexed, arms bent at the elbows, and the level of the arms raised.

TABLE 6-12	Assessing Range of Motion (ROM)*	
Body Part	**Assessment Procedure**	**ROM**
Upper Extremities		
Shoulders	Raise both arms to a vertical position level at the sides of the head.	Flexion.
	Place both hands behind the neck, with elbows out to the sides.	External rotation and abduction.
	Place both hands behind the small of the back (internal rotation).	Internal rotation.
	Have patient make small circles with hands with arms extended at shoulder level.	Circumduction.
Elbows	Bend and straighten the elbows.	Flexion and extension.
	Place hands at waist with elbows flexed.	Internal rotation.
Wrist	Flex and extend wrist.	Flexion and extension.
	Bend wrist to radial then ulnar side.	Radial and ulnar deviation.
	Turn palm upward, then downward.	Supination and pronation.
Hand	Make a fist with both hands; open hand.	Flexion and extension.
	Extend and spread fingers and thumb outward; bring back together.	Adduction and abduction.
Lower Extremities		
Hips (with patient supine)	With knees extended, raise one leg upward.	Flexion: Expect 90 degrees.
	Repeat with knee flexed.	Abduction: Expect 45 degrees.
	Swing legs laterally.	Adduction: Expect 30 degrees.
	With knee flexed, hold the ankle, and rotate the leg inward and outward.	Internal and external rotation: Expect 40-45 degrees.
Knees (with patient sitting)	Raise the foot, keeping the knee in place.	Extension: Expect full extension and up to 15 degrees hyperextension.
Ankles	With foot held off the floor, point toes, and then bring toes back toward the knee.	Plantar flexion: Expect 45 degrees.
		Dorsiflexion: Expect 20 degrees.
	Turn foot inward and then outward.	Inversion and eversion: Expect to reach 5 degrees.
Toes	Bend toes down and back.	Expect to reach 40 degrees.

*This may be done actively by the patient (AROM) or passively by the nurse (PROM).

SKILL 6-7   Assessing Intake and Output

 Basic Skills / Nutrition and Fluids / Measuring Intake and Output

Measuring and recording intake and output (I&O) during a 24-hour period helps to complete the assessment database for fluid and electrolyte balance. You are responsible for accurate recording of all intake (liquids taken orally, by enteral feedings, and parenterally) and all output (urine, diarrhea, vomitus, gastric suction, and drainage from surgical tubes). Placing a patient on I&O requires cooperation and assistance from the patient and family.

Monitoring I&O is an independent or a dependent nursing intervention. Keeping records of I&O is appropriate if a patient has a fever, has edema, is receiving intravenous or diuretic therapy, or is on restricted fluids. It is also important when a patient has electrolyte losses associated with vomiting, diarrhea, gastrointestinal drainage, or extensive open wounds such as burns. Evaluate general monitoring of I&O for all patients, although measuring and documentation on the chart is not required in some situations.

When indicated, you total and evaluate I&O at the end of each shift or at specified times, usually 8 hours. Significant alterations are apparent by comparing 24-hour totals over several days. Because fluid imbalance occurs at any time, be aware of I&O for all patients, even when documentation is not required.

Delegation Considerations

The skill of assessing I&O totals at the end of each shift, comparing 24-hour totals over several days, and monitoring and recording of intravenous therapy, wound or chest tube drainage, and tube feedings cannot be delegated to NAP. The nurse directs the NAP to:

- Measure and record oral intake.
- Measure and record urinary output and wound drainage device output.
- Report changes in patient's condition such as significant alteration in intake or changes in color, amount, or odor of output.

The nurse emphasizes maintaining standard precautions relating to body fluids, accurately measuring and recording I&O, and using the metric system with standard containers.

Equipment

- ❑ Sign alerting all personnel of I&O measurement
- ❑ Daily I&O record
- ❑ Graduated measuring container
- ❑ Bedpan, urinal, bedside commode, or urine "hat" (a receptacle that fits under the toilet seat)
- ❑ Clean gloves

STEP	RATIONALE

ASSESSMENT

1 Identify patients with conditions that increase fluid loss:

a Fever — Prolonged fever diminishes body fluids by increasing insensible water losses from lungs through increased respiratory rate and from diaphoresis.

b Diarrhea and/or vomiting — Diarrhea and vomiting leads to fluid and electrolyte imbalances, especially in the very young and frail older adults. Loss of potassium and chloride ions and excretion of hydrogen ions alter acid-base balance.

c Surgical wound drainage or chest tube drainage — Wound drainage represents plasma or whole blood loss. If significant amounts are lost, fluid loss needs to be replaced.

d Gastric suction — Hydrochloric acid, potassium, and fluids from the stomach are removed.

e Major burns — Fluid volume loss is directly proportional to amount and depth of injury. Major fluid shifts can occur at specific intervals following severe burns.

f Severe trauma (especially crushing injuries) — Hyperkalemia results from release of intracellular potassium from injured cells.

g Endocrine imbalance
   (1) Cushing's disease — Corticosteroids cause sodium and water retention with potassium excretion.
   (2) Addison's disease — Deficiency of corticosteroids causes sodium and water excretion.
   (3) Diabetic ketoacidosis — Osmotic diuresis from increased blood glucose levels causes fluid volume deficit.

2 Identify patients with impaired swallowing, unconscious patients, and patients with impaired mobility. — These patients have risk of insufficient fluid intake.

3 Identify patients who are taking medications that influence fluid balance, including diuretics and steroids. — Synthetic steroid preparations, such as prednisone, cause fluid retention, whereas diuretics cause a fluid deficit.

4 Assess signs and symptoms of dehydration and fluid overload (e.g., bradycardia versus tachycardia, hypotension versus hypertension, reduced skin turgor versus edema). — Signs of dehydration result from reduction of fluid within tissues and circulatory system. Compensation for overhydration results in a fluid shift into tissues, causing edema.

5 Weigh patients daily, and observe for dehydration or fluid volume excess. — Kidneys attempt to excrete excess fluid during periods of overhydration and conserve body water during periods of dehydration.

Critical Decision Point *Obtain daily weights with the same scale, at the same time of day, and with comparable articles of clothing.*

6 Monitor laboratory reports: — Patients' condition and therapies such as parenteral fluid replacement can alter laboratory values.

a Urine specific gravity (normal is 1.010 to 1.030) — Increased urine specific gravity suggests dehydration.

b Hematocrit (Hct) (normal range is 38% to 47% for females and 40% to 54% for males). — Increased hematocrit suggests dehydration. Low hematocrit suggests blood loss/hemorrhage or anemia.

7 Assess patient and family's knowledge of the purpose and process of I&O measurement. — Improves cooperation in reporting intake and output to nurse.

NURSING DIAGNOSES

- Deficient fluid volume
- Diarrhea
- Excess fluid volume
- Urinary incontinence (functional, stress, reflex, or urge)
- Urinary retention

Individualize related factors based on patient's condition or needs.

PLANNING

1 Expected outcomes following completion of procedure:
- Oral intake is 600 to 900 mL greater than output and at least 1500 mL per 24 hours. — Normal oral intake maintained.
- Weight remains within 2% of baseline. — Indicates stable fluid balance.
- Hematocrit and urine specific gravity are within normal limits (WNL). — Normal hydration achieved without fluid alterations.

STEP	RATIONALE
2 Post sign alerting personnel that I&O measurement is required.	Ensures that staff will measure all sources of intake and output.
3 Place I&O record in established location at the bedside or at the door.	Provides access to record for timely recording.

IMPLEMENTATION

STEP	RATIONALE
1 Explain to patient and family the reasons I&O are important.	Encouraging fluids is a nursing responsibility. Encourage any patient not restricted in total fluid intake to consume at least 1500 mL/day. Postoperative patients are frequently prescribed clear liquid diets and advanced to solid fluids as you determine that they are able to tolerate it.

2 Measure and record all intake of fluid:
  a Liquids with meals, gelatin, custards, ice cream, popsicles, sherbets, ice chips (recorded as 50% of measured volume [e.g., 100 mL of ice chips equals 50 mL of water]). Convert household measures to the metric system: 1 ounce equals 30 mL, therefore 12 ounces (soda can) equals 360 mL.
  b Count liquid medicines such as antacids as fluid intake, as are fluids with medications.
  c Calculate fluid intake from tube feedings (see Chapter 31).
  d Calculate fluid intake from parenteral fluids, blood components, and total parenteral nutrition solutions (see Chapters 28 and 29).
	Provides comprehensive and accurate assessment.

Critical Decision Point *Record intake as soon as you measure it to maintain accuracy. If more than one patient is in the same room, each must have urine receptacles labeled with name and bed location.*

STEP	RATIONALE
3 Instruct patient and family to call you or NAP to empty contents of urinal, urine hat, or commode each time patient uses it. Patient and family also need to monitor incontinence, vomiting, and excessive perspiration and report it to the nurse.	You can weigh urine leakage on a pad (1 mL of urine weighs 1 g), and count the number of pads used in 24 hours.
4 Inform patient and family that Foley catheter drainage bag and wound, gastric, or chest tube drainage are closely monitored, measured, and recorded and who is responsible for this. Each patient must have a graduated container clearly marked with name and bed location and used only for the patient indicated.	Prevents patient or family from disrupting drainage systems.
5 Measure drainage at the end of the shift, using appropriate containers and noting color and characteristics. NOTE: Apply clean gloves. If splashing is anticipated, wear mask, eye protection, and/or gown. a Measure urine drainage using a "hat" into which patient voids or a graduated container (see illustration).	Provides comprehensive and accurate assessment over standard time frames. Prevents transmission of infection.

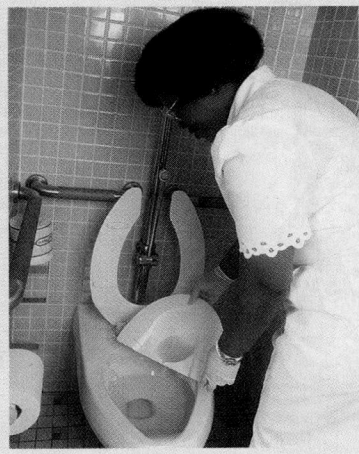

STEP 5a Measuring and emptying the urine "hat."

STEP	RATIONALE

b Observe color and characteristics of urine in Foley tubing. Sometimes you will measure hourly urine output using a special device (see illustration).

Drainage in the tubing is representative of current output. Characteristics of drainage in the bag are often very noticeably different based on changes over time.

c Measure chest tube drainage by marking and recording the time on the collection chamber at specified intervals (see illustration) (see Chapter 26).

Critical Decision Point   *Empty chest tube drainage ONLY when container is nearly full. A closed system is necessary to maintain lung reexpansion.*

Critical Decision Point   *In adults, urine output less than 30 mL/hr indicates decreased renal perfusion and is reported. When output is low, use a special device that facilitates measuring hourly output.*

d Measure Jackson-Pratt/Hemovac drainage using a medicine cup (see illustration) (see Chapter 38).

Drainage is usually less than 30 mL in volume.

e Measure gastric drainage or larger drainage pouches by opening clamp and pouring into graduated cup with a 240-mL capacity (see illustration).

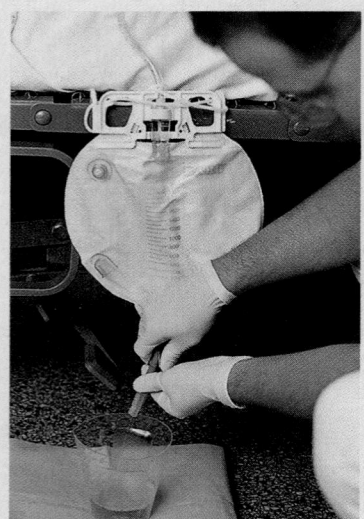

STEP 5b   Device for monitoring hourly urine output.

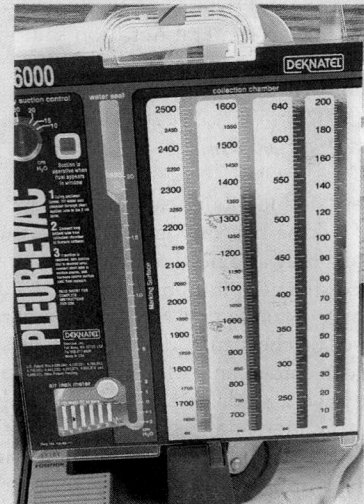

STEP 5c   Collection chamber for measuring chest tube drainage.

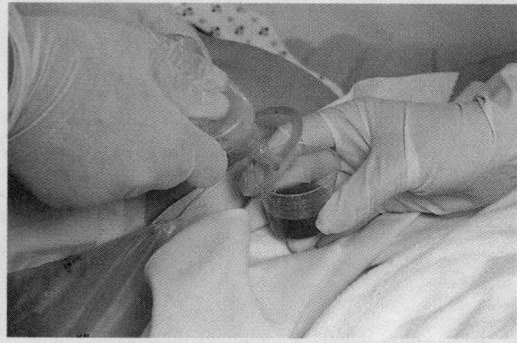

STEP 5d   Measuring wound drainage through a Jackson-Pratt drain.

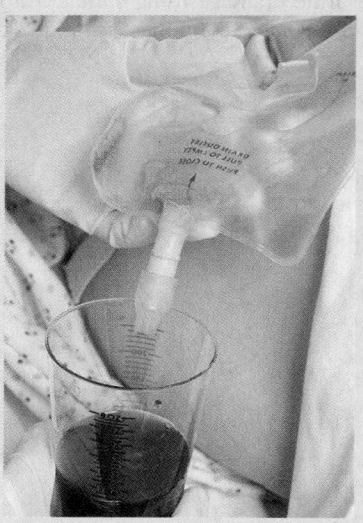

STEP 5e   Measuring drainage from large drainage pouch.

STEP	RATIONALE

EVALUATION

1 Observe condition of skin and mucous membranes.

Condition reflects hydration status.

2 Observe color, characteristics, and amount of urine and wound drainage.

Presence of sudden increase in bright red blood indicates hemorrhage, which leads to hypovolemic shock. Certain medication and some foods (beets, rhubarb, blackberries) cause color changes in the urine.

3 Note I&O balance or imbalance (Table 6-13, p. 170).

Indicates patient's overall fluid status.

Unexpected Outcomes

1 Prolonged fluid loss without adequate replacement of fluid as evidenced by output greater than intake, weight loss greater than 2% over 24 to 48 hours, and an increased hematocrit value.

2 Chemical or physiological imbalance results in fluid retention evidenced by intake greater than output.

Related Interventions

- Obtain frequent vital signs.
- Observe for orthostatic hypotension when sitting patient up in bed or assisting with ambulation (see Chapters 5 and 10).
- Administer fluid replacement as ordered.
- Notify health care provider of changes in patient's physical assessment status.

- Notify health care provider.
- Weigh patient.
- Place patient on fluid restrictions.
- Administer diuretics as ordered.

Recording and Reporting

- At specified time according to agency policy, calculate total I&O on the specified intake and output record at the bedside or at the door.
- Document the total on the patient's record (Fig. 6-6).
- Report immediately to health care provider any urine output less than 30 mL/hr or significant changes in daily weight, which suggest fluid volume deficit or excess.

Teaching Considerations

- Some patients who are able to ambulate need to be reminded of need to measure and record all liquid I&O.
- Severely ill or disoriented patients are sometimes unable to understand reasons for I&O measurement or to participate in measuring and recording. Family members often are able to help maintain accurate records.
- Patients who have fluid restriction (e.g., renal failure, congestive heart failure) need strict I&O because fluid imbalance quickly results in serious physiological changes. Remove water pitcher from bedside.

Pediatric Considerations

- Infants and young children have a greater need for water and are more vulnerable to alterations in fluid and electrolyte balance from conditions such as vomiting and diarrhea (Hockenberry and Wilson, 2007).

- You can measure output in infants by weighing diapers; 1 g of diaper weight is equal to 1 mL of urine.
- Infants need to ingest a greater amount of fluid per kilogram of body weight than do older children (Hockenberry and Wilson, 2007).

Gerontological Considerations

- With age, bladder capacity decreases, the prevalence of involuntary bladder contractions increases, and more urine is produced at night (Meiner and Lueckenotte, 2006).
- Urinary incontinence is not a function of age and should be thoroughly evaluated (Meiner and Lueckenotte, 2006).
- Patients with chronic illness and/or older than age 60 are at greater risk of fluid and electrolyte imbalances secondary to gastroenteritis.
- Older adults are more susceptible to fluid and electrolyte imbalances with prolonged fever.

Home Care Considerations

- Have patient and caregiver practice measuring I&O correctly using I&O chart and available containers. Provide more appropriate measuring devices if needed.
- Instruct patient and caregiver regarding daily weights as an important adjunct to monitoring I&O. Stress the importance of using the same scale, same time of day, and similar clothing.

TABLE 6-13 | Assessing for Fluid Imbalances

Fluid Volume Deficit	Fluid Volume Excess
• Output greater than intake	• Intake greater than output
• Decreased blood pressure	• Crackles (pulmonary edema)
• Increased pulse	• Bounding pulse
• Fever	
• Flat neck veins when supine	• Jugular venous distention (JVD)
• Slow venous filling of dependent hands	
• Rapid weight loss >5%	• Rapid weight gain
• Dry mouth	
• Dry skin	
• Tenting	• Pitting edema

? CRITICAL THINKING EXERCISES

You are caring for Mrs. Williams, a 73-year-old retired schoolteacher who underwent a right hip arthroplasty. This is her first postoperative day on your clinical unit. The night nurse reported that patient had an "uneventful" night. She has an intravenous infusion, right hip dressing, Foley catheter to gravity, and a Jackson-Pratt drain in place.

1 What body systems would you assess for this patient?
   a Describe key elements in these assessments.
2 Upon auscultation of her posterior lung field bases, you hear a crackling noise upon inspiration. You also assess and note her breathing is shallow. What is this sound, and what does it indicate? What nursing diagnosis is a priority to consider at this time?
3 You next assess her cardiac status, and she has a heart rate of 86 beats per minute, rhythm regular. What does this assessment indicate?
4 Mrs. Williams complains of right hip pain and requests pain medication. After you administer the medication, you inspect and then auscultate her abdomen. After listening for 60 seconds at a site below and to the right of the umbilicus, you are unable to hear bowel sounds. What is the best assessment of this situation?
5 While assisting Mrs. Williams with the bath, you assess the peripheral neurovascular status of her lower extremities. What key elements are included in this assessment? What findings indicate deep vein thrombosis?
6 Mrs. Williams' history reveals osteoporosis. List the risk factors predisposing a patient to osteoporosis. What specific teaching regarding musculoskeletal health should be employed?

✓ REVIEW QUESTIONS

1 A nurse, in orientation, is performing an abdominal assessment. Which action would indicate that further practice and study is indicated?
   1 The bowel is auscultated before being palpated.
   2 The nurse determines any tenderness before touching the patient.
   3 Inspection is done before percussion.
   4 The abdomen is palpated before auscultation is done.

2 A nurse is performing a neurological assessment. Which approach is most effective in obtaining accurate data when testing sensory pathways?
   1 Perform each test quickly.
   2 Have the patient as relaxed as possible.
   3 Compare symmetrical areas.
   4 Use a predictable order of assessment.
3 An older adult female patient presents with a history of vomiting and diarrhea. Assessment findings reveal lethargy, decreased skin turgor, a weight loss of 5 pounds in 3 days, and a hematocrit of 51%. What other assessment data would the nurse expect to find?
   1 Hypoactive bowel sounds and an elevated urine specific gravity of 1.026
   2 Concentrated urine and hyperactive bowel sounds
   3 Moist mucous membranes and a low urine specific gravity of 1.008
   4 Increased capillary refill time and brisk reactive pupils
4 During the respiratory assessment, the nurse thinks he hears some crackles in his older adult patient. What should the nurse do to ensure that the assessment is correct?
   1 Ask the patient if he has ever had crackles in his lungs.
   2 Ask the patient to breathe in through his nose.
   3 Have the patient breathe in deeper when the bases are auscultated.
   4 Check the patient's medical record to determine if they were previously heard on auscultation.
5 Calculate the patient's intake based on the following amounts: 3 ounces of orange juice, half carton of milk (240 mL per carton), 3-ounce popsicle, 12 ounces of cola, and an 8-ounce cup of ice.

REFERENCES

Anbarghalami R and others: When to suspect child abuse, *RN* 70(4):34, 2007.
Ball JW, Bindler RC: *Child health nursing: partnering with children and families*, Upper Saddle River, NJ, 2006, Pearson Prentice Hall.
Bartley MK: Preventing venous thromboembolism in medical/surgical patients, *Nurs Manage* 36:16, 2005.
Bartley MK: Keep venous thromboembolism at bay, *Nursing* 36(10):36, 2006.
Dougherty K: Recognizing signs of child abuse, *Nursing 2006 Critical Care* 1(6):45, 2006.
Elkin M and others: *Nursing interventions and clinical skills*, ed 4, St. Louis, 2007, Mosby.
Engel JK: *Pediatric assessment*, ed 5, St. Louis, 2006, Mosby.
Frakes MA, Evans T: TB: your vigilance is VITAL, *RN* 67(11):30, 2004.
Geroff AD, Olshaker JS: Elder abuse, *Emerg Med Clin North Am* 24(2):491, 2006.

Glover AL: How to detect and defend against DVI, *Nursing* 35(10):32, 2005.

Gray-Vickrey P: What's behind acute delirium? *Nursing Made Incredibly Easy!* 3(1):20, 2005.

Hockenberry MJ, Wilson D: *Wong's nursing care of infants and children*, ed 8, St. Louis, 2007, Mosby.

Holcomb S: Boning up on osteoporosis, *Nursing Made Incredibly Easy!* 3(2):7, 2005.

Holcomb SM: Osteoporosis, *Nursing* 36(4):48, 2006.

Kovach K: Intimate partner violence, *RN* 67(8):38, 2004.

Meiner SE, Lueckenotte A: *Gerontologic nursing*, ed 3, St. Louis, 2006, Mosby.

Monahan FD and others: *Phipps' medical-surgical nursing: health and illness perspectives*, ed 8, St. Louis, 2007, Mosby.

Moore MC: *Pocket guide to nutritional care*, ed 5, St. Louis, 2005, Mosby.

Mosby's expert 10 minute physical examinations, St. Louis, 2005, Mosby.

Muehlbauer M, Crane PA: Elder abuse and neglect, *J Psychosoc Nurs Ment Health Serv* 44(11):43, 2006.

Reuben DB and others: *2005 Geriatrics at your fingertips*, ed 7, Williston, Vt, 2005, Blackwell.

Roberts S: Insulin shots: choosing the right spot, *Diabetes Forecast* 60(8):43, 2007.

Seidel HM and others: *Mosby's guide to physical examination*, ed 6, St. Louis, 2006, Mosby.

Truscott W: The role of PPE in contact transfer, *Infection Control Today*, October 18, 2005.

Zitelli B, Davis H: *Atlas of pediatric physical diagnosis*, ed 5, St. Louis, 2007, Mosby.

RESEARCH REFERENCES

American Cancer Society: *Cancer facts and figures 2008*, Atlanta, 2008a, The Society.

American Cancer Society: *Cancer prevention and early detection facts and figures 2008*, Atlanta, 2008b, The Society.

North American Menopause Society. Management of osteoporosis in post menopausal women: 2006 position statement of the North American Menopause Society, *Menopause* 13(3):340, 2006.

Medical Asepsis

KEY TERMS

Asepsis
Aseptic technique
Colonized
Contamination
Immunocompro-
  mised
Infection
Invasive procedure
Isolation
Medical asepsis
Microorganism

Health care–
  acquired
  infection
Pathogen
Standard
  precautions
Surgical asepsis
Transmission-
  based
  precautions

MEDIA RESOURCES

- **evolve** learning system   http://evolve.elsevier.com/Perry/skills
  - Video Clips
  - Review Questions

- View Video!   Mosby's Nursing Video Skills, 3.0

- NSO   Nursing Skills Online

OBJECTIVES

Mastery of content in this chapter will enable the nurse to:

- Discuss how to apply critical thinking in the prevention of the transmission of infection.
- Explain the difference between medical and surgical asepsis.
- Identify nursing care measures intended to break the chain of infection.
- Explain how each element of the infection chain contributes to infection.
- Describe factors that can influence nursing staff compliance with hand hygiene.
- Perform proper procedures for hand hygiene.
- Perform correct isolation techniques.

Infection control practices that reduce and eliminate sources and transmission of infection help to protect patients and health care providers from disease. Patients in all health care settings are at risk of becoming colonized or infected as a result of an impaired immune response, exposure to an increased number of pathogenic organisms, and performance of invasive procedures. Health care–acquired infections (HAIs) are those that develop as a result of contact with a health care facility/provider, and the infection was not present or incubating at the time of admission. A hospital is one of the most likely settings for acquiring an HAI because of staff, patients, and environmental factors that support a high population of pathogens that are resistant to antibiotics. Health care workers transmit many HAIs by direct contact during the delivery of care. Although protection of the patient from HAIs is an obvious priority, nurses are also at risk because of contact with infectious materials or exposure to a communicable disease.

As a nurse, you are responsible for educating patients about infection control. Patient and family teaching needs to include information concerning signs and symptoms of infection, modes of transmission, and methods of prevention. Knowledge of the infectious process, disease transmission, and critical thinking skills associated with use of aseptic techniques and barrier protection are essential. The Joint Commission's (TJC's) new Speak Up Program (2007) encourages patients to ask questions about their rights, including questions about infection control. For example, it is believed that if patients ask health care providers if they have washed their hands, compliance by health care providers will increase. Through education you play a vital role in the prevention and control of infections.

The mere presence of a pathogen does not mean that an infection will begin. Development of an infection occurs in a cyclical process, often referred to as the chain of infection, which depends on the following six elements:

1. An infectious agent or pathogen
2. A reservoir or source for pathogen growth
3. A portal of exit from the reservoir
4. A mode of transmission
5. A portal of entry to the host
6. A susceptible host

An infection develops if this chain remains intact (Fig. 7-1). Nurses use infection control practices to break an element of the chain so as not to transmit infection (Table 7-1). The nurse's efforts to minimize the onset and spread of infection are based upon asepsis and the principles of aseptic technique. Asepsis is the absence of pathogenic (disease-producing) microorganisms (DeCastro, 2005). The two types of aseptic technique nurses practice are medical and surgical asepsis.

Medical asepsis, or clean technique, includes procedures used to reduce the number of and prevent the spread of microorganisms. Hand hygiene, barrier techniques, and routine environmental cleaning are examples of medical asepsis. Principles of medical asepsis are common in the home, as in the case of washing hands before preparing food.

Surgical asepsis, or sterile technique, includes procedures used to eliminate all microorganisms from an area. Sterilization destroys all microorganisms and their spores (Rutala, 2005). Nurses in the operating room (OR), labor and delivery area, and procedural areas practice sterile technique when using sterile instruments and supplies.

Nurses also use sterile technique on nursing units during performance of certain invasive procedures (e.g., insertion of a central line or an indwelling urinary catheter). The techniques for maintaining surgical asepsis are more rigid than those performed under medical asepsis (see Chapter 8).

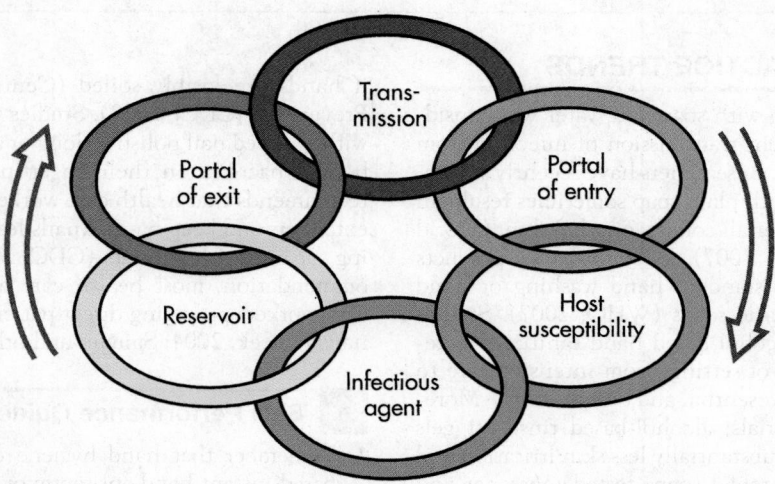

FIG 7-1 Chain of infection.

TABLE 7-1	Breaking the Chain of Infection
Element of Infection Chain	**Medical Aseptic Practices**
Infectious agent (pathogenic organism capable of causing disease)	Cleanse contaminated objects. Perform cleaning, disinfection, and sterilization.
Reservoir (site or source of microorganism growth)	Control sources of body fluids and drainage. Perform hand hygiene. Bathe patient with soap and water or with disposable bath. Change soiled dressings. Dispose of soiled tissues, dressings, or linen in moisture-resistant bags. Place syringes, uncapped hypodermic needles, and intravenous needles in designated puncture-proof containers. Keep table surfaces clean and dry. Do not leave bottled solutions open for prolonged periods. Keep solutions tightly capped. Keep surgical wound drainage tubes and collection bags patent. Empty and dispose of drainage suction bottles according to agency policy.

Portal of exit (means by which microorganisms leave a site)	Respiratory
	   Avoid talking, sneezing, or coughing directly over wound or sterile dressing field.
	   Cover nose and mouth when sneezing or coughing.
	   Wear mask if suffering respiratory tract infection.
	Urine, feces, emesis, and blood
	   Wear clean gloves when handling blood and body fluids.
	   Wear gowns and eyewear if there is a chance of splashing fluids.
	   Handle all laboratory specimens as if infectious.

Transmission (means of spread)	Reduce microorganism spread.
	   Perform hand hygiene.
	   Use personal set of care items for each patient.
	   Avoid shaking bed linen or clothes; dust with damp cloth.
	   Avoid contact of soiled item with uniform.
	   Discard any item that touches the floor.
	   Follow standard precautions or select transmission-based isolation precautions.

Portal of entry (site through which microorganism enters a host)	Skin and mucosa
	   Maintain skin and mucous membrane integrity, lubricate skin, offer frequent hygiene, turn and position.
	   Cover wounds as needed.
	   Clean wound sites thoroughly.
	   Dispose of used needles in puncture-proof container.
	Urinary
	   Keep all drainage systems closed and intact, maintaining downward flow.

Host (patient)	Reduce susceptibility to infection.
	   Provide adequate nutrition.
	   Ensure adequate rest.
	   Promote body defenses against infection.
	   Provide immunization.

EVIDENCE-BASED PRACTICE TRENDS

For generations, hand washing with soap and water was considered the best method to prevent transmission of infection from health care workers to patients. Researchers have recently shown, however, that hand washing with plain soap sometimes results in paradoxical increases in bacterial counts on the skin (World Health Organization [WHO], 2007). Alcohol-based products have been more effective for standard hand washing or hand antisepsis than soap or antiseptic soaps (WHO, 2007). Studies have shown the efficacy of alcohol-based hand sanitizers in reducing infections in a variety of settings from intensive care to long-term care (Jagger, 2007; Rosenthal and others, 2005). Moreover, in several prospective trials, alcohol-based rinses or gels containing emollients caused substantially less skin irritation and dryness than plain or antimicrobial soaps tested (Visscher and others, 2006). Soap and water is still necessary for hand hygiene

if hands are visibly soiled (Centers for Disease Control and Prevention [CDC], 2002). Studies show that health care workers with chipped nail polish or long or artificial nails have high numbers of bacteria on their fingertips. For this reason, the CDC recommends that health care workers not wear artificial nails and extenders and keep natural nails less than ¼ inch long when caring for high-risk patients (CDC, 2002). In response to this recommendation, most health care agencies now prohibit health care workers providing direct patient care from wearing artificial nails (Micek, 2004; Saiman and others, 2002).

 Skill Performance Guidelines

1 Remember that hand hygiene using an appropriate alcohol-based instant hand antiseptic or soap and water is an essential part of patient care and infection prevention.

2 Always know a patient's susceptibility to infection. Age, nutritional status, stress, disease processes, and forms of medical therapy can place patients at risk.
3 Recognize the elements of the chain of infection, and initiate measures to prevent the onset and spread of infection.
4 Incorporate consistently the basic principles of asepsis into patient care.

5 Protect fellow health care workers from exposure to infectious agents through proper use and disposal of equipment.
6 Be aware of body sites where nosocomial infections are most likely to develop (e.g., urinary or respiratory tract). This enables the nurse to direct preventive measures.

SKILL 7-1   Hand Hygiene

 Basic / Basic Infection Control / Performing Hand Hygiene

NSO Infection Control Module / Lessons 1 and 2

The most important and most basic technique in preventing and controlling transmission of infection is hand hygiene. Hand hygiene is a general term that applies to hand washing, antiseptic hand wash, antiseptic hand rub, or surgical hand antisepsis. Hand washing refers to washing hands with plain soap and water. An antiseptic hand wash is defined as washing hands with water and soap or other detergents containing an antiseptic agent. An antiseptic hand rub means to apply an antiseptic hand rub product to all surfaces of the hands to reduce the number of microorganisms present. Surgical hand antisepsis is an antiseptic hand wash or antiseptic hand rub performed preoperatively by surgical personnel to eliminate transient and reduce resident hand flora. Antiseptic detergent preparations often have persistent antimicrobial activity (WHO, 2007).

The most common means of transmitting infection between patients is contact with the health care worker's hands. For example, a nurse caring for a patient who has excessive pulmonary secretions assists the patient in expectorating mucus and disposes of the tissues in a bedside container. The patient's roommate asks the nurse to open containers of food on the meal tray. The nurse then leaves the patient's room to pour a dose of medication due in 5 minutes. If the nurse fails to perform hand hygiene before each of these actions, organisms from the first patient's mucus are transmitted to the roommate's food and to the medication container. Kim and others (2003) have found that hand-hygiene compliance among health care workers who work in patient isolation is low. An observational study conducted in two intensive care units at a tertiary care hospital found an overall compliance rate of 22.1%. *Hand hygiene is not optional.* It is a critical responsibility for all health care workers.

When hands are visibly dirty or contaminated with proteinaceous material or visibly soiled with blood or other body fluids,

you need to wash your hands with either a nonantimicrobial soap and water or an antimicrobial soap and water. If hands are not visibly soiled, use an alcohol-based hand rub for routinely decontaminating hands in the following situations:
1 Before having direct contact with patients
2 Before putting on sterile gloves and before inserting indwelling urinary catheters, peripheral vascular catheters, or other invasive devices
3 After contact with a patient's intact skin (e.g., when taking a pulse or blood pressure, and lifting a patient)
4 After contact with body fluids or excretions, mucous membranes, nonintact skin, and wound dressings if hands are not visibly soiled
5 When moving from a contaminated body site to a clean body site during care
6 After contact with inanimate objects (including medical equipment) in the immediate vicinity of a patient
7 After removing gloves (CDC, 2002)
   You may also wash hands with an antimicrobial soap and water in these situations.

Delegation Considerations
The skill of hand hygiene can be delegated to nursing assistive personnel (NAP). The nurse supervises and evaluates performance of NAP in proper hand hygiene.

Equipment
- ❏ Alcohol-based waterless antiseptic containing emollients
- ❏ Easy-to-reach sink with warm running water
- ❏ Antimicrobial or regular soap
- ❏ Paper towels or air dryer
- ❏ Disposable nail cleaner (optional)

STEP	RATIONALE

ASSESSMENT

1 Inspect surface of hands for breaks or cuts in skin or cuticles. Avoid long or artificial nails. Report and cover any skin lesions before providing patient care.

Open cuts or wounds can harbor high concentrations of microorganisms. Agency policy may prevent nurses from caring for high-risk patients if open lesions are present on hands or if artificial or long nails are worn. Artificial nails increase the microbial load on hands (WHO, 2007).

2 Inspect hands for visible soiling.

Visible soiling requires hand washing with soap and water.

3 Note condition of nails. Be sure fingernails are short, filed, and smooth.

Subungual region (beneath fingernails) harbors microorganisms. Natural nails should be no more than 1/4 inch long when caring for high-risk patients (CDC, 2002).

NURSING DIAGNOSES

This skill is required for patients having a variety of nursing diagnoses. Individualize related factors based on patient's condition or needs.

STEP	RATIONALE

PLANNING

1 Expected outcomes following completion of procedure:
  • Hands and areas under fingernails are clean and free of debris.

Transient bacteria have been removed.

IMPLEMENTATION

1 Push wristwatch and long uniform sleeves above wrists. Avoid wearing rings. If worn, remove during hand hygiene.

Provides complete access to fingers, hands, and wrists. Wearing of rings increases number of microorganisms on hands (CDC, 2002).

2 Hand antisepsis using an instant alcohol waterless antiseptic rub
  a Dispense ample amount of product into palm of one hand (see illustration).

Many microorganisms on hands come from the subungual region (beneath the fingernails). Enough product is needed to thoroughly cover the hands.

  b Rub hands together, covering all surfaces of hands and fingers with antiseptic (see illustration).

Provides enough time for product to work.

  c Rub hands together until the alcohol is dry. Allow hands to completely dry before applying gloves.

Ensures complete antimicrobial action.

3 Hand washing using plain or antimicrobial soap and water
  a Stand in front of sink, keeping hands and uniform away from sink surface. (If hands touch sink during hand washing, repeat.)

Inside of sink is a contaminated area. Reaching over sink increases risk of touching edge, which is contaminated.

  b Turn on water. Turn faucet on (see illustration), or push knee pedals laterally, or press pedals with foot to regulate flow and temperature.

  c Avoid splashing water against uniform.

Microorganisms travel and grow in moisture.

  d Regulate flow of water so that temperature is warm.

Warm water removes less of the protective oils on hands than hot water.

  e Wet hands and wrists thoroughly under running water. Keep hands and forearms lower than the elbows during washing.

Hands are the most contaminated parts to wash. Water flows from least to most contaminated area, rinsing microorganisms into sink.

  f Apply a small amount of soap or antiseptic, lathering thoroughly (see illustration). Soap granules and leaflet preparations are an option to use.

The use of antiseptic exclusively can be drying to the hands and cause skin irritations.

Critical Decision Point   *The decision whether to use an antiseptic soap or not depends on the procedure to be performed and the patient's immune status.*

  g Perform hand hygiene using plenty of lather and friction for at least 10 to 15 seconds. Interlace fingers and rub palms and back of hands with circular motion at least 5 times each. Keep fingertips down to facilitate removal of microorganisms.

Soap cleanses by emulsifying fat and oil and lowering surface tension. Friction and rubbing mechanically loosen and remove dirt and transient bacteria. Interlacing fingers and thumbs ensures that all surfaces are cleansed.

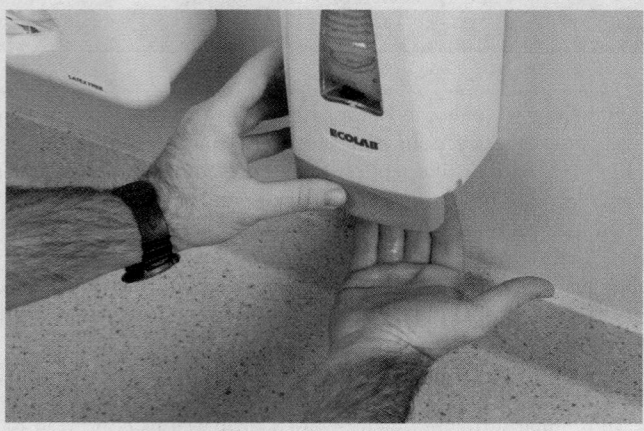

STEP 2a   Apply waterless antiseptic to hands.

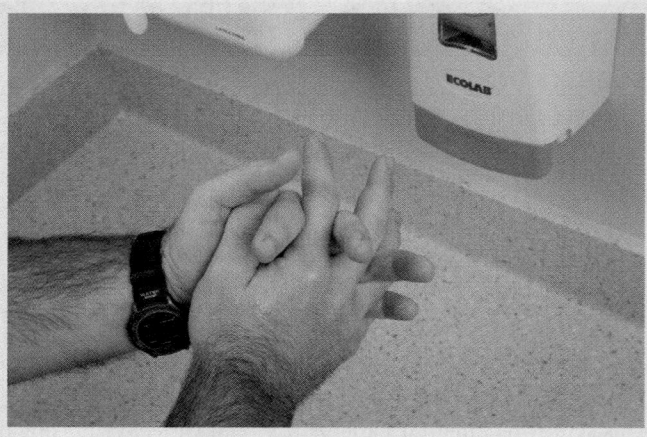

STEP 2b   Rub hands thoroughly.

STEP	RATIONALE

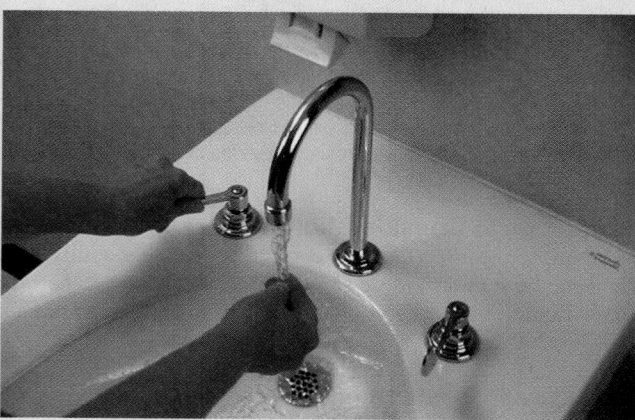

STEP 3b   Turning on water.

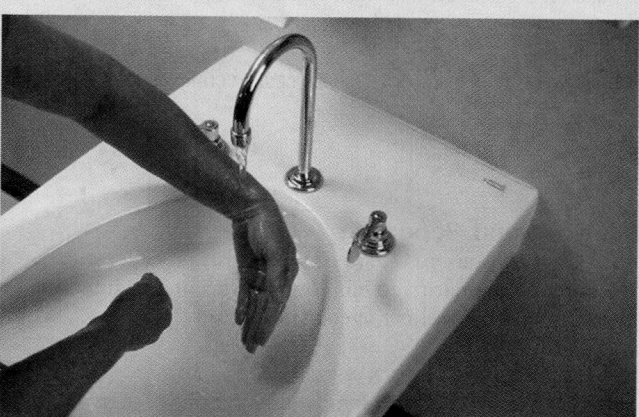

STEP 3i   Rinsing hands.

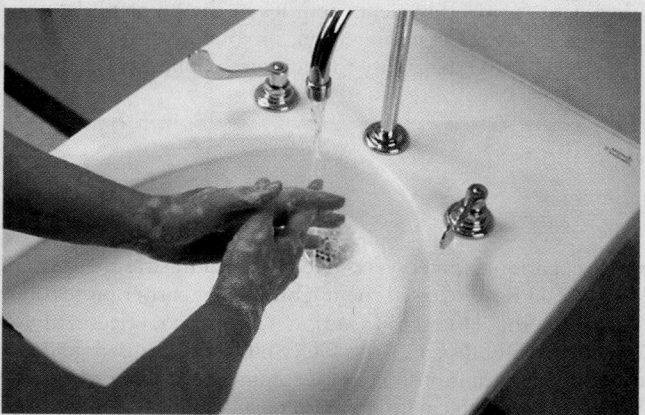

STEP 3f   Lathering hands thoroughly.

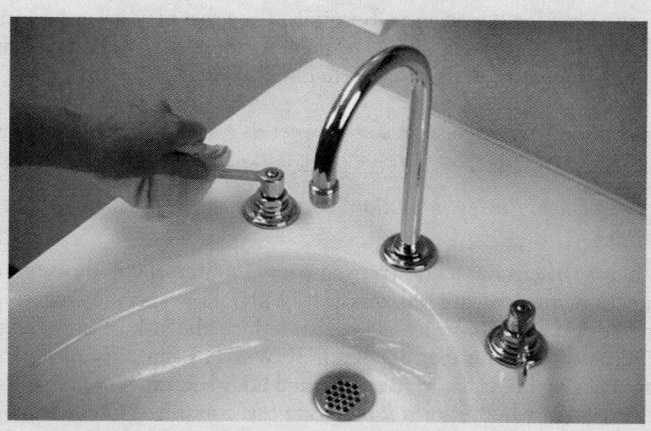

STEP 3l   Turning off faucet.

h   Areas underlying fingernails are often soiled. Clean them with the fingernails of other hand and additional soap, or clean with a disposable nail cleaner.

Area under nails can be highly contaminated, which will increase the risk for transmission of infection from the nurse to the patient.

Critical Decision Point   *Do not tear or cut skin under or around nail.*

i   Rinse hands and wrists thoroughly, keeping hands down and elbows up (see illustration).

Rinsing mechanically washes away dirt and microorganisms.

j   Dry hands thoroughly from fingers to wrists with paper towel, single-use cloth, or warm air dryer.

Drying from cleanest (fingertips) to least clean (wrist) avoids contamination. Drying hands prevents chapping and roughened skin.

k   If used, discard paper towel in proper receptacle.

Prevents transfer of microorganisms.

l   To turn off hand faucet, use clean, dry paper towel, avoiding touching handles with hands (see illustration). Turn off water with foot or knee pedals (if applicable).

Wet towel and hands allow transfer of pathogens from the faucet by capillary action.

m   Apply lotion to hands. Use the facility-provided lotion if one is provided. Avoid petroleum-based lotions.

Helps to minimize skin dryness. The provided lotion will be compatible with antimicrobial soaps and latex.

EVALUATION

1   Inspect surface of hands for obvious signs of dirt or other contaminants.

Determines if hand hygiene is adequate.

Unexpected Outcomes

1 Hands or areas under fingernails remain soiled.

2 Repeated use of soaps or antiseptic cause dermatitis or cracked skin.

Related Interventions

- Repeat hand washing with soap and water.
- Use the alcohol-based hand antiseptic rub whenever hands are not visibly soiled.
- Rinse and dry hands thoroughly after using soap and water; avoid excessive amounts of soap or antiseptic; try various products.
- Use hand lotions or barrier creams (small individual-use containers are preferred because large containers have been found to harbor pathogens).

Recording and Reporting

- It is not necessary to record or report this procedure.
- Report any dermatitis to employee health and/or infection prevention and control per agency policy.

Teaching Considerations

- Instruct the patient and family caregiver in proper techniques and situations for hand hygiene.
- Patients are aware of the importance of hand hygiene (TJC, 2007). It has been shown that when patients are educated about the risks for infection in hospitals, they can play an important role in improving hand hygiene compliance by reminding health care workers to perform hand hygiene.

Gerontological Considerations

- The impact of infections is much greater in older adults. Hand hygiene by staff attending older adults is of utmost importance and should be an ongoing continuing education requirement (CDC, 2007b).

Home Care Considerations

- Evaluate patient and primary caregiver to determine their understanding of the transmission of microorganisms and their ability and motivation to perform hand hygiene correctly.
- Evaluate the hand hygiene facilities in the home to determine the possibility of contamination, proximity of the facilities to the patient, and the ability to maintain supplies and equipment.

SKILL 7-2 Caring for Patients Under Isolation Precautions

 Basic / Basic Infection Control / Using Personal Protective Equipment

When a patient has a known or suspected source of colonization or infection, health care workers (HCWs) follow specific infection prevention and control practices to reduce the risk of cross contamination to other patients and HCWs. The majority of organisms causing HAIs are in the colonized body substances of patients, regardless of whether or not a culture has confirmed infection and a diagnosis has been made (Saint and others, 2008). Body substances such as feces, urine, mucus, and wound drainage contain potentially infectious organisms. Isolation or barrier precautions include the appropriate use of personal protective equipment including gowns, masks, eyewear, and gloves. Assess the need for barrier precautions for each task you plan and for all patients regardless of their diagnoses. Because of increased attention to the prevention of blood-borne pathogens and tuberculosis (TB), the Centers for Disease Control and Prevention (CDC) (2005) and the Occupational Safety and Health Administration (OSHA) (1994, 2001) have stressed the importance of barrier protection.

In 2007 the Hospital Infection Control Practices Advisory Committee (HICPAC) of the CDC published revised guidelines for isolation precautions. These recommendations were based on current epidemiological information regarding disease transmission in health care settings. Although primarily intended for care of patients in acute care, you can apply the recommendations to patients in subacute care or long-term care facilities. HICPAC recommends that hospitals modify the recommendations according to their needs and as dictated by federal, state, or local regulations (CDC, 2007b).

The new guidelines contain recommendations for respiratory hygiene/cough etiquette as part of standard precautions. Standard precautions, or tier one precautions, are for the care of all patients

---

BOX 7-1 Centers for Disease Control and Prevention Isolation Guidelines

Standard Precautions (Tier One)* for Use With All Patients

- Standard precautions apply to blood, all body fluids, secretions, excretions, nonintact skin, and mucous membranes.
- During the delivery of health care, avoid unnecessary touching of surfaces in close proximity to the patient to prevent both contamination of clean hands from environmental surfaces and transmission of pathogens from contaminated hands to surfaces.
- When hands are visibly dirty, contaminated with proteinaceous material, or visibly soiled with blood or body fluids, wash hands with either a nonantimicrobial soap and water or an antimicrobial soap and water.
- If hands are not visibly soiled, or after removing visible material with nonantimicrobial soap and water, perform hand hygiene in the following situations:
  - Before having direct contact with patients
  - After contact with blood, body fluids or excretions, mucous membranes, nonintact skin, or wound dressings

- After contact with a patient's intact skin (e.g., when taking a pulse or blood pressure)
- If hands will be moving from a contaminated body site to a clean body site during patient care
- After contact with inanimate objects (including medical equipment) in the immediate vicinity of the patient
- After removing gloves
- Wash hands with nonantimicrobial soap and water if contact with spores (e.g., *Clostridium difficile*) is likely to have occurred.
- Do not wear artificial fingernails or extenders if duties include direct contact with patients at high risk for infection and associated adverse outcomes.
- Wear PPE when the nature of the anticipated patient interaction indicates that contact with blood or body fluids may occur.
- Wear gloves when it can be reasonably anticipated that contact with blood or other potentially infectious materials, mucous membranes, nonintact skin, or potentially contaminated intact skin (e.g., of a patient incontinent of stool or urine) could occur.

BOX 7-1	Centers for Disease Control and Prevention Isolation Guidelines—cont'd

- Wear gloves with fit and durability appropriate to the task. Wear disposable medical examination gloves for providing direct patient care.
- Remove gloves after contact with a patient and/or the surrounding environment (including medical equipment) using proper technique to prevent hand contamination. Do not wear the same pair of gloves for the care of more than one patient.
- Change gloves during patient care if the hands will move from a contaminated body site to a clean body site.
- Wear masks, eye protection, or face shields if patient care activities may generate splashes or sprays of blood or body fluid.
- Wear a gown appropriate to the task, to protect skin and prevent soiling or contamination of clothing during procedures and patient-care activities when contact with blood, bloody fluids, secretions, or excretions is anticipated. Wear a gown for direct patient contact if the patient has uncontained secretions or excretions.
- Remove gown and perform hand hygiene before leaving the patient's environment. Do not reuse gowns, even for repeated contacts with the same patient.
- Properly clean and reprocess patient care equipment; discard single-use items.
- Place contaminated linen in leakproof bag and handle to prevent skin and mucous membrane exposure.
- Discard all sharp instruments and needles in a puncture-resistant container. OSHA recommends that needles be disposed of uncapped or a mechanical device be used for recapping. Sharps with built-in safety features must be used when available, and these safety features must be activated after use.
- A private room is unnecessary unless the patient's hygiene is unacceptable. Check with infection control professional.
- Respiratory hygiene/cough etiquette: Have patients cover the nose/mouth when coughing or sneezing; use tissues to contain respiratory secretions and dispose in nearest waste container; perform hand hygiene after contacting respiratory secretions and contaminated objects/materials; contain respiratory secretions with procedure or surgical mask; sit at least 3 feet away from others if coughing.

Transmission-Based Precautions (Tier Two) for Use With Specific Types of Patients
Airborne Precautions

In addition to Standard Precautions, use Airborne Precautions for patients known or suspected to have serious illnesses transmitted by airborne droplet nuclei. Examples of such illnesses include:
(1) Measles
(2) Varicella (including disseminated zoster)[†]
(3) Tuberculosis

Droplet Precautions

In addition to Standard Precautions, use Droplet Precautions for patients known or suspected to have serious illnesses transmitted by large particle droplets. Examples of such illnesses include:

(1) Invasive *Haemophilus influenzae* type b disease, including meningitis, pneumonia, epiglottitis, and sepsis
(2) Invasive *Neisseria meningitidis* disease, including meningitis, pneumonia, and sepsis
(3) Other serious bacterial respiratory infections spread by droplet transmission, including:
  (a) Diphtheria (pharyngeal)
  (b) Mycoplasma pneumonia
  (c) Pertussis
  (d) Pneumonic plague
  (e) Streptococcal pharyngitis, pneumonia, or scarlet fever in infants and young children
(4) Serious viral infections spread by droplet transmission, including:
  (a) Adenovirus[†]
  (b) Influenza
  (c) Mumps
  (d) Parvovirus B19
  (e) Rubella

Contact Precautions

In addition to Standard Precautions, use Contact Precautions for patients known or suspected to have serious illnesses easily transmitted by direct patient contact or by contact with items in the patient's environment. Examples of such illnesses include:

(1) Gastrointestinal, respiratory, skin, or wound infections or colonization with multidrug-resistant bacteria judged by the infection control program, based on current state, regional, or national recommendations, to be of special clinical and epidemiological significance
(2) Enteric with a low infectious dose or prolonged environmental survival, including:
  (a) *Clostridium difficile*
  (b) For diapered or incontinent patients: enterohemorrhagic *Escherichia coli* 0157:H7, *Shigella,* hepatitis A, or rotavirus
(3) Respiratory syncytial virus, parainfluenza virus, or enteroviral infections in infants and young children
(4) Skin infections that are highly contagious or that may occur on dry skin, including:
  (a) Diphtheria (cutaneous)
  (b) Herpes simplex virus (neonatal or mucocutaneous)
  (c) Impetigo
  (d) Major (noncontained) abscesses, cellulitis, or decubiti
  (e) Pediculosis (until appropriately treated)
  (f) Scabies (until appropriately treated)
  (g) Staphylococcal furunculosis in infants and young children
  (h) Zoster (disseminated or in the immunocompromised host)
(5) Viral/hemorrhagic conjunctivitis
(6) Viral hemorrhagic infections (Ebola, Lassa, or Marburg)

Modified from Centers for Disease Control and Prevention: *Guideline for isolation precautions: preventing transmission of infectious agents in healthcare settings,* 2007, http://www.cdc.gov/ncidod/dhqp/gl_isolation.html, accessed January 8, 2008.
PPE, Personal protective equipment; *OSHA,* Occupational Safety and Health Administration.
*Formerly universal precautions and body substance isolation.
[†]Certain infections require more than one type of precaution.

regardless of risk or presumed infection status (Box 7-1). Standard precautions are the primary strategies for prevention of infection transmission and apply to contact with (1) blood, (2) body fluids, (3) nonintact skin, and (4) mucous membranes, as well as contact with equipment or surfaces contaminated with these potentially infectious materials. The strategy of respiratory hygiene/cough etiquette applies to any person with signs of respiratory infection, including cough, congestion, rhinorrhea, or increased production

of respiratory secretions when entering a health care site. Educating health care staff, patients, and visitors to cover the mouth and nose with a tissue when coughing and to dispose properly of used tissues are among the elements of respiratory hygiene.

The second tier (see Box 7-1) includes precautions designed for care of patients who are known or suspected to be infected, or colonized, with microorganisms transmitted by the contact, droplet, or airborne route (Siegel, 2005) or by contact with contaminated sur-

STEP	RATIONALE

faces. The three types of transmission-based precautions—airborne, droplet, and contact—may be combined for diseases that have multiple routes of transmission, for example, chickenpox. When used either singly or in combination, you use them in addition to standard precautions. Box 7-1 summarizes the types of patients who are cared for under transmission-based precautions.

When a patient requires isolation in a private room, remember that loneliness can easily develop. Isolation disrupts normal social relationships with visitors and caregivers. Some patients who suffer from an infectious disease also experience self-concept or body image changes. When a patient from another culture requires isolation, use extra caution to be sure the patient and family understand the therapeutic purpose of isolation. For example, the isolation of a loved one is considered disrespectful and uncaring behavior in collectivistic cultures (Hispanics, Africans, and Asians) (Mashaba, 2002). Unless you act to minimize feelings of psychological and physical isolation, the patient's emotional state will interfere with recovery.

Delegation Considerations

The skill of caring for patients under isolation precautions can be delegated to NAP. The nurse directs the NAP by:
- Reviewing the reason a patient is on isolation precautions.
- Warning of high-risk factors for infection transmission that pertain to the assigned patient.

Equipment

- ❑ Clean gloves, mask, eyewear or goggles, and gown. Gowns may be either disposable or reusable depending upon facility's protocol.
- ❑ Other patient care equipment (as appropriate) (e.g., hygiene, medications, dressing change)
- ❑ Soiled linen and trash receptacle
- ❑ Sign for door indicating type of isolation and/or for visitors to come to the nurses' station before entering room

ASSESSMENT

1 Assess patient, and review medical history for possible indications for isolation, for example, risk factors for TB, major draining wound, or purulent productive cough. Review the precautions for the specific isolation system, including appropriate barriers to apply (Table 7-2, p. 184).

Mode of transmission for infectious microorganism determines type and degree of precautions followed. Ensures adequate protection.

2 Review laboratory test results.

Informs nurse of type of microorganism for which patient is being isolated, body fluid in which it was identified, and whether patient is immunosuppressed.

3 Consider types of care measures you will perform while in patient's room (e.g., medication administration or dressing change).

Enables nurse to organize care items for procedures and time spent in patient's room.

4 Review nursing care plan notes, or confer with colleagues regarding patient's emotional state and reaction/adjustment to isolation. Determine from nursing care plan, medical record, or significant other if patient and family understand the purpose of isolation procedures.

Determines patient's need for emotional support and teaching.

5 Determine from nursing care plan, medical record, or significant other if patient and family understand the purpose of isolation procedures.

Determines patient's level of knowledge and need for instruction/reinforcement.

6 Before applying latex gloves, assess if the patient has a known latex allergy (see Chapter 8).

Patient with latex allergy can have a serious allergic or sensitivity reaction after even brief exposure to gloves.

NURSING DIAGNOSES

- Deficient knowledge regarding purpose of isolation
- Impaired social interaction
- Ineffective protection
- Risk for infection

Individualize related factors based on patient's condition or needs.

PLANNING

1 Expected outcomes following completion of procedure:
   - Patient spontaneously engages in discussions with nurse and family. Patient asks for information about disease transmission.

   Active interaction reveals patient's willingness and/or ability to communicate and to be taught and to understand information.

   - Patient explains purpose of isolation.

   Instruction about precautions improves patient's ability to cooperate in care.

STEP	RATIONALE

IMPLEMENTATION

1 Perform hand hygiene (see Skill 7-1).

Reduces transmission of microorganisms.

2 Prepare all equipment needed in patient's room.

Prevents nurse from making more than one trip into room.

3 Prepare for entrance into isolation room. Choice of barrier protection depends on type of isolation and agency policy. For example, if patient is on airborne precautions, apply only a special mask and keep room door closed.

Proper preparation ensures nurse is protected from microorganism exposure.

  a Apply gown, being sure it covers all outer garments. Pull sleeves down to wrist. Tie securely at neck and waist (see illustration).

Prevents transmission of infection and protects nurse when patient has excessive drainage, discharges.

  b Apply either surgical mask or a fitted respirator around mouth and nose (type and fit-testing will depend on type of isolation and facility policy).

Prevents exposure to airborne microorganisms or exposure to microorganisms from splashing of fluids.

  c Apply eyewear or goggles snugly around face and eyes (when needed).

Protects nurse from exposure to microorganisms that may occur during splashing of fluids.

  d Apply clean gloves. (NOTE: Provide a latex-free environment if the patient or the health care worker has a latex allergy.) Bring glove cuffs over edge of gown sleeves (see illustration).

Reduces transmission of microorganisms.

4 Enter patient's room. Arrange supplies and equipment.

Prevents extra trips entering and leaving room.

5 Explain purpose of isolation and precautions for patient and family to take. Offer opportunity to ask questions. Assess for emotions that are related to being on isolation, such as loneliness or boredom, and for signs or symptoms of depression, for example, lack of appetite or difficulty sleeping.

Improves patient's and family's ability to participate in care and minimizes anxiety. Identifies opportunity for planning social interaction and diversional activities.

6 Obtain vital sign measurements:

  a Reusable equipment brought into the room must be thoroughly disinfected when removed from the room.

If used later on other patients, increases risk of infection being transmitted. Dedicated equipment used only with patient on isolation precautions is preferable.

  b If stethoscope is to be reused, clean earpieces and diaphragm or bell with 70% alcohol or facility-approved germicide. Set aside on clean surface.

Systematic disinfection of stethoscopes with 70% alcohol or approved germicide will minimize chance of spreading infectious agents between patients (CDC, 2007b).

  c Use individual or disposable thermometers.

Prevents cross contamination.

7 Administer medications (see Chapters 20, 21, and 22):

  a Give oral medication in wrapper or cup.

Handle and discard supplies to minimize transfer of microorganisms.

  b Dispose of wrapper or cup in plastic-lined receptacle.

  c Administer injection, being sure to wear gloves.

Reduces the risk of exposure to blood.

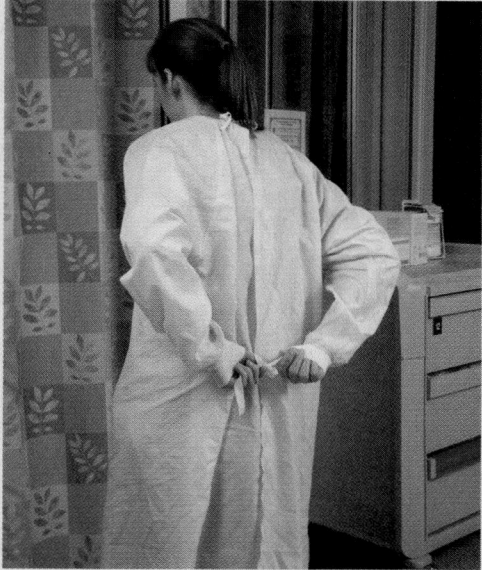

STEP 3a Nurse ties isolation gown.

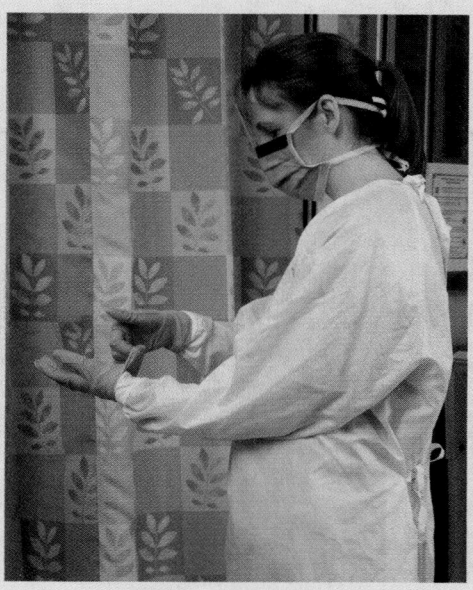

STEP 3d Bring glove cuffs over edge of gown sleeves.

STEP	RATIONALE
d Discard disposable syringe and uncapped or sheathed needle into designated sharps container.	Reduces risk of needle-stick injury.
e Place reusable plastic syringe (e.g., Carpuject) on clean towel for eventual removal and disinfection.	Prevents added contamination of syringe.
8 Administer hygiene, encouraging the patient to ask any questions or express concerns about isolation. Provide informal teaching at this time.	Hygiene practices further minimize transfer of microorganisms. Quality time should be spent with the patient when in the room.
a Avoid allowing isolation gown to become wet; carry wash basin outward away from gown; avoid leaning against wet tabletop.	Moisture allows organisms to travel through gown to uniform.

Critical Decision Point   *When there is a of risk for excess soiling, wear a gown impervious to moisture.*

STEP	RATIONALE
b Assist patient in removing own gown; discard in impervious linen bag.	Reduces transfer of microorganisms.
c Remove linen from bed; avoid contact with isolation gown. Place in impervious linen bag.	Handle linen soiled by patient's body fluids so as to prevent contact with clean items.
d Provide clean bed linen and set of towels.	
e Change gloves and perform hand hygiene if gloves become excessively soiled and further care is necessary.	
9 Collect specimens (see Chapter 43):	
a Place specimen containers on clean paper towel in patient's bathroom.	Container will be taken out of patient's room; prevents contamination of outer surface.
b Follow procedure for collecting specimen of body fluids (see Chapter 43).	
c Transfer specimen to container without soiling outside of container. Place container in a plastic bag, and label the outside of the bag or as per agency policy.	Specimens of blood and body fluids are placed in well-constructed containers with secure lids to prevent leaks during transport.
d Check label on specimen for accuracy. Send to laboratory (warning labels are often used, depending on hospital policy). Label containers of blood or body fluids with a biohazard sticker (see illustration).	Ensures that health care providers who transport or handle containers are aware of infectious contents.
10 Dispose of linen, trash, and disposable items:	
a Use single bags that are impervious to moisture and sturdy to contain soiled articles. Use double bag if necessary for heavily soiled linen or heavy wet trash.	Linen or refuse should be totally contained to prevent exposure of personnel to infective material.
b Tie bags securely at top in knot (see illustration).	

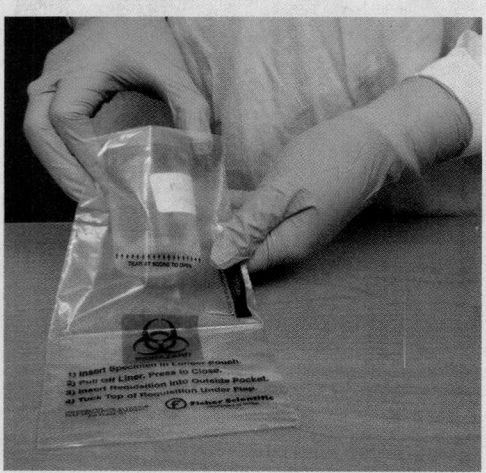

STEP 9d   Specimen container placed in biohazard bag.

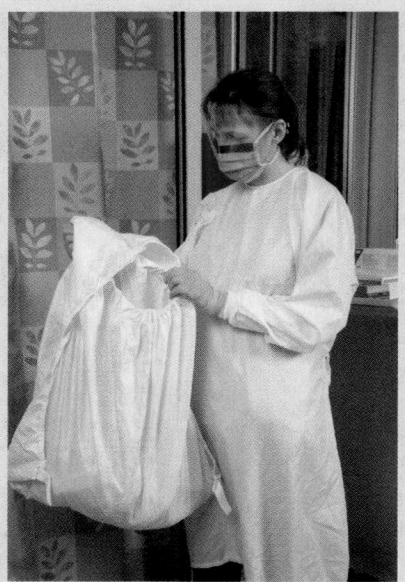

STEP 10b   Nurse ties bag securely.

STEP	RATIONALE
11 Remove all reusable pieces of equipment. Clean any contaminated surfaces with hospital-approved disinfectant (CDC, 2007b) (see agency policy).	All items must be properly cleaned, disinfected, or sterilized for reuse.
12 Resupply room as needed. Have staff colleague hand new supplies to you.	Limiting trips of personnel into and out of room reduces nurse's and patient's exposure to microorganisms.
13 Leave isolation room. Remember, order of removal of protective barriers depends on what you wear in room. This sequence describes steps to take if all barriers are worn:	
a Remove gloves. Remove one glove by grasping cuff and pulling glove inside out over hand. Hold removed glove in gloved hand (see illustration). Slide fingers of ungloved hand under remaining glove at wrist. Peel glove off over first glove. Discard gloves in proper container (CDC, 2004).	Technique prevents contact with contaminated glove's outer surface.
b Remove eyewear or goggles. Handle by headband or earpieces. Discard in proper container.	Outside of goggles is contaminated. Hands have not been soiled.
c Untie neck strings, and then untie back strings of gown. Allow gown to fall from shoulders (see illustration); touch inside of gown only. Remove hands from sleeves without touching outside of gown. Hold gown inside at shoulder seams, and fold inside out into a bundle; discard in laundry bag (CDC, 2004).	Hands do not come in contact with soiled front of gown.
d Remove mask. If the mask secures over the ears, remove elastic from ears, pull mask away from face (see illustration). For a tie-on mask, untie *bottom* mask string and then top strings, pull mask away from face and drop into trash receptacle. (Do not touch outer surface of mask.) (CDC, 2004).	Ungloved hands will not be contaminated by touching only elastic or mask strings. Prevents top part of mask from falling down over nurse's uniform.
e Perform hand hygiene.	Reduces transmission of microorganisms.
f Retrieve wristwatch and stethoscope (unless it must remain in room), and record vital sign values on notepaper.	Clean hands can contact clean items.
g Explain to patient when you plan to return to room. Ask whether patient requires any personal care items. Offer books, magazines, audiotapes.	Diversions can help to minimize boredom and feeling of social isolation.
h Leave room and close door, if necessary. Close door if patient is in negative airflow room.	

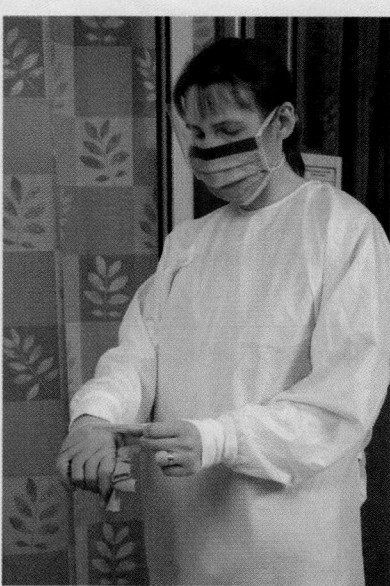

STEP 13a Hold removed glove in gloved hand and pull remaining glove.

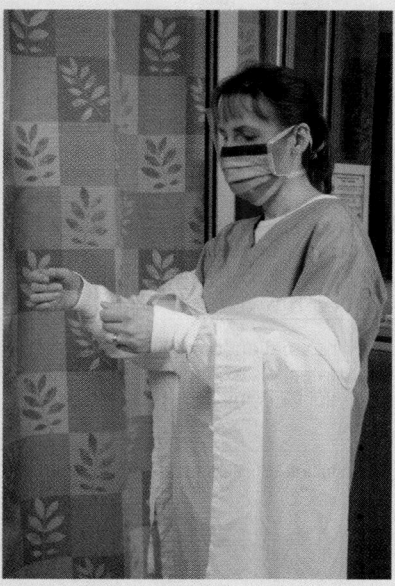

STEP 13c Remove gown by allowing it to fall from shoulders.

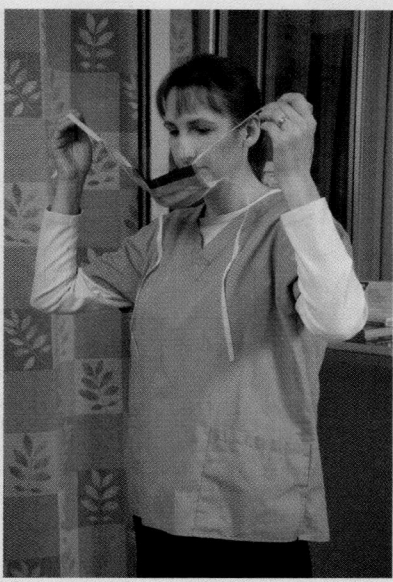

STEP 13d Pull mask away from face.

STEP	RATIONALE

EVALUATION

1 While in room, ask if patient has had sufficient opportunity to discuss health problems, course of treatment, or other topics important to patient.

Measures patient's perception of the adequacy of discussions with caregivers.

2 Ask patient to describe purpose of isolation and offer chance to ask questions.

Feedback demonstrates learning.

Unexpected Outcomes

1 Patient avoids social and therapeutic discussions.

2 Patient or health care worker may have an allergy to latex gloves.

Related Interventions

• Confer with family and/or significant other, and determine best approach to reduce patient's sense of loneliness and depression.
• Notify physician/employee health, and treat sensitivity or allergic reaction appropriately.
• Use latex-free gloves for future care activities.

Recording and Reporting

• Document procedures performed and patient's response to social isolation in nurses' progress notes. Also document any patient education performed and reinforced.

Teaching Considerations

• Teach visitors and family members how to follow the recommended isolation precautions when visiting patient. Teach the appropriate use of barrier techniques for home caregiving as appropriate.

Pediatric Considerations

• Isolation creates a sense of separation from family and loss of control. Strange environment adds to confusion child feels during isolation. Preschoolers are unable to understand cause-effect relationship for isolation. Older children may be able to understand cause but still fantasize.
• Children require simple explanations; for example, "You need to be in this room to help you get better." Show all barriers to a child. Actively involve parents in any explanations. Nurses let

child see their faces before applying masks so that child does not become frightened.

Gerontological Considerations

• Isolation can be a particular concern for older adults, especially those who have signs and symptoms of confusion or depression. Many times patients become more confused when they are confronted with a nurse using barrier precautions or when they are left in a room with the door closed. Nurses must assess need for closing door (negative airflow room) along with safety of patient and additional safety measures that may need to be taken.
• Assess older adults for signs of depression such as loss of appetite or decrease in verbal communications. If necessary, report to the health care team for appropriate interventions.

Home Care Considerations

• Although isolation precautions followed in the hospital are not directly applicable to home care, caregivers should be aware of potential sources of contamination in home.

TABLE 7-2	Transmission Categories (Tier Two) (For Use With Patients Infected or Colonized With Specific Organisms)	
Category	**Disease**	**Barrier Protection**
Airborne precautions	For diseases transmitted by small droplet nuclei (smaller than 5 μm), such as measles, chickenpox, disseminated varicella-zoster, pulmonary or laryngeal TB*	Private room, negative airflow of at least six air exchanges per hour; respirator or mask*
Droplet precautions	For diseases transmitted by large droplets (larger than 5 μm), such as streptococcal pharyngitis, pneumonia, and scarlet fever in infants or small children, pertussis, mumps, meningococcal pneumonia or sepsis, pneumonic plague	Private room or cohort patient; mask when closer than 3 ft from patient
Contact precautions	For diseases transmitted by direct patient or environmental contact, such as colonization or infection with multidrug-resistant organisms, respiratory syncytial virus, major wound infections, herpes simplex, and scabies	Private room or cohort patient; gloves, gowns

Modified from Centers for Disease Control and Prevention, Hospital Infection Control Practice Advisory Committee: Guidelines for isolation precautions in hospitals, *MMWR Morbid Mortal Wkly Rep* 57(RR-16), 2007.
TB, Tuberculosis.
*See CDC TB guidelines 2005.

PROCEDURAL GUIDELINE 7-1   Special Tuberculosis Precautions

In 1994 the CDC published guidelines for preventing TB transmission in health care facilities in response to a resurgence of TB in the United States associated with the increasing incidence of human immunodeficiency virus (HIV) infection, TB infection transmission in health care settings, and increasing immigration from countries with a high incidence of TB (CDC, 2005). The current CDC guidelines for preventing and controlling TB focus on early detection of infection, preventing close contact with patients with active TB disease, and applying effective infection control measures in health care settings. Suspect TB in any patient with respiratory symptoms lasting longer than 3 weeks accompanied by other suspicious symptoms such as unexplained weight loss, night sweats, fever, and a productive cough often streaked with blood. Isolation for patients with suspected or confirmed TB includes placing the patient on airborne precautions in a single-patient negative-pressure room.

OSHA and CDC guidelines require health care workers who care for patients with suspected or confirmed TB to wear special respirators (e.g., N95 or P100). These respirators are high-efficiency particulate masks that have the ability to filter particles at a 95% or better efficiency. Health care workers who use these respirators must be fit-tested in a reliable way to obtain a face-seal leakage of 10% or less (Roberge, 2008). OSHA also requires employers to provide training concerning transmission of TB, especially in areas where the risk of exposure is high. In addition, the CDC now recommends the use of the QuantiFERON-TB Gold test (QFT-G) (CDC, 2005), a blood test, in place of the traditional TB skin test. The advantages of the QFT-G test are that it does not boost responses measured by subsequent tests and the results are not subject to reader bias.

Delegation Considerations

Assessment of a patient's status and type of care to perform cannot be delegated. Basic care procedures performed under TB isolation can be delegated to NAP. The nurse directs the NAP by:

- Clarifying personnel precautions used under TB isolation, including fitting of mask.
- Instructing personnel in the types of clinical changes to report.

Equipment

- TB isolation room with negative airflow
- N95 or P100 respirator
- Clean gloves, gown, protective eyewear (based on patient's clinical condition)
- Basic care items (e.g., medication equipment, hygiene items)

Procedural Steps

1 Assess potential for infectious pulmonary or laryngeal TB (e.g., documentation of positive acid-fast bacilli [AFB] smear or culture, signs or symptoms of TB, cavitation on chest x-ray study, history of recent exposure, physician progress notes indicating plan to rule out TB).

2 Perform hand hygiene.

3 Before entering room, apply recommended mask. Be sure it fits snugly.

4 Explain purpose of TB isolation to patient, family, and others.

5 Instruct patient to cover mouth with tissue when coughing and to wear disposable surgical mask when leaving the room.

6 Provide care (see Skill 7-2).

7 Leave the room and close the door.

8 Remove mask; dispose in proper receptacle.

9 Place reusable mask in labeled paper bag for storage, being careful not to crush mask. (Check agency policy for number of times it can be used.)

10 Assess patient's laboratory data for repeated AFB smears that may be negative.

11 Ask patient/family to identify method of transmission for TB.

12 Be alert, and assess any suspected respiratory symptoms in neighboring patients.

CRITICAL THINKING EXERCISES

Joe is assigned to Mr. Nesbitt, a 78-year-old nursing home resident. When Joe enters Mr. Nesbitt's room, he begins to conduct a physical assessment.

1 As Joe turns Mr. Nesbitt to check the condition of his skin, he notices moisture on his own hand. Joe looks more closely and realizes the moisture is from an open, oozing lesion on Mr. Nesbitt's sacral area. What should Joe do next?

2 Using gloves, Joe assesses the wound. Joe then quickly checks the position and function of Mr. Nesbitt's indwelling urinary catheter and then performs hand hygiene before leaving Mr. Nesbitt's room. Critique Joe's approach. Did he use correct aseptic technique?

3 After Joe places Mr. Nesbitt on contact precautions, he observes a student nurse preparing to go into the patient's room with a mask. Is the student nurse's use of a mask appropriate?

✓ REVIEW QUESTIONS

1 A health care worker has visible dirt on his hands. Which method of cleaning his hands is most appropriate?
   1 An alcohol-based disinfectant
   2 Water, then an alcohol-based hand rub
   3 An alcohol gel containing an emollient
   ④ Soap and water

2 Which aspect of hand washing is most effective to loosen dirt and transient bacteria?
   1 Using hot water instead of warm water
   ② Using plenty of lather with friction
   3 Drying the hands vigorously from wrists to fingers
   4 Applying lotion to the hands

3 When a patient is to be placed on isolation precautions, there are many factors to consider regarding his or her care. Select all that apply.
   ① The need for social interaction
   ② The type of isolation required
   ③ The patient's cultural background
   ④ Education of family and friends regarding the isolation
   ⑤ Organization of care to minimize trips in and out of the isolation room
   6 How the patient contracted an infection

4 The use of a mask when the nurse is closer than 3 feet to a patient involves which type of precautions?
   ① Airborne
   ✓→ 2 Droplet
   3 Contact
   4 Standard

5 A nurse goes in and out of a patient's room and only needs a gown when coming into contact with the patient. What should the nurse do on leaving the room? Select all that apply.
   1 Leave the used gown hanging on the hook for the next time it is needed.
   2 Put a mask on whenever entering the room.
   ③ Discard the gown after using it.
   ④ Perform hand hygiene before and after going into the patient's room.

REFERENCES

Centers for Disease Control and Prevention: Guidelines for preventing the transmission of Mycobacterium tuberculosis in health care facilities, MMWR Morb Mortal Wkly Rep 43(No. RR-13), 1994.

Centers for Disease Control and Prevention, Hospital Infection Control Practice Advisory Committee and the HICPAC/ SHEA/APIC/IDSA Hand Hygiene Task Force: Guideline for hand hygiene in health-care settings, MMWR Recomm Rep 51(No. RR-16), 2002.

Centers for Disease Control and Prevention: Guidance for the selection and use of personal protective equipment (PPE) in healthcare settings, 2004, http://www.cdc.gov/ncidod/dhqp/ppe.html, accessed January 8, 2008.

Centers for Disease Control and Prevention: Guidelines for preventing the transmission of Mycobacterium tuberculosis in health-care facilities, MMWR Morb Mortal Wkly Rep 54(RR-17), 2005.

Centers for Disease Control and Prevention: Guideline for isolation precautions: preventing transmission of infectious agents in healthcare settings, 2007a, http://www.cdc.gov/ncidod/dhqp/gl_isolation.html, accessed January 8, 2008.

Centers for Disease Control and Prevention, Hospital Infection Control Practices Advisory Committee: Guidelines for isolation precautions in hospitals, MMWR Morb Mortal Wkly Rep 57(RR-16), 2007b.

DeCastro M: Aseptic technique. In APIC text of infection control and epidemiology, Washington, DC, revised 2005, Association for Professionals in Infection Control and Epidemiology Inc.

Jackson M, Lynch P: Body substance isolation, Infect Control Hosp Epidemiol 13(14):191, 1992.

Micek, J: Greater KC APIC chapter taking the lead in collaborative efforts regarding artificial nails with metropolitan area healthcare facilities, Am J Infect Control 32(3):E81, 2004.

Occupational Safety and Health Administration: Respiratory protection, Fed Regist 59(219):58884, 1994.

Occupational Safety and Health Administration: Occupational exposure to bloodborne pathogens, needlesticks and other sharps injuries; final rule, 29 CFR Part 1910, Fed Regist 66:5318, 2001.

Roberge R: Evaluation of the rationale for concurrent use of N95 filtering facepiece respirators with loose-fitting powered air-purifying respirators during aerosol generating medical procedures, J Infect Control 36(2):135, 2008.

Rutala W: Disinfection and sterilization of patient-care items. In APIC text of infection control and epidemiology, Washington, DC, revised 2005, Association for Professionals in Infection Control and Epidemiology Inc.

Saiman L and others: Banning artificial nails from health care settings, Am J Infect Control 30(4):252, 2002.

Siegel J: Isolation systems. In APIC text of infection control and epidemiology, Washington, DC, revised 2005, Association for Professionals in Infection Control and Epidemiology Inc.

The Joint Commission: The Joint Commission's new Speak Up program urges patients to know your rights [news release], Oakbrook Terrace, Ill, 2007, The Joint Commission.

Visscher M and others: Effects of hand hygiene regimens on skin conditions in health care workers, Am J Infect Control 34(10, suppl):S111, 2006.

WHO guidelines on hand hygiene care, Geneva, Switzerland, 2007, WHO Press.

RESEARCH REFERENCES

Fendler EJ and others: The impact of alcohol hand sanitizer use on infection rates in an extended care facility, Am J Infect Control 30(4):226, 2002

Hilburn J and others: Use of alcohol hand sanitizer as an infection control strategy in an acute care facility, Am J Infect Control 31(2):109, 2003.

Jagger J: Caring for healthcare workers: A global perspective, Infect Control Hosp Epidemiol 28(1):1, 2007.

Kim P and others: Rates of hand disinfection associated with glove use, patient isolation, and changes between exposure to various body sites, Am J Infect Control 31(2):97, 2003.

Mashaba G: South African culturally based health-illness patterns and humanistic care practices. In Leininger M, McFarland M: Transcultural nursing, New York, 2002, McGraw-Hill.

Rosenthal V and others: Reduction in nosocomial infection with improved hand hygiene in intensive care units of a tertiary care hospital in Argentina, Am J Infect Control 33(7):392, 2005.

Saint S and others: Preventing hospital-acquired urinary tract infection in the United States: A national study, Clinical Infectious Disease 46: 243, 2008.

Sterile Technique

MEDIA RESOURCES

- **evolve** http://evolve.elsevier.com/Perry/skills
  learning system
  - Review Questions
  - Video Clips

- **View Video!** Mosby's Nursing Video Skills, 3.0

- **NSO** Nursing Skills Online

KEY TERMS

Asepsis

Latex allergy reaction

Microorganisms

Pathogenic microorganisms

Standard precautions

Sterile

Sterile field

Strike through

Surgical asepsis

Transmission-based precautions

OBJECTIVES

Mastery of content in this chapter will enable the nurse to:

- Discuss settings where surgical aseptic techniques are used.
- Describe conditions when surgical asepsis is used.
- Identify principles of surgical asepsis.
- Explain the importance of organization and caution when using surgical aseptic techniques.

- Apply and remove a cap, mask, and eyewear correctly.
- Identify individuals at risk for latex allergy.
- Perform the following skills: applying sterile gloves using open glove method, preparing a sterile field, applying a sterile drape correctly.

Surgical asepsis or aseptic techniques and practices are designed to make and maintain objects and areas free from pathogenic microorganisms (DeCastro, 2005). As in medical asepsis, hand hygiene with an appropriate cleanser or antiseptic is essential before the initiation of an aseptic procedure. Although nurses commonly practice surgical asepsis in operating rooms (ORs), labor and delivery areas, and major diagnostic or special procedure areas, nurses use surgical aseptic techniques at the patient's bedside (Box 8-1) in three primary situations:

- During procedures that require intentional perforation of a patient's skin (e.g., insertion of intravenous [IV] catheters [see Chapter 31])
- When the skin's integrity is broken due to a surgical incision or burns (see Chapters 38 and 39)
- During procedures that involve insertion of devices or surgical instruments into normally sterile body cavities (e.g., insertion of a urinary catheter [see Chapter 33])

A nurse in an OR follows a series of steps toward sterile technique, such as applying a mask, protective eyewear, and a cap; performing a surgical hand scrub; applying a sterile gown; and applying sterile gloves. In contrast, a nurse performing a sterile dressing change at a patient's bedside or in the home setting may only wash his or her hands and apply sterile gloves. Regardless of the procedures followed or the setting, the nurse needs to recognize the importance of following strict aseptic principles (DeCastro, 2005). All individuals involved in surgical asepsis have a responsibility to provide and maintain a safe environment by following aseptic principles (Association of periOperative Registered Nurses [AORN], 2007).

In treatment areas and at the bedside, it is important to have a patient's full cooperation to minimize contamination of a work area. Be sure to prepare a patient before any procedure. Certain patients may fear moving or touching objects during a sterile procedure, whereas others even try to assist. Explain how you will perform a procedure and what a patient can do to avoid contaminating sterile items, including avoiding sudden body movement, refraining from touching sterile supplies, and avoiding coughing or talking over a sterile area.

The Centers for Disease Control and Prevention (CDC) (2007) has established standard precautions as the minimum standard for infection control (see Chapter 7). Standard precautions are used for potential contact with blood and all body fluids. The use of standard precautions calls for the wearing of masks in combination with eye protection devices such as goggles or glasses with solid side shields whenever splashes, spray, splatter, or droplets of blood or other potentially infectious fluids may occur. These barriers keep the eyes, nose, and mouth free from exposure. Similarly, you wear gowns when there is risk for being splattered with blood or other infectious materials. All health care institutions need to provide personal protective equipment and instructions for their use to all employees at risk for exposure (Occupational Safety and Health Administration [OSHA], 1991, 1994).

EVIDENCE-BASED PRACTICE TRENDS

In 1860 Joseph Lister promoted the use of carbolic acid as a surgical hand scrub. Since then, using an antiseptic on the hands of surgical team members has been an accepted practice. Bacteria on the hands of health care workers sometimes lead to wound infections when introduced into surgical wounds. Studies show that antiseptics containing 60% to 95% alcohol alone, or 50% to 95% alcohol when combined with other selected antiseptics (e.g., chlorhexidine), lower bacterial counts on the skin more effectively then do other antiseptics without alcohol (CDC, 2002). In addition, bacteria appear to reproduce slowly on the hands after a surgical scrub with alcohol. After a nurse wears gloves for 1 to 3 hours, bacterial counts on hands seldom exceed prescrub values (CDC, 2002). For this reason, an alcohol-based hand rub may be used as a preoperative hand scrub after an initial 15-second prewash with plain soap and water (AORN, 2007; CDC, 2002).

The subungual area (under a fingernail) of the hand is a source of high concentrations of bacteria, most frequently coagulase-negative staphylococci and gram-negative rods. Even after careful performance of hand hygiene, large numbers of potential pathogens exist under the subungual spaces. Health care workers who wear artificial nails or nail extenders are more likely to harbor gram-negative pathogens on their fingertips, both before and after hand hygiene (CDC, 2002). Numerous reports identify that fungal growth frequently occurs under artificial nails as a result of moisture becoming trapped between the natural and artificial nail (AORN, 2007). Because of the risk for infection posed by artificial nail use, health care workers having direct contact with patients at high risk (e.g., those in intensive care units or operating rooms) should not wear artificial nails (Church, 2005). Many health care institutions have chosen to ban artificial nails and extenders in all clinical areas, with the rationale that all patients are at risk for infection.

| **BOX 8-1** | Principles of Surgical Asepsis |

1. All items used within a sterile field must be sterile.
2. A sterile barrier that has been permeated by punctures, tears, or moisture must be considered contaminated.
3. Once a sterile package is opened, a 2.5-cm (1-inch) border around the edges is considered unsterile.
4. Tables draped as part of a sterile field are considered sterile only at table level.
5. If there is any question or doubt about an item's sterility, the item is considered to be unsterile.
6. Sterile persons or items contact only sterile areas; unsterile persons or items contact only unsterile areas.
7. Movement around in and in the sterile field must not compromise or contaminate the sterile field.
8. A sterile object or field out of the range of vision or an object held below a person's waist is contaminated.
9. A sterile object or field becomes contaminated by prolonged exposure to air; stay organized, and complete any procedure as soon as possible.

Skill Performance Guidelines

1 Follow standard precautions with all patients.
2 Review your agency's policies and procedures before conducting a sterile procedure.
3 Assess the patient's potential for infection before choosing the barrier to be used, such as masks or eye wear.
4 Use barrier techniques to decrease the transmission of microorganisms from health care personnel and the environment to the patient.
5 Remember that hand hygiene is essential before initiating any sterile procedure.
6 Incorporate the principles of surgical asepsis when conducting any sterile procedure.

SKILL 8-1 Applying and Removing Cap, Mask, and Protective Eyewear

 Basic / Basic Infection Control / Using Personal Protective Equipment

NSO *Infection Control Module / Lesson 1*

Although masks and caps are usually worn in surgical procedure areas (e.g., the operating room), there are certain aseptic procedures performed at a patient's bedside that also might require these barriers. For example, it may be an agency's policy for a nurse to wear a mask during the changing of a central line dressing or insertion of a peripherally inserted central catheter (PICC). Other policies might require that a nurse wear a mask and a cap to secure hair during dressing changes on a patient with extensive burns or with a central line (Lynn-McHale and Carlson, 2005). When there is a risk for splattering of blood or body fluid, there is also the need to apply protective eyewear (OSHA, 2001).

Assess a patient's potential for acquiring an infection before applying a mask (e.g., does the patient have a large open wound? do you have a respiratory infection? is the patient immunosuppressed?). If you wear a mask, change it when it becomes moist or soiled (e.g., splattered with blood). Some nurses choose to wear a surgical cap to secure loose hair that might contaminate a sterile area (Carrico, 2005). Wear eyewear when there is a risk for body fluids splashing into your eyes. As in all situations that require protection from splatters from blood or body fluid, follow standard precautions (see Chapter 7).

Delegation Considerations

The skill of applying and removing cap, mask, and protective eyewear can be delegated to nursing assistive personnel (NAP). However, the procedures performed at a patient's bedside that require cap and mask generally cannot be delegated (refer to specific skill for recommendations). The nurse determines if protective barriers are necessary for the other staff. The nurse directs the NAP by:

• Explaining the procedure to be performed and how to assist with positioning and obtaining supplies.

Equipment

❑ Surgical mask (different types are available for people with different skin sensitivities)
❑ Surgical cap (NOTE: Use only if hospital policy requires, or use to secure hair if there is a possibility of contamination of a sterile field.)
❑ Hairpins, rubber bands, or both
❑ Protective eyewear (e.g., goggles or glasses with appropriate side shields)

STEP	RATIONALE

ASSESSMENT

1 Consider type of sterile procedure to be performed, and consult agency's policy for use of mask/caps/eyewear.

Not all sterile procedures require mask, cap, or eyewear.
Ensures patient and nurse will be properly protected.

2 If you have symptoms of a cold or respiratory infection, either avoid participating in procedure or apply a mask.

A greater number of pathogenic microorganisms reside within the respiratory tract when infection is present.

3 Assess the patient's actual or potential risk for infection when choosing barriers for surgical asepsis (e.g., older adult, neonatal patient, or immunocompromised patient).

Some patients are at a greater risk for acquiring an infection, so nurse uses additional barriers.

NURSING DIAGNOSES

• Ineffective protection
• Risk for infection

Individualize related factors based on patient's condition or needs.

PLANNING

1 Expected outcome following completion of procedure:
• Patient will not develop signs of localized infection.

Indicates lack of microorganism transfer to patient and sterile field.

2 Prepare equipment, and inspect packaging for integrity and exposure to sterilization.

Ensures availability of equipment and sterility of supplies before procedure begins.

STEP	RATIONALE

IMPLEMENTATION

1 Applying cap:
  a If hair is long, comb back behind ears and secure.
  b Secure hair in place with pins.

  c Apply cap over head as you would apply hairnet. Be sure all hair fits under edges of cap (see illustration).

2 Applying mask:
  a Find top edge of mask, which usually has a thin metal strip along edge.
  b Hold mask by top two strings or loops, keeping top edge above bridge of nose.
  c Tie two top strings at top of back of head, over cap (if worn), with strings above ears (see illustration).
  d Tie two lower ties snugly around neck with mask well under chin (see illustration).
  e Gently pinch upper metal band around bridge of nose.

3 Applying protective eyewear:
  a Apply protective glasses, goggles, or face shield comfortably over eyes, and check that vision is clear (see illustration).
  b Be sure eyewear fits snugly around forehead and face.

4 Apply sterile gloves if needed (see Skill 8-3).

5 Removing eyewear:
  a Remove gloves first, if worn (see Skill 8-3).

Cap must cover all hair entirely.
Ensures that long hair does not fall down or cause cap to slip and expose hair.
Loose hair hanging over sterile field or falling dander contaminates objects on sterile field.

Pliable metal fits snugly against bridge of nose.

Prevents contact of hands with clean facial portion of mask. Mask will cover all of nose.
Position of ties at top of head provides tight fit. Strings over ears may cause irritation.
Prevents escape of microorganisms through sides of mask as nurse talks and breathes.
Prevents microorganisms from escaping around nose.

Positioning affects clarity of vision.

Ensures eyes are fully protected.

Prevents contamination of hair, neck, and facial area.

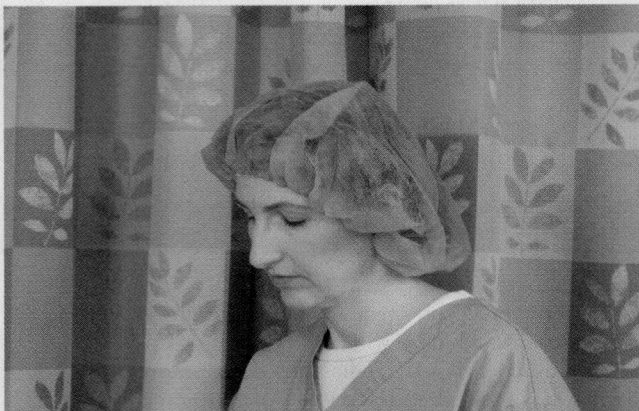

STEP 1c Nurse applies cap over head, covering all hair.

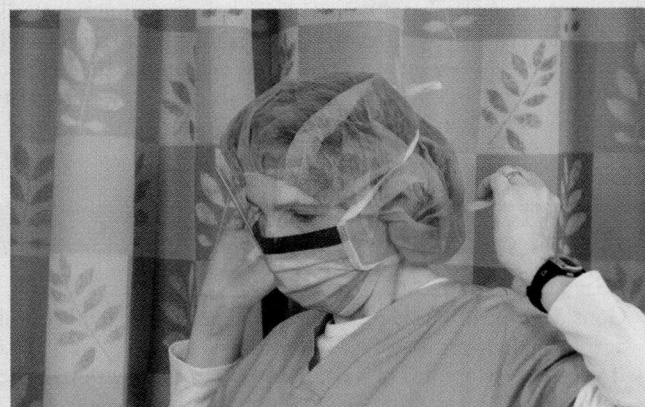

STEP 2d Tie bottom strings of mask.

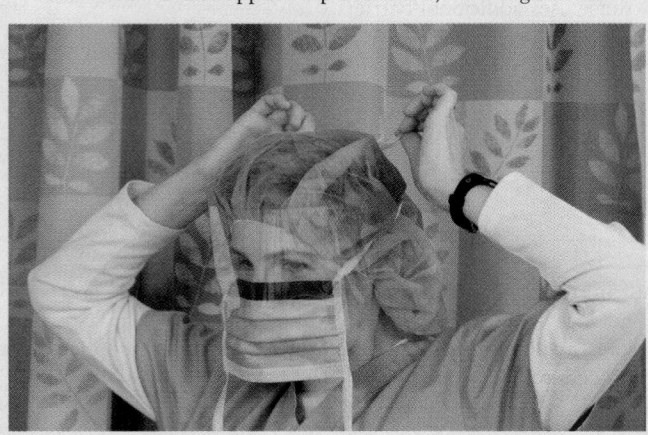

STEP 2c Tie top strings of mask.

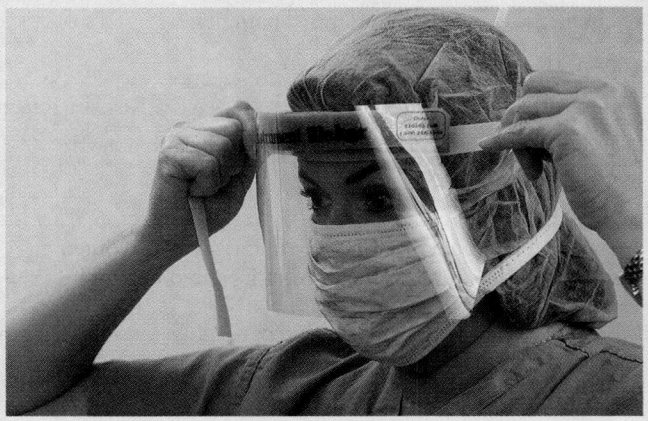

STEP 3a Apply face shield over cap.

STEP	RATIONALE
b Untie bottom strings of mask.	Prevents top part of mask from falling down over the uniform. If mask falls and touches uniform, it will be contaminated.
c Untie top strings of mask, and remove mask from face, holding ties securely. Discard mask in proper receptacle (see illustrations).	Avoids contact of nurse's hands with contaminated mask.
d Remove eyewear, avoiding placing hands over soiled lens. **If wearing face shield, remove it before removal of mask.** NOTE: **A combination mask and eyewear is available in some institutions.**	Prevents transmission of microorganisms.
e Grasp outer surface of cap, and lift from hair.	Minimizes contact of hands with hair.
f Discard cap in proper receptacle, and perform hand hygiene.	Reduces transmission of infection.

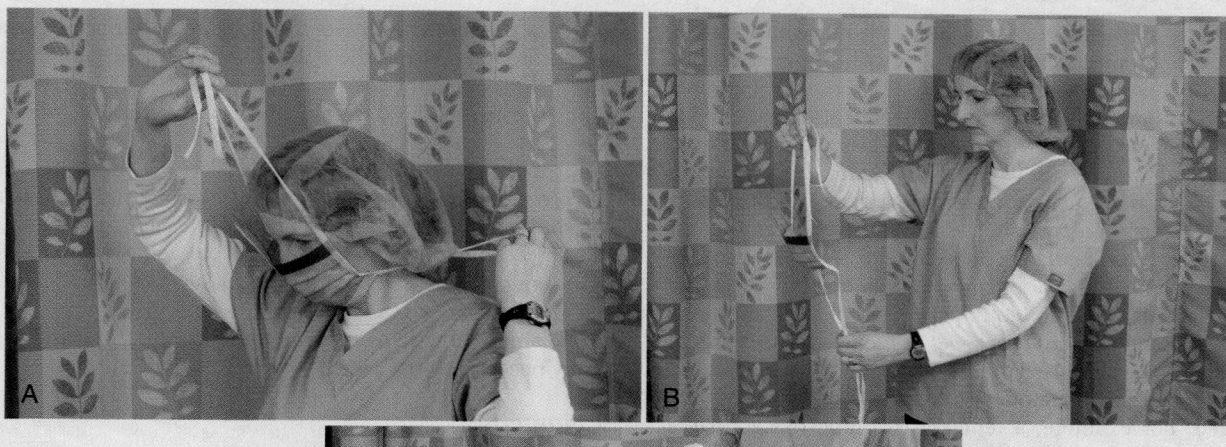

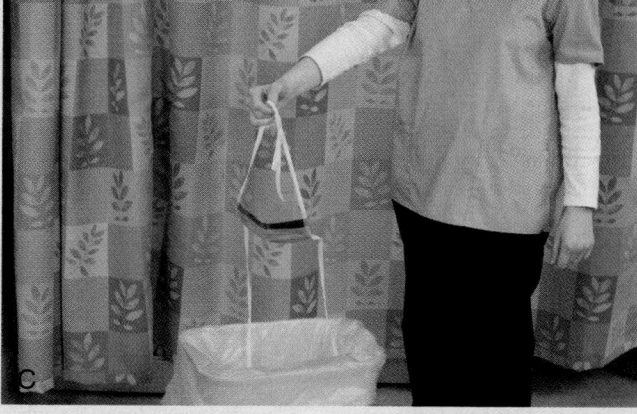

STEP 5c   **A,** Untying top mask strings. **B,** Removing mask from face. **C,** Discarding mask. *(From Phipps W and others:* Medical-surgical nursing: concepts and clinical practice, *ed 6, St. Louis, 1999, Mosby.)*

EVALUATION

1 Following procedure, assess area of body treated for drainage, tenderness, edema, or change in temperature or color of skin.	Rules out presence of localized infection.

Unexpected Outcomes	Related Interventions
1 Redness, heat, edema, pain, or purulent drainage develops at wound or treatment site, indicating possible infection.	• Notify health care provider of change in condition of affected area, and initiate appropriate treatments as ordered. • If there is a pattern or trend in patients developing similar infection, infection prevention and control team will investigate.

Recording and Reporting
- No recording or reporting is required for this set of skills. Record specific procedure performed in nurses' progress notes, and describe patient's status.

Home Care Considerations
- Instruct family caregiver as to specifics of when to apply cap, mask, and protective eyewear.
- Determine ability of family caregiver to safely implement sterile procedure.
- Instruct patient and family caregiver to observe for signs of infection.

SKILL 8-2   Preparing a Sterile Field

*Intermediate / Infection Control / Establishing
     and Maintaining a Sterile Field
Adding Items to a Sterile Field
Pouring a Sterile Solution
Using a Prepackaged Sterile Kit*

NSO *Infection Control Module / Lesson 3*

When performing sterile aseptic procedures, the nurse must have a work area in which objects can be handled with minimal risk for contamination. A sterile field serves such a purpose. It is an area considered free of microorganisms and may consist of a sterile kit or tray, a work surface draped with a sterile towel or wrapper, or a table covered with a large sterile drape (DeCastro, 2005). Sterile drapes establish a sterile field around a treatment site, such as a surgical incision, venipuncture site, or site for introduction of an indwelling urinary catheter. Drapes also provide a work surface for placing sterile supplies and for manipulating items with sterile gloves. Drapes are available in cloth, paper, and plastic. They may be wrapped in individual sterile packages or included within sterile kits or trays. Most are fluid resistant. Many styles, shapes, and sizes are available to accommodate different areas or body parts to be covered. For example, a fenestrated drape has a slitlike opening in it to expose only the perineal area during urinary catheter insertion.

Many sterile items come prepackaged within containers that serve as both sterile fields and work areas for the nurse. For example, bladder catheterization kits and tracheal suction kits contain sterile items that can be moved within the tray and containers into which sterile solutions can be poured. Once a sterile field is cre-

ated, it is the responsibility of the nurse to perform the procedure without contaminating the field. The skill of preparing a sterile field includes opening sterile packages, preparing a sterile drape, adding sterile supplies to a field, and pouring sterile solutions.

Delegation Considerations
The procedures performed at patients' bedsides that require use of a sterile field generally should not be delegated (refer to specific skill for recommendations) to NAP. However, NAP may assist in positioning patients and obtaining extra supplies. The nurse directs the NAP by:
- Explaining how to assist with patient positioning and to hand any necessary supplies

Equipment
- ☐ Sterile gloves
- ☐ Sterile drape or kit that is to be used as a sterile field
- ☐ Sterile gown (see agency policy)
- ☐ Disposable cap and mask (see agency policy)
- ☐ Sterile supplies and solutions specific to the procedure
- ☐ Waist-high table/countertop surface
- ☐ Protective eyewear

STEP	RATIONALE
ASSESSMENT	
1 Verify that procedure requires surgical aseptic technique.	Some procedures require medical rather than surgical aseptic technique.
2 Assess patient's comfort, oxygen requirements, and elimination needs before preparing for procedure.	Certain procedures for which sterile field is prepared may last a long time. Nurse anticipates patient's needs so that patient can relax and avoid any unnecessary movement that might disrupt procedure.
3 Position patient for maximum comfort and ease of breathing.	Additional staff may be needed to assist with positioning so patient does not contaminate sterile field.
4 Check sterile package integrity for punctures, tears, discoloration, moisture, or any other signs of contamination. If using commercially packaged supplies or those prepared by agency, check for sterilization indicator (a marker that changes color when exposed to heat or steam).	The inspection of packaging ensures that only sterile items are presented to sterile field (AORN, 2007).
5 Anticipate number and variety of supplies needed for procedure.	Not all sterile kits contain sufficient amounts or types of supplies. Failure to have necessary supplies causes nurse to leave sterile field, increasing risk for contamination.

NURSING DIAGNOSES
- Ineffective protection
- Risk for infection

Individualize related factors based on patient's condition or needs.

STEP	RATIONALE

PLANNING

1 Expected outcomes following completion of procedure:
- The sterile field is not contaminated.
- Patient is not exposed to microorganisms.

Nurse uses correct surgical aseptic practice.

2 Complete all other priority tasks (e.g., medication administration, suctioning patient) before beginning procedure.

Sterile fields should be prepared as close as possible to time of use to reduce potential for contamination (AORN, 2007).

3 Ask visitors to step out briefly during procedure. Discourage movement by staff who will assist with procedure.

Traffic or movement can increase potential for contamination through spread of microorganisms by air currents.

4 Prepare equipment at bedside.

Ensures availability before the procedure and prevents break in sterile technique. (NOTE: Povidone-iodine and chlorhexidine are not considered sterile solutions and require separate work surfaces for prepping.)

5 Position patient comfortably for specific procedure to be performed. If a body part is to be examined or treated, position patient so area is accessible. Have NAP assist with positioning as needed.

Patient should be able to lie still in one position comfortably during procedure. Movement can cause contamination of sterile items.

6 Explain to patient purpose of procedure and importance of sterile technique.

Ensures patient's ability to cooperate. Teaching before procedure eliminates need to talk during procedure, which can cause air droplet contamination of sterile area.

IMPLEMENTATION

1 Apply gloves, cap, mask, protective eyewear, as needed (consult agency policy) (see Skills 8-1 and 8-3).

Controls spread of airborne microorganisms.

2 Select a clean, flat, dry work surface above waist level.

A sterile object below a person's waist is considered contaminated.

3 Perform hand hygiene thoroughly using an alcohol-based hand rub or an antimicrobial soap and water (CDC, 2002).

Reduces carriage of microorganisms on hands, which may be transmitted to the patient.

4 Preparing a sterile work surface

  a Using a sterile commercial kit or tray containing sterile items:

    (1) Place sterile kit or package containing sterile items on clean, dry, flat work surface above waist level.

Items placed below waist level are considered contaminated.

    (2) Open outside cover (see illustration), and remove kit from dust cover. Place on work surface.

Inner kit remains sterile.

    (3) Grasp outer surface of tip of outermost flap.

Outer surface of package is considered unsterile. There is a 2.5-cm (1-inch) border around any sterile drape or wrap that is considered contaminated.

    (4) Open outermost flap away from body, keeping arm outstretched and away from sterile field (see illustration).

Reaching over sterile field contaminates it.

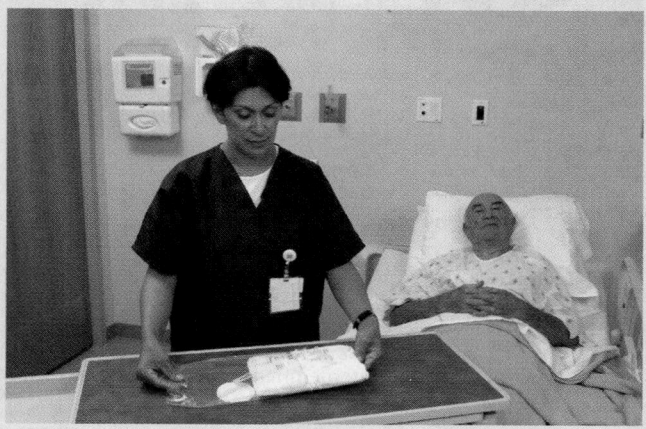

STEP 4a(2) Open outside cover of sterile kit.

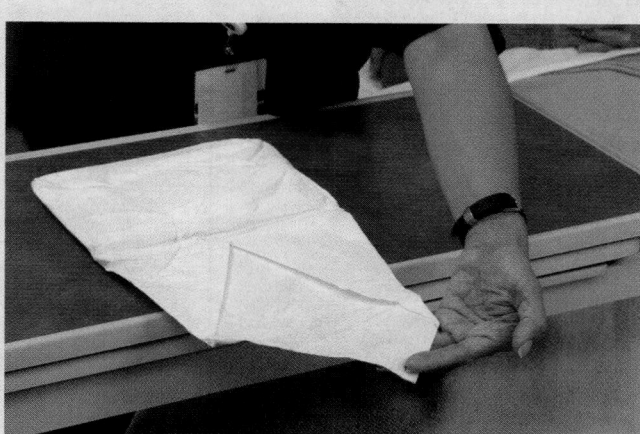

STEP 4a(4) Open outermost flap of sterile kit away from body.

STEP	RATIONALE

(5) Grasp outside surface of edge of first side flap. Open side flap, pulling to side, allowing it to lie flat on table surface. Keep your arm to side and not over sterile surface (see illustration).

Outer border is considered unsterile.
Drape or wrapper should lie flat so it will not accidentally rise up and contaminate inner surface or sterile contents.

(6) Repeat Step (5) for second side flap (see illustration).

(7) Grasp outside border of last and innermost flap (see illustration). Stand away from sterile package, and pull flap back, allowing it to fall flat on table.

Outer border is considered unsterile.
Never reach over a sterile field.

b Using a sterile linen-wrapped package:

(1) Place package on clean, dry, flat work surface above waist level.

Items placed below waist level are considered contaminated.

(2) Remove tape seal, and unwrap both layers following same steps (see Steps 4a(2) through 4a(7)) as with sterile kit above (see illustration).

Linen-wrapped items have two layers. The first is a dust cover. The second layer must be opened to view chemical indicator. If item is dropped on floor, it is considered contaminated.

(3) Use opened package wrapper as sterile field.

Inner surface of wrapper is considered sterile.

c Using a sterile drape:

(1) Place pack containing sterile drape on flat, dry surface and open as described (see Steps 4a(2) through 4a(7)) for sterile package.

Ensures sterility of packaged drape.

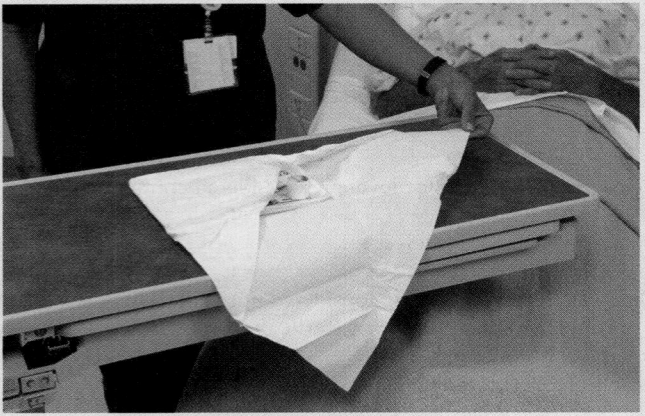

STEP 4a(5)   Open first side flap, pulling to side.

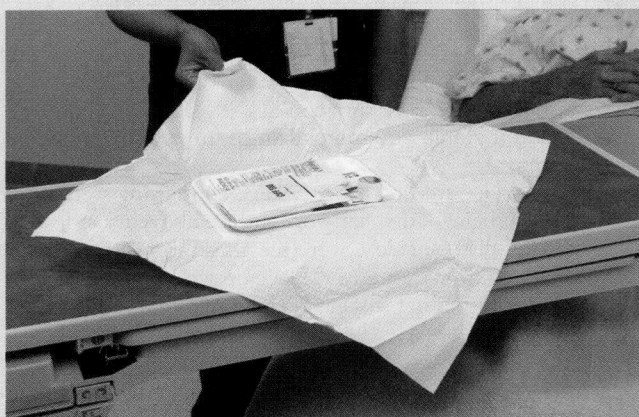

STEP 4a(7)   Open last and innermost flap.

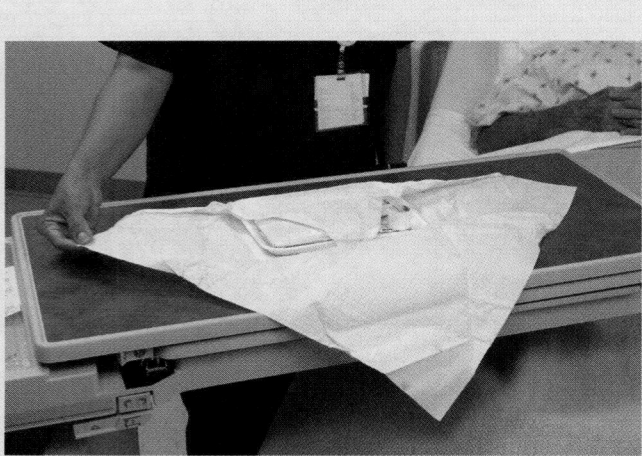

STEP 4a(6)   Open second side flap, pulling to side.

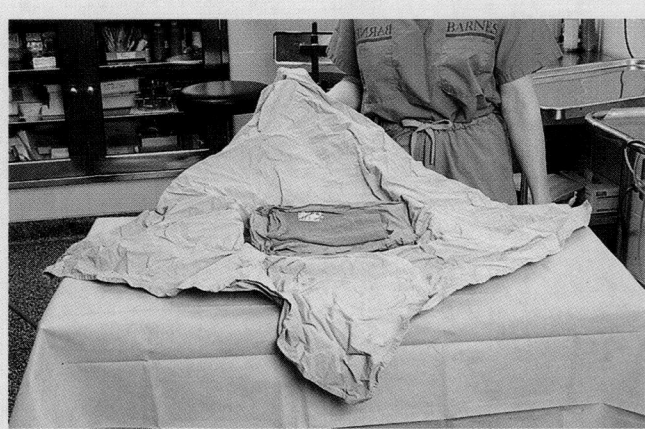

STEP 4b(2)   Open sterile linen-wrapped package.

STEP	RATIONALE

(2)   Apply sterile gloves (*optional*, see agency policy).

A sterile object remains sterile only when touched by another sterile object. Gloves are not necessary as long as fingers grasp the one inch unsterile border of the drape.

(3)   Grasp folded top edge of drape with fingertips of one hand. Gently lift drape up from its wrapper without touching any object.

If a sterile object touches any nonsterile object, it becomes contaminated.

(4)   Allow drape to unfold, keeping it above waist and work surface and away from body. (Discard wrapper with other hand.)

Object held below the waist is contaminated.

(5)   With other hand, grasp adjacent corner of drape. Hold drape straight over work surface (see illustration).

Drape can now be properly placed with two hands.

(6)   Holding drape, first position the bottom half over top half of intended work surface (see illustration).

Prevents nurse from reaching over sterile field.

(7)   Then allow top half of drape to be placed over bottom half of work surface (see illustration). A flat draped area is now available for placement of sterile supplies.

Creates flat sterile work surface.

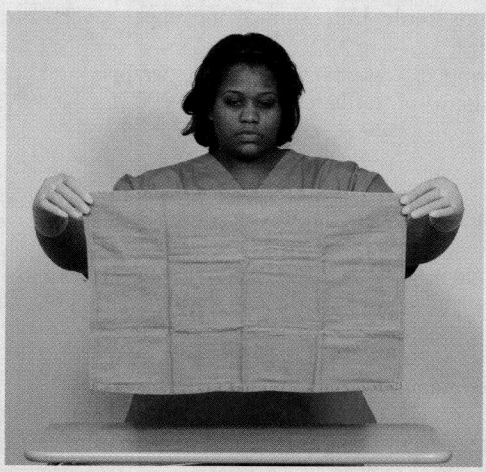

STEP 4c(5)   Hold corners of sterile drape up and away from body.

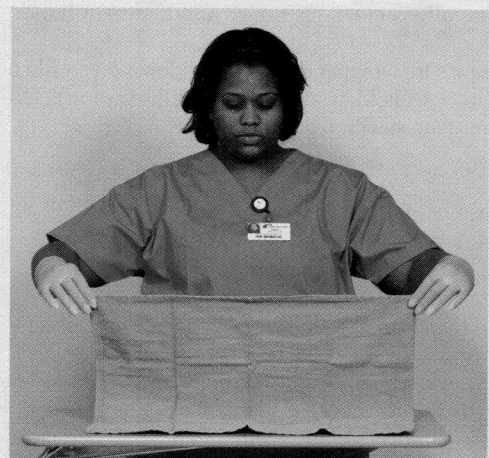

STEP 4c(6)   Position bottom half of sterile drape over top half of work surface.

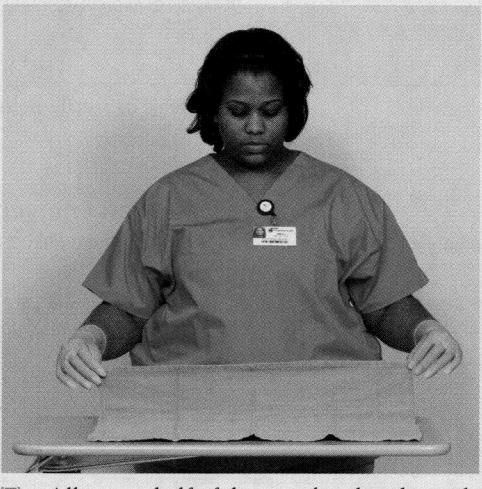

STEP 4c(7)   Allow top half of drape to be placed over bottom half of work surface.

STEP	RATIONALE

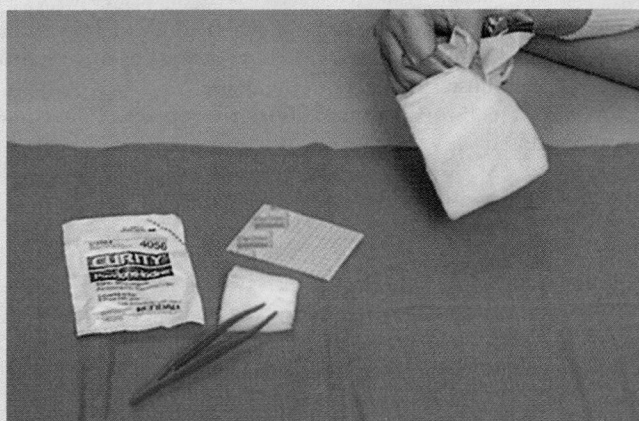

STEP 5c   Adding items to sterile field.

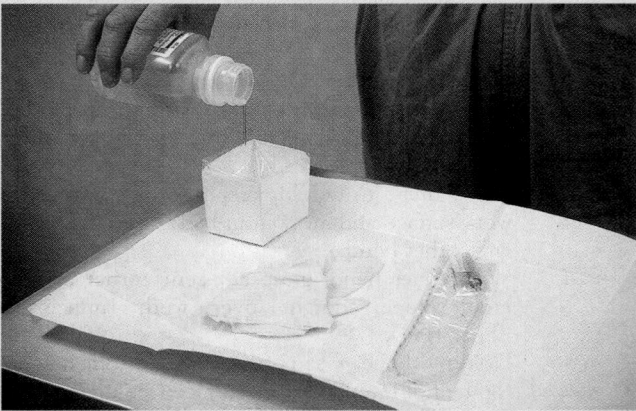

STEP 6d   Pouring solution into receiving container on sterile field.

5   Adding sterile items to the field:

a   Open sterile item (following package directions) while holding outside wrapper in nondominant hand.

Frees dominant hand for unwrapping outer wrapper.

b   Carefully peel wrapper over nondominant hand.

Item remains sterile. Inner surface of wrapper covers hand, making it sterile.

c   Being sure wrapper does not fall down on sterile field, place item onto field at an angle (see illustration). **Do not hold arm over sterile field.**

Secured wrapper edges prevent flipping wrapper and contaminating contents of sterile field (AORN, 2007).

Critical Decision Point   *Do not flip or toss objects onto sterile field.*

d   Dispose of outer wrapper.

Prevents accidental contamination of sterile field.

6   Pouring sterile solutions:

a   Verify contents and expiration date of solution.

Ensures proper solution and sterility of contents.

b   Be sure receptacle for solution is located near table/work surface edge. Sterile kits have cups or plastic molded sections into which fluids can be poured.

Prevents reaching over sterile field during pouring of solution.

c   Remove seal and cap from bottle in an upward motion.

Prevents contamination of the bottle lip.

d   With solution bottle held away from field and bottle lip 1 to 2 inches above inside of sterile receiving container, slowly pour entire contents of solution container. Hold bottle with the label facing the palm of the hand (see illustration).

Edge and outside of bottle are considered contaminated. Slow pouring prevents splashing. Sterility of contents cannot be ensured if cap is replaced.

Prevents label from becoming wet and illegible.

Critical Decision Point   *When liquids permeate sterile field or barrier, it is called strike through, resulting in contamination.*

EVALUATION

1   Observe for break in sterile technique.

Break in sterile field requires the nurse to set up new sterile field.

Unexpected Outcomes

1   Sterile field comes in contact with contaminated object, or liquid splatters onto drape, causing strike through.

2   Sterile item falls off sterile field.

Related Interventions

- Discontinue field preparation, and start over with new equipment.

- Open package containing new sterile item, and add to field, unless field becomes contaminated.

Recording and Reporting

- No recording or reporting is required for this set of skills. Record sterile procedure performed in nurses' progress notes, and describe patient's status.

Home Care Considerations

- Most care procedures in the home setting involve clean technique. In the event that a sterile environment is ordered, patient and family need to be aware of the principles that apply to the sterile environment. For example, teach family how to correctly use package wrapper as a sterile drape/barrier when applying a sterile dressing, or teach family the correct procedure for removing sterile item from package.
- Assess patient's and family's understanding and ability to provide a sterile environment when needed to perform a specific procedure.

SKILL 8-3   Sterile Gloving

 Intermediate/ Infection Control / Performing Sterile Gloving

NSO *Infection Control Module / Lesson 4*

Gloves help prevent the transmission of pathogens by direct and indirect contact. Nurses apply sterile gloves before performing sterile procedures such as inserting urinary catheters, changing dressings on central IV catheters, or applying sterile dressings. It is important to select the proper-size glove. The gloves should not stretch so tightly over the fingers that they can easily tear, yet they need to be tight enough that objects can be picked up easily. Sterile gloves are available in various sizes, such as 6, 6½, and 7. However, in most clinical areas sterile gloves in "one size fits all" are available.

It is important to choose not only the right size of glove but also the correct material. Many patients and health care workers are allergic to latex, the natural rubber used in most gloves and in other medical products (Church, 2005). Box 8-2 lists individuals who are at risk for latex allergy. Latex proteins enter the body through skin or mucous membranes, intravascularly, or via inhalation. The powder used to make latex gloves slip on easily is a carrier of the latex proteins (AORN, 2007; Molinari, 2005). When applying or removing gloves, the powder particles become airborne and can remain so for hours. The latex can then be inhaled or settle on clothing, skin, or mucous membranes. Reactions to latex can be mild to severe (Box 8-3). For individuals at high risk or with suspected sensitivity to latex, it is important to choose latex-free or synthetic gloves. More health care institutions are implementing latex-safe environments for workers (AORN, 2007).

Once you apply gloves, always be conscious of the position of your hands during procedures. If a sterile glove touches a clean, contaminated, or questionably contaminated object, it becomes unsterile and a new sterile glove must be applied. It is helpful to interlock the fingers and hold the hands together in front of the body and above waist level while waiting to handle sterile items. If a tear develops in a sterile glove, apply a new glove immediately.

Delegation Considerations

The skill of applying and removing sterile gloves can be delegated to NAP. However, many procedures that require the use of sterile gloves cannot be delegated to NAP. (Refer to specific skill for recommendations.) The nurse directs the NAP by:

- Explaining the reason for using sterile gloves for a specific procedure.

Equipment

- ☐ Package of proper-size sterile gloves, latex or synthetic nonlatex (NOTE: Hypoallergenic, low-powder, and low-protein latex gloves may still contain enough latex protein to cause an allergic reaction [Molinari, 2005].)

BOX 8-2   Individuals at Risk for Latex Allergy

- Spina bifida
- Congenital or urogenital defects
- History of indwelling catheters or repeated catheterizations
- History of using condom catheters

- High latex exposure (e.g., health care workers, housekeepers, food handlers, tire manufacturers, workers in industries that use gloves routinely)
- History of multiple childhood surgeries
- History of food allergies

Modified from Molinari J: Dental services. In *APIC text of infection control and epidemiology*, Washington, DC, revised 2005, Association for Professionals in Infection Control and Epidemiology Inc.

BOX 8-3   Levels of Latex Reactions

There are three types of common latex reactions which, in order of severity, include:

1 *Irritant dermatitis:* A nonallergic response characterized by skin redness and itching.
2 *Type IV hypersensitivity:* Cell-mediated allergic reaction to chemicals used in latex processing. Reaction can be delayed up to 48 hours, including redness, itching, and hives. Localized swelling, red and itchy or runny eyes and nose, and coughing may develop.

3 *Type I allergic reaction:* A true latex allergy that can be life-threatening. Reactions vary based on type of latex protein and degree of individual sensitivity, including local and systemic. Symptoms include hives, generalized edema, itching, rash, wheezing, bronchospasm, difficulty breathing, laryngeal edema, diarrhea, nausea, hypotension, tachycardia, and respiratory or cardiac arrest.

Modified from Gritter M: The latex threat, *Am J Nurs* 98(9):26, 1998.

STEP	RATIONALE

ASSESSMENT

1 Consider the type of procedure to be performed, and consult institutional policy on use of sterile gloves.

Ensures proper use of sterile gloves when needed.

2 Consider patient's risk for infection. For example, preexisting condition and size or extent of area being treated.

Directs nurse to follow added precautions (e.g., use of additional protective barriers) if necessary.

3 Examine glove package to determine if it is dry and intact with no water stains.

Torn or wet package is considered contaminated. Signs of water stains on the package indicate previous contamination by water.

4 Inspect condition of hands for cuts, hang nails, open lesions, or abrasions. In some settings you are allowed to cover any open lesion with a sterile, impervious transparent dressing (check agency policy).

Cuts, abrasions, and hang nails tend to ooze serum, which possibly contains pathogens. Breaks in skin integrity permit microorganisms to enter and increase the risk for infection for both patient and nurse (AORN, 2007). Presence of such lesions may prevent nurse from participating in procedure.

5 Assess patient for the following risk factors before applying latex gloves:

Determines level of patient's risk for latex allergy.

   a Previous reaction to the following items within hours of exposure: adhesive tape, dental or face mask, golf club grip, ostomy bag, rubber band, balloon, bandage, elastic underwear, IV tubing, rubber gloves, condom.

Items known to lead to latex allergy.

   b Personal history of asthma, contact dermatitis, eczema, urticaria, rhinitis.

   c History of food allergies, especially avocado, banana, peach, chestnut, raw potato, kiwi, tomato, papaya.

   d Previous history of adverse reactions during surgery, dental procedure.

Suggests allergic response.

   e Previous reaction to latex product.

Suggests allergic response.

NURSING DIAGNOSES

- Ineffective protection
- Risk for infection
- Risk for injury

Individualize related factors based on patient's condition or needs.

PLANNING

1 Expected outcomes following completion of procedure:
   - Patient will not develop signs or symptoms of infection after procedure.

Indicates microorganisms not introduced into sterile body cavities or sites (such as skin or urinary tract).

   - Patient will not develop latex sensitivity or latex allergy reaction.

Patient at risk for latex allergy is not exposed to latex proteins.

2 Select correct size and type of gloves.

There is less chance of contamination if correct size of gloves is worn.

Critical Decision Point *Synthetic nonlatex gloves are necessary for patients at risk or if nurse has sensitivity or allergy to latex.*

3 Place glove package near work area.

Ensures availability before procedure.

IMPLEMENTATION

1 Applying gloves:
   a Perform thorough hand hygiene.

Reduces number of bacteria on skin surfaces and reduces transmission of infection.

STEP	RATIONALE
b Remove outer glove package wrapper by carefully separating and peeling apart sides (see illustration).	Prevents inner glove package from accidentally opening and touching contaminated objects.
c Grasp inner package, and lay it on clean, dry, flat surface at waist level. Open package, keeping gloves on inside surface of wrapper (see illustration).	Sterile object held below waist is contaminated. Inner surface of glove package is sterile.
d Identify right and left glove. Each glove has a cuff approximately 5 cm (2 inches) wide. Glove dominant hand first.	Proper identification of gloves prevents contamination by improper fit. Gloving of dominant hand first improves dexterity.
e With thumb and first two fingers of nondominant hand, grasp glove for dominant hand by touching only glove's inside surface (see illustration).	Inner edge of cuff will lie against skin and thus is not sterile.
f Carefully pull glove over dominant hand, leaving cuff and being sure cuff does not roll up wrist. Be sure thumb and fingers are in proper spaces.	If glove's outer surface touches hand or wrist, it is contaminated.
g With gloved dominant hand, slip fingers underneath second glove's cuff (see illustration).	Cuff protects gloved fingers. Sterile touching sterile prevents glove contamination.

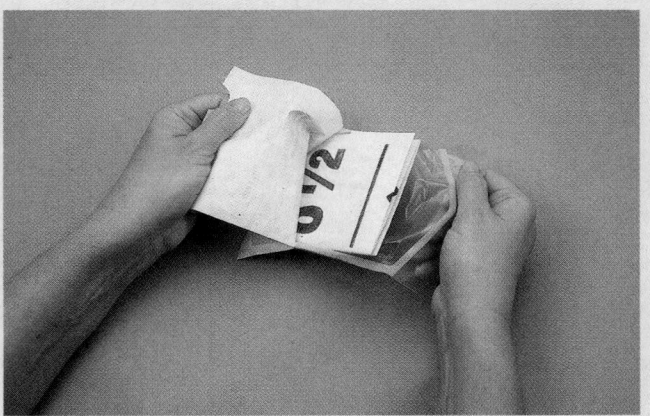

STEP 1b   Open outer glove package wrapper.

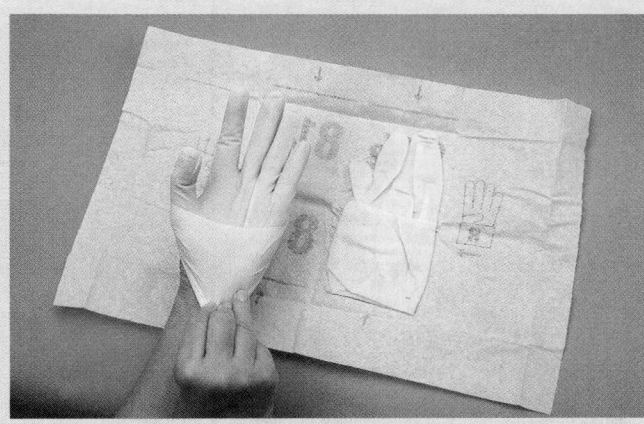

STEP 1e   Pick up glove at cuff for dominant hand, and insert fingers; pull glove completely over dominant hand (example is for left-handed person).

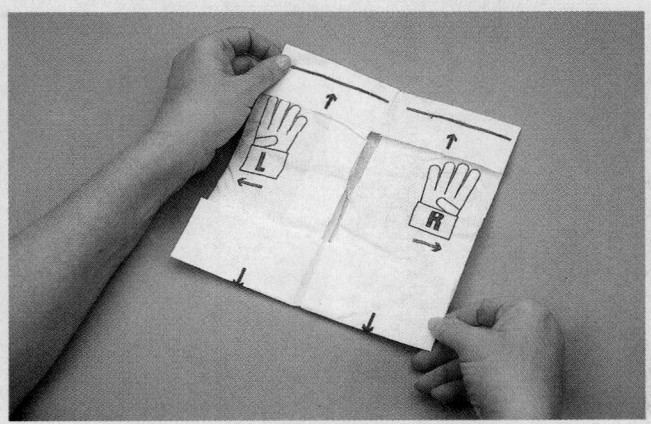

STEP 1c   Open inner glove package on work surface.

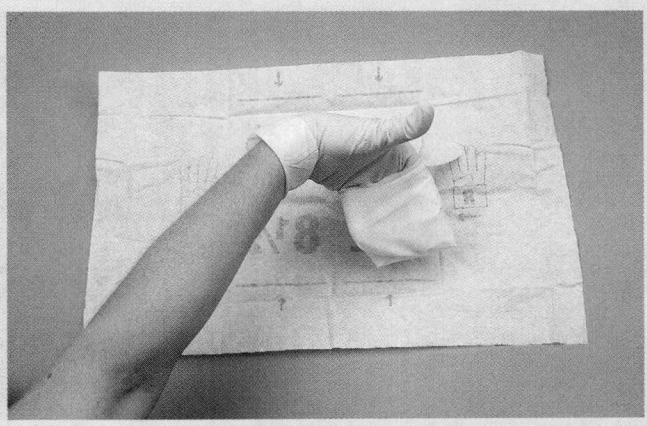

STEP 1g   Pick up glove for nondominant hand.

STEP	RATIONALE
h Carefully pull second glove over nondominant hand (see illustration).	Contact of gloved hand with exposed hand results in contamination.

Critical Decision Point   *Do not allow fingers and thumb of gloved dominant hand to touch any part of exposed nondominant hand. Keep thumb of dominant hand abducted back.*

STEP	RATIONALE
i After second glove is on, interlock hands together, above waist level. The cuffs usually fall down after application. Be sure to touch only sterile sides (see illustration).	Ensures smooth fit over fingers.
2 Disposing of gloves:	
a Grasp outside of one cuff with other gloved hand; avoid touching wrist.	Minimizes contamination of underlying skin.
b Pull glove off, turning it inside out and place it in gloved hand.	Outside of glove does not touch skin surface.
c Take fingers of bare hand and tuck inside remaining glove cuff (see illustration). Peel glove off inside out and over the previously removed glove. Discard both gloves in receptacle	Fingers do not touch contaminated glove surface.
d Perform thorough hand hygiene.	This protects health care worker from contamination resulting from any unseen tears or pinholes in gloves; also removing powder from hands helps to prevent skin irritations.

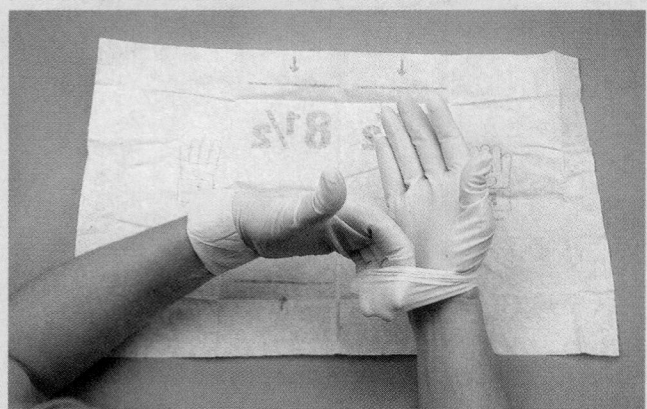

STEP 1h   Pull second glove over nondominant hand.

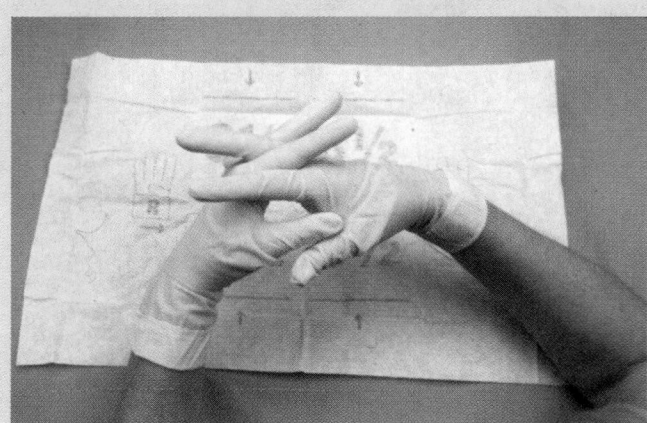

STEP 1i   Interlock gloved hands.

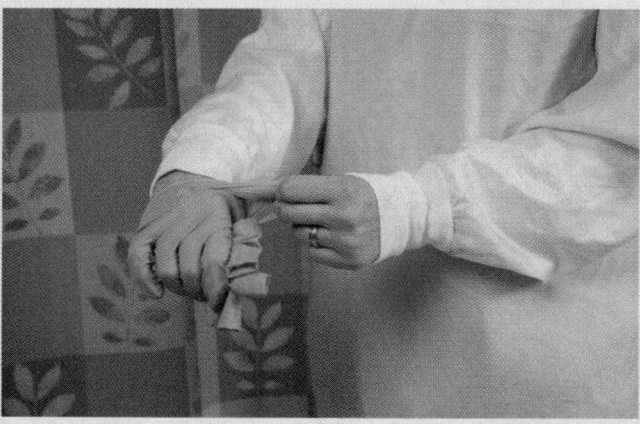

STEP 2c   Remove second glove by turning it inside out.

STEP	RATIONALE

EVALUATION

1 Assess patient for signs of infection, focusing on area treated.

Improper technique contributes to development of an infection.

Unexpected Outcomes

1 Patient develops localized signs of infection (e.g., urine becomes cloudy or odorous; wound becomes painful, edematous, reddened with purulent drainage).

2 Patient develops systemic signs of infection (e.g., fever, malaise, increased white blood cell count).

3 Patient develops allergic reaction to latex (see Box 8-3).

Related Interventions

• Contact health care provider, and implement appropriate treatments as ordered.

• Contact health care provider, and implement appropriate treatments as ordered.

• Immediately remove source of latex.
• Bring emergency equipment to bedside. Have epinephrine injection ready for administration, and be prepared to initiate IV fluids and oxygen.

Recording and Reporting

• It is not necessary to record application of gloves. Record specific procedure performed and patient's response and status.

• In the event of a latex allergy reaction, record patient's response in nurses' notes and vital sign flow sheet. Note type of response and patient's reaction to emergency treatment.

Teaching Considerations

• Nurse or patient with a known latex allergy should wear a medical alert bracelet or tag and carry a wallet card stating "latex allergy."

• Individuals with known latex allergies should carry a quick-acting oral antihistamine and an epinephrine autoinjector at all times.

[?] CRITICAL THINKING EXERCISES

1 You are assigned to Mrs. Lorenzo, a 78-year-old grandmother who is blind and is being admitted to the facility for a cholecystectomy. You enter her room to begin a series of procedures: insertion of an indwelling urinary catheter, irrigation of a nasogastric tube, insertion of a peripheral intravenous catheter, and measurement of the patient's blood pressure. Which procedure requires use of sterile gloves?

2 You prepared the peripheral site for Mrs. Lorenzo's intravenous catheter, then attempted to insert the catheter without success, and you need to try another location. What would you do next?

3 Mrs. Lorenzo tells you she has allergic reactions when she eats bananas or tomatoes. Based on this information, what would you ask Mrs. Lorenzo, and what actions would you take?

4 Mrs. Lorenzo's physician is planning to insert a central venous line. You obtained the necessary equipment, prepared a sterile drape, and opened the sterile pack. You removed the outer wrapper and placed the item on the sterile field. While doing this, you noticed the item touched the drape 2 inches from the border of the drape. What would you do next?

2 When opening a sterile pack, which action will compromise the sterility of the contents?
   1 Keeping the contents of the pack away from the table edge
   2 Holding or moving the object below the waist
   3 Opening the pack just before the procedure
   4 Allowing movement around the sterile field that does not touch near the sterile field

3 A nurse is preparing to change a dressing using sterile gloves. It is most important to remember which concept when putting them on?
   1 Grab only the inside of the glove with the ungloved hand.
   2 Grab only the cuffs of the gloves with the bare hand.
   3 Wear a glove that is as tight as possible.
   4 Keep the glove fingertips parallel to the body.

4 A teenager with spina bifida is to have a catheter inserted. Which action is most important before performing this procedure?
   1 Wash the insertion area with soap and water before insertion of the catheter.
   2 Position the patient as comfortably as possible.
   3 Ask the patient if the patient is allergic to eggs.
   4 Obtain a nonlatex catheter for the procedure.

5 A nurse is supervising a nursing student setting up for a sterile dressing change. Which action by the nursing student would require intervention from the nurse?
   1 The first flap of the sterile package is opened away from the student's body.
   2 The glove for the dominant hand is pulled on first.
   3 During pouring the label of the solution bottle is facing the floor.
   4 The bottle of solution is kept above the student's waist.

[✓] REVIEW QUESTIONS

1 Contamination of the nurse can occur if used isolation items are not removed properly. To maintain the nurse's protection, sterile barriers are removed in what order?
   1 Gloves, mask, eyewear, then cap
   2 Mask, eyewear, cap, then gloves
   3 Eyewear, cap, mask, then gloves
   4 Gloves, eyewear, cap, then mask

REFERENCES

Association of periOperative Registered Nurses: *Standards, recommended practices, and guidelines*, Denver, 2007, The Association.

Carrico R, ed: *APCC text of infection control & epidemiology*, Washington, DC, 2008, Association for Professionals in Infection Control & Epidemiology.

Centers for Disease Control and Prevention, Hospital Infection Control Practice Advisory Committee and the HICPAC/SHEA/APIC/IDSA Hand Hygiene Task Force: Guideline for hand hygiene in health-care settings, *MMWR Recomm Rep* 51(No. RR-16), 2002.

Centers for Disease Control and Prevention, Hospital Infection Control Practice Advisory Committee: *Guidelines for isolation precautions in healthcare settings 2007,* http://www.cdc.gov/ncidod/dhap/pdf/guidelines/Isolation2007.

Church N: Surgical services. In *APIC text of infection control and epidemiology,* Washington, DC, revised 2005, Association for Professionals in Infection Control and Epidemiology Inc.

DeCastro M: Aseptic technique. In *APIC text of infection control and epidemiology,* Washington, DC, revised 2005, Association for Professionals in Infection Control and Epidemiology Inc.

Gritter M: The latex threat, *Am J Nurs* 98(9):26, 1998.

Lynn-McHale D, Carlson KK, eds: AACN *procedure manual for critical care,* ed 5, Philadelphia, 2005, WB Saunders.

Molinari J: Dental services. In *APIC text of infection control and epidemiology,* Washington, DC, revised 2005, Association for Professionals in Infection Control and Epidemiology Inc.

Occupational Safety and Health Administration: enforcement procedures for the occupational exposure to blood-borne injury final rule *Fed Reg* 66:5318, 2001.

Occupational Safety and Health Administration: Respiratory protection: proposed rule, *Fed Regist* 59(219):58884, 1994.

Phipps W and others: *Medical-surgical nursing: concepts and clinical practice,* ed 6, St. Louis, 1999, Mosby.

Safe Patient Handling, Transfer, and Positioning

MEDIA RESOURCES

-  http://evolve.elsevier.com/Perry/skills
  - Review Questions
  - Video Clips

- Mosby's Nursing Video Skills, 3.0

KEY TERMS

Balance
Base of support
Body alignment
Body mechanics
Center of gravity
Drawsheet
Footdrop
Friction
Hand rolls
Hemiparesis
Hemiplegia
Hoyer lift
  (mechanical/
  hydraulic lift)
Leverage
Line of gravity
Logrolling
Orthostatic
  hypotension
Paralysis
Paresis
Posture
Proprioceptive
  function
Weight

OBJECTIVES

Mastery of content in this chapter will enable the nurse to:
- Describe body mechanics and its importance in caring for patients.
- Describe principles of safe patient transfer and positioning.
- Describe normal body alignment for standing, sitting, and lying down.
- Assess for alterations in body alignment.

- Describe procedures for safely lifting patients.
- Describe positioning techniques for the supported Fowler's, supine, prone, 30-degree lateral side-lying, and Sims' positions.
- Describe the procedures for helping a patient to move up in bed, helping a patient to a sitting position, logrolling a patient, and transferring a patient from a bed to a chair.

Health care providers are required to provide employees with safety information and training to use when transferring, positioning, and lifting patients. Refer to the policies and procedures in the institution where you work. The Occupational Safety and Health Administration (OSHA) has identified guidelines on back safety and the prevention of musculoskeletal injuries (OSHA, 2005; U.S. Department of Labor, 2003).

Before lifting or transferring patients, consider principles of safe patient transfer and positioning (Box 9-1). Before lifting, assess the weight to be lifted and what assistance, if any, is needed (Nelson, 2006; U.S. Department of Labor, 2003). If help is needed, assess if a second person is adequate or if mechanical assistance is needed. Once the amount of assistance is determined, use the following steps for proper body mechanics:
- Keep back, neck, pelvis, and feet aligned and avoid twisting. Twisting your spine can lead to serious injury.
- Tighten stomach muscles and tuck pelvis; this provides balance and protects the back.
- Bend at the knees; this helps to maintain your center of gravity and lets the strong muscles of the legs do the lifting.
- Keep the weight to be lifted as close to the body as possible; this action places the weight in the same plane as the lifter and close to the center of gravity for balance.
- Maintain the trunk erect and knees bent so that multiple muscle groups work together in a synchronized manner.
- The best height for lifting vertically is approximately 2 feet off the ground and close to the lifter's center of gravity.
- Person with the heaviest load coordinates efforts of the personnel involved in lifting or transferring.

Body mechanics is the coordinated effort of the musculoskeletal and nervous systems to maintain balance, posture, and body alignment during lifting, bending, moving, and performing activities of daily living. Body mechanics also facilitates body movement so that a person can carry out a physical activity without using excessive muscle energy.

Many patients have conditions resulting in immobility or require limitations in activity imposed by their treatment plan. It is an important nursing role to safely position and move patients effectively to reduce the risks related to immobilization. Positioning of patients to maintain correct body alignment is essential to preventing complications. These complications include pressure ulcers (see Chapter 18), which can develop in 24 hours and require months to heal (Groeneveld and others, 2004); and contractures, which can occur within a few days when muscles, tendons, and joints become less flexible because of lack of mobility and incorrect alignment. For example, plantar flexion contracture or footdrop is a complication seen in bedridden patients. It is caused when the force of gravity pulls an unsupported, weakened foot into a plantar-flexed position, and calf muscles and heel cords shorten, complicating future attempts at walking. Pillows placed under the knees or an elevated knee gatch can produce knee and hip contractures and increase pressure on the sacrum, thus creating risk for pressure ulcers.

Some patients are at high risk for complications from improper positioning and have increased risk for injury during transfer. Examples include patients with poor nutrition, poor circulation, loss of sensation, alterations in bone formation or joint mobility, and impaired muscle development. Central nervous system (CNS) damage may result in motor impairment, proprioceptive loss, or cognitive dysfunction, all of which affect mobility. The application of proper body mechanics, alignment, and the use of safe patient transfer and positioning techniques assists patients in achieving an optimal level of independence without resultant injury to health care providers.

EVIDENCE-BASED PRACTICE TRENDS

Musculoskeletal disorders are the most prevalent and debilitating occupational health hazard among nurses. There has been little improvement in the incidence of musculoskeletal injuries in health care workers. In 1989, 4.2 lost-workday injury cases per 100 were reported; in 2000 there were 4.1 cases per 100 (Baptiste and others, 2006; Bureau of Labor Statistics, 2003; Nelson and Baptiste, 2004). Because of the risk for injury to nurses and their patients, the American Nurses Association (ANA) developed position statements calling for the use of assistive equipment and devices to safely reposition and transfer patients (ANA, 2003, 2007). The use of assistive equipment and consistent use of proper body mechanics significantly reduces the risk for musculoskeletal injuries (ANA, 2003, 2007). In addition, OSHA recommends that manual lifting of patients be minimized in all cases and eliminated when feasible (OSHA, 2005). Many facilities are moving toward limited lift policies that minimize patient handling by nurses (de Castro and others, 2006; Miami Valley Hospital, 2007; UC Davis Health System, 2005). Instead, lift devices reduce on-the-job injuries (Nelson and Baptiste, 2004; Nelson and others, 2003; Pelczarski, 2007). Knowledge about safe, efficient lifting techniques and

BOX 9-1	Principles of Safe Patient Transfer and Positioning

Mechanical lifts and lift teams are essential when the client is unable to assist.

When a client is able to assist, remember these principles:
- The wider the base of support, the greater the stability of the nurse.
- The lower the center of gravity, the greater the stability of the nurse.
- The equilibrium of an object is maintained as long as the line of gravity passes through its base of support.
- Facing the direction of movement prevents abnormal twisting of the spine.
- Dividing balanced activity between arms and legs reduces the risk for back injury.
- Leverage, rolling, turning, or pivoting requires less work than lifting.
- When friction is reduced between the object to be moved and the surface on which it is moved, less force is required to move it.

proper use of assistive equipment and devices promotes safe patient transfer without injury to the patient or the nurse.

Skill Performance Guidelines

1 Know how physiological influences on body alignment and mobility affect patients throughout the life span. In the child the major consequences of decreased muscle activity are loss of muscle strength, endurance, muscle mass, and joint mobility; bone demineralization; and contracture (Hockenberry and Wilson, 2007). Inactive older adults are at risk for muscle atrophy, loss of bony mass, contractures of joints, and pressure ulcers (Meiner and Lueckenotte, 2006).

2 Know the pathological conditions that affect a patient's body alignment and mobility (Nelson, 2006). Postural abnormalities affect body mechanics. For example, a patient with severe kyphosis cannot lie supine or lift an object safely because the center of gravity is not aligned. Diseases affecting bone formation (e.g., osteoporosis) alter body alignment and mobility. Degenerative joint diseases (e.g., osteoarthritis), impaired muscle development (e.g., muscular dystrophy), and central nervous system damage (e.g., paralysis) interfere with normal body alignment and mobility. Therefore the patient's risk for musculoskeletal injury is increased.

3 Know the history of underlying conditions such as chronic disease (e.g., diabetes, chronic obstructive pulmonary disease) or malnutrition. Patients with underlying chronic conditions are at risk for skin breakdown and other hazards of immobility and as a result require more frequent position changes.

4 Control factors that indirectly affect body mechanics by altering the safety of the environment. Cluttered hallways and bedside areas increase the patient's risk for falling (see Chapters 13 and 41).

5 Know the patient's fluid balance status. Dehydration or edema may require more frequent position changes because patients are prone to skin breakdown. Dehydration also predisposes a patient to orthostatic hypotension. Identify patients with incontinence or profuse sweating. Moisture from incontinence or sweating can decrease tensile strength and alter skin resiliency to external forces (Fader and others, 2004).

6 Know the patient's range of motion (ROM). Contractures or spasticity limit joint and muscle mobility; the nurse must take care not to position the limb in an unnatural way. This could result in injury to or dysfunction of the affected limb (see Chapter 10).

7 Determine the patient's level of sensory perception. Loss of sensation increases vulnerability to the hazards of immobility because of the inability to sense pain or need for repositioning. Patients with decreased sensation must have their positions evaluated and changed frequently to avoid damage to the integumentary and musculoskeletal systems.

SKILL 9-1   Using Safe and Effective Transfer Techniques

Basic / Safe Patient Handling
Transferring From a Bed to a Wheelchair
*   With a Transfer Belt*
Transferring From a Bed to a Stretcher

NSO *Safety Module / Lesson 3*

Transferring is a nursing skill that helps weakened or dependent patients or patients with restricted mobility attain positions to regain optimal independence as quickly as possible. Physical activity maintains and improves joint motion, increases strength, promotes circulation, relieves pressure on skin, and improves urinary and respiratory functions. It also benefits a patient psychologically by increasing social activity and mental stimulation and providing a change in environment (Lampinen and others, 2006). As a result, mobilization plays a crucial role in a patient's rehabilitation.

One of the major concerns during transfer is the safety of the patient and the nurse. The nurse prevents self-injury by using correct posture, minimal muscle strength, effective body mechanics and lifting techniques, and appropriate lift devices (see Figure 9-1, p. 216). Consider individual patient problems during transfer. For example, a patient who has been immobile for several days or longer may be weak or dizzy or may develop orthostatic hypotension (a drop in blood pressure) when transferred. As a rule of thumb, use a transfer belt and obtain assistance when transferring patients if there is any doubt about safe transfer.

Delegation Considerations

The skill of effective transfer techniques can be delegated to nursing assistive personnel (NAP). The nurse directs the NAP by:

- Assisting and supervising when moving patients who are transferred for the first time after prolonged bed rest, extensive surgery, critical illness, or spinal cord trauma.
- Explaining the patient's mobility restrictions, changes in blood pressure, or sensory alterations that may affect safe transfer.

Equipment

☐ Transfer belt, sling, or lap board (as needed)
☐ Nonskid shoes, bath blankets, pillows
☐ Slide board (friction-reducing board)
☐ *Wheelchair:* Position chair at 45-degree angle to bed, lock brakes, remove footrests, lock bed brakes
☐ *Stretcher:* Position next to bed, lock brakes on stretcher, lock brakes on bed
☐ *Optional:* Mechanical/hydraulic lift: Use frame, canvas strips or chains, and hammock or canvas strips; stand assist lift device

RATIONALE

ASSESSMENT

1 Assess physiological capacity to transfer:

   Determines patient's ability to tolerate and assist with transfer and whether special adaptive techniques are necessary.

   a Muscle strength (legs and upper arms)

   Immobile patients have decreased muscle strength, tone, and mass. Affects ability to bear weight or raise body.

   b Joint mobility and contracture formation

   Immobility or inflammatory processes (i.e., arthritis) may lead to contracture formation and impaired joint mobility.

STEP	RATIONALE
c Paralysis or paresis (spastic or flaccid)	Patient with CNS damage may have bilateral paralysis (requiring transfer by swivel bar, sliding bar, mechanical lift) or unilateral paralysis, which requires belt transfer to strong side. Weakness (paresis) requires stabilization of knee while transferring. Flaccid arm must be supported with sling during transfer.
d Bone continuity (trauma, amputation)	Patients with trauma to one leg or hip may be non–weight bearing when transferred. Amputees may use sliding board to transfer.
2 Assess presence of weakness, dizziness, or postural hypotension.	Determines risk for fainting or falling during transfer. The move from a supine to a vertical position redistributes about 500 mL of blood; immobile patients may have decreased autonomic nervous system response to equalize blood supply, resulting in orthostatic hypotension (Phipps and others, 2007).
3 Assess level of endurance: a Assess level of fatigue during activity.	Ability to transfer may be limited by fatigue. Estimates ability to participate in transfer. Assess endurance by patient's participation in activities of daily living (ADLs). Planned rest periods before transfer may enhance function.
b Assess vital signs.	Vital sign changes such as increased pulse and respiration may indicate activity intolerance (see Chapter 5). Patient with low blood pressure may not tolerate sudden position change and is at risk for orthostatic hypotension.
4 Assess patient's proprioceptive function (awareness of posture and changes in equilibrium): a Ability to maintain balance while sitting in bed or on side of bed	Determines stability of patient's balance for transfer. Determines risk for fainting or falling during transfer.
b Tendency to sway to or position self to one side	Patients with brain dysfunction may have proprioceptive losses. This may cause them to lean to one side or lose balance during transfer.
5 Assess patient's sensory status, including adequacy of central and peripheral vision, adequacy of hearing, and presence of peripheral sensation loss.	Determines influence of sensory loss on ability to make transfer. Visual field loss decreases patient's ability to see in direction of transfer. Peripheral sensation loss decreases proprioception. Patients with visual and hearing losses need transfer techniques adapted to deficits. Patients with cerebrovascular accident (CVA) may lose area of visual field, which profoundly affects vision and perception.

Critical Decision Point *Patients with hemiplegia may "neglect" one side of the body (inattention to or unawareness of one side of body or environment), which distorts perceptions of the visual field.*

STEP	RATIONALE
6 Assess patient's level of comfort: a Pain b Muscle spasm	Pain reduces patient's motivation and ability to be mobile. Pain relief before transfer enhances patient participation (Pasero and McCaffery, 2004).
7 Assess patient's cognitive status:	Determines patient's ability to follow directions and learn transfer techniques.

Critical Decision Point *Patients with head trauma or CVA may have perceptual cognitive deficits that create safety risks. If patient has difficulty in comprehension, simplify instructions by providing one step at a time and maintain consistency.*

STEP	RATIONALE
a Ability to follow verbal instructions	May indicate patients at risk for injury.
b Short-term memory	Patients with short-term memory deficits may have difficulty with transfer, initial learning, or consistent performance.
c Recognition of physical deficits and limitations to movement	Patient's knowledge of deficits can help the nurse plan a safe transfer.
8 Assess patient's level of motivation such as patient's eagerness versus unwillingness to be mobile.	Altered psychological states often reduce patient's desire to engage in activity.
9 Assess patient for specific risks of falling when transferred: neuromuscular deficits, motor weakness, calcium loss from long bones, cognitive and visual dysfunction, and altered balance (see Chapter 13).	Certain conditions increase patient's risk for falling or potential for injury.

STEP	**RATIONALE**
10 Determine need for special transfer equipment necessary for home setting. Assess home environment for hazards (see Chapter 41) and family's ability to assist.	Ensures continuity of care in the home. A safe home environment will lessen chance of accidental injury.
11 Assess previous mode of transfer (if applicable).	Determines mode of transfer and assistance required to provide continuity. Transfer (gait) belts should be used with patients who need assistance (Hignett, 2003; Nelson, 2006; Nelson and Baptiste, 2004).
12 Determine the number of people needed to assist with transfer. Do not start procedure until all required caregivers are available.	Ensures safe patient transfer.

NURSING DIAGNOSES

- Activity intolerance
- Acute or chronic pain
- Confusion

- Disturbed thought processes
- Impaired physical mobility
- Impaired skin integrity

- Risk for falls
- Risk for injury

Individualize related factors based on patient's condition or needs.

PLANNING

1 Expected outcomes following completion of procedure:	
• Patient dangles legs or sits without dizziness, weakness, or orthostatic hypotension.	Precautions during transferring prevent vascular compromise.
• Patient tolerates increased activity.	Gradual increase in number of transfers and period of time out of bed increases tolerance and endurance.
• Patient can bear more weight.	Repeated transfers usually result in improved endurance and greater independence of patient.
• Patient transfers without injury.	Proper techniques avoid injury.
• Patient is more motivated to be mobile.	
• Patient transfers with minimal discomfort.	Transfer procedures performed correctly.
2 Explain procedure to patient. Repeat instructions simply and with continuity to patient with cognitive dysfunction.	Promotes understanding and cooperation, reducing anxiety.

IMPLEMENTATION

1 Perform hand hygiene.	Reduces transfer of microorganisms.
2 Assist patient to sitting position (bed at waist level):	

Critical Decision Point *If patient is in hospital bed, use electrical controls instead to raise patient to a sitting position in bed.*

a Place patient in supine position.	Enables nurse to assess patient's body alignment continually and to administer additional care, such as suctioning or hygiene needs.
b Face head of the bed at a 45-degree angle, and remove pillows.	Proper positioning reduces twisting of the nurse's body when moving the patient. Pillows may cause interference when the patient is sitting up in bed.
c Place feet in a wide base of support with foot closer to head of bed in front of other foot.	Improves nurse's balance and allows transfer of body weight as patient is moved to sitting position.
d Place hand nearer head of bed under patient's shoulders, supporting patient's head and cervical vertebrae.	Maintains alignment of head and cervical vertebrae and allows for even lifting of patient's upper trunk.
e Place other hand on bed surface.	Provides support and balance.
f Raise patient to sitting position by shifting weight from front to back leg.	Improves nurse's balance, overcomes inertia, and transfers weight in direction in which patient is moved.
g Push against bed using arm that is placed on bed surface.	Divides activity between nurse's arms and legs and protects back from strain. By bracing one hand against mattress and pushing against it as patient is lifted, part of weight that would be lifted by nurse's back muscles is transferred through nurse's arms onto mattress.
3 Assist patient to sitting position on side of bed with bed in low position, using electrical bed:	
a With patient in supine position, raise head of bed 30 degrees.	Decreases amount of work needed by patient and nurse to raise patient to sitting position.

STEP	RATIONALE
b Turn patient onto side, facing nurse on side of bed on which patient will be sitting (see illustration).	Prepares patient to move to side of bed and protects from falling.
c Stand opposite patient's hips. Turn diagonally so you face patient and far corner of foot of bed.	Places nurse's center of gravity nearer patient. Reduces twisting of nurse's body because nurse is facing direction of movement.
d Place feet apart in a wide base of support with foot closer to head of bed in front of other foot (see illustration).	Increases balance and allows nurse to transfer weight as patient is brought to sitting position on side of bed.
e Place arm nearer head of bed under patient's shoulders, supporting head and neck.	Maintains alignment of head and neck as nurse brings patient to sitting position.
f Place other arm over patient's thighs (see illustration).	Supports hip and prevents patient from falling backward during procedure.
g Move patient's lower legs and feet over side of bed. Pivot toward rear leg, allowing patient's upper legs to swing downward.	Decreases friction and resistance. Weight of patient's legs when off bed allows gravity to lower legs, and weight of legs assists in pulling upper body into sitting position.
h At same time, shift weight to rear leg and elevate patient (see illustration).	Allows nurse to transfer weight in direction of motion.

Critical Decision Point   *Remain in front until patient regains balance, and continue to provide physical support to weak or cognitively impaired patient.*

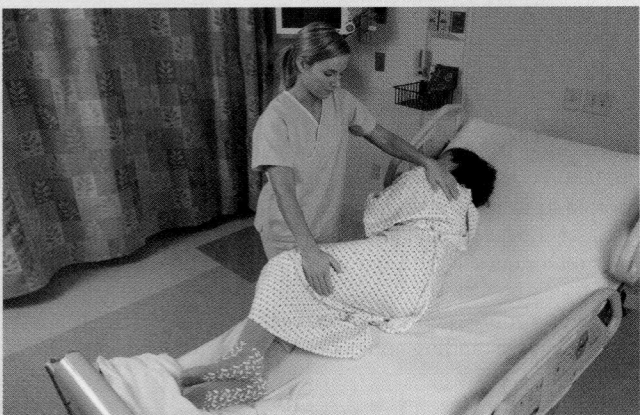

STEP 3b   Side-lying position.

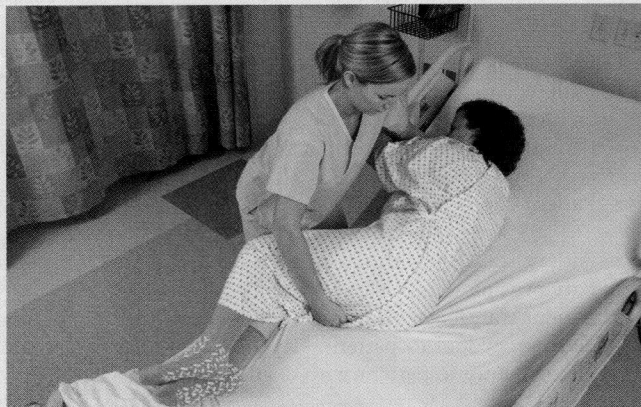

STEP 3f   Nurse places arm over patient's thigh.

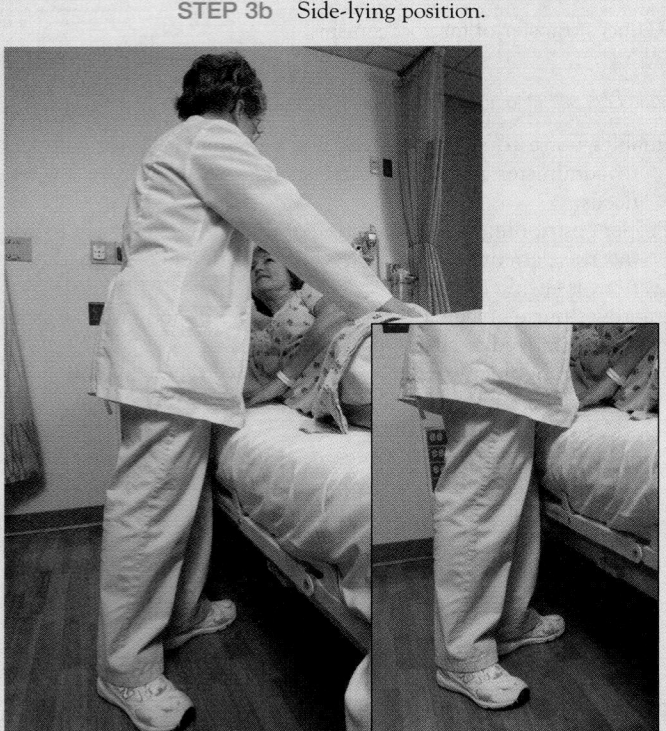

STEP 3d   Proper foot placement.

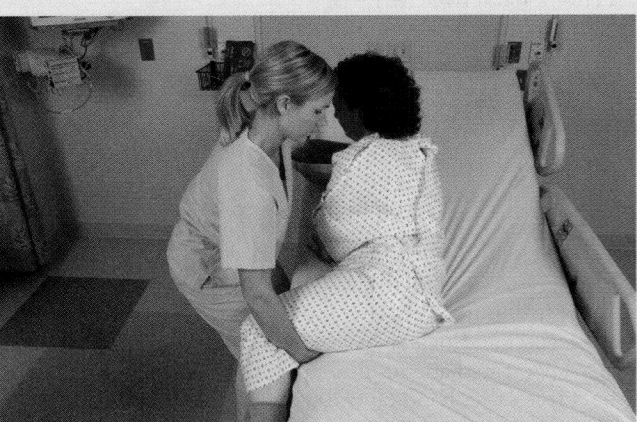

STEP 3h   Nurse shifts weight to rear leg and elevates patient.

STEP	RATIONALE

4 Transferring patient from bed to chair with bed in the low position:

  a If patient has partial weight bearing with upper body strength, use bariatric transfer aid with minimum of two or three caregivers (see illustration).

The use of mechanical lift devices are strongly recommended to transfer a patient to reduce risk for musculoskeletal injury (Nelson, 2006; Nelson and Baptiste, 2004).

Critical Decision Point   *If patient demonstrates weakness or paralysis of one side of the body, place chair on patient's strong side.*

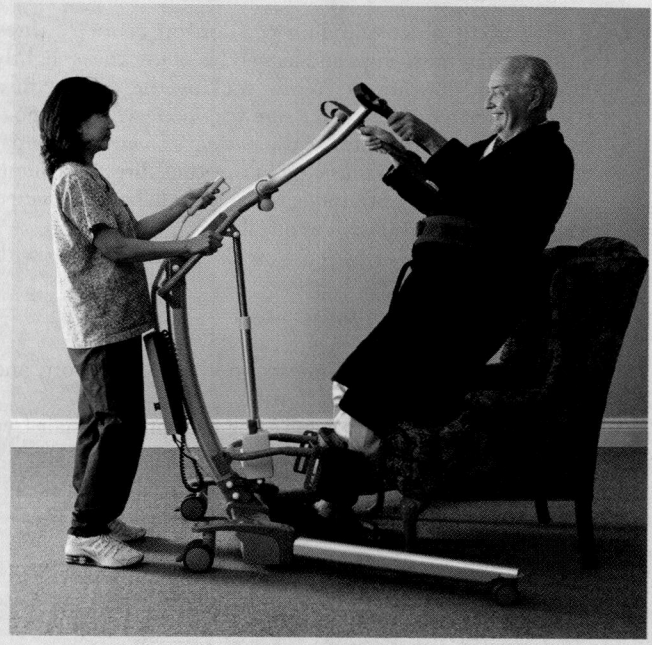

STEP 4a   Stand assist lift device. (*Courtesy Waverly Glen Systems, a Prism Medical Company.*)

  b If patient has normal weight bearing and upper body strength, assist patient to sitting position on side of bed (see Steps 3a through 3h). Have chair in position at 45-degree angle to bed. Allow patient to sit on side of the bed (dangling) for a few minutes before transferring to chair. Ask if patient feels dizzy. Do not leave patient unattended during dangling.

Position chair within easy access for transfer. Dangling or allowing a patient to sit on the side of the bed before transfer helps equilibrate blood pressure, reducing the risk for dizziness or fainting when standing (Koval, 2004).

  c Apply transfer belt (see illustration) or use transfer board. The board is placed across bed to chair so patient can slide across board.

Transfer belt allows nurse to maintain stability of patient during transfer and reduces risk for falling (Hignett, 2003; Nelson, 2006). Patient's arm should be in sling if flaccid paralysis is present. Transfer board makes sliding over to chair easy with less physical effort.

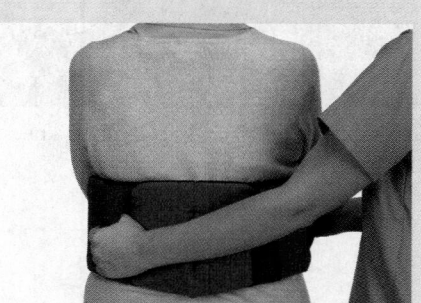

STEP 4c   Transfer belt with handles.

STEP	RATIONALE
d Assist patient with applying stable nonskid shoes. Place the patient's weight-bearing, or strong, leg forward, with weak foot back.	Nonskid soles decrease risk for slipping during transfer. Always have patient wear shoes during transfer; bare feet increase risk for falls. Patient will stand on stronger, or weight-bearing, leg.
e Spread your feet apart.	Ensures balance with wide base of support.
f Flex hips and knees, aligning knees with patient's knees (see illustration).	Flexion of knees and hips lowers nurse's center of gravity to object to be raised; aligning knees with patient's allows for stabilization of knees when patient stands.
g Grasp transfer belt along patient's sides.	Transfer belt provides movement of patient at center of gravity. Patients should never be lifted by or under arms.
h Rock patient up to standing position on count of three while straightening hips and legs and keeping knees slightly flexed (see illustration). While rocking the patient in a back and forth motion, make sure your body weight is moving in the same direction as the patient's to ensure the patient and caregiver are moving in the same direction simultaneously. Unless contraindicated, patient may be instructed to use hands to push up if applicable.	Rocking motion gives patient's body momentum and requires less muscular effort to lift patient.
i Maintain stability of patient's weak or paralyzed leg with your knee.	Ability to stand can often be maintained in paralyzed or weak limb with support of knee to stabilize.
j Pivot on foot farther from chair.	Maintains support of patient while allowing adequate space for patient to move.
k Instruct patient to use armrests on chair for support, and ease into chair (see illustration).	Increases patient stability.
l Flex hips and knees while lowering patient into chair (see illustration).	Prevents injury to nurse from poor body mechanics.

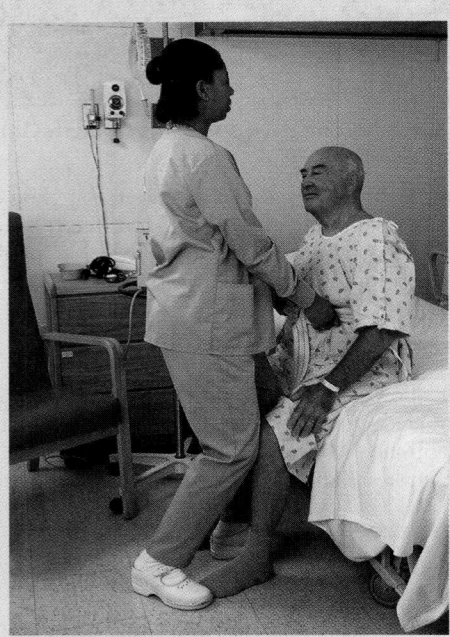

STEP 4f Nurse flexes hips and knees, aligns knees with patient's knee, and grasps transfer belt.

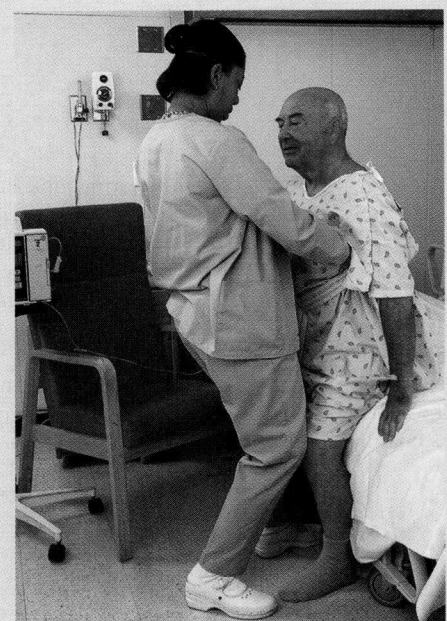

STEP 4h Nurse rocks patient to standing position.

STEP	RATIONALE

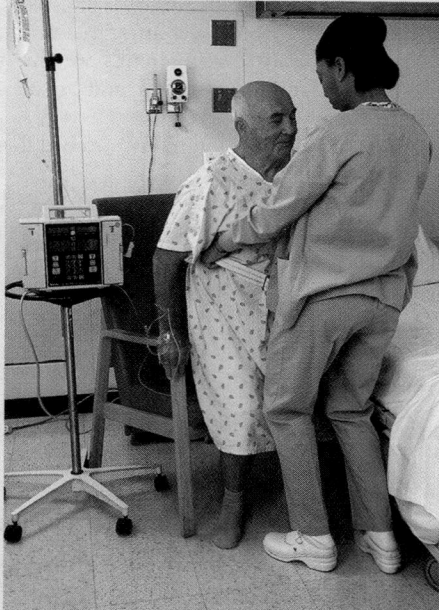

STEP 4k   Patient uses armrests for support.

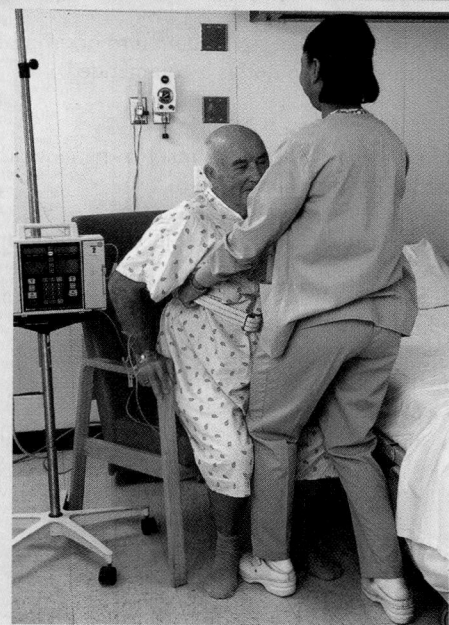

STEP 4l   Nurse eases patient into chair.

m   Assess patient for proper alignment in sitting position. Provide support for paralyzed extremities. Lap board or sling will support flaccid arm. Stabilize leg with bath blanket or pillow.

Prevents injury to patient from poor body alignment.

n   Proper alignment for sitting position: head is erect, and vertebrae are in straight alignment. Body weight is evenly distributed on buttocks and thighs. Thighs are parallel and in horizontal plane. Both feet are supported on floor, and ankles are comfortably flexed. A 2.5- to 5-cm (1- to 2-inch) space is maintained between edge of seat and popliteal space on posterior surface of knee.

Prevents stress on intravertebral joints. Prevents increased pressure over bony prominences and reduces damage to underlying musculoskeletal system.

o   Praise patient's progress, effort, and performance.

Continued support and encouragement provide incentive for patient perseverance.

5   Perform horizontal transfer from bed to stretcher using slide board or friction-reducing board (see illustration):

The three-person lift for horizontal transfer from bed to stretcher is no longer recommended and in fact is discouraged (Baptiste and others, 2006; OSHA, 2005). Physical stress can be decreased significantly by the use of a slide board or friction-reducing board positioned under a drawsheet beneath the patient. In addition, the patient is more comfortable using this method.

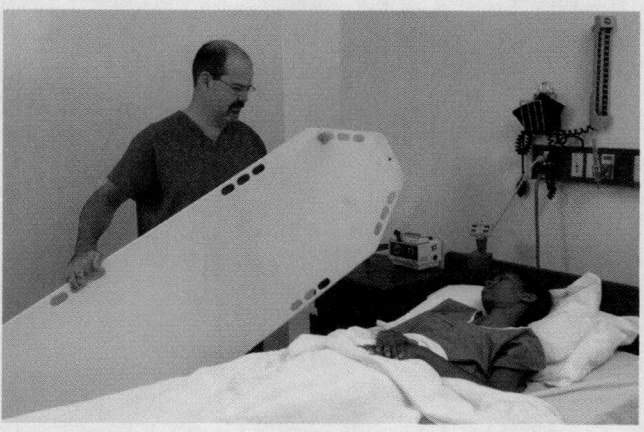

STEP 5   Slide board.

STEP	RATIONALE
a Determine number of staff required to horizontally transfer patient safely (three nurses recommended).	During any patient transferring task, if any caregiver is required to lift more than 35 pounds of a patient's weight, the patient should be considered fully dependent and an assist device is used (Nelson, 2006).
b Lower the head of the bed as much as patient can tolerate. Ensure bed brakes are locked.	Maintains alignment of spinal column. Ensures bed does not inadvertently move.
c Cross patient's arms on chest.	Prevents injury to arms during transfer.
d Lower side rails. To place slide board under patient, position two nurses on side of bed to which the patient will be turned. Position third nurse on the other side of bed.	Distributes weight equally between nurses.
e Fanfold the drawsheet on both sides.	Provides strong handles in order to grip the drawsheet without slipping.
f Using the count of three, turn patient onto side as one unit with a smooth, continuous motion.	Maintains body in alignment, preventing stress on any part of the body.
g Place slide board under drawsheet (see illustration).	Prevents friction from contact of skin with board.

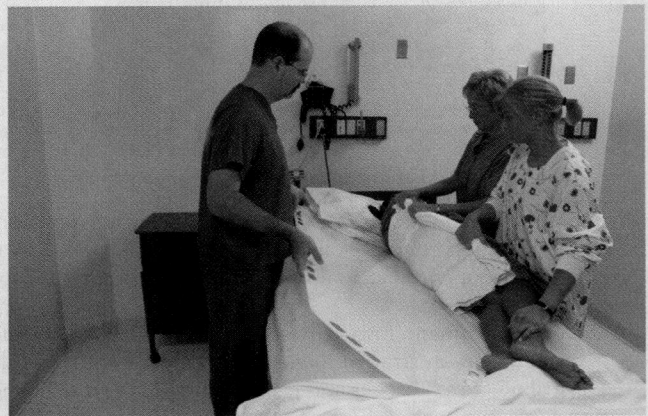

STEP 5g   Placing slide board under drawsheet.

STEP	RATIONALE
h Gently roll the patient back onto the slide board.	
i Line up the stretcher with the bed. Lock brakes on stretcher.	Ensures the stretcher does not inadvertently move during transfer.
j Two nurses position themselves on the side of the stretcher, while the third nurse positions self on the side of the bed without the stretcher.	

Critical Decision Point   *A nurse may also be positioned at the head of the patient's bed to protect and support the patient's head and neck if patient is weak or unable to assist.*

STEP	RATIONALE

k Fanfold drawsheet; using the count of three, the two nurses pull drawsheet with patient onto stretcher while the third nurse holds the slide board in place (see illustration).

The slide board remains stationary and provides a slippery surface to reduce friction and allows the patient to transfer easily to the stretcher.

l Position patient in center of stretcher. Raise head of stretcher if not contraindicated. Raise stretcher side rails. Cover patient with blanket.

Provides for patient comfort.

6 Use mechanical/hydraulic lift to transfer patient from bed to chair (before using lift, be thoroughly familiar with its operation):

Research supports the use of mechanical lifts to prevent musculoskeletal injuries (Hignett, 2003; Nelson, 2006; Nelson and Baptiste, 2004). The use of ceiling-mounted lifts is becoming a more popular choice because of the availability of the lift in each patient's room (see illustration) (Nelson and Baptiste, 2004).

a Bring lift to bedside or lower ceiling lift and position properly.

Ensures safe elevation of patient off bed.

b Position chair near bed, and allow adequate space to maneuver lift.

Prepares environment for safe use of lift and subsequent transfer.

c Raise bed to high position with mattress flat. Lower side rail on side near chair.

Allows nurse to use proper body mechanics.

d Raise opposite side rail unless a second nurse is assisting.

Maintains patient safety.

e Roll patient on side away from you.

Positions patient for placement of lift sling.

f Place hammock or canvas strips under patient to form sling. With two canvas pieces, lower edge fits under patient's knees (wide piece), and upper edge fits under patient's shoulders (narrow piece).

Two types of seats are supplied with mechanical/hydraulic lift: hammock style is better for patients who are flaccid, weak, and need support; canvas strips can be used for patients with normal muscle tone. Hooks should face away from patient's skin. Place sling under patient's center of gravity and greatest portion of body weight.

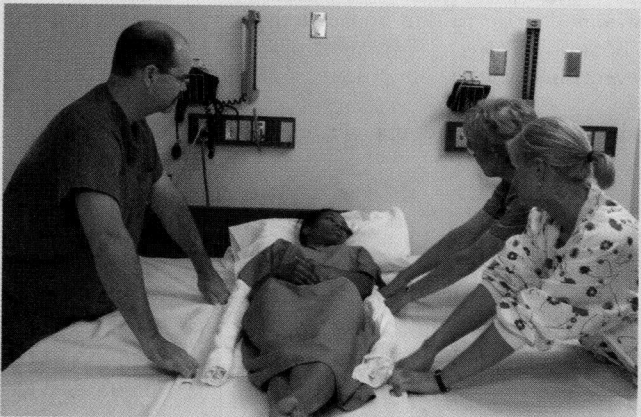

STEP 5k   Transfer of patient to stretcher using slide board.

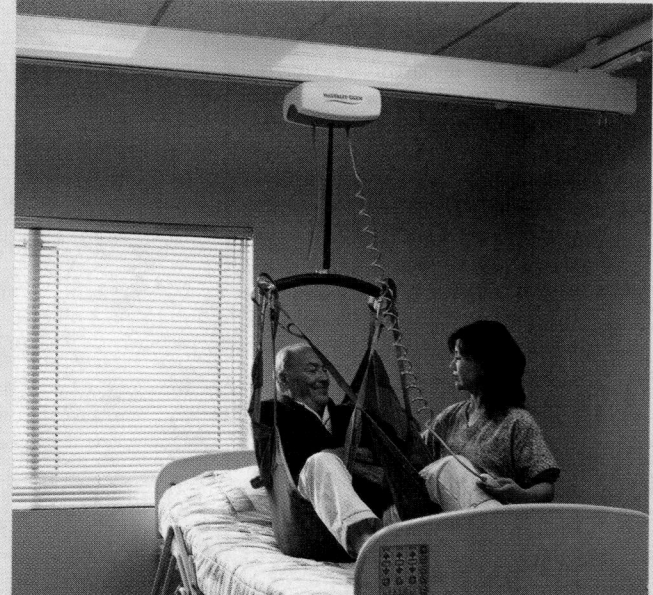

STEP 6   Ceiling lift. (*Courtesy Waverly Glen Systems, a Prism Medical Company.*)

STEP	RATIONALE
g Raise bed rail.	Maintains patient safety.
h Go to opposite side of bed, and lower side rail.	
i Roll patient to opposite side, and pull hammock (strips) through and smooth over bed surface.	Completes positioning of patient on mechanical/hydraulic sling.
j Roll patient supine onto canvas hammock.	Sling should extend from shoulders to knees (hammock) to support patient's body weight equally.
k Remove patient's glasses, if appropriate.	Swivel bar is close to patient's head and could break eyeglasses.
l Place lift's horseshoe bar under side of bed (on side with chair).	Positions lift efficiently and promotes smooth transfer.
m Lower horizontal bar to sling level by following manufacturer's directions. Lock valve if required.	Positions hydraulic lift close to patient. Locking valve prevents injury to patient.
n Attach hooks on strap (chain) to holes in sling. Short chains or straps hook to top holes of sling; longer chains hook to bottom of sling.	Secures hydraulic lift to sling.
o Elevate head of bed.	Positions patient in sitting position.
p Fold patient's arms over chest.	Prevents injury to patient's arms.
q Pump hydraulic handle using long, slow, even strokes until patient is raised off bed (see illustration). For ceiling lift turn on control device to move lift.	Ensures safe support of patient during elevation.
r Use steering handle to pull lift from bed and maneuver to chair.	Moves patient from bed to chair.
s Roll base around chair.	Positions lift in front of the chair in which patient is to be transferred.
t Release check valve slowly (turn to left), and lower patient into chair (see illustration). For ceiling lift again use control device to lower patient.	Safely guides patient into back of chair as seat descends.
u Close check valve or turn off control device as soon as patient is down and straps can be released.	If valve is left open or device left on, boom may continue to lower and injure patient.
v Remove straps and mechanical/hydraulic lift.	Prevents damage to skin and underlying tissues from canvas or hooks.
w Check patient's sitting alignment, and correct if necessary (see Step 4n).	Prevents injury from poor posture.
7 Perform hand hygiene.	Reduces transmission of microorganisms.

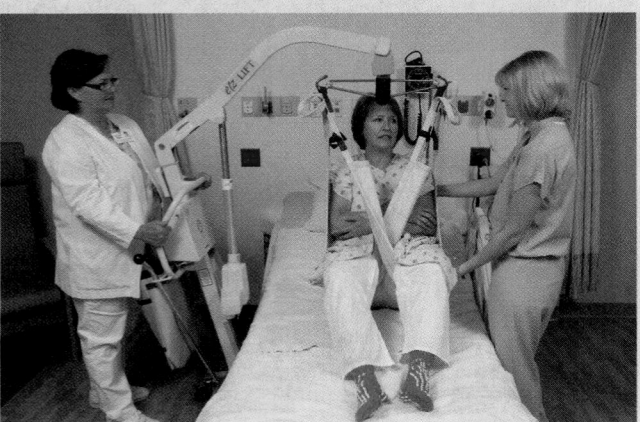

STEP 6q   Sling under patient and attached to lift.

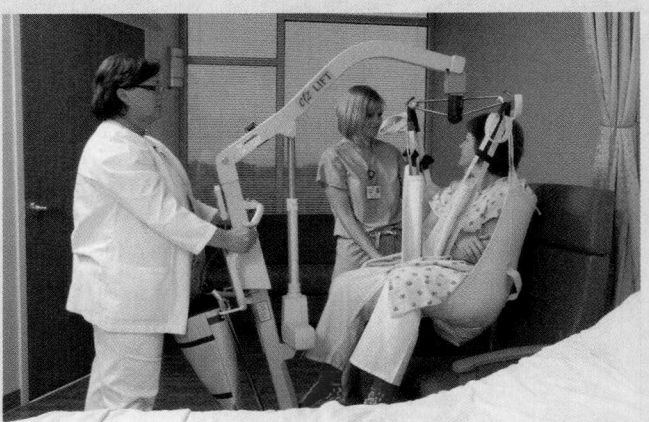

STEP 6t   Use of hydraulic lift to lower patient into chair.

STEP	RATIONALE

EVALUATION

1 Monitor vital signs. Ask if patient feels dizzy or fatigued.	Evaluates patient's response to postural changes and activity.
2 Note patient's behavioral response to transfer.	Reveals level of motivation and self-care potential.
3 Ask if patient experienced pain during transfer.	Determines need for additional pain control or alteration in technique of transferring (e.g., additional assistance).
4 Have patient who transfers to chair attempt to bear weight with nurse at side.	Determines tolerance to weight bearing.

Unexpected Outcomes

1 Patient is unable to comprehend and follow directions for transfer.

2 Patient sustains injury on transfer

3 Patient's level of weakness does not permit active transfer.
4 Patient continues to bear weight on non–weight-bearing limb.
5 Patient is unable to stand for time required to transfer.

Related Interventions

- Reassess continuity and simplicity of instruction.
- Transfers may be difficult when patient is fatigued or in pain; assess before transfer (allow for a rest period before transferring, or medicate for pain if indicated).
- Evaluate incident that caused injury (e.g., assessment was inadequate, change in patient status, improper use of equipment).
- Complete incident report according to institution policy.
- Increase bed activity and exercise to heighten tolerance.
- Reassess patient's understanding of weight-bearing status.
- Provide for additional nurses to provide adequate assistance during transfer.

Recording and Reporting

- Record procedure, including pertinent observations: weakness, ability to follow directions, weight-bearing ability, balance, ability to pivot, number of personnel needed to assist, and amount of assistance (muscle strength) required.
- Report transfer ability and assistance needed to next shift or other caregivers. Report progress or remission to rehabilitation staff (physical therapist, occupational therapist).

Teaching Considerations

- For many patients, returning home enhances psychological well-being and increases motivation and ability for self-care function. Appropriate teaching of self-care skills and use of aids enhance patient's outcomes.
- Teach family and patient transfer skills, including principles of body mechanics and hazards of immobility. Incorporate return demonstration in discharge planning.

Pediatric Considerations

- Whenever possible, transporting child by stretcher, stroller, or wheelchair outside confines of room will increase environmental stimuli and provide social contact with others (Hockenberry and others, 2007).
- Children confined to bed for any length of time, such as those in traction, need to have dependent skin surfaces assessed at least three times in a 24-hour period.

Gerontological Considerations

- A major health concern that threatens the function of an older adult is the risk for falls (Meiner and Lueckenotte, 2006). Concern increases when an older adult enters a hospital. Assess the patient for the risk for falls upon admission, and implement a protocol to prevent falls (Phipps and others, 2007) (see Chapter 13).
- Use a drawsheet to avoid shearing force during repositioning in bed. This protects an older adult patient who has fragile skin.

Home Care Considerations

- Have family or support person practice transfer in hospital to achieve success before taking patient home. Alternatively, have patient (if living alone) practice transfer skills in bed that will be used at home. Teach patient to transfer to chair with arms for ease of rising and sitting.
- Home should be free of hazards (e.g., throw rugs, electric cords, slippery floors). If wheelchair is used, access must be possible through all doors, and space for transfer must be available in bedroom and bathroom (see Chapter 41).
- Aids that enhance transfer ability are shower stools, commode elevators, handrails on tub, and nonskid shower surface. Many self-care devices are available for wheelchair-bound patients or patients with weak or poor muscle function. Medical supply stores provide excellent information and catalogs of such supplies.

SKILL 9-2   Moving and Positioning Patients in Bed

 Basic/ Safe Patient Handling / Assisting With Moving and Positioning a Patient in Bed

NSO   *Safety Module / Lesson 4*

Correct positioning of patients is crucial for maintaining body alignment and comfort, preventing injury to the musculoskeletal and integumentary systems, and providing sensory, motor, and cognitive stimulation. A patient with impaired mobility, decreased sensation, impaired circulation, or lack of voluntary muscle control can develop damage to the musculoskeletal and integumentary systems while lying down. The nurse must minimize this risk by maintaining unrestricted circulation and correct body alignment while moving, turning, or positioning a patient. The term *body alignment* refers to the conditions of the joints, tendons, ligaments, and muscles in various body positions. When the body is aligned, whether standing, sitting, or lying, no excessive strain is placed on these structures. Body alignment means the body is in line with the pull of gravity and contributes to body balance. Without this balance, the center of gravity is displaced, which increases the force of gravity and predisposes the person to falls and injuries. Body balance is achieved when a wide base of support exists, the center of gravity falls within the base of support, and a vertical line can be drawn from the center of gravity through the base of support (Fig. 9-1).

Delegation Considerations

The skills of moving and positioning patients in bed and maintaining correct body alignment can be delegated to NAP. The nurse directs the NAP by:

- Instructing about any moving and positioning restrictions (e.g., avoid prone position, patient has one-sided weakness).
- Designating specific times throughout the shift that NAP must reposition the patient.
- Providing information regarding patient's individual needs for body alignment (i.e., patient with spinal cord injury).

Equipment

- ❑ Pillows
- ❑ Therapeutic boots/splints (*optional*)
- ❑ Trochanter roll
- ❑ Sandbag
- ❑ Hand rolls
- ❑ Side rails

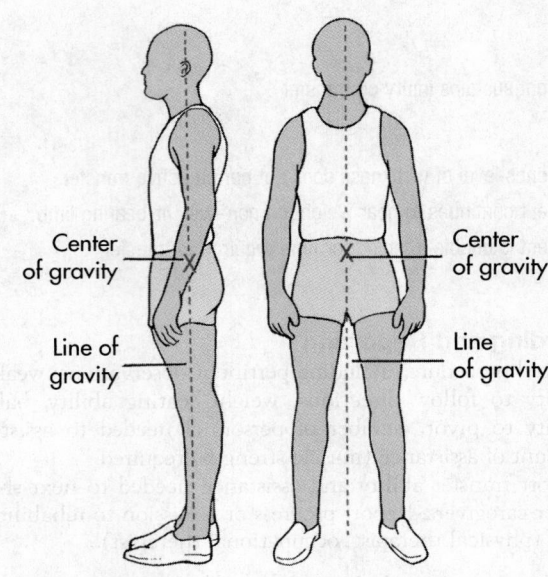

Center of gravity

Center of gravity

Line of gravity

Line of gravity

FIG 9-1   Body alignment when standing.

STEP	RATIONALE

ASSESSMENT

1 Assess patient's ROM (see Chapter 10), body alignment, and comfort level while patient is lying down.	Provides baseline data for later comparisons. Determines ways to improve position and alignment.
2 Assess for risk factors that contribute to complications of immobility:	Increased risk factors require patient to be repositioned more frequently.
a *Paralysis:* Hemiparesis resulting from CVA; decreased sensation	Paralysis impairs movement; muscle tone changes; sensation is affected. Because of difficulty in moving and poor awareness of involved body part, patient is unable to protect and position body part for self.
b *Impaired mobility:* Traction, arthritis, hip fracture, joint surgery, or other contributing disease processes	Traction, bone fractures, surgery, or arthritic changes of affected extremity result in decreased ROM.
c *Impaired circulation:* Arterial insufficiency	Decreased circulation predisposes patient to pressure ulcers.
d *Age:* Very young, older adult	Premature and young infants require frequent turning because their skin is fragile. Normal physiological changes associated with aging predispose older adults to greater risks for developing complications of immobility.
3 Assess patient's level of consciousness.	Determines need for special aids or devices. Patients with altered levels of consciousness may not understand instructions and may be unable to help.
4 Assess condition of patient's skin.	Provides a baseline to determine effects of positioning.

STEP	RATIONALE
5 Assess patient's physical ability to help with moving and positioning, which may be affected by age, level of consciousness, disease process, strength, ROM, and coordination.	Enables nurse to use patient's mobility, strength, and coordination. Determines need for additional help. Ensures patient and nurse safety.
6 Assess for presence of tubes, incisions, and equipment (e.g., traction).	Will alter positioning procedure and type of positions to use. Determines approach needed for instruction.
7 Assess motivation of patient and ability of family members to participate in moving and positioning.	Indicates whether instruction is necessary before discharge.
8 Check physician's or health care provider's orders before positioning patient.	Some positions may be contraindicated in certain situations (e.g., spinal cord injury; hip fracture; respiratory difficulties; certain neurological conditions; presence of incisions, drains, or tubing).

NURSING DIAGNOSES

- Activity intolerance
- Confusion
- Impaired physical mobility
- Impaired skin integrity
- Impaired thought processes
- Risk for impaired skin integrity

Individualize related factors based on patient's condition or needs.

PLANNING

1 Expected outcomes following completion of procedure:	
• Patient retains ROM.	Correct positioning allows patient to achieve optimal joint mobility and alignment.
• Patient's skin shows no evidence of breakdown.	Frequent position changes decrease risk for skin breakdown.
• Patient's comfort level increases.	Proper positioning reduces stress on joints.
• Patient's level of independence in completing ADLs increases.	Maintaining good body alignment and joint mobility increases patient's overall mobility. Patient with inadequate joint mobility may need assistance to carry out ADLs.
2 Raise level of bed to comfortable working height.	Raises level of work toward nurse's center of gravity and reduces the risk for back injuries.
3 Remove all pillows and devices used in previous position.	Reduces interference from bedding during positioning procedure.
4 Get extra help as needed.	Provides for patient and nurse safety.
5 Explain procedure to patient.	Helps to decrease anxiety and increase cooperation.

IMPLEMENTATION

1 Perform hand hygiene.	Reduces transmission of infection.
2 Close door to room, or close bedside curtains.	Provides for patient privacy.
3 Put bed in flat position.	Provides easy access to patient and allows nurses to reposition patient to any position without working against gravity.

Critical Decision Point   *Before flattening bed, account for all tubing drains and equipment to prevent dislodgment or spillage if caught in mattress or bed frame as bed is lowered.*

4 Assist patient in moving up in bed (two nurses):	This task is not a one-person task unless patient can fully assist (Nelson, 2006; U.S. Department of Labor, 2003).
a Place patient on back with head of bed flat. Place height of bed appropriate for all staff.	Enables nurse to assess body alignment. Reduces gravity's pull on patient's upper body.
b Remove pillow from under head and shoulders, and place pillow at head of bed.	Prevents striking patient's head against head of bed.
c Face head of bed.	Facing direction of movement prevents twisting of nurse's body while moving patient.
(1) Each nurse should have one arm under patient's head and shoulders and one arm under patient's thighs.	Provides support across length of patient's body.
(2) *Alternative position if patient can assist:* Position one nurse at patient's upper body. Nurse's arm nearest head of bed should be under patient's head and opposite shoulder; other arm should be under patient's closest arm and shoulder. Position other nurse at patient's lower torso. The nurse's arms should be under patient's lower back and torso.	Prevents trauma to patient's musculoskeletal system by supporting shoulder and hip joints and evenly distributing weight.

STEP	RATIONALE
d Place feet apart, with foot nearest head of bed in front of other foot (forward-backward stance).	Wide base of support increases nurse's balance. Stance enables nurse to shift body weight as patient is moved up in bed, thereby reducing force needed to move load.
e When possible, ask patient to flex knees with feet flat on bed.	Decreases friction and enables patient to use leg muscles during movement.
f Instruct patient to flex neck, tilting chin toward chest.	Prevents hyperextension of neck when moving patient up in bed.
g Instruct patient to assist moving by pushing down with feet on bed surface.	Reduces friction. Increases patient mobility. Decreases nurse's workload.
h Flex knees and hips, bringing forearms closer to level of bed.	Increases balance and strength by bringing nurse's center of gravity closer to patient. Uses thighs instead of back muscles.
i Warn patient to push with heels and elevate trunk while breathing out, thus moving toward head of bed on count of three.	Prepares patient for move. Reinforces assistance in moving up in bed. Increases patient cooperation. Breathing out avoids Valsalva maneuver.
j On count of three, rock and shift weight from front to back leg. At the same time patient pushes with heels and elevates trunk.	Rocking enables nurse to improve balance and overcome inertia. Shifting nurse's weight counteracts patient's weight and reduces force needed to move load. Patient's assistance reduces friction and nurse's workload.
5 Move immobile patient up in bed with drawsheet (two nurses):	Depending upon the patient's weight, it may take more than two nurses to move patient. Patients over 200 lb require three caregivers to assist with move.
a Place drawsheet under patient, extending from shoulders to thighs.	Supports patient's body weight and reduces friction during movement.
b Place patient on back with head of bed flat.	Even distribution of weight makes lift easier.
c Position one nurse at each side of patient.	Distributes weight equally between nurses.
d Fanfold the drawsheet on both sides, and grasp firmly near patient.	Provides strong handles in order to grip the drawsheet without slipping.

Critical Decision Point   *Protect patient's heels from shearing force by having another caregiver lift heels while moving patient up in bed.*

STEP	RATIONALE
e Place feet apart with forward-backward stance. Flex knees and hips. On count of three shift weight from front to back leg, and move patient and drawsheet to desired position in bed (see illustrations).	Facing direction of movement ensures proper balance. Shifting weight reduces force needed to move load. Flexing knees lowers nurses' center of gravity and uses thighs instead of back muscles.

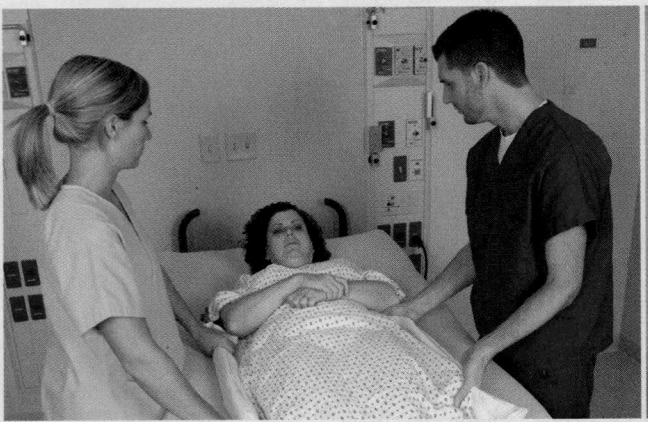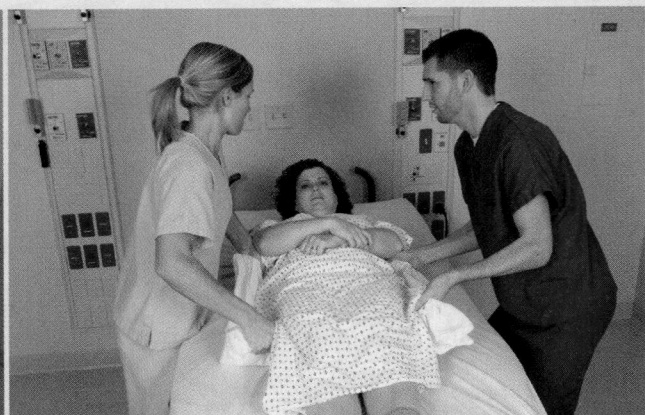

STEP 5e   Moving immobile patient up in bed with drawsheet.

6 Realign patient in correct body alignment and protect pressure areas. Nurses assist patient to one of the positions listed below.	Prevents injury to musculoskeletal system.

STEP	RATIONALE

a Position patient in supported Fowler's position (see illustration):

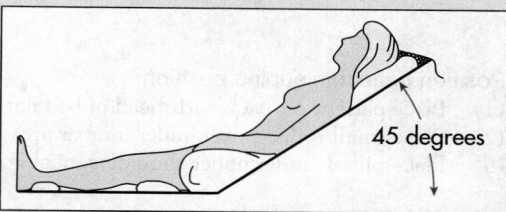

STEP 6a Supported Fowler's position.

(1) Elevate head of bed 45 to 60 degrees if not contra-indicated.

Increases comfort, improves ventilation, and increases patient's opportunity to socialize or relax.

(2) Rest head against mattress or on small pillow.

Prevents flexion contractures of cervical vertebrae.

(3) Use pillows to support arms and hands if patient does not have voluntary control or use of hands and arms.

Prevents shoulder dislocation from effect of downward pull of unsupported arms, promotes circulation by preventing venous pooling, and prevents flexion contractures of arms and wrists.

(4) Position pillow at lower back.

Supports lumbar vertebrae and decreases flexion of vertebrae.

(5) Place small pillow or roll under thigh.

Prevents hyperextension of knee and occlusion of popliteal artery from pressure from body weight.

(6) Support calves with pillows.

Heels should not be in contact with the bed, to prevent prolonged pressure of mattress on heels. This is sometimes referred to as "floating" heels.

b Position hemiplegic patient in supported Fowler's position:

(1) Position patient in supine position. Elevate head of bed 45 to 60 degrees.

Increases comfort, improves ventilation, and increases patient's opportunity to relax. Adjust head of bed according to patient's condition. For example, those with increased risk for pressure ulcers will remain at 30-degree angle (see Chapter 18).

(2) Position patient in straight alignment.

Counteracts tendency to slump toward affected side. Improves ventilation and cardiac output; decreases intracranial pressure. Improves patient's ability to swallow and helps to prevent aspiration of food, liquids, and gastric secretions.

(3) Position head on small pillow with chin slightly forward. If patient is totally unable to control head movement, avoid hyperextension of the neck.

Prevents hyperextension of neck. Too many pillows under head may cause or worsen neck flexion contracture.

(4) Provide support for involved arm and hand by placing arm away from patient's side and supporting elbow with pillow.

Paralyzed muscles do not automatically resist pull of gravity as they do normally. As a result, shoulder subluxation, pain, and edema may occur.

Critical Decision Point *Position flaccid hand in normal resting position with wrist slightly extended, arches of hand maintained, and fingers partially flexed; may use section of rubber ball cut in half; clasp patient's hands together. Position spastic hand with wrist in neutral position or slightly extended; fingers should be extended with palm down or may be left in relaxed position with palm up.*

(5) Place trochanter rolls alongside the patient's legs.

Ensures proper alignment. Prevents external rotation of hips that contributes to contractures.

STEP	RATIONALE
(6) Support feet in dorsiflexion with therapeutic boots or splints.	Prevents plantar flexion contractures or footdrop by positioning the patient's ankle in neutral dorsiflexion. Position foot so that heel is aligned in the opening of the splint to prevent pressure. Other therapeutic boots or splints are manufactured with thick padding to cushion the heel and prevent pressure ulcers.
c Position patient in supine position:	
(1) Place patient on back with head of bed flat.	Necessary for placing patient in supine position.
(2) Place small rolled towel under lumbar area of back.	Provides support for lumbar spine.
(3) Place pillow under upper shoulders, neck, or head.	Maintains correct alignment and prevents flexion contractures of cervical vertebrae.
(4) Place trochanter rolls or sandbags parallel to lateral surface of patient's thighs.	Reduces external rotation of hip.
(5) Place patient's feet in therapeutic boots or splints.	Maintains feet in dorsiflexion. Prevents plantar flexion contractures or footdrop.
(6) Place pillows under pronated forearms, keeping upper arms parallel to patient's body (see illustration).	Reduces internal rotation of shoulder and prevents extension of elbows. Maintains correct body alignment.

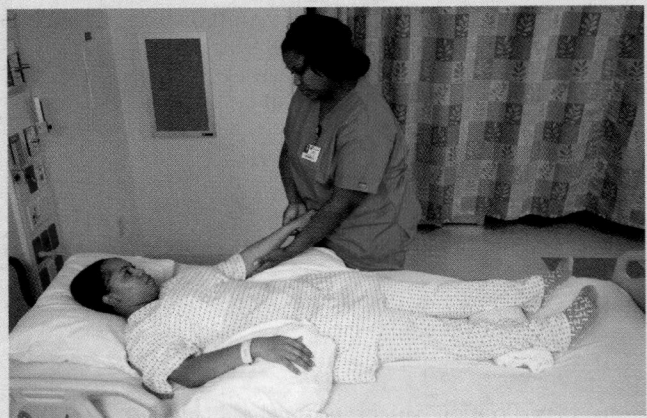

STEP 6c(6)   Supine position with pillows in place.

STEP	RATIONALE
(7) Place hand rolls in patient's hands. Consider physical therapy referral for use of hand splints.	Reduces extension of fingers and abduction of thumb. Maintains thumb slightly adducted and in opposition to fingers.
d Position hemiplegic patient in supine position:	
(1) Place head of bed flat.	Necessary for positioning in supine position.
(2) Place folded towel or small pillow under shoulder or affected side.	Decreases possibility of pain, joint contracture, and subluxation. Maintains mobility in muscles around shoulder to permit normal movement patterns.
(3) Keep affected arm away from body with elbow extended and palm up. Position affected hand in one of recommended positions for flaccid or spastic hand. (Alternative is to place arm out to side, with elbow bent and hand toward head of bed.)	Maintains mobility in arm, joints, and shoulder to permit normal movement patterns. (Alternative position counteracts limitation of ability of arm to rotate outward at shoulder [external rotation]. External rotation must be present to raise arm over head without pain.)
(4) Place folded towel under hip of involved side.	Diminishes the effect of spasticity in entire leg by controlling hip position.
(5) Flex affected knee 30 degrees by supporting it on pillow or folded blanket.	Slight flexion breaks up abnormal extension pattern of leg. Extensor spasticity is most severe when patient is supine.
(6) Support feet with soft pillows at right angle to leg.	Maintains foot in dorsiflexion and prevents footdrop. Pillows prevent stimulation to ball of foot by hard surface, which has tendency to increase muscle tone in patient with extensor spasticity of lower extremity.
e Position patient in prone position:	In certain patients with pulmonary conditions, such as acute respiratory distress syndrome (ARDS), the use of the prone position can help improve oxygenation.

STEP	RATIONALE
(1) With patient supine, roll patient to one side while placing arm on side to be turned, alongside of the body.	Prepares patient for positioning.
(2) Roll patient over arm positioned close to body, with elbow straight and hand under hip. Position on abdomen in center of bed.	Positions patient correctly so alignment can be maintained.
(3) Turn patient's head to one side, and support head with small pillow.	Reduces flexion or hyperextension of cervical vertebrae.
(4) Place small pillow under patient's abdomen below level of diaphragm.	Reduces pressure on breasts of some female patients and decreases hyperextension of lumbar vertebrae and strain on lower back. Improves breathing by reducing mattress pressure on diaphragm.
(5) Support arms in flexed position level at shoulders.	Maintains proper body alignment. Support reduces risk for joint dislocation.
(6) Support lower legs with pillow to elevate toes (see illustration).	Prevents footdrop. Reduces external rotation of legs. Reduces mattress pressure on toes.

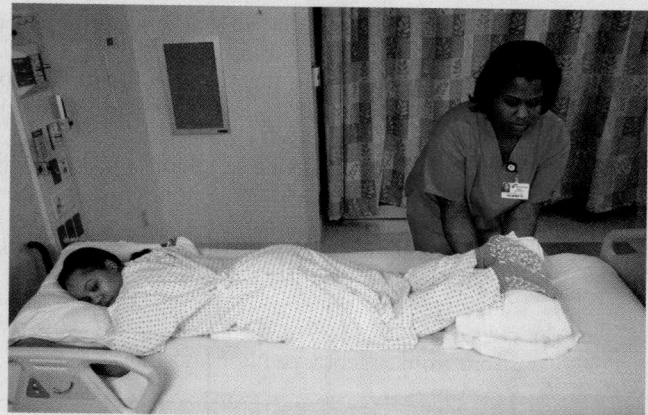

STEP 6e(6) Prone position with pillows supporting lower legs.

f Position hemiplegic patient in prone position:

Critical Decision Point   *Increase frequency of positioning if pressure areas begin to appear, joint mobility becomes impaired or worsened, or patient complains of discomfort. Consult with physical and occupational therapists as needed.*

STEP	RATIONALE
(1) Move patient toward unaffected side.	Ensures proper alignment in center of bed when patient is rolled onto abdomen.
(2) While rolling patient onto side, place pillow on patient's abdomen.	Prevents sagging of abdomen when patient is rolled over; decreases hyperextension of lumbar vertebrae and strain on lower back.
(3) Roll patient onto abdomen by positioning involved arm close to patient's body, with elbow straight and hand under hip. Roll patient carefully over arm.	Prevents injury to affected side.
(4) Turn head toward involved side.	Promotes development of neck and trunk extension, which is necessary for standing and walking.
(5) Position involved arm out to side, with elbow bent, hand toward head of bed, and fingers extended (if possible).	Counteracts limitation of arm's ability to rotate outward at shoulder (external rotation). External rotation must be present to raise arm over head without pain.
(6) Flex knees slightly by placing pillow under legs from knees to ankles.	Flexion prevents prolonged hyperextension, which could impair joint mobility.
(7) Keep feet at right angle to legs by using pillow high enough to keep toes off mattress.	Maintains feet in dorsiflexion.

STEP	RATIONALE

g   Position patient in 30-degree lateral (side-lying) position:

(1)   Lower head of bed completely or as low as patient can tolerate.

Provides position of comfort for patient and removes pressure from bony prominences on back.

(2)   Lower side rail, and position patient toward you, which is toward the side of bed opposite direction patient is to be turned.

Provides room for patient to turn to side.

(3)   Raise side rail and go to opposite side of bed.

(4)   Flex patient's knee that will not be next to mattress. Place one hand on patient's hip and one hand on patient's shoulder.

Use of leverage makes turning to side easy.

Critical Decision Point   *Patient at risk for pressure ulcer development requires the 30-degree lateral position (see Chapter 18).*

(5)   Roll patient onto side toward you.

Rolling decreases trauma to tissues. In addition, patient is positioned so leverage on hip makes turning easy.

(6)   Place pillow under patient's head and neck.

Maintains alignment. Reduces lateral neck flexion. Decreases strain on sternocleidomastoid muscle.

(7)   Place hands under patient's dependent shoulder, and bring shoulder blade forward.

Prevents patient's weight from resting directly on shoulder joint.

(8)   Position both arms in slightly flexed position. Support upper arm with pillow level with shoulder; other arm, by mattress.

Decreases internal rotation and adduction of shoulder. Supporting both arms in slightly flexed position protects joint. Ventilation is improved because chest is able to expand more easily.

(9)   Place hands under dependent hip and bring hip slightly forward so that angle from hip to mattress is approximately 30 degrees.

The 30-degree lateral position reduces pressure on trochanter.

(10)   Place small tuck-back pillow behind patient's back. (Make by folding pillow lengthwise. Smooth area is slightly tucked under patient's back.)

Provides support to maintain patient on side.

(11)   Place pillow under semiflexed upper leg level at hip from groin to foot (see illustration).

Flexion prevents hyperextension of leg. Maintains leg in correct alignment. Prevents pressure on bony prominences.

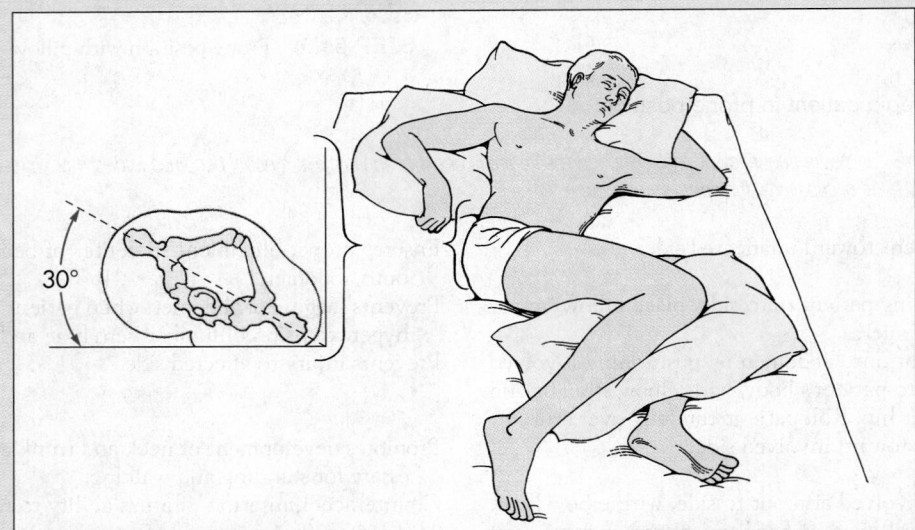

STEP 6g(11)   Thirty-degree lateral position with pillows in place.

STEP	RATIONALE

(12) Place sandbag parallel to plantar surface of dependent foot. May use ankle-foot orthotic on feet if available.

Maintains dorsiflexion of foot.

h   Position patient in Sims' (semiprone) position:
  (1) Lower head of bed completely.
  (2) Place patient in supine position.
  (3) Roll patient on side, and position in lateral position, lying partially on abdomen, with dependent shoulder lifted out and arm placed at patient's side.
  (4) Place small pillow under patient's head.
  (5) Place pillow under flexed upper arm, supporting arm level with shoulder.

Provides for proper body alignment while patient is lying down.
Prepares patient for position.
Patient is rolled only partially on abdomen.

Maintains proper alignment and prevents lateral neck flexion.
Prevents internal rotation of shoulder. Maintains alignment.

  (6) Place pillow under flexed upper legs, supporting leg level with hip.

Prevents internal rotation of hip and adduction of leg. Flexion prevents hyperextension of leg. Reduces mattress pressure on knees and ankles.

  (7) Place sandbags parallel to plantar surface of foot (see illustration).

Maintains foot in dorsiflexion. Prevents plantar flexion contractures or footdrop.

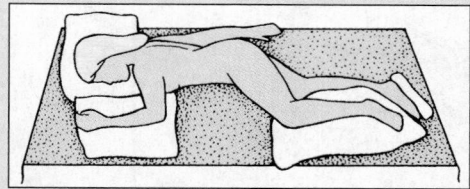

STEP 6h(7)   Sandbag supporting right foot in dorsiflexion.

i   Logrolling the patient (three nurses):

Critical Decision Point   *A nurse should supervise and aid nursing assistive personnel when there is a physician's or health care provider's order to logroll a patient. Patients who have suffered from a spinal cord injury or are recovering from neck, back, or spinal surgery often need to keep the spinal column in straight alignment to prevent further injury.*

  (1) Place small pillow between patient's knees.
  (2) Cross patient's arms on chest.
  (3) Position two nurses on the side the patient is to be turned toward; and one nurse on the side where pillows are to be placed (see illustration).

Prevents tension on the spinal column and adduction of the hip.
Prevents injury to arms.
Distributes weight equally between nurses during turning.

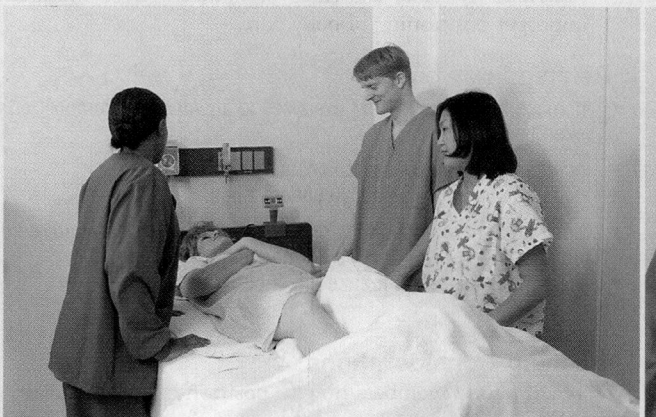 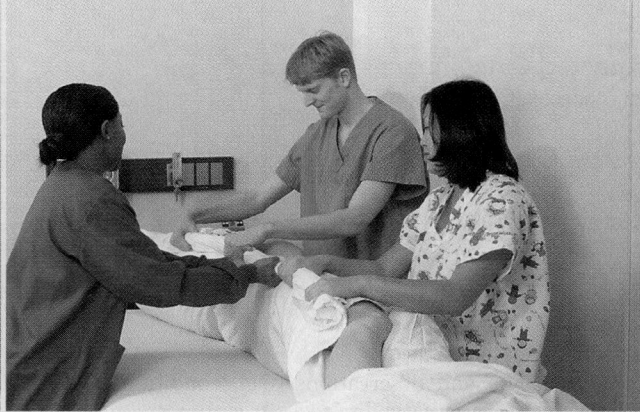

STEP 6i(3-5)   Logrolling a patient.

STEP	RATIONALE
(4) Fanfold the drawsheet along side of patient that will be turning.	Provides strong handles to grip the drawsheet without slipping.
(5) With one nurse grasping drawsheet at lower hips and thighs, and the other nurse grasping drawsheet at patient's shoulders and lower back; roll the patient as one unit in a smooth, continuous motion on the count of three (see illustration).	Maintains proper alignment by moving all body parts at the same time, preventing tension or twisting of the spinal column.
(6) Nurse on the opposite side of the bed places pillows along the length of the patient for support (see illustration).	Maintains patient in side-lying position.

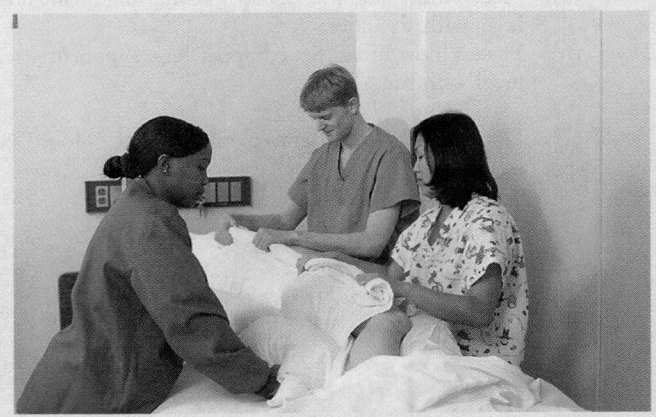

STEP 6i(6)   Place pillows along patient's back for support.

STEP	RATIONALE
(7) Gently lean the patient as a unit back toward the pillows for support.	Ensures continued straight alignment of spinal column, preventing injury.
7 Perform hand hygiene.	Reduces transmission of microorganisms.

EVALUATION

1 Assess patient's body alignment, position, and level of comfort. Patient's body should be supported by adequate mattress, and vertebral column should be without observable curves.	Determines effectiveness of positioning. Additional supports (e.g., pillows, bath blankets) may be added or removed to promote comfort and correct body alignment.
2 Measure ROM.	Determines if joint contracture is developing.
3 Observe for areas of erythema or breakdown involving skin.	Provides ongoing observation regarding patient's skin and musculoskeletal systems. Indicates complications of immobility or improper positioning of body part.

Unexpected Outcomes	Related Interventions
1 Joint contractures develop or worsen.	• Increase frequency of ROM exercises to affected and immobilized areas (see Chapter 10).
2 Skin shows localized areas of erythema and breakdown.	• Increase frequency of repositioning. • Place turning schedule above patient's bed.
3 Patient avoids moving.	• Medicate with analgesia as ordered by physician or health care provider to ensure patient's comfort before moving. • Allow pain medication to take effect before proceeding.

Recording and Reporting

- Record procedure and observations (e.g., condition of skin, joint movement, patient's ability to assist with positioning).
- Report observations at change of shift, and document in nurses' notes.
- Record time and position change of patient throughout shift.

Teaching Considerations

- Teach family members how to position client, especially when caring for infant, young child, or confused or unconscious patient.
- Teach patient ways to assist with positioning, and provide opportunity for return demonstration.
- Teach patient and family signs and symptoms of pressure ulcers and contractures.

STEP	RATIONALE

Pediatric Considerations

- Encourage children to be as active as their condition and restrictive devices allow. Make materials or objects to stimulate activity, and encourage participation of others available (Hockenberry and others, 2007).
- Children who are unable to move require passive exercise and movement (see Chapter 10).

Gerontological Considerations

- Reposition older adult patients at least every 1 to 2 hours, and maintain a regular program of ROM exercises (Meiner and Lueckenotte, 2006).

Home Care Considerations

- Assess ability and motivation of patient, family members, and primary caregiver to participate in moving and positioning patient in bed.

- Assess home to determine compatibility of environment with assistive devices (e.g., over-bed trapeze, Hoyer lift, hospital bed).

Long-Term Care Considerations

- Patients who have maintained bed rest for a long period may revert back to a favorite position. Frequently assess these patients, and turn more often as needed.
- Use drawsheet to prevent shearing force on fragile skin (Hignett, 2003; Nelson, 2006).
- Allow patient to assist with moving and positioning whenever possible to promote independence.

? CRITICAL THINKING EXERCISES

Mr. Clark is a 37-year-old man who suffered a spinal cord injury in a motor vehicle accident. He is admitted on your shift. He has sustained multiple deep lacerations on his face and trunk and facial fractures of maxillary and zygomatic bones. He rates his pain at 9 on a scale of 0 to 10. You are preparing to transfer him to a stretcher.

1 The emergency department nurse was extremely busy and was unable to provide a complete report. What other information would you obtain about this patient?

2 Mr. Clark is scheduled immediately for a computed tomography (CT) scan of the head and spine. He refuses to allow you to move him onto the stretcher. What interventions would you select to elicit his cooperation? Select all that apply.
   A Administer pain medication as ordered by the physician.
   B Explain the purpose and importance of the CT scan.
   C Describe the method by which you will move him onto the stretcher.
   D Tell him it is a physician's or health care provider's order and must be carried out.
   Explain your choice(s).

3 Mr. Clark has returned from the CT scan. The physician or health care provider has ordered Mr. Clark to be turned and positioned every 1 to 2 hours until he is taken to surgery to stabilize his spinal fracture. What do you think would be the safest technique to move Mr. Clark from side to side? Explain your answer.

4 You are very busy, and the nursing assistive personnel state that they will turn Mr. Clark. What is the appropriate, safe action in response to their turning Mr. Clark? Explain your answer.

✓ REVIEW QUESTIONS

1 A 65-year-old patient who weighs 260 lb is to be transferred from his bed to a chair. The patient is unable to bear full weight on one leg. His upper body strength is good. Which technique is the most appropriate technique for transfer?
   1 Use of a transfer board
   2 Use of a bariatric transfer device
   3 Use of a three-person carry
   4 Use of a ceiling lift

2 A patient who has suffered a stroke will be taken care of by his daughter at home. Which statement by the daughter regarding body mechanics indicates that learning has occurred?
   1 "I'm glad I have a strong back."
   2 "As I twist to place my father in his chair, I'll make sure he doesn't fall."
   3 "I will keep my knees bent and trunk erect so my muscles work together."
   4 "I will tighten my back muscles and push my pelvis forward to provide balance when lifting my father."

3 The nurse is transferring a patient, after abdominal surgery, from the bed to the chair for the first time. Which step in the transfer is most appropriate for the nurse and the patient?
   1 Apply a transfer belt around the patient's waist.
   2 Use the under-axilla support technique to prevent pulling on the abdominal area.
   3 Have the patient sit on the side of the bed and dangle for a few minutes.
   4 Observe this patient's response while she transfers to increase her independence.

4 A patient has arrived on the unit after undergoing extensive abdominal surgery. He is awake and alert but is refusing to be repositioned in bed. What should the nurse assess first to determine the reason for his refusal to move?
   1 His oxygen saturation level
   2 His pain level
   3 His level of consciousness
   4 The amount of equipment he has

5 A young adult is admitted with an unstable spinal cord injury. What is the most appropriate method of moving this patient from her side to her back?
   1 Use a slide board to move her from side to side.
   2 Logroll the patient using three people.
   3 Allow the patient to move herself to promote independence.
   4 Use a step-by-step method: move the trunk, then hips, and finally the leg.

REFERENCES

American Nurses Association: *Position statement on elimination of manual patient handling to prevent work-related musculoskeletal disorders*, June 2003, http://www.nursingworld.org.readroom/position/workplac/athand.htm.

American Nurses Association: *Nursing's legislative and regulatory initiatives for the 110th congress: workplace health and safety*, Department of Government Affairs, 2007, http://www.anapoliticalpower.org.

Bureau of Labor Statistics: *Occupational industries and illnesses: industry data*, 2003, http://stats.bls.gov/bls/occupation.htm.

de Castro A and others: Prioritizing safe patient handling: the American Nurses Association's Handle With Care Campaign, *Am J Nurs Adm* 36(7/8):363, 2006.

Fader M and others: Effects of absorbent incontinence pads on pressure management mattresses, *J Adv Nurs* 48(6):569, 2004.

Hockenberry MJ, Wilson D: *Wong's nursing care of infants and children*, ed 8, St. Louis, 2007, Mosby.

Koval K: A clinical pathway for hip factures in the elderly, *Tech Orthop* 19(3):181, 2004.

Meiner S, Lueckenotte A: *Gerontologic Nursing*, ed 3, St. Louis, 2006, Mosby.

Nelson A: *Safe patient handling and movement algorithms*, 2006, VISN Patient Safety Center, http://visn8med.va.gov/patientsafetycenter/.

Nelson A and others: Safe patient handling and movement: preventing back injury among nurses requires careful selection of the safest equipment and techniques, *Am J Nurs* 103(3):32, 2003.

Occupational Health and Safety Administration: Ergonomics standard proposal, *Fed Regist* 29 CFR Part 1910, 70(14), January 24, 2005, http://www.osha-slc.gov/SLTC/ergonomics/index.html.

Pasero C, McCaffery M: Comfort-function goals, *Am J Nurs* 104(9):77, 2004.

Pelczarski K: Take a proactive approach to bariatric patient needs, *Mater Manag Health Care* 16(6):24, 2007.

Phipps W and others: *Medical-surgical nursing: health and illness perspectives*, ed 8, St. Louis, 2007, Mosby.

UC Davis Health System: *New team gives nurses a lift in handling patients*, March 2005, http:ucdmc.ucdavis.edu/.

U.S. Department of Labor, Occupational Safety and Health Administration: *Guidelines for nursing homes: ergonomics for the prevention of musculoskeletal disorders*, Washington, DC, 2003.

RESEARCH REFERENCES

Baptiste A and others: Friction-reducing devices for lateral patient transfers: a clinical evaluation, *AAOHN J* 54(4):173, 2006.

Groeneveld A and others: The prevalence of pressure ulcers in a tertiary care pediatric and adult hospital, *J Wound Ostomy Continence Nurs* 31(3):108, 2004.

Hignett S: Systematic review of patient handling activities starting in lying, sitting and standing positions, *J Adv Nurs* 41(6):545, 2003.

Lampinen P and others: Activity as a predictor of mental well-being among older adults, *Aging Ment Health* 10(5):454, 2006.

Miami Valley Hospital: *Lift team case study*, June 2007, http://www.miamivalleyhospital.com/.

Nelson A, Baptiste A: Evidence-based practices for safe patient handling and moving, *Online J Issues Nurs* 9(3):4, 2004.

Exercise and Ambulation

10

MEDIA RESOURCES

- **evolve** http://evolve.elsevier.com/Perry/skills
  learning system

- Mosby's Nursing Video Skills, 3.0

KEY TERMS

Abduction	Foot pump
Active range-of-motion exercises	Gait
	Gait belt
Active-assisted range-of-motion exercises	Hyperextension
	Immobility
	Internal rotation
Activity tolerance	Inversion
Adduction	Isometric contraction
Atrophy	
Bed rest	Isometric exercise
Circumduction	Joint
Contractures	Lateral flexion
Crutch gait	Mobility
Crutch palsy	Opposition
Dangling	Orthostatic hypotension
Deep vein thrombosis (DVT)	
	Osteoblastic
Dorsal	Osteoclastic
Dorsiflexion	Passive range-of-motion exercises
Eversion	
Exercise	Plantar flexion
Extension	Pronation
External rotation	Rotation
Flexion	Supination
Footboard	Thrombus

OBJECTIVES

Mastery of content in this chapter will enable the nurse to:

- Discuss indications for assisting with ambulation or using devices to assist with ambulation.
- Discuss indications for performing range-of-motion and isometric exercises.
- Identify complications that may develop in a patient wearing either elastic stockings or a sequential compression device.
- Identify significant assessment data to be noted before and during the use of a continuous passive motion machine.
- Identify significant assessment data to be noted before assisting with ambulation and range-of-motion and isometric exercises.

- Demonstrate the following skills on selected patients: assisting with ambulation, assisting with ambulation with the use of an ambulation aid, assisting with range-of-motion exercises, assisting with isometric exercises, applying a continuous passive motion machine, and applying elastic stockings and sequential compression device.
- Develop teaching plans for selected patients for safety precautions to use at home while using an ambulation aid, applying and monitoring effects of elastic stockings and sequential compression devices, using the CPM machine, and performing range-of-motion and isometric exercises.

Mobility refers to an ability to move about freely, whereas immobility refers to a person's inability to move about freely. Mobility and immobility are best understood as the end points on a continuum, with many degrees of partial mobility in between. Some patients move back and forth on the mobility-immobility continuum as a result of disease or injury. Other patients experience immobility for an indefinite period.

The level of mobility has a significant impact on an individual's physiological, psychosocial, and developmental well-being (Hur and others, 2005; Padilla and others, 2005; Turvey and others, 2006). When mobility is altered, many body systems are at risk for impairment. Impaired mobility can result in altered cardiovascular functioning, disruption of normal metabolic functioning, increased risk for pulmonary complications, the development of pressure ulcers, and urinary elimination alterations (Huether and McCance 2008; Monahan and others, 2007).

The severity of mobility impairment depends on a patient's age, overall health status, nutritional status, and the degree of immobility experienced. For example, pronounced effects of immobility develop more quickly in older adult patients with chronic illnesses than in younger patients (Meiner and Lueckenotte, 2006). Older adults are at greater risk for developing orthostatic hypotension, syncope, confusion, increased risk for fractures, and functional incontinence as a result of decreased mobility from bed rest (Liu-Ambrose and others, 2004; Schneider and others, 2004). Increase in activity and exercise may reduce length of stay and cost for acutely hospitalized older adult patients (de Morton and others, 2007).

Alterations in mobility also have profound psychosocial and developmental effects. Immobilization may lead to emotional, intellectual, sensory, and sociocultural alterations. For adults and older adults, immobility may alter employment, family role functions, and social interactions. Such changes can lead to altered self-concept, lowered self-esteem, and depression. Children also are affected by immobility. Activity for them is a way of releasing energy and expressing themselves. When deprived of physical activity, children become restless and may even show signs of anger and aggression (Hockenberry and Wilson, 2007).

Changes in a patient's mobility result from various health problems. Examples of medical conditions that can alter mobility are musculoskeletal conditions such as fractured extremities or muscle sprains, neurological conditions such as spinal cord trauma, degenerative neurological conditions such as myasthenia gravis, and head injuries. Some patients may actually be immobilized for therapeutic reasons (e.g., prescribed bed rest or reduced activity). Nursing measures attempt to maintain and/or restore optimal mobility, as well as to decrease the hazards associated with immobility. Frequent repositioning, deep breathing and coughing exercises, muscle and joint exercises, increased fluid intake, and dietary intake of foods containing fiber are examples of measures that help to reduce the hazards of immobility.

EVIDENCE-BASED PRACTICE TRENDS

Orthostatic hypotension is a drop in blood pressure that occurs when a patient changes position from a horizontal to a vertical position (Eanarroch, 2007; Ejaz and others, 2004). It is traditionally defined as a drop in systolic or diastolic blood pressure of greater than 20 mm Hg or greater than 10 mm Hg, respectively (Mauer and others, 2004). Those at higher risk are immobilized patients, those undergoing prolonged bed rest, older adult patients, those patients receiving antihypertensive medications, and those patients with chronic illnesses such as diabetes mellitus and cardiovascular disease (Vara-González and others, 2006). Signs and symptoms of orthostatic hypotension include dizziness, light-headedness, nausea, tachycardia, pallor, and even fainting (Schrezenmaier and others, 2005).

Physiological changes associated with aging and prolonged bed rest may influence the effectiveness of the baroreceptors. In these patients, moving to the dangling position may cause a gravity-induced drop in blood pressure; thus it is recommended to raise the head of the bed and allow a few minutes before dangling (Eanarroch, 2007). This allows a less dramatic shift in blood volume and provides a gradual adjustment to the upright position. Other interventions to minimize orthostatic hypotension include movement of the legs and feet in the dangling position to promote venous return via intermittent contraction and relaxation of the skeletal leg muscles and asking the patient to take several deep breaths before and during dangling (Akyal, 2007). Dangling a patient before standing is an intermediate step that allows assessment of the individual before changing positions to maintain the safety and prevent injury to the patient.

CULTURAL CONSIDERATIONS

The techniques for promoting exercise and ambulation pose implications for the nurse's ability to give culturally appropriate care. Assisting with exercises and applying compression hose, for example, may place patients in positions that can be embarrassing. Follow these cultural guidelines:

- Collaborate with family members in teaching elder patients from Asian, Hispanic, and African cultures about the concept of active participation in their rehabilitation.
- Most elders expect to remain in bed until healing is completed.
- Accommodate religious practices that limit use of certain rehabilitation appliances:

- Orthodox Jews may not be able to operate a continuous passive motion (CPM) machine during Sabbath and Holy Days.
- Consult the rabbi to obtain permission for the patient to use the CPM machine.
- Nurses should be responsible for turning the CPM machine on and off during the Sabbath and Holy Days (Galanti, 2003).
- Use gender-congruent care to apply elastic stockings and sequential compression devices for women from cultures that emphasize female modesty. Hindus, Muslims, and Orthodox women may not comply with the treatment measure for fear of being exposed to the opposite sex.
- Most elder Asian, Hispanic, and African women prefer to bare their legs and thighs only to other women.
- Provide for female privacy when assisting patients with ambulation.
- Muslim females need to be fully covered when in public because of the emphasis on *hijab*, or female modesty (Simpson and others, 2008).
- Southeast Asian women such as Cambodians, Vietnamese, and Laotians severely restrict exposure of their lower torso and will not likely ambulate unless properly dressed.

Skill Performance Guidelines

1 Check the physician's orders to determine the patient's activity level and type of exercises or assistive device.

2 Know the patient's past medical history. Know why the patient needs assistance with ambulation and any contraindications or limits to exercise.

3 Know the patient's normal range for vital signs. Vital signs vary. Exercise and mobility can be fatiguing and stressful, so a set of baseline vital signs is necessary.

4 Assess baseline muscle strength. The patient may need muscle-strengthening exercises before ambulation.

5 Assess baseline joint function. This determines whether range-of-motion (ROM) exercises are needed and provides a baseline for comparison of joint function after ROM exercises are performed.

6 Obtain and become familiar with the type of assistive device to be used. Knowledge of proper preparation and use of devices is needed to be able to teach patients to use them safely and correctly.

7 Prepare the patient. Make sure the patient is rested and not fatigued. Obtain extra personnel to assist, safety devices, and flat, nonskid shoes for the patient.

8 Address the patient's fear of falling if present.

9 Determine the type and frequency of intervention. Activity that is appropriate for one day or one shift can change, resulting in an increased or decreased need for assistance with ambulation or a change in the type of intervention.

10 Know the patient's home care plan. The patient may need to continue the exercise regimen or use an assistive device at home.

PROCEDURAL GUIDELINE 10-1 Performing Range-of-Motion Exercises

Basic / Safe Patient Handling / Performing Range-of-Motion Exercises

ROM exercises may be active, passive, or active assisted. They are active if the patient is able to perform the exercise independently and passive if the exercises are performed for the patient by the caregiver. In every aspect of activities of daily living (ADLs), encourage the patient to be as independent as possible. Active and passive ROM exercises are encouraged and supervised every day by the nurse. Incorporate active ROM exercises in the patient's ADLs (Table 10-1, p. 231). Incorporate passive ROM into bathing and feeding activities. Collaborate with the patient to develop a schedule for ROM activities.

Delegation Considerations

The skill of performing ROM exercises can be delegated to nursing assistive personnel (NAP). Patients with spinal cord or orthopedic trauma usually require exercise by professional nurses or physical therapists. The nurse directs the NAP by:

- Reminding to perform exercises slowly and to provide adequate support to each joint being exercised.
- Cautioning not to exercise joints beyond the point of resistance or to the point of fatigue or pain.
- Discussing the patient's individual limitations or preexisting conditions such as arthritis that may affect ROM.

Equipment
- ❑ No mechanical or physical equipment needed
- ❑ Clean gloves (*optional*)

Procedural Steps
1 Review patient's chart for physical assessment findings, physician's orders, medical diagnosis, medical history, and progress.

2 Obtain data on patient's baseline joint function. Observe for limitations in joint mobility, redness, or warmth over joints, joint tenderness, deformities, or crepitus produced by joint motion.

3 Determine patient's or caregiver's readiness to learn. Explain all rationales for the ROM exercises, and describe and demonstrate exercises to be performed.

4 Assess patient's level of comfort (on a scale of 0 to 10 with 10 being the worst pain) before exercises. Determine if patient would benefit from pain medication before beginning ROM exercises.

5 Wear clean gloves if wound drainage or skin lesions are present.

6 Assist the patient to a comfortable position, preferably sitting or lying down.

Continued

PROCEDURAL GUIDELINE 10-1   Performing Range-of-Motion Exercises—cont'd

7   When performing active-assisted or passive ROM exercises (Table 10-2, p. 232), support joint by holding distal portion of extremity or using cupped hand to support joint (see illustration).

8   Complete exercises in head-to-toe sequence. Each movement should be repeated 5 times during exercise period. Inform patient how these exercises can be incorporated into ADLs (see Table 10-1).

Critical Decision Point   *When resistance is noted within a joint, do not force joint motion. Consult with physician or physical therapist.*

9   Observe patient performing ROM activities.
10   Measure joint motion as needed.
11   Monitor pain throughout ROM exercise period.

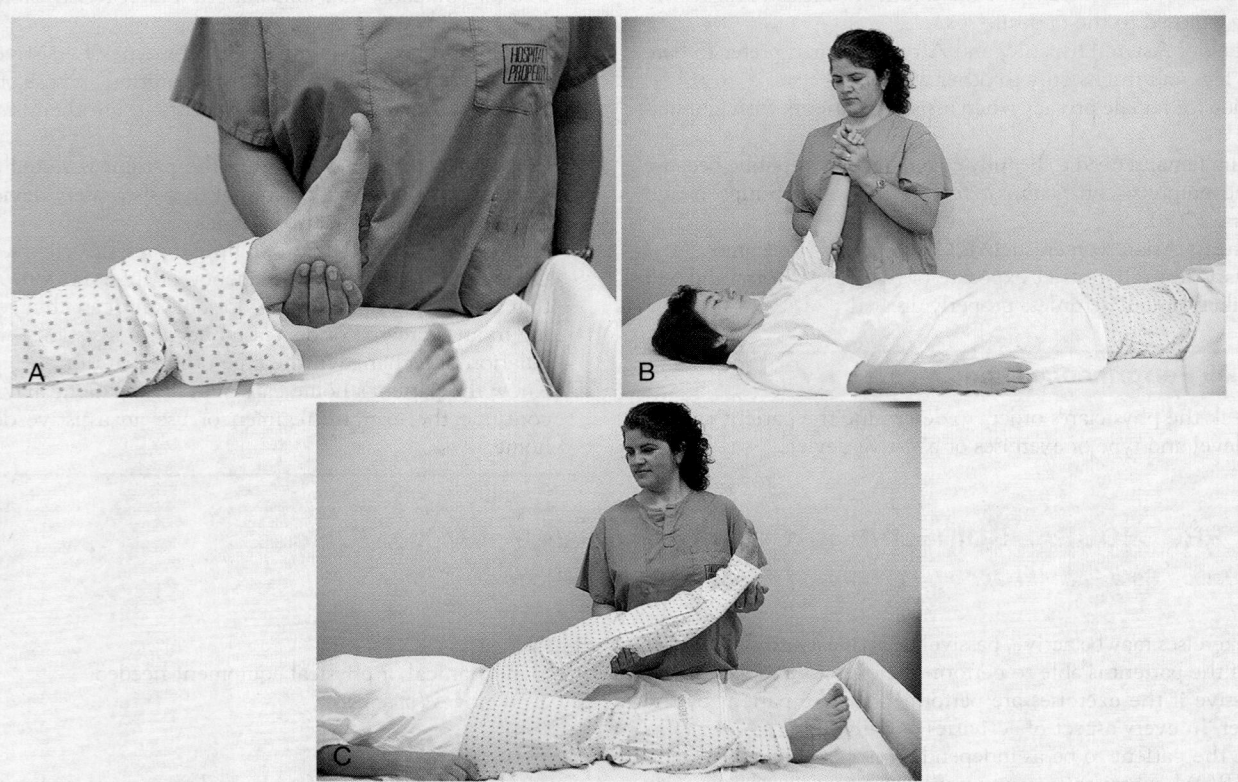

STEP 7   A, Support joint by holding distal and proximal areas adjacent to joint. **B,** Support joint by cradling distal portion of extremity. **C,** Use cupped hand to support joint.

TABLE 10-1	Incorporating Active Range-of-Motion Exercises Into Activities of Daily Living	
Joint Exercised	**Activity of Daily Living**	**Movement**
Neck	Nodding head yes	Flexion
	Shaking head no	Rotation
	Moving right ear to right shoulder	Lateral flexion
	Moving left ear to left shoulder	Lateral flexion
Shoulder	Reaching to turn on overhead light	Flexion, extension
	Reaching to bedside stand for book	Hyperextension
	Rotating shoulders toward chest	Abduction
	Rotating shoulders toward back	Adduction
Elbow	Eating, bathing, shaving, grooming	Flexion, extension
Wrist	Eating, bathing, shaving, grooming	Flexion, extension, ulnar/radial deviation
Fingers and thumb	All activities requiring fine motor coordination (e.g., writing, eating, painting)	Flexion, extension, abduction, adduction, opposition
Hip	Walking	Flexion, extension, hyperextension
	Moving to side-lying position	Flexion, extension, abduction
	Moving from side-lying position	Extension, adduction
	Rolling feet inward	Internal rotation
	Rolling feet outward	External rotation
Knee	Walking	Flexion, extension
	Moving to and from side-lying position	Flexion, extension
Ankle	Walking	Dorsiflexion, plantar flexion
	Moving toe toward head of bed	Dorsiflexion
	Moving toe toward foot of bed	Plantar flexion
Toes	Walking	Extension, hyperextension
	Wiggling toes	Abduction, adduction

TABLE 10-2 | Range-of-Motion Exercises

Body Part	Type of Joint	Type of Movement	Range (Degrees)	Primary Muscles
Neck, cervical spine	Pivotal	Flexion: Bring chin to rest on chest	45	Sternocleidomastoid
		Extension: Return head to erect position	45	Trapezius
		Hyperextension: Bend head back as far as possible	10	Trapezius
		Lateral flexion: Tilt head as far as possible toward each shoulder	40-45	Sternocleidomastoid
		Rotation: Turn head as far as possible in circular movement	180	Sternocleidomastoid, trapezius
Shoulder	Ball and socket	Flexion: Raise arm from side position forward to position above head	45-60	Coracobrachialis, deltoid, pectoralis major
		Extension: Return arm to position at side of body	180	Latissimus dorsi, teres major, triceps brachii
		Hyperextension: Move arm behind body, keeping elbow straight	45-60	Latissimus dorsi, teres major, deltoid
		Abduction: Raise arm to side to position above head with palm away from head	180	Deltoid, supraspinatus
		Adduction: Lower arm sideways and across body as far as possible	320	Pectoralis major

TABLE 10-2 | Range-of-Motion Exercises—cont'd

Body Part	Type of Joint	Type of Movement	Range (Degrees)	Primary Muscles
		Internal rotation: With elbow flexed, rotate shoulder by moving arm until thumb is turned inward and toward back	90	Pectoralis major, latissimus dorsi, teres major, subscapularis
		External rotation: With elbow flexed, move arm until thumb is upward and lateral to head	90	Infraspinatus, teres major, deltoid
		Circumduction: Move arm in full circle, (circumduction is combination of all movements of ball-and-socket joint)	360	Deltoid, coracobrachialis, latissimus dorsi, teres major
Elbow	Hinge	Flexion: Bend elbow so that lower arm moves toward its shoulder joint and hand is level with shoulder	150	Biceps brachii, brachialis, brachioradialis
		Extension: Straighten elbow by lowering hand	150	Triceps brachii
Forearm	Pivotal	Supination: Turn lower arm and hand so that palm is up	70-90	Supinator, biceps brachii
		Pronation: Turn lower arm so that palm is down	70-90	Pronator teres, pronator quadratus
Wrist	Condyloid	Flexion, move palm toward inner aspect of forearm	80-90	Flexor carpi ulnaris, flexor carpi radialis
		Extension: Move fingers and hand posterior to midline	80-90	Extensor carpi radialis brevis, extensor carpi radialis longus, extensor carpi ulnaris
		Hyperextension: Bring dorsal surface of hand back as far as possible	80-90	Extensor carpi radialis brevis, extensor carpi radialis longus, extensor carpi ulnaris
		Radial deviation: Bend wrist medially toward thumb	Up to 30	Flexor carpi radialis brevis, extensor carpi radialis brevis, extensor carpi radialis longus
		Ulnar deviation: Bend wrist laterally toward fifth finger	30-50	Flexor carpi ulnaris, extensor carpi ulnaris

Continued

TABLE 10-2 | Range-of-Motion Exercises—cont'd

Body Part	Type of Joint	Type of Movement	Range (Degrees)	Primary Muscles
Fingers	Condyloid hinge	Flexion: Make fist	90	Lumbricales, interosseus volaris, interosseus dorsalis
		Extension: Straighten fingers	90	Extensor digiti quinti proprius, extensor digitorum communis, extensor indicis proprius
		Hyperextension: Bend fingers back as far as possible	30-60	Extensor digitorum
		Abduction: Spread fingers apart	30	Interosseus dorsalis
		Adduction: Bring fingers together	30	Interosseus volaris
Thumb:	Saddle	Flexion: Move thumb across palmar surface of hand	90	Flexor pollicis brevis
		Extension: Move thumb straight away from hand	90	Extensor pollicis longus, extensor pollicis brevis
		Abduction: Extend thumb laterally (usually done when placing fingers in abduction and adduction)	30	Abductor pollicis brevis and longus
		Adduction: Move thumb back toward hand	30	Adductor pollicis obliquus, adductor pollicis transversus
		Opposition: Touch thumb to each finger of same hand		Opponens pollicis, opponens digiti minimi
Hip	Ball and socket	Flexion: Move leg forward and up	90-120	Psoas major, iliacus, sartorius
		Extension: Move leg back beside other leg	90-120	Gluteus maximus, semitendinosus, semimembranosus
		Hyperextension: Move leg behind body as far as possible	30-50	Gluteus maximus, semitendinosus, semimembranosus

TABLE 10-2 | Range-of-Motion Exercises—cont'd

Body Part	Type of Joint	Type of Movement	Range (Degrees)	Primary Muscles
Hip, cont'd	Ball and socket, cont'd			
		Abduction: Move leg laterally away from body	30-50	Gluteus medius, gluteus minimus
		Adduction: Move leg back toward medial position and beyond if possible	30-50	Adductor longus, adductor brevis, adductor magnus
		Internal rotation: Turn foot and leg toward other leg	90	Gluteus medius, gluteus minimus, tensor fasciae latae
		External rotation: Turn foot and leg away from other leg	90	Obturatorius internus, obturatorius externus, quadratus femoris, piriformis, gemellus superior and inferior, gluteus maximus
		Circumduction: Move leg in circle	120-130	Psoas major, gluteus maximus, gluteus medius, adductor magnus
Knee	Hinge	Flexion: Bring heel back toward back of thigh	120-130	Biceps femoris, semitendinosus, semimembranosus, sartorius
		Extension: Return leg to floor	120-130	Rectus femoris, vastus lateralis, vastus medialis, vastus intermedius

Continued

TABLE 10-2 | Range-of-Motion Exercises—cont'd

Body Part	Type of Joint	Type of Movement	Range (Degrees)	Primary Muscles
Ankle	Hinge	Dorsal flexion: Move foot so that toes are pointed upward	20-30	Tibialis anterior
		Plantar flexion: Move foot so that toes are pointed downward	45-50	Gastrocnemius, soleus
Foot	Gliding	Inversion: Turn sole of foot medially	10 or less	Tibialis anterior, tibialis posterior
		Eversion: Turn sole of foot laterally	10 or less	Peroneus longus, peroneus brevis
Toes	Condyloid	Flexion: Curl toes downward	30-60	Flexor digitorum, lumbricalis pedis, flexor hallucis brevis
		Extension: Straighten toes	30-60	Extensor digitorum longus, extensor digitorum brevis, extensor hallucis longus
		Abduction: Spread toes apart	15 or less	Abductor hallucis, interosseus dorsalis
		Adduction: Bring toes together	15 or less	Adductor hallucis, interosseus plantaris

SKILL 10-1 Performing Isometric Exercises

In addition to ROM exercises, some immobilized patients are able to perform muscle-strengthening exercises. Isotonic muscle contractions cause a change in muscle length. Examples of exercises that cause isotonic muscle contractions are walking, performing aerobics, and moving arms and legs against light resistance. Performing these types of exercises regularly positively affects heart and lung function, improves muscle tone, and has beneficial effects on the entire body if performed properly. Some individuals, however, are unable to tolerate such increases in activity. For these individuals, isometric exercises are more appropriate and are easily accomplished by an immobilized patient in bed (Kasper and others, 2005; Rydwik and others, 2005). Isometric or static exercises involve tightening or tensing of muscles without moving body parts (isometric contractions). They increase muscle tension but do not change the length of muscle fibers.

Isometric exercises involve the contraction of a muscle while pushing against a stationary object or resisting the movement of an object. Examples of isometric exercises are performing push-ups and hip lifting. In hip lifting, the individual, who is in a sitting position, pushes with the hands against a sitting surface such as a chair to raise the hips. Isometric exercises help to promote muscular strength and provide the necessary stress for bone maintenance and growth. Without sufficient stress against bone, osteoclastic activity (activity by cells responsible for bone tissue absorption) increases over osteoblastic activity (activity by bone-forming cells) (Huether and McCance, 2008). The result is demineralization of the bone and eventual osteoporosis.

Delegation Considerations

The skill of performing isometric exercises can be delegated to NAP. However, patients with cardiovascular disease or musculoskeletal disorders require assessment by a nurse when initially performing these exercises. The nurse directs the NAP by:

- Discussing the amount of time and frequency of the prescribed isometric exercises.
- Reminding to perform exercises slowly at patient's pace.
- Discussing the patient's individual limitations or preexisting conditions such as arthritis that may affect ROM needed for isometric exercises.

STEP	RATIONALE

ASSESSMENT

1 Review patient's chart for contraindications to isometric exercises such as cardiovascular disease.	Isometric exercises raise blood pressure and pulse. The presence of a preexisting medical condition, such as a history of cardiac problems, may be a contraindication.
2 Assess patient's baseline vital signs.	Isometric exercises may raise blood pressure. Documentation of baseline vital signs is necessary to determine whether exercises cause deterioration in vital signs (Huether and McCance, 2008).
3 Assess patient's baseline muscle strength:	Enables nurse to compare muscle strength before and after exercise.
a Ask patient to perform task against resistance (e.g., push one foot against palm of hand).	
b Assess grasp strength by having patient grasp nurse's hands. Note whether hand grasps are equal.	
c Have patient grasp two fingers of nurse's right hand with patient's left hand and two fingers of nurse's left hand with patient's right hand.	
d Observe patient's ability to do daily activities (e.g., whether patient has adequate strength to bathe self, pull self up in bed, move from bed to chair).	
e Obtain patient's subjective statements related to muscle strength. Does patient feel weaker?	
4 Assess patient's nutritional status.	Proper nutrition is essential if patient is to be able to perform exercises. Promotion of protein anabolism involves conservation and replenishment of energy stores (Meiner and Lueckenotte, 2006).
5 Assess level of comfort: pain severity.	Pain may reduce patient's motivation to perform isometric exercises. Pain relief before attempting exercises may enhance patient's participation.
6 Assess patient's or caregiver's understanding of isometric exercises to be used.	Allows patient to verbalize concerns and identifies educational needs of patient or caregiver.

NURSING DIAGNOSES

- Activity intolerance
- Deficient knowledge regarding exercises
- Fatigue
- Impaired physical mobility
- Pain (acute, chronic)

Individualize related factors based on patient's condition or needs.

STEP	RATIONALE

PLANNING

1 Expected outcomes following completion of procedure:
- Patient will gradually increase number of exercise repetitions.
- Vital signs will remain stable.

2 Explain procedure, and demonstrate exercises.
3 Assist patient to comfortable position.

Patient gradually becomes stronger and is able to increase number of repetitions.
Documents patient's activity tolerance.
Relieves anxiety and encourages patient cooperation.
Reduces stress and promotes patient participation.

IMPLEMENTATION

1 Provide privacy.
2 Instruct patient to perform the following isometric exercises as prescribed. Each exercise prescription is individualized according to the patient's needs and limitations. Exercises are as follows:

Prevents patient embarrassment.
Gradual build-up of exercise repetitions improves both muscle strength and endurance (Gillespie, 2006).

Critical Decision Point   *Teach patients to exhale while exerting effort during isometric exercises. Many persons hold their breath (Valsalva maneuver), which increases intrathoracic pressure, causing a decrease in venous return to heart.*

   a Quadriceps isometric exercises:

     (1) Assist patient to supine recumbent position.
     (2) Instruct patient to press back of the knee against mattress while trying to lift heel from bed (see illustration).

Quadriceps muscles enable a person to ambulate and get out of chair; large muscles of thigh (quadriceps) must be strong enough for patient to extend knees and stabilize them.

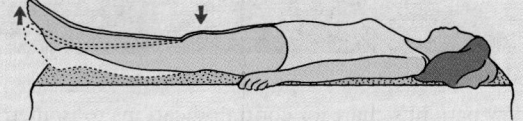

STEP 2a(2)   Lift heels while pressing back of knees against mattress.

     (3) Hold muscles tightly contracted for 5 to 15 seconds, and then relax completely for several seconds.

Nurse can assist patient in learning this exercise by placing hand between the back of patient's knee and mattress and asking patient to press hand against mattress with the back of the knee.

     (4) Repeat exercise.
   b Gluteal muscle isometric exercises:
     (1) Assist patient to supine position.
     (2) Instruct patient to pinch buttocks muscles together and hold for 5 to 15 seconds and then relax completely for several seconds (see illustration).

Improves patient's balance when sitting.

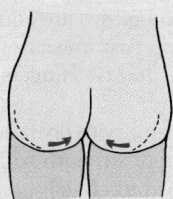

STEP 2b(2)   Pinch gluteal muscles together.

     (3) Repeat exercise.
   c Abdominal muscle isometric exercises:
     (1) Have patient pull abdominal muscles in as tightly as possible (see illustration).
     (2) Hold for 5 to 15 seconds. Release muscles gradually.
     (3) Repeat exercise.

Improves trunk stability.

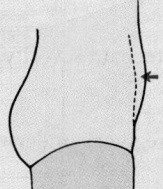

STEP 2c(1)   Pull abdominal muscles in tightly.

   d Foot muscle isometric exercises:

Increases muscle activity in leg and thereby promotes venous return to heart.

STEP	RATIONALE

(1) Instruct patient to flex foot toward and away from knee, holding muscles tightly in each position for 5 to 15 seconds.

(2) Repeat exercise.

e Hand muscle isometric exercises:

(1) Obtain sponge rubber ball. (Size of ball depends on size of patient's hand.)

(2) Have patient grip ball with entire hand 5 to 10 times.

(3) Dig each fingertip, one at a time, into ball 5 to 10 times each.

(4) Gradually increase frequency of exercise until patient can grip ball and exercise once or twice a day.

Strengthens grip to hold onto crutch or walker more effectively.

f Biceps isometric exercises:

(1) Have patient raise arms to shoulder height and interlock fingertips of both hands.

(2) Use arm muscles to try to pull hands apart.

(3) Hold for 5 to 15 seconds.

(4) Relax muscles.

(5) Repeat exercise.

Strengthens biceps and thereby helps with ambulation if ambulatory assistive device is used.

g Triceps muscle isometric exercises:

(1) Arm exercises (see illustration)

(a) Have patient raise arms to shoulder height.

(b) Make fist with one hand and place against palm of other hand.

(c) Push hands together as hard as possible and hold for 5 to 15 seconds.

(d) Relax and repeat exercise.

Strengthens triceps to assist with transfer techniques and use of crutches or walker. Patient must have enough strength to extend and stabilize the elbows when lifting or shifting body weight.

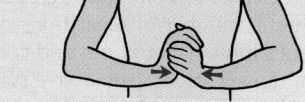

STEP 2g(1) Triceps muscle isometric exercises.

(2) Sitting exercises (see illustration)

(a) Assist patient to sitting position on edge of bed or in chair. If mattress is soft, blocks or books are placed on bed under patient's hands.

(b) Instruct patient to try to lift buttocks off bed or seat of chair by pressing down on mattress or chair seat with hands.

(c) Hold muscles tight for 5 to 15 seconds, and then relax.

(d) Repeat exercise.

To use crutches or walker effectively, patient must have enough strength in the triceps to extend and stabilize the elbows while lifting or shifting body weight.

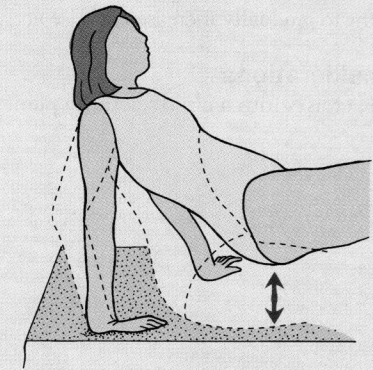

STEP 2g(2) Triceps muscle resistive isometric exercises.

STEP	RATIONALE

EVALUATION

1 Observe patient's ability to perform exercises.	Demonstrates patient's learning.
2 Evaluate patient's level of energy, muscular strength, and comfort following exercises.	Determines whether patient is performing exercises accurately and whether the exercises are increasing muscle strength.
3 Obtain vital signs after one or two repetitions.	Determines patient's tolerance to activity.

Unexpected Outcomes	Related Interventions
1 Patient is unable to perform exercises. Patient may be too weak.	• Continue ROM exercises, and reposition patient to try to increase strength. • Make sure nutrition and rest are adequate.
2 Patient is unwilling to perform exercises.	• Lack of understanding of significance of exercises may be the problem. • Stress importance of the exercises. • Be sure patient is not experiencing distracting symptoms such as nausea or pain.
3 Muscular strength is not increasing.	• Patient may not be performing exercises as described or as often as instructed. • Stress importance of following routine.
4 Patient's blood pressure and heart rate increase significantly during exercises.	• Patient may not be able to tolerate procedure. • Discontinue exercises, and consult physician.

Recording and Reporting

• Record in nurses' notes type of isometric exercises used, length of time contractions held, number of repetitions of each exercise, assessment of patient's muscular strength and comfort after exercises, patient's vital signs, patient's subjective statements regarding muscular strength, and patient's ability to perform exercises.

Teaching Considerations

• Instruct patient to perform exercises before regular activities, such as breakfast or work. Building exercises into routine activities increases likelihood of adherence to exercise program.
• Instruct patient to gradually increase exercise activity each day.

Pediatric Considerations

• Incorporate exercises into a child's activity plan.

• Children are more likely to exercise as part of a game or in groups as opposed to exercising alone (Hockenberry and Wilson, 2007).

Gerontological Considerations

• Physical exercise is important for older adults to maintain health, preserve functional status, and improve general quality of life (Gillespie, 2006; Meiner and Lueckenotte, 2006).
• For the older adult who has not previously participated in exercise, it is important to start with only 5 minutes of exercise and gradually work up to a 20- to 30-minute daily routine (Meiner and Lueckenotte, 2006).
• Encourage older adults to drink water before and after exercising (Gillespie, 2006).

SKILL 10-2   Continuous Passive Motion Machine

The continuous passive motion (CPM) machine is designed to exercise varying joints such as the hip, ankle, knee, shoulder, and wrist. The CPM machine is most commonly used after knee surgery. The CPM machine is usually prescribed on the day of surgery or the first postoperative day, depending on the surgeon's preference and patient's condition (Monohan and others, 2007). A typical initial setting is 20 to 30 degrees of flexion and full extension (0 degrees) at two cycles per minute. However, this setting varies according to the patient's condition and physician's preference (Ignatavicius and Workman, 2006). The purpose of the CPM machine is to mobilize the joint to prevent contractures, muscle atrophy, venous stasis, and thromboembolism. The CPM machine can aid in alleviating pain, edema, stiffness, and dislocation and potentially can shorten a patient's hospital stay.

The electronically controlled CPM machine flexes and extends the joint to a prescribed degree and at a set speed as ordered by the physician. Velcro straps secure the extremity. When the device is turned on, the frame slides slowly back and forth, gently moving the joint through a preset ROM. The CPM machine can weigh up to 25 lb. Using two hospital personnel to lift the machine reduces the risk for caregiver back strain and prevents risk for damage to the patient's extremity.

Delegation Considerations
The skill of using the CPM machine cannot be delegated to NAP. The nurse directs the NAP by:
- Instructing to immediately report increase in patient's pain, skin breakdown, or joint inflammation.

Equipment
❏ CPM machine
❏ Clean gloves

STEP	RATIONALE
ASSESSMENT	
1 Assess the CPM machine for electrical safety.	All electrical equipment in health care settings is routinely checked for safety. Routine observation of electrical cord and functioning of equipment each time it is used further monitors safety.
2 Assess the setup of the machine before placing on bed: check the stability of the frame, the flexion/extension controls, padding of exposed metal parts or hard surfaces, and the on/off switch.	Ensures that all pieces of the equipment are operational and will prevent damage to the patient's joint. Ensures metal parts are padded to prevent skin breakdown or chafing of skin rubbing against metal or hard surfaces.
3 Assess the patient's pain on a scale of 0 to 10 (10 being the worst pain) before and during use.	Establishes comfort baseline (Berry and others, 2006). Determines how the patient tolerates the CPM machine and the need for analgesia.
4 Assess patient's baseline vital signs.	Provides baseline to measure exercise tolerance.
5 Assess the patient's ability and willingness to learn about the CPM machine.	Determines readiness to learn, reduces anxiety, and promotes patient participation.
6 Assess the nature of the patient's condition and ROM limits prescribed by health care provider.	Procedure must be orderd by a physician or licensed primary health care provider.

NURSING DIAGNOSES

- Activity intolerance
- Deficient knowledge regarding CPM machine

- Fatigue
- Impaired mobility

- Pain (acute)

Individualize related factors based on patient's condition or needs.

PLANNING	
1 Expected outcomes following completion of the procedure:	
• Patient will increase length of time and flexion of joint as prescribed by physician.	CPM machine facilitates joint range of motion, prevents formation of adhesions, edema, stiffness, deformity.
• Patient's vital signs will remain stable.	Documents patient's activity tolerance.
• Patient denies increased discomfort during or after CPM exercise.	Providing analgesia for patient assists in tolerating exercise.
2 Explain procedure, and demonstrate CPM machine.	Relieves anxiety and encourages patient cooperation.
3 Assist patient to comfortable position.	Reduces stress and promotes patient participation.

IMPLEMENTATION	
1 Perform hand hygiene.	Reduces transmission of microorganisms.
2 Provide analgesia 20 to 30 minutes before CPM machine is needed.	Pain control assists patient in tolerating exercise (Pasero and McCaffery, 2004).

STEP	RATIONALE
3 Wear clean gloves if wound drainage is present.	Reduces nurse's risk for exposure to blood-borne viruses or bacteria.
4 Place elastic hose on patient if ordered (see Skill 10-3).	Elastic hose promote venous return from lower extremities.
5 Place CPM machine on bed.	
6 Set limits of flexion and extension as prescribed by physician and set speed control to slow or moderate range.	Prevents injury by setting machine at safe limits.
7 Put machine through one full cycle.	Ensures CPM machine is working properly.
8 Stop CPM machine when in extension. Place sheepskin on CPM machine.	Ensures all exposed hard surfaces are padded to prevent rubbing and chafing of patient's skin.
9 Place patient's extremity in CPM machine (see illustration).	
10 Adjust CPM machine to patient's extremity. Lengthen and shorten appropriate sections of frame.	
11 Center patient's extremity on frame.	Avoids pressure areas on extremity.
12 Align patient's joint with mechanical joint of CPM.	
13 Secure patient's extremity on CPM machine with Velcro straps (see illustration). Apply loosely.	
14 Start machine. When it reaches flexed position, stop machine and check degree of flexion.	Prevents possible complications and ensures correct settings.
15 Start CPM machine, and observe for two full cycles.	Ensures CPM machine is fully operational at the preset extension and flexion modes.
16 Make sure patient is comfortable.	
17 Provide patient with on/off switch.	Allows patient to turn on and off CPM machine if malfunctions or if discomfort develops.
18 Instruct patient to turn CPM machine off if malfunctioning or experiencing pain. Instruct patient to notify nurse immediately.	
19 Discard gloves, and perform hand hygiene.	Prevents transmission of microorganisms.

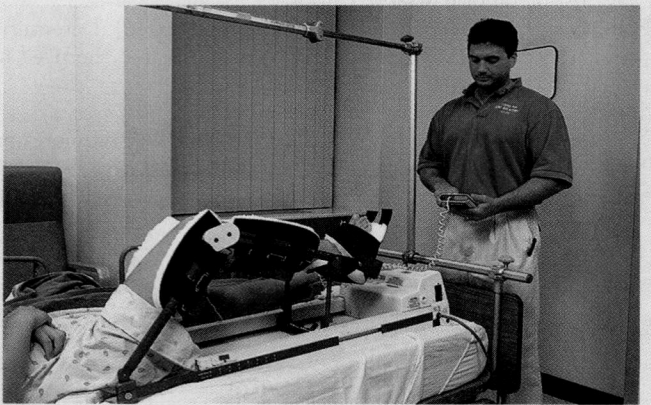

STEP 9   Leg positioned in CPM cradle.

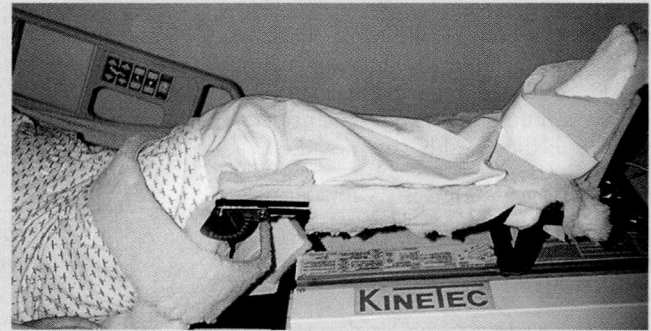

STEP 13   Patient's extremity properly placed and secured on CPM machine.

EVALUATION

1 Inspect bony prominences and areas of skin in contact with machine at least every 2 hours.	Identifies potential skin breakdown.
2 Ask patient to rate pain on a scale of 0 to 10.	Determines if analgesia is effective.
3 Check patient's alignment and positioning at least every 2 hours.	Promotes comfort and ensures proper extension and flexion of joint.
4 Observe patient and CPM machine with each increase in flexion and extension.	Prevents complications and ensures CPM machine is functioning properly.

Unexpected Outcomes	Related Interventions
1 Patient does not tolerate increase in flexion or extension.	• Consult with physician and physical therapist to plan additional therapies to increase flexion and extension of joint. • Provide rest periods throughout day to rest the joint. • Consider need for analgesia before CPM machine is used.

Unexpected Outcomes	Related Interventions
2 Patient experiences increased pain when using CPM machine.	• Determine efficacy of current analgesia, and obtain new orders to change dosage or medication. • Determine cause of increased pain.
3 Patient develops reddened areas on bony prominences or extremity.	• Determine if hard surfaces on CPM machine are well padded. • Monitor patient's alignment and positioning at least every 2 hours. • Provide skin care at least every 2 hours.

Recording and Reporting

- Record in nurses' notes the patient's tolerance for CPM machine, rate of cycles per minute, degree of flexion and extension used, condition of extremity and skin, condition of operative site if present, length of time CPM machine in use.
- Report immediately to nurse in charge or physician any resistance to range of motion; increased pain; swelling, heat, or redness in joint.

Teaching Considerations

- Instruct patient in the use and importance of the CPM machine.

Pediatric Considerations

- During therapy, arrange for social or creative activities that are developmentally appropriate for the child's age (Lassetter, 2006).
- Demonstrate use of CPM machine using a large doll or stuffed animal before applying to child's extremity to relieve anxiety.

Gerontological Considerations

- Older adults have increased risk for skin breakdown because of decreased elasticity and fragility of the skin. Pressure from the CPM machine increases the risk for pressure ulcers, especially on the heel (Meiner and Lueckenotte, 2006).
- Encourage the older adult to move at his or her own speed. Relaxation exercises decrease anxiety, ease muscle tension, and assist with some pain relief (Dossey, 2005). Special attention to nonverbal cues and additional instruction in pain management is often necessary to ensure the older adult's comfort.

Home Care Considerations

- Home care physical therapist may assist patient/family in continuing CPM machine in the home.
- Patient/family must have specific instructions regarding the use of the CPM machine, length of time for each session, expected outcomes, and what to do if the patient experiences increased pain or does not tolerate the CPM sessions or if the equipment malfunctions.

SKILL 10-3   Applying Elastic Stockings and Sequential Compression Device

 Basic / Safe Patient Handling / Applying Elastic Stocking Using a Sequential Compression Device

Prevention is the best method for reducing the risk for deep vein thrombosis (DVT) secondary to immobility. Early ambulation remains the most effective preventive measure (Monohan and others, 2007). However, there are times when early ambulation is not an option, particularly in the critically ill patient. Early application of elastic stockings, sequential compression device (SCD), or foot pumps along with low-molecular-weight or low-dose heparin therapy is reported to be successful in preventing the development of deep vein thrombosis (Grande and Caparro, 2005; Kehl-Pruett, 2006; Monohan and others, 2007; Rawat and others, 2008).

Three factors (commonly referred to as Virchow's triad) contribute to the development of DVT: hypercoagulability of the blood, venous wall damage, and stasis of blood flow (Monohan and others, 2007). Elastic stockings help reduce two of the factors: blood stasis and venous wall injury. First, they promote venous return by maintaining pressure on superficial veins to prevent venous pooling, thereby reducing the risk for clot formation in the lower extremities. Second, it is suggested that elastic stockings prevent passive dilation of the veins, thereby decreasing the risk for endothelial tears. An increased incidence of DVT is found in patients with increased venous diameter. In such cases the endothelial layer can tear.

Sequential compression devices are used alone or in conjunction with elastic stockings, depending upon the physician's preference. These devices consist of an air pump, connecting tubing, and extremity sleeves that sequentially inflate and deflate chambers within the sleeve. The intermittent pumping action drives superficial blood into deep veins, where it is evacuated proximally by the venous valves, thus removing pooled blood and preventing both venous stasis and the accumulation of clotting factors. Another device

that promotes venous return is the venous plexus foot pump (Fig. 10-1). Venous plexus foot pumps promote circulation by mimicking the natural action of walking by intermittently compressing the sole of the foot and then relaxing it, so the venous plexus can fill with blood. Foot pumps increase circulation in the lower extremities.

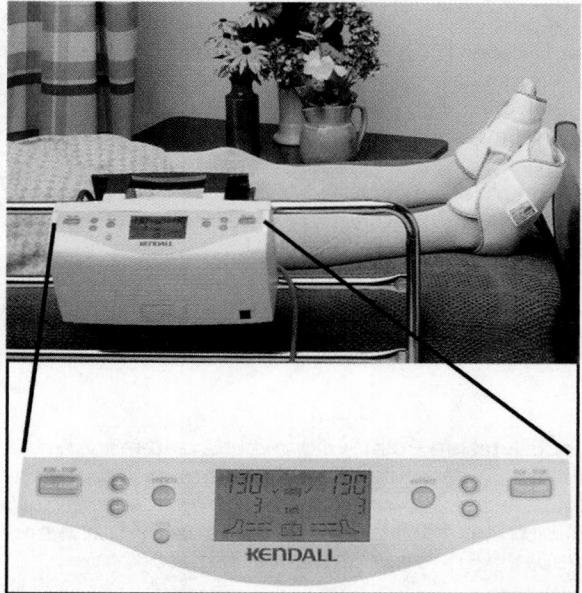

FIG 10-1 Venous plexus foot pump with bedside controls. (*Courtesy Tyco Healthcare Group LP.*)

Delegation Considerations

The skill of applying elastic stockings and sequential compression device (SCD) can be delegated to NAP. Initially determine the size of elastic stockings and accurate application of the SCD, and assess the patient's lower extremities for any signs and symptoms of impaired circulation. The nurse directs the NAP to:

- Remove the SCD sleeves from the legs before allowing patient to get out of bed. This ensures patient's safety and avoids patient's becoming tangled in SCD sleeves and connectors.
- Observe for signs and symptoms of allergic reactions to elastic (e.g., redness, itching, irritation) and report finding immediately.

- Inform the nurse if one calf appears larger than the other, a calf is red and/or warm to the touch, or the calf is painful.

Equipment

- ❏ Tape measure (to measure patient's legs for size selection of elastic stockings and SCDs)
- ❏ Powder or cornstarch if patient not allergic (*optional*)
- ❏ Elastic support stockings
- ❏ Disposable SDC sleeve(s)
- ❏ Tubing assembly
- ❏ Sequential compression device (motor)

STEP	RATIONALE

ASSESSMENT

1　Assess patient for risk factors in Virchow's triad:	Potential candidates for elastic stockings and/or SCD are patients who have an alteration in one of the elements of Virchow's triad. Risk assessment for DVT is crucial to prevent this complication of immobility (Hums and Blostein, 2006; Monohan and others, 2007).
a　*Hypercoagulability:* All patients with clotting disorders, fever, dehydration, pregnancy and/or first 6 weeks post partum if the woman was confined to bed, or oral contraceptive use (especially if patient smokes).	Hypercoagulability increases tendency for blood to clot.
b　*Venous wall abnormalities:* Local trauma, orthopedic surgeries, major abdominal surgery, varicose veins, and atherosclerosis.	Venous wall abnormalities can impair circulation or traumatize blood cells, both of which increase patient's risk for clotting.
c　*Blood stasis:* Immobility, obesity, pregnancy.	Stasis facilitates clotting.

Critical Decision Point　*Discourage patients from activities that promote venous stasis (e.g., crossing legs, placing pillows under knee). When possible, have patient elevate legs on a stool while sitting to improve venous return.*

2　Observe for signs, symptoms, and conditions that might contraindicate use of elastic stockings or SCD:	
a　Dermatitis or open skin lesion	Elastic stockings and SCD sleeves may aggravate a skin condition or cause it to spread. Also the physician may want medication and dressing applied to the lesion.
b　Recent skin graft	Recent skin grafts are delicate, and application of elastic stockings or SCD increases the risk for the graft's becoming dislodged (Monohan and others, 2007).
c　Decreased circulation in lower extremities as evidenced by cyanotic, cool extremities and/or gangrenous conditions affecting the lower limb(s)	Elastic stockings and SCD may further impede circulation (Monohan and others, 2007).
d　Neurovascular impairment such as decreased sensation or paralysis.	Improperly fitting elastic stockings and SCD may cause further constriction or pressure and cause further neurovascular dysfunction.
3　Obtain physician's order.	May be needed for reimbursement.
4　Assess patient's or caregiver's understanding of application of elastic stockings and SCD sleeves.	Identifies potential educational needs of patient or caregiver.
5　Assess the condition of patient's skin and circulation to the legs (i.e., presence of pedal pulses, edema, temperature, discoloration of the skin, lesions, cuts).	Identifies a baseline for skin integrity and the quality of peripheral pulses in lower extremities. Prevention is the best medicine to avoid the development of thrombophlebitis. Early application of elastic stockings and SCD sleeves can be instrumental in preventing this complication.

Critical Decision Point　*Thrombophlebitis can develop in the lower extremities. Clinical manifestations of thrombophlebitis vary according to the size and location of the thrombus. Signs and symptoms of superficial thrombosis include palpable veins and the surrounding area being tender to touch, reddened, and warm. There may be a slight temperature elevation. Edema of the extremity may or may not occur. Signs and symptoms of DVT include a swollen extremity; pain; warm, cyanotic skin; and temperature elevation. Although Homans' sign (pain in calf on dorsiflexion of foot) was an assessment parameter in the past, it is no longer a reliable sign. Fewer than 20% of patients exhibit a positive Homans' sign (Monohan and others, 2007).*

6　Assess patient's or caregiver's understanding of proper care of elastic stockings.	Identifies potential educational needs of patient or caregiver.

STEP	RATIONALE

NURSING DIAGNOSES

- Decreased cardiac output
- Deficient knowledge regarding application of elastic stockings

- Impaired physical mobility
- Ineffective peripheral tissue perfusion

- Risk for impaired skin integrity

Individualize related factors based on patient's condition or needs.

PLANNING

1   Expected outcomes following completion of procedure:
- Patient shows no evidence of skin irritation.

Proper application ensures no side effects that would impair skin integrity.

- Patient shows no evidence of thrombophlebitis.
- Patient demonstrates application of elastic stockings.
- Patient has decreased edema in lower extremities.

Proper application prevents trauma to venous walls.
Verifies correct psychomotor learning.
Decreases venous pooling in lower extremities.

2   Explain procedure and reasons for applying elastic stockings and SCD.

Reduces anxiety and encourages patient cooperation.

3   Use tape measure to measure patient's legs to determine proper size for elastic stockings and SCD sleeve (see illustrations).

Stockings must be measured according to manufacturer's directions. The choice of length depends on the physician's order. However, knee length is more comfortable for the patient and results in better adherence to therapy (Brady and others, 2007). If too large, stockings will not adequately support extremities. If too small, stockings may impede circulation.

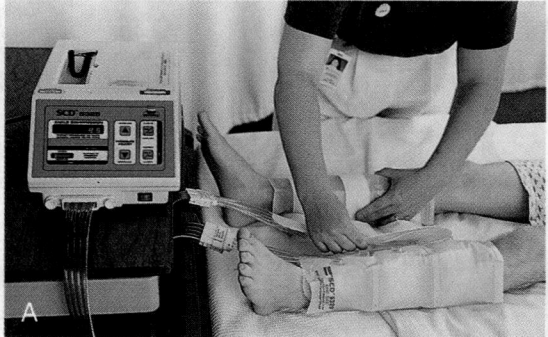 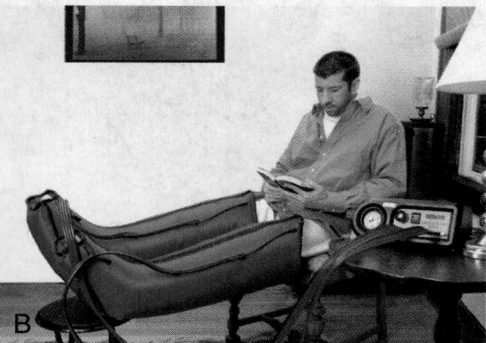

STEP 3   **A,** Knee-length SCD. (Copyright © 2008 Covidien AG or an affiliate. All rights reserved. Reprinted with permission. **B,** Thigh-length SCD. (*Courtesy Bio Compression Systems, Inc., Moonachie, NJ.*)

IMPLEMENTATION

1   Perform hand hygiene.

Reduces transmission of microorganisms.

2   Position patient in supine position. Elevate head of bed to comfortable level.

Promotes good body mechanics for nurse. Patient position eases application. Also the elastic stockings are applied before the patient stands to prevent stagnation of blood in the lower extremities.

3   If necessary, bathe legs and dry thoroughly. It is optional to apply a small amount of powder to legs and feet, provided patient does not have sensitivity to either.

Powder reduces friction and allows for easier application of stockings. Use powder sparingly to prevent caking.

STEP	RATIONALE

4 Applying elastic stockings:

a Turn elastic stocking inside out by placing one hand into sock, holding toe of sock with other hand, and pulling (see illustration).

Allows easier application of stocking.

b Place patient's toes into foot of elastic stocking, making sure that sock is smooth (see illustration).

Wrinkles in elastic stocking can cause constrictions and impede circulation to lower region of extremity.

c Slide remaining portion of sock over patient's foot, being sure that the toes are covered. Make sure the foot fits into the toe and heel position of the sock. Sock will now be right side out (see illustration).

If toes remain uncovered, they will become constricted by elastic, and their circulation can be reduced.

d Slide sock up over patient's calf until sock is completely extended up leg. Be sure sock is smooth and no ridges or wrinkles are present (see illustration).

e Instruct patient not to roll socks partially down.

Rolling sock partially down has a constricting effect and impedes venous return.

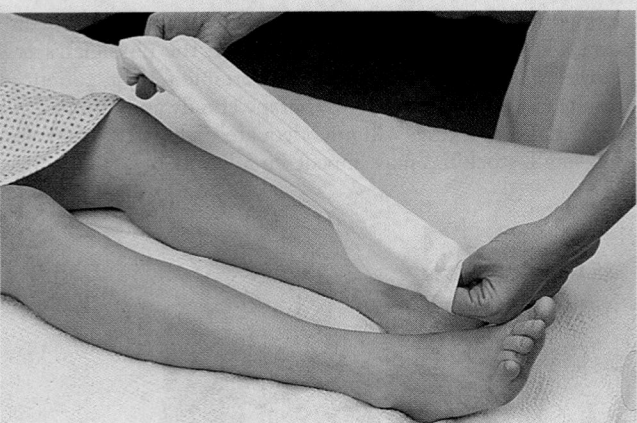

STEP 4a   Turn stocking inside out; hold toe and pull through.

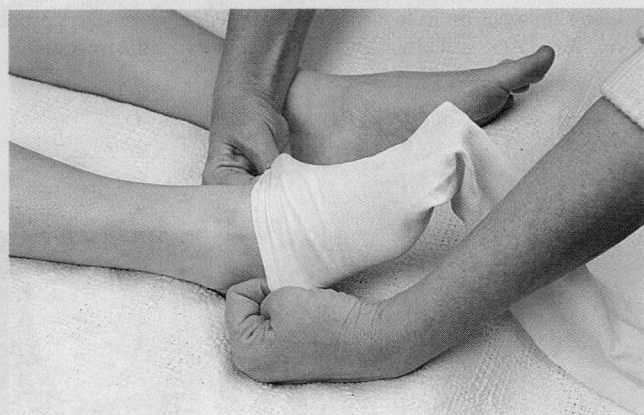

STEP 4c   Slide remaining portion of sock over foot.

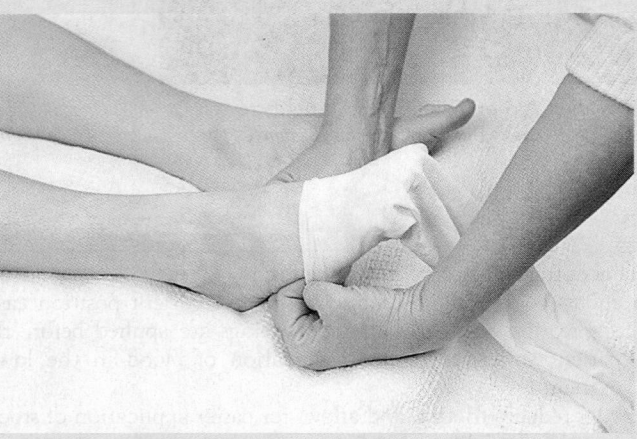

STEP 4b   Place toes into foot of stocking.

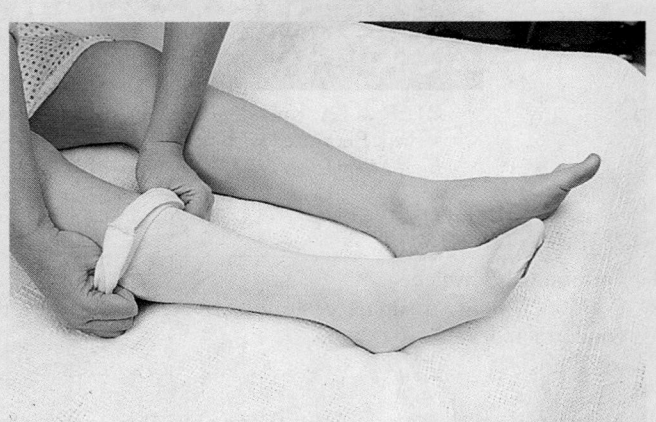

STEP 4d   Slide sock up leg until completely extended.

STEP	RATIONALE

5 Applying SCD sleeves:
   a Remove SCD sleeves from plastic, unfold, and flatten.
   b Arrange the SCD sleeve under the patient's leg according to the leg position indicated on the inner lining of the sleeve (see illustration).

Ensures straight and even application.

   c Place patient's leg on SCD sleeve.
     (1) Back of ankle should line up with the ankle marking on inner lining of sleeve.

Correct application of SCD sleeve is important for proper functioning.

   d Position back of knee with the popliteal opening (see illustration).

Prevents pressure on popliteal artery.

Critical Decision Point   *If patient is wearing elastic stockings, eliminate any wrinkles and folds before applying SCD sleeves.*

   e Wrap SCD sleeve securely around patient's leg.

Secure fit needed for adequate compression.

   f Check fit of SCD sleeve by placing two fingers between patient's leg and sleeve (see illustration).

Ensures proper fit and prevents constriction, which impedes circulation.

   g Attach connector of SCD sleeve to plug on mechanical unit. Arrows on connector line up with arrows on plug from mechanical unit (see illustration).

Critical Decision Point   *Make sure tubing and connection site are visible. Check for kinks or twisting of tubing to avoid a potential pressure ulcer.*

   h Turn mechanical unit on. Green light indicates unit is functioning.

Power source initiates sequential compression cycle.

   i Monitor functioning of SCD through one full cycle of inflation and deflation.

Ensures proper functioning of unit and determines if SCD sleeves are too loose or constricting.

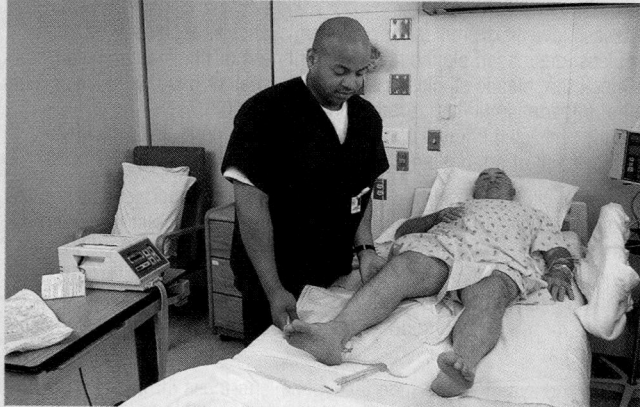

STEP 5b   Correct positioning of leg on inner lining of SCD.

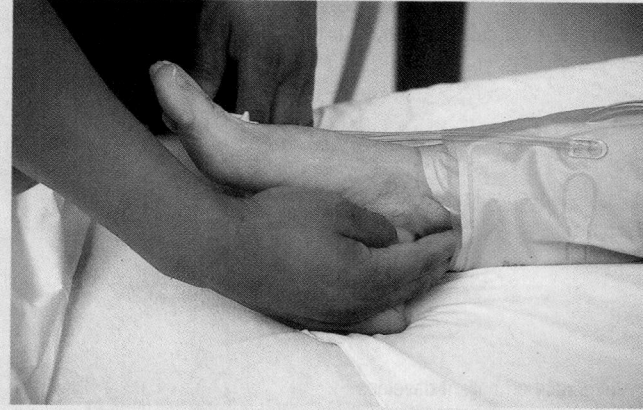

STEP 5f   Check fit of SCD sleeve.

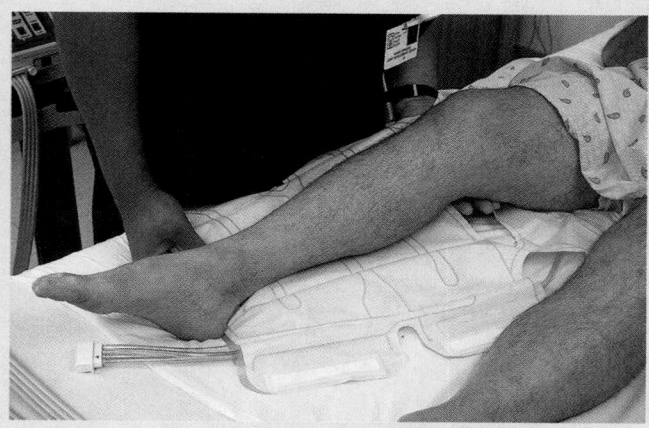

STEP 5d   Position back of patient's knee with the popliteal opening.

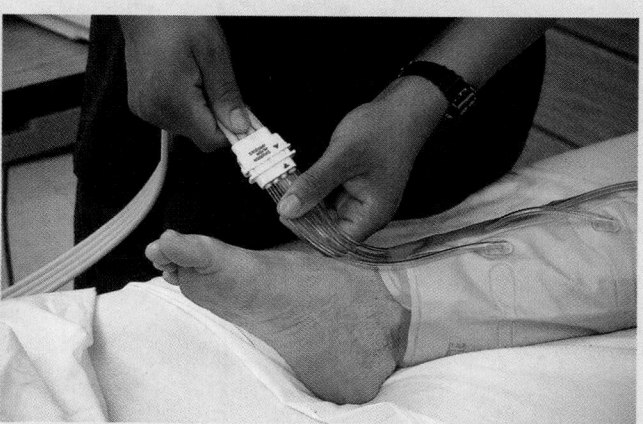

STEP 5g   Align arrows when connecting to mechanical unit.

STEP	RATIONALE
6 Reposition patient to position of comfort.	Maintains proper body alignment and promotes comfort.

Critical Decision Point *Remove SCD sleeves when transferring patient in and out of bed to prevent injury.*

STEP	RATIONALE
7 Perform hand hygiene.	Reduces transmission of microorganisms.
8 Remove elastic stockings or SCD sleeves at least once per shift long enough to inspect skin for irritation or breakdown.	Compliance with wearing elastic stockings and SCD poses an issue when patients find them to be uncomfortable or applied incorrectly. Elastic stockings and SCDs are removed long enough to perform an assessment and/or hygiene measures and replaced as soon as possible (Brady and others, 2007).

EVALUATION

1 Inspect elastic stockings to make sure there are no wrinkles or binding at top of stocking.	Wrinkles lead to increased pressure and alter circulation.
2 Observe circulatory status of lower extremities. Observe color, temperature, and condition of skin.	Ensures circulatory status in lower extremities has not been compromised.
3 Observe patient's reaction to elastic stockings and/or SCD sleeves.	Ensures patient is adapting to elastic stockings and/or SCD sleeves.
4 Observe patient or caregiver apply elastic stockings.	Determines ability to perform skill accurately.
5 Inspect SCD for kinks or twisting in tubing.	Ensures proper functioning of unit.

Unexpected Outcomes	Related Interventions
1 Skin reaction to elastic stockings or SCD.	• Observe for evidence of redness, skin lesions, and patient's subjective report of itching or burning. • Some patients may have an allergic skin reaction to material used in elastic stockings or SCD.
2 Decrease in circulation in lower extremities.	• Assess lower extremities for coolness, cyanosis, decreased pedal pulses, decreased blanching, and numbness or tingling sensation. • Check that elastic stockings are not too small or have wrinkles or folds that impede circulation (Brady and others, 2007). • Notify physician immediately; signs and symptoms may indicate obstruction of arterial blood flow.
3 Possible deep vein thrombosis.	• Because clinical signs may be vague, an order for more sensitive radiology tests should be obtained from a physician. Doppler compression ultrasonogram (also known as Doppler duplex) or impedance plethysmography may be carried out to rule out the presence of thrombosis (Monohan and others, 2007). • Do not massage lower extremities because of potential for dislodging thrombus.
4 Pulmonary embolism develops.	• Signs and symptoms include tachypnea, shortness of breath, anxiety, pleuritic chest pain, cough, hemoptysis, tachycardia, and signs of right ventricular failure (i.e., distended neck veins) (Monohan and others, 2007). • Notify physician immediately. • Monitor vital signs. • Administer supplemental oxygen as ordered.
5 Alarm on SCD mechanical unit is activated.	• Troubleshoot: check for kinks in tubing, air leaks, and that all connections are secure. • Get a new mechanical unit if there is failure to find reason for alarm.

STEP	RATIONALE

Recording and Reporting

- Record in nurses' notes date and time of elastic stockings and/or SCD sleeves application, condition of skin and circulatory status of lower extremities before application, length and size of elastic stockings and SCD sleeves, time elastic stockings and SCD sleeves are removed, condition of skin and circulatory status after removal.
- Immediately report signs of thrombophlebitis or impeded circulation in lower extremities to charge nurse or physician.

Teaching Considerations

- Provide time for patient to perform return demonstration of application of elastic stockings.
- Instruct patient to launder elastic stockings every 2 days with mild detergent and lay flat to dry.
- Recommend that patient have two pair of elastic stockings so that a clean set is available at all times.
- Instruct patient to wear nonskid shoes when getting up with elastic stockings to prevent risk for falls.

Pediatric Considerations

- Elastic stockings are not generally used with younger children. However, they are used when their condition warrants and sizes are available for their needs. When the size is not available, elastic wraps may sometimes be used. Extra caution is needed to monitor elastic wrap application to ensure bandage is not constricting circulation in leg.
- SCD may be used occasionally in this patient population.
- Observe younger children frequently because of the potential for an electrical hazard. Keep mechanical unit out of reach of child (Hockenberry and Wilson, 2007).

Gerontological Considerations

- Perform comprehensive assessment of older adults. Normal physiological aging can mask the signs and symptoms of venous insufficiency.
- Older adults may need assistance in applying elastic stockings because of decreased strength or arthritic changes in the hands.
- Older adults may experience wasting of muscles because of the aging process; therefore it is essential to measure these patients carefully to ensure proper fit.
- Reinforce need for the older patient to call for help before transferring from bed to prevent entanglement with cord or tubing from SCD mechanical unit.

Home Care Considerations

- Assess if patient is adhering to prescribed use of elastic stockings. Potential reasons for discontinuing use are the expense, cosmetic concerns, discomfort, and difficulty with application.
- Elastic stockings should be removed at least twice a day, and inspection of the skin and circulation of the extremities should be carried out by the patient.
- Instruct caregiver or patient in troubleshooting when SCD mechanical unit alarms.
- SCD sleeves should be checked periodically for air leaks and wear and tear.

Long-Term Care Considerations

- Elastic stockings will lose elasticity over time and should be replaced at least every 6 months.
- SCD sleeves may lose their elasticity from long-term use. Check frequently for wear and tear.
- Check for proper fit. Elastic stockings and SCD sleeves may become too tight or loose if patient's weight fluctuates.

SKILL 10-4   Assisting With Ambulation and Use of Canes, Crutches, and Walker

Patients who are immobile for even a short time may require assistance with ambulation. Assistance may mean walking alongside a patient while providing support, or a patient may require the use of an assistive device to aid in ambulation. Whenever assisting a patient up and out of bed or a chair there is a risk for orthostatic hypotension. Orthostatic hypotension or postural hypotension is a drop in blood pressure that occurs when a patient changes from a horizontal to a vertical position. A drop in blood pressure greater than 20 mm Hg in systolic pressure or 10 mm Hg in diastolic pressure with symptoms of dizziness, light-headedness, nausea, tachycardia, pallor, and fainting indicates orthostatic hypotension. Before ambulating patients, use interventions to maintain muscle tone, increase venous return to the heart, and decrease stasis of blood in the lower extremities. Use safety precautions before and during ambulation to control for orthostatic hypotension and subsequent falling.

An assistive device may be ordered to increase stability, to support a weak extremity, or to reduce the load on weight-bearing structures such as hips, knees, or ankles. These devices range from standard canes, which provide minimal support, to crutches and walkers, which are often used by patients who are unable to bear complete weight on the lower extremities or who bear weight on only one lower extremity. When assisting a patient with weight bearing restrictions to walk, position yourself on the patient's stronger side. Then, if the patient begins to fall, you can pull the patient toward you on the stronger side.

Selection of the appropriate device depends on the patient's age, diagnosis, muscular coordination, and ease of maneuverability (Hoeman, 2007). Use of assistive devices may be temporary, such as during recuperation from a fractured extremity or orthopedic surgery, or permanent, as in the case of a patient with paralysis or permanent weakness of the lower extremities.

Canes are lightweight, easily movable devices that extend about waist high and are made of wood or metal. Canes help to maintain balance by widening the base of support. They are indicated for patients with hemiparesis and are used to ease the strain on weight-bearing joints. Canes are not recommended for patients with bilateral leg weakness; for such patients, crutches or a walker are more appropriate (Hoeman, 2007). There are three types of commonly used canes. The *standard crook* cane provides the least support and is used by patients requiring only minimal assistance to walk. It has a half-circle handle, which allows it to be hooked over chairs. The *tripod cane* (pyramid cane) has three legs, and the *quad cane* has four legs; the additional legs provide a wide base of support. These types of canes are useful for patients with unilateral, partial, or complete leg paralysis. They also have the advantage of standing alone, freeing the arms to help the patient rise from a chair.

A crutch is a wooden or metal staff that reaches from the ground almost to the axilla. Crutches are used to remove weight from one or both legs. They are used by patients who must transfer more weight to their arms than is possible with canes. There are three types of crutches: *axillary*, *Lofstrand*, and *platform*. The axillary crutch is frequently used by patients of all ages on a short-term basis. The Lofstrand crutch has a hand grip and a metal band that fits around a patient's forearm. Both the metal band and the hand grip are adjusted to fit the patient's height. This type of crutch is useful for patients with a permanent disability, such as paraplegia. The metal arm band stabilizes and assists in guiding the crutch. The band offers other advantages as well. First, the encircling arm band allows patients to use their hands for other activities, such as opening doors, without dropping the crutches. Second, the anterior opening of the band allows patients to free themselves of the crutches if a fall occurs. The platform crutch is used by patients who are unable to bear weight on their wrists. It has a horizontal trough on which patients can rest their forearms and wrists and a vertical handle for the patient to grip.

A walker is an extremely light, movable device, about waist high, consisting of a metal frame with handgrips, four widely placed, sturdy legs, and one open side. Because it has a wide base of support, the walker provides great stability and security. A walker can be used by a patient who is weak or who has problems with balance (Hoeman, 2007). In addition to the standard walker,

there are several other models available: a foldable version that is easy to transport, one with a fold-down seat, and one with wheels on the front legs. Walkers with wheels are useful for patients who have difficulty lifting the walker as they walk because of limited balance or endurance. The disadvantage, however, is that the walker can roll forward when weight is applied (Hoeman, 2007).

Delegation Considerations

The skill of assisting patients with ambulation can be delegated to NAP. The nurse directs the NAP by:
- Instructing to have the patient dangle following lying in bed before ambulation.
- Instructing to immediately return the patient to the bed or chair if the patient is nauseated, dizzy, pale, or diaphoretic. Report these signs and symptoms immediately.
- Discussing the importance of applying safe, nonskid shoes and ensuring that the environment is free of clutter and there is no moisture on the floor before ambulating patient.

Equipment
- ❑ Ambulation device (crutch, walker, cane)
- ❑ Safety device (gait belt)
- ❑ Well-fitting, flat, nonskid shoes for patient
- ❑ Robe
- ❑ Goniometer (*optional*)

STEP	RATIONALE

ASSESSMENT

1 Review patient's chart, including:
  a Patient's medical history

  b Patient's previous activity level

  c Current activity order

2 Assess patient's physical readiness:
  a Obtain patient's heart rate, blood pressure, and orientation to time, place, and person.

  b Observe ROM, muscle strength, coordination, and whether there is the presence of foot deformities.

  c Assess patient for any visual, perceptual, or sensory deficits.
  d Assess environment for potential threats to patient safety.
  e Assess patient for discomfort.

3 Determine patient's or caregiver's understanding of technique of ambulation to be used.

4 Determine optimal time for ambulation.

5 Assess degree of assistance patient needs.

Certain medications, chronic illness, and history of falling may influence patient's ability to ambulate independently.
Identifies patient's previous activity level. Patient may tire easily or be prone to orthostatic hypotension if bed rest has been prolonged.
Verifies if an ambulation aid is needed and specifies amount of activity permitted.

Ambulation following immobility can be fatiguing and stressful. Baseline is needed to detect orthostatic hypotension. Baseline vital signs also offer a means for comparison after exercise. The oriented patient is able to understand instructions.
Determines if patient has enough flexibility and muscle strength to ambulate safely and if patient needs muscle-strengthening exercises. Determines the presence of foot deformities affecting ambulation.
Determines if patient can use assistive device safely. Ambulation after immobility can be fatiguing and stressful.
Protects patient from potential injury.
Patient may be in pain or may fear pain resulting from exercise. If necessary, administer analgesic before exercise.
Allows patient to verbalize concerns. Patients who have been immobile for a long time may be hesitant to ambulate. Caregiver may be hesitant to learn how to assist with ambulation.
Patient's personal habits must be considered when planning activities.
For safety, another person may be needed initially to assist with patient ambulation. Allow patient as much independence as possible.

STEP	RATIONALE

NURSING DIAGNOSES

- Activity intolerance
- Decreased cardiac output
- Fatigue

- Impaired physical mobility
- Ineffective peripheral tissue perfusion
- Risk for fall

- Risk for impaired skin integrity
- Risk for injury

Individualize related factors based on patient's condition or needs.

PLANNING

1 Expected outcomes following completion of procedure:
- Patient ambulates without injury.

- Patient is able to ambulate without excessive fatigue or dizziness.
- Patient demonstrates correct gait.
- Patient resumes social and self-care activities.

Precautions prevent orthostatic hypotension. Appropriate level of assistance on device ensures patient's safety.
Assistive device chosen requires minimal exertion.

Demonstrates learning.
Progressive ambulating activities increase patient's endurance and independence.

2 Preparing patient for ambulation:
- **a** Explain reasons for exercise, and demonstrate specific gait technique to patient or caregiver.
- **b** Decide with patient how far to ambulate.
- **c** Schedule ambulation around patient's other activities.

- **d** Place bed in low position, and slowly assist patient to Fowler's upright position. If in chair, have patient sit upright with feet flat on floor.
- **e** Assist patient in bed to a dangling position on side of bed (see illustration). Let patient sit for a few minutes, taking a few deep breaths, until balance is gained. Have patient move legs and feet while dangling. Assist the sitting patient to a standing position and allow to stand until balance is gained.

Teaching and demonstration enhance learning, reduce anxiety, and encourage cooperation.
Determines mutual goal.
Taking scheduled rest periods between activities reduces patient fatigue.
Allows a few minutes for circulation to equilibrate. Prevents orthostatic hypotension and potential injuries.

Movement of legs in dangling position promotes venous return (Eanarroch, 2007).

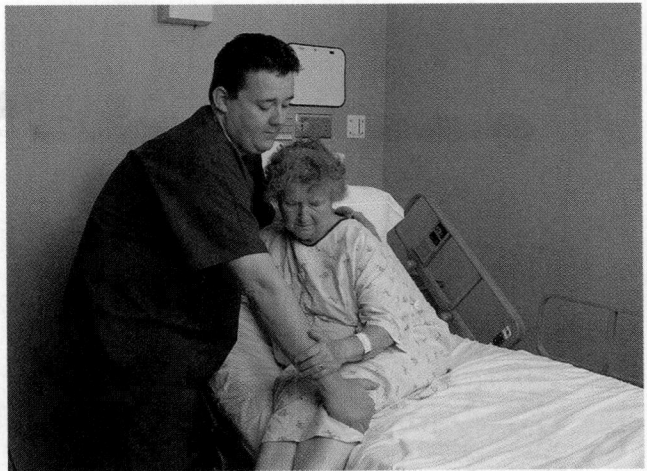

STEP 2e   Assisting patient to side of bed. (*From DeWit SC:* Fundamental concepts and skills for nursing, *ed 2, Philadelphia, 2005, Saunders.*)

- **f** Ask if patient feels dizzy or light-headed. If patient appears light-headed, sit patient back down and recheck blood pressure.

Allows nurse to detect orthostatic hypotension before ambulation begins.

STEP	RATIONALE

g   Care must be taken if patient has intravenous (IV) tubing or a Foley catheter. Obtain an IV pole with wheels that can be pushed as patient walks. Urinary catheter drainage bags must stay at or below the level of the bladder, so a second person may be needed to assist.

Allows patient to ambulate unencumbered.
Urine in tubing must not reenter bladder, which would increase infection risk.

Critical Decision Point   *Remove obstacles from pathways, including throw rugs, and wipe up any spills immediately. Avoid crowds. Crowds increase the risk for the crutch, cane, or walker being kicked or jarred and patient losing balance.*

3   Determining appropriate height of ambulation device, if used:

a   *Crutch measurement:* Includes three areas: patient's height, distance between crutch pad and axilla, and angle of elbow flexion. Use one of two methods:

(1)   *Standing:* Position crutches with crutch tips at 15 cm (6 inches) to side and 15 cm in front of patient's feet and crutch pads 5 cm (2 inches) below axilla (Hoeman, 2007).

Promotes optimal support and stability.

Radial nerve passes under axillary area superficially. If crutch is too long, it can cause pressure on axilla and radial nerve. Injury to radial nerve causes paralysis of elbow and wrist extensors, commonly called crutch palsy. Also, if crutch is too long, shoulders are forced upward and patient cannot push body off the ground. If ambulation device is too short, patient will be bent over and uncomfortable.

(2)   *Supine:* Crutch pad is approximately 5 cm or two to three finger widths under axilla with crutch tips positioned 15 cm (6 inches) lateral to patient's heel (Hoeman, 2007) (see illustration).

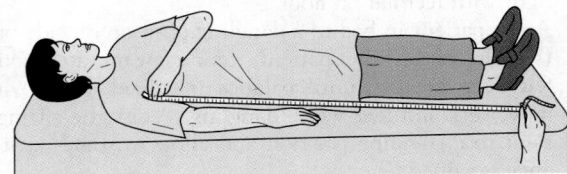

STEP 3a(2)   Supine method.

(3)   Instruct patient to report any tingling or numbness in the upper torso.

(4)   Following correct crutch adjustment, two to three fingers must fit between top of crutch and axilla (see illustration).

May mean crutches are being used incorrectly or that they are wrong size.
Adequate space prevents crutch palsy.

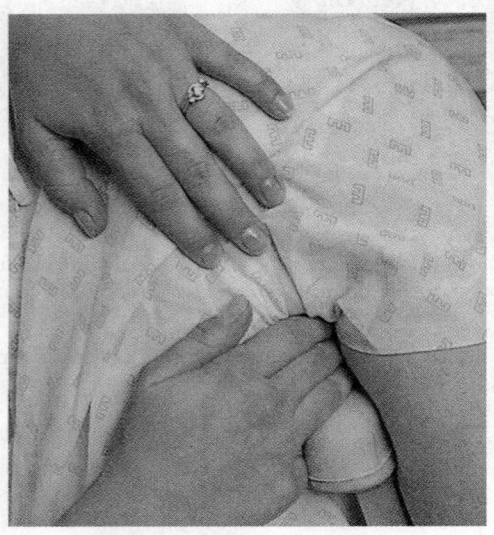

STEP 3a(4)   Top of crutch.

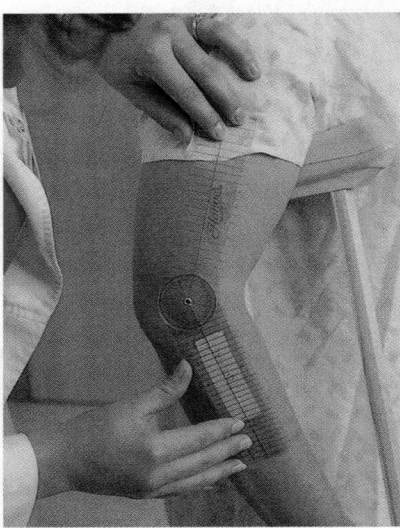

STEP 3a(5)   Elbows flexed. Verification of elbow flexion.

STEP	RATIONALE
(5) With either measurement method, elbows are flexed 15 to 30 degrees. Verify elbow flexion with goniometer (see illustration).	Angle ensures arms can push body off ground. Goniometer can be obtained from physical therapy department.
(6) In addition to overall *length* of axillary crutch, *height* of handgrip is important. Both dimensions are adjustable on a well-made crutch, and the ability to adjust these dimensions is an important feature for a growing child. Adjust handgrip so that patient's elbow is slightly flexed.	If handgrip is too low, radial nerve damage can occur even if overall crutch length is correct because the extra length between handgrip and axillary bar can force bar up into axilla as patient stretches down to reach handgrip. If handgrip is too high, patient's elbow is sharply flexed, and strength and stability of arms are decreased.
b *Cane measurement:* Patient holds cane on uninvolved side 10 to 15 cm (4 to 6 inches) to side of foot. Cane extends from greater trochanter to floor while cane is held 15 cm (6 inches) from foot (Hoeman, 2007). Allow approximately 15 to 30 degrees of elbow flexion.	Offers most support when cane is placed on stronger side of body. Cane and weaker leg work together with each step. If cane is too short, patient will have difficulty supporting weight and be bent over and uncomfortable. As weight is taken on by hand and affected leg is lifted off floor, complete extension of elbow is necessary.
c *Walker measurement:* Upper bar of walker is slightly below patient's waist. Elbows are flexed at approximately 15 to 30 degrees when patient is standing inside walker with hands on handgrips.	
4 Make sure the ambulation device has rubber tips.	Rubber tips prevent the device from slipping.
5 Make sure the surface patient will walk on is clean and dry. Remove any objects that might obstruct the pathway.	Prevents injuries.

IMPLEMENTATION

1 Assisted ambulation with one nurse:	
a Before beginning ambulation, confirm that patient does not feel light-headed.	Helps patient gain balance before attempting ambulation and ensures that patient will not become faint while walking.
b Apply gait belt, and assist patient to standing position; observe balance.	Prevents injury. Gait belt encircles patient's waist and has space for nurse to hold while patient walks. If patient appears weak or unsteady, return patient to bed.
c Have patient take a few steps while nurse is positioned on patient's stronger side. If an assistive device (e.g., cane, walker) is used, then nurse stands on patient's weak side.	If patient has hemiplegia (one-sided paralysis) or hemiparesis (one-sided weakness), stand next to patient's unaffected side, and support patient by placing arm closest to patient on the walking belt.
d Stand on patient's stronger or uninjured side and grasp gait belt in middle of patient's back.	If patient begins to fall, this position allows the caregiver to move the patient to the stronger side and reduce injury. Provides support at waist so patient's center of gravity remains midline.
e Take a few steps forward with patient. Then assess for strength and balance.	Ensures patient has satisfactory strength and balance to continue.
f If patient becomes weak or dizzy, return patient to bed or chair, whichever is closer.	Allows patient to rest.

STEP	RATIONALE

g If patient begins to fall, gently ease patient to floor by holding firmly onto gait belt, stand with feet apart to provide broad base of support, extend leg, and let patient gently slide to the floor. As patient slides, nurse bends knees to lower body (see illustrations).

Nurse can cause more damage to self and patient by trying to catch patient.

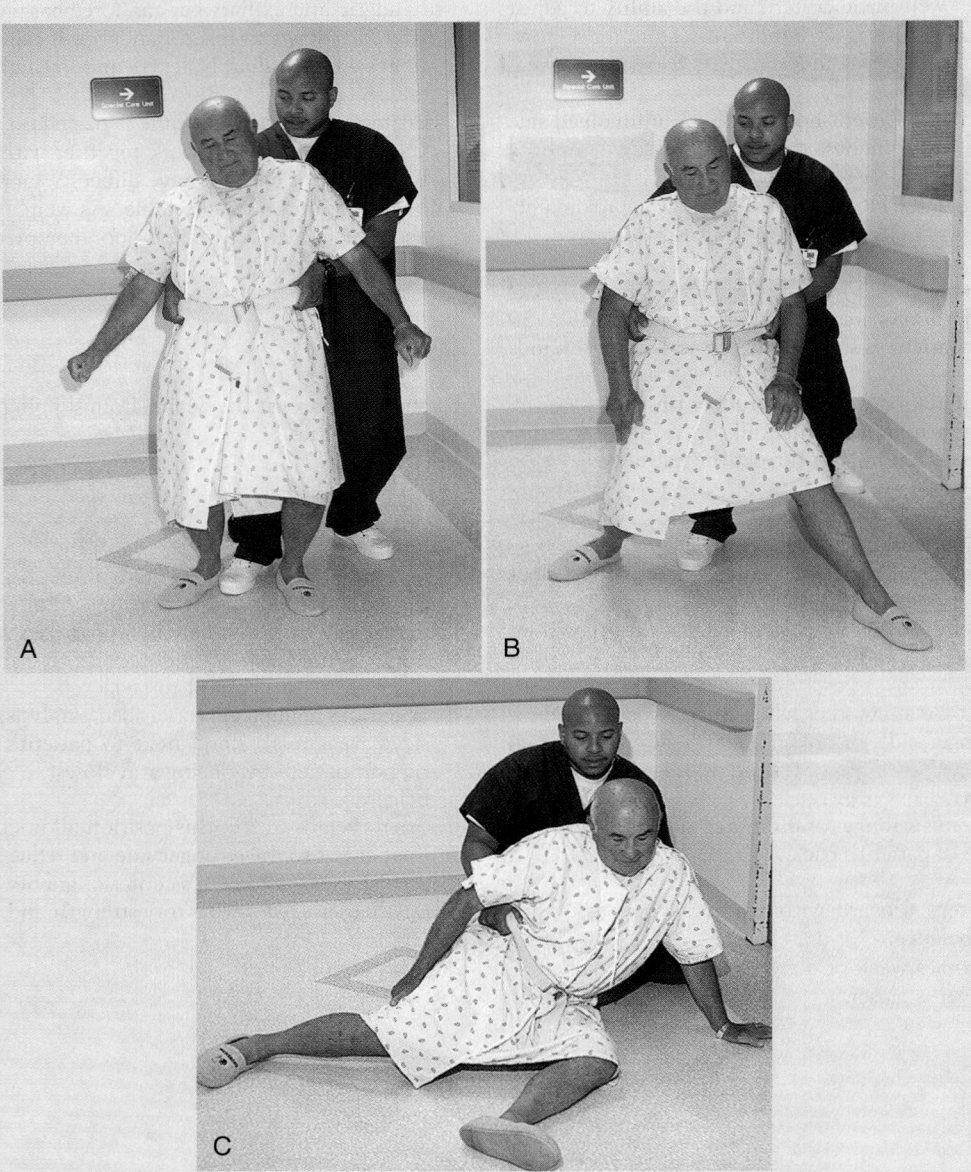

STEP 1g   **A,** Stand with feet apart to provide broad base of support. **B,** Extend one leg, and let patient slide against it to the floor. **C,** Bend knees to lower body as patient slides to floor.

STEP	RATIONALE
2 Assisted ambulation with two nurses:	
a Follow Steps 1a and 1b.	
b Have a nurse stand on either side of patient.	
c Both nurses grasp walking belt in middle of patient's back.	Provides secure grip for each nurse.
d Step forward in unison with patient, keeping speed and step size same as patient's.	Ensures stability of patient.
e Gradually increase distance walked.	Strengthens muscles, increases endurance, and prevents patient from becoming too fatigued.
f If patient becomes weak or dizzy, follow Steps 1f and g.	
3 Ambulation with assistive devices:	
a Assisting patient in crutch walking by choosing appropriate crutch gait:	To use crutches, patient supports self with hands and arms; therefore strength in arm and shoulder muscles, ability to balance body in upright position, and stamina are necessary. Exercises such as squeezing a rubber ball, raising and lowering both arms in a slow and rhythmic manner while holding weights, push-ups, and pull-ups will assist in strengthening the upper extremities. The type of gait patient uses in crutch walking depends on amount of weight patient is able to support with one or both legs.
(1) Four-point gait:	This is the most stable of crutch gaits because it provides at least three points of support at all times. Patient must be able to bear weight on both legs. Each leg is moved alternately with each opposing crutch so that three points of support are on the floor all the time. Often used when patient has some form of paralysis, such as for spastic children with spastic cerebral palsy (Hockenberry and Wilson, 2007). May also be used for arthritic patients.
(a) Begin in tripod position. Place crutches 15 cm (6 inches) in front and 6 inches to side of each foot. Have the patient place weight on the handgrips, not under the arms (see illustration).	Improves patient's balance by providing wide base of support. Patient should have a posture of erect head and neck, straight vertebrae, and extended hips and knees.

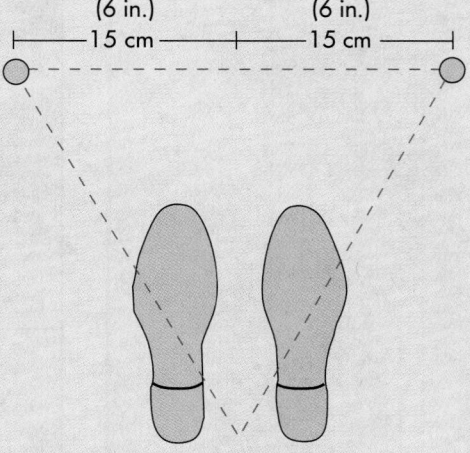

STEP 3a(1)(a)   Tripod position.

STEP	RATIONALE

(b) Move right crutch forward 10 to 15 cm (4 to 6 inches) (see illustration A).

(c) Move left foot forward to level of left crutch (see illustration B).

(d) Move left crutch forward 10 to 15 cm (4 to 6 inches) (see illustration C).

(e) Move right foot forward to level of right crutch (see illustration D).

(f) Repeat above sequence.

Crutch and foot position is similar to arm and foot position during normal walking.

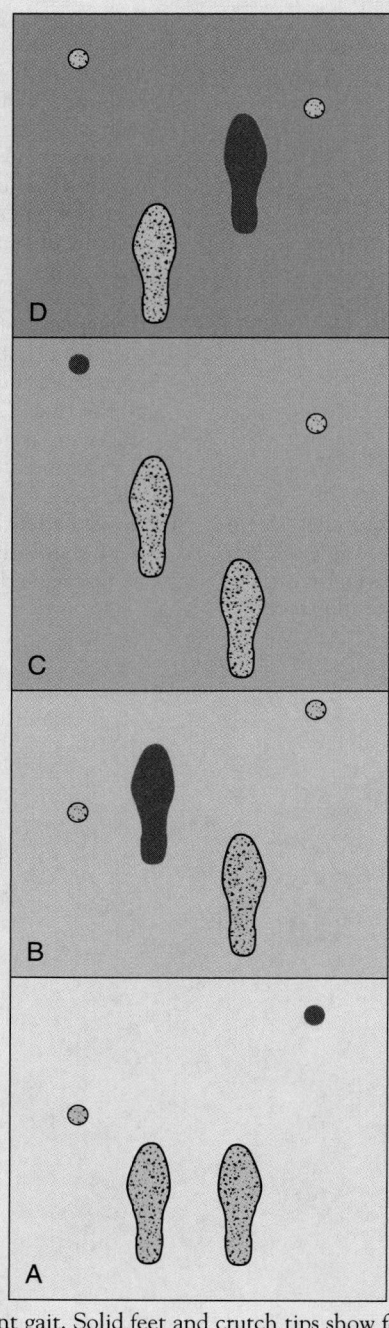

STEP 3a(1)(b-e) Four-point gait. Solid feet and crutch tips show foot and crutch tip movement in each of the four phases. (Read from bottom to top.) **A,** Right tip moves forward. **B,** Left foot moves toward left crutch. **C,** Left crutch tip moves forward. **D,** Right foot moves toward right crutch.

STEP	RATIONALE
(2) Three-point gait:	Requires patient to bear all weight on one foot. Weight is borne on uninvolved leg and then on both crutches. Affected leg does not touch ground during early phase of three-point gait. May be useful for patient with broken leg or sprained ankle.
(a) Begin in tripod position (see illustration A).	Improves patient's balance by providing wide base of support.
(b) Advance both crutches and affected leg (see illustration B).	
(c) Move stronger leg forward, stepping on floor (see illustration C).	
(d) Repeat sequence.	
(3) Two-point gait:	Requires at least partial weight bearing on each foot. Is faster than the four-point gait. Requires more balance because only two points support body at one time (Hoeman, 2007).
(a) Begin in tripod position (see illustration A).	Improves patient's balance by providing wide base of support.
(b) Move left crutch and right foot forward (see illustration B).	Crutch movements are similar to arm movement during normal walking as patient moves a crutch at the same time as the opposing leg.
(c) Move right crutch and left foot forward (see illustration C).	
(d) Repeat sequence.	

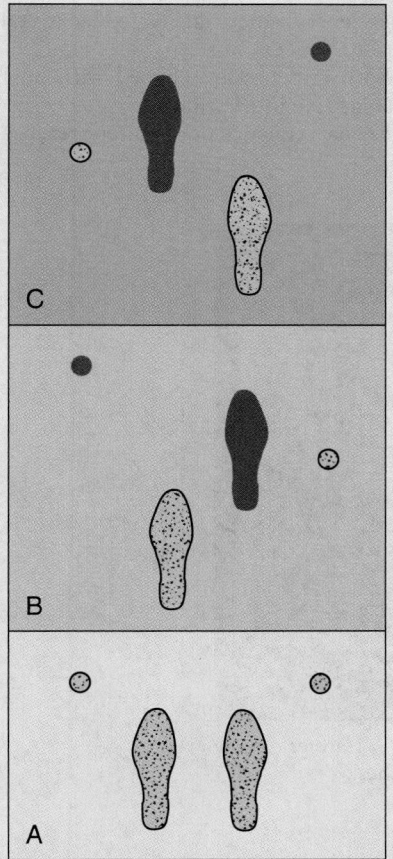

STEP 3a(2)(a-c) Three-point gait with weight borne on unaffected right leg. Solid foot and crutch tips show weight bearing in each phase. (Read from bottom to top.)

STEP 3a(3)(a-c) Two-point gait. Solid areas indicate weight-bearing leg and crutch tips. (Read from bottom to top.)

STEP	RATIONALE

(4) Swing-to gait:

Frequently used by patients whose lower extremities are paralyzed or who wear weight-supporting braces on their legs.

    (a) Begin in tripod position.

This is the easier of the two swinging gaits. It requires the ability to partially bear body weight on both legs.

    (b) Move both crutches forward.
    (c) Lift and swing legs to crutches, letting crutches support body weight.
    (d) Repeat two previous steps.

(5) Swing-through gait:

Requires that patient have the ability to bear partial weight on both feet.

    (a) Begin in tripod position.

Improves patient's balance by providing wide base of support.

    (b) Move both crutches forward.

Initial placement of crutches is to increase patient's base of support so that when the body swings forward, patient is moving the center of gravity toward the additional support provided by the crutches.

    (c) Lift and swing legs through and beyond crutches.

b Assisting patient in climbing stairs with crutches:

(1) Begin in tripod position.

Improves patient's balance by providing wide base of support.

(2) Patient transfers body weight to crutches (see illustration).

Prepares patient to transfer weight to unaffected leg when ascending first stair.

(3) Patient advances unaffected leg to stair (see illustration).

Crutch adds support to affected leg. Patient then shifts weight from crutches to unaffected leg.

(4) Both crutches are aligned with unaffected leg on stairs (see illustration).

Maintains balance and provides wide base of support.

(5) Repeat sequence until patient reaches top of stairs.

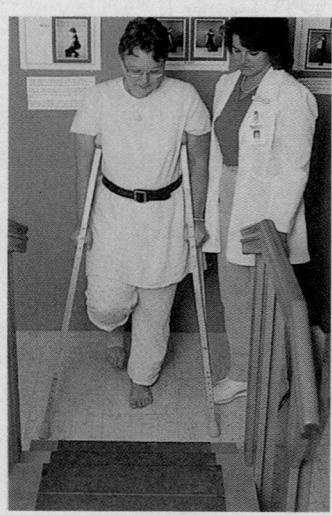

STEP 3b(2) Transfer body weight to crutches.

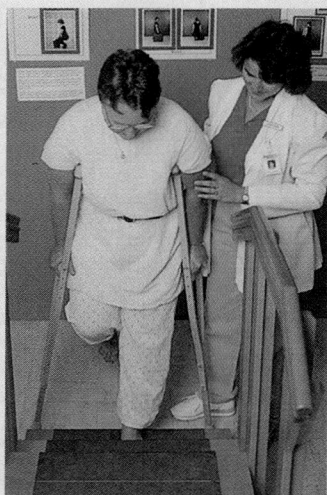

STEP 3b(3) Advance unaffected leg to stair.

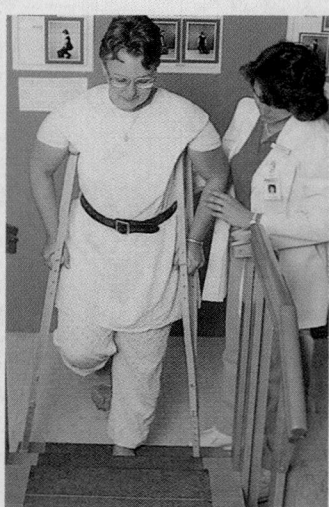

STEP 3b(4) Align crutches with unaffected leg.

STEP	RATIONALE

c   Assisting patient in descending stairs with crutches:

(1)   Begin in tripod position.

(2)   Patient transfers body weight to unaffected leg (see illustration).

(3)   Move crutches to stair, and instruct patient to begin to transfer body weight to crutches (see illustration) and move affected leg forward.

(4)   Patient moves unaffected leg to stair and aligns with crutches (see illustration).

(5)   Repeat sequence until stairs are descended.

Improves patient's balance by providing wide base of support.

Prepares patient to release support of body weight maintained by crutches.

Maintains patient's balance and base of support.

Maintains balance and provides base of support.

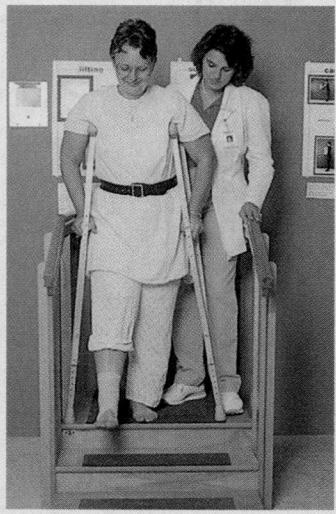

STEP 3c(2) Body weight is transferred to unaffected leg.

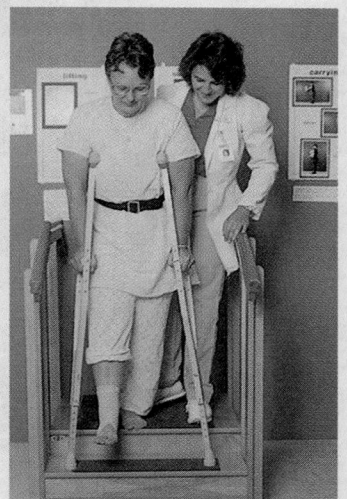

STEP 3c(3) Transfer weight to crutches.

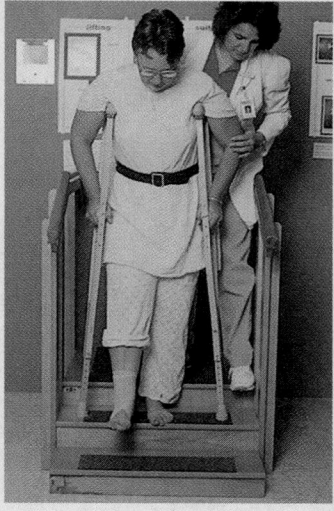

STEP 3c(4) Move unaffected leg, and align crutches.

STEP	RATIONALE

d   Assisting patient in ambulating with walker (see illustration):

Walker is used by patients who are able to bear partial weight. Walkers do need to be picked up, so patient does need sufficient strength to be able to pick up walker. Four-wheeled model does not need to be picked up; however, it is not as stable (Hoeman, 2007).

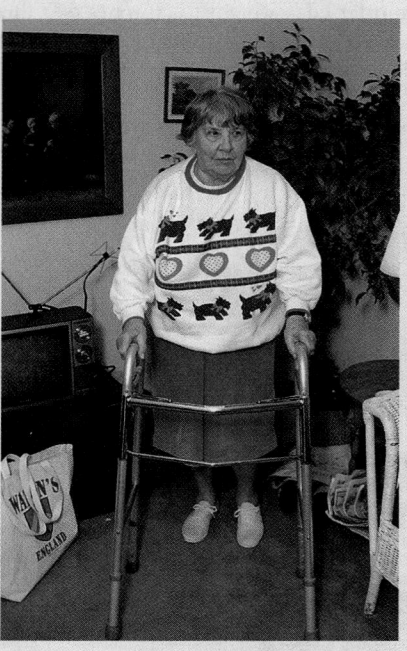

STEP 3d   Walker.

(1)   Have patient stand in center of walker and grasp handgrips on upper bars.

Patient balances self before attempting to walk.

(2)   Lift walker, move it 15 to 20 cm (6 to 8 inches) forward, and then set it down, making sure all four feet of the walker stay on the floor. Take a step forward with either foot. Then follow through with the other leg.

Provides broad base of support between walker and patient. Patient then moves center of gravity toward the walker. Keeping all four feet of the walker on the floor is necessary to prevent tipping of the walker.

(3)   If there is unilateral weakness, after the walker is advanced, instruct patient to step forward with the weaker leg, support self with the arms, and follow through with the uninvolved leg. If patient is unable to bear weight on one leg, after advancing walker have patient swing onto it, supporting weight on hands.

STEP	RATIONALE

e Assisting patient in ambulating with cane (same steps are taught whether standard or quad canes are used) (see illustrations):

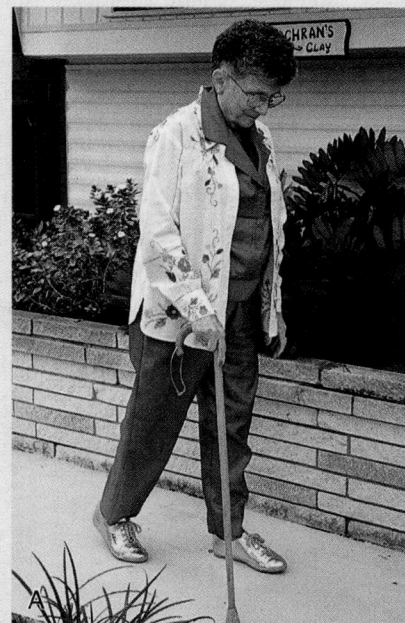
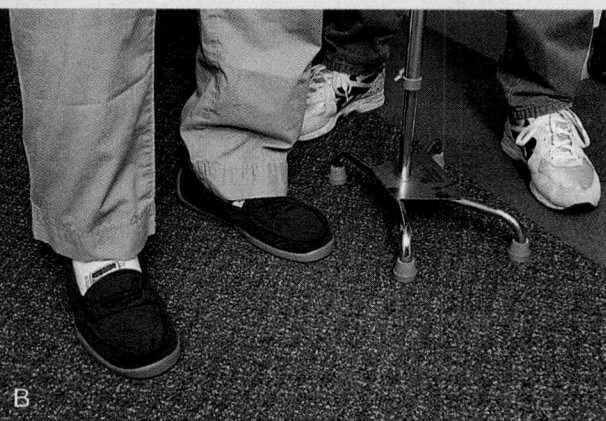

STEP 3e   **A,** Standard cane. **B,** Quad cane.

(1) Begin by placing cane on the side opposite the involved leg.	Provides added support for the weak or impaired side.
(2) Place cane forward 15 to 25 cm (6 to 10 inches), keeping body weight on both legs.	Distributes body weight equally.
(3) Move involved leg forward, even with the cane.	Body weight is supported by cane and uninvolved leg.
(4) Advance uninvolved leg past cane.	Body weight is supported by cane and involved leg.
(5) Move involved leg forward, even with uninvolved leg.	Aligns patient's center of gravity. Returns patient's body weight to equal distribution.
(6) Repeat these steps.	

EVALUATION

1 After ambulation, obtain patient's vital signs, observe skin color, and ask about patient's energy level.	Evaluates how patient tolerated procedure and evaluates whether there was progress in ambulation. Assesses stage of patient's illness and degree of convalescence when evaluating the process.
2 Evaluate patient's subjective statements regarding experience.	Evaluates activity tolerance.
3 Evaluate gait of patient, observing body alignment in standing position and balance.	Determines if patient is correctly using supportive aids for ambulation. Keep in mind patient's previous manner of ambulating when assessing gait.
4 Observe patient's ability to perform self-care activities.	

Unexpected Outcomes	Related Interventions
1 Patient is unable to ambulate because of fear of falling, physical discomfort, upper body muscles that are too weak to use ambulation device, and lower extremities that are too weak to support body.	• Initiate isometric exercise program to strengthen upper body muscles. • Provide analgesia if needed.
2 Patient sustains injury.	• Notify physician. Return patient to bed if injury stable.

Recording and Reporting

- Record in nurses' notes the type of gait patient used, amount of assistance required, distance walked, and activity tolerance.
- Immediately report any injury sustained during attempts to ambulate, alteration in vital signs, or inability to ambulate to nurse in charge or physician.

Teaching Considerations

- Teach patients using walkers to examine the frame daily. When inspecting a walker, the patient should observe for signs of bending or deformation of the frame, protruding screws that can scratch, and loose or missing screws that weaken the joints of the frame. Assess handgrips for any cracks or signs of being loose.
- Instruct patients to use the arms of a chair rather than the walker to give them leverage when getting up from a chair; the walker is likely to tip if used for this purpose.
- Blistering or soreness of the hands can result from continual pressure between the hand and the handle of a crutch. Advise patient to release pressure intermittently and wear gloves or pad the handle to reduce friction.

Pediatric Considerations

- For rehabilitation of a small child who has not yet learned to walk or who is unsteady, special crutches with three or four legs provide needed stability to allow the child to maintain an upright posture and learn to walk (Hockenberry and Wilson, 2007).
- Another option for children who are just learning to walk would be front- or rear-rolling walkers.

Gerontological Considerations

- The older adult may require additional time in the morning before resuming activities.

Home Care Considerations

- Instruct patient in how to use the ambulation aid on various terrains (e.g., carpet, stairs, rough ground, inclines). Instruct patient in how to maneuver around obstacles such as doors and how to use the aid when transferring to and from a chair, toilet, and tub.

Long-Term Care Considerations

- Conduct safety and maintenance checks of ambulation devices on a routine basis.
- Perform periodic assessments to ensure that the patient is using the ambulation device properly.

 CRITICAL THINKING EXERCISES

Mr. Timber, 78 years old, is hospitalized for a right total knee replacement. He has a medical history of diabetes mellitus. He is now 1 day postoperative following right knee replacement. He rates his pain as 8 on a 10-point scale. Postoperative orders include ambulating with crutches today and using the CPM machine 4 times a day.

1 As you discuss the plan of care with Mr. Timber for the day, you include the need for ambulation with crutches. He states, "I'm not getting out of bed; I hurt and just had surgery." Discuss nursing interventions that will facilitate this patient's cooperation and participation.

2 Mr. Timber has several risk factors associated with the occurrence of orthostatic hypotension. Identify these risk factors and the nursing interventions needed to minimize orthostatic hypotension.

3 You are applying the CPM machine to Mr. Timber's right leg. Discuss several measures to ensure proper and safe functioning of this machine.

4 Mr. Timber needs crutches for approximately 4 to 6 weeks during his recovery. He is allowed no weight bearing on his right leg for the first week. What is the appropriate crutch gait for Mr. Timbers? Discuss several teaching considerations associated with the use of crutches.

REVIEW QUESTIONS

1 The nurse notes a patient's left elbow is resistant to extension and flexion while performing range-of-motion exercises. What is the appropriate nursing action at this time?
   1 Move the joint through the full range of motion.
   ② Perform range-of-motion to the left elbow only until resistance is met.

   3 Omit all the range-of-motion exercises until the physician is notified.
   4 Tell the physician that the patient is uncooperative with exercising.

2 A patient who has been immobile for more than 2 weeks is now able to begin performing isometric exercises. Which nursing diagnosis best relates to the safety of this patient?
   1 Disturbed thought processes
   2 Impaired skin integrity
   3 Disturbed body image
   ④ Risk for activity intolerance

3 The nurse suspects that a patient has deep vein thrombosis in the left lower leg. What is the priority nursing intervention at this time?
   1 Perform test for Homans' sign immediately.
   2 Massage the area gently to promote circulation.
   3 Keep the patient calm and quiet in bed.
   4 Apply the ordered elastic stockings and sequential compression devices.

4 Which of the following activities may be delegated to nursing assistive personnel in regard to assisting patients with ambulation?
   1 Check the patient's medications to determine if they may influence the ability to ambulate independently.
   2 Instruct the patient concerning the correct use of a walker.
   3 Inspect the environment for potential threats to patient safety.
   ④ Evaluate the patient's ability to perform crutch walking.

5 The nurse is preparing to ambulate a married, female Muslim patient with left-sided weakness. Which action demonstrates appropriate care of this patient during ambulation?
   1 Assign the strongest health care worker to ambulate her.
   2 Stand on the left side of the patient during ambulation.
   3 The patient will hold her cane in her left hand while the nurse is behind her during ambulation.
   ④ A female caregiver should walk on the patient's right side.

REFERENCES

Eanarroch E: Orthostatic and postprandial hypotension. In J Biller, editor: *The interface of neurology & internal medicine*, Hagerstown, Md, 2007, Lippincott Williams and Wilkins.

Galanti G: *Caring for patients from different cultures*, Philadelphia, 2003, University of Pennsylvania Press.

Gillespie HO: Exercise. In Edelman CL, Mandle CL, editors: *Health promotion throughout the lifespan*, ed 6, St. Louis, 2006, Mosby.

Grande C, Caparro M: Use of low-molecular-weight heparins in the treatment and secondary prevention of cancer-associated thrombosis, *Semin Oncol Nurs* 21(4):41, 2005.

Hockenberry MJ, Wilson D: *Wong's nursing care of infants and children*, ed 8, St. Louis, 2007, Mosby.

Hoeman S: *Rehabilitation prevention, intervention, and outcomes*, ed 4, St. Louis, 2007, Mosby.

Huether S, McCance K: *Understanding pathophysiology*, ed 4, St. Louis, 2008, Mosby.

Hums W, Blostein P: A comparative approach to deep vein thrombosis risk assessment, *J Trauma Nurs* 13(1):28, 2006.

Ignatavicius D, Workman L: *Medical surgical nursing: critical thinking for collaborative care*, ed 5, St. Louis, 2006, Mosby.

Kasper D and others, editors: *Harrison's principles of internal medicine*, ed 16, New York, 2005, McGraw-Hill.

Meiner S, Lueckenotte A: *Gerontologic Nursing*, ed 3, St. Louis, 2006, Mosby.

Monohan WJ and others: *Phipps' medical-surgical nursing: health and illness perspectives*, ed 8, St. Louis, 2007, Mosby.

Pasero D, McCaffery M: Comfort-function goals, *Am J Nurs* 104(9):77, 2004.

Rashidi A, Rajaram S: Culture care conflicts among Asian-Islamic immigrant women in U.S. hospitals, *Holist Nurse Pract* 16(1):55, 2001.

RESEARCH REFERENCES

Akyol A: Falls in the elderly: what can be done? *Int Nurs Rev* 54(2):191, 2007.

Berry PH and others: *Pain: current understanding of assessment, management, and treatment*, Reston, Va, 2006, National Pharmaceutical Council.

Brady D and others: The use of knee-length versus thigh-length compression stockings and sequential compression devices, *Crit Care Nurs Q* 30(3):255, 2007.

de Morton and others: Exercise for acutely hospitalized older medical patients, *Cochrane Database Sys Rev* (1)CD005955, 2007.

DeWit SC: *Fundamental concepts and skills for nursing*, ed 2, Philadelphia, 2005, Saunders.

Dossey B: *Holistic nursing: a handbook for practice*, ed 4, Boston, 2005, Jones & Bartlett.

Ejaz and others: Characteristics of 100 consecutive patients presenting with orthostatic hypotension, *Mayo Clin Proc* 79(7):890, 2004.

Hur H and others: Activity intolerance and impaired physical mobility in elders, *Int J Nurs Terminol Classif* 16(3-4):47, 2005.

Kehl-Pruett W: Deep vein thrombosis in hospitalized patients: a review of evidence based guidelines for prevention, *Dimens Crit Care Nurs* 25(2):53, 2006.

Lassetter J: The effectiveness of complementary therapies on the pain experience of hospitalized children, *J Holist Nurs* 24(3):196, 2006.

Liu-Ambrose T and others: Resistance and agility training reduce fall risk in women aged 75 to 85 with low bone mass: a 6-month randomized, controlled trial, *J Am Geriatr Soc* 52(5):657, 2004.

Mauer M and others: The degree and timing of orthostatic blood pressure changes in relation to falls in nursing home residents, *J Am Med Dir Assoc* 5(4):233, 2004.

Padilla J and others: Accumulation of physical activity reduces blood pressure in pre- and hypertension, *Med Sci Sports Exerc* 37(8):1264, 2005.

Rawat A and others: Primary prophylaxis of venous thromboembolism in surgical patients, *Vasc Endovasc Surg* 43(3):205, 2008.

Rydwik E and others: Physical training in institutionalized elderly people with multiple diagnoses—a controlled pilot study, *Arch Gerontol Geriatr* 40(1):29, 2005.

Schneider JK and others: Promoting exercise behavior in older adults, *J Gerontol Nurs* 30(4):45, 2004.

Schrezenmaier C and others: Evaluation of orthostatic hypotension: relationship of a new self-report instrument to laboratory-based measures, *Mayo Clin Proc* 80(3):330, 2005.

Simpson J and others: Muslim women's experience with health care providers in a rural area of the United States, *J Transcult Health Care* 19(1):16, 2008.

Turvey C and others: Depression, physical impairment, and treatment of depression in chronic heart failure, *J Cardiovasc Nurs* 21(3):178, 2006.

Vara-González L and others: Reproducibility of postural changes of blood pressure in hypertensive elderly patients in primary care, *Blood Press Monit* (11)1:17, 2006.

Orthopedic Measures

KEY TERMS

Cast
Cast brace
Cast saw
Cast syndrome
Comminuted
  fracture
Compartment
  syndrome
Countertraction
Crepitation
External fixation
Harris splint
Neurovascular
  assessment

Pearson
  attachment
Petaling
Pulleys
Reduction
Spica cast
Spreader bar
Stockinette
Thomas splint
Traction
Traction boot
Walking heel

MEDIA RESOURCES

- **e**volve http://evolve.elsevier.com/Perry/skills
  learning system
  - Review Questions

OBJECTIVES

Mastery of content in this chapter will enable the nurse to:

- Explain benefits of the use of casts for patients with musculoskeletal injuries.
- Describe how to assist in application of casts.
- Describe neurovascular assessments of a patient with an orthopedic injury.
- Describe techniques for drying casts.
- Describe toileting techniques for patients in casts and traction.
- Describe turning and positioning techniques for patients in casts.

- Describe elements of patient education for a patient with a cast and after removal of a cast.
- Explain the purposes of placing patients in skin or skeletal traction.
- Describe patient conditions requiring the use of each form of skin or skeletal traction.
- Describe steps for applying each form of skin or skeletal traction.
- Explain nursing measures for preventing complications from traction.

Patients in a cast, traction, or other immobilization device are susceptible to problems that affect all body systems. Depending on the extent of a patient's injury or illness, an orthopedic device may affect a single body part or the entire body. Alterations in the patient's level of mobility require extensive nursing care.

The adequacy of central and peripheral circulation to the injured area is carefully assessed, because delivery of oxygen and removal of wastes are vital for bone healing, muscle growth and strength, and regaining mobility. Color, temperature, and capillary refill assessments provide data about the adequacy of circulation to the injured extremity. Inflammation, cellulitis, or edema indicates venous stasis or infection.

Integumentary tissues inside and outside a cast must remain healthy and well nourished. Assessment of the tissues includes detection of pressure, inflammation, or lesions that could lead to infection or pressure ulcers. Turning, positioning, and range-of-motion (ROM) exercises help to maintain the health of integumentary and musculoskeletal tissues of individuals in casts (Fig. 11-1). Turning

also aids circulation throughout the body, decreases the development of renal calculi, and prevents the development of pressure ulcers. In addition, musculoskeletal tissues maintain strength through regularly performed active ROM exercises with or without resistance or weight. Quadriceps-, gluteus-, triceps-, biceps-, and hamstring-setting exercises, performed routinely and steadily, help to maintain muscle mass and tone (see Chapter 10).

A challenge for nurses caring for patients in body or spica casts is to maintain respiratory function. Although turning facilitates lung expansion and removal of secretions from the airways, it also encourages patients to breathe deeply and cough. Bed rest over time affects respiration, resulting in decreased ventilation and alveolar collapse. Patients with altered mobility who develop respiratory complications require respiratory therapy and at times administration of antibiotics.

Additional challenges center on intake and maintenance of functions of the gastrointestinal and genitourinary systems. Patients in casts or traction who are confined to bed frequently

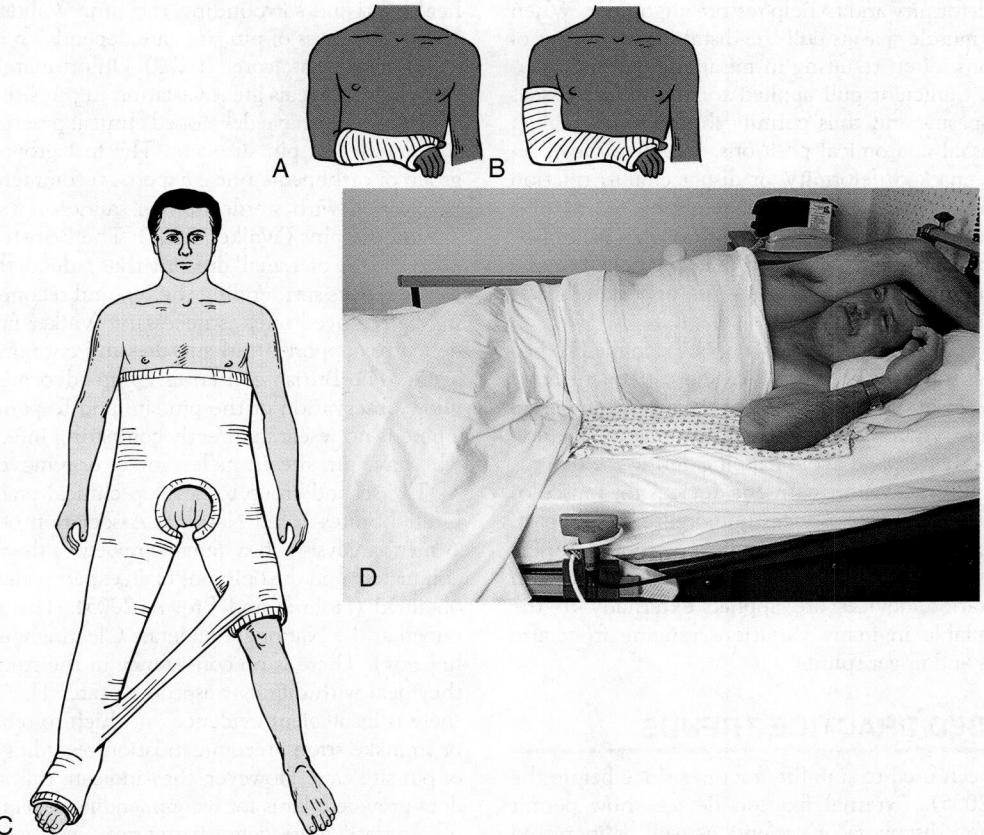

FIG 11-1   Types of casts. **A,** Short arm cast. **B,** Long arm cast. **C,** One-and-a-half hip spica cast. **D,** Body cast.

develop anorexia, constipation, and fecal impaction. Maintaining a high (3000 mL or more) fluid intake plus a high-bulk or high-residue diet fosters proper bowel elimination. Fluid intake also facilitates renal circulation and urinary output to lessen the possibility of a urinary tract infection or development of renal calculi. Diets should be high in protein, carbohydrates, vitamins, fiber, and fluids and should contain a moderate amount of fat, unless contraindicated. Because of individual metabolic and endocrine stress responses, a patient will experience catabolism with muscle mass loss for a period of 10 to 20 or more days. Bone remodeling, the process of bone resorption and bone deposit, is governed by hormones and stress placed on the bone. When serum calcium levels decrease, parathyroid hormone is released. This stimulates bone resorption, calcium is released from the bone, and the serum calcium level rises. This can lead to poor bone replacement and the development of osteoporosis and renal calculi. With an elevated serum calcium level, calcitonin from the thyroid gland is released, bone resorption is suppressed, and calcium salts are deposited in the bone matrix.

Casts, slings, and splints affect motor and sensory functions. Motor changes include muscle and joint weakness from disuse or pressure. Sensory changes from pressure or trauma include complaints of pain, numbness, and tingling. When such sensory signs are present, changing the patient's position may relieve them. It is essential to monitor for the five P's (pain, pallor, pulselessness, paresthesia, and paralysis) of neurovascular status, because permanent damage may result if circulation is not restored or pressure is not removed (Judge, 2007). Bivalving, cutting the cast, or loosening the immobilizer removes the pressure or tightness and increases circulation. Motor weakness can be restored to normal ranges through ROM exercises and physical therapy.

Traction is a force or pull applied to the bones directly or indirectly to overcome deformity and to help restore alignment. When bones are fractured, muscle spasms pull the distal fragments out of their normal positions, often resulting in misalignment and overriding of the bones. Sufficient pull applied to the injured tissues overcomes muscle spasms and thus permits the bones to realign themselves in the usual anatomical positions. In situations of severe muscle spasms, marked deformity, or displacement, traction must be applied directly to the distal fragments by means of a strong wire or pin to which traction is applied through a bar, ropes, pulleys, and weights. Such skeletal traction may be applied to one or more bones, including the bones of the skull, upper and lower extremities, and pelvic bones.

Patients in traction or those with casts who are confined to bed may easily tire during the day and often take short, frequent naps. Thus they are less sleepy at night and may lie awake past their usual bedtime. To offset this syndrome, have patients remain active, engage in stimulating activities, and avoid napping during the day.

Slings, splints, and braces are treatment devices for musculoskeletal injury or disorder. These devices immobilize a body part, prevent deformity, protect against injury, relieve pain and muscle spasm, maintain position until healing is complete, or assist with function. Immobilization devices are applied externally to the body. They are available in many variations ranging from arm slings to back braces and finger splints.

EVIDENCE-BASED PRACTICE TRENDS

Skeletal pins have been used to stabilize fractures since before the 1800s (Patterson, 2005). External fixation devices now permit early mobilization and discharge of patients as well as increased comfort. They are the treatment of choice for stabilization of open,

comminuted, unstable long bone fractures and for lengthening bones (Has and others, 2006). The pins are generally larger and have a high incidence of infection, with pin tract infection being one of the most common complications. Infection leading to osteomyelitis (infection of the bone) is a serious complication of skeletal traction.

Pin site care includes cleaning, dressing, and crust removal (Williams and Griffiths, 2004). Traditionally nurses performed pin site care to decrease the incidence of pin site infections. The recommendations for pin site care varied in the frequency of care, the cleansing agents used, the removal of crusts, and the application of dressings. Some clinicians recommended no pin site care as a method of reducing the incidence of infection. Often the protocol was physician or nurse preference. Until recently there was no uniform, consistent, research-based regimen accepted as the standard of care (Dahl and others, 2003; Patterson, 2005; Walker, 2007; Williams and Griffiths, 2004).

A Cochrane review of published research related to pin site care indicates that there is little evidence to support a specific protocol for pin site care (Temple and Santy, 2004). Williams and Griffiths (2004) also analyze the literature for research relating to cleansing of pin sites, dressing application, or crust removal in comparison to a control group with no pin site care. They find only one study meeting the criteria. In that study, one group was treated with 0.9% normal saline, another group with 70% alcohol, and the control group had no cleansing. In this small study, the normal saline group had the most positive outcome. They conclude that there is insufficient evidence to support daily treatment or no treatment of pin sites. More recently, Walker (2007) examines pin site care practices. Several studies find that although hydrogen peroxide is a common cleansing agent, it may cause damage to the healthy tissue surrounding the pin. Walker concludes that the "...effectiveness of pin site care depends on assessment and delivery of appropriate care" (p. 70). Unfortunately, the author's literature review reveals great variation in pin site care.

Two groups have developed clinical practice guidelines to direct the practice of pin site care. The first group, a British consensus group of orthopedic nurse experts, recommends that pin sites only be cleaned with sterile normal saline or water to remove crusts around the pins (Walker, 2007). The British consensus group supports the use of a small dressing that reduces the amount of pressure to the tissues surrounding the pin and recommends that the dressing be removed only as necessary. Walker finds no definitive evidence to support a pin site dressing containing an antimicrobial agent. The British consensus group advocates removal of crust to allow observation of the pin site and to permit exudate drainage. There is no research directly comparing infection rates in patients who have pin site crusts left intact or removed (Walker, 2007).

The second group to develop clinical practice guidelines is the United States–based National Association of Orthopaedic Nurses. A meta-analysis and systematic review of the research literature was conducted, and the opinions of an expert panel of five members were obtained (Holmes and Brown, 2005). This guideline can be obtained at the National Guideline Clearinghouse (http://www.guideline.gov). There is no consistency in the studies addressed because they deal with different aspects of care. The experts conclude that there is insufficient evidence on which to recommend pin site care or to make strong recommendation regarding any particular aspect of pin site care. However, they indicate that the research evidence does provide a basis for recommending several specific actions over others until more definitive answers become available. There are four recommendations (Holmes and Brown, 2005):

BOX 11-1	Levels of Evidence Support
Level 1	Supported by main finding from one randomized, experimental study with statistically significant difference in group outcomes
Level 2	Supported by one comparative case series study with a statistically significant difference in group outcomes
Level 3	Supported by a descriptive finding of a least one single case series study
Level 4	Reported as an incidental finding in at least one study and endorsed by two thirds of the panel
Level 5	Supported by endorsement of two thirds of the panel

Modified from National Guideline Clearinghouse: *Skeletal pin site care clinical practice guideline,* 2005, http://www.guideline.gov, accessed September 12, 2007.

1 Pins located in areas of considerable soft tissue should be considered at greater risk for infection (levels of support: 3, 4, 5) (Box 11-1).
2 At sites with mechanically stable bone-pin interfaces, pin site care should be done on a daily or weekly basis (after the first 48 to 72 hours) (levels of support: 1 and 5).
3 Chlorhexidine 2 mg/mL solution is possibly the most effective cleansing solution for pin site care (level of support: 2).
4 Patients and/or their families need to demonstrate how to care for the pin site before discharge from the hospital. Health care organizations need to provide patients with written instructions that include signs and symptoms of infection (level of support: 5).

CULTURAL CONSIDERATIONS

Assess underlying cultural and religious beliefs that affect a person's mobility. Consider the affected body part in relation to the patient's occupation or livelihood. Depression or feelings of uselessness may ensue within some cultures if the patient's ability to be the breadwinner is affected. Some Muslim patients do not accept instructions regarding the use of the alternative hand for eating and/or personal hygiene after elimination. The right hand is traditionally used for clean tasks, whereas the left is for dirty tasks. Muslim patients may need assistance to wash to perform their ritualized cleansing before prayers when family members are not present. Collaborate with family, religious, and community leaders to promote patients' understanding.

Some cultural groups may be threatened by application of traction directly to the head. For example, Southeast Asians consider the head as the seat of life, and only family members are allowed to touch it. In addition, some Africans believe that the individual's power and soul reside in the head. Some believe that procedures that puncture the skin of the head allow the individual's essence or spirit to escape.

When monitoring neurovascular status for patients with casted extremities, ashen-gray appearance of the skin and nail beds indicates poor circulation in dark-skinned patients instead of pallor, mottling, or bluish discoloration (see Chapter 6). Careful assessment is critical.

Maintain privacy of patients with a cast or traction by closing the bedside curtains and adequately draping the patient. Some cultures such as Asians, Hispanics, and Africans value female modesty (Spector, 2008). Hindus, Muslims, Amish, and Orthodox Jews emphasize female modesty especially in the presence of males.

When rehabilitative care is necessary, collaborate with family members in implementing a rehabilitative regimen for the patient. For example, some cultures (Asians, Hispanics, and Africans) do not define caring as allowing the patient to do things on his or her own, especially elders. It is beneficial for the patient to allow family to perform direct caring tasks for the patient (Andrews and Boyle, 2003). However, the care the family provides should not impede the rehabilitation goals and return of function.

Skill Performance Guidelines

1 Identify the patient's dietary preferences. Wound healing and repair of bone and tissues require additional nutritional intake. Providing foods the patient enjoys meets these additional nutritional needs.
2 Determine the limits of ROM to the casted extremity or extremity in traction. Although it is important to maintain joint mobility, do not move the affected extremity beyond the limits imposed by the cast or traction. Excessive movement will impair wound healing, extremity alignment, and new bone growth.
3 Determine the patient's level of independent functioning. Knowing what the patient is capable of doing enables you to properly assist the patient with activities of daily living (ADLs) such as bathing and eating.
4 Identify the patient's normal elimination patterns. Restrictions on mobility imposed by the cast, traction, or use of analgesics can alter elimination patterns.
5 Determine that the patient understands the normal bone-healing process. This knowledge assists in developing a teaching plan for the patient to care for the casted extremity at home.
6 Review the results of recent laboratory tests. Serum calcium and phosphorus are two minerals that compose callus, the precursor to bone ossification. Hemoglobin, hematocrit, and red blood cell levels will decrease in blood loss anemia as a result of bone fractures.
7 Assess the frequency and type of analgesics ordered for the patient by the physician. The patient may experience acute, continuous pain and/or muscle spasms during the first 4 to 7 days (the acute inflammatory stage) and thus require 24-hour administration of analgesics and/or muscle relaxants during this time.

SKILL 11-1   Assisting With Cast Application

A cast is an externally applied structure that holds musculoskeletal tissues and bones in a specific position to permit healing of injuries or fractures or to align malpositioned tissues, such as in clubfoot or congenital hip dislocation. The rigidity of the cast holds the bones in place for the time required to heal or align the diseased or injured tissues. Because a cast holds tissue in the position in which it is applied, you must apply it carefully and properly to achieve the goals for its use.

Casts are made from plaster of Paris or synthetic materials. A plaster of Paris cast has multiple rolls of open-weave cotton saturated with calcium sulfate crystals. These casts are heavier than synthetic casts and take 24 to 72 hours with no weight bearing or application of pressure while drying. Plaster of Paris is easy to mold and shape around unstable fractures. Synthetic casts are composed of polyester and cotton material, which is impregnated with a water-activated polyurethane resin. Synthetic casts are also made of fiberglass or plastic. Although the newer synthetic casts are more expensive than plaster, they can withstand contact with water without crumbling. These casts are lightweight, set in 15 minutes, and can sustain weight bearing or pressure in 15 to 30 minutes.

Optimal skin care is important as the cast is applied. Clean the extremity, removing dirt, glass, or debris from areas beneath the cast. After application of the cast, ensure that plaster crumbs are removed and rough edges are "petaled" to prevent skin breakdown.

Delegation Considerations

The skill of assisting with cast application can be delegated to nursing assistive personnel (NAP); however, the nurse is responsible for assessment of the patient's condition. The nurse directs the NAP by:

- Informing NAP to avoid patient positioning that increases patient discomfort.
- Informing and assisting NAP, as needed, in the proper method of assisting with cast application.

Equipment

NOTE: Equipment may be preassembled on "cast cart."
- ❏ Plaster rolls (sizes include 2-, 3-, 4-, and 6-inch rolls) or cast materials such as fiberglass, casting tape, or plastic (Fig. 11-2), depending on purpose of cast or specific patient condition
- ❏ Padding material (felt, stockinette, sheet wadding, Webril,

or other material; available in various thicknesses and lengths)
- ❏ Plastic-lined bucket or basin filled three-fourths full with warm water
- ❏ Clean gloves and aprons
- ❏ Scissors
- ❏ Paper or plastic sheets
- ❏ Cast saw (if old cast is to be removed)
- ❏ Cart, chair, fracture table

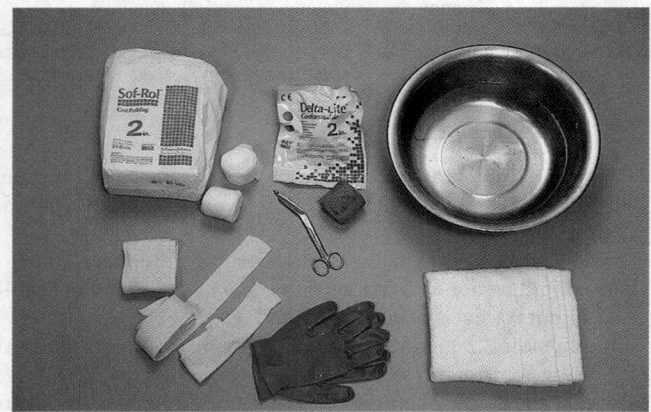

FIG 11-2 Plaster roll and padding material.

STEP	RATIONALE

ASSESSMENT

1 Assess patient's health status, including conditions affecting wound healing (e.g., diabetes, peripheral vascular disease, malnutrition, age) and allergy to latex.	Health status influences healing of tissues enclosed by cast. History of latex allergy influences type of equipment to use.
2 Assess patient's understanding of upcoming cast application.	Relieves patient's anxiety and helps determine whether additional information is needed.
3 Assess condition of tissues to be in the cast, including circulation (pulse, color, temperature) to extremities, ROM, sensation, and amount of subcutaneous fat. Note presence of skin breakdown, bruising, rash, and irritation.	Determines need for additional skin care before cast application. Provides baseline for close observation after cast is applied. Skin of infants, children, and older adults may contain less subcutaneous fat.

Critical Decision Point *Patients with skin breakdown or skin lesions may not be candidates for casting.*

4 Assess patient's pain severity on a scale of 0 to 10.	Fractures are painful; patient responses vary. Provides baseline to determine efficacy of cast application.
5 Determine extent to which patient will be able to use casted extremity.	Predicts the degree of assistance that is needed for self-care and/or ambulation.

NURSING DIAGNOSES

- Acute pain
- Bathing/hygiene, dressing/grooming, and toileting self-care deficit

- Deficient knowledge regarding casting procedure
- Impaired home maintenance
- Impaired physical mobility

- Ineffective tissue perfusion
- Risk for impaired skin integrity
- Risk for injury
- Risk for peripheral neurovascular dysfunction

Individualize related factors based on patient's condition or needs.

STEP	RATIONALE

PLANNING

1 Expected outcomes following completion of procedure:

- Patient initially experiences only slight edema, soreness, mild pain, and some limitation of active ROM from being in cast.

  Cast limits normal function of affected tissues.

- Skin of tissues below cast is warm with normal color and a capillary refill of 3 seconds or less.

  Neurovascular function to body part is maintained (Judge, 2007).

- Patient verbalizes no abnormal or unusual sensations and is able to move fingers or toes below casted part.

- Skin around proximal and distal cast edges remains intact without irritation.

  Skin is free of pressure and friction from cast edges (Altizer, 2004).

- Patient is able to perform limited ROM actively on those joints not involved.

  Other joints move without impairment.

- Patient has some impaired mobility in standing, turning, or ambulating.

  Cast is heavy, or it impairs mobility because of size or area of body in cast.

- Patient uses assistance with usual ADLs if head, neck, or upper extremity is in cast.

  Cast sometimes interferes with ability to dress, feed, or bathe oneself.

- Patient verbalizes increase in comfort after cast in place. Rates pain less than 4 on a scale of 0 to 10.

  Injured tissues and bone are stabilized.

- Patient demonstrates cast-care techniques.

  Demonstrates learning.

2 Instruct patient, parent, and other assistants in how they can facilitate application of cast by maintaining affected part in desired position.

  Cast will hold tissues in the position in which they are held during cast application. Patient teaching reduces anxiety and increases cooperation.

IMPLEMENTATION

1 Administer analgesic per order before cast application: by mouth (PO), 30 to 40 minutes before; intramuscularly (IM), 20 to 30 minutes before; intravenously (IV), 2 to 5 minutes before. Administer muscle relaxant 30 minutes before cast application if spasms are present.

  Reduces pain during cast application. Provides optimal analgesic effect. Often, muscle spasms are treated more effectively with skeletal muscle relaxants than with opioids (Lehne, 2004).

2 Perform hand hygiene, and apply clean gloves. Use latex-free gloves if there is risk for an allergic reaction.

  Reduces transmission of microorganisms. Synthetic cast can leave gluelike resin on hands. Prevents exposure to latex allergen (Barker and Montagna, 2005).

3 Position patient as needed; patient may be lying, sitting, or standing, depending on type of cast and tissues to be casted.

  Parts to be put in cast must be supported and in optimal position of function for cast application.

4 Prepare skin for cast if necessary; may involve cleansing with soap and water, changing dressing, and trimming long hair. Use gentle strokes to maintain skin integrity.

  Reduces complications to underlying tissues after casting. Gentle manipulation prevents pain or additional injury.

5 Explain that patient may experience warmth during the cast application process.

  Plaster gives off heat from a chemical reaction when drying.

Critical Decision Point   *Keep cast exposed to permit maximum dissipation of the heat. Most casts cool in about 15 minutes.*

6 Depending on type of cast material, do *one* of the following:

a With the thumb under the outer edge, submerge plaster roll under water in a casting bucket or plastic basin until bubbles stop, then squeeze slightly and give roll to person applying cast.

  Dampened plaster rolls are unrolled and molded to fit part being casted. Some have resin for easy moldability.

b Submerge synthetic cast roll in lukewarm water for 10 to 15 seconds. Squeeze to remove excess water.

  Initiates chemical reaction that produces heat and hardens tape (Altizer, 2004).

STEP	RATIONALE

7   Hold body part(s) to be put in cast in position requested by person applying cast (see illustrations).

Support of body part involves applying slight manual traction, if desired, to maintain optimal position.

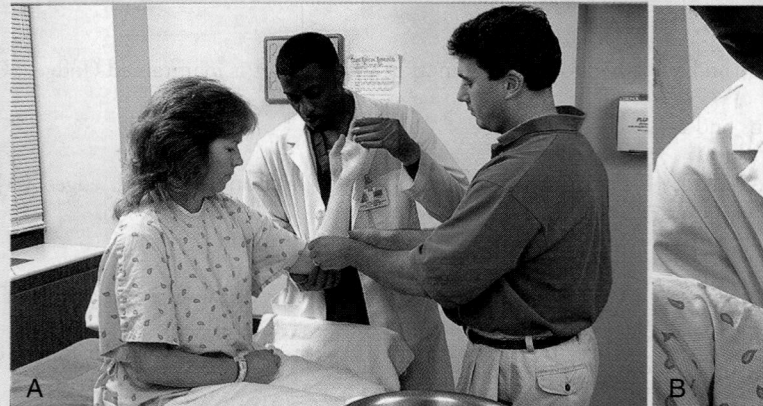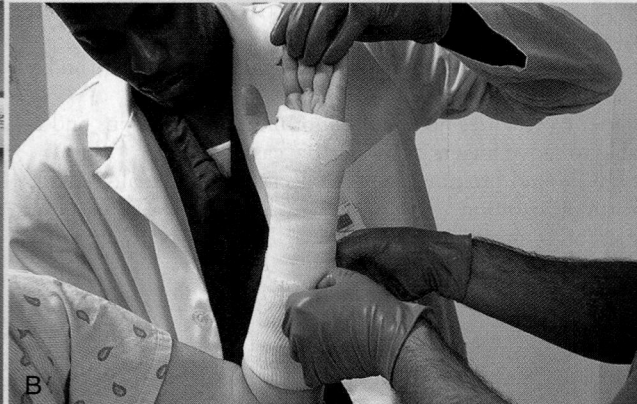

STEP 7   **A** and **B,** Assistant supports patient's extremity as cast is applied.

8   Hold body part while casting tape is applied and molded. Synthetic tape is applied with slight tension. When wrapping is completed, gently compress with hands (see illustration).

Casting tape has synthetic adhesive or glass-fiber materials that dry quickly and are lightweight. Compression promotes bonding of cast layers (Altizer, 2004).

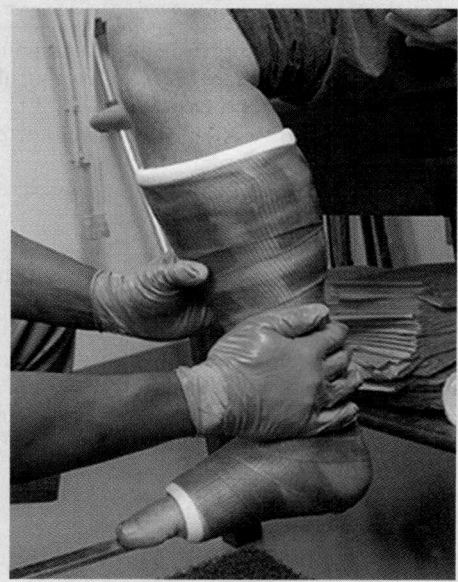

STEP 8   Applying synthetic cast roll.

9   Continue to supply dampened rolls of plaster, synthetic cast roll, or cast tape or hold parts as necessary until cast is finished. You should be able to insert two fingers between cast and limb.

10   Supply walking heel cast, cast brace, bar, or other cast stabilization material as requested by physician or health care practitioner.

Plaster must be of sufficient thickness to give strength to cast. More than two fingers' space in cast indicates cast is too loose and will not support limb, and less than two fingers' space indicates cast may be too tight and inhibit circulation.

Ambulation (after cast dries) may be permitted with partial weight bearing (see Chapter 10), which is facilitated by walking cast shoe, heel, or sole. Bars stabilize spica cast, or "posts" (metal poles) stabilize four-poster cast. Brace can be incorporated into cast to aid in maintaining joint motion and mobility.

STEP	RATIONALE
11 Ensure that the stockinette, Webril, or other casting material is applied evenly and smoothly to prevent wadding and lumping. Damp plaster is then unrolled over padding to hold it securely outside cast. Assist with "finishing" by folding stockinette or other padding down over outer edge of cast to provide smooth edge.	Smooth edges lessen possible skin irritation. By finishing cast with stockinette, later petaling with tape is not required when cast is dry (Altizer, 2004).
12 Supply scissors to trim plaster rolls around thumb, fingers, and toes as necessary.	Cast should be snug but should not constrict uninvolved joint movement or circulation.
13 Depending on tissues casted:	
a Place damp plaster cast on cloth-covered pillows (two to three) to prevent deformation or pressure points as it sets. Maintain elevation at or above heart level (see Evaluation section). If ice is applied, place to the side rather than the top of the cast to prevent indentations.	Pillows prevent cast from hardening in undesirable position. Elevation of both plaster and synthetic casts enhances venous return and decreases edema. Elevation above heart level can compromise arterial blood flow if circulation is diminished (Bongiovanni and others, 2005).

Critical Decision Point   *Handle casted extremity with palms only until the cast is dry. Fingers can cause indentations that lead to pressures areas.*

STEP	RATIONALE
b Place casted tissues in sling, making sure sling just holds, and does not encase, cast.	Covering (encasing) impedes air movements and delays drying.
14 Remove and dispose of gloves into appropriate receptacle. Perform hand hygiene.	Reduces transmission of microorganisms.
15 Cover patient, or reclothe as needed, leaving damp, casted areas uncovered.	Covering blocks air movement, delays drying, and retains heat, which leads to skin damage with plaster (Altizer, 2004).
16 Assist with transfer of patient to stretcher or wheelchair for return to nursing unit, to prepare patient for discharge. May accompany patient to room and assist with transfer to bed if necessary. Patient may have cast applied in room.	Safety in transfer requires use of pillows to support cast, side rails, restraints, and sufficient personnel to support patient and cast. Safety in transfer requires more than one person to accompany patient in body, spica, long arm, and long leg casts to prevent falls.
17 Clean equipment (bucket, scissors, cast saw), and return to storage area; discard used materials. Perform hand hygiene.	Facilitates use of equipment and treatment area for next patient. Reduces transmission of infection.
18 Explain purposes of exposure for faster drying, use of fans or lights to facilitate drying, use of elevation if pertinent, or application of ice bags if ordered.	Casts must dry from inside out for thorough drying. Do not use fans in open areas or under cast; organisms can be blown into cast and cause infection. Hot blow dryers or heat lamps can burn tissues. Elevation and use of ice decrease edema formation (Bongiovanni and others, 2005).

Critical Decision Point   *Synthetic casts are dry or set in 7 to 15 minutes. Soft tissues around affected area may swell from processes of "reducing" or manipulating before cast was applied.*

STEP	RATIONALE
19 Reposition patient every 2 hours. Do not rest cast heel on pillow.	Prevents any one area of the cast from receiving continuous pressure. Avoids indentation of cast.
20 Inform patient to notify personnel of any alteration in sensation, abnormal sensation, pain that persists regardless of interventions or that is out of proportion, or inability to move fingers or toes in affected extremity.	When pressure within a casted extremity increases, it may lead to compartment syndrome, which occurs when pressure within the muscle compartment increases as a result of edema, bleeding, or decreased venous return. The fascia covering the muscle group acts as a tourniquet on structures within the compartment: nerves, blood vessels, and muscle tissue. Neurovascular assessments determine development of syndrome (Judge, 2007).
21 Cover cast with watertight plastic when bathing patient. Use blow dryer on cool setting to dry damp areas of synthetic cast.	Plaster of Paris cast will crumble if wet. If a blow dryer is on hot setting, it will cause the outer portion to dry while the inner section of the cast remains wet, leading to mildew development.

STEP	RATIONALE

EVALUATION

1. Observe patient for signs of pain or anxiety: ask patient to rate pain on a scale of 0 to 10, observe for inability to move body parts distal to cast, pain on passive motion of distal body parts, hyperventilation, swallowing air (aerophagia), nausea and/or vomiting, tachycardia, and blood pressure elevation.

These are signs of development of compartment syndrome, cast syndrome, or severe claustrophobia from snugness of cast, common for patients in spica or body cast (Judge, 2007).

2. Perform neurovascular assessment every 1 to 2 hours for the first 24 hours. Assess for pain, pallor, pulselessness, paresthesia, and paralysis (Table 11-1, p. 274). Compare findings with preapplication neurovascular assessment (see illustration).

Neurovascular status reflects vascular supply or pressure to tissues that indicates functioning and viability of tissues (Judge, 2007).

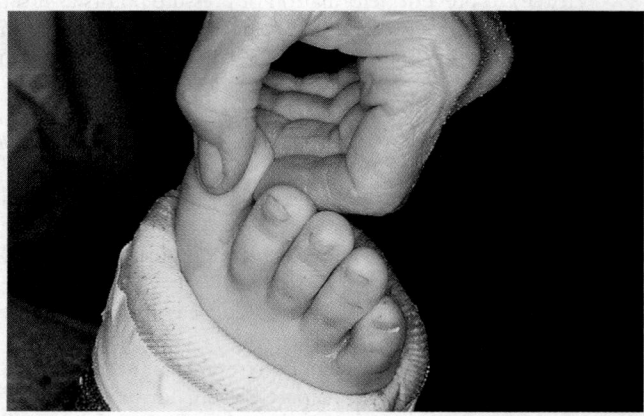

STEP 2   Assessing capillary refill. The nail bed is compressed. When released it should "pink up" in 3 seconds or less.

Critical Decision Point   *Deterioration in neurovascular status requires immediate action, because irreversible tissue death occurs within 4 to 12 hours of inadequate oxygenation.*

3. Observe for edema distal to cast. Some older adults have concurrent dependent edema because of health state.

Edema results from trauma or venous stasis. Rarely, heat of plaster drying contributes to development of edema.

4. Evaluate temperature of tissues above and below cast. Older adult patients frequently have cooler-than-usual extremities because of decreased peripheral circulation.

Warmth of tissues distal to the cast usually indicates adequate perfusion.

Critical Decision Point   *Some older adult patients have slow or even poor capillary refill because of peripheral vascular conditions; use more than one neurovascular assessment to determine circulatory adequacy.*

5. Compare tissues in cast with contralateral tissues to determine current condition.

Comparison with normal tissues assists in forming judgment of neurovascular status.

6. Inspect condition of skin around edges of cast. If skin irritation is evident, "petal" the edge of the cast by overlapping strips of tape or moleskin over the edge.

This area is susceptible to pressure and friction.

7. Ask patient to perform ROM if possible; note if patient is unable to do active ROM of uncasted areas. Some older adult patients have stiffness of joints or edema from other health conditions.

Perform range of motion within limitations imposed by cast. Only exercise tissues out of cast.

8. If patient cannot do *active* ROM to contiguous tissues, perform *passive* ROM on these joints, noting responses or complaints of increased pain.

Passive movements decrease edema and demonstrate ability of part you will move. However, inability to perform active ROM and increased pain during passive movement may mean development of compartment syndrome; report this immediately (Judge, 2007; Solomon and others, 2005).

9. Ask patient to describe sensations or feelings of tissues in cast. Listen for descriptions such as "pins and needles," "asleep," "numb," "burning," "tingling," or "throbbing"; do not prompt patient by using those words.

Signifies pressure or hypoxia to neurological tissues, affecting normal transmission of nerve impulses (Judge, 2007; Lucas and Davis, 2005).

STEP	RATIONALE
10 Smell the cast edges; a sour, musty smell is normal as a result of sweat and skin cells that accumulate under the cast.	Detects early sign of infection (foul odor).
11 After cast is dry and set, observe patient perform and verbalize knowledge of cast care.	Return demonstration objectively measures patient's learning.

Unexpected Outcomes

Related Interventions

1. Malunion, delayed union, or nonunion of affected parts occurs because of insufficient reduction (placement) in cast or factors such as infection or foreign objects.

- Ensure that cast is snug and not loose.
- Report loose cast to health care provider; reapplication will likely be needed.
- Treat infection, maintain normal blood glucose level, and provide adequate nutrition.

2. Osteomyelitis develops if open wound was present at time of casting.

- A window may be cut in cast to inspect and dress wound. *Do not* discard window cutout. Tape in place (Altizer, 2004; Lucas and Davis, 2005).

3. Pressure ulcer develops over bony prominence, or skin irritation occurs at cast edges.

- Physician may split, window, bivalve, or remove cast (Altizer, 2004; Lucas and Davis, 2005).
- Cut small pieces (petals) of adhesive tape or moleskin 2.5 to 5.0 cm (1 to 2 inches), and tape smoothly over edge of cast.

4. Muscle weakness occurs.

- Exercise limb within limits of cast. Health care provider may order physical therapy.

5. Compartment syndrome that manifests as cold extremity, decreased capillary refill, swelling, pallor, diminished pulse, numbness, tingling, or altered motion of distal parts occurs.

- Notify health care provider.
- Bivalving and cutting underlying soft dressing with spreading the cast open may be necessary to prevent permanent damage (Altizer, 2004; Judge, 2007; Lucas and Davis, 2005).

6. Nausea, vomiting, feeling of abdominal fullness or pain is experienced by patient in body or hip spica cast, indicating cast syndrome (superior mesenteric artery syndrome) where the duodenum is compressed between the superior mesenteric artery and the spine

- Change the patient from the supine to the prone position.
- Give nothing by mouth.
- Notify health care provider, and prepare to cut abdominal window, bivalve cast, and/or insert nasogastric tube (Braun and others, 2006).

7. Patient is unable to demonstrate cast care.

- Reinstruction is necessary.

Recording and Reporting

- Record application of cast, condition of skin, circulation, and instructions given to patient and family.
- Report immediately abnormal or unusual findings from neurovascular assessments such as bluish color to distal parts, marked increase in edema or pain, delayed capillary refill (longer than 3 seconds), inability to palpate distal peripheral pulses if originally palpable, increased numbness or tingling, cold tissues, and inability to move tissues actively.
- Record odor and drainage from cast. Report to health care provider. Draw circle on cast around drainage site. Record time and date on circle.

Teaching Considerations

- Teach patient to realign pillows to promote cast drying when patient is repositioned.
- Teach patient about effects of pressure from cast on underlying skin and tissue.
- Prepare patient for itching sensations under cast. Patient should avoid sticking objects down or in cast to scratch, because these objects can cause breaks in underlying skin and subsequent infections. May require medication to control the itching.
- If patient must use crutches, instruct in crutch-walking techniques (see Chapter 10).
- Teach patient proper ROM and isometric exercises for affected extremity.
- Caution patient against drying wet cast with hair dryer; this can cause plaster to crack or skin underneath to be damaged.

Pediatric Considerations

- Synthetic casts come in a variety of colors. Allow child to choose color.
- Teach parents or other caregivers to protect cast from moisture or unnecessary wear. Plastic wrap placed around perineal area during urination or defecation prevents soiling. Protect the cast with a plastic bag or plastic wrap when the child bathes or showers. With a spica cast, tuck the ends of a small disposable diaper around the edges of the casted area to cover and protect the perineum in babies (Hockenberry and Wilson, 2007; London and others, 2007).
- If child has clubfoot, frequent cast changes are necessary. Cast changes accommodate normal bone and tissue growth and correction of abnormality (London and others, 2007).
- Children are particularly prone to placing objects into cast to scratch. Monitor them closely. Assess edges of cast to ensure that the child has not inserted small objects into cast (Hockenberry and Wilson, 2007; London and others, 2007).
- Use antihistamines and a hair dryer set to *cool* to control itching (Hockenberry and Wilson, 2007).
- Infants or children signify pain through crying or restlessness. Gastric distention may occur in child who repeatedly screams and cries with fracture and cast application (Hockenberry and Wilson, 2007).
- Child in body cast or spica cast often finds it easier to self-feed from prone position with tray adjacent to child or on floor (Hockenberry and Wilson, 2007).

Gerontological Considerations

- Some older nonverbal patients do not express pain, leading you to believe that there is no pain. Patients may express pain through crying, agitation, or restlessness (Ebersole and others, 2008; Tabloski, 2006).
- Lightweight, synthetic casts are better for older adult patients. Cast is less restrictive, and light weight helps patients maintain better balance.
- Age-related decreased muscle strength in older adults is a result of loss of skeletal muscle (Mauk, 2006), and it sometimes causes difficulty in ambulating with a cast.
- Some older adult patients have reduced sensation as a result of decreased skin receptors and are less able to detect compression (Mauk, 2006).
- Bone healing (remodeling cycle) takes longer to complete, and rate of mineralization slows down (Mauk, 2006).

Home Care Considerations

- Instruct patient that rest, ice, and elevation of affected extremity will help reduce swelling.
- Inform patient to inspect cast and petal rough edges to reduce risk for trauma to underlying skin and need for cast changes.
- Have patient inspect cast daily for foul odor, which indicates skin excoriation or infection under cast; monitor neurovascular status, paying particular attention to blueness or paleness of nails, pain, feeling of tightness, numbness, or tingling sensation.
- Instruct patient to keep plaster of Paris cast dry. When bathing, patient will not submerge casted extremity because cast absorbs water, loses structural integrity, and crumbles. If cast becomes wet, dry immediately.
- Clean synthetic casts with warm water and mild soap.
- Patient must notify physician of any clinical manifestation of complications: fever, unrelieved pain, foul odor, or complaints that cast is too tight or rubbing skin.

TABLE 11-1 | Five Ps of Neurovascular Assessment

Criteria	Assessment	Rationale
Pain	Determine amount and severity of pain if present. Ask patient for descriptions; avoid coaching patient with words to describe pain.	Manipulation and reduction may produce dull, aching pain as a result of pressure on nerve endings. Patients vary in perception and tolerance of pain. Further assess pain on passive motion, unrelenting pain, or pain out of proportion because it may signify compartment syndrome. Sudden increase in pain may signify thrombus formation (Judge, 2007; Lucas and Davis, 2005).
Pallor	Observe color of tissues distal to cast. Older adult patients may have bluish color normally; however, no other signs of circulatory compromise should be present.	Pink indicates arterial pressure is normal, whitish color signifies decreased arterial supply, and bluish color signifies venous stasis.
Pulselessness	When possible, palpate distal pulse of casted extremity; note presence and strength of pulse. Assess capillary refill by pressing on toenail or fingernail (if cast is on extremity), releasing, and noting "pinking" of nail; nail should "pink up" in 3 seconds or less (see illustration for Skill 11-1, Evaluation, Step 2).	Weak or absent pulse may indicate decreased circulation to casted area. Blanching on pressure with subsequent capillary refill is indicative of arterial perfusion. Capillary refill is too sluggish if refill takes more than 3 seconds. It takes 2 seconds to say "capillary refill" slowly and 4 seconds to repeat it once (Judge 2007).
Paresthesia	Assess for numbness, tingling, or abnormal sensations.	May indicate nerve damage and/or development of compartment syndrome (Lucas and Davis, 2005).
Paralysis	Assess for motion.	May indicate nerve damage and/or development of compartment syndrome (Judge, 2007; Solomon and others, 2005).

SKILL 11-2 Assisting With Cast Removal

Cast removal consists of removing the cast and padding with a mechanical device such as a cast saw (Fig. 11-3). Prepare for this procedure, so the patient remains still and cooperates during cast removal. Cast removal is painless but can be noisy. Occasionally you will have to gently restrain a child or confused patient during the procedure to prevent injury by the equipment. After the cast is removed, you will provide appropriate skin care.

Delegation Considerations

The skill of assisting with cast removal can be delegated to NAP; however, the nurse is responsible for assessment of the patient's condition. The nurse directs the NAP by:

- Informing about the proper method of treating skin tissues following cast removal.

Equipment

- ❑ Cast saw
- ❑ Plastic sheets or papers
- ❑ Cold water enzyme wash
- ❑ Skin lotion
- ❑ Basin, water, washcloths, and towels
- ❑ Scissors
- ❑ Clean gloves
- ❑ Eye protection for patient and health care professional

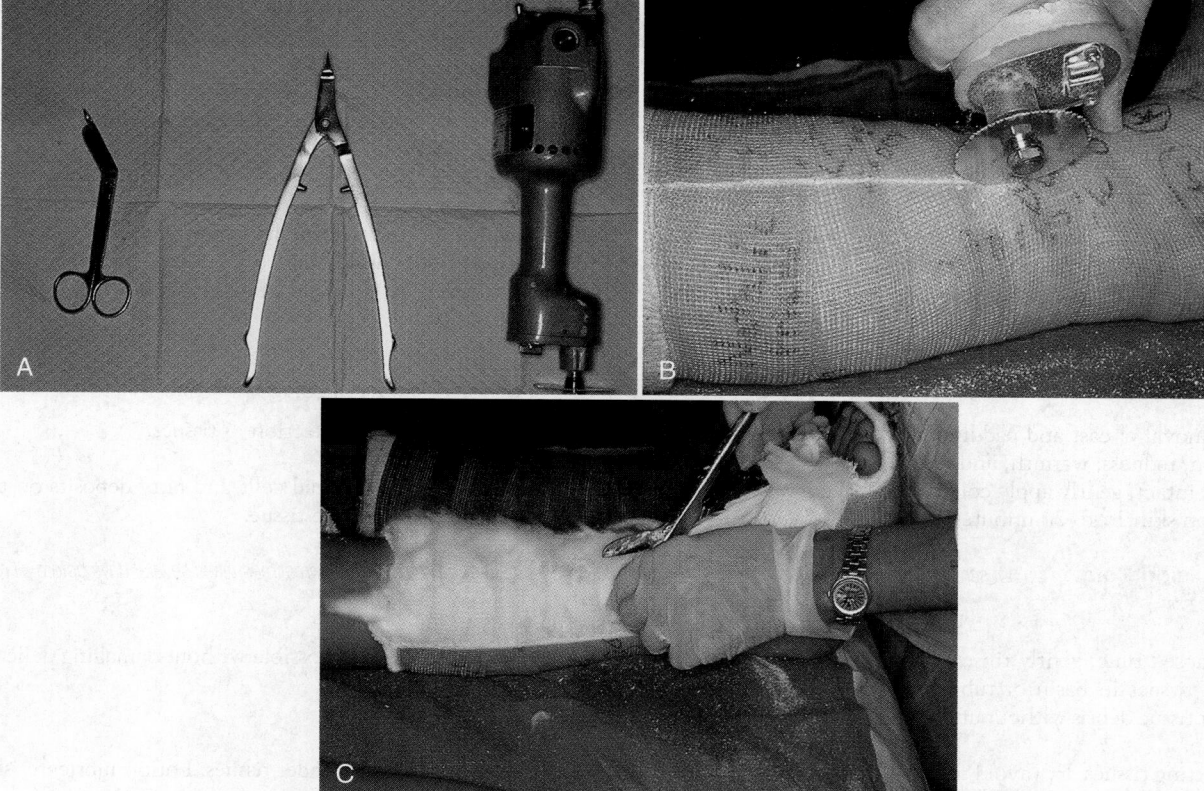

FIG 11-3 Equipment for removing a cast. **A,** *Left to right:* Scissors, cast spreader, cast saw. **B,** Cast saw is used to remove cast. To bivalve a cast, it is cut longitudinally on either side and the wadding is cut with scissors. The two halves may be secured together with an elastic wrap, or the top is removed and the bottom shell of the cast becomes a posterior splint. **C,** Cutting through wadding under cast with scissors.

STEP	RATIONALE

ASSESSMENT

1 Assess patient's understanding of and response to upcoming cast removal.

Helps develop a teaching plan that aids in reducing anxiety.

2 Consult with health care provider regarding physical readiness for cast removal (patient's physical findings, health care provider's orders, x-ray examination results).

Determines level of healing, readiness to remove cast, and need for supportive care after removal.

3 Ask if patient feels any itching or irritation under cast.

Indicates healing and accumulation of dried skin layers.

NURSING DIAGNOSES

- Anxiety
- Deficient knowledge regarding cast removal
- Risk for impaired skin integrity
- Risk for injury

Individualize related factors based on patient's condition or needs.

PLANNING

1 Expected outcomes following completion of procedure:
- Patient incurs no underlying tissue or skin injury; there is buildup of dry, dead skin. Patient's skin remains intact.

Cast is removed safely. Layers of dead skin cells that accumulate are removed over time without scrubbing.

- Patient verbalizes understanding of normal physical sensations and procedural steps of cast removal.

Understanding lessens anticipatory anxiety.

- Patient is able to describe and demonstrate level of activity and weight bearing allowed following cast removal.

Allows patient to safely assume activity at home.

- Patient is able to explain skin care measures.

Allows patient to assume self-care.

2 Explain physical sensations to expect during cast removal. Cast saw vibrates cast loose; patient will feel heat and vibration; and cast cutter is noisy.

Explanation minimizes fear of possible injury.

STEP	RATIONALE
3 Describe procedural steps: appearance of saw, vibration sensations, removal of outer cast, appearance of padding and skin, cleansing of skin.	Patient is prepared to witness and participate in procedure. The skin will be dry and scaly, and the extremity will appear "thin" from disuse (Altizer, 2004).

IMPLEMENTATION

STEP	RATIONALE
1 Apply eye protection on patient and health care provider.	Prevents accidental injury form flying cast particles.
2 Apply clean gloves if drainage is anticipated, and assist person removing cast by positioning, turning, and holding cast and tissues in cast.	Prevents injury from saw. Use latex-free gloves if there is risk for an allergic reaction (Barker and Montagna, 2005).

Critical Decision Point   *Instruct patient to remain still during cast removal.*

STEP	RATIONALE
3 After removal of cast and padding, inspect tissues for general condition, redness, warmth, and drainage.	Indicates inflammation or infection of tissues.
4 If skin is intact, gently apply cold water enzyme wash to skin; let stay on skin 15 to 20 minutes.	Helps dissolve or emulsify dead cells and fatty deposits on tissues. Prevents injury to delicate tissue.

Critical Decision Point   *Do not scrub skin, because this traumatizes delicate tissue and leads to skin breakdown. It sometimes takes several days before all residue is removed from skin.*

STEP	RATIONALE
5 After elapsed time, gently rinse off enzyme wash; if possible, immerse tissues in basin or tub of warm water to aid in removal of tissue debris without undue rubbing or pressure using mild soap.	Removes as much debris as possible without damaging delicate tissues (Altizer, 2004).
6 After patting tissues dry (avoid rubbing), apply generous coating of skin lotion, gently massaging into skin.	Rubbing could traumatize tender tissues. Lotion lubricates skin.
7 Obtain order to gently put joints through active and passive ROM. Clarify level of activity allowed.	Joints and muscles will be stiff and weak. Activity is resumed slowly to avoid reinjury.
8 Assist in transfer of patient for return to room or for discharge if anticipated.	
9 Instruct patient to observe for swelling and to continue to elevate the extremity to control swelling.	Elevation promotes venous return.
10 Cleanse all equipment and casts, or discard them according to standard precautions. Remove gloves. If cast is soiled with blood, discard as biohazard waste.	Reduces transmission of microorganisms.

EVALUATION

STEP	RATIONALE
1 Observe underlying skin.	Reveals condition of skin.
2 Assess patient's verbal and nonverbal responses.	Expressions, tone of voice, and movement reveal level of anxiety or fear.
3 Ask patient to explain ordered exercise plan and demonstrate exercises.	Demonstrates learning.
4 Have patient explain and perform skin care.	Demonstrates learning of self-care.

Unexpected Outcomes	Related Interventions
1 Underlying skin becomes scratched from friction of saw.	• Remind patient to remain still during cast removal. • Apply antibiotic ointment per order.
2 Patient is tense, anxious, restless, and withdraws from cast saw.	• Provide further explanation and support.
3 Affected tissues develop extensive edema, pain, or limited use.	• Instruct patient to: • Elevate body part if edema returns. • Use nonopioid analgesics every 4 hours for up to 24 hours if needed. • Slowly perform ROM exercises every 4 hours. (If marked weakness exists, physician may order patient to receive physical therapy or to use sling or immobilizer for 1 to 2 days for continued rest.)
4 Patient is unable to perform ADLs and exercises because of nonunion or pain.	• Physician will assess the fracture site by radiographic film.
5 Patient is unable to explain self-care measures.	• Reinstruct or clarify as needed.

Recording and Reporting

- Record cast removal, condition of tissues formerly in cast, person removing cast, instructions given to patient and family and their verbalization/demonstration of knowledge.
- Report changes in movement, severe swelling, and increased pain to physician.

Teaching Considerations

- Inform patient to expect the muscle will be atrophied, there will be noticeable hair growth, the skin will be dry and flaky following cast removal, and the joints will be stiff and smaller because of lack of muscular use (Altizer, 2004). Consult with physical therapy, and recommend patient follow scheduled exercises to increase mobility and muscle strength. Inform that the amount of cellular debris under cast depends on length of time tissues are in cast and overall skin integrity.
- Instruct patient to use caution with tender skin areas or joints and to control swelling by elevating the extremity.
- Instruct patient to call physician if unable to perform ADLs, if excessive edema occurs, if patient experiences limited use of joints or muscles, or if mobility is affected. If treating patient for congenital deformity with repeated cast changes, instruct when next cast change is due; give patient written appointment.

Pediatric Considerations

- Many young children come to regard the cast as part of them, which intensifies their fear of removal. Preparation for the procedure reduces anxiety (Hockenberry and Wilson, 2007). Using the analogy of having fingernails or hair cut sometimes helps reduce their anxiety.
- Some infants and children are frightened of cast saw. Demonstration of saw before removal of cast will help alleviate anxiety. Children describe the sensation as a "tickly" one (Hockenberry and Wilson, 2007).
- After cast removal, allow the child to soak in a bathtub to remove desquamated skin and sebaceous secretions. Inform parents that it may take several days to eliminate this completely and not to forcibly remove skin debris (Hockenberry and Wilson, 2007).

Gerontological Considerations

- Some older adult patients experience marked stiffness or weakened muscles, depending on length of time in cast.
- Some older adults' skin is drier, thinner, and more fragile (Mauk, 2006).

Home Care Considerations

- Instruct patient to use chair or bed with pillows to elevate extremity for intermittent edema.
- Suggest regular use of moisturizers for dry, scaly skin of casted extremity.
- Assess patient's environment for potential safety risks.
- After cast is removed, teach patient to dangle before ambulation, to proceed slowly with ambulation, and to gradually increase the time and distance ambulated.
- Provide patient with instructions regarding muscle relaxants and analgesics if prescribed.

SKILL 11-3   Care of a Patient in Skin Traction

Skin traction is one of the two basic types of traction used to treat fractured bones and correct orthopedic abnormalities. Skin traction applies pull indirectly to the bones by straps attached to the skin around the structure. Skin traction is typically between 5 and 7 pounds and is commonly used for minor trauma or immediate immobilization before surgery. Because of the lower tolerance of skin tissues to the pressure exerted, this traction is applied for shorter periods, with less weight, and at times can be interrupted. Skeletal traction, when used for severe trauma, is applied for longer periods, requires much heavier weights, and is never interrupted. Effective traction requires you to implement six general principles of care (Box 11-2). You facilitate recovery through immobilization and alignment of body parts. You provide safe care through skillful application of traction. The following are the major forms of skin traction, with some variation within some of the types.

1 *Bryant's traction:* Vertically held type of bilateral traction to the legs. It was used for children under 3 years of age and weighing less than 35 to 40 pounds (Hockenberry and Wilson, 2008). Current evidence-based evidence suggests that for infants and children under the age of 2, fractured femurs can be effectively treated with application of a hip spica cast or Pavlik harness (Wheeler, 2008). Clinical practice guidelines have been developed by Cincinnati Children's Hospital Medical Center and can be obtained at the National Guideline Clearinghouse (http://www.guideline.gov).

2 *Buck's extension:* Horizontally applied unilateral or bilateral traction (Fig. 11-4, A). You apply Buck's traction in one of two ways: apply adhesive strips to the lateral surfaces of the limb or limbs (usually one leg or forearm) and wrap with elastic bandages, or apply a commercially prepared foam boot with Velcro straps. Attach a spreader bar to the adhesive strips as in Bryant's traction or to the foam boot and then to ropes, pulleys, and weights. Buck's extension provides temporary immobilization of hip fracture until open reduction and internal fixation (ORIF) can be performed. It also reduces muscle spasms, contractures, and dislocations and is occasionally an interim treatment for lumbosacral muscle spasms causing low back pain.

3 *Dunlop's traction:* Simultaneous horizontal form of Buck's extension to the humerus with an accompanying vertical Buck's extension to the forearm (Fig. 11-4, B). The horizontal Buck's extension is the "treating" traction for fractures of the humerus, whereas the vertical Buck's extension maintains the forearm in the desired position relative to the humerus.

4 *Russell's traction:* Modification of Buck's extension using Newton's third law of motion (for each force in one direction there is an equal force in the opposite direction). Doubles the amount of pull through the arrangement of ropes, pulleys, and weights (Fig. 11-5, p. 279). It also is used in skeletal traction.

Because skin tissues and subcutaneous attachments cannot tolerate great amounts of weight without losing strength and continuity,

BOX 11-2   Six General Principles of Traction Care

1 Maintain the Established Line of Pull

This line is along the axis of the bone. Weights will hang freely, not hitting the bed or resting on the floor. Recheck the position of the weights if the level of the bed is altered. Avoid (1) bumping against the weights when walking near the bed and (2) allowing the weights to sway; both movements can cause pain for the patient in traction. It is preferred that the weights not hang over the patient; if this is necessary, tape the ropes so the weights will not fall on the patient.

2 Maintain Traction Equipment

Traction rope rests in the groove of the pulley and moves easily. Monitor the rope for fraying. Securely tie the knots in the traction rope, and tape the rope ends well. The rope knots are not lodged against the pulley because this will interfere with the line of pull. For the same reason, ensure that the pulley, spreader bar, and foot plate do not rest against the foot of the bed.

3 Maintain Countertraction

To provide traction ensure that countertraction is maintained by the weight of the patient's body, the pull of the weights in the opposite direction, or elevation of the bed. For instance, the feet of a patient in Buck's traction will not touch the foot of the bed; or if the patient is in cervical traction, the head will not touch the head of the bed.

4 Maintain Continuous Traction Unless Ordered Otherwise

Maintain continuous traction unless the physician orders intermittent traction. To change the patient's position in bed, do not lift or adjust the weights if traction is continuous. Ensure the correct amount of weight is used. For intermittent traction gently place and slowly remove the weights, avoiding jerking or suddenly moving the weights that could jar the patient.

5 Maintain Correct Body Alignment

The patient will have correct body alignment while lying centered in the bed. The patient will be instructed regarding any restricted positions. The nurse must ensure that the patient does not angle the body or lean off the side of the bed because the line of traction pull would then be changed or interrupted.

6 Prevent Friction to the Skin

Remove skin traction and reapply daily. Five to eight pounds is the usual amount of weight used for skin traction in adult patients. With any traction monitor the skin for evidence of redness, bruising, or skin breakdown. Avoid friction or pressure from the equipment.

Modified from Maher AB and others: *Orthopaedic nursing,* ed 3, Philadelphia, 2002, Saunders.

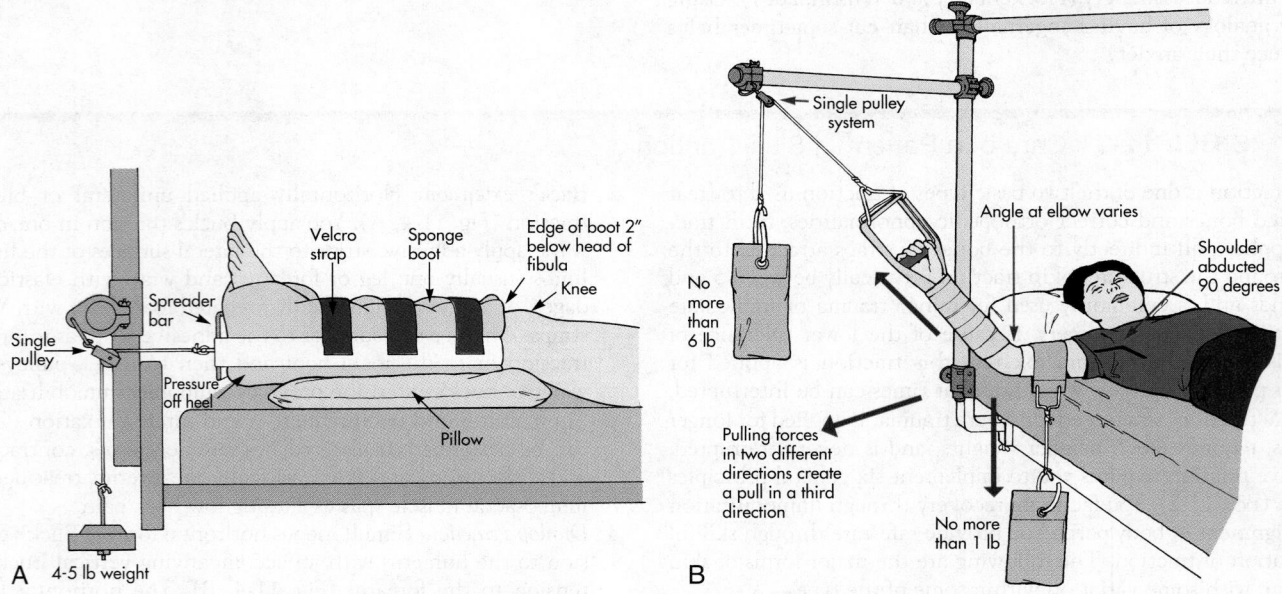

FIG 11-4   A, Buck's extension. **B,** Dunlop's traction. (*From Folcik M and others:* Traction: assessment and management, *St. Louis, 1994, Mosby.*)

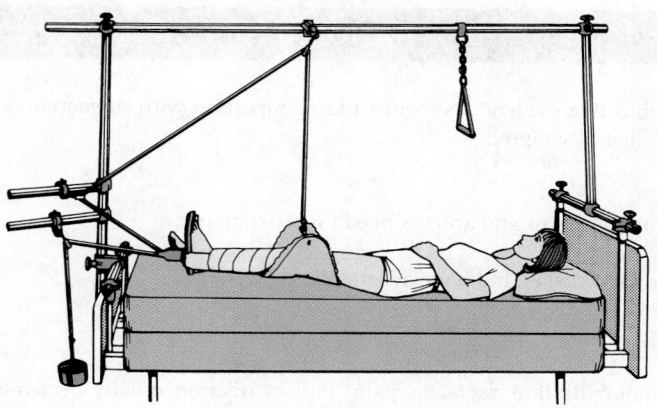

FIG 11-5 Russell's traction. *(From Phipps W and others: Medical-surgical nursing: health and illness perspectives, ed 7, St. Louis, 2003, Mosby.)*

skin traction uses weights varying from 5 to 7 lb for Buck's extension and 7 to 10 lb for Dunlop's traction. Each form of skin traction has a usual or "classic" position used for the majority of patients in that traction. Variations may be needed to treat a specific injury or condition. If pertinent, these variations are noted in the discussion of each type of traction.

Delegation Considerations

The skill of assessment of the patient and the status of traction cannot be delegated to NAP. However, the skill of assisting with application of skin traction can be delegated to NAP. The nurse directs the NAP by:

- Discussing any of the necessary restrictions in positioning patient and in application/removal of weights.
- Instructing the NAP to report any change in patient's skin condition or complaints of pain.

Equipment

- ❑ Ropes, pulleys, weights, weight holder (Ropes are nylon for strength; weights vary from 1 to 5 lb—have several of each weight.) (Children and older adults require less weight than do young adults.)
- ❑ Bed frame for attachment of traction or portable frames that attach to bed
- ❑ One or more spreader bars
- ❑ Adhesive-backed moleskin
- ❑ Elastic bandages
- ❑ Heel or elbow protectors *(optional)*
- ❑ Knee sling for Russell's traction, traction boot for Buck's extension
- ❑ Wastebasket with plastic bag liner

STEP	RATIONALE
ASSESSMENT	
1 Assess condition of patient's overall health, including degree of mobility and current medical conditions such as diabetes, peripheral vascular disease, or peripheral neuropathy.	Determines patient's health state and ability to tolerate traction.
2 Assess condition of specific tissues to be placed in traction; skin, excessive hair, bruises, rash, varicose veins, ulcers, dermatitis, or other lesions.	Determines ability of local tissues to tolerate traction (Resch and others, 2005).

Critical Decision Point   *Do not place traction over irritated or broken skin.*

a *Buck's extension:* Assess one or both legs.	Each type of traction predisposes patient to area at risk for skin breakdown.
b *Dunlop's traction:* Assess arm and forearm.	
c *Russell's traction:* Assess lower limbs.	
3 Assess patient's understanding of reason for traction.	Determines concerns, acceptance, and need for instruction.
4 Assess patient's severity of pain on a scale of 0 to 10.	Serves as baseline for later comparison and evaluation. Traction usually relieves pain and spasms.
5 Assess patient's neurovascular status.	Serves as baseline for later comparison and evaluation.

NURSING DIAGNOSES

- Acute pain
- Bathing/hygiene, dressing/grooming, and toileting self-care deficit
- Deficient knowledge regarding the type and use of traction
- Impaired physical mobility
- Ineffective peripheral tissue perfusion
- Risk for impaired skin integrity
- Risk for peripheral neurovascular dysfunction

Individualize related factors based on patient's condition or needs.

PLANNING

1 Expected outcomes following completion of procedure:	
• Patient participates in bathing and feeding.	Activities are performed safely and without injury.
• Skin around straps and moleskin or boot remains intact, without irritation.	Skin is free of pressure and/or pulling.

STEP	RATIONALE
• X-ray studies confirm satisfactory alignment of fracture fragments with or without evidence of beginning callus formation (evidence of callus may not become apparent for 7 to 10 days or longer) if patient is in traction for fracture.	Objective evidence is required for comparison with subjective relief of symptoms.
• Patient describes purpose of traction and follows activity restrictions.	Patient learns and accepts need for restrictions.
• Patient verbalizes increase in comfort after traction application and rates pain as 4 or lower on a scale of 0 to 10.	Injured tissues and bone are stabilized.
• As a result of being in one specific type of skin traction, one of the following occurs.	
a *Buck's extension:* Patient is able to maintain leg in alignment. Older adult patients with severe hip pain noticeably relax.	Immobilization decreases pain. Pull of traction usually decreases muscle spasms.
b *Dunlop's traction:* Same result occurs as for Buck's extension (used for upper extremity).	
c *Russell's traction:* Patient notes lessening of pain in hip area (if traction is for hip trauma), relief of muscle spasms, and ease in ability to maintain more normal anatomical position of leg and thigh.	Russell's traction exerts double pull with less weight than Buck's extension because of pulley arrangement.
• Sufficient time in traction (varying from 1 to 10 or more days) elicits symptom relief. Continuous skin traction is limited to 7 to 10 days.	It takes time for inflammation to decrease and tissues to regain more normal functions. Prolonged continuous skin traction leads to skin breakdown.
• Neurovascular status remains stable. Distal skin tissue remains warm and of a normal color with capillary refill of 3 seconds or less. Patient verbalizes no abnormal sensations and is able to move fingers or toes distal to fracture site.	There is no evidence of increased pressure within the muscle compartment and no neurovascular deficit (Judge, 2007).
• Patient verbalizes understanding of procedure, including traction setup and mobility restrictions.	Promotes cooperation and reduces anxiety.

IMPLEMENTATION

1 Administer opioid for acute pain and muscle relaxant for spasms in advance of traction application (see Skill 11-1).	Allowing drugs to reach peak effect at time of traction application will reduce pain and resultant muscle spasm.
2 Prepare patient and area of body to be in traction:	
a *Buck's extension:* Wash affected leg (or legs) very gently, and dry carefully. Do not shave legs.	Shaving creates micronicks that will become inflamed under traction strips.
b *Dunlop's traction:* Cleanse arm and forearm gently as needed.	Prevents irritation under straps and bandages.
c *Russell's traction:* Cleanse lower extremity to knee as needed.	Prevents irritation under bandages.
3 Position patient as requested by physician:	Position varies depending on the body part in traction, plus effects of weight and gravity. Body parts are kept anatomically aligned.
a *Buck's extension:* Patient on back; head of bed flat or elevated no more than 30 degrees.	
b *Dunlop's traction:* Patient flat on back.	
c *Russell's traction:* Patient on back; head of bed slightly elevated.	
4 Assist with application of adhesive strips and elastic bandages or commercially prepared Buck's traction boot as needed. NOTE: You may need to hold patient in desired position or apply strips or elastic bandages while physician and other assistants hold patient's tissues in desired positions.	Ensures proper alignment of body parts under traction.
a For lower extremity, apply adhesive strips beginning below head of fibula on lateral surface of leg.	To avoid pressure over superficial peroneal nerve located on the outer part of the leg and over the proximal fibula.
b Apply elastic bandages from distal to proximal.	To prevent trapping of blood and to promote venous return (see Chapter 39).

Critical Decision Point   *Pain or tingling on the anterior surface of the leg and dorsum of the foot indicates pressure on peroneal nerve as a result of bandages or traction boot. This can cause footdrop.*

STEP	RATIONALE
c Ensure that boot size is correct. Traction boot should fit snugly (not too tight or too loose).	Boot that is too tight leads to pressure to skin, peroneal nerve, and vascular structures. A traction boot that is too loose leads to slipping and lack of traction force.
d Properly seat heel in traction boot. Do not pad at heel. Cut out heel section of foam boot if necessary.	Prevents pressure over heel.
e Do not apply traction boot over pneumatic compression devices. You may use foot pumps (see Chapter 10).	Causes undue pressure on tissues and negates effects of compression device.
5 Assist with attachment of spreader bars, ropes, and pulleys. Tie ropes securely in knots, pass ropes in grooves of pulleys to weights, and make sure they are not frayed (see Box 11-2).	Provides proper weighted traction for extremity alignment.
6 When all traction materials and spreader bars are in place, weights are placed on weight holder and attached to loop in rope. The weights are then *lowered slowly and gently* until rope is taut. Physician orders exact amount of weight to be applied, position patient will maintain for majority of time, and turning regimen when pertinent.	Traction is slowly established to avoid involuntary muscle spasms or pain for patient. Weight should be sufficient to create enough pull to overcome muscle spasms but not to cause distraction or marked increase in pain.
7 Before physician leaves, assess patient's position and ask about additional permissible positions for patient and bed.	Ensures patient's safety and position for effective traction.
a *Buck's extension:* Patient is primarily on back; may be allowed to turn to unaffected side for brief periods (10 to 15 minutes).	Positioning on side permits back care and rest to tissues.
b *Dunlop's traction:* Patient must lie on back. Bed may be tilted on low shock blocks toward side opposite traction. Head of bed is kept flat.	Tilting uses body for some countertraction.
c *Russell's traction:* Patient lies on back; head of bed may be elevated 30 to 45 degrees, depending on injury.	Low-Fowler's position creates most effective traction pull.
8 For safety, raise upper side rails as appropriate. Patients in Bryant's traction should always have someone in attendance.	Promotes patient safety.
9 Gather unused materials, and return to storage areas. Perform hand hygiene.	Promotes safety and cleanliness. Reduces transmission of microorganisms.

EVALUATION

1 Observe patient's participation in self-care.	Some patients avoid activity unnecessarily, whereas others try to do too much.
2 Assess condition of skin around traction straps or bandages.	Ensures early identification of irritation or breakdown.
3 Inspect entire traction setup and functioning: observe all knots, ropes in pulleys, correct weights on weight holder; note whether apparatus is hanging freely and not resting on floor; position any material for specific traction; ensure sheets/blankets not interfering with traction apparatus; and ensure patient is in proper body alignment.	Evaluation is necessary to determine if traction is functioning as designed or desired or to make needed adjustments. Malfunctioning traction interferes with healing.
4 Ask if patient understands mobility restrictions.	Feedback demonstrates learning.
5 Ask patient to rate pain on a scale of 0 to 10, and assess if patient is experiencing spasm or muscle burning.	Indicates misalignment of bones or presence of muscle spasms. Initial reaction may be slight increase in soreness or pain until patient is able to relax and allow traction to perform as designed.
6 Assess neurovascular status 15 minutes after application of skin traction and every 1 to 2 hours for 24 hours, then extend to every 4 hours if patient is stabilizing (see Skill 11-1, Evaluation, Step 2).	Provides objective data concerning peripheral perfusion to tissues. A circumferential dressing applied too tightly can cause pressure applied to nerves and vascular structures, resulting in a potentially irreversible deficit (Judge, 2007).
7 Skin traction is released every 4 to 8 hours, with skin condition assessed and care given. Wash, pat dry, lubricate skin, and apply a light dusting of powder before reapplication of traction.	Prevents pressure ulcers and gives early feedback regarding skin condition. *Skin traction may not be removed if it is immobilizing a fracture.*

STEP	RATIONALE

Unexpected Outcomes

1. Patient experiences increased pain, soreness, or stiffness from pull applied to injured tissues.

2. Patient experiences muscle spasms from muscle irritation.

3. Patient experiences displaced alignment (evident on radiographic film) if fracture is present.

4. Patient experiences sense of claustrophobia or being "held down" in traction.

5. *Buck's extension:* Patient develops pressure area on heel or inability to dorsiflex or evert foot in traction if traction boot, adhesive straps, or elastic bandages exert pressure over head of fibula.

6. *Dunlop's traction:* Patient experiences pressure on elbow, or patient is unable to approximate thumb to rest of fingers or experiences feeling of numbness of thumb or tingling along sides of thumb and index finger, or capillary refill is over 3 seconds in nail beds.

7. *Russell's traction:* Patient has pain behind knee or nonpalpable popliteal pulse.

8. Patient experiences burning, weeping, or drainage under adhesive strips or moleskin because of possible allergy or hypersensitivity.

Related Interventions

• Medicate with analgesics.

• Administer skeletal muscle relaxants.
• Maintain proper weights, alignment, and positioning.

• Explain intervention to patient, and monitor patient frequently.
• Administer antianxiety medication.
• Reapply traction, and evaluate neurovascular status within 15 minutes.

• Elastic bandage is too tight over radial nerve at wrist.
• Remove elastic bandage from forearm only, and rewrap more loosely; then reevaluate symptoms for alleviation or continuance.

• Readjust to prevent pressure to popliteal area.

• Remove traction, and notify health care provider.

Recording and Reporting

• Record assessment of skin underneath traction apparatus and nursing interventions to maintain skin integrity.
• Record neurovascular assessment of bilateral body parts (see Skill 11-1, Evaluation, Step 2).
• Record length of time patient is in or out of specific traction.
• Document instructions given to patient and family.

Teaching Considerations

• Explain that traction increases muscle weakness, spasms, and pain in older adult patients.
• When traction time is decreased or discontinued, teach patient to ambulate slowly within medical guidelines, gradually increasing length of time out of bed and distance walked.
• Teach patient to notify physician of undesirable signs, such as marked increase in pain, muscle spasms, and increased numbness. Symptoms may signify reinjury or insufficient healing.

Pediatric Considerations

• Infants and children have immature musculoskeletal tissues and are almost constant "movers."
• Always assess the skin under child for small misplaced objects such as toys.
• Young children may cry when weights are initially applied but usually stop crying soon.
• Modified Bryant's traction may be used occasionally with the thighs at 45 degrees of flexion and hips at 30 degrees abduction (Wilson and Scott, 2007).

Gerontological Considerations

• Some older adults have keratoses, rashes, or other lesions that become irritated in skin traction (Miller, 2004).
• Some older adults have long-standing conditions of musculoskeletal tissues such as arthritis or gout that could lead to inflamed tissues and skin breakdown.
• Older and chronically ill patients may have increased need for position changes resulting from limitations due to osteoporosis, osteomalacia, weakened muscles, or increased risk for skin breakdown (Miller, 2004).
• Older adults' skin heals more slowly, tears more easily, loses its elasticity, and becomes thinner than that of a younger adult (Tabloski, 2006). Use an alternating air pressure mattress or foam overlay on the bed to decrease the risk for skin breakdown.

Home Care Considerations

• If patient is to be discharged to home, instruct family or caregivers in care needs (including home traction) and mode of ambulation.
• After discontinuing traction, teach patient to dangle before ambulation, to proceed slowly with ambulation, and to gradually increase the time and distance ambulated.
• Assess the home environment, and adapt it to accommodate hospital bed and traction.
• Inspect integrity of traction daily—weights hang freely, traction ropes rest in groove of pulley, and patient's body is not allowed to interfere with countertraction. In many cases the patient's body is the countertraction.
• Instruct patient about use of muscle relaxants and analgesics if prescribed.

SKILL 11-4 Care of a Patient in Skeletal Traction and Pin Site Care

Skeletal traction is the second kind of traction used for the treatment of fractures or correction of orthopedic abnormalities. As with skin traction, you apply skeletal traction to one or several bones. Skeletal traction begins externally but continues internally directly through the bones. You attach weights to the skeletal pin, wire, or nail via ropes and pulleys. Amounts of weights for skeletal traction vary from 10 lb for Dunlop's skeletal traction, to 20 to 25 lb for cervical traction, to 30 to 40 lb for balanced suspension to the femur. Amounts of weights used are also dictated by age, overall condition of the patient in traction, and the purpose of the traction.

The procedure can also involve external fixation, which consists of a metal frame that secures pins inserted through the bone above and below a fracture site. The external fixation stabilizes a fracture with hardware visible outside the body. It fosters the healing of complex fractured bones, usually in the lower extremities.

Skeletal traction is often used when continuous traction is desired to properly immobilize, position, and align a fractured bone during the healing process. You provide safe care after skillful application of traction. Common forms of skeletal traction include the following:

1 *Balanced-suspension skeletal traction (BSST) to the femur:* Traction used for displaced or overriding fractures of the femur. Balanced suspension relieves muscle spasms and improves realignment of the fracture fragments and callus formation (Fig. 11-6). It is used less frequently because of the length of time required for hospitalization when it is used as the major form of treatment. It is now used primarily before surgical implantation of an internal fixation pin, plate, or nail until the patient's condition stabilizes to permit surgery. Balanced suspension involves the use of splints under the thigh and leg to suspend them off the bed, with a Kirschner wire or Steinmann pin supplying the traction

(Fig. 11-7, A and B). The pin or wire is drilled through the upper tibia and attached to a spreader, which is then attached to ropes, pulleys, and weights (Fig. 11-7, C). Sufficient weights are hung to overcome the quadriceps and hamstring muscle spasms; sometimes weights of 30 to 40 lb or more may be required initially. Suspension weights may be 7 to 8 lb, and they are balanced by 7 to 8 lb of countertraction.

2 Upper extremity traction:

Side-arm traction: Skeletal form of Dunlop's traction (Fig. 11-8, A). The difference consists mainly of a pin drilled through the lower humerus and attached to a spreader, ropes, pulleys, and weights. The forearm is held in vertical Buck's extension, as it would be in Dunlop's skin traction. Side-arm skeletal traction is for severe fractures, in which the greater pull permitted with the skeletal pin overcomes muscle spasms, resulting in effective alignment and union.

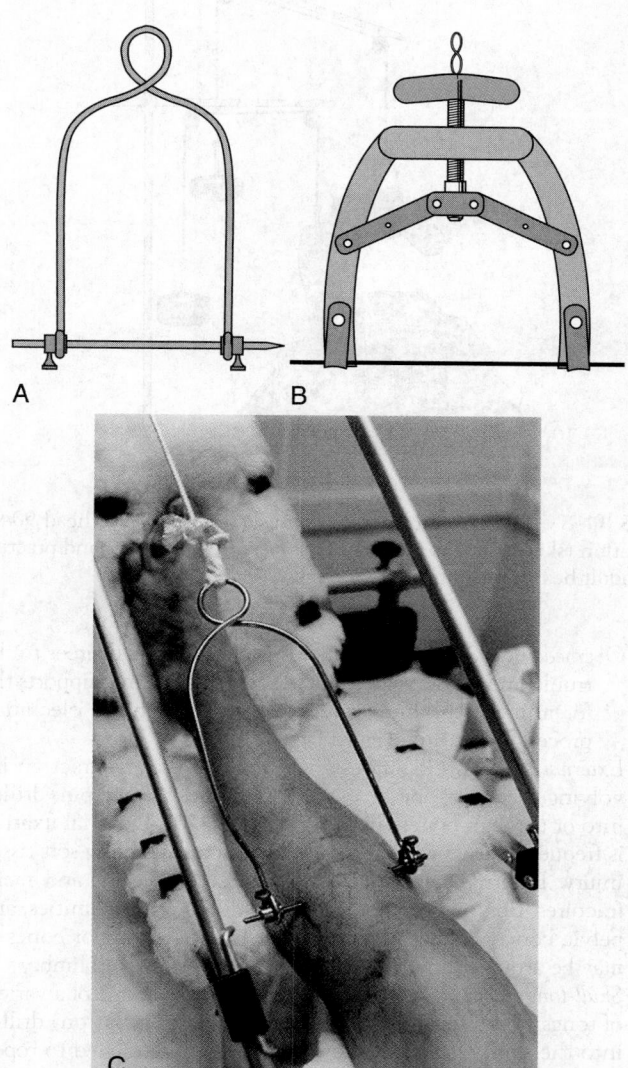

A   B

C

FIG 11-7 **A,** Steinmann pin and holder. **B,** Kirschner wire and tractor. **C,** Steinmann pin placed in tibial plateau for treatment of distal femoral fracture. (*C from Phipps W and others:* Medical-surgical nursing: concepts and clinical practice, *ed 6, St. Louis, 1995, Mosby.*)

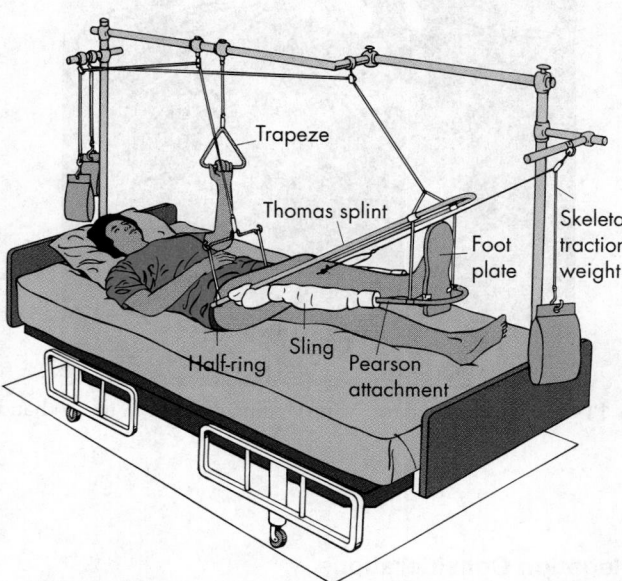

Trapeze

Thomas splint

Foot plate

Skeletal traction weight

Half-ring

Sling

Pearson attachment

FIG 11-6 Balanced-suspension skeletal traction. Traction is applied via Kirschner wire through proximal portion of tibia. Limb is supported by Thomas splint beneath thigh and Pearson attachment beneath lower leg. Foot plate attachment prevents footdrop. Weights apply countertraction to Thomas splint and suspend its lower end. Patient can shift position of the hips without change in amount of traction.

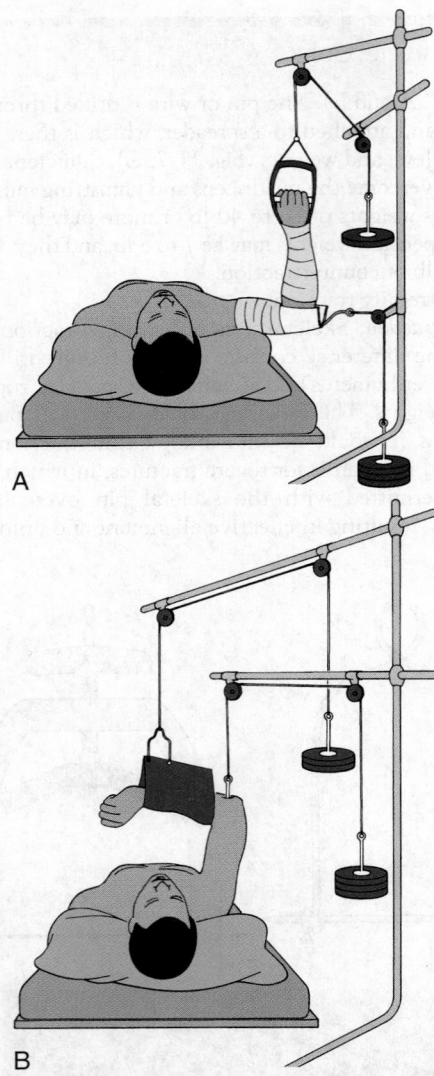

FIG 11-8 **A,** Side-arm traction (skin/skeletal). **B,** Overhead 90-90 traction (skeletal). *(From Beare PG, Myers JL: Principles and practice of adult health nursing, ed 3, St. Louis, 1998, Mosby.)*

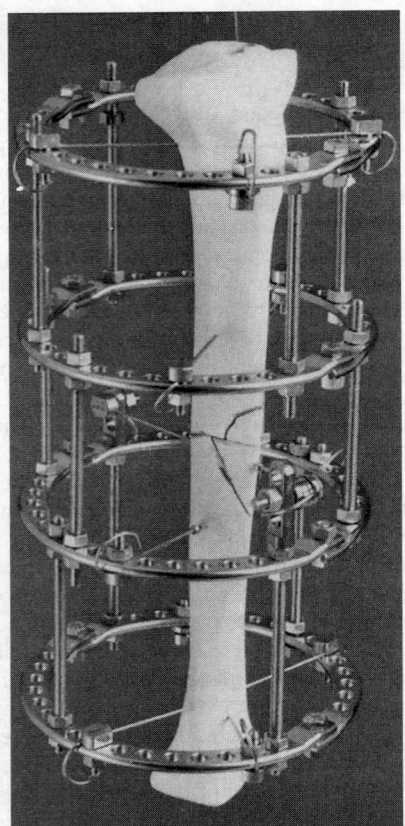

FIG 11-9 External fixator. Ilizarov external fixator for treatment of comminuted fractures. *(From Phipps W and others: Medical-surgical nursing: health and illness perspectives, ed 7, St. Louis, 2003, Mosby.)*

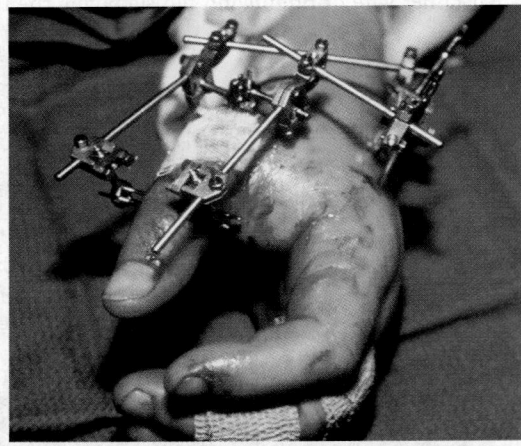

FIG 11-10 External fixator. Mini-Hoffman system in use on hand.

> *Overhead 90-90 traction:* Humerus is placed at 90 degrees to the trunk, and elbow is flexed at 90 degrees. A sling supports the forearm. A Kirschner wire is placed through the olecranon process of the ulna (Fig. 11-8, *B*).

3 *External fixation:* Commonly used form of skeletal traction involving the use of one of a variety of frames to hold pins drilled into or through bones (Figs. 11-9 and 11-10). External fixation is frequently used with comminuted fractures having soft tissue injury. External fixation frames are used for skull and facial fractures, ribs, all bones of the upper and lower extremities, and pelvic bones. Frames may fit on one side of a bone or bones or may be attached to pins on either side of an injured limb.

4 *Skull-tong traction:* Traction involving the use of one of a variety of tongs (Crutchfield, Vinke, Gardner-Wells, or Barton) drilled into the skull or placed below the scalp and attached to ropes, pulleys, and weights (Fig. 11-11). This type of traction is for fractures of cervical vertebrae and involves the use of special beds or turning frames to facilitate nursing care. Halo traction is for neurologically intact patients to prevent further spinal cord damage (Fig. 11-12).

Delegation Considerations

The skill of assessment of the patient's condition and status of traction cannot be delegated to NAP. However, the skills of assisting with insertion of skeletal pins and pin site care can be delegated to NAP who are adequately trained in principles of surgical asepsis. The nurse directs the NAP by:

- Instructing to report any signs and symptoms associated with infection or inflammation at pin insertion site.

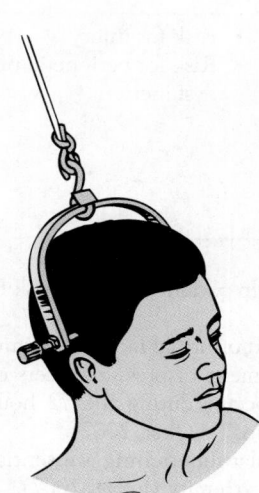

FIG 11-11   Gardner-Wells tongs for stabilization of cervical vertebral fractures.

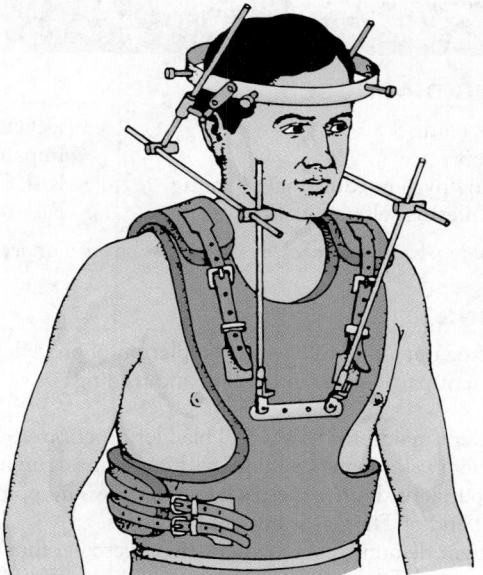

FIG 11-12   Halo vest. (*From Beare PG, Meyers JL: Principles and practice of adult health nursing, ed 3, 1998, Mosby.*)

Equipment
- ❏ Sterile gloves for physician
- ❏ Wastebasket with plastic liner
- ❏ Antiseptic ointment
- ❏ Skin preparation solutions as desired

Balanced-Suspension Skeletal Traction
- ❏ Sterile tray for insertion of Kirschner wire or Steinmann pin (secure from operating suite)
- ❏ Local anesthetic of physician's choice, usually 1% to 2% lidocaine
- ❏ Thomas splint or Harris splint
- ❏ Pearson attachment
- ❏ Foot support
- ❏ Trapeze bar
- ❏ Ropes, pulleys, weights, weight holders
- ❏ Towels, felt, stockinette
- ❏ Drill and extension cord if needed
- ❏ Adhesive tape

Upper Extremity Skeletal Traction
- ❏ Sterile tray with Kirschner wire or Steinmann pin (secure from operating suite)
- ❏ Adhesive strips or moleskin
- ❏ Elastic bandages
- ❏ Handgrip bar

- ❏ Ropes, pulley, weights, and weight holders
- ❏ Low shock blocks (*optional*)
- ❏ Local anesthetic of physician's choice, usually 1% to 2% lidocaine

External Fixation
- ❏ External fixator, usually Hoffman or Roger Anderson apparatus, Vital fixator, AO fixator, Ilizarov, or other fixator (see Figs. 11-9 and 11-10)
- ❏ Sterile tray with pins for insertion (secure from operating room)

Skull-Tong Traction
- ❏ Tongs: Crutchfield, Vinke, Gardner-Wells, Barton, or halo traction frame (see Figs. 11-11 and 11-12)
- ❏ Sterile tray: Usually traction is applied in operating room
- ❏ Drill and extension cord if needed
- ❏ Thomas cervical collar

Pin Care
- ❏ Sterile applicators
- ❏ Chlorhexidine 2 mg/mL
- ❏ Sterile containers
- ❏ Manufactured split sterile gauze barrier (*optional*)
- ❏ Topical antibiotic ointment (*optional*)
- ❏ Clean gloves, sterile gloves (*optional*)

STEP	RATIONALE

ASSESSMENT

1 Assess overall health condition of patient, including mobility status.	Determines patient's ability to tolerate both bed rest and skeletal traction.
2 Carefully assess specific tissues you will place in skeletal traction. Note marked edema, rash, or other open lesions.	Determines ability of tissues to tolerate traction. Skeletal pin goes through skin to bone and out through skin.
3 Assess patient's knowledge of upcoming traction, application, and purposes.	Determines willingness and ability to participate in care.
4 Assess patient's severity of pain on a scale of 0 to 10.	Used as baseline for later comparisons.
5 Observe patient's nonverbal behaviors, and encourage patient questions.	Reveals anxiety about impending procedure.

STEP	RATIONALE

NURSING DIAGNOSES

- Acute pain
- Anxiety
- Bathing/hygiene, dressing/grooming, and toileting self-care deficit
- Deficient knowledge regarding traction
- Impaired physical mobility
- Risk for impaired skin integrity
- Risk for infection
- Risk for injury
- Risk for peripheral neurovascular dysfunction

Individualize related factors based on patient's condition or needs.

PLANNING

1 Expected outcomes following completion of procedure:
- Patient participates in bathing and feeding.

  Self-care activities help patient to reduce risk for complications of immobility.

- Patient maintains bowel and bladder function.

  A fracture bedpan and/or urinal facilitate elimination functions.

- Patient's skin remains intact without redness, inflammation, or purulent drainage, especially over pressure points, proximal end of Thomas splint, and pin sites.

  Indicates no development of pressure ulcers or infection. Serous drainage usually occurs during the 72 hours following placement of skeletal pins (Walker, 2007).

- Patient demonstrates adequate neurovascular functioning in extremity. Distal skin tissues remain warm and of a normal skin color with capillary refill of 3 seconds or less. Patient verbalizes no abnormal sensations and is able to move fingers or toes below fracture site.

  Adequate neurovascular functioning is essential to the health and well-being of the extremity (Judge, 2007).

- Patient retains ROM in unaffected extremities.

  Routine exercise prevents contractures and muscle wasting.

- Patient demonstrates correct use of trapeze.

  Prevents injury.

- Patient describes purpose of skeletal traction and follows activity restrictions.

  Demonstrates learning and acceptance of restrictions.

- Patient experiences reduced pain and muscle spasm.

  Alignment of fracture reduces stress on bone fragments and adjoining muscle groups.

- Patient does not become tense or withdrawn.

  Demonstrates absence of anxiety.

- Patient complies with restrictions imposed by traction apparatus.

  No injury is sustained.

IMPLEMENTATION

1 Prepare initial traction setup:
  a Position patient according to physician's request. You may need assistance to support tissues to be placed in traction. Patient will most often be on back with head of bed slightly elevated. Patient will be flat in bed for Dunlop's skeletal traction.

  Ensures proper alignment during and after traction application.

  b Physician performs skin preparation and discards materials in wastebasket. Applies sterile gloves and gown using surgical asepsis.

  Reduces possibility of wound and bone infection.

  c Physician injects local anesthetic into sites as desired. Nurse and other assistants support patient, limb, or other tissues to be placed in traction. Burr holes may be drilled in the outer layer of the skull for placement of tongs.

  Anesthetic acts quickly to create painless area. Patient will feel pressure of pin being drilled through or into bones and will hear drill but should feel no pain.

  d Provide encouragement and praise during drilling of pin tracts.

  Reduces patient anxiety.

  e Assist (usually by holding spreader bar, splint, or Pearson attachment) while physician continues to use drill to insert number of pins or nails desired for traction. Support area of joints not at injury site. Do not move distal portion unnecessarily.

  Movement can cause severe pain or additional trauma.

2 Prepare specific traction setups:
  a Balanced-suspension skeletal traction (BSST)

STEP	RATIONALE
(1) *For lower extremity traction:* Assist with placement of Thomas or Harris splint, Pearson attachment, foot support, ropes, pulleys, and weights. Gently lower weights to establish traction. Apply antiseptic ointment to pin exit sites, and cover with sterile manufactured split dressing.	Splint and attachment are usually previously prepared for quick use. Foot plate prevents footdrop. Apply ointment and dressings to cover open wounds to prevent infection.
(2) *For side-arm traction:* Assist with application of Buck's extension to forearm, place handgrip, and establish skin traction by *slowly* lowering weights until rope is taut (see Fig. 11-8, A).	Skin traction allows forearm to remain in vertical position without undue effort from patient.
(3) *For 90-90 traction:* Assist with preparing sling for forearm (see Fig. 11-8, B).	
(4) Assist with application of spreader to hold skeletal pin; tie rope to spreader, and thread through pulleys to weight holder and weights. Slowly lower weights until rope is taut. Place shock blocks if requested. Apply antiseptic ointment to pin exit sites, and cover with sterile manufactured split dressing.	Amount of weight depends on severity of patient's injury. Amounts vary from 5 to 10 lb or more. Shock blocks allow one side of bed to be raised to help patient maintain desired position. Ointment and sterile split dressings prevent infection.
(5) Cover ends of pins (wires) with corks or tape.	Prevents injury to patient or caregivers.
(6) Attach trapeze bar, and instruct in use.	Allows the patient to assist in movement and to maintain upper body muscle tone.
b External fixation	
(1) Hold affected tissues or limb while physician attaches and tightens fixator screws or clamps. Apply antiseptic ointment to pin exit sites, and cover with sterile manufactured split dressing.	Proper tension or tightness to pins is vital to prevent twist or torque, which will delay healing. Ointment and sterile split dressings prevent infection.
c Skull-tong traction	
(1) Patient's cervical vertebrae are maintained in proper alignment with a Thomas cervical collar. Collar remains in place until skull-tong traction is surgically placed. Traction is applied by weights ordered by physician.	Maintains proper cervical vertebrae alignment, thus reducing further injury and/or paralysis to the cervical segment of the spinal cord.
3 Assess patient's initial reaction or response to traction before physician leaves.	Adjustments may be required immediately.
4 Raise side rails as appropriate without inappropriately restraining patient.	Provides for patient's safety.
5 Gather equipment and supplies, and return to proper storage places. Perform hand hygiene.	Provides for safety and cleanliness and prevents transmission of infection.
6 Ensure that skeletal traction is maintained continuously	Prevents overriding of bones that causes soft tissue damage and prevents misalignment (Hockenberry and Wilson, 2007).
7 Perform pin site care on a daily or weekly basis after the first 48 to 72 hours:	The National Association of Orthopaedic Nurses' expert panel found little research evidence to support a specific protocol for management of skeletal pin sites. Four evidenced-based recommendations are provided earlier in the chapter (Holmes and Brown, 2005). Some institutions have policies outlining pin site care, and others permit pin site care only with a physician's orders.
NOTE: After traction procedure, discuss with physician whether pin care will be performed. Type and frequency of pin site care varies according to physician preference and institutional policy.	
a Perform hand hygiene, and apply clean gloves.	Reduces transmission of infection. Use latex-free gloves if there is risk for an allergic reaction (Barker and Montagna, 2005).
b Remove old split gauze dressing around pins, and discard in receptacle. Note condition of tissues around pin site.	Evaluates ongoing condition of tissues. Ensures early identification of infection.
c Prepare supplies, and apply new gloves (sterile gloves are optional, see agency policy).	Aseptic technique reduces infection transmission.

STEP	RATIONALE
d Begin by cleaning pins on one side of extremity, and then do same on other side. Never touch one pin site with material used on another.	Prevents cross contamination.
e Dip sterile cotton-tipped applicator into sterile container of chlorhexidine 2 mg/mL solution. Place sterile applicator by the pin, and roll it along the skin, away from insertion site. Clean outward in a circular fashion from the pin. Dispose of applicator.	Remove crusts from pin site when signs of infection are present. Chlorhexidine 2 mg/mL is the most effective cleansing solution for pin site care (Holmes and Brown, 2005).
f Dip a new sterile applicator in chlorhexidine solution; roll applicator across skin away from pin.	Removes cleansing solution to reduce skin irritation.
g Using a sterile applicator, apply a small amount of topical antibiotic ointment to pin site, and cover with a sterile 2 × 2 inch manufactured split gauze dressing. (NOTE: Some physicians do not use antibiotic ointment, and some leave site uncovered.)	Antiinfective reduces bacterial growth.
h Repeat procedure for other pin site.	
8 Discard supplies. Remove and dispose of gloves. Perform hand hygiene.	Reduces transmission of infection.

EVALUATION

1 Evaluate entire traction setup and functioning:	Determines if traction is functioning as desired.
a Observe that knots are not caught in pulleys and that ropes are running straight through pulleys.	Anything that inhibits the smooth movement of the traction rope in the pulley will disrupt the traction and may lead to nonunion.
b Observe ropes for fraying.	
c Evaluate that correct weight is hanging (do not add or remove weight without physician order) and dangling freely.	
d Determine that linens are not interfering with traction apparatus.	
e Observe patient's body alignment.	Poor body alignment leads to discomfort and affects proper bone healing (Hockenberry and Wilson, 2007).
2 Determine patient's response to traction; evaluate for presence of pain and muscle spasms on a scale of 0 to 10.	Skeletal traction takes longer for patient to note relief of symptoms because of increased tissue trauma. Determines need for analgesics, muscle relaxants, and success of traction in stabilizing fracture.
3 Inspect pin sites for drainage, tenderness, or inflammation.	Early signs of infection (Holmes and Brown, 2005).
4 Evaluate for other indicators of infection, such as fever; elevated white blood cell count; continuous, dull, aching pain; redness; or warmth in extremity.	Early signs of osteomyelitis (Huether and McCance, 2004).
5 Perform neurovascular assessment (see Skill 11-1, Evaluation, Step 2).	Determines peripheral perfusion to tissues, as well as patient's sensation and voluntary motor activity (Judge, 2007).
6 Assess for indicators of hypoxemia, such as restlessness or agitation.	Recognizes early signs of fat embolism syndrome (FES) (Porth, 2005).
7 Inspect skin, especially around ankle, elbow, foot, or distal tibia, for fracture blisters. Do not rupture blister. Apply hydrocolloid dressing to ruptured blister.	Fracture blisters are associated with increased interstitial pressure from posttraumatic edema. Intact skin provides a barrier to prevent infection (Porth, 2005). Covering the blister with a dressing maintains a clean environment.

Unexpected Outcomes

1 Skeletal pin moves or slides in pin tract, leading to increased risk for infection or nonunion.

2 Patient experiences delayed union, malunion, or nonunion.

3 Patient has severe edema, marked increase in pain, inability to actively move joints, or increased pain on passive movement, indicating compartment syndrome.

4 Patient develops infection at pin site or at fracture site with development of osteomyelitis.

5 Patient experiences prolonged bleeding or frank hemorrhage.

6 Patient experiences nerve damage:

   a Peroneal nerve: footdrop with inability to evert and dorsiflex foot

   b Radial or median nerve at wrist with inability to approximate thumb and fingers (radial) and numbness and tingling of thumb, index, middle fingers (median) with wrist drop

7 Patient experiences FES (more common in fractures of long bones) with symptoms of hypoxemia: restlessness, decreased level of orientation, disorientation, tachycardia, tachypnea, dyspnea, hypotension, and petechial rash over upper chest and neck.

8 Patient experiences deep vein thrombosis with possible pulmonary embolus, including clinical manifestations of dyspnea, chest pain, tachypnea, apprehension, tachycardia, cyanosis, and circulatory collapse.

9 Patient experiences declining voluntary motor responses.

Related Interventions

- Notify health care provider.

- Ensure that proper amount of weight is continuously maintained.
- Provide proper nutrition.
- Notify health care provider of infection.
- Notify physician or health care provider immediately.

- Maintain aseptic technique.
- Notify health care provider.
- Administer ordered antibiotics.
- Some chronically ill or older patients have preexistent iron deficiency anemia made worse by bleeding or hemorrhage. Replacement of blood loss is often required.

- Notify physician.
- Loosen boot or circumferential dressings.
- Notify physician.
- Loosen elastic bandage at wrist for side-arm traction.
- Reposition sling at wrist for overhead 90-90 traction.
- Notify physician, treat with oxygen, elevate head of bed.

- Do not massage lower extremity.
- If symptoms of pulmonary embolus are evident, elevate head of bed (if conscious), administer oxygen, and notify physician *immediately*.

- Notify physician.

Recording and Reporting

- Record in nurses' notes type of traction applied, persons applying traction, site to which traction was applied, time of application, amount of weights, and patient's initial response.
- Record all findings of neurovascular assessment (see Skill 11-1, Evaluation, Step 2) every 1 to 2 hours or as ordered.
- Document patient teaching and verbalization of understanding.

Teaching Considerations

- Before discharge, teach patient use of ambulatory aid (cane, walker, or crutches); give written instructions to patient and significant others.
- Provide patient written instructions for home care maintenance, especially if being discharged with external fixation (pin site care, elevate extremity when sitting or lying to prevent edema formation). Have patient and/or family demonstrate whatever care needs to be done (Holmes and Brown, 2005).
- Supply patient with dietary instructions if necessary.
- Teach patient to notify physician of undesirable signs, including increase in pain, muscle spasms, increased numbness or tingling, appearance of drainage, redness, or soreness at operative or traction pin sites.

Pediatric Considerations

- Teach families proper care of the external fixator devices (Holmes and Brown, 2005), and prepare them for the reactions of others regarding the devices.
- Blood loss from a fracture can become critical more quickly in the child than the adult because the relationship of blood volume to total body weight is greater in the child.

- Bone remodeling is rapid in children because of the thickened periosteum and liberal blood supply (Hockenberry and Wilson, 2007).
- Teach parents that infants may cry when establishing traction.
- Some children may experience boredom, regression, and interference with schoolwork. Parents and other caregivers must look for ways to divert the child's attention and support the child. Obtain schoolwork and assist the child, when able, in performing tasks. Counsel parents regarding regression to decrease their anxiety.
- Physical activity is essential for growth and development. Immobility often results in increased anxiety. Some behaviors children demonstrate include restlessness, depression, regression, lack of concentration, dependence, acting out, and outbursts of crying or temper tantrums (Hockenberry and Wilson, 2007).
- Assure children that someone will always be available to assist them while they are in traction.

Gerontological Considerations

- Some older adult patients suffer from diabetes or peripheral vascular disease, adding risks to use of traction.
- An overhead trapeze assists the older patient in maintaining upper body strength and in facilitating hygiene and repositioning.

Home Care Considerations

- After traction is discontinued, teach patient to dangle before ambulation, to proceed slowly with ambulation, and to gradually increase the time and distance ambulated.
- Provide patient instructions regarding use of muscle relaxants and analgesics if prescribed.

SKILL 11-5   Care of a Patient With Immobilization Devices

Immobilization devices increase stability, support weak extremities, or reduce the load on weight-bearing structures such as hips, knees, or ankles. A splint immobilizes and protects a body part. Temporary splints reduce pain and prevent tissue damage from further motion immediately after an injury such as a fracture or sprain. Air splints, Thomas splints, and improvised splints from material on hand are examples of temporary splints applied in emergency situations. Upper extremity fractures are sometimes managed using splints such as hand and digital splints or sugar-tong splints.

Slings support splints, casts, or injured upper extremities (Fig. 11-13). They are commercially available or are made. They are available for almost any body part. Velcro or buckle closures permit these devices to be adjusted to fit a body part of almost any size and shape.

The abduction splint or pillow, used after hip replacement surgery, maintains the patient's legs in an abducted position (Fig. 11-14). This permits the patient to be turned without changing the healing limb's position and prevents dislocation of the hip prosthesis. The device is easy to remove for skin care, dressing changes, or neurovascular assessments. A posterior splint with elastic wraps is sometimes used to support an extremity.

Cloth and foam splints, known as immobilizers, provide long-term immobilization (Fig. 11-15). Immobilizers treat sprains and dislocations that do not require complete and continuous immobilization in a cast or traction. Immobilizers are often used following orthopedic surgery. Other common types of immobilizers include cervical collars (soft or hard), belt-type shoulder immobilizers, and vinyl wrist forearm splints. Molded splints, made of plastic, provide support to patients with chronic injuries or diseases such as arthritis. They maintain the body part in a functional position to prevent contractures and muscle atrophy. A splint goes into place and removes quickly and easily when assessing skin or a wound.

Braces support weakened structures during weight bearing or to prevent postural deformity. They are made of sturdy materials such as leather, metal, and molded plastic. Chest and abdominal braces immobilize the thoracic and lumbar vertebral column to treat scoliosis (lateral curvature of the spine) or kyphosis (convex curvature of the spine) (Hockenberry and Wilson, 2007). The brace does not correct the curve but instead prevents its progression. Lumbar braces support lumbar and sacral tissues after spinal surgery or fusion. Leg braces hold the thigh, leg, and foot in functional positions for weight bearing and ambulation. Both short leg and long leg braces support weak leg muscles, aid in control of involuntary muscle movement, or maintain surgical correction during the postoperative healing process.

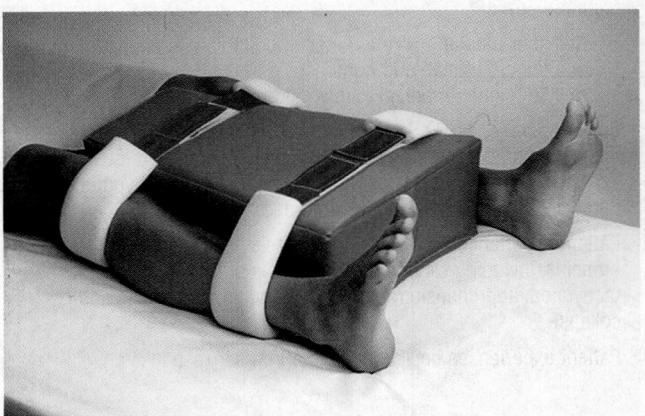

FIG 11-14   Abduction pillow.

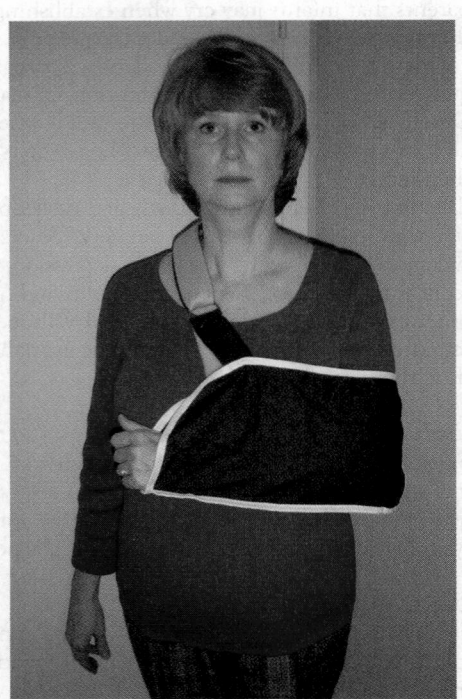

FIG 11-13   Sling for shoulder/arm immobilization. (*Courtesy Wanda Dubuisson.*)

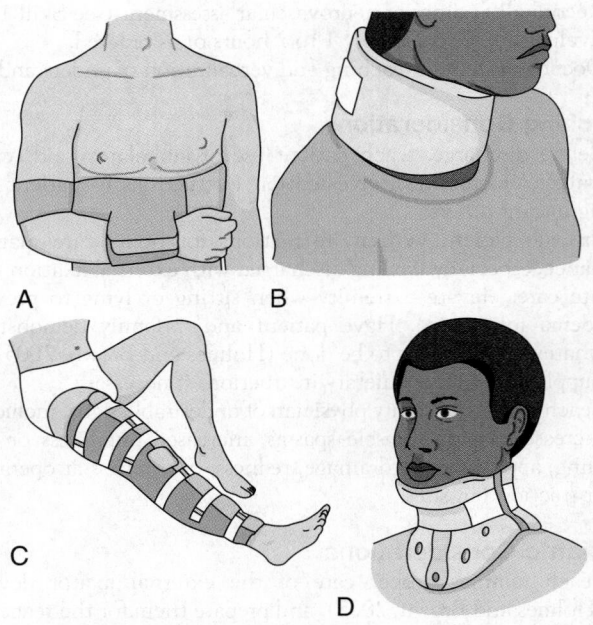

FIG 11-15   Examples of immobilizers. **A,** Shoulder immobilizer. **B,** Soft cervical collar. **C,** Knee immobilizer. **D,** Hard cervical collar. (*From Beare PG, Meyers JL: Principles and practice of adult health nursing, ed 3, 1998, Mosby.*)

Delegation Considerations

The skill of assessment of a patient's condition cannot be delegated to NAP. However, the skill of caring for a patient wearing a brace, splint, or sling may be delegated to NAP or family members. The nurse directs the family members and NAP by:

- Reviewing the purpose of the brace/splint/sling as it applies to the patient.
- Reviewing correct application of the brace/splint/sling and positioning of any ties or straps.
- Reviewing prescribed schedule of wear and activities permitted while in the brace/splint/sling.

- Informing the nurse if the patient complains of pain, rubbing, or pressure from the brace/splint/sling or if a change occurs in the patient's skin condition.

Equipment

- ❏ Brace/splint/commercially prepared sling or triangular bandage and safety pin
- ❏ Cotton shirt or gown

STEP	RATIONALE
ASSESSMENT	
1 Review patient's chart, including medical history, previous and current activity level, and description of the condition requiring immobilization.	Reveals patient's current and previous health status and purpose for the brace/splint/sling.
2 Assess patient's previous experience with braces/splints/slings.	Reveals patient's baseline knowledge.
3 Assess patient's pain severity on scale of 0 to 10.	Provides baseline to determine efficacy of device.
4 Assess patient's understanding of reason for, care of, application of, and schedule of wear for brace/splint/sling.	Determines level of instruction needed.
5 Assess patient's risk for skin breakdown because of brace/splint/sling or immobilization. Look at area of skin to be in contact with support device.	Immobilized and older patients are particularly vulnerable to skin breakdown (Miller, 2004).
6 Refer to occupational or physical therapy consultation to determine type of brace to be used, desired position, and amount of activity and movement permitted.	
7 Assess patient's additional need for an assistive device such as a cane, walker, or crutches.	An assistive device is often necessary to provide support and promote balance during ambulation.

NURSING DIAGNOSES

- Acute pain
- Bathing/hygiene and dressing/grooming self-care deficit
- Deficient knowledge regarding immobilization device

- Disturbed body image
- Impaired home maintenance
- Impaired physical mobility
- Risk for impaired skin integrity
- Risk for ineffective tissue perfusion

- Risk for injury
- Risk for peripheral neurovascular dysfunction

Individualize related factors based on patient's condition or needs.

PLANNING	
1 Expected outcomes following completion of procedure:	
• Patient's skin remains in good condition without circulatory impairment.	Indicates no friction or pressure from device.
• Patient and significant other, if any, verbalize purpose, correct application, and care of the device.	Encourages cooperation and minimizes risks and anxiety of the procedure.
• Patient rates pain less than 4 on a scale of 0 to 10.	Indicates proper fit of device and permits safer ambulation.
• Circulation and sensation distal to brace/splint is maintained.	Reveals there are no changes in neurovascular status following application (Judge, 2007).
• Patient uses the device correctly, including schedule of wear, activity limitations, and positioning.	Demonstrates learning.
• Patient demonstrates adjustment to changes in physical appearance or function	Reveals that patient is confident in abilities and willing to try different strategies to enhance appearance (London and others, 2007).

IMPLEMENTATION	
1 Preparing to apply a splint/brace/sling:	
a Perform hand hygiene.	Reduces transmission of microorganisms.
b Explain reasons for the brace/splint/sling, and demonstrate how the device works.	Teaching and demonstration enhance learning, reduce anxiety, and encourage cooperation.

STEP	RATIONALE
c Assist the patient to a comfortable position, preferably sitting or lying down.	Patient's position will depend on the type of brace/splint/sling being used. Apply upper-extremity braces/splints/slings with the patient sitting upright. Apply lower-extremity braces with the patient lying down.
d Prepare the skin that will be enclosed in the brace/splint/sling by cleaning the skin with soap and water, rinsing, patting dry, and changing any dressings (if present). If applying a back brace, put a thin cotton shirt or gown on the patient. Ensure that there are no wrinkles causing pressure.	This protects the skin, absorbs moisture, and keeps the brace/splint/sling clean (London and others, 2007).

Critical Decision Point *Instruct patient to inform the health care provider if there is a feeling of pressure, pain, numbness, rubbing, or if the skin becomes reddened.*

STEP	RATIONALE
e Inspect the device for wear, damage, or rough edges.	Decreases potential for skin breakdown and maintains correct alignment.
2 Apply the brace/splint/sling as directed by physician, orthotist, physical therapist, or occupational therapist.	Proper application of the brace/splint/sling is important to avoid skin breakdown, pressure ulcers, neurovascular compromise, calluses, or worsening of the deformity.
a Securing splint with elastic bandage: (1) Apply even tension while wrapping bandage for splint from distal to proximal. (2) Prevent padding from gathering or bunching.	Prevents trapping of blood distal to immobilization device.
b Applying sling using triangular bandage: (1) Position one end of the bandage over the shoulder of the unaffected arm. (2) Take the remaining bandage, and place the material against the chest, then under and over the affected arm, cradling the arm.	
(3) Position the pointed end of the triangle toward the elbow.	This position cradles the arm.
(4) Tie the two ends of the triangle at the side of the neck.	This prevents skin irritation and pressure to the back of the neck.
(5) Fold the pointed end of the sling at the elbow in the front, and secure with a safety pin, closing the end of the sling.	Provides full support of extremity
(6) Adjust the length of the sling by adjusting the amount of material in the knot.	
(7) Ensure the sling supports the limb comfortably without interfering with circulation.	This prevents pressure on the radial artery, which will impair circulation.
3 Teach patient the prescribed schedule of wear and allowed activities while in the brace/splint/sling as directed by physician, physical therapist, or occupational therapist.	Proper use of the brace/splint/sling will facilitate healing and mobility and reduce pain and stress.
4 Reinforce the signs of skin breakdown, pressure, or rubbing to report.	Brace/splint/sling may need to be adjusted. Sometimes changes are necessary because of growth or atrophy, when muscles regain or lose strength, or after reconstructive surgery. Pay particular attention to insensitive areas of the body (London and others, 2007).
5 Assist patient with finding attractive clothes to fit over immobilizing device.	Improves body image and decreases feeling of alienation.
6 Teaching patient how to care for the brace/splint/sling:	Ensures that the device is in optimum working order. If the device is broken, or out of alignment, notify the orthotist (Hockenberry and Wilson, 2007).
a Store metal braces upright. Keep joints well oiled.	
b Clean splints of molded materials with soap and water, dry thoroughly, and store away from heat.	
c Treat leather materials with a leather preservative to prevent drying or cracking.	
d Most slings can be gently washed to remove any soiling.	

STEP	RATIONALE

e When not in use, store brace/splint/sling in a safe but easily accessible location.

f Keep the brace clean and dry. Clean plastic parts with a damp cloth and thoroughly dry. Clean metal joints with a pipe cleaner and oil weekly. Remove rust with steel wool, and clean metal parts with a solvent.
 | Keeps brace in good working order.

7 Assist patient with ambulating with brace/splint/sling in place. | Ensures patient safety during ambulation.

Critical Decision Point *Let the patient know that although the brace/splint/sling seems awkward at first, after practice, the patient will feel more comfortable and better able to move about.*

8 Have patient apply and remove the brace/splint/sling. Some patients need assistance with application and removal of sling. | Promotes patient independence; demonstration confirms level of learning skill.

EVALUATION

1 Inspect areas of the skin underneath the brace/splint/sling for signs of pressure, including redness or breakdown. | Ensures early identification of irritation or breakdown.

2 Observe patient using the brace/splint/sling. | Some patients avoid activity unnecessarily, whereas others may try to do too much.

3 Ask the patient to rate level of comfort on scale of 0 to 10 while the brace/splint/sling is in place. | Indicates proper fit of device to ensure safe ambulation.

4 Palpate pulse and test sensation of extremity distal to position of brace/splint/sling. | Neurovascular status reflects vascular supply or pressure on tissues.

5 Ask patient/family how easy ADLs are to perform while wearing the brace/splint/sling. | Determines if alternative self-care approaches are necessary

6 Patient states confidence in physical and social abilities related to wearing immobilizing device and is willing to try different strategies to enhance appearance. | Reveals confidence in ability and willingness to try different strategies to enhance appearance.

Unexpected Outcomes

1 Patient is unable to use the brace/splint/sling correctly.

2 Patient develops areas of pressure, redness, or skin breakdown.

3 Circulation to the affected extremity is altered because of improper fit.

Related Interventions

- Reassess patient for correct fit.
- Reassess level of comfort.
- Reassess muscle strength in uninvolved extremities.
- Obtain referral for physical or occupational therapy.

- Assess device for proper fit and positioning.
- Inspect brace/splint/sling for damage, wear, or rough edges.
- Inform the health care provider.
- Inform the orthotist, physical therapist, or occupational therapist so that adjustments to brace/splint can be made.
- Do not allow patient to use the brace/splint until adjustments are made.
- If necessary, *temporarily* pad the area of incorrect fit rather than the reddened or irritated area.

- Remove the device immediately.
- Notify health care provider.

Recording and Reporting

- Record specific assessments related to skin integrity, neurovascular status, type of brace/splint/sling applied, schedule of wear, activity level and movement permitted, and patient's tolerance of procedure in progress notes.
- Document instructions given to patient and family.
- Record observations regarding patient's ability to apply, ambulate with, and remove the brace/splint/sling.
- Immediately report any injury sustained while using the brace/splint/sling.

Teaching Considerations

- Teach parents how to apply and maintain the brace/splint/sling. Place cotton T-shirt under upper extremity brace and long, cotton tube socks under lower extremity brace.
- Avoid lotions or powders that may irritate skin.
- Teach family exercises to perform when child is out of brace (e.g., Boston brace).
- Teach patient appropriate ROM exercises within limitation of device.
- Advise patient and caregiver of signs and symptoms of impaired skin integrity to report.

Pediatric Considerations

- Recognize that bracing in an adolescent often affects body image and self-esteem.
- Encourage adolescent to engage in conversation that focuses on body perception and to discuss experiences with peers (Hockenberry and Wilson, 2007).

Geriatric Considerations

- With aging there is decreased rate of epidermal proliferation, decreased skin moisture, thinner dermis, and decreased dermal blood supply (Miller, 2004).
- The older patient experiences diminished muscle mass, degenerative connective tissue changes, and progressive decline in bone mass (Ebersole and others, 2008).
- Some older patients have limited mobility as a result of postural deviations such as increased kyphosis and decreased lordosis (Ebersole and others, 2008).

Home Care Considerations

- Recognize that prolonged immobility in a brace/splint/sling may cause decreased ROM or contractures.
- Assess the ability and willingness of the patient and primary caregiver to perform care required for the brace/splint/sling.
- Remove the brace/splint/sling when bathing or showering.
- Assess for environmental factors in the home that will interfere with safe ambulation.
- Inspect and clean braces/splints/slings weekly.
- Assist patients with adapting clothing so they can maintain an acceptable appearance.
- Assist patient or parents with developing plan to manage ADLs while braced.
- Enlist occupational therapy in helping patient develop the highest quality of life possible.

? CRITICAL THINKING EXERCISES

Mrs. Cleveland, age 85, fell while coming down the steps at her church. She is admitted to the orthopedic unit, where you are assigned as her primary nurse. She sustained an intertrochanteric fracture of the right femur and a fracture of her right wrist as she tried to catch herself. She has a fiberglass cast on her right forearm and Buck's extension traction boot on her right leg. It is anticipated that she will go to surgery within 24 hours for an open reduction and internal fixation of her femur.

1   Position Mrs. Cleveland's casted arm:
   A Carefully with palms of your hands to ensure that there are no indentations
   B On a plastic-covered pillow to prevent the linens from becoming damp
   C On several pillows, elevate the casted extremity with the hand higher than the elbow to decrease swelling
   D With a cradle over it to ensure air flow for proper drying

2   Mrs. Cleveland is receiving an opioid analgesic intravenously via a patient-controlled analgesia (PCA) pump. As the afternoon progresses, Mrs. Cleveland complains of pain and a squeezing, jumpy feeling in her right thigh. You will first:
   A Massage her right thigh to relax her muscles
   B Medicate her with a muscle relaxant to decrease muscle spasms
   C Medicate her with a bolus dose of opioid analgesic for breakthrough pain
   D Release the Buck's traction briefly to decrease the pain

3   It has been 12 hours, and Mrs. Cleveland's fingers on her right hand are swelling. Her cast has been elevated to heart level and ice packs have been applied to the sides of the cast. In spite of these measures and liberal doses of opioid analgesics, the pain continues. What action should you take?
   A Apply a heating pad circumferentially.
   B Apply additional ice packs to the top and bottom of the cast.
   C Obtain an order to change the analgesic to another one.
   D Notify the physician, and prepare for bivalving the cast.

4   The linens are soiled and need to be changed. You and the NAP will:
   A Change the linens as you remove the boot and maintain manual traction
   B Leave the traction in place and briefly roll Mrs. Cleveland to the unaffected side to change the linens
   C Remove the traction long enough to change the linens
   D Wait until the morning to change the linens when Mrs. Cleveland goes to surgery

---

✓ REVIEW QUESTIONS

1   A patient is in balanced skeletal traction because of a fractured femur. What should be included in the patient's nursing care?
   1 Keeping the head of the bed elevated between 10 and 20 degrees to prevent hypostatic pneumonia
   2 Eliminating the pillow under the affected part if the patient lies perfectly still
   3 Teaching the patient how to use the trapeze bar
   4 Removing some of the weights if the patient complains of periodic pain

2   The nurse is planning care of a young man with a newly fractured left leg with a cast. What is the most effective way to control swelling of the fractured extremity?
   1 Apply the ordered ice bag to the left leg.
   2 Elevate the casted extremity on one pillow.
   3 Use a cooling blanket under the patient.
   4 Reposition the patient's hip every 2 hours.

3   A patient is having her long arm cast removed. Which activities should the patient be expected to perform after the cast is removed? Select all that apply.
   1 Inspect the underlying skin for redness or drainage
   2 Apply emollient lotion to soften the skin
   3 Begin full activities and exercise
   4 Use friction to remove dead skin by rubbing the area with a towel
   5 Wash the skin gently with mild soap and hot water
   6 Keep the arm elevated as needed to control swelling

4   The nurse suspects that a patient might be developing clinical manifestations of neurovascular deficit following application of Buck's skin traction. Which of the following neurovascular assessments is the most significant?
   1 Capillary refill of 3 seconds in the affected foot
   2 Diminished posterior tibial pulse of the affected foot
   3 Numbness and tingling in the affected foot
   4 Pain on passive motion of the affected foot

5   The nurse has four patients, each in a different type of traction. During the assessment of the patients, nursing care would be correct if the head of the bed was raised to 45 degrees for the patient in which traction?
   1 Modified Bryant's traction
   2 Dunlop's traction
   3 Russell's traction
   4 Buck's traction

REFERENCES

Altizer L: Casting for immobilization, *Orthop Nurs* 23(2):136, 2004.

Andrews M, Boyle J: *Transcultural concepts in nursing care*, Philadelphia, 2003, Lippincott.

Barker P, Montagna D: It's just "balloon-acy"! The hidden dangers of latex allergy, *AAOHN J* 53(6):241, 2005.

Beare PG, Meyers JL: *Principles and practice of adult health nursing*, ed 3, 1998, Mosby.

Bongiovanni MS and others: Orthopedic trauma: critical care nursing issues, *Crit Care Nurs Q* 28(1):60, 2005.

Braun SV and others: Superior mesenteric artery syndrome following spinal deformity correction, *J Bone Joint Surg* 88(10):2252, 2006.

Ebersole P and others: *Geriatric nursing and healthy aging*, ed 3, St. Louis, 2008, Mosby.

Folcik M and others: *Traction: assessment and management*, St. Louis, 1994, Mosby.

Hockenberry MJ, Wilson, D: *Wong's nursing care of infants and children*, ed 8, St. Louis, 2007, Mosby.

Huether SE, McCance KL: *Understanding pathophysiology*, ed 3, St. Louis, 2004, Mosby.

Judge NL: Neurovascular assessment, *Nurs Stand* 21(45):39, 2007.

Lehne RA: *Pharmacology for nursing care*, ed 5, St Louis, 2004, Saunders.

London ML and others: *Maternal and child nursing care*, ed 2, Upper Saddle River, NJ, 2007, Prentice Hall.

Lucas B, Davis P: Why restricting movement is important. In Kneal J, Davis P, editors: *Orthopaedic and trauma nursing*, ed 2, Edinburgh, 2005, Churchill Livingstone.

Maher AB and others: *Orthopaedic nursing*, ed 3, Philadelphia, 2002, Saunders.

Mauk KL: *Gerontological nursing: competencies for care*, Boston, 2006, Jones & Bartlett.

Miller CA: *Nursing for wellness in older adults: theory and practice*, ed 4, Philadelphia, 2004, Lippincott Williams & Wilkins.

National Guideline Clearinghouse: *Evidence-based care guidelines for femoral shaft fractures in children*, http://www.guideline.gov, accessed September 12, 2008.

Phipps W and others: *Medical-surgical nursing: concepts and clinical practice*, ed 6, St. Louis, 1995, Mosby.

Phipps W and others: *Medical-surgical nursing: health and illness perspectives*, ed 7, St. Louis, 2003, Mosby.

Porth CM: *Pathophysiology: concepts of altered health states*, ed 7, Philadelphia, 2005, Lippincott Williams & Wilkins.

Resch S and others: Preoperative skin traction or pillow nursing in hip fractures: a prospective, randomized study in 123 patients, *Disabil Rehabil* 27(18-19):1191, 2005.

Solomon L and others: *Apley's concise system of orthopaedics and fractures*, ed 3, London, 2005, Hodder Arnold.

Spector R: *Cultural diversity in health and illness*, ed 7, Upper Saddle River, NJ, 2008, Prentice Hall.

Tabloski PA: *Gerontological nursing*, Upper Saddle River, NJ, 2006, Prentice Hall.

Wheeles C: *Wheeles's textbook of orthopaedics*, Durham, 2008, Data Trace Publishing.

RESEARCH REFERENCES

Dahl AW and others: No difference between daily and weekly pin-site care: a randomized study of 50 patients with external fixation, *Acta Orthop Scand* 74(6):704, 2003.

Has B and others: External fixation and infection of soft tissues close to fracture localization, *Mil Med* 171(10):88, 2006.

Holmes SB, Brown SJ: Skeletal pin site care: National Association of Orthopaedic Nurses guidelines for orthopaedic nursing, *Orthop Nurs* 24(2):99, 2005.

National Guideline Clearinghouse: *Skeletal pin site care clinical practice guideline*, http://www.guideline.gov, accessed September 12, 2007.

Patterson MM: Multicenter pin care study, *Orthop Nurs* 24(5):349, 2005.

Temple J, Santy J: Pin site care for preventing infection associated with external bone fixators and pins, *Cochrane Database Syst Rev* (1):CD004551, 2004.

Walker JA: Evidence for skeletal pin site care, *Nurs Stand* 21(45):70, 2007.

Williams H, Griffiths P: The effectiveness of pin site care for patients with external fixators, *Br J Community Nurs* 9(5):206, 2004.

Wilson N, Stott N: Paediatric femoral fractures: factors influencing length of stay and readmission rate, *Injury* 38(8):931, 2007.

12

Support Surfaces and Special Beds

MEDIA RESOURCES

- evolve *learning system*   http://evolve.elsevier.com/Perry/skills
  - Review Questions
  - Audio Glossary

OBJECTIVES

Mastery of content in this chapter will enable the nurse to:

- Identify the different types of support surfaces and specialty beds used for pressure redistribution.
- Explain why preventive nursing care is still essential when using support surfaces and special beds.
- Describe guidelines to follow when placing patients on support surfaces and special beds.
- Compare and contrast differences between mattress overlays and mattress replacements.
- Describe mechanisms by which skin breakdown can occur on an air-suspension or an air-fluidized bed, a bariatric bed, a Rotokinetic bed, or a support surface mattress.
- Describe correct placement of a patient on an air-fluidized bed, an air-suspension bed, a bariatric bed, a Rotokinetic bed, or a support surface mattress.

Despite increasing technological advances in health care, pressure ulcers remain a major problem that increases patient suffering, length of stay in a hospital or long-term care facility, and health care costs. Although a multidisciplinary team approach is key to reducing pressure ulcers, all agree that nurses are at the forefront of prevention and treatment of pressure ulcers in health care settings (Wound, Ostomy and Continence Nurses Society [WOCN], 2003). The National Pressure Ulcer Advisory Panel (NPUAP) (2007a) defines pressure ulcers as localized injury to the skin and/or underlying tissue, usually over a bony prominence, as a result of pressure or pressure in combination with shear and/or friction. Pressure ulcers occur in any age-group or ethnic population, regardless of socioeconomic status. The occurrence of pressure ulcers is a serious and expensive health care problem in the United States. Estimated costs for treatment of one full-thickness pressure ulcer can be as high as $70,000. The total cost for treatment of pressure ulcers in the United States is estimated at $11 billion per year (Reddy and others, 2006).

The pressure ulcer objective in *Healthy People 2010* is to reduce the prevalence of pressure ulcer diagnosis in nursing home residents from the current rate of 0.16% to 0.08% (NPUAP, 2004). To meet this challenge, along with the challenges of health care reform to improve quality while reducing costs, it is essential to identify patients at risk for breakdown. Factors contributing to pressure ulcer formation are both extrinsic (e.g., moisture, friction, and shear) and intrinsic (e.g., malnutrition, loss of sensation, impaired mobility, aging skin, impaired mental status, infection, incontinence, and low arteriolar pressure).

The major cause of pressure ulcers is unrelieved pressure. The greater the pressure and the longer the pressure is applied, the greater the likelihood that a pressure ulcer will develop. To stay healthy, body tissues require an adequate supply of oxygen and nutrients and removal of carbon dioxide and other waste products of metabolism. This requires maintenance of adequate blood flow through the capillaries, which is normally 12 to 32 mm Hg. When external pressure on the tissues exceeds 32 mm Hg (the capillary closing pressure), the network of capillaries collapses, and the supply of oxygen and nutrients to the cells, as well as removal of metabolic waste products, is interrupted. As a result, there is tissue ischemia and, if unrelieved, tissue death or necrosis. A classic study determined that pressures in excess of 20 to 40 mm Hg for prolonged periods cause tissue injury (Koziak, 1961).

Support surfaces have differing purposes, including pressure redistribution, repositioning, and support of a morbidly obese patient. They are used in acute, rehabilitative, long-term, and home care settings. Support surfaces are essential to helping prevent pressure ulcers or promote wound healing by reducing capillary closing pressure. The support surfaces reduce pressure by redistributing pressure over a larger surface area. The extent to which a support surface reduces pressure is characterized in two ways. The first is preventive, in which pressure is not consistently reduced below

32 mm Hg, for example, foam, air, or gel overlay. The second is therapeutic, in which pressure is consistently reduced below 32 mm Hg, for example, a powered overlay air mattress or low-air-loss mattress. Preventive surfaces are for patients at risk for skin breakdown and partial-thickness ulcers. Therapeutic surfaces are for patients with stage III and stage IV pressure ulcers (Mackey, 2005; NPUAP, 2007b). However, the use of support surfaces is one intervention to redistribute pressure, and you use this in conjunction with other pressure ulcer risk reduction strategies (see Chapter 18).

At-risk patients left sitting in chairs sometimes develop deeper and more serious pressure ulcers than patients left in a bed because the patient's body is exerting greater pressure on a smaller surface area, the buttocks. A patient lying in bed has the pressure distributed over a greater surface area but is also at risk for developing pressure ulcers over bony prominences because they receive greater pressure than other parts of the body. Never place patients at high risk for pressure ulcer development on ordinary hospital mattresses. Use specialized support surfaces (such as foam, air, or gel mattresses, beds, and cushions) to reduce pressure. Pressure-redistribution surfaces are classified as nonpowered (formerly called static) support surfaces or powered (formerly called dynamic) support surfaces (NPUAP, 2007b). Nonpowered support surfaces include mattresses or mattress overlays filled with air, water, gel, foam, or a combination of any of these. Powered support surfaces change the pressure beneath the patient, reducing the duration of any applied pressure. Many studies have examined the benefits demonstrated by pressure-redistribution surfaces in the prevention of pressure ulcers. (Courtney and others, 2006; Gibbons and others, 2006; Reddy and others, 2006).

Several support surfaces reduce friction, shear, and moisture (Table 12-1). Mattresses or beds with a slick surface help decrease friction and shear. Surfaces with porous covers allow airflow, which reduces moisture, resulting in decreased risk for skin maceration.

Frequent repositioning, which temporarily relieves pressure, is the backbone of preventive protocols. No bed or mattress totally eliminates the need for competent nursing care. It is the nurse's responsibility to use appropriate turning schedules for patients in bed or in a chair. Use lift teams and lifting devices to transfer patients from a regular bed to a special support surface (see Chapter 9). Although useful, turning devices still injure soft tissues, requiring a nurse to be especially observant for signs of pressure formation.

EVIDENCE-BASED PRACTICE TRENDS

Sustained pressure on areas that support the body leads to reduced blood supply and eventually necrosis of the skin and underlying muscles. Pressure reduction and relief is a major nursing intervention for the prevention of pressure ulcers (WOCN, 2003). There are two main approaches to pressure redistribution. The first approach is the use of support surfaces to distribute the body weight

TABLE 12-1 | Support Surfaces

Category and Mechanism of Action	Indications for Use	Advantages	Disadvantages
Support Surfaces and Overlays			
Foam Overlays (available as an overlay or in a full mattress)			
Reduces pressure and the cover (top) can reduce friction and shear. Base height of 3-4 inches; see manufacturer's guidelines regarding the amount of body weight supported.	Use for moderate- to high-risk patients.	One-time charge. No setup fee. Cannot be punctured. Available in various sizes (e.g., bed, chair, operating room table). Little maintenance. Does not need electricity.	Hot and may trap moisture. Limited life span. Plastic protective sheet needed for incontinent patients or patients with draining wounds.
Water Overlays (available as an overlay or in a full mattress)			
Reduces pressure and pressure points because these surfaces provide flotation with pressure reduction by evenly redistributing patient's weight over the entire support surface.	Use for high-risk patients.	Readily available. Some control over motion sensations. Easy to clean.	Easily punctured. Heavy. Fluid motion may make procedures (e.g., dressing changes, CPR) difficult. Maintenance needed to prevent microorganism growth. Patient transfers out of bed are difficult. Difficult to raise and lower head of bed.
Gel Overlays			
Reduces pressure and pressure points because these surfaces provide flotation with pressure reduction by evenly redistributing patient's weight over the entire support surface.	Use for moderate- to high-risk patients. Useful for patients who are wheelchair dependent.	Low maintenance. Easy to clean. Multiple-patient use. Impermeable to needle punctures.	Heavy. Expensive. Lacks air flow for moisture control. Variable friction control.
Nonpowered Air-Filled Overlays			
Overlays are pressure reducing and can lower the mean interface pressure between the patient's tissue and the mattress.	Use for moderate- to high-risk patients. Use for patients who can reposition themselves.	Easy to clean. Multiple-patient use. Low maintenance. Potential repair of some air-filled products. Durable.	Damaged by punctures from needles and sharps. Requires routine monitoring to determine adequate inflation pressure. Patient transfers out of bed are difficult.
Low-Air-Loss Overlay (available in a full bed or overlay)			
Maintains a constant and slight air movement against the skin to prevent moisture buildup.	Use for moderate- to high-risk patients.	Easy to clean. Maintains a constant inflation. Deflates to facilitate transfer and CPR. Moisture control. Fabric covering the overlay is air permeable, bacteria impermeable, and waterproof. Reduces shear and friction. Setup provided by the manufacturer.	Damaged by needles and sharps. Noisy. Requires electricity.
Specialty Beds			
Air-Fluidized Beds			
Bed frame contains silicone-coated beads and incorporates both air and fluid support. The silicone-coated beads become fluidized when air is pumped through the beads.	Use for high-risk patients. Use with patients with stage III or IV pressure ulcers or burns.	Less frequent turning or repositioning. Improved patient comfort. Quickly becomes firm for CPR or other treatments when the device is turned "off." Reduces shear, friction, and edema to site. May facilitate management of copious wound drainage or incontinence. Setup provided by the manufacturer.	Continuous circulation of warm, dry air may increase patient risk for dehydration. Bed may increase room temperature. Patient may experience disorientation. Transfer of patients is difficult. Heavy. Expensive. Width of bed may preclude care to obese patients or patients with contractures.

TABLE 12-1	Support Surfaces—cont'd		
Category and Mechanism of Action	**Indications for Use**	**Advantages**	**Disadvantages**
Low-Air-Loss Beds Bed frame with a series of connected air-filled pillows. The amount of pressure in each pillow is controlled and can be calibrated to patient need.	Indicated in patients who need pressure relief, those who cannot be frequently repositioned, or those who have skin breakdown on more than one surface. Contraindicated in patients with unstable spinal column.	Head and foot of bed can be raised and lowered. Easy transfer in and out of bed. Less frequent turning schedule. Pillows can be transferred to stretcher with patient. Setup provided by the manufacturer.	Portable motor is noisy. Bed surface material is slippery, and patients can easily slide down mattress or out of bed when being transferred. Needs a portable motor.
Kinetic Therapy Provides continuous passive motion to promote mobilization of pulmonary secretions and also provides low air loss, which provides pressure relief.	Primarily indicated for patients needing spinal stabilization. Should not be used when the patient is hemodynamically unstable.	Reduces pulmonary complications associated with restricted mobility. Reduces the risk for urinary stasis and urinary tract infections. Reduces venous stasis.	Does not reduce shear or moisture. Cannot be used with cervical or skeletal traction. Patients may have some motion sickness initially. Patients may have sensations of claustrophobia.

Data from Wound, Ostomy and Continence Nurses Society: *Guideline for prevention and management of pressure ulcers,* Glenview, Ill, 2003, The Society; Bryant RA: *Acute and chronic wounds: current management concepts,* ed 3, St. Louis, 2007, Mosby; Morrison MJ: *The prevention and treatment of pressure ulcers,* St. Louis, 2001, Mosby.
CPR, Cardiopulmonary resuscitation.

over a large area. The second approach is to use an alternating support surface where inflatable cells alternately inflate and deflate. Pressure-redistribution surfaces need to serve as adjuncts and not replacements for repositioning protocols (WOCN, 2003).

Pressure redistribution occurs through immersion and envelopment. Immersion refers to pressure being spread out over the surrounding area instead of directly over a bony prominence. It is dependent on the stiffness and thickness of the support surface and flexibility of the cover. Envelopment is the ability of the support surface to conform to irregularities such as clothing, bedding, and bony prominences without causing a substantial increase in pressure (Brienza and Geyer, 2005; NPUAP, 2007b; Posthauer and others, 2006; WOCN, 2003).

Cullum and others (2004) conclude that "interface pressure measurements (force per unit area that acts perpendicularly between the body and the support surface) do not demonstrate reliable clinical performance of support surfaces." However, tissue interface pressure is still the current method to evaluate the ability of support surfaces to reduce pressure (Nix, 2007).

Research provides good evidence to support the effectiveness of high-specification foam over standard hospital foam. High-specification foam evenly distributes the patient's body weight over the foam surface and as a result reduces pressure. Alternating or powered mattresses are also associated with lower incidence of pressure ulcers compared with standard hospital mattresses (WOCN, 2003). In addition, there is evidence to support the use of air-fluidized and low-air-loss devices as treatments to reduce pressure ulcer risk (Cullum and others, 2003). However, there is limited evidence that low-air-loss beds reduce the incidence of pressure ulcers in intensive care units (WOCN, 2003).

Pressure ulcers can occur in any setting. Patients in the operating room are also at risk for injury to the skin and underlying tissue. This injury occurs from a combination of factors such as surgical positioning and the effects of anesthetic agents. Because the damage resulting from intraoperative pressure develops in the muscle and subcutaneous tissues and progresses outward, damage is sometimes not visible for several days (Courtney and others, 2006). Use support surfaces in the operating room for patients at high risk for pressure ulcer development. Pressure redistribution is associated with a decreased incidence of postoperative pressure ulcers (WOCN, 2003).

When you care for postoperative patients, observe the skin for signs of injury or breakdown, even when a patient is ambulatory in the postoperative setting. In addition, instruct patients who had their surgeries in ambulatory care settings to observe for signs of skin breakdown.

Choosing a support surface is a dynamic process that changes according to a patient's condition and setting, and it is important to consider cost and product availability. Evidence is lacking as to the choice of one specific support surface over another for prevention of pressure ulcers. Regardless, it is important to place at-risk patients on redistribution surfaces (WOCN, 2003).

CULTURAL CONSIDERATIONS

- Ethnically diverse groups may not have any experience with the type of technology used in the Western health care system.
- Some cultural groups may hesitate to ask for help or questions, especially when they have limited English communication. In addition, Asians may hesitate to ask questions for fear of embarrassment.
- Give opportunities for a patient and family members to manipulate the equipment/appliance when an interpreter is present.
- Accommodate cultural rituals and practices when scheduling turning of a patient.
- Schedule turning to maximize contact between patients and visitors.
- Many cultures value female modesty highly, including Amish, Muslims, Hindus, and Orthodox Jews. Use gender-congruent caregivers as needed.

 Skill Performance Guidelines

1 Perform complete assessment to determine patient's risk for pressure ulcers and selection of appropriate special mattresses and beds. A complete patient assessment includes use of appropriate pressure ulcer risk scales, which include factors such as presence of shear and friction, and a patient's mobility and continence status (see Chapter 18).
2 Know the reason for and extent of a patient's reduced mobility. A patient who is not easy to reposition or who has pressure ulcers involving multiple surfaces benefits from pressure-redistribution support devices other than those used for a partially immobile patient.
3 Determine if the patient needs a pressure-redistribution support device for a short-term or long-term basis. Some patients in acute care settings need the device only during the acute phase of the illness. However, patients with chronic altered mobility or decreased sensation or patients who are discharged to long-term care or home care often require long-term pressure redistribution.
4 Continue to provide basic preventive care measures against the hazards of immobility, for example, regular skin assessment, turning, correct positioning, or range-of-motion (ROM) exercises (when not contraindicated).
5 Use safe patient-handling techniques and proper body mechanics when positioning or working with patients (see Chapter 9).
6 Follow all safety measures to prevent injury to patients from accidental falls or improper positioning when placing them on special beds or mattresses.
7 Encourage patients to remain as mobile as possible within the limits of their physical conditions and prescribed activity levels.
8 Educate care provider about the advantages/disadvantages and methods of operation of all support devices to ensure their proper use in all settings.
9 Collaborate and consult with health care professionals who have expertise in this area.
10 Anticipate need to consult with social service or home care department regarding product durability, third-party reimbursement, and arrangements for delivery to and care of special beds in the home.

PROCEDURAL GUIDELINE 12-1 Selection of Pressure-Reducing Support Surfaces

Delegation Considerations

The selection of a pressure-reducing support device cannot be delegated to nursing assistive personnel (NAP).

Equipment

☐ Agency's pressure ulcer risk assessment tool (see Chapter 18)
☐ Body chart, tape measure, and/or camera to document existing areas of impaired skin integrity
☐ Documentation record
☐ Skin care products

Procedural Steps

1 Assess patient's risk for skin breakdown using a risk assessment tool (e.g., Braden Scale).
2 Assess patient's existing pressure ulcers, including areas of blistering, abnormal reactive hyperemia, and abrasion.
3 Determine need for pressure-reduction surface from assessment data, such as the Braden risk score.
   a Place "at-risk" patients on a pressure-reduction surface and not an ordinary hospital mattress (WOCN, 2003).
4 Identify patient factors when selecting an appropriate surface (see Fig. 12-6, p. 303) (Nix, 2007):
   a Does the patient need pressure redistribution? If you cannot reposition the patient, or if there is a pressure ulcer, the patient requires pressure redistribution.
   b Is the surface needed for short- or long-term care? A short-term surface is usually needed for the acute illness and hospitalization. A long-term surface is usually needed for extended or home care.
   c What is the potential comfort level achieved by the surface? If the patient is sensitive to noise, then a device with a loud motor will increase the patient's discomfort.
   d Are the patient, family, and caregivers adherent to repositioning? In addition, are they aware that a support surface should never replace repositioning? In a home setting, a support surface is often necessary when the family, caregiver, or patient is unable to independently reposition or assist with repositioning.
   e Does the support surface have a potential to interfere with the patient's independent functioning? The height of the overlay and its soft edge may affect the patient's ability to transfer, and a high-air-loss bed is not appropriate for a patient who needs to get in and out of bed frequently.
   f What are the patient's financial limitations?
   g If the patient is using the device in the home, what are the environmental limitations? Will the home and existing electrical service accommodate the surface selected? Can the caregivers and family in the home manage the surface, and does the surface have a service contract to assist the family?
   h What is the durability of the product? Is the surface easily subjected to puncture? What is the ease of cleaning the surface?
5 Determine the specific device (see Table 12-1).
   a Pressure-redistribution devices redistribute pressure over bony prominences. Surfaces providing pressure redistribution include therapeutic mattress replacements, nonpowered and powered (i.e., moving) surfaces, low-air-loss beds and mattresses, and air-fluidized beds (WOCN, 2003).

PROCEDURAL GUIDELINE 12-1   Selection of Pressure-Reducing Support Surfaces—cont'd

Pressure-redistribution surfaces are also used in the operating room for individuals who are at high risk or for lengthy procedures (Cullum and others, 2004).

b Use a nonpowered support surface if the patient can assume a variety of positions without bearing weight on a pressure ulcer without bottoming out (Agency for Health Care Policy and Research [AHCPR], 1994). Bottoming out makes the support surface ineffective. To assess for bottoming out, place a hand (palm up) under the mattress or cushion below the area of risk for pressure areas (e.g., patient's pressure points when lying or sitting on surface). If there is less than 1 inch of support material felt, the patient has bottomed out (WOCN, 2003).

c Select a powered support surface when the patient cannot assume a variety of positions without bearing weight on a pressure ulcer, if the patient fully compresses the static support surface, or if the pressure ulcer does not show evidence of healing (AHCPR, 1994). Alternating or powered mattresses are associated with lower incidence of pressure ulcers compared with standard mattresses (WOCN, 2003).

d High-specification foam has demonstrated effectiveness in decreasing the incidence of pressure ulcers in fairly high-risk patients, including older adults and patients with fractures of the neck of the femur (WOCN, 2003).

e Patients with stage III or IV pressure ulcers on multiple turning surfaces often benefit from an air-fluidized bed (AHCPR, 1994; WOCN, 2003).

f There is limited evidence that low-air-loss beds reduce the incidence of pressure ulcers in intensive care (WOCN, 2003).

g When excess moisture or intact skin is a potential risk, a support surface that provides airflow is important in drying the skin and reducing the incidence of pressure ulcers (NPUAP, 2007b).

6 Check agency policy regarding implementing support surface.

a Obtain a health care provider's order. This is usually required for a patient to obtain third-party reimbursement.

b Consult with agency's case manager or social worker to assist with the patient's financial eligibility and terms and length of third-party reimbursement for the surface.

c Consult with agency's home care or discharge planning if the device is anticipated for long-term use. Specific procedures and evaluations are needed for continuity of surface when the patient is transferred to extended care or discharged home.

7 Document pressure ulcer risk assessment and skin assessment in the patient's record. Document the support surface selected and patient response to the surface (see specific skills for recording and reporting details).

SKILL 12-1   Placing a Patient on a Support Surface

Numerous support surfaces are designed to reduce pressure on tissues overlying bony prominences. These devices are recommended for preventive measures for patients with reduced mobility and risk for developing pressure ulcers. Most of the devices are easy to apply and keep clean. The extent to which the devices actually reduce pressure and prevent skin breakdown is highly variable. Few systematic studies exist that consistently find one surface better than others (Cullum and others, 2003).

Support surfaces are categorized as mattress (or wheelchair) overlays, mattress replacements, or specialty beds. An overlay rests on top of the hospital mattress and uses foam, air, water, gel, or combinations of these products to provide pressure relief. Mattress overlays and mattress replacements are either nonpowered (e.g., foam, gels) or powered (e.g., alternating-pressure surfaces).

A flotation pad is made of a silicone or polyvinyl chloride gel enclosed in a vinyl-covered square. The pad serves as an artificial layer of fat to protect bony surfaces such as the sacrum and greater trochanters. These flotation pads are available for the bed or for wheelchair patients.

One type of air mattress is fully integrated into the hospital bed. You can adjust this bed surface to a patient's comfort level by adding or removing air through buttons within the patient's reach, or you can automatically adjust pressures to a patient's position and movement when in the automatic mode. Always use a bed sheet to cover an air mattress to prevent skin from touching the plastic surface.

There are two types of foam mattresses. One is the foam mattress overlay, which has a flat smooth surface, foam rubber peaks ("egg-crate" variety, shown in Fig. 12-1) or a cut surface. Place it on top of the bed mattress, and place a sheet over the foam mattress pad overlay to prevent soiling and provide ease of cleaning. The second type is the foam specialty mattress, which completely replaces the hospital mattress and is covered by a loose-fitting cover intended to protect the mattress and minimize friction and shear. The foam mattresses are used more for comfort than for pressure redistribution. Some of the newer foam mattresses have memory and an increased life span. The memory foam molds to the shape of the body and reduces pressure to the area in contact with the foam.

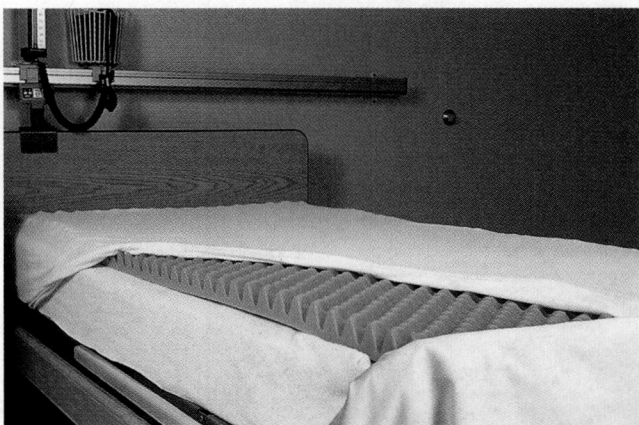

FIG 12-1   "Egg-crate" foam overlay is primarily for comfort.

Air mattress overlays are either nonpowered or powered and consist of interconnected air cells or cushions inflated by the use of a motorized blower (Fig. 12-2). More complex air mattresses contain several layers of tubes or support cells. These mattresses use a pressure-cycling device to intermittently inflate and deflate or to maintain a constant inflation and slight air movement in the mattress.

A nonpowered mattress is inflated with a simple air blower after placing the mattress on a bed. An integrated air mattress connects with a pressure-cycling device that intermittently inflates and deflates sections of the mattress, creating a cycling effect that minimizes pressure on bony prominences (Fig. 12-3).

Replacement mattresses have foam, gel, air, or fluid sections that you can customize to the needs of a specific patient with moderate to high risk for skin breakdown. Another available option is an air-integrated replacement mattress instead of the conventional mattress. These mattresses may also be fully integrated into the bed. Air mattresses are usually for patients with moderate to high risk for skin breakdown. You must deflate air mattresses before

initiating cardiopulmonary resuscitation (CPR). Many facilities have purchased replacement mattresses to replace their standard hospital mattresses because of improved skin and wound outcomes (Cullum and others, 2004).

Another intervention is a low-pressure seat cushion (Fig. 12-4) overlaid on a wheelchair or a dry nonpowered flotation mattress system (Fig. 12-5) that you overlay on the bed or wheelchair. Through a system of controlled dynamics, the cushion maintains low pressures by distributing pressure across a patient's body surface. This minimizes friction and shear.

Support surfaces aid in reducing pressure on a patient's skin. They do not replace regular repositioning, meticulous skin care, or range-of-motion (ROM) exercises. The decision to place a patient on a pressure-redistribution surface and the selection of this surface is a nursing responsibility (see Procedural Guideline 12-1). Factors guiding the selection of support surfaces for an individual patient include wound extent and location, mobility/activity, comfort, and body size (Nix, 2007) (Fig. 12-6).

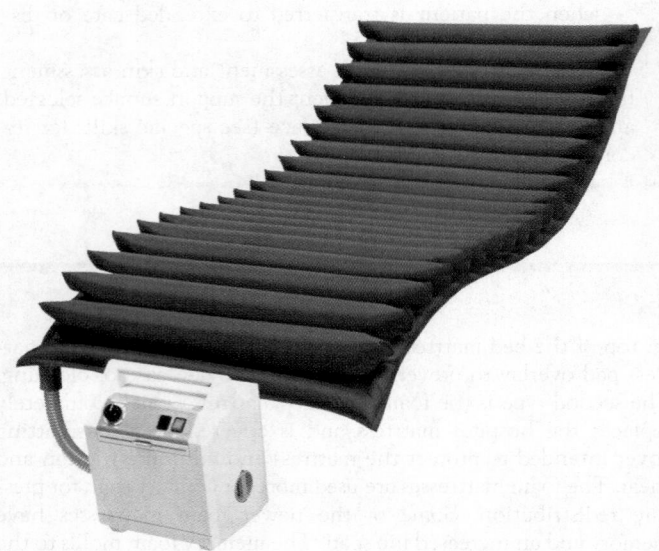

FIG 12-2   Dynamic air mattress overlay. (© 2002 Hill-Rom Services, Inc. Reprinted with permission. All rights reserved.)

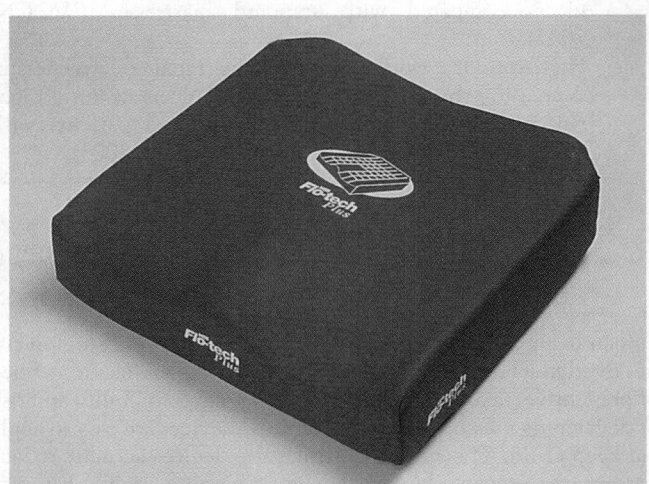

FIG 12-4   Low-pressure seat cushion. (*Reproduced with permission from medical Support Systems Ltd.*)

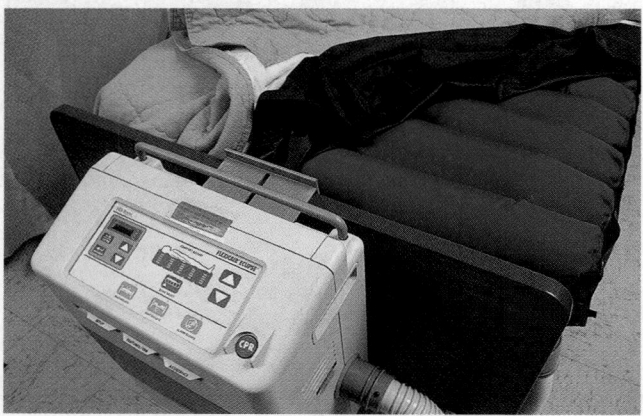

FIG 12-3   Motor for integrated air mattress.

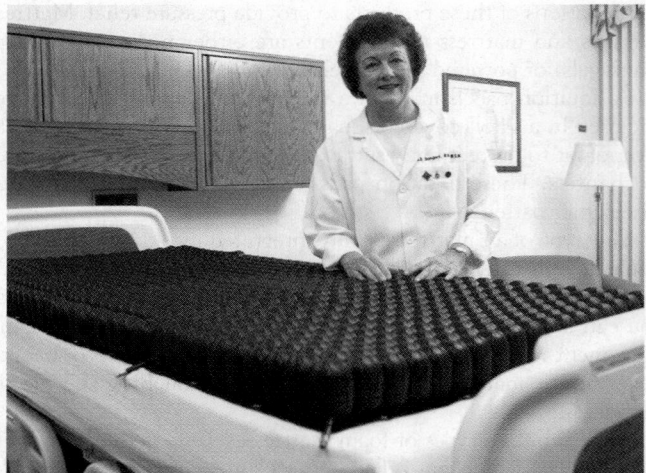

FIG 12-5   ROHO Dry Floatation mattress for a bed. (*Courtesy the ROHO Group, Belleville, Ill.*)

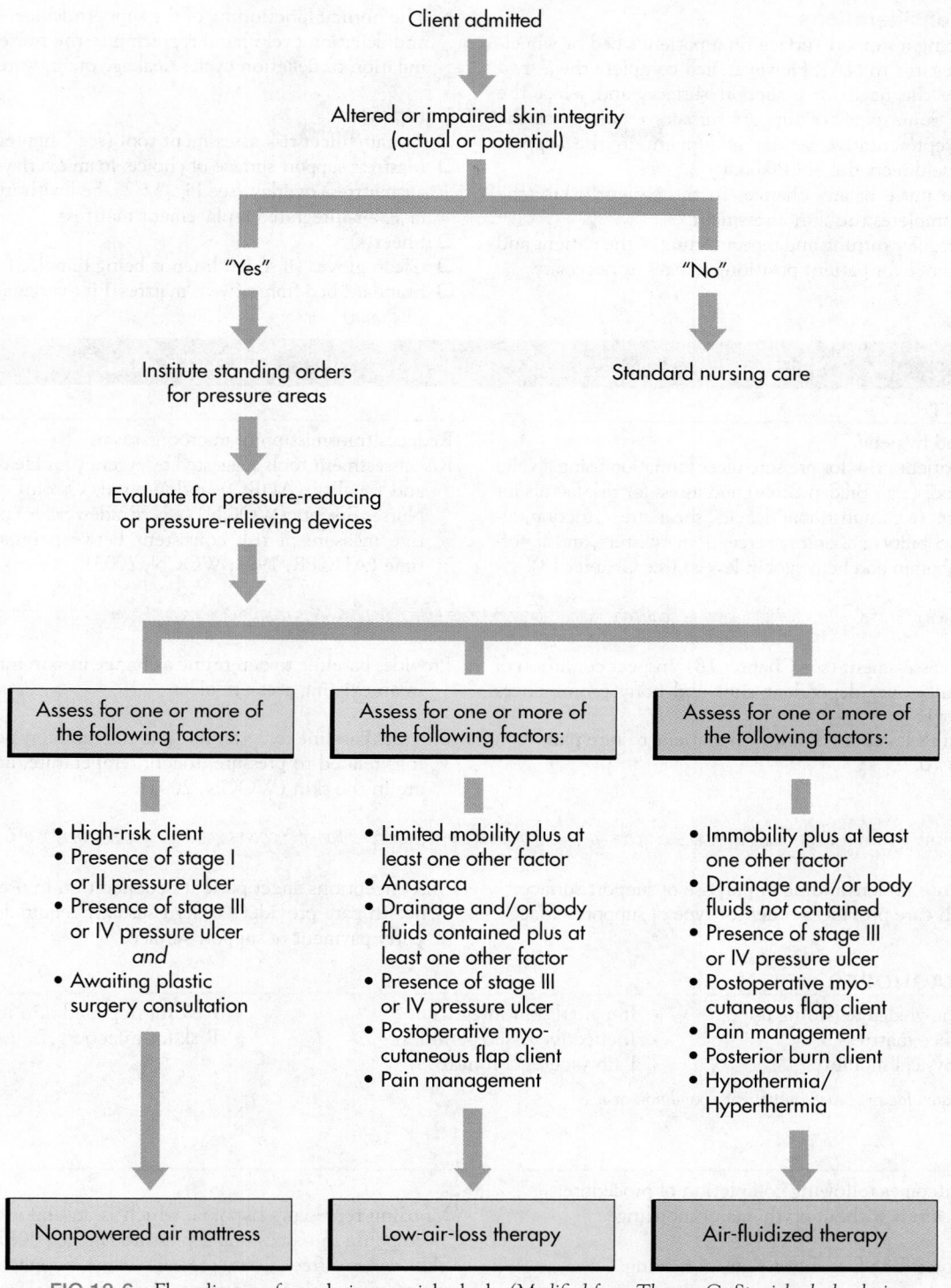

Client admitted

Altered or impaired skin integrity
(actual or potential)

"Yes"

"No"

Institute standing orders
for pressure areas

Standard nursing care

Evaluate for pressure-reducing
or pressure-relieving devices

Assess for one or more of
the following factors:

- High-risk client
- Presence of stage I
  or II pressure ulcer
- Presence of stage III
  or IV pressure ulcer
  and
- Awaiting plastic
  surgery consultation

Assess for one or more of
the following factors:

- Limited mobility plus at
  least one other factor
- Anasarca
- Drainage and/or body
  fluids contained plus at
  least one other factor
- Presence of stage III
  or IV pressure ulcer
- Postoperative myo-
  cutaneous flap client
- Pain management

Assess for one or more of
the following factors:

- Immobility plus at least
  one other factor
- Drainage and/or body
  fluids *not* contained
- Presence of stage III
  or IV pressure ulcer
- Postoperative myo-
  cutaneous flap client
- Pain management
- Posterior burn client
- Hypothermia/
  Hyperthermia

Nonpowered air mattress

Low-air-loss therapy

Air-fluidized therapy

FIG 12-6   Flow diagram for ordering specialty beds. (*Modified from Thomas C: Specialty beds: decision making made easy,* Ostomy Wound Manage *23:51, 1989. Information from Nix N: Support surfaces. In Bryant RA, Nix N: Acute and chronic wounds: current management concepts, ed 3, St. Louis, 2007, Mosby.*)

Delegation Considerations

The skill of placing a support surface on a patient's bed or wheelchair can be delegated to NAP. However, first complete the assessment, determine the need for a support surface, and select the specific surface. Some types of support surfaces require that the manufacturer's representative set up and maintain the support system. The nurse directs the NAP about:

- Notifying the nurse of any changes in the patient's skin; the nurse then completes the skin assessment.
- Continuing regular turning and repositioning of the patient and seeking assistance for patient position changes as necessary.

- The normal functioning of the support device, such as inflation and deflation cycles, and reporting to the nurse any changes in inflation or deflation cycles, leakage of air, water, or gel.

Equipment

- ❏ Pressure ulcer risk assessment tool (see Chapter 18)
- ❏ Mattress support surface of choice: foam overlays (see Fig. 12-1), air mattress overlay (see Fig. 12-2), bed with integrated surface, air-integrated replacement mattress
- ❏ Sheet(s)
- ❏ Clean gloves (if soiled linen is being handled)
- ❏ Standard bed frame (with mattress) if overlay is to be used (*optional*)

STEP	RATIONALE

ASSESSMENT

1. Perform hand hygiene.
2. Determine patient's risk for pressure ulcer formation using a valid assessment tool (e.g., Braden Scale) and assess for risk factors for pressure ulcers (e.g., nutritional deficits, shear stress, friction, alterations in mobility and sensory perception, moisture, and abnormal serum albumin and hemoglobin levels) (see Chapter 18).

Reduces transmission of microorganisms.

Risk assessment tools suggested by Agency for Healthcare Research and Quality (AHRQ) and Wound, Ostomy and Continence Nurses Society (WOCN) (e.g., Braden Scale) provide an objective measure of risk consistent between nurse assessors over time (AHCPR, 1992; WOCN, 2003).

Critical Decision Point *Patients with unstable conditions do not always tolerate turning or positioning required for the application of a support surface mattress.*

3. Perform skin assessment (see Chapter 18). Inspect condition of skin, especially over dependent sites and bony prominences (see Chapter 18).
4. Assess patient's level of comfort; ask patient to rate pain on a scale of 0 to 10.

Provides baseline to determine a change in skin integrity or change in an existing pressure ulcer.

Provides baseline to determine patient's comfort needs. Nerve endings related to pressure, touch, temperature, and limb position are in the skin (WOCN, 2003).

Critical Decision Point *Some patients experiencing pain need pain medication before application of support surface of choice or transfer to another bed.*

5. Assess patient's understanding of purpose of support surface.
6. Verify health care provider's order for type of support surface.

Misconceptions affect patient's cooperation in use of mattress.

A health care provider's order is usually required to ensure third-party payment of support surface.

NURSING DIAGNOSES

- Deficient knowledge regarding use of support surface mattress
- Impaired physical mobility

- Impaired skin integrity
- Ineffective tissue perfusion
- Pain (acute, chronic)

- Risk for impaired skin integrity
- Risk for infection

Individualize related factors based on patient's condition or needs.

PLANNING

1. Expected outcomes following completion of procedure:
   - Patient's skin is without erythema or mottling.

   - Existing pressure ulcer shows signs of healing.

   - Patient expresses improved level of comfort.
   - Patient is removed from therapeutic surface when risk for pressure ulcers decreases.
2. Explain the purpose of mattress and method of application to patient.

Mottling represents hypoxia, which is an abnormal physiological response in tissues under pressure (Pieper, 2007).

Skin remains free of new pressure ulcers. Support surface does not interfere with circulation to dependent areas.

Equalized pressures have eliminated localized areas of discomfort.

Provides for efficient, cost-effective care while maintaining high-quality outcomes.

Reduces anxiety and promotes cooperation.

IMPLEMENTATION

Critical Decision Point *Perform application of support surface mattress or transfer to bed in an organized, efficient manner or when a patient is out of bed for surgery or diagnostic testing. Some patients whose medical conditions are unstable do not tolerate prolonged periods of position changes (i.e., lying flat or turning from side to side). Turning an acutely ill patient to the lateral side sometimes causes complications, such as increased oxygen demand and hypotension.*

STEP	RATIONALE
1 Close room door or bedside curtain.	Provides patient privacy and considerate care during application of mattress to bed or transfer to alternative bed.
2 Perform hand hygiene. Apply clean gloves (if linens are soiled or wet). Obtain assistance to position patient and/or mattress as needed.	Gloves prevent contact with body fluids. Assistance from other caregivers reduces risk for friction and shear in transfer to new surface.
3 Apply support surface to bed or prepare alternative bed (bed may be occupied or unoccupied). Keep sharp objects away from air mattress or air-surface bed.	
a Replacing mattress:	
(1) Apply mattress to bed frame after removing standard hospital mattress.	Hospital mattress needs to be stored. In some instances, mattress replacements are standard procedure.
(2) Apply sheet over mattress. Keep linens between surfaces to a minimum.	Sheet reduces soiling. Multiple layers decrease surface effectiveness in reducing pressure (WOCN, 2003).
b Preparing an air mattress/overlay:	
(1) Apply deflated mattress flat over surface of bed mattress. (There may be directions on pad indicating which side to place up.)	Provides smooth, even surface.
(2) Bring any plastic strips or flaps around corners of bed mattress.	Secures air mattress in place.
(3) Attach connector on air mattress to inflation device. Inflate mattress to proper air pressure determined by air pump or blower.	Mattresses vary as to requiring one-time or continuous inflation cycle. Inflation must be checked daily (Nix, 2007). Manufacturer's directions indicate desired air pressure designed to distribute patient's body weight evenly. Directions are included with each mattress.
(4) Place sheet over air mattress, being sure to eliminate all wrinkles.	Prevents soiling of mattress, reduces direct contact of skin with plastic surface. Wrinkles can cause pressure.
(5) Check air pumps to be sure pressure cycle alternates.	Alternating airflow mattress produces intermittent cycling, inflating only parts of mattress at any one time. Intermittent cycle continually alternates pressure against skin and soft tissue (Nix, 2007).
(6) Assist patient with transferring in and out of bed.	Mattress surface is less firm and slippery. This makes it difficult for some patients to transfer from bed to chair/stretcher.
c Using an air-surface bed:	
(1) Obtain and place linen on bed.	In some instances, an air-surface bed is available in patient rooms. If not, an ordering system exists to obtain one as needed (see agency policy).
(2) Place switch in the "prevention" mode.	In the "prevention" mode, surface pressures change automatically with patient position to equalize pressure and eliminate points of pressure.

Critical Decision Point *Beds are equipped with a CPR switch to instantly lower head section from an elevated position and to deflate the mattress to provide a firm surface for chest compressions (see illustration). Note this on the Kardex. Some patients have difficulty tolerating the firm surface.*

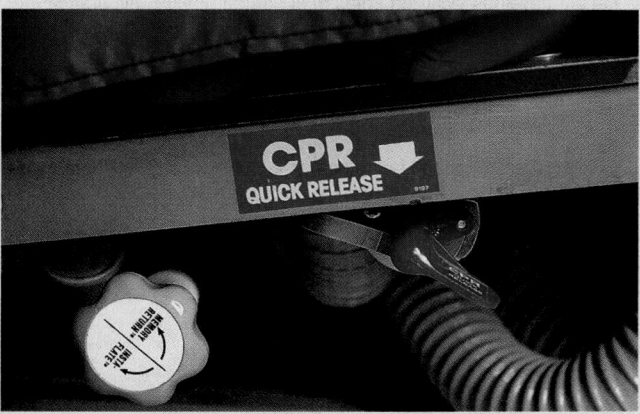

STEP 3c(2) Cardiopulmonary resuscitation switch deflates low-air-loss bed to provide hard surface.

STEP	RATIONALE

d Preparing a water mattress (supplemental and self-contained):

Critical Decision Point   *There is considerable reduction in the use of water mattresses because they harbor organisms in the water, leaks in the mattress are risky for patients with open wounds, and the structural integrity of the building does not always support the weight of the mattress.*

STEP	RATIONALE
(1) Apply unfilled supplemental mattress flat over the surface of standard bed mattress. (Self-contained water mattress would replace bed mattress.)	Provides a smooth, even surface.
(2) Bring any plastic strips or flaps around corners of bed mattress.	Secures water mattress in place.
(3) Attach connector on water mattress to water source, and fill mattress to level recommended by manufacturer. Follow manufacturer's directions regarding temperature of water. Mattress should be filled in close proximity to water source. Manufacturer's directions (enclosed with mattress) indicate desired water level designed to distribute patient's body weight evenly (usually determined by patient weight or height and weight).	Proper water temperature prevents loss of body heat as patient lies on mattress (Nix, 2007).
(4) Place sheet over water mattress, being sure to eliminate all wrinkles.	Reduces soiling of mattress and prevents direct contact of skin with plastic surface. Wrinkles can cause pressure.
(5) Keep sharp objects away from mattress.	Tears and punctures result in loss of water, making the mattress ineffective.
4 Position patient comfortably as desired over support surface. Reposition routinely.	Location of existing pressure ulcer might influence type of positioning (WOCN, 2003).
5 Remove gloves and perform hand hygiene.	Reduces transmission of microorganisms.

EVALUATION

STEP	RATIONALE
1 Reassess patient's risk for pressure ulcer formation at routine intervals.	Documents change in status, which is critical for evaluating continued need for therapeutic surface.
2 Inspect and compare condition of patient's skin every 8 hours or according to agency policy to determine changes in skin integrity, pressure ulcer status, and effectiveness of support surface.	Determines if pressure sores develop or if the condition of existing sores changes.
3 Ask patient to rate comfort on a scale of 0 to 10.	If pressure-relief mattress is effective, patient generally experiences less discomfort.
4 Evaluate functioning of support surface periodically.	Regular inspection of mechanical components of mattress ensures proper functioning.

Unexpected Outcomes	Related Interventions
1 Patient develops localized areas of abnormal reactive hyperemia for longer than 30 minutes (WOCN, 2003), mottling, swelling, and tenderness with evidence of breakdown.	• Modify skin care regimen. • Increase frequency of skin assessment. • Increase types of pressure-relief interventions. • Revise turning schedule. • Consult with skin care expert. • Notify health care provider.
2 Existing pressure areas fail to heal or increase in size or depth.	• Modify skin care regimen. • Revise turning schedule. • Consult with skin care expert. • Notify health care provider.
3 Patient expresses discomfort while on support surface.	• Evaluate need for analgesia or mild sedation. • Evaluate need to modify support surface. • Reposition patient more frequently. • Unless contraindicated, provide back massage. Do not massage reddened areas or bony prominences because massage to these areas contributes to skin breakdown (WOCN, 2003).
4 Bed or mattress develops leak (air, water, gel).	• Take corrective action according to agency or manufacturer's policies/directions.

Recording and Reporting

- Record type of support surface applied, extent to which patient tolerated procedure, and condition of patient's skin in nurses' notes or skin assessment flow sheet.
- Report evidence of pressure ulcer formation to nurse in charge or to health care provider.

Teaching Considerations

- Explain risks of immobility and pressure ulcer formation to patient and family members (see Chapter 18).
- Instruct in proper body mechanics, positioning, and pressure relief (see Chapter 9).
- Explain purpose and function of the pressure-redistribution surface. Include reminder that the surface augments care and does not replace the need for turning and pressure-relief maneuvers.
- Explain precautions regarding sharp objects, fire hazard, and other concerns.

Pediatric Considerations

- Various pain assessment tools have been developed specifically for use in children (see Chapter 15).

- Parents are also helpful in assisting the child in expressing pain and treatment preferences (Hockenberry and Wilson, 2007).

Gerontological Considerations

- Implement preventive measures because aging skin is drier, thinner, and less pressure sensitive, increasing the risk for skin breakdown (Wysocki, 2007).
- Adding mattress overlays changes the bed height. Use care when transferring and teaching family members to transfer from bed to chair.

Home Care Considerations

- Most of the devices covered in this section may be adapted for home use on a standard twin bed or hospital bed.
- Base selection on patient needs and environmental audit. For example, a patient on total bed rest who smokes is not an ideal candidate for a foam mattress because of the potential for fire; a patient with pets that sleep in the bed is not suited for a water- or air-filled mattress because of the risk for puncture.
- Reimbursement varies by surface type and payer source.

SKILL 12-2   Placing a Patient on an Air-Suspension Bed

Air-suspension beds are for patients who are immobile or otherwise confined to the bed. The air-suspension bed supports a patient's weight on air-filled cushions. There are two types of systems: low-air-loss and high-air-loss. A low-air-loss system minimizes pressure and reduces shear (Fig. 12-7). If a patient has large stage III or stage IV pressure ulcers on multiple turning surfaces of the skin, a low-air-loss bed or air-fluidized bed may be indicated (AHCPR, 1994; WOCN, 2003).

High air loss provides for selective drying while not having the effect of substantially increasing insensible fluid losses. For patients requiring high air loss under a given body part, for example, under

the buttocks, you can substitute high-air-loss cushions. It is also possible to adapt the air-suspension beds to individual patient needs with specialty cushions for positioning, foot support, and lateral arm supports.

Another adaptation of the air-suspension bed is the kinetic low-air-loss bed (Fig. 12-8). This bed is marketed widely to intensive care areas and has the ability to provide a pressure-relief surface while rotating continuously approximately 30 to 35 degrees. Do not use this surface with a patient who has an unstable spine or who is in traction (see Chapter 11).

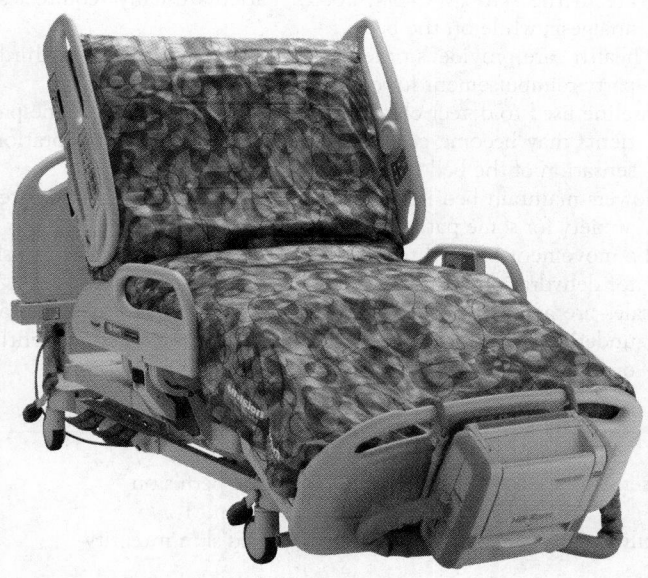

FIG 12-7   Low-air-loss bed. (© 2002 Hill-Rom Services, Inc. Reprinted with permission. All rights reserved.)

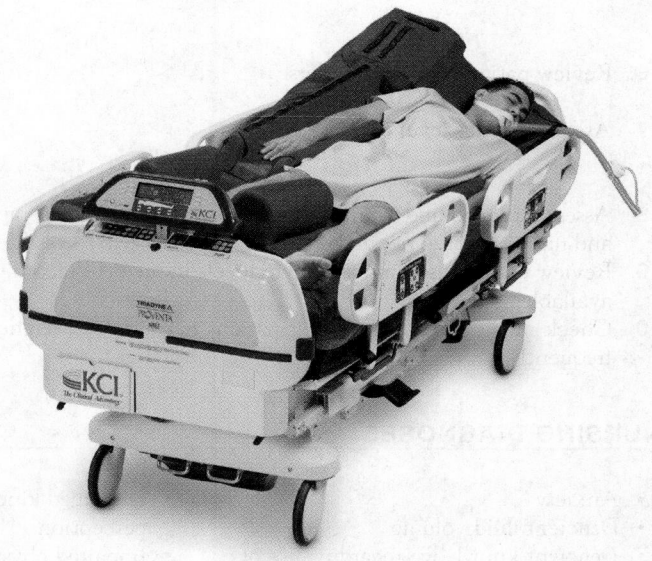

FIG 12-8   Lateral rotation bed. (TRIA Dyne Proventa Courtesy Kinetic Concepts, Inc, San Antonio, Tex.)

Delegation Considerations

The skill of placing a patient on an air-suspension bed can be delegated to NAP. However, first complete the assessment, determine the need for a support surface, and select the specific surface. Some types of support surfaces require that the manufacturer's representative set up and maintain the support system. When delegating aspects of care for a patient on a support surface, the nurse directs the NAP about:

- Notifying the nurse of any changes in the patient's skin. The nurse then completes the skin assessment.
- Continuing regular turning and repositioning of the patient and seeking assistance for patient position changes as necessary. This is not always necessary for patients placed on a lateral rotation air-suspension bed.

- The normal functioning of the air-suspension bed, such as inflation and deflation cycles, and reporting to the nurse any changes in inflation or deflation cycles.
- Notifying the nurse if the patient becomes disoriented, becomes restless, or complains of nausea.

Equipment

- ❏ Air-suspension bed
- ❏ Gore-Tex sheet (supplied by manufacturer)
- ❏ Disposable bed pads, if indicated
- ❏ Clean gloves (optional)

STEP	RATIONALE
ASSESSMENT	
1 Perform hand hygiene.	Reduces transmission of microorganisms.
2 Determine patient's risk for pressure ulcer formation using a valid assessment tool (e.g., Braden Scale) and assess for risk factors for pressure ulcers include nutritional deficits, shear stress, friction, alterations in mobility and sensory perception, moisture, and abnormal serum albumin and hemoglobin levels (see Chapter 18).	Risk assessment tools as suggested by AHRQ and WOCN (e.g., Braden Scale) provide an objective measure of risk consistent between nurse assessors over time (AHCPR, 1992; WOCN, 2003).
3 Identify patients who will benefit from air-suspension therapy, such as immobilized or burn patients.	Beds effectively minimize pressure on fragile tissues and dependent body parts. Selected for patients who require pressure relief for treatment of or prevention of pressure ulcers.

Critical Decision Point *Do not use this surface with a patient who has an unstable spine or who is in traction.*

STEP	RATIONALE
4 Perform skin assessment. Inspect condition of skin, especially over dependent sites and bony prominences. Note appearance of existing ulcers and determine stage of ulcer (see Chapter 18).	Provides baseline to determine a change in skin integrity or change in an existing pressure ulcer over time.
5 Assess patient's level of comfort; ask patient to rate pain on a scale of 0 to 10.	Provides baseline to determine patient's comfort needs. Nerve endings related to pressure, touch, temperature, and limb position are in the skin (WOCN, 2003). Patients usually require less analgesia while on the bed.
6 Review patient's medical orders.	A health care provider's order is usually required to obtain third-party reimbursement for cost of bed.
7 Assess patient's level of consciousness.	Baseline used to detect change while patient is on bed. Some patients may become confused or disoriented from the flotation sensation of the bed (WOCN, 2003).
8 Assess patient's and family members' feelings about therapy and understanding of purpose of bed.	Blowers maintain bed inflation, which make a sound that creates anxiety for some patients.
9 Review patient's serum electrolyte levels in medical record, if available.	The movement of air through the mattress increases patient's risk for dehydration (WOCN, 2003).
10 Check medical record to see if patient needs to be weighed frequently.	Scales are available in some air-suspension beds and available as underbed units for patients who need to be weighed frequently or for those who cannot be moved for weighing.

NURSING DIAGNOSES

- Anxiety
- Deficient fluid volume
- Deficient knowledge regarding use of support surface mattress

- Disturbed kinesthetic sensory perception
- Impaired physical mobility
- Impaired skin integrity

- Ineffective tissue perfusion
- Pain (acute, chronic)
- Risk for impaired skin integrity

Individualize related factors based on patient's condition or needs.

STEP	RATIONALE

PLANNING

1 Expected outcomes following completion of procedure:
- Patient's skin remains warm, clean, and intact, or existing lesions show evidence of healing. — Skin is free from pressure effects of immobility.
- Existing pressure ulcers show evidence of healing by formulation of granulation tissue. — Bed's low-pressure surface facilitates healing of existing pressure ulcers (Nix, 2007).
- Patient expresses improved sense of comfort. — Bed's surface is soft, minimizing pain stimulation.
- Patient remains alert and oriented or shows no change in level of orientation. — Patient does not experience sensory perceptual changes from flotation.

2 Explain procedure and purpose of bed to patient and caregiver. — Reduces anxiety and promotes patient's cooperation.

3 Prepare necessary equipment and supplies. — Promotes organized transfer of patient to specialty bed.

4 Review instructions supplied by bed manufacturer. — Promotes safe and correct use of bed.

5 For patients with severe to moderate pain, premedicate approximately 30 minutes before transfer. — Promotes patient's comfort and ability to cooperate during transfer to bed. Decreases patient's energy expenditure (WOCN, 2003).

6 Obtain any additional personnel needed to transfer patient to bed (see Chapter 9). — Ensures patient's safety by having sufficient personnel to assist in transferring.

IMPLEMENTATION

1 Close patient's room door or bedside curtain. Perform hand hygiene. — Maintains patient's privacy during transfer.

2 Apply clean gloves (if linen or surface is soiled or wet).

3 Explain steps of transfer. — Reduces anxiety and helps patient be a part of decision making during maneuvering.

4 Transfer patient to bed using appropriate transfer techniques (see Chapters 9 and 10). Bed surface is sometimes slippery, so do not attempt transfers without assistance. — Appropriate safe patient handling techniques maintain alignment and reduce risk for injury during procedure. Company representative will adjust bed to patient's height and weight.

5 Once patient has been transferred, release Instaflate or turn bed on by depressing switch; regulate temperature. — Releasing Instaflate or turning on bed allows pressure cushions to automatically adjust to preset levels to minimize pressure, friction, and shear (Nix, 2007).

6 Position patient, and perform ROM exercises as appropriate. — Promotes comfort and reduces contracture formation. The bed reduces pressure on skin, but patients must still be turned and exercised to avoid joint deformity or contractures (AHCPR, 1994).

7 To turn patient, position bedpans, or perform other therapies, turn on Instaflate setting. Once you have completed the procedure, release Instaflate. — Instaflate firms the bed surface to facilitate turning and handling patient. Patient will not receive pressure relief while bed is in this mode.

Critical Decision Point *Patient will NOT receive pressure relief when the bed is firm. Activate CPR switch to quickly deflate bed/mattress in an emergency (see Skill 12-1).*

8 Become familiar with bed's special features, and use as needed.
- a Scales — Facilitates ease of routine weights.
- b Portable transport units to maintain inflation when primary power is interrupted — Provides for continuous pressure reduction.
- c Availability of specialty cushions for prone positioning, providing pressure relief, reducing moisture, preventing the patient from sliding down in bed, or relieving weight from orthopedic devices — Reduces pressure, friction, and shearing forces.
- d Lateral rotation (see Fig. 12-8), which allows approximately 30 degrees of turning — Helps to reduce risk and prevent pulmonary and urinary complications of reduced mobility (Cullum and others, 2003; WOCN, 2003).

9 Remove gloves. Perform hand hygiene. — Reduces transmission of microorganisms.

EVALUATION

1 Inspect condition of patient's skin periodically while patient is on bed. — Determines if any new pressure areas are forming.

2 Observe existing pressure ulcers for evidence of healing. — Evaluates healing progress of any existing pressure ulcers.

3 Ask patient to rate level of comfort on a scale of 0 to 10. — Flotation effects of bed minimize pain stimuli.

4 Assess patient's level of orientation. — Determines onset of perceptual changes.

Unexpected Outcomes	Related Interventions
1 Existing areas of skin breakdown or pressure areas fail to heal or increase in size or depth.	• Modify skin care regimen. • Revise turning schedule. • Consult with skin care expert. • Notify health care provider.
2 Patient is restless, confused, or agitated.	• Determine need for antianxiety medication and consult with physician. • Evaluate alternative pressure-relief devices.
3 Patient becomes nauseated.	• Provide short-term antiemetic. • Notify health care provider. • If using lateral rotation, decrease the cycle frequency.
4 Bed malfunctions.	• Maintain patient safety. • Follow agency or manufacturer's policy.

Recording and Reporting

- Record transfer of patient to bed, tolerance of procedure, and condition of skin in nurses' notes or skin assessment flow sheet.
- Report changes in condition of skin, level of orientation, and electrolyte levels to health care provider.
- Record teaching provided and patient and/or caregiver response.
- Report restlessness or change in orientation.

Teaching Considerations

- Explain function and purpose of air-suspension therapy.
- Explain the need to continue to change position at intervals to diminish the effects of immobility.
- Explain the need for adequate fluid intake, because bed surface sometimes causes dehydration.

Pediatric Considerations

- This bed is used commonly with older children. Make sure instructions are age appropriate and include any restrictions, such as raising the head of the bed, positioning.

- Younger children are usually easier to position, and thus the risk for pressure ulcers is easier to control.

Gerontological Considerations

- When hospitalized, some older adult patients experience misperceptions of their environment that are intensified by the constant flotation of the air-suspension bed. Proprioception abnormalities affecting older adults are the result of nervous system and muscle changes (WOCN, 2003).

Home Care Considerations

- A version of the bed is available for home use for rent or purchase; the bed rental company is responsible for proper cleaning.
- Instruct family in importance of maintaining patient hydration.
- Instruct family regarding the need to provide patient's skin care.

SKILL 12-3   Placing a Patient on an Air-Fluidized Bed

An air-fluidized bed is a powered device designed to distribute a patient's weight evenly over its support surface (Fig. 12-9). The contact pressure of the patient's body against the filter sheet stays at 11 to 16 mm Hg. The bed minimizes pressure and reduces shearing force and friction through the principle of fluidization. Fluidization is created by forcing a gentle flow of temperature-controlled air upward through a mass of fine ceramic microspheres. The microspheres fluidize and take on the appearance of boiling milk and all the properties of a fluid. The patient lies directly on a polyester filter sheet that allows air to pass through but does not allow the microspheres to escape. Patients feel as though they are floating on a surface like a warm waterbed.

Air-fluidized beds are useful in the care of patients who require minimal movement to prevent skin damage by shearing force and for patients who experience significant pain when being turned or positioned. Patients who benefit from the bed include burn patients, those who have undergone extensive skin grafts or who have existing pressure ulcers, and victims of multiple trauma. Patients tend to perspire and lose body fluids while on the bed (Bryant, 2007). The surface of the filter sheet warms; as patients perspire, moisture is quickly absorbed into the circulating microspheres. Diaphoresis often goes undetected, and thus insensible fluid loss is not always evident until a patient develops fluid and electrolyte imbalances. This individual is often already compro-

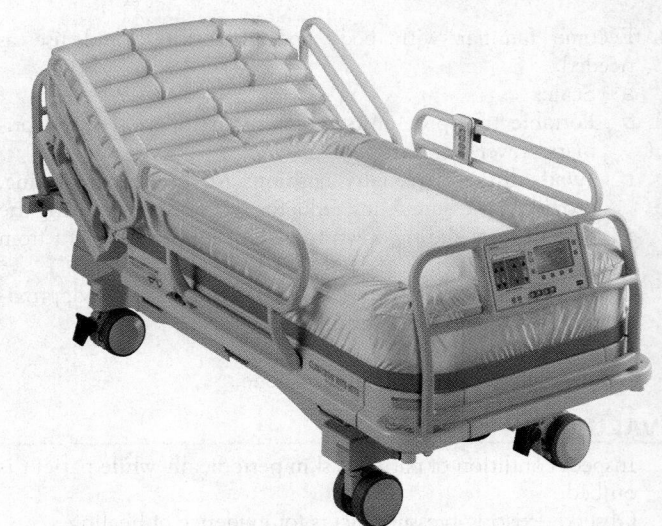

FIG 12-9   Combination air-fluidized, low-air-loss bed. (© 2008 Hill-Rom Services, Inc. Reprinted with permission. All rights reserved.)

mised in relation to hydration, fluids, and electrolytes; therefore you need to monitor the patient's fluid balance status carefully.

Conventional fluidized beds do not allow for head-of-bed position changes. Use foam wedges to elevate the head. There are also combinations of fluidized-low-air-loss beds that allow head-of-bed elevation. These beds use air to lift the upper body, while the lower body stays on a fluidized bed surface. The weight of the bed structure makes transport extremely difficult. A pediatric version of this bed is available.

Delegation Considerations

The skill of placing a patient on an air-fluidized bed can be delegated to NAP. However, first complete the assessment, determine the need for a support surface, and select the specific surface. Some types of support surfaces require that the manufacturer's representative set up and maintain the support system. The nurse directs the NAP about:

- Notifying the nurse of any changes in the patient's skin. The nurse then completes the skin assessment.
- Continuing regular turning and repositioning of the patient and seeking assistance for patient position changes as necessary. This is not always necessary for patients placed on a lateral rotation air-suspension bed.
- The normal functioning of the air-suspension bed, such as inflation and deflation cycles, and reporting to the nurse any changes in inflation or deflation cycles.
- Notifying the nurse if the patient becomes disoriented, becomes restless, or complains of nausea.

Equipment

- ❏ Air-fluidized bed
- ❏ Foam positioning wedges, if indicated
- ❏ Filter sheet (supplied by rental company)
- ❏ Clean gloves (*optional*)

STEP	RATIONALE

ASSESSMENT

1 Perform hand hygiene.

2 Determine patient's risk for pressure ulcer formation using a valid assessment tool (e.g., the Braden Scale) and assess additional risk factors for pressure ulcers including nutritional deficits, shear stress, friction, alterations in mobility and sensory perception, moisture, and abnormal serum albumin and hemoglobin levels (see Chapter 18).

Reduces transmission of microorganisms.

Risk assessment tools suggested by AHRQ and WOCN (e.g., Braden Scale) provide an objective measure of risk consistent between nurse assessors over time (AHCPR, 1992, WOCN, 2003).

Critical Decision Point *The bed does not always provide a stable surface for patients requiring skeletal traction.*

3 Perform skin assessment. If there is wound drainage, apply gloves. Inspect condition of skin, especially over dependent sites and bony prominences. Note appearance of existing ulcers and determine stage of ulcer (see Chapter 18). Pay particular attention to potential pressure sites and any existing pressure ulcers.

Data provide baseline to determine any change in patient's condition while on bed.

4 Assess patient's level of comfort; ask patient to rate pain on a scale of 0 to 10.

Provides baseline to determine patient's comfort needs. Nerve endings related to pressure, touch, temperature, and limb position are in the skin (WOCN, 2003).

5 Assess patient's level of orientation.

Baseline used to detect change while patient is on bed. Flotation effect causes altered sensory perceptions (WOCN, 2003).

6 Assess patient's and family members' feelings about therapy and understanding of purpose of bed.

Bed is large and makes sound when air blower is operating, which creates anxiety for patient.

7 Review patient's serum electrolyte levels in medical record (if available).

There is a tendency for patients to lose body fluids through diaphoresis. Use baseline data to compare with subsequent laboratory results to determine electrolyte imbalances (WOCN, 2003).

8 Identify patients at risk for complications of air-fluidized therapy:

Allows nurse to anticipate need for frequent monitoring once patient is placed on support surface.

  a Some older adult patients become dehydrated from the airflow, which may increase insensible fluid losses.

  b Patients receiving enteric tube feedings are at risk for aspiration due to the inability to elevate head of bed, which is limited to placing foam wedges under patient's head and shoulders.

  c Patients who have limited ability to change positions and who are susceptible to dehydration sometimes have pulmonary secretions that are difficult to remove.

  d Patients with specific positioning requirements such as elevating head of bed are limited to use of foam wedges.

9 Review patient's medical orders.

Health care provider's order is usually required to obtain third-party reimbursement for cost of bed.

STEP	RATIONALE

NURSING DIAGNOSES

- Anxiety
- Deficient knowledge regarding use of support surface mattress
- Disturbed kinesthetic sensory perception

- Impaired physical mobility
- Impaired skin integrity
- Ineffective peripheral tissue perfusion
- Pain (acute, chronic)
- Risk for deficient fluid volume

- Risk for imbalanced body temperature
- Risk for impaired skin integrity
- Risk for infection

Individualize related factors based on patient's condition or needs.

PLANNING

1 Expected outcomes following completion of procedure: • Patient's skin remains warm, clean, and intact, or there is evidence of healing of pressure ulcers. • Patient expresses improved sense of comfort. • Skin remains well hydrated, with good turgor; mucous membranes are moist; and electrolyte levels are in normal range. • Patient remains alert and oriented or shows no change in level of consciousness.	Skin is free from pressure effects of immobility. Bed's surface effective in promoting comfort. Patient's fluid and nutrient intake balance any insensible fluid loss from being on bed (WOCN, 2003). Patient does not experience sensory perceptual changes from flotation (WOCN, 2003).
2 Explain procedure and purpose of bed to patient and family.	Reduces anxiety and promotes patient's cooperation.
3 Review instructions supplied by bed manufacturer.	Promotes safe and correct use of bed.
4 For patients with severe to moderate pain, premedicate approximately 30 minutes before transfer.	Promotes patient's comfort and ability to cooperate during transfer to bed. Decreases patient's energy expenditure (WOCN, 2003).
5 Obtain any additional personnel needed to transfer patient to bed.	Ensures patient's safety by having sufficient personnel to assist in transferring.

IMPLEMENTATION

1 Close patient's room door or bedside curtain.	Maintains patient's privacy during transfer.
2 Explain steps of transfer.	Reduces anxiety and helps patient be a part of decision making during maneuvering.
3 Perform hand hygiene. Apply gloves (if bed linens or surface is soiled).	Reduces transmission of microorganisms.
4 Transfer patient to bed using appropriate transfer techniques (see Chapter 9).	Appropriate transfer techniques maintain alignment and reduce risk for injury during procedure.

Critical Decision Point   *Do not position a patient in a prone (face down) position on an air-fluidized bed. Suffocation may occur.*

5 Turn fluidization cycle on by depressing the switch; regulate temperature.	Fluidization minimizes pressure against skin's surface and reduces friction and shear force when patient moves.
6 Position patient for comfort, and perform ROM exercises as appropriate.	Promotes comfort and reduces contracture formation. The bed reduces pressure on skin, but you still need to turn patients and perform exercises to avoid joint deformity or contractures (WOCN, 2003).
7 Use foam wedges as needed (e.g., elevating the head of a patient for position changes).	Areas supported by the foam wedges do not benefit from the pressure relief of the bed's surface.
8 To turn patient, position bedpans, or perform other therapies, stop fluidization. Once procedure is complete, set to continuous fluidization.	Stopping fluidization provides firm, molded support that facilitates turning and handling patient. Continuous fluidization provides permanent fluid support.

Critical Decision Point   *In emergencies when resuscitation is required, press CPR switch and unplug unit to defluidize bed immediately (see Skill 12-1).*

9 Remove gloves, and perform hand hygiene.	Reduces transmission of microorganisms.

EVALUATION

1 Inspect condition of patient's skin, including bony prominences, heels, and occipital area, according to agency policy while on bed, and monitor risk assessment.	Evaluates healing progress of any existing pressure ulcers. Determines if any new pressure areas are forming.
2 Ask patient to rate level of comfort on a scale of 0 to 10.	Bed surface is soft and conforming and should assist with minimizing pain (WOCN, 2003).

STEP	RATIONALE
3 Review patient's serum electrolyte levels, monitor body temperature, and note the hydration status of skin and mucous membranes.	Reveals fluid and electrolyte losses.
4 Measure patient's level of orientation.	Determines onset of perceptual changes.

Unexpected Outcomes	Related Interventions
1 Existing areas of skin breakdown or pressure areas fail to heal or increase in size or depth.	• Modify skin care regimen. • Consult with skin care expert. • Reevaluate patient's risk factors affecting wound healing. • Notify health care provider.
2 Patient's skin and mucous membranes are dehydrated.	• Provide oral fluids unless contraindicated. • If electrolyte levels are also abnormal, notify health care provider. • Monitor patient's intake and output. • Provide intravenous fluids as ordered.
3 Patient is restless or agitated or complains of nausea.	• Administer sedation or antiemetic. • Modify support surface selected. • Notify health care provider.
4 The filter sheet develops a tear.	• Mend tears with adhesive tape as per manufacturer's guidelines until a new bed is available. • Avoid use of additional sheets because they interfere with optimal bed performance.

Recording and Reporting

- Record transfer of patient to bed, tolerance to procedure, condition of skin, and orientation level in nurses' notes or on assessment flow sheet.
- Report changes in condition of skin and electrolyte levels to nurse in charge or to health care provider.
- Report teaching provided and patient and/or caregiver response.
- Report changes in patient's level of orientation.

Teaching Considerations

- Explain function and purpose of air-fluidized therapy.
- Explain that patient will require assistance to change positions.
- Explain the need to maintain adequate hydration of patient.

Pediatric Considerations

- This bed is used commonly with children who are burn victims. Make sure instructions are age appropriate and include any restrictions, such as raising the head of the bed, positioning.

- Parents need to know that the child will initially have some dizziness or nausea when first placed on the bed. This is due to the flotation sensation and will disappear as the child gets adjusted to the bed.

Gerontological Considerations

- Older adult patients are at increased risk for dehydration.
- When hospitalized, some older adult patients may experience significant misperceptions of their environment that may be intensified by the flotation of the air-fluidized bed.

Home Care Considerations

- Beds weigh between 1700 and 2100 pounds; therefore the company leasing the bed needs to inspect the home for accessibility and structural support.
- Consult with social worker or case manager to determine third-party reimbursement.

SKILL 12-4 Placing a Patient on a Bariatric Bed

A valuable resource in the care of a morbidly obese patient (a person who weighs more than 100 lb above ideal weight) is the bariatric bed (Fig. 12-10), a safe, adaptable surface. The bariatric bed is capable of allowing upright or sitting positions, patient transport, and in-bed scale use. The bed is equipped with hand controls that allow self-positioning and facilitate independence for an obese patient. The full-function hand controls also allow the nurse caring for an obese patient to change the bed position and thus facilitate care while reducing risk for staff injury while moving the patient. The in-bed scale provides the nurse with a means of obtaining accurate weights and thus improves health care and patient dignity. The bed is slightly wider than a standard hospital bed, yet it is within the guidelines for standard door width, which allows movement into and out of a room without difficulty.

Because the bariatric bed is capable of supporting weights up to 850 pounds, it provides a stable balanced surface that limits hospital liability should the standard bed frame collapse or the electric motor burn out.

A full- or double-wide bariatric bed can accommodate a patient up to 1000 lb. However, when using a full- or double-wide bariatric bed, you must assemble it in the patient's room and not use it for transfers because this bed is too large to fit through standard hospital doorways.

A limitation of this bed is the lack of pressure reduction or relief in the mattress. An at-risk obese patient needs to have some type of pressure-redistribution mattress placed on the bariatric bed. Choices for pressure redistribution include air or gel type of mattresses and low-air-loss replacement systems. These beds also have CPR switches, which permit an immediate hard surface for chest compressions.

Delegation Considerations

The skill of placing a patient on a bariatric bed can be delegated to NAP. However, first complete the assessment, determine the need for a support surface, and select the specific surface. Determine the number of people needed to assist in safe patient transfer from traditional to bariatric bed. Some types of specialty beds require that the manufacturer's representative set up and maintain the system. The nurse directs the NAP about:

- Notifying the nurse of any changes in the patient's skin; the nurse then completes the skin assessment.
- Continuing regular turning and repositioning of the patient and the number of people needed to assist with patient position changes.
- Specifics on applying, cleaning, and maintaining support surface.

Equipment

- ☐ Bariatric bed
- ☐ Pressure-relief mattress overlay
- ☐ Sheets
- ☐ Overhead frame (*optional*)
- ☐ Heavy-duty lift
- ☐ Clean gloves

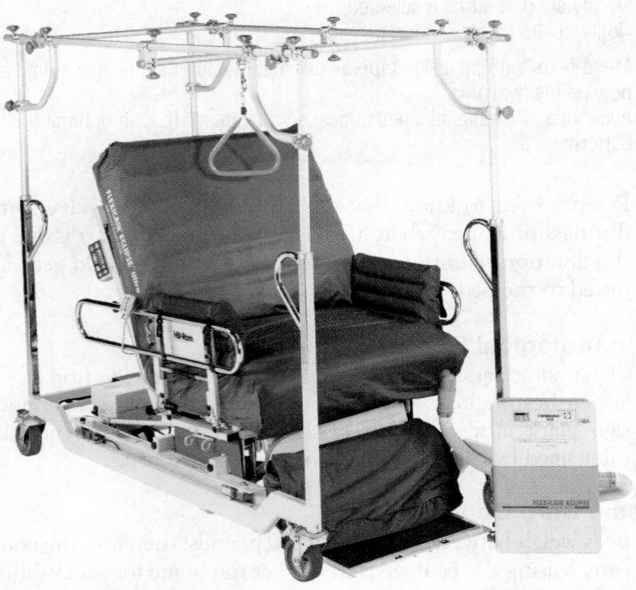

FIG 12-10 Bariatric bed with low-air-loss mattress replacement. (© 2008 Hill-Rom Services, Inc. Reprinted with permission. All rights reserved.)

STEP	RATIONALE
ASSESSMENT	
1 Perform hand hygiene.	Reduces transmission of microorganisms.
2 Determine patient's risk for pressure ulcer formation using a valid assessment tool (e.g., Braden Scale) and assess for risk factors for pressure ulcers, including nutritional deficits, shear stress, friction alterations in mobility and sensory perception, moisture, and abnormal serum albumin and hemoglobin levels (see Chapter 18).	Provides an objective measure of risk consistent between nurse assessors over time (AHCPR, 1992, WOCN, 2003).
3 Identify patients who will benefit from the bariatric bed system; assess their mobility status.	Selected for patients who are morbidly obese and who have the potential of being independent in positioning with assistance of a stable surface.
4 Assess condition of patient's skin, paying particular attention to potential pressure sites and skinfolds. Assistance may be needed to turn patient so as to observe all skin surfaces. Determine the need for patient to have pressure-redistribution mattress placed on the bariatric bed.	Data provide baseline to determine any change in patient's condition while on the bed (Gallagher-Camden, 2007).

STEP	RATIONALE
5 Assess patient's and family members' understanding of purpose of bed.	Improves patient and family cooperation.
6 Review patient's medical orders.	A health care provider's order is usually needed to obtain third-party reimbursement for cost of bed.
7 Assess need for patient to be weighed.	Scales are available in many bariatric beds or as underbed scales for beds without in-bed scales.

NURSING DIAGNOSES

- Deficient knowledge regarding use of support surface mattress
- Impaired physical mobility

- Impaired skin integrity
- Ineffective tissue perfusion

- Pain (acute, chronic)
- Risk for impaired skin integrity

Individualize related factors based on patient's condition or needs.

PLANNING

1 Expected outcomes following completion of procedure:	
• Patient is independent for position changes.	Bed surface is adaptable by hand-operated controls.
• Patient's skin remains intact, or existing lesions show evidence of healing.	Skin is free from pressure effects of immobility.
• Patient remains free of injury.	Bed is stable to allow for positioning without tipping or bending.
2 Explain procedure and purpose of bed to patient and family.	Reduces anxiety and promotes patient's cooperation.
3 Review instructions supplied by bed manufacturer.	Promotes safe and correct use of bed.

Critical Decision Point *Do not exceed weight limits indicated by the manufacturer.*

4 For patients with severe to moderate pain, medicate approximately 30 minutes before transfer.	Promotes patient's comfort and ability to cooperate during transfer to bed. Decreases patient's energy expenditure (WOCN, 2003).
5 Obtain any additional personnel identified during assessment to transfer patient to bed.	Ensures safety of patient and staff by having sufficient personnel to assist in transferring.

IMPLEMENTATION

Critical Decision Point *Use of this bed is contraindicated in patients with spinal cord injuries.*

1 Close patient's room door or bedside curtain.	Maintains patient's privacy during transfer.
2 Perform hand hygiene. Apply clean gloves.	Reduces transmission of microorganisms.
3 Explain steps of transfer.	Reduces anxiety and helps patient be part of decision making during maneuvering.
4 Put on clean gloves (if needed) before assisting patient to bed using appropriate transfer techniques (see Chapter 9). Depending on patient's mobility status, it is sometimes necessary to call for assistance and use a heavy-duty lift.	Appropriate transfer techniques maintain alignment and reduce risk for injury to patient and health care workers during the procedure.
5 Place pull sheet, slide board, hydraulic lifts, or other assistive devices under the patient, and transfer safely.	Reduces trauma from friction and shear to patient's skin (Pieper, 2007).
6 Cover and position patient, and place hand controls within reach. Be certain that the out-of-bed alarm is on, if needed. Attach overhead frame if needed.	Allows for maximal patient independence. Alarm alerts caregiver that patient has left the bed surface.
7 Encourage patient to initiate frequent position changes and move in the bed as much as possible.	Morbidly obese patients quickly increase pressure over bony prominences. Frequent removal (e.g., every 30 to 60 minutes) of pressure from these points assists in reducing the risk for pressure ulcer formation.
8 Remove gloves, and perform hand hygiene.	Reduces transmission of microorganisms.

EVALUATION

1 Inspect condition of patient's skin according to agency policy while patient is on bed.	Evaluates healing of any existing pressure ulcers. Determines if any new pressure areas are forming.
2 Ask patient to rate sense of comfort and safety.	Bed frame is stable for movement and position changes.
3 Evaluate patient's risk for injury.	Surface is balanced and allows maximal patient independence.
4 Evaluate patient's ability to move in bed.	Evaluates effectiveness of bed and education to promote independence.

Unexpected Outcomes	Related Interventions
1 Existing areas of skin breakdown or pressure areas fail to heal or increase in size or depth.	• Modify skin care regimen. • Consult with skin care expert. • Notify health care provider.
2 Patient is unable to operate bed for position changes independently.	• Reassess patient's level of independence and ability to understand instructions. • Reinstruct patient and family in how to operate the bed. • Provide for return demonstration regarding bed operation.

Recording and Reporting

• Record transfer of patient to bed, tolerance of procedure, and condition of skin in nurses' notes or skin assessment flow sheet.
• Report changes in condition of skin to nurse in charge or health care provider.

Teaching Considerations

• Explain function and purpose of bariatric bed.
• Explain function and purpose of pressure-relief mattress overlay used.
• Explain the need to continue to change position at intervals to diminish effects of immobility.

SKILL 12-5   Placing a Patient on a Rotokinetic Bed

The Rotokinetic bed helps maintain skeletal alignment while providing constant rotation (Fig. 12-11). It is used in the care of patients with spinal cord injuries or multiple trauma. The support structure of the bed outlines the body parts and maintains proper alignment when secured properly. This bed improves skeletal alignment with constant side-to-side rotation up to 90 degrees (Tomaselli and others, 2005). The bed rotates from side to side at a 60- to 90-degree angle every 7 minutes. You may adjust turning angles to meet the patient's needs. Constant rotation reduces pressure ulcer development and stimulates body systems. It is recommended that the bed stay in the rotation mode for at least 20 hours a day. There is an emergency lever that can quickly interrupt rotation when needed. To initiate CPR, return the bed to the horizontal position and lock in place.

The constant motion often leads to sensory distress for the patient, especially older adults. This is associated with the constant kinetic stimulation, the limited visual field, and inner ear disequilibrium. Be aware of these complications, and provide necessary emotional support. A health care provider's order is required for third-party payment.

Delegation Considerations

The skill of placing a patient on a Rotokinetic bed cannot be delegated to NAP. This type of bed is frequently used for patients with multiple trauma or spinal cord injuries, and you need to carefully determine what aspects of the patient's care to delegate to the appropriately skilled personnel. The nurse directs the NAP about:
• Notifying the nurse of any changes in the patient's skin; the nurse then completes the skin assessment.
• The exact rotation frequency of the bed.
• Stopping the rotation only for selected aspects of care determined by the nurse (e.g., bathing, oral hygiene, enemas).
• Immediately notifying the nurse if the patient experiences confusion, nausea, and pain.

Equipment

❑ Rotokinetic bed with support packs, bolsters, and safety straps
❑ Top sheet
❑ Pillowcases for bolsters

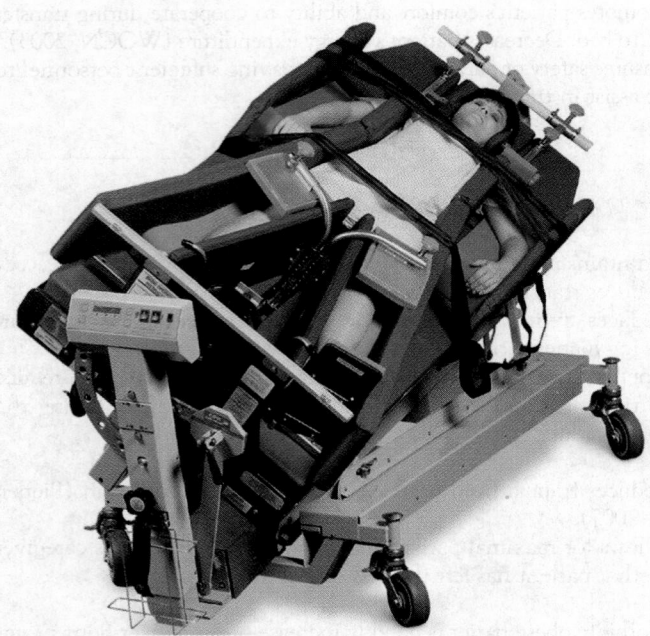

FIG 12-11   Rotokinetic bed. (*RotoRest, Courtesy Kinetic Concepts, Inc, San Antonio, Tex.*)

ASSESSMENT

1 Perform hand hygiene.
2 Determine patient's risk for pressure ulcer formation using a validated assessment tool (e.g., Braden Scale) and assess for risk factors for pressure ulcers including nutritional deficits, shear stress, friction, alterations in mobility and perception, moisture, and abnormal serum albumin and hemoglobin levels (see Chapter 18).

Reduces transmission of microorganisms.
Risk assessment tools suggested by AHCPR and WOCN (e.g., Braden Scale) provide an objective measure of risk consistent between nurse assessors over time (AHCPR, 1992; WOCN, 2003).

STEP	RATIONALE
3 Perform skin assessment. Inspect condition of skin, especially over dependent sites and bony prominences (see Chapter 18).	Provides baseline to measure ongoing data to determine a change in skin integrity or change in an existing pressure ulcer.
4 Review patient's medical orders.	Health care provider's order is needed to receive third-party reimbursement for cost of bed (not required in Canada).
5 Assess patient's level of comfort; ask patient to rate pain on a scale of 0 to 10.	Provides baseline to determine the patient's comfort needs. Nerve endings related to pressure, touch, temperature, and limb position are located in the skin (WOCN, 2003).
6 Assess patient's level of orientation.	Baseline used to detect change while patient is on bed. Constant motion often leads to sensory distress.
7 Perform pulmonary assessment, and obtain vital signs.	Provides baseline of patient's pulmonary status and vital signs. Patients with severe injuries or spinal cord injuries are at risk for accumulation of pulmonary secretions. In addition, when these patients are first placed on the bed, they are at risk for changes in pulse and blood pressure due to the motion of the bed.
8 Assess patient's and family members' feelings about and understanding of purpose of bed.	Appearance and movement of bed creates anxiety for patient and family members.

NURSING DIAGNOSES

- Anxiety
- Deficient knowledge regarding the use of Rotokinetic bed
- Disturbed kinesthetic sensory perception
- Impaired physical mobility
- Impaired skin integrity
- Ineffective tissue perfusion
- Pain (acute, chronic)
- Risk for impaired skin integrity
- Risk for infection

Individualize related factors based on patient's condition or needs.

PLANNING

1 Expected outcomes following completion of procedure:	
• Patient's skin remains intact without evidence of abnormal reactive hyperemia or mottling.	Skin is free from pressure effects of immobility (Peiper, 2007).
• Existing pressure ulcers show evidence of healing.	Patient is experiencing benefits of bed.
• Patient's musculoskeletal system is properly aligned and free of contractures.	Device provides support and alignment to trunk and extremities.
• Patient's breath sounds improve from baseline assessment or remain clear to auscultation.	Patient's pulmonary congestion is improving or absent.
• Patient remains alert, oriented, and cooperative.	Patient does not experience sensory perceptual changes from bed positions.
• Patient denies nausea or dizziness.	Motion of bed is not negatively affecting patient.
• Patient's blood pressure remains consistent with baseline vital signs.	Patient not experiencing cardiovascular disturbances (Nix, 2007).
2 Explain procedure and purpose of bed to patient and family.	Reduces anxiety and promotes cooperation.
3 Review instructions supplied by bed manufacturer.	Promotes safe and correct use of bed.
4 Premedicate approximately 30 minutes before transfer.	Promotes patient's comfort and ability to cooperate during transfer to bed. Decreases patient's energy expenditure (WOCN, 2003).
5 Obtain any additional personnel needed to transfer patient to bed.	Ensures patient's safety.

IMPLEMENTATION

1 Close patient's room door or bedside curtain.	Maintains patient's privacy during transfer.
2 Place Rotokinetic bed in horizontal position, and remove all bolsters, straps, and supports. Close posterior hatches.	
3 Unplug electrical cord. Lock gatch.	Prevents accidental rotation during transfer.
4 Perform hand hygiene and apply gloves.	Reduces transmission of microorganisms.
5 Maintaining proper alignment of the patient and using appropriate transfer techniques (see Chapter 9), transfer patient to Rotokinetic bed.	Reduces risk for further tissue injury during transfer. May need health care provider available to assist in transfer.
6 Secure thoracic panels, bolsters, head and knee packs, and safety straps.	Maintains proper alignment and prevents sliding during rotation.
7 Cover patient with top sheet.	Prevents unnecessary exposure.
8 Plug bed in.	

STEP	RATIONALE
9 Have company representative set optional angle as ordered by health care provider. Gradually increase rotation.	Health care provider determines rotational angle based on the patient's overall condition and tolerance to constant motion.
10 Increase degree of rotation gradually according to patient's tolerance.	Gradually increasing rotation reduces or prevents nausea, dizziness, and orthostatic hypotension (Tomaselli and others, 2005).
11 It is difficult to maintain eye contact when talking with patients during rotation. Provide space for caregivers and family to move around the bed to facilitate communication.	Allows opportunity to meet patient's psychosocial needs.
12 You may stop the bed for assessment and procedures. To stop the bed, permit bed to rotate to the desired position, turn the motor off, and push knob into a lock position. If necessary, you can manually reposition the bed.	Allows nurse to assess patient.
13 Inform patient that there will be a sensation of light-headedness or falling. However, reassure patient that he or she will not fall because the pads will prevent this and are checked by two people to ensure proper placement.	Informing patient of what to expect will decrease anxiety.

EVALUATION

1 Inspect condition of skin (occipital region, ears, axillae, elbows, sacrum, groin, heels) and musculoskeletal alignment every 2 hours or more often if indicated by patient's condition.	Evaluates healing process of any existing pressure ulcers and determines effectiveness of Rotokinetic therapy.
2 Inspect patient's pressure ulcers for evidence of healing.	Evaluates healing process.
3 Observe alignment and range of motion of all joints.	Determines if complications (e.g., atelectasis) have developed.
4 Auscultate lung sounds every shift, and compare with baseline.	Provides ongoing pulmonary assessment.
5 Determine patient's level of orientation once per shift while on bed.	Evaluates if sensory overload has developed from excess kinetic stimulation.
6 Ask whether patient is experiencing nausea or dizziness.	Determines if patient is having inner ear disturbance.
7 Monitor blood pressure.	Determines if patient experiences orthostatic hypotension from position rotation.

Unexpected Outcomes	Related Interventions
1 Existing areas of skin breakdown or pressure areas fail to heal or increase in size or depth.	• Evaluate rotation schedule; bed needs to remain in rotation 20 hours per day to prevent skin breakdown. • Modify skin care regimen.
2 Patient experiences hypotension.	• If severe drop in blood pressure, stop rotation, notify health care provider, remain with patient, and monitor vital signs every 5 minutes. • For less severe blood pressure changes, decrease rotational angle. Gradually increase the rotation angle as patient adjusts to rotation.
3 Patient becomes disoriented, confused, and anxious.	• Reorient patient to person, place, time. • Provide audio stimulation, via radio or tapes. • Provide television adapted to Rotokinetic bed (available from manufacturer). • Hang mirror on ceiling so patient is able to view surroundings. • Provide symptomatic relief of motion sickness.
4 Patient develops abnormal lung sounds.	• Increase frequency of pulmonary hygiene measures (e.g., cough and deep breathe, suctioning). • Have patient use incentive spirometry.
5 Bed fails to rotate.	• Provide for patient safety. • Position bed flat. • Follow manufacturer's/agency policies.

Recording and Reporting

- Describe condition of skin before placement on the Rotokinetic bed. Take a photograph to document skin condition and provide a baseline for later assessments for progress in healing.
- Record and report time of transfer to Rotokinetic bed and degree of rotation.
- Record and report subjective data indicating response to the constant rotation and presence/absence of dizziness, nausea, or blood pressure changes.
- Use a flow sheet to document routine assessment and care, including the length of time the bed rotation stopped. The bed needs to be rotating at least 20 hours out of every 24 hours and stopped for no more than 30 minutes at a time.

Teaching Considerations

- Explain function and purpose of Rotokinetic bed.
- Explain that patient will feel sensation of light-headedness or falling. However, patient will not fall because pads are positioned to prevent this.

Pediatric Considerations

- Provide age-appropriate education for the child. It is important that the child understand that he or she is secure in the bed and will not fall out as the bed turns.
- Distraction, such as talking books, videos, and music, help the older child adjust to the bed and the restricted mobility.

Gerontological Considerations

- Older adults are at increased risk for sensation of light-headedness or dizziness.

 CRITICAL THINKING EXERCISES

You are assigned to admit Mr. Sachiko Hoji, a 48-year-old Asian male, following a motor vehicle accident, which resulted in quadriplegia. The patient is unable to change positions or transfer without assistance. He also has a language barrier, and communicating instructions about his care is difficult. He lives with his wife of 20 years, who interprets for him.

1 You anticipate that this patient will need a support surface. Before selecting this surface, what assessments will you make?

2 What category of support surface will you select? What is your rationale for this selection?

3 Following consultation with physical therapy and social service, the health care provider orders an air-suspension bed with lateral rotation because Mr. Hoji does have some blistering over bony prominences and his impaired mobility and sensation increase his risk for developing pressure ulcers. Mr. Hoji begins experiencing a small amount of nausea and restlessness when initially placed on the air-suspension bed. He tells his wife, "I am afraid that I will fall out of this bed when it tilts. Will I?" What actions should you implement for Mr. Hoji's nausea and anxiety?

REVIEW QUESTIONS

1 A patient at risk for pressure areas is placed on a specialty bed. Dehydration and/or electrolyte imbalances can occur with which type of specialty bed/mattress?
1 Egg-crate mattress
2 Air-suspension bed
3 Aid-fluidized bed
4 Bariatric bed

2 The nurse is caring for a patient on a Rotokinetic type of bed when the patient complains of sudden dizziness. The nurse checks his blood pressure and notes that on lateral rotation the patient develops orthostatic hypotension. What should be the nurse's initial actions?
1 Have the nursing assistive personnel notify the health care provider while the nurse assesses the patient.
2 Stop the rotation of the bed for a few minutes while the nurse assesses the patient.
3 Talk to the patient, and assess for other factors that can make him hypotensive.
4 Increase his oral fluids, and assess the patient again after he has been hydrated.

3 The nurse is caring for a patient, who can change position independently, on an air-filled overlay on the mattress. While conducting a skin assessment, the nurse notices skin breakdown over the coccyx and left hip, even though this patient has received meticulous skin care and routine repositioning. What is the appropriate nursing action?
1 Maintain the present mattress.
2 Increase repositioning frequency.
3 Check functioning and filling of the mattress.
4 Consider changing to a pressure-relief device.

4 A patient needs to be placed on a bariatric bed. Which factor would be least considered when determining the need for the larger bed?
1 The patient's ability to assist with transfer to the bed
2 Availability of personnel to reposition the patient
3 The ability of the environment to accommodate the bed
4 The integrity of the skin on pressure areas and in skinfold regions

5 A patient on an air-fluidized bed needs to be turned. Which nursing intervention indicates the nurse needs additional teaching about using this type of bed?
1 The nurse prepares to place the patient in prone position on the bed.
2 The nurse uses foam wedges to support the patient's head for comfort.
3 The nurse asks the patient how much she can do before turning her.
4 The nurse assess visible skin areas before and after turning the patient.

REFERENCES

Agency for Health Care Policy and Research: *Pressure ulcers in adults: prediction and prevention*, Clinical Practice Guideline No. 3, Rockville, Md, 1992, U.S. Department of Health and Human Services.

Agency for Health Care Policy and Research, Panel for the Treatment of Pressure Ulcers: *Treatment of pressure ulcers*, Clinical Practice Guideline No. 15, AHCPR Pub No. 95-0652, Rockville, Md, 1994, U.S. Department of Health and Human Services.

Bryant RA: *Acute and chronic wounds: current management concepts*, ed 3, St. Louis, 2007, Mosby.

Gallagher-Camden S: Skin care needs of the obese patient. In Bryant RA, Nix DP: *Acute and chronic wounds: current management concepts*, ed 3, St. Louis, 2007, Mosby.

Hockenberry MJ, Wilson J: *Wong's nursing care of infants and children*, ed 8, St. Louis, 2007, Mosby.

Mackey D: Support surfaces: beds, mattresses, overlays—oh my! *Nurs Clin North Am* 40(2):251, 2005.

Morrison MJ: *The prevention and treatment of pressure ulcers*, St. Louis, 2001, Mosby.

National Pressure Ulcer Advisory Panel: *Healthy people 2010: ulcer prevention objective*, http://www.npuap.org/HP 2010.html, accessed July 2004.

Nix D: Support surfaces. In Bryant RA, Nix DP: *Acute and chronic wounds: current management concepts,* ed 3, St. Louis, 2007, Mosby.

Pieper B: Mechanical forces: pressure, shear, and friction. In Bryant RA, Nix DP: *Acute and chronic wounds: current management concepts,* ed 3, St. Louis, 2007, Mosby.

Thomas C: Specialty beds: decision making made easy, *Ostomy Wound Manage* 23:51, 1989.

Tomaselli N and others: Pressure-reducing devices: lateral rotation therapy. In Lynn-McHale Wiegand DJ, Carlson KK, editors: *AACN procedure manual for critical care,* ed 5, Philadelphia, 2005, WB Saunders.

Wound, Ostomy and Continence Nurses Society: *Guideline for prevention and management of pressure ulcers,* Glenview, Ill, 2003, The Society.

Wysocki AB: Anatomy and physiology of skin and soft tissues. In Bryant RA, Nix DP: *Acute and chronic wounds: current management concepts,* ed 3, St. Louis, 2007, Mosby.

RESEARCH REFERENCES

Brienza DM, Geyer MJ: Using support surfaces to manage tissue integrity, *Adv Skin Wound Care* 18(3):151, 2005.

Courtney BA and others: Save our skin: initiative cuts pressure ulcer incidence in half, *Nurs Manage* 37(4):35, 2006.

Cullum N and others: Beds, mattresses and cushions for pressure sore preventions and treatment, *Cochrane Database Syst Rev* 1(1), most recent update April 2003.

Cullum N and others: *Beds, mattresses and cushions for pressure sore prevention and treatment* (Cochrane Review) The Cochrane Library, No. 2, Chichester, UK, 2004, John Wiley & Sons.

Gibbons W and others: Eliminating facility-acquired pressure ulcers at Ascension Health, *Jt Comm J Qual Patient Saf* 32:488, 2006.

Koziak M: Etiology of decubitus ulcers, *Arch Phys Med Rehabil* 42:19, 1961.

National Pressure Ulcer Advisory Panel: *Pressure ulcer definition and stages,* 2007a, http://www.npuap.org/documents/PU_Definition_Stages.pdf, accessed July 2007.

National Pressure Ulcer Advisory Panel: *Support surface standards initiative: terms and definitions related to support surfaces,* 2007b, http://www.npuap.org/NPUAP_S3I_TD.pdf, accessed July 2007.

Posthauer ME and others: Support service initiative: terms, definitions, and patient care, *Adv Skin Wound Care* 19(9):487, 2006.

Reddy M and others: Preventing pressure ulcers: a systemic review, JAMA 296:274, 2006.

Rithalia S: Assessment of patient support surfaces: principal, practice and limitations, *J Med Eng Technol* 29(4):163, 2005.

Safety

13

SKILLS AND PROCEDURES

KEY TERMS

Aspiration
Belt restraints
Extremity restraints
Material safety data sheet (MSDS)
Mitten restraints
Mummy restraints
Physical restraint
Seizure
Seizure precautions
Sentinel event

MEDIA RESOURCES

- evolve learning system http://evolve.elsevier.com/Perry/skills
  - Review Questions
  - Video Clips
- View Video! Mosby's Nursing Video Skills, 3.0
- NSO Nursing Skills Online

Accrediting and governmental agencies support initiatives to maintain patient safety within health care organizations. In addition, patient safety is clearly stipulated as a standard in both ethical and professional practice guidelines. In July of 2002, The Joint Commission established its first set of national patient safety goals for improving the safety of patient care in health care organizations. Since then, The Joint Commission has annually updated its patient safety goals. The 2009 patient safety goals include reducing the risk for harm resulting from falls and encouraging patients' active involvement in their own care (The Joint Commission [TJC], 2008c). Each patient safety goal has a set of requirements that a health care organization must meet to gain The Joint Commission accreditation, unless the goal does not pertain to the agency. Nurses are accountable within their institutions for following the safety goal requirements. Chapter 20 discusses the patient safety goals pertaining to medication administration.

In a recent study, researchers interviewed inpatients from 12 Midwestern hospitals to identify patients' perceptions of medical errors (Burroughs and others, 2007). The study reveals that hospital patients define medical errors more broadly than traditional clinical definitions of medical errors. Patients consider falls, communication problems, and lack of nurse responsiveness as errors, along with medication errors and injury from medical equipment. It is important for nurses to understand what patients perceive as errors so that patients will become partners in programs to prevent errors. More hospitals are involving patients in safety interventions. The Joint Commission requires hospitals to have a way for patients and their families to report concerns about safety, such as asking caregivers if they have washed their hands. Recently The Joint Commission launched a national campaign, urging patients to "Know Your Rights," part of the Commission's Speak Up program (TJC, 2007b). The program encourages people to take an active role in their own health care by speaking up if they have questions, paying attention to the care they receive, educating themselves about their diagnosis and treatment plan, and knowing the medications they are on. In addition, The Joint Commission encourages patients to participate in all decisions about their treatment.

Within a safety-conscious health care system, fall prevention is a priority. More than one third of adults 65 years of age and older fall annually in the United States (CDC, 2007). However, younger patients fall as well, because of the effects of medications, such as analgesics and sedatives, or weakness from their illness. Often younger patients disregard their risks for falls and try to ambulate or get out of their hospital bed on their own. In 2000, direct medical costs totaled $179 million for fatal falls and $19 billion for nonfatal falls (Stevens and others, 2006). Falls lead to traumatic brain injury and fractures, all of which extend hospital length of stay and lead to ongoing health problems. Many patients who do fall later develop a fear of falling, which then limits their activity, resulting in reduced mobility and physical fitness.

In addition to fall prevention, nurses protect patients from self-injury. Patients with serious psychosocial health problems are at risk for injury. Accidents classified as patient-inherent accidents include self-inflicted cuts, injuries, and burns; ingestion or injection of foreign substances; and self-mutilation or setting fires. Patient-inherent accidents occur in persons of all ages, requiring nurses to always be attentive and know which patients are at risk.

A nurse's assessment findings and critical thinking direct the actions needed to promote a patient's safety. For example, knowing a patient's medical condition, the patient's risks for injury, and the actions and side effects of medications, coupled with assessment findings lead you to select interventions for a safe environment. A thorough assessment helps you to anticipate ways to prevent patient injury. A safe environment is one in which patients meet basic needs, physical hazards are reduced or eliminated, transmission of microorganisms is reduced, and sanitary measures are carried out.

EVIDENCE-BASED PRACTICE TRENDS

There continues to be significant research in the area of fall prevention. In a review of studies designed to reduce the fear of falling in community-living older adults, it appears that multifactorial programs show good success (Zijlstra and others, 2007a). A multifactorial program is one that uses multiple interventions because individuals are at risk for falls for a variety of reasons. Well-designed research studies show that home-based exercise, fall-related multifactorial programs, and community-based tai chi delivered in a group format are effective in reducing the fear of falling in community-living older adults. Studies also show that tai chi improves body balance and ambulation (Greenspan and others, 2007; Maciaszek and others, 2007). Tai chi is an internal Chinese martial art practiced with the aim of promoting health and longevity. Tinetti (2003) warns that effective home-based exercise programs are only short term, usually lasting 1 year or less.

Safety research has focused primarily on ambulatory older adults. However, wheelchair-related falls are a serious problem for persons with disabilities. For a patient who relies on a wheelchair for mobility, a tip or fall will possibly affect morbidity and mortality (Gavin-Dreschnack and others, 2005). Wheelchair-related injuries from falls include factures, concussions, dislocations, amputations, and serious head and spinal injuries. Gavin-Dreschnack and others (2005) developed a model for examining wheelchair-related falls. It proposes that an interaction of the following promotes falls: characteristics of users, wheelchair type and features, health care practices, wheelchair activities, and environmental characteristics. Risks associated with users include younger individuals, males, paraplegia or spina bifida, daily use of wheelchair, and propelling with both hands. An example of a wheelchair characteristic that increases risk for falls is having smaller and harder front wheels, which contribute to forward tips when striking uneven terrain. Caregivers are at risk for injury by not handling patients correctly or not asking for assistance. Injuries occur while caregivers transfer patients who are agitated, fearful, unsteady, or too weak to transfer. Tripping over the front foot or leg rest is a common source of injury, as well as leaning over the back of the wheelchair to engage or disengage the wheel lock. Patients are at risk for falls during transfer tasks and reaching while seated in the wheelchair. Most wheelchair accidents occur outdoors because of uneven terrain, stairs, and wet or icy surfaces.

CULTURAL CONSIDERATIONS

- Become aware of ethnoreligious rituals such as use of open flame and burning that create a risk for fire. Buddhists and Hindus (Pacquiao, 2003) burn incense at the bedside. Hindus light an eternal flame at the bedside at the time of the patient's death. Orthodox Jews light candles throughout Sabbath (Robinson, 2000). Native Americans have cleansing or smudging ceremonies using fire and smoke.
- Negotiate with patients to find an alternative because you cannot have an open flame at the bedside.
- Battery-operated candles are appropriate for observant Jews who avoid use of electrical appliances during Sabbath. Select an area designated for burning incense, herbs, and candles in close proximity to the patient's bedside.
- When restraints are needed, assess the meaning of restraints to the patient and the family. Some Asian families, for example, view the restraining of elders as disrespectful. Similarly, some survivors of war or persecution view restraints as imprisonment or punishment.
- Collaborate with family members in accommodating a patient's cultural perspectives about restraints. Removing the restraints when family members are present will show respect and caring for the patient.
- Define the unit's protocol on the use of restraints. Identify potential areas for negotiation with the patient/family's preferences such as using a jacket versus arm restraints.
- When seizure precautions are necessary, explain and demonstrate the therapeutic regimen to the patient/family. Some cultures observe different caring practices for a person with seizures. Hmongs often observe surveillance and protection of the patient.

 Skill Performance Guidelines

1. Know risk factors for injury such as a patient's age, level of awareness, anxiety, orientation, ability to process information and make judgments, ability to communicate, sensory and motor status, and usual daily activity pattern.
2. Assess a patient's medical history and present therapies. Certain illnesses, such as stroke, and medications, such as sedatives or tranquilizers, cause physical or cognitive impairment that increases the risk for injury.
3. Always be alert to conditions within a patient's environment that pose risk for patient injury.
4. Know the proper indications and institutional policy for and use of physical restraints for a patient receiving nursing care in a hospital or extended care facility.

PROCEDURAL GUIDELINE 13-1   Fire, Electrical, Radiation, and Chemical Safety

NSO *Safety Module / Lesson 1*

Fires in health care settings are typically electrical or anesthetic related. Although smoking is usually not allowed in the hospital setting, smoking-related fires continue to pose a significant risk because of unauthorized smoking in bed or the bathroom. In the home setting, oxygen-related fires are a risk for patients requiring continuous oxygen therapy (see Chapter 23). Health care agencies need to routinely check and maintain all electrical devices. Each biomedical device (e.g., suction machine, infusion pump, or ventilator) needs to have a safety inspection sticker with an expiration date. Electrical equipment in good working order requires proper grounding. The third (longer) prong in an electrical plug is the ground. If a patient brings an electrical device to the hospital, an engineer inspects the device for safe wiring and function before use. Always discourage patients from bringing nonessential electrical devices (e.g., hair dryers or electric toothbrushes) to a health care setting. Many patients with disabilities use battery chargers for mobility equipment function. These devices need to be inspected by hospital engineers as well.

If a fire occurs in a health care agency, the first priority is to protect patients from immediate injury. Health care personnel report the exact location of the fire, contain it, and extinguish it if possible. All personnel then work together to evacuate patients. The best intervention is to prevent fires. Nursing measures include complying with the agency's smoking policies and keeping combustible materials away from heat sources. Some agencies have fire doors that are held open by magnets and close automatically when a fire alarm sounds. It is important to keep equipment away from these doors.

Diagnostic radioactive materials and radiation therapy are health hazards. Hospitals have strict guidelines on the care of patients who receive radiation or who have radioactive implants. The Nuclear Regulatory Commission strictly regulates safe handling, use, and disposal of radioactive materials. Be familiar with agency policies governing use of these materials. Safety measures related to time, distance, and shielding aim to reduce exposure of patients, visitors, and staff to radiation. Nursing staff need to strictly follow radiation safety procedures. Often patients are restricted to specific floors of a hospital where radioactive materials are used (e.g., oncology units). Always know established agency protocols and policies.

Chemicals in medications (e.g., chemotherapeutic agents), anesthetic gases, cleaning solutions, and disinfectants are toxic. Chemicals cause injury to the body after skin contact, mucous membrane (e.g., eyes) contact, ingestion, or when vapors are inhaled. Health care facilities provide employees access to a material safety data sheet (MSDS) for each hazardous chemical. An MSDS is a form containing data about the properties of the particular chemical and information for handling the substance in a safe manner (e.g., storage, disposal, protective equipment, and spill-handling procedures).

Continued

PROCEDURAL GUIDELINE 13-1   Fire, Electrical, Radiation, and Chemical Safety—cont'd

Delegation Considerations

The skill of protecting patients from fire, electrical, radiation, and chemical hazards can be delegated to nursing assistive personnel (NAP). The nurse leads the health care team in an emergency response. The nurse directs the NAP by:

- Identifying patients requiring the most assistance to evacuate or protect.
- Alerting to any risk for chemical exposure.

Equipment

Fire

❑ Appropriate fire extinguisher for fire: Type A, B, C, or ABC

Radiation

❑ Protective radiation shields (lead apron)
❑ Lead-shielded container if required
❑ Radiation exposure badge or dosimeter
❑ Clean gloves
❑ Radioactive materials caution sign for patient's door

Chemical

❑ Appropriate personal protective equipment: clean gloves, mask, gown
❑ MSDS form

Procedural Steps

1 Review agency guidelines for rapid response to fire, electrical, radiation, and chemical emergency. Know your responsibilities such as initiating fire alarm, patient evacuation, and shielding radioactive sources.

2 Familiarize yourself with location of fire alarms, emergency equipment (e.g., fire extinguishers), MSDS forms, emergency eye wash stations, and emergency exit routes.

3 Assess a patient's mental status and ability to ambulate, transfer, or move to anticipate the procedures that will be needed to evacuate the patient.

4 For patients receiving radioactive implants, assess their knowledge of the risks of radiation exposure and purpose of safety precautions. Assess family members' knowledge as well.

5 Assess if patient receiving radioactive implants is pregnant. Explain the risk for radiation exposure to fetuses, and determine if the patient plans to have any visitors who are pregnant or 18 years of age or younger.

6 Fire safety
  a Follow the acronym RACE
    (1) **R**escue patient from immediate injury by removing from area or shielding from the fire hazard.
    (2) **A**ctivate the fire alarm. Follow agency policy for alerting staff to respond. (Perform Steps (1) and (2) simultaneously by using the call system to alert staff while you help patients at risk.)
    (3) **C**ontain the fire:
      (a) Close all doors and windows.
      (b) Turn off oxygen and electrical equipment.
      (c) Place wet towels along base of doors.
    (4) **E**vacuate patients:
      (a) Direct ambulatory patients to walk by themselves to a safe area. Know the fire exits and emergency evacuation route.
      (b) If patient is on life support, maintain respiratory status manually until you remove patient from fire area.
      (c) Move bedridden patients by stretcher, bed, or wheelchair.
      (d) For patients who cannot walk or ambulate themselves:
        i Place on blanket, and drag patient out of area of danger.
        ii *Use two-person swing:* Place patient in sitting position, and have two staff members form a seat by clasping forearms together. Lift patient into "seat," and carry out of area of danger (see illustrations).
        iii *Use a "back-strap" method:* Stand in front of patient, and place patient's arms around your neck. Grasp patient's wrists firmly against your chest. Pull patient onto your back, and carry out of danger.
    (5) If fire department personnel are on the scene, they will help evacuate patients.

> **Critical Decision Point**   *Know the weight and size of patients and their self-help ability when choosing evacuation carry. Use safe patient-handling techniques. Use of a two-person carry versus trying to carry patient independently reduces risk for injury.*

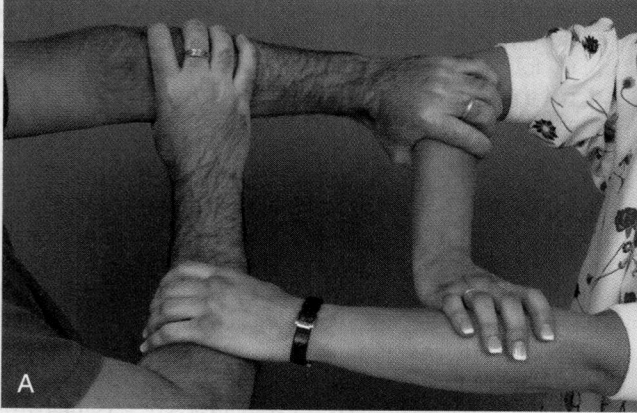
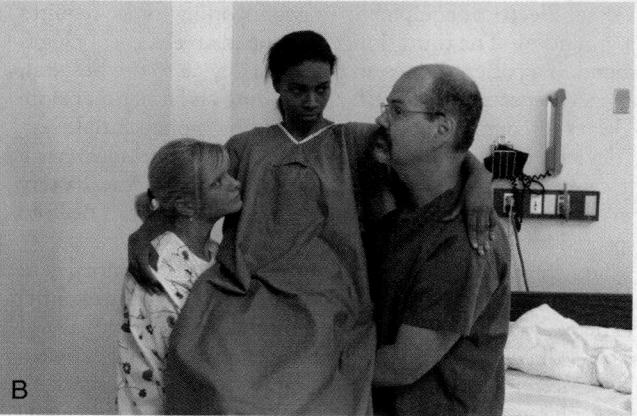

STEP 6a(4)(d)ii   **A,** Hands positioned to form two-person evacuation swing. **B,** Patient seated firmly on swing and holding shoulders of nurses for evacuation.

PROCEDURAL GUIDELINE 13-1   Fire, Electrical, Radiation, and Chemical Safety—cont'd

b Use appropriate fire extinguisher to put out fire: Type A for ordinary combustibles (e.g., wood, cloth, paper, most plastics), Type B for flammable liquids (e.g., gasoline, grease, paint, anesthetic gas), Type C for electrical equipment, Type ABC for any type of fire (most common extinguisher in use).

  (1) To use an extinguisher, pull the pin (see illustration A).

  (2) Aim the nozzle at the base of the fire (see illustration B), squeeze the extinguisher handles, and sweep from side to side to coat the area evenly.

7 Electrical safety

a If patient receives an electrical shock, immediately disengage electrical source, then assess for presence of a pulse to detect asystole or an arrhythmia. CAUTION: When disengaging electrical source, check for presence of water on floor.

  (1) If patient does not have a pulse, begin cardiopulmonary resuscitation (see Chapter 27).

  (2) Notify emergency personnel and patient's physician.

  (3) If patient has a pulse and remains alert and oriented, obtain vital signs and assess the skin for signs of thermal injury.

8 Radiation safety

a When caring for patients receiving radiation therapy or who have radioactive implants, wear a radiation exposure dosimeter to track cumulative radiation exposure (see illustration).

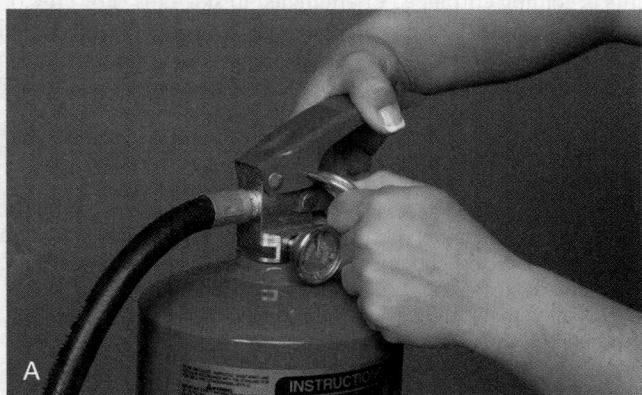

STEP 6b(1)   Remove safety pin from fire extinguisher.

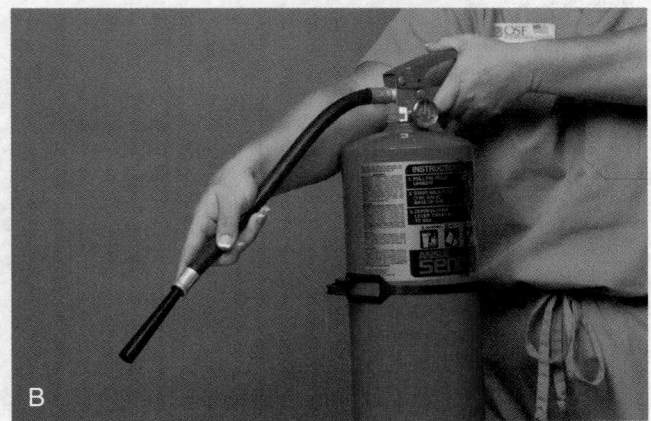

STEP 6b(2)   Aim hose at base of fire, and squeeze handles, sweeping from side to side.

b Explain treatment plan to patient and family, including activity limitations, safety regulations, and time and distance limits. (For example, there can be no pregnant visitors, visitors are usually limited to 30 minutes per day and must stay 6 feet away from radiation source.)

c Place patient in a private room with private bath, and place sign ("Caution: Radioactive Material") on door, indicating radioactive materials are in room.

d Provide activities and distractions for patient (e.g., music, reading materials, planned calls from family members).

e Rotate care providers during patient's length of stay on unit to minimize their exposure to radiation.

f When entering patient's room, wear a protective lead apron and gloves. Have family members wear protective gear as well.

g Follow agency policy for removal of laboratory specimens, dietary tray, dressings, linens, trash, and body fluids. Body excretions and secretions and items in contact with patient will carry radiation.

h After caring for patient, wash gloves before removing, and dispose of them in designated waste container. Perform thorough hand hygiene.

i When patient is discharged from facility, request a radiation safety officer to conduct a survey of sources of radiation.

9 Chemical safety

a Attend to any person exposed to a chemical. Treat chemical splashes to the eyes immediately; flush eyes with water. Use clean, lukewarm tap water for at least 20 minutes; stand under a shower, or place head under running faucet. Remove contact lenses if flushing does not remove them.

b Notify persons in the immediate area of the spill, and evacuate all nonessential personnel from spill area.

c Refer to MSDS, and if spilled material is flammable, turn off electrical and heat sources.

d Avoid breathing vapors of spilled material; apply appropriate respirator.

e Use appropriate personal protective equipment (see MSDS) for cleanup of spill.

f Dispose of any materials used in cleanup as hazardous waste.

10 Regularly inspect patient's room for fire or electrical hazards.

11 Have patient describe steps used to minimize radiation exposure and associated risks of exposure.

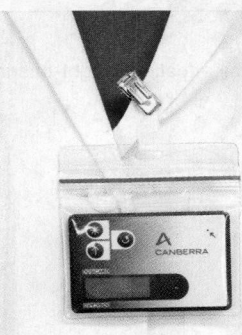

STEP 8a   Radiation dosimeter. (*Courtesy Canberra Industries.*)

SKILL 13-1 Fall Prevention in a Health Care Facility

NSO *Safety Module / Lessons 1 and 2*

Falls are the most common type of inpatient accident. Approximately 30% of hospital patient falls result in physical injury, and most are multifactorial in cause (Krauss and others, 2005). In a study of falls occurring within an acute care hospital, Krauss and others found that gait or lower extremity problems, urinary/stool frequency or incontinence, and use of certain medications (e.g., sedatives/hypnotics or diabetes medications) increased the likelihood of patient falls. The circumstances of patient falls have patterns, many occurring unassisted while patients ambulate, get out of bed, or are toileting. In addition, having side rails raised increases the occurrence of falling because patients try to climb over the rails to reach a chair or bathroom, and often fall further as a result (U.S. Department of Veterans Affairs, 2004).

The Joint Commission currently recommends that health care organizations have a formal fall reduction program, which includes an evaluation of the effectiveness of the program (TJC, 2007c). There is evidence to show that hospital-based fall-prevention programs that focus on a multifactorial approach, reduce fall rates (CDC, 2006). Effective fall-prevention programs include a risk assessment, medication reviews with necessary modifications, use of assistive devices, exercise and strength training, and education for home safety (CDC, 2006). A recent study shows that hourly nurse rounds are an effective strategy to reduce falls (Meade and others, 2006). This strategy makes sense because research has also shown that when there is a reduction in total nursing care hours (fewer total staff), there is an increase in falls (Potter and others, 2003). Combining hourly rounds with activities such as regular toileting and assessing patients' comfort needs manages those factors that often prompt patients to get out of bed without assistance.

Fall risk assessment is critical to successful fall prevention. Frail older adults are especially at risk because of impaired strength, mobility, balance, and endurance. They are twice as likely to fall as healthier persons of the same age (CDC, 2007). However, patients of all ages are at risk for falling when they receive care in a health care facility. In the hospital setting there are a variety of fall risk factor screening tools. Because there are multiple known risk factors for falls, no single assessment tool is sensitive and specific to analyze fall risk (Registered Nurses' Association of Ontario [RNAO], 2002). The Risk Assessment Tool for Falls (Box 13-1) includes a patient's physical and mental status, medications, and devices used to ambulate to determine the degree of fall risk. Choose measures based on a patient's risk score, medical condition, and the environment.

Nurses are responsible for making a patient's bedside safe. In Fig. 13-1 there are a variety of environmental interventions for patient safety. The call light/bed control system allows patients to adjust a bed's position and to signal caregivers when they need assistance. Explain how to operate the system to patients and family, and place the device within a patient's reach, whether in a bed or chair (Fig. 13-2). A full set of raised side rails (two to a bed or four to a bed) is a physical restraint. Traditionally, health care providers used side rails for patient protection. However, recent research by Krauss and others (2005) shows that having side rails raised increases the occurrence of falls. There have also been cases of patients becoming entrapped or entangled in side rails (Powell-Cope and others, 2005). Side rails consist of one full-length rail per side or one or more shorter rails per side. A rail is set at a fixed height or is adjustable. Depending on a bed's design or age, the position of

---

BOX 13-1 | Risk for Falls Assessment Tools

Tool 1: Risk Assessment Tool for Falls
Directions: Place a check mark in front of elements that apply to your patient. The decision of whether a patient is at risk for falls is based on your nursing judgment. Guideline: A patient who has a check mark in front of an element with an asterisk (*) or four or more of the other elements would be identified as at risk for falls.

General Data
- Age over 60
- History of falls before admission*
- Postoperative/admitted for surgery
- Smoker

Physical Condition
- Dizziness/imbalance
- Unsteady gait
- Diseases/other problems affecting weight-bearing joints
- Weakness
- Paresis
- Seizure disorder
- Impairment of vision
- Impairment of hearing
- Diarrhea
- Urinary frequency

Mental Status
- Confusion/disorientation*
- Impaired memory or judgment
- Inability to understand or follow directions

Medications
- Diuretics or diuretic effects
- Hypotensive or central nervous system suppressants (e.g., narcotic, sedative, psychotropic, hypnotic, tranquilizer, antihypertensive, antidepressant)
- Medication that increases gastrointestinal motility (e.g., laxative, enema)

Ambulatory Devices Used
- Cane
- Crutches
- Walker
- Wheelchair
- Geriatric (Geri) chair
- Braces

Tool 2: Reassessment Is Safe "Kare" (Risk) Tool
Directions: Place a check mark in front of any element that applies to your patient. A patient who has a check mark in front of any of the first four elements would be identified as at risk for falls. In addition, when a high-risk patient has a check mark in front of the element "Use of a wheelchair," the patient is considered to be at greater risk for falls.
- Unsteady gait/dizziness/imbalance
- Impaired memory or judgment
- Weakness
- History of falls
- Use of a wheelchair

Modified from Brians LK and others: The development of the RISK tool for fall prevention, *Rehabil Nurs* 16(2):67, 1991.

mattresses, side rails and head boards can increase or create gaps or spaces where patients can become entrapped. For example, when there is a space or gap left between a side rail and mattress edge, a patient's head, neck, or chest can become entrapped when the patient tries to exit the bed, often leading to fatal injuries. Raising only one of two, or three of four, side rails gives patients room to exit a bed safely and move around within the bed. It is also important to keep a bed in low position with wheels locked when stationary. Finally, always check a bed for structural risks (e.g., wobbly rails, damaged rails, or soft mattresses) (U.S. Food and Drug Administration [FDA], 2006).

Electronic bed and chair alarms are available to warn nursing staff when a patient who needs assistance tries to leave the bed or chair on his or her own. One example is pressure-sensitive strips placed beneath a patient and under the buttocks on a bed or chair. As a patient rises off the sensor, an alarm sounds to alert staff.

Another device is a tab alarm that connects to a patient in a chair or bed by a wire tether. When a patient moves beyond the length of the tether, the alarm sounds. An Ambularm is another device that is worn on the leg. It signals when the leg is in a dependent position, such as over a side rail or on the floor. Additional devices to use at a patient's bedside are a bedside commode, a nonskid floor mat, an overhead trapeze, and a movable hand rail (hemi-walker) (see Fig. 13-1). All of these devices help patients either move in bed or transfer out of bed more safely.

An alternative to a physical restraint is the Posey Bed Canopy System (Fig. 13-3). The canopy is a bed enclosure that allows a patient freedom of movement within a protected environment. The enclosure bed is designed for use with side rails down to reduce risk for entrapment. It allows freedom of movement, thus reducing the side effects caused by physical restraints. The bed works particularly well with the cognitively impaired.

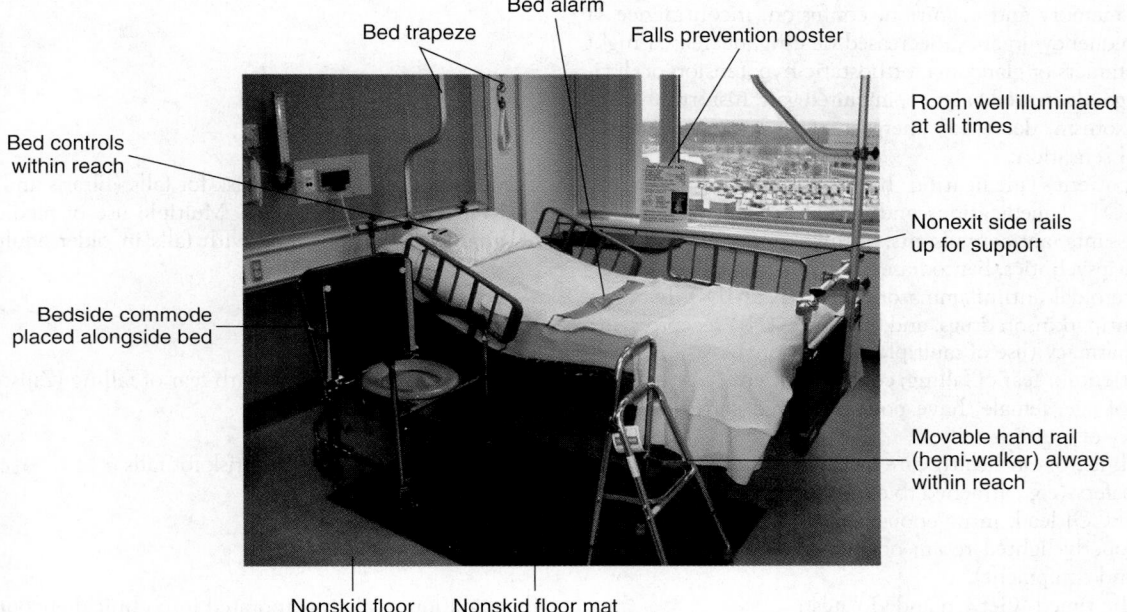

Fig. 13-1   Making the hospital patient's environment safe. (*From U.S. Department of Veterans Affairs, National Center for Patient Safety: 2004 Falls toolkit, falls notebook interventions, 2004, http://www.patientsafety.gov/Safetytopics/fallstoolkit/index.html, accessed June 25, 2007.*)

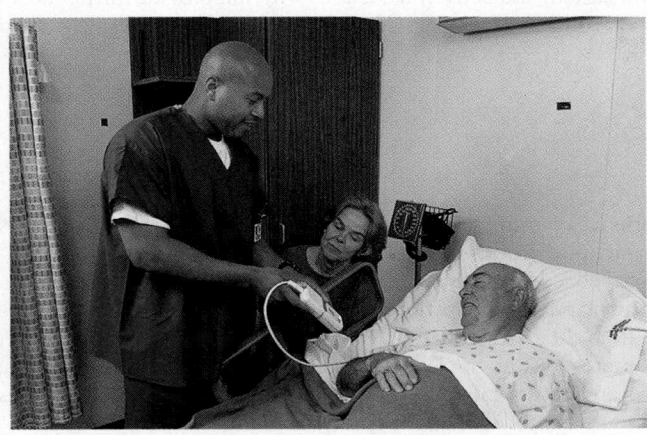

Fig. 13-2   Nurse demonstrates use of call light to a patient.

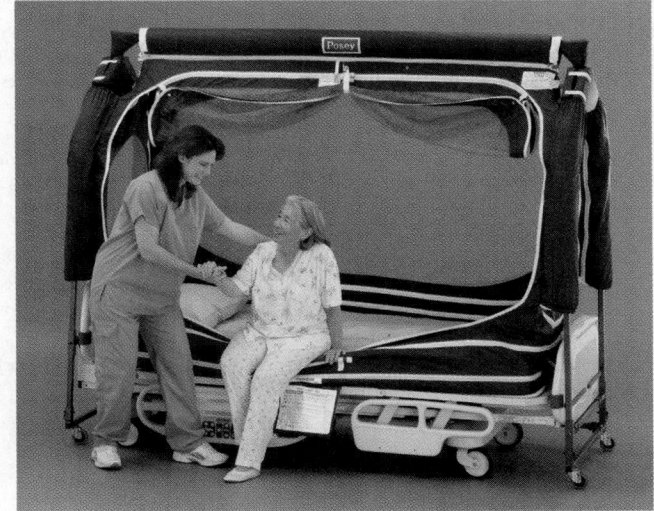

Fig. 13-3   An enclosure bed system. (*Courtesy J.T. Posey Co., Arcadia, Calif.*)

Delegation Considerations

The skill of assessment of a patient's risk for falling cannot be delegated to NAP. However, the skills necessary to prevent falls can be delegated. The nurse directs the NAP by:

- Explaining a patient's mobility limitations and specific measures needed to minimize risks.
- Explaining patient behaviors (e.g., disorientation, wandering, anxiety) that are precursors to falls and that should be reported immediately.

Equipment

- ❑ A risk assessment tool for falls
- ❑ Hospital bed with side rails
- ❑ Wedge cushion
- ❑ Call light
- ❑ Seat belt
- ❑ Gait belt
- ❑ Wheelchair

STEP	RATIONALE

ASSESSMENT

STEP	RATIONALE
1 Assess patient's motor, sensory, balance, and cognitive status (see Chapter 6), including ability to follow directions and cooperate. Focus on fall risks including: age greater than 65 years, impaired memory and cognition, confusion, incontinence or urinary frequency/urgency, decreased hearing, decreased night vision, cataracts or glaucoma, orthostatic hypotension or dizziness/vertigo, decreased balance, impaired gait, history of stroke or parkinsonism, decreased energy or fatigue, and decreased peripheral sensation.	Certain physiological factors predispose patients to fall.
2 Review patient's medication history (including over-the-counter [OTC] medications and herbal products) for use of antidepressants, anticonvulsants, antihypertensives, antihistamines, antipsychotics, benzodiazepines, corticosteroids, diuretics, nonsteroidal antiinflammatory drugs (NSAIDs), hypoglycemics, antiparkinson drugs, and histamine (H_2) receptors and for polypharmacy (use of multiple medications).	Some medications increase risk for falls (Elzaris and others, 2003; Krauss and others, 2005). Multiple use of medications (polypharmacy) is associated with falls in older adults (McCarter-Bayer and others, 2005).
3 Assess patient for fear of falling; consider patients who are over 80 years of age, female, have poor perceived general health, and history of multiple falls.	Factors shown to correlate with fear of falling (Zijlstra and others, 2007b).
4 Assess risk factors in health care facility that pose a threat to patient's safety (e.g., attached to equipment such as electrocardiogram [ECG] lead, intravenous [IV] tubing, or oxygen tubing; improperly lighted room; obstructed walkway; clutter of supplies and equipment).	Environmental barriers pose risk for falls.
5 Perform the timed "Get Up and Go" test: • Have patient rise from sitting position without using arms for support. • Instruct patient to walk 10 feet (3 m), turn around, and walk back to the chair. • Have patient return to chair and sit down without using arms for support. Look for unsteadiness in patient's gait.	Examination easily incorporated into clinical encounters with patient is useful in screening for altered balance and gait (Tinetti, 2003). Patient's taking less than 20 seconds to complete test is adequate for independent mobility. Patient who takes longer than 30 seconds is dependent and at risk for fall.
6 Determine if patient has had a history of falls (TJC, 2007a) or other injuries within the home. Be specific, and follow the acronym SPLATT (Meiner and Lueckenotte, 2006): • **S**ymptoms at time of fall • **P**revious fall • **L**ocation of fall • **A**ctivity at time of fall • **T**ime of fall • **T**rauma post fall	Key symptoms are often helpful in identifying cause for fall. Onset, location, and activity associated with fall provide further details on causative factors and how to prevent future falls.
7 Determine what patient knows about risks for falling and steps he or she takes to prevent falls.	Patient's own knowledge of risks influences ability to take necessary precautions in reducing falls.
8 After assessment apply a color-coded wristband (e.g., yellow) for patients at risk for falling.	Color-coded bands are easily recognizable. A national effort aimed at standardizing patient wristband colors has gained support from 20 states and the American Hospital Association. Eight States within the United States are implementing wristband standards for falls, allergy warning, and do not resuscitate (Missouri Center for Patient Safety, 2007).

STEP	RATIONALE

NURSING DIAGNOSES

- Activity intolerance
- Deficient knowledge related to safety precautions
- Disturbed sensory perception

- Impaired memory
- Impaired physical mobility
- Impaired transfer ability
- Impaired urinary elimination

- Impaired walking
- Risk for falls
- Risk for injury

Individualize related factors based on patient's condition or needs.

PLANNING

STEP	RATIONALE
1 Expected outcomes following completion of procedure:	
• Patient's environment is free of hazards.	Environmental hazards predispose patient to potential injury.
• Patient or family member is able to identify safety risks.	Patient awareness of risks promotes cooperation and an understanding of treatment plan.
• Patient does not suffer a fall or injury.	Fall precautions are successful in preventing a fall.

IMPLEMENTATION

STEP	RATIONALE
1 Introduce yourself to patient, including both name and title or role.	Reduces patient uncertainty.
2 Identify patient by checking armband and having patient state name, if possible. Use two patient identifiers.	Prevents patient care errors.
3 Explain the plan of care.	Promotes patient cooperation.
4 Gather equipment, and perform hand hygiene.	Promotes organization and reduces transmission of microorganisms.
5 Provide privacy. Assign patient to bed that allows the patient to exit toward his or her stronger side. Position and drape patient as needed.	Maintains patient's self-esteem. Enhances patient's ability to move in bed and transfer out of bed.
6 Adjust bed to low position with wheels locked.	Allows for proper body mechanics. Height of bed allows ambulatory patient to easily get in and out of bed safely.
7 Orient patient to call light/bed control system:	
a Provide patient's hearing aid and glasses.	Enables patient to remain alert to conditions in environment.
b Explain and demonstrate how to turn call light/intercom system on and off at bedside and in bathroom.	Knowledge of location and use of call light is essential to patient safety.

Critical Decision Point *Observe patient in a return demonstration to ensure learning has taken place.*

STEP	RATIONALE
c Explain best times for patient/family to use call/bell/intercom (e.g., to get out of bed, go to bathroom, report pain).	Increases likelihood of nurse being able to respond before patient tries to get out of bed unassisted.
d Consistently secure call light/bed control system to an accessible location within patient's reach.	Ensures patient is able to reach device immediately when needed.
8 Adjust side rails (see Fig. 13-1):	
a Check agency policies regarding side rail use.	Side rails are a restraint device if they immobilize or reduce the ability of a patient to move his or her arms, legs, body, or head freely (Centers for Medicaid and Medicare Services [CMS], 2007).
b Explain to patient and family the main reason for using side rails: moving and turning self in bed.	Promotes patient and family cooperation.
c Keep one side rail up in a two-rail system, and keep three of four rails up (one lower rail down) in a four-rail system, with bed in low position and wheels locked when you are not administering patient care.	Allows patient to maneuver and get out of bed safely.

Critical Decision Point *Assess for excessive gaps and openings between bed frame and mattress. Use side rail netting or protective padding to prevent mattress from being pushed to one side.*

STEP	RATIONALE
9 Provide environmental interventions:	
a Place nonslip padded floor mat on exit side of bed.	Prevents falls from slipping on floor.
b Have assistive devices (e.g., walking aids, bedside commodes) located on exit side of bed.	Provides added support when transferring out of bed. Commode eliminates need to get up to walk to bathroom.
c Have patient's bedside table, water, and personal care items (e.g., eyeglasses, dentures, telephone) within easy reach.	Prevents patient from reaching and allows patient to perform self-care activities safely.

STEP	RATIONALE
10 Explain to patient that you will conduct hourly rounds to re-assess for fall risks, provide toileting needs, and attend to symptom management.	Use of hourly rounds has been shown to reduce incidence of falls (Meade and others, 2006).
11 Provide clear instructions to patient and family regarding any mobility restrictions, ambulation and transfer techniques (see Chapter 9).	Promotes patient independence and understanding of treatment plan.
12 When ambulating a patient, have patient wear a gait belt, and walk along patient's strong side (see Chapter 10).	Gait belt gives nurse a secure hold on patient during ambulation.
13 Explain to patient specific safety measures to prevent falls (e.g., wear well-fitting, flat footwear with nonskid soles; dangle feet for a few minutes before standing; walk slowly; ask for help if dizzy or weak).	Promotes patient understanding and cooperation. Dangling provides adjustment to orthostatic hypotension, allowing blood pressure to stabilize before ambulating (see Chapter 10).
14 Offer a hip protector to patients who are fearful of falling.	Hip protectors reduce fear of falling in community-living older adults (Zijlstra and others, 2007a).
15 Make sure ambulatory patient's pathway to bathroom facilities is clear.	Eliminates potential hazards and promotes patient independence.
16 Provide adequate, nonglare lighting throughout room. Have night-light in room.	Reduces likelihood of bumping into or falling over objects. Glare is a major problem for older adults. Ensures room is illuminated at all times.
17 Remove unnecessary objects or equipment from room.	Eliminates potential hazards when patient gets out of bed or ambulates.
18 Meet with physical therapist about the possibility of gait training and muscle-strengthening exercise.	Gait and exercise training are single interventions that are effective among older adults at risk for falling (Tinetti, 2003).
19 Discuss with physician or primary care provider the possibility of adjusting the number of medications patient receives to reduce side effects and interactions.	You can reduce the number of medications a patient receives safely by balancing the benefits of the medications and risk for adverse events (Tinetti, 2003).
20 Safe transport using a wheelchair:	
a During transfer, position wheelchair on same side of bed as patient's strong or unaffected side (see Chapter 9).	Facilitates patient's ability to assist in transfer to chair.
b Place wedge cushion in chair (see illustration).	Wedge cushion prevents slipping out of chair.

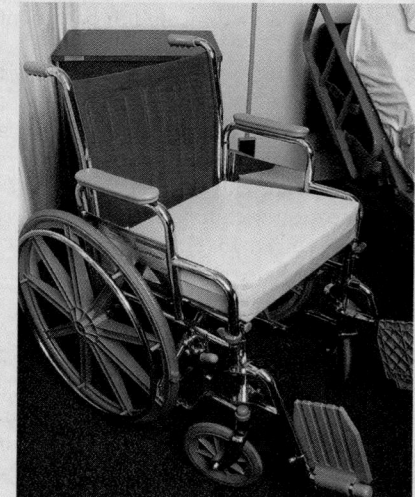

STEP 20b   Wheelchair with foot plates raised and wedge cushion in place.

STEP	RATIONALE
c Securely lock brakes on both wheels when transferring patient into or out of wheelchair.	Keeps chair steady and secure.
d Raise foot plates before transfer (see illustration for Step b); lower foot plates, placing patients feet on them after patient is seated.	Prevents tripping over foot plate.
e Have patient sit with buttocks well back in seat. *Option:* Apply a quick-release seat belt.	Prevents patient from sliding out of chair.

STEP	RATIONALE

f Back wheelchair into and out of elevator or door, leading with large rear wheels first.

Prevents smaller front wheels from catching in the crack between elevator and floor, causing chair to tip.

EVALUATION

1 Conduct hourly rounds.

Monitors patient for ongoing risks for falling.

2 Observe patient's immediate environment for presence of hazards.

Ensures there are no obstacles or barriers to patient's freedom of movement.

3 Evaluate patient's ability to use assistive devices.

Determines if instruction or clarification needed.

4 Ask patient or family member to identify safety risks.

Determines level of patient learning.

5 Reassess motor, sensory, and cognitive status. Determine that no falls or injuries occur.

Determines how effective nursing interventions were in reducing actual or potential threats to patient's safety.

Unexpected Outcomes

1 Patient is unable to identify safety risks.

2 Patient starts to fall while ambulating with a caregiver.

Related Interventions

• Reinforce identified risks with patient, or review needed safety measures with family.

• Put both arms around patient's waist or grasp gait belt.
• Stand with feet apart to provide broad base of support.
• Extend one leg, and let patient slide against it to the floor (Fig. 13-4).
• Bend knees and lower body as patient slides to floor (Fig. 13-5).

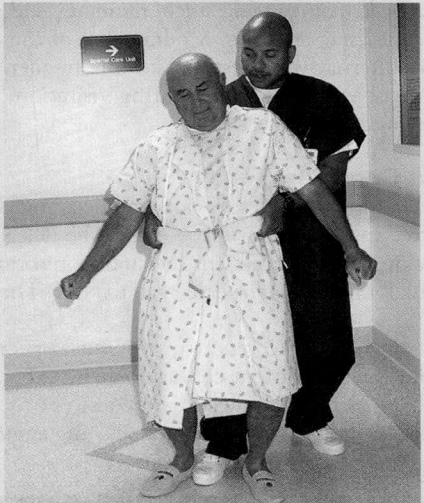

Fig. 13-4   Stand with feet apart to provide broad base of support; extend one leg for patient to slide against to the floor.

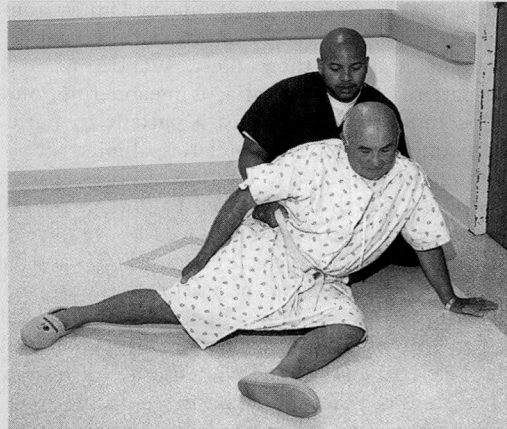

Fig. 13-5   Bend knees and lower body as patient slides to floor.

3 Patient found after suffering a fall.

• Call for assistance.
• Assess patient for injury, and stay with patient until assistance arrives.
• Notify physician.
• Follow institution's incident/occurrence reporting policy.
• Evaluate patient and environment; determine whether fall could have been prevented.
• Reinforce identified risks with patient and measures recommended to prevent recurrent fall.

Recording and Reporting

• Record risk assessment findings and specific interventions (including instructions) risk assessment tool, nurses' notes, or care plan.
• Report to health care personnel specific risks to patient's safety and measures taken to minimize risks.
• If patient suffers a fall, inform physician. Document what occurred, including description of fall as given by patient or witness. Be sure to include baseline assessment, any injuries noted,

tests or treatments given, follow-up care, and additional safety precautions taken after fall.

Teaching Considerations

• Make available to patients and families the Centers for Disease Control and Prevention's (CDC's) *Tool Kit to Prevent Senior Falls*. It contains fact sheets, health education materials, and a home assessment checklist. Materials are research based and sponsored by the CDC. Information is available at http://www.cdc.gov/ncipc/pub-res/toolkit/.

- Encourage patients to have yearly vision and hearing examinations. Adaptive devices, such as a hearing aid or glasses, are sometimes necessary or need modification.
- Emphasize to patient the need to always look ahead when ambulating and to use good posture.
- Instruct patients on how to use assistive devices, and ensure they understand.

Pediatric Considerations

- Children's activity levels and curiosity increase risk for falls. Eliminate places for the child to climb. Consider use of crib hoods.
- Keep side rails of hospital beds down to allow toddlers and pre-schoolers easy exit without feeling the need to crawl over the rails (Hockenberry and Wilson, 2007).
- When caring for infants, keep a hand on a child when you turn away from the bedside, even for a second.

Gerontological Considerations

- Fear of falling and avoidance of activities due to fear of falling are highly prevalent in older adults, especially those 80 years of age and older (Zijlstra and others, 2007b).
- Increasing lower body strength and improving dynamic balance through regular physical activity will reduce risk for falling. Tai chi is one type of exercise program that has been effective (Greenspan and others, 2007; Maciaszek and others, 2007).

Home Care Considerations

- See Chapter 41.

Long-Term Care Considerations

- Patients who wander from a facility are at risk for injury. Use specific interventions such as electronic wandering devices to reduce this risk (see Chapter 41).

SKILL 13-2   Designing a Restraint-Free Environment

 Basic / Restraints and Alternatives / Using Restraint Alternatives

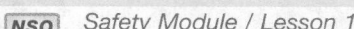

NSO   *Safety Module / Lesson 1*

Patients who are at risk for falling, self-inflected injury from pulling out tubes or removing dressings, or wandering, present special challenges in maintaining their safety. Wandering, a common problem in patients with dementia, is meandering, aimless, or repetitive locomotion that exposes a patient to harm and is frequently incongruent with boundaries, limits, or obstacles (NANDA International, 2007). The use of physical restraints is one safety strategy that has been used to protect patients from injury. However, efforts have been in place for several years by the Centers for Medicare and Medicaid Services (2007) and The Joint Commission (2007b) to reduce the use of restraints and to use them only with extreme caution. Physical restraints are the last resort and used only when reasonable alternatives have failed.

Because of the risks associated with the use of restraints (see Skill 13-3), current legislation emphasizes reducing their use. A restraint-free environment is the first goal of care for all patients.

There are many alternatives to the use of restraints, and you should try all of them before using restraints. Modification of the environment is an effective alternative to restraints. More frequent observation of patients, involvement of family during visitation, and frequent reorientation are helpful measures.

Delegation Considerations

The skill of assessing patient behaviors and deciding about the type of restraint-free interventions to use cannot be delegated to NAP. However, making the environment safe and monitoring patient behaviors for risk for injury can be delegated to NAP. The nurse directs the NAP by:

- Instructing personnel to report to the nurse specific behaviors and actions, such as patient confusion, getting out of bed unassisted, pulling at tubes, and combativeness.
- Advising NAP on measures to use to make the environment safe.

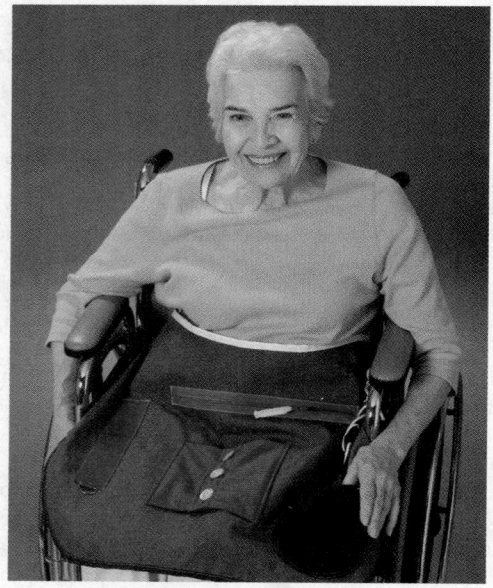

Fig. 13-6   Activity apron. (*Courtesy Posey Company, Arcadia, Calif.*)

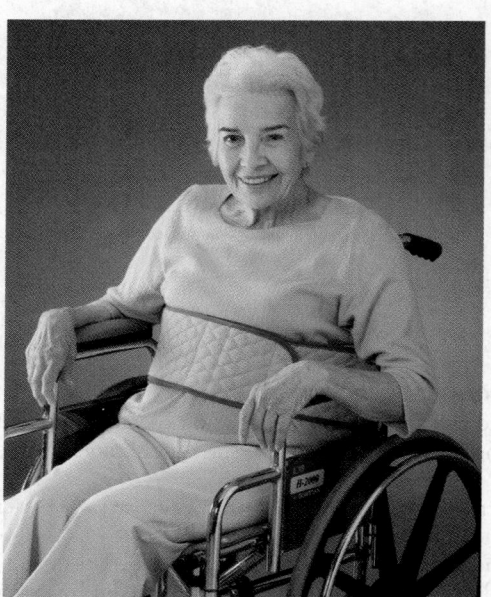

Fig. 13-7   Wrap-around belt. (*Courtesy Posey Company, Arcadia, Calif.*)

STEP	RATIONALE

Equipment

- ❑ Visual or auditory stimuli (e.g., calendar, clock, radio, television, pictures)
- ❑ Diversional activities (e.g., puzzle, game, music, stuffed animal) or activity apron (Fig. 13-6)
- ❑ Wedge cushion
- ❑ Wrap-around belt (Fig. 13-7)
- ❑ Ambularm or pressure-sensitive bed or chair alarm

ASSESSMENT

1 Assess patient's physical and mental status, including orientation; level of consciousness; ability to understand, remember, and follow directions; level of combativeness; balance; gait; vision; hearing; bowel/bladder routine; level of pain; laboratory values; and presence of orthostatic hypotension.	Accurate assessment identifies safety risks and the physiological causes for behaviors that increase risks. Ensures proper selection of intervention.
2 Review prescribed medications (e.g., sedatives, hypnotics, analgesics, diuretics) for interactions and untoward effects.	Medication interactions or side effects often contribute to falling or altered mental status.
3 Assess patient's knowledge of condition and treatment.	Knowledge of treatment protocols and rationales will increase patient's cooperation.
4 For patients who wander, assess for cognitive decline (Mini-Mental State Examination [MMSE], see Chapter 6) and wandering patterns (e.g., continuous movement from place to place, inability to locate significant landmarks in a familiar setting, haphazard locomotion) (Algase Wandering Scale) (Algase and others, 2001, 2004). Also assess for boredom, looking for something that is "lost," overstimulation.	Confirms risk for wandering. Determines cause and nature of wandering, which will lead to effective intervention selection.

NURSING DIAGNOSES

- Deficient knowledge regarding need for restricted activity
- Risk for falls
- Risk for injury
- Risk for trauma
- Wandering

Individualize related factors based on patient's condition or needs.

PLANNING

1 Expected outcomes following completion of procedure.	
• Patient will be injury free and/or will not inflict injury on others while in a restraint-free environment.	Restraints and/or alternatives are successful in preventing injury.

IMPLEMENTATION

1 Orient patient and family to surroundings, introduce to staff, and explain all treatments and procedures. Be sure patient is able to read your name badge.	Promotes patient understanding and cooperation.
2 Provide the same caregivers to the extent possible. Encourage family and friends to stay with patient. Companions are often helpful. In some institutions, volunteers are effective companions. Prevent patient from being alone as much as possible.	Increases familiarity with individuals in patient's environment, decreasing anxiety and restlessness.
3 Place patient in a room that is easily accessible to caregivers, close to nurses' station.	Allows for frequent observation to reduce falls in high-risk patients (U.S. Department of Veterans Affairs, 2004).
4 Be sure patient has glasses, hearing aid, or other sensory-aid devices on and functioning.	Improves patient's level of orientation to environment.
5 Provide visual and auditory stimuli meaningful to patient (e.g., clock, calendar, radio [with patient's choice of music], television, and family pictures).	Orients patient to day, time, and physical surroundings. Nurse must individualize stimuli for this to be effective.
6 Meet patient's basic needs (e.g., toileting, relief of pain, relief of hunger) as quickly as possible.	Basic needs provided in a timely fashion decreases patient discomfort, anxiety, and restlessness.

Critical Decision Point   *Getting out of bed for toileting purposes is one of the most common events leading to a patient's fall, especially during evening or night hours, when rooms are often dark.*

STEP	RATIONALE

7 Provide scheduled ambulation, chair activity, and toileting (e.g., ask patient every hour if needing to void). Organize treatments so patient has long uninterrupted periods throughout the day.

Regular opportunity to void avoids risk for patient trying to reach bathroom alone. Provides for sleep and rest periods. Constant activity overstimulates patients.

8 Position IV catheters, urinary catheters, and tubes/drains out of patient view. Use camouflage by wrapping IV site with bandage or stockinette. Place undergarments on patient with urinary catheter, or cover abdominal feeding tubes/drains with loose abdominal binder.

Maintains medical treatment and reduces patient access to tubes/lines.

9 Use stress reduction techniques, such as back rub, massage, and guided imagery (see Chapter 15).

Reduced stress allows patient's energy to be channeled more appropriately.

10 Use diversional activities such as puzzles, games, books, pet therapy, folding towels, drawing/coloring, or an object to hold. Place an activity apron over patient's lap. Be sure it is an activity in which patient has interest. Involve a family member in the activity.

Meaningful diversional activities provide distraction, help to reduce boredom, and provide tactile stimulation. Minimize occurrences of wandering. Activity apron offers color and texture variations and buttons for the patient to manipulate, all of which stimulates the patient's interest.

11 Position patient on a wedge cushion, and apply a wrap-around belt.

The wedge cushion prevents slipping in chair and makes it difficult for patient to get out of chair without assistance. The wrap-around belt allows patient to lift flap for self-release.

12 Use a pressure-sensitive bed or chair pad with alarms or an Ambularm. To apply an Ambularm monitor:

Alarms alert staff to patient who is standing or rising without assistance.

   a Explain use of device.

   b Measure patient's thigh circumference just above knee to determine appropriate size. Leg circumference less than 18 inches requires regular size; 18 inches or greater requires large size

Band that is too loose will slip off; one that is too tight will irritate skin or interfere with circulation.

   c Test battery and alarm by touching snaps to corresponding snaps on leg band.

   d Apply leg band just above knee, and snap battery securely in place (see illustration).

   e Instruct patient that alarm will sound unless he or she keeps leg in horizontal position (see illustration).

   f Deactivate alarm to ambulate patient; unsnap device from leg band.

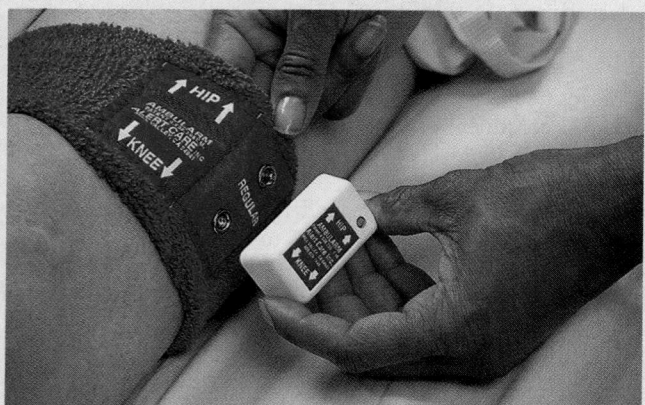

STEP 12d Snap battery in place to activate alarm. (*Courtesy Alert Care, Tiburon, Calif.*)

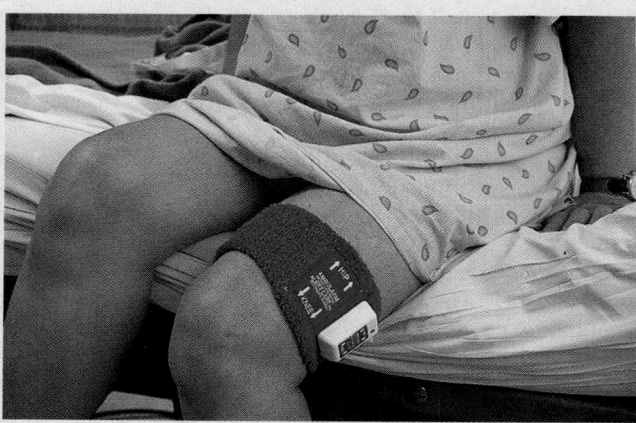

STEP 12e Audio alarm will sound when patient approaches a near-vertical position when getting out of bed. (*Courtesy Alert Care, Tiburon, Calif.*)

STEP	RATIONALE
13 Consult with physical therapy, speech therapy, and occupational therapy for activities that provide stimulation and exercise.	Involvement in meaningful and purposeful activities reduces tendency to wander. Exercise improves balance and coordination.
14 Eliminate invasive treatments (e.g., tube feedings, blood sampling) as soon as possible.	Stimuli increase patients' restlessness
15 For patients who wander, remove items from view that are used while walking (e.g., shoes, cane, keys).	Removes stimuli that prompt the person to wander.

EVALUATION

1 Observe patient for any injuries.	Patient should be injury free.
2 Observe patient's behavior toward staff, visitors, and other patients.	Ensures that patient's behavior does not cause injury to others.
3 Determine need for continuation of invasive treatments and whether you can substitute less invasive treatment.	Eliminates cause and reason for restraint.

Unexpected Outcomes

1 Patient displays behaviors that increase risk for injury to self or others.

2 Patient sustains an injury or is out of control, placing others at risk for injury.

Related Interventions

- Review episodes for a pattern (e.g., activity, time of day) that indicates alternatives that would eliminate behavior.
- Discuss with all caregivers alternative interventions.
- Notify health care provider, and complete an incident or occurrence report according to agency policy.
- Identify alternative measures for safety or behavioral control
- As a last resort, apply physical restraint (see Skill 13-3)

Recording and Reporting

- Record restraint alternatives attempted, patient behaviors, and interventions to mediate these behaviors in nurses' notes and/or care plan.

Teaching Considerations

- Teach family members ways to involve patient in their visits, keeping the patient appropriately stimulated.
- Teach the family how to adapt the home environment to minimize patient wandering (see Chapter 42).

Gerontological Considerations

- Keep older adults active and moving about to increase endurance and function.

Home Care Considerations

- Patients at risk for self-injury or violence to others need intensive supervision. Family and/or caregiver need to recognize this and be able to provide it.
- Have family members set up area in the home where it is safe for an older adult to wander.

Long-Term Care Considerations

- Develop a buddy system for patients with individuals who are able to provide companionship for varying periods. This increases socialization, protects the wanderer, and enhances ego of the "buddy" (Ebersole and others, 2008).
- Reminisce with patient to help maintain orientation.

SKILL 13-3 Applying Physical Restraints

 Basic / Restraints and Alternatives / Applying Restraints

NSO *Safety Module / Lesson 2*

A restraint is any manual method, physical or mechanical device, material, or equipment that immobilizes or reduces the ability of a patient to move his or her arms, legs, body, or head freely (CMS, 2007). In a study of 40 U.S. hospitals, restraints were most commonly used to prevent the disruption of therapy, such as pulling out IV tubes or removing urinary catheters (Minnick and others, 2007). Recently the Centers for Medicaid and Medicare Services (2007) released revisions to the Medicare conditions of participation, outlining standards for the safe use of restraints in hospitals. The agency also defines patients' rights and choices regarding restraints. The Centers for Medicaid and Medicare Services (2007) requires that a restraint be used only under the following circumstances: (1) to ensure the immediate physical safety of the patient, a staff member, or others; (2) when less restrictive interventions have been ineffective; (3) in accordance with a written modification to the patient's plan of care; (4) when it is the least restrictive intervention that will be effective to protect the patient, staff member, or others from harm; (5) in accordance with safe and appropriate restraint techniques as determined by a hospital's policies; and (6) it is discontinued at the earliest possible time.

Restraints are not a solution for a patient problem; they are a temporary means to control behavior. Restraints do not necessarily prevent falls. Research has shown that patients suffer fewer injuries if left unrestrained (Park and Tang, 2007). The use of mechanical or physical restraints needs to be part of a patient's prescribed medical treatment. A physician's time-limited order is necessary, and you must use the appropriate restraint and apply it correctly. The patient's or family member's informed consent is necessary in the long-term care setting. You need to try all less restrictive interventions first. Consult with occupational and physical therapists for activity interventions, and provide supporting documentation. For example, a nurse caring for a patient who repeatedly tries to pull out an IV line must try less restrictive measures first, such as camouflage or diversional activity. If the alternatives fail, the nurse then considers use of a restraint to prevent injury. In addition, the nurse takes measures to prevent the hazards of immobility and other complications.

The use of restraints is associated with several serious complications, including pressure ulcers, hypostatic pneumonia, constipation, incontinence, and death. The Food and Drug Administration (FDA), which regulates restraints as medical devices and requires manufacturers to label them "prescription only," estimates that hundreds of restraint-related injuries occur each year. Most patient deaths from use of restraints have resulted from strangulation from a vest or jacket restraint. Numerous institutions have stopped using vest restraints. For these reasons this text will not describe the use of vest restraints.

Delegation Considerations

The skill of assessment of patient's behavior, level of orientation, need for restraints, appropriate type to use, and the assessments while restraint is in place cannot be delegated to NAP. However, restraint application and supportive care can be delegated to NAP. The nurse directs NAP by:

- Reviewing correct placement of the restraint.
- Reviewing when and how to change patient's position.
- Instructing NAP to notify nurse if there is a change in skin integrity, circulation of extremities, or patient's breathing.
- Instructing to provide range of motion (ROM), nutrition and hydration, skin care, toileting, and opportunities for socialization.

Equipment

- ☐ Proper restraint
- ☐ Padding (if needed)

STEP	RATIONALE
ASSESSMENT	
1 Assess patient's behavior, such as confusion; disorientation; agitation; restlessness; combativeness; repeated removal of tubing, dressings, or other therapeutic devices; and inability to follow directions.	If patient's behavior continues despite treatment or restraint alternatives, use of restraint will be indicated.
2 Review agency policies regarding restraints. Check physician's order for purpose, type, location, and time or duration of restraint. Determine if signed consent for use of restraint is necessary.	A physician or licensed independent practitioner who is responsible for the care of the patient orders restraints. The physician must be authorized to order restraints by the hospital's policy. You need to consult the attending physician as soon as possible if the attending physician did not write the original order. Each original restraint order and renewal is limited to 4 hours for adults, 2 hours for children ages 9 through 17, and 1 hour for children under age 9 (CMS, 2007). The least restrictive type of restraint should be ordered. Original orders may be renewed up to a maximum of 24 hours (CMS, 2007).

Critical Decision Point   *If a nurse or qualified health practitioner (see hospital policy) restrains a patient in an emergency situation because of violent or aggressive behavior that presents an immediate danger, a face-to-face physician assessment within 1 hour is necessary (TJC, 2007a).*

3 Review manufacturer's instructions for restraint application before entering patient's room. Determine the most appropriate size restraint.	Nurse needs to be familiar with all devices used for patient care and protection. Incorrect application of restraint device will possibly result in patient injury or death.

STEP	RATIONALE

4 Inspect area where restraint is to be placed. Note if there is any nearby tubing or devices. Assess condition of skin, sensation, adequacy of circulation, and range of joint motion.

Restraints sometimes compress and interfere with functioning of devices or tubes. Assessment provides baseline to monitor patient's response to restraint.

NURSING DIAGNOSES

- Anxiety
- Impaired physical mobility
- Risk for impaired skin integrity

- Risk for injury
- Risk for peripheral neurovascular dysfunction

- Risk for self-directed or other-directed violence
- Risk for situational low self-esteem

Individualize related factors based on patient's condition or needs.

PLANNING

1 Expected outcomes following completion of procedure:
- Patient will maintain intact skin integrity, pulses, temperature, color, and sensation of restrained body part.
- Patient will be free from injury.
- Patient's therapy (e.g., IV tube, catheters) is uninterrupted.

- Patient's self-esteem and dignity are maintained.

Restraints applied and monitored correctly.

Restraints removed in timely manner.
Disruption of therapy causes patient injury, pain, or discomfort and increases risk for infection.
Physical restraints have a detrimental effect on psychosocial well-being of patient.

IMPLEMENTATION

1 Gather equipment, and perform hand hygiene.
2 Approach patient in a calm, confident manner. Check patient's identification using two identifiers. Explain what you plan to do.

3 Provide privacy. Be sure patient is comfortable and in correct anatomical position.
4 Adjust bed to proper height, and lower side rail on side of patient contact.
5 Pad skin and bony prominences (as necessary) that will be under the restraint.

6 Apply proper-size restraint:
NOTE: Refer to manufacturer's directions.
  a *Belt restraint:* Have patient in a sitting position. Apply belt over clothes, gown, or pajamas. Make sure you place restraint at the waist, not the chest or abdomen. Remove wrinkles or creases in clothing. Bring ties through slots in belt. Help patient lie down if in bed. Avoid applying the belt too tightly (see illustrations).

Promotes organization and reduces transmission of microorganisms.
Ensures correct patient is restrained. Approach reduces patient anxiety and promotes cooperation.

Positioning prevents contractures and neurovascular impairment.

Allows nurse to use proper body mechanics and prevent injury.

Reduces friction and pressure from restraint to skin and underlying tissue.

Restrains center of gravity and prevents patient from rolling off stretcher or sitting up while on stretcher or from falling out of bed. Tight application interferes with ventilation if belt moves up over abdomen or chest.

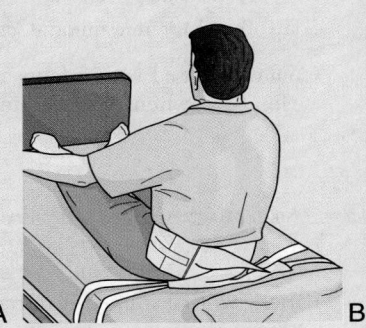 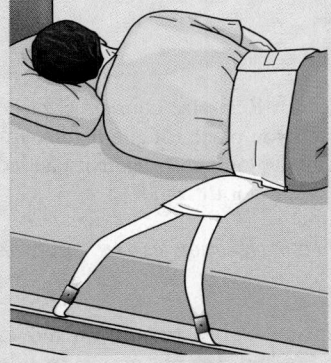

STEP 6a **A,** Apply belt restraint with patient sitting. **B,** A properly applied belt restraint allows patient to turn in bed. (**A** *from Sorrentino SA: Mosby's textbook for nursing assistants, ed 7, St. Louis, 2008, Mosby.*)

STEP	RATIONALE

b *Extremity (ankle or wrist) restraint:* Restraint designed to immobilize one or all extremities. Commercially available limb restraints are composed of sheepskin with foam padding. Wrap limb restraint around wrist or ankle with soft part toward skin, and secure snugly (not tightly) in place by Velcro straps. Insert two fingers under secured restraint (see illustration).

Maintains immobilization of extremity to protect patient from fall or accidental removal of therapeutic device (e.g., IV tube, Foley catheter).

Tight application will interfere with circulation and cause neurovascular injury.

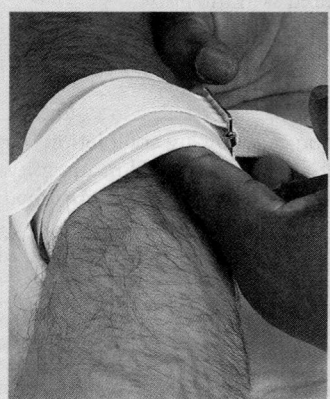

STEP 6b   Securing an extremity restraint. Check restraint for constriction by inserting two fingers under restraint. (*From Sorrentino SA: Mosby's textbook for nursing assistants, ed 7, St. Louis, 2008, Mosby.*)

Critical Decision Point   *Patient with wrist and ankle restraints is at risk for aspiration if placed in supine position. Place patient in lateral position rather than supine.*

c *Mitten restraint:* Thumbless mitten device restrains patient's hands. Place hand in mitten, being sure Velcro strap(s) are around the wrist and not the forearm (see illustration).

Prevents patients from dislodging invasive equipment, removing dressings, or scratching, yet allows greater movement than a wrist restraint.

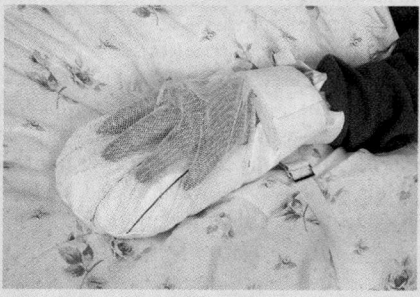

STEP 6c   Mitten restraint. (*Courtesy Posey Company, Arcadia, Calif.*)

d *Elbow restraint (freedom splint):* Restraint consists of piece of fabric with slots in which you place tongue blades. Insert patient's arm so that elbow joint rests against padded area with tongue blades, keeping joint rigid.

Commonly used with infants and children to prevent elbow flexion (e.g., when IV placed in antecubital fossa).

Critical Decision Point   *This text does not address application of vest restraints. Many health care agencies have banned the use of jacket (vest) restraints because of their association with fatal injuries.*

7 Attach restraint straps to portion of bed frame that moves when raising or lowering head of bed. **Do not attach to side rails.** Attach a restraint to chair frame for patient in chair or wheelchair, being sure tie is out of patient's reach.

Patient will be injured if restraint is secured to side rail and it is lowered.

STEP	RATIONALE

8 Secure restraints with a quick-release tie (see illustrations). Do not tie in a knot.

Allows for quick release in an emergency.

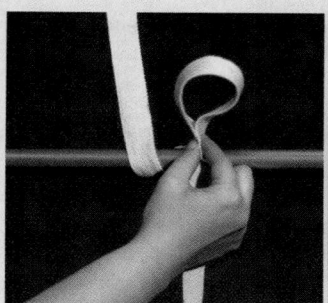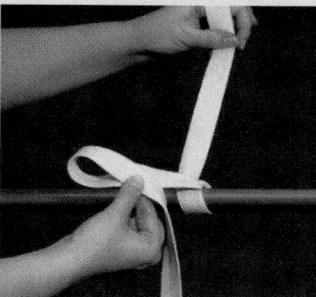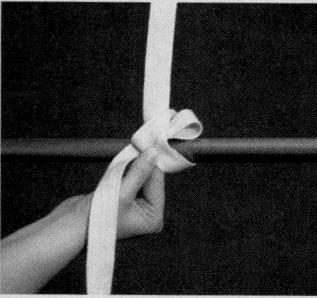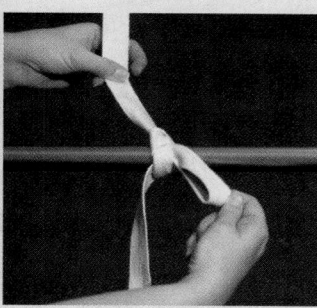

STEP 8   The Posey quick-release tie. (*Courtesy Posey Company, Arcadia, Calif.*)

9 Insert two fingers under secured restraint.

Checking for constriction prevents neurovascular injury.

10 Assess proper placement of restraint, including skin integrity, pulses, temperature, color, and sensation of the restrained body part.

Provides baseline to later evaluate if injury develops from restraint.

11 Remove restraints at least every 2 hours (TJC, 2007a). If patient is violent or noncompliant, remove one restraint at a time and/or have staff assistance while removing restraints.

Removal provides opportunity to change patient's position, offer nutrients, perform full ROM, toilet and exercise patient.

Critical Decision Point   *Do not leave violent or aggressive patient unattended while restraints are off.*

12 Secure call light or intercom system within reach.

Allows patient, family, or caregiver to obtain assistance quickly.

13 Leave bed or chair with wheels locked. Keep bed in lowest position.

Locked wheels prevent bed or chair from moving if patient tries to get out. If patient falls when bed is in lowest position, this will reduce chance of injury.

14 Perform hand hygiene.

Reduces transmission of microorganisms.

EVALUATION

1 Following application, evaluate patient's condition for signs of injury every 15 minutes (TJC, 2007a). Use judgment, and consider the patient's condition and the type of restraint when selecting physical assessment measures (e.g., circulation, nutrition and hydration, ROM in extremities, vital signs, hygiene and elimination, physical and psychological status, and readiness for discontinuation). Visual checks can be performed if the patient is too agitated to approach (TJC, 2007a).

Frequent assessments prevent injury to patient and removal of restraint at earliest possible time.

2 The physician, licensed independent practitioner (LIP), or RN trained according to CMS requirements needs to evaluate the patient within either 1 or 4 hours after initiation of restraints, depending on hospital's Medicare status (see agency policy).

Determines patient's immediate situation, reaction to restraints, medical and behavioral condition, and need to continue or terminate restraints (CMS, 2007).

3 After 24 hours, before writing a new order, a physician or LIP who is responsible for the patient's care must see and assess the patient.

Ensures that restraint application continues to be medically appropriate.

4 Observe IV catheters, urinary catheters, and drainage tubes to determine that they are positioned correctly and that therapy remains uninterrupted.

Reinsertion can be uncomfortable and can increase risk for infection or interrupt therapy.

Unexpected Outcomes

1 Patient experiences impaired skin integrity related to improper or prolonged use of restraint.

2 Patient has altered neurovascular status of an extremity, such as cyanosis, pallor and coldness of skin, or complaints of tingling, pain, or numbness.

3 Patient exhibits increased confusion and disorientation.

4 Patient releases restraint and suffers a fall or other traumatic injury.

Related Interventions

• Reassess need for continued use of restraint and if you can use alternative measures. If restraint is necessary to protect patient or others from injury, ensure you applied restraint correctly and provide adequate padding.
• Check skin under restraint for abrasions, and remove restraints more frequently.
• Institute appropriate skin/wound care.
• Change wet or soiled restraints to prevent skin maceration.
• Remove restraint immediately, and notify physician.

• Evaluate cause for altered behavior, and attempt to eliminate cause.
• Provide appropriate sensory stimulation, reorient as needed, and attempt restraint alternatives.

• Attend to patient's immediate physical needs, inform physician of fall or injury, and reassess type of restraint and its correct application.

Recording and Reporting

• Record patient's behavior before restraints were applied, level of orientation, and patient's or family member's understanding of purpose of restraint and consent (when required).
• Record the reason for the restraint, the type of restraint used, the time of starting and ending the restraints, and the routine observations every 15 minutes (e.g., skin color, pulses, sensation, vital signs, behavior) in the nurses' notes and flow sheets.

Teaching Considerations

• Explain thoroughly the use of restraints. Caution family against removing, repositioning, or retying restraint.

Pediatric Considerations

• Limit the use of restraints to clinically appropriate and adequately justified situations after using all appropriate alternatives. Restrain a child only to restrict movement when the patient is at risk for injuring self or others.
• When a child needs to be restrained for a procedure, it is best that the person applying the restraint not be the child's parent or guardian.
• A mummy restraint is a safe, efficient, short-term method to restrain a small child or infant for examination or treatment. Open a blanket, and fold one corner toward the center. Place child on blanket with shoulders at fold and feet toward opposite corner (Fig. 13-8, A). With child's right arm straight down against body, pull right side of blanket firmly across right shoulder and chest and secure beneath left side of body (Fig. 13-8, B). Place left arm straight against body, and bring left side of blanket across shoulder and chest and lock beneath child's body on right side (Fig. 13-8, C). Fold lower corner and bring over body, and tuck or fasten securely with safety pins (Fig. 13-8, D) (Hockenberry and others, 2007).

Gerontological Considerations

• Restrained older adults respond with anger, fear, humiliation, demoralization, discomfort, and resignation (Ebersole and others, 2004).

Home Care Considerations

• A physical restraint is a device that requires a physician's order. Do not send it home with family unless device is necessary to protect patient from injury. If patient's family wishes to use restraint at home, a physician's order is required and you need to give clear instructions regarding proper application, care needed while in restraints, and complications to look for. Carefully assess the family for competency and understanding of intent for using restraint.

Long-Term Care Considerations

• Unnecessary restraint is false imprisonment. The person needs to understand reason for restraint. Inform the person how the restraint will help planned medical treatment and risk of restraint use.

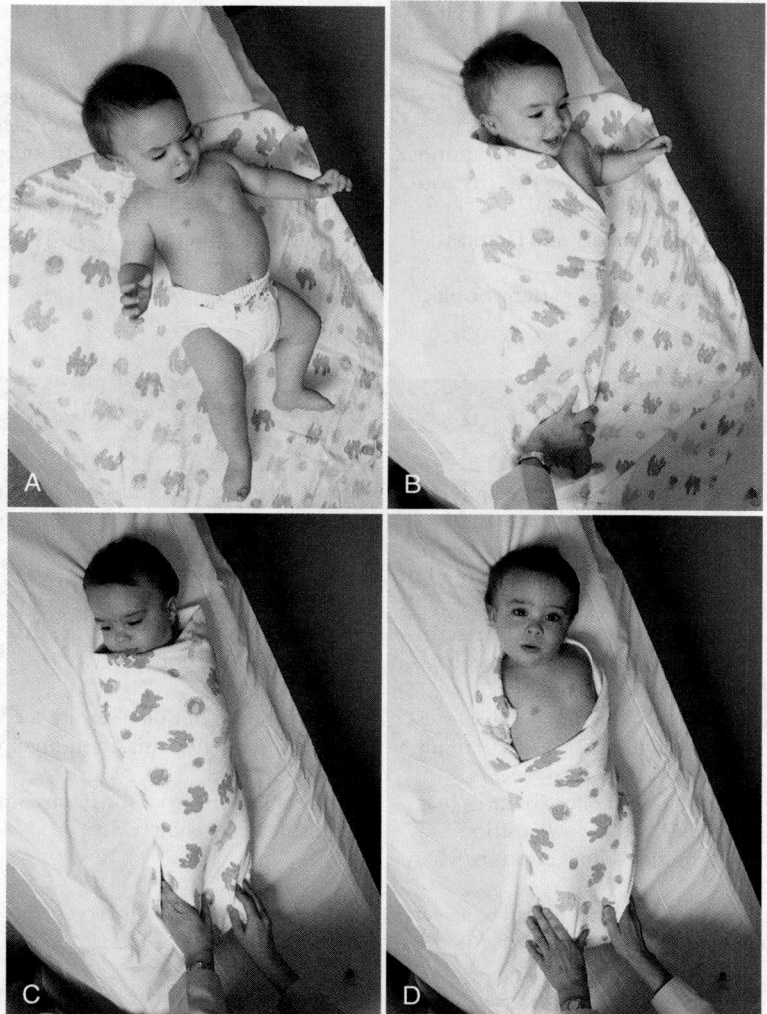

Fig. 13-8   Application of mummy restraint. **A,** Infant placed on folded corner of blanket. **B,** One corner of blanket brought across body and secured beneath body. **C,** Second corner brought across body and secured, and lower corner folded and tucked or pinned in place. **D,** Modified mummy restraint with chest uncovered. *(From Hockenberry MJ and others: Wong's essentials of pediatric nursing, ed 7, St. Louis, 2005, Mosby.)*

SKILL 13-4   Seizure Precautions

Seizures are sudden, abnormal, and excessive electrical discharges from the brain that change motor or autonomic function, consciousness, or sensation. The unpredictability of seizures profoundly affects persons' lives (Pena, 2003). Seizures are epileptic and nonepileptic. Epileptic seizures result from epilepsy, a neurological condition in which a brain abnormality causes recurrent seizure activity. Nonepileptic seizures are a response to a stimulus outside of the central nervous system, such as alcohol withdrawal, high fever, drug toxicity, and poisoning. The two basic types of seizures are partial (simple and complex) and generalized. A partial seizure starts in a specific part of the brain. In a simple seizure, the patient does not lose consciousness. In a partial complex seizure, a patient loses consciousness. Generalized seizures, of which there are several types, affect the whole brain and cause both nonconvulsive and convulsive seizures. Continuous seizure activity that lasts more than 30 minutes is status epilepticus, which is a medical emergency (Gambrell and Flynn, 2004).

Patients who have a seizure disorder require a safe hospital environment. Each type of seizure has a unique combination of clinical features. It is very important to assess a patient carefully if you witness a seizure. A generalized convulsive tonic-clonic or grand mal seizure lasts from 1 to 2 minutes. A cry, loss of consciousness, tonicity (muscle rigidity), clonicity (rhythmic muscle jerking), and incontinence are all characteristic of these seizures. Your priority becomes protecting the patient from injury. Following the seizure there is a postictal phase, which lasts for up to an hour. During this phase the patient lies very still, has flaccid muscles, excessive salivation, confusion, and fatigue (Gambrell and Flynn, 2004).

During a seizure, take steps to keep the patient's airway open. Traditionally nurses have used oral airways to maintain the patient's airway. However, forcing something in the patient's mouth will possibly result in injury to the jaw, tongue, or teeth and cause stimulation of the gag reflex, causing vomiting, aspiration, and respiratory distress (National Institute of Neurological Disorders and

Stroke, 2004). Forcing an airway into a patient's mouth is no longer recommended. You insert an airway only when there is clear access for insertion.

Delegation Considerations

The skill of assessment of a patient on seizure precautions cannot be delegated to NAP. However, the skills for making the environment safe can be delegated. The nurse directs NAP by:

- Alerting NAP to a patient's prior seizure history and factors that may trigger a seizure.
- Emphasizing that NAP not try to restrain the patient or place anything in the patient's mouth.

Equipment

- ❑ Suction machine
- ❑ Oral airway
- ❑ Oral Yankauer suction catheter
- ❑ Oxygen via nasal cannula or face mask
- ❑ Stethoscope, sphygmomanometer, pulse oximeter
- ❑ Equipment for intravenous access (see Chapter 31)
- ❑ Emergency medications (e.g., IV diazepam, lorazepam, valproate, phenytoin)
- ❑ Clean gloves

STEP	RATIONALE
ASSESSMENT	
1 Assess patient's seizure history and knowledge of precipitating factors. Note the frequency of past seizures, presence and type of aura (e.g. metallic taste, perception of breeze blowing on face, or noxious odor), and body parts affected, if known. Use family as resource if necessary.	Knowledge about seizure history enables nurse to anticipate onset of seizure activity and take appropriate safety measures.
2 Assess for medical and surgical conditions, including electrolyte disturbances such as hypoglycemia, hyperkalemia; heart disease; excess fatigue; alcohol or caffeine consumption.	Common conditions that lead to seizures or exacerbate existing seizure condition.
3 Assess medication history and patient's adherence. Also assess therapeutic drug levels of anticonvulsants if test results available.	If patient does not take seizure medications as prescribed and stops them suddenly, this often precipitates seizure activity.
4 Inspect patient's environment for potential safety hazards (e.g., extra furniture) if seizure occurs. Keep bed in low position, side rails up at head of bed, patient in side-lying position when possible.	Protects patient from injury sustained by striking head or body on furniture or equipment.
5 For patients with a history of generalized seizures, have oxygen setup, suction apparatus, and clean gloves available for immediate use.	This ensures prompt intervention directed toward maintaining a patent airway.
6 Assess a patient's cultural perspective about the meaning of seizures and their treatment.	Some cultures follow different caring practices for a person with seizures.

NURSING DIAGNOSES

- Deficient knowledge regarding safety precautions during seizure activity
- Ineffective airway clearance
- Noncompliance with medications
- Risk for aspiration
- Situational low self-esteem

Individualize related factors based on patient's condition or needs.

PLANNING	
1 Expected outcomes following completion of procedure:	
• Patient remains free of traumatic injury while experiencing seizure.	Seizure precautions prevent patients from incurring injury from a fall or the tonic-clonic seizure activity.
• Patient's airway remains patent during seizure activity.	Airway occlusion and aspiration are potential complications of seizure activity.
• Patient does not experience a lowered sense of self-esteem following seizure episode.	Loss of bowel or bladder control is common in tonic-clonic seizures, causing patient to feel embarrassment or shame.

IMPLEMENTATION	
1 When seizure begins, note the time, stay with patient, and call for help. Track the duration of seizure. Have health care provider notified immediately. Have staff member bring emergency cart to bedside.	If tonic-clonic seizure develops, assistance is sometimes needed to control patient's movements to prevent injury (Pena, 2003). Provides access to emergency medications and IV equipment as needed.
2 Position patient safely. If standing or sitting, guide patient to floor and protect head by cradling in nurse's lap or placing a pad under head. Do not lift patient from floor to bed while seizure is in progress. Clear surrounding area of furniture. If patient is in bed, remove pillows and raise side rails.	Measures to prevent traumatic injury. Suffocation will possibly occur with use of pillow.

STEP	RATIONALE

3 If possible, turn patient onto one side, head tilted slightly forward.

Allows tongue to fall away from the airway and allows drainage of saliva.

4 If possible, provide privacy. Have staff control flow of visitors in area.

Embarrassment is common after a seizure, especially if others witnessed the seizure.

5 Do not restrain patient; if patient is flailing the limbs, hold limbs loosely. Place something soft under the head. Loosen clothing such as a collar or belt.

Prevents musculoskeletal injury. Promotes free ventilatory movement of chest and abdomen.

6 Never force apart a patient's clenched teeth. Do not place any objects into patient's mouth such as fingers, medicine, tongue depressor, or airway when teeth are clenched.

Prevents injury to mouth and possible aspiration.

Critical Decision Point *Injury will possibly result from forcible insertion of hard object. Soft objects will break and become aspirated. Insert a bite block or oral airway in advance if you recognize the possibility of a tonic-clonic seizure.*

7 Maintain the patient's airway, and suction as needed. Check patient's level of consciousness and oxygen saturation. Check vital signs. Provide oxygen by nasal cannula or mask if ordered. *Use oral airway only if you can easily access oral cavity.*

Prevents hypoxia during seizure activity.

8 Stay with patient, observing sequence and timing of seizure activity. Note the following: type of seizure; parts of body affected; if there was a loss of consciousness; presence of autonomic signs of lip smacking, mastication, or grimacing; rolling of eyes; presence of incontinence or diaphoresis; presence of apnea.

Continued observation assists in documentation, diagnosis, and treatment of seizure disorder.

9 As patient regains consciousness, reorient and reassure. Explain what happened and answer patient's questions. Stay with patient until full recovery.

Informing patients of type of seizure activity experienced will assist them in participating knowledgeably in their care. Some patients remain confused for a period or become violent.

10 Following seizure, assist patient to position of comfort in bed with side rails up (one rail down for easy exit) and bed in lowest position (see illustration). Place call light or intercom system within reach, and provide a quiet, nonstimulating environment.

Provides for continued safety. Patients are often confused and sleepy following a seizure.

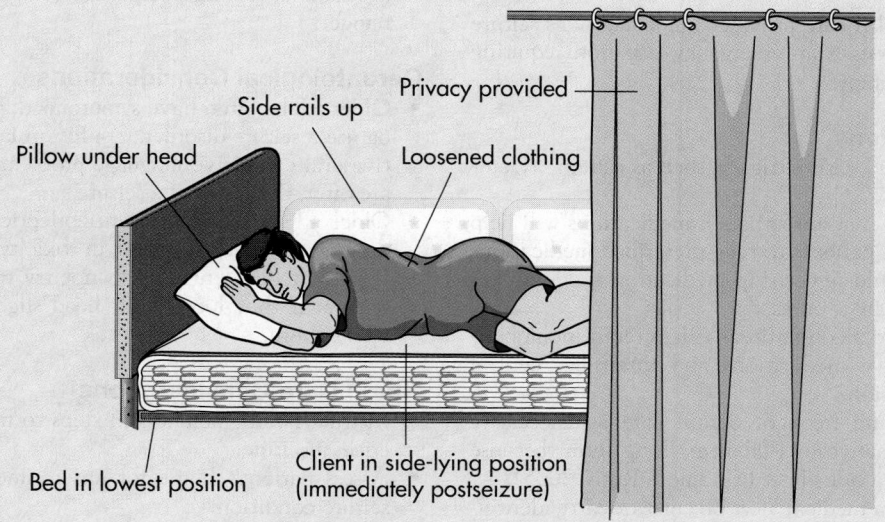

Side rails up
Pillow under head
Privacy provided
Loosened clothing
Bed in lowest position
Client in side-lying position (immediately postseizure)

STEP 10 Position of patient following seizure and when on seizure precautions.

11 Offer psychosocial support; provide time for patient to express feelings and concerns.

Patients who accept the reality of their disease integrate it into their own self-concept and have higher levels of self-esteem.

12 Perform hand hygiene.

Reduces transmission of microorganisms.

EVALUATION

1 Conduct a head-to-toe assessment, including an inspection of oral cavity for breaks in mucous membranes from bites or broken teeth.

Determines presence of any traumatic injuries resulting from seizure activity.

STEP	RATIONALE

Critical Decision Point   *If onset of seizure was not witnessed and you suspect patient fell and struck head, treat as a closed head injury or spinal injury. Place a cervical collar on patient before attempting to turn.*

2   Evaluate patient's mental status after seizure (level of consciousness, confusion, hallucinations).

Temporary mental status changes are common following a seizure.

3   Check patient's oxygen saturation and vital signs.

Determines stability of oxygenation and circulation.

4   If possible, ask patient to verbalize feelings after seizure.

Therapeutic interaction enables patient to recognize feelings associated with having a seizure disorder.

Unexpected Outcomes

1   Patient suffers traumatic injury.

2   Patient's airway becomes occluded, and materials are aspirated.

3   Patient develops status epilepticus.

Related Interventions

- Attend to patient's immediate physical needs, inform physician of injury, reassess patient's environment to ensure that environment is free of safety hazards, complete incident/occurrence report, and communicate to other care providers the measures you took to reduce risk for further injury.
- Turn onto side, insert oral airway (if possible), and apply suction to remove materials and maintain patent airway.
- Maintain nasal oxygen.
- Maintain airway, and insert oral airway if possible.
- Administer oxygen.
- Prepare for IV insertion, 0.9% sodium chloride.
- Administer IV lorazepam, phenytoin, or fosphenytoin as ordered (Gambrell and Flynn, 2004).

Recording and Reporting

- Record thoroughly in nurses' notes what you observed before, during, and after seizure. Provide detailed description of type of seizure activity and sequence of events (e.g., presence of aura [if any], level of consciousness, posture, color, movement of extremities, incontinence, and patient's status immediately following seizure).
- Report to primary health care provider immediately as seizure begins. Status epilepticus is an emergency situation requiring immediate medical therapy.

Teaching Considerations

- Instruct patient to avoid seizure triggers such as caffeine (Gambrell and Flynn, 2004).
- Patients need to know that antiepileptic medications will help control epilepsy. Warn patients to take prescribed medications regularly. Patients should never stop medication suddenly because this will precipitate seizures.
- Advise patient to avoid alcohol, because it is often incompatible with anticonvulsive medications and intensifies central nervous system depression.
- Proper oral hygiene and frequent dental care are necessary when patient takes phenytoin (Dilantin) long term, because gingival hyperplasia is a side effect (Skidmore-Roth, 2005).
- Patient needs to wear a medical alert bracelet or carry identification card noting presence of seizure disorder and listing medications taken.
- Fatigue, stress, and illness can potentiate seizures. Therefore patients need to eat a balanced diet at regular intervals, get enough sleep, and consult their physician promptly when ill.
- A seizure condition usually imposes driving limitations. It is recommended that a waiting period of 1 seizure-free year elapse before patient attempts to drive or operate dangerous equipment.

Pediatric Considerations

- Teach parents what to observe for in seizures because many times they are present at the onset.
- Encourage children with severe atonic seizures to wear a helmet to protect them when they fall. A child with tonic-clonic seizures should have side rails padded and suction and oxygen available to manage respiratory secretions for airway maintenance.

Gerontological Considerations

- Older adults often have symptoms that make it difficult to recognize a seizure disorder. Confusion lasting several days, receptive and expressive language problems, and unusual behaviors are often the result of a seizure.
- Older adults metabolize antiepileptics more slowly; therefore drugs accumulate, resulting in toxicity.
- If patient has dentures, do not try to remove them during a seizure. If they loosen, tilt head slightly forward and remove after seizure.

Home Care Considerations

- Instruct family members in steps to take when patient experiences a seizure.
- Assess patient's home for environmental hazards in light of seizure condition.
- Until seizure condition is well controlled (usually for at least 1 year), make sure patient does not take a tub bath or engage in activities such as swimming unless knowledgeable family member is present.
- Refer patient to the Epilepsy Foundation or a similar community resource for support groups.

CRITICAL THINKING EXERCISES

Daniel Werneck is a 78-year-old patient who entered the hospital for lower gastrointestinal bleeding. During the morning, nurses administered a series of enemas to Mr. Werneck before diagnostic tests of the colon. Mr. Werneck has a history of high blood pressure, but it has been controlled on medications. He has some weakness in his left leg due to an old back injury. As the evening nurse, you assess Mr. Werneck and find he is having diarrheal stools. You also learn that he is having some abdominal cramping. His wife stays with him until visiting hours conclude. He is alert and tells you, "I'm fine. I just feel a bit worn out from the testing today."

1 What factors in Mr. Werneck's case place him at risk for falling?
2 What interventions can you implement for fall prevention?
3 At midnight you enter Mr. Werneck's room and find him lying on the floor. What are your first two actions?

 REVIEW QUESTIONS

1 A nurse is conducting a class on fall prevention for the rest of the staff. Which statement is appropriate to include in the presentation?
1 Falls are most successfully prevented by making the patient's environment safe.
2 The early use of restraints in a suddenly restless patient will effectively reduce falls.
3 A bed alarm even when used alone will generally prevent falls in most patients.
4 The fall prevention strategies used should be appropriate for the patient's behaviors.

2 A nurse is caring for a patient who has a radioactive implant. Which strategies would be appropriate for the nurse to implement while caring for this patient? Select all that apply.
1 Organize the patient's care so the nurse is in the room for crucial activities only.
2 Educate the patient's visitors to limit their visitation to 2 hours per day.
3 Wear a dosimeter and designated radiation protection during direct care.
4 Ask the patient what kinds of magazines and books she enjoys reading.
5 Rotate with other nurses to care for this patient while maintaining continuity of care.
6 Protect the patient's privacy by not placing a "Radiation in Use" sign on the door.

3 A fire begins in the bathroom of a 200-pound patient who has a cast that extends from his hip to his ankle. What is the best method for evacuating this patient?
1 Place him on a blanket on the floor, and drag him out of the room.
2 Get another staff member to help using the "seat" carry technique.
3 Use the "back-strap" method to get him out of his room.
4 Leave him in bed, and push the bed out of the room.

4 The physician writes an order restraining one of the patients. What information would the nurse expect to find in the order? Select all that apply.
1 The time limitation for application of the restraint
2 The type of restraint to be applied
3 Alternative strategies to be used before a restraint is used
4 A list of behaviors that require using restraints
5 The documentation required while the patient is restrained
6 To notify the patient's next of kin that restraints were applied

5 A fire is discovered in a trash can in a patient's room. Which action by the nurse should be questioned?
1 Turning off the oxygen sources
2 Getting the patient out of the room
3 Asking the patient to place her blanket over the trash can
4 Calling for help

REFERENCES

Centers for Disease Control and Prevention, Injury Center: *Falls among older adults: an overview*, Atlanta, 2007, http://www.cdc.gov/ncipc/factsheets/adultfalls.htm, accessed June 16, 2007.

Centers for Disease Control and Prevention, National Center for Injury Prevention and Control: *A toolkit to prevent senior falls*, Atlanta, 2007, http://www.cdc.gov/ncipc/pub-res/toolkit/toolkit.htm, accessed April 24, 2007.

Centers for Medicare and Medicaid Services: *Revisions to Medicare conditions of participation, 482.13*, Bethesda, Md, 2007, US Department of Health and Human Services.

Ebersole P and others: *Toward healthy aging: human needs and nursing process*, ed 7, St. Louis, 2008, Mosby.

Gambrell M, Flynn N: Seizures 101, *Nursing* 34(8):36, 2004.

Hockenberry MJ and others: *Wong's essentials of pediatric nursing*, ed 7, St. Louis, 2005, Mosby.

Hockenberry MJ, Wilson D: *Wong's nursing care of infants and children*, ed 8, St. Louis, 2007, Mosby.

McCarter-Bayer A and others: Preventing falls in acute care: an innovative approach, *J Gerontol Nurs* 31(3):25, 2005.

Meade CM and others: Effects of nursing rounds on patients' call light use, satisfaction, and safety, *Am J Nurs* 106(9):58, 2006.

Meiner SE, Lueckenotte AG: *Gerontologic nursing*, ed 3, St. Louis, 2006, Mosby.

Missouri Center for Patient Safety: *Banding together for patient safety* [press release], Jefferson City, Mo, 2007, The Center.

NANDA International: *NANDA-I nursing diagnoses: definitions and classification, 2007-2008*, Philadelphia, 2007, NANDA International.

National Institute of Neurological Disorders and Stroke: *Seizures and epilepsy: hope through research*, Bethesda, Md, 2004, National Institutes of Health.

Pacquiao DF: Cultural competence in ethical decision-making. In Andres M, Boyle J: *Concepts in transcultural nursing*, Philadelphia, 2003, Lippincott, Williams, & Wilkins.

Park M, Tang J: Changing the practice of physical restraint use in acute care, *J Gerontol Nurs* 33(2):9, 2007.

Pena CG: Seizure: a calm response and careful observation are crucial. *Am J Nurs* 103(11):73, 2003.

Registered Nurses' Association of Ontario: *Nursing best practice guideline: prevention of falls and fall injuries in the older adult*, Toronto, Ontario, January 2002, The Association.

Robinson G: *Essential Judaism: a complete guide to beliefs, customs, and rituals*, New York, 2000, Pocket Books.

Skidmore-Roth L: *Mosby's drug guide for nurses*, ed 6, St. Louis, 2005, Mosby.

Sorrentino SA: *Mosby's textbook for nursing assistants*, ed 6, St. Louis, 2000, Mosby.

The Joint Commission: *Comprehensive accreditation manual for hospitals*, Chicago, 2007a, The Joint Commission.

The Joint Commission: The Joint Commission's New Speak Up™ program urges patients to "know your rights," *The Joint Commission News Release*, June 8, 2007b.

The Joint Commission: *2009 National patient safety goals*, Chicago, 2008, The Joint Commission.

U.S. Department of Veterans Affairs, National Center for Patient Safety: *2004 Falls toolkit, falls notebook interventions*, 2004, http://www.patientsafety.gov/Safetytopics/fallstoolkit/index.html, accessed June 25, 2007.

U.S. Food and Drug Administration: *Hospital bed system dimensional and assessment guidance to reduce entrapment—guidance for industry and FDA staff*, 2006, http://www.fda.gov/cdrh/beds/guidance/1537.html, accessed November 10, 2007.

RESEARCH REFERENCES

Algase DL and others: The Algase Wandering Scale: initial psychometrics of a new caregiver reporting tool, *Am J Alzheimer's Dis Other Demen* 16(3):141, 2001.

Algase DL and others: Validation of the Algase Wandering Scale (version 2) in a cross cultural sample, *Aging Ment Health* 8(2):133, 2004.

Brians LK and others: The development of the RISK tool for fall prevention, *Rehabil Nurs* 16(2):67, 1991.

Burroughs TE and others: Patients' concerns about medical errors during hospitalization, *Jt Comm J Qual Patient Saf* 33(1):5, 2007.

Elzaris ZR and others: Medications and falls in the elderly: a review of the evidence and practical considerations, *P&T* 28(11):724, 2003.

Gavin-Dreschnack, D and others: Wheelchair-related falls: current evidence and directions for improved quality care, *J Nurs Care Qual* 20(2):119, 2005.

Greenspan AI and others: Tai chi and perceived health status in older adults who are transitionally frail: a randomized controlled trial, *Phys Ther* 87(5):525, 2007.

Krauss MJ and others: A case-control study of patient, medication, and care-related risk factors for inpatient falls, *J Gen Intern Med* 20:116, 2005.

Infect Control Hosp Epidemiol 28(5):544, 2007.

Maciaszek J and others: Effect of tai chi on body balance: randomized controlled trial in men with osteopenia or osteoporosis, *Am J Chin Med* 35(1):1, 2007.

Minnick AF and others: Prevalence and variation of physical restraint use in acute care settings in the US, *J Nurs Scholarsh* 39(1):30, 2007.

Potter P and others: Identifying nurse staffing and patient outcome relationships: a guide for change in care delivery, *Nurs Econ* 21(4):158, 2003.

Powell-Cope G and others: Modification of bed systems and use of accessories to reduce the risk of hospital-bed entrapment, *Rehabil Nurs* 30(1):9, 2005.

Stevens JA and others: The cost of fatal and nonfatal falls among older adults. *Inj Prev* 12:290, 2006.

Tinetti ME: Preventing falls in elderly persons, *N Engl J Med* 348(1):42, 2003.

Wolf SL and others: Reducing frailty and falls in older persons: an investigation of tai chi and computerized balance training—Atlanta FICSIT Group: Frailty and injuries—cooperative studies of intervention techniques, *J Am Geriatr Soc* 44(5):489, 1996.

Zijlstra GA and others: Interventions to reduce fear of falling in community-living older people: a systematic review, *J Am Geriatr Soc* 55(4):603, 2007a.

Zijlstra GA and others: Prevalence and correlates of fear of falling, and associated avoidance of activity in the general population of community-living older people, *Age Ageing* 36(3):304, 2007b.

Disaster Preparedness

MEDIA RESOURCES

- **evolve** *learning system* http://evolve.elsevier.com/Perry/skills
  - Review Questions
  - Audio Glossary

KEY TERMS

Biological agent
Biological disaster
Bioterrorism/
  bioterrorist attack
Chemical warfare
  agent
Decontamination
Department of
  Homeland
  Security (DHS)
Detection and
  surveillance
Disaster response
Epidemic
Field triage tag
First responders
Hazard/hazard
  identification
Incident Command
  System (ICS)

International
  Nursing Coalition
  for Mass
  Casualty
  Education
  (INCMCE)
Mutual aid
  agreement
Nuclear event
Pandemic
Shelter-in-place
Strategic national
  stockpile (SNS)
Triage
Weapons of mass
  destruction
  (WMD)

Mastery of content in this chapter will enable the nurse to:
- Describe elements of the Centers for Disease Control and Prevention's strategic plan for disasters.
- Discuss the characteristics of different types of disasters.
- Identify actions to take in the event of biological, chemical, and radiation exposure.
- Discuss guidelines for patient care in the event of a mass casualty incident.
- Describe psychosocial effects of disasters on patients.

Although disaster preparedness and the possibility of terrorist attacks have been a subject of discussion and research for over 20 years, the attacks on the World Trade Center and Pentagon on September 11, 2001, forever changed the reality and sense of security felt by citizens of the United States. The attacks demonstrated the vulnerabilities, including the lack of preparedness of the health care community, in the event of a mass casualty incident (MCI). The attacks increased public awareness of not only probable future terrorist attacks but also the more common natural or environmental disasters affecting individuals on a more regular basis.

Throughout history nurses played a role in the multidisciplinary team approach in preparing for and responding to disasters. Information gathered from postdisaster evaluations have provided a considerable body of knowledge and experience to improve the response of the entire health care team and the many agencies/individuals involved in disaster response (e.g., police, firefighters, administrators, and paramedics). The Department of Homeland Security has identified preparedness and education of the nation as an essential component to national security against domestic and foreign threats.

HOMELAND SECURITY

The National Strategy for Homeland Security and the Homeland Security Act of 2002 were enacted to secure the homeland from terrorist attack. The Department of Homeland Security (DHS) was established to provide a unifying core as the basis for efforts to prevent and discourage terrorist attacks. This governmental agency coordinates the efforts of multiple organizations to secure and maintain the safety of our nation. The DHS has several strategic goals: awareness, prevention, protection, response, recovery, service, and organizational excellence (DHS, 2007).

Terrorism Preparedness

In addition to the activities of the DHS, the Centers for Disease Control and Prevention (CDC) is a leading federal agency designed to protect the health and safety of people at home and abroad. The mission of the CDC's Coordinating Office for Terrorism Preparedness and Emergency Response (COTPER) is to protect the health and enhance living of all people related to community preparedness and response (CDC, March, 2008). The CDC's strategic plan in the event of a disaster first focuses on preparedness, which is key to the impact any disaster has on the individuals or communities involved. Preparedness requires that nurses have a basic understanding of the science of a disaster and an understanding of the key components of any plan to deal with an MCI (CDC, March, 2008).

In the event of a biological, chemical, or radiation attack the CDC's strategic plan includes the following:
- *Preparedness and prevention:* The comprehensive preparedness required to manage self, family, and/or the community when an event occurs that is likely to result from a catastrophic and or destructive event that disrupts normal functioning.
- *Detection and surveillance:* Awareness of the environment, recognizing what is unusual or different, and knowing what these differences possibly mean for purpose of mitigation or prevention.
- *Diagnosis and characterization of biological, chemical, and radiological agents:* The ability of an individual to recognize or identify clusters of data indicating a biological, chemical, or radiological MCI event has occurred.
- *Response:* The systematic, coordinated, and effective delivery of services when disaster strikes.
- *Communication:* The establishment of protocols and standing orders in the event of a disaster to successfully manage health care and to use the media for communicating information to the public (e.g., directions to treatment facilities, evacuation routes). Traditional modes of communication will likely be interrupted in the event of an MCI; therefore part of disaster preparedness involves backup plans for maintaining public and intraagency/interagency communication (e.g., use of two-way radios and satellite phones).

Although the CDC's plan is for mass casualty disaster events or community-wide incidents, the plan clearly applies to any disaster event.

The CDC and the American Red Cross advocate preparedness and coordination of prompt, effective emergency efforts. This preparedness coordination includes outreach to other agencies or groups through mutual aid agreements. These agreements might include the willingness of one agency to provide shelter (e.g., a church, school, or recreation center), while other agencies provide clothing (e.g., department stores, the Salvation Army, or Goodwill). Some agreements might also include identifying and caring for the deceased (e.g., funeral homes), and still other agencies agree to provide vehicular support in the time of a disaster. Disaster planning is not only a multidisciplinary task but also a multiagency task. Although the average citizen, government agency, and other health care workers play a vital role in disaster preparedness, nurses will always have unique responsibilities within this multidisciplinary and multiagency coalition.

DISASTER DEFINED

A disaster is any unexpected event whose effect leads to significant destruction and/or adverse consequences. More specifically, a disaster is any event in which needs exceed available resources. Box 14-1 provides common disaster terminology definitions. Although these definitions standardize the events of an MCI, it is important to understand that each disaster is unique in the way it affects individuals, families, and communities.

When most Americans hear the term *disaster*, they immediately think terrorist attack. In reality the most common forms of disaster are natural or manmade (e.g., major fires, hurricanes, tornadoes, and floods). Disasters often occur with the spread of natural-borne disease if the public is not adequately protected and prepared.

An epidemic is an infectious disease or condition that attacks many people at the same time in the same geographical area. A pandemic is an epidemic that occurs in many parts of the world. History tells us there are approximately three influenza pandemics every 100 years that result in the deaths of millions of people. Experts believe we are due for another pandemic influenza virus to which virtually no one in the world is immune. A pandemic flu is highly contagious from person to person. Surveillance by the

World Health Organization (WHO) continues with such infections as severe acute respiratory syndrome (SARS) and avian influenza (bird flu) for indications of mutations and increased transmission (Boxes 14-2 and 14-3). If a pandemic flu occurs, it will take months for a vaccine to be developed, and once manufactured, doses would first be rationed to persons with a compromised immune system, older adults, and health care workers (Vaccine Education Center, 2006). To be adequately prepared, citizens need education on preventing the spread of influenza (see Chapter 7).

Disaster Preparedness

To further support the need for health care providers to increase their preparedness, some states are enacting new laws that require disaster training as part of the continuing education requirement for licensure. However, only disaster planning, education, training, and drills on a local, national, and global level will effectively prepare health care providers, volunteers, and other individuals

needed in the event of an MCI. Nurses need to influence, develop, and practice policies that will improve the safety and quality of health care at the time of an MCI.

Alerting the Public

The DHS established a color-coded national framework to provide officials and citizens with information regarding the nature and degree of terrorist threat (Fig. 14-1). To determine the current advisory level for the nation, visit the DHS website at http://white-house.gov/homeland. Green designates a low risk level for terrorist attacks. At the green level, government agencies are to ensure personnel receive proper training and to regularly assess facilities for vulnerability to terrorist attack. At the same time citizens are encouraged to develop and share family emergency plans, create emergency supply kits, become informed, and know how to "shelter-in-place." Shelter-in-place is a precaution designed to keep individuals safe while remaining indoors. Sheltering-in-place does

---

BOX 14-1 | Disaster Definitions and Types

- **Disaster:** A catastrophic and/or destructive event that disrupts normal functioning; it may include any anticipated or unexpected event whose effects lead to significant destruction and/or adverse consequences
- **Mass casualty incident or event (MCI):** Any event or situation that results in multiple casualties and/or deaths; an MCI exists when health care needs exceed health care resources
- **All-hazards event:** Multiple manmade or natural events with destructive capacity to cause multiple casualties
- **All-hazards preparedness:** The comprehensive preparedness necessary to manage casualties resulting from a disaster regardless of etiology
- **Casualty:** Any individual who is ill, injured, missing, or killed as a result of an MCI

- **Medical disasters:** Catastrophic events that result in human casualties that overwhelm the available health care resources
- **Natural/environmental disasters:** Catastrophic events that result from an ecological event that exceeds the capacity of the community (e.g., the impact of hurricanes or tornados on a community)
- **Manmade disasters:** Catastrophic events whose principal direct cause is attributable to human action
- **Technological disasters:** Catastrophic events in which people, property, community infrastructure, and economic welfare are adversely affected by the disruption of technology (e.g., industrial accidents, unplanned release of nuclear waste)

BOX 14-2 | Severe Acute Respiratory Syndrome (SARS)

- A viral respiratory illness caused by a coronavirus (SARS-CoV).
- Spread by close person-to-person contact through respiratory droplets. Strict adherence to contact and droplet precautions, along with eye protection, seems to prevent SARS-CoV transmission in most instances.
- In 2003, 8,098 people worldwide became sick with SARS; of these, 774 died.
- Onset of a high fever; other symptoms include headache and body aches.

- About 10% to 20% have diarrhea. After 2 to 7 days, SARS patients may develop a dry cough.
- Most SARS patients develop pneumonia.
- Treatment may consist of various therapies, including antibiotics, antivirals, corticosteroids, alternative medicine (i.e., glycyrrhizin), and assisted ventilation.
- Ongoing research for vaccine development.

Data from Centers for Disease Control and Prevention (n.d.), http://www.cdc.gov/ncidod/sars, accessed August 6, 2008.

BOX 14-3 | Avian Influenza ("Bird Flu")

- An infectious disease of birds that is highly contagious among poultry; has also been documented in pigs, tigers, leopards, ferrets, domestic cats, and the stone marten (a weasel-like animal).
- More than 200 cases among humans reported worldwide; approximately half of the people reported as infected have died.
- Believed to be primarily transmitted through close contact with diseased birds or contaminated surfaces; person-to-person transmission is rare.
- Incubation period 2 to 8 days; possibly as long as 17 days.
- Initial symptoms include a high fever and flulike symptoms (i.e., fever, cough, sore throat, and muscle aches). Watery diarrhea and vomiting have also been reported as early symptoms. Eye infection (conjunctivitis) and pneumonia may occur. Clinical deterioration is rapid, with respiratory distress and multiorgan dysfunction.

- Antiviral drugs (e.g., oseltamivir [Tamiflu]) can improve survival when administered within 48 hours of symptom onset.
- On April 17, 2007, the U.S. Food and Drug Administration announced approval of a vaccine against one strain of the avian flu H5N1 virus. The vaccine has been purchased by the federal government and is being held in the strategic national stockpile. Research continues for vaccines against other strains of the H5N1 virus.
- Concern is that the virus could start a pandemic; however, currently the virus does not spread easily from person to person and is not sustainable among humans.

Data from *WHO avian influenza fact sheet*, Feb 2006, http://www.who.int/mediacentre/factsheets/avian_influenza/en/, accessed August 6, 2008; U.S. Department of Health and Human Services, Centers for Disease Control and Prevention, May 2007.

HOMELAND SECURITY
ADVISORY SYSTEM

SEVERE   **SEVERE RISK OF**   **TERRORIST ATTACKS**
HIGH   **HIGH RISK OF**   **TERRORIST ATTACKS**
ELEVATED   **SIGNIFICANT RISK OF**   **TERRORIST ATTACKS**
GUARDED   **GENERAL RISK OF**   **TERRORIST ATTACKS**
LOW   **LOW RISK OF**   **TERRORIST ATTACKS**

FIG 14-1 The Homeland Security Advisory System indicates the potential risk level for serious terrorist activity.

not mean seeking a shelter, but rather taking refuge in a small interior room with no or few windows. It does not require sealing an entire home or office. When the security alert is at the green level, individuals should learn how to turn off utilities, examine volunteer opportunities, provide community service, and consider completing emergency preparation courses (e.g., cardiopulmonary resuscitation [CPR] and first aid).

Condition blue (guarded) occurs when there is a general risk for terrorist attack. In addition to the green level activities, government agencies communicate with designated emergency response or command locations, review and update emergency response procedures, and provide the public with information to strengthen the ability to act appropriately. Citizens are to review stored disaster supplies, replace outdated items, and be alert to suspicious activity.

Condition yellow (elevated) signifies there is a significant risk for terrorist attacks. Government agencies continue previously listed activities and also increase surveillance of critical locations, coordinate emergency plans, assess the characteristics of the threat, and implement appropriate contingency and emergency response plans. Individuals need to ensure their disaster supply kit is stocked and ready, and they should check important telephone numbers. Individuals also need to review their family emergency plan, practice alternative routes to and from school and work, and continue to be alert to suspicious activity, which should be reported to authorities (e.g., calling 9-1-1).

Condition orange indicates a high risk for terrorist attack. Government agencies continue previously listed activities and begin coordinating necessary security, take additional precautions at public events, prepare to execute contingency procedures, and restrict access to a threatened facility to essential personnel only. Individuals continue to complete recommendations at the lower levels of alert, exercise caution when traveling, be patient and expect delays, and check on neighbors or others who need assistance in an emergency.

Red is the highest level of alert, which suggests a severe risk for terrorist attacks. Generally this level of alert does not last for extended periods. Increased numbers of emergency personnel will need to respond to critical emergency needs; to assign emergency personnel to monitor, redirect, and constrain transportations systems; and to close public and government facilities, as needed.

Citizens need to listen to local emergency management officials, stay tuned to TV or radio for current information, prepare to shelter-in-place or evacuate, expect delays and restrictions, provide volunteer services only as requested, and contact schools and/or businesses to determine the status of the school or workplace.

When alerting the public, it is important that all messages be consistent, immediate, accurate, and open. Working closely with the media is important, because members of the media play a key role in providing accurate information and possibly reducing the number of concerned individuals who unnecessarily come to hospitals. Key message topics include the following (CDC, March, 2008):

If you think you are exposed, take these steps . . .

If you are injured . . .

Likely effects of biological or chemical exposure/radiation contamination include . . .

To avoid contamination . . .

Available resources, experts/contacts for medical information include . . .

The D-I-S-A-S-T-E-R Paradigm

In 2003 the American Medical Association (AMA) developed a series of National Disaster Life Support (NDLS) courses to provide coordinated training with an all-hazards approach to mass casualty incidents (AMA, 2007). The D-I-S-A-S-T-E-R model put forth in the training program standardizes methods for recognizing a disaster, managing the scene, and providing care to disaster victims.

Detection

Detection is the first goal in an MCI and includes (a) determining the presence of an MCI or public health emergency (PHE), (b) recognizing the cause of the incident, and (c) becoming aware of the environment or more specifically changes in the environment (e.g., an unusual pattern of patient presentation, unusual smells, or suspicious individuals). Although many events will probably have a clear cause, others will have an insidious onset. For example, if a large number of otherwise healthy young adults start showing up in an emergency department (ED) with similar but unexplained symptoms, the nurse and other health care providers should begin to suspect something is not right. Detection is sometimes simply the awareness of an unusual health care situation.

Remember, to be able to provide care, you first need to ensure personal safety. It is essential that rescue and health care workers avoid becoming victims, which may go against your initial instinct to help others. When the scene of a disaster is in a clearly designated area outside the health care agency, you need to determine the security of the scene. Always consider external scenes of disasters, such as sites of explosions or severe storm damage, unsafe until trained professionals arrive and determine the scene is safe.

The use of biological agents is a considerable terrorist threat because they are easy to disperse and will affect large numbers of people at a relatively low cost (Box 14-4). Incubation periods and common initial clinical symptoms make detection of a biological attack difficult.

Another form of MCI is the dissemination, or spreading, of a toxic chemical agent. There are a number of methods for spreading toxic chemical agents (e.g., fire or explosion). Health care providers are often at risk for becoming secondary victims when chemical agents create an MCI. Chemical agents are categorized based on their mechanism of injury. These include pulmonary agents, blistering agents, blood agents, and nerve agents.

The thought of nuclear and radiological incidents creates considerable fear for many individuals. Most often, the cause for disseminating radioactive material is generally known. A fire or an

BOX 14-4	Potential Organisms for Bioterrorism by CDC Category

Category A—Greatest Threat
- Can be easily disseminated or transmitted person to person
- Cause high mortality with a potential for major public health impact

Anthrax (*Bacillus anthracis*)
Botulism (*Clostridium botulinum* toxin)
Plague (*Yersinia pestis*)
Smallpox (variola major)
Viral hemorrhagic fevers (Ebola, Marburg, Lassa, Machupo)

Category B—High Risk
- Moderately easy to disseminate
- Cause moderate morbidity and low mortality

Brucellosis (*Brucella* species)
Epsilon toxin of *Clostridium perfringens*
Food safety threats (e.g., *Salmonella*, *Escherichia coli*, *Shigella*)
Ricin toxin from *Ricinus communis* (castor beans)
Staphylococcal enterotoxin B
Water safety threats (e.g., *Vibrio cholerae*, *Cryptosporidium parvum*)

Category C—Emerging Biological Weapons for Terrorist Use
- Pathogens that could be engineered for mass dissemination

Nipah virus
Hantavirus

CDC, Centers for Disease Control and Prevention.

explosion is often associated with nuclear attacks; however, devices designed to disseminate radioactive material are not always obvious (i.e., a "dirty bomb"). The effects of nuclear and radiological events depend on the amount of radiation exposure. Most victims will have delayed onset of symptoms (including nausea, vomiting, and diarrhea), whereas some will have obvious burns. Generally the sooner symptoms appear, the greater the exposure to radioactive material.

Incident Command

Incident command is the need for the emergency system to be activated when a threat or hazard is suspected. For most individuals this means activating the 9-1-1 system, so that emergency responders can be brought in to assume command. Emergency responders initially remain outside the possible contaminated area. Therefore the impact of the disaster on roads, traffic, and availability of resources will possibly delay or prevent their arrival. An Incident Command System (ICS), also referred to as an incident management system (IMS), provides a standard approach to managing emergencies where multiple agencies are involved (Boatright and McGlown, 2005). Fig. 14-2 offers an example of a general chain of command in an MCI.

Scene Security and Safety

Nurses are not responsible for determining the security and safety of a disaster scene. This task is the responsibility of trained emergency personnel (e.g., firefighters and police). When a health care agency is the scene of the disaster or a secondary site for a disaster, trained personnel determine scene security and safety. A health care agency becomes a secondary disaster site when contaminated by the agent from the original disaster scene. For example, a patient has been exposed to mustard gas, an oily chemical that is difficult to remove from a patient's body. If not properly decontaminated, the victim contaminated by the mustard gas will inadvertently contaminate

health care providers and others. The same is true for many biological agents. The first priority at any disaster scene is to protect yourself and other team members. The second priority is to protect the public, patients, and the environment (Box 14-5).

You need to know which personal protective equipment (PPE) will minimize the risk for contact with contaminated materials or individuals. Proper use of many advanced forms of PPE requires training and fitting and an understanding that not all PPE will protect against all potential hazards. When used inappropriately, PPE becomes a hazard (e.g., dehydration and decreased vision, mobility, and ability to communicate). Some of these hazards result because while using advanced forms of PPE the user is unable to eat, drink, or go to the bathroom.

Personal protective equipment is categorized by the level of safety provided. Level A protection provides maximum protection because it offers a self-contained breathing apparatus, fully encloses the individual, and includes chemical-resistant boots and gloves (Fig. 14-3, p. 353). Highly trained personnel use Level A protection in heavily contaminated areas. If you are not wearing this type of protection and you are near an area where level A PPE is being used, the general rule is to get out or do not enter. Level B protection provides respiratory protection but less skin protection. Used by trained responders, this PPE includes a self-contained breathing apparatus, hooded chemical-resistant suit, and face, boot, and glove protection. Level B protection also requires training and fitting. First responders (those emergency personnel first on the scene) and hospital personnel are trained and fitted to use Level C protection. As with Level A and B protection, Level C protection presents danger to the user, primarily dehydration and hyperthermia. Standard work uniform or work clothes offer Level D protection. There is no respiratory protection. Standard precautions are important to take when using Level D protection. Depending on the circumstances, some health care providers will also choose to use a fluid-impermeable gown, cap, eye protection, mask, gloves, and shoe covers.

The most recently labeled level of protection is BioPPE. BioPPE requires the use of standard work clothes along with contact and respiratory protection. Double gloving and an N95 mask (see Chapter 7) or better respirator is recommended. Hand hygiene that includes washing with soap and water followed by use of an alcohol gel is important not only at this level but at all other levels. BioPPE protection is not adequate when caring for patients exposed to toxic chemicals; however, it provides adequate protection against radiological and biological agents.

Assessment

Assessing hazards is more important than knowing the exact cause of a disaster. By allowing trained individuals to assess a disaster scene, you will avoid becoming a victim. Health care providers and volunteers need to learn to shift thinking and realize that the MCI will possibly result in secondary hazards that come in many forms (Box 14-6, p. 353).

Support

In terms of a disaster, *support* means, "Give me what I need to get the job done." The earlier you ask for support, the better. Support varies with the situation and task at hand. Support resources necessary during a disaster include human resources, agencies, facilities, supplies, and vehicles. For example, although there are not enough hospitals to accommodate all victims, a school or recreation center could easily be turned into a makeshift hospital if there has been preparation for unforeseen disasters.

The CDC has developed a strategic national stockpile (SNS) that contains large numbers of medical equipment in the event of

HOSPITAL EMERGENCY INCIDENT COMMAND SYSTEM

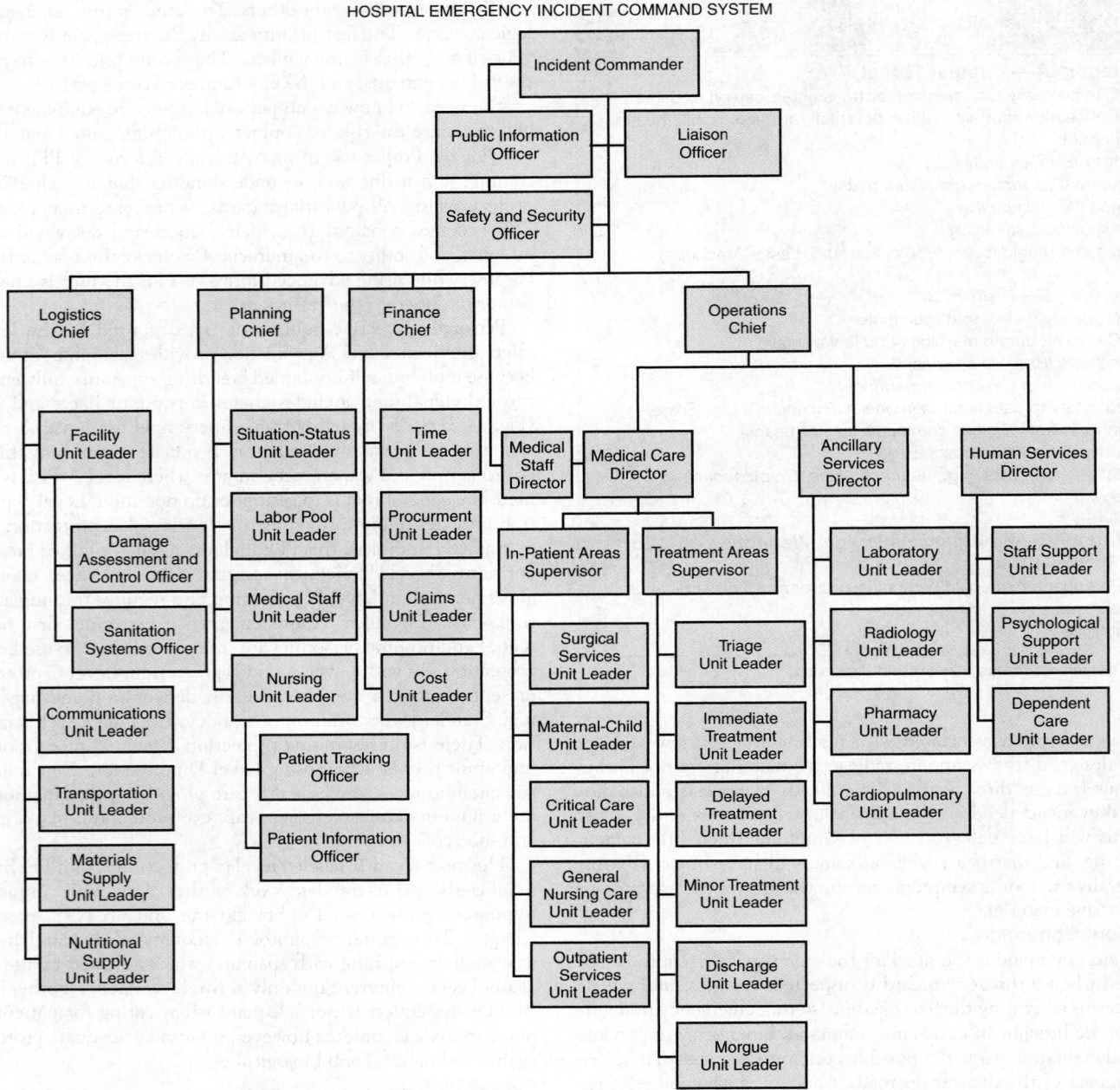

FIG 14-2 The Hospital Emergency Incident Command System prepares all response teams to work smoothly in a disaster situation.

BOX 14-5	The Do's and Don'ts of Scene Safety and Security
Do	**Don't**
• Stay out of a disaster scene unless well trained and invited. • Call 9-1-1.	• Don't enter the scene unless invited. • Don't needlessly disturb the scene; important evidence could be lost or contaminated by an eager but untrained helper. • Don't interfere with the services of other emergency personnel when uninvited or untrained. • Don't open suspicious packages.

a disaster (CDC, June, 2008). Most local communities will be prepared to provide essential resources for up to 72 hours (via hospitals, pharmacies, etc.) to support local needs. Once local and federal authorities confirm the need for the SNS and upon request of the affected state's governor's office, the 12-hour push package is flown or transported within 12 hours to any state in the United States. The 12-hour push package contains approximately 100 steel containers that hold pharmaceuticals (prepackaged 10-day supplies of antibiotics, antidotes, narcotics, epinephrine, albuterol, prednisone, etc.), intravenous (IV) fluids and IV supplies, ventilators, suction equipment, airway supplies, tablet-counting machines, and other emergency provisions (CDC, June, 2008).

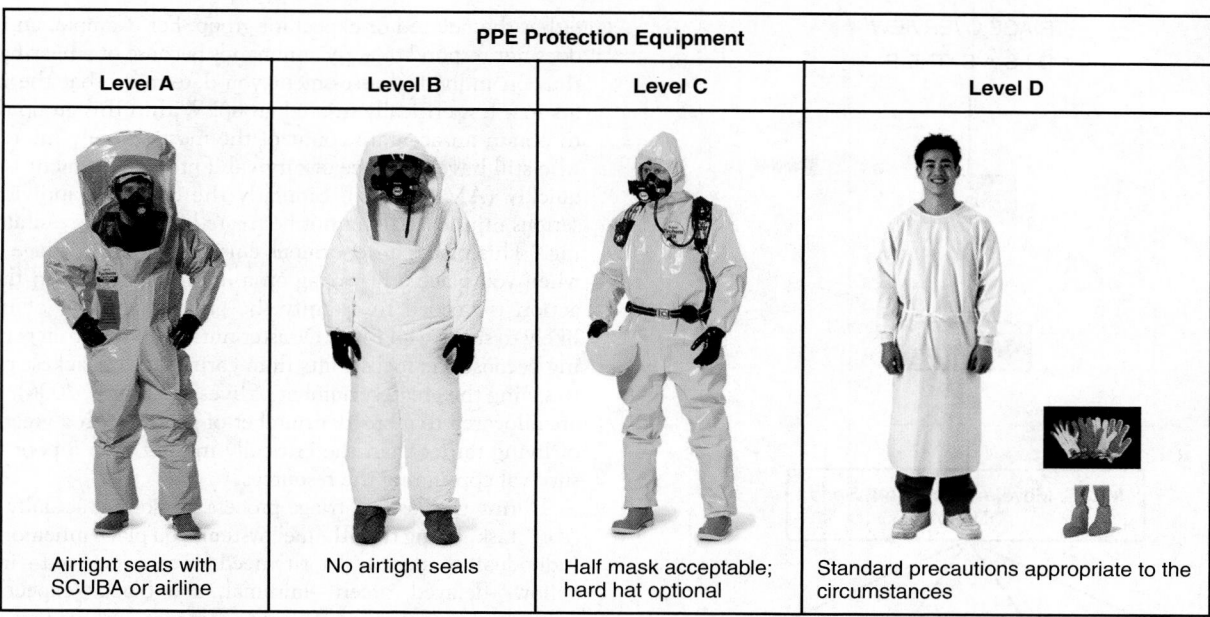

PPE Protection Equipment			
Level A	**Level B**	**Level C**	**Level D**
Airtight seals with SCUBA or airline	No airtight seals	Half mask acceptable; hard hat optional	Standard precautions appropriate to the circumstances

FIG 14-3   The Occupational Safety and Health Administration (OSHA) defines personal protective equipment for the four levels of hazardous exposure. (**A, B, C** *courtesy DuPont Personal Protection, Wilmington, Del;* **D** *courtesy Kappler, Guntersville, Ariz.*)

BOX 14-6 | Potential Hazards at the Scene of a Disaster

- Downed power lines
- Smoke/toxic gases
- Debris that can result in trauma
- Fractured/leaking gas lines
- Fire resulting in burns
- Structural collapse
- Blood and other body fluids
- Inclement weather
- Hazardous materials
- Nuclear, biological, or chemical exposure

- Flooding and the threat of drowning
- Radiation exposure
- Explosion, particularly secondary explosions
- Snipers
- Darkness
- Infection
- High-velocity projectiles and the pressure wave after an explosion
- Becoming incapacitated and unable to protect yourself or your patient

---

Chaos is common in every disaster. Chaos is manageable, but it is difficult to control. In the event of a disaster many "worried well" (injured individuals who are able to transport themselves to a health care facility or even frightened individuals who fear contamination) will leave a disaster scene. Within 30 minutes these individuals will overrun the hospital nearest the disaster scene, leaving the most highly injured individuals at the site of the disaster. Added to the chaos at the health care facility is the responsibility to care for sick and injured individuals already admitted to the hospital or emergency department.

First responders must quickly distinguish between actual victims with exposure to the weapon (chemical, biological, or nuclear) of mass destruction that led to the MCI. Regardless of the lethality of any biological, nuclear, or chemical terrorist attack, the "shock" to the community and society will often serve the intended purpose of the terrorist. You also need to recognize the worried well as victims because they are obviously suffering fear and anxiety. However, do not let them distract you from the job of rescuing as many potential survivors as possible. Quickly differentiating worried well from actual injured patients will prevent wasting valuable time. Furthermore, it will help alleviate community-wide hysteria and unnecessary, costly, and potentially humiliating decontamination procedures (Croddy and Ackerman, 2007).

Also, consider the security of a health care facility in disaster planning. Health care providers offer a valuable resource and cannot spend time maintaining the security of the health care facility. The local police in collaboration with agency administration and security personnel are responsible to maximize the protection of lives and assets of the health care agency. Keep security officers informed as to the incident history, current status, and potential problems. As part of this protection, roadblocks, checkpoints, and facility lockdown procedures are often put in place.

Triage, Treat, and Evacuate

Triage is the sorting of individuals by the seriousness of their condition and the likelihood of their survival. There are many different modern triage systems to classify, tag, and treat victims of MCI. These systems use a variety of symbols, colors, and other devices to classify individuals as to the need for treatment. The disaster triage model described here is the MASS triage system adopted by the NDLS Family of Courses (AMA, 2007). Mass casualty triage is an initial sorting of victims into groups. Victims are then individually assessed, sorted into "ID-me" victim categories, and evacuated for treatment. Fig. 14-4 provides an overview of this triage system. Color-coded teams provide a systematic response. The ultimate goal is to move, assess, sort, and send victims for treatment. The initial assessment is a very crude form of assessment, yet health

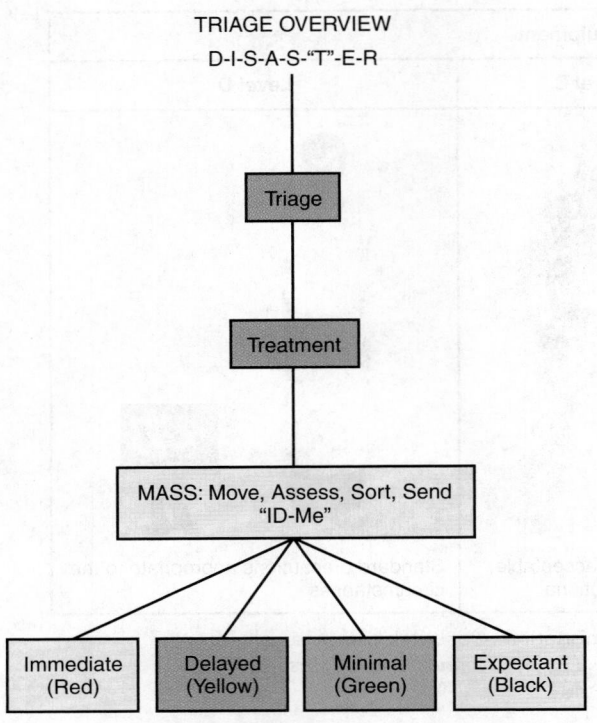

TRIAGE OVERVIEW
D-I-S-A-S-"T"-E-R

Triage

Treatment

MASS: Move, Assess, Sort, Send
"ID-Me"

Immediate (Red) · Delayed (Yellow) · Minimal (Green) · Expectant (Black)

FIG 14-4   MASS triage system.

care providers remain constantly vigilant because some victims will quickly deteriorate and require immediate health care.

At a disaster, step one of this triage system, "move," requires victims who are able to walk to move to a specified collection area. Personnel identify these patients as minimally injured and requiring the least amount of care. A brief screening of these individuals will reveal that their airway, breathing, and circulation are intact; their mental status is intact to the extent that they are able to follow directions; and they are not likely to have low blood pressure or have difficulty breathing. Although you will constantly monitor this group, the individuals in the green or minimal group are those who will undergo formal individualized medical assessment last. These individuals will probably wait more than 2 hours for treatment without immediate risk. By managing this group first, (1) it is less likely individuals will transport themselves to the nearest hospital, thus immediately overwhelming that hospital, which needs to be used for the most injured victims, and therefore (2) reserve limited hospital resources for the more injured individuals.

The "move" phase also allows rescue workers to identify those individuals who can follow commands but are not able to walk. This group becomes the yellow or delayed group. Some of these victims have injuries with systemic effects but are not currently experiencing shock and will likely withstand a 2-hour wait. These injuries vary from low blood pressure to broken bones or lost limbs. Rescue workers recognize that this group is at greater risk than the green group and the classification is not based on individual assessment. The injuries of these individuals may quickly deteriorate, requiring you to triage them to a more critical group.

The second step of the triage process, "assess," allows rescue workers to focus on the remaining victims, who are presumed more critically injured. This group is now the red, immediate, group. Rescuers immediately assess these individuals and provide potentially lifesaving interventions focusing priorities on airway, breathing, circulation, mental status, and level of consciousness (LOC). As you assess individuals in this group, you may restore them into

either the delayed or expectant group. For example, an individual does not respond to early commands because of a hearing loss, and thus on individual assessment you determine that the individual fits in a less critically injured group. Within this group the goal is to obtain an accurate count of the most severely injured victims who still have a chance of survival if proper treatment is delivered quickly (AMA, 2005). Similarly the dead and individuals with serious injuries that cannot be treated quickly necessitate a "black tag." This places an enormous emotional toll on triage personnel when you place a black tag on a living human, even though this action is needed to identify the greatest number of individuals likely to survive an MCI. Disaster nursing differs from general nursing because the focus shifts from caring for the sickest people first to saving the greatest number of lives (NeSmith, 2006). Resources are allocated to a broader number of people with a greater chance of living rather than the critically injured with a poor chance of survival consuming the resources.

During the "assess" triage process, personnel actually begin the "sort" task. Using the "ID-me" system, you place mnemonic tags on individuals to identify priority need for care (e.g., red—immediate, yellow—delayed, green—minimal, and black—expectant). Box 14-7 provides examples of how to sort victims based on injury.

During the third step of the triage process, you sort or triage an individual into a group and securely tie a tag to the person's body. Do not tie a tag to the clothing because clothing is removed for decontamination, evaluation, or treatment. At this point workers obtain an accurate count of victims in the red group. You send this information to the incident commander, who will alert receiving hospitals of the expected number of casualties they will receive. These victims are then transported to receiving hospitals. You can then reassess victims remaining from the other triage groups and retriage them.

The final step in the MASS triage system is "send." Rescue workers evacuate, transport, or release all living patients as soon as possible. Immediate (red) patients are first, then delayed (yellow), followed by minimal (green), and then expectant (black). The dead are not initially moved. Movement of these individuals is the responsibility of law enforcement officials.

EVIDENCE-BASED PRACTICE

When the first plane hit the World Trade Center in 2001, calls overwhelmed hospital telephone systems. Collapse of the World Trade Center towers included destruction of a cell phone tower and a local telephone company. Further compounding the problem for those with generator backup systems or Blackberries was that many resource numbers had failed to be updated (Magee, 2005). After the Madrid, Spain, terrorist bombing in 2004, the CDC developed a disaster plan designed to treat 300 injured patients for up to 72 hours (National Center for Injury Prevention and Control, 2007). This plan includes the following:

• The need for maintenance of updated call lists and identification of staff by proximity to the hospital
• A centralized database with staff competency skills (e.g., Advanced Cardiac Life Support certification) so staff are used efficiently
• Names of retired or unemployed staff
• A plan for hospitals to implement a drill with emergency medical services (EMS) at least once a year in order to prepare for an MCI

On an individual basis, the American Red Cross suggests that families create a plan that not only identifies where they will meet

BOX 14-7 | ID-Me—Assess, Treat, and Send

Immediate (Red)	Delayed (Yellow)	Minimal (Green)	Expectant (Black)
• Unconscious or unresponsive • Altered mental status • Experiencing hypoxia or near-hypoxia • Chest pain • Chest wounds • Full-thickness burns over 20% to 60% of the body • Uncontrollable bleeding • Amputations above elbow or knee • Rapid or weak pulse • Open abdominal wounds	• Deep lacerations • Open fractures with controlled bleeding and strong pulses • Multiple fractures • Finger amputations • Abdominal injuries with stable vital signs • Closed head injuries without altered level of consciousness	• Abrasions • Contusions • Sprains • Minor lacerations • No apparent injuries • Other injuries of similar severity	• Victims still alive but so severely injured as to have little chance of survival • Victims who have died

in the event of a disaster, but also specifies a contact person. The contact person should live out-of-state, and all members of the family should know the contact person's phone number in case of an evacuation (Johnson, 2007).

Lessons were learned following Hurricane Katrina. E-mail was a reliable method of communication, and therefore it is recommended that e-mail addresses be maintained for hospital staff (Ellis, 2007). When it becomes necessary to evacuate patients urgently in the case of a storm, each patient should be given a copy of his or her medication record in a waterproof bag. Other lessons learned during Katrina include the difficulty some staff had passing through roadblocks, so now it is recommended that all staff keep their hospital ID with them. And finally, the need for diversional activities to reduce stress deserves important consideration. Musical instruments or a DVD player and movies are some items that staff could share.

CULTURAL CONSIDERATIONS

To provide the highest standard of care while in a disaster situation it is essential to acknowledge the local culture. A lack of cultural consideration of the victim leads to the impression of insensitivity and racism by emergency responders (Clemons, 2006). Regardless of cultural differences and perhaps language difficulties, it is important to convey compassion and to work closely with people within the community for disaster recovery. As noted with bereavement counseling, existing support networks are often more effective.

Emergency responders need to support them rather than further disrupt these networks (Deeny and McFetridge, 2005). Some disaster events result in a changed culture for individuals, families, and communities.

Skill Performance Guidelines

When considering all forms of disaster, there are basic guidelines for a nurse or other health care provider to follow:
1 Rapid response is crucial. Know your agency's policies for disaster response and the specific role each member must perform.
2 Health care providers are responsible for ensuring that the contaminated, the injured, and those concerned about potential exposure to a hazardous agent are medically treated in an efficient manner.
3 The potential for public alarm and major disruption of everyday life is enormous because of widespread fear of the unknown. Know crisis intervention and stress management techniques.
4 A health care agency such as a hospital is part of a community. Hospitals and other agencies need to work with their communities in developing and instituting plans for notification and communication.
5 In an MCI the majority of people will self-triage and go directly to a local hospital, bypassing triage and treatment whether contaminated, exposed, or not. Plans are needed to transfer patients to other medical facilities.

SKILL 14-1   Care of a Patient After Biological Exposure

Bioterrorism or a biological attack is the result of the release of a biological agent into a specified environment. Some biological attacks are unannounced or covert and the onset of symptoms is delayed by an incubation period, the time between exposure and onset of symptoms. Differing biological agents have incubation periods from 1 or 2 days to several weeks. During incubation periods, some of these biological agents may be transmitted as the infected patient exposes others. The mode of transmission of the biological agent determines the severity of the disaster. Recognition of bioterrorism is a challenge because early signs and symptoms mimic the flu or

produce a rash mistaken for a viral illness (Fig. 14-5). Sometimes several biological agents are disseminated at the same time, further confusing the issue. In order to understand how to protect yourself from becoming a victim, you need to understand the mode of transmission and precautions to take for biosafety (Table 14-1, p. 359).

Delegation Considerations

The skill of assessment of a patient exposed to a biological agent cannot be delegated to nursing assistive personnel (NAP). The nurse directs the NAP to:

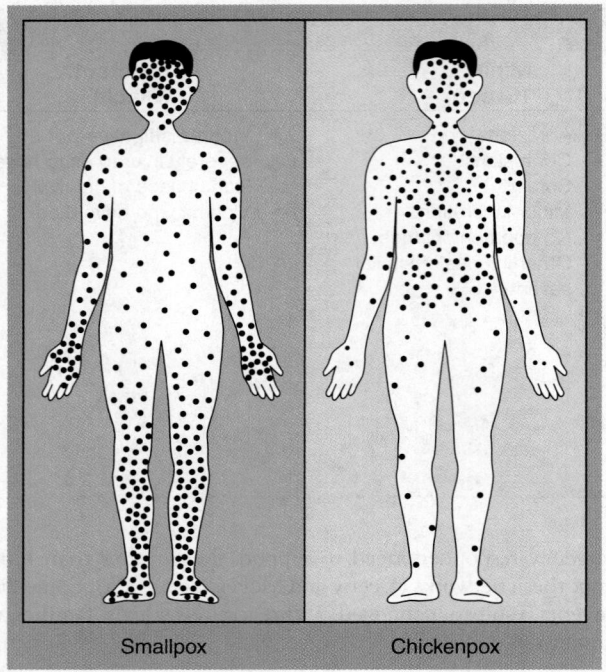

Smallpox | Chickenpox

FIG 14-5 Differences in distribution of smallpox versus chickenpox. (*Courtesy Centers for Disease Control and Prevention.*)

- Use appropriate PPE to prevent exposure.
- Use proper techniques for handling a body after death to prevent contamination.

Equipment

Choice of equipment depends on the route of transmission of the infecting agent. The following is a general list of supplies needed in the event of release of the most contagious biological agents. Not all of the following equipment will be needed in all situations.

- ❑ Biohazard bags with label
- ❑ Soap and water
- ❑ 0.5% diluted bleach or Environmental Protection Agency (EPA)–approved germicidal agent
- ❑ Negative-pressure room (high-efficiency particulate air [HEPA] filtration may be required) with anteroom
- ❑ Clean gloves
- ❑ Gown
- ❑ Shoe covers
- ❑ Head covers
- ❑ Mask
- ❑ Standard face mask
- ❑ N95 mask
- ❑ Face shield
- ❑ Equipment for physical examination

STEP	RATIONALE
ASSESSMENT	
1 Conduct a focused health history and physical examination (e.g., pulmonary assessment—oxygen saturation, lung sounds, sputum character; cardiac—heart sounds; neurological—Glasgow Coma Scale, reflexes). Review history of patient's presenting symptoms, and determine pattern.	Symptom identification and clustering of data is the first step to accurately determining exposure to type of biological agent and patient's response.
2 Measure patient's vital signs.	Provides baseline to later evaluate patient's response to therapy.
3 Review results of diagnostic tests, and consult with physician or primary care provider.	Initial signs and symptoms of exposure to biological agent suggest common disorders (e.g., flu). Further review of diagnostic findings helps to rule out other common disorders.
4 Assess the patient for health risks (e.g., history of heart disease, pulmonary disease, cancer) that complicate the effects of exposure to a biological agent.	Patients with preexisting medical conditions often require additional treatment or are at greater risk for death.
5 Stay calm, and assess patient's immediate psychological response after exposure. Some patients will present with dissociative symptoms (e.g., feeling as though "not there" or sensing everything is outside of the person): disorientation, depression, anxiety, psychosis, and an inability to care for self. Even without direct exposure to a biological agent many individuals, spurred by feelings of fear and doom, will present for emergency services.	Aids the nurse to be able to provide appropriate crisis intervention and stress management. Remaining calm and projecting confidence while assessing individuals for clinical symptoms versus feelings of panic will go a long way toward reducing the anxiety of the ill and worried well as they experience the general sense of panic associated with a biological event.
6 Identify resources available (e.g., critical incident stress debriefing teams, counselors, psychiatric/mental health nurse practitioners).	Expert resources will help assess extent of psychological impact of disaster.

> **Critical Decision Point**   *You should consider a biological event when large numbers of ill persons present who have unexplained yet similar symptoms; when there are unexplained deaths, particularly among young and healthy populations; when there is an unusual pattern associated with the symptoms (e.g., geographical, season, patient population); when the patient fails to respond to traditional therapy; when a single patient presents with symptoms suggestive of an uncommon agent (e.g., anthrax or smallpox). Once you suspect a biological event, notify incident command immediately.*

STEP	RATIONALE

NURSING DIAGNOSES

- Acute confusion
- Acute pain
- Anxiety/fear
- Decreased cardiac output
- Impaired gas exchange

- Impaired oral mucous membrane
- Impaired skin integrity
- Impaired swallowing
- Ineffective airway clearance
- Nausea

- Post-trauma syndrome
- Risk for imbalanced body temperature
- Risk for imbalanced fluid volume
- Risk for peripheral neurovascular dysfunction

Individualize related factors based on patient's condition or needs.

PLANNING

1 Expected outcomes following completion of procedure:
- Patient will be comforted.

- Patient's vital signs will return to baseline.

- Patient's work of breathing will decrease.
- Patient's skin integrity will return to baseline.

- Patient's LOC will return to baseline.

- Patient's mental health status will return to a pretrauma level of functioning.

2 Dispense timely and accurate information, including an accurate description of the agent patient is exposed to and implications, to the patient and family.

In some cases, care is only palliative, with comfort as the focus. Do not underestimate the value of COMFORT as CARE.

When there are no underlying medical conditions and *if* the patient's disease process is responsive to treatment (when available), vital signs will return to normal, taking days or weeks.

Indicates improved gas exchange and cardiac output.

Antibiotic and antitoxin therapy will aid in resolution/healing of lesions over time.

Treatment measures restore neurological function and oxygenation status.

Crisis intervention is successful in reducing patient's anxiety, fear, and dissociative symptoms.

Information helps to relieve anxiety and fear.

IMPLEMENTATION

1 Perform hand hygiene.

2 Institute transmission-based isolation precautions (see Chapter 7). (Refer to Table 14-1, p. 359, for mode of transmission of category A biological agents.) Use strict isolation with smallpox because of its communicability from person to person. Use airborne precautions, contact precautions, and a negative pressure room for patients suspected of having smallpox (Siegel, and others, 2007).

3 Decontaminate if indicated. If you suspect anthrax, have the patient remove clothing and place in a labeled plastic biohazard bag. Do not have the patient pull clothing off over the head, but rather cut off clothing. Instruct the patient to shower thoroughly using soap and water.

4 Administer appropriate antibiotics and/or antitoxins.

5 Administer immunizations (e.g., smallpox).

6 Administer fluid and nutrition therapy.

7 Administer oxygen therapy.

8 Provide supportive care (e.g., comfort measures, including pain management).

Reduces transmission of microorganisms.

Reduces transmission of microorganisms and the likelihood of additional secondary sites of contamination.

Handle clothing minimally to avoid agitation. Showering with soap and water will aid in decontamination and reducing exposure (CDC, April, 2000).

Various biological agents are commonly treated with ciprofloxacin and/or doxycycline (e.g., anthrax, plague, typhoidal tularemia), and botulism requires supportive care and use of an antitoxin. For some viral pathogens, treatment is only supportive.

In the event smallpox is the biological weapon, the best treatment is prevention by immunization with vaccinia vaccine before the onset of symptoms. Vaccination within 3 days of exposure will completely prevent the disease or significantly reduce its effect. Vaccination 4 to 7 days post exposure offers some protection from disease or will decrease the severity of disease (CDC, 2007a).

Biological agents commonly cause gastrointestinal (GI) disturbances that sometimes result in dehydration.

Various biological agents (e.g., pulmonary anthrax) commonly cause respiratory symptoms that will result in an altered gas exchange.

Some victims of a biological attack will not survive; palliative care is essential (see Chapter 16).

STEP	RATIONALE
9 Identify all patient contacts (names, addresses, phone numbers) in the emergency department waiting room.	All patient contacts need to be identified for proper follow-up by the public health department. Often patients will self-triage and transport to the emergency department (Auf der Heide, 2006).
10 Counsel patient and family on acute and potential long-term psychological effects of exposure. Offer access to trained counselors. Support the survivors of a disaster by identifying resources available.	Reaction of patients will include shock, fear, and immobilization. Long-term psychological effects will possibly arise without proper counseling. Social support networks foster coping in the days following a disaster event (Mitchell and others, 2005).

Critical Decision Point   *Collaborate with the physician and other rescue workers for an ongoing plan for managing the patient exposed to a biological agent. You will need to do this while caring for other patients who are already present in the health care agency seeking care for illness unrelated to the current MCI.*

EVALUATION

1 Observe for improved airway maintenance, breathing, circulation, level of consciousness, and neurological functioning.	Evaluates the patient's response to available treatment and/or supportive care.
2 Evaluate vital signs.	Evaluates patient's response to treatment.
3 Inspect the condition of patient's skin; note character of remaining lesions.	Evaluates patient's response to antibiotic therapy.
4 Ask patient, "How do you feel right now?" Check level of orientation and ability to conduct conversation.	Evaluates the patient for changes that suggest either improvement or deterioration of psychological status.

Unexpected Outcomes

1   Patient's physical symptoms progress despite appropriate treatment.

2   Patient becomes more anxious or delusional or develops suicidal ideations.

3   Patient death.

4   Secondary contamination of rescue workers.

Related Interventions

- Notify physician or nurse in charge.
- Continue to provide comfort care.
- Notify mental health treatment team.
- Remain calm, offer reassurance, and protect self and others from physical harm.
- Continue to provide comfort measures.
- When handling bodies, take into account continued risk for contamination; make sure everyone is fully informed regarding proper procedure.
- Rescue workers immediately report symptoms to a physician or nursing supervisor.

Recording and Reporting

- Report suspected cases of a biological incident to physician or ED officer. In the event of an ED exposure to a communicable disease, the department will be locked down immediately. Public health officials (e.g., the emergency officer) will determine if the hospital should be locked down.
- Create and utilize checklists that can be used quickly in a disaster event to record specific data regarding patient status and response to treatment and/or comfort measures.
- Report any unexpected outcome to physician or nurse in charge.

Teaching Considerations

- Preparation for an MCI will go a long way toward preventing casualties and chaos. Public education of the likelihood of a mass casualty biological event is necessary and includes information about types of biological agents, mode of transmission, symptoms, treatment, and locations of shelters and disaster treatment sites.
- Encourage families to prepare for the unexpected (see Home Care Considerations).

Pediatric Considerations

- "Children are vulnerable to the stresses of evacuation, which include living in shelters and losing their homes, schools, parents, pets, and loved ones" (Bernardo, 2001).
- Some disasters result in relocation of children and their families to new homes. When this new home is located in an area of differing culture, customs, or other life patterns, the child is further exposed to stress (Bernardo, 2001).
- Children are particularly vulnerable to environmental toxins because (1) they are closer to the ground and thus more likely to inhale the toxin, (2) they have an increased respiratory rate, (3) their organ systems tend to be more sensitive than those of adults, and (4) they have more years of life expectancy over which to develop complications from the toxic exposure (Langan and James, 2005).
- Children are vulnerable to communicable diseases and more likely to develop infections following a disaster due to exposure to pollutants and waterborne and airborne infectious agents (Brandenburg, 2007).
- Avoid separating parents from their children, because their presence is reassuring to the child (Plum and Veneema, 2007).

- The death of a child as a result of a disaster is always traumatic; if a parent wants to be present during pediatric resuscitation, ideally you should allow it; make sure a nurse is available to explain to the parent what is happening.

Gerontological Considerations

- Under disaster conditions, triage older adults according to injuries, not age.
- Because the older adult often has several concurrent illnesses, possible exposure to a biological agent will often worsen those conditions and result in the need for more immediate care than an initial triage may suggest.

Home Care Considerations

- Preparing for a biological disaster
  - Assemble a disaster kit before disaster strikes. The Federal Emergency Management Agency (FEMA) and the American Red Cross offer free literature on establishing home care preparedness (Boxes 14-8 and 14-9, p. 361).
  - Individuals with special needs (e.g., hearing impairment, impaired mobility, individuals without vehicles, individuals with special diets) will require additional planning to be prepared in the event of a disaster.
  - One of the most important steps to prepare for a disaster is to have a household disaster plan.
  - In case of a disaster many schools and employers have disaster plans; individuals need to familiarize themselves with these plans along with their own home disaster plan.
  - Post emergency telephone numbers by the telephone, and teach children how and when to call 9-1-1.
  - Family members need to have a mechanism in place to ensure they are able to stay in contact in case they are separated (e.g., a designated meeting place, a friend to call to notify when separated from the family).
  - An individual of the family needs to know how to turn off water, gas, and electricity in case of a disaster because emergency management personnel often make this request of civilians in the event of a disaster.
  - Install a HEPA filter in the return duct of the furnace. These filters will filter out most biological agents but will not filter out chemical agents (FEMA, 2007).
  - Have as many members of the family as possible take a first aid class to reduce the risk of complications from a biological infectious agent during a disaster. Individuals need to maintain a first aid kit in an accessible location in the home and know what type of PPE will protect the family from secondary exposure.
- When biological disaster becomes a reality
  - Listen to the radio or television for instructions. However, limit media exposure to reduce reliving of the event and further traumatization. Children and older adults are prone to the emotional stressors of such continuous reporting, which will lead to a sense of helplessness (Langan and James, 2005).
  - Remain isolated, and advise friends and relatives not to visit if family members are symptomatic.
  - Use the appropriate PPE needed to protect the family; this will possibly include sheltering-in-place.
  - Maintain strict hand hygiene for both well and symptomatic family members after using the bathroom, before eating and drinking, and after contact with pets.
  - Wear gloves (vinyl or latex) when in contact with a sick individual's blood or body fluids.
  - When a sick individual's symptoms worsen, transport to the nearest designated hospital.
  - Monitor the temperature of symptomatic individuals. Provide them with plenty of food and fluids.
  - Change the sick person's clothing and bed linens frequently; wash them separately from those of other family members, using any commercial detergent.
  - Disinfect any surfaces the symptomatic person comes in contact with, using an appropriate disinfectant (e.g., Lysol), especially when soiled by blood or other body fluids.
  - The caregiver's highest priority is to avoid becoming a victim. This individual needs to get plenty of rest, drink fluids frequently, and eat a healthy diet. If the caregiver develops symptoms, obtain the appropriate medical care immediately.

TABLE 14-1 Summary of Selected Class A Biological Warfare Agents

| Disease/Infectious Agent | Form and Incubation/Onset of Symptoms | Untreated Course of Disease | | Probable Route of Contamination for Use as a Biological Warfare Agent | Treatment of Mass Casualties | Prophylaxis/ Vaccine |
		Early-Onset Symptoms	Late-Onset Symptoms			
Bacterial Biological Agents						
Anthrax *Bacillus anthracis*, a gram-positive bacillus that can remain stable in spore form	Inhalation or pulmonary (usually within 48 hours but may incubate for up to 60 days)	Febrile flulike symptoms (malaise, low-grade fever, dry cough, and headache)	Severe respiratory distress, hemodynamic failure, and death	Aerosol; no person-to-person transmission	Ciprofloxacin or doxycycline	Ciprofloxacin or, if susceptible, doxycycline; vaccine available, but in short supply
	Cutaneous (1-12 days)	Local urticaria; painless papular lesions usually located on head, forearms, or hands	Papular lesions become vesicular, later developing black eschar and edema	Person-to-person transmission with direct contact with skin lesions		

Continued

TABLE 14-1 Summary of Selected Class A Biological Warfare Agents—cont'd

Disease/Infectious Agent	Form and Incubation/Onset of Symptoms	Untreated Course of Disease		Probable Route of Contamination for Use as a Biological Warfare Agent	Treatment of Mass Casualties	Prophylaxis/ Vaccine
		Early-Onset Symptoms	Late-Onset Symptoms			
Anthrax—cont'd	Gastrointestinal (1-7 days)	Abdominal pain, nausea, vomiting, and diarrhea	Gastrointestinal bleeding, fever; usually followed by toxic sepsis and death	Contaminated food and/or water		
Plague Acute, severe bacterial infection secondary to a gram-negative bacillus, *Yersinia pestis*	Bubonic Onset of symptoms dependent upon route of transmission (1-6 days)	Swollen, tender lymph nodes (most notable femoral and inguinal), high fever, rapid pulse	Hypotension, extreme exhaustion, death	Aerosol and then human-to-human by droplet inhalation	Ciprofloxacin or doxycycline	Ciprofloxacin or doxycycline; no vaccine available at the present time
	Pneumonic (1-6 days)	High fever, chills, tachycardia, headache	Fulminate pneumonia (foamy hemoptysis, tachypnea, and dyspnea), sepsis, and death			
Botulism Anaerobic gram-positive bacillus that produces a potent muscle-paralyzing neurotoxin	Food borne (12-36 hours)	Nausea, vomiting, diarrhea	Symmetrical cranial nerve paralysis, descending flaccid paralysis (progressive paralysis of arms, respiratory muscles, and legs), and death	Contaminated food	Passive immunization (antitoxin); supportive care	Passive immunization (antitoxin); antitoxin available in short supply
	Inhalational (2 hours-8 days)	No fever, no changes in mental status	Symmetrical cranial nerve paralysis, descending flaccid paralysis (progressive paralysis of arms, respiratory muscles, and legs), and death	Inhalation of aerosolized toxin		
Typhoidal tularemia *Francisella tularensis*, an extremely infectious bacteria	Contaminated water, food or via aerosol distribution (1-14 days)	Flulike symptoms (headache, cough, fever and chills, malaise)	Pharyngeal ulcers, pleuritic chest pain, pneumonia, pericarditis, respiratory failure, sepsis, and death	Inhalation of aerosolized bacteria	Ciprofloxacin or doxycycline	Ciprofloxacin or doxycycline; vaccine available, only limited supply; vaccine offers incomplete protection

Major Viral Biological Agent of Concern—Smallpox

Disease/Infectious Agent	Form and Incubation/Onset of Symptoms	Early-Onset Symptoms	Late-Onset Symptoms	Probable Route of Contamination for Use as a Biological Warfare Agent	Treatment of Mass Casualties	Prophylaxis/ Vaccine
Smallpox Variola virus	Distribution via airborne droplets, aerosols, and fomites (7-17 days; weaponized smallpox when delivered aerosolized has an incubation period of only 3-5 days)	Acute viral symptoms (high fever, myalgia, headache, and backache)	Continued viral symptoms, high fever, prostration, and synchronous onset of rash progressing from macules to papules to vesicles, and eschar formation. The vesicles are more abundant on the extremities and face and all develop at the same time; pustules appear on the palms of hands and soles of feet (unlike chickenpox)	Transmitted person to person by large droplets; therefore spread may be by inhalation of aerosolized virus, oral secretions, by infected human vector exposure, or by exposure to contaminated objects	Supportive therapy only (ventilator)	None; vaccine available in short supply

BOX 14-8	Basic Disaster Supply Kit

- Water: 1 gallon of water per person per day (minimum of 3-day supply)
- Food: minimum of 3-day supply
- Manual can opener
- Plastic resealable bags
- Utility knife
- Disposable cups, plates, and utensils
- Several flashlights
- Battery-powered radio or TV
- Fresh batteries
- Matches in a waterproof container
- First-aid kit
- One complete change of clothing and footwear for each person
- Blankets
- Sanitation and hygiene items (hand sanitizer, toilet paper, etc.)
- Small fire extinguisher
- Shut-off valve wrench

Additional Considerations
- Items for infants, seniors, or disabled persons
- Pet-care items
- Entertainment items for small children
- An extra set of keys and IDs
- Copies of medical prescriptions in plastic sealable bags

Additional Supplies for Sheltering-in-Place (in the Event of a Chemical or Radiological Hazard)
- Roll of duct tape and scissors
- Plastic sheeting precut to fit shelter-in-place room openings (10 square feet per person will provide sufficient air to prevent carbon dioxide buildup for up to 5 hours)
- Additional supplies in preparation for a pandemic flu: Have a 2-week supply of basic items so that you can survive without outside help or going out in public.
- Thermometer, nonaspirin pain reliever, prescription medication
- Household-cleaning supplies (disinfectant sprays, bleach, etc.)
- Extra bath and hand soap

Data from American Red Cross and Centers for Disease Control and Prevention: *Preparedness today: what you need to do*, http://www.redcross.org/preparedness/cdc_english/kit.asp.

BOX 14-9	Suggested Foods for a Disaster Supply Kit

- Ready-to-eat canned meats, fruits, and vegetables
- Protein or fruit bars
- Peanut butter
- Dry cereal or granola
- Nuts
- Dried fruit
- Canned juices
- Nonperishable pasteurized milk
- Comfort/stress foods

Data from American Red Cross and Centers for Disease Control and Prevention: *Preparedness today: what you need to do*, http://www.redcross.org/preparedness/cdc_english/kit.asp.

SKILL 14-2 Care of a Patient After Chemical Exposure

A chemical disaster is the dispersal of a toxic chemical agent into the environment. The mechanism of dispersal is not always known. In fact, the dispersal mechanism such as an explosion or fire will possibly be a secondary terrorist attack designed to create greater fatalities. Explosions spread a toxic chemical in uncontrolled directions, creating more victims. Symptoms from chemical exposure are usually apparent within minutes, but some are delayed up to 24 hours. Early recognition of a chemical event is a priority because you will need to administer many chemical antidotes quickly. Toxic chemical incidents, like biological events, are often unannounced or overt. Terrorists often intend for chemical agents to cause mass casualties and induce fear and/or mass hysteria.

Chemical events are generally confined to small areas, though larger dispersal of these agents may occur (e.g., via a crop duster). The nature and scale of contamination depends on the state of the agent used (e.g., gas versus liquid), characteristics of the chemical used (e.g., heavy or lighter than air), and where the event occurs (e.g., indoors, where ventilation systems affect dispersal, or out-

doors, where wind and velocity affect speed and direction of dispersal). For safety reasons, rescue workers should be upwind and uphill from a toxic chemical disaster scene to avoid exposure. The exception is when cyanide gas has been released. Cyanide is lighter than air and will thus travel uphill. It has the unique smell of bitter almonds. If you detect the smell, evacuate the area immediately, though exposure may have already occurred (CDC, 2004).

Because symptoms are almost immediate, it is important to evacuate victims as quickly as possible from the contaminated zone to a decontamination zone. Special respiratory and skin PPE prevents contamination of rescue workers. In addition, before decontamination, victims are a potential source of contamination for rescue workers. It is imperative that the nurse protect against toxic chemical contamination when in contact with a contaminated patient. Secondary contamination is high with toxic chemical incidents. Table 14-2 summarizes common chemical warfare agents, presenting symptoms, and untreated course of exposure.

TABLE 14-2 | Summary of Selected Chemical Warfare Agents

Chemical Agent	Onset of Symptoms	Untreated Course of Chemical Exposure
"Lethal" agents—nerve agents (tabun, sarin, soman, and VX)	Symptoms are generally immediate.	Pinpoint pupils and shortly thereafter salivation, runny nose, dyspnea, chest tightness, nausea, muscle twitching, coma, seizures, and death
"Blood" agents—hydrogen cyanide	Rapid onset of symptoms though cyanide poisoning is often associated with the smell of bitter almonds.	Death due to asphyxiation
"Blister" agents—mustard and lewisite	Symptoms may be immediate or delayed.	Skin irritation and blistering
"Choking" agents—phosgene and chlorine	Symptoms can be immediate or delayed up to 24 hours.	Coughing, choking, and disruption in pulmonary function that can lead to death

The rapid chemical decontamination of victims of a toxic chemical incident is more important than determining the exact toxic chemical. When decontamination is necessary, trained personnel are required. Decontamination is either gross or technical, which generally occurs at the scene. The hospital also provides decontamination when a contaminated individual presents for treatment. The nurse and all other health care personnel need to use appropriate precautions to avoid becoming victims.

Delegation Considerations
The skill of assessment of a patient exposed to a biological agent cannot be delegated to NAP. The nurse directs the NAP to:
- Use appropriate PPE to prevent exposure.
- Use techniques for handling a body after death to prevent contamination.

Equipment
The following is a general list of supplies needed in the event of release of the most toxic chemical agents:
- ❏ Decontamination room or area (adult decontamination rooms may not meet the needs of children requiring decontamination; decontamination areas for ambulatory victims will not meet the needs of those who are not ambulatory)
- ❏ Scissors or a tool to cut off clothing
- ❏ Biohazard bags with labels
- ❏ Large volumes of water, decontamination shower (Fig. 14-6)
- ❏ Appropriate PPE
- ❏ Equipment for physical examination

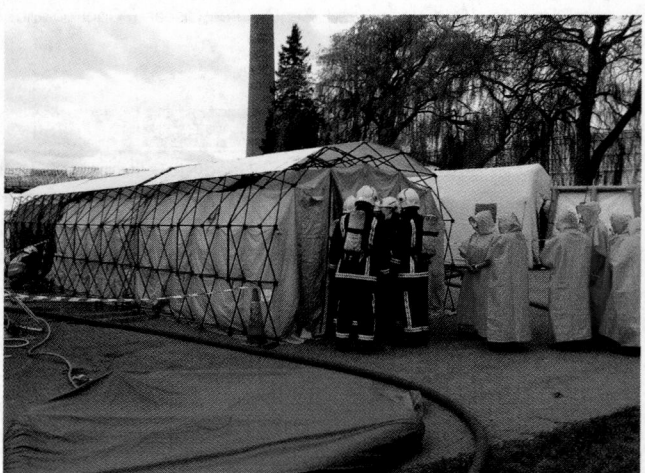

FIG 14-6   Inflatable decontamination shower for ambulatory victims. (*Courtesy Professional Protection Systems, Ltd.*)

STEP	RATIONALE

ASSESSMENT

STEP	RATIONALE
1 Assess the patient's symptoms. Perform appropriate focused physical examination (see Skill 14-1).	Symptom identification and clustering of data accurately identifies patient's problem and response.
2 Observe for presence of liquid on patient's skin or clothing and odor (e.g., chlorine).	Common conditions present when chemical exposure has occurred.
3 Assess the patient for preexisting medical conditions that will complicate the effects of the toxic chemical exposure.	Patients with preexisting medical conditions will likely require additional treatment and sometimes are at greater risk for death.

Critical Decision Point   *Consider a toxic chemical event when large numbers of ill persons present who have unexplained yet similar symptoms. The primary objective for initial care is decontamination, the process used to remove harmful contaminants from the surface of the skin. You achieve this by removing clothing, by scrubbing the skin, and by hydrolysis, a process of chemical dilution using large volumes of water.*

STEP	RATIONALE
4 Calmly assess patient's immediate psychological response following exposure. Some patients present with dissociative symptoms, disorientation, depression, anxiety, psychosis, and inability to care for self. Even without direct exposure to a chemical agent many individuals, spurred by feelings of fear and doom, will present for emergency services and quickly overwhelm available emergency services.	Aids the nurse in being able to provide appropriate crisis intervention and stress management. Remaining calm and projecting confidence versus showing feelings of panic will go a long way toward reducing the anxiety of the ill and worried well as they experience the general sense of panic associated with chemical exposure.

STEP	RATIONALE
5 Identify resources available (e.g., critical incident stress debriefing teams, counselors, psychiatric/mental health nurse practitioners).	• Expert resources will assess extent of psychological impact of disorders.

NURSING DIAGNOSES

• Acute confusion	• Impaired oral mucous membrane	• Nausea
• Acute pain	• Impaired skin integrity	• Post-trauma syndrome
• Anxiety/fear	• Impaired swallowing	• Risk for imbalanced fluid volume
• Decreased cardiac output	• Impaired verbal communication	• Risk for peripheral neurovascular
• Impaired gas exchange	• Ineffective airway clearance	dysfunction

Individualize related factors based on patient's condition or needs.

PLANNING

1 Expected outcomes following completion of procedure:	
• Patient will be comforted.	Because of the fatal nature of many chemical agents, the only care available is palliative.
• Patient's vital signs will return to baseline.	When there are no underlying medical conditions and *if* the patient's condition is responsive to treatment (when available), vital signs will return to normal within days or weeks.
• Patient's work of breathing will decrease.	Indicates improved gas exchange and cardiac output.
• Patient's skin integrity will return to baseline.	Minimizing exposure of skin to chemical agent will reduce severity and extent of skin lesions.
• Patient's LOC will return to baseline.	Neurological stability is achieved by minimizing exposure to chemical and giving antitoxin quickly.
• Patient's mental health status will return to a pretrauma level of functioning.	Crisis intervention is successful in reducing patient's anxiety, fear, and dissociative symptoms.
2 Explain care to patient and family, including decontamination and treatment. Explain your role, orient to location and activities to perform, explain what patient has experienced, and ask, "How are you feeling right now?" Assure them that a medical professional will see them shortly.	Information helps to calm anxiety and fear.

IMPLEMENTATION

1 Perform hand hygiene.	Reduces transmission of and injury from toxic chemicals.
2 Only trained personnel using required PPE may decontaminate patients with toxic chemical contamination.	Reduces likelihood of secondary toxic chemical contamination to untrained personnel attempting decontamination.

Critical Decision Point *Hold victim outside decontamination area until preparations are completed for decontamination procedure. If patient is grossly contaminated, consider decontamination before entry into building.*

3 Provide for patient privacy by closing room curtains or closing door.	Prevents discomfort and embarrassment when clothing is removed.
4 Decontaminate the patient:	
a Act quickly; avoid touching contaminated parts of clothing as much as possible.	
b Remove all of patient's clothing. **Caution: Do not pull over patient's head; instead, cut garments off.**	Cutting off clothing prevents contamination of head and hair.
c Use large amounts of soap and water to wash patient thoroughly.	Will lead to chemical dilution (CDC, 2006a) and in some cases will prevent patient death.
d If eyes are burning or vision is blurred, rinse eyes with plain water for 10 to 15 minutes. If patient wears contacts, remove and place with contaminated clothing; do not reinsert in eyes. Wash eyeglasses with soap and water; reapply when completed (CDC, 2006a).	Flushes toxins from the eye.
5 Dispose of patient's contaminated clothing in an appropriate biohazard bag and seal. Then place bag in another plastic bag and seal (see agency policy).	Reduces the likelihood of secondary chemical contamination.

STEP	RATIONALE
6 Initiate treatment for chemical agent using appropriate chemical agent protocol.	Appropriate chemical agent protocol will vary with patient exposure (e.g., linesterase, nerve agent, chlorine, lewisite) (Box 14-10).
7 Establish airway if needed; administer oxygen therapy.	Various chemical agents commonly cause respiratory problems that will result in altered gas exchange.
8 Control bleeding.	Various chemical agents cause extensive bleeding.
9 Administer fluid and nutrition therapy.	Various chemical agents commonly cause GI disturbances that will possibly result in dehydration.
10 Provide supportive care (e.g., comfort measures, including pain management).	Some victims will not survive; it is essential for the nurse to provide palliative symptom control.
11 Counsel patient and family on both acute and potential long-term psychological effects of exposure. Offer access to trained counselors.	Reaction of patients to exposure will include shock, immobilization, and fear. Long-term psychological effects will possibly arise without proper counseling (CDC, 2006a).

Critical Decision Point *Collaborate with the physician and other rescue workers for an ongoing plan to manage patients exposed to a toxic chemical agent. You will need to do this while also caring for other patients who are already present in the health care agency seeking care for illness unrelated to the current MCI.*

EVALUATION

1 Observe status of airway maintenance, breathing, circulation, level of consciousness, and neurological functioning. Assess vital signs.	Evaluates the patient's physical response to available treatment and/or supportive care.
2 Inspect condition of skin; note extent of blistering.	Determines extent of healing.
3 Evaluate patient's level of orientation, ability to problem solve, and perception of condition.	Evaluates the patient's psychological status and ability to make decisions.

Unexpected Outcomes	Related Interventions
1 Secondary contamination of rescue workers.	• Rescue workers immediately remove their clothing, scrub their bodies, and use copious amounts of soap and water. • Contain clothes in appropriate biohazard bags. • Provide clean clothes.
2 Patient's physical symptoms progress despite appropriate treatment.	• Notify physician or nurse in charge. • Continue to provide comfort care.
3 Patient's psychological symptoms progress despite appropriate treatment. Patient exhibits anxiety, disorientation, and suicidal ideation.	• Notify mental health treatment team. • Remain calm, offer reassurance, and protect self and others from physical harm. • Continue to provide comfort measures.
4 Patient death.	• When handling bodies take into account continued risk for contamination; make sure everyone is fully informed regarding proper procedures. When delegating preparation of the deceased, always take into account the level of training of those managing the body.

Recording and Reporting

- Report suspected cases of a toxic chemical event to physician or emergency officer.
- Record in nurses' notes patient's status and response to treatment and/or comfort measures.
- Report any unexpected outcome to physician or nurse in charge.

Teaching Considerations

- Preparation for an MCI goes a long way toward preventing casualties and chaos. Public education about the likelihood of a mass casualty chemical event is necessary. This education needs to include information regarding types of chemical agents, mode of dissemination, symptoms, and treatment.
- Education of the public needs to include locations of shelters and disaster treatment sites.

- See Skill 14-1 for family disaster plan and preparation.

Pediatric Considerations

- To avoid becoming a secondary victim, emergency responders need to consider potential contamination of children before picking up and holding them. Often decontamination will consist of providing fresh air and a large volume of low pressure, warm water. Observe children for potential hypothermia because they are more susceptible (Hohenhaus, 2005).
- Adult decontamination facilities are not always appropriate to meet the needs of children. The special protective equipment worn by rescue workers may frighten young children. The cleaning process and possible separation from uncontaminated parents will likely cause considerable stress and anxiety. Additional health care workers are often necessary to ensure adequate decontamination has taken place. Verbal encouragement

and praise will be effective in facilitating the process (Langan and James, 2005).

- See Skill 14-1 for further pediatric considerations.

Gerontological Considerations

- See Skill 14-1 for gerontological considerations.

Home Care Considerations

- Keep upwind and uphill from the release of the toxic chemical unless it is cyanide.
- Use appropriate PPE needed to protect the family; this includes sheltering-in-place (CDC, 2006b).
- See Skill 14-1 for further home care considerations.

BOX 14-10	**Examples of Chemical Exposure Protocols**

Chlorine Protocol

1. Dyspnea?
   - Try bronchodilators
   - Admit to hospital
   - Oxygen by mask
   - Chest x-ray examination
2. Treat other problems and reevaluate (consider phosgene)
3. Respiratory system OK?
   - Yes—go to 5
4. Is phosgene poisoning possible?
   - Yes—go to Phosgene Protocol on the CDC website
5. Give supportive therapy: treat other problems or discharge

Mustard Protocol

1. Airway obstruction?
   - Yes—tracheostomy
2. If there are large burns:
   - Establish IV line—do not push fluids as for thermal burns
   - Drain vesicles—unroof large blisters and irrigate area with topical antibiotics
3. Treat other symptoms appropriately:
   - Antibiotic eye ointment
   - Sterile precautions prn
   - Morphine prn

Modified from Centers for Disease Control and Prevention: *Emergency room procedures in chemical hazard emergencies: a job aid*, (n.d.) http://www.cdc.gov/nech/demil/articles/initialtreat.htm, accessed August 6, 2008.
CDC, Centers for Disease Control and Prevention; *IV*, intravenous; *prn*, as needed.

SKILL 14-3   Care of a Patient After Radiation Exposure

Radiological events differ from nuclear events. A radiological event is the dispersal of radioactive material via a "dirty bomb" or by deliberate contamination of food supplies, water supplies, or over the terrain. A nuclear event involves a device that releases nuclear energy in an explosive manner as a result of a nuclear chain reaction. Early symptoms of radiation exposure are similar to those experienced by anxious individuals. Thus once radiation release becomes publicly recognized, an enormous number of worried well will compromise incident management, scene security, and triage (Veenema, 2007).

Radiation comes in a variety of forms. Alpha particles are the least dangerous, traveling only a few centimeters. They do not penetrate materials easily and are harmful only if ingested. An individual's clothing will block alpha particles from reaching the skin. Beta particles penetrate a short distance into the skin. Protective clothing is necessary for protection. Gamma rays pose the greatest health risk because the waves penetrate deeply, causing severe burns and internal injury. Lead shielding protects against gamma rays. Blasts caused by a nuclear explosion not only cause injury resulting from radiation exposure but also traumatic injuries and burns. Some victims will present with many combined forms of injury requiring treatment. The sooner symptoms begin to appear, the greater the patient's exposure to the radiation. Early symptoms, within a few hours, suggest the individual has received a lethal dose of radiation. Early symptoms include nausea, vomiting, diarrhea, and a possible burn. For some, hair begins to fall out, and the victim quickly becomes immunocompromised.

Nuclear incidents usually result in wide destruction requiring specialized equipment and resources at the scene to assess structural damage and levels of radioactivity. Radiological events usually cover much smaller areas, but they are often difficult to define.

Table 14-3 presents characteristic differences between a nuclear event and a radiological event. Specialized equipment and training are required to assess the source of radioactivity, determine the scope of contamination, and perform decontamination. Decontamination is important with radiation exposure; however, it needs to occur in an area where there is not continued radiological release. The principles to follow to protect individuals from exposure involve distance, time, and shielding.

Delegation Considerations

The skill of assessment of a patient exposed to a biological agent cannot be delegated to NAP. The nurse directs the NAP to:

- Use appropriate PPE to prevent exposure.
- Use techniques for handling a body after death to prevent contamination.

TABLE 14-3	**Characteristics of a Nuclear Event and a Radiological Event**	
Characteristics	**Nuclear Event**	**Radiological Event**
Event recognition	Obvious	Not obvious
Thermonuclear explosion	Yes	No
Casualties	Large	Small
Amount of radiation release and contamination	Large	Small
Likelihood of terrorism	No	Yes

From American Medical Association: *Core Disaster Life Support: provider manual*, version 1.01, Chicago, 2002, The Association. Used with permission of the American Medical Association.

Equipment

The following is a general list of supplies needed in the event of release of the most radiological exposure:

❑ Decontamination room or area (adult decontamination rooms do not always meet the needs of children requiring decontamination; decontamination of ambulatory victims will not meet the needs of those who are not ambulatory)

❑ Scissors or some other tool to cut off clothing

❑ Clothing containers, type depends on the kind of radiological exposure

❑ Appropriate PPE for use by personnel in area of radiation release

❑ Appropriate PPE for health care workers in hospital setting (i.e., surgical masks, N95 masks, recommended if available)

❑ Radiation meter available to survey hands and clothing at frequent intervals (CDC, 2006d)

❑ Equipment for select specimen collection

❑ Equipment for physical examination.

STEP	RATIONALE

ASSESSMENT

1 Assess the patient's symptoms by performing a focused physical examination (see Skill 14-1).

Symptom identification and clustering of data is the first step to determining patient's condition and response.

Critical Decision Point   *Before assessment a specially trained technician will conduct a radiation survey of the patient, initially conducting a scan of the face, hands, and feet using a radiation survey instrument. If meter results are positive, a thorough survey (5 to 8 minutes per person) is conducted (CDC, 2007b).*

2 Assess the patient for secondary traumatic wounds: location, drainage, size, appearance.

Radioactive fragments are sometimes imbedded in a wound. Very high, localized levels of internal contamination indicate radioactive fragments (CDC, 2006d).

Critical Decision Point   *Do not touch the wound if you suspect that radioactive fragments are present.*

3 Assess the patient for preexisting medical conditions that will complicate the effects of the radiological exposure.

4 Determine patient's allergies, specifically allergy for iodine sensitivity.

5 Assess individual psychological response to radiological event. Some patients present with dissociative symptoms (e.g., feeling as though "not there," sensing that experiences are outside the person), disorientation, depression, anxiety, psychosis, and an inability to care for self. Ask the patient, "How do you feel now?" Determine level of orientation, ability to follow conversation.

6 Identify resources available (e.g., critical incident stress debriefing teams, counselors, psychiatric/mental health nurse practitioners).

Patients with preexisting medical conditions will possibly require additional treatment or are at greater risk for death.

Patients with iodine sensitivity need to avoid taking potassium iodide, the treatment of choice for radioactive iodine exposure.

Aids the nurse in being able to provide appropriate crisis intervention and stress management. Remaining calm and projecting confidence while assessing individuals for clinical symptoms versus feelings of panic will go a long way toward reducing the anxiety of the ill and worried well as they experience the general sense of panic associated with a radiological event.

Expert resources assess extent of psychological impact of disaster.

Critical Decision Point   *A radiological event is the event most feared by most individuals. Many are uneducated regarding the dangers of and differences between radiation materials. Health care agencies will likely have many anxious, frightened individuals who can potentially create a danger to the environment.*

NURSING DIAGNOSES

- Acute pain
- Anxiety
- Deficient fluid volume

- Diarrhea
- Fear
- Impaired tissue integrity

- Nausea
- Post-trauma syndrome
- Risk for infection

Individualize related factors based on patient's condition or needs.

PLANNING

1 Expected outcomes following completion of procedure:
- Patient will be comforted.
- Patient will be successfully decontaminated.

- Patient's vital signs will return to baseline.

- Patient will be free of nausea and diarrhea.

- Patient's skin integrity will return to baseline.

In some cases the only care that is available is palliative.

Decontamination procedures remove radioactive materials from patient's skin.

When there are no underlying medical conditions and *if* the patient's disease process is responsive to treatment (when available), vital signs will return to normal within days or weeks.

GI alterations following radiation exposure typically respond to antidiarrheal and antiemetic medications.

Radiological burns are minimized through successful decontamination procedures.

STEP	RATIONALE
• Patient's immune system (e.g., complete blood count [CBC]) will return to baseline.	Exposure to radiation successfully minimized.
• Patient's work of breathing will decrease.	Indicates improved gas exchange and cardiac output.
2 Explain care to patient and family. Explain your role, orient to location and activities to perform, explain what patient has experienced, and ask, "How are you feeling right now?" Assure them that medical personnel will see them shortly.	Crisis intervention reestablishes patient's orientation and sense of reality.

IMPLEMENTATION

1 Perform hand hygiene.	Reduces transmission of microorganisms.
2 Only trained personnel use required PPE to decontaminate patients with radiological contamination.	Reduces likelihood of secondary radiological contamination to untrained personnel attempting decontamination.
3 Provide for patient privacy by closing room curtains or door.	Prevents anxiety or embarrassment when clothes are removed.
4 Decontaminate the patient:	
a Remove patient's clothing.	Normally eliminates up to 90% of contamination (CDC, 2006d).
b Wash patient's skin thoroughly with water and soap, taking care not to abrade or irritate the skin. Do not allow radioactive material to be incorporated into any wounds.	Use of large amounts of water is critical in decontamination.
c Have radiation technician resurvey the patient after washing. Rewash as necessary.	Determines if radiation residual is present.
d Isolate and cover any area of the skin that is still positive for radiation by using a plastic bag or wrap (CDC, 2003).	The area is washed until no further reduction in contamination is achieved (verified by survey instrumentation) and then covered to reduce exposure of health care workers.
5 Bag and tag patient's contaminated clothing for further evaluation, and place in an appropriate biohazard container (CDC, 2006d).	Reduces the likelihood of secondary contamination when you use containers designed to contain the radiological particle.

Critical Decision Point *Collaborate with the physician and other rescue workers for an ongoing plan to manage patients exposed to radiological materials. You will need to do this while also caring for other patients who are already present in the health care agency seeking care for illness unrelated to the current nuclear or radiological event.*

6 Prepare for possibly obtaining a complete blood count (CBC), urinalysis, fecal specimen, and swabs of body orifices (see Chapter 43).	CBC establishes baseline to determine patient's immunological status over time. A physician who suspects internal contamination will order collection of urine, feces, and body orifice swabs to analyze for radionuclides (CDC, 2006d).
7 Treat symptoms according to ordinary treatment practices: provide IV fluid support, antidiarrheal therapies, antiemetic medications, and potassium iodide tablets (CDC, 2006d).	Patient exposed to radiation is at risk for GI alterations and fluid imbalance. Potassium iodide reduces risk for thyroid cancer from radioactive iodine exposure.

EVALUATION

1 Observe skin integrity, fluid balance, respiratory and GI status, level of consciousness, and neurological functioning. Look for improvement of other radiological agent–specific symptoms. Evaluate vital signs.	Evaluates the patient's physical response to available treatment and/or supportive care.
2 Monitor CBC and other laboratory tests.	Determines patient's immune response.
3 Evaluate patient's level of consciousness, orientation, and ability to relate events. Ask if patient remembers what has occurred; observe affect.	Determines if psychological status has improved.

Unexpected Outcomes	Related Interventions
1 Secondary contamination of rescue workers.	• Institute appropriate decontamination of worker.
2 Patient's symptoms progress despite appropriate treatment.	• Notify physician or nurse in charge.
	• Continue to provide comfort care.
3 Patient's psychological state deteriorates with development of disorientation, suicidal ideation, violence toward others.	• Notify mental health treatment team.
	• Remain calm, offer reassurance, and protect self and others from physical harm.
	• Continue to provide comfort care.
4 Patient death.	• When handling bodies, take into account continued risk for contamination; make sure everyone is fully informed about proper procedure. When delegating preparation of the deceased, take into account the level of training of those managing the body.

Recording and Reporting

- Record in nurses' notes patient's status and response to treatment and/or comfort measures.
- Report presence of open wound and any suspected radioactive fragment to physician or nurse in charge.
- Report any unexpected outcomes to physician.

Teaching Considerations

- See Skill 14-1.

Pediatric Considerations

- Children are vulnerable to radiation because (1) their organ systems are more sensitive than those of adults and (2) they have more years of life expectancy over which to develop complications from the radiological exposure (Claudio and others, 2003).
- See Skills 14-1 and 14-2 for further pediatric considerations.

Gerontological Considerations

- Because some older adults have many concurrent illnesses, it is possible radiological agents will worsen these conditions and result in the older adult needing more immediate care than an initial triage had indicated.
- See Skill 14-1 for further gerontological considerations.

Home Care Considerations

- When a radiological or nuclear event becomes reality, listen to the radio or television for special instructions, including appropriate means for maintaining a safe shelter.
- Keep upwind and uphill from the release of the radioactive materials (CDC, 2006c).
- See Skill 14-1 for further home care considerations.

? CRITICAL THINKING EXERCISES

Victims of an explosion involving a chemical are arriving in the emergency department. Authorities state the substance is unknown at this time, but there were reports by people in the area of a "funny smell" earlier in the day.

1 Enrique is a rescue worker on the scene. What are some safety measures he should take to avoid exposure?

2 Victims on the scene are triaged. How would the following patients be color coded, and which would receive the highest priority? A 22-year-old with cyanosis, a respiratory rate of 35, and confusion; a 14-year-old with a diffuse red rash on the extremities; a 56-year-old with controlled bleeding of deep lacerations received from falling debris; a 41-year-old with burns on 50% of the body.

3 What should the nurse working in the emergency department expect the initial care to be, and how is it achieved?

4 Yvette is an 18-year-old patient who arrived in the emergency department for treatment. Her clothing appears to be saturated with the unknown chemical. How should Yvette's clothing be handled?

5 Among the victims to be treated is a 3-year-old. What special considerations need to be taken when decontaminating children?

✓ REVIEW QUESTIONS

1 A hospital committee formed to work on an emergency response plan is meeting initially to discuss how to proceed with the process. Why is a clearly defined, executable, and practiced emergency response plan the best indicator that an institution is more likely to be successful in a disaster situation?
1 Practice makes staff more familiar with disaster protocols in the event of a true disaster.
2 Practice of protocols helps to meet all of the regulatory agency guidelines.
3 Practice prevents the likelihood of acute traumatic stress disorder in the staff.
4 Practice is cost-effective in the long term because fewer staff will be required to handle the disaster as a result of the staff members' being better prepared.

2 A major traffic accident involving multiple vehicles and an explosion has sent numerous patients to the local emergency department. Which experienced nurse has the most difficult assignment and a greater chance for demonstrating signs and symptoms of acute traumatic stress disorder?

1 A nurse who has been delegated to care for the community patients currently admitted to the emergency department
2 A nurse assigned to triage disaster victims transported to the emergency department but able to walk in to the triage area
3 A nurse who is assigned to care for patients on an as-needed basis
4 A nurse who must inform a mother that her three children did not survive

3 Four victims from a disaster arrive at the emergency department at the same time. Which victim should receive the highest level of priority for care?
1 A disaster victim who arrives at the emergency department without a pulse
2 A disaster victim who arrives at the emergency department with labored respirations, cool skin, a pulse of 120 beats per minute, and a blood pressure of 90/60 mm Hg
3 A disaster victim who is a noted politician with an open fracture of his left arm
4 A disaster victim who is under the age of 6 years, regardless of the extent of his injuries

4 A patient arrives at the ED with suspected cutaneous anthrax. What type of precautions should be used with this patient?
1 Standard
2 Contact
3 Respiratory
4 Airborne

5 A practice emergency drill is being held in the emergency department. The drill would be considered successful if which group of people were initially protected at the disaster scene?
1 The health care workers
2 The patient(s)
3 The news crews reporting the event
4 The family members of the victim(s)

REFERENCES

American Red Cross: Counseling materials, http://www.redcross.org/services/disaster/keepsafe/unexpected.html, accessed June 25, 2007.

American Red Cross and Centers for Disease Control and Prevention: *Preparedness today: what you need to do,* http://www.redcross.org/services/prepare/0,1082,0_239_,00.html, accessed August 18, 2008.

Auf der Heide E: *The importance of evidence based disaster planning, Ann Emerg Med* 47:34, 2006, http://www.atsdr.cdc.gov/emergency_response/importance_disaster_planning.pdf, accessed July 1, 2007.

Bernardo L: Pediatric implications in bioterrorism. I. Physiologic and psychosocial differences, *Int J Trauma Nurs* 7(1):14, 2001.

Boatright C, McGlown KJ: Homeland security challenges in nursing practice, *Nurs Clin North Am* 40(3):481, 2005.

Brandenburg M: Pediatric considerations in disasters. In Hogan D, Burstein J, editors: *Disaster medicine*, ed 2, Philadelphia, 2007, Lippincott, Williams & Wilkins.

Centers for Disease Control and Prevention: *Interim guidelines for hospital response to mass casualties from a radiological incident*, 2003, http://www.bt.cdc.gov/radiation/pdf/MassCasualtiesGuidelines.pdf, accessed August 6, 2008.

Centers for Disease Control and Prevention: *About CDC organization COTPER*, http://www.cdc.gov/about/organization/cotper.htm March, 2008, accessed June 24, 2007.

Centers for Disease Control and Prevention: *Biological and chemical terrorism: strategic plan for preparedness and response*, April, 2000, http://www.cdc.gov/mmwr/preview/mmwrhtml/rr4904a1.htm, accessed July 1, 2007.

Centers for Disease Control and Prevention: *Bioterrorism: frequently asked questions about smallpox vaccine*, 2007a, http://www.bt.cdc.gov/agent/smallpox/vaccination/faq.asp#vaccine, accessed October 31, 2007.

Centers for Disease Control and Prevention: *Casualty management after a deliberate release of radioactive material*, 2007b, http://www.bt.cdc.gov/radiation/casualties-radioactive.asp, accessed July 7, 2007.

Centers for Disease Control and Prevention: *Chemical agents: facts about personal cleaning and disposal of contaminated clothing*, 2006a, http://www.bt.cdc.gov/planning/personalcleaningfacts.asp, accessed July 1, 2007.

Centers for Disease Control and Prevention: *Chemical agents: facts about sheltering in place*, http://www.bt.cdc.gov/planning/shelteringfacts.asp, 2006b, accessed June 28, 2007.

Centers for Disease Control and Prevention: *Chemical emergencies: facts about cyanide*, http://www.bt.cdc.gov/agent/cyanide/basics/facts.asp, 2004, accessed June 28, 2007.

Centers for Disease Control and Prevention: *Emergency room procedures in chemical hazard emergencies: a job aid* (n.d.), http://www.cdc.gov/nech/demil/articles/initialtreat.htm, accessed July 7, 2007.

Centers for Disease Control and Prevention: *Radiation emergencies: sheltering in place during a radiation emergency*, 2006c, http://www.bt.cdc.gov/radiation/shelter.asp, accessed July 2, 2007.

Centers for Disease Control and Prevention: *Radiological terrorism: emergency management pocket guide for clinicians*, June, 2008, http://www.bt.cdc.gov/radiation/pocket.asp, accessed June 26, 2007.

Centers for Disease Control and Prevention: *Strategic national stockpile*, http://www.bt.cdc.gov/stockpile, accessed May 9, 2007k.

Centers for Disease Control and Prevention, http://www.cdc.gov/ncidod/sars.

Claudio L and others: Addressing environmental health issues. In Levy BS, Sidel VW, editors: *Terrorism and public health: a balanced approach to strengthening systems and protecting people*, New York, 2003, Oxford Press.

Clemons L: *Culturally competent: disaster nursing*, 2006, http://www.minoritynurse.com/features/health/06-06-06-3.html, accessed June 14, 2007.

Croddy E, Ackerman G: Biological and chemical terrorism: a unique threat. In Veenema TG, editor: *Disaster nursing and emergency preparedness for chemical, bio-logical, and radiological terrorism and other hazards*, ed 2, New York, 2007, Springer Publishing.

Department of Homeland Security: *Strategic Plan—securing our homeland*, http://www.dhs.gov/xabout/strategicplan/, accessed June 17, 2007.

Ellis KJ: Disaster readiness: lessons from Katrina, *Nephrol Nurs J* 34(1):82, 2007.

Federal Emergency Management Agency: *Before a biological attack*, http://www.fema.gov/hazard/terrorism/bio/bio_before.shtm, accessed May 9, 2007.

HEICS III: Hospital emergency incident command system update project: a project of the San Mateo County Emergency Medical Services Agency with support and funding from the California Emergency Medical Services Authority, http://www.emsa.ca.gov/ Dms2/heics3.htm, accessed July 7, 2007.

Hohenhaus SM: Practical considerations for providing pediatric care in a mass casualty incident, *Nurs Clin North Am* 40(3):523, 2005.

Johnson TD: Preparedness: better to be safe than sorry, *Nations Health* 37(2):28, 2007.

Langan JC, James DC: *Preparing nurses for disaster management*, Upper Saddle River, NJ, 2005, Pearson Prentice Hall.

Magee M: *Health politics: power, populism, and health*, New York, 2005, Spencer Books.

Mitchell AM and others: Disaster care: psychological considerations, *Nurs Clin North Am* 40(3):535, 2005.

National Center for Injury Prevention and Control: *In a moment's notice: surge capacity for terrorist bombings—challenges and proposed solutions*, Atlanta, 2007, Centers for Disease Control and Prevention; http://www.bt.gov/masscasualties/pdf/surge-capacity_cover.pdf, p. 50, accessed May 9, 2007.

NeSmith EG: Defining "disasters" with implications for nursing scholarship and practice, *Disaster Manag Response*, 4(2):59, 2006.

Plum KC, Veenema TG: Management of psychosocial effects. In Veenema TG, editor: *Disaster nursing and emergency preparedness for chemical, biological, and radiological terrorism and other hazards*, ed 2, New York, 2007, Springer Publishing.

Rebmann T: *Preparing nurses for disaster management*, 2005, Pearson Prentice Hall, Upper Saddle River, NJ.

Siegel JD and others: *2007 Guideline for isolation precautions: preventing transmission of infectious agents in healthcare settings*, http://www.cdc.gov/ncidod/dhgp/pdf/guidelines/Isolation2007.pdf, p. 123, accessed July 1, 2007.

U.S. Department of Health and Human Services, Centers for Disease Control and Prevention: *Avian influenza*, May 2007.

Vaccine Education Center at the Children's Hospital of Philadelphia: *Pandemic flu: what you should know*, vol 1, Winter 2006, Philadelphia.

Veenema TG, editor: *Disaster nursing and emergency preparedness for chemical, biological, and radiological terrorism and other hazards*, ed 2, New York, 2007, Springer Publishing.

WHO *avian influenza fact sheet*, February 2006, Geneva, http://www.who_int/mediacentre/factsheets/avian_influence/en, accessed August 8, 2008.

15

Pain Assessment and Basic Comfort Measures

MEDIA RESOURCES

- evolve *learning system* http://evolve.elsevier.com/Perry/skills

  - Review Questions
  - Video Clips

- View Video! Mosby's Nursing Video Skills, 3.0

OBJECTIVES

Mastery of content in this chapter will enable the nurse to:
- Assess a patient's level of comfort.
- Assess a patient's level of pain.
- Identify skills appropriate for relieving a patient's reported pain.
- Plan care based on a patient's history, including pain history, and physical assessment.
- Describe delivery of medication through a patient-controlled analgesia (PCA) device.
- Teach a patient to use a PCA device.
- Monitor and manage a patient receiving epidural analgesia.
- Monitor and manage a patient receiving a local anesthetic infusion pump.
- Identify and discuss various nonpharmacological pain-relief measures.
- Monitor and manage a patient receiving nonpharmacological measures to relieve pain.
- Evaluate the effectiveness of pain-management techniques.

Pain is a complex phenomenon that is physical and/or mental in nature. Pain is subjective and highly individualized. Pain is tiring and demands a person's physical, emotional, and mental energy. It interferes with personal relationships and even influences the meaning of life. Although certain types of pain create predictable signs and symptoms, nurses primarily assess pain by relying on the patient's report. The patient is the only one who knows whether pain is present and what the experience is like. McCaffery and Pasero (1999) state, "Pain is whatever the experiencing person says it is, existing when she/he says it does." It is not patients' responsibility to convince nurses that they have pain; it is nurses' responsibility to believe them.

Pain is difficult to categorize on duration or pathological condition alone. However, the literature commonly identifies three types of pain: acute, chronic/persistent, and cancer pain (American Pain Society [APS], 2003). Because cancer pain differs from chronic noncancer pain in significant ways (time frame, pathology, treatment strategies), currently it is in a different category entirely.

Acute pain or transient pain
- Has an identifiable cause
- Has a rapid onset
- Varies in intensity
- Is of short duration
- Generally disappears with healing

Chronic pain or persistent pain
- Extends beyond the period of healing
- Often lacks identified pathology
- Rarely has autonomic signs
- Does not provide a protective function
- Disrupts sleep and activities of daily living (ADLs)
- Degrades health and function of individual

Cancer pain
- May be acute, chronic, or intermittent
- Is usually related to tumor recurrence or treatment

The most effective pain management involves a combined approach of nonpharmacological strategies with the administration of pharmacological agents: nonopioids and opioids (Table 15-1). Timely administration before a patient's pain becomes severe is crucial for optimal relief. Pain is easier to prevent than to treat. In most situations, administration of pharmacological agents "around-the-clock" rather than on an "as-needed" (prn) basis is preferable. This approach alleviates pain before it becomes severe and facilitates an earlier recovery (Gordon and others, 2005).

Often a combination of nonopioids and opioids is effective in managing pain. Although patients, family members, and caregivers fear that frequent administration of pain medications will result in a patient's psychological dependence (addiction) on the opioid, such dependence is actually rare (APS, 2003). Some patients exhibit drug-seeking behaviors when in fact they are seeking pain relief. This is termed pseudoaddiction. Occasionally a physician will order a placebo to discredit a patient's report of pain. This is unethical and should be avoided (American Pain Society Consensus Statement on Placebo, 2005). Patients are also concerned about drug tolerance. It is important for you to understand the differences between addiction, pseudoaddiction, physical dependence, and drug tolerance (Box 15-1).

Complementary strategies for pain relief provide an opportunity for a patient to assume an active role in achieving a higher level of comfort and, in some instances, freedom from pain. Using an integrated approach that considers both pharmacological and nonpharmacological therapies in managing pain is recommended

TABLE 15-1	Two Analgesic Groups: Examples Within Each Group	
Nonopioids		**Opioids**
a *Acetaminophen* (Tylenol)		a *Mu agonists** (full agonists)— Examples:
b *NSAIDs*—Short acting— Examples:		Codeine
Aspirin		Fentanyl (Duragesic patch)
Trisalicylate (Trilisate)		Hydrocodone
Ibuprofen (Motrin, Advil)		Hydromorphone (Dilaudid)
Ketorolac (Toradol)		Levorphanol (Levo-Dromoran)
Ketoprofen (Orudis)		Meperidine (Demerol)
Naproxen (Naprosyn)		Methadone
Piroxicam (Feldene)		Morphine
c *NSAIDS*—Long acting— Examples:		Oxycodone
Bextra		Propoxyphene (Darvon)
Celebrex		Tramadol hydrochloride (Ultram)
Vioxx		b *Agonist-antagonists*—Examples:
d *Topicals*—Examples:		Buprenorphine (Buprenex)
Lidocaine (Lidoderm)		Nalbuphine (Nubain)
Eutectic mixture of lidocaine and prilocaine (EMLA)		Pentazocine (Talwin)
ELA-MAX (OTC)		
Capsaicin		

Modified from McCaffery M, Pasero C: *Pain: clinical manual,* ed 2, St. Louis, 1999, Mosby.
NSAID, Nonsteroidal antiinflammatory drug; *OTC,* over-the-counter.
*Many of the pure opioids are also found in combination with nonopioids. Several are also available in long-acting formulations.

BOX 15-1	Terminology Related to the Use of Opioids in Pain Treatment

Physical Dependence

"Physical dependence is a state of adaptation that often includes tolerance and is manifested by a drug class specific withdrawal syndrome that can be produced by abrupt cessation, rapid dose reduction, decreasing blood level of the drug, and/or administration of an antagonist."

Addiction

"Is a primary, chronic, neurobiologic disease, with genetic, psychosocial, and environmental factors influencing its development and manifestations. It is characterized by behaviors that include one or more of the following: impaired control over drug use, compulsive use, continued use despite harm, and craving."

Pseudoaddiction

"A term that describes patient behavior that may occur when pain is undertreated. Patients with unrelieved pain may focus on obtaining medications, may 'clock watch,' may otherwise seem inappropriately 'drug seeking.' Even such behaviors as illicit drug use and deception can occur in the patient's efforts to obtain relief. Pseudoaddiction can be distinguished from true addiction in that behaviors resolve when pain is effectively treated."

Drug Tolerance

"A state of adaptation in which exposure to a drug induces changes that result in a diminution of one or more of the drug's effects over time."

"Definitions Related to the Use of Opioids for the Treatment of Pain" is a copyrighted work of the American Pain Society and American Society of Addiction Medicine, © 2001, Reviewed July, 2004.

(King and Pettigrew, 2004; Lewandowski and others, 2005; Mitchell and McDonald, 2006).

A patient's age, level of cognition, and personality influence the experience of pain. Culture and ethnicity; coping style; emotional, physical, and spiritual needs; state of health; and past pain experiences also influence pain. It is important for patients to actively participate in any therapies aimed at alleviating discomfort; they are the best authority on their pain (McCaffery and Pasero, 1999).

EVIDENCE-BASED PRACTICE TRENDS

As with every aspect of nursing practice, it is vital for the professional nurse to use current evidence, especially research, to practice excellent pain management. Systematic reviews of research trials are especially valuable to the nurse searching for the latest and most valid research information. Because pain is currently considered a comorbid medical condition and not simply a symptom of a pathological state, the trend is to try to prevent pain. Preemptive analgesia is a method of preventing pain while reducing overall opioid use. Consumption of opioids and the implication of addiction are of major concern to patients in pain, health care providers, and the judicial system. Understanding the influence of genes (Iohom and Fitzgerald, 2004; Prows and Prows, 2004) and gender (Miller and Newton, 2006) in pain management has just begun. The use of herbals, homeopathy (Austin, 2004; Soeken, 2004; Tracy and others, 2006), and dietary therapies (Caprotti, 2004; Tall and Raja, 2004) to treat pain is evolving. The goal is to develop an individualized pain management plan that provides optimum pain relief with minimal adverse effects.

The concept of patients as authoritative participants makes pain control an ethical and legal issue. Pain can dehumanize, destroy autonomy, and create a sense of hopelessness and powerlessness in a patient, yet the treatment of pain is regularly and systematically inadequate. Although pain is strictly subjective and qualitative, health care providers often treat it objectively and quantitatively (Ferrell, 2005; Larsson and Wijik, 2007). Patients unable to report pain (e.g., young children, critically ill patients, and patients with dementia) are at highest risk for undertreatment (Herr, and others, 2006). Pain that is caused by or persists as a result of nurses' or physicians' attitudes and outdated practices therefore becomes a matter of ethics. For example, a nurse who does not believe that patients have pain because they are watching TV or visiting with friends or a physician who orders only a mild analgesic such as Darvocet for a dying patient with intractable pain is not using current evidence on which to base his or her practice. Table 15-2 summarizes common misconceptions about pain that all health care professionals need to consider when planning patient care.

In the early 1990s the Agency for Healthcare Policy and Research (AHCPR) issued guidelines for effective pain management for patients with acute and cancer pain (Agency for Healthcare Policy and Research, 1992). These guidelines help caregivers, patients, and patients' families understand the nature and treatment of pain. A few minor changes have been made (APS, 2003), but the guidelines are still consistent with current research. In 1999 The Joint Commission (then known as the Joint Commission on Accreditation of Healthcare Organizations [JCAHO]), which accredits 80% of the nation's hospitals, encompassing 98% of hospital beds, set standards for the assessment and treatment of patients in pain (JCAHO, 2003). Since then, health care organizations have been encouraged to change policies that prevent adequate pain management for patients (Box 15-2). The pain management skills in this text are for use alone or in combination, depending on patient needs. You can teach many of these measures to a patient and family for use in the home.

CULTURAL CONSIDERATIONS

- Understand cultural differences in pain expression.
- Cultures vary in when to recognize pain, what words to use in expressing pain, when to seek treatment, and what treatments are desirable. Russians, Asians, and American Indians tend to be stoic, whereas Italians, Puerto Ricans, and Jews tend to be more expressive (Spector, 2004).
- Explore beliefs about pain/discomfort with a patient. Cultures with a holistic worldview of health and illness mix religious/spiritual, natural (hot and cold), and the supernatural in their belief systems.
- Assess the meaning of pain to a patient.
- Some Hindu patients believe that suffering is a consequence of actions in previous life. For example, a belief in the concept of Karma motivates the patient to bear the pain, refuse pain medications, and suffer in silence. Some Jews view pain as a communal suffering that they should share with others to affirm one's life experience (Spector, 2004).
- Assess multiple modalities used by a patient/family for relief of pain.
- Individuals and cultural groups use complementary and alternative modalities of pain relief such as aromatherapy, imagery, and acupressure along with biomedical interventions (King and Pettigrew, 2004).

TABLE 15-2	Misconceptions: Barriers to the Assessment and Treatment of Pain
Misconception	**Correction**
1 The best judge of the existence and severity of a patient's pain is the physician or nurse caring for the patient.	The patient's self-report is the most reliable indicator of the existence and intensity of pain.
2 Clinicians should use their personal opinions and beliefs about the truthfulness of the patient to determine the patient's true pain status.	Allowing each clinician to act on personal beliefs presents the potential for different pain assessments by different clinicians, leading to different interventions from each clinician. This results in inconsistent and often inadequate pain management. It is essential to establish the patient's self-report of pain as the standard for pain assessment.
3 Visible signs, either physiological or behavioral, always accompany pain and can be used to verify its existence and severity.	Even with severe pain, periods of physiological and behavioral adaptation occur, leading to periods of minimal or no observable signs of pain. Lack of pain expression does not necessarily mean lack of pain.
4 The pain rating scale preferred for use in daily clinical practice is the visual analog scale (VAS).	The preferred pain rating scale depends on the patient's cognitive and physical ability, culture, developmental level, and availability.
5 Cognitively impaired older adult patients are unable to use pain rating scales.	When an appropriate pain rating scale is used and the patient is given sufficient time to process information and respond, many cognitively impaired older adults can use a pain rating scale.
6 If patients hurt enough, they will tell you.	Patients are often hesitant to report pain for fear of being labeled as complainers, hypochondriacs, or addicts.
7 Psychosocial interventions alone will reduce or alleviate pain.	Nonpharmacological interventions are synergistic with medications, but are not a substitute for pharmacological management of pain.

Modified from McCaffery M, Pasero C: *Pain: clinical manual*, ed 2, St. Louis, 1999, Mosby.

BOX 15-2	The Joint Commission Pain Standards

The 2003 standards issued by The Joint Commission (then known as JCAHO, the Joint Commission on Accreditation of Healthcare Organizations) called on health care organizations to do the following:
- Recognize the right of patients to appropriate assessment and management of pain
- Assess pain in all patients
- Record the assessment in a way that facilitates regular reassessment and follow-up

- Educate providers/patients and families
- Establish policies that support appropriate prescription or ordering of pain medicines
- Include patient needs for symptom control in discharge planning
- Collect data to monitor effectiveness and appropriateness of pain management

From Joint Commission on Accreditation of Healthcare Organizations: *Comprehensive accreditation manual for hospitals: the official handbook*, Oak Brook Terrace, Ill, 2003, The Commission.

- Assess meanings of cultural artifacts that patients bring with them. Do not move or remove these objects without the patient's consent (Spector, 2004).
- Collaborate with a patient's identified religious or cultural healers in planning holistic interventions for the patient. Hispanics often consult a *curandero,* who empowers people to look at their emotional, physical, and spiritual life so that their bodies might heal; Southeast Asians may consult a shaman or faith healers (King and Pettigrew, 2004; Spector, 2004).
- Recognize cultural variations in tolerance and metabolism of analgesics and central nervous system (CNS) depressants. Asians require much smaller doses of analgesics (Prows and Prows, 2004).
- Assess cultural variables influencing the operation of patient-controlled analgesia (PCA). Orthodox or observant Jews may not use electrical equipment during the Sabbath and Holy Days; therefore the staff should program the PCA to achieve optimum pain relief. Alternative methods will be needed during these times.
- Some groups may refuse invasive pain-relief measures because of their cultural and religious beliefs (Monsevais and McNeill, 2007; Spector, 2004).

Skill Performance Guidelines

1 Know a patient's past and current medical history, type of therapy, and current medications, including over-the-counter products. Some patients with prior pain conditions can alert the nurse to successful pain-relieving measures. Patients with chronic/persistent pain are often familiar with the names and actions of medications, including opioid medications. This should not cause you to view a patient negatively or with suspicion. Patients currently receiving opioids for chronic pain often require higher doses of analgesics to alleviate new pain. Drug-drug interactions, including enhanced or reduced effects or side effects, often occur with polypharmacy.

2 Determine a patient's perception of the pain experience. A thorough assessment of factors contributing to a patient's pain enables you to select or assist the prescriber in selecting appropriate therapies.

3 Demonstrate respect for a patient's evaluation of the quality and quantity of pain experienced and the response to methods of pain management. It is important to assess a patient's acceptable level of comfort so that both you and the patient are striving for the same outcome.

4 Control environmental factors that influence a patient's response to discomfort, such as excess environmental stimuli or fatigue.

5 Decide the frequency for assessing a patient's comfort, and write it on the plan of care. It is a nurse's responsibility to assess the patient's response to comfort measures. Identifying pain trends and comparing changes in pain patterns is useful in making therapeutic decisions.

6 Communicate to the health care provider significant changes in a patient's comfort level and need for changes in the pain management regimen.

7 Know your institution's policy for frequency of pain assessment and timing for follow-up assessment. The nurse who knows a patient well and evaluates a patient's response to the pain management interventions can identify along with the patient when pain-relieving measures are no longer effective or no longer necessary and when the type and quality of pain have changed. Do not accept "there is nothing that will help this patient's pain." Learn the institutional policy for how to proceed in this situation.

SKILL 15-1 Providing Pain Relief

Basic Skills / Vital Signs / Assessing Pain
Intermediate Skills / Postoperative Nursing Care / Managing Pain

Alleviating suffering is a major nursing responsibility. Because pain is often an element of suffering, promoting optimal pain relief is a primary goal. Through a comprehensive pain assessment you can begin to understand the impact of pain on a patient's life. Effectively managing a patient's pain does not necessarily mean eliminating pain. Pain management requires you to work with the patient and family, to identify an acceptable intensity of pain that allows maximum patient function. Further, collaboration with other health care providers is essential for the best possible pain relief.

The nursing process offers a systematic method of pain management that results in improved pain relief for most patients. This process recognizes distinct differences in patient perceptions and responses to pain. Acknowledging the patient as a unique person is essential to optimal pain management. Use the nursing process to come to know the patient and develop an individualized plan. Management of pain is such a priority that the American Society for Pain Management Nursing (ASPMN), in cooperation with the American Nurses Association (ANA), rewrote its *Scope and Standards* of pain management for the nurse generalist and the nurse specialist. From these standards, a certification examination in pain management was initially offered in October 2005. Both examinations are now available through the American Nurses Credentialing Association (ASPMN, 2004).

Delegation Considerations

The skill of pain assessment cannot be delegated. Nursing assistive personnel (NAP) may screen patients for pain and provide selected nonpharmacological strategies (e.g., back rubs, heat, cold, elevation) as instructed by the nurse. The nurse directs the NAP to:

- Eliminate environmental conditions that aggravate pain (e.g., an excessively warm, noisy room).
- Provide maximum rest periods; a written schedule for all to follow is ideal.
- Turn and place patients in positions of comfort at least every 2 hours or remind patients to turn themselves that frequently.
- Ask patient to report pain using the same pain-intensity scale—chosen by patient with the nurse.
- Report, in a timely manner, any patient reports of pain intensity above predetermined goal and nonverbal behaviors suggestive of pain.
- Screen for pain during patient transfer or other activity that might provoke pain.

Equipment

- ☐ Pain-intensity scale (check institutional policy for recommended instruments)

STEP	RATIONALE

ASSESSMENT

1 Assess patient's risk for pain (e.g., those undergoing invasive procedures, anxious patients, patients unable to communicate).

Allows nurse to anticipate patient's needs and to intervene in a timely manner, possibly preventing pain.

2 Ask patients if they are in pain. However, older adult patients or patients from various cultures may not admit to having pain; thus additional pain assessment techniques are necessary. Some people use the word *pain* only for severe pain. You may need to try other terms such as *hurt* or *discomfort*.

There is no objective test to measure pain. Accept the patient's report of pain (APS, 2003; Institute for Clinical Systems, 2006). In patients of differing cultures, watch for nonverbal indicators of pain; ask significant others if they believe the patient is in pain. Many see increasing pain as a sign of advancing disease (Hadjistaviapoulos and others, 2007).

3 Assess patient's response to previous pharmacological interventions, especially ability to function (e.g., sleeping, eating and other ADLs). Determine if analgesic side effects are likely based on medication and patient's previous responses (e.g., itching and nausea with morphine).

Determines extent to which therapies have been successful or not successful. (Hansson and others, 2006).

STEP	RATIONALE
4 Examine site of patient's pain or discomfort. Include inspection (discoloration, swelling, drainage), palpation (change in temperature, area of altered sensation, painful area, areas that trigger pain, areas that reduce pain), and range of motion of involved joints (if applicable). Percussion and auscultation help to identify abnormalities (e.g., underlying mass or lung crackles) and determine cause of pain. Remember: when examining the abdomen, auscultate first, then inspect and palpate.	Clinical observations clarify information from patient. Site of discomfort will possibly direct you to specific types of pain-relief measures.
5 Assess for physical, behavioral, and emotional signs and symptoms of pain:	Combination of signs and symptoms reveal source and nature of pain (Bedard and others, 2006; Bucknall and others, 2007; Herr and others, 2006).
a Moaning, crying, whimpering, vocalizations ("Stop, stop!")	
b Decreased activity	
c Facial expressions (e.g., grimace, clenched teeth)	
d Change in usual behavior	
e Abnormal gait	
f Irritability	
g Guarding of body part	
h Increased blood glucose level	The stress of unrelieved pain causes the endocrine system to release excessive amounts of hormones and decreased insulin levels (McCaffery and Pasero, 1999). The metabolic responses can include hyperglycemia.
i Diaphoresis	
j Change in mental status (e.g., confusion)	Confusion is often a sign of unrelieved pain and not opioids, as is commonly assumed (Mansfield, 2006).
k Decreased gastrointestinal (GI) motility, nausea, and vomiting	Signs and symptoms of pain originate from involvement of visceral organs with stimulation of the parasympathetic nervous system.
l Muscle tension, restlessness, exhaustion	Continued stimulation of sympathetic nervous system depletes energy stores (Baird and Sands, 2004).
m Insomnia, anorexia, fatigue	These physical manifestations may in turn increase the perception of pain (Onen and others, 2005).
n Depression, hopelessness, anger, fear, social withdrawal, powerlessness, stoicism	Depression frequently occurs in patients with chronic pain and increases perception and intensity of pain (Larsson and Wijik, 2007; McDonald and others, 2005; Vallerand and others, 2007).
o Concomitant symptoms: symptoms that often occur with pain (e.g., headache, constipation, restlessness)	Signs and symptoms of sympathetic nervous system stimulation (Bruchi and others, 2005; Onen and others, 2005).

Critical Decision Point *Physiological responses (e.g., tachycardia, hypertension) to acute pain are of short duration and return to normal within minutes. Be aware that with persistent pain, a patient will not usually exhibit physical signs and symptoms. Never use physiological responses alone to determine pain therapy selected. Patient self-report is the "gold standard."*

STEP	RATIONALE
6 Assess characteristics of pain, using the PQRSTU of pain assessment:	Guides clinician in collecting complete information about patient's pain experience.
a **P**rovocative/**P**alliative factors (For example, "What makes your pain better or worse?")	Select factors precipitate certain types of pain. Identifies the nature and source of discomfort, which helps determine best intervention. A combination of interventions is often the most effective approach to pain relief (APS, 2003; Mitchell and McDonald, 2006; Whitehead-Pleaux and others, 2006).
b **Q**uality (For example, use open-ended questions such as "Tell me what your pain feels like.")	Assists in identifying the underlying pain mechanism (e.g., somatic or neuropathic pain) necessary for determining appropriate treatment (McCaffery and Pasero, 1999).
c **R**egion/**R**adiation (For example, "Show me where your pain is.")	Identify possible causative factors.
d **S**everity: Using a pain-intensity scale appropriate to patient's age, developmental level, and comprehension, ask the patient to rate pain (see illustrations). Be sure to assess patients' pain when they are moving, not just lying in bed or sitting in a chair. Pain intensity often changes with movement.	Pain is a subjective experience, so you should accept a patient's evaluation. An appropriate pain rating scale is reliable, easily understood, easy to use, and reflects changes in pain intensity (Beyer and others, 2005; Ware and others, 2006).

STEP   RATIONALE

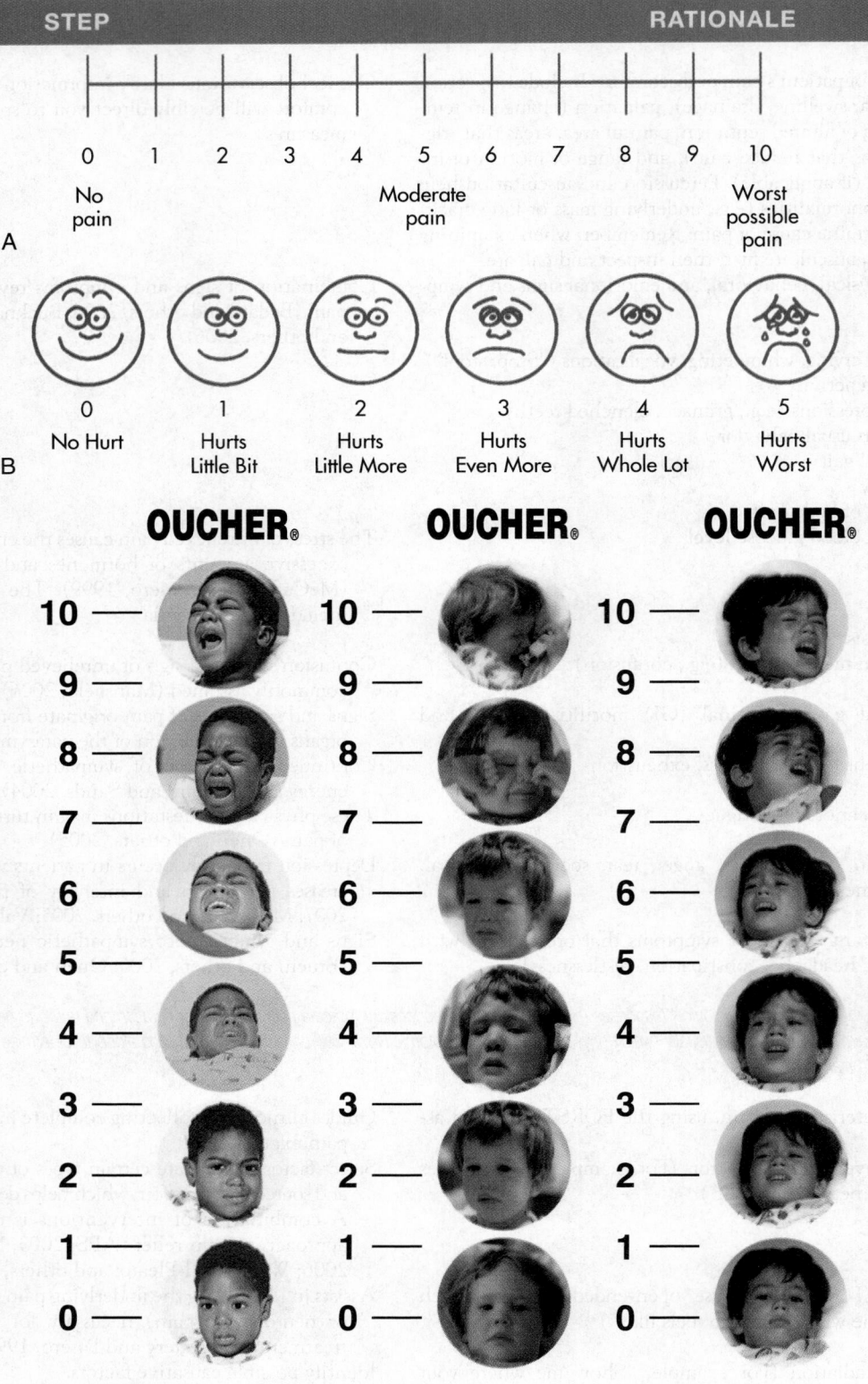

A, Pain rating scale.

| 0 | 1 | 2 | 3 | 4 | 5 | 6 | 7 | 8 | 9 | 10 |

No pain   Moderate pain   Worst possible pain

A

B

| 0 | 1 | 2 | 3 | 4 | 5 |

No Hurt   Hurts Little Bit   Hurts Little More   Hurts Even More   Hurts Whole Lot   Hurts Worst

OUCHER.   **OUCHER.**   **OUCHER.**

C   African-American   Caucasian   Hispanic

STEP 6d **A,** Pain rating scale. (*From McCaffery M, Pasero C: Pain: clinical manual, ed 2, St. Louis, 1999, Mosby.*) **B,** Wong-Baker FACES Pain Rating Scale. (*From Wong DL and others:* Whaley and Wong's nursing care of infants and children, *ed 7, St. Louis, 2003, Mosby.*) **C,** African-American version of the Oucher Pain Scale. (*Developed and copyrighted in 1990 by Mary J. Denyes, PhD, RN, Wayne State University and Antonia M. Villarruel, PhD, RN, University of Michigan. Cornelia P. Porter, PhD, RN, and Charlotta Marshall, RN, MSN, contributed to the development.*) Caucasian version of the Oucher Pain Scale. (*Developed and copyrighted in 1983 by Judith E. Beyer, PhD, RN, University of Missouri-Kansas City School of Nursing, Kansas City, Mo.*) Hispanic version of the Oucher Pain Scale. (*Developed and copyrighted in 1990 by Antonia M. Villarruel, PhD, University of Michigan, and Mary J. Denyes, PhD, RN, Wayne State University.*)

STEP	RATIONALE

Critical Decision Point   *It is important to consistently use the same pain-intensity scale with the same patient. You will use different instruments (visual analog scale [VAS], numerical rating scale [NRS], colors, FACES, etc.) with different patients depending on their preference, age, developmental level, and/or comprehension ability (Beyer and others, 2005; Ware and others, 2006).*

Critical Decision Point   *Occasionally a patient will be unable to report the pain intensity. In this situation, ask if the pain is "a lot, a little, or in between?" Many geriatric patients understand a categorical pain scale such as none, mild, moderate, severe more than they do a numerical scale (Mansfield, 2006; Ware and others, 2006).*

e Timing: Ask patient if pain is constant, intermittent, continuous, or a combination. Also ask if pain increases during specific times of the day, with particular activities, or in specific locations.

Environmental stimuli, such as loud noises, bright lights, strong odors, or temperature extremes, sometimes alter patient's response to pain.

f Ask patient, "How is the pain affecting you **(U)** in regard to ADLs, work, relationships, and enjoyment of life?"

A critical assessment factor, even mild to moderate pain may significantly interfere with function (McCaffery and Pasero, 1999).

NURSING DIAGNOSES

- Activity intolerance
- Anxiety
- Deficient knowledge
- Disturbed sleep pattern
- Fatigue
- Fear
- Hopelessness
- Ineffective breathing pattern

- Ineffective coping
- Ineffective role performance
- Ineffective therapeutic regimen management
- Impaired home maintenance
- Impaired physical mobility
- Insomnia
- Interrupted family processes

- Pain (acute, chronic)
- Powerlessness
- Readiness for enhanced comfort
- Risk for constipation
- Risk for impaired skin integrity
- Self-care deficit
- Situational low self-esteem

Individualize related factors based on patient's condition or needs.

PLANNING

1 Expected outcomes following completion of procedure:
- Patient verbalizes full or partial relief from pain.

The patient's self-report of pain is the single most reliable indicator of pain (Institute for Clinical Systems Improvement, 2006; Miakowski and others, 2005).

- Nonverbal behaviors, such as relaxed face and absence of squinting, reflect a reduction in pain

Nonverbal behaviors are valid and reliable indicators of pain, especially in the cognitively impaired patient (Bucknall and others, 2007; Herr and others, 2006; Mansfield, 2006).

- Patient's function improves in sleep, nutrition, physical activity, and personal relationships.

Adequate pain relief permits patient to participate in usual ADLs (Bucknall and others, 2007; Vallerand and others, 2007).

2 Prepare patient's environment:

a Temperature suited to patient

Temperature extremes alter patient's responses to pain.

b Lighting

Bright or very dim lighting aggravates pain sensation.

c Sound

Loud or irritating sounds aggravate pain.

d Activity. Prevent unnecessary interruptions, coordinate activities, and plan for rest periods.

Fatigue accentuates perception of pain.

e Close room door or curtain.

Provides privacy and reduces stimuli that increase pain.

3 Explain steps to be taken to minimize pain stimuli.

Reduces fear and anxiety.

IMPLEMENTATION

1 Perform hand hygiene, and apply clean gloves if indicated.

Reduces transmission of infection.

2 Administer pain-relieving medications as ordered.

Analgesics are the cornerstone of pain management.

3 Obtain order for pain-relieving medications if none are ordered.

Nurse advocates for patient to have appropriate pain relief.

4 Administer medications for analgesic side effects known to be a problem for this patient.

Preemptive action will prevent or minimize unpleasant problems. When a side effect is common to the patient, do not make patient wait to ask for treatment.

5 Remove painful stimuli:

Reduces stimulation of pain and pressure receptors. Also maximizes response to pain-relieving interventions.

STEP	RATIONALE

a   Assist patient with turning and repositioning to a comfortable position in normal body alignment.

b   Smooth wrinkles in bed linens.   Reduces pressure and irritation to skin.

c   Loosen any constrictive bandage or device: blood pressure cuff, elastic wrap bandages, band of elastic hose, intravenous (IV) dressings, and identification bands.   Bandage or device encircling extremity will restrict circulation.

d   Reposition underlying tubes or equipment.

6   Apply splinting (e.g., pillow or folded blanket):

a   Explain purpose of splinting to patient.   Promotes patient's cooperation.

b   Assist patient in placing hands firmly over area of discomfort (see illustration).   Splinting immobilizes painful area.

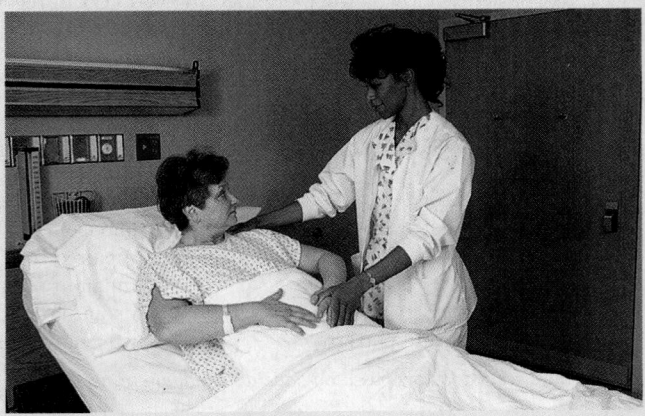

STEP 6b   Patient splinting painful area.

c   Assist patient in splinting during coughing, deep breathing, and turning.   Splinting decreases movement and subsequent pain during activity.

d   Assist patient in attaining comfortable position within normal body alignment.   Turning and repositioning reduce stimulation of pain and pressure receptors.

e   Use pillow to support body position.

7   Provide psychosocial interventions such as reducing environmental stimuli, alleviating anxiety by giving information, praying with patient, or providing distraction through watching TV or listening to music. Perform these interventions only after patient starts to obtain relief for severe pain with administered medication. These are supplements to pain relief, not substitutes.   Assists patients in relaxing. Thoughts influence feelings, which change perception and behaviors, including a perception of pain relief (Austin, 2004; McCaffery and Pasero, 1999).

8   If used, remove and dispose of gloves. Perform hand hygiene.   Reduces transmission of infection.

EVALUATION

1   Within 1 hour of an intervention (e.g., when the drug used is at its peak effect) ask patient to verbalize how well the pain has been relieved. Have patient rate pain intensity now on a scale of 0 to 10.   Evaluates effectiveness of pain-relieving interventions in a timely manner after each intervention (Bucknall and others, 2007; McDonald and others, 2007).

2   Compare patient's current pain intensity with personally set pain-intensity goal.   Assists in determining appropriate changes to the pain-management plan.

3   Compare the patient's ability to function and perform ADLs before and after pain interventions.   Contributes to determining effectiveness of pain-relieving interventions, especially in nonverbal patients.

4   Observe patient's nonverbal behaviors.   Determines effectiveness of pain-relieving interventions.

5   Evaluate for analgesic side effects.   Side effects of analgesics may be controlled by reducing the dose, increasing time intervals, or administering other medications (e.g., stimulant laxative for opioid-induced constipation) (Whilear and Maxwell, 2004).

Unexpected Outcomes

1 Patient verbalizes continued pain that exceeds pain-intensity goal, describes worsening of pain, displays nonverbal behavior reflecting pain, or identifies pain in a different location.

2 Patient experiences unexpected reaction to medication.

Related Interventions

- Perform another complete pain assessment (Bucknall and others, 2007; Sloman and Wruble, 2006).
- Implement nonpharmacological pain-relief measures (see Skill 15-5) (Mitchell and McDonald, 2006; Soeken, 2004).
- Ask family members what might be helpful (Mansfield, 2006).
- Notify physician.

- Assess unexpected effects on patient.
- Notify physician.
- Be prepared to administer antidote (e.g., antiemetic, antihistamine, opioid-reversing agent).
- Monitor for effectiveness of antidote; antidote may have a shorter half-life than the pain medication. A repeat dose of the antidote may be necessary.
- Complete adverse reaction documentation, and record in patient's medical record according to agency policy.

Recording and Reporting

- Record and report character of pain before intervention, therapies used, and patient response.
- Record and report inadequate pain relief (not reaching goal), a reduction in patient function, and/or adverse effects from pain interventions (pharmacological and nonpharmacological).

Teaching Considerations

- Review patient's and family's understanding of the pain-intensity scale used to rate the pain.
- Explain to patient and family about behavioral changes that may result from pain.
- Ask patient and family about fear of addiction, a common primary concern, or other misconceptions (Hadjistaviapoulos and others, 2007; Larsson and Wijik, 2007; Miller and Newton, 2006).

Pediatric Considerations

- Although validity and reliability scores of pain rating scales generally increase with age, you can use some rating scales with a child as young as 3 years of age (Beyer and others, 2005; Chambers and others, 2005; Wilson and Helgadotter, 2006).
- Some children are reluctant to report pain because they have misconceptions about the cause of their pain or they fear the consequences (e.g., another painful procedure or an injection).
- Infants and children experience pain but respond to pain differently than adults do because of their different developmental levels. For example, they cry and thrash about, have sleep disturbances, have a shortened attention span, suck or rock, refuse to eat or play, or are quiet and withdrawn. Still others become active when they are in pain; variations in activity levels are related to the child's personality, developmental level, and previous pain experiences (Chambers and others, 2005; Wilson and Helgadotter, 2006).
- Parents are a helpful source of information when assessing a child's pain and when planning pain-relief therapies. Most parents know how their child exhibits pain and which pain-relief interventions have been successful or unsuccessful.
- Children with verbal skills can rate their level of pain on the Wong-Baker FACES Pain Rating Scale or the Oucher Pain Scale (Beyer and others, 2005; Chambers and others, 2005).

- Additional pain assessment scales for neonates, newborns, and nonverbal children are available.

Gerontological Considerations

- Older patients tend to have inadequately managed pain because of concerns regarding adverse effect of pharmacological treatments (American Geriatrics Society, 2002/2005; Hadjistaviapoulos and others, 2007; Larsson and Wijik, 2007).
- Some older adults require more time to explain the pain management instrument you select.
- Pain is not a natural occurrence of aging, although older adult patients are at risk for experiencing more pain-causing conditions (American Geriatrics Society, 2002/2005).
- Older adult patients with pain may underreport pain (Clark and others, 2006; Higgins and others, 2004). As the nurse, explain the importance of honesty in reporting their pain.
- Older adult patients who are nonverbal with conditions that are painful receive fewer analgesics than similar patients who are able to report their pain (Higgins and others, 2004; Larson and Wijik, 2007).
- A strategy for assessing pain in older adults or nonverbal patients with painful conditions is an around-the-clock analgesia trial and observation of their behaviors (Mansfield, 2006; Won and Lapane, 2004).

Home Care Considerations

- Consider home living conditions, such as type of bed, stairs, and environmental stimuli. A supportive bed and quiet environment will enhance sleep and promote pain management.
- Pain management attitudes of the primary care provider (significant other) require investigation, because without his or her participation successful pain management in the patient experiencing pain will not be realized (Larsson and Wijik, 2007).
- Administration (around-the-clock versus prn) and storing of analgesics requires planning.
- Assess situation for others in environment who might take the medications.

SKILL 15-2 Patient-Controlled Analgesia

Intermediate / Postoperative Nursing Care / Managing Pain

Patient-controlled analgesia (PCA) is an interactive method of pain management that permits patient control over pain through self-administration of analgesics (ASPMN, 2006; Kastanias and Smith, 2006). Commonly prescribed medications delivered via PCA include morphine sulfate, hydromorphone (Dilaudid) and fentanyl. A patient simply depresses the button on a PCA device to receive a regulated dose of analgesic. It is crucial that candidates for PCA be able to understand how, why, and when to self-administer the medication (APS, 2003). Patients with acute (e.g., postoperative) and chronic (e.g., cancer) pain extensively use it. Available routes of PCA administration include subcutaneous, intravenous (IV), and epidural, and now oral PCA and transdermal PCA are available as well (Kastanias and Smith, 2006; Pasero and others, 2007). Though a controversial practice, nurse-controlled analgesia (NCA) occasionally is ordered, whereby the nurse depresses the button after first assessing the patient. This is called PCA by proxy. In addition, family-controlled analgesia (FCA) is used in children with cognitive or physical disabilities (ASPMN, 2006). PCA is not recommended in situations in which oral analgesics could easily manage pain (APS, 2003).

A PCA may be electronic (Fig. 15-1) or nonelectronic, consisting of an infusion device, a prefilled drug reservoir, and tubing that delivers the medication from the infuser through the patient-control module to tubing connected to IV fluid, which runs at a continuous rate. PCAs are individually programmed to automatically deliver a specific physician-prescribed continuous infusion (basal rate) of medication, a bolus dose (patient initiated), or both. The PCA prevents overdosing by interposing a preprogrammed delay time or "lockout" (usually 6 to 16 minutes) between patient-initiated doses. In addition, the prescriber may limit the total amount of opioid that the patient may receive in 1 to 4 hours. Use basal (continuous) infusions cautiously because studies have not shown superior analgesic benefit. Continuous infusion increases the risk for opioid overdose (APS, 2003).

The PCA has several advantages. It allows more constant serum levels of the opioid and, as a result, avoids the peaks and troughs of a large bolus. Because the blood level stays within a narrow range of the minimum effective analgesia concentration for the individual, pain relief is enhanced and the incidence of side effects, such as sedation and respiratory depression, is decreased (Pasero, 2003b). A second advantage is that when used postoperatively, fewer complications arise because earlier and easier ambulation occurs as a result of effective pain relief. Increased patient control and independence are other advantages. Because the device provides medication on demand as soon as the patient feels the need, the total amount of opioid use is reduced. PCA allows the patient to manage pain with minimal nursing intervention and therefore also saves nursing time. Patients are not as dependent on the nursing staff for pain medication administration. The fact that the patient must be awake to push the button to receive a dose also makes overdosing unlikely.

Concerns involving PCA use are patient-related, pump failure, or operator errors. Patients may misunderstand how PCA therapy works, mistake the PCA button for the nurse call button, or have family members who operate the demand button (ASPMN, 2006).

The pump may fail to deliver the drug on demand, have a faulty alarm or low battery, or lack free-flow protection. Operators may incorrectly program the dose, concentration, or rate. Other errors include failing to clamp or unclamp tubing, improperly loading syringe or cartridge, failing to monitor for side effects/overdose, and not responding to alarms (Leavitt, 2003). A PCA requires careful monitoring; never try to operate the PCA without fully understanding the particular model in use.

Delegation Considerations

The skill of administration of patient-controlled analgesia (PCA) cannot be delegated to NAP. The nurse directs the NAP to:
- Immediately report any new symptom or change in patient status, including unrelieved pain or oversedation, to the nurse.
- Never administer a PCA dose for the patient (ASPMN, 2006).

Equipment

- ❏ PCA system
- ❏ Identification label and time tape (may already be attached and completed by pharmacy)
- ❏ Alcohol swab
- ❏ Adhesive tape
- ❏ Clean gloves, when applicable
- ❏ Equipment for vital signs and pulse oximeter.

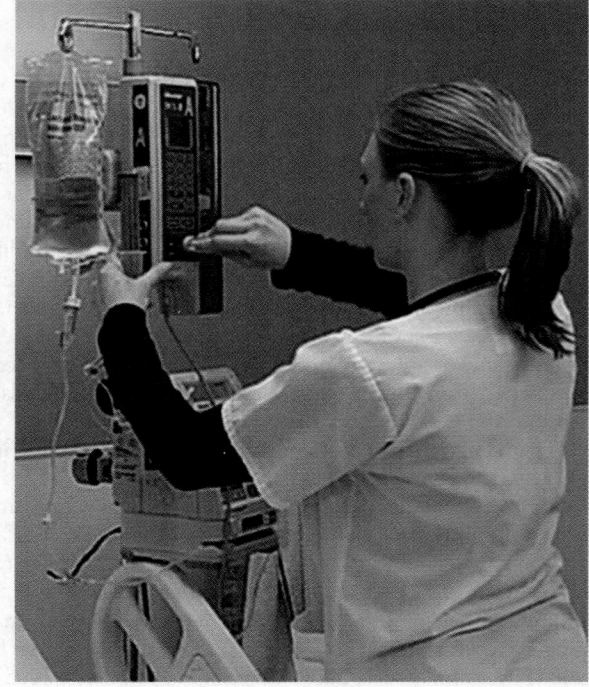

FIG 15-1 Patient-controlled analgesia (PCA) device.

STEP	RATIONALE

ASSESSMENT

1 Assess patient's cognitive ability.

2 Assess for physical, behavioral, and emotional signs and symptoms of pain or discomfort (see Skill 15-1).

3 Assess characteristics of pain (see Skill 15-1).

4 Assess environment for factors that contribute to pain.

5 If patient has had surgery, apply clean gloves and inspect incision. Palpate gently around the area for tenderness. Use sterile gloves if handling the incision.

6 Assess patency of existing IV infusion line and surrounding tissue for inflammation or swelling (see Chapter 31).

7 Assess knowledge and effectiveness of previous pain management strategies, especially previous PCA use.

8 Check physician's order for name of medication, dose, frequency of medication (continuous or demand or both), and lockout period.

9 Identify patient using at least two identifiers.

10 Have a second registered nurse (RN) confirm physician's order and the correct setup of the PCA. The second RN should independently check the physician's order and the machine, not just simply look at the first RN's setup.

11 Check patient's history of drug allergies. Be aware that nausea is not an allergic reaction and can be treated. Itching alone is not an allergic reaction and is common to opioid use. Itching is also treatable and should not preclude use of PCA.

Rationale column:

Determines if patient is able to use PCA for pain management.

Combination of signs and symptoms reveals source and nature of pain.

Guides clinician in collecting information about patient's pain experience.

Factors may increase pain perception.

Reveals evidence of tissue trauma or damage, which stimulates peripheral pain receptors to transmit impulses to cortex to create conscious awareness of pain (McCaffery and Pasero, 1999).

IV line must be patent with fluid infusing for medication to reach venous circulation. Confirmation of placement of IV catheter and integrity of surrounding tissues ensures medication is administered safely.

Response to pain-control strategies assists in identifying learning needs and affects patient's willingness to try therapy.

Opioid medication administration is a dependent nursing function and requires physician's prescription.

Complies with The Joint Commission (2009) requirements to ensure right patient receives right medication.

Prevents medication errors.

Avoids placing patient at risk for allergic reaction.

NURSING DIAGNOSES

- Activity intolerance
- Acute confusion (contraindicates use of PCA)
- Anxiety
- Deficient knowledge regarding use of patient-controlled analgesia
- Fear
- Ineffective coping
- Pain (acute, chronic)
- Risk for infection

Individualize related factors based on patient's condition or needs.

PLANNING

1 Expected outcomes following completion of procedure:
   - Patient verbalizes pain relief.
   - Patient exhibits a relaxed facial expression and body position.
   - Patient remains alert and oriented.

   - Patient increasingly participates in self-care activities.
   - Patient correctly operates PCA device.

2 Explain purpose and demonstrate function of PCA to patient and family:

   a Device is programmed to deliver ordered type and dose of pain medication, lockout interval, and 1- or 4-hour maximum dose limit.

Rationale column:

Drug is given safely and is effective in providing pain control.

Points to successful pain relief.

Indicates freedom from overly sedating effects of opioids. Sleepiness is usually from fatigue and is not necessarily a sign of oversedation.

Suggests successful pain relief.

Demonstrates learning and appropriate operation of PCA device.

Effective explanations allow patient participation in care and independence in pain control. Preoperative education about PCA therapy improves postoperative pain relief (ASPMN, 2006; Pasero, 2003b).

Ensures safety by implementing parts of the six rights of drug administration.

Critical Decision Point *Teach the family not to push the button for the patient unless directed to do so by a nurse or physician.*

STEP	RATIONALE

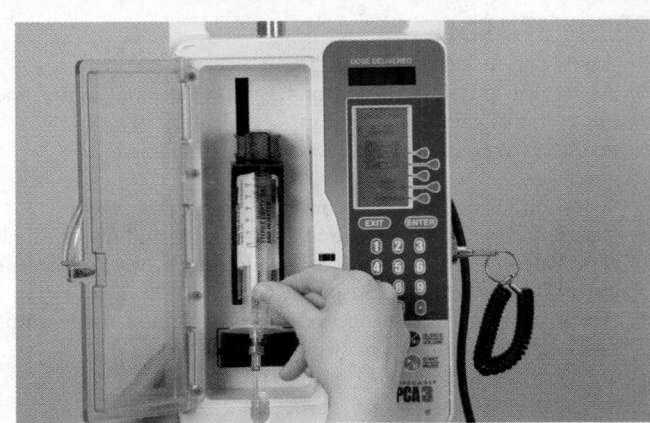

STEP 3   Nurse inserting drug cartridge into PCA device.

b Device allows patient to push medication demand button on timing unit instead of calling nurse.	Gives patient control of pain. Patient does not have to call and wait for nurse to prepare and deliver medication.
c Provides lockout time between demand doses to prevent overdose.	Relieves patient's fear of possible overdose. System has built-in safeguards to help prevent accidental administration of doses or overdosing.
d Infuser will be on IV pole or attached to bed clothing or wrist.	
e Device administers small but frequent amounts of medication as needed to provide comfort and minimize side effects.	Small dosing with patient-controlled administration produces constant serum drug levels rather than peaks and troughs associated with prn nurse-administered therapy (Pasero, 2003b).

Critical Decision Point   *Instruct patient to check with nurse or physician with questions and concerns or if medication is not controlling pain. Drug may need to be changed, or dosage may need to be adjusted.*

3 Check infuser and patient-control module for accurate labeling or evidence of leaking.	Avoids medication error. Damage to system can occur in shipping and handling; inspect to avoid injury or harm to patient, self, or others.
4 Program computerized PCA pump to deliver prescribed medication dose and lockout interval.	Ensures safe, therapeutic drug administration.
5 Draw curtains around patient's bed, or close door to room.	Maintains patient's privacy.
6 Position patient comfortably for procedure. Maintain any position restrictions. Venipuncture or central line site needs to be accessible.	Comfortable position enhances effectiveness of analgesia.

IMPLEMENTATION

1 Perform hand hygiene.	Reduces transmission of infection.
2 Follow the "six rights" to be sure of correct medication (see Chapter 20). Check patient's identification band, and ask patient to state name.	Minimizes risk for medication error and harm to patient. The Joint Commission (2008) requires two types of identifiers. To initiate or change PCA administration programming, two nurses must check system.
3 Attach drug reservoir to infusion device (see illustration), and prime tubing.	Locks system and prevents air from infusing into IV tubing.
4 Apply clean gloves.	Reduces potential contact with blood when working with IV line.
5 Attach needleless adapter to tubing adapter of patient-control module.	Needed to connect with IV line.
6 Wipe injection port of maintenance IV line with alcohol if using a closed port.	Alcohol is a topical antiseptic that minimizes entry of surface microorganisms during needle insertion.
7 Insert needleless adapter into injection port nearest patient.	Establishes route for medication to enter main IV line. Prevents delay of medication delivery to patient.
8 Secure connections with tape, and anchor PCA tubing.	Prevents dislodging of needle from port. Facilitates ambulation.
9 Administer loading dose of analgesia as prescribed.	A one-time dose may be given manually by nurse or programmed into PCA pump.

STEP	RATIONALE
10 Discard gloves and supplies in appropriate containers. Perform hand hygiene.	Reduces transmission of microorganisms.
11 If patient is experiencing pain, have patient demonstrate use of PCA system (see illustration); if not, have patient repeat instructions given earlier by nurse.	Repeating instructions reinforces learning. Checking patient's understanding through return demonstration helps nurse determine patient's level of understanding and ability to manipulate device.

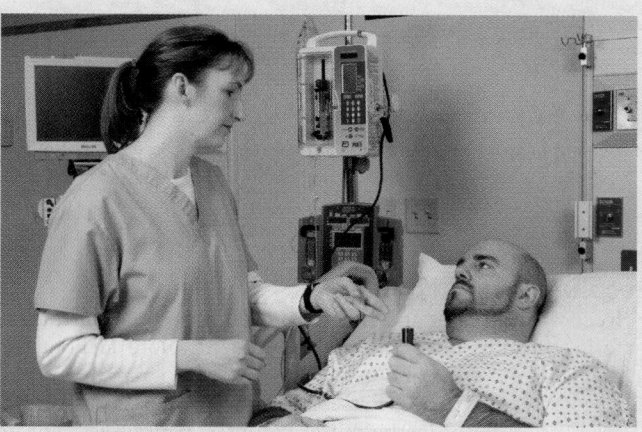

STEP 11   Patient learns to use PCA pump.

STEP	RATIONALE
12 Dispose of empty cassette or syringe in compliance with institutional policy.	The federal Controlled Substances Act regulates the control and dispensation of opioids for all institutions.
13 If PCA is discontinued before device is completely empty, record drug wastage on PCA medication record per institutional policy. Note date, time, amount of drug wasted, and reason for wastage.	Two registered nurses must witness wastage of opioids (narcotics) and sign the record to meet requirements of the Controlled Substances Act for scheduled drugs
14 Most PCA systems need a secondary IV infusion running at TKO (to keep open rate). Be sure infusion is running properly.	To maintain patency of vein between PCA intermittent (bolus) doses.

EVALUATION

1 Use pain rating scale to evaluate patient's pain intensity according to agency policy.	Determines response to PCA dosing. Documenting "PCA in use" or "PCA effective" is not an adequate record of the patient's pain level.
2 Observe patient for nausea or itching.	Common side effects of opioid.
3 Observe for signs of adverse reactions, especially excessive sedation (Box 15-3, p. 384). Monitor level of sedation, vital signs, and pulse oximetry every 2 hours for the first 12 hours (APS, 2003).	Patient is at highest risk the first 12 hours of use, more if they have additional risk factors (e.g., advanced age, sleep apnea, obesity, being opioid naive) (DeJongue and others, 2000). Excess sedation precedes respiratory depression.
4 Have patient demonstrate dose delivery.	Evaluates skill in use of PCA.
5 According to agency policy, evaluate number of attempts (number of times patient pushed the button) and delivery of demand doses (number of times drug actually given), as well as basal dose, if ordered.	Assists in evaluating effectiveness of PCA dose and frequency in relieving pain. Maintains compliance with Controlled Substances Act.

Unexpected Outcomes	Related Interventions
1 Patient verbalizes continued or worsening discomfort, or displays nonverbal behaviors indicative of pain. Suggests underlying condition has changed or patient is undermedicated.	• Perform complete pain assessment. • Assess for possible complications. • Inspect IV site for possible catheter occlusion or infiltration. • Evaluate number of attempts and deliveries initiated by patient. • Check that maintenance IV fluid is continuously running. • Evaluate pump for operational problems. • Consult with physician.

Unexpected Outcomes	Related Interventions
2 Patient is not readily arousable.	• Stop PCA. • Notify physician. • Elevate head of bed 30 degrees, unless contraindicated. • Instruct patient to take deep breaths. • Apply oxygen at 2 L/min per nasal cannula. • Assess vital signs. • Evaluate amount of opioid delivered within past 4 to 8 hours. • Ask family members if they pressed the button without patient's knowledge. • Review medication administration record for other possible sedating drugs. • Prepare to administer an opioid-reversing agent. • Observe patient frequently.
3 Patient unable to manipulate PCA device to maintain pain control.	• Consult with physician regarding alternative medication route. • Discuss with physician possible basal (continuous) dose. • Assess patient support system for significant other who can responsibly manipulate PCA device (ASPMN, 2006).

Recording and Reporting

• Record drug, dose, and time begun on appropriate medication form. Specify concentration and diluent. Note lockout time, demand, and/or basal dose.

• Record regular periodic assessments of patient status on PCA medication form, in the narrative notes, pain assessment flow sheet, or other documentation, according to institutional policy. Forms vary from institution to institution, but information required is similar. Detailed recording complies with required documentation of schedule II drugs. Indicate vital signs, if appropriate; sedation status; pain rating; status of vascular access site; amount of solution infused; amount of solution remaining; amount of drug received.

Teaching Considerations

• Give instructions during pain-free or pain-reduced states and before initiating therapy. Instruct surgical patients preoperatively.

• Encourage patients to push button on timing unit whenever they feel pain. Tell a patient not to delay if he or she is experiencing pain. Pain is easier to prevent than to treat.

• Explain regimen to family so that they can support and assist patient.

• Inform patient of nonpharmacological pain management strategies that supplement or enhance pharmacological intervention.

• Inform patient and family that patient cannot overdose with PCA if only the patient pushes the button.

Pediatric Considerations

• Patient-controlled analgesia is an effective means of pain control in children who can understand the concept. When selecting children for PCA use, consider the patient's developmental level, cognitive level, and motor skills. Ordinarily PCA use is safe and effective for patients as young as 5 years old (Pasero 2003b). From a developmental perspective, use of PCA is particularly effective with adolescents, because it leads to feeling of control.

• Patients as young as 5 years of age can use PCA, depending on their ability to understand the concept and physically push the button. Instruct family members not to push the button for the child. Some facilities have provided specific guidelines and training to allow parents to push the button for children too young or unable to use the device on their own. This practice is controversial because it may increase the risk for overdosing (ASPMN, 2006).

• Pharmacological pain support is safe and effective in pediatric patients when dose is calibrated according to child's weight (Lehr and BeVier, 2003). As with adults, doses may need adjusting after initiation of medication to obtain optimal analgesia with minimal side effects (Gordon and others, 2005).

• There are no reports of addiction secondary to the use of PCA in pediatric patients (American Society of Addiction Medicine, 2004).

Gerontological Considerations

• Older patients appear more sensitive to analgesic properties and side effects of opioids (American Geriatrics Society, 2002/2005). Older adults' reduced renal and liver function slows opioid metabolism and excretion. This causes a faster peak effect and a longer duration of action of the opioid (APS, 2003). In addition, their decrease in water concentrates hydrophilic opioids, possibly resulting in increased side effects. Thus start with a low dose, and titrate upward slowly.

• If confusion occurs while using a PCA, lower the dose, lengthen the lockout, or add a nonopioid analgesic to reduce the opioid dose (Pasero, 1999). Nurse-activated around-the-clock dosing is another alternative (ASPMN, 2006).

BOX 15-3	Sedation Scale

S = Sleep, easy to arouse
1 = Awake and alert
2 = Slightly drowsy, easily aroused
3 = Frequently drowsy, arousable, drifts off to sleep during
    conversation
4 = Somnolent, minimal or no response to physical stimulation

From McCaffery M, Pasero C: *Pain: clinical manual,* St. Louis, 1999, Mosby.

SKILL 15-3   Epidural Analgesia

The epidural space (Fig. 15-2) is a potential space between the vertebral bones and the dura mater, the outermost meninges covering the brain and spinal cord. Analgesic medication delivered into this space creates epidural analgesia. The intrathecal/subarachnoid space is just around the spinal cord and contains cerebrospinal fluid (CSF). Only physicians and nurse anesthetists administer intrathecal (spinal) drugs. Registered nurses, as regulated by their State Boards of Nursing, are not allowed to administer analgesics into the intrathecal space. However, intrathecal pumps are available. With the consent of the admitting physician, contact the pain clinic for instructions if you have a patient who is admitted with an intrathecal pump in place. This skill focuses on epidural analgesia only.

Drugs administered in the epidural space spread (1) by diffusion through the dura mater into the CSF, where they act directly on receptors in the dorsal horn of the spinal cord, (2) via blood vessels in the epidural space and delivered systemically, and/or (3) by means of absorption by fat in the epidural space, creating a depot where the drug is slowly released into the systemic circulation (Pasero, 2003a).

Opioids and local anesthetics, separately or in combination, are often used in epidural analgesia, although adjuvants are also given (Chang and others, 2006). An infusion delivers opioids close to their site of action (CNS), where they have greater bioavailability than IV or oral opioids and thus require much smaller doses to achieve adequate pain relief. Common opioids given via the epidural route are morphine, hydromorphone (Dilaudid), fentanyl, and sufentanil. These opioids vary in their lipophilic (fat-loving) and hydrophilic (water-loving) properties, which alter absorption rate and duration of action. Fentanyl and sufentanil are lipophilic, causing them to have a quicker onset and shorter duration of action (2 hours). Morphine and hydromorphone are hydrophilic, resulting in a longer onset and duration of action (up to 24 hours with a single bolus dose). Epidural local anesthetics such as bupivacaine (Marcaine) and ropivacaine (Naropin) (Pasero, 2003a) block generation and conduction of pain nerve impulses in the CNS. These local anesthetics significantly block sensory nerves while having a minimal effect on motor nerves. Thus the patient is able to ambulate. Combining opioids with local anesthetics improves pain control and reduces complications (CNS and cardiotoxicity) while lowering opioid doses (Pasero, 2003a). Research

shows the epidural route to be the most effective in managing postoperative pain from thoracic and abdominal surgeries (Chang and others, 2006).

For epidural catheter placement, the patient is in the lateral decubitus or sitting position with shoulders and hips squared and hips and head flexed (McCaffery and Pasero, 1999). Usually an anesthesiologist or nurse anesthetist places a catheter into the epidural space (Fig. 15-3) below the second lumbar vertebra, where the spinal cord ends; however, thoracic epidurals may also be inserted. When the catheter is for temporary or short-term use, it is usually not sutured in place and exits from the insertion site on the back (Fig. 15-4). By contrast, a catheter intended for permanent or long-term use is "tunneled" subcutaneously and exits on the side of the body or on the abdomen. Tunneling decreases the chance of infection or dislodging of the catheter. In both cases a sterile occlusive dressing covers the catheter and it is secured to the patient. The only way to ensure proper placement of an epidural catheter is by x-ray.

Epidural medication is administered either intermittently via bolus injection through an epidural catheter by the clinician, demand injection by the patient (patient-controlled epidural analgesia [PCEA]), or continuously via a controlled delivery system such as an implanted infusion pump (Fig. 15-5). With a continuous device in place, the implanted epidural pump can be injected with drugs intermittently as well as deliver continuous infusions.

The use of epidural opioids for pain control requires astute nursing observation and care. The catheter poses a threat to patient safety because of its anatomical location, its potential for migration through the dura, and its proximity to spinal nerves and vessels.

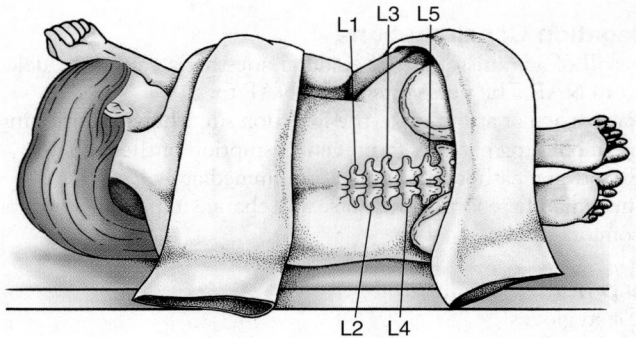

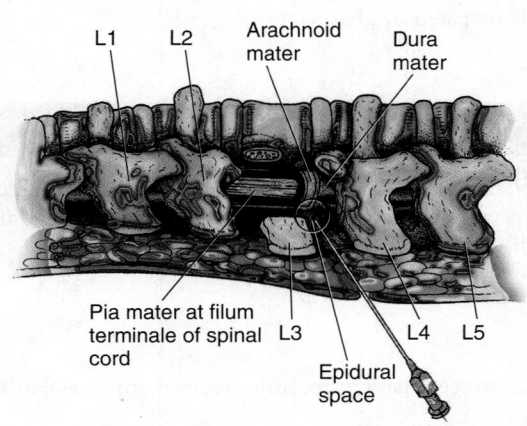

FIG 15-2   Anatomical drawing of epidural space. (*From Sinatra S: Spinal opioid analgesia: an overview. In Sinatra RS and others, editors: Acute pain management, St. Louis, 1992, Mosby.*)

FIG 15-3   Insertion of epidural catheter.

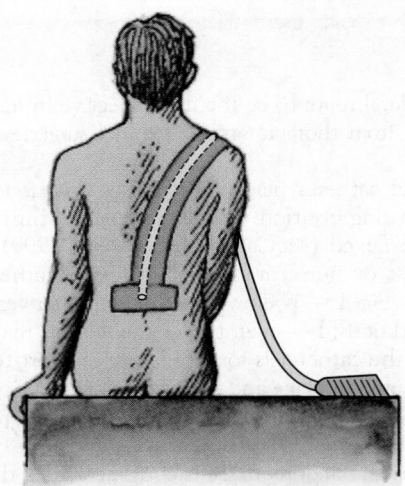

FIG 15-4   Epidural catheter taped in place. (*Courtesy Astra Zeneca Pharmaceuticals, Wilmington, Del.*)

An epidural catheter migration into the subarachnoid space produces medication levels too large for epidural use. Epidural and intrathecal doses are not equivalent. Intrathecal doses are much smaller than epidural doses. As an example, the epidural dose of morphine is 10 to 20 times greater than that required for an intrathecal dose. Question orders for administering concurrent oral medications that often cause oversedation and/or respiratory depression (e.g., muscle relaxants or anxiolytics). Obtain approval for use of any CNS depressant medications from the health care professional managing the epidural analgesia (Chang and others, 2006).

Delegation Considerations

The skill of administration of epidural anesthesia cannot be delegated to NAP. The nurse directs the NAP to:

- Pay particular attention to the insertion site when repositioning or ambulating patients to prevent disruption of the catheter.
- Report any catheter disconnection immediately.
- Immediately report to the nurse any change in patient status or comfort level.

Equipment

- ❑ Clean gloves
- ❑ Prediluted preservative-free opioid or local anesthetic as prescribed by physician and prepared for use in IV infusion pump (usually prepared by pharmacy)

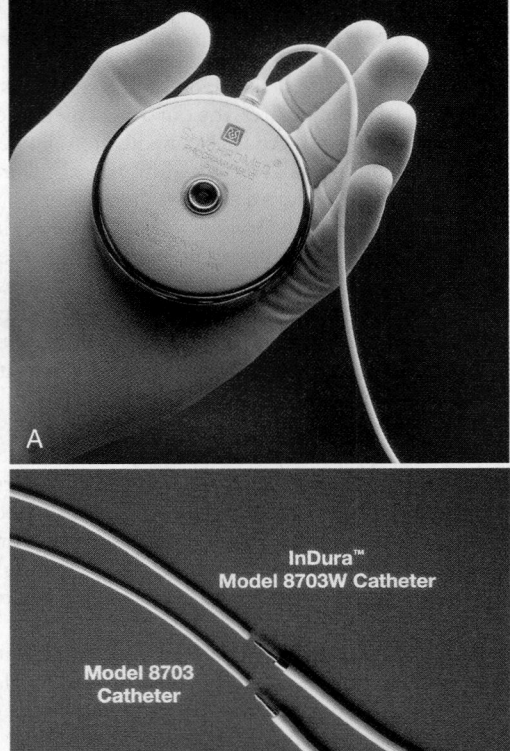

FIG 15-5   A SynchroMed implantable pump (**A**) and spinal catheters (**B**) for delivery of a precise volume of long-term intraspinal analgesia each day. (*Courtesy Medtronic, Inc., Columbia Heights, Minn.*)

- ❑ Infusion pump
- ❑ Infusion pump compatible tubing without Y-ports; some infusion pumps have tubing color coded for intraspinal use
- ❑ Filter needle, per institutional policy
- ❑ Tape
- ❑ Label (for tubing)
- ❑ Equipment for vital signs

STEP	RATIONALE

ASSESSMENT

1   Assess patient's comfort level, presenting medical/surgical condition, and appropriateness for epidural analgesia.

Certain conditions make epidural analgesia the method of choice for pain control: postoperative states, patients with trauma or advanced cancer that is not responsive to other pain management modalities, and those predisposed to cardiopulmonary complications because of preexisting medical condition or surgery.

2   Check to see if patient recently received anticoagulants.

Recent anticoagulants sometimes contraindicate the placement of epidural catheter because of risk for epidural hematoma at the insertion site (Regional anesthesia, 2003).

STEP	RATIONALE
3 Check to see if patient routinely takes herbal medications and, if so, which ones.	Some herbals interfere with the clotting mechanism, which could cause bleeding at the epidural insertion site, but currently there is no contraindication to their use (Regional anesthesia, 2003). It is prudent to recognize herbs a patient uses to check for drug-drug interactions (Capriotti, 2004; King and Pettigrew, 2004; Soeken, 2004).

Critical Decision Point   *Contraindications to epidural analgesia include coagulopathies, abnormal clotting studies, history of multiple abscesses, and sepsis (Regional anesthesia, 2003). Additional contraindications include skeletal or spinal abnormalities.*

STEP	RATIONALE
4 Check patient's history of drug allergies.	Avoids placing patient at risk for allergic reaction.
5 Assess for physical, behavior, and emotional signs and symptoms of pain (see Skill 15-1).	Combination of signs and symptoms provides baseline to later determine efficacy of analgesia.
6 Assess characteristics and intensity of pain (see Skill 15-1).	Serves as a baseline to later determine efficacy of analgesia.
7 Assess environment for factors that are contributing to pain.	Helps identify stimuli that aggravate patient's response to pain.
8 Assess sedation level of patient by assessing level of wakefulness or alertness, ability to follow commands, and drowsiness (see Box 15-3).	Establishes a baseline before first dose. Sedation always precedes respiratory depression from opioids (Chang and others, 2006).
9 Assess rate, pattern, and depth of respirations (see Chapter 5).	Establishes a baseline.
10 Assess blood pressure (see Chapter 5).	Establishes a baseline. Vasodilation can occur, and hypotension, including orthostatic hypotension, is common (Bruchi and Chung, 2005).
11 Assess initial motor and sensory function of lower extremities (see Chapter 6).	Establishes a baseline. Excess analgesia causes adverse neurological effects (Pasero and others, 2007).
12 Check to see if catheter is secured to patient's skin from the back or front (see illustration).	Aids in preventing dislodging or migration of catheter.

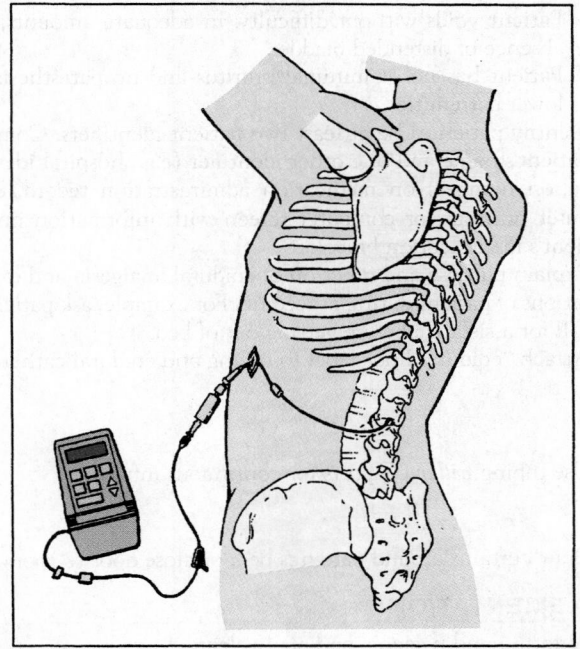

STEP 12   External epidural catheter attached to ambulatory infusion pump. (*Courtesy SIMS Deltec, Inc., St. Paul, Minn.*)

STEP	RATIONALE
13 Check medication administration record (MAR) against physician's order for medication, dosage, and infusion method.	Medication administration is a dependent nursing function and requires physician's prescription.
14 If you plan a continuous infusion, check patency of IV tubing.	Kinked or clamped tubing will interrupt analgesic infusion.

STEP	RATIONALE
15 Keep a patent IV in place until 24 hours after epidural analgesia has ended.	Allows for IV access in case IV medications have to be given to counteract adverse reactions.

NURSING DIAGNOSES

- Activity intolerance
- Anxiety
- Deficient knowledge regarding epidural analgesia

- Disturbed sensory perception
- Impaired physical mobility
- Pain (acute, chronic)

- Risk for infection
- Risk for injury

Individualize related factors based on patient's condition or needs.

PLANNING

STEP	RATIONALE
1 Expected outcomes following completion of procedure: • Patient verbalizes pain relief.	Indicates drug and dose are effective in relieving pain, catheter is intact, and equipment is functioning properly in compliance with physician's order.
• Catheter and injection cap or infusion pump tubing are securely taped and labeled.	Closed, intact system prevents entry of pathogens and disruption of flow of medication.
• Patient remains normotensive, and heart rate stays in normal range.	Indicates absence of potential side effects of epidural opioids.
• Patient is alert and oriented.	Indicates absence of excessive sedation.
• Respirations are regular, of adequate depth, and 8 breaths per minute or greater.	Indicates adequate ventilation and reduced risk for respiratory depression from opioids.
• Patient does not experience headache.	Indicates catheter in epidural space.
• Epidural dressing is dry and intact.	No cerebrospinal fluid leakage.
• Catheter and infusion tubing are free of knots and kinks.	Infusion system is patent.
• No redness, warmth, exudate, tenderness, or swelling is evident at catheter insertion site. Patient is afebrile.	Indicates absence of inflammation or infection.
• Patient voids without difficulty, in adequate amounts, and absence of distended bladder.	Indicates absence of urinary retention (a potential side effect).
• Patient has no or minimal pruritus and no paresthesias of lower extremities.	Indicates absence of potential side effect of epidural medications.
2 Identify patient. Use at least two patient identifiers. Compare patient's name and one other identifier (e.g., hospital identification number) on medication administration record, computer printout, or computer screen with information on patient's identification bracelet.	Ensures correct patient receives analgesia. Complies with The Joint Commission's requirements (2008) and improves medication safety.
3 Explain purpose and function of epidural analgesia and expectations of patient during procedure. For example, ask patient to call for assistance before getting out of bed.	Proper explanation enhances patient cooperation and effective results.
4 Attach "epidural line" label to tubing and epidural catheter.	Labeling helps to ensure medication analgesic is administered into correct line and into epidural space. Labeling of high-risk catheters prevents connection with an inappropriate tube or catheter (The Joint Commission [TJC], 2006).
5 Use tubing *without* Y-ports for continuous infusions.	Use of tubing without Y-ports prevents accidental injection or infusion of other medication meant for vascular space into epidural space.
6 Draw curtains around patient's bed, or close door to room.	Maintains patient's privacy.

IMPLEMENTATION

STEP	RATIONALE
1 Perform hand hygiene, and apply clean gloves.	Reduces transmission of microorganisms.
2 Administer continuous infusion: a Attach container of diluted preservative-free medication to infusion pump tubing and prime tubing (see Chapter 31).	Tubing should be filled with solution and free of air bubbles to avoid air embolus.

STEP	RATIONALE
b Insert tubing into infusion pump, then attach distal end of tubing to epidural catheter.	Infusion pumps propel fluid through tubing.
c Check infusion pump for proper calibration and operation. Many nurses have two nurses check settings.	Ensures patient is receiving proper dose and pain relief.
d Tape all tubing connections. Give ordered bolus or start infusion. (See Chapter 22 for use of infusion pump.)	Taping maintains a secure, closed system to help prevent infection. Sometimes a filter is necessary in the tubing, depending on institutional policy.
3 Administer bolus dose of medication:	
a Draw up prediluted, preservative-free opioid solution through filter needle.	Preservative may be toxic to nerve tissue (Chang and others, 2006).
b Change from filter needle to regular 20-gauge needleless adapter.	Prevents infusion of microscopic glass particles and allows medication to be injected.
c Clean injection cap of epidural catheter with povidone-iodine or substitute antiinfective according to agency policy. **(Do not use alcohol.)**	Sterilizing injection port prevents inadvertent introduction of microorganisms into CNS. Alcohol causes pain and is toxic to neural tissue (Pasero, 2003a).
d Allow to dry, or dry injection cap with sterile gauze.	Reduces possible injection of povidone-iodine.
e Attach syringe directly to injection cap. Aspirate.	Aspiration of more than 1 mL of clear fluid or bloody return means catheter may have migrated into subarachnoid space or into a vessel (Pasero, 1999). Do not inject drug. Notify physician.
f Inject opioid at a rate of 1 mL over 30 seconds.	Slow injection prevents discomfort by lowering the pressure exerted by fluid as it enters the epidural space.
g Remove syringe from injection cap. There is no need to flush with saline.	The catheter is in a space, not a blood vessel, thus flushing with saline is not required (McCaffery and Pasero, 1999).
h Dispose of syringe in sharps container.	Prevents possible exposure to blood.
4 Remove and dispose of gloves. Perform hand hygiene.	Reduces transmission of microorganisms.
5 Before removal of epidural catheter, check for presence of therapeutic anticoagulation. Check agency policy for removal while patient is receiving anticoagulation therapy.	Removal of epidural catheter while a patient is anticoagulated increases the risk for spinal hematoma because of anticoagulation and inability to compress vessels (Regional anesthesia, 2003).

EVALUATION

1 Assess catheter insertion site every 2 to 4 hours for redness, warmth, tenderness, swelling, or drainage.	Local inflammation and superficial skin infection at insertion site may occur. Purulent drainage indicates infection, clear drainage indicates puncture of dura, causing medication to be delivered into the intrathecal space or causing cerebrospinal fluid leakage. Bloody drainage may indicate the catheter entered a blood vessel. Report any of these immediately to the physician managing the epidural catheter—treat as an emergency.
2 Observe sedation level and respiratory rate, rhythm, and pattern every 2 hours for 12 to 24 hours after an epidural bolus of opioid is given to an opioid-naive patient (someone who has not received opioids on an around-the-clock basis for more than 5 to 7 days). Also, closely monitor a patient who is not opioid naive but who is receiving a larger dose of opioid than usual or who has other risk factors (e.g., sleep apnea) (Pasero and others, 2007).	Sedation occurs before respiratory depression and should be closely monitored to prevent respiratory depression (Kabeli, 2005), especially in patients at higher risk for respiratory depression.

Critical Decision Point   *Be prepared to deliver an ampule of naloxone (Narcan), a strong opioid antagonist, 0.4 mg diluted in 9 mL of saline at 1 to 2 mL/min (for adults), if respirations fall below 8 breaths per minute and are shallow. Desired effect is to increase respirations, not reverse analgesia. Rapid reversal of opioids by Narcan could result in profound withdrawal, seizures, dysrhythmias, pulmonary edema, and severe pain (APS, 2003). Continue to assess respiratory status after Narcan administration because renarcotization with resulting respiratory depression could occur (APS, 2003).*

3 Monitor blood pressure and pulse. Assist patient when changing positions.	Postural hypotension, vasodilation, and heart rate changes may occur.
4 Monitor intake and output. Assess for bladder distention. Observe for frequency or urgency.	Urinary retention may occur as a result of effects of medication on spinal nerves innervating the bladder.
5 Observe for pruritus, especially of face, head, neck, and torso. Inform the patient that this is a side effect but is not an allergic response.	Itching is the most common side effect when opioids are delivered via the intraspinal route It is not an indication of an allergic response (McCaffery and Pasero, 1999).

STEP	RATIONALE
6 Observe for nausea and vomiting.	Nausea and vomiting can begin 4 to 6 hours after a bolus because of time needed for drug to reach chemoreceptor trigger zone. Nausea from epidural analgesia worsens by movement.
7 Check insertion site for clear or bloody drainage. Assess for reports of headache.	Headache and cerebrospinal fluid leakage occur from a dural puncture. Bloody drainage may occur if catheter has migrated into a vessel.
8 Monitor temperature. Observe insertion site for signs of inflammation.	Infection can occur from poor sterile technique or systemic bacteremia.
9 Evaluate for motor weakness or numbness and tingling of lower extremities (paresthesias).	Excessive analgesia, infusion of drugs toxic to central nervous system, or contact of catheter with neural tissue may cause adverse sensory deficits (Chang and others, 2006). Indicates need to notify physician immediately. Reducing epidural dose helps eliminate unwanted motor and sensory deficits.
10 After removal of epidural catheter, evaluate for signs and symptoms of hematoma formation: motor or sensory changes below level of catheter.	Although rare, unrecognized spinal hematoma formation could result in permanent neurological damage.

Unexpected Outcomes	Related Interventions
1 Patient states pain is still present or has increased. Primary causes are insufficient drug dose or catheter blockage, breakage, or improper position.	• Check all tubing, connections, medication doses, and pump settings.
2 Patient is not readily arousable.	• Stop epidural infusion. • Prepare to administer opioid reversing agent per physician order. • Monitor continuously until patient is easily arousable.
3 Patient experiences periods of apnea or respirations are less than 8 breaths per minute, shallow, or irregular.	• Instruct patient to take deep breaths. • Stop or reduce rate of epidural infusion. • Notify physician. • Prepare to administer opioid-reversing agent per physician order. • Monitor every 30 minutes until respirations are 8 or above and of adequate depth.
4 Patient reports sudden headache. Clear drainage is present on epidural dressing or more than 1 mL of fluid is aspirated from catheter. Possible indication that catheter has migrated into the subarachnoid space.	• Stop infusion. • If receiving bolus doses, do not administer. • Notify physician.
5 Blood is present on epidural dressing or is aspirated from the catheter. Probable indication that catheter has punctured a blood vessel.	• Stop infusion. • Notify physician.
6 Redness, warmth, tenderness, swelling, or exudate at catheter insertion site. Patient is febrile. Signs and symptoms of infection.	• Notify physician.
7 Patient experiences minimal urinary output, urinary frequency or urgency, bladder distention, pruritus, or nausea and vomiting.	• Consult with physician about reducing the dose of opioid. • Discuss treatment for side effects.

Reporting and Recording

- Record drug, dose, and time given (if injection) or time begun and ended (if continuous infusion) on appropriate medication record. Specify concentration and diluent
- With continuous infusion, obtain and record pump readout hourly for first 24 hours after infusion is begun and then every 4 hours. Review pump settings and usage with staff on next shift.
- Record regular periodic assessments of patient's status in nurse's notes or on appropriate flow sheet, including vital signs, I&O, sedation level, pain severity score, neurological status, appearance of epidural site, presence or absence of adverse reactions to medication, and presence or absence of complications resulting from placement and maintenance of epidural catheter.
- Report any adverse reactions or complications to health care provider.

Teaching Considerations

- Describe catheter placement and use to patient as appropriate. Drawing or showing pictures helps.
- Teach patient the purpose, action, and signs and symptoms of adverse reactions to opioid or local anesthetic. Teach patient when and what signs and symptoms to report to the nurse.
- Teach patient to report pain level using mutually acceptable pain scale.
- Inform patient of other pain-management strategies that supplement or enhance pharmacological intervention (e.g., imagery, distraction, relaxation).
- Tell patient of pain-management strategies that interfere with pharmacological interventions such as over-the-counter medications and herbals.
- Explain that pain relief begins within 30 to 60 minutes of initiation of epidural infusion.
- Explain therapy to family or significant others so that they can support and assist patient.

- Explain the first attempt to sit or stand may cause orthostatic hypotension, and patient will need to rise very slowly to compensate.
- Some patients may feel so much better after obtaining pain relief that they attempt to ambulate without assistance or to overdo their activities. Caution them to begin slowly to avoid injury and to always call for nurse to assist with any activity. Also explain that the first attempt to ambulate may feel strange secondary to decreased sensation, but motor function should be unaffected.

Pediatric Considerations

- Apply EMLA cream to the epidural site 2 hours before catheter insertion. Children are at risk for the same side effects and adverse reactions as adults (McCaffery and Pasero, 1999).

Gerontological Considerations

- Older adults are at the same risk for complications and medication adverse effects as other adult patients. Careful assessment remains key.

Home Care Considerations

- Patients needing long-term or permanent therapy are discharged with a tunneled catheter. Before considering catheter placement and care in the home, assess several variables including fine motor skills, cognitive ability, stage of disease and prognosis, and degree of involvement of family caregiver (Pasero and others, 2007)

- Teach patient and caregiver proper dosage and administration of medication. Evaluating patient's technique for catheter care and administering medication, as well as reinforcing instructions, are priorities.
- Explain available drug and dosage for breakthrough pain. Inform patient how to contact clinician for increase in dosage if highest level prescribed is ineffective.
- Teach patient and caregiver aseptic technique for medication administration as needed and for all catheter care procedures, including dressing changes. Instruct patient to change dressing every week (policy will vary with home care agency). Teach signs and symptoms of infection, and instruct patient to report to nurse or physician immediately should signs and symptoms appear.
- Teach patient and caregiver about signs and symptoms of adverse reactions to medication being used and interventions to alleviate side effects in the home.
  - *Urinary retention:* Teach patient or caregiver how to perform straight catheterization (see Chapter 33).
  - *Pruritus:* Advise patient to wear clean, lightweight, cotton clothing; keep room cool; use cool moist compresses; lubricate skin.
- Teach patient and caregivers about medications to control side effects.
- Give phone numbers of clinicians to contact in emergency and resources in the community.

SKILL 15-4   Local Infusion Pump Analgesia

During surgery for joint replacement, some surgeons will insert an infusion pump (Fig. 15-6) to deliver a local anesthetic (Marcaine, lidocaine, ropivacaine, or mepivacaine) to the surgical site through a one-way catheter. Pain relief is provided directly to the surgical site. Some patients will need oral analgesics as well, but the total dose is often reduced (Regional anesthesia, 2003). The pump has both a demand (4 to 6 mL per bolus) and a continuous rate (2 to 4 mL/hr) feature. Continuous reservoirs hold 100 mL, whereas the patient-controlled units have a 60-mL reservoir. The device remains in place for about 48 hours. Rarely is the pump removed during hospitalization; the patient learns to remove the catheter at home. This device is for one-time use only. Nursing care focuses on assessment of catheter connections, evaluation of local anesthetic side effects, and patient teaching.

Delegation Considerations

The skill of administration of a local anesthetic infusion cannot be delegated to NAP. The nurse directs the NAP to:
- Pay particular attention to the insertion site when providing care, to avoid dislocation.
- Report any catheter disconnection immediately.
- Notify nurse immediately of a change in patient's status or level of comfort.

Equipment
- ❏ Pump in place from surgery (see Fig. 15-6)

Home Catheter Removal
- ❏ Clean gloves
- ❏ Sterile gauze dressing
- ❏ Tape

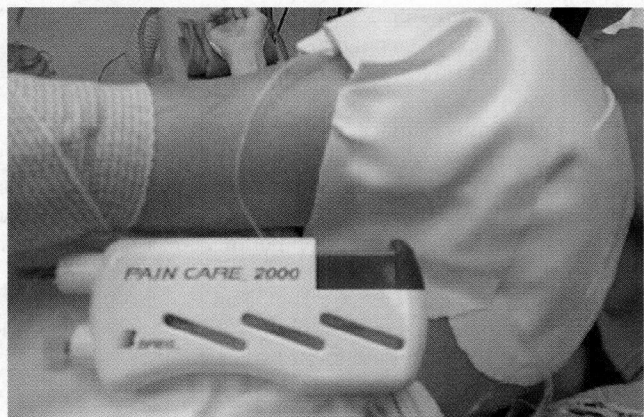

FIG 15-6   Local anesthetic infusion pump in use after shoulder surgery. (*Courtesy Breg, Inc., Vista, Calif.*)

STEP	RATIONALE

ASSESSMENT

1 Assess surgical dressing and site of catheter insertion. Dressing should be dry and intact.	Determines if catheter properly placed.
2 Assess catheter connections. If connections become detached, do NOT reattach, instead notify physician.	Intact system prevents entrance of microorganisms.
3 Assess characteristics of patient's pain (see Skill 15-1).	Provides baseline to determine efficacy of analgesia.

STEP	RATIONALE
4 Assess for blood backing up in tubing.	Indicates possible displacement of catheter into blood vessel.
5 Read label on device and compare to medication administration record (MAR) or physician's order.	Provides information regarding type of anesthetic, concentration, volume, flow rate, date and time prepared, and name of person who prepared it.
6 Determine the level of extremity activity patient can perform per physician orders.	Excessive activity causes displacement of catheter.
7 Assess for signs of local anesthetic toxicity: hypotension, dizziness, tremor, severe itching, swelling of the skin or throat, irregular heartbeat, palpitations, confusion, ringing in the ears, muscle twitching, numbness around the mouth, metallic taste, seizures.	Early identification of toxicity prevents or lessens the possibility of complications.
8 Determine patient's knowledge of infusion pump.	Assesses level of teaching and support required by patient.

NURSING DIAGNOSES

- Anxiety
- Deficient knowledge regarding purpose of infusion pump
- Disturbed sensory perception
- Impaired physical mobility
- Pain (acute, chronic)

Individualize related factors based on patient's condition or needs.

PLANNING

1 Expected outcomes following completion of procedure:	
• Patient verbalizes full or partial relief from pain.	The patient's self-report of pain is the single most reliable indicator of pain.
• Reduction of nonverbal pain behaviors indicative of pain, such as grimacing, clenching teeth, rocking.	Nonverbal behaviors are valid and reliable indicators of pain, especially in the cognitively impaired patient (Cohen-Mansfield, 2006; Herr and others, 2006).
• Patient moves about in bed, sleeps and eats better; is more active, and communicates easily with family and friends.	Adequate pain relief allows patient to participate in ADLs.
• Catheter removed correctly without injury to patient.	Patient and family are able to follow instructions for catheter removal.

IMPLEMENTATION

1 Teach patient or family how to remove catheter (may also be done by home care nurse):	
a Perform hand hygiene, and apply clean gloves.	Decreases transmission of microorganisms.
b Place patient in relaxed position.	Relaxes joint muscles, reducing traction from muscle tension, and provides distraction.
c Gently remove surgical dressing.	Provides access to infusion catheter.
d Grasp catheter firmly, and pull outward from skin with steady motion. If resistance occurs, stop pulling. Reposition extremity, and try again. If tubing continues to stretch and demonstrates resistance, stop pulling, cover area with sterile dressing, and notify physician.	Approach designed to minimize tissue trauma.
e Look for mark on end of catheter tip.	Indicates complete removal of catheter.
f Once catheter is removed, place a sterile dressing over the area and apply pressure for at least 2 minutes.	Prevents hematoma formation.
g Discard soiled dressing and gloves. Perform hand hygiene.	Reduces transmission of microorganisms.

EVALUATION

1 During infusion, ask patient to rate pain intensity using appropriate scale.	Determines patient response to local injection of medication.
2 Observe for signs of adverse drug reaction.	Local analgesics can result in systemic adverse effects if absorbed by veins.
3 Observe patient's position, mobility, relaxation, participation in ADLs, and any nonverbal behaviors (see Skill 15-1).	Indicates successful pain management.
4 Inspect condition of surgical dressing.	A wet dressing indicates possible catheter migration out of wound.
5 During follow-up visit inspect catheter exit site.	Determines if area has healed without infection.

Unexpected Outcomes

1 Patient verbalizes pain intensity greater than previously determined goal or demonstrates nonverbal behaviors indicative of pain. Catheter may be displaced or clogged, or surgical site may be developing complications.

2 Patient reports symptoms of local anesthetic adverse reaction. Possible hypersensitivity to local anesthetic, displacement of catheter into vein, pump failure (releasing too much drug into site).

Related Interventions

- Check reservoir for presence of medication.
- Check patency of tubing.
- Notify physician.

- Notify physician.
- Stop infusion.

Reporting and Recording

- Record drug, concentration, date inserted, and type of demand feature (continuous or demand) in medication record.
- Record location of catheter, patient's pain rating, response to anesthetic, and additional comfort measures given in nurses notes.
- Record additional analgesics necessary to control pain.
- Record any adverse reactions to local anesthetic.
- Report damp dressing and /or displaced catheter to surgeon.

Teaching Considerations

- It is best to teach patients preoperatively because patients emerge from operating room with device in place.
- If device is on demand (not continuous), instruct patient to depress button every 6 hours.
- Instruct patient to inform nurse if pain meets or exceeds pain-intensity goal because additional oral and/or IV analgesics are available for breakthrough pain.
- Instruct patient to notify physician if excessive fluid or bleeding on the dressing occurs.
- Provide written instructions regarding the possible adverse reactions to Marcaine and to report these to the physician immediately.

- Provide verbal and written instructions as to how and when to discontinue device when at home. Remind patient to place catheter in a plastic bag and bring it to first follow-up visit with physician.
- Provide instructions regarding extremity movement.

Pediatric Considerations

- Local continuous infusion pumps have been used for children undergoing orthopedic surgery. Instruct parents and the child as described under Teaching Considerations. Explain special precautions not to dislodge the catheter.

Gerontological Considerations

- No special considerations except if patient is mentally compromised. Continuous dosing is sometimes administered, but demand doses require a mentally competent adult. In addition, take special precautions to protect the catheter.

Home Care Considerations

- Provide instructions as described under Teaching Considerations.

SKILL 15-5   Nonpharmacological Aids to Promote Comfort

Basic / Bathing / Performing a Back Massage
Intermediate / Preoperative Nursing Care / Teaching About Pain Management

There are a variety of nonpharmacological interventions to lessen a patient's pain in any health care setting. You use these pain-relief measures in combination with pharmacological interventions, not in place of medications. Nonpharmacological techniques help diminish the physical effects of pain, alter a patient's perception of pain, and provide a patient with a greater sense of control. Distraction, relaxation, guided imagery, and cutaneous stimulation such as massage and acupressure are examples of effective nonpharmacological measures. Many of these techniques trigger a relaxation response by stimulating the parasympathetic nervous system (PNS). Because pain often causes muscle tension and anxiety, PNS stimulation relieves these disturbing responses. Austin (2004) reviews the evidence for several mind-body therapies. The Agency for Health Care Policy and Research (Jacox and others, 1994) guidelines for acute pain management cite that nonpharmacological interventions are appropriate for patients who find such interventions appealing, express anxiety or fear, may benefit from avoiding or reducing drug therapy, and have incomplete pain relief with pharmacological interventions alone (Arthritis Foundation,

2007; King and Pettigrew, 2004; Werth and Praise, 2005; Whitehead-Pleaux and others, 2006).

Patients experience a number of painful diagnostic and therapeutic procedures. The degree of discomfort depends in large part on a patient's knowledge and perceptions of the experience. Because higher centers in the brain influence perception greatly, the pain experience is a product of a person's past pain experiences, values, cultural expectations, and emotions. A variety of nonpharmacological interventions to relieve pain (e.g., biofeedback, therapeutic touch, physical therapy, and transcutaneous electrical nerve stimulation) also augment medications (Tracy and others, 2006). You will have an excellent opportunity to assist patients in controlling their pain by teaching them a variety of nonpharmacological techniques (Box 15-4) that will possibly modify their view of and reaction to pain. By participating in the pain management plan, a patient takes an important step in achieving pain relief. Because everyone responds differently to these techniques, finding those that work best for a patient will take time. A combination of nonpharmacological techniques is often beneficial.

BOX 15-4 | Nonpharmacological Strategies for Pain Management

Relaxation and Power of the Mind
- Self-comfort
- Muscle relaxation
- Autogenics training
- Breathing exercises
- Music relaxation
- Visual imagery

Put Your Body to Work
- Exercise
- Pacing
- Energy conservation
- Body mechanics

Spirituality and Reflection
- Enhancing spirituality
- Humor medicine
- Set aside time to focus on what is
- Share your stress
- Journaling

What to Do When Your Pain Flares
- Cultivating endorphins
- Cold and hot packs
- Ball therapy
- Contrast baths
- Hand massage

Modified from *When your pain flares up*, Pain Management Center, Fairview Health Services, Minneapolis, 2002, Fairview Press.

CUTANEOUS STIMULATION

Massage

A gentle massage, a form of cutaneous stimulation, is the application of touch and movement to muscles, tendons, and ligaments without manipulation of the joints. A proper massage not only blocks perception of pain impulses but also helps relax muscle tension and spasm that otherwise might increase pain. Massage hastens the elimination of wastes stored in muscles, improves oxygenation of tissues, and stimulates the relaxation response in the nervous system. A superficial massage of the back, shoulders, and lower part of the neck is sometimes referred to as a back rub. Offer a back rub after a bath or before a patient prepares for sleep to promote relaxation and comfort, to relieve muscle tension, and to stimulate circulation. An effective back rub takes 3 to 6 minutes and is an important intervention for decreasing pain and improving sense of well-being. Massage also involves the feet and hands. Do not perform massage over bruised, swollen, or inflamed areas or bones of spine.

Heat/Cold

Heat and cold applications relieve pain and promote healing. The selection of heat versus cold varies with a patient's preference and condition. Although the physiological responses to heat and cold differ, superficial heat or cold applications provide comfort in similar conditions such as muscle spasms, strains, and localized joint pain. See Chapter 40 for a review of warm and cold therapy.

RELAXATION

Relaxation is a cognitive and/or physical strategy that provides pain relief or reduces pain to an acceptable level. A patient's full participation and cooperation are necessary for relaxation techniques to be effective. The techniques are particularly useful for chronic pain, labor pain, and relief of procedure-related pain. Relaxation interventions involve progressive muscle relaxation, massage, quiet breathing, deep breathing, guided imagery, or a combination (Austin, 2004; Baird and Sands, 2004).

GUIDED IMAGERY

Guided imagery is a creative sensory experience that effectively reduces pain perception and minimizes reaction to pain. It draws on internal experience of memories, dreams, fantasies, and visions; explores the inner world of experience; protects the privacy of a patient; and fosters the imagination. The goal of imagery is to have a patient use one or several of the senses to create an image of a desired result. This image creates a positive psychophysiological response. Focus of the imagination helps patients change their perceptions about their disease, treatment, and healing ability, which helps relieve pain, tension, or stress. Choosing images that patients find pleasant requires a careful assessment by the nurse. Otherwise, the nurse may mistakenly describe images of objects or things that a patient fears or dislikes. For example, a scene of rolling waves at the seashore is restful to one patient but desolate or frightening to another (Lewandowski and Good, 2005; Soeken, 2004).

DISTRACTION

Distraction is a technique that diverts an individual's attention away from the pain sensation. By introducing meaningful stimuli, you help a patient refocus attention. Some believe that a person can consciously attend to only one stimulus, thus diverting the attention away from pain (McCaffery and Pasero, 1999). Distraction strategies you can offer a patient include changing activity, listening to music (Mitchell and McDonald, 2006; Whitehead-Pleaux and others, 2006), reading, focusing on another person, walking, napping, writing, concentrating on a mental and physical activity simultaneously (playing a musical instrument), learning something new (completing a crossword puzzle), and listening to or watching a comedy program. Therapeutic communication with the nurse is another example of distraction. When the distraction is removed, a patient may have a heightened awareness of pain.

Delegation Considerations

Selected nonpharmacological pain-relieving strategies can be delegated to NAP. The nurse directs the NAP by:
- Identifying and explaining which nonpharmacological measures work best for the patient.
- Making clear the expected patient response.
- Instructing to report a worsening of patient's pain.

Equipment
- ❏ *Massage:* Lotion or oil, folded sheet, bath towel
- ❏ *Relaxation:* Relaxation tape and tape player
- ❏ *Distraction:* Based on type of distraction (e.g., tape player, assorted music tapes, puzzles, video games, other games)

STEP	RATIONALE

ASSESSMENT

1 Using pain scale, have patient identify intensity of discomfort.

Pain score establishes baseline to determine effects of interventions (APS, 2003).

2 Assess physiological, behavioral, and emotional signs and symptoms of pain (see Skill 15-1, Assessment, Step 5).

Responses serve as means to evaluate effectiveness of pain-relief measures. Overt signs and symptoms are not always present with chronic pain. Physical signs and symptoms indicate change in comfort level.

3 Assess characteristics of pain and underlying probable cause (see Skill 15-1, Assessment, Step 6).

Establishes baseline to determine if nonpharmacological approaches are appropriate. Massage is contraindicated in cases of muscle, bone, or joint injury.

Critical Decision Point   *It helps to administer an analgesic before implementing a nonpharmacological strategy so that the patient is able to gain a level of comfort needed to practice noninvasive approaches.*

4 Examine the site of patient's pain or discomfort. Include inspection (discoloration, swelling, drainage), palpation (change in temperature, area of altered sensation, painful area, areas that trigger pain, areas that reduce pain), and range of motion of involved joints (if applicable).

Clinical observations clarify information from patient. Site of discomfort may direct nurse to specific types of pain-relief measures.

5 Review physician's orders for pain relief.

In some acute care settings, a medical order is necessary to perform nonpharmacological therapies.

6 Assess patient's understanding of pain and willingness to receive nonpharmacological pain-relief measures.

Patients have the right to decide about their own care. Participation increases effectiveness. If patient is reluctant to try activity, accept this uncertainty and provide information about suggested therapy so that patient can make decision.

7 Assess activities patient participates in at home that serve as distraction (e.g., jigsaw puzzles, crocheting or knitting, board games, music, imagery, and relaxation tapes).

Doing these activities in health care setting increases likelihood that patient will participate.

8 Assess patient's language level, and identify descriptive terms to use when employing nonpharmacological pain-relieving strategies.

Provides clarification of information.

NURSING DIAGNOSES

- Activity intolerance
- Anxiety

- Deficient knowledge regarding non-pharmacological methods of pain control

- Ineffective coping
- Pain (acute, chronic)
- Powerlessness

Individualize related factors based on patient's condition or needs.

PLANNING

1 Expected outcomes following completion of procedures:
- Patient demonstrates and describes pain-relief measures.
- Patient is relaxed and comfortable after technique as evidenced by slow, deep respirations; calm facial expressions; calm tone of voice; relaxed muscles; relaxed posture.
- Patient verbalizes pain relief.

Demonstrates patient learning.

Nonpharmacological strategies assist patient with relaxing and experiencing less discomfort. Physiological response to relaxation procedures and massage is deep relaxation.

Patient's subjective expression is the most reliable indicator of the presence of pain (APS, 2003).

2 Explain purpose of technique and what you expect of patient during activity.

Proper explanation of activity enhances patient participation.

3 Plan time to perform technique when patient is able to concentrate (e.g., after voiding, awakening from a nap).

Increases opportunity for success.

4 Prepare environment by:
a Controlling lighting in room

Darkened room is relaxing.

b Controlling distractions by visitors or staff

Distractions prevent patient from attending to pain-reduction or pain-control techniques.

c Maintaining comfortable room temperature (sheet or light blanket prevents chilling)

Temperature extremes alter patient's response to pain.

d Closing curtains around patient's bed or closing door

Maintains patient's privacy, helps control lighting, and reduces anxiety.

5 Assist patient to comfortable position for technique chosen, such as semi-Fowler's or Sims' position.

Patient comfort enhances relaxation and participation in skills.

STEP	RATIONALE

IMPLEMENTATION

1 Massage:
  a Perform hand hygiene.

  b Adjust bed to high, comfortable position, and lower upper side rail on side where nurse is standing.

  c Place patient in comfortable position such as prone or side-lying position. Have patients with respiratory difficulties lie on side with head of bed elevated.

  d Drape patient, only exposing the area you will massage.

  e Ensure patient is not allergic to lotion. Then warm lotion in hands or in basin of warm water.

  f Choose stroke technique based on desired effect:
     (1) Effleurage (Massaging upward and outward from vertebral column, and back again) (see illustration)

     (2) Pétrissage (see illustration)

     (3) Friction

  g Encourage patient to breathe deeply and relax during massage.

  h Standing behind patient, stimulate scalp and temples.

  i Supporting patient's head, rub muscles at base of head.

  j With patient in supine position, massage hands and arms, as appropriate:

     (1) Support hand, and apply friction to palm using both thumbs.
     (2) Support base of finger, and work each finger in corkscrewlike motion.
     (3) Complete hand massage using effleurage strokes from fingertips to wrist.
     (4) Knead muscles of forearm and upper arm between thumb and forefinger, as appropriate.

  k After determining patient has no neck injury or condition that contraindicates neck manipulation, massage neck as appropriate:
     (1) Place patient in the prone position unless contraindicated.

Reduces transmission of microorganisms.

Ensures proper body mechanics and prevents strain on nurse's back muscles.

Enhances relaxation and exposes area to be massaged.

Maintains patient's privacy and warmth.

Warm lotion is soothing, and warmth helps to produce local muscle relaxation.

Gliding stroke, used without manipulating deep muscles, smoothes and extends muscles, increases nutrient absorption, improves lymphatic and venous circulation.

Use on tense muscle groups to "knead" muscles, promote relaxation, and stimulate local circulation.

Strong circular strokes bring blood to surface of skin, thereby increasing local circulation and loosening tight muscle groups.

Potentiates effects of massage.

Strong circular strokes (friction) stimulate local circulation and relaxation.

Releases tension in hands and arms. Studies indicate that anxious behaviors may be significantly reduced with hand massage (Mok and Woo, 2004).

Encourages relaxation; enhances circulation and venous return.

Provides access to neck muscles.

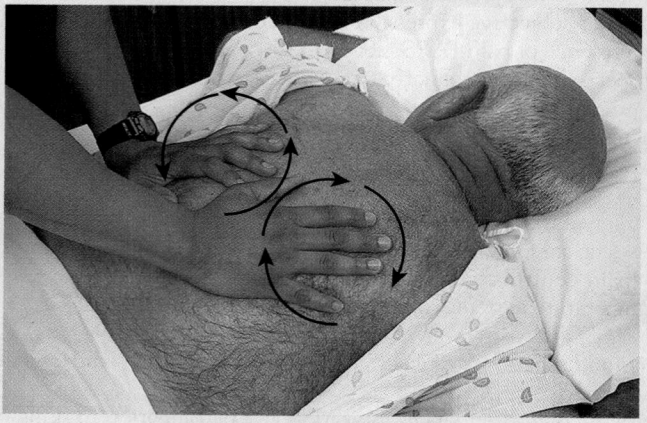

STEP 1f(1) Effleurage.

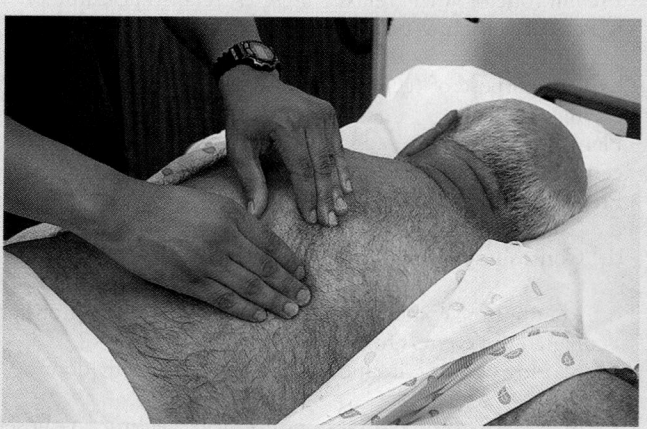

STEP 1f(2) Pétrissage.

STEP	RATIONALE

(2) Knead each neck muscle between the thumb and the forefinger.

Reduces tension that often localizes in neck muscles.

(3) Gently stretch neck by placing one hand on top of shoulders and other at base of head. Gently move hands away from each other.

Helps relax muscle body.

l Massage back, as appropriate:

(1) Keep patient in prone position unless contraindicated; side-lying position is an option.

(2) Do not allow hands to leave patient's skin.

Continuous contact with skin's surface is soothing and stimulates circulation to tissues. Breaking contact with skin can startle patient.

(3) Apply hands first to sacral area; massage in circular motion. Stroke upward from buttocks to shoulders. Massage over scapulas with smooth, firm stroke. Continue in one smooth stroke to upper arms and laterally along sides of back down to iliac crests (see illustration). Continue massage pattern for 3 minutes.

General, firm pressure applied to all muscle groups promotes relaxation.

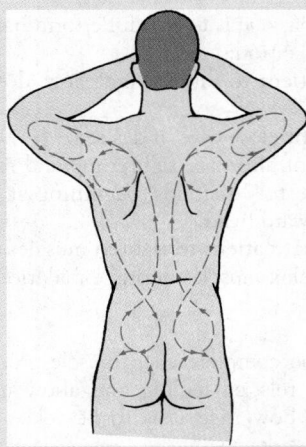

STEP 1l(3)   Circular massage.

(4) Use effleurage along muscles of spine in upward and outward motion.

Massage follows distribution of major muscle groups.

(5) Use pétrissage on muscles of each shoulder toward front of patient.

Area often tightens because of tension.

(6) Use palms in upward and outward circular motion from lower buttocks to neck.

Brings blood to surface of skin.

(7) Knead muscles of upper back and shoulder between thumb and forefinger.

These muscles are thick and can be vigorously massaged.

(8) Use both hands to knead muscles up one side of back, then the other.

(9) End massage with long stroking effleurage movements.

Most soothing of massage movements.

m Massage feet, as appropriate:

(1) Place patient in supine position.

Returns patient to comfortable anatomical position.

(2) Hold foot firmly. Support ankle with one hand, or support sides of foot with each hand while performing massage.

Maintains joint stability during massage.

STEP	RATIONALE
(3) Make circular motions with thumb and fingers around bones of ankle and top of foot.	Relaxes muscles.
(4) Trace space between tendons with firm finger pressure, moving from toe to ankle.	
(5) Massage sides and top of each toe.	
(6) Use top of fist to make circular motions on bottom of foot.	
(7) Knead sides of foot between index finger and thumb.	
(8) Conclude with firm, sweeping motions over top and bottom of foot.	Light strokes tickle.
n Tell patient you are ending massage.	Informs and prepares patient for inhalation and exhalation (next step).
o When procedure is complete, instruct patient to inhale deeply, exhale, and then initially move about slowly after resting a few minutes.	Returns patient to more awake and alert state. When deeply relaxed, patient may experience dizziness on arising too rapidly.
p Wipe excess lotion or oil from patient's body, where applied, with bath towel.	Excess lotion or oil can irritate skin and lead to breakdown.
q Return bed to low position, and raise side rails as appropriate when massage is finished. Perform hand hygiene.	Reduces spread of microorganisms. Side rails cannot be used as a restraint.
2 Progressive relaxation:	
a Instruct patient to take several slow, deep, diaphragmatic breaths.	Increased oxygen lessens anxiety and prevents shortness of breath with relaxation. Breathing technique avoids hyperventilation.
b Have patient close eyes, if desired.	Helps patient maintain focus.
c Have patient alternate tightening and relaxing all muscle groups for 6 to 7 seconds, beginning at feet and working upwards toward head.	Alternating tension and relaxation in muscle groups allows patient to feel difference.
(1) Instruct patient to tighten muscles during inhalation and relax muscles during exhalation.	Relaxation is an integrated response associated with diminished sympathetic nervous system arousal; decreased muscle tension is desired outcome. Relaxation decreases pulse and respiration rates and blood pressure and reduces anxiety.
(2) As you complete each muscle group, ask patient to enjoy relaxed feeling and allow mind to drift and think how nice it is to be relaxed; ask patient to breathe deeply.	Distracts patient from perceiving pain. Enhances the relaxation response. Breathing deeply prevents Valsalva response, which increases intrathoracic pressure and compromises cardiac function.
d Calmly explain during exercise that patient will feel sensations of tingling, heaviness, floating, or warmth as relaxation occurs.	Prevents anxiety if sensation occurs without warning.
e Ask patient to continue slow, deep breaths.	Allows opportunity to enjoy feelings of relaxation.
f When exercise is complete, instruct patient to inhale deeply, exhale, and then initially move about slowly after resting a few minutes.	Returns patient to more awake and alert state. Rising too rapidly will cause dizziness.
3 Deep breathing:	
a Instruct patient to sit comfortably with feet uncrossed. If patient is unable to sit, move to a supine position with small pillow under head.	Encourages relaxation.
b Place one hand on the chest and the other on the abdomen.	Allows patient to focus on chest and then abdomen.
c Inhale deeply through the nose, allowing the abdomen to rise and the hand to move outward.	Provides steady timing of inhalation and focuses the patient on stretching abdominal muscles.
d When the abdomen is partially expanded, continue to breathe and allow chest to expand, moving the upper hand outward.	Affords maximal inhalation.

STEP	RATIONALE
e Pause for a few seconds.	Permits optimal exchange of oxygen and carbon dioxide.
f Exhale slowly through pursed lips.	Provides slow, controlled release of air.
g Repeat for 4 to 6 minutes.	
4 Guided imagery:	
a Direct patient through guided imagery exercise:	
(1) Instruct patient to imagine that inhaled air is ball of healing energy.	Development of specific images assists in removal of pain perception.
(2) Imagine inhaled air travels to area of pain.	Patient's ability to concentrate decreases pain perception.
b Alternatively nurse may direct imagery:	
(1) Ask patient to imagine a pleasant place such as beach or mountains.	Directs imagery after selection of restful place by the nurse and patient.
(2) Direct patient to experience all sensory aspects of restful place (e.g., for beach: warm breeze, warm sand between toes, warmth of sunshine, rhythmic sound of waves, smell of salt air, gulls gliding and swooping in air).	Helps patient concentrate and relax through stimulation of numerous senses.
(3) Direct patient to continue deep, slow, rhythmic breathing.	Promotes relaxation through muscle relaxation.
(4) Direct patient to count to three, inhale, and open eyes. Suggest patient move about slowly initially.	
c Provide patient time to practice exercise without interruption.	Guided imagery requires an intense level of concentration that takes time to achieve.
5 Distraction:	
a Direct patient's attention away from pain with distraction techniques.	Redirection of attention alters emotional or cognitive aspects of pain.
b Ask patient to close eyes or to focus on single object in room.	Directs attention inward and protects patient from external distraction.
c Instruct patient to concentrate on slow, rhythmic breathing. Guide breathing, or instruct patient to control and concentrate on breathing by thinking: "in, one, two; out, one, two."	Promotes relaxation by concentrating on kinesthetic action, thus reducing ability to concentrate on pain.
d Continue distraction using chosen activity.	
(1) Use music of patient's choosing. Emphasize listening to rhythm, and adjust volume as pain increases or decreases.	Focusing on an activity diverts attention from painful sensation.
(2) Direct patient to give detailed account of an event or story.	Stress details of event to enhance distraction from pain stimulus.
(3) Engage patient in conversation; encourage participation of family members and visitors.	Visitors can help direct attention away from mild to moderate pain.

EVALUATION

1 Observe character of respirations, body position, facial expression, tone of voice, mood, mannerisms, verbalization of discomfort.	Determines effectiveness of procedure, level of relaxation, degree of pain relief achieved, and which procedures were the most effective.
2 Ask patient to use pain rating scale to rate comfort level.	Objectively measures change in pain intensity.
3 Observe patient perform pain-control measures.	Confirms learning.

Unexpected Outcomes

1 Patient is not able to concentrate on technique because of intense pain.

2 Patient states pain intensity unchanged or escalating, or patient is demonstrating nonverbal behaviors indicative of pain.

Related Interventions

- Administer analgesics before nonpharmacological strategy.
- Ensure environment is conducive to technique.

- Fully assess pain.
- Consider administering analgesics before technique, or consult with physician on an alternative analgesic.
- Consider a different technique or a combination (e.g., elevation and cold) of nonpharmacological strategies.
- Focus on helping patient to relax.
- Answer any questions or concerns.

Recording and Reporting

- Record in nurses' notes patient's assessment findings, procedure and technique, preparation given to patient, patient's response to procedure or technique, and further comfort needs related to event. Incorporate pain-relief technique into nursing care plan.
- Record alterations in patient's condition (e.g., changes in blood pressure, pulse, respiration, condition of patient's skin, complaints of dizziness).
- Report patient's response to nonpharmacological interventions to the staff at change of shift.
- Report any unusual responses to techniques (e.g., uncontrolled or aggravated pain) to nurse in charge or physician.

Teaching Considerations

- Provide patients information about each nonpharmacological therapy, including purpose, rationale for how pain is relieved, how patient can maximize benefits.
- Some techniques require more practice before patients achieve results. Pharmacological intervention is sometimes required to lessen pain so that patient can relax and to augment other methods of pain control.
- Teach patient to rest between periods of activity because fatigue increases pain perception.
- Discuss and practice with patient techniques to use at home. Upon discharge, include written instructions.
- If appropriate, teach family member how to perform massage (if not contraindicated) as part of home care.

Pediatric Considerations

- You can use a number of nonpharmacological pain-management therapies successfully with children. Adopt distraction and relaxation strategies to the developmental level of the child (e.g., use a pacifier for the infant, offer reading or playing a recording of a favorite story for the preschooler, encourage a teenager to listen to music on a CD player with headphones). Play therapists are usually available at pediatric hospitals and are good resources for appropriate distraction techniques.
- Because children have an active imagination, relaxation is often a powerful adjuvant in pain control.
- Parents are very helpful in providing pain relief. They provide comfort, for example, by their presence, their conversation, and by holding and cuddling their child (Murray, 2004; Whitehead-Pleaux and others, 2006).

Gerontological Considerations

- Visual, hearing, cognitive, and motor impairments make it difficult for older adults to be able to effectively use procedures such as distraction, relaxation, or guided imagery. Make certain glasses, hearing aids, etc. are in place. Do not assume these techniques will not work (American Pain Foundation, 2007; Tracy and others, 2006).
- Ask the patient what other interventions have helped relieve pain in the past.

Home Care Considerations

- Family members need to collaborate planning time to reduce noise and other stimuli in the home to promote patient's relaxation.
- Discuss nonpharmacological interventions with patient's family and friends.

❓ CRITICAL THINKING EXERCISES

You are caring for Mrs. Koby, a 69-year-old woman who has been diagnosed with ovarian cancer. She was admitted last night, and she has elected to start radiation therapy treatment rather than have surgery. Her sister had surgery for ovarian cancer 3 years ago and died of complications right after she had the surgery for ovarian cancer. She has a student nurse assigned to help with her care. You notice that Mrs. Koby is lying rigid in her bed when you rush by her room to deal with a crisis of another of your patients. The student reports to you that Mrs. Koby has a pain-intensity level of 9 on a 0 to 10 scale. The student thinks the patient may even be underreporting the pain because she lies stiff and barely moves, her breath is shallow, and she has tears in her eyes. Mrs. Koby informed the student that she cannot take anything for pain yet because the radiation oncologist told her she should take pain medication only when the pain became too severe to tolerate and then should take it only at night to help her sleep. The only medication ordered is Darvocet-N 100, one or two capsules every 6 hours prn for pain. Mrs. Koby has no other chronic disease. She reports she has not had a bowel movement for 3 days; she says it is too painful to try to have a bowel movement. Her vital signs are within normal range, she has hypoactive bowel sounds, and her abdomen is soft. Her lungs are clear.

1 What is your **first** action to assist this patient?
   A Give a dose of a mild pain reliever (e.g., Darvocet) first, and then call the patient's physician if it does not work within an hour.
   B Conduct a thorough pain assessment and call the patient's physician to request an IV pain medication.

   C Conduct a thorough pain assessment and call the physician to request a strong oral medication (e.g., liquid morphine) every 6 hours prn.
   D Give a dose of mild pain reliever (e.g., Darvocet) first and then conduct a pain assessment.

2 How and when will you assess this patient's pain intensity?
   A Assess pain hourly using the 0 to 10 scale until her pain reaches her goal level, then assess with each vital sign.
   B Use the 0 to 10 pain scale, and assess pain intensity with each vital sign.
   C Use the FACES pain scale, and assess every 8 hours.
   D Observe for nonverbal pain behaviors during activity; assess pain level every 12 hours.
   Explain your choice.

3 Mrs. Koby's family is concerned about her getting an overdose of medication if a PCA is ordered for her. To reassure the family and the patient you explain:
   A The physician and staff are not very concerned about an overdose because Mrs. Koby has late-stage ovarian cancer.
   B Two nurses will be in Mrs. Koby's room every 2 hours to check the PCA and make sure she has not received too much medication.
   C Mrs. Koby will be taught to check the PCA hourly to make sure she is not giving herself too much medication.
   D The PCA computer has a built-in mechanism that is programmed not to deliver too much medication.

4 When you discontinue a PCA, what steps must be taken to be in compliance with the federal Controlled Substances Act as well as your agency policy?

REVIEW QUESTIONS

1. A 72-year-old man with a 4-year history of severe osteoarthritis comes to the medical clinic, reporting that his hip pain has increased, limiting his ability to do activities he enjoys. When beginning the assessment, the nurse should remember:
   1. Patients with chronic pain usually require lower doses of analgesics for relief.
   2. Patients with chronic pain are usually familiar with the names and actions of their medications.
   3. Patients with chronic pain do not typically benefit from relaxation therapies.
   4. Patients with chronic pain usually have autonomic signs and symptoms.

2. The patient had extensive abdominal surgery for colon cancer. It is the evening of the day of surgery. She has patient-controlled analgesia (PCA), with morphine sulfate being delivered via an intravenous infusion in her left arm. Her husband has repeatedly asked if there is any way to make her more comfortable. Currently the patient reports that her pain is at a level of 5 out of 10. The nurse instructs the patient's husband to:
   1. Alert the nurse when the patient appears to be sleeping.
   2. Push the button for the patient when she appears uncomfortable.
   3. Encourage the patient to depress the button when she feels discomfort.
   4. Caution patient against overuse, because this could lead to an overdose of morphine.

3. A patient is receiving opioids via the epidural route and is experiencing pruritus of the head, neck, and torso. What nursing intervention is indicated?
   1. Stop the epidural medication infusion after checking the patient's vital signs.
   2. Explain to the patient that this is a frequent side effect, not an allergic reaction.
   3. Turn down slightly the infusion rate of the epidural medication.
   4. Notify the health care provider of the patient's pruritus so the medication can be changed.

4. The patient has pain following a traumatic injury to her left leg. She is in traction and receiving PCA administration. The nurse is assessing her to determine the likelihood of nonpharmacological pain therapies being effective. Which statement from the patient suggests that nonpharmacological therapies will be beneficial to her:
   1. "I have a cousin who used relaxation when she had her back pain, I always though it seemed a waste of time."
   2. "I am so afraid I will not walk normally again, I can't imagine having to use a cane or even worse, a wheelchair"
   3. You know, this PCA seems to make me pretty comfortable. The pain is less now."
   4. "I think something other than this medication would be good, I would prefer massage"

5. A patient is to have an epidural catheter placed for pain management. The nurse should ask which of the following questions to evaluate the patient for a history of condition that could contraindicate the procedure?
   1. "Have you had a recent lumbar puncture?"
   2. "Do you ever have migraine headaches?"
   3. "Have you taken anticoagulants recently?"
   4. "Do you have an allergy to latex?"

REFERENCES

Acute Pain Management Guideline Panel: *Acute pain management: operative or medical procedures and trauma.* AHCPR Clinical Practice Guideline No. 1, AHCPR Publication No. 92-0032 (revised 2003), The Panel.

Agency for Healthcare Policy and Research, Acute Pain Management Guideline Panel, *Acute pain managment operative or medical procedures and trauma, Clinical practice guideline,* AHCPR, Pub. No. 92-0032, Rockville Md, 1992, Agency for Health Care Policy and Research, Public Health Service, US Department of Health and Human Services.

American Pain Society: Position statement on the use of placebos in pain management, *J Pain* 6(4):215, 2005.

American Geriatrics Society Panel on Persistent Pain in Older Persons: The management of persistent pain in older persons, *J Am Geriatric Soc* 50(6 suppl):S205, 2002 (updated with FDA Regulatory Warnings 2005).

American Pain Foundation: *Treatment options: a guide for people living with pain,* 2004, from http://www.painfoundation.org, accessed January 5, 2007.

American Pain Society: *Analgesic use in the treatment of acute pain and cancer pain,* ed 6, Glenview, Ill, 2003, American Pain Society.

American Society for Pain Management Nursing: Patient controlled analgesia: authorized agent controlled analgesia, a position statement, *Pain Manag Nurs* 7(4):134, 2006.

American Society of Addiction Medicine: *Consensus document,* 2001, http://www.asam.org/ppol/paindef.html, accessed September 15, 2007.

Arthritis Foundation: *Pain center: heat and cold,* 2003, http://www.arthritisfoundation.com, accessed September 15, 2007.

Austin J: Mind-body therapies for the management of pain, *Clin J Pain* 20(1):27, 2004.

Bruchi S and others: Prevalence of clinical hypertension in patients with pain compared to nonpain general patients, *Clin J Pain* 21(2):147, 2003.

Capriotti T: Any science behind the hype of "natural" dietary supplements? *Medsurg Nurs* 13(5):339, 2004.

DeJongue B and others: Using and understanding sedation scoring systems: a systematic review, *Intensive Care Med* 26:275, 2000.

Ferrell B: Ethical perspectives on pain and suffering, *Pain Manag Nurs* 6(3):83, 2005.

Gordon DB and others: American Pain Society recommendations for improving quality of acute and cancer pain management: American Pain Society Quality of Care Task Force, *Arch Intern Med* 165:1574, 2005.

Hadjistaviapoulos T and others: An interdisciplinary expert consensus statement on assessment of pain in older persons, *Clin J Pain* 23(1, 2007 suppl):S1, 2007.

Herr K and others: Pain assessment in the nonverbal patient: position statement with clinical practice recommendations, *Pain Manag Nurs* 7(2):44, 2006.

Jacox A and others: *Management of cancer pain,* Clinical practice guideline No. 9, Rockville, Md, 1994, Agency for Health Care Policy and Research, Public Health Service, U.S. Department of Health and Human Services.

Joint Commission on Accreditation of Healthcare Organizations: *Comprehensive accreditation manual for hospitals: the official handbook,* Oak Brook Terrace, Ill, 2003, The Commission.

Kabeli C: Obstructive sleep apnea and modifications in sedation, *Crit Care Nurs Clin North Am* 17:269, 2005.

Kastanias P and others: Patient-controlled oral analgesia: a low-tech solution in a high-tech world, *Pain Manag Nurs* 7(3):126, 2006.

Lehr V, BeVier P: Patient-controlled analgesia for the pediatric patient, *Orthop Nurs* 22(4):298, 2003.

Lewandowski W and others: Changes in the meaning of pain and the use of guided imagery, *Pain Manag Nurs* 6(2):58, 2005.

McCaffery M, Pasero C: *Pain: clinical manual,* ed 2, St. Louis, 1999, Mosby.

Miakowski C and others: *Guideline for management of cancer pain in adults and children,* 2005, National Guideline Clearinghouse, American Pain Society, http://www.guideline.gov, accessed September 5, 2007.

Miller C, Newton S: Pain perception and expression: the influence of gender, personal self-efficacy, and lifespan socialization, *Pain Manag Nurs* 7(4):148, 2006.

Mok E, Woo P: The effects of slow-stroke back massage on anxiety and shoulder pain in elderly stroke patients, *Complement Ther Nurs Midwifery* 10(4):209, 2004.

Monsevais D, McNeill J: Multicultural influences on pain medication attitudes and beliefs in patients with nonmalignant chronic pain syndromes, *Pain Manag Nurs* 8(2):64, 2007.

Murray G: Managing acute pain in children, *World Ir Nurs* 12(11):35, 2004.

Pasero C: *Epidural analgesia for acute pain management,* self-learning module, Pensacola, Fla, 1999, American Society for Pain Management Nursing.

Pasero C: Epidural analgesia for postoperative pain, *Am J Nurs* 103(10):62, 2003a.

Pasero C: *Intravenous patient-controlled analgesia for acute pain management,* self-directed learning module, Pensacola, Fla, 2003b, American Society for Pain Management Nursing.

Pasero C and others: Registered nurse management and monitoring of analgesia by catheter techniques: position statement, *Pain Manag Nurs* 8(2):48, 2007.

Prows C, Prows D: Medication selection by genotype: how genetics is changing drug prescribing and efficacy, *Am J Nurs* 104(5):60, 2004.

Regional anesthesia in the anticoagulated patient: defining the risks, 2003, http://www.asra.com/Concensus_Conferences/ConsensusStatements.shtml, accessed December 20, 2003.

Sinatra S: Spinal opioid analgesia: an overview. In Sinatra RS and others, editors: *Acute pain management*, St. Louis, 1992, Mosby.

Spector R: *Cultural diversity in health and illness*, ed 6, Upper Saddle River, NJ, 2004, Pearson Prentice Hall.

Sucka L: The basic science mechanisms of TENS and clinical applications, *APS Bull* 11(2):10, 2001.

The Joint Commission: Tubing misconnections, a persistent and potentially deadly occurrence, *Sentinel Event Alert*, issue 36, April 3, 2006.

The Joint Commission: *2008 National patient safety goals hospital program*, 2007, Oakbrook Terrace, Ill, The Commission, http://www.jointcommission.org, accessed July 2007.

The Joint Commission: *National patient safety goals, 2009*, Oakbrook Terrace, Ill, 2008, The Commission, http://www.jointcommission.org.

When your pain flares up, Pain Management Center, Fairview Health Services, Minneapolis, 2002, Fairview Press.

Whilear P and others: Principles of palliative care medicine. Part 2: Pain and symptom management, *Adv Stud Med* 4(2):69-70, 88-100, 2004.

RESEARCH REFERENCES

Baird C, Sands L: A pilot study of the effectiveness of guided imagery with progressive muscle relaxation to reduce chronic pain and mobility difficulties of osteoarthritis, *Pain Manag Nurs* 5(3):97, 2004.

Bedard D, Purden M: The pain experience of post-surgical patients following the implementation of an evidence-based approach, *Pain Manag Nurs* 7(3):80, 2006.

Beyer J and others: The alternate faces reliability of the OUCHER pain scale, *Pain Manag Nurs* 6(1):10, 2005.

Bruchi S and others: Prevalence of clinical hypertension in patients with pain compared to general medical patients, *Clin J Pain* 21(2):147, 2005.

Bucknall T and others: Nurses' assessment of postoperative pain after analgesic administration, *Clin J Pain* 23(1):1, 2007.

Chambers C and others: FACES scale for measurement of postoperative pain intensity in children following minor surgery, *Clin J Pain* 21(2):277, 2005.

Chang K and others: Determination of patient controlled epidural analgesic requirements, *Clin J Pain* 22(9):751, 2006.

Clark L and others: Nurses' reflections on pain management in a nursing home setting, *Pain Manag Nurs* 7(2):71, 2006.

Cohen-Mansfield J: Pain assessment in noncommunicative elderly persons: PAINE, *Clin J Pain* 22(6):569, 2006.

Hansson E and others: Effects of quality improvement program in acute care evaluated by patients, nurses, and physicians, *Pain Manag Nurs* 7(3):93, 2006.

Higgins I and others: Chronic pain in nursing home residents: the need for nursing leadership, *J Nurs Manag* 12(3):167, 2004.

King M, Pettigrew A: Complementary and alternative therapy use by older adults in three ethnically diverse populations: a pilot study, *Geriatric Nurs* 25(1):30, 2004.

Larsson A, Wijik H: Patient experiences of pain and pain management at the end of life: a pilot study, *Pain Manag Nurs* 8(1):12, 2007.

Lusher J and others: Analgesic addiction and pseudoaddiction in painful chronic illness, *Clin J Pain* 22(3):316, 2006.

Mansfield J: Pain assessment in noncommunicative elderly persons—PAINE, *Clin J Pain* 22(6):569, 2006.

McDonald D and others: Nurses' response to pain communication from patients: a post-test experimental study, *Int J Nurs Stud* 44:29, 2005.

Mitchell LA, McDonald RA: An experimental investigation of the effects of preferred and relaxing music listening on pain perception, *J Music Ther* 43(4):295, 2006.

Onen S and others: How pain and analgesics disturb sleep, *Clin J Pain* 21(5):422, 2005.

Soeken K: Selected CAM therapies for arthritis-related pain: the evidence from systematic reviews, *Clin J Pain* 20(1):13, 2004.

Tall J, Raja S: Dietary constituents as novel therapies for pain, *Clin J Pain* 20(1):19, 2004.

Tracy S and others: Translating best practices in nondrug postoperative pain management, *Nurs Res* 55(2):557, 2006.

Vallerand A and others: Perceptions of control over pain by patients with cancer and their caregivers, *Pain Manag Nurs* 8(2):55, 2007.

Ware L and others: Evaluation of the revised FACES pain scale, verbal descriptor scale, numeric rating scale, and Iowa pain thermometer in older, minority adults, *Pain Manag Nurs* 7(3):11, 2006.

Werth J, Paise J: Use of herbal therapies to relieve pain: a review of efficacy and adverse effects, *Pain Manag Nurs* 6(4):145, 2005.

Whitehead-Pleaux AM and others: The effects of music therapy on pediatric patients' pain and anxiety during donor site dressing change, *J Music Ther* 43(2):136, 2006.

Wilson M, Helgadotter H: Patterns of pain and analgesic use in 3- to 7-year-old children after tonsillectomy, *Pain Manag Nurs* 7(4):159, 2006.

Won AB, Lapane KL: Persistent nonmalignant pain and analgesic prescribing patterns in elderly nursing home residents, *J Am Geriatric Soc* 52(6):867, 2004.

Palliative Care

MEDIA RESOURCES

- **evolve** http://evolve.elsevier.com/Perry/skills

  learning system

  - Review Questions
  - Checklists

KEY TERMS

Advance directives
Autopsy
Brain death
Hospice
Loss

Organ/tissue
  donation
Palliative care
Postmortem care

OBJECTIVES

Mastery of content in this chapter will enable the nurse to:

- Identify the nurse's role in assisting patients and families in grief and at the end of life.
- Discuss principles of palliative care.
- Describe hospice care.
- Describe symptom management at the end of life.
- Discuss the nurse's role in facilitating autopsy and organ and tissue donation requests.
- Describe physiological changes in impending death.
- Describe postmortem care.

Nurses have historically played a vital role in the care of patients and families facing serious, life-limiting illness and death. They continue to expand their knowledge, leading the way in the development of compassionate, evidence-based palliative care (Blum, 2006; Wilson and others, 2006). The World Health Organization (2002) defines palliative care as an "approach that improves the quality of life of individuals and their families facing life-threatening illness, through the prevention and relief of suffering by means of early identification and impeccable assessment and treatment of pain and other physical, psychological and spiritual problems." When patients receive relief from the symptoms caused by disease or treatment, they have a higher quality of life and are empowered to participate more fully in health care decisions. Although this chapter focuses on end-of-life care, patients of all ages with any diagnosis receive palliative care, even as they seek treatment and cure for their illness.

At the end of life, palliative care helps patients experience a "good death," often through hospice care (Kehl, 2006). Hospice, an interdisciplinary, patient- and family-centered program of total palliative care, helps people live as well as possible through the dying process. Patients are eligible for hospice care as a Medicare or Medicaid benefit during the final phase of a terminal illness, usually the last 6 months of life. Because hospice is a philosophy of care, not necessarily a place, the services are sometimes provided at home, in freestanding hospice facilities, or nursing home, extended care, or acute care settings. Hospice benefits include respite for family caregivers, limited hospitalization for acute symptom management, and bereavement care after death (National Hospice and Palliative Care Organization, 2005). Unfortunately, many patients enter into hospice care only a few days or weeks before death, limiting the time they have to benefit from the nurses, physicians, social workers, volunteers, and spiritual care providers who make up the interdisciplinary team (Hill, 2005). Be familiar with the scope of hospice services, and ask patients and family members if they know about this option for end-of-life care.

Palliative and hospice care place a primary focus on a patient's values, quality of life, and care preferences. Advance directives offer a legal means by which patients communicate their values to others if they are unable to participate in making decisions. The Patient Self-Determination Act of 1991 requires that all health care agencies serving Medicaid and Medicare patients provide patients with information regarding advance directives. In an advance directive, patients indicate in writing what types of treatments are acceptable or unacceptable to them, describe their life values, or designate a person to speak for them as their durable power of attorney (DPOA) for health care decisions. Advance directives specify medical interventions a patient does not want in certain situations, such as mechanical ventilation, and are also used to communicate the care a patient wants, for example, pain relief to the fullest extent possible. Instruct patients to have a copy of their advance directive placed in their agency medical record and to give copies to their physician and family members. Be familiar with your agency's policies and state laws, because they often differ from place to place.

Family members often face difficult decisions at the time of death, and some experience stress when deciding to withdraw life-sustaining treatments, which may complicate their grief (Doka, 2005). In a study by Davis and colleagues (2005), family members who had access to an advance directive experienced less stress when making decisions for their loved one than family members who did not have one. As helpful as advance directives often are, many people do not have one and need help understanding their usefulness and how to prepare one. Discussions about advance directives and goals of care involve the patient, DPOA, family members, and the interdisciplinary health care team.

Cardiopulmonary resuscitation (CPR), an emergency procedure providing artificial ventilation and manual external cardiac massage, is used in cases of cardiac and/or pulmonary arrest. CPR is performed on a patient who has a cardiopulmonary arrest unless the patient's physician has written and signed a "do not resuscitate" (DNR) or "no CPR" order. Adults, in consultation with the health care team, may consent to a DNR status verbally or in writing. Assure patients who choose not to be resuscitated that they will continue to receive full palliative care and symptom relief.

Grief experiences at the end of life have profound physical, psychological, social, and spiritual effects on dying persons, family members, friends, and caregivers. The first of the three skills in this chapter discusses how nurses help patients and family members identify and express their feelings of loss and grief. The grief associated with dying arises from many sources: fear of the unknown, pain, sadness about leaving loved ones behind, loss of control, or unresolved guilt. Some patients have concern about being a burden on others, and family members often feel overwhelmed (McPherson and others, 2007). A nurse listens carefully in order to understand the significance of the loss to the patient or family members, identifies concerns, and assesses their ability to sustain hope and move forward in life.

The second skill in this chapter describes how to help patients and family members manage the many symptoms caused by grief, disease, or medical treatments at the end of life. Examples of the patient's physical symptoms include pain, shortness of breath, fatigue, loss of appetite, mental status changes, and constipation. Patients or family members also experience psychological symptoms, such as anxiety, depression, or uncertainty because of lack of understanding of the disease, prognosis, or treatment plan (Block, 2006). Spiritual distress often heightens a patient's perceptions of discomfort. Assess a patient's or family member's needs and strengths, and initiate a plan of care for symptom management (Fig. 16-1).

At the time of death, nurses provide compassionate care to the patient and family by offering information, guidance, and support and by acting as a liaison to facilitate communication. As described in the third skill, nurses provide postmortem care, care of the body after death, in a manner consistent with the patient's religious and cultural beliefs.

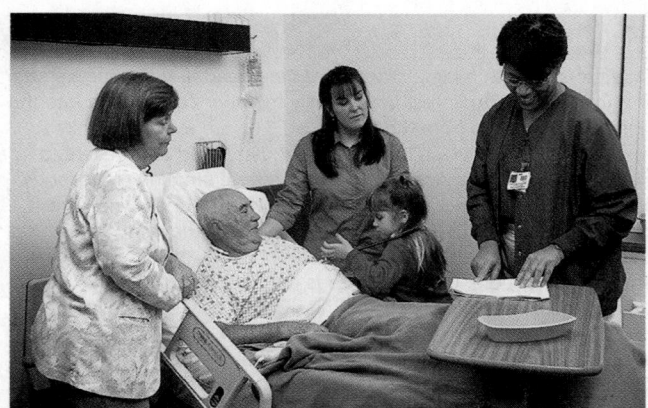

FIG 16-1 The nurse collaborates to develop an effective approach to symptom management.

EVIDENCE-BASED PRACTICE TRENDS

An extensive body of research over the past 20 years supports the development of evidence-based palliative care. Research continues on every aspect of care, including the type and prevalence of symptoms, symptom management, pharmacological interventions, use of advance directives, caregiver and nurse coping, and family decision making. Palliative care places primary emphasis on patient and family needs and experiences. Knowledge gained from studying their perceptions of care in a variety of settings helps identify best palliative care practices (Bray and Goodyear-Smith, 2007; Lee and others, 2006; London and Lundstedt, 2007).

Harstäde and Andershed (2004) discuss three themes that patients identify as essential to good palliative care: safety, trust, and participation. Patients regard continuity of care and clinical competence as components of safety. Trust in the judgments made by staff and in the treatments given facilitate a patient's sense of receiving good care. When patients in the study were invited to participate in discussions and decisions, they reported a sense of safety and trust.

Research helps nurses identify how to improve practice. One study of palliative care in an acute setting reports poor recognition and documentation of patients' psychological, social, and spiritual needs at the end of life. Nurses and other health care providers did not recognize imminent death and did not inform family members in a timely manner. Professional caregivers seemed more focused on tasks than on spending time with patients and family members (Parish and others, 2007). This research helps nurses develop specific documentation and communication strategies, consistent with patient needs and preferences.

As the number of older adult or cognitively impaired patients receiving palliative care increases, research must expand to provide evidence-based care for these patients (Brandt and others, 2005; Kelly and others, 2006). A qualitative study of older adults with advanced cancer identified genuine caring, cautious hopefulness, involvement in desired activities, and positive interactions with caregivers as meaningful to patients (Ryan, 2005). Findings from a study such as this can be used to develop effective palliative interventions. Another study identified barriers to pain management experienced by nursing home residents. Patients in the study identified medication concerns, staff reactions to their request for pain medication, and their perception that staff members were too busy

(Jones and others, 2005). Clinical practice recommendations for assessing pain in nonverbal patients provide nurses with evidence-based assessment guidelines (Herr and others, 2006).

CULTURAL CONSIDERATIONS

Human responses to illness, death, and grief are transmitted from generation to generation through family and culture. Cultural norms influence family, gender, and community roles at the time of death. Culture also affects the meaning of pain and suffering, how one expresses grief and emotion, and ideas about an afterlife. Given the wide range of cultural beliefs, first engage in self-reflection on your own cultural and personal beliefs regarding loss and death (Jenko and Moffitt, 2006). Gather knowledge on common end-of-life cultural or religious practices, and then validate, through nurse-patient discussions, the relevance of those practices for a particular patient of that culture or religion.

In the United States, technical Western medicine has influenced professional caregivers' values, which sometimes conflict with others' cultural values. For example, some members of the Jewish faith stay with the dying person until burial. Make sure you accommodate this need, even in a busy hospital setting. Some Hindu families support their elders' refusal of nourishment and pain medication, based on their belief of continuing life cycles. The refusal of pain medication is often upsetting to caregivers who believe they should reduce pain whenever possible. Many communally oriented cultures actively involve others in their grief rituals and behaviors. For example, many African Americans find comfort in the presence of an extended family, friends, and spiritual leaders at the bedside of a dying family member and need the nurse's support to accommodate large gatherings of people.

Cultural differences influence communication at the end of life. In some cultures, discussing death is taboo. Some cultures believe in the authority of the healer or the power of words and fear that informing a patient that he or she has a serious disease brings about a poor outcome. Contrast this belief with a Western bias for disclosure and informed consent or the belief that "talking through" things helps with emotional adjustment. Caregivers who rely on biomedical approaches to serious illness feel conflict with patients and families who rely mainly on spiritual interventions or afterlife considerations. Religious and cultural practices also govern how to care for a body near or after death (Box 16-1).

Skill Performance Guidelines

1 Consider the patient and family as the unit of care.
2 Provide individualized, holistic, culturally sensitive care throughout the grief process, dying experience, and bereavement period. Integrate objective data with subjective data, based on the patient's experience.
3 Perform skills and select interventions in collaboration with the patient, family, and interdisciplinary team. Patients and family members best know their needs and should be given control and options.
4 Determine if the patient has an advance directive. Assist patients and family members in preparing one if they wish, and make existing advance directives available to care providers and family members.

BOX 16-1 | Religious and Cultural Considerations in Care of the Body Near and After Death

Buddhism—Persons prefer a quiet place for death. A Buddhist monk may chant to promote a peaceful, accepting mind in the dying person. Incense may be used. When the person has died, the body should be covered with a cotton sheet. Others should not touch the body, and the deceased's mouth and eyes are left open. Maintain strict silence after death. Autopsy and organ donation are permitted.

Christianity—Christianity has many denominations with varying practices, as do other world religions. Bible texts may be read near or at the time of death. Protestant Christians receive the sacraments of Holy Communion or sometimes baptism. Christians in the Roman Catholic tradition often request sacraments of Penance and Anointing of the Sick and Holy Communion at the end of life. African American Christians often want prayers and anointing and view death as "going home" to Jesus. There are no prescribed rituals for body preparation, and autopsy and organ donation are usually permissible.

Hinduism—Persons prefer to die at home or in a quiet setting. Because of a belief in reincarnation, efforts are made to resolve relationships before death. The head of a person close to death should face the east with a lamp placed near the head. If the dying person is unable to chant his mantra, a family member can chant it into the right ear. Passages from the Bhagavad Gita are recited. Family members prefer to wash the body after death and are present to chant, pray, and use incense. Hindus prefer cremation of the body.

Islam—A Muslim reader recites verses from the Qur'an when the person is near death. Family members prepare the body, and non-Muslims should not touch the body. After death the person's eyes should be closed and arms and legs straightened. Autopsy or organ donation is generally not permissible, except as required by law.

Judaism—Deathbed confessional, blessings, and readings from the Torah are traditional. In Orthodox Judaism, a family member remains with the body until burial, which takes place within 24 hours, not on the Sabbath. A family member closes the deceased's eyes upon death. Synagogue burial societies may prepare the body, which is wrapped in white linen. Organ donation prohibitions may exist in Orthodox Judaism, but not for all Jews. Autopsies may be considered if organs are not removed.

SKILL 16-1   Supporting Patients and Families in Grief

People suffer losses and experience grief throughout life. Losses are described in several ways: necessary, actual, perceived, maturational, and situational. Necessary losses, such as leaving friends after high school graduation, are a natural part of life. Such losses are usually replaced by something different or better. Some necessary losses are more difficult and never seem acceptable, such as the loss of a loved one through death. Life goes on, but replacements for these losses do not appear. A person experiences an actual loss when an object or person can no longer be felt, heard, or experienced. Examples include the loss of person, a body part, or a destroyed home. Perceived losses are uniquely interpreted by the individual and are often not obvious to others. For example, one person perceives failure to get into a preferred college as a loss of all opportunity, whereas another person views the same experience as a relief. Maturational losses include changes that occur as a part of normal life development. For instance, a parent feels loss when a child marries and moves away from home. Situational losses include loss from sudden, unpredictable external events such as a hurricane that destroys one's home or city. All types of loss can cause grief and a need for adjustment.

Hospitalization, chronic illness, and disability involve multiple losses. Upon entering a hospital, a patient loses privacy and control over normal routines. With chronic illness, a person's body no longer functions as it once did, leading to a loss of self-esteem and important social roles. Disability adds concern over financial security and often threatens the stability of relationships at home and work. Death, the ultimate loss, ends relationships that bind people together and separates people from the physical presence of a significant person in their lives.

GRIEF

A person's psychological makeup, personal experiences, family, cultural expectations, and spiritual beliefs influence how that person grieves (Potter, 2006). The depth and duration of grief, one's inner emotional response to loss, depends on the type of loss and the person's perception of the loss, as described above. People respond differently to loss and therefore grieve differently. Grief also involves mourning, the outward, social expressions after loss. Mourning behaviors and rituals help grieving individuals adapt to the loss, receive social support, adjust expectations, and go forward in life. Bereavement includes grief and mourning, the inner emotional responses and the outward behaviors in response to loss.

A nurse helps patients by understanding types of grief (Corless, 2006). Normal or uncomplicated grief consists of those feelings, behaviors, and reactions commonly associated with loss, such as sadness, anger, crying, resentment, and loneliness. Although difficult, an uncomplicated grief experience often helps a person mature and develop life perspective. Anticipatory grief occurs before an actual loss or death and involves the process of gradually disengaging from what is being lost. For example, if the dying process extends over a long period of time, the patient and family prepare for death before it occurs and sometimes, but not always, display fewer common grief responses at the time of death. Complicated grief occurs when a person has difficulty moving through the grief experience. It may become chronic (lasting over long periods of time), delayed (suppressing grief until a much later and unexpected time), exaggerated (overwhelming grief that is expressed in self-destructive behaviors), or masked (unaware that disruptions in normal functions are a result of the loss).

Many theories describe grief or mourning as "stages" or "tasks" experienced or undertaken by people during and after a loss. These theories provide useful frameworks for understanding a patient's emotions and behaviors during a loss. They help the nurse select appropriate interventions and evaluate how a patient copes with loss. Although grief theories describe stages and tasks, actual grief experiences rarely involve these stages in a set order. Grieving people often move back and forth through the stages or tasks, perhaps over a period of several years. Table 16-1 summarizes some classic grief theories (Bowlby, 1980; Kübler-Ross, 1969; Worden, 1982).

Nurses use basic knowledge of grief responses to support patients and their families and to address other common psychosocial and spiritual symptoms at the end of life, such as fear, loneliness, or hopelessness. Personality type and culture influence the extent to which individuals share emotions or find it helpful to talk about their grief (Stroebe and others, 2005). Some patients openly talk about their approaching death, and others choose not to acknowledge it. Health care providers often avoid initiating conversations on these difficult topics (Shubha, 2007). When possible, provide opportunities for discussion, paying close attention to the patient's response and indications of a desire to talk further (see Chapter 3).

Delegation Considerations

The skill of assessing patient or family member's grief reactions and designing appropriate interventions cannot be delegated to nursing assistive personnel (NAP). The nurse directs the NAP to:

- Inform the nurse when the patient or family member exhibits behavior commonly associated with grief (e.g., crying, anger, withdrawal).
- Form supportive relationships with patients and families and inform the nurse when patients or family members have questions or concerns.
- Alert the nurse to the arrival of family members so the nurse can discuss the plan of care and offer support.

TABLE 16-1	Comparison of Grief and Mourning Theories
Theory	**Stages**
Kübler-Ross' Stages of Dying	A behavioral-oriented theory that includes five stages:
	Denial—Individual acts as though nothing has happened and may be unable to believe or understand loss has occurred.
	Anger—Individual resists the loss and may express anger toward others.
	Bargaining—Individual tries to postpone awareness of reality of the loss and may act in subtle or overt ways to try to prevent the loss.
	Depression—Individual feels overwhelmingly sad and withdraws from interpersonal interactions.
	Acceptance—Individual accepts reality of the loss and looks to the future.
Bowlby's Phases of Mourning	A behavior theory that includes four phases:
	Numbing—Individual feels "stunned" or "unreal." Numbing protects the person from consequences of loss and intense emotions. Lasts from a few hours to a week or more.
	Yearning and searching—Individuals in this acutely distressful, painful phase may experience physical symptoms such as tightness in the chest and throat, shortness of breath, a feeling of weakness and lethargy, insomnia, and anorexia. Phase may last for months or years.
	Disorganization and despair—Individual endlessly examines how and why the loss occurred. Common time for person to express anger. Gradually this phase gives way to an acceptance that loss is permanent.
	Reorganization—Individual begins to accept unaccustomed roles, acquires new skills, and builds new relationships. Individual needs support to separate from the loss. Phase may last a year or more.
Worden's Tasks of Mourning	A behavioral theory that includes four tasks:
	Accept reality of loss—Individual is in a process to accept the reality that the person or object is gone and will not return.
	Work through pain and grief—Emotional pain comes as a natural part of loss. Identifying, feeling, and expressing emotions characterize this task.
	Adjust to environment in which the deceased is missing—Individual does not realize the full impact of loss for at least 3 months. The person feels the impact of loneliness and considers how to take on the deceased's roles.
	Emotionally relocate the deceased and move on with life—Individual does not forget the deceased but places his or her relationship with the loss in a less prominent place in his or her life. People fear they might forget the deceased.

STEP	RATIONALE

ASSESSMENT

1 Sit near patient in a quiet, private location. Center yourself, and establish a quiet presence. Establish eye contact. Be aware that use of eye contact conveys different messages, depending on patient's culture.

2 Consider the influence of patient's age, gender, race, language, religion, culture, and socioeconomic status on communication.

Presence expresses caring and creates healing moments (Rushton and others, 2007). Privacy protects confidentiality and promotes a sense of safety for patient when expressing thoughts and emotions.

Age, gender, race, language, religion, culture, and socioeconomic status influence patient's grief response and communication style (Kemp, 2005).

STEP	RATIONALE
3 Listen carefully, observing patient responses. Use open communication to develop a genuine, caring nurse-patient relationship.	A nurse establishes trust in a caring relationship, listens to the patient, and demonstrates a desire for communication (Green, 2006).
4 Determine meaning of the loss to patient and its type, suddenness, and when it occurred. To do so, use questions such as the following: • "Tell me about your sister." • "What concerns do you have about how your illness will affect your family?"	The type, meaning, suddenness, and time elapsed since the loss influence the grief experience and coping methods.
5 Use knowledge of grief theory, and observe patient behaviors. Validate observations by sharing them with patient; paraphrase, clarify, or summarize, as in the following examples: • "You look sad. Is there something in particular that brought on your tears?" • "It seems this is hard for you to talk about." • "You've mentioned several times that you feel hopeless."	Use information about type and stage of grief to guide discussion, not to judge patient's responses. Confirms accuracy of your observations and validates patient's feelings. Prompts patient to continue.
6 Encourage patient to describe the loss and its impact on daily life, for instance: "You said your illness has ruined your life. Tell me more."	Listening to patient's description helps to minimize assumptions.
7 Ask patient to describe the coping strategies he or she uses most often in difficult times, for example: "What or who helped you get through the death of your father?"	Familiar, effective coping strategies are often helpful in the current crisis, loss, or grief experience.
8 Assess family caregivers' unique needs and resources. Determine how patient's situation affects daily routines. Note if patient receives care at home and who gives the care.	Illness significantly affects family relationships. Although many family caregivers experience similar issues (fear and emotional burden), diversity in caregivers' needs also exist (Osse and others, 2006).
9 Assess patient's spiritual needs and resources, focusing on those aspects likely to be involved (e.g., trust, life purpose, faith/belief, and hope).	Situations of loss and grief often challenge or strengthen spiritual concepts, such as meaning, hope, community, and a sense of God's presence (Oates, 2004).

NURSING DIAGNOSES

- Caregiver role strain
- Complicated grieving
- Compromised family coping
- Death anxiety
- Fear

- Grieving
- Ineffective coping
- Ineffective denial
- Readiness for enhanced family coping
- Readiness for enhanced hope

- Readiness for enhanced spiritual well-being
- Risk for caregiver role strain
- Risk for complicated grieving
- Risk for spiritual distress

Individualize related factors based on patient's condition or needs.

PLANNING

1 Expected outcomes following completion of interventions: • Patient will maintain relationships with most important people. • Patient will express grief, in keeping with his or her cultural and religious practices. • Patient will use effective coping strategies. • Patient will achieve short-term goals for maintaining normal life routines.	Patient in grief or loss retains connections with social network. Patient receives support necessary to retain cherished values and ways of being. Patient identifies a sense of relief. Patient adjusts to life-changing circumstances and maintains a sense of control.

IMPLEMENTATION

1 Show an empathic understanding of patient's strengths and needs.	Promotes nurse-patient trust, caring, and reciprocity (Mok and Chiu, 2004).
2 Offer information about patient's illness, and clarify misunderstandings or misinformation.	Misunderstanding adds to patient's uncertainty, anxiety, and suffering.
3 Encourage patient to sustain relationships with others to help maintain independence and still get necessary help. Include patient-identified support persons in discussions.	Affiliation with others offers support and helps patient stay engaged in life.

STEP	RATIONALE
4 Assist patient in achieving short-term goals (e.g., symptom relief, completion of tasks, resolution of relational problems).	Helping patients identify and meet their personal goals contributes to their quality of life (Quill and others, 2006).
5 Provide frequent opportunities for patient and family members to express their fears and concerns. Be attentive to expressions of intense emotions.	Emotions change quickly and frequently at stressful times and complicate communication for nurses and patients (Sheldon and others, 2006).
6 Help patients and family members identify and solve caregiving problems. Encourage use of available resources (e.g., hospice, respite care, palliative care team members, and support groups).	Facilitates family grief resolution and reduces caregiving stress. Solving caregiving problems results in better patient care (Forest, 2004).
7 Instruct patient in relaxation strategies, guided imagery, meditation, massage, healing touch, or acupressure.	Complementary therapies effectively reduce stress and provide useful coping strategies (Mariano, 2006).
8 Encourage visits with loved ones, life review with stories or photographs, or projects such as organizing photo albums or journal writing.	Patient sees that life still has meaning and dignity and is able to "create a legacy" (Colye, 2006; Jenko and others, 2007).
9 Address patient's spiritual needs by facilitating religious/spiritual practices and connections with religious community, prayer, music, providing a listening presence. Make a referral to a spiritual care provider.	Spiritual interventions help patients connect with those things at the core of their identity. Caregivers who connect meaningfully with a patient need to initiate interventions (Chochinov and Cann, 2005).

EVALUATION

1 Note patient descriptions of relationships and activities with others.	Provides information on the extent to which patient retains relational ties.
2 Observe patient's behaviors during ongoing interactions.	Demonstrates patient's ability to express grief and coping.
3 Elicit patient perceptions of benefit gained from stress management and coping interventions.	Evaluates efficacy of interventions.
4 Discuss progress toward meeting short-term goals with patient.	Evaluates patient's achievement of desired goals or need for revision.

Unexpected Outcomes

1 Patient does not acknowledge loss and shows signs of extreme sorrow, anger, withdrawal, or denial.
2 Family and patient relationships do not give patient needed support.

Related Interventions

- Consider referral to a grief specialist professional (e.g., nurse practitioner, psychologist, spiritual care provider).
- Share and validate observations of family strain or patient concern over family interactions.
- Consider a family-patient discussion with nurse or health care professional.

Recording and Reporting

- Record interventions used to support patient coping, and note patient's verbal and nonverbal responses.
- Report patient's grief reactions to members of the interdisciplinary team, noting especially those behaviors that affect health outcomes, such as treatment refusals or prolonged inactivity.

Teaching Considerations

- Give family members basic information about common grief responses and how to offer support. Coach family members on ways to provide emotional and spiritual support to patient and each other (e.g., attentive listening, avoiding false reassurances, allowing for the expression of difficult emotions, talking about normal family activities).

Pediatric Considerations

- Children's understandings of death, influenced by age and developmental level, differ from adults'. Respect parents' wishes about when and what to tell children about illness or death. When discussing sensitive topics with children, encourage parents to be honest and give straightforward, caring explanations in language a child is able to understand.

- Play therapy or drawing helps children express thoughts, emotions, or fears about illness or death.
- Be alert to all family members' grief reactions, because they may feel guilt, resentment, or helplessness with the illness or death of a sibling, child, or grandchild. Facilitate communication with family members who, due to circumstances, must be separated from the child.
- Surrogate decision makers, usually the parents, need to make health care decisions for infants and young children. Some decisions are difficult, because outcomes in children are often unpredictable.

Gerontological Considerations

- Many older adults have coexisting medical conditions that add to their symptom burden. They have also lived long enough to have experienced cumulative losses, including members of their family and support group, which complicates their grief experience (Murphy-Ende, 2006).

SKILL 16-2 Symptom Management at the End of Life

Quality palliative care centers on vigilant symptom management. Coyle (2006) describes the "hard work" of dying and the physical and emotional stressors of living with multiple symptoms. Managing patients' symptoms at the end of life begins by understanding the impact those symptoms have on patients' lives from their point of view (Fig. 16-2). Assess all symptoms thoroughly, because a patient's fear of not being heard or believed compounds the magnitude of symptoms, particularly pain and air hunger.

Forest (2004) describes many of the symptoms experienced by patients at the end of life. Patients identify pain as their most common and severe symptom (Kwon and others, 2007). Refer to Chapter 15 for a discussion of pain, a complex area of symptom management. Nursing interventions for addressing other symptoms common at the end of life follow.

Delegation Considerations

The skill of symptom management cannot be delegated to NAP. The nurse directs the NAP to:

- Notify the nurse if patient reports new symptoms or if existing symptoms worsen or change.
- Provide basic comfort care such as positioning, room temperature control, hygiene, and mouth care.

- Report possible adverse effects of drug therapy, as instructed by the nurse.
- Speak to unconscious or dying patients because sometimes they are still able to hear.

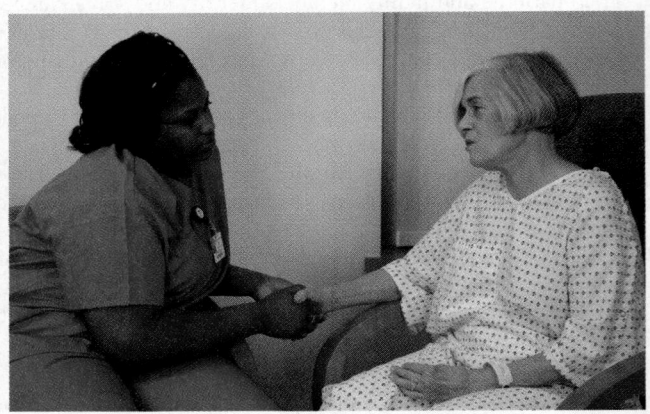

FIG 16-2 Nurses use their presence and therapeutic communication to assess how symptoms affect a patient's life.

STEP	RATIONALE

ASSESSMENT

1 Ask patients to describe symptoms in their own words. Use open-ended prompts, such as "Describe your leg pain to me" and "Tell me about your sleeping patterns since you started taking this medication."

Allows patients to describe their personal perceptions and experiences of symptoms.

2 Allow sufficient time for patients to describe their symptoms, and encourage them to say more with questions like the following:
- "Is there anything else bothering you?"
- "You've told me about your _____ pain. Do you have pain anywhere else?"

Ensures a more complete assessment. Prevents nurse from making assumptions about the patient's symptoms and prematurely stopping the assessment process.

3 Assess patient's pain severity on a scale of 0 to 10 and assess other characteristics of pain routinely and with all new reports of pain (see Chapter 15).

Consistent use of a standard pain scale helps assess changes in patient pain levels and evaluate effectiveness of pain interventions.

4 Assess respiratory rate, breathing patterns, and lung sounds. Ask if patient feels he or she is getting enough air. Assess for presence of airway secretions.

Dyspnea or air hunger results from metabolic or respiratory changes. Changes in breathing patterns include increased use of accessory muscles, or Cheyne-Stokes respiration, which is alternating periods of apnea and hyperpnea (Plonk and Arnold, 2005).

5 Observe the condition of the skin, especially the back, heels, and buttocks (see Chapter 18).

Decreased peripheral circulation and activity level contributes to skin breakdown.

6 Inspect the patient's oral cavity, including the mucosa, tongue, and teeth (see Chapter 6).

Dehydration, difficulty swallowing, and inflammation of the mouth are common. Bacterial colonization of the mouth increases with age, reduced salivary flow, medications, and immunosuppression (Dahlin, 2004).

7 Assess bowel function (see Chapter 6):

Patients receiving palliative care commonly experience constipation because of decreased intestinal motility, fluid intake, and activity and increased anal sphincter tone from pain medications, especially opioids (Whitecar and others, 2004).

a Determine usual bowel elimination pattern (frequency, character, usual time of day).

Diarrhea results from infections, diseases, or medications (e.g., antibiotics or chemotherapy). Watery stool leaking around the blockage indicates fecal impaction.

STEP	RATIONALE

   b Identify typical food and fluid intake over 1 week.

   c Ask about current activity level.

   d Determine usual bowel management routines and success of those approaches.

   e Review medication regimens, prescription and over-the-counter drugs known to cause constipation (e.g., opioids, antacids).

   f If patient is passing liquid stool, assess for presence of a fecal impaction.

8 Assess urinary elimination (see Chapter 33) and ability to control urination. If incontinent, assess for potential complications (e.g., skin breakdown or patient discomfort).

> Urinary incontinence results from progressive disease (e.g., spinal cord involvement and reduced level of consciousness).

9 Ask if patient is experiencing nausea, vomiting, or decreased appetite.

> Medications, pain, depression, disease progression, or decreased blood flow to digestive organs near death often contribute to nausea, vomiting, and decreased appetite.

10 Assess daily food and fluid intake in relation to patient's condition and preferences.

> Near death, patients have little desire for food and water as body functions slow. Little evidence exists that anorexia or dehydration cause patient discomfort (Plonk and Arnold, 2005).

11 Assess fatigue using a general scale in patients near the end of life (none, moderate, severe). Ask if fatigue limits patient's ability to perform desired activities (see Chapter 10).

> Metabolic demands of a disease and treatments cause weakness and fatigue. Exhaustion phase of the general adaptation syndrome causes energy depletion (Anderson and Dean, 2006).

12 Assess for excessive restlessness in a patient near death.

> Terminal restlessness (delirium), common in patients near the end of life, causes significant patient and caregiver stress (Brajtman, 2005).

   a Assess for conditions that cause restlessness, such as pain, nausea, dyspnea, full bladder or bowel, poor sleep patterns, anxiety, or joint pain from immobility.

> Determines presence of common physical problems that need to be treated or ruled out as causative factors.

   b Review medical record for hypercalcemia, hypoglycemia, hyponatremia, or dehydration.

> Metabolic imbalances cause restlessness or delirium (Emanuel and others, 2005).

   c Review patient's medications.

> Unintended responses to medications result in hypoactive or hyperactive activity states.

   d Determine if patient has unresolved emotional or spiritual issues.

> Spiritual distress contributes to restlessness or increased pain (Scobie and Caddell, 2005).

NURSING DIAGNOSES

- Acute pain
- Anxiety
- Chronic pain
- Constipation
- Deficient fluid volume

- Diarrhea
- Fatigue
- Nausea
- Impaired oral mucous membrane
- Impaired swallowing

- Ineffective breathing pattern
- Ineffective tissue perfusion
- Risk for constipation
- Total urinary incontinence

Individualize related factors based on patient's condition or needs.

PLANNING

1 Expected outcomes following completion of interventions:

- Patient will report acceptable level of pain.

> Indicates pain control.

- Patient will report feeling warm and comfortable.

> Warming interventions help reverse effects of reduced peripheral circulation.

- Patient will report comfortable eating and drinking patterns.

> Optimal food and fluid intake based on patient preferences and comfort.

- Patient will have soft, formed bowel movements.

> Indicates adequate bowel function and peristaltic activity.

- Skin will remain free of irritation or breakdown.

> Interventions to protect the skin from bowel or urinary incontinence are effective.

- Patient will not be restless.

> Therapies effect calming.

- Patient reports less distress from fatigue.

> Energy conservation methods are effective; patient adjusts to changes in activity level.

- Patient experiences less respiratory distress.

> Patient less apprehensive and is able to breathe.

2 Explain care activities before performing, and include patient in setting the daily schedule.

> Minimizes anxiety and maintains patient's autonomy and patient's involvement.

STEP	RATIONALE

IMPLEMENTATION

1 Administer medications, and initiate nonpharmacological pain management interventions (see Chapter 15):

   a Provide patient education on the causes and patterns of pain, and explain interventions.

2 Provide general comfort measures:

   a Provide bath and skin care based on patient's preferences and hygiene needs (see Chapters 17 and 18).

   b Provide eye care, and use artificial tears in patients with decreased consciousness (see Chapter 17).

   c Reposition frequently; do not position on tubes or other objects.

3 Provide oral hygiene after meals and at bedtime while awake and more frequently in mouth-breathing or unconscious patients (see Chapter 17).

   a Use antifungal oral rinses as prescribed or sodium bicarbonate or normal saline rinses.

   b Moisten lips with nonpetroleum balm.

4 Administer antiemetics rectally, as prescribed. As nausea subsides, offer clear liquids and ice chips. Avoid liquids such as coffee, milk, and fruit juices. Consider presence of nausea in patients receiving enteral feedings who have decreased consciousness or are unable to report.

Well-timed interventions keep pain from escalating. Pain decreases patient's sense of well-being and activity.

Patient's knowledge of pain and interventions allows the patient to maintain some control (Paice and Fine, 2006).

Daily baths are not always desired or necessary at end of life if they cause discomfort, fatigue, or increased pain (Lentz, 2003).

Eye irritation causes pain. Blink reflex diminishes near death, causing drying of cornea (Marthaler, 2005).

Prolonged, even slight pressure from weight of patient's body or objects causes skin injury.

Mouth rinses are effective in removing oral debris and cleaning the mouth. (Stricker and Sullivan, 2003). Dehydration develops as patient experiences metabolic changes and fluid intake declines. Patients near death breathe through the mouth, drying oral mucosa.

Gastrointestinal (GI) mucosa tolerates clear liquids more readily. Certain liquids increase stomach acidity.

Critical Decision Point *Do not force patients at the end of life to eat or drink if they do not want food or water.*

5 Initiate a bowel management regimen to reduce the risk for constipation:

   a Increase fluid intake if medically tolerated and preferred by patient.

   b Encourage physical activity (e.g., walking), if tolerated.

   c Administer daily stool softener or laxative as prescribed; give enemas as needed.

   d Patients using opioids for pain take a stool softener and a stimulant laxative to prevent constipation (Economou, 2006).

6 Provide low-residue diet for diarrhea; treat infections or discontinue medications, if possible. Administer antidiarrheal medications.

7 Address urinary incontinence with intervention appropriate for patient's conditions (e.g., condom catheter, indwelling urinary catheter, adult incontinence pads [see Chapter 33]).

8 Have patient identify what he or she wants to accomplish, and use strategies to conserve energy for meeting those goals:

   a Allow for frequent rest periods during day, identify times when patient has energy, and eliminate extra steps in activities.

   b Assist ambulatory patients with physical activity.

9 Support patient's ventilatory efforts:

   a Position patient in semi-Fowler's or Fowler's position.

   b Position patient near death on side to decrease noisy respirations. Scopolamine patches reduce saliva and excessive secretions. Suction only if necessary.

   c Stay near patients experiencing dyspnea or air hunger. Use interventions patients perceive relieve their shortness of breath (choice of oxygen delivery modes, fan near face, position). Administer opioids or anxiolytics as prescribed. Keep room cool with low humidity.

Interventions improve peristalsis and soften fecal mass.

Patients with chronic diarrhea require rigorous skin care to promote comfort. They are also at risk for dehydration and thirst.

Enteral feedings benefit a few patients but often add a burden at the end of life. Help family members consider both the benefits and burdens of enteral feedings (Amella and others, 2005).

Urinary output declines near death, making it possible to manage incontinence without an indwelling catheter. Consider an indwelling catheter if skin integrity, patient preference, or fatigue from bed changes become an issue.

Provides patient with a sense of well-being and purpose to meet important personal goals (Quill and others, 2006).

Strategies to conserve energy and reduce fatigue allow for completion of desired activities.

Fatigued patients may need assistance and monitoring through activities.

Promotes maximal ventilation, lung expansion, and drainage of secretions.

Deep airway suctioning causes discomfort and is not effective in reducing airway noise or secretion clearance (Emanual and others, 2005).

Sharing control with patients reduces anxiety that contributes to feelings of air hunger. Morphine relieves perception of dyspnea and dries secretions. Anxiolytics relieve anxiety (Pitorak, 2005). Use of oxygen has little benefit unless the patient feels better using it.

STEP	RATIONALE
10 Manage restlessness through environmental manipulation and pharmacological intervention:	
a Keep patient's room quiet with soft lighting and at a comfortable temperature. Offer family members opportunities to maintain close contact. Encourage use of soft music, prayer, or reading from patient's favorite book.	Reduces unnecessary external stimulation and provides a comforting space. Privacy allows family members chance to provide verbal assurances and touch. The presence of a family member to hold a hand provides a calming effect (Wheeler, 2004).
b Use least-sedating pharmacological means possible to control restlessness. Consult with interdisciplinary team for titration of medication (haloperidol or lorazepam). Discontinue all nonessential medication. Use subcutaneous, transdermal, sublingual, or rectal medication delivery routes.	Reduce delirium without making the patient unconscious. Control of restlessness relieves family's concern that patient is in pain or distress. Discontinuation of unnecessary medications makes drug interactions less likely. Use least-invasive route for patient comfort (Plonk and Arnold, 2005).

EVALUATION

1 Ask patient to rate pain on scale of 0 to 10 (see Chapter 15) and evaluate pain characteristics.	Patient will report a reduced pain severity and increased comfort.
2 Ask patient to describe mouth comfort, and inspect oral cavity.	Mucosa is moist. Alert patient denies difficulty or pain with chewing or swallowing.
3 After patient defecates, inspect feces.	Feces will be soft and formed, and bowel movement will occur at least every 3 days.
4 Observe skin condition.	Skin is intact and without lesions.
5 Ask patient to rate fatigue (scale of 0 to 10). Observe for fatigue or shortness of breath when patient performs activities.	Patient will be less distressed with activity and will be able to perform desired activities. Simple rating scale easily used by patient.
6 Observe patient's respiratory patterns, and ask patient to describe how his or her breathing feels.	Patient will breathe quietly, at a normal respiratory rate, with no shortness of breath.
7 Observe patient's behavior, or ask family to report on patient's behavior. Note level of restlessness.	Patient will appear comfortable and less restless.

Unexpected Outcomes	Related Interventions
1 One or several symptoms remain unresolved, with patient reporting little or no relief.	• Increase the frequency of or change an intervention. Try combination therapies.
2 Patient becomes anxious, fearful, or exhausted as a result of continued symptoms.	• Give patients therapy choices, and try different interventions. Explain goals of therapies and possible reasons for symptoms. • Answer call lights quickly, and explain plan of care throughout the day.

Recording and Reporting

- Record detailed description of patient symptoms in nurses' notes or appropriate flow sheets. Use consistent descriptors for comparison over time.
- Report unexpected new symptoms or uncontrolled existing symptoms to physician or nurse practitioner.
- Record type of interventions used and patient's response in nurses' notes. Note successful interventions in the care plan.

Teaching Considerations

- Involve family members in the patient's care (Fig. 16-3). With proper instruction, they can perform most symptom management interventions, deliver personal care (e.g., bathing, oral hygiene), and administer medications in the home setting.

Pediatric Considerations

- Allow young children to visit a dying parent or grandparent, if desired. Encourage parents to express their concerns regarding how to talk about death and loss with their child.

- Teach parents how to recognize and assess pain in a nonverbal child.
- Encourage involvement of siblings of a child who is dying, based on their needs and readiness.

Gerontological Considerations

- Include older adults in conversations, and accommodate communication limits (e.g., hearing deficits).
- Older adults need companionship and maintenance of self-esteem. Detached caregiver behaviors, such as being slow to respond to physical discomforts, failing to keep room odor free, and speaking in hushed tones of voice are often perceived by the person as abandonment. Encourage a family member, friend, sitter, or hospice volunteer to stay with the patient during the night. Some older adults who have developed a lifestyle around aloneness prefer solitude. Be sensitive to the patient's preferences (Ebersole and others, 2008).

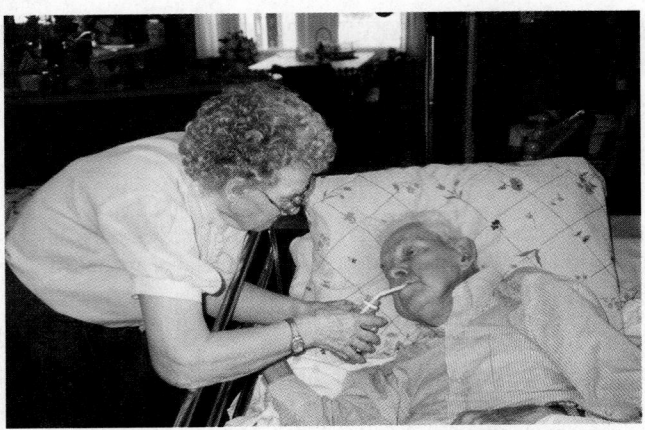

FIG 16-3   Involve family in patient's care.

- Assessing and addressing pain in an older adult, cognitively impaired, or nonverbal patient is sometimes difficult and involves proactive symptom management (Herr and others, 2006).

Home Care Considerations
- Recommend that family members monitor their own energy levels and request respite care when they need relief. Suggest resources for help with meals, shopping, or staying with the patient while family goes out.

SKILL 16-3   Care of a Body After Death

Nurses provide postmortem care in home and institutional settings, caring for a deceased person's body with sensitivity and in a manner consistent with the patient's religious or cultural beliefs. Maintaining the integrity of rituals and mourning practices gives families a sense of some familiarity and control in the face of death. Individual variations exist within cultural and religious groups. Box 16-1, p. 406 describes general preferences.

Two legal considerations arise at the time of death. First, the 1986 Omnibus Budget Reconciliation Act (OBRA) legally requires that a patient's survivors be made aware of the option of organ and tissue donation. In most states citizens can sign the back of their driver's license if they wish to be an organ or tissue donor. However, a family member still usually gives consent for donation at the time of death. Patients may indicate their wish to donate organs and tissue in an advance directive.

In the case of vital organ donation (e.g., heart, lungs, liver, pancreas, or kidneys), a patient must remain on life support until the organs are surgically removed. The nurse's role in organ procurement includes helping to identify potential organ donors, providing care for the donor's body, and caring for the family throughout the donation process (Peiffer, 2007). Family members often need help understanding what "brain death," the irreversible absence all brain function (including the brain stem), means for a person who has died. Patients appear to still be alive, because life support keeps the deceased's organs functioning until they can be retrieved. Tissues such as eyes, bone, and skin are retrieved from deceased patients not on life support. Because of the sensitive nature of making requests for organ donation, professionals educated in organ procurement often assume that responsibility. They inform family members of their options for donation, provide information about costs (no cost to the family), and inform them that donation does not delay funeral arrangements.

Nurses also play a role in the donation request process. Facilitate the conversation by providing a private place and by helping to identify the surrogate to be involved in the request. Sometimes you notify the local donor registry to determine if a patient qualifies for organ donation, because certain medical conditions prohibit donation. Reinforce explanations of the procedure, and inform the family about how you will care for the deceased's body. Above all, honor the family's cultural and religious practices concerning organ and tissue donation, and support their final decision. Donor families often report that donating organs helped them in their grief and that they felt positive about the experience.

The second procedure of legal and medical significance often performed after a death is an autopsy, or postmortem examination. An autopsy, the surgical dissection of a body after death, helps determine the exact cause and circumstances of a death, discover the pathway of a disease, or provide data for research purposes. An autopsy is not performed in every death. State laws determine when autopsies are required, but they are usually performed in circumstances of unusual death (e.g., violent trauma, unattended, unexpected death in the home) and when death occurs within 24 hours of hospital admission (American Medical Association, 2004). Be available to answer questions and support the family's choices. Autopsies normally do not delay burial or change the appearance of the deceased, but there may be a cost to families. The patient's legal representative and the physician or designated requester must sign a consent form. If appropriate, explain the value autopsies have for advancing medical knowledge.

After death the body undergoes many physical changes, including loss of skin elasticity and change in body temperature (algor mortis), purple discoloration of the skin (livor mortis), and a stiffening of the body (rigor mortis). Provide postmortem care as soon as possible to prevent tissue damage or disfigurement (Marthaler, 2005). To prevent livor mortis of the face, elevate the head of the bed 30 degrees immediately after death and before beginning other activities.

Delegation Considerations
The skill of care of a body after death can be delegated to NAP. However, it is often best for the nurse and NAP to work together in providing postmortem care. The nurse directs the NAP to:
- Follow agency policy in cases of autopsy or organ and tissue donation.
- Gather necessary equipment so postmortem care can proceed with minimal interruptions.
- Honor family cultural or religious rituals when performing postmortem care.
- Handle the body with dignity and respect for privacy.

Equipment

- ❑ Clean gloves and isolation gown
- ❑ Plastic bag for hazardous waste disposal
- ❑ Washbasin, washcloth, warm water, and bath towel
- ❑ Clean gown or disposable gown for body as indicated by agency policy
- ❑ Shroud kit with name tags

- ❑ Syringes for removing urinary catheter
- ❑ Scissors
- ❑ Small pillow or towel
- ❑ Paper tape, gauze dressings
- ❑ Paper bag, plastic bag, or other suitable receptacle for patient's belongings, to be returned to family members.
- ❑ Valuables envelope

STEP	RATIONALE

ASSESSMENT

1. Ask physician or other designated care provider to establish time of death, and determine if the physician has requested an autopsy.

   Certifies patient's death. Autopsy requested to determine cause of death and learn more about a disease. If an autopsy is planned or a possible crime is involved, special precautions, as determined by agency policy, must be taken to preserve evidence.

2. Determine if family members or significant others are present and if they have been informed of the death. Identify the patient's surrogate (next of kin or DPOA).

   Verifies that the family has been notified of the patient's death to avoid inappropriate communication of this sensitive information.

3. Determine if patient's surrogate has been asked about organ and tissue donation, and validate that the donation request form has been signed. Notify the organ request team, per policy.

   Federal guidelines require documentation that request has been made.

4. Give family members and friends a private place to gather. Allow them time to ask questions or discuss grief.

   Creates a safe environment for the grieving family. Questions provide information about how they are coping with loss and their needs.

5. Ask family members if they have requests for preparation or viewing of the body (such as position of body, special clothing, shaving). Determine if they wish to be present or assist with care of the body.

   Respects the individuality of the patient and family and supports their right to having cultural or religious values and beliefs upheld (Jenko and Moffitt, 2006). Provides closure for those who wish to assist with body preparation.

6. Contact a support person (spiritual care provider or staff member) to stay with family members not helping to prepare the body.

   Provides family support during an emotional time.

7. Consult physician's orders for special care directives or specimens that are to be collected.

   Specimens may be used in determining cause of death.

8. Assess the general condition of the body, and note presence of dressings, tubes, and medical equipment.

   Validates if tissue damage was present before postmortem care.

NURSING DIAGNOSES

For patients: • Risk for impaired skin integrity	For family members and significant others: • Compromised family coping • Ineffective coping • Knowledge deficit • Powerlessness

Individualize related factors based on the patient's, family's, and significant others' needs.

PLANNING

1. Expected outcomes following completion of procedure:
   - Body will be free of new skin damage.

     Careful handling of body prevents lacerations, bruises, or abrasions during postmortem care.

   - Significant others will express grief.

     Significant others feel supported through their loss.

> **Critical Decision Point**   *Immediately after death and before proceeding with other activities, place body in supine position and elevate head of bed 30 degrees to decrease livor mortis.*

2. Place body in a private room, if possible. If the patient has a roommate, explain and move roommate to another location temporarily.

   Provides staff with a larger area for postmortem care and for family members to gather in a private setting.

3. Direct NAP to gather needed equipment and arrange at bedside.

   Because this is often an emotional time for family members, organized care is important.

STEP	RATIONALE

IMPLEMENTATION

1 Assist family members in notifying others of the death. Notify the mortuary, as chosen by the family, and discuss plans for postmortem care.

Following a death, grieving persons have difficulty focusing on details and often need guidance. Notify mortuary to pick up body promptly. Being informed increases a sense of control.

2 If patient has made tissue donation, consult agency policy for care of the body guidelines.

Retrieval of tissues (e.g., eyes, bone, skin) may require special procedures.

3 Perform hand hygiene; apply clean gloves, gown, or protective barriers.

Reduces transmission of microorganisms.

Critical Decision Point *If family members are assisting in postmortem care, be sure they, too, are protected from body fluids. Have them apply gown and gloves.*

4 Identify and tag the body, leaving identification on the body as directed by agency policy.

Ensures proper identification of the body for delivery to morgue or mortuary.

5 Remove indwelling devices (e.g., urinary catheter, endotracheal tube). Disconnect and cap off (no need to remove) intravenous lines. Do not remove indwelling devices in cases of autopsy, and follow agency policy for body preparation.

Creates a normal appearance for family viewing of the body. Removing intravenous catheters allows fluids to leak out. Mortuary personnel remove lines after embalming (Marthaler, 2005). Removal of tubes and lines is contraindicated if an autopsy is planned.

6 Place dentures in mouth for viewing. If dentures do not stay securely in mouth, place in denture cup and transport with body to mortuary. If culturally appropriate, close the mouth with a rolled-up towel under the chin.

Gives the face a moral natural appearance.

Jaw muscles relax after death, making it difficult to keep dentures in place. Mortuary personnel remove dentures to clean and seal mouth.

7 Place small pillow under the head, or position according to cultural preferences. Do not tie hands together on top of body. Check agency policy regarding need to secure hands and feet. Use only circular gauge bandaging on body.

Patient appears natural.

Weight of limp arms causes skin damage and discoloration if tied. Some agencies require securing of appendages to prevent tissue damage when body is being moved.

8 Close eyes by gently pulling eyelids over eyes. Some cultures prefer that eyes remain open.

Closed eyes convey to some people a more peaceful and natural appearance.

9 Shave male facial hair, unless prohibited by cultural practices or if the patient wore a beard.

Presents patient in his normal appearance. Honors cultural or religious preferences.

10 Wash soiled body parts. Some cultural practices require that family members cleanse the body.

Prepares body for viewing and reduces odors. Mortuary personnel provide a complete bath.

11 Remove soiled dressings, and replace with clean dressings, using paper tape or circular gauze bandaging.

Changing dressings helps to control odors and creates more acceptable appearance. Paper tape minimizes skin damage when tape is removed.

Critical Decision Point *Turning a recently dead body to the side sometimes causes the flow of exhaled air. This is a normal event and not a sign of life.*

12 Place an absorbent pad under the buttocks.

Relaxation of sphincter muscles at time of death causes release of urine or feces.

13 Place a clean gown on the body. Some agencies require gown removal before placing body in the shroud.

Provides privacy and prepares body for viewing.

14 Brush and comb hair. Remove any clips, hairpins, or rubber bands.

The deceased appears cared for. Hard objects damage or discolor the face and scalp.

15 Identify the personal belongings that stay with the body and those to be given to the family.

Prevents loss of valuable or meaningful property.

16 If family requests viewing, place a clean sheet over the body up to the chin with arms outside covers, if desirable. Remove unneeded medical equipment from the room. Provide soft lighting and chairs for family.

Maintains respect for the patient and those viewing the body. Prevents exposure of body parts. Removing medical equipment provides a more peaceful, natural setting (Marthaler, 2005).

17 Allow family time alone with the body and encourage them to say goodbye with religious rituals and in a culturally expected manner. Some cultures require silence at the time of death, whereas others express grief with loud wailing, "falling out," or hysteria. Do not rush any grieving process.

Compassionate care provides family members with a meaningful experience during the early phase of grief.

Ensure privacy and a safe environment. Provide a chair at bedside for family member who might collapse.

18 After viewing, remove linens and gown, per agency policy. Place body in shroud provided by the agency (see illustration).

The shroud protects injury to skin, avoids exposure of body, and provides a barrier against potentially contaminated body fluids.

STEP	RATIONALE

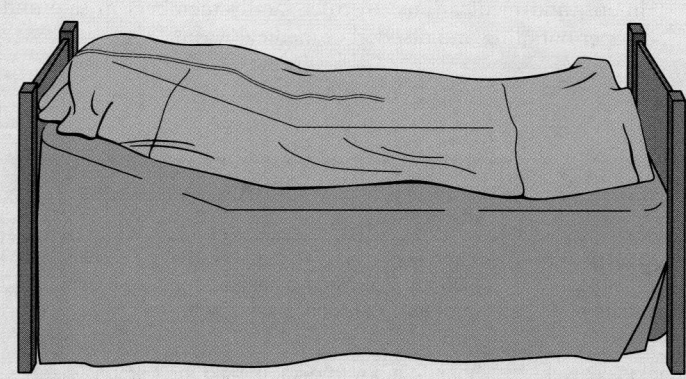 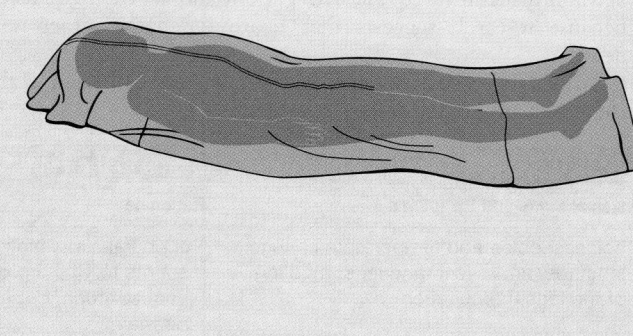

STEP 18   Body in the shroud.

19 Place an identification label on the outside of the shroud if required by agency policy. Follow agency policy for marking a body that poses an infectious risk to others.	Ensures proper identification of the body. Reduces exposure of morgue and mortuary staff to contamination.
20 Arrange prompt transportation of the body to the mortuary. If you anticipate a delay, transport body to the morgue.	Mortuary personnel get the best results if embalming occurs before full rigor mortis, stiffening of the body after death, occurs.

EVALUATION

1 Observe family members', friends', and significant others' response to the loss.	The need for referral or assistance is based on evaluation of a person's unique response to loss.
2 Note appearance and condition of patient's skin during preparation of the body.	Provides information for postmortem care documentation.

Unexpected Outcomes	Related Interventions
1 A person becomes immobilized by grief and has difficulty functioning.	• Enlist the help of a trusted friend or family member to provide direction and support. • Call for assistance from a psychiatric nurse practitioner, spiritual care provider, or social worker who has a relationship with the family.
2 A grieving person becomes very agitated and threatens or strikes out against others.	• Enlist help of security staff or crisis intervention professional if safety is a concern.
3 Lacerations, bruises, or abrasions are noted on the body. Positioning or preparation of the body results in skin injury.	• Document according to policy.

Recording and Reporting

- Record time of death in the nurses' notes and other appropriate forms, describe any resuscitative measures taken (if applicable), and note the name of the professional certifying the death.
- Record any special preparation of the body for autopsy or organ/tissue donation. Note whom you called and who made the request for organ/tissue donation.
- Record names of mortuary and names of family members consulted at the time of death and their relationship to the deceased.
- Record on appropriate form personal articles left on the body (e.g., teeth or glasses), jewelry taped to skin, or tubes and lines left in place. Note how valuables and personal belongings were handled and who received them. Secure signatures as required by agency policy.
- Record time the body was transported and its destination. Note the location of body identification tags.

Pediatric Considerations

- Arrange for family members, especially parents, to be with the child throughout the dying process and at the time of death, if they wish.
- Parents frequently want to hold their child's body after death. Parents of deceased newborns often want a memento of their baby (picture, article of clothing, footprint, or lock of hair). Make every effort to honor parent requests (Romesberg, 2004).

Gerontological Considerations

- Some older adults have very small families and surviving circles of friends. Nurses and other care providers are sometimes the only human presence during death. Arrange for someone to be with the person when death is imminent.

Home Care Considerations

- Educate family members caring for a patient dying at home about what to expect at the time of death (Table 16-2). Encourage family members to talk with patient and say their goodbyes, because research suggests that hearing remains intact near death.
- Consider the type of support family members will need at the time of death, and make arrangements.

- After death in the home, follow agency guidelines for body preparation and transfer and for disposal of durable medical equipment (e.g., tubing, needles, syringes), soiled dressings or linens, and medications. Instruct family members in safe and proper handling and disposal of medical waste.

TABLE 16-2　Physical Signs and Symptoms in the Final Stages of Dying

Physical Signs and Symptoms	Rationale	Intervention
Coolness, color, and temperature change in hands, arms, feet, and legs; mottling of the legs; perspiration	Peripheral circulation diminished as blood shunts to vital organs. Patient may feel cool to touch, but core temperature is normal.	Place socks on feet. Cover with light blanket. Do not use electric blanket because person not able to report excess heat.
Increased sleeping	Conservation of energy, psychological withdrawal, medications.	Spend time with person; hold the person's hand. Speak to the person, even if no response.
Disorientation, confusion of time, place, person	Metabolic changes, medications, changing sleep/wake cycles, decreased oxygenation.	Identify self by name; reorient person to time and place. Decrease environmental stimuli.
Incontinence of urine, and/or bowel	Decreased muscle tone and consciousness.	Change bedding as appropriate. Use bed pads; try not to use indwelling catheters.
Upper airway secretions; noisy respirations	Decreased cough reflex, inability to expectorate secretions or clear throat, relaxation of glottis, decreased muscle tone.	Elevate head with pillow or raise head of bed; turn head to side to drain secretions. Minimal suctioning.
Restlessness	Metabolic changes and decrease in oxygen to the brain.	Calm patient by speech and action; reduce light, back rub, stroke arms, or read aloud. Do not use restraints.
Decreased intake of food and fluids, nausea	Blood shunted away from gastrointestinal (GI) tract causing decreased GI motility and anorexia; ketosis.	Do not force patient to eat or drink; give ice chips or popsicles, if desired. Provide mouth care.

Modified from Ebersole P and others: *Toward healthy aging,* ed 7, St. Louis, 2008, Mosby.

❓ CRITICAL THINKING EXERCISES

You are caring for Mr. Lange, a 79-year-old man hospitalized for abdominal pain, anorexia, weight loss, and weakness. He was treated 10 years earlier for prostate cancer. Test results now confirm that he has a large tumor in his abdomen and the cancer has spread to the lymph nodes. No medical interventions are available to cure or slow his disease progression. When you enter the room, Mr. Lange tells you in an angry voice that he wants to transfer to a different hospital where people will help him fight his cancer. Explain your choice.

1 What should you do first in response to Mr. Lange's statement?

2 Later in the day, Mr. Lange continues to express anger at you and other caregivers and asks you to help him "get out of here." Which statement best supports your use of grief theory in this case?

   A Grief theory does not apply, because Mr. Lange is not at the end of life.

   B He does not fit Kübler-Ross' stage theory because anger is not the first reaction to loss.

   C Kübler-Ross' theory explains that Mr. Lange's anger is a response to his loss of ability to function normally and fear about his future.

3 The next day, Mr. Lange reports mild abdominal pain and mentions that he has not had a bowel movement for 3 days. His wife reports to you that he has not had anything to eat or drink for 24 hours. What action will you take first, based on this information?

   A Administer an as-needed (prn) medication for constipation.

   B Further assess Mr. Lange's pain and bowel patterns.

   C Ask Mr. Lange's wife to describe what his pain was like when he first came to the hospital.

   D Encourage Mr. Lange to increase his fluid consumption and activity to increase peristalsis.

4 Four weeks later, you take care of Mr. Lange again. His symptoms include weight loss, anorexia, abdominal pain, depression, and anxiety. His wife tells you that the nurse practitioner told them about home hospice care. His wife says to you, "I'm still not sure if hospice would be best for us." What key points would you include in a discussion with Mr. Lange and his wife about hospice care?

5 Mrs. Lange asks you for advice on how she might get her husband to eat more. She believes that if he ate more he would get stronger and enjoy life more. She feels sad that he refuses the meals she prepares. How would you best begin your conversation with Mrs. Lange?

   A "You might let him plan the menu so he can select what he wants."

   B "There are several nutritional supplements that might help him gain weight."

   C "His appetite is decreased because he is not getting enough activity. If you encourage him to walk more, he might feel hungry at mealtimes."

   D "It must be distressing to see him lose his interest in eating. Loss of appetite is common and normal in people with serious illness."

REVIEW QUESTIONS

1 A patient with cancer is being admitted into hospice care. Which question by the nurse would best demonstrate one of the three themes found in good palliative care?
   1 "What arrangements have been made for your funeral and burial?"
   2 "How has your family been dealing with the changes in your health?"
   3 "What are the most important things we can do to help during this time?"
   4 "Is pain your primary problem at the current time?"

2 A mother who lost her only son recently as a result of a motorcycle accident has been unable to go back to work after the funeral and is seeking advice from her family physician. Which type of grief would the nurse suspect the mother is experiencing?
   1 Chronic
   2 Anticipatory
   3 Complicated
   4 Overwhelming

3 A new nurse in hospice is working with a patient dying with a tumor pressing on his spine. Which symptom would the nurse expect the patient to state as his most common and severe?
   1 Loss of independence
   2 Pain
   3 Incontinence
   4 Lack of appetite

4 A patient in hospice care becomes very restless even with his intravenous (IV) pain medication. What is the appropriate nursing intervention?
   1 Tell the patient's family that excessive restlessness occurs near death.
   2 Increase the IV pain medication slowly.
   3 Notify the physician of the change in the patient's condition.
   4 Determine if there is something responsible for the sudden restlessness.

5 A dying patient wants to have an open casket at his funeral. After the patient's death, which action by the nurse is most critical in maintaining his appearance?
   1 Tape his eyelids down so the eyeballs maintain their moisture and shape.
   2 Place him supine with the head of the bed elevated 30 degrees.
   3 Bathe him gently so skin sloughing does not occur during hygienic care.
   4 Remove all the indwelling devices and bandages before bathing the patient.

REFERENCES

Amella E and others: Tube feeding: prolonging life or death in vulnerable populations? *Mortality* 10(1):69, 2005.

American Medical Association: *Autopsy: life's final chapter,* 2004, http://www.ama-assn.org/ama/pub/category/7635.html#7.

Anderson P and others. In Ferrell B, Coyle N, editors, *Textbook of palliative nursing,* New York, 2006, Oxford University Press.

Block S: Psychological issues in end of life care. *J Palliat Med* 9(3):751, 2006.

Blum C: "Till death do us part?" the nurse's role in the care of the dead a historical perspective: 1850-2004, *Geriat Nurs* 27(1):58, 2006.

Bowlby J: *Attachment and loss,* vol 3, Loss, sadness, and depression, New York, 1980, Basic Books.

Chochinov H, Cann B: Interventions to enhance the spiritual aspects of dying, *J Palliat Med* 8(1): S103, 2005.

Corless I: Bereavement. In Ferrell B, Coyle N, editors, *Textbook of palliative nursing,* New York, 2006, Oxford University Press.

Dahlin C: Oral complications at the end of life, *Am J Nurs* 104(7):40, 2004.

Doka K: Ethics, end of life decisions and grief, *Mortality* 10(1):83, 2005.

Ebersole P and others: *Toward healthy aging,* ed 7, St. Louis, 2008, Mosby.

Economou D: Bowel management: constipation, diarrhea, obstruction and ascites. In Ferrell B, Coyle N, editors, *Textbook of palliative nursing,* New York, 2006, Oxford University Press.

Emanuel L and others: *Education in palliative and end of life care for oncology: module 6,* Chicago, 2005, The EPEC Project.

Forest P: Being there: the essence of end of life nursing care, *Urol Nurs* 24(4):270, 2004.

Green A: A person-centered approach to palliative care nursing, *J Hospice Palliat Nurs* 8(5):294, 2006.

Herr K and others: Tools for assessment of pain in nonverbal older adults with dementia: a state of the science review, *J Pain Symptom Manage* 31(2):170, 2006.

Hill J: Hospice utilization: political, cultural and legal issues, *J Nurs Law* 10(4):216, 2005.

Jenko M, Moffitt S: Transcultural nursing principles, *J Hospice Palliat Nurs* 8(3):173, 2006.

Jenko M and others: Life review with the terminally ill, *J Hospice Palliat Nurs* 9(3):159, 2007.

Kehl K: Moving toward peace: an analysis of the concept of a good death, *Am J Hospice Palliat Med* 23(4):2006.

Kemp C: Cultural issues in palliative care, *Semin Oncol Nurs* 21(1): 44, 2005.

Kübler-Ross E: *On death and dying,* New York, 1969, Macmillan.

Kwon Y and others: Symptoms in the lives of terminal cancer patients: which is the most important? *Oncology* 71(1-2):69, 2007.

Lentz J: Daily baths: torment or comfort at the end of life, *J Hospice Palliat Nurs* 5(1):34, 2003.

Mariano C: Holistic integrative therapies in palliative care. In Matzo M, Sherman D, editors, *Palliative care nursing: quality care to the end of life,* New York, 2006, Springer.

Marthaler M: End of life care: practical tips, *Dimens Crit Care Nurs* 24(5):215, 2005.

Murphy-Ende K: Palliative care in the older adult. In Cope D, Reb A, editors, *An evidence based approach to the treatment and care of the older adult with cancer,* Pittsburgh, 2006, Oncology Nursing Society.

National Hospice and Palliative Care Organization: *Facts and figures,* 2005, http://www.nhpco.org/files/public/2005-facts-and-figures.pdf, accessed September 13, 2007.

Oates L: Providing spiritual care in end-stage cardiac failure, *Int J Palliat Nurs* 10(10):485, 2004.

Paice J, Fine P: Pain at the end of life. In Ferrell B, Coyle N, editors, *Textbook of palliative nursing,* New York, 2006, Oxford University Press.

Peiffer K: Brain death and organ procurement, *Am J Nurs* 107(3):58, 2007.

Pitorak E: Care at the time of death, *Home Healthc Nurse* 23(5):318, 2005.

Plonk W, Arnold R: Terminal care: the last weeks of life, *J Palliat Care* 8(5):1042, 2005.

Potter M: Loss, suffering, bereavement, and grief. In Matzo M, Sherman D, editors, *Palliative care nursing: quality care to the end of life,* New York, 2006, Springer.

Romesberg T: Understanding grief: a component of neonatal palliative care, *J Hospice Palliat Nurs* 6(3):161, 2004.

Rushton C and others: Compassionate end-of-life-care: the power of your presence, *Am Nurs Today* 2(9):16, 2007.

Shubha R: Psychological issues in end of life care, *J Psychosoc Nurs Ment Health Serv* 45(8):25, 2007.

Stricker CT, Sullivan J: Evidence-based oncology oral care practice guidelines: development implementation and evaluation, *Clin J Oncol Nurs* 7(2):222, 2003.

Stroebe W and others: Grief work, disclosure and counseling: do they help the bereaved? *Clin Psychol Rev* 25(4):395, 2005.

Wheeler M: Palliative care is more than pain management, *Home Healthc Nurs* 22(4):251, 2004.

Whitecar P and others: Principles of palliative care medicine. II. Pain and symptom management, *Adv St Med* 4(2):88, 2004.

Wilson S and others: Dignified dying as a nursing phenomenon in the United States, *J Hospice Palliat Nurs* 8(1):34, 2006

Worden JW: *Grief counseling and grief therapy,* New York, 1982, Springer.

World Health Organization National Cancer Control Programs: *Policies and managerial guidelines,* ed 2, Geneva, 2002, World Health Organization.

RESEARCH REFERENCES

Brajtman S: Helping the family through the experience of terminal restlessness, *J Hospice Palliat Nurs* 7(2):73, 2005.

Brandt H and others: The last days of life of nursing home patients with and without dementia assessed with the palliative care outcome scale, *Palliat Med* 19(4):334, 2005.

Bray Y, Goodyear-Smith F: A migrant family's experience of palliative care, *J Hospice Palliat Care* 9(2):92, 2007.

Byock I and others: Promoting excellence in end of life care: a report on innovative models of palliative care, *J Palliat Med* 9(1):137, 2006.

Coyle N: The hard work of living in the face of death, *J Pain Symptom Manage* 32(3):266, 2006.

Davis B and others: Family stress and advance directives, *J Hospice Palliative Nurs* 7(4):219, 2005.

Harstäde C, Andershed B: Good palliative care: how and where? the patient's opinions, *J Hospice Palliative Nurs* 6(1):27, 2004.

Jones K and others: Nursing home resident barriers to effective pain management: why nursing home residents may not seek pain medication, *J Am Med Dir* 6(1):10, 2005.

Kelly S and others: Terminal geriatrics patients in the critical care unit: the impact of a palliative care team, *Am J Crit Care* 15(3):343, 2006.

Lee S and others. Decision making in palliative care: the patient's perspective, *J Palliat Care* 22(3):198, 2006.

London R, Lundstedt J: Families speak about inpatient end of life care, *J Nurse Care Qual* 22(2):152, 2007.

McPherson C and others: Feeling like a burden: exploring the perspectives of patients at the end of life, *Soc Sci Med* 64:417, 2007.

Mok E, Chiu P: Nurse-patient relationships in palliative care, *J Adv Nurs* 48(5):475, 2004.

Osse B and others: Problems experienced by the informal caregivers of cancer patients and their needs for support, *Cancer Nurs* 29(5):378, 2006.

Parish K and others: Dying for attention: palliative care in the acute setting, *Aust J Adv Nurs* 24(2):21, 2007.

Quill T and others: What is most important to you to achieve? an analysis of patient responses when receiving palliative care consultation, *J Palliat Med* 9(2):382, 2006.

Ryan P: Approaching death: a phenomenologic study of five older adults with advanced cancer, *Oncol Nurs Forum* 32(6):1101, 2005.

Scobie G, Caddell C: Quality of life at end of life: spirituality and coping mechanisms in terminally ill patients, *Internet J Pain Symptom Control Palliat Care* 4(1), 2005.

Sheldon L and others: Difficult communication in nursing, *J Nurs Scholarsh* 38(2):141, 2006.

Personal Hygiene and Bed Making

17

KEY TERMS

Alopecia	Mastication
Aspiration	Necrotic
Buccal	Neuropathy
Cheilosis	NPO
Cuticle	Periodontal
Dental caries	Periodontitis
Dermatitis	Plaque
Eschar	Podiatrist
Flossing	Pruritus
Gag reflex	Sebaceous gland
Gingivae	Sebum
Gingivitis	Slough
Halitosis	Stomatitis
Hygiene	Tartar
Maceration	Tepid

MEDIA RESOURCES

- **evolve** *learning system* http://evolve.elsevier.com/Perry/skills
  - Review Questions
  - Video Clips

- [View Video!] Mosby's Nursing Video Skills, 3.0

Mastery of content in this chapter will enable the nurse to:

- Discuss guidelines used to provide personal hygiene to patients.
- Identify principles of aseptic technique applied while administering a bed bath.
- Administer a complete bed bath.
- Explain precautions to take when assisting patients with a tub bath or shower.
- Discuss precautions used to minimize transmission of infection during perineal care.
- Identify guidelines to follow when administering oral hygiene.
- Explain differences in providing oral hygiene to dependent versus unconscious patients.
- Administer oral hygiene correctly to a patient.
- Discuss precautions used to prevent breakage of dentures.
- Identify guidelines for administering hair, nail, and foot care.
- Comb, brush, and shampoo the hair of a bedridden patient.
- Shave a male or female patient.
- Identify risk factors for foot and nail problems.
- Safely administer nail care.
- Change the linen on an occupied bed.

Many patients who are totally dependent on someone else require assistance with personal hygiene or must learn or adapt new hygiene techniques. Hygiene is important for promoting and preserving health. Maintenance of personal hygiene is necessary for an individual's health, comfort, safety, and sense of well-being. When performing hygiene, you have the opportunity to interact with patients to discuss emotional, social, and health-related concerns. Always convey sensitivity and respect for a patient's personal beliefs and habits, and ensure a patient as much privacy as possible. In addition, performing hygiene is an excellent time to conduct a physical assessment.

THE SKIN

Skin, the largest human body organ, protects us from heat, light, injury and infection and serves to (1) help regulate body temperature; (2) store water, vitamin D, and fat; (3) help sense pain and other stimuli; and (4) prevent the entry of bacteria. Three primary layers make up the skin: the epidermis, dermis, and subcutaneous tissue. The skin covers the entire surface of the body and is continuous with mucous membranes of the mouth, eyes, ears, nose, vagina, and rectum. Thorough hygiene is essential for the integrity and function of each layer.

The epidermis, or outer skin layer, is the first line of defense against external injury and infection. It contains several thin layers of cells undergoing different stages of maturation. Sebum, secreted from hair follicles from sebaceous glands, provides an acidic coating. This acidic coating protects the epidermis against penetration by chemicals and microorganisms. It also minimizes loss of water and plasma proteins.

Bacteria reside on the skin's outer surface. The resident bacteria are normal flora that do not cause disease but prevent disease-causing microorganisms from reproducing. Bathing removes dead cells and bacteria and helps maintain skin integrity.

The dermis contains bundles of collagen and elastic fibers to support the epidermis. The dermis contains nerve fibers, blood vessels, sweat glands, sebaceous glands, and hair follicles. Sebum lubricates skin and hair. Two types of sweat glands, the eccrine and the apocrine glands, are distributed over the skin's surface. Eccrine glands secrete a watery fluid (sweat) that assists in temperature control through evaporation. The apocrine glands secrete sweat in the axillary and genital areas. Bacterial decomposition of sweat from the apocrine glands causes body odor.

The subcutaneous tissue layer contains blood vessels, nerves, lymph tissue, and loose connective tissue filled with fat cells. Fatty tissue insulates the body. Subcutaneous tissue also provides support for upper skin layers.

Because a portion of the skin is usually exposed to environmental irritants and is an active organ sensitive to physiological changes within the body, some skin problems commonly occur (Table 17-1). You will assess for the presence of such conditions while providing hygiene and suggest measures to alleviate these conditions. The patient is always the best resource to explain the nature and course of skin problems as they develop. Skin problems cause changes that affect a patient's appearance and body image. Be sensitive to a patient's feelings while attempting to care for a skin problem.

THE MOUTH

The oral cavity, which is lined with a normally moist, intact light pink mucous membrane, contains the teeth and gums. The membranous lining protects underlying organs, secretes mucus to keep the oral cavity lubricated, and absorbs water, salts, and other solutes. Saliva, a clear viscous fluid secreted by the mucous and salivary glands of the mouth, moistens the oral cavity and begins the digestion of starches. Saliva also provides a means for removing cellular and bacterial debris and aids in the chewing and swallowing of food. Saliva is an important factor in oral health. It removes plaque and microorganisms as it circulates in the oral cavity. If the production of saliva is interrupted through disease, such as Sjögren syndrome, or medical equipment, such as oral or nasal endotracheal intubations, the oral cavity becomes dry. This can result in an increase in bacteria, plaque formation, and dental caries (Munro and Grap, 2004).

The teeth are organs of chewing, or mastication. Dentin, a hard, ivory-like substance that surrounds the pulp cavity, forms the major part of a tooth (Fig. 17-1, p. 424). A layer of enamel, visible in the oral cavity, covers the upper portion of the tooth, or crown. The periodontal membrane, just below the gum margins, surrounds the tooth root and holds it firmly in place. A tooth receives its blood, lymph, and nerve supply from the base of the tooth socket within the jaw. Healthy teeth are smooth, shiny, and properly aligned.

The gums, or gingival tissue, are mucous membranes with underlying supportive fibrous tissue. They encircle the necks of erupted teeth to hold them firmly in place. The gums are normally pink, moist, firm, and relatively inelastic. Regular oral hygiene is necessary to maintain the integrity of teeth surfaces and to prevent gingivitis, or gum inflammation.

THE HAIR

Hair grows from follicles located within the dermis of the skin (Fig. 17-2, p. 424). Tiny blood vessels supply each follicle with nourishment necessary for normal hair growth. Each hair has a shaft extending from the follicle. Sebaceous glands secrete the oily substance sebum into each follicle, which lubricates the hair and scalp. The hair shaft is normally shiny and pliant and is not excessively oily, dry, or brittle.

TABLE 17-1 | Common Skin Problems

Problem	Characteristics	Implications	Interventions
Dry skin	Flaky, rough texture resulting from lack of moisture in the outer stratum corneum, resulting in a less pliable epidermis. Most common on anterior surfaces of lower legs, knees, elbows, and backs of hands.	Skin may crack, bleed, and become inflamed. As a result, redness, pruritus, and discomfort may develop.	Effective treatment of dry skin does not include limiting frequency of bathing, but lies in bathing with warm water not hot and the use of moisturizers. Use superfatted soap (e.g., Dove) for cleansing. Rinse body of all soap well, because residue left can cause irritation and breakdown. Add moisture to air through use of humidifier. Increase fluid intake when skin is dry.
Acne	Inflammatory, papulopustular skin eruption, usually involving bacterial breakdown of sebum; appears on face, neck, shoulders, and back.	Infected material within pustule can spread if area is squeezed or picked. Permanent scarring can result.	Wash hair and skin each day with warm water and soap to remove oil. Use cosmetics sparingly because oily cosmetics or creams accumulate in pores and tend to make condition worse. Implement necessary dietary restrictions by eliminating foods found to aggravate condition. Use prescribed topical antibiotics for severe acne.
Hirsutism	Excessive growth of body and facial hair, especially in women.	Hirsutism may cause negative body image by giving female a male appearance.	Shaving is safest method to remove hair. Electrolysis and laser permanently remove hair. Tweezing and bleaching are temporary.
Skin rashes	Skin eruption that results from overexposure to sun or moisture or from allergic reaction; may be flat or raised, localized or systemic, pruritic or nonpruritic.	If skin is continually scratched, inflammation and infection may occur. Rashes also cause discomfort.	Wash area thoroughly, and apply antiseptic spray or lotion to prevent further itching and aid healing process. Warm or cold soaks may relieve inflammation.
Contact dermatitis	Acute or chronic eczematous rash characterized by abrupt onset with well-defined geometric margins of erythema, pruritus, pain, and appearance of scaly oozing lesions. Appears on head, neck, scalp, hands, legs, dorsum of feet, and trunk.	Dermatitis is often difficult to eliminate because person is usually in continual contact with substance causing skin reaction. Substance may be hard to identify.	Identify and avoid contributing agents (e.g., cleansers, poison ivy or oak, cosmetics, latex, shoes/rubber). Treatment consists of removing contributing agent, if identified, and applying over-the-counter topical steroids or calamine lotion. In some cases prescription steroids may be ordered. Patients may also find comfort with tepid baths.
Abrasion	Scraping or rubbing away of epidermis; may result in localized bleeding and later weeping of serous fluid.	Infection occurs easily as result of loss of protective skin layer.	Nurses should always be careful not to scratch patients with their jewelry or fingernails. Wash abrasions with mild soap and water. Dressing or bandage could increase risk for infection because of retained moisture.

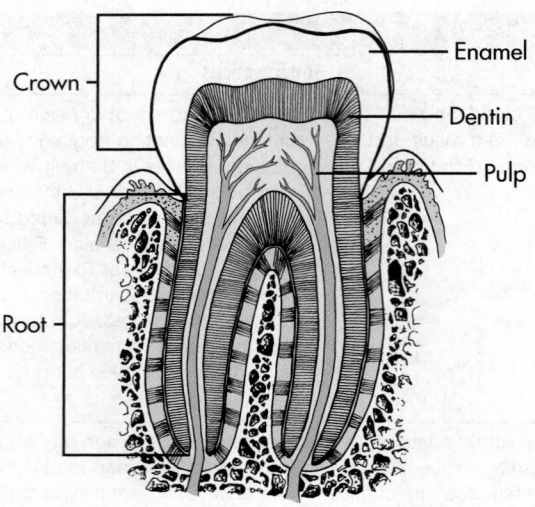

FIG 17-1   Normal tooth.

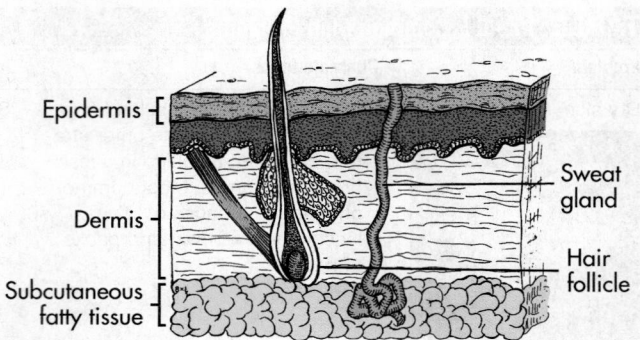

FIG 17-2   Cross section of hair follicle and supporting structures.

The primary function of hair is protection. For example, hair protects the scalp from injury. Eyebrows and eyelashes protect the eyes from foreign particles. Special hair care practices focus primarily on care for scalp, axilla, and pubic areas. Hair growth, distribution, and pattern are indicators of a person's health status. Hormonal changes, emotional and physical stress, aging, intake of toxins (e.g., arsenic, cocaine), gender, race, nutrition, infection, and certain diseases affect hair characteristics. The hair shaft is lifeless; any change in its color or condition occurs as a result of changes in hormonal activity and nutrient supply to the hair follicle.

A person's appearance and sense of well-being often depend on the way the hair looks and feels. Illness or disability sometimes prevents patients from maintaining daily hair care. An immobilized patient's hair soon becomes tangled if not brushed or combed regularly. Dressings may leave sticky adhesive, blood, or antiseptic solutions on the hair. Diaphoresis leaves hair oily and unmanageable. Proper hair care is important to a person's body image.

THE NAILS

The nails are epithelial tissues that grow from the root of the nail bed, located in the skin at the nail groove. A normal healthy nail is transparent, smooth, and convex, with a pink nail bed and translucent white tip. A normal color indicates adequate oxygenation to peripheral tissues. Pigment deposits or bands are common in nail beds of patients with dark skin. The nail is surrounded by a cuticle, which slowly grows over the nail and must be regularly pushed back, using a soft nail brush. Take care to not break the skin around the nail. Breaks in the skin allow the entry of bacteria. The skin around the nail beds and cuticles is normally smooth and without inflammation. Disease causes changes in the shape, thickness, and curvature of the nails.

The feet and nails require special care to prevent infection, odor, and injury. Problems typically result from abuse or poor care. Foot pain can often change a walking gait, causing strain on different muscle groups.

EVIDENCE-BASED PRACTICE TRENDS

In 1994 Skewes developed a concept of a disposable bath in a bag. This product continues to be a mainstay in providing hygiene to critically ill and dependent patients. A study compares the tradi-tional basin bed bath with a prepackaged disposable bed bath in terms of four outcomes: time and quality of bath, microbial counts on the skin, nurses' satisfaction, and costs. The study reveals that the disposable bath is a desirable form of bathing for patients who are unable to bathe themselves in critical care and long-term care settings, and it is even preferable to the traditional basin bath (Larson and others, 2004).

Another area of evidence-based practice is oral hygiene practice guidelines. Critically ill mechanically ventilated patients are at risk for ventilator-associated pneumonia (VAP). Ventilator-associated pneumonia results from the colonization of bacteria in the oral pharynx. These microorganism then translocate from the mouth into the lungs. Dental plaque is also a reservoir for microorganisms causing VAP (Munro and Grap, 2006; Munro and others; 2004). Because of this evidence, guidelines for oral care in ventilator patients and those who need assistance with oral hygiene often include the use of a chlorhexidine rinse as a part of oral hygiene. Chlorhexidine early in the postintubation period may help delay the onset or development of VAP (Grap and others, 2004). Presently chlorhexidine is recommended during the postoperative period for patients undergoing cardiac surgery (American Association of Critical-Care Nurses [AACN], 2006).

CULTURAL CONSIDERATIONS

Each culture is unique in the way members perform personal hygiene. In addition, because hygiene is a personal matter, patients from different cultures will vary in their perceptions of who can assist in their care and what type of care is acceptable (Galanti, 2004):
- For Middle Eastern and East Asian women, avoid uncovering the lower torso and exposing the arms.
- Orthodox Jews, Amish, Hindus, and Muslims consider touching unrelated males and females taboo. Use gender-congruent caregivers whenever possible.
- Among Hindus and Muslims, the right hand is for eating and praying and the left hand is for cleaning gender-private areas.
- Chinese, Japanese, Koreans, and Hindus consider the upper body cleaner than the lower body.
- Hindus consider it irreverent to show any negative nonverbal communication when washing older adults' feet.

▉ Skill Performance Guidelines

1   Consider patients' cultural preferences in regard to hygiene.
2   Consider patients' normal oral and bathing hygiene routines, including type of products used and the time of day when hygiene is routinely performed. Individualize your care based on patients' preferences.

3 Wear gloves whenever there is risk for contacting body fluids.

4 Control environmental factors that alter skin integrity, such as moisture, heat, and external sources of pressure such as wrinkled bed linen and improperly placed external medical devices/equipment.

5 Encourage patients and family or significant other to participate in hygienic care.

6 Establish a regular oral hygiene routine that is easy for a patient to follow at home. The American Dental Association (ADA) currently recommends brushing at least twice per day and flossing daily.

7 Dental hygiene improves a patient's comfort level. Patients who are mouth breathers and those who are using oxygen, are unable to eat or drink, have nasogastric tubes inserted, or have had trauma or surgery of the mouth benefit from frequent oral care (e.g., every 2 hours).

SKILL 17-1   Bathing and Personal Hygiene

 Basic Skills / Bathing / Performing a Complete or Partial Bed Bath Assisting With a Tub Bath or Shower

Bathing removes sweat, oil, dirt, and microorganisms from the skin. It also stimulates circulation and provides a refreshed and relaxed feeling. For some patients, a bath is a time for socialization and pleasure, especially for those who are bedridden or seriously disabled.

In 2007 the National Pressure Ulcer Advisory Panel (NPUAP) identified important points for skin care (Black and others, 2007). Although these were intended for pressure ulcer prevention, they provide sound principles for good bathing techniques.

• Clean the skin at the time of soiling and at routine intervals. Individualize frequency of cleansing according to patient need and preference. Problems such as incontinence, wound drainage, or excessive diaphoresis often require bathing several times a day.

• Avoid hot or excessively cold water, and use a mild cleansing agent that minimizes irritation.

• Avoid use of force and friction when bathing a patient. Avoid massaging reddened areas, especially over bony prominences.

• Minimize environmental factors that lead to skin drying, such as low humidity (less than 40%) and exposure to cold. Additional guidelines to apply in bathing include:

  • Protect patients from injury by assessing and controlling the bathwater temperature. This is especially important for older adults and others with reduced sensation such as patients with diabetes with peripheral neuropathy or spinal cord–injured patients. This is also important for patients who are unable to speak for themselves because of disease processes.

  • Use bathing as a time to interact with and assess a patient. When giving a complete bath, perform a physical assessment of all body systems and discuss issues of concern for the patient.

  • During bathing, assist patients through normal joint range-of-motion (ROM) exercises to promote circulation and joint integrity.

  • For patients who fatigue easily, consider administering a partial versus complete bed bath.

There are two categories of baths: cleansing and therapeutic. Cleansing baths include the bed bath, tub bath, sponge bath at the sink, shower, and the prepackaged disposable bed bath (Box 17-1). The type of cleansing bath depends on the assessment of a patient's physical capabilities and the degree of hygiene required. When a person is unable to perform personal care because of illness or disability, you are responsible for assisting with bathing. This includes time for cleaning and grooming hair, shaving, and cleansing of nails. You can perform many of these procedures during or immediately after a bath.

Physicians generally order therapeutic baths for a specific effect, such as soothing the skin or promoting healing. Types of therapeutic baths include:

1 *Sitz bath:* Cleanses and reduces pain and inflammation of perineal and anal areas. Used for a patient who has undergone rectal or perineal surgery or childbirth or has local irritation from hemorrhoids or fissures. The patient sits in a special tub or basin (see Chapter 40).

2 *Medicated bath (addition of over-the-counter, herbal, or physician-ordered ingredient to the bath):* Aids in relief of skin irritation and creates an antibacterial and drying effect.

Perineal care (see Procedural Guideline 17-1, p. 433) involves thorough cleansing of a patient's external genitalia and surrounding skin. A patient routinely receives perineal care during a bath. However, there are patients at risk for acquiring an infection who need more frequent perineal care. These patients include those who have fecal incontinence, an indwelling Foley catheter, or who are recovering from rectal or genital surgery or childbirth.

BOX 17-1   Types of Baths

Complete bed bath: Bath administered to totally dependent patient in bed.

Partial bed bath: Bed bath that consists of bathing only body parts that would cause discomfort if left unbathed, such as the hands, face, axilla, and perineal area. Partial bath also includes washing back and providing back rub. Dependent patients in need of partial hygiene or self-sufficient bedridden patients who are unable to reach all body parts receive a partial bed bath.

Sponge bath at the sink: Involves bathing from a bath basin or sink with patient sitting in a chair. Patient is able to perform a portion of the bath independently. Assistance is needed from a nurse for hard-to-reach areas.

Tub bath: Involves immersion in a tub of water that allows more thorough washing and rinsing than a bed bath. Patients may require the nurse's assistance. Some institutions have tubs equipped with lifting devices that facilitate positioning dependent patients in the tub.

Shower: Patient sits or stands under a continuous stream of water. The shower provides more thorough cleansing than a bed bath but can be fatiguing.

Disposable bed bath/travel bath: The Bag Bath contains several soft, nonwoven cotton cloths that are premoistened in a solution of no-rinse surfactant cleanser and emollient. The Bag Bath offers an alternative because of the ease of use, reduced time bathing, and patient comfort (Larson and others, 2004). There are now several commercial body cleansing systems available that contain the same ingredients as the Bag Bath.

Delegation Considerations

The skill of bathing can be delegated to nursing assistive personnel (NAP). The nurse directs the NAP about:

- Not massaging reddened skin areas during bathing.
- Reporting any signs of impaired skin integrity.
- Proper ways to position male and female patients with musculoskeletal limitations or an indwelling Foley catheter or other equipment (e.g., intravenous tubing).

Equipment

- ❏ Washcloths and bath towels
- ❏ Bath blanket
- ❏ Soap and soap dish
- ❏ Toiletry items (deodorant, powder, lotion)
- ❏ Toilet tissue or hygiene wipes
- ❏ Warm water
- ❏ Clean hospital gown or patient's own pajamas or gown
- ❏ Laundry bag
- ❏ Clean gloves (when risk for contacting body fluids)
- ❏ Washbasin

STEP	RATIONALE

ASSESSMENT

1 Assess patient's tolerance for bathing, activity tolerance, comfort level, cognitive ability, musculoskeletal function, and presence of shortness of breath.	Determines patient's ability to perform bathing. Also determines type of bath to administer (e.g., tub bath, partial bed bath).
2 Assess patient's visual status, ability to sit without support, hand grasp, ROM of extremities (see Chapter 6).	Determines degree of assistance needed for bathing.
3 Assess for presence of external medical device/equipment (e.g., intravenous [IV] line or oxygen tubing).	Affects how nurse will plan bathing activities.
4 Assess patient's bathing preferences: frequency and time of day bathing preferred, type of hygiene products used, and other factors related to cultural diversity.	Patient participates in plan of care. Promotes patient's comfort and willingness to cooperate.
5 Ask if patient has noticed any problems related to condition of skin and genitalia.	Provides information to direct physical assessment of skin and genitalia during bathing. Also influences selection of skin care products.
6 Before or during bath, assess condition of patient's skin. Note the presence of dryness, indicated by flaking, redness, scaling, and cracking, or excessive moisture, inflammation, or pressure ulcers (see Chapter 18).	Provides a baseline for comparison over time in determining if bathing improves condition of skin.

Critical Decision Point *The NPUAP revised pressure ulcer staging. The stages I to IV go from a reddened area with open or intact skin, advancing through ulcers affecting subcutaneous fat, bone, tendon, or muscle and ending with eschar (necrotic tissue) and slough (necrotic tissue separating from body) in an unstageable wound (NPUAP 2007).*

7 Identify risks for skin impairment. *Option:* Use a pressure ulcer assessment tool (e.g. Braden Scale; see Chapter 18) 　a Immobilization (e.g., patients with paralysis, immobilized extremities, traction; weakened or disabled patients) 　b Reduced sensation (e.g., paresthesias, circulatory insufficiency, neuropathies)	Risk factors increase the likelihood of injury to the skin because of pressure, impaired tissue synthesis, softening of or friction on tissues, and impaired circulation. Incorporate pressure ulcer assessment tool (see Chapter 18).
c Nutritional and hydration alterations	Decrease in nutrition and hydration affect the condition of the skin with decreases in skin turgor, thickness, and elasticity. The skin integrity is easily susceptible to infections or breaks in the skin.
d Excessive moisture on skin, particularly on skin surfaces that rub against each other (e.g., under breasts, in perineal area)	Skin folds trap moisture and cause friction between surfaces, which can lead to breaks in the skin integrity and can result in infection.
e Vascular insufficiencies	Result in poor circulation to the skin.
f External devices applied to or around skin (e.g., casts, braces, restraints, dressings, catheters, tubes)	Improperly placed medical devices or those that move after placement provide pressure or friction that can result in a wound.
g Older adult patients	Older adults have a decreased appetite, which contributes to deficits in caloric intake, nutrients, vitamins, and fluids. This can predispose a patient to breaks in the skin integrity.
h Shear or friction (sliding down in bed)	Causes damage to skin and underlying tissues.
i Incontinence (bowel or bladder)	Accumulation of fluid causes skin maceration.

STEP	RATIONALE
8 Assess patient's knowledge of skin hygiene in terms of its importance, preventive measures to take, and common problems encountered (see Table 17-1).	Determines patient's learning needs.
9 Check physician's therapeutic bath order for type of solution, length of time for bath, body part you will bathe.	Therapeutic baths are usually for specific physical effect, which often includes promotion of healing or soothing effect.
10 Review orders for specific precautions concerning patient's movement or positioning.	Prevents accidental injury to patient during bathing activities. Determines level of assistance required by patient.

NURSING DIAGNOSES

- Activity intolerance
- Bathing/hygiene self-care deficit
- Deficient knowledge regarding skin care
- Impaired physical mobility
- Impaired skin integrity
- Risk for impaired skin integrity
- Risk for infection

Individualize related factors based on patient's condition or needs.

PLANNING

1 Expected outcomes following completion of procedure:	
• Skin is free of excretions, drainage, or odor.	Skin is clean.
• Skin shows decreased redness, cracking, flaking, and scaling over subsequent baths.	Indicates reduction in skin dryness.
• Joint ROM remains same or improves from previous measurement.	Repeated ROM exercise during bathing helps prevent contractures and promotes joint movement.
• Patient expresses sense of comfort and relaxation.	Bath relaxes patient and removes sources of discomfort.
• Patient tolerates bath without fatigue or chilling.	Fatigue during bathing indicates worsening of chronic cardiopulmonary conditions.
• Patient describes benefits and techniques of proper hygiene and skin care.	Demonstrates learning with ability to repeat back to demonstrate understanding.
2 Explain procedure, and ask patient for suggestions on how to prepare supplies. If partial bath, ask how much of bath patient wishes to complete.	Promotes patient's cooperation and participation and promotion of self-care as appropriate.
3 Adjust room temperature and ventilation, close room doors and windows, and draw room divider curtain.	Warm room that is free of drafts prevents rapid loss of body heat during bathing. Privacy ensures patient's mental and physical comfort.
4 Prepare equipment and supplies.	Avoids interrupting procedure or leaving patient unattended to retrieve missing equipment.
5 If it is necessary to leave the room, be sure call light is within reach of patient, the bed is in low position, and the wheels are locked	Provides for patient's safety.

IMPLEMENTATION

1 Complete or partial bath:

Critical Decision Point *If patient is at risk for falling, be sure side rails are up before obtaining fresh water. Also lower bed when it is necessary to leave bedside.* NOTE: *Having all side rails raised is considered a restraint. Check agency policy.*

a Offer patient bedpan or urinal. Provide towel and washcloth.	Patient will feel more comfortable after voiding. Prevents interruption of bath.
b Perform hand hygiene. Apply clean gloves.	Reduces transmission of microorganisms.
c Raise bed to comfortable working height. Lower side rail closest to you, and assist patient in assuming comfortable supine position, maintaining body alignment. Bring patient toward side closest to you.	Aids nurse's access to patient. Maintains patient's comfort throughout procedure. Uses proper body mechanics, thus minimizing strain on back muscles.
d Place bath blanket over patient. Have patient hold top of bath blanket, and remove top sheet from under bath blanket without exposing patient. Place soiled linen in laundry bag.	Blanket provides warmth and privacy. Take care to not allow linen to contact uniform.
e Remove patient's gown or pajamas:	Provides full exposure of body parts during bathing.
(1) If gown has snaps at sleeves, simply unsnap and remove gown without pulling the IV tubing.	
(2) If an extremity is *injured* or has reduced mobility, begin removal from *unaffected* side first.	Undressing unaffected side first allows easier manipulation of gown over body part with reduced ROM.

STEP	RATIONALE

(3) If patient has IV line and gown with no snaps, remove gown from arm *without* IV first. Then remove gown from arm with IV (see illustrations). Remove IV from pole, and slide IV container and tubing through arm of patient's gown. Rehang IV container; check flow rate, and regulate if necessary.

Manipulation of IV tubing and container will possibly disrupt flow rate.

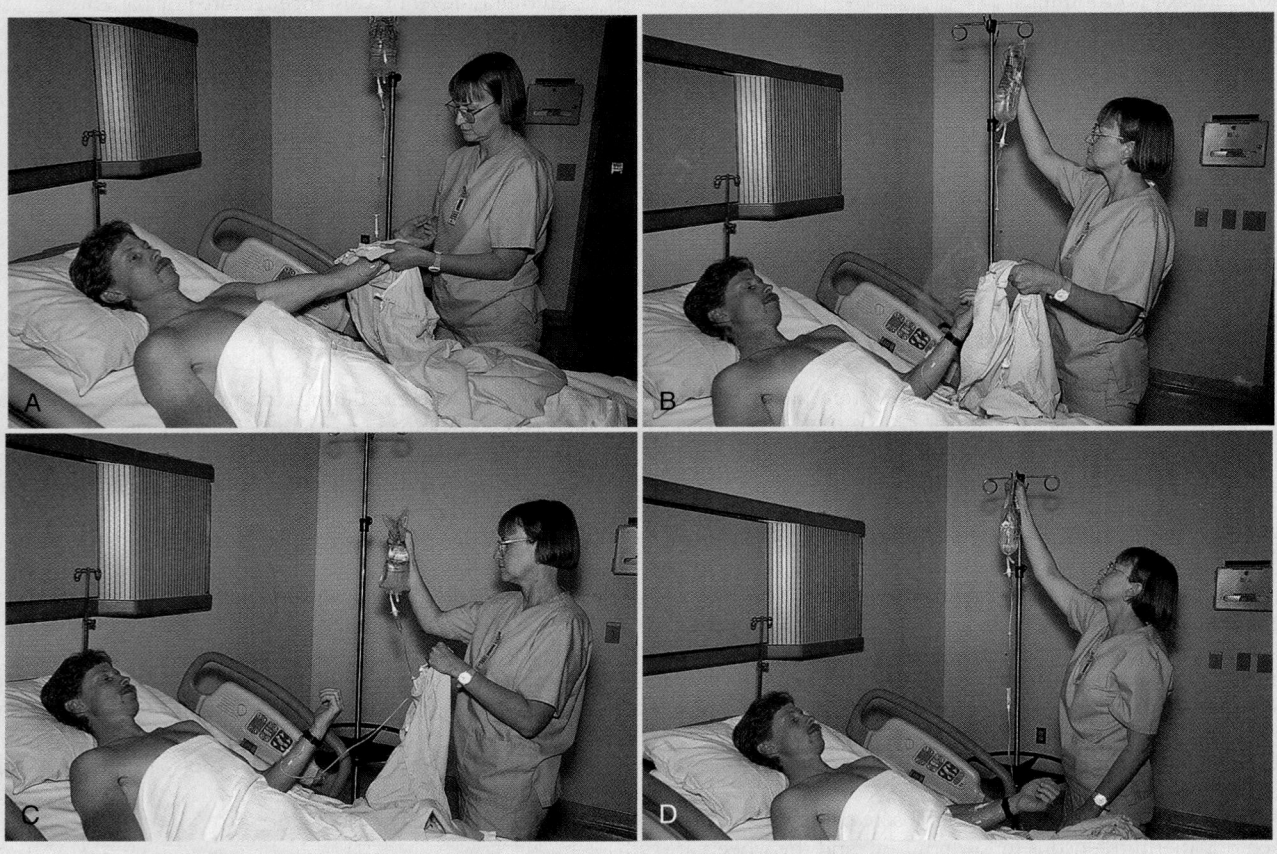

STEP 1e(2)   **A,** Remove patient's gown. **B,** Remove IV bag from pole. **C,** Slide IV tubing and bag through arm of patient's gown. **D,** Rehang IV bag.

(4) If IV pump is in use, turn pump off, clamp tubing, remove tubing from pump, and proceed as in Step 1e(3). Insert tubing into pump, unclamp tubing, and turn pump on at correct rate. Observe flow rate, and regulate if necessary. **Do not disconnect tubing.**

Regulation is necessary to prevent improper infusion of fluids.

f   Raise side rail and fill washbasin two-thirds full with warm water. Check water temperature, and then bring to bedside and have patient place fingers in water to test temperature tolerance. Place plastic container of bath lotion in bathwater to warm, if desired.

Warm water promotes comfort, relaxes muscles, and prevents unnecessary chilling. Testing temperature prevents accidental burns. Bathwater warms lotion for application to patient's skin.

g   Place bath basin and supplies on over-bed table over bed. Lower side rail, and remove pillow if allowed. Raise head of bed 30 to 45 degrees. Place bath towel under patient's head. Place second bath towel over patient's chest.

Allows nurse to move to opposite side of bed without having to move equipment. Removal of pillow makes it easier to wash patient's ears and neck. Placement of towels prevents soiling of bed linen and bath blanket.

h   Wash face:

(1) Inquire if patient is wearing contact lenses. If possible, have the patient care for the contact lenses (see Chapter 19).

Prevents accidental injury to eyes.

STEP	**RATIONALE**
(2) Form mitt with washcloth (see illustration). Immerse in water, and wring thoroughly.	Mitt retains water and heat better than loosely held washcloth; keeps cold edges from brushing against patient, and prevents splashing.

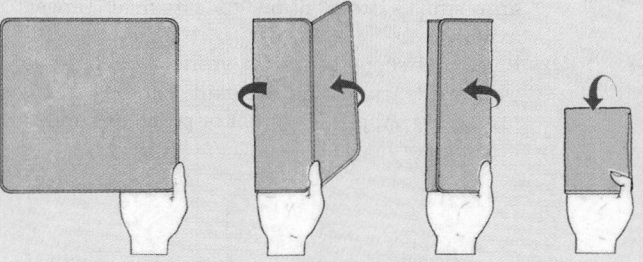

STEP 1h(2)   Steps for folding washcloth to form a mitt.

(3) Wash patient's eyes with plain warm water, using a clean area of cloth for each eye, bathing from inner to outer canthus (see illustration). Soak any crusts on eyelid for 2 to 3 minutes with damp cloth before attempting removal. Dry around eyes gently and thoroughly.	Soap irritates eyes. Use of separate sections of mitt reduces infection transmission. Bathing eye gently from inner to outer canthus prevents secretions from entering nasolacrimal duct. Pressure causes internal injury.

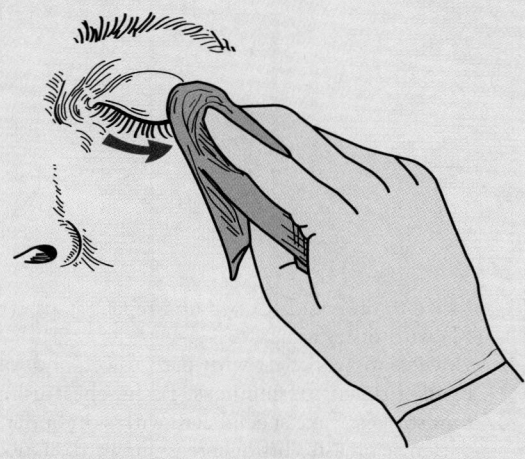

STEP 1h(3)   Wash eye from inner to outer canthus.

(4) Ask if patient prefers to use soap on face. Wash, rinse, and dry forehead, cheeks, nose, neck, and ears without using soap. Ask men if they want to be shaved (see Skill 17-4).	Soap tends to dry face, which is exposed to air more than other body parts.
i Provide eye care for the unconscious patient:	
(1) Cleanse the eyelids with a washcloth from the inner to outer canthus using plain warm water.	Patients who are unconscious have lost the normal protective corneal reflex of blinking, increasing the risk for corneal drying, abrasions, and eye infection.
(2) Instill prescribed eye drops or ointment if appropriate per physician's order (see Chapter 21).	
(3) In the absence of a blink reflex, keep the eyelids closed. Close the eye gently using the back of your fingertip, before placing the eye patch or shield. Place tape over the patch or shield. Do not tape the eyelid. Check physician's order or agency policy regarding taping eyelid without presence of patch or shield.	When the blink reflex is absent, the patient looses a protective mechanism. Keeping the eyelids closed maintains eye moisture and prevents injury.
j Wash upper extremities and trunk:	

STEP	RATIONALE

(1) Remove bath blanket from patient's arm that is closest to the nurse. Place bath towel lengthwise under arm. Bathe with minimal soap and water using long, firm strokes from distal to proximal (fingers to axilla).

Long, firm strokes promote venous return.

(2) Raise and support arm above head (if possible) to wash axilla, rinse, and dry axilla thoroughly (see illustration). Apply deodorant or powder to underarms if desired or needed.

Movement of arm exposes axilla and exercises joint's normal ROM. Deodorant controls body odor.

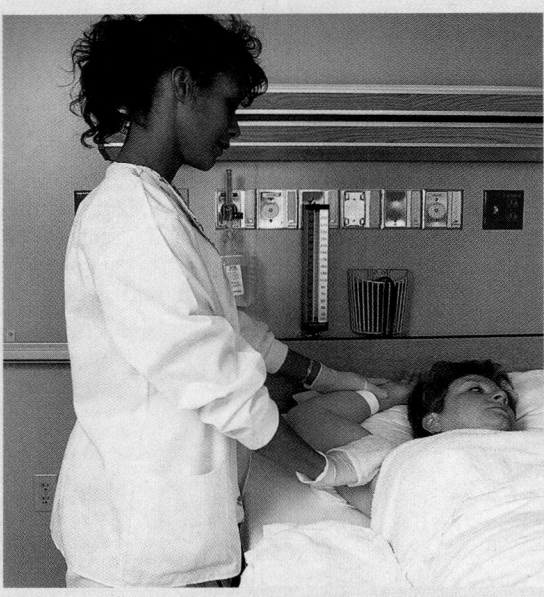

STEP 1j(2)   Positioning the arm to wash the axilla.

(3) Move to other side of bed and repeat steps 1j(1) and (2) with other arm.

(4) Cover patient's chest with bath towel, and fold bath blanket down to umbilicus. Bathe chest using long, firm strokes. Take special care with skin under female patient's breasts, lifting breast upward, if necessary, using back of the hand. Rinse and dry well.

Draping prevents unnecessary exposure of body parts. Towel maintains warmth and privacy. Secretions and dirt collect easily in areas of tight skin folds. Skin under breasts is vulnerable to excoriation if not kept clean and dry.

k Wash hands and nails:

(1) Fold bath towel in half, and lay it on bed beside patient. Place basin on towel. Immerse patient's hand in water. Allow hand to soak for 3 to 5 minutes (if appropriate) before cleansing fingernails (see Skill 17-5). Remove basin, and dry hand well. Repeat for other hand.

Soaking softens cuticles and calluses of hand, loosens debris beneath nails, and enhances feeling of cleanliness. Thorough drying removes moisture from between fingers.

l Check temperature of bathwater, and change water if necessary; otherwise continue.

Warm water maintains patient's comfort.

m Wash the abdomen:

(1) Place bath towel lengthwise over chest and abdomen. (You may need two towels.) Fold bath blanket down to just above pubic region. Bathe, rinse, and dry abdomen with special attention to umbilicus and skin folds of abdomen and groin. Keep abdomen covered between washing and rinsing. Dry well.

Keeping skin folds clean and dry helps prevent odor and skin irritation. Moisture and sediment that collect in skin folds predispose skin to maceration.

(2) Apply clean gown or pajama top. *Option:* You may omit this step until completion of bath.

Maintains patient's warmth and comfort. Dressing affected side first allows easier manipulation of gown over body part with reduced ROM.

STEP	RATIONALE

Critical Decision Point *If one extremity is injured or immobilized, always dress affected side first.*

n Wash the lower extremities:

(1) Cover chest and abdomen with top of bath blanket. Expose near leg by folding blanket toward midline. Be sure other leg and perineum are draped.

Prevents overexposure.

(2) Wash leg using long, firm strokes from ankle to knee, then knee to thigh (see illustration). Assess for signs of redness, swelling, or pain.

Promotes circulation and venous return. Assessment is a key intervention to identification of risk factors for venous thrombosis emboli.

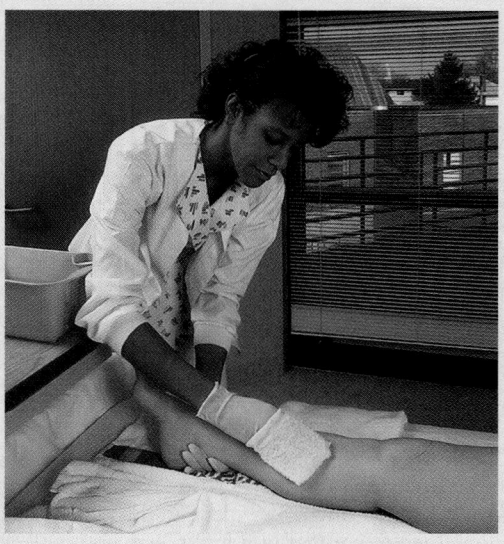

STEP 1n(2) Wash patient's leg.

(3) Cleanse foot, making sure to bathe between toes. Clean and file nails as needed (check agency policy) (see Skill 17-5). Dry toes and feet completely. Remove and discard towel.

Secretions and moisture are often present between toes, predisposing patient to maceration and breakdown.

Critical Decision Point *During the bath assess for signs of warmth, redness, swelling, tenderness, and pain in the lower extremities because these might be early signs of deep vein thrombosis (DVT) (Beck, 2006).*

(4) Raise side rail, move to opposite side of bed, lower side rail, and repeat Steps 1n(2) and (3) for other leg and foot. If skin is dry, apply moisturizing lotion. When finished, cover patient with bath blanket.

Moisturizers are effective in reducing dry skin.

(5) Cover patient with bath blanket, raise side rail, and change bathwater.

Decreased bathwater temperature causes chilling. Clean water reduces microorganism transmission.

o Wash back:

(1) Apply clean pair of gloves. Lower side rail. Assist patient in assuming prone or side-lying position (as applicable). Place towel lengthwise along patient's side.

Exposes back and buttocks for bathing.

(2) If fecal material is present, enclose in a fold of under pad or toilet tissue, and remove with disposable wipes.

Skin folds near buttocks and anus may contain fecal secretions and microorganisms.

(3) Keep patient draped by sliding bath blanket over shoulders and thighs during bathing. Wash, rinse, and dry back from neck to buttocks using long, firm strokes. Pay special attention to folds of buttocks and anus.

Maintains warmth and prevents unnecessary exposure.

(4) Cleanse buttocks and anus, washing front to back (see illustration). Cleanse, rinse, and dry area thoroughly. If needed, place a clean absorbent pad under patient's buttocks.

Cleansing buttocks after back prevents contamination of water.

STEP	RATIONALE

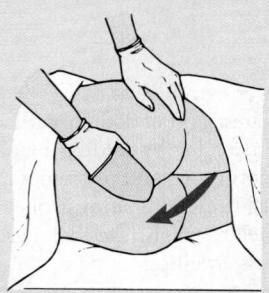

STEP 1o(4)   Cleanse from perineum to rectum (front to back).

p Remove gloves, and give a back rub if patient desires (see Chapter 15).	Promotes patient relaxation.
q Apply body lotion to skin as needed and topical moisturizing agents to dry, flaky, reddened, or scaling areas. When finished, cover patient with bath blanket.	Dry skin results in reduced pliability and cracking. Moisturizers help to prevent skin breakdown.

Critical Decision Point   *Do not massage any reddened area on patient's skin. Reddened areas, especially over bony prominences, indicate localized injury to skin and/or underlying tissue (NPUAP, 2007).*

r Assist patient in grooming. Comb patient's hair. Women may want to apply makeup.	Promotes patient's body image.
s Make patient's bed (Procedural Guidelines 17-6, p. 459, and 17-7, p. 460).	Provides clean environment.
t Check the function and position of external devices (e.g., indwelling catheters, nasogastric tubes, IV tubes, braces).	Ensures that bathing activities did not disrupt systems.
u Remove soiled linen, and place in dirty-linen bag. Do not allow linen to contact uniform. Clean and replace bathing equipment. Replace call light and personal possessions. Place bed in low position with side rails raised as appropriate. Leave room as clean and comfortable as possible.	Prevents transmission of infection. Clean environment promotes patient's comfort. Keeping call light and articles of care within reach promotes patient's safety.
v Perform hand hygiene.	Reduces transmission of microorganisms.

EVALUATION

1 Observe skin; pay particular attention to areas that were previously soiled, reddened, flaking, scaling, or cracking or that showed early signs of breakdown.	Bathing should leave the skin clean and clear. If the are signs of skin irritation (e.g., redness, blistering), use the Braden Scale to measure patient's risk for pressure ulcers (see Chapter 18).
2 Observe ROM during bathing.	Measures joint mobility.
3 Ask patient to rate level of comfort.	Determines changes in level of comfort during bathing.
4 Ask if patient is fatigued.	Determines patient's tolerance of bathing activities.

Unexpected Outcomes	Related Interventions
1 Areas of excessive dryness, rashes, irritation, or pressure ulcer appear on skin.	• Review agency skin care policy regarding special cleansing and moisturizing products. • Limit frequency of complete baths. • Complete pressure ulcer assessment (see Chapter 18). • Institute turning and positioning measures to keep client off pressure ulcer. • Obtain special bed surface if client is at risk for skin breakdown.
2 Client becomes excessively fatigued and unable to cooperate or participate in bathing.	• Reschedule bathing to a time when client is more rested. • Clients with cardiopulmonary conditions and breathing difficulties require pillow or elevated head of bed during bathing. • Notify health care provider about changes in client's fatigue level. • Perform hygiene measures in stages between scheduled rest periods.
3 Client seems unusually restless or complains of discomfort.	• Consider analgesia before bathing. • Schedule rest periods before bathing.

Recording and Reporting

- Record procedure on flow sheet if appropriate and amount of assistance, client participation.
- Record condition of skin and any significant findings (e.g., reddened areas, bruises, nevi, joint or muscle pain) in nurses' notes.
- Report evidence of alterations in skin integrity, break in suture line, or increased wound secretions to nurse in charge or health care provider.

Teaching Considerations

- Instruct patients with decreased sensation to be cautious when entering warm bathwater. Whenever possible they need to use unaffected extremity to test water temperature to avoid accidental scalding.
- Instruct patients in how to inspect surfaces between skin folds for signs of irritation or breakdown.

Pediatric Considerations

- Some adolescents require and/or prefer more frequent bathing as a result of more active sebaceous glands.
- Young adolescent girls should learn basic perineal hygiene measures and know why they are predisposed to urinary tract infections.

Gerontological Considerations

- When caring for cognitively impaired older adults, approach bathing in a calm manner, use the same bathing method, and when possible use the same caregiver. It is best to use the least-distressing method first, such as soaking feet in bathtub or using a disposable bag bath. These approaches must be modified for each patient (Hoeffer and others, 2006; Mahoney and others, 2006).
- Older adults with incontinence need meticulous skin care to reduce skin irritation from urine and feces.

Home Care Considerations

- Type of bath chosen depends on assessment of the home, availability of running water, and condition of bathing facilities.
- In the home setting, set up equipment according to established routines. Patient is the best resource for what works in terms of convenience and saving time.
- Patients at risk for falls may benefit from the following:
  - Installation of grab bars in shower
  - Adhesive strips applied to shower or tub floor
  - Addition of a shower chair or placement of a chair or stool

Long-Term Care Considerations

- Tubs in long-term care settings frequently come equipped with electronic thermometers to measure water temperature. The tubs also have hydraulic lifts to assist residents into the tub.

PROCEDURAL GUIDELINE 17-1 Perineal Care

 Basic Skills / Bathing / Performing Perineal Care for a Female Patient
Performing Perineal Care for a Male Patient

Delegation Considerations

The skill of perineal care can be delegated to NAP. The nurse directs the NAP about:

- Any physical restriction that affects proper positioning.
- The proper ways to position male and female patients with an indwelling Foley catheter during perineal care.
- Informing the nurse of any perineal drainage, excoriation, or rash observed.

Equipment

- ❏ Washcloths and bath towels
- ❏ Bath blanket
- ❏ Soap and soap dish
- ❏ Toilet tissue or hygiene wipes
- ❏ Warm water
- ❏ Laundry bag
- ❏ Washbasin
- ❏ Waterproof pad or bedpan
- ❏ Clean gloves
- ❏ Additional supplies when perineal care is given other than during a bath:
  - Cotton balls or swabs
  - Solution bottle or container filled with warm water or prescribed rinsing solution
  - Waterproof bag

Procedural Steps

1 Perform hand hygiene. Apply gloves.
2 Perineal care for a female:
  a If patient is able to maneuver and handle washcloth, allow cleansing perineum on own.
  b Assist patient in assuming dorsal recumbent position. Note restrictions or a limitation in patient's positioning. Be sure to position waterproof pad under patient's buttocks.
  c Drape patient with bath blanket placed in the shape of a diamond. Lift lower edge of bath blanket to expose perineum.
  d Fold lower corner of bath blanket up between patient's legs onto abdomen and under hip (see illustration). Wash and dry patient's upper thighs.

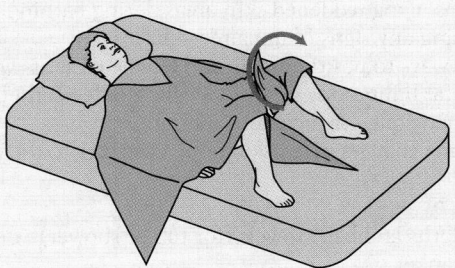

STEP 1d Drape patient for perineal care.

Continued

PROCEDURAL GUIDELINE 17-1 Perineal Care—cont'd

e Wash labia majora. Use nondominant hand to gently retract labia from thigh; with dominant hand, wash carefully in skin folds. Wipe in direction from perineum to rectum (front to back). Repeat on opposite side using separate section of washcloth. Rinse and dry area thoroughly.

f Gently separate labia with nondominant hand to expose urethral meatus and vaginal orifice. With dominant hand, wash downward from pubic area toward rectum in one smooth stroke (see illustration). Use separate section of cloth for each stroke. Cleanse thoroughly over labia minora, clitoris, and vaginal orifice. Avoid tension on indwelling catheter if present, and clean area around it thoroughly.

g Rinse area thoroughly. If patient uses bedpan, pour warm water over perineal area. Dry thoroughly, using front-to-back method.

h Fold lower corner of bath blanket back between patient's legs and over perineum. Ask patient to lower legs and assume comfortable position.

3 Perineal care for a male:

a If patient is able to maneuver and handle washcloth, allow cleansing perineum on own.

b Assist patient to supine position. Note restriction in mobility.

c Fold lower half of bath blanket up to expose upper thighs. Wash and dry thighs.

d Cover thighs with bath towels. Raise bath blanket to expose genitalia. Gently raise penis, and place bath towel underneath. Gently grasp shaft of penis. If patient is uncircumcised, retract foreskin. If patient has an erection, defer procedure until later.

e Wash tip of penis at urethral meatus first. Using circular motion, cleanse from meatus outward (see illustration). Discard washcloth, and repeat with clean cloth until penis is clean. Rinse and dry gently.

f Return foreskin to its natural position.

Critical Decision Point *After administering male perineal care for uncircumcised males, make sure the foreskin is in its natural position. This is extremely important in those patients with decreased sensation in their lower extremities. Tightening of foreskin around shaft of penis causes local edema, discomfort, and if not corrected, permanent urethral damage.*

g Gently cleanse shaft of penis and scrotum by having patient abduct legs. Pay special attention to underlying surface of penis. Lift scrotum carefully, and wash underlying skin folds. Rinse and dry thoroughly.

h Fold bath blanket back over patient's perineum, and assist patient to comfortable position.

4 Observe perineal area for any irritation, redness, or drainage that persists after perineal hygiene.

5 Dispose of gloves in receptacle.

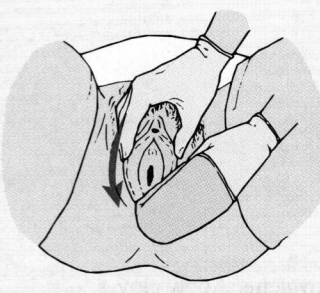

STEP 2f Cleanse from perineum to rectum (front to back).

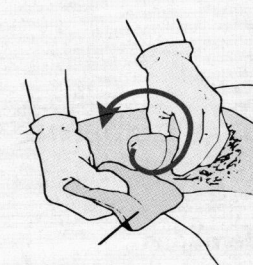

STEP 3e Use circular motion to cleanse tip of penis.

PROCEDURAL GUIDELINE 17-2 Use of Disposable Bed Bath, Tub, or Shower

Basic Skills / Bathing/ Assisting With Tub Bath or Shower

Delegation Considerations

The skill of bathing and perineal care can be delegated to NAP. The nurse directs the NAP about:

• Not massaging reddened skin areas during bathing.
• Reporting any signs of impaired skin integrity.
• Proper ways to position male and female patients with musculoskeletal limitations or an indwelling Foley catheter or other equipment (e.g., intravenous tubing).
• Reporting changes in the skin or perineal area to the nurse.

Equipment
☐ Washcloths and bath towels (for tub or shower)
☐ Bath blanket
☐ Soap and soap dish

☐ Toiletry items (deodorant, powder, lotion)
☐ Toilet tissue or hygiene wipes
☐ Clean hospital gown or patient's own pajamas or gown
☐ Laundry bag
☐ Disposable bed bath or cleansing pack (alternative to soap and water)
☐ Clean gloves (when risk for contacting body fluids)

Procedural Steps

1 Disposable bed bath:

a Warm the package contents in a microwave following package directions. The cleansing pack contains 8 to 10 premoistened towels.

PROCEDURAL GUIDELINE 17-2   Use of Disposable Bed Bath, Tub, or Shower—cont'd

b Use a single towel for each general body part cleansed. Follow the same order of cleansing as the total or partial bed bath (see illustration).

c Allow the skin to air dry for 30 seconds. It is permissible to lightly cover patient with a bath towel to prevent chilling.

d Note: If there is excessive soiling (e.g., in the perineal region), an extra cleansing pack or conventional washcloths, soap and water, and towels.

2 Tub bath or shower:

a Consider patient's condition, and review orders for precautions concerning patient's movement or positioning. Physician's order usually is needed for a tub bath or shower.

b Schedule use of shower or tub.

c Check tub or shower for cleanliness. Use cleaning techniques outlined in agency policy. Place rubber mat on tub or shower bottom. Place disposable bath mat or towel on floor in front of tub or shower.

d Collect all hygienic aids, toiletry items, and linens requested by patient. Place within easy reach of tub or shower.

e Assist patient to bathroom if necessary. Have patient wear robe and slippers to bathroom.

f Demonstrate how to use call signal for assistance. Place "occupied" sign on bathroom door.

g Fill bathtub halfway with warm water. Check temperature of bathwater, then have patient test water, and adjust temperature if water is too warm or too cold. Explain which faucet controls hot water.

h If patient is taking shower, turn shower on and adjust water temperature before patient enters shower stall. Use shower seat or tub chair if needed (see illustration).

i Instruct patient to use safety bars when getting in and out of tub or shower. Caution patient against use of bath oil in tub water.

j Instruct patient not to remain in tub longer than 20 minutes. Check on patient every 5 minutes.

k Return to bathroom when patient signals, and knock before entering.

l For patient who is unsteady, drain tub of water before patient attempts to get out. Place bath towel over patient's shoulders. Assist patient in getting out of tub as needed, and assist with drying.

m Assist patient as needed in donning clean gown or pajamas, slippers, and robe. (In home, extended care, or rehabilitation setting encourage patient to wear regular clothing.)

n Assist patient to room and comfortable position in bed or chair.

o Clean tub or shower according to agency policy. Remove soiled linen, and place in dirty-linen bag. Discard disposable equipment in proper receptacle. Place "unoccupied" sign on bathroom door. Return supplies to storage area.

p Perform hand hygiene.

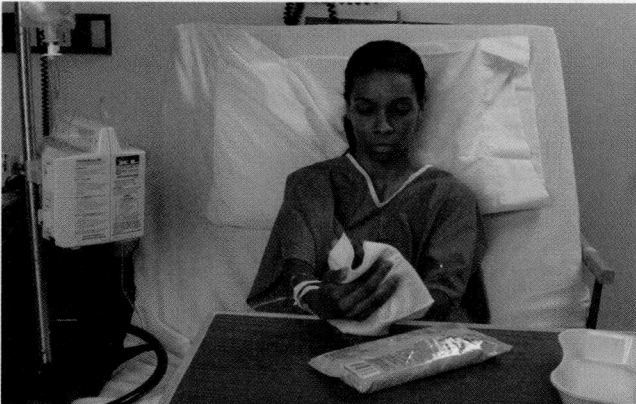

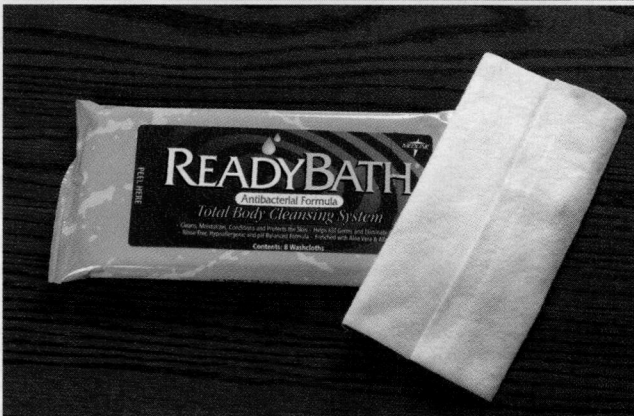

STEP 1b   Disposable bed bath packet.

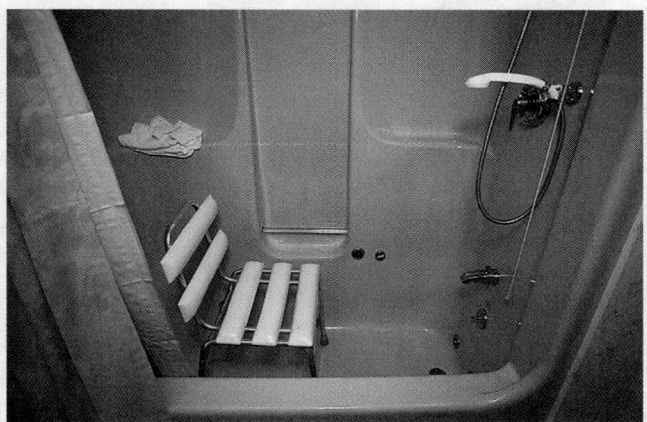

STEP 2h   Shower seat for patient safety.

SKILL 17-2 Oral Hygiene

Maintenance of daily oral hygiene, including brushing, flossing, and rinsing, is essential for the prevention and control of plaque-associated oral diseases. In addition to preventing inflammation and infection, oral hygiene promotes comfort, nutrition, and verbal communication. Brushing cleanses the teeth of food particles, plaque (the cause of dental caries), and bacteria; massages the gums; and relieves discomfort from unpleasant odors and tastes. Flossing removes tartar that collects at the gum line. Rinsing removes dislodged food particles and excess toothpaste.

When a patient becomes ill, many factors influence the need for oral hygiene. Offer oral hygiene assistance as required, from preparing needed supplies to actually brushing a patient's teeth. It is also your responsibility to determine the frequency with which patients require oral hygiene. Base frequency of care on the condition of the oral cavity and the patient's level of comfort.

Encourage patients who wear dentures to continue to care for them and to provide this care as frequently as with natural teeth. Routine denture care reduces the risk for gingival infection. Dentures also harbor bacteria that have been associated with pneumonia (Paju and Scannapieco, 2007). However, when patients are unable to care for their own dentures, you need to provide this care (Procedural Guideline 17-3). Dentures are a patient's personal property, so be sure to handle them with care because they are easy to break. When a patient is not wearing dentures, store them in water in an enclosed cup labeled with the patient's name.

DELEGATION CONSIDERATIONS

The skill of oral hygiene (including toothbrushing, flossing, and rinsing) can be delegated to NAP. However, the nurse is responsible for the assessment of the patient's gag reflex to determine if the patient is at risk for aspiration. The nurse directs the NAP by:

- Explaining what changes in oral mucosa (e.g., patient's report of oral discomfort, presence of lesions or open areas) to observe for and report to the nurse.
- Explaining need to report excessive coughing or choking during or after oral care.

Equipment

- ❑ Soft-bristled toothbrush (hard toothbrush damages enamel and gums)
- ❑ Nonabrasive fluoride toothpaste or dentifrice
- ❑ Dental floss
- ❑ Tongue depressor
- ❑ Water glass with cool water, straw
- ❑ Normal saline or an essential oil antiseptic mouthwash (*optional*)
- ❑ Emesis basin antiseptic mouthwash (*optional*)
- ❑ Face towel
- ❑ Paper towels
- ❑ Clean gloves

STEP	RATIONALE

ASSESSMENT

	STEP	RATIONALE
1	Perform hand hygiene, and apply clean gloves.	Reduces transmission of microorganisms. Gloves prevent contact with microorganisms in blood or saliva.
2	Instruct patient not to bite down. Then, using a tongue depressor, inspect integrity of lips, teeth, buccal mucosa, gums, palate, and tongue (see Chapter 6).	Determines status of patient's oral cavity and extent of need for oral hygiene.
3	Identify presence of common oral problems:	Helps determine type of hygiene patient requires and information patient requires for self-care.
a	*Dental caries:* Chalky white discoloration of tooth or presence of brown or black discoloration	
b	*Gingivitis:* Inflammation of gums	
c	*Periodontitis:* Receding gum lines, inflammation, gaps between teeth	
d	*Halitosis:* Bad breath	
e	*Cheilosis:* Cracking of lips	
f	*Stomatitis:* Inflammation of the mouth	
g	Dry, cracked, coated tongue	
4	Remove gloves, and perform hand hygiene.	Prevents spread of microorganisms.
5	Assess risk for oral hygiene problems:	Certain conditions increase likelihood of impaired oral cavity integrity and need for preventive care.
a	Dehydration, inability to take fluids or food by mouth (NPO)	Causes excess drying and fragility of mucous membranes and lips; increases accumulation of secretions on tongue and gums.
b	Presence of nasogastric or oxygen tubes; mouth breathers	Causes drying of mucosa.
c	Chemotherapeutic drugs	Drugs kill rapidly multiplying cells, including normal cells lining oral cavity. Mucositis, with ulcers and inflammation, can develop.
d	Radiation therapy to head and neck	Reduces salivary flow and lowers pH of saliva; leads to stomatitis and tooth decay (Munro and others, 2006).
e	Presence of artificial airway (e.g., endotracheal tube)	Increases irritation to gums and mucosa. Excess secretions accumulate on teeth and tongue.
f	Blood-clotting disorders (e.g., leukemia, aplastic anemia)	Predisposes to inflammation and bleeding of gums.

STEP	RATIONALE
g Oral surgery, trauma to mouth	Break in mucosa increases risk for infection. Vigorous brushing can disrupt suture lines.
h Aging	With advancing age, mucosa becomes thin and less elastic.
i Chemical injury	Results from irritants such as alcohol, tobacco, acidic foods, or side effects of medications (e.g., antibiotics, steroids, antidepressants).
j Diabetes mellitus	Prone to dryness of mouth, gingivitis, periodontal disease, and loss of teeth.
6 Determine patient's oral hygiene practices and willingness to attend to hygiene needs:	Identifies errors in patient's technique, deficiencies in preventive oral hygiene, and patient's level of knowledge regarding dental care.
a Frequency of toothbrushing and flossing	American Dental Association (2008) recommends twice-a-day brushing and once-a-day flossing.
b Type of toothpaste, dentrifice used	Antimicrobial mouth rinses and toothpastes reduce the bacterial count and inhibit bacterial activity in dental plaque, which can cause gingivitis, an early reversible form of periodontal (gum) disease.
c Last dental visit	
d Frequency of dental visits	
e Type of mouthwash	
7 Assess patient's ability to grasp and manipulate toothbrush. Assessment determines level of assistance required from nurse.	Some older adult patients or persons with musculoskeletal or nervous system alterations are unable to hold toothbrush with firm grip or manipulate brush. Large-handled toothbrushes or a toothbrush handle pushed through a small rubber ball may be of assistance.

NURSING DIAGNOSES

- Bathing/hygiene self-care deficit
- Deficient knowledge regarding oral hygiene care
- Impaired oral mucous membrane
- Risk for infection

Individualize related factors based on patient's condition or needs.

PLANNING

1 Expected outcomes following completion of procedure:	
• Patient expresses feeling of cleanliness.	Hygiene measures remove secretions and thickened mucosa.
• Oral cavity structures have normal characteristics:	Maintains integrity of teeth and healthy oral mucosa.
• Oral mucosa is moist, intact, and of normal color.	
• Gums are pink, firm, and adherent to neck of teeth.	
• Teeth are clean, smooth, and shiny.	
• Tongue is pink and without secretions or coating.	
• Patient describes correct oral hygiene techniques and necessary frequency.	Demonstrates understanding of instruction.
• Patient makes choices regarding hygiene procedure and assists by flossing and brushing.	Patient is able to manage self-care.
2 Prepare equipment at bedside.	
3 Explain procedure to patient, and discuss preferences regarding use of hygienic aids.	Some patients feel uncomfortable about having the nurse care for their basic needs. Patient involvement with procedure minimizes anxiety.

IMPLEMENTATION

1 Place paper towels on over-bed table, and arrange other equipment within easy reach.	Creates organized workspace.
2 Raise bed to comfortable working position. Raise head of bed (if allowed), and lower side rail. Move patient, or help patient move closer. Side-lying position can be used.	Raising bed and positioning patient prevent nurse from straining muscles. Semi-Fowler's position helps prevent patient from choking or aspirating.
3 Place paper towel over patient's chest.	Prevents soiling of patient's gown.
4 Apply clean gloves.	Prevents contact with microorganisms or blood in saliva.
5 Apply toothpaste to brush bristles. Hold brush over emesis basin. Pour small amount of water over toothpaste.	Moisture aids in distribution of toothpaste over tooth surfaces.

STEP	RATIONALE

6   Patient may assist by brushing. Hold toothbrush bristles at 45-degree angle to gum line (see illustration). Be sure tips of bristles rest against and penetrate under gum line. Brush inner and outer surfaces of upper and lower teeth by brushing from gum to crown of each tooth. Clean biting surfaces of teeth by holding top of bristles parallel with teeth and brushing gently back and forth (see illustration). Brush sides of teeth by moving bristles back and forth (see illustration).

Angle allows brush to reach all tooth surfaces and to clean under gum line where plaque and tartar accumulate. Back-and-forth motion loosens food particles caught between teeth and along chewing surfaces.

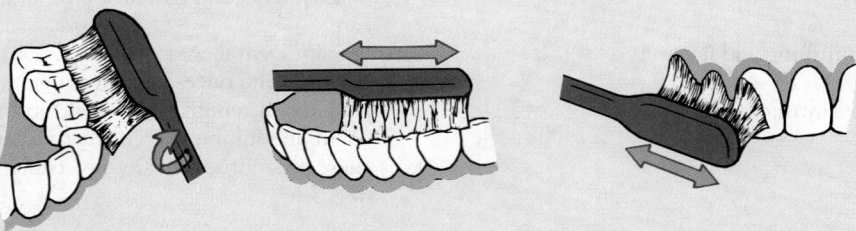

STEP 6   Directions of brush for toothbrushing.

7   Have patient hold brush at 45-degree angle and lightly brush over surface and sides of tongue (see illustration). Avoid initiating gag reflex.

Microorganisms collect and grow on tongue's surface and contribute to bad breath. Gagging may cause aspiration of toothpaste.

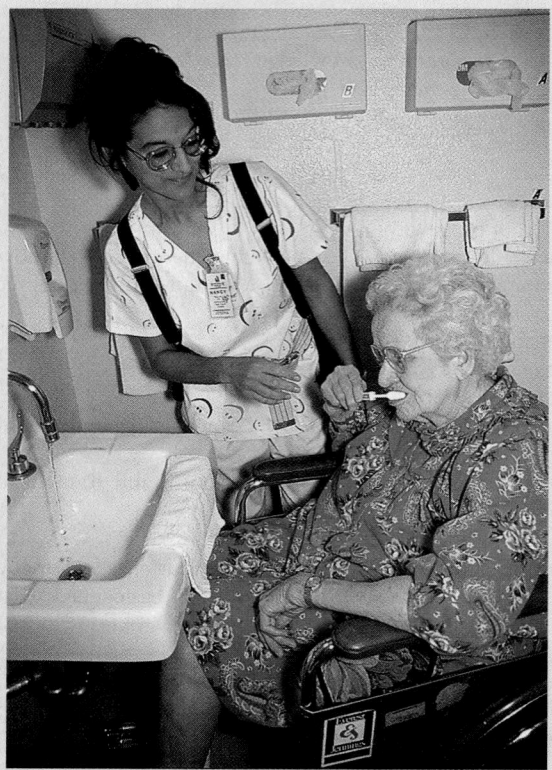

STEP 7   Nurse observes patient's toothbrushing technique.

STEP	**RATIONALE**
8 Allow patient to rinse mouth thoroughly with water by taking several sips of water (may use straw), swishing water across all tooth surfaces, and spitting into emesis basin. Use this time to teach patient importance of brushing teeth twice a day	Rinsing removes food particles. The ADA (2008) recommends persons brush their teeth twice a day with fluoride toothpaste.
9 Have patient rinse teeth with antiseptic mouth rinse for 30 seconds. Then have patient spit rinse into emesis basin.	The ADA (2008) recommends that antiseptic mouth rinse is as effective as flossing for reducing plaque and gingivitis between teeth; the effect on dental caries prevention has not been determined.
10 Assist in wiping patient's mouth.	Promotes sense of comfort.
11 Allow patient to floss. Floss between all teeth. Hold floss against tooth while moving floss up and down sides of teeth. Instruct patient in importance of daily flossing (see illustrations).	Removes plaque and prevents gum disease. The ADA (2008) recommends flossing once daily to remove decay-causing bacteria between teeth and under gum line.
12 Allow patient to rinse mouth thoroughly with cool water and spit into emesis basin. Assist in wiping patient's mouth.	Rinsing removes plaque and tartar from oral cavity.
13 Assist patient to comfortable position, remove emesis basin and over-bed table, raise side rail, if appropriate, and lower bed to original position.	Provides for patient comfort and safety.
14 Wipe off over-bed table, discard soiled linen and paper towels in appropriate containers, remove soiled gloves, and return equipment to proper place.	Proper disposal of soiled equipment prevents spread of infection.
15 Perform hand hygiene.	Reduces transmission of microorganisms.

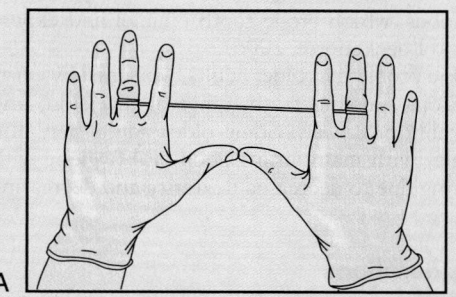 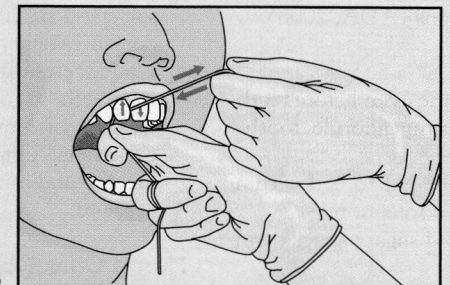 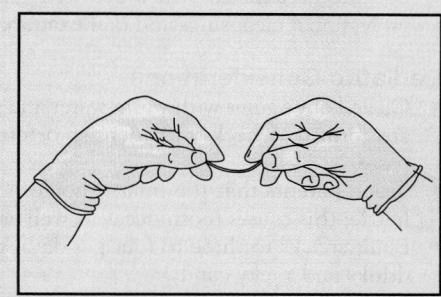

STEP 11 Flossing. **A,** Dental floss is held between the middle fingers to floss the upper teeth. **B,** Floss is moved in up-and-down motions between the teeth. Floss is moved up and down from the crown to the gum line. **C,** Floss is held with the index fingers to floss the lower teeth.

EVALUATION

1 Ask patient if any area of oral cavity feels uncomfortable or irritated.	Pain indicates more chronic problem.
2 Apply clean gloves, and inspect condition of oral cavity.	Determines effectiveness of hygiene and rinsing.
3 Ask patient to describe proper hygiene techniques and recommended frequency.	Evaluates patient's learning.
4 Observe patient brushing and flossing.	Evaluates patient's ability to demonstrate correct technique.

Unexpected Outcomes	Related Interventions
1 Mucosa is dry and inflamed. Tongue has thick coating.	• Increase patient's hydration. • Increase frequency of tongue brushing. • Apply moisturizing lubricant to patient's lips.
2 Gum margins are retracted from teeth, with localized areas of inflammation. Bleeding occurs around gum margins.	• Report findings because patient may have an underlying bleeding tendency. • Switch to a softer-bristled toothbrush. • Avoid vigorous brushing and flossing.
3 Mucosa becomes inflamed from repeated chemotherapy administration, and sores develop.	• Refer patient to dentist. • Teach patient oral hygiene.

Recording and Reporting

• Record procedure and note condition of oral cavity in nurses' notes.
• Report bleeding, pain, or presence of lesions to nurse in charge or physician.

Teaching Considerations

• Educate patients about methods to prevent tooth decay (e.g., reduce intake of carbohydrates, especially sweet sticky snacks between meals; brush within 30 minutes of eating sweets; rinse mouth thoroughly with water or alcohol-free antiseptic mouth rinse. Use fluoride toothpaste.
• Educate patients to visit a dentist regularly (twice a year) for professional cleansings and oral examinations (ADA, 2008).

Pediatric Considerations

• Clean baby's gums with warm water and gauze even before teeth are formed. Check with dentist before using fluoride toothpaste.
• Teach parents that the infant should not be put to bed with a bottle; this causes tooth decay as well as ear infections.
• Limit snacks to three to four per day. Avoid sugary snacks and drinks and sticky candy.
• Notify dentist if family uses bottled or well water. Prescription for fluoride may be ordered.
• Dentist will evaluate for the need of sealants for molars.
• Flossing requires parental supervision until at least 8 years of age.

• Children should have their first dental examination at 1 year, or sooner if needed. Then children need to have a dental examination every 6 months.

Gerontological Considerations

• A number of normal age-related changes occur in the oral cavity. Thinning of the oral mucosa and decreased vascularity of the gingivae predispose older adults to injury and periodontal disease. Loss of tissue elasticity and decreased mass and strength of the muscles make chewing more difficult. Loss of the alveolar bone can loosen natural teeth.
• The number of taste buds declines with advancing age. In an attempt to enhance the taste of food, some older adults choose salty and sugary foods, which erode tooth enamel and expose dentin (Meiner and Lueckenotte, 2006).
• Plaque retention is a problem in older adults, worsened by existing teeth restorations, missing teeth, gingival recession, and wearing of removable prosthesis. Some older adults may also experience difficulty with maintaining good oral hygiene with flossing and brushing due to decreased dexterity and decreasing eyesight.

Home Care Considerations

• During the initial admission visit, document the condition of the patient's mouth, teeth, and gums, thus providing a baseline for assessment of the patient's ability to comply with special diets and fluid intake and to carry out oral hygiene practices.

PROCEDURAL GUIDELINE 17-3 Care of Dentures

Basic Skills / Personal Hygiene and Grooming / Cleaning Dentures

Delegation Considerations

The skill of denture care can be delegated to NAP. The nurse directs NAP to:

- Inform the nurse if there are cracks in dentures.
- Inform the nurse if the patient has any oral discomfort.

Equipment

- ☐ Soft-bristled toothbrush or denture toothbrush
- ☐ Emesis basin or sink
- ☐ Denture dentifrice or toothpaste
- ☐ Denture adhesive *(optional)*
- ☐ Glass of water
- ☐ 4 × 4 inch gauze
- ☐ Washcloth
- ☐ Denture cup
- ☐ Clean gloves

Procedural Steps

1 Determine if patient can clean dentures independently or requires assistance. Dentures need cleaning as often as natural teeth.

2 Fill emesis basin with tepid water. (If using sink, place washcloth in bottom of sink, and fill sink with approximately 1 inch of water.)

3 Apply clean gloves.

4 Remove dentures: If patient is unable to do this independently, grasp upper plate at front with thumb and index finger wrapped in gauze, and pull downward. Gently lift lower denture from jaw, and rotate one side downward to remove from patient's mouth. Place dentures in emesis basin or sink.

5 Apply cleaning agent to brush, and brush surfaces of dentures (see illustration). Hold dentures close to water. Hold brush horizontally, and use back-and-forth motion to cleanse biting surfaces. Use short strokes from top of denture to biting surfaces to clean outer teeth surfaces. Hold brush vertically, and use short strokes to clean inner teeth surfaces. Hold brush horizontally, and use back-and-forth motion to clean undersurface of dentures.

6 Rinse thoroughly in tepid water.

7 Some patients use an adhesive to seal dentures in place. Apply a thin layer to undersurface before inserting.

8 If patient needs assistance with insertion of dentures, moisten upper denture and press firmly to seal it in place. Then insert moistened lower denture. Ask if denture feels comfortable.

9 Some patients prefer to store their dentures to give the gums a rest and to reduce risk for infection. Store in tepid water in denture cup. Keep denture cup in a secure place and labeled with patient's name to prevent loss.

10 Dispose of supplies. Remove and discard gloves and perform hand hygiene.

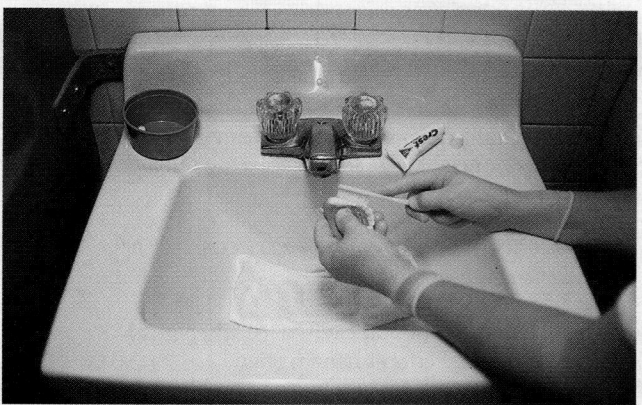

STEP 5 Brushing surface of dentures.

SKILL 17-3 Performing Mouth Care for an Unconscious or Debilitated Patient

Basic Skills / Personal Hygiene and Grooming / Performing Oral Hygiene for an Unconscious Patient

Unconscious or debilitated patients pose challenges because of their risk for having alterations of the oral cavity. Unconscious and orally intubated patients are susceptible to drying of mucousthickened salivary secretions because they are unable to eat or drink, frequently breathe through the mouth, and often receive oxygen therapy. The unconscious patient cannot swallow salivary secretions that accumulate in the mouth. These secretions often contain gram-negative bacteria that cause pneumonia if aspirated into the lungs.

The critically ill patient faces the same risk factors for oral problems as other patients, such as dehydration, mouth breathing, chemical injury to the mucosa, and oral trauma. Some patients require mouth care as often as every 1 to 2 hours until the mucosa returns to normal. Optimal oral care should focus on plaque removal and stimulation of salivary flow (Munro and others, 2006).

Chlorhexidine rinse is an antibacterial solution widely accepted for use in oral care.

Many patients have no gag reflex as a result of change in consciousness or a neurological injury. While providing hygiene to an unconscious patient, protect the patient from choking and aspiration. The safest technique is to have two nurses provide care. One can be a NAP. The nurse does cleansing while the NAP suctions secretions. Proper oral hygiene requires keeping the oral mucosa moist and removing secretions that lead to infection.

Evaluate the level and frequency of oral care on a daily basis during assessment of the oral cavity. Some debilitated patients require mouth care every hour, but normally at least every 2 hours. Routine suctioning of the mouth and pharynx is required to manage oral secretions to reduce the risk for aspiration. Research also recommends routine brushing of teeth with a soft-bristled brush to prevent dental plaque and the use of alcohol-free antiseptic oral rinse and an application of a water-based mouth moisturizer to provide moisture and maintain the integrity of the oral mucosa (Cutler and others, 2005).

Delegation Considerations

The skill of providing oral care to an unconcious or debilitated patient can be delegated to NAP. The nurse must first assess patient for gag reflex. The nurse directs the NAP about:

- Proper way to position patients for mouth care.
- Use of an oral suction catheter for clearing oral secretions (see Procedural Guideline 25-1).
- Signs of impaired integrity of oral mucosa to report to nurse.
- Reporting any bleeding of mucosa or gums or excessive coughing or choking to the nurse.

Equipment

- ❑ Antiinfective solution (e.g., commercial diluted hydrogen peroxide and sodium bicarbonate solution) that loosens crusts; check agency policy
- ❑ Small pediatric soft-bristled toothbrush or a foam toothette for patients with sensitive gums.
- ❑ Antibacterial solution (e.g., chlorhexidine) rinse
- ❑ Fluoride toothpaste
- ❑ Water-based mouth moisturizer
- ❑ Tongue blade
- ❑ Small bulb syringe or suction catheter and machine (*optional*)
- ❑ Oral airway (uncooperative patient or patient who shows bite reflex)
- ❑ Water-soluble lip lubricant
- ❑ Waterglass with cool water
- ❑ Face towel
- ❑ Paper towels
- ❑ Emesis basin
- ❑ Clean gloves

STEP	RATIONALE

ASSESSMENT

1 Perform hand hygiene, and apply clean gloves. — Reduces transmission of microorganisms in blood or saliva.
2 Test for presence of gag reflex by placing tongue blade on back half of tongue. — Reveals whether patient is at risk for aspiration.

Critical Decision Point   *Patients with impaired gag reflex require oral care as well. Determine the type of suction apparatus needed at the bedside to protect a patient's airway against aspiration.*

3 Inspect condition of oral cavity (see Chapter 6). — Determines condition of oral cavity and need for hygiene.
4 Remove gloves. Perform hand hygiene. — Prevents spread of infection.
5 Assess patient's risk for oral hygiene problems (see Skill 17-2). — Certain conditions increase likelihood of alterations in integrity of oral cavity structures. May require more frequent care.

NURSING DIAGNOSES

- Impaired oral mucous membrane
- Risk for aspiration

Individualize related factors based on patient's condition or needs.

PLANNING

1 Expected outcomes following completion of procedure:
   - Buccal mucosa and tongue are pink, moist, and intact. Gums are moist and intact. Teeth are clean, smooth, and shiny. Tongue is pink and without coating. Lips are moist, smooth, and without cracks. — Degree of improvement in condition of oral cavity structures will depend on extent of secretions or changes that existed before care.
   - Debilitated patient expresses feeling of cleanliness. — Comfort achieved.
   - Oral pharynx remains clear of secretions. — Secretions removed, thus avoiding aspiration.
2 Unless contraindicated (e.g., head injury, neck trauma), lower side rail and position patient on side (Sims' position) with head turned well toward dependent side and head of bed lowered. Raise side rail. — Allows secretions to drain from mouth instead of collecting in back of pharynx. Prevents aspiration.
3 Explain procedure to patient, even if patient is unconscious. — Allows debilitated patient to anticipate procedure without anxiety. Some unconscious patients retain ability to hear.
4 Perform hand hygiene, and apply clean gloves. — Reduces transfer of microorganisms.
5 Place paper towels on over-bed table, and arrange equipment. If needed, turn on suction machine, and connect tubing to suction catheter. — Prevents soiling of tabletop. Equipment prepared in advance ensures smooth, safe procedure.
6 Pull curtain around bed, or close room door. — Provides privacy.

STEP	RATIONALE

IMPLEMENTATION

1 Raise bed to appropriate height for nurse; lower side rail.

Use of good body mechanics with bed in high position prevents injury.

2 Position patient on side close to side of bed; turn patient's head turned toward mattress.

Proper positioning of head prevents aspiration.

3 Remove dentures or partial plates if present.

Allows for thorough cleansing of prosthetics later (see Procedural Guideline 17-3). Provides clearer access to oral cavity.

4 Place towel under patient's head and emesis basin under chin.

Prevents soiling of bed linen.

5 If patient is uncooperative or having difficulty keeping mouth open, insert an oral airway. Insert upside down, then turn the airway sideways and then over tongue to keep teeth apart. Insert when patient is relaxed, if possible. Do not use force (see illustration).

Prevents patient from biting down on nurse's fingers and provides access to oral cavity.

Critical Decision Point *Never place fingers into the mouth of an unconscious or debilitated patient. The normal response is to bite down.*

6 Clean mouth using brush moistened in water. Apply toothpaste or use antiinfective solution first to loosen crusts. Cleanse tooth surfaces using an up-and-down gentle motion. A toothette may be used for patients with sensitive gums. Clean chewing and inner tooth surfaces first. Clean outer tooth surfaces (see Skill 17-2). Moisten brush with chlorhexidine solution to rinse. Use brush or toothette to clean roof of mouth, gums, and inside cheeks. Gently brush tongue but avoid stimulating gag reflex (if present). Repeat rinsing several times. Use brush or toothette to apply water-based mouth moisturizer..

Brushing action removes food particles between teeth, along chewing surfaces and crusts for mucosa. Do not use commercial swabs because they do not clean teeth. Repeated rinsing removes all debris and aids in moistening mucosa.

7 Suction secretions as they accumulate, if necessary.

Suction removes secretions and fluid that collect in posterior pharynx. Reduces risk for aspiration.

8 Apply thin layer of water-soluble moisturizer to lips (see illustration).

Lubricates lips to prevent drying and cracking.

9 Inform patient that procedure is completed.

Provides meaningful stimulation to unconscious or less-responsive patient.

10 Raise side rails as appropriate. Remove gloves, and dispose of in proper receptacle.

Prevents transmission of microorganisms.

11 Lower side rails. Reposition patient comfortably, and return bed and side rail to original position.

Maintains patient's comfort and safety.

12 Clean equipment, and return to its proper place. Place soiled linen in proper receptacle.

Proper disposal of soiled equipment prevents spread of infection.

13 Perform hand hygiene.

Reduces transmission of microorganisms.

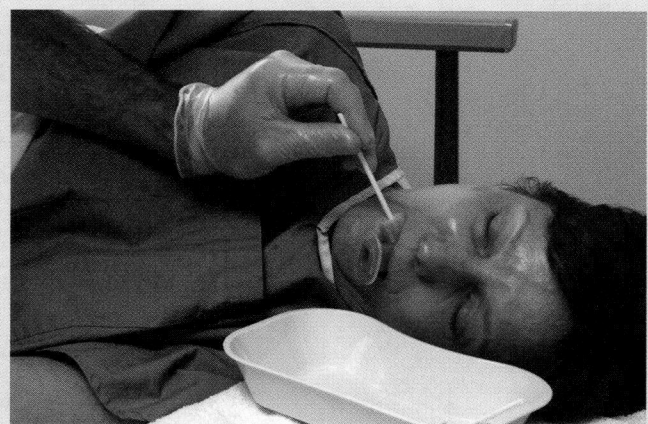

STEP 5 Cleansing around oral airway with toothette.

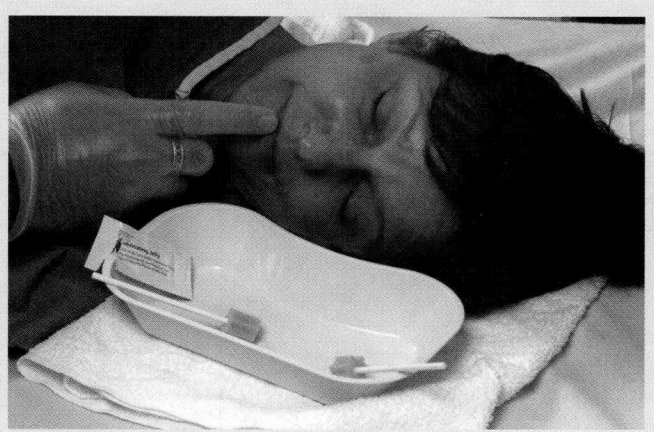

STEP 8 Application of water-soluble moisturizer to lips.

STEP	RATIONALE

EVALUATION

1 Apply clean gloves, and inspect oral cavity.

Determines efficacy of cleansing. Once thick secretions are removed, underlying inflammation or lesions may be revealed.

2 Ask debilitated patient if mouth feels clean.

Evaluates level of comfort.

3 Assess patient's respirations on an ongoing basis.

Ensures early recognition of aspiration.

Unexpected Outcomes

1 Secretions or crusts remain on mucosa, tongue, or gums.

2 Localized inflammation of gums or mucosa is present.

3 Lips are cracked or inflamed.

4 Patient aspirates secretions.

Related Interventions

- More frequent oral hygiene is needed.
- More frequent oral hygiene with soft-bristled toothbrush is needed.
- Apply a water-based mouth moisturizer to provide moisture and maintain the integrity of the oral mucosa.
- Chemotherapy and radiation can cause stomatitis. Patients should rinse mouth before and after meals and at bedtime using normal saline (½ teaspoon of salt in 8 ounces of water). This is economical, appears to be safe, is readily available, and is tolerated by most patients (Brown and Wingard, 2004).
- Apply moisturizing gel or water-soluble lubricant to lips.
- If present, suction oral airways as secretions accumulate to maintain patent airway (see Chapter 25).
- Elevate patient's head of bed to facilitate breathing.
- If aspiration is suspected, notify the physician. Prepare patient for a chest x-ray examination.

Recording and Reporting

- Record procedure on documentation record.
- Include patient's ability to cooperate and whether suction is necessary for oral care.
- Document any pertinent observations (e.g., presence of gag reflex, presence of bleeding gums, dry mucosa, ulcerations, and crusts on tongue).
- Report any unusual findings to nurse in charge or health care provider.

Teaching Considerations

- Family members may care for debilitated patient in the home. Instruction in mouth care is necessary so that family understands how to protect patient from aspirating, while thoroughly cleansing oral cavity. Observe family caregiver perform mouth care procedure.

Home Care Considerations

- Irrigate oral cavity with bulb syringe; if unavailable, substitute gravy baster or large syringe. Caution family caregiver against instilling a large amount of solution.
- Encourage primary caregiver to cleanse patient's mouth at least twice a day. If patient breathes through mouth, a soft-bristled toothbrush moistened, and used every 1 to 2 hours will keep mouth moist and fresh.

SKILL 17-4 Hair Care (Combing and Shaving)

*Basic Skills / Personal Hygiene and Grooming / Performing Hair Care and Shampooing in Bed
Shaving a Male Patient*

A person's appearance and sense of well-being are influenced by how the hair looks and feels. Brushing, combing, and shampooing are basic measures for all patients unable to provide self-care. Male patients should be offered the opportunity to shave or be shaved daily when their condition allows. Most men prefer to shave themselves. Most long-term care facilities have beauty shops where patients can go for professional hair care.

Fever, malnutrition, emotional stress, and depression affect the condition of the hair. Diaphoresis leaves the hair oily and unmanageable. Excessively dry or oily hair may be associated with hormone changes. Dry, brittle hair occurs with aging and excessive use of shampoo.

Certain chemotherapy agents and radiation therapy cause loss of hair (alopecia). Many patients choose to wear a wig; however, some choose to wear hair scarves or turbans (Fig. 17-3). Table 17-2 describes common hair and scalp conditions and nursing interventions.

The frequency of shampooing depends on the condition of the hair and the person's daily routines and cultural preferences. Because everyone's hair varies according to condition, gender, and race, you will need to develop an individualized plan of care, including preferred products for hair care. Dry hair, which commonly results from aging and protein deficiency, requires less frequent shampooing than oily hair or the hair of people who exercise actively.

Remind hospitalized patients that more frequent shampooing is necessary when a patient remains in bed for extended periods of time, has excessive perspiration, or has treatments that leave blood or solutions in the hair. Two types of shampooing are available for a patient: traditional shampoo using water and newer disposable shampoo and conditioner. In a hospital setting it is often necessary to transport a patient by stretcher to a special area where a spray nozzle and sink are available for shampooing.

You can shampoo patients who are allowed to sit in a chair in front of a sink. Also, make sure that a patient's condition does not contraindicate neck hyperextension. Caution is needed with patients who have suffered neck injuries, because flexion and hyperextension of the neck could cause further injury. In addition, patients with positional vertigo are not able to tolerate neck hyperextension if it increases their dizziness. A folded towel placed under the neck on the edge of the sink provides added comfort. If a patient cannot sit in a chair or be transferred to a stretcher, you will have to shampoo with the patient in bed, using traditional shampoo and water or disposable shampoo (Procedural Guidelines 17-4, p. 449, and 17-5, p. 451). You can do this after the bath (common in the care of infants) or later as a separate procedure.

Delegation Considerations

The skill of hair care can be delegated to NAP. The nurse directs the NAP about:

- Proper ways to position patient with head or neck mobility restrictions.
- Procedures for use of medicated shampoo for lice, stressing the steps to take to prevent transmission to other patients.
- Patient being at risk for bleeding tendencies and the need to use an electric razor.

Equipment

- ❑ Hair care: Wide-tooth comb
- ❑ Hairbrush
- ❑ Conditioner (*optional*)
- ❑ Shaving: New disposable razor: clean gloves (*optional*), bath towel(s), mirror, washcloth, washbasin, shaving cream or soap, aftershave lotion (if patient desires)
- ❑ Shaving: Electric razor: razor (with clean cutting heads), bath towel, skin or beard conditioner, mirror, aftershave lotion (if patient desires)
- ❑ Mustache care: Scissors, brush or comb, bath towel, gooseneck lamp or overhead light, mirror

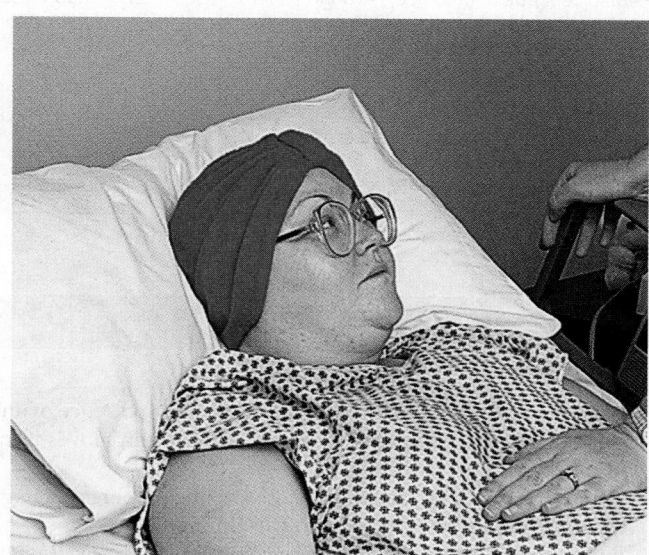

FIG 17-3 Patients may choose to wear a turban because of hair loss.

TABLE 17-2 | Hair and Scalp Problems

Characteristics	Implications	Interventions
Dandruff—Scaling of the scalp accompanied by itching; in severe cases, dandruff on eyebrows.	Dandruff causes embarrassment; if dandruff enters eyes, conjunctivitis may develop.	Shampoo regularly with medicated shampoo; in severe cases obtain health care provider's advice.
Ticks—Small gray-brown parasites that burrow into skin and suck blood.	Ticks transmit several diseases, including Rocky Mountain spotted fever, Lyme disease, and tularemia.	Do not pull ticks from skin because sucking apparatus remains and may become infected; placing drop of oil or ether on tick or covering it with petrolatum eases removal; oil suffocates tick.
Pediculosis capitis (head lice)—Tiny grayish/brown/white parasitic insects that attach to hair strands; about size of a sesame seed; nits or eggs look like oval particles attached at an angle to hair shaft; bites or pustules may be observed behind ears and at hairline.	Head lice are difficult to remove and, if not treated, may spread to furniture and other people.	Check entire scalp. Use medicated shampoo for eliminating lice or permethrin (Nix), available as a crème rinse. **Caution against use of products containing Lindane, because the ingredient is toxic and known to cause adverse reactions** (National Pediculosis Association, 2007). Remove patient's clothing before treatment, and apply new clothing following treatment. Repeat treatment according to product directions. Check the hair for nits, and comb with a nit comb for 2 to 3 days until sure all lice and nits have been removed. Manual removal of lice is best option when treatment has failed. Vacuum infested areas of home. Wash linens in hot water, and dry for at least 30 minutes.
Pediculosis corporis (body lice)—Tend to cling to clothing, so may not be easily seen; body lice suck blood and lay eggs on clothing and furniture.	Patient itches constantly; scratches on skin may become infected; hemorrhagic spots may appear on skin where lice are sucking blood. May spread to other people.	Patient should bathe or shower thoroughly; after skin is dried, apply lotion for eliminating lice; after 12 to 24 hours another bath or shower should be taken; bag infested clothing or linen until laundered. Vacuum items that cannot be washed.
Pediculosis pubis (crab lice)—Found in pubic hair; crab lice are grayish white with red legs.	Lice may spread through bed linen, clothing, furniture, or sexual contact.	Shave hair off affected area; cleanse as for body lice; if lice were sexually transmitted, partner must be notified.
Hair loss (alopecia)—Balding patches in periphery of hairline; hair becomes brittle and broken; caused by diseases, medication side effects, and improper use of hair care products and hair styling devices.	Patches of uneven hair growth and loss alter patient's appearance.	Offer patients access to scarves, hairpieces, or wigs. Stop hair care practices that damage hair.

STEP	RATIONALE

ASSESSMENT

1 Inspect condition of hair and scalp. Inspect for presence of any infestation (e.g., pediculosis). NOTE: Apply clean gloves if infestation is suspected.	Indicates need for medicated applications or shampoo.
2 Assess patient's hair care and shaving product preferences (e.g., shampoo, aftershave lotion, skin conditioner).	Influences approach to grooming. Promotes patient's independence through decision making.
3 Before shaving, assess if patient has bleeding tendency. Review medical history or laboratory values (e.g., platelet counts, prothrombin time).	Determines need to use electric razor for patient's safety because of potential for bleeding.
4 Assess patient's ability to manipulate razor.	Determines level of assistance required.

NURSING DIAGNOSES

- Bathing/hygiene self-care deficit
- Dressing/grooming self-care deficit
- Impaired physical mobility
- Risk for injury

Individualize related factors based on patient's condition or needs.

STEP	RATIONALE

PLANNING

1 Expected outcomes following completion of procedure:

   • Patient expresses sense of comfort with hair and scalp grooming.

   • Patient expresses sense of comfort, with sensation of face feeling clean and refreshed.

   • Skin surface is smooth, well hydrated, and free of cuts.

   • Patient assists with procedure as tolerated.

2 While performing procedure, ask patient to explain steps he or she uses to comb hair and/or shave. Ask patient to indicate if becomes uncomfortable.

3 Position patient sitting in chair or in bed with head elevated 45 to 90 degrees (as tolerated).

4 Arrange supplies at bedside table, and adjust lighting. Perform hand hygiene.

Rationale column:

Scalp stimulated and areas of matted or tangled hair removed.

Hair and soap lather are removed.

Patient is free from injury.
Participation provides sense of control.
Patient involvement will lessen anxiety.

Elevation of head of bed makes it easier to access all sides of head and face.

Easy access to supplies prevents interruption of procedure. Lighting provides clear view of patient's face.

IMPLEMENTATION

1 Combing and brushing hair:

   a Part the hair into two sections, then separate hair into two more sections (see illustration).

   Rationale: Brushing and combing are more effective when small areas of hair are groomed at any one time.

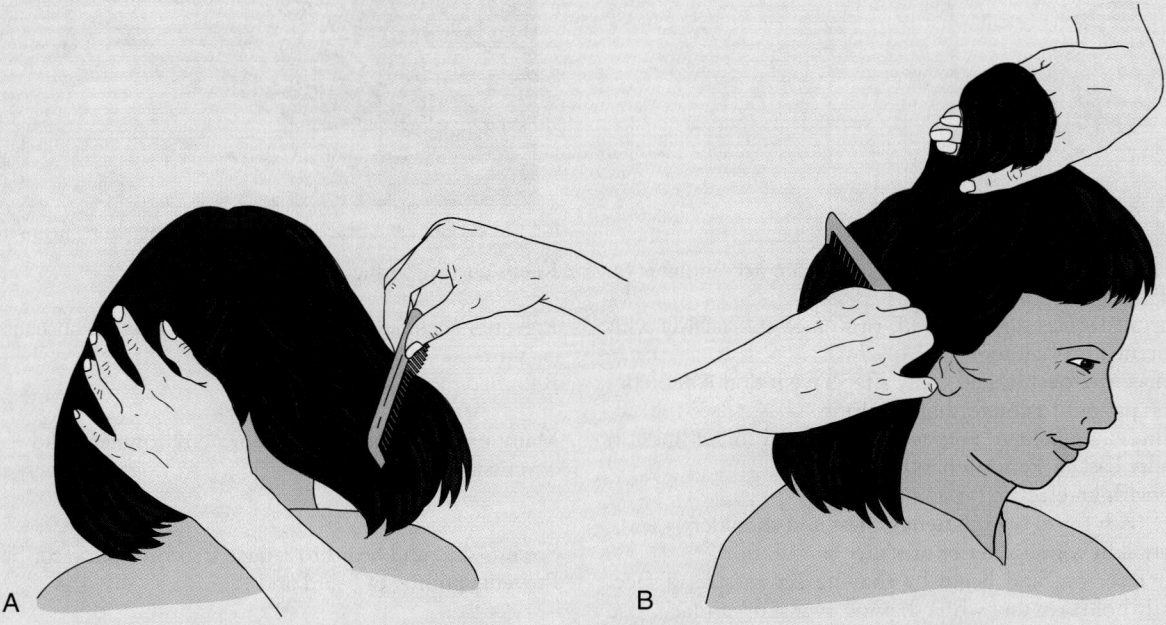

STEP 1a Parting hair. **A,** Part hair down the middle, and divide it into two main sections. **B,** Then part the main section into two smaller sections.

   b Brush or comb from the scalp toward the hair ends.

   c Moisten hair lightly with water, conditioner, or an alcohol-free detangle product before combing.

   d Move fingers through hair to loosen any larger tangles.

   e Using a wide-tooth comb, start on either side of the head, and insert the comb with the teeth upward to the hair near the scalp. Comb through the hair in a circular motion by turning the wrist while lifting up and out. Continue until all hair is combed through, and then comb into place to shape and style.

2 Shaving with a disposable razor:

   a Place bath towel over patient's chest and shoulders.

   b Run warm water in washbasin. Check water temperature.

Rationale column:

Minimizes pulling.
Makes hair easier to comb.

Lessens pulling.
Moves comb evenly through hair without pulling.

Prevents shaving cream or water from soiling gown.
Warm water will soften beard. Proper temperature prevents accidental burns.

STEP	RATIONALE

c Place washcloth in basin, and wring out thoroughly. Apply cloth over patient's entire face for several seconds.

Warm cloth helps soften skin and beard. Sensation of warmth can be relaxing.

Critical Decision Point *If patient has sores, open lesions, or a tendency to bleed, apply clean gloves.*

d Apply shaving cream or soap to patient's face. Smooth cream evenly over sides of face, chin, and under nose.

e Hold razor in dominant hand at 45-degree angle to the patient's skin. Begin by shaving across one side of patient's face using short, firm strokes in direction hair grows (see illustration). Use nondominant hand to gently pull skin taut while shaving. Check with patient, and ask if he feels comfortable.

Cream creates additional softening effect and lubricates skin for application of razor.

Technique facilitates shaving of facial hair. Short downward strokes work best over upper lip. Holding skin taut prevents razor cuts and discomfort during shaving. Patient is best resource to confirm if shaving technique causes discomfort.

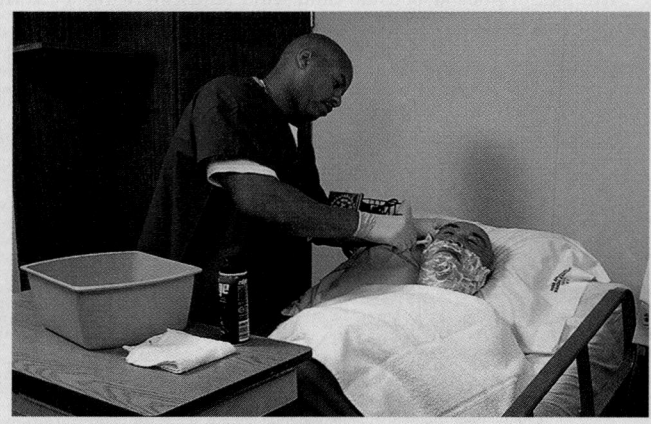

STEP 2e Shaving a patient using short, firm strokes.

f Dip razor blade in water as shaving cream accumulates on blade's edge.

Keeps cutting surface of razor blade clean.

g After all facial hair is shaved, rinse face thoroughly with moistened washcloth.

Prevents accumulation of shaving cream, which causes drying of skin.

h Dry face thoroughly, and apply aftershave lotion if desired.

Retained moisture will chap skin.

i Assist patient to comfortable position.

j Return equipment to proper place. Discard soiled linen in laundry basket. Perform hand hygiene.

Maintains cleanliness of patient's environment and reduces transmission of infection.

3 Shaving with an electric razor:
a Place bath towel over patient's chest and shoulders.
b Apply skin conditioner or preshave preparation.
c Turn razor on, and begin by shaving across side of face. Gently hold skin taut while shaving over skin's surface. Use gentle downward stroke of razor in direction of hair growth.

Softens skin and beard to reduce friction from razor head.
Prevents pulling of beard and skin.

d After completing shave, apply aftershave lotion as desired.

Stimulates and lubricates skin.

e Perform steps 2i and j (for disposable razor).

4 Moustache and beard care:
a Place bath towel over patient's chest and shoulders.
b If necessary, gently comb moustache or beard.

Straightens hair that requires trimming.

c Allow patient to use mirror and direct areas to trim with scissors.

Allows patient to make decisions about care; maintains sense of independence.

EVALUATION

1 Ask patient how hair and scalp feel.

Evaluates patient's satisfaction with grooming

2 Inspect condition of shaved area and skin underneath beard or mustache.

Nurse looks for areas of localized bleeding from cuts and for areas of dryness.

3 Ask patient if face feels clean and comfortable.

Evaluates level of patient's comfort.

4 Ask if patient is satisfied with degree of participation.

Patient maintains sense of control.

Unexpected Outcomes

1 Patient senses tangles or discomfort in scalp.

2 Small isolated nicks or cuts appear on skin.

3 Skin surface appears dry.

Related Interventions

- Inspect scalp area. Repeat brushing/combing as needed.

- Obtain a new disposable razor, or change the blade. If razor is reusable, be sure to clean according to agency policy.
- Change technique so as to glide razor over the patient's skin.

- This is a result of soap drying skin; use moisturizing shaving foam.
- Apply moisturizing lotion to patient's skin after shave.

Recording and Reporting

- It is not necessary to record shaving procedure unless it is included on the agency's checklist. However, record any complications such as bleeding in nurses' notes.

Teaching Considerations

- Shaving is a simple procedure that you can teach to a family member. Instruct primary caregiver in safety precautions for shaving, especially if patient is receiving anticoagulant therapy.
- Instruct family member in technique to follow in the event the patient is accidentally nicked.

Pediatric Considerations

- Usually the facial hair of adolescents does not grow quickly, so shaving daily is not necessary.
- Adolescents who shave should be asked about the frequency and allowed to perform activity as desired. Family members may wish to be involved in shaving their adolescent child if the child is unable to perform the activity.

- Young girls with long hair may not tolerate brushing tangles out of hair. Tangling occurs easily in children restricted to bed. Once tangles are removed, it may be helpful to braid the hair.
- Children with lice should use the appropriate shampoo, followed with a visual examination for nits (see Table 17-2, p. 446).

Gerontological Considerations

- Usually the facial hair of older patients does not grow quickly, so shaving daily is not necessary.

Home Care Considerations

- Provide adequate towels around patient's neck to avoid spilling shaving cream or water on chest or bed.
- Provide adequate lighting for procedure.
- Perform procedure in comfortable setting, such as bathroom or bedroom.

PROCEDURAL GUIDELINE 17-4   Shampooing Hair of a Bed-Bound Patient

Basic Skills / Personal Hygiene and Grooming / Performing Hair Care and Shampooing in Bed

Delegation Considerations

The skill of shampooing the hair of bed-bound patients can be delegated to NAP. The nurse directs the NAP about:

- Proper way to position a patient with a head or neck mobility restriction.
- Knowledge of care for lice, stressing steps to take to prevent transmission to other patients

Equipment

- ❑ Clean gloves
- ❑ Bath towels (two or more)
- ❑ Washcloths
- ❑ Shampoo and hair conditioner (*optional*)
- ❑ Hydrogen peroxide (*optional*)
- ❑ Water pitcher with warm water
- ❑ Plastic shampoo board
- ❑ Washbasin
- ❑ Bath blanket
- ❑ Waterproof pad
- ❑ Clean comb and brush
- ❑ Hair dryer (*optional*)
- ❑ Disposable gown (*optional*)
- ❑ Option: Saline

Procedural Steps

1 Before washing patient's hair, determine that there are no contraindications to procedure. Certain medical conditions, such as head and neck injuries, spinal cord injuries, and arthritis, place patient at risk for injury during shampooing because of positioning and manipulation of patient's head and neck.

2 Apply clean gloves, if needed. Inspect the hair and scalp before beginning shampoo. This determines if special shampoos or treatments are necessary (e.g., dandruff, lice, removal of blood). If lice are present, wear disposable gown and gloves during procedure.

3 Place waterproof pad under patient's shoulders, neck, and head. Position patient supine, with head and shoulders at top edge of bed. Place shampoo board under patient's head and washbasin under end of trough spout (see illustration). Be sure trough spout extends beyond edge of mattress.

4 Place rolled towel under patient's neck and bath towel over patient's shoulders.

5 Brush and comb patient's hair.

6 Obtain pitcher with warm water.

7 Ask patient to hold face towel or washcloth over eyes.

8 Slowly pour water from pitcher over hair until it is completely wet (see illustration). If hair contains matted blood, apply gloves, apply hydrogen peroxide to dissolve clots, and then rinse hair with saline. Apply small amount of shampoo.

9 Work up lather with both hands. Start at hairline, and work toward back of neck. Lift head slightly with one hand to wash back of head. Shampoo sides of head. Massage scalp by

PROCEDURAL GUIDELINE 17-4   Shampooing Hair of a Bed-Bound Patient—cont'd

applying pressure with fingertips.

10 Rinse hair with water. Make sure water drains into basin. Repeat rinsing until hair is free of soap.

11 Apply conditioner or créme rinse if requested, and rinse hair thoroughly.

12 Wrap patient's head in bath towel. Dry patient's face with cloth used to protect eyes. Dry off any moisture along neck or shoulders.

13 Dry patient's hair and scalp. Use second towel if first becomes saturated.

14 Comb hair to remove tangles, and dry with dryer if desired.

15 Apply oil preparation or conditioning product to hair, if desired by patient.

16 Variation for patients with coarse, curly hair: Condition hair after washing. To untangle hair, use the wide teeth of a comb. Beginning at the nape of the neck, comb small subsections of the hair starting at the hair ends. Continue to work through small sections until hair is free of tangles.

17 Assist patient to comfortable position, and complete styling of hair.

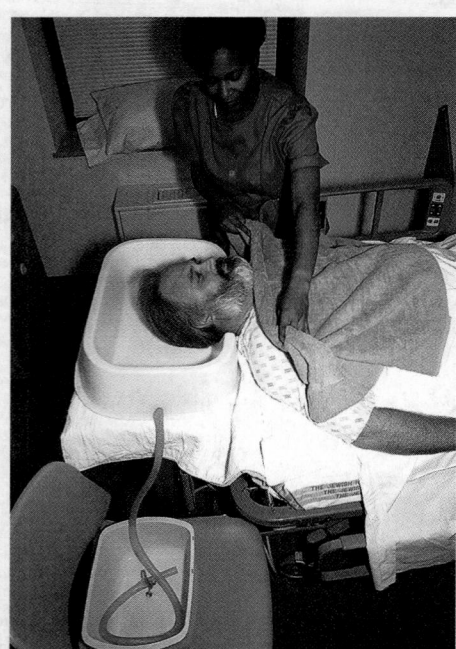

STEP 3   Patient positioned over shampoo board.

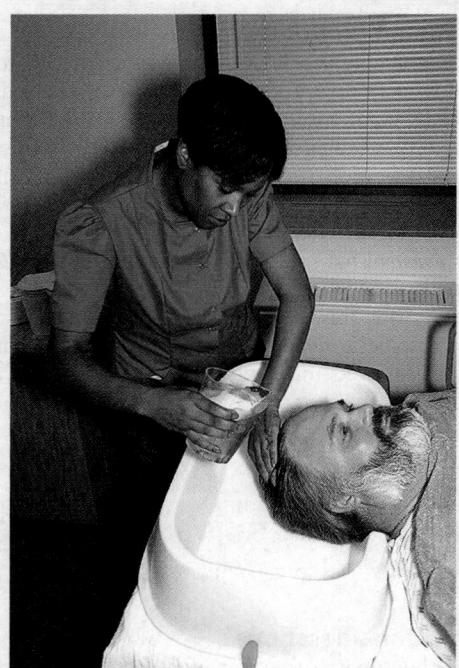

STEP 8   Pour water over hair.

PROCEDURAL GUIDELINE 17-5 Shampooing Hair Using a Disposable Shampoo Product

Delegation Considerations
The skill of shampooing the hair of patients using a disposable shampoo product can be delegated to NAP. The nurse directs the NAP about:
- Proper way to position patient with head or neck mobility restriction.

Equipment
- ❏ Disposable shampoo product
- ❏ Comb or brush
- ❏ Towel
- ❏ Clean gloves

Procedural Steps
1 Explain procedure to patient.
2 Patient can be either in bed or sitting in chair
3 Perform hand hygiene.
4 Comb hair to remove any tangles or debris.
5 Open package, apply cap to head, and secure all hair beneath cap.
6 Massage head through cap. Check fitting around head to maintain correct fit.
7 Massage 2 to 4 minutes; additional time may be required for longer hair or hair matted with blood.
8 Discard cap in trash; do not dispose of in toilet because it may clog plumbing.
9 If patient desires, towel dry hair.
10 Brush or comb patient's hair.
11 Perform hand hygiene.

SKILL 17-5 Performing Nail and Foot Care

Basic Skills / Personal Hygiene and Grooming / Performing Nail and Foot Care

Include nail and foot care in a patient's daily hygiene; the best time is during the patient's bath. Many agencies require a health care provider's order before a nurse can trim nails. Feet and nails often require special care to prevent infection, odors, pain, and injury to soft tissues. Often people are unaware of foot or nail problems until discomfort or pain occurs. Common foot and nail problems are presented in Table 17-3, p. 452. For proper foot and nail care, instruct patients to protect the feet from injury, keep the feet clean and dry, and wear appropriate footwear. Instruct patients in the proper way to inspect the feet for lesions, dryness, or signs of infection. To maintain and promote foot and nail health, patients should visit a podiatrist when necessary. This is especially important for patients with peripheral vascular diseases, diabetes mellitus, older adults, and patients whose immune system is suppressed.

Patients most at risk for developing serious foot problems are those with peripheral neuropathy and peripheral vascular disease. These two disorders, commonly found in patients with diabetes, cause a reduction in blood flow to the extremities and a loss of sensory, motor, and autonomic nerve function. As a result, a patient is unable to feel heat and cold, pain, pressure, and position of the foot. The reduction in blood flow impairs healing and promotes risk for infection. The development of diabetic foot ulcers has three contributing factors, including (1) peripheral neuropathy (changes in the function and efficiency of the nerves), (2) ischemia (decrease in the blood flow related to plaque formation in arteries), and (3) a pivotal event (trauma caused by banging the toe or stepping on a foreign object). However, 55% of foot ulcers are due to repeat trauma over time, such as ill-fitting shoes (Delmas, 2006). If foot ulcers do not heal, they can quickly become infected and lead to gangrene and, in turn, amputation.

Delegation Considerations
The skill of nail and foot care of patients without diabetes or circulatory compromise can be delegated to NAP. The nurse directs the NAP about:
- Not clipping patient's nails.
- Any special considerations for patient positioning.

Equipment
- ❏ Washbasin
- ❏ Emesis basin
- ❏ Washcloth
- ❏ Bath or face towel
- ❏ Nail clippers (check agency policy)
- ❏ Soft nail or cuticle brush
- ❏ Plastic applicator stick
- ❏ Emery board or nail file
- ❏ Body lotion
- ❏ Disposable bath mat
- ❏ Paper towels
- ❏ Clean gloves if drainage present

TABLE 17-3 | Common Foot and Nail Problems

Condition	Characteristics	Implications	Interventions
Callus	Thickened portion of epidermis, consisting of mass of horny, keratotic cells; usually flat, painless, and found on undersurface of foot or on palm of hand; caused by local friction or pressure.	Foot calluses may cause discomfort when wearing tight-fitting shoes.	Refer patient to podiatrist and do not self-treat. Use of orthotic devices cushions and redistributes weight and pressure off calluses.
Corns	Keratosis caused by friction and pressure from shoes; mainly on toes, over bony prominence; usually cone-shaped, round, and raised. Calluses with painful core.	Conical shape compresses underlying dermis, making it thin and tender. Pain is aggravated by tight-fitting shoes. Patients may suffer alteration in gait because of pain.	Refer patient to podiatrist. Avoid use of oval corn pads, which increase pressure on toes. Use wider, softer shoes.
Plantar warts	Fungating lesions on sole of foot caused by papillomavirus.	Warts may be contagious, are painful, and make walking difficult.	Refer patient to podiatrist.
Athlete's foot (tinea pedis)	Fungal infection of foot; scaliness and cracking of skin between toes and on soles of feet; small blisters containing fluid may appear, apparently induced by constricting footwear.	Athlete's foot can spread to other body parts, especially hands. It is contagious and frequently recurs.	Feet should be well ventilated. Drying feet well after bathing and applying powder help prevent infection. Wearing clean socks or stockings reduces incidence. Health care provider orders application of griseofulvin, miconazole nitrate, or tolnaftate.
Ingrown nails	Toenail or fingernail growing inward into soft tissue around nail; results from improper nail trimming, poor shoe fit, or heredity.	Ingrown nails can cause localized pain when pressure is applied.	Treatment is frequent warm soaks (*exception:* diabetic patient) in antiseptic solution and removal of portion of nail that has grown into skin. Instruct patient in proper nail-trimming techniques. Refer to podiatrist.
Paronychia	Inflammation of tissue surrounding nail after hangnail or other injury; occurs in people who frequently have their hands in water; common in diabetic patients.	Area can become infected.	Treatment is warm compresses or soaks (*exception:* diabetic patient) and local application of antibiotic ointments. Paronychia can be prevented by careful manicuring.
Foot odors	Result of excess perspiration promoting microorganism growth. Faulty foot hygiene or improper footwear may also contribute.	Cause discomfort from excess perspiration.	Frequent washing, use of foot deodorants and powders and clean footwear will prevent or reduce this problem.

STEP	RATIONALE

ASSESSMENT

1 Inspect all surfaces of fingers, toes, feet, and nails. Pay particular attention to areas of dryness, inflammation, or cracking. Also inspect areas between toes, heels, and soles of feet. Inspect socks for stains.

Integrity of feet and nails determines frequency and level of hygiene required. Heels, soles, and sides of feet are prone to irritation from ill-fitting shoes. Socks may become stained from bleeding or draining ulcer.

2 Assess color and temperature of toes, feet, and fingers. Assess capillary refill of nails. Palpate radial and ulnar pulse of each hand and dorsalis pedis pulse of foot; note character of pulses (see Chapter 6).

Assess circulation to extremities. Plaque buildup decreases blood flow to the distal extremities, especially in the lower extremities of a diabetic patient (Delmas, 2006).

3 Observe patient's walking gait. Have patient walk down hall or walk straight line while wearing comfortable shoes or slippers (if able).

Alterations in the bony structures of the feet may cause pain, imbalance, and unsteady gait.

4 Ask if patient has history of leg pain upon walking that is relieved with rest.

Claudicating pain is related to ischemia with diabetic and neuropathic disorders.

5 Ask female patients about whether they use nail polish and polish remover frequently.

Chemicals in these products cause excessive dryness.

6 Assess type of footwear patient wears: Does patient wear socks? Are shoes tight or ill fitting? Are garters or knee-high nylons worn? Is footwear clean?

Some types of shoes and footwear predispose patient to foot and nail problems (e.g., infection, areas of friction, ulcerations).

7 Identify patient's risk for foot or nail problems:

Certain conditions increase likelihood of foot or nail problems.

   a Older adult

Poor vision, lack of coordination, or inability to bend over contributes to difficulty among older adults in performing foot and nail care. Normal physiological changes of aging also result in dry, brittle nails.

   b Diabetes mellitus

Vascular changes associated with diabetes reduce blood flow to peripheral tissues. Break in skin integrity places patient with diabetes at high risk for skin infection.

   c Heart failure, renal disease

Both conditions increase tissue edema, particularly in dependent areas (e.g., feet). Edema reduces blood flow to neighboring tissues.

   d Cerebrovascular accident (stroke)

Presence of residual foot or leg weakness or paralysis results in altered walking patterns. Altered gait pattern causes increased friction and pressure on feet.

8 Assess type of home remedies patients use for existing foot problems:

Certain preparations or applications cause more injury to soft tissue than initial foot problem.

   a Over-the-counter liquid preparations to remove corns or warts

Advise patient not to self-treat corns or calluses, but to seek professional treatment.

   b Cutting of corns or calluses with razor blade or scissors

Carries risk for cutting skin, which can lead to infection.

   c Use of oval corn pads

Advise patients not use oval pads, which may exert pressure on toes, thereby decreasing circulation to surrounding tissues. Seek professional treatment.

   d Application of adhesive tape

Skin of older adult is thin and delicate and prone to tearing when adhesive tape is removed.

9 Assess patient's ability to care for nails or feet: visual alterations, fatigue, and musculoskeletal weakness.

Extent of patient's ability to perform self-care determines degree of assistance required from nurse.

10 Assess patient's knowledge of foot and nail care practices.

Level of patient's knowledge determines patient's need for health teaching.

NURSING DIAGNOSES

- Bathing/hygiene self-care deficit
- Deficient knowledge regarding foot and nail care
- Impaired physical mobility
- Impaired skin integrity
- Ineffective tissue perfusion
- Risk for infection

Individualize related factors based on patient's condition or needs.

PLANNING

1 Expected outcomes following completion of procedure:
- Nails are smooth. Cuticles and tissues surrounding nail are clear and of normal color. Surfaces of feet are smooth.
- Patient walks freely, without pain or unusual gait.

Excess skin layers are removed. Nail integrity and cleanliness are maintained.
Patient understands the importance of proper fitting footwear.

STEP	RATIONALE

• Patient explains or demonstrates nail care correctly.	Patient learns skill.
2 Explain procedure to patient, including fact that proper soaking requires several minutes in warm water.	Patient must be willing to place fingers and feet in basins up to 10 minutes. Patient may become anxious or fatigued.
3 Obtain health care provider's order for cutting nails (required by most agencies).	Patient's skin may be accidentally cut. Certain patients are more at risk for infection, depending on their medical condition.

IMPLEMENTATION

1 Perform hand hygiene. Arrange equipment on over-bed table.	Easy access to equipment prevents delays.
2 Pull curtain around bed, or close room door (if desired).	Maintaining patient's privacy reduces anxiety.
3 Assist ambulatory patient with sitting in bedside chair. Help bedfast patient to supine position with head of bed elevated. Place disposable bath mat on floor under patient's feet, or place towel on mattress.	Sitting in chair facilitates immersing feet in basin. Bath mat protects feet from exposure to soil or debris.
4 Fill washbasin with warm water. Test water temperature.	Prevents accidental burns to patient's skin. Diabetic patients have peripheral neuropathy with decreased sensation.
5 Place basin on bath mat or towel, and help patient place feet in basin. Place call light within patient's reach.	Patients with muscular weakness or tremors may have difficulty positioning feet. Maintains patient's safety.

Critical Decision Point   *Patients who have diabetes mellitus or peripheral vascular disease (PVD) should **not** soak their feet because of potential of increased dryness of skin and decrease in ability to sense temperature variations related to decreased sensations (ADA, 2007).*

6 Adjust over-bed table to low position, and place it over patient's lap. (Patient may sit in chair or lie in bed.)	Easy access prevents accidental spills.
7 Fill emesis basin with warm water, and place basin on paper towels on over-bed table.	Warm water softens nails and thickened epidermal cells.
8 Instruct patient to place fingers in emesis basin and place arms in comfortable position.	Prolonged positioning causes discomfort unless normal anatomical alignment is maintained.
9 Unless patient has diabetes mellitus or PVD, allow patient's feet and fingernails to soak 10 minutes.	Goal is to soften skin and debris beneath nails but not cause excessive dryness.
10 Clean gently under fingernails with end of plastic applicator stick while fingers are immersed.	Removes debris under nails that harbors microorganisms.
11 Remove emesis basin, and dry fingers thoroughly.	Thorough drying impedes fungal growth and prevents maceration of tissues.

Critical Decision Point   *Check agency policy for appropriate process for cleaning beneath nails. Do not use an orange stick or end of cotton swab; these splinter and can cause injury.*

12 File fingernails straight across and even with tops of fingers. *Option* (check agency policy): Use nail clippers to clip nails straight across, then shape with nail file (see illustration).	Filing cutting straight across avoids skin overgrowth at the nail edges, which leads to ingrown toenails or infection. If nails become thick, a professional should provide nail care (Pinzur and others, 2005).

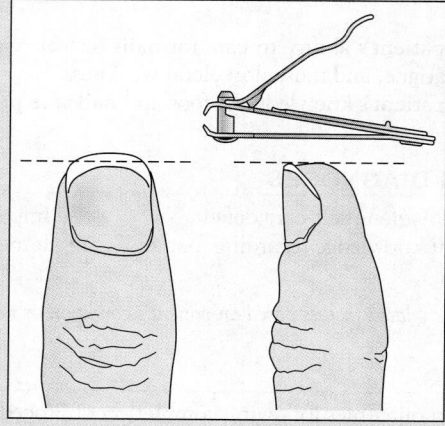

STEP 12   Clip nails straight across when using a nail clipper.

STEP	RATIONALE

Critical Decision Point   *If patient has diabetes mellitus or circulatory problems, do not cut nails. Check agency policy; refer to professional.*

STEP	RATIONALE
13 Use a soft cuticle brush or nail brush to clean around cuticles to decrease overgrowth.	Nail brush avoids causing inflamed cuticles.
14 Move over-bed table away from patient. Apply clean gloves, and scrub callused areas of feet with washcloth.	Provides easier access to feet. Gloves prevent transmission of fungal infection. Friction removes dead skin layers.
15 Clean, file, and trim toenails using procedures in Steps 12 and 13.	Prevent damage to tissue surrounding nails.
16 Apply lotion to feet and hands, and assist patient back to bed and into comfortable position.	Lotion lubricates dry skin by helping to retain moisture.
17 Remove gloves, and place in receptacle. Clean and return equipment and supplies to proper place. Dispose of soiled linen in hamper. Perform hand hygiene.	Reduces transmission of infection.

EVALUATION

STEP	RATIONALE
1 Inspect nails, areas between toes, and surrounding skin surfaces.	Inspection enables nurse to evaluate condition of skin and nails and allows nurse to note any remaining rough nail edges.
2 Ask patient to explain or demonstrate nail care.	Demonstration allows nurse to evaluate patient's level of learning techniques.
3 Observe patient's walk after toenail care.	Observation allows nurse to evaluate level of comfort and mobility achieved.

Unexpected Outcomes

1 Cuticles and surrounding tissues are inflamed and tender to touch.

2 Localized areas of tenderness occur on feet with calluses or corns at point of friction.

3 Ulcerations involving toes or feet may remain.

Related Interventions

- Repeat nail care.
- Evaluate need for antifungal cream.
- Change in footwear or corrective foot surgery may be needed for permanent improvement in calluses or corns.
- Refer patient to podiatrist.
- Institute wound care policies (see Chapters 18 and 38).
- Consult with wound care specialist and/or podiatrist.
- Increase frequency of assessment and hygiene.

Recording and Reporting

- Record procedure and observations in medical record (e.g., breaks in skin, inflammation, ulcerations).
- Report any breaks in skin or ulcerations to nurse in charge or physician.

Teaching Considerations

- Instruct patient not to walk barefoot or use corn or callus products.
- Instruct a patient with diabetes or peripheral vascular disease to do the following:
  - Inspect and bathe feet daily.
  - Inspect all surfaces of the foot.
  - Use a mirror to view bottom of foot.
  - Clean around nails with a soft brush.
  - Dry the feet, and pay special attention to drying between the toes.
  - Use lambs wool between the toes if the skin stays moist or becomes macerated.
  - Wear socks that absorb perspiration and "breathe."
  - Wear nonconstricting shoes with soft leather and an adequate toe box.
  - See a podiatrist annually (Pinzur and others, 2005).

Pediatric Considerations

- Children's nails should be assessed and clipped to prevent them from scratching themselves. Check agency policy. Use appropriate-size clippers when clipping the nails of infants and small children. Do not use scissors.

Gerontological Considerations

- Changes in aging skin include thinning of epidermis and subcutaneous fat and dryness because of decreased activity of oil and sweat glands. These changes are often evident in the feet. In addition, nails become opaque, tough, scaly, brittle, and hypertrophied.
- A lifetime of limited exercise can result in laxity of foot ligaments and musculature and lead to instability and impaired mobility.

Home Care Considerations

- Assess the home for any areas that could cause accidental injury to foot through bumping foot.
- *Alternative therapies:* Moleskin application to area of feet under friction or wrapping small pieces of lamb's wool around toes to reduce irritation from corns.

SKILL 17-6   Care of a Patient's Environment

When caring for patients who need to remain in or near their bed for an extended period, it is important to try to make that environment as comfortable as possible. A calm, comfortable restorative environment can be maintained in a hospital, extended care facility, or a patient's home. Rooms should be well-ventilated, safe, and large enough to allow patients, visitors, and care providers to move about freely. The care provider should be able to control temperature, noise, and odors easily.

Although there are variations across health care settings, a typical hospital room contains the following basic pieces of furniture: over-bed table, bedside stand, chairs, lamp, and bed. Long-term care and rehabilitation facilities often have similar equipment. The over-bed table rolls on wheels, and can be adjusted to various heights over the bed or chair. The table provides ideal working space for the nurse performing procedures. It also provides a surface on which to place meal trays, toiletry items, and objects frequently used by a patient. Do not place the bedpan and urinal on the over-bed table. The bedside stand is for storing a patient's personal possessions and hygiene equipment. The telephone, water pitcher, and drinking cup are usually on top of the bedside stand.

Most hospital rooms contain an armless straight-backed chair or an upholstered lounge chair with arms. Straight-backed chairs are convenient when temporarily transferring a patient from the bed, such as during bed making. Lounge chairs tend to be more comfortable when a patient is willing and able to sit for an extended period.

Proper lighting is necessary for everyone's safety and comfort. A brightly lit room is usually stimulating, but a darkened room is best for rest and sleep. Adjust room lighting by closing or opening drapes, regulating over-bed and floor lights, and closing or opening room doors. When entering a patient's room at night, refrain from abruptly turning on an overhead light unless necessary.

Each room usually has an over-bed light and a floor or table lamp. Position movable lights that extend over the bed from the wall for easy reach, but move them aside when not in use. Additional portable lighting provides extra light during bedside procedures.

Other equipment usually found in a patient's room includes a call light, a television set, a wall-mounted blood pressure gauge, oxygen and vacuum wall outlets, and personal care items. Special mattresses and bed boards are designed for comfort or positioning. Whenever using comfort and positioning equipment, check agency policy and manufacturer's directions before application.

BEDS

Because the bed is the most used piece of equipment by a patient, it should be comfortable, safe, and adaptable to various positions. The typical hospital bed consists of a firm mattress on a metal frame that you can raise or lower horizontally. The frame is divided into three sections so that the operator can raise and lower the head and foot of the bed separately, in addition to inclining the entire bed with the head up or down. Each bed sits on four rollers, or casters, that allow you to move the bed easily. Table 17-4 lists common bed positions.

Often patients who are critically ill or who are immobilized in traction are transported to different locations, such as the radiology department, in bed. There are beds in which scales are incorporated to facilitate routine weighing of a patient.

The position of a bed is usually changed by electric controls built into the side of the bed, at the foot of the bed, or on a bedside

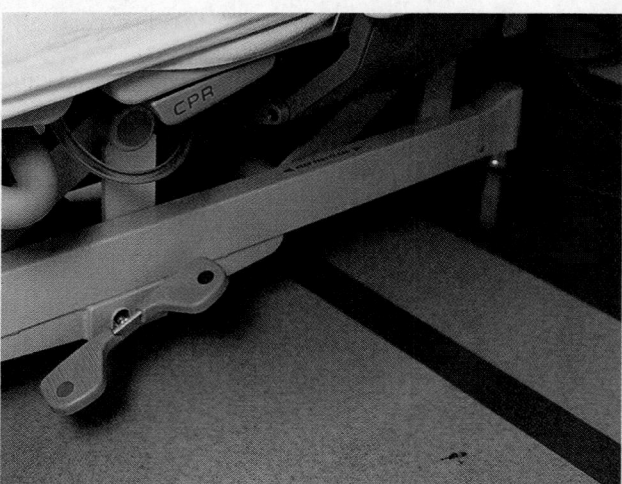

FIG 17-4   Lock on bed wheels.

cable. Patients can raise or lower sections of the bed without expending much energy. It is important for you to instruct patients in the proper use of the controls and to caution them against positions that will cause harm.

Beds contain a number of safety features. Use locks located on the wheels, casters, or at the center of the bed frame (Fig. 17-4) whenever the bed is stationary to prevent accidental movement during performance of a procedure (e.g., transferring a patient from bed to a stretcher). Side rails (either four or two depending on bed design), located on both sides of a bed, help patients position themselves and provide upper extremity support as a patient gets out of bed. Use caution when raising side rails. Research suggests that the risk for patient falls is greater when side rails on both sides of the bed are raised because patients try to climb over the rails to exit the bed. Raising only one rail (when there are only two) or three (when there are four rails) gives patients an exit route if they are able to move independently. Use of all side rails is considered a physical restraint (see Chapter 13). Side rails are adjustable metal frames that you can raise or lower by pushing or pulling a knob. When a side rail has been lowered, do not leave the bedside with a patient still in bed. Each bed has a special headboard that is removable. This feature is important in emergency situations when the medical team must have easy access to a patient's head during cardiopulmonary resuscitation (see Chapter 27).

MATTRESSES

Most beds have firm, water-repellent mattresses. A mattress should have an even surface for a patient's comfort. A rubber or plastic surface permits easy cleaning. Special mattresses provide extra comfort and support for patients and relieve pressure on bony prominences. Chapter 12 reviews a variety of special mattresses and support surfaces and indications for their use.

SPECIAL EQUIPMENT

Some rooms or beds have special equipment. Examples include IV pumps and poles and overhead trays. The nurse is responsible for knowing how to use all equipment safely.

Skill Performance Guidelines

1 Keep the environment as comfortable as possible. Depending on a patient's age and physical condition, maintain room temperature between 20° C and 23° C (68° F and 74° F). Infants, older adults, and the acutely ill may need a warmer temperature. However, certain critically ill patients require cooler room temperatures to lower the body's metabolic demands. Controlling drafts and eliminating lingering odors from draining wounds, vomitus, bedpans, or urinals will also improve a patient's comfort. Hospitals now prohibit smoking in patients' rooms.

2 Control extraneous noises in a patient's room. Ill patients are sensitive to noises in a hospital environment. Try to control noise level by handling equipment properly; making sure equipment is in proper working order; controlling voice volume; and, unless contraindicated, closing a patient's room door.

3 Make the environment as safe as possible. Keep all personal care items within a patient's reach. When the head of the bed is raised, the bedside stand is usually not within easy reach and must be moved forward. If a patient must leave the bed to go to the bathroom, be sure there are no objects obstructing the way.

4 Make the environment personal for a patient. A picture of family members, some get well cards, or a small radio may help a patient to relax. However, do not clutter a patient's room with unnecessary equipment and supplies. Whenever possible, remove equipment and supplies after treatments are complete.

5 Be sure the call light is easily accessible to a patient at all times. Often a patient will have numerous IV lines and drainage tubes connected to portable poles and suction machines.

MAKING AN UNOCCUPIED BED

Patients spend much of their time in bed, eating, bathing, using bedpans or urinals, and undergoing numerous therapeutic procedures. It is essential for you to keep the bed as clean and comfortable as possible. Frequent inspections are necessary to be sure that the linen is clean, dry, and wrinkle free. Change bed linen that becomes wet or soiled immediately.

Whenever possible, make the bed while it is unoccupied. Having the patient get out of bed is an ideal way to promote ambulation. You will usually make a bed after the patient's bed bath or while the patient is up bathing and showering. Another convenient time for bed making is when the patient is out of the room for tests or procedures.

By making an unoccupied bed you can ensure that the linen is smooth and free of wrinkles. It is also easier to insert any extra waterproof pads or special mattresses (see Chapter 12) when the bed is unoccupied.

TABLE 17-4	Common Bed Positions	
Position	**Description**	**Uses**
Fowler's 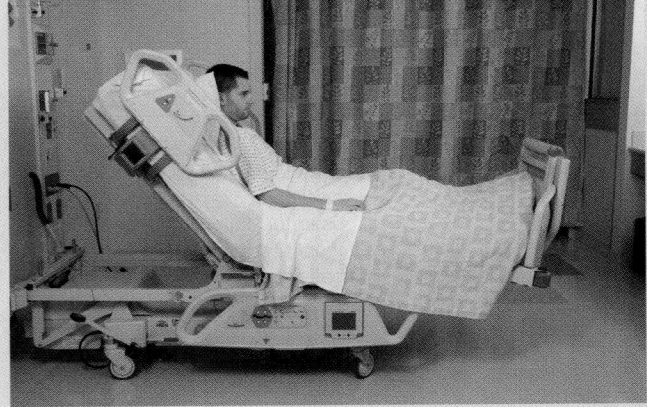	Head of bed raised to angle of 45 to 90 degrees; semisitting position; foot of bed may also raise at knee	Preferred while patient eats; used during nasogastric tube insertion and nasotracheal suction; promotes lung expansion.
Semi-Fowler's 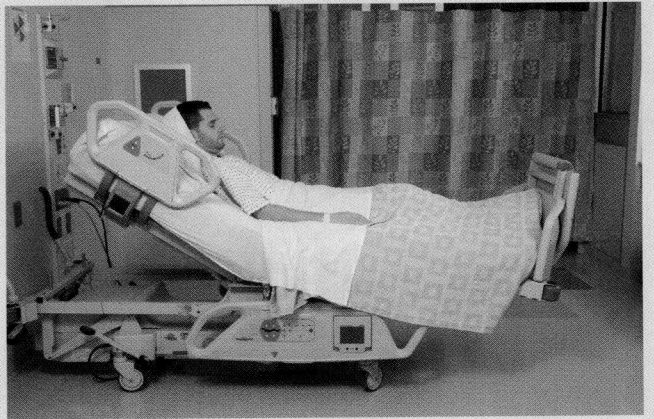	Head of bed raised approximately 30 to 40 degrees; incline is less than Fowler's position; foot of bed may also raise at knee.	Promotes lung expansion; relieves strain on abdominal muscles. Used when patients receive gastric feedings to reduce risk for aspiration.

Continued

TABLE 17-4 | Common Bed Positions—cont'd

Position	Description	Uses
Trendelenburg's 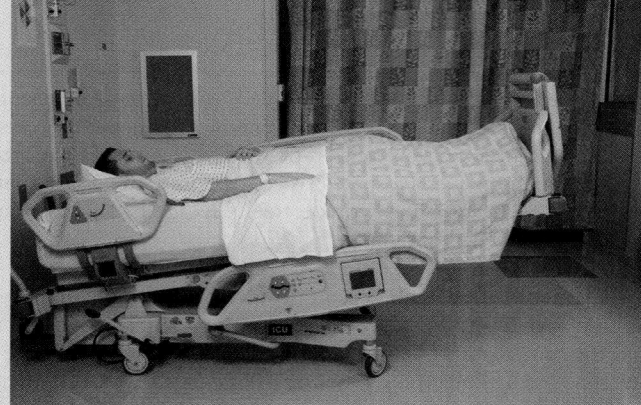	Entire bed frame tilted, with head of bed down.	For postural drainage; facilitates venous return in patients with poor peripheral perfusion.
Reverse Trendelenburg's 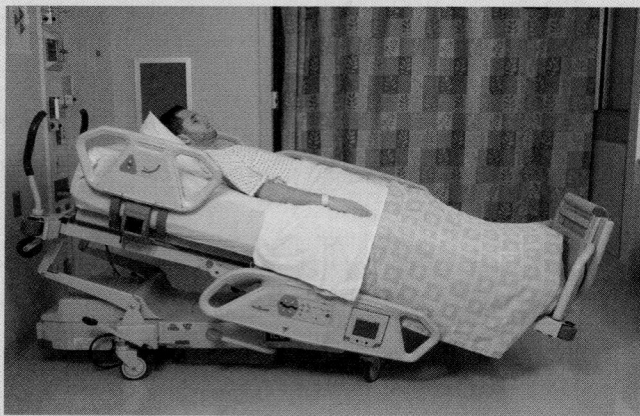	Entire bed frame tilted, with foot of bed down.	Used infrequently; promotes gastric emptying and prevents esophageal reflux.
Supine or flat 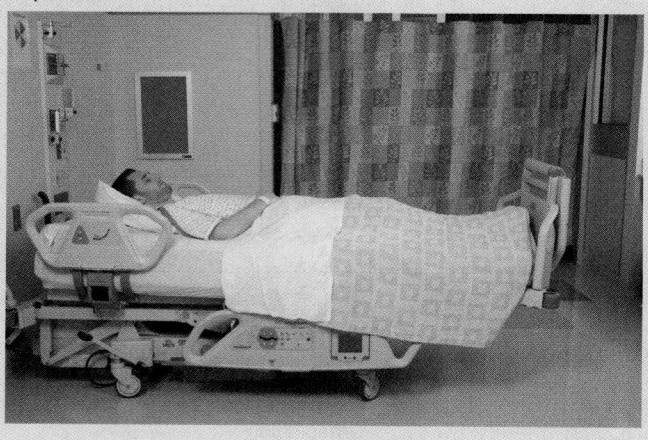	Entire bed frame horizontally parallel with floor.	For patients with vertebral injuries and in cervical traction. Position used for patients who are hypotensive and generally preferred by patients for sleeping.

PROCEDURAL GUIDELINE 17-6 Making an Unoccupied Bed

Basic Skills / Bedmaking / Making an Unoccupied Bed

Delegation Considerations

The skill of making an unoccupied bed can be delegated to NAP. Inform NAP of any position or activity restrictions that apply to patient's ability to get out of bed.

Equipment

- ❏ Linen bag
- ❏ Mattress pad (change only when soiled)
- ❏ Bottom sheet (flat or fitted)
- ❏ Drawsheet (*optional*)
- ❏ Top sheet, blanket
- ❏ Bedspread
- ❏ Waterproof pads (*optional*)
- ❏ Pillowcases
- ❏ Bedside chair or table
- ❏ Clean gloves (if linen is soiled)
- ❏ Washcloth
- ❏ Antiseptic cleanser

Procedural Steps

1. Determine if patient has been incontinent or if excess drainage is on linen. Gloves will be necessary.
2. Assess activity orders or restrictions in mobility in planning if patient can get out of bed for procedure. Assist to bedside chair or recliner.
3. Lower side rails on both sides of bed, and raise bed to comfortable working position.
4. Remove soiled linen, hold away from uniform and place in laundry bag. Avoid shaking or fanning linen.
5. Reposition mattress, and wipe off any moisture using a washcloth moistened in antiseptic solution (consult agency housekeeping guidelines). Dry thoroughly.
6. Apply all bottom linen on one side of bed before moving to opposite side.
   a. *For fitted sheet:* Make sure fitted sheet is placed smoothly over mattress and top and bottom mattress edge.
   b. *For flat sheet:* Place sheet over mattress. Allow about 25 cm (10 inches) to hang over side mattress edge. Lower hem of sheet should lie seam down, even with bottom edge of mattress. Pull remaining top portion of sheet over top edge of mattress. While standing at head of bed, miter top corner of bottom sheet (see Procedural Guideline 17-7, Steps 13 to 15). Tuck remaining portion of unfitted sheet under mattress.
7. *Optional:* Apply drawsheet, laying center fold along middle of bed lengthwise. Smooth drawsheet over mattress, and tuck excess edge under mattress, keeping palms down.
8. Move to opposite side of bed, and spread bottom sheet smoothly over edge of mattress from head to foot of bed.
   a. *For fitted sheet:* Make sure fitted sheet is placed smoothly over mattress from head to foot of bed, and over mattress edges.

   b. *For a flat sheet:* Miter top corner of bottom sheet, making sure corner is taut. Grasp remaining edge of flat bottom sheet, and tuck tightly under mattress while moving from head to foot of bed.
9. Smooth folded drawsheet over bottom sheet, and tuck under mattress, first at middle, then at top, and then at bottom.
10. If needed, apply waterproof pad over bottom sheet or drawsheet.
11. Place top sheet over bed with vertical center fold lengthwise down middle of bed. Open sheet out from head to foot, being sure top edge of sheet is even with top edge of mattress.
12. Make horizontal toe pleat; stand at foot of bed, and fanfold in sheet 5 to 10 cm (2 to 4 inches) across bed. Pull sheet up from bottom to make fold approximately 15 cm (6 inches) from bottom edge of mattress.
13. Tuck in remaining portion of sheet under foot of mattress. Then place blanket over bed with top edge parallel to top edge of sheet and 15 to 20 cm (6 to 8 inches) down from edge of sheet. (*Optional:* Apply additional spread over bed.)
14. Make cuff by turning edge of top sheet down over top edge of blanket and spread.
15. Standing on one side at foot of bed, lift mattress corner slightly with one hand, and with other hand tuck top sheet, blanket, and spread under mattress. Be sure toe pleats are not pulled out.
16. Make modified mitered corner with top sheet, blanket, and spread. After making triangular fold, do not tuck tip of triangle (see illustration).
17. Go to other side of bed. Spread sheet, blanket, and spread out evenly. Make cuff with top sheet and blanket (closed bed). Make modified corner at foot of bed. Alternatively, fanfold sheet, blanket, and spread at the foot of the bed, with top layer ready to be pulled up (this leaves an open bed).
18. Apply clean pillowcase.
19. Place call light within patient's reach on bed rail or pillow, and return bed to lowest position allowing for patient transfer. Assist patient to bed.
20. Arrange patient's room. Remove and discard supplies. Perform hand hygiene.

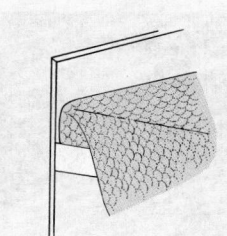

STEP 16 Modified mitered corner.

PROCEDURAL GUIDELINE 17-7 Making an Occupied Bed

Basic Skills / Bedmaking / Making an Occupied Bed

At times it is necessary to make a bed that is occupied by a patient. If a patient is confined to bed, you should make the bed in a way that conserves time and the patient's energy. In addition, you need to know what position the patient can safely assume while the bed linens are changed. Also, try to keep the patient as comfortable as possible. In cases in which a patient experiences severe pain, an analgesic administered 30 to 60 minutes before the procedure is helpful in controlling pain and maintaining comfort.

Even though a patient is unable to get out of bed, encourage self-help as much as possible. For example, the patient can turn, assist in moving up in bed, or hold top sheets while linen is applied. These activities help maintain the patient's strength and mobility and allow participation in hygiene care.

Making an occupied bed poses some difficulties. It is harder to prevent transfer of organisms from soiled linens to clean linens and to keep newly applied linen smooth and wrinkle-free. If organized, you can do this procedure quickly.

Delegation Considerations

The skill of making an occupied bed can be delegated to NAP. Inform NAP of any position or activity restrictions that apply to patient's ability to get out of bed. The nurse directs NAP about:

- Looking for wound drainage, drainage tubes, or IV tubing that is found in the linens.

Equipment

- ❑ Linen bags
- ❑ Mattress pad (change only when soiled)
- ❑ Bottom sheet (flat or fitted)
- ❑ Drawsheet (*optional*)
- ❑ Top sheet, blanket
- ❑ Bedspread
- ❑ Waterproof pads (*optional*)
- ❑ Pillowcases
- ❑ Bedside chair or table
- ❑ Clean gloves (if linen is soiled)
- ❑ Washcloth
- ❑ Antiseptic cleanser

Procedural Steps

1 Determine if patient has been incontinent or if excess drainage is on linen.

2 Assess restrictions in mobility/positioning of patient. Explain procedure to patient, noting that patient will be asked to turn over layers of linen.

3 Perform hand hygiene and apply gloves if linen is soiled or there is risk of contacting body fluids.

4 Assemble all equipment on bedside table. Draw room curtain around bed. Lower side rail from side where you are standing.

5 Raise bed to a comfortable working level; lower head of bed, keeping patient comfortable. Remove call light.

6 Loosen top linen at foot of bed.

7 Remove bedspread and blanket separately. If soiled, place in linen bag. If to be reused, fold into square and place over back of chair.

8 Cover patient with bath blanket, placing over top sheet. Have patient hold top edge of bath blanket, or tuck blanket under shoulders. Reach beneath blanket, and remove top sheet. Discard in linen bag.

9 Assist patient to side-lying position facing away from you. Encourage use of side rail to aid in turning. Adjust pillow under patient's head.

10 Assess to make sure that there is no tension on any external medical devices.

11 Loosen bottom linens, moving from head to foot. Fanfold bottom sheet, drawsheet, and any cloth pads toward and under patient. Tuck edges of old bottom linen alongside patient's buttocks, back, and shoulders (see illustration).

12 Clean, disinfect, and dry mattress surface if needed.

13 Apply clean linens to exposed half of bed in separate layers. Start with mattress pad by placing lengthwise with center crease in middle of bed. Fanfold layer to center of bed alongside patient. Repeat process with bottom sheet and drawsheet.

14 Pull fitted sheet smoothly over mattress ends. Allow edge of flat sheet to hang about 25 cm (10 inches) over mattress edge. Be sure lower hem of bottom sheet lies seam down and even with bottom edge of mattress (see illustration).

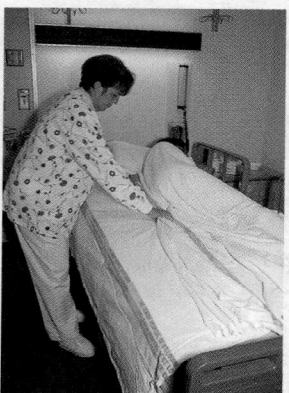

STEP 11 Old linen tucked alongside patient.

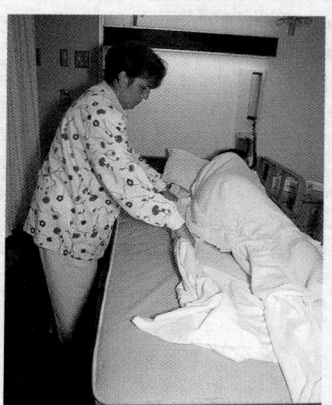

STEP 14 Clean linen applied to bed and fan-folded alongside patient.

PROCEDURAL GUIDELINE 17-7   Making an Occupied Bed—cont'd

15 If bottom sheet is not fitted, miter top corner of bottom sheet at head of bed. Face head of bed diagonally. Place hand away from head of bed under top corner of mattress, lift and with other hand tuck edge of bottom sheet smoothly under mattress so that side edges of sheet above and below mattress meet when brought together.

16 Pick up top of sheet at about 45 cm (18 inches) from top of mattress (see illustration A). Lift sheet and lay it on top of mattress to form a triangular fold with lower base of triangle even with mattress side edges (see illustration B).

17 Tuck lower edge of sheet, which is hanging free under mattress. Hold portion of sheet covering side of mattress in place with one hand (see illustrations). With the other hand, pick up triangular linen fold and bring it down over side of mattress. Tuck with palms down, without pulling triangular fold. Tuck this portion under mattress (see illustrations).

18 Tuck remaining portion of sheet under mattress, moving toward foot of bed. Keep linen smooth.

19 Place open drawsheet along middle of bed lengthwise and tuck remainder under patient's buttocks and torso. You may also place a waterproof pad under drawsheet.

20 Raise side rail, and ask patient to turn toward you; assist as needed. Tell patient that he or she will be rolling over layers of linen. Make sure patient turns slowly.

21 Move to opposite side of bed; lower side rail. Assist patient in positioning on other side over folds of linen (see illustration).

22 Loosen edges of soiled linen from under mattress. Remove soiled linen by folding into a bundle or square.

23 Hold linen away from your body, and place soiled linen in laundry bag.

24 Clean, disinfect, and dry other half of mattress as needed.

25 Pull clean, fanfolded linen over edge of mattress from head to foot of bed.

26 Assist patient in rolling back into supine position. Pull fitted sheet over mattress ends.

27 Miter top corner of bottom flat sheet (see Steps 15 to 17).

28 Facing side of bed, grasp remaining edge of bottom flat sheet. Lean back, keep back straight, and pull while tucking excess linen under mattress, from head to foot of bed.

29 Smooth fanfolded drawsheet over bottom sheet. (Tucking is optional.) Also smooth out waterproof pad.

30 Place top sheet over patient with vertical centerfold lengthwise down middle of bed. Open sheet out from head to foot and unfold over patient. Be sure top edge of sheet is even with top edge of mattress.

31 Ask patient to hold clean top sheet. Remove bath blanket and discard in linen bag.

32 Place clean or reused bed blanket on bed over patient. Make sure top edge is parallel with top edge of sheet and 15 to 20 cm (6 to 8 inches) from top sheet's edge.

33 Make cuff by turning edge of top sheet down over top edge of blanket.

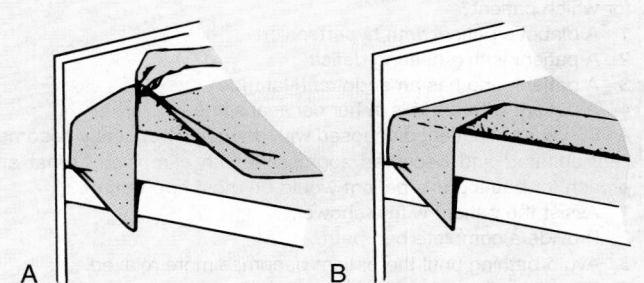

STEP 16   **A,** Top edge of sheet picked up. **B,** Sheet on top of mattress in triangular fold.

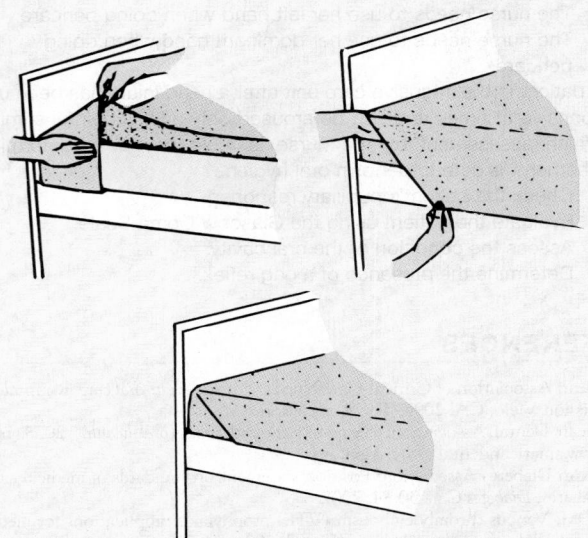

STEP 17   Triangular fold placed over side of mattress; linen tucked under mattress.

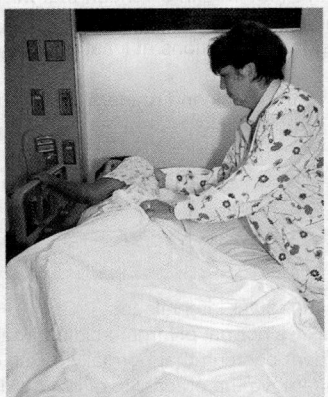

STEP 21   Patient rolling over layers of linen.

Continued

PROCEDURAL GUIDELINE 17-7   Making an Occupied Bed—cont'd

34 Make horizontal toe pleat; stand at foot of bed, and fanfold in sheet and blanket 5 to 10 cm (2 to 4 inches) across bed. Pull sheet and blanket up from bottom to make fold approximately 15 cm (6 inches) from bottom edge of mattress.

35 Tuck in remaining portion of sheet and blanket under foot of mattress. Tuck top sheet and blanket together. Be sure toe pleats are not pulled out.

36 Make modified mitered corner with top sheet and blanket. After making triangular fold, do not tuck tip of triangle (see illustration).

37 Go to other side of bed. Spread sheet and blanket out evenly. Repeat Steps 34 to 36.

38 Apply clean pillowcase.

39 Place call light within patient's reach on bed rail or pillow, and return bed to lowest position.

40 Arrange patient's room. Remove and discard supplies. Perform hand hygiene.

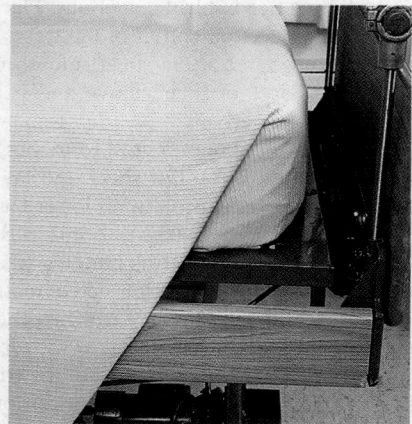

STEP 36 Modified mitered corner.

❓ CRITICAL THINKING EXERCISES

Mr. Bank is a 78-year-old male with a 3-year history of type 1 diabetes mellitus and hypertension. He was just discharged after 5 days of hospitalization with a diagnosis of healing right-heel ulcer, controlled hypertension, and assistance required with daily dressing changes. Mr. Bank lives alone and is able to perform all routine activities of daily living (ADLs). During the initial home visit you assess that although he understands the need for the daily dressing changes, he is not able to state what precautions are needed to prevent any reoccurrence. Select all that apply.

1 Describe the abnormal physical changes that Mr. Bank should look for that require professional evaluation.
   A Dry, cracked skin on feet
   B Reddened or open areas on any portion of feet
   C Nails that are transparent, smooth, and convex; with a pink nail bed and translucent white tip
   D Inflamed cuticles around nail bed edges

2 What three actions should Mr. Bank do to maintain good foot care?
   A Wear properly fitting shoes
   B Wear clean nylon socks
   C Inspect feet daily, both top and bottom
   D Have nails trimmed by professional
   E Soak feet daily in warm water for 15 minutes

3 Identify a proactive foot care intervention that Mr. Bank should do.
   A Self-treat corns and callus with over-the-counter products
   B Seek professional evaluations at least once a year and as needed
   C Cut toenails to the quick and round all nail edges
   D Wear shoes without socks

✔ REVIEW QUESTIONS

1 Provide bathing at regular intervals to:
   1 Restore the skin's normal pH from acidic to basic
   2 Remove resident bacteria that normally cause disease
   3 Cleanse and remove the outer skin of dead skin cells
   4 Promote the maturation of new skin cells

2 Some patients require special positioning precautions when the hair is shampooed. Special positioning precautions are most appropriate for which patient?
   1 A diabetic patient with hypertension
   2 A patient with a hearing deficit
   3 A patient who has an endotracheal tube
   4 A patient with arthritis in her cervical spine

3 An 88-year-old patient diagnosed with dementia frequently becomes very agitated and becomes aggressive with caregivers. What approach for bathing this patient would be most appropriate?
   1 Assist the patient with a shower.
   2 Provide a complete bed bath.
   3 Avoid bathing until the patient becomes more relaxed.
   4 Provide a disposable bed bath in bed.

4 A Muslim woman needs to have a bed bath. What adjustment does the female nurse need to make when performing pericare?
   1 The nurse needs to use gloves when performing pericare.
   2 The nurse needs to have another nurse in attendance while doing pericare.
   3 The nurse needs to use her left hand when doing pericare.
   4 The nurse needs to use her dominant hand when doing pericare.

5 A patient in the intensive care unit after a head injury has been unresponsive at times and can be aroused only after a painful stimulus. Which assessment by the nurse is most crucial in determining whether it is safe to perform oral hygiene?
   1 Check the patient's pupillary response.
   2 Evaluate the patient using the Glascow Coma Scale.
   3 Assess the condition of the oral cavity.
   4 Determine the presence of a gag reflex.

REFERENCES

American Association of Critical-Care Nurses: *Practice alert: oral care in critical care*, Mission Viejo, CA, 2006, The Association.

American Dental Association: *Cleaning teeth and gums (oral health)*, 2008, http://www.americandental association.org.

American Diabetes Association: Position statement on standards of medical care in diabetes, *Diabetes Care* 30:S4, 2007.

Beck DM: Venous thromboembolism (VTE) prophylaxis: implications for medical-surgical nurses, *Medsurg Nurs* 15(5):282, 2006.

Brown C, Wingard J: Clinical consequences of oral mucositis, *Semin Oncol Nurs* 20(1):16, 2004.

Delmas L: Best practice in the assessment and management of diabetic foot ulcers, *Rehabil Nurs* 31(6):228, 2006.

Galanti G: *Caring for patients from different cultures*, ed 3, Philadelphia, 2004, University of Pennsylvania Press.

Meiner S, Lueckenotte AG: *Gerontologic nursing*, ed 3, St. Louis, 2006, Mosby.

National Pediculosis Association: *Child care provider's guide to controlling head lice*, 2007, http://www.headlice.org.

National Pressure Ulcer Advisory Panel: *Updated staging systems*, 2007, http://www.npuap.org.

Paju S, Scannapieco FA: Oral biofilms, periodontitis, and pulmonary infections, *Oral Dis* 13:508, 2007.

Pinzur MS and others: Guidelines for diabetic foot care, The Diabetes Committee of the American Orthopaedic Foot and Ankle Society, *Foot Ankle Int* 20:1, 2005.

Skewes SM: No more bed baths! *RN* 57(1):34, 1994.

RESEARCH REFERENCES

Black J and others: National Pressure Ulcer Advisory Panel's updated pressure ulcer staging system, *Dermatol Nurs* 19(4):343, 2007.

Cutler C and others: Improving oral care in patients receiving mechanical ventilation, *Am J Crit Care* 13(3):389, 2005.

Furr L and others: Factors affecting quality of oral care in intensive care units, *J Adv Nurs* 48(5):454, 2004.

Grap MJ and others: Duration of action of a single, early oral application of chlorhexidine on oral microbial flora in mechanically ventilated patients: a pilot study, *Heart Lung* 33(2):83, 2004.

Hoeffer B and others: Assisting cognitively impaired nursing home residents with bathing: effects of two bathing interventions on caregiving, *Gerontologist* 46(4):524, 2006.

Larson E and others: Comparison of traditional and disposable bed baths in critically ill patients, *Am J Crit Care* 13(3):235, 2004.

Mahoney E and others: Challenges to intervention implementation: lessons learned in the Bathing Persons With Alzheimer's Disease at Home study, *Nurs Res* 55(2 suppl):S10, 2006.

Munro C, Grap M: Oral health and care in the intensive care unit: state of the science, *Am J Crit Care* 13(1):25, 2004.

Munro C and others: Oral health status and development of ventilator-associated pneumonia: a descriptive study, *Am J Crit Care* 15(5):453, 2006.

Pressure Ulcer Care

MEDIA RESOURCES

- evolve http://evolve.elsevier.com/Perry/skills
  - Review Questions
  - Video Clips

- Mosby's Nursing Video Skills, 3.0

- NSO Nursing Skills Online

OBJECTIVES

Mastery of content in this chapter will enable the nurse to:

- Describe guidelines for the prevention of pressure ulcers.
- Identify risk factors for development of pressure ulcers.
- Identify outcome criteria for patients at risk for pressure ulcers or impaired skin integrity.
- Discuss the use of risk assessment tools commonly used in assessment of pressure ulcer risk.
- Describe patient characteristics, as well as the characteristics of pressure ulcer itself, to include in an assessment.
- Discuss indications for the use of topical agents in the treatment of pressure ulcers.
- Use topical agents correctly in the management of a pressure ulcer.
- Discuss teaching needs of a patient and family regarding pressure ulcers.

A pressure ulcer is a localized injury to the skin and/or underlying tissue, usually over a bony prominence as a result of pressure or pressure in combination with shear and/or friction (National Pressure Ulcer Advisor Panel [NPUAP], 2007). Pressure ulcers are inaccurately called decubitus ulcers or bedsores by some. Many used to believe that only bed-bound persons developed these ulcers; however, we now know that pressure ulcers occur from any position that causes soft tissue compression. Compression of soft tissue interferes with the blood flow to the tissue; if this compression continues for a prolonged period of time, the tissue dies from lack of blood flow, or ischemia. Ischemia develops when pressure on the skin is greater than the pressure inside the vessels, causing the vessels to collapse, preventing the blood from reaching the tissue. The tissue dies from ischemic injury. Initially ischemia is often evident by skin discoloration such as redness and warmth in patients with light skin or purple and warmth in patients with darkly pigmented skin. If pressure is unrelieved or repeated, tissue will continue to break down relative to a patient's general health and tolerance for pressure. This pressure, if not relieved, can cause irreversible tissue damage in as little as 90 minutes (Kosiak, 1959).

Fig. 18-1 shows pressure points over bony prominences where pressure ulcers can occur. The most common sites are the sacrum, coccyx, ischial tuberosities, greater trochanters, elbows, heels, scapulas, ileal crests, and lateral and medial malleoli (Pieper, 2007). Pressure ulcers can occur on any area of skin subjected to pressure. Nonbony locations in which pressure ulcers can occur include the nares, usually related to pressure caused from nasogastric (NG) tubes or oxygen cannulas; the ears, resulting from an oxygen cannula; or the genitalia, with ulcers resulting from Foley catheter tension.

Other factors such as incontinence, friction and shear, immobility, loss of sensory perception, level of activity and poor nutrition contribute to pressure ulcer formation. Moisture and ammonia from incontinence soften the skin, allowing the skin to become susceptible to breakdown. Friction, the mechanical force of two surfaces moving over each other, causes surface damage such as blisters. Shear is any tension that stretches the skin during turning or moving in bed. This force causes reduced blood flow to the tissues.

Immobility often restricts a patient's ability to change and control body position, thus increasing the pressure over bony prominences. Loss of sensory perception decreases the individual's ability to respond to increased, prolonged pressure in an area of the body and change positions accordingly. Level of activity refers to the person's normal physical movement. A person who is bed bound is at greater risk for skin breakdown than a person who is fully or

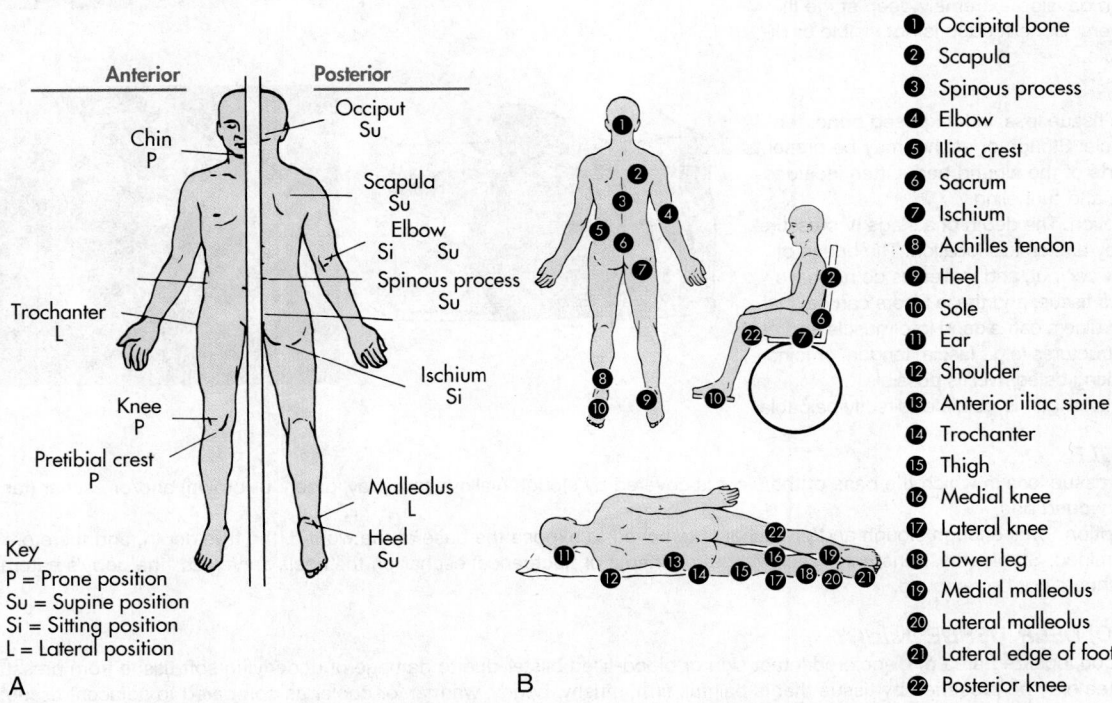

Pressure ulcer sites

1. Occipital bone
2. Scapula
3. Spinous process
4. Elbow
5. Iliac crest
6. Sacrum
7. Ischium
8. Achilles tendon
9. Heel
10. Sole
11. Ear
12. Shoulder
13. Anterior iliac spine
14. Trochanter
15. Thigh
16. Medial knee
17. Lateral knee
18. Lower leg
19. Medial malleolus
20. Lateral malleolus
21. Lateral edge of foot
22. Posterior knee

Anterior | **Posterior**

Chin P
Occiput Su
Scapula Su
Elbow Si Su
Spinous process Su
Trochanter L
Ischium Si
Knee P
Pretibial crest P
Malleolus L
Heel Su

Key
P = Prone position
Su = Supine position
Si = Sitting position
L = Lateral position

A   B

FIG 18-1 **A,** Bony prominences most frequently underlying pressure ulcers. **B,** Pressure ulcer sites.
(From Trelease CC: Developing standards for wound care, Ostomy Wound Manage 26:50, 1988.)

BOX 18-1 | Staging of Pressure Ulcers

Staging Definition

Stage I

Intact skin with nonblanchable redness of a localized area usually over a bony prominence. Darkly pigmented skin may not have visible blanching; its color may differ from the surrounding area.

Further description: The area may be painful, firm, soft, warmer or cooler as compared to adjacent tissue. Stage I may be difficult to detect in individuals with dark skin tones. May indicate "at risk" person (a heralding risk).

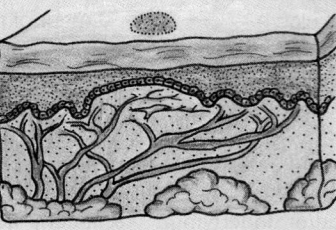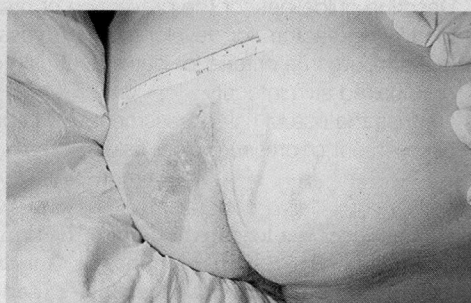

Stage II

Partial-thickness loss presenting as a shallow open ulcer with a red-pink wound bed, without slough. May also present as an intact or open/ruptured serum-filled blister.

Further description: Presents as a shiny or dry shallow ulcer without sloughing or bruising. (Bruising indicates suspected deep tissue injury). This stage should not be used to describe skin tears, tape burns, perineal dermatitis, maceration, or excoriation.

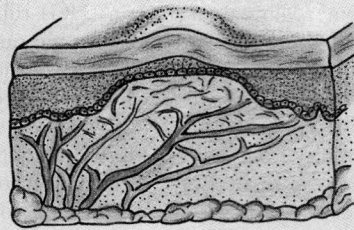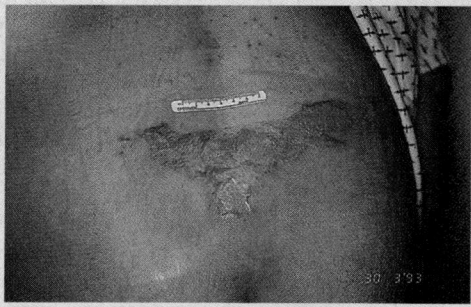

Stage III

Full-thickness skin loss. Subcutaneous fat may be visible, but bone, tendon, or muscle is not exposed. Slough may be present but does not obscure the depth of tissue loss. May include undermining and tunneling.

Further description: The depth of a stage III pressure ulcer varies by anatomical location. The bridge of the nose, ear, occiput, and malleolus do not have subcutaneous tissue, and stage III ulcers can be shallow. In contrast, areas of significant adiposity can develop extremely deep stage III pressure ulcers. Bone/tendon is not visible or directly palpable.

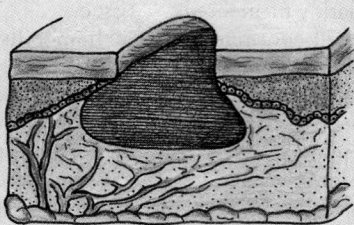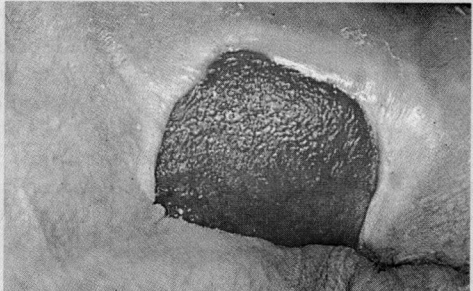

Stage IV

Full-thickness tissue loss with exposed bone, tendon, or muscle. Slough or eschar may be present on some parts of the wound bed. Often includes undermining and tunneling.

Further description: The depth of a stage IV pressure ulcer varies by anatomical location. The bridge of the nose, ear, occiput, and malleolus do not have subcutaneous tissue, and these ulcers can be shallow. Stage IV ulcers can extend into muscle and/or supporting structures (e.g., fascia, tendon, or joint capsule), making osteomyelitis possible. Exposed bone/tendon is visible or directly palpable.

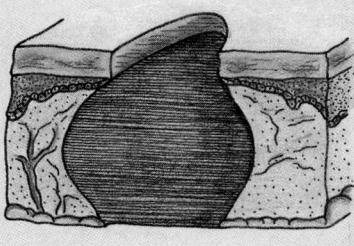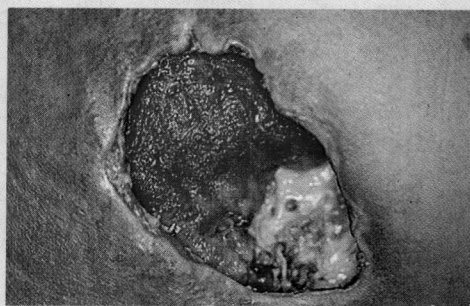

UNSTAGEABLE

Full-thickness tissue loss in which the base of the ulcer is covered by slough (yellow, tan, gray, green, or brown) and/or eschar (tan, brown, black) in the wound bed.

Further description: Until enough slough and/or eschar is removed to expose the base of the wound, the true depth, and therefore stage, cannot be determined. Stable (dry, adherent, intact without erythema or fluctuance) eschar on the heels serves as "the body's natural (biological) cover" and should not be removed.

(SUSPECTED) DEEP TISSUE INJURY

Purple or maroon localized area of discolored intact skin or blood-filled blister due to damage of underlying soft tissue from pressure and/or shear. The area may be preceded by tissue that is painful, firm, mushy, boggy, warmer, or cooler as compared to adjacent tissue.

Further description: Deep tissue injury may be difficult to detect in individuals with dark skin tones. Evolution may include a thin blister over a dark wound bed. The wound may further evolve and become covered by thin eschar. Evolution may be rapid, exposing additional layers of tissue even with optimal treatment.

Data from National Pressure Ulcer Advisory Panel: *NPUAP pressure ulcer definition and stages,* 2007, http://www.npuap.org/pr2.htm, accessed August 19, 2007.

partially mobile. Research indicates that malnutrition contributes to the development of pressure ulcers (Wound, Ostomy and Continence Nurses Society [WOCN], 2003). Pressure ulcers pose serious risks to a patient's health. A break in the skin, seen in stages II to IV pressure ulcers (Box 18-1), eliminates the body's first line of defense against infection.

The numbers of patients who develop pressure ulcers are significant. Reports vary as to the number of patients who are at risk for and develop pressure ulcers. Patients are now older and sicker; they are hospitalized for shorter periods of time and are discharged to home or intermediate or long-term care facilities at a more acute stage of illness (Pieper, 2007). These changes will contribute to an increased number of patients at risk for developing pressure ulcers. It is thus critical to respond with an aggressive preventive approach. It is imperative that you identify the factors that place a patient at risk for the development of pressure ulcers. Once you identify the factors, begin interventions to reduce or relieve the negative effects of each factor. When a pressure ulcer develops, explore the factors that contributed to the skin breakdown, vigorously attempt to minimize the effects of these variables, and use current wound-healing principles in the management of the ulcer (see Chapters 38 and 39).

EVIDENCE-BASED PRACTICE TRENDS

Perform risk assessments on patients entering a health care setting, and repeat them when there is a significant change in a patient's health status and on a regularly scheduled basis (Fig. 18-2). Base skin assessment on patient acuity (Ayello and Braden, 2002; WOCN, 2003). When you look at the overall score on the Braden Scale, a patient will fall within one of these categories: mild risk, 16 to 18; moderate risk, 13 to 14; high risk, 9 or less (Braden and Bergstrom, 1994). Use these risk scores to plan care by looking at the individual risk factors that place a patient at risk and developing a care plan to decrease or eliminate the identified risk factors (Bolton and others, 2007).

In the acute care setting, 7% to 17% of the patients have pressure ulcers (Whittington and Briones, 2004) and 15% of older adults will develop pressure ulcers within the first week of hospitalization (Lyder, 2004). Therefore with patients in high-risk settings, it is important to target prevention efforts to minimize risk (Reddy and others, 2006; WOCN, 2003).

The risk assessment findings indicate interventions to reduce the risk associated with pressure ulcer development. For example, a patient who is incontinent of stool and urine requires a plan that includes the use of a perineal cleanser and a skin barrier. Use absorbent products to wick the drainage away from the skin. When patients are at risk for skin breakdown related to immobility, the plan of care usually includes the use a pressure-redistribution surface, a turning schedule, and regular skin assessments (WOCN, 2003).

The treatment plan for a patient with a pressure ulcer needs to include elimination or reduction of the factors that have caused the pressure ulcer. You plan topical care based upon the principle of moist wound healing. A moist wound environment supports the growth of new tissue. If the wound is not free of necrotic tissue, you need to choose topical wound care that will clean the wound bed of devitalized tissue. Make sure to address infection or colonization. Treat infection both systematically and topically. Prevent colonization by using topical dressings and medications (Jones and Fennie, 2007). Wound healing in a patient with a pressure ulcer progresses if the patient has an adequate nutritional status, as well as control over preexisting conditions such as diabetes and cardiovascular and pulmonary disease (Doughty and Sparks-Defriese, 2007).

CULTURAL CONSIDERATIONS

Persons with a pressure ulcer report that the ulcer and the treatment affect their lives emotionally, mentally, physically, and socially (Spilsbury and others, 2007). Patients are aware of the amount and quality of care they receive, including levels of comfort during dressing changes and the timing of interventions. The presence of a pressure ulcer increases hospital stay and results in ongoing treatments. Given that the presence of a pressure ulcer affects a patient's quality of life, providing culturally appropriate information about treatment and wound-healing expectations is an important aspect of care.

When planning care for a patient with a pressure ulcer, consider cultural issues such as skin tones, the issues related to patient and caregiver education, the need for a gender-congruent caregiver, as well as the social effects of a pressure ulcer. The assessment of the skin will depend on skin color. For example, redness in a dark-skinned patient is difficult to determine without the use of palpation and a comparison to other, nonaffected body parts (Box 18-2). When providing pressure ulcer care, remember that in some cultures hair has significance and should not be shaved (Galanti, 2004). If shaving is absolutely necessary for wound healing, you may need the assistance of the patient's family or cultural elder.

When providing patient and caregiver education, consider the primary language and reading ability of the patient and caregiver when using printed materials. Frequently the initial use of pictures with labels can help determine if reading skills are adequate to use printed patient educational materials. Part of the overall assessment of a patient includes how the presence of a pressure ulcer will affect the social situation, for example, if a wound would prevent a patient from socializing in the community. Also the presence of a pressure ulcer can cause pain and resultant disability, which affects family dynamics.

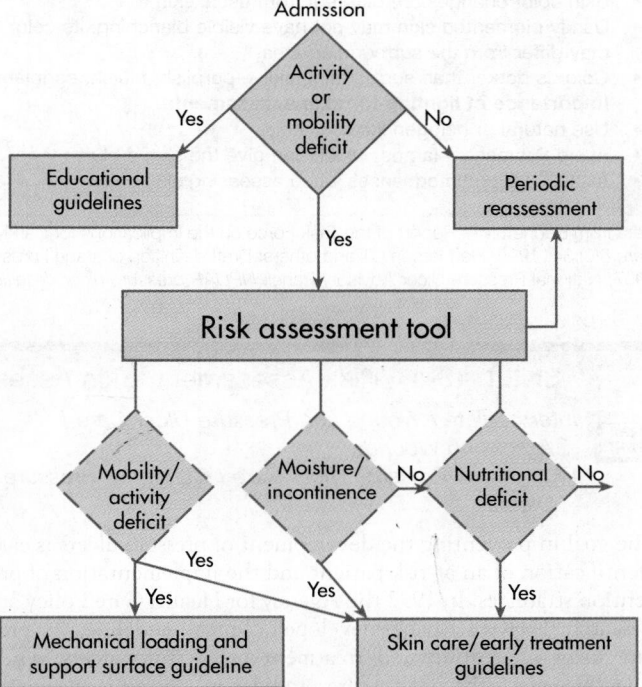

FIG 18-2 Risk assessment tool. (*Modified from Panel for the Prediction and Prevention of Pressure Ulcers in Adults: Pressure ulcers in adults: prediction and prevention, Clinical practice guideline No. 3, Pub No. 92-0047, Rockville, Md, 1992, Agency for Health Care Policy and Research, Public Health Service, U.S. Department of Health and Human Services.*)

Skill Performance Guidelines

1 Routinely assess patients for individual risks for developing pressure ulcers. Select and use a risk assessment tool; the Braden and Norton scales have the most clinical validity. Perform risk assessment on entry to a health care setting, and repeat it on a regularly scheduled basis or when there is a significant change in a patient's condition (Pieper, 2007).

2 Assess and inspect skin at least daily. Note all pressure points; document results.

3 Redistribute the amount and duration of pressure to prevent ischemic tissue injury. Frequently turn and reposition a patient to redistribute pressure from the superficial capillaries and allow tissues to compensate for temporary ischemia. Classic research finds that tissue ischemia begins within 1 to 2 hours after onset of pressure (Kosiak, 1959). Use safe patient handling measures to turn and reposition patients at a minimum of every 1 to 2 hours. Proper positioning helps minimize formation of pressure ulcers (see Chapter 9).

4 Specialized beds, overlays, and mattresses (see Chapter 12) redistribute pressure over dependent body parts. By distributing pressure evenly over a patient's body surface, less pressure is applied at the skin level. Place patients at high risk for pressure ulcer formation on these devices as soon as possible. Consider the use of a chair cushion to redistribute pressure when a patient is seated.

5 Cleanse patients who are incontinent of stool or urine as soon as possible. Skin moisture and wetness from incontinence is often a risk factor for skin breakdown (Gray and others, 2007). Protect areas subjected to repeated episodes of incontinence with a barrier ointment or barrier paste.

6 Institute interventions to minimize friction and shear. Use lift sheets when repositioning a patient because this will reduce the amount of rubbing of the skin against the sheets. Raise the head of the bed no more than 30 degrees (unless medically contraindicated) to prevent sliding and shear injury (WOCN, 2003).

7 Adequate nutrition is important in the prevention and treatment of pressure ulcers (WOCN, 2003). A diet high in protein with enough calories, vitamins, and minerals helps maintain normal tissue status and promotes healing. With tissue injury the body needs more calories for healing; deficiencies in any nutrients may result in impaired or delayed healing. Make sure monitoring the nutritional status is part of the total assessment (WOCN, 2003).

8 If a patient develops a pressure ulcer, routinely assess the ulcer to determine progress toward healing. Base interventions to support healing upon the assessment.

BOX 18-2 | Cultural Considerations for Skin Assessment of Pressure Ulcers: Patients With Darkly Pigmented Skin

Patients with darkly pigmented skin cannot be assessed for pressure ulcer risk by examining only skin color. Follow these recommended guidelines:

Assess Localized Skin Color Changes
Any of the following may appear:
- Skin color changes are different from usual skin tone.
- Darkly pigmented skin may not have visible blanching; its color may differ from the surrounding area.
- Color is darker than surrounding skin—purplish, bluish, eggplant.
Importance of lighting for skin assessment:
- Use natural or halogen light.
- Avoid fluorescent lamps, which can give the skin a bluish tone.
- Avoid wearing tinted lenses when assessing skin color.

Tissue Consistency
- Assess for edema, swelling.
- Assess for firm or boggy feel.

Sensation
- Assess for pain or changes in skin sensation such as itching.

Skin Temperature
- Initially skin in the area of pressure ulcer may feel warmer than surrounding skin.
- Subsequently skin may feel cooler than surrounding skin.
- Feel areas of skin that are not involved in or around a pressure point to serve as a point of temperature reference.

Data from Bennett MA: Report of the Task Force on the Implications for Darkly Pigmented Intact Skin in the Prediction and Prevention of Pressure Ulcers, *Adv Wound Care* 8(6):34, 1995; Henderson CT and others: Draft definition of stage I pressure ulcers: inclusion of persons with darkly pigmented skin, *Adv Wound Care* 10(5):16, 1997; National Pressure Ulcer Advisory Panel: *NPUAP pressure ulcer definition and stages,* 2007, http://www.npuap.org/pr2.htm, accessed August 19, 2007.

SKILL 18-1   Risk Assessment, Skin Assessment, and Prevention Strategies

Intermediate / Wound and Pressure Ulcer Care / Assessing Wounds
Wound and Pressure Ulcer Care / Caring for Pressure Ulcers

NSO *Wound Care Module / Lessons 1 and 4*

The goal in preventing the development of pressure ulcers is early identification of an at-risk patient and the implementation of prevention strategies. In 1992 the Agency for Health Care Policy and Research (AHCPR) panel developed clinical guidelines for pressure ulcer prevention and treatment of pressure ulcers. These guidelines assist the health care provider in planning and implementing care for both prevention and treatment of a patient with a pressure ulcer (Bergstrom and others, 1994). In 2003 the Wound, Ostomy and Continence Nurses Society (WOCN) developed the *Guideline for Prevention and Management of Pressure Ulcers.* Much like the process used to develop the AHCPR guidelines, a panel of experts performed extensive searches on available literature on pressure ulcers. The panel then established a level of evidence rating that provides the best available evidence in the prevention and management of pressure ulcers. The Agency for Healthcare Research and Quality, which has replaced the AHCPR, accepted the WOCN guidelines as a part of their resource component.

The overall management goals suggested by WOCN (2003) include:

1 Identify individuals at risk for developing pressure ulcers, and initiate an early prevention program

2 Implement appropriate strategies/plans to:
  a Attain/maintain intact skin
  b Prevent complications
  c Promptly identify or manage complications
  d Involve the patient and caregiver in self-management
3 Implement cost-effective strategies/plans that prevent and treat pressure ulcers

The WOCN 2003 panel recommends performing a risk assessment on entry to a health care setting and repeating this on a regularly scheduled basis or when there is a significant change in an individual's condition. For example, if a patient who was ambulatory becomes bed bound because of a surgical procedure, this person is potentially at higher risk for skin breakdown than when first admitted when ambulatory. The WOCN suggests the use of risk assessment tools such as the Braden Scale or the Norton Scale. The Norton Scale, developed in 1962, has five risk factors: physical condition, mental state, activity, mobility, and incontinence (Norton and others, 1975). The Braden Scale (Table 18-1) has six parameters: sensory perception (ability to respond meaningfully to pressure-related discomfort), moisture (degree to which skin is exposed to moisture), activity (degree of physical activity), mobility (ability to change and control body position), nutrition (usual food intake pattern), and friction and shear (Ayello and Braden, 2002; Braden and Bergstrom, 1989, 1994). Risk cutoff scores vary for specific patient populations (Table 18-2). It is important to understand how to interpret the meaning of a patient's total score on whatever scale you use.

Inspect patient's skin and bony prominences at least daily. Remove devices, shoes, socks, antiembolic stockings and heel and elbow protectors for the skin inspection. Inspect all bony prominences, including back of head, shoulders, rib cage, elbows, hips, ischium, sacrum, coccyx, knees, ankles, and heels (see Fig. 18-1). Palpate any reddened or discolored areas with a gloved finger to determine if the erythema (redness of the skin caused by dilatation and congestion of the capillaries) blanches. Blanching is normal. If you palpate an area that does not blanch (abnormal reactive hyperemia), this area is a site for potential skin breakdown.

Delegation Considerations
The skill of assessment of pressure ulcer risk cannot be delegated to nursing assistive personnel (NAP). The nurse directs the NAP to:
• Report any redness or break in patient's skin.
• Report any abrasion from assistive devices.

Equipment
❑ Risk assessment tool
❑ Documentation record
❑ Pressure-redistribution mattress, bed, and/or chair cushion
❑ Positioning aids
❑ Gloves

TABLE 18-1	Braden Scale for Predicting Pressure Ulcer Risk*			
Sensory Perception Ability to respond meaningfully to pressure-related discomfort	1. *Completely limited:* Unresponsive (does not moan, flinch, or grasp) to painful stimuli due to diminished level of consciousness or sedation. OR Limited ability to feel pain over most of body.	2. *Very limited:* Responds only to painful stimuli. Cannot communicate discomfort except by moaning or restlessness. OR Has a sensory impairment that limits the ability to feel pain or discomfort over half of body.	3. *Slightly limited:* Responds to verbal commands but cannot always communicate discomfort or need to be turned. OR Has some sensory impairment, which limits ability to feel pain or discomfort in one or two extremities.	4. *No impairment:* Responds to verbal commands. Has no sensory deficit that would limit ability to feel or voice pain or discomfort.
Moisture Degree to which skin is exposed to moisture	1. *Constantly moist:* Skin is kept moist almost constantly by perspiration, urine, etc. Dampness is detected every time patient is moved or turned.	2. *Very moist:* Skin is often, but not always, moist. Linen must be changed at least once a shift.	3. *Occasionally moist:* Skin is occasionally moist, requiring an extra linen change approximately once a day.	4. *Rarely moist:* Skin is usually dry; linen requires changing only at routine intervals.
Activity Degree of physical activity	1. *Bedfast:* Confined to bed.	2. *Chair fast:* Ability to walk severely limited or nonexistent. Cannot bear own weight and/or must be assisted into chair or wheelchair.	3. *Walks occasionally:* Walks occasionally during day, but for very short distances, with or without assistance. Spends majority of each shift in bed or chair.	4. *Walks frequently:* Walks outside the room at least twice a day and inside room at least once every 2 hours during waking hours.

Continued

| **TABLE 18-1** | Braden Scale for Predicting Pressure Ulcer Risk*—cont'd | | | |

Mobility

Ability to change and control body position

| 1. *Completely immobile:* Does not make even slight changes in body or extremity position without assistance. | 2. *Very limited:* Makes occasional slight changes in body or extremity position but unable to make frequent or significant changes independently. | 3. *Slightly limited:* Makes frequent though slight changes in body or extremity position independently. | 4. *No limitations:* Makes major and frequent changes in position without assistance. |

Nutrition

Usual food intake pattern

1. *Very poor:* Never eats a complete meal. Rarely eats more than one third of any food offered. Eats 2 servings or less of protein (meat or dairy products) per day. Takes fluids poorly. Does not take a liquid dietary supplement.	2. *Probably inadequate:* Rarely eats a complete meal and generally eats only about half of any food offered. Protein intake includes only 3 servings of meat or dairy products per day. Occasionally will take a dietary supplement.	3. *Adequate:* Eats over half of most meals. Eats a total of 4 servings of protein (meat, dairy products) each day. Occasionally will refuse a meal, but will usually take a supplement when offered.	4. *Excellent:* Eats most of every meal. Never refuses a meal. Usually eats a total of 4 or more servings of meat and dairy products. Occasionally eats between meals. Does not require supplementation.
OR	OR	OR	
Is NPO and/or maintained on clear liquids or IVs for more than 5 days.	Receives less than optimal amount of liquid diet or tube feeding.	Is on a tube-feeding or TPN regimen that probably meets most of nutritional needs.	

Friction and Shear

| 1. *Problem:* Requires moderate to maximum assistance in moving. Complete lifting without sliding against sheets is impossible. Frequently slides down in bed or chair; repositioning with maximal assistance. Spasticity, contractions, or agitation leads to almost constant friction. | 2. *Potential problem:* Moves feebly or requires minimal assistance. During a move skin probably slides to some extent against sheets, chair, restraints, or other devices. Maintains relatively good position in chair or bed most of the time but occasionally slides down. | 3. *No apparent problem:* Moves in bed and in chair independently and has sufficient muscle strength to sit up completely during move. Maintains good position in bed or chair. | |

From Barbara Braden, PhD, RN, Creighton University School of Nursing, Omaha, Neb.

NPO, Nothing by mouth; *IV,* intravenous; *TPN,* total parenteral nutrition.

*Score patient in each of the six subscales. Maximum score is 23, indicating little or no risk. A score of ≤16 indicates "at risk"; ≤9 indicates high risk.

TABLE 18-2	Pressure Ulcer Braden Risk Cutoff Scores by Patient Population
Patient Population	**Risk Cutoff Scores**
General population	≤16
Intensive care unit patients	≤15
Older adult patients	≤18
Black and Latino patients	≤18

Data from Braden BJ, Bergstrom N: Clinical utility of the Braden Scale for predicting pressure sore risk, *Decubitus* 2(3):44, 1989; Bergstrom N, Braden BJ: Predictive validity of the Braden Scale among black and white subjects, *Nurs Res* 51(6):398, 2002; Lyder CH and others: The Braden Scale for pressure ulcer risk: evaluating the predictive validity in black and Latino/Hispanic elders, *Appl Nurs Res* 12(2):60, 1999.

STEP	RATIONALE

ASSESSMENT

1 Identify any patient characteristics that might be risk factors for pressure ulcer formation:

Determines need to administer preventive care and identifies specific factors placing patient at risk.

a Paralysis, or immobilization caused by restrictive devices

Patient is unable to turn or reposition independently to relieve pressure.

b Sensory loss (e.g., hemiplegia, spinal cord injury)

When sensory loss is present, a patient feels no discomfort from pressure and does not independently change position.

c Circulatory disorders (e.g., diabetes mellitus)

Reduce perfusion of skin's tissue layers.

d Fever

Increases metabolic demands of tissues. Accompanying diaphoresis leaves skin moist.

e Anemia

Decreased hemoglobin level reduces oxygen-carrying capacity of blood and amount of oxygen available to tissues.

f Malnutrition

Inadequate nutrition leads to weight loss, muscle atrophy, and reduced tissue mass. Deficiencies in any of the nutrients will result in impaired or delayed healing (Stotts, 2007).

g Incontinence

Skin becomes exposed to moist environment containing bacteria. Moisture causes skin maceration.

h Heavy sedation and anesthesia

Patient is not mentally alert and does not turn or change position independently. Sedation also alters sensory perception.

i Age

Neonates and very young children are at high risk, with the head being the most common site of pressure ulcer occurrence (WOCN, 2003). There is a loss of dermal thickness in the older individual, impairing the ability to distribute pressure (Pieper, 2007).

j Dehydration

Results in decreased skin elasticity and turgor.

k Edema

Edematous tissues are less tolerant of pressure, friction, and shear.

l Existing pressure ulcers

Limits surfaces available for position changes, placing available tissues at increased risk.

m History of pressure ulcer

Tensile strength of the skin from a previously healed pressure ulcer is about 80%; therefore this area cannot tolerate pressure as much as undamaged skin (Doughty and Sparks-Defriese, 2007).

2 Select a risk assessment tool such as the Braden Scale or Norton Scale. Perform the risk assessment on entry to the health care setting, and repeat on a regularly scheduled basis or when there is a significant change in an individual's condition (WOCN, 2003).

Valid and reliable risk assessment tools evaluate patient's risk for developing a pressure ulcer. Using the risk assessment will identify risk factors that contribute to the potential for skin breakdown and pinpoint specific areas to target interventions to decrease the risk for skin breakdown.

3 Obtain risk score (see Tables 18-1 and 18-2, pp. 469 to 470 and Table 18-3, p. 474), and evaluate its meaning based on patient's unique characteristics.

The risk cutoff score will depend on the instrument used. In addition, the score involves identifying the risk factors that contributed to the score and minimizing those specific deficits.

4 Assess condition of patient's skin over regions of pressure (see Fig. 18-1, p. 465).

Body weight against bony prominences places underlying skin at risk for breakdown.

a Inspect for skin discoloration (redness in light-tone skin; purplish or bluish in darkly pigmented skin); tissue consistency (firm or boggy feel), and/or palpate for abnormal sensations (Lyder and others, 2001; Nix, 2007). See Box 18-2, p. 468, for cultural considerations in assessing patients with darkly pigmented skin.

Indicates that tissue was under pressure; hyperemia is a normal physiological response to hypoxemia in tissues.

b Palpate discolored area for blanching.

If on palpation an area of redness blanches (lightens in color), this indicates normal reactive hyperemia; the tissue is not at risk for skin breakdown. Tissue that does not blanch when palpated indicates abnormal reactive hyperemia; there is ischemic injury.

c Inspect for pallor and mottling.

Persistent hypoxia in tissues that were under pressure; an abnormal physiological response.

d Inspect for absence of superficial skin layers.

Represents early pressure ulcer formation, usually a partial-thickness wound that may have resulted from friction and/or shear.

e Palpate for skin temperature differences (warmth or coolness) (Bennett, 1995; Henderson and others, 1997).

Palpation of differences in temperature between the area of a stage I pressure ulcer and adjacent skin area may be an initial indicator of ischemia (Sprigle and others, 2001).

5 Assess patient for additional areas of potential pressure:

Patients at high risk have multiple sites for pressure necrosis (tissue death), in addition to bony prominences.

a Nares: NG tube, oxygen cannula

STEP	RATIONALE
b Tongue and lips: oral airway, endotracheal (ET) tube	
c Ears: oxygen cannula, pillow	
d Drainage tubes	Stress against tissue at exit site or if tubing is caught under any part of the body.
e Wound drainage	Wound drainage is caustic to skin and underlying tissues, thereby increasing risk for skin breakdown.
f Indwelling urethral (Foley) catheter	For female patients, the catheter can put pressure on the labia, especially when edematous. For male patients, pressure from a catheter not properly anchored can put pressure on the tip of the penis and urethra.
g Orthopedic and positioning devices	Improperly fitted or applied devices have the potential to cause pressure on adjacent skin and underlying tissue.

Critical Decision Point *Inspect skin around and beneath orthopedic devices, such as cervical collar, braces, or cast. Note any abrasions or warmth in areas where devices can rub against the skin.*

STEP	RATIONALE
6 Observe patient for preferred positions when in bed or chair.	Preferred positions result in weight of body being placed on certain bony prominences. Presence of contractures may result in pressure exerted in unexpected places.
7 Observe ability of patient to initiate and assist with position changes.	Potential for friction and shear increases when patient is completely dependent on others for position changes.
8 Assess patient and caregiver understanding of risks for the development of pressure ulcers.	Determines baseline knowledge for pressure ulcer risk and identifies areas for patient teaching.

NURSING DIAGNOSES

- Deficient knowledge related to pressure ulcer prevention
- Imbalanced nutrition: less than body requirements
- Impaired physical mobility
- Impaired skin integrity
- Ineffective tissue perfusion
- Risk for impaired skin integrity

Individualize related factors based on patient's condition or needs.

PLANNING

STEP	RATIONALE
1 Expected outcomes following completion of procedure:	
• No change from baseline skin assessment.	The systematic use of a risk assessment scale will identify risk factors and target treatment efforts.
• Skin is intact with no evidence of erythema or no signs of breakdown.	Prevention strategies reduce risk factors.
2 Explain procedure(s) and purpose to patient and caregiver.	Relieves anxiety and provides opportunity for education.
3 Perform hand hygiene, and prepare equipment and supplies.	Reduces transmission of microorganisms.

IMPLEMENTATION

STEP	RATIONALE
1 Implement the prevention guidelines adapted from the Wound, Ostomy and Continence Nurses Society's *Guideline for Prevention and Management of Pressure Ulcers* (2003).	Reduces patient's risk for developing a pressure ulcer.
2 Close room door or bedside curtain.	Maintains patient privacy.
3 If patient has open, draining wounds, use clean gloves.	Use of standard precautions prevents accidental exposure to body fluids.
4 Assist patient with changing position. Place in the following positions (see Chapter 9):	Avoid positions that place patient directly on an area of existing skin breakdown. It is often helpful to use a schedule for position changes.
a Supine	Protects shoulders, trochanter, and malleolus.
b Prone	Used only in patients who are able to tolerate this position; breathing difficulty is normal.
c 30-degree lateral (see illustration)	Achieved with one pillow under shoulder and one pillow under leg on the same side. The 30-degree lateral position should provide pressure relief from the sacrum and the trochanter (WOCN, 2003).

STEP	RATIONALE

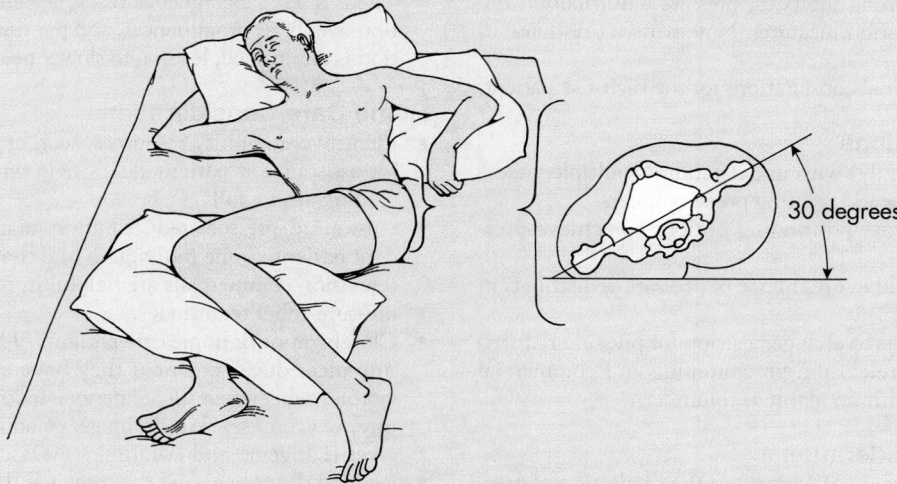

STEP 4c Thirty-degree lateral position.

Critical Decision Point *When repositioning a patient, observe for skin discoloration in area that was under pressure. In light-skinned patients, expect redness from initial flushing. Darkly pigmented skin does not always have visible "blanching"; its color differs from the surrounding skin (NPUAP, 2007). Bennett also suggests using natural or halogen light sources when assessing for discoloration on patients with darkly pigmented skin. Avoid using fluorescent lighting because it gives a bluish tint to skin that interferes with accurate assessment of skin coloring (see Box 18-2).*

5 Palpate any area of discoloration or mottling. Note if the involved area blanches with palpation or remains discolored or red. Nonblanchable erythema or skin temperature changes may be an important early indicator of a stage I pressure ulcer (see Box 18-1).	Early detection of pressure indicates need for more frequent position changes or the use of a pressure-redistribution device.
6 Do not massage any reddened or discolored pressure points.	Areas of nonblanchable erythema or discolored areas may indicate that deeper tissue damage is present. Massage in this area may worsen the inflammation by damaging underlying damaged blood vessels.
7 When positioning patient in bed, keep the head of the bed at a 30-degree angle or lower if patient's medical condition allows.	Pressure is reduced to the sacral area when the head of the bed is not at a high elevation.

Critical Decision Point *If patient requires a pressure-redistribution surface for the bed, consider an appropriate pressure-redistribution surface for the chair.*

8 Remove gloves, discard appropriately, and perform hand hygiene.	Reduces spread of microorganisms.

EVALUATION

1 Observe a patient's skin for areas at risk for change in color or texture.	Enables nurse to evaluate success of prevention techniques.
2 Observe tolerance of patient for position change.	Position changes sometimes interfere with patient's sleep and rest pattern.
3 Compare subsequent risk assessment scores.	Provides ongoing comparison of patient's risk level to facilitate appropriateness of plan of care.

Unexpected Outcomes	Related Interventions
1 Skin becomes mottled, reddened, purplish, or bluish.	• Refer patient to wound, ostomy, and continence nurse; dietitian; clinical nurse specialist (CNS); and physical therapist as necessary. Reevaluate position changes.
2 Patient reports sense of fatigue and inability to sleep.	• Modify patient's positioning and turning schedule to promote sleep.
3 Areas under pressure develop persistent discoloration, induration, or temperature changes.	• Refer patient to wound, ostomy, and continence nurse; dietitian; CNS; and physical therapist as necessary. • Modify patient's poistioning and turning schedule.

Recording and Reporting

- Record any skin changes, patient's risk score, and skin assessment. Describe positions, turning intervals, pressure-redistribution devices, and other prevention measures. Note patient's response to the interventions.
- Report need for additional consultations for the high-risk patient.

Teaching Considerations

- Assist patient (and family) with understanding multiple factors involved in preventing and treating pressure ulcers.
- Explain and demonstrate positioning options to achieve pressure redistribution.
- Explain the purpose and maintenance of pressure-redistribution devices (see Chapter 12).
- When teaching patients to change position for pressure redistribution, suggest using television programming and commercial intervals or a watch with an alarm as reminders.

Gerontological Considerations

- In older adults, a risk score of 18 is often the prediction of pressure ulcer risk on the Braden Scale (Bergstrom and others, 1998; Pieper, 2007).
- Reevaluate sitting posture and position because body weight and muscle tone change with age.

- In an older patient, the dermis demonstrates decreased thickness, causing thinning of the skin, especially over the legs and forearms. There is less subcutaneous tissue, leading to less padding protection over bony prominences, and the time for epidermal regeneration is diminished, leading to slower healing (Lyder, 2004).

Home Care Considerations

- Identify community resources, such as neighbors and relatives, for assistance if patient needs help with position changes, including after a fall.
- Customize pressure-redistribution maneuvers to an independent patient. Some individuals find that a watch with a timer or television commercials are helpful in remembering to complete pressure-relief techniques.
- Closely monitor home care patients older than 60 years for pressure ulcer development if they have any of the following risk factors: wheelchair dependence, incontinence, anemia, fracture, oxygen use, skin drainage, or adult child as primary caregiver (Langemo and Baranoski, 2003).
- Remind the patient and the caregiver that position changes need to occur while a patient is sitting in a chair. Consider shifts every 15 minutes. Small shifts such as moving or repositioning the legs redistributes pressure over bony prominences (WOCN, 2003).

TABLE 18-3	Guidelines for Pressure Ulcer Risk Assessment	
Level of Care	**Initial**	**Reassessment**
Acute care	On admission	• At least every day • Whenever a major change in patient's condition occurs • Intervals will vary depending upon how rapidly patient's condition is changing
Long-term care	On admission	• Weekly for first 4 weeks after admission • Routinely on quarterly basis • Whenever the patient's condition changes or deteriorates
Home care	On admission	• Every RN visit

Modified from Ayello EA, Braden B: How and why to do pressure ulcer risk assessment, *Adv Wound Care* 15(3):125, 2002.
RN, Registered nurse.

SKILL 18-2   Treatment of Pressure Ulcers

 Intermediate / Wound and Pressure Ulcer Care / Caring for Pressure Ulcers

Treatment of patients with pressure ulcers requires a holistic approach. You need to conduct a thorough assessment of the patient and the patient's ability to heal and have a good understanding of the identified goal for the patient's overall care before implementing topical pressure ulcer treatment. The first principle of managing a patient with a pressure ulcer is to relieve or control the contributing factors. Once you find the cause of the pressure ulcer, take steps to control or eliminate those factors. For example, if the ulcer is related to unrelieved pressure, choose the appropriate pressure-redistribution surface, develop a turning schedule, or choose the appropriate chair pad. Next perform an assessment to determine the patient's wound-healing abilities: cardiovascular and pulmonary function, nutritional status, and other conditions that interfere with wound healing, such as diabetes, steroid administration, and immunosuppression (Doughty and Sparks-Defriese, 2007).

The principle that guides the selection and use of topical dressings is to provide a wound environment that supports wound healing (Rolstad and Ovington, 2007). The best wound environment for healing is moist and free of necrotic tissue and infection. Interventions and dressings that support a clean, moist wound bed are

appropriate. An important assessment before initiating wound therapy is a thorough assessment of the wound and the periwound skin. Data from this assessment assist in planning the appropriate care for a patient with a pressure ulcer.

No specific studies demonstrate the benefit of using one cleanser over another for pressure ulcers. In the majority of cases, water or saline is sufficient for cleansing a clean wound (WOCN, 2003). When the wound is contaminated with debris or necrotic tissue or heavy drainage, use a commercial cleanser that is noncytotoxic to healthy tissue (e.g., Shur Clens). If the tissue in the wound is devitalized, consult with the patient's health care provider to consider debridement, which is the removal of devitalized tissue. Debridement is accomplished by the choice of dressing, the use of enzyme preparations, or surgical or laser techniques. The choice of the type of debridement will depend upon the condition of the wound, the type of devitalized tissue, and the pain tolerance of the patient.

Choose wound dressings to meet the characteristics of the wound bed (Rolstad and Ovington, 2007). The choice of a wound dressing depends on the type of wound tissue in the base of the wound, the amount of wound drainage, the presence or absence of infection, the location of the wound, the size of the wound, the ease of use, the cost-effectiveness, and comfort for the patient. Some categories of wound dressings include transparent films, hydrocolloids, hydrogels, foams, calcium alginates, gauze, and antimicrobial dressings (see Chapter 39). The use of dressings in the management of a pressure ulcer will change as the wound characteristics change; thus frequent wound evaluation is key.

Advanced wound care products used in select cases include growth factors, electrical stimulation, hyperbaric therapy, negative-pressure wound therapy, and tissue-engineered skin. Growth factors occur naturally in wound fluid and stimulate both granulation and epithelialization when applied topically. Pulsed electrical stimulation is a procedure usually performed by physical therapists with the goal of increased wound healing. Hyperbaric oxygen therapy uses increased amounts of pressurized oxygen delivered to patients in a variety of specialized methods. Negative-pressure wound therapy (such as the Wound V.A.C.) applies suction to remove excess fluid from the wound bed. The Wound V.A.C. works via a tubing system placed into a foam dressing placed into the wound and covered with a semiocclusive dressing. This therapy supports the proliferation of granulation tissue (see Chapter 39). Tissue-engineered skin develops living cells that you place over a clean wound bed to facilitate wound closure. Advanced wound therapies play an important role in pressure ulcer healing, but use only after consultation with a wound care expert.

Delegation Considerations

The skill of changing the pressure ulcer dressing cannot be delegated to the NAP. The nurse directs the NAP to:

- Report any wound drainage that might be on linens or intact skin, which indicates the need to change the dressing or to use an alternative dressing.
- Report any new areas of redness, blistering, or skin irritation.

Equipment

- ❑ Protective equipment: clean gloves, goggles, cover gown
- ❑ Plastic bag for dressing disposal
- ❑ Measuring device
- ❑ Sterile cotton-tipped applicators (check agency policy for use of sterile applicators)
- ❑ Topical agent (as ordered)
- ❑ Cleansing agent (as ordered)
- ❑ Sterile solution container
- ❑ Washbasin, washcloths, towels
- ❑ Dressing of choice
- ❑ Hypoallergenic tape (if needed)
- ❑ Documentation records

STEP	RATIONALE
ASSESSMENT	
1 Assess patient's level of comfort and need for pain medication (Dallan and others, 2004).	The dressing change should not be a traumatic event for a patient; evaluate wound pain before, during, and after wound care management (Krasner and others, 2007).
2 Determine if patient has allergies to topical agents or latex.	Latex gloves and topical agents contain elements that cause localized skin reactions.
3 Review the order for topical agent or dressing.	Ensures administration of proper medication and treatment.

Critical Decision Point *Determine if the order is consistent with established wound care guidelines and outcomes for the patient. If the order is not consistent with guidelines or varies from the identified outcome for the patient, review the order with the health care team.*

STEP	RATIONALE
4 Close room door or bedside curtains. Perform hand hygiene, and apply clean gloves.	Provides privacy. Reduces transmission of microorganisms and prevents accidental exposure to body fluids.
5 Position patient to allow dressing removal, and position plastic bag for dressing disposal.	Provides an area accessible for dressing change. Proper disposal of old dressing promotes proper handling of contaminated waste.
6 Assess each of patient's pressure ulcers and surrounding skin to determine ulcer characteristics, including the stage (see Box 18-1).	Staging is a way of assessing a pressure ulcer, based on the depth of tissue destruction.

Critical Decision Point *To correctly stage a pressure ulcer, you must be able to see the base of the wound. Therefore you cannot stage pressure ulcers that are covered with necrotic tissue until the eschar is debrided and the base of the wound is visible (NPUAP, 2007). Until debridement, document that the ulcer is unstageable. The staging system as recommended by the WOCN and the NPUAP does not include a stage for granulating wounds. "Downstaging" of granulating wounds is NOT appropriate because the full-thickness repair process involves replacement of the lost normal tissue with granulation tissue. For example, a granulating stage IV wound should NOT be "downstaged" to a stage III, because a stage III wound by definition is one with exposed subcutaneous tissue. Therefore a granulating stage IV wound is most appropriately classified as a "granulating stage IV" or "healing stage IV." If the stage IV wound is completely healed, it can be classified as a "healed stage IV," which conveys that the wound is now filled with granulation tissue and resurfaced with epithelium.*

STEP	RATIONALE
7 Assess the type of tissue in the wound bed. Color type will indicate the type of tissue. Black tissue is necrotic tissue, yellow or gray tissue is slough, and red tissue is granulation tissue. Record the approximate amount of each tissue in centimeters found in the wound bed using approximate percentages of each type of tissue.	The approximate percentage of each type of tissue in the wound will provide critical information on the progress of wound healing and the choice of dressing. A wound with a high percentage of black tissue will require debridement, yellow tissue or slough tissue indicates the presence of an infection or colonization, and granulation tissue will indicate a wound moving toward healing.

| STEP | RATIONALE |

8 Assess wounds on a frequent basis:

   a Consider using an assessment tool such as the Bates-Jensen Wound Assessment Tool (BWAT) (Bolton and others, 2004) (Fig. 18-3). Reassess the wound at each dressing change to determine whether modifications are necessary (WOCN, 2003).

Changes in the appearance of a wound indicate that you need to adjust the topical therapy to continue to move the wound toward healing.

BATES-JENSEN WOUND ASSESSMENT TOOL   NAME _____

Complete the rating sheet to assess pressure sore status. Evaluate each item by picking the response that best describes the wound and entering the score in the item score column for the appropriate date.

Location: Anatomic site. Circle, identify right (**R**) or left (**L**) and use "**X**" to mark site on body diagrams:

_____	Sacrum & coccyx	_____	Lateral ankle
_____	Trochanter	_____	Medial ankle
_____	Ischial tuberosity	_____	Heel Other Site _____

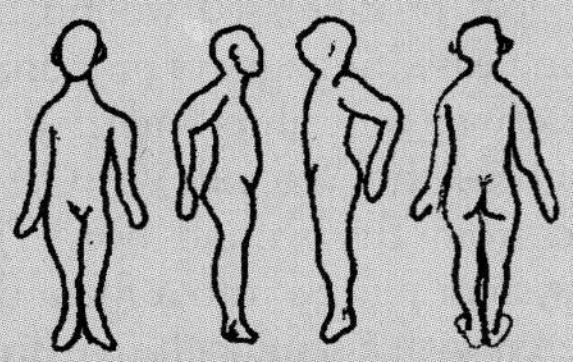

Shape: Overall wound pattern; assess by observing perimeter and depth.

Circle and <u>date</u> appropriate description:

_____	Irregular	_____	Linear or elongated
_____	Round/oval	_____	Bowl/boat
_____	Square/rectangle	_____	Butterfly Other Shape _____

Item	Assessment	Date	Date	Date
		Score	Score	Score
1. Size	1 = Length x width < 4 sq cm 2 = Length x width 4-16 sq cm 3 = Length x width 16.1-36 sq cm 4 = Length x width 36.1-80 sq cm 5 = Length x width > 80 sq cm			
2. Depth	1 = Non-blanchable erythema on intact skin 2 = Partial thickness skin loss involving epidermis &/or dermis 3 = Full thickness skin loss involving damage or necrosis of subcutaneous tissue; may extend down to but not through underlying fascia; &/or mixed partial & full thickness &/or tissue layers obscured by granulation tissue 4 = Obscured by necrosis 5 = Full thickness skin loss with extensive destruction, tissue necrosis or damage to muscle, bone or supporting structures			
3. Edges	1 = Indistinct, diffuse, none clearly visible 2 = Distinct, outline clearly visible, attached, even with wound base 3 = Well-defined, not attached to wound base 4 = Well-defined, not attached to base, rolled under, thickened 5 = Well-defined, fibrotic, scarred or hyperkeratotic			
4. Under-mining	1 = None present 2 = Undermining < 2 cm in any area 3 = Undermining 2-4 cm involving < 50% wound margins 4 = Undermining 2-4 cm involving > 50% wound margins 5 = Undermining > 4 cm in any area or tunneling in any area			
5. Necrotic Tissue Type	1 = None visible 2 = White/grey non-viable tissue &/or non-adherent yellow slough 3 = Loosely adherent yellow slough 4 = Adherent, soft, black eschar 5 = Firmly adherent, hard, black eschar			
6. Necrotic Tissue Amount	1 = None visible 2 = < 25% of wound bed covered 3 = 25% to 50% of wound covered 4 = > 50% and < 75% of wound covered 5 = 75% to 100% of wound covered			

© 2001 Barbara Bates-Jensen

FIG 18-3   Bates-Jensen Wound Assessment Tool. (*Courtesy Barbara Bates-Jensen.*)

STEP	RATIONALE

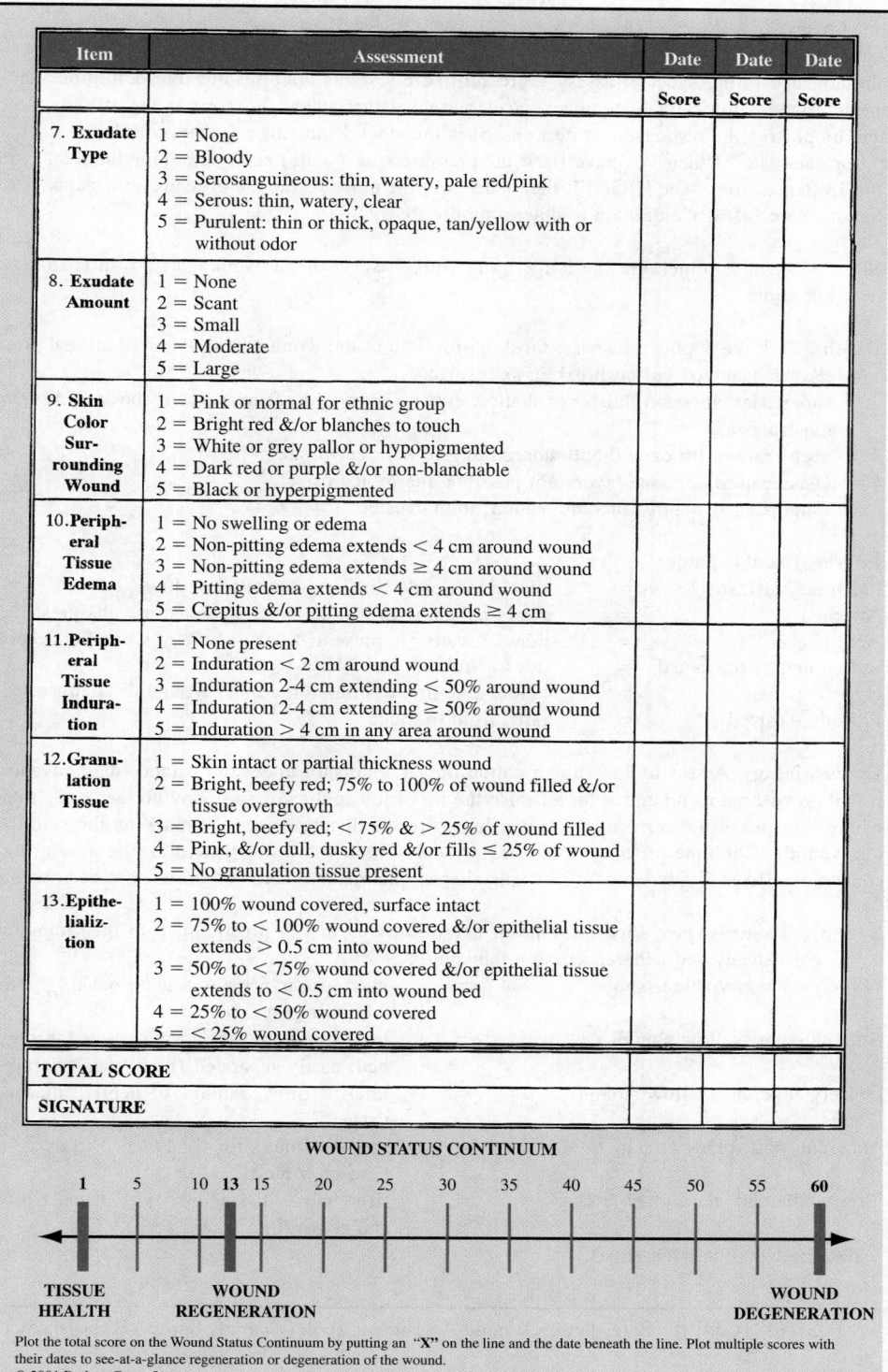

Item	Assessment	Date Score	Date Score	Date Score
7. **Exudate Type**	1 = None 2 = Bloody 3 = Serosanguineous: thin, watery, pale red/pink 4 = Serous: thin, watery, clear 5 = Purulent: thin or thick, opaque, tan/yellow with or without odor			
8. **Exudate Amount**	1 = None 2 = Scant 3 = Small 4 = Moderate 5 = Large			
9. **Skin Color Surrounding Wound**	1 = Pink or normal for ethnic group 2 = Bright red &/or blanches to touch 3 = White or grey pallor or hypopigmented 4 = Dark red or purple &/or non-blanchable 5 = Black or hyperpigmented			
10. **Peripheral Tissue Edema**	1 = No swelling or edema 2 = Non-pitting edema extends < 4 cm around wound 3 = Non-pitting edema extends ≥ 4 cm around wound 4 = Pitting edema extends < 4 cm around wound 5 = Crepitus &/or pitting edema extends ≥ 4 cm			
11. **Peripheral Tissue Induration**	1 = None present 2 = Induration < 2 cm around wound 3 = Induration 2-4 cm extending < 50% around wound 4 = Induration 2-4 cm extending ≥ 50% around wound 5 = Induration > 4 cm in any area around wound			
12. **Granulation Tissue**	1 = Skin intact or partial thickness wound 2 = Bright, beefy red; 75% to 100% of wound filled &/or tissue overgrowth 3 = Bright, beefy red; < 75% & > 25% of wound filled 4 = Pink, &/or dull, dusky red &/or fills ≤ 25% of wound 5 = No granulation tissue present			
13. **Epithelialization**	1 = 100% wound covered, surface intact 2 = 75% to < 100% wound covered &/or epithelial tissue extends > 0.5 cm into wound bed 3 = 50% to < 75% wound covered &/or epithelial tissue extends to < 0.5 cm into wound bed 4 = 25% to < 50% wound covered 5 = < 25% wound covered			
TOTAL SCORE				
SIGNATURE				

WOUND STATUS CONTINUUM

1   5   10 **13** 15   20   25   30   35   40   45   50   55   **60**

←———————————————————————————————————→

TISSUE HEALTH   WOUND REGENERATION   WOUND DEGENERATION

Plot the total score on the Wound Status Continuum by putting an "**X**" on the line and the date beneath the line. Plot multiple scores with their dates to see-at-a-glance regeneration or degeneration of the wound.
© 2001 Barbara Bates-Jensen

FIG 18-3, cont'd   For legend see opposite page.   *Continued*

WOUND ASSESSMENT TOOL

Instructions for use
General Guidelines:
Fill out the attached rating sheet to assess a pressure sore's status after reading the definitions and methods of assessment described below. Evaluate once a week and whenever a change occurs in the wound. Rate according to each item by picking the response that best describes the wound and entering that score in the item score column for the appropriate date. When you have rated the pressure sore on all items, determine the total score by adding together the 13-item scores. The HIGHER the total score, the more severe the pressure sore status. Plot total score on the Pressure Sore Status Continuum to determine progress.

Specific Instructions:

1. **Size**: Use ruler to measure the longest and widest aspect of the wound surface in centimeters; multiply length x width.

2. **Depth**: Pick the depth, thickness, most appropriate to the wound using these additional descriptions:
   1 = tissues damaged but no break in skin surface.
   2 = superficial, abrasion, blister or shallow crater. Even with, &/or elevated above skin surface (e.g., hyperplasia).
   3 = deep crater with or without undermining of adjacent tissue.
   4 = visualization of tissue layers not possible due to necrosis.
   5 = supporting structures include tendon, joint capsule.

3. **Edges**: Use this guide:
Indistinct, diffuse	=	unable to clearly distinguish wound outline.
Attached	=	even or flush with wound base, <u>no</u> sides or walls present; flat.
Not attached	=	sides or walls <u>are</u> present; floor or base of wound is deeper than edge.
Rolled under, thickened	=	soft to firm and flexible to touch.
Hyperkeratosis	=	callous-like tissue formation around wound & at edges.
Fibrotic, scarred	=	hard, rigid to touch.

4. **Undermining**: Assess by inserting a cotton tipped applicator under the wound edge; advance it as far as it will go without using undue force; raise the tip of the applicator so it may be seen or felt on the surface of the skin; mark the surface with a pen; measure the distance from the mark on the skin to the edge of the wound. Continue process around the wound. Then use a transparent metric measuring guide with concentric circles divided into 4 (25%) pie-shaped quadrants to help determine percent of wound involved.

5. **Necrotic Tissue Type**: Pick the type of necrotic tissue that is <u>predominant</u> in the wound according to color, consistency and adherence using this guide:
White/gray non-viable tissue	=	may appear prior to wound opening; skin surface is white or gray.
Non-adherent, yellow slough	=	thin, mucinous substance; scattered throughout wound bed; easily separated from wound tissue.
Loosely adherent, yellow slough	=	thick, stringy, clumps of debris; attached to wound tissue.
Adherent, soft, black eschar	=	soggy tissue; strongly attached to tissue in center or base of wound.
Firmly adherent, hard/black eschar	=	firm, crusty tissue; strongly attached to wound base <u>and</u> edges (like a hard scab).

© 2001 Barbara Bates-Jensen

FIG 18-3, cont'd Bates-Jensen Wound Assessment Tool. (*Courtesy Barbara Bates-Jensen.*)

STEP	RATIONALE

6. **Necrotic Tissue Amount**: Use a transparent metric measuring guide with concentric circles divided into 4 (25%) pie-shaped quadrants to help determine percent of wound involved.

7. **Exudate Type**: Some dressings interact with wound drainage to produce a gel or trap liquid. Before assessing exudate type, gently cleanse wound with normal saline or water. Pick the exudate type that is <u>predominant</u> in the wound according to color and consistency, using this guide:

Bloody	=	thin, bright red
Serosanguineous	=	thin, watery pale red to pink
Serous	=	thin, watery, clear
Purulent	=	thin or thick, opaque tan to yellow
Foul purulent	=	thick, opaque yellow to green with offensive odor

8. **Exudate Amount**: Use a transparent metric measuring guide with concentric circles divided into 4 (25%) pie-shaped quadrants to determine percent of dressing involved with exudate. Use this guide:

None	=	wound tissues dry.
Scant	=	wound tissues moist; no measurable exudate.
Small	=	wound tissues wet; moisture evenly distributed in wound; drainage involves $\leq$ 25% dressing.
Moderate	=	wound tissues saturated; drainage may or may not be evenly distributed in wound; drainage involves > 25% to $\leq$ 75% dressing.
Large	=	wound tissues bathed in fluid; drainage freely expressed; may or may not be evenly distributed in wound; drainage involves > 75% of dressing.

9. **Skin Color Surrounding Wound**: Assess tissues within 4 cm of wound edge. Dark-skinned persons show the colors "bright red" and "dark red" as a deepening of normal ethnic skin color or a purple hue. As healing occurs in dark-skinned persons, the new skin is pink and may never darken.

10. **Peripheral Tissue Edema**: Assess tissues within 4 cm of wound edge. Non-pitting edema appears as skin that is shiny and taut. Identify pitting edema by firmly pressing a finger down into the tissues and waiting for 5 seconds, on release of pressure, tissues fail to resume previous position and an indentation appears. Crepitus is accumulation of air or gas in tissues. Use a transparent metric measuring guide to determine how far edema extends beyond wound.

11. **Peripheral Tissue Induration**: Assess tissues within 4 cm of wound edge. Induration is abnormal firmness of tissues with margins. Assess by gently pinching the tissues. Induration results in an inability to pinch the tissues. Use a transparent metric measuring guide with concentric circles divided into 4 (25%) pie-shaped quadrants to determine percent of wound and area involved.

12. **Granulation Tissue**: Granulation tissue is the growth of small blood vessels and connective tissue to fill in full thickness wounds. Tissue is healthy when bright, beefy red, shiny and granular with a velvety appearance. Poor vascular supply appears as pale pink or blanched to dull, dusky red color.

13. **Epithelialization**: Epithelialization is the process of epidermal resurfacing and appears as pink or red skin. In partial thickness wounds it can occur throughout the wound bed as well as from the wound edges. In full thickness wounds it occurs from the edges only. Use a transparent metric measuring guide with concentric circles divided into 4 (25%) pie-shaped quadrants to help determine percent of wound involved and to measure the distance the epithelial tissue extends into the wound.

© 2001 Barbara Bates-Jensen

FIG 18-3, cont'd For legend see opposite page.

b   Note color, temperature, edema, moisture, and condition of skin around the ulcer. Remember to modify the assessment technique based on patient's individual skin color (see Box 18-2).

Skin condition at the ulcer edge indicates progressive tissue damage. Maceration on the periwound skin shows the need to alter the choice of the wound dressing.

STEP	RATIONALE

c Measure the wound dimensions in centimeters. Measure using a wound measurement guide (see illustration); measure two dimensions, length and width, per the facility's protocol.

Consistency in how you measure the wound is important for determining wound progress.

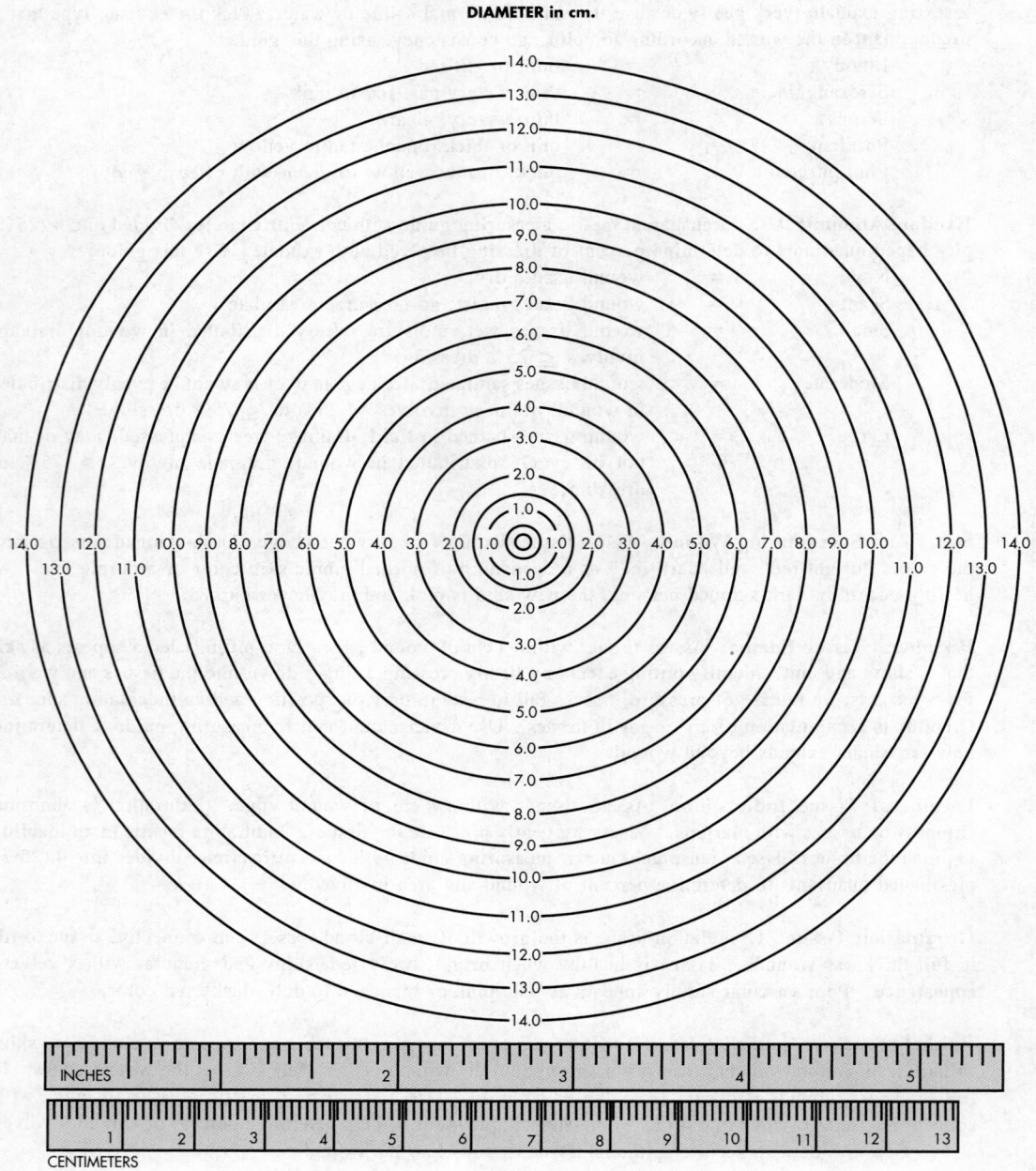

DIAMETER in cm.

DISCARD AFTER USE

STEP 8c   Measuring guide. Center over wound to be measured. (*Modified from Maklebust J, Sieggreen M: Pressure ulcers: guidelines for prevention and nursing management, ed 2, Springhouse, Pa, 1996, Springhouse.*)

d Measure the depth of the pressure ulcer using a sterile, cotton-tipped applicator or other device that will allow measurement of wound depth.

  (1) Place the applicator *gently* into the pressure ulcer until it touches the bottom.

Depth measure is important for determining the amount of tissue loss.

STEP	RATIONALE

(2) Mark the place on the applicator where it reaches the top of the wound, and then remove the applicator from the ulcer.

(3) Measure the distance from the tip of the applicator to the mark using a measuring tape or ruler to determine the depth of the pressure ulcer.

e Measure depth of undermining tissue. Use a cotton-tipped applicator, and gently probe under skin edges (see illustration).

Undermining represents the loss of the underlying tissue. Undermining may indicate progressive tissue necrosis, or the ongoing injury from shearing.

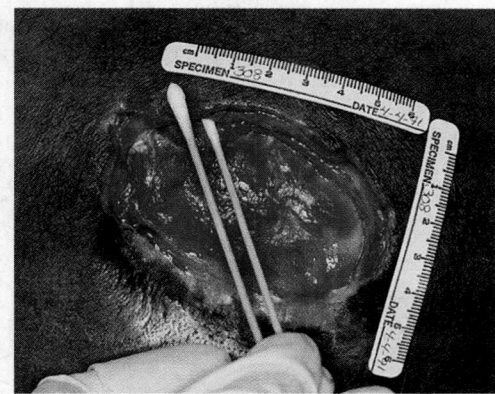

STEP 8e Measuring depth of undermining of skin.

9 Remove gloves, discard appropriately, and perform hand hygiene.

Reduces transmission of microorganisms. Repeated hand hygiene is necessary as the nurse assesses other pressure areas. Different organisms contaminate different wounds. Failure to repeatedly perform hand hygiene and use standard precautions causes cross-wound contamination.

10 Assessment of the entire patient is necessary in developing a pressure ulcer treatment plan. Include in this assessment the identification of complications and comorbid conditions, a nutritional assessment, an assessment of pain, a psychosocial assessment, and an evaluation of the individual's risks for additional pressure ulcers (see Skill 18-1).

Critical Decision Point *When you suspect malnutrition, consider a nutritional consultation to modify patient's diet to promote wound healing.*

11 Educate patient and caregiver about prevention, treatment, and factors contributing to the recurrence of pressure ulcers (AHCPR, 1994; WOCN, 2003).

Explanations relieve anxiety and promote cooperation during procedure. Patient and caregiver need to partner with the health care providers to prevent further skin breakdown.

NURSING DIAGNOSES

- Deficient knowledge regarding pressure ulcer treatment plan
- Imbalanced nutrition: less than body requirements
- Impaired physical mobility
- Impaired skin integrity
- Ineffective tissue perfusion
- Pain (acute, chronic)

Individualize related factors based on patient's condition or needs.

PLANNING

1 Expected outcomes following completion of procedure:
- Ulcer drainage decreases.

- Granulation tissue is present in wound base.
- Skin surrounding ulcer remains healthy and intact.

- Nutrition is adequate to compensate for wound fluid losses and wound repair (see illustration).

Less drainage from the ulcer reflects a decrease in the inflammatory process and progress toward healing.
Evidence that wound is moving toward healing.
No additional damage is evident; the dressing is appropriate to contain wound drainage.
Nutritional therapy provides adequate protein to support wound healing.

STEP	RATIONALE

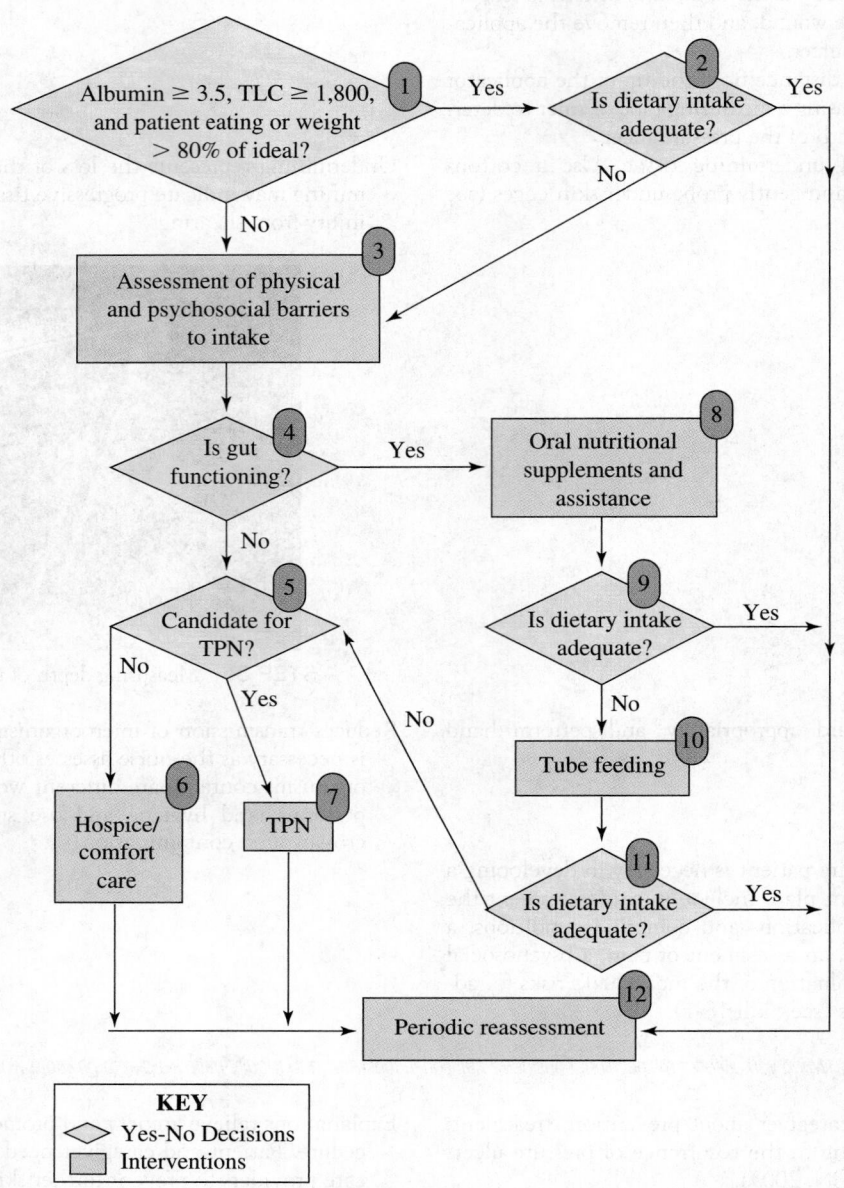

STEP 1   Nutritional assessment and support. *TLC*, Total lymphacyte count; *TPN*, total parenteral nutrition. *(From Bergstrom N and others: Treatment of pressure ulcers, AHCPR Pub No. 95-0652, Rockville, Md, 1994, Agency for Health Care Policy and Research, Public Health Service, U.S. Department of Health and Human Services.)*

- Patient's overall skin is protected from further breakdown.

Patient remains at risk for further breakdown while existing ulcer heals.

2   Explain procedure to patient and family. Individualize the teaching plan for older adult patients, taking into account the normal aging changes that affect learning.

Preparatory explanations relieve anxiety, correct any misconceptions about the ulcer and its treatment, and offer an opportunity for patient and family education.

3   Prepare the following necessary equipment and supplies:
   a   Washbasin, warm water, soap, washcloth, and bath towel
   b   Normal saline or other wound-cleansing agent in sterile solution container

Used to bathe surrounding skin.

Cleanse ulcer surface before the application of topical agents and a new dressing.

Critical Decision Point   *Use only noncytotoxic agents to clean ulcers, such as Shur Clens.*

STEP	RATIONALE
c Prescribed topical agent:	
(1) Enzymatic agents: Be sure to follow the manufacturer's specific directions for the frequency of application.	Enzymes debride dead tissue to clean ulcer surface. Enzymes are not applied to healthy tissue.
OR	
(2) Topical antibiotics.	Topical antibiotics are used to decrease the bioburden of the wound and should be considered for use if no healing is noted after 2 to 4 weeks of optimal care (AHCPR, 1994; WOCN, 2003).

Critical Decision Point *If using an enzymatic debriding agent, do not use wound-cleansing agents with metals.*

STEP	RATIONALE
d Dressing (Table 18-4) (see also Chapter 39)	The dressing should maintain a moist environment for the wound while keeping the surrounding skin dry (AHCPR, 1994).
(1) Select an appropriate dressing based on the pressure ulcer characteristics, purpose for which the dressing is intended, and patient care setting.	
(2) Gauze. Apply as a moist-to-dry dressing, a dry cover dressing when using enzymatic agent or topical antibiotics, or as a means to deliver solution to a wound (see Chapter 39).	Gauze protects a wound and is highly absorptive.

Critical Decision Point *Make sure the dressing's absorbency is adequate for the amount of wound drainage. Check that wound does not dry out or that surrounding skin does not become macerated.*

STEP	RATIONALE
(3) Transparent dressing. Apply over superficial ulcers and skin subjected to friction.	Maintains a moist environment.

Critical Decision Point *Use transparent dressings for autolytic debridement of noninfected pressure ulcers.*

STEP	RATIONALE
(4) Hydrocolloid dressing.	Maintains moist environment to facilitate wound healing while protecting the wound base.

Critical Decision Point *Use a hydrocolloid to protect skin from friction and shear injury. Some brands have custom shapes available for specific anatomical parts such as heel, elbows, and sacrum.*

STEP	RATIONALE
(5) Hydrogel. Available in a sheet or in a tube.	Maintains moist environment to facilitate wound healing.
(6) Calcium alginate.	Highly absorbent of wound exudate in heavily draining wounds.
(7) Foam.	Protective and will prevent wound dehydration; also absorbs small to moderate amounts of drainage.
e Hypoallergenic tape or adhesive dressing sheet.	Used to secure nonadherent dressing. Prevents skin irritation and tearing.

IMPLEMENTATION

STEP	RATIONALE
1 Assemble needed supplies at beside. Close room door or bedside curtains. Perform hand hygiene, and apply gloves. Open sterile packages and topical solution containers. (Wear goggles and moisture-proof cover gown if potential for contamination from spray exists when cleansing the wound.)	Maintains patient privacy. Reduces transmission of microorganisms.
2 Remove bed linen and patient's gown to expose ulcer and surrounding skin. Keep remaining body parts draped.	Prevents unnecessary exposure of body parts.
3 Gently wash skin surrounding ulcer with warm water and soap.	Cleansing of skin surface reduces bacteria.
4 Rinse area thoroughly with water.	Soap can be irritating to skin.
5 Gently dry skin thoroughly by patting lightly with towel.	Retained moisture causes maceration of skin layers.
6 Perform hand hygiene, and change gloves.	Maintains aseptic technique during cleansing, measuring, and application of dressings. Refer to institutional policy regarding use of clean or sterile gloves.
7 Cleanse ulcer thoroughly with normal saline or prescribed wound-cleansing agent.	Cleansing wound at each dressing change minimizes the trauma to the wound (WOCN, 2003).

STEP	RATIONALE
8 Apply topical agents, if prescribed: a Enzymes:	Follow manufacturer's directions for frequency of application. Be aware of what solutions inactivate the enzymes, and avoid their use in wound cleansing.
(1) Using a sterile cotton-tipped applicator (check agency policy), apply a small amount of enzyme debridement ointment directly to the necrotic areas on the base of pressure ulcer. Avoid getting the enzyme on the surrounding skin. Apply per manufacturer's directions. **Do not apply enzyme to surrounding skin.**	Proper distribution of ointment ensures effective action. Some enzymes can cause burning, paresthesia, and dermatitis to surrounding skin.
(2) Place gauze dressing directly over ulcer, and tape in place. Follow specific manufacturer's recommendation for type of dressing material to use to cover a pressure ulcer when using enzymatic agent.	Protects wound and prevents removal of ointment during turning or repositioning.
b Hydrogel agents:	
(1) Cover surface of ulcer with hydrogel using sterile cotton-tipped applicator or gloved finger.	Provides a moist environment.
(2) Apply a secondary dressing, such as dry gauze, hydrocolloid, or transparent dressing over gel to completely cover ulcer.	Holds hydrogel against wound surface because amorphous hydrogel (in tube) or sheet form does not adhere to the wound and requires a secondary dressing to hold it in place.
c Calcium alginate dressings:	Use in heavily draining wounds.
(1) Pack wound with alginate using sterile cotton-tipped applicator or gloved finger.	
(2) Apply a secondary dressing, such as dry gauze, foam, or hydrocolloid over alginate.	Holds alginate against wound surface.
9 Reposition patient comfortably off pressure ulcer.	Avoids accidental removal of dressings. Guards against contamination of dressing.
10 Remove gloves, and dispose of soiled supplies. Perform hand hygiene.	Reduces transmission of microorganisms.

EVALUATION

1 Observe skin surrounding ulcer for inflammation, edema, and tenderness.	A clean pressure ulcer shows evidence of movement toward healing within 2 to 4 weeks.
2 Inspect dressings and exposed ulcers, observing for drainage, foul odor, and tissue necrosis. Monitor patient for signs and symptoms of infection, including fever and elevated white blood cell (WBC) count.	Ulcers can become infected.
3 Compare subsequent ulcer measurements.	Allows comparison of serial measurements to assess wound healing.
4 Use one of the scales designed to measure wound healing, such as the PUSH Tool (Box 18-3) (Nix, 2007) or the BWAT (Bates-Jensen, 1990).	Provides a standard method of data collection that will demonstrate wound progress or lack thereof.

Critical Decision Point *Deterioration of a patient's condition or an ulcer's condition indicates the need for reevaluation of the treatment plan (AHCPR, 1994).*

Unexpected Outcomes	Related Interventions
1 Skin surrounding ulcer becomes macerated.	• Reduce exposure of surrounding skin to topical agents and moisture. • Select a dressing that has increased moisture-absorbing capacity.
2 Ulcer becomes deeper with increased drainage and/or development of necrotic tissue.	• Review current wound care management. • Consult with multidisciplinary team regarding changes in wound care regimen. • Obtain wound cultures (see Chapter 43).
3 Pressure ulcer extends beyond original margins.	• Monitor for systemic signs and symptoms of poor wound healing, such as abnormal laboratory results (WBC count, levels of hemoglobin/hematocrit, serum albumin, serum prealbumin, total proteins), weight loss, and fluid imbalances. • Assess and revise current turning schedule. • Consider further pressure-redistribution devices.

Recording and Reporting

- Record appearance of ulcer in patient's record.
- Describe type of topical agent used, dressing applied, and patient's response.
- Report any deterioration in ulcer appearance to nurse in charge or health care provider.

Teaching Considerations

- Discuss treatment, and identify individual(s) who will assist with care at home.
- Discuss process of wound healing and expected wound appearance. For example, discuss patient's perception about appearance of the pressure ulcer. Sometimes eschar looks like a scab that indicates wound healing.
- Discuss with patient and support persons perceptions about size of pressure ulcer. Many people think that a "bedsore" is small, about 1 inch. Some of the larger wounds, especially after debridement, are very troublesome to patients and support persons.
- Discuss with patient and support persons perceptions about treatment. Some patients and caregivers believe it is cruel for staff to keep turning and positioning the patient every 2 hours. Some misunderstand some dressing change techniques such as pulling out the dried gauze dressing used for mechanical debridement.
- Identify the signs, symptoms, and four stages of ulcers to report to the health care team.
- Review prevention guidelines to prevent further breakdown.
- Discuss options for maintaining good nutrition.

Gerontological Considerations

- Wound healing is often slower in the older adult (Doughty and Sparks-Defriese, 2007).

- The normal reduction in the Langerhans cells in the older adult's epidermis causes a decrease in T-cell function and immunity.
- Because older skin has a slower and less intense inflammatory reaction, monitor older patients more closely for altered responses to skin irritants.

Home Care Considerations

- Consider caregiver time when selecting a dressing. In the home care setting, caregivers may sometimes choose more expensive dressing materials to reduce the frequency of dressing changes (AHCPR, 1994).
- Some patients have more time than financial resources. Some choose a less expensive treatment option such as dressing material, especially if there is no third-party reimbursement. Another example is teaching the family to make a normal saline solution rather than buying it ready-made.
- Identify clean storage area for dressing supplies. Determine availability of required supplies. Discuss need for home care nurse.
- Discuss need for home pressure-redistribution surface or bed. Identify adaptive equipment needed to care for patient at home.
- Medicare regulations limit reimbursement of some types of support surfaces in the treatment of pressure ulcers.

Long-Term Care Considerations

- Rehabilitation units often use a variety of support surfaces and beds.
- Some patients may be discharged to long-term care facilities that specialize in pressure ulcer and wound care.

TABLE 18-4	Treatment Options by Ulcer Stage				
Ulcer Stage	**Ulcer Status**	**Dressing**	**Comments***	**Expected Change**	**Adjuvants**
I	Intact	None	Allows visual assessment.	Resolves slowly without epidermal loss over 7 to 14 days.	Turning schedule. Support hydration. Nutritional support. Pressure-redistribution mattress or chair cushion.
		Transparent dressing	Protects from shear. Do not use in the presence of excessive moisture.		
		Hydrocolloid	May not allow visual assessment.		
II	Clean	Hydrocolloid	Limits shear. Change when seal of dressing breaks, maximal wear time 7 days.	Heals through reepithelialization.	See previous stage. Manage incontinence.
		Hydrogel	Provides a moist environment.		
III	Clean	Hydrocolloid	See stage II clean.	Heals through granulation and reepithelialization.	See previous stages. Evaluate pressure-redistribution needs.
		Hydrogel foam	Apply over wound to protect and absorb moisture.		
		Calcium alginate	Use when there is significant exudate. Cover with secondary dressing.		
		Gauze	Use with normal saline or other prescribed solution. Wring out excess solution; unfold to make contact with wound.		
		Growth factors	Use with gauze per manufacturer's instructions.		

Continued

TABLE 18-4 | Treatment Options by Ulcer Stage—cont'd

Ulcer Stage	Ulcer Status	Dressing	Comments*	Expected Change	Adjuvants
IV	Clean	Hydrogel	See stage III clean.	Heals through granulation, scar tissue development and reepithelialization.	Surgical consultation may be necessary for closure. See stages I, II, and III.
	Eschar	Calcium alginate	See stage III clean.		
		Gauze	See stage III clean.		
		Growth factors	Use with gauze.		
		Adherent film	Will facilitate softening of eschar.	Eschar will lift at the edges as healing progresses.	See previous stages. Surgical consultation may be considered for debridement.
		Hydrocolloid	Will facilitate softening of eschar.		
		Gauze plus ordered solution	Will deliver solution and wick wound drainage.		May be considered for slow debridement.
		Enzymes	Will break down eschar, providing debridement.	Eschar will loosen over time.	
		None	Rarely, if eschar is dry and intact, no dressing is used, allowing eschar to act as physiological cover.		

*As with *all* occlusive dressings, wounds should not be clinically infected.

BOX 18-3 | PUSH Tool 3.0

Patient Name: _____   Patient ID#: _____
Ulcer Location: _____   Date: _____

Directions:

Observe and measure the pressure ulcer. Categorize the ulcer with respect to surface area, exudate, and type of wound tissue. Record a sub-score for each of these ulcer characteristics. Add the sub-scores to obtain the total score. A comparison of total scores measured over time provides an indication of the improvement or deterioration in pressure ulcer healing.

Length × width	0	1	2	3	4	5	Sub-score
	0 cm²	<0.3 cm²	0.3-0.6 cm²	0.7-1.0 cm²	1.1-2.0 cm²	2.1-3.0 cm²	
	6	**7**	**8**	**9**	**10**		
	3.1-4.0 cm²	4.1-8.0 cm²	8.1-12.0 cm²	12.1-24.0 cm²	>24.0 cm²		
Exudate amount	**0** None	**1** Light	**2** Moderate	**3** Heavy			Sub-score
Tissue type	**0** Closed	**1** Epithelial tissue	**2** Granulation tissue	**3** Slough	**4** Necrotic tissue		Sub-score
							Total score

Length × Width: Measure the greatest length (head to toe) and the greatest width (side to side) using a centimeter ruler. Multiply these two measurements (length × width) to obtain an estimate of surface area in square centimeters (cm²) *Caveat:* Always use a centimeter ruler and always use the same method each time the ulcer is measured.

Exudate amount: Estimate the amount of exudate (drainage) present after removal of the dressing and before applying any topical agent to the ulcer. Estimate the exudate (drainage) as none, light, moderate, or heavy.

Tissue type: This refers to the types of tissue that are present in the wound (ulcer) bed. Score as a "4" if there is any necrotic tissue present. Score as a "3" if there is any amount of slough present and necrotic tissue is absent. Score as a "2" if the wound is clean and contains granulation tissue. A superficial wound that is re-epithelizing is scored as a "1." When the wound is closed, score as a "0."

4—Necrotic Tissue (Eschar): black, brown, or tan tissue that adheres firmly to the wound bed or ulcer edges and may be either firmer or softer than surrounding skin.

3—Slough: Yellow or white tissue that adheres to the ulcer bed in strings or thick clumps, or is mucinous.

2—Granulation Tissue: pink or beefy red tissue with a shiny, moist, granular appearance.

1—Epithelial Tissue: for superficial ulcers, new pink or shiny tissue (skin) that grows in from the edges or as islands on the ulcer surface.

0—Closed/Resurfaced: The wound is completely covered with epithelium (new skin).

Version 3.0: 2004 National Pressure Ulcer Advisory Panel.

CRITICAL THINKING EXERCISES

Ms. Willet is a 72-year-old white woman who recently underwent a total hip replacement, left side. Her significant medical history includes rheumatoid arthritis and coronary artery disease. This is her first postoperative day, and she is resting in bed with an immobilizer (a foam wedge that is placed between her thighs to keep her hip in position) in place. She weights 200 pounds and is approximately 5 feet 6 inches tall. A physical therapist is scheduled to see her today to assist her into a sitting position. When the physical therapist is not available, Ms. Willet is on bed rest. Skin assessment reveals a 2.5-cm, round, black right heel ulcer, as well as a 2-cm red warm spot located over the sacrum.

1 The Braden risk assessment tool was used to determine the risk factors that place Ms. Willet at risk for skin breakdown. What factors in the above scenario may contribute to the potential for skin breakdown?
2 The black tissue on Ms. Willet's heel is best described as:
   a Granulation
   b Eschar
   c Slough
   d Induration
3 The red warm spot noted over her sacrum is described as:
   a Erythema
   b Sheet burn
   c Blistering
   d Bruising
   Explain your choice.
4 Identify the likely cause of the red warm area over Ms. Willett's sacrum, and name one approach to determine if there is skin breakdown. Explain your choice.

REVIEW QUESTIONS

1 A nurse on a surgical unit is providing care to patients who have recently undergone major abdominal procedures. How often should a pressure ulcer risk assessment be performed for these patients?
   1 At least every day of their hospital stay
   2 Upon admission to the unit, on a regularly scheduled basis, and as their condition changes
   3 Every other day until the fifth postoperative day
   4 If indicated by the presence of a history of pressure ulcers
2 A patient who is completely immobile and who does not make even slight changes in body or extremity position without assistance is being assessed for the risk for developing a pressure ulcer using the Braden scale. What would be the appropriate intervention to prevent pressure ulcers in this patient?
   1 Use a moisture barrier ointment at least 3 times per day.
   2 Consult with the wound clinical nurse specialist about the most appropriate bed surface to reduce pressure.
   3 Order a nutrition consultation to be sure that the patient has adequate vitamin and mineral intake.
   4 Consult with the physical therapy staff to determine exercises to increase muscle strength.
3 When the patient's skin integrity is assessed, an ulcer is noted over the sacral area. This ulcer is approximately 2 cm wide and 3 cm long, with the base of the ulcer covered with dark, hard, adherent tissue. What stage is this pressure ulcer?
   1 Stage II, a partial-thickness ulcer
   2 Stage III, a full-thickness ulcer because of the involvement of all tissue layers
   3 Stage IV, a full-thickness ulcer that must be involving supporting tissue because of the hard dark tissue, which is defined as eschar

4 This pressure ulcer cannot be staged because the wound base must be visible to assess the depth of tissue destruction.
4 An order for a hydrocolloid dressing is written for a patient with a pressure ulcer. What is the rationale for using a hydrocolloid dressing?
   1 It provides an antibiotic solution to decrease surface bacteria, which helps healing.
   2 It protects the wound base and provides a moist environment.
   3 It can be changed several times per day without damaging the wound bed.
   4 It contains a debriding agent to clean a wound environment.
5 The pediatric nursing team is orienting new nurses on preventing pressure ulcers in neonates and young children. Where should the nurses check frequently for the occurrence of these ulcerations in these children?
   1 Shoulders
   2 Head
   3 Sacrum
   4 Heels

REFERENCES

AHCPR Panel for the Prediction and Prevention of Pressure Ulcers in Adults: *Pressure ulcers in adults: prediction and prevention,* Clinical practice guideline No. 3, Pub No. 92-0047, Rockville, Md, 1992, Public Health Service, U.S. Department of Health and Human Services.

Ayello EA, Braden B: How and why do pressure ulcer risk assessment, *Adv Wound Care* 15(3):125, 2002.

Bates-Jensen B: New pressure ulcer status tool, *Decubitus* 3:14, 1990.

Bennett MA: Report of the Task Force on the Implications for Darkly Pigmented Intact Skin in the Prediction and Prevention of Pressure Ulcers, *Adv Wound Care* 8(6):34, 1995.

Bergstrom N and others: *Treatment of pressure ulcers,* AHCPR Pub No. 95-0652, Rockville, Md, 1994, Agency for Health Care Policy and Research, Public Health Service, U.S. Department of Health and Human Services,

Bolton L and others: Wound-healing outcomes using a standardized assessment and care in clinical practice, *J Wound Ostomy Continence Nurs* 31(2):65, 2004.

Dallan LE and others: Pain management and wounds. In Baranoski S, Ayello EA, editors: *Wound care essentials: practice principles,* Philadelphia, 2004, Lippincott, Williams.

Doughty DB, Sparks-Defriese B: Wound-healing physiology. In Bryant RA, Nix DP, editors: *Acute and chronic wounds: current management concepts,* ed 3, St. Louis, 2007, Mosby.

Henderson CT and others: Draft definition of stage I pressure ulcers: inclusion of persons with darkly pigmented skin, *Adv Wound Care* 10(5):16, 1997.

Galanti GA: *Caring for patients from different cultures,* ed 3, Philadelphia, 2004, University of Pennsylvania Press.

Gray M and others. Moisture vs. pressure: making sense out of perineal wounds, *J Wound Ostomy Continence Nurs* 34:134, 2007.

Langemo D, Baranoski S: Key points on caring for pressure ulcer in home care, *Home Healthc Nurse* 21:309, 2003.

Lyder CH: Regulation and wound care. In Baranoski S, Ayello EA, editors: *Wound care essentials: practice principles,* Philadelphia, 2004, Lippincott, Williams.

Krasner DL and others: Managing wound pain. In Bryant RA, Nix DP, editors: Acute and chronic wounds: current management concepts, ed 3, St. Louis, 2007, Mosby.

Maklebust J, Sieggreen M: *Pressure ulcers: guidelines for prevention and nursing management,* ed 2, Springhouse, Pa, 1996, Springhouse.

National Pressure Ulcer Advisory Panel: *NPUAP pressure ulcer definition and stages,* 2007, http://www.npuap.org/pr2.htm, accessed August 19, 2007.

Nix DP: Patient assessment and evaluation of healing. In Bryant RA, Nix DP, editors: *Acute and chronic wounds: current management concepts,* ed 3, St. Louis, 2007, Mosby.

Norton D and others: An *investigation of geriatric nursing problems in hospital,* 1962, reissue, Edinburgh, 1975, Churchill Livingstone.

Panel for the Prediction and Prevention of Pressure Ulcers in Adults: Pressure ulcers in adults: prediction and prevention, Clinical practice guideline No. 3, Pub No. 92-0047, Rockville, Md, 1992, Agency for Health Care Policy and Research, Public Health Service, U.S. Department of Health and Human Services.

Pieper B: Mechanical forces: pressure, shear and friction. In Bryant RA, Nix DP, editors: *Acute and chronic wounds: current management concepts,* ed 3, St. Louis, 2007, Mosby.

Rolstad BS, Ovington LG: Principles of wound management. In Bryant RA, Nix DP, editors: *Acute and chronic wounds: current management concepts,* ed 3, St. Louis, 2007, Mosby.

Stotts N: Nutritional assessment and support. In Bryant RA, Nix DP, editors: *Acute and chronic wounds: current management concepts,* ed 3, St. Louis, 2007, Mosby.

Trelease CC: Developing standards for wound care, *Ostomy Wound Manage* 26:50, 1988.

Whittington KT, Briones R. National Prevalence and Incidence Study: 6-year sequential acute care data, *Adv Skin Wound Care* 17:490, 2004.

Wound, Ostomy and Continence Nurses Society: *Guideline for prevention and management of pressure ulcers,* WOCN clinical practice guidelines series, Glenview, Ill, 2003, The Association.

RESEARCH REFERENCES

Bergstrom N, Braden, BJ: Predictive validity of the Braden scale among black and white subjects, *Nurs Res* 51(6):398, 2002.

Bergstrom N and others: Predicting pressure ulcer risk: a multisite study of the predictive validity of the Braden scale, *Nur Res* 47:261, 1998.

Bolton LB and others: The impact of nursing interventions: overview of effective interventions, outcomes, measures, and priorities for future research, *Med Care Res Rev* 64:123S, 2007.

Braden BJ, Bergstrom N: Clinical utility of the Braden scale for predicting pressure sore risk, *Decubitus* 2(3):44, 1989.

Braden BJ, Bergstrom N: Predictive utility of the Braden scale for predicting pressure sore risk, *Res Nurs Health* 17:459, 1994.

Jones KR, Fennie K. Factors influencing pressure ulcer healing in adults over 50: an exploratory study, *J Am Med Dir Assoc* 8:378, 2007.

Kosiak M: Etiology and pathology of decubitus ulcers, *Arch Phys Med Rehabil* 40:62, 1959.

Lyder CH and others: The Braden scale for pressure ulcer risk: evaluating the predictive validity in black and Latino/Hispanic elders, *Appl Nurs Res* 12(2):60, 1999.

Lyder CH and others: Quality of care for hospitalized Medicare patients at risk for pressure ulcers, *Arch Intern Med* 161:1549, 2001.

Reddy M and others: Preventing pressure ulcers: a systematic review, *JAMA* 296:974, 2006.

Spilsbury K and others: Pressure ulcers and their treatment and effects on quality of life: hospital inpatient perspectives, *J Adv Nurs* 57:494, 2007.

Sprigle S and others: Clinical skin temperature measurement to predict incipient pressure ulcers, *Adv Skin Wound Care* 14:133, 2001.

Care of Eye and Ear Prostheses

19

KEY TERMS

Audiologist

Cerumen

Enucleation

Prosthesis

Refractive error

MEDIA RESOURCES

- evolve http://evolve.elsevier.com/Perry/skills
  learning system
  - Review Questions

OBJECTIVES

Mastery of content in this chapter will enable the nurse to:
- Explain proper care of eye and ear prostheses.
- Identify guidelines used in caring for eye and ear prostheses.
- Correctly remove, store, clean, and insert a contact lens.
- Explain the rationale for maintaining aseptic technique during care of an artificial eye.
- Correctly perform eye and ear irrigations.
- Describe techniques that determine whether a hearing aid functions properly.
- Correctly remove, clean, and reinsert a hearing aid.

Artificial sensory devices, known as prostheses, replace or restore sensory function to diseased or lost body parts. Eyeglasses and contact lenses help to restore visual loss, and hearing aids improve sound reception. A patient may also depend on a prosthetic device to maintain an attractive appearance. Artificial eyes in particular help patients maintain a normal appearance when an eye is lost as a result of injury or disease.

Any prosthesis must fit and work properly if patients are to function optimally within their environment. Breakage or loss may result in serious impairment that can put a patient at risk for injury and interfere with communication, isolate the patient socially, and increase patient dependence and thereby threaten self-esteem. Understandably, patients are especially sensitive about care of contact lenses, hearing aids, or artificial eyes.

Prosthetic devices require regular cleaning to ensure function and prevent injury. Most patients have an established routine for cleaning their prostheses. When patients are unable to care for their prostheses, you must understand the correct way to clean, handle, and store contact lenses, hearing aids, and artificial eyes. Careful handling of prostheses is vital to avoiding damage to these devices or to a patients' eyes or ears.

EVIDENCE-BASED PRACTICE TRENDS

Vision and hearing impairments, either as separate problems or in combination, have the potential to cause cognitive function decline or contribute to acute confusion, especially in older adults (Crews and others, 2006; Ebersole and others, 2008). In determining risk factors associated with acute confusion in the long-term care setting, both vision and hearing deficits are significant risk factors (Cacchione and others, 2003a; Cacchione and others, 2003b).

Early identification of sensory loss and prompt interventions to improve vision and/or hearing loss is beneficial in reducing confusion, improving orientation, and increasing patient independence. In some instances hearing loss is related to a buildup of cerumen. Once this buildup is removed, hearing improves and the patient's cognitive function improves. In addition, these patients are better able to hear, understand, and follow health care instructions relating to self–medication administration, symptom management, and when to return to the health care provider.

In community settings sensory impairments negatively impact the use of community support services and health-related quality of life (Tay and others, 2007). The decline in health-related quality is especially problematic in the older adult population. As a result of this decline, older adults are at risk for a decline in function, independence, and socialization.

CULTURAL CONSIDERATIONS

Communication is vital to all people from all cultures. When vision and/or hearing is threatened or impaired, that change must be understood in terms of the patient's culture. In cultures such as the Navaho Indian and in some Asian and Middle Eastern cultures, limited eye contact is the norm and is a nonverbal form of respect (Galanti, 2004). Changes in the ability to move the eyes, as with a prosthesis, present a social difficulty because the patient is unable to lower the eyes.

The Navajo are comfortable with the soft-spoken word and silence (Galanti, 2004). Hearing impairments may force a patient's family and friends to speak more loudly. In addition, because of the comfort with silence, one can easily mistake a patient's silence for a measure of comfort and never correctly assess what the patient is able to hear or if the information is heard correctly. At times you will use touch to get the attention of a patient with decreased hearing. In some cultures, such as Muslim, same-sex caregivers are required in order to use touch. Remember this before using touch to gain a patient's attention.

Skill Performance Guidelines

1. Let the patient be a resource in the care of each device. Although it is the nurse's responsibility to ensure patients do not damage the devices or injure themselves, patients familiar with their devices are likely to have an established routine and helpful tips.
2. Always protect the device from breakage. In addition to the patient dependence caused by loss of the prosthesis, replacement or repair is very expensive.
3. When a sensory loss exists, use techniques that facilitate interaction with the patient. Be sensitive to the degree of loss that may remain when a device is used.
4. Encourage patients to express feelings related to reliance on an artificial device for function or appearance. Be supportive and teach patients and their families methods for interacting more effectively.

PROCEDURAL GUIDELINE 19-1   Eye Care for Comatose Patients

Comatose patients do not have the natural protective mechanisms to protect the cornea. These protective mechanisms include blinking and lubrication of the eye. When patients are in a coma, the nurse is responsible for providing this care. Left unprotected, damage to the cornea can occur. These damages range from corneal scarring to premature cataract formation or vision changes. Simple nursing measures, such as protecting the eyes or administering sterile lubricant, decrease the risk for or prevent damage to the cornea.

PROCEDURAL GUIDELINE 19-1 Eye Care for Comatose Patients—cont'd

Delegation Considerations

The skill of eye care for a comatose patient can be delegated to nursing assistive personnel (NAP). However, it is the nurse's responsibility to assess a patient's eyes and administer the sterile lubricant. The nurse directs the NAP by:

- Explaining how to adapt the skill for specific patients (e.g., using skin-sensitive tape to affix eye pads for patients with sensitive skin).
- Instructing the NAP to immediately report any eye drainage or irritation to the nurse for further assessment.

Equipment

- ❑ Clean gloves
- ❑ Water or normal saline solution
- ❑ Clean washcloth
- ❑ Cotton balls
- ❑ Eye pads or patches
- ❑ Paper tape
- ❑ Eyedropper bulb syringe
- ❑ Sterile lubricant or eye preparations as ordered

Procedural Steps

1 Observe patient's eyes for drainage, irritation, redness, and lesions.

2 Assess for blink reflex.
3 Perform pupillary examination: determine if pupils are equal, round, and react to light and accommodation (PERRLA) (see Chapter 6).
4 Observe patient's eye movements, noting symmetry of eye movement.
5 Explain procedure to patient and family members.
6 Position patient in supine position.
7 Perform hand hygiene, and apply clean gloves.
8 Use clean washcloth or cotton balls moistened with water or saline, and gently wipe each eye from inner to outer canthus. Use a separate, clean cotton ball or corner of the washcloth for each eye.
9 Use an eyedropper to instill the prescribed lubricant (e.g., saline, methylcellulose, liquid tears) as ordered.
10 If blink reflex is absent, gently close patient's eyes and apply eye patches or pads. Secure patch, being careful not to tape patient's eyes.
11 Dispose of excess material, remove gloves, and perform hand hygiene.
12 Remove eye pads/patches every 4 hours or as ordered, and observe condition of patient's eye for drainage, irritation, redness, and lesions.
13 Notify physician if signs of irritation or infection are present.

PROCEDURAL GUIDELINE 19-2 Taking Care of Contact Lenses

A contact lens is a thin, concave disk that fits directly over the cornea of the eye. It is transparent over at least the pupil and may be colorless or tinted. Contact lenses correct refractive errors of the eye or abnormalities in the cornea's shape that distort vision. They are relatively easy to apply and remove.

All modern contact lenses are gas (oxygen) permeable and adhere to the cornea by surface tension. There are two basic types of contact lenses in use today: rigid gas permeable (RGP) and soft. They differ primarily in size, flexibility, and durability. Rigid contact lenses are made of firm, durable plastic and are smaller than the cornea. Soft contact lenses are made of a flexible hydrogel plastic and cover the entire cornea and a small rim of the sclera. There are many different kinds of both RGP and soft lenses to accommodate patient needs for comfort, vision correction, and convenience. Specific lenses have prescribed wear and replacement schedules.

The wear schedule determines how long the lens may be kept in the eye after insertion. Most contact lens wearers use daily wear lenses (American Optometric Association, 2007). Patients wear these lenses only while awake and then discard them or clean them for reinsertion. Others use extended-wear lenses, which are worn continuously for several days before removal and may be soft or RGP. Although the limit for extended wear lenses is usually 6 nights, certain soft lenses have been approved for continuous wear up to 30 nights.

It is important to remember that all lenses must be removed periodically to prevent infection and corneal damage and that proper cleaning is necessary before reinserting a lens. As contact lenses are worn, secretions and foreign matter adhere to the lens surfaces (American Optometric Association, 2007). It is extremely important to determine whether patients wear contact lenses, particularly when patients are admitted to hospitals or agencies in unresponsive or confused states. If a seriously ill patient is wearing contact lenses and this fact goes undetected, severe corneal injury can result.

Delegation Considerations

The skill of taking care of contact lenses can be delegated to NAP. The nurse directs the NAP about:

- Patient's specific type of contact lens, including cleaning solutions and routine, wear schedule, and replacement schedule.
- Reporting immediately to the nurse any eye pain or discomfort, redness, swelling, tearing, or drainage.
- Careful handling of the lens to prevent damage and injury.

Equipment

- ❑ Bath towels or waterproof pads
- ❑ Sterile saline solution
- ❑ Sterile lens care solution(s) for cleaning, disinfecting, and rinsing
- ❑ Sterile wetting or conditioning solution (depends on care regimen)
- ❑ Sterile enzyme solution (depends on care regimen)
- ❑ Clean lens storage container
- ❑ Suction cup (optional)
- ❑ Powder-free, clean gloves

Procedural Steps

1 Observe patient's eye, or ask patient if contact lens is in place.

Critical Decision Point *Carefully assess unconscious or confused patients who enter the health care setting; lenses are often difficult to detect if colorless (untinted).*

Continued

PROCEDURAL GUIDELINE 19-2   Taking Care of Contact Lenses—cont'd

2 Ask if patient is able to manipulate and hold contact lenses and if glasses are available for periods when contacts are not in use, and determine patient's usual routine for wearing, cleansing, and storing lenses.

3 Assess patient for any unusual visual signs/symptoms (e.g., change in visual acuity, blurred vision, halos, photophobia).

4 Review types of medication prescribed for patient: sedatives, hypnotics, muscle relaxants, antihistamines, etc., or another medication that decreases blink reflex and subsequent lubrication of cornea.

5 Explain procedure to patient.

6 Verify expiration date of all solutions, and assemble equipment at bedside.

7 Be sure that fingernails are short and smooth.

8 Position patient in supine or high-Fowler's position in bed.

9 Removing lenses:
  a Perform hand hygiene. Apply snug, powder-free, clean gloves, and place towel just below patient's face.
  b Removal of soft lens: Follow Steps (1) through (4) for each eye.
    (1) Add 2 to 3 drops of sterile saline solution to patient's eye.
    (2) Ask patient to look up to expose lower eyeball to which lens will be displaced.
    (3) Use middle finger of dominant hand, and gently retract lower lid.
    (4) With pad of index finger of same hand, slide lens off cornea down onto lower sclera. *Use of pad rather than fingernail prevents injury to cornea and damage to lens.*

Critical Decision Point   *If lens edges stick together, place lens in palm and soak thoroughly with sterile saline solution. Gently roll lens with index finger in back-and-forth motion. If necessary, soak lens in storage solution, which may return lens to normal shape.*

  c Removal of hard lenses (Repeat steps (1) through (5) for each eye.)
    (1) Inspect the eye to be sure lens is positioned directly over the cornea.

Critical Decision Point   *If lens is not positioned directly over the cornea, have patient close eyelid, place index and middle fingers of one hand on eyelid just beside the lens and beneath, and gently attempt to massage lens back into place. If lens cannot be repositioned, an immediate referral to an ophthalmologist is needed.*

    (2) Place index finger on outer corner of patient's eye, and draw skin gently back toward ear.
    (3) Ask patient to open eye wide.

Critical Decision Point   *For patients unable to open eye or blink on command, a lens suction cup can be used to remove lens from eye. Gently apply suction cup to lens surface and lift out.*

    (4) Ask patient to blink. Do not release pressure on eyelid until blink is completed. If lens does not dislodge, gently retract eyelid beyond edge of lens. Press lower eyelid gently against lower edge of lens to dislodge lens.

    (5) Allow both eyelids to close slightly, and grasp lens as it rises from eye. Cup lens in hand.

  d After lenses are removed, inspect eye for redness, pain, swelling of eyelids or conjunctivae, discharge, or excess tearing.

10 Cleaning and storage: Typical cleaning and disinfecting of contact lenses (verify specific method for lenses):
  a Apply 1 or 2 drops of cleaning solution to lens in palm of hand. Using index finger (soft lenses) or little finger (rigid lenses), rub lens gently but thoroughly on both sides for 20 to 30 seconds.
  b Holding lens over emesis basin, rinse thoroughly with recommended rinsing solution.

Critical Decision Point   *Do not use tap water for cleaning, rinsing, or storage. Tap water contains microbes and may be absorbed into the lens, making it uncomfortable to wear. Periodic cleaning with enzymatic cleaner and/or heat disinfecting may be part of the prescribed regimen. Follow prescriber's instructions and schedules.*

  c Place lens in proper storage case compartment: "R" for right lens and "L" for left. Rigid lenses are placed inside up.
  d Fill with recommended disinfectant or storage solution.
  e Secure cover(s) over storage case. Label case with patient's name, identification number, and room number.

11 Inserting lenses:
  a Perform hand hygiene. Apply snug, powder-free, clean gloves.
  b Place towel just below patient's face.
  c Inserting a soft lens: Follow Steps (1) through (5) for each eye.
    (1) Remove right lens from storage case, and rinse with recommended rinsing solution; inspect lens for foreign materials, tears, and other damage.
    (2) Hold lens on tip of index finger of dominant hand with concave side up.
    (3) Inspect lens from side at eye level to ensure that lens is not inverted (see illustration).

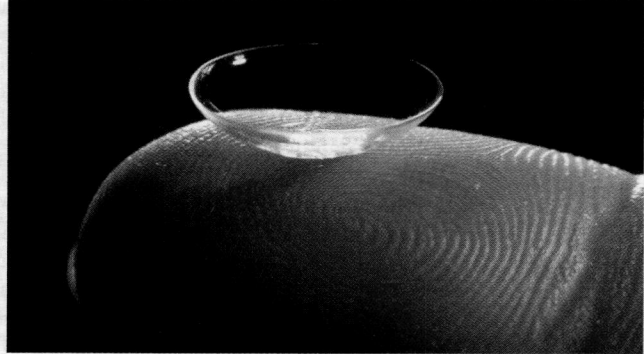

STEP 11c(3)   Correct position of soft lens before insertion.

    (4) Using middle or index finger of opposite hand, retract upper lid until iris is exposed (see illustration). Using middle finger of the hand holding the lens, pull down lower lid.

Continued

PROCEDURAL GUIDELINE 19-2 Taking Care of Contact Lenses—cont'd

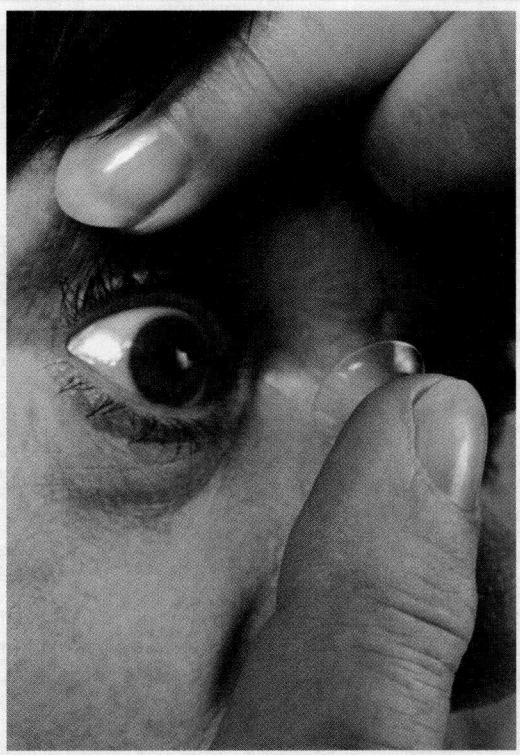

STEP 11c(4)   Correct position of hands for soft lens insertion.

   (5) Instruct patient to look straight ahead and focus on an object in the distance. Gently place lens directly on cornea, and release lids slowly, starting with lower lid.

  d Inserting a rigid lens: Follow Steps (1) through (6) for each eye.

   (1) Remove right lens from storage case; attempt to lift lens straight up.

   (2) Hold lens on tip of index finger of dominant hand with concave side up.

   (3) Inspect the lens to ensure that it is moist, clean, clear, and free of chips or cracks.

   (4) Wet the lens surfaces using a few drops of prescribed wetting solution.

   (5) Using middle finger of the hand holding the lens, pull down lower lid (see illustration).

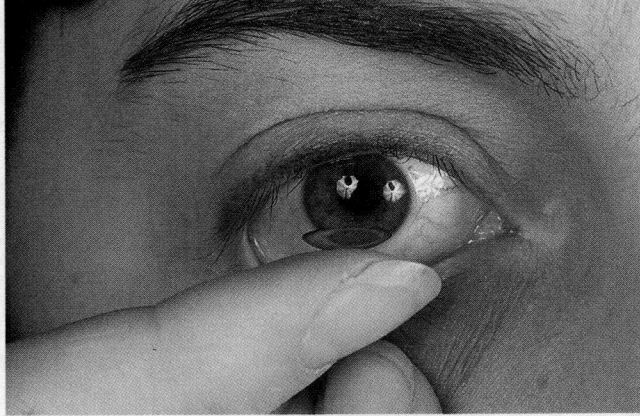

STEP 11d(5)   Hand position for rigid lens insertion.

   (6) Instruct patient to look straight ahead and focus on an object in the distance (see illustration). Gently place lens directly on cornea, and release lids slowly, starting with lower lid.

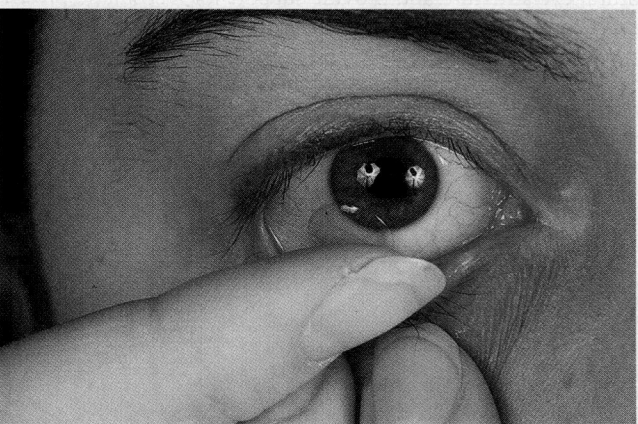

STEP 11d(6)   Instruct patient to look straight ahead and focus on an object in the distance.

  e Ask patient to close eyes briefly and to avoid blinking.

12 Inspect eye to ensure lens is on cornea.

> **Critical Decision Point**   *If lens is on sclera rather than cornea, ask patient to slowly close eye and look toward the lens. Gentle pressure on the eyelid may help to center the lens on the cornea. Ask patient to blink a few times.*

13 Ask patient to cover other eye with hand and report if vision is clear and lens is comfortable.

14 Repeat procedure to insert lens in other eye.

15 Discard solution from storage case, and rinse case thoroughly with sterile lens storage solution. Sterilize or replace case as recommended by manufacturer. Allow case to air dry. Dispose of towel, remove gloves, and perform hand hygiene.

16 Ask patient if lens feels comfortable after removal and reinsertion of lenses.

17 Observe for unexpected outcomes (e.g., blurred vision, burning, pain, foreign body sensation).

PROCEDURAL GUIDELINE 19-3   Taking Care of an Artificial Eye

As a result of tumor, infection, congenital blindness, or severe trauma to the eye, patients may undergo **enucleation,** the complete surgical removal of the eyeball. During this surgical procedure a spherical implant is placed in the orbit to maintain the natural eye structure and provide support for a cosmetic prosthesis. The muscles and other tissues of the eye are sewn around the implant, holding it in place. The implant therefore is not visible (Fig. 19-1). Modern implants are made of glass or plastic and are porous so that the tissues of the eye grow into the sphere (Center for Ocular Prosthetics, 2007). Like a healthy eye, this integrated implant moves as the companion eye moves.

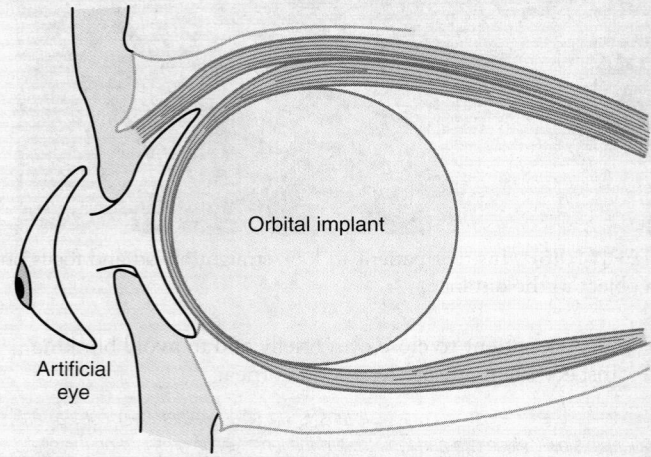

FIG 19-1   Side view of orbital implant, artificial eye removed.

A concave cosmetic prosthesis is placed over the implant, resulting in a nearly normal appearance. Some implants are fitted with a peg that secures and optimally transfers implant movement to the prosthesis. The prosthesis, the artificial eye, is glass or plastic and colored to match the companion eye.

Prostheses are relatively easy to remove and insert and are usually worn day and night. Cleaning with sterile saline or soap and water is done at intervals of up to a year based on ocularist recommendations and the patient's preference (Kolberg Ocular Prosthetics, 2007).

Delegation Considerations
The skill of taking care of an artificial eye can be delegated to NAP. The nurse directs the NAP by:
- Instructing to report eye pain or discomfort, inflammation, drainage, or odor.
- Reinforcing the importance of careful handling of the prosthesis to prevent damage or injury.

Equipment
- ❏ Bath towels or waterproof pads
- ❏ Sterile saline for washing prosthesis
- ❏ Irrigation bulb or large syringe (without needle)
- ❏ Sterile saline: 30 to 180 mL at 90° to 100° F (about 32° to 38° C)
- ❏ Emesis basin
- ❏ 4 × 4 inch gauze pads
- ❏ Clean gloves
- ❏ Facial tissues *(optional)*
- ❏ Washbasin with warm water and mild soap *(optional)*
- ❏ Suction device (or medicine dropper bulb) *(optional)*
- ❏ Covered plastic storage case *(optional)*

Procedural Steps
1 Ask patient or inspect eyes to determine which is artificial. Some implants allow movement of the prosthesis and can make distinguishing it from the natural eye difficult. An artificial eye pupil does not react to changes in light.
2 Assess patient's frequency and method of cleaning and length of time since last cleaning.

Critical Decision Point   *Unless the patient's eye care practitioner advises otherwise, the prosthesis is usually not removed unless the patient experiences discomfort because excessive handling may cause irritation and increased secretions (Kolberg Ocular Prosthetics, 2007).*

3 Assess patient's ability to remove, clean, and reinsert prosthesis.
4 Before and after removal of prosthesis, assess eyelids and socket for inflammation, tenderness, swelling, drainage, or odor. Pay particular attention to the implant peg if present. Assess patient's pain or other symptoms.

Critical Decision Point   *Signs/symptoms may indicate infection or injury. Infection can spread easily to neighboring eye, underlying sinuses, or brain tissue. The implant peg is a common site of infection.*

5 Discuss procedure with patient.
6 Assemble supplies at bedside. Place one towel over work area.
7 Removing prosthesis:
   a Position in sitting or supine position with head elevated. Provide privacy.
   b Perform hand hygiene. Apply clean gloves.
   c Place towel just below patient's face.
   d With thumb or forefinger of dominant hand gently retract lower eyelid against lower orbital ridge (see illustration).

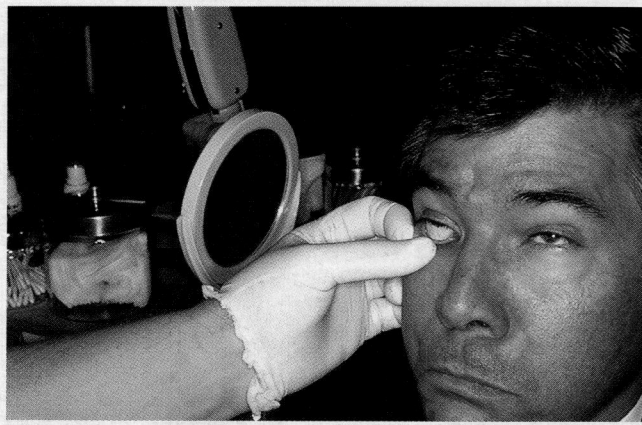

STEP 7d   Retraction of lower lid to aid removal of eye prosthesis.

PROCEDURAL GUIDELINE 19-3   Taking Care of an Artificial Eye—cont'd

e   Exert slight pressure below eyelid, and slide prosthesis out (see illustration).

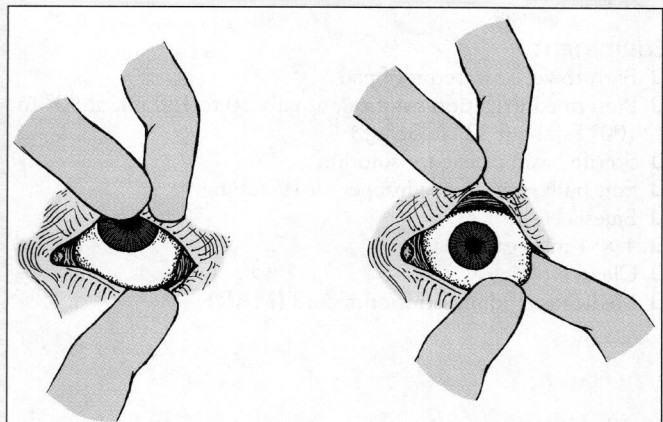

STEP 7e   Exertion of pressure below eyelid and removal of prosthesis.

> **Critical Decision Point**   *If prosthesis does not slide out, use moistened suction device to apply direct suction to prosthesis (Kolberg Ocular Prosthetics, 2007).*

f   Note presence and orientation of colored dot at margin of prosthesis.

g   Place prosthesis in palm of hand.

h   Clean prosthesis by washing with mild soap and warm water or plain saline solution by rubbing well between thumb and index finger (see manufacturer's instructions). NOTE: Never use alcohol or other products because they are harmful to the prosthesis (Erickson Laboratories, 2007).

i   Inspect prosthesis for rough edges or surfaces. Set aside on towel.

> **Critical Decision Point**   *Patients are instructed to have artificial eye checked and polished at least twice a year to avoid unnecessary discomfort to the patient as a result of protein deposits or scratches on the surface of the artificial eye. An artificial eye is usually replaced every 5 years (Erickson Laboratories, 2007).*

8   If prosthesis will not be reinserted immediately, store in sterile saline in a labeled case in a documented location (see manufacturer's instructions).

9   Cleaning eyelid margins and socket:

a   Wash and rinse eyelid margins with mild soap and water. Wipe from inner to outer canthus using a clean section of cloth with each wipe.

b   Retract upper and lower eyelid margins with thumb and index finger.

c   Gently irrigate socket with sterile saline solution. Note presence of discharge or odor.

d   Remove excess moisture with gauze pads by wiping from inner to outer canthus.

10   Inserting prosthesis:

a   Moisten prosthesis in water or sterile saline.

b   Retract patient's upper eyelid with index finger or thumb of nondominant hand.

c   With dominant hand, hold prosthesis so that iris faces outward and colored dot is properly oriented (see illustration).

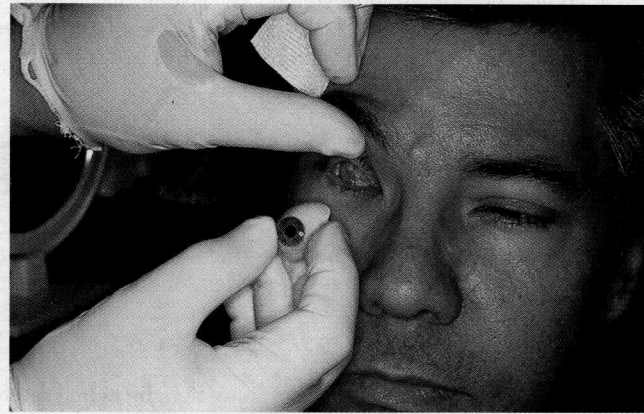

STEP 10c   Prosthesis must be oriented for correct insertion.

d   Gently slide prosthesis up under upper eyelid, and then push down lower lid to allow prosthesis to slip into place.

e   Ask patient if prosthesis fits comfortably and without pain.

11   Inspect eyelids and socket for signs of infection (such as excessive, purulent, or foul drainage), excessive tearing or clear discharge, excessive itching, or lashes turned toward prosthesis.

12   Observe patient removing, cleaning, and reinserting the prosthesis.

13   Teach patient to inspect eye socket for redness, drainage, or excessive dryness. Teach patient to inspect artificial eye for damage, scratches, or areas of roughness. Alert patient to report any odor noted on eye or prosthesis to the health care provider.

SKILL 19-1   Eye Irrigation

Eye irrigation is performed to flush out exudates, irritating solutions, or foreign particles. This irrigation is performed in an emergency attempt to preserve vision. When a chemical or irritating substance contaminates the eyes, irrigate immediately with copious amounts of cool water for at least 15 minutes to minimize corneal damage (U.S. National Library of Medicine, 2007). Users of contact lenses or artificial eyes may need eye irrigation to flush out particles of dust or fibers from the eye or socket.

Often cool tap water is recommended for emergency eye flushing because it is effective and immediately available for first aid. Nevertheless, controversy remains over the best solution for irrigating the eye in a health care setting (Segal, 2007). When faced with a choice of normal intravenous (IV) solutions, lactated Ringer's is more effective than normal saline in restoring pH after a chemical burn to the eye (Kuckelkorn and others, 2002).

Delegation Considerations
The skill of eye irrigation cannot be delegated to NAP.

Equipment
- ❑ Bath towel or waterproof pad
- ❑ Prescribed irrigation solution, usually 30 to 180 mL at 90° to 100° F (about 32° to 38° C)
- ❑ Sterile basin or bag for solution
- ❑ Soft bulb syringe, eyedropper, or IV tubing
- ❑ Emesis basin
- ❑ 4 × 4 inch gauze pads
- ❑ Clean gloves
- ❑ Medication administration record (MAR)

STEP	RATIONALE

ASSESSMENT

1 Review prescriber's medication order, including solution to be instilled and the affected eye(s) (right, left, or both) to receive irrigation.	Ensures safe and correct administration of irrigant.
2 Assess reason for eye irrigation.	Determines the amount and type of solution and the immediacy of the need for treatment.
3 If time permits, do a complete eye examination, including determining if pupils are equal, round, and react to light and accommodation (PERRLA) (Boyd-Monk, 2005) (see Chapter 6).	Provides a baseline.
4 Assess the eye for redness, tearing, discharge, and swelling. Ask patient about symptoms of itching, burning, pain, blurred vision, or photophobia.	Establishes baseline signs and symptoms.
5 Ask patient to rate level of pain. Use a scale of 0 to 10.	Established baseline for level of pain.
6 Assess patient's ability to cooperate.	Determines level of assistance needed.

Critical Decision Point   *Spasm of the eyelid or pain may make opening the eye difficult. Local anesthetics, such as proparacaine or tetracaine, cause topical numbness and are used before certain eye examination procedures (Hoyt and Haley, 2005).*

NURSING DIAGNOSES

- Acute pain
- Disturbed sensory perception (visual)
- Risk for infection
- Risk for injury

Individualize related factors based on patient's condition or needs.

PLANNING

1 Expected outcomes following completion of procedure:	
• Patient demonstrates minimal anxiety during irrigation.	Potential for anxiety and pain is high during emergency.
• Patient verbalizes reduced pain, burning, or itching and improved visual acuity after irrigation.	Reflects effectiveness of procedure in removing irritant.
• Patient maintains normal pupillary reaction and eye movement after irrigation.	Reflects effectiveness of procedure in minimizing exposure to irritant and preventing eye damage.
2 Discuss procedure with patient.	Decreases patient anxiety.
3 Check accuracy and completeness of each MAR with prescriber's written medication or procedure order. Check patient's name, drug name and dosage, route of administration, and time for administration. Compare MAR with label of eye irrigation solution.	The order sheet is the most reliable source and only legal record of drugs or procedure patient is to receive. Ensures patient receives correct medication.

STEP	RATIONALE
4 Check patient's identification by reading identification bracelet and asking name.	Ensures correct patient receives medication. At least two patient identifiers (neither to be patient's room number) are to be used whenever administering medications (The Joint Commission [TJC], 2008).
5 Assemble supplies at bedside.	Provides easy access to supplies.
6 Assist patient to side-lying position on side of affected eye or supine position for simultaneous irrigation of both eyes.	Position facilitates flow of solution from inner to outer canthus, preventing contamination of unaffected eye and nasolacrimal duct (Emergencies in the field, 2007).

IMPLEMENTATION

1 Perform hand hygiene. Apply clean gloves.	Reduces transmission of microorganisms. Protects hands from chemical irritants.
2 Remove any contact lens if possible.	Contact lens may have absorbed irritant, or it may prevent a thorough irrigation. Lens may be lost if flushed out by irrigation.

Critical Decision Point   *In an emergency such as first aid for a chemical burn, do not delay by removing patient's contact lens before irrigation. Do not remove contact unless rapid swelling is occurring. Flush eye, from the inner to outer canthus, with cool tap water immediately (U.S. National Library of Medicine, 2007). Advise patient to consult prescriber before reusing contact lens.*

3 Place towel just below patient's face and emesis basin just below patient's cheek.	Catches irrigation fluid.
4 Clean visible secretions or foreign material from eyelids and lashes, wiping from inner to outer canthus.	Minimizes transfer of material into eye during irrigation. Prevents secretions from entering nasolacrimal duct.
5 Gently retract eyelids. Hold open by applying pressure to orbit, not to eyeball.	Exposes eye and minimizes blinking.
6 Hold solution-filled bulb, dropper, or tubing approximately 2.5 cm (1 inch) from inner canthus.	Direct contact with irrigation equipment may injure the eye.
7 Ask patient to look toward brow. Gently irrigate with a steady stream toward the lower conjunctival sac (see illustration).	Minimizes force of stream on cornea. Flushes irritant out of eye and away from other eye and nasolacrimal duct.

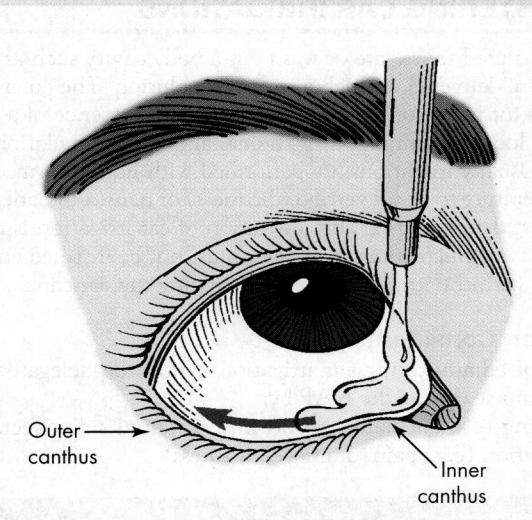

Outer canthus

Inner canthus

STEP 7   Irrigation of eye from inner to outer canthus.

8 Reinforce the importance of the procedure, and encourage patient using calm, confident, soft voice.	Reduces anxiety.
9 Allow patient to blink periodically.	Moves irritant from upper conjunctival sac.
10 Continue for prescribed volume and/or time or until secretions have been cleared.	Ensures complete removal of irritant.
11 Blot excess moisture from eyelids and face with gauze or towel.	Removes moisture that may contain microbes or irritant. Promotes patient comfort.
12 Dispose of soiled supplies, remove gloves, and perform hand hygiene.	Reduces transmission of microorganisms.

STEP	RATIONALE

EVALUATION

1. Observe for verbal and nonverbal signs of anxiety during irrigation.

Verifies patient is adequately comforted.

2. Assess patient's comfort level after irrigation.

Verifies effective removal of irritant.

3. Inspect eye for movement and to determine if pupils are equal, round, react to light and accommodation (PERRLA).

Impaired reaction to light, accommodation, or movement may indicate injury.

4. Ask patient about improved visual acuity.

Corneal damage from the irritant can result in altered visual acuity (e.g., blurred vision, cloudiness).

Unexpected Outcomes	Related Interventions
1 Anxiety	• Reinforce rationale for irrigation. • Allow patient to close eye periodically during irrigation. • Instruct patient to take slow, deep breaths.
2 Pain or foreign body sensation	• Advise patient to close eye and avoid eye movement. • Immediately notify physician or eye care practitioner.

Recording and Reporting
• Record in nurses' notes condition of eye and patient's report of pain and visual symptoms. Record amount and type of irrigation on patient's MAR.
• Report continuing symptoms of pain or blurred vision.

Teaching Considerations
• Assist patient with identifying potential hazards at home and work and taking steps to prevent accidents, such as use of safety goggles while working with dust or chemicals.

• Review first aid procedures for eye emergencies with patient and/or caregiver.
• Instruct patient to not press or rub an injured eye.

Pediatric Considerations
• A child with a foreign body or chemical in the eye may panic. It may be necessary to restrain the child to safely and quickly irrigate the eye.

SKILL 19-2	Ear Irrigation

ADMINISTERING EAR IRRIGATIONS

Medications used to irrigate or wash out a body cavity such as the ear (otic) are delivered through a stream of solution. The common indications for irrigation of the external ear are presence of a foreign body, local inflammation of the canal, and accumulation of cerumen. Usually irrigations are performed with liquid warmed to body temperature to avoid vertigo (dizziness) or nausea in patients. The greatest danger during administration of ear irrigation is rupture of the tympanic membrane. Fluids must not be instilled under pressure or with the irrigating device occluding the ear canal.

Delegation Considerations
The skill of administering ear irrigation cannot be delegated to NAP. The nurse directs the NAP by:
• Instructing to immediately report any potential side effects of ear irrigation (e.g., pain, drainage, dizziness).

• Instructing to assist the patient when ambulating because some light-headedness may be present, which increases the patient's risk for falling.

Equipment
❑ Clean gloves
❑ Otoscope (optional)
❑ Irrigation syringe
❑ Basin (Sterile basin may be required if a sterile irrigating solution is used.)
❑ Emesis basis or other receptacle to collect drainage or irrigating solution exiting the ear
❑ Towel
❑ Cotton balls
❑ Prescribed irrigation solution warmed to body temperature, or mineral oil, or over-the-counter softener
❑ Medication administration record (MAR)

STEP	RATIONALE

ASSESSMENT

1. Review prescriber's medication order, including solution to be instilled and the affected ear(s) (right, left, or both) to receive irrigation.

Ensures safe and correct administration of medication.

2. Review medical record for history of ruptured tympanic membrane, or visualize patient's tympanic membrane using an otoscope.

Ruptured membrane contraindicates irrigation.

3. Inspect the pinna and external auditory meatus for redness, swelling, drainage, abrasions, and presence of cerumen or foreign objects.

Findings provide baseline to monitor effects of medication or solution.

STEP	RATIONALE
a Always attempt to remove foreign objects in the ear by first simply straightening the ear canal.	This may cause the object to fall out.
b If vegetable matter (such as a dried bean or pea) is occluded in the canal, do not perform irrigation.	Children often place vegetable matter in the ear. The material can swell on contact with water, and cause further damage to the canal.
4 Ask if patient is experiencing discomfort. Note patient's ability to hear clearly.	Pain is symptomatic of external ear infection or inflammation. Occlusion of auditory canal by cerumen or foreign object can impair hearing.
5 Review patient's knowledge of purpose for irrigation and of normal care of the ears.	May indicate need for instruction regarding hygiene.

NURSING DIAGNOSES

- Deficient knowledge (regarding purpose for irrigation)
- Disturbed sensory perception (auditory)
- Pain (acute or chronic)
- Risk for injury

Individualize related factors based on patient's condition or needs.

PLANNING

1 Expected outcomes following completion of procedure:	
• Patient denies pain during instillation.	Fluid is properly instilled.
• Patient hears conversation more clearly.	Obstruction in ear canal is resolved.
• Patient is able to discuss purpose of irrigation and describe correct ear care techniques.	Feedback reflects patient's learning.
• Skin overlying meatus and canal becomes clear, without redness, swelling, tenderness, or discharge. Canal is clear of cerumen and foreign material.	Inflammation, irritation, and occlusion of canal are relieved.
2 Check accuracy and completeness of each MAR with prescriber's written medication or procedure order. Check patient's name, drug name and dosage, route of administration, and time for administration. Compare MAR with label of ear irrigation solution.	The order sheet is the most reliable source and only legal record of drugs or procedure patient is to receive. Ensures patient receives correct medication.
3 Check patient's identification by reading identification bracelet and asking name.	Ensures correct patient receives medication. At least two patient identifiers (neither to be patient's room number) are to be used whenever administering medications (TJC, 2008).
4 If patient is found to have impacted cerumen, instill 1 to 2 drops of mineral oil or over-the-counter softener into ear twice a day for 2 to 3 days before irrigation.	Loosens cerumen and ensures easier removal during irrigation.
5 Explain procedure. Warn that the irrigation may cause sensation of dizziness, ear fullness, and warmth.	Prepares patient to anticipate effects of irrigation and promotes cooperation.

IMPLEMENTATION

1 Perform hand hygiene, arrange supplies at bedside, and apply gloves.	Reduces transfer of microorganisms; helps nurse to perform procedure smoothly.
2 Close curtain or room door.	Maintains privacy.
3 Assist patient to a sitting or lying position with head turned toward affected ear. Place towel under patient's head and shoulder, and have patient, if able, hold emesis basin under affected ear.	Position minimizes leakage of fluids around neck and facial area. Solution will flow from ear canal to basin.
4 Pour irrigating solution into basin.	
NOTE: *If a sterile irrigating solution is used, a sterile basin is required.*	
5 Gently clean auricle and outer ear canal with moistened cotton applicator. Do *not* force drainage or cerumen into the ear canal.	Prevents infected material from reentering ear canal. Forceful instillation of solution into occluded canal can cause injury to eardrum.
6 Fill irrigating syringe with solution (approximately 50 mL).	Enough fluid is needed to provide a steady irrigating stream.
7 For adults and children over age 3 years, gently pull pinna up and back; in children age 3 years or younger, pull the pinna down and back (Hockenberry and Wilson, 2007).	Straightening of ear canal provides direct access to deeper external ear structures. Developmental differences in younger children and infants necessitate different techniques. Allows fluid to flow through length of canal.

STEP	RATIONALE
8 Slowly instill irrigating solution by holding tip of syringe 1 cm (½ inch) above opening to ear canal. Direct the fluid toward the superior aspect of ear canal. Allow fluid to drain out during instillation into the basin. Continue until canal is cleansed or solution is used (see illustration).	Slow instillation prevents buildup of pressure in ear canal and ensures contact of solution with all canal surfaces.

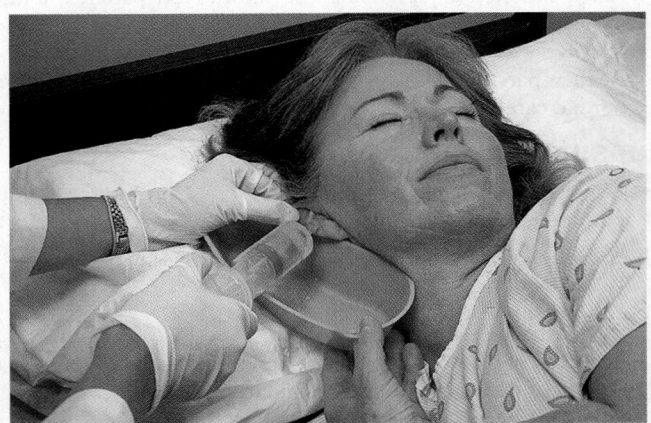

STEP 8 Tip of syringe does not occlude ear canal during irrigation.

STEP	RATIONALE
9 Do *not* occlude ear canal with tip of syringe.	Buildup of fluid in ear canal under forced pressure may cause rupture of tympanic membrane.
10 Dry outer ear canal with cotton ball. Leave cotton loosely in place for 5 to 10 minutes.	Maintains comfort. Absorbs excess moisture in ear canal.
11 Assist patient to a sitting position.	Maintains comfort.
12 Remove gloves, dispose of supplies, and perform hand hygiene.	Reduces transmission of infection.

EVALUATION

1 Ask patient if discomfort is noted during instillation of solution.	Fluid instilled improperly under pressure causes discomfort.
2 Ask patient about sensations of light-headedness or dizziness.	Instillation of fluid into the ear can cause some light-headedness or dizziness, which can put patient at risk for falling.
3 Reinspect condition of meatus and canal.	Determines if solution relieves symptoms and removes foreign materials.
4 Measure patient's hearing acuity.	Determines if conduction deafness is relieved.
5 Ask patient to describe purpose of irrigation and proper techniques for ear care.	Reflects patient's understanding of procedure and proper hygiene.

Unexpected Outcomes	Related Interventions
1 Patient experiences increased ear pain.	• Rupture of eardrum may have occurred. Stop irrigations immediately, and notify prescriber immediately.
2 Ear canal remains occluded with cerumen.	• Repeat irrigation.
3 Foreign body remains in ear canal.	• Refer patient to an otolaryngologist if a foreign object remains after irrigation.
4 Patient is unable to explain ear care practices.	• Reinstruction is necessary.
	• Include family members or caregivers if possible.

Recording and Reporting

- Record in nurses' notes and/or MAR the procedure, amount of solution instilled, time of administration, and ear receiving irrigation.
- Record appearance of external ear and patient's hearing acuity in nurses' notes.
- Report adverse effects/patient response and/or withheld drugs to nurse in charge or physician.

Teaching Considerations

- Instruct patient that cerumen has an antibacterial effect that maintains an acid pH in the auditory canal.
- Instruct patients to clean ears daily with a washcloth, soap, and warm water.
- Warn patients against placing objects (including cotton swabs) in ears.

Pediatric Considerations

- When cleansing the ear of a small child, be certain child's head is immobilized to prevent puncturing eardrum. It may be necessary to have child's parent participate in this procedure.

Home Care Considerations

- Instruct patient to use a clean bulb syringe for irrigation. Mineral oil drops or over-the-counter otic preparations can help with removal of cerumen.

SKILL 19-3   Care of Hearing Aids

Hearing is vital for normal communication and orientation to sounds in the environment. Hearing loss is common but not limited to older adults. However, when hearing loss occurs, it is difficult to hear doorbells, car horns, sirens, and alarms. In addition, it is difficult for people with hearing loss to follow patient education (Rados, 2005). For people with hearing loss, hearing aids may improve the ability to hear and understand spoken words. A hearing aid is a small, battery-powered, electronic device that amplifies sound. All parts of the hearing aid work together. The microphone changes sound waves to electrical signals. These signals pass through the amplifier and are made louder. The receiver changes the amplified electrical signals back into sound waves. Finally, the amplified sound waves are channeled into the ear through the hearing aid ear mold (air conduction) or as vibrations through the skull (bone conduction) (Boys Town National Research Hospital, 2007). These prostheses are limited by the function of the ear structures.

For patients with profound damage to the structures of the inner ear (sensorineural deafness), a cochlear implant is used. This internal implant receives signals from a separate external processor and transmits them electrically to the auditory nerve. The external processor looks similar to a conventional hearing aid and has a microphone but does not produce sound (Advanced Bionics Corporation, 2007).

Conventional hearing aids are analog or digital. Digital technology uses a tiny processor to convert the sound before it is amplified (Fransman and Walker, 2007). This allows the signal to be analyzed to remove background noise and automatically adjust volume. Some hearing aids are programmable by the audiologist to amplify some sound frequencies more than others. Patients often experience greater hearing loss at higher frequencies; in speech this represents consonant sounds like *p*, *k*, *f*, *th*, and *s*. A programmable aid can accommodate differences in hearing loss and help make speech understandable. *Programmable* may also be used to refer to a patient's ability to set the aid for different listening situations, or "programs," such as music, conversation, or telephone.

There are many styles of hearing aids to accommodate patient needs for comfort, appearance, amplification, and versatility. Smaller, in-the-canal (ITC) and completely-in-canal (CIC) hearing aids are most discreet but tend to accumulate the most cerumen and are difficult to handle because of their size (Fig. 19-2). In-the-ear (ITE) aids are larger and can hold more internal circuitry and external controls (Fig. 19-3). All of the circuitry for these hearing aids is contained within the custom-made, rigid ear mold. The circuitry for behind-the-ear (BTE) or postaural aids is better protected from earwax, and the separate ear mold easily adjusts to changes in ear shape (Fig. 19-4). With any style, controls for adjusting volume and programs are on the aid itself or on a separate remote control. The circuitry and battery pack may also be separate and worn at the chest or waist or even on eyeglasses.

It is a challenge to adjust one's communication style to accommodate a patient with a hearing impairment. Use the patient as a resource for communication techniques that are generally helpful. Briefly, be sure that the patient can see your face, speak slowly in a

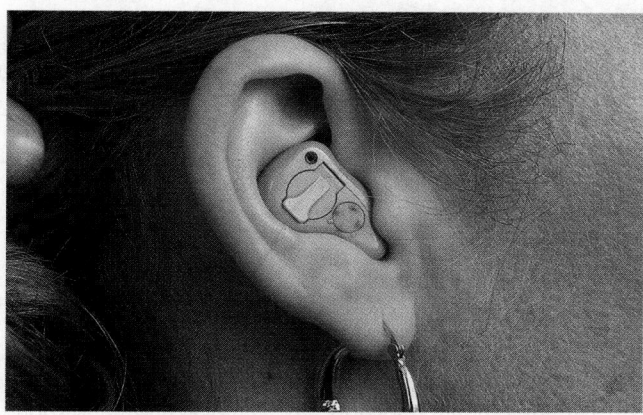

FIG 19-3   In-the-ear (ITE) hearing aid.

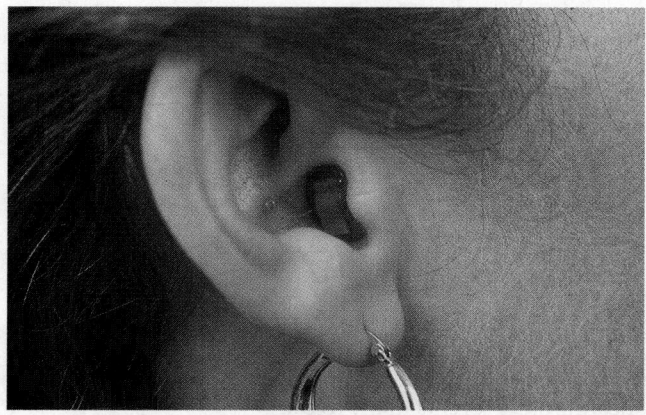

FIG 19-2   Completely-in-canal (CIC) hearing aid.

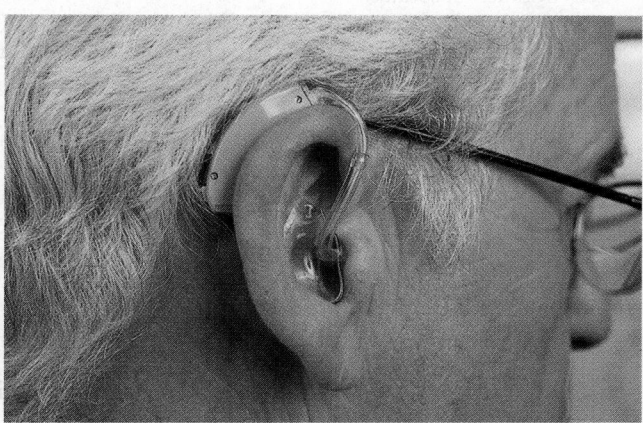

FIG 19-4   Behind-the-ear (BTE) hearing aid.

normal tone, and rephrase rather than repeat if the patient cannot understand you. Also, remember that the patient is unable to hear alerts such as fire alarms or overhead announcements.

Hearing aids are usually worn only while a patient is awake and are cleaned as needed after removal. Remember that a hearing aid is delicate and must be protected from moisture, heat, and breakage.

Delegation Considerations

This skill can be delegated to NAP. The nurse directs the NAP by:

- Instructing to report ear pain, inflammation, drainage, odor, or changes in hearing.
- Identifying alternative ways to communicate with the patient while the aid is not in use.
- Instructing how to carefully handle the aid to prevent damage or injury.

Equipment

- ❑ Bath towels (2)
- ❑ Facial tissues
- ❑ Wax loop
- ❑ Storage case
- ❑ Washcloth
- ❑ Warm water and soap
- ❑ Spare battery, size depends on aid (optional)
- ❑ Dryer, desiccant or electronic (optional)
- ❑ Clean gloves (if drainage present)

STEP	RATIONALE
ASSESSMENT	
1 Determine whether patient can hear clearly with use of aid. With your back to the patient, ask a question slowly and clearly in a normal tone of voice.	Confused facial expression, reaction incongruent with the conversation, verbalization of inability to hear, or movement to better see your face indicate uncompensated impairment or a malfunctioning hearing aid. Prevents lipreading.
2 Ask if patient is able to manipulate and hold hearing aid, or observe patient insert aid independently.	Determines level of assistance required in care.
3 Assess patient's knowledge of and routines for cleaning and caring for hearing aid.	Determines compliance with and knowledge of self-care.
4 Assess patient for any unusual physical or auditory signs/symptoms (pain, itching, redness, discharge, odor, tinnitus, decreased acuity).	May indicate injury, infection, or cerumen accumulation.
5 Assess patient for perceived ability to deal with situations and events such as conversing in a group, going to a social event, being in a lecture audience, or talking on the phone.	May indicate situational low self-esteem related to hearing impairment, which affects social interaction.

NURSING DIAGNOSES

- Bathing/hygiene self-care deficit
- Deficient knowledge regarding hearing aid care
- Disturbed sensory perception (auditory)
- Impaired verbal communication
- Risk for injury
- Risk for situational low self-esteem

Individualize related factors based on patient's condition or needs.

PLANNING	
1 Expected outcomes following completion of procedure:	
• Patient verbalizes comfort after removal and reinsertion of hearing aid.	Hearing aid is removed or inserted properly and positioned correctly.
• Patient responds appropriately to normal conversation and environmental sounds.	Hearing aid and batteries are operational. Aid is secure and unobstructed.
• Patient demonstrates proper care of hearing aid.	Learning is achieved.
2 Discuss procedure with patient. Explain all steps before removing aid.	Patient can assist in planning by explaining additional tips for care. Patient may be confused or anxious if verbal instructions are given after removal of hearing aid.
3 Assemble supplies at bedside. Place towel over work area.	Provides easy access to supplies. Towel catches aid if accidentally dropped and avoids breakage.
4 Have patient assume supine, side-lying, or sitting position in bed or chair.	Provides easy access for nurse. Promotes patient comfort.

IMPLEMENTATION	
1 Removing and cleaning hearing aid:	
a Perform hand hygiene. Apply clean gloves if drainage is present.	Reduces transmission of microorganisms.
b Turn hearing aid volume off. Grasp aid securely, and gently remove device following natural ear contour.	Prevents feedback (whistling) during removal. Prevents dropping hearing aid. Prevents injury to ear.

STEP	RATIONALE
c Some ITC and CIC devices have no volume control but are turned off by opening the battery door. Ask patient if this is necessary. CIC devices have a clear plastic, fiber handle for removal. Firmly grasp handle, and gently pull straight out.	
d Hold aid over towel, and wipe exterior with tissue to remove cerumen.	Prevents breakage if dropped. Cerumen may irritate canal and interfere with fit.
e Inspect all openings in aid for accumulated cerumen. Carefully remove cerumen with wax loop or other device supplied with the hearing aid.	Cerumen may block sound from receiver. Cerumen may block pressure equalization channel and create feeling of ear pressure. Makeshift tools may damage hearing aid.

Critical Decision Point *The pressure equalization channel is a tiny hole through the entire length of the ear mold and should be clear for the entire length. The receiver points into the ear through another opening.* **It is easily damaged. NEVER insert anything into the receiver port!**

STEP	RATIONALE
f Inspect ear mold for rough edges.	May irritate ear canal.
g Open battery door, and place hearing aid in labeled storage container.	Allows drying of internal components. Protects against breakage and loss.
h Repeat Steps 1b through 1g for other aid.	
i Assess ear for redness, tenderness, discharge, or odor.	Signs may indicate injury or infection.
j Place towel beneath patient's ear(s). Wash ear canal(s) with washcloth moistened in soap and water. Rinse and dry.	Absorbs excess water. Removes cerumen from ear canal. Removes soap residue and water that may harbor microbes or damage aid.
k Dispose of towels, remove gloves, and perform hand hygiene.	Reduces transmission of microorganisms.
2 Inserting hearing aid:	
a Perform hand hygiene, and apply gloves if drainage is present.	Reduces transmission of microorganisms.
b Remove hearing aid from storage case, and check battery.	
(1) Close battery door.	Door must be closed to turn on hearing aid.
(2) Turn volume slowly to high.	Prevents damage to hearing aid.
(3) Cup hand over hearing aid, and listen for feedback (whistle or squeal).	Feedback occurs when hearing aid is working but not in correct position.
c Turn hearing aid volume off.	Prevents feedback (whistling) during insertion.
d Identify hearing aid as either right (marked "R" or red color coded) or left (marked "L" or blue color coded).	Proper orientation prevents damage and injury.
e Hold hearing aid with thumb and index finger of dominant hand. Insert pointed end of ear mold into ear canal. Follow natural ear contours to guide aid into place.	Prevents dropping. Proper positioning prevents injury. Pulling on ear may distort canal and make insertion more difficult.
f Anchor any separate pieces, as in case of BTE aid or body aid.	Prevents pieces from falling and breaking.
g Slowly turn on volume to comfortable level for patient.	Gradual adjustment prevents discomfort and injury to ear.
h Close and store case. Perform hand hygiene.	Preserves desiccant. Prevents loss. Reduces transmission of microorganisms.

EVALUATION

1 Ask patient to rate level of comfort after removal or insertion.	Verifies proper technique and positioning.
2 Observe patient during normal conversation and in response to environmental sounds.	Verifies aid is operational, correctly positioned, unobstructed, and effective.
3 Observe patient removing, cleaning, and reinserting hearing aid.	Demonstrates patient's understanding of techniques.

Unexpected Outcomes	Related Interventions
1 Whistling or squealing from inserted hearing aid	• Reposition hearing aid. • Reduce volume if adjustable. • Assess ear for inflammation or blockage.
2 Inability to understand conversations or hear environmental sounds	• Check function, type, and placement of battery, and replace battery if indicated. • Increase volume if adjustable. • Inspect aid and ear canal for cerumen blockage. • Refer to audiologist for reassessment.

Unexpected Outcomes

3 Patient experiences discomfort or pain, inflammation, drainage, or odor from affected ear.

4 Patient lacks knowledge and/or skills to perform hearing aid care properly.

Related Interventions

- Remove aid, and inspect for sharp or rough edges. Refer to provider for repair.
- Assess ear for signs of injury or infection.
- Confirm R or L. Reposition hearing aid (pain).
- If sensation remains, remove aid, and report to physician.
- Be prepared to collect sample of exudate for culture (inflammation, drainage, or odor).
- Teach patient and home care provider hearing aid care skills.
- Provide written instructions and brochures with needed information.

Recording and Reporting

- Record removal of hearing aid, storage location if not reinserted after cleaning, and patient's preferred communication techniques.
- Report any signs or symptoms of infection or injury or sudden decrease in hearing acuity.

Teaching Considerations

- Batteries are toxic if swallowed; keep them away from pets and children.
- Encourage patients to visit hearing aid specialist or audiologist at least annually.
- Encourage patients to identify helpful communication tips and teach them to others. Many patients find facial cues informative. Speakers must:
  - Face the patient, stay within 3 to 4 feet away, and keep hands away from the mouth
  - Get the patient's attention before speaking
  - Rephrase rather than repeat when the patient cannot understand
  - Reduce background noise or move to a quiet area

Pediatric Considerations

- Children are more often fitted with BTE hearing aids because the ear canal is still growing.
- The aid is made less conspicuous with hair styling or becomes a statement of fashion and personality with a brightly colored or transparent case.
- Assistance is needed by children to prevent acoustic feedback (whistling), which they are unable to hear. This is usually elimi-

nated by removing and reinserting the device and making sure no hair is caught between the ear mold and canal, or lowering the volume of the device (Hockenberry and Wilson, 2007).

Gerontological Considerations

- Advise patient to protect the hearing aid from water, alcohol, hairspray or cologne, perspiration, rain, and snow. Advise patient to avoid exposing the hearing aid to extremes of temperature.
- Encourage patient to store hearing aids and batteries with desiccant or in an electronic dryer to prolong life, minimize repairs, and preserve batteries.
- Dogs in particular are attracted to the smell of used hearing aids. Advise patient to protect the hearing aids and their pets by properly storing the aids out of reach.
- The small size of some hearing aids may make them difficult to manipulate, particularly for individuals with decreased dexterity or visual acuity. Consult an audiologist to identify an aid that accommodates the patient's particular need.
- Instruct patients and caregivers to be alert for and report signs of decreased auditory acuity such as inappropriate responses to questions, inattentiveness, decreased socialization, difficulty following oral instructions, or monopolizing conversation.

Home Care Considerations

- Determine presence and willingness of caregiver to perform necessary care of hearing aid.
- Assess patient's home, and determine need for special precautions given patient's limited hearing.

CRITICAL THINKING EXERCISES

1 Mr. Ojo is a 19-year-old Hispanic American college student admitted to the emergency department following a fall during which he fractured his right wrist. He is right handed and wears RGP contact lenses. In preparing to assist with contact lens care, what data will you be collecting in your examination of Mr. Ojo's eyes?

2 Mrs. Wong is being discharged following removal of her left eye. She has an eye prosthesis and demonstrates correct care. What does Mrs. Wong need to know about any unexpected outcomes?

3 Katherine Davis is an independent 50-year-old grandmother who frequently watches her grandchildren; she lives alone with two dogs. Because of increased hearing loss, she is fitted with bilateral in-the-canal hearing aids. Given her family lifestyle, what will you teach her about these aids?

REVIEW QUESTIONS

1 A patient who wears contact lenses for 20/150 vision in each eye is scheduled for hand surgery and will have her hand in a cast for 6 weeks. What is the priority nursing diagnosis for this patient?
   1 Anxiety
   2 Self-care deficit
   3 Imbalanced nutrition: less than body requirements
   4 Disturbed sensory perception

2 A patient is being discharged following care for severe conjunctivitis related to noncompliance with the prescribed lens care regimen. Which patient statement indicates a need for further teaching?
   1 "I should discard my open lens care solutions when I get home."
   2 "Cloudy solutions should be discarded even if they haven't expired."
   3 "Plain soap is the best thing for washing my hands before I touch my contacts."
   4 "I'm switching to disposable contacts so I won't have to worry about getting another infection."

3 A nurse who wears contact lenses splashes rubbing alcohol into his right eye. What is the priority action to take?
  1 Carefully remove the contact lens from the affected eye.
  2 Gently cover the eye with a comfortable patch.
  3 Test the pH of the secretions with litmus paper.
  4 Irrigate the eye with water or prescribed solution.

4 A patient is being discharged home after having an enucleation and an artificial eye placed. Which statement by the patient indicates a need for further teaching?
  1 "I will clean the eye at least once a week."
  2 "I don't have to use sterile solutions for cleaning the eye."
  3 "The colored dot is there to show me which way to put it in."
  4 "Rubbing alcohol and fingernail polish remover are bad for the eye."

5 You are caring for a patient who is hearing impaired. Which approach is most appropriate to best facilitate communication? Select all that apply.
  1 Speak slightly more loudly than usual.
  2 Speak slightly more slowly using a normal tone.
  3 Stand where the patient can see your face.
  4 Use hand gestures to help explain what is being said.

REFERENCES

Advanced Bionics Corporation: *Hearing health: hearing loss*, 2003, http://www.bionicear.com, retrieved September 20, 2007.

American Optometric Association: *What you need to know about contact lens hygiene and compliance*, http://www.aoa.org/documents/AOA-Contact-lens-hygiene.pdf, accessed September 2, 2007.

Boyd-Monk H: Bringing common eye emergencies into focus, *Nursing* 35(12):46, 2005.

Boys Town National Research Hospital: *About hearing aids: hearing aids and how they work*, http://www.boystownhospital.org/parents/hearingaids/how.asp, retrieved September 20, 2007.

Center for Ocular Prosthetics-Custom Made Artificial Plastic Eyes. http://www.artificialeyesplastic.com/new-eye-care.htm, accessed August 2, 2007.

Ebersole P and others: *Toward healthy aging*, ed 7, St. Louis, 2008, Mosby.

Emergencies in the Field: Focusing on eye emergencies, *Nursing* 37(2):46, 2007.

Erickson Laboratories: *Prosthetic care*, http://www.ericksonlaboratories.com/care.html, accessed August 2, 2007.

Fransman BA, Walker S: Digital hearing aids: a life transformation, *Learning Disability Practice* 10(3):16, 2007.

Galanti GA: *Caring for patients from different cultures*, ed 3, Philadelphia, 2004, University of Pennsylvania Press.

Hockenberry MJ, Wilson D: *Wong's nursing care of infants and children*, ed 8, St. Louis, 2007, Mosby.

Hoyt KS, Haley RJ: Innovations in advanced practice assessment and management of eye emergencies, *Top Emerg Med* 27(2):101, 2005.

Kolberg Ocular Prosthetics: *Artificial eye information and patient support page*, 2007, http://www.artificialeye.net, accessed September 2, 2007.

Rados C: Sound advice about hearing aids, *FDA Consumer*, p 20, May-June 2005.

The Joint Commission: *2008 National patient safety goals*, 2008, http://www.jointcommission.org/PatientSafety/NationalPatientSafetyGoals, accessed September 2, 2007.

U.S. National Library of Medicine: Medline Plus: *Eye emergencies*, 2007, http://www.nlm.nih.gov/medlineplus/ency/article/000054.htm, updated February 2007, accessed September 2, 2007.

RESEARCH REFERENCES

Cacchione PZ and others: Clinical profile of acute confusion in the long-term care setting, *Clin Nurs Res* 12(2):145, 2003a.

Cacchione PZ and others: Risk for acute confusion in sensory impaired, rural, long-term care elders, *Clin Nurs Res* 12(4):340, 2003b.

Crews JE and others: Double jeopardy: the effects of co-morbid conditions among older people with vision loss, *J Vis Impair Blind* 100(special suppl):824, 2006.

Segal E: First aid for skin/eye decontamination: are present practices effective? *J Chem Health Safety* 14(4):16, 2007.

Tay T and others: Sensory impairment, use of community support services, and quality of life in aged care clients, *J Aging Health* 19(2):229, 2007.

20

Safe Medication Preparation

MEDIA RESOURCES

- **evolve** *learning system* http://evolve.elsevier.com/Perry/skills
  - Review Questions
  - Video Clips

- **View Video!** Mosby's Nursing Video Skills, 3.0

- **NSO** Nursing Skills Online

OBJECTIVES

Mastery of content in this chapter will enable the nurse to:
- Discuss The Joint Commission's National Patient Safety Goals for medication administration.
- Discuss factors that contribute to medication errors.
- Discuss the types of medication actions.
- Identify the system of measurement for a given prescribed medication.
- Accurately calculate medication doses.
- Describe the safety features of medication delivery systems.
- List and discuss the six rights of medication administration.
- Identify guidelines for safe administration of medications.
- Identify steps to take in reporting medication errors.

Medication administration is a difficult and challenging nursing responsibility. Consider the situation of a nurse who works on a hospital's acute medical unit. It is not unusual for a patient on such a unit to receive 8 to 10 different medications daily, with each medication given more than once. Add the fact that the nurse cares for a minimum of four to six patients, and you begin to realize that medication administration is a challenging task. The nurse must be able to know the purpose of all those medications, the potential side effects, the normal dosages and routes of administration, the time each medication is due, and the patients' allergies.

When the Institute of Medicine (IOM) published the book *To Err Is Human: Building a Safer Health System,* the book created a national awareness of problems within the health care system (Kohn and others, 2000). The IOM estimates that medical errors are the eighth leading cause of death in this country annually. Medication errors are the most common types of such errors, accounting for more than 7,000 deaths each year. Of medication errors considered preventable, over half result in an adverse drug effect (ADE). An ADE is any response to a drug that is harmful, unintended, and that occurs at doses normally used in humans for the prophylaxis, diagnosis, or therapy of disease. The IOM has a national agenda for reducing medical errors and improving patient safety. One essential recommendation made by the IOM is to develop standards for patient safety to establish minimum levels of performance and set expectations for health professionals (IOM, 2003).

Multiple factors contribute to medication errors. Most medication errors occur at patient care–transition points such as during hospital admission, transfer from one unit to another, and discharge to home or another facility (Burke, 2005). One of every three ADEs results from omission or commission (Hughes and Ortiz, 2005). Omission errors result when a drug is not prescribed, dispensed, administered, or taken by a patient appropriately. Commission errors

occur while a nurse performs the six rights of medication administration (see p. 515) (McIntyre and Courey, 2007). In a study conducted in Taiwan, researchers asked registered nurses (RNs) to recall one of the most significant medication errors that they had experienced and to identify the contributing factors (Tang and others, 2007). The nurses reported more than one factor caused medication errors, including personal neglect, heavy workload, and new staff. The nurses also identified the need to solve other problems while administering drugs and advanced drug preparation without rechecking as critical factors. The Taiwan nurses identified issues no different from those identified by U.S. nurses. In many cases, drug errors occur as a result of failure of nurses to follow policy (Fitzpatrick and others, 2006). However, some policies promote unthinking rather than a rigorous problem-solving approach. Nurses need to make clinical judgments when administering medications and not simply give drugs automatically. This means thorough patient assessment and review of the pharmacokinetics and purpose of a medication are critical for safe medication administration.

The Joint Commission (TJC) accredits health care organizations across the United States. Improving patient safety is one commitment of the organization. The Joint Commission's accreditation program is a risk-reduction activity in that compliance with its standards is intended to reduce the risk for adverse outcomes for patients (TJC, 2007a). It established its first set of National Patient Safety Goals for improving the safety of patient care in health care organizations in 1992. All accredited health care organizations are surveyed for implementation of the goals and requirements. Each year The Joint Commission publishes a new set of goals. Failure of organizations to comply with the goal requirements leads to penalties and delayed accreditation approval. Medication safety has consistently been one of the National Patient Safety Goals (Box 20-1).

BOX 20-1 Joint Commission 2008 National Patient Safety Goals—Implications for Medication Administration

- Improve the accuracy of patient identification.
  - Use at least two patient identifiers (neither to be patient's room number) when providing care, treatment (e.g., medications) or services.
- Improve the effectiveness of communication among caregivers.
  - Verbal or telephone orders require a verification "read-back" of the complete order or test result by the person receiving the order/test result.
  - Standardize a list of abbreviations, acronyms, symbols, and dose designations that are **not** to be used throughout an organization.
- Improve the safety of using medications.
  - Identify and at a minimum, annually review a list of look-alike/sound-alike drugs used by the organization.
  - Label all medications, medication containers (e.g., syringes, medicine cups) on and off the sterile field. Labels include drug name, strength, amount, expiration date when not used within

24 hours, and expiration time when expiration occurs in less than 24 hours.
  - Reduce the likelihood of patient harm associated with the use of anticoagulation therapy. Use only oral unit-dose products and premixed infusions. When heparin is administered intravenously and continuously, use programmable infusion pumps.
- Accurately and completely reconcile medications across the continuum of care.
  - There is a process for comparing the patient's current medications with those ordered for the patient while under the care of the health care organization.
  - Communicate a complete list of the patient's medications to the next provider of service when a patient is referred or transferred to another setting, service, or level of care. Also provide the complete list to the patient upon discharge from the facility.
  - Encourage patients' active involvement in their own care as a patient safety strategy.

Modified from The Joint Commission: *2008 National patient safety goals,* http://www.jointcommission.org/PatientSafety/NationalPatientSafetyGoals/08_npsg_facts. htm, accessed August 5, 2007b.

All professional nurses need to take seriously the implications involved in medication administration. Safe medication administration requires good judgment with critical thinking. RNs and licensed practical nurses (LPNs) are able to administer medications under the direction of a licensed physician. Advanced practice nurses (APNs) have some prescriptive authority in almost every state, but the degree of required physician involvement varies. In some states and settings, medication can be delegated to nursing assistive personnel with nurse oversight.

PHARMACOLOGICAL CONCEPTS

Medication Names

Some medications have as many as three different names. The chemical name describes the medication's composition and molecular structure, such as *N*-acetyl-para-aminophenol, commonly known as Tylenol. The chemical name is rarely used in clinical

TABLE 20-1	Forms of Medication
Form	**Description**

Medication Forms Commonly Prepared for Administration by Oral Route

Solid Forms

Form	Description
Caplet	Shaped like a capsule and coated for ease of swallowing.
Capsule	Medication encased in a gelatin shell.
Tablet	Powdered medication compressed into a hard disk or cylinder.
Enteric coated	Tablet that is coated so that it does not dissolve in stomach; meant for intestinal absorption.

Liquid Forms

Form	Description
Elixir	Clear fluid containing water and alcohol; usually has sweetener added.
Extract	Concentrated medication form made by removing the active portion of medication from its other components.
Aqueous solution	Substance dissolved in water and syrups.
Suspension	Finely dissolved drug particles in a liquid medium must be shaken. When left standing, particles settle to bottom of container; not used intravenously.
Syrup	Medication dissolved in a concentrated sugar solution.
Tincture	Alcohol extract from plant or vegetable.

Other Oral Forms and Terms Associated With Oral Preparations

Form	Description
Troche (lozenge)	Flat, round dosage form containing medication that dissolves in mouth; not meant for ingestion.
Aerosol	Aqueous medication sprayed and absorbed in the mouth and upper airway; not meant for ingestion.
Sustained release	Tablet or capsule that contains small particles of a medication coated with material that requires a varying amount of time to dissolve.

Medication Forms Commonly Prepared for Administration by Topical Route

Form	Description
Ointment (salve or cream)	Semisolid, externally applied preparation, usually containing one or more medications.
Liniment	Oily liquid applied to the skin.
Lotion	Emollient liquid that can be clear solution, suspension, or emulsion. Applied externally.
Paste	Medication preparation that is thicker than ointment; absorbed through the skin more slowly than ointment. Applied externally.
Transdermal patch or disk	Disk or patch embedded with a medication that is applied to the skin. Drug is absorbed through the skin over a designated period of time.

Medication Forms Commonly Prepared for Administration by Parenteral Route

Form	Description
Solution	Sterile preparation that contains water/normal saline with one or more dissolved compounds. The solution must be sterile.
Powder	Sterile particles of medication that are reconstituted with water/saline, dissolved, and administered parenterally. The solution must be sterile.

Medication Forms Commonly Prepared for Instillation Into Body Cavities

Form	Description
Suppository	Solid dosage form mixed with gelatin and shaped in the form of a pellet for insertion into a body cavity (rectum or vagina). The suppository melts when it reaches body temperature and is then absorbed.
Intraocular disk	Disk (similar to a contact lens) embedded with a medication that is inserted into the patient's eye. The medication is absorbed over a designated period of time.
Solution	Substance dissolved in water or other liquid.

practice. A manufacturer who first develops a medication gives the generic name of a medication. Acetaminophen is the generic name for Tylenol. The generic name is the official name that is listed in official publications such as the *United States Pharmacopeia* (USP). A medication trade name or brand name is used to market the medication. The trade name has the symbol ™ at the upper right of the name, indicating a manufacturer's trademark of the name (e.g., Panadol™, Tempra™, Tylenol™).

Problematic brand and generic names contribute to medication errors (McIntyre and Courey, 2007). Names of drugs not only sound alike and have similar pronunciations, but some have similar spelling. The USP identifies several problematic medications with similar names, such as Lamictal for epilepsy and Lamisil for fungal infections; Levoxine for hypothyroidism and Lanoxin for heart failure. The IOM recommends that the Food and Drug Administration (FDA) give increased attention to the safe use of medications (IOM, 2003). This includes developing standards for the design of medication packaging and labeling. The IOM also recommends identifying and correcting potential sound-alike and look-alike confusion with medication names. The appearance of some drugs is deceiving. Similar color, size, and shape have led to medication errors. For example, St. Joseph's aspirin and Crestor, a lipid-lowering agent, have a similar peach color, size, and circular shape. Look-alike drugs cause problems especially for patients with visual or cognitive impairment (McIntyre and Courey, 2007). Hospital and clinic pharmacies try to consistently dispense medications with the same trade names so nurses will become familiar with them. However, nurses find medications under a variety of different names and must be careful to obtain the exact name and spelling before administering a medication. TJC publishes on its website (http://www.jointcommision.org) a look-alike/sound-alike drug list and recommendations for nurses, prescribers, and health care organizations to prevent mixing up look-alike/sound-alike medications (TJC, 2007b).

Classification

Medications with similar characteristics are categorized by their class. Medication classification indicates the effect of a medication on a body system, the symptoms the medication relieves, or the medication's desired effect. For example, patients with type 2 diabetes often take oral medications to control their blood glucose levels. The sulfonylureas are one classification of medications used by these patients. There are at least seven different medications in the sulfonylurea classification (McKenry and others, 2006). Some medications are part of more than one class. For example, aspirin is an analgesic, an antipyretic, and an antiinflammatory medication.

Medication Forms

Medications are available in a variety of forms or preparations. The form of the medication determines its route of administration. The composition of a medication influences its absorption and metabolism. Many medications are made in several forms (Table 20-1). When administering a medication, be certain to use the proper form.

Pharmacokinetics

A medication must enter a patient's body, be absorbed and distributed to cells, tissues, or a specific organ, and then alter physiological function to be therapeutic. Pharmacokinetics is the study of how medications enter the body, reach their site of action, are metabolized, and exit the body. Understanding pharmacokinetics allows nurses to properly time medication administration, select an administration route, and judge a patient's response to medications.

Absorption is the passage of medication molecules into the blood from the site of administration. Factors that influence the rate of absorption include the administration route, ability of a medication to dissolve, blood flow to the administration site, body surface area, and lipid solubility of a medication (Table 20-2). After a medication is absorbed, it is distributed to tissues and organs and finally to the site of drug action. The rate and extent of distribution depends on circulation, cell membrane permeability, and protein binding. When there is poor perfusion, as in the case of heart failure, this alters medication distribution. A medication must pass through biological membranes to reach certain organs. Some membranes are barriers to the passage of medications. For example, the blood-brain barrier allows only fat-soluble medications to pass into the brain and cerebrospinal fluid. The degree to which medications bind to serum proteins such as albumin affects distribution. Most medications bind to albumin to some extent. When medications bind to albumin, they are unable to exert pharmacological activity. Only the unbound, or "free," medication is active. Older adults and patients with liver disease or malnutrition have reduced albumin, which increases their risk for medication toxicity.

After a medication reaches its site of action, it becomes metabolized into a less active or inactive form. Biotransformation occurs under the influence of enzymes that detoxify, degrade (break down), and remove biologically active chemicals. Most biotransformation occurs in the liver, although the lungs, kidneys, blood,

TABLE 20-2	Medication Absorption
Absorption Factor	**Physiological Effects**
Route of administration	Topical applications on skin absorb slowly. Medications applied to mucous membranes and respiratory airways absorb quickly. Oral medications pass through the gastrointestinal tract and absorb slowly. The IV route absorbs most rapidly.
Ability to dissolve	Solutions and liquid suspensions absorb more readily than tablets or capsules. Acidic medications absorb rapidly, whereas basic medications (pH >7.0) do not absorb before reaching the small intestine.
Blood flow	When the administration site contains a rich blood supply, medications absorb rapidly.
Body surface area	A medication in contact with a large surface area (e.g., small intestine) will absorb faster than those in contact with smaller surface area (e.g., stomach).
Lipid solubility	Medications that are highly lipid soluble absorb more readily.

- Patients taking a medication for the first time
- Very young and elderly
- Women
- Patients taking more than four to five medications (polypharmacy)
- Patients extremely underweight or overweight
- Patients with renal and/or hepatic disease
- Patients with altered blood flow conditions
- Patients with a past history of an ADR
- Patients with depression or anxiety
- Patients with sensory deprivation or overload
- Patients who abuse alcohol, nicotine, or street medications
- Patients who treat selves with over-the-counter medications

Modified from Arnold GJ: Clinical recognition of adverse medication reactions: obstacles and opportunities for the nursing profession, *J Nurs Care Qual* 13(2):45, 1998.
ADR, Adverse drug reaction.

and intestines also play a role. Patients (e.g., older adults and those with chronic disease) are at risk for medication toxicity if their organs that metabolize medications do not function correctly.

The final aspect of pharmacokinetics is excretion, the process of medications exiting the body through the lungs, exocrine glands, bowel, kidneys, and liver. A medication's chemical makeup determines the organ of excretion. For example, gaseous and volatile compounds, such as alcohol and nitrous oxide, exit through the lungs. The site of excretion poses implications for nursing care. For example, when medications exit through sweat glands, you provide hygiene to reduce skin irritation. You must know if a drug is excreted through the intestines, because the administration of laxatives or enemas increases peristalsis, accelerates excretion, and thus lessens the time for drug effects. When patients have reduced renal function, they are at risk for medication toxicity.

TYPES OF MEDICATION ACTION

Medications vary in the way they act and their types of action. Patients do not always respond in the same way to each successive dose of a medication. Sometimes the same medication causes very different responses in different patients. Therefore it is essential to understand all the effects that medications have on patients.

Therapeutic Effects

Each medication has a therapeutic effect, the intended or desired physiological response of a medication. For example, you administer morphine sulfate, an analgesic, to relieve a patient's pain. Sometimes a single medication has many therapeutic effects. For example, aspirin relieves pain and reduces fever and tissue inflammation. It is important to know the exact therapeutic effect for which a medication is prescribed so you can properly teach patients about a medication's intended effect and to accurately evaluate the medication's desired effect.

Side Effects/Adverse Effects

Some medications react in the body to produce unpredictable and sometimes unexplainable responses (McKenry and others, 2006). No medication is totally safe and absolutely free of nontherapeutic effects. Side effects are predictable and often unavoidable secondary effects produced at a usual therapeutic drug dose. For example,

some antihypertensive medications cause impotence in male patients. Side effects are either harmless or injurious. The intensity of side effects is often dose dependent (McKenry and others, 2006). If the side effects are serious enough to outweigh the benefits of a medication's therapeutic action, the prescriber will likely discontinue the medication. Patients commonly stop taking medications because of side effects such as anorexia, nausea, vomiting, dizziness, drowsiness, dry mouth, constipation, and diarrhea. Report any side effect to the prescriber to ensure that it is not incorrectly interpreted as a more serious adverse medication reaction.

Adverse drug effects are unintended, undesirable, and often unpredictable. Every medication has a potential to harm a patient (McKenry and others, 2006). Unfortunately, although ADEs are sometimes immediately apparent, they often take weeks or months to develop. Early clinical recognition of ADEs is the important first step in identification. Be alert to assess any unusual individual responses to drugs, especially with newly released medications (McKenry and others, 2006). Adverse drug events range from mild (e.g., rashes or photosensitivity to light) to potentially fatal (anaphylaxis). Prompt recognition and reporting of ADEs will prevent serious injury to patients. Box 20-2 highlights patients most at risk for ADEs. Patients falling into one or more risk categories require close monitoring. Health care agencies have specific policies for reporting ADEs (U.S. Food and Drug Administration, 2007).

Toxic Effects

Toxic effects develop after prolonged intake of a medication, when a medication accumulates in the blood because of impaired metabolism or excretion, or when too high a dose is given. Excess amounts of a medication within the body sometimes have lethal effects, depending on the medication's action. For example, toxic levels of morphine, an opioid, cause severe respiratory depression and death. Antidotes are available to treat specific types of medication toxicity.

Idiosyncratic Reactions

Medications often cause unpredictable effects such as an idiosyncratic reaction, in which a patient overreacts or underreacts to a medication or has a reaction different from normal. Predicting which patients will have an idiosyncratic response is impossible. For example, Ativan, an antianxiety medication, when given to an older adult may cause agitation and delirium.

Allergic Reactions

Allergic reactions also are unpredictable responses to a medication. Exposure to an initial dose of a medication causes a patient to become sensitized immunologically. The medication acts as an antigen, which causes antibodies to be produced. With repeated administration, the patient develops an allergic response to the drug, its chemical preservatives, or a metabolite. An allergic reaction ranges from mild to severe, depending on the patient and the medication. Among the different classes of medications, antibiotics cause a high incidence of allergic reactions. Table 20-3 summarizes common, mild allergy symptoms. Sudden constriction of bronchiolar muscles, edema of the pharynx and larynx, severe wheezing, and shortness of breath are characteristic of severe or anaphylactic reactions. Some patients become severely hypotensive, necessitating emergency resuscitation measures. Anaphylaxis is potentially fatal.

It is common practice at the time of a patient's admission to a health care facility to have any known medication allergies identified and recorded in a clearly identifiable place that is easy for all those involved in the patient's care to see. Nurses record allergy information on the front of the patient's medical record, in the

TABLE 20-3	Mild Allergic Reactions
Symptom	**Description**
Urticaria (hives)	Raised, irregularly shaped skin eruptions with varying sizes and shapes; eruptions have reddened margins and pale centers.
Eczema (rash)	Small, raised vesicles that are usually reddened; often distributed over the entire body.
Pruritus	Itching of the skin; accompanies most rashes.
Rhinitis	Inflammation of mucous membranes lining the nose, causing swelling and a clear watery discharge.

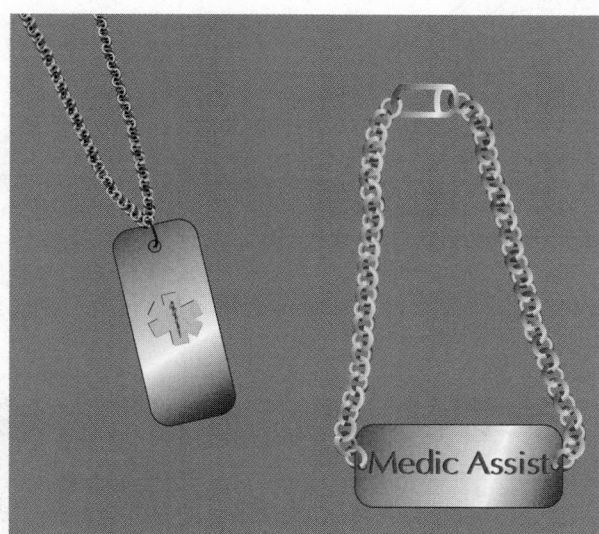

Fig. 20-1　Identification bracelet and medal.

medication administration record (MAR), or on a specially designed label that is applied to the front of the patient's chart. Patients also receive color-coded allergy identification bands to wear around the wrist. **Always record a patient's allergies in the MAR.** Patients in other settings (e.g., home or community clinics) who have a known allergy to a medication or substance should wear an identification bracelet or medical alert medal, which alerts all health care providers to the allergies in case the patient is found unconscious or is unable to communicate (Fig. 20-1).

Medication Tolerance and Dependence

Medication tolerance is a decreased physiological response that occurs after repeated administration of a medication (McKenry and others, 2006). It is usually noted clinically when patients receive the same medication for long periods and require higher doses to produce the desired therapeutic effect. Medications known to produce tolerance include opium alkaloids (e.g., morphine), nitrates, and ethyl alcohol. Recently, researchers have found that a substance, peroxynitrite, builds up in the spinal cord after repeated doses of morphine, making the drug less effective (Fernandes, 2007). Patients hospitalized for acute episodes of illness usually do not develop tolerance. It sometimes takes months for tolerance to occur. Cross-tolerance, the development of tolerance to pharmacologically similar drugs, occurs following tolerance to a medication (McKenry and others, 2006).

Drug dependence, described in the past as addiction and habituation, can be physical or psychological. In psychological dependence, patients have an emotional desire for a drug to maintain an effect (McKenry and others, 2006). A person believes a desirable effect will result when taking the medication. An example is the medication marijuana, which many individuals use to cause relaxation. Physical dependence is a physiological adaptation to a medication that manifests itself by intense physical disturbance when the medication is withdrawn. An example is the repeated use of codeine for reducing mild to moderate pain. When patients receive medications for a short term (such as for postoperative pain), dependence is rare. If a patient is dependent on alcohol, a higher-than-usual medication dose is necessary for the desired effect of the medication.

Medication Interactions

When one medication modifies the action of another medication, a medication interaction occurs. The effect is an increase or decrease in the pharmacological action of each medication. Medication interactions are common in individuals taking many medications. Some medications intensify or diminish the action of other medications and alter the way in which another medication is absorbed, metabolized, or eliminated from the body. This is a common problem in older adults; they tend to have multiple physicians who are prescribing a variety of medications without discontinuing any previous medications or are unaware of the other physicians. A medication interaction is sometimes desirable. A health care provider will order combination medication therapy to create an interaction for therapeutic benefit.

Summation occurs when the combined effect of two drugs produces a result that equals the sum of the individual effects of each drug (McKenry and others, 2006). In other words 1 + 1 = 2. For example, codeine and aspirin both act as analgesics. Given together, the two drugs provide greater pain relief than when a patient uses either one alone. Summation allows the administration of a lower dose of each drug with less risk for adverse effects. A synergistic effect is a drug interaction in which the combined effect of drugs is greater than the sum of each individual agent acting independently (McKenry and others, 2006). In other words, 1 + 1 = 3 or more. The use of a combination of drugs to treat hypertension is an example of synergism. Each drug lowers blood pressure but in a different way; the summed effect produces a greater reduction in hypertension than the sum of each medication.

Medication Dose Responses

After administration, a medication undergoes absorption, distribution, metabolism, and excretion. Except when administered intravenously, medications take time to enter the bloodstream. The quantity and distribution of a medication in different body compartments change constantly. When a medication is prescribed, the goal is a constant blood level within a safe therapeutic range. Repeated doses are necessary to achieve a constant therapeutic

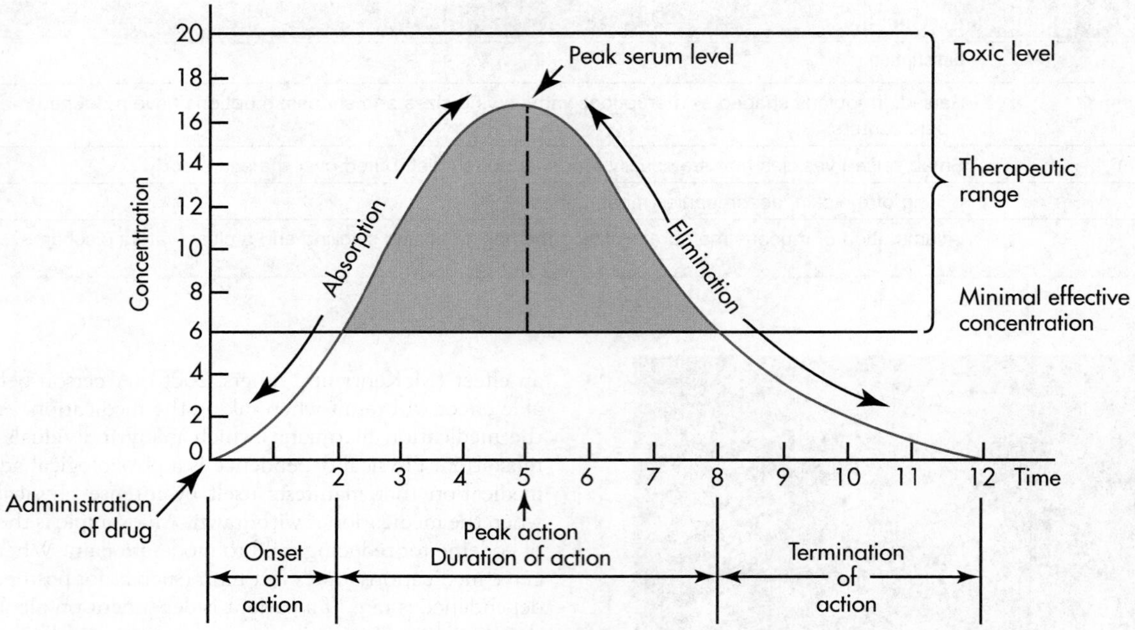

Fig. 20-2 Plasma level profile of a drug. (*From McKenry LM, Salerno E*: Mosby's pharmacology in nursing, *ed 22, St. Louis, 2006, Mosby.*)

concentration of a medication because a portion of a medication is always being excreted. The highest serum concentration (peak concentration) of a medication usually occurs just before the body absorbs the last of the medication (McKenry and others, 2006) (Fig. 20-2). After peaking, the serum concentration falls progressively. With intravenous (IV) infusions, the peak concentration occurs quickly, but the serum level also begins to fall immediately. The point at which the lowest amount of drug is in the serum is the trough concentration. Some medication doses (e.g., vancomycin or gentamycin) are based on peak and trough serum levels. A patient's trough level is drawn as a blood sample 30 minutes before administering the drug, and the peak level is drawn whenever the drug is expected to reach its peak concentration. The results of the blood test reveal if the drug is reaching its therapeutic blood level.

All medications have a serum half-life, which is the time it takes for excretion processes to lower the serum medication concentration by half. To maintain a therapeutic plateau, a patient needs to receive regular fixed doses. For example, current evidence shows that pain medications are most effective when they are given around-the-clock rather than when the patient intermittently complains of pain because the body maintains an almost constant level of pain medication. After an initial medication dose, the patient receives each successive dose when the previous dose reaches its half-life. The patient and nurse need to follow regular dosage schedules and administer prescribed doses at correct intervals. Know the following time intervals of medication action to anticipate a medication's effect:

1 *Onset of medication action:* Period of time it takes after you administer a medication for it to produce a therapeutic effect
2 *Peak action:* Time it takes for a medication to reach its highest effective peak concentration
3 *Duration of action:* Length of time during which the medication is present in a concentration great enough to produce a therapeutic effect
4 *Plateau:* Blood serum concentration reached and maintained after repeated, fixed doses

TABLE 20-4	Routes of Medication Administration
Route	**Description**
Nonparenteral	
Oral, buccal	By mouth
Sublingual	Under the tongue
Topical	On the skin (as a cream or patch) and eyedrops/eardrops
Suppository	Into the rectum or vagina
Parenteral	
Intramuscular (IM)	Into a muscle
Subcutaneous	Into the subcutaneous tissue of the skin
Intradermal (ID)	Into the dermis of the skin
Epidural	Into the epidural space
Intravenous (IV)	Into a vein

ROUTES OF ADMINISTRATION

The route prescribed for administering a medication (Table 20-4) depends on its properties and desired effect and on a patient's physical and mental condition. Because of what you know about your patients, you need to collaborate with a prescriber in determining the best route for a patient's medical condition. Table 20-5 summarizes the factors that influence the choice of administration routes.

MEDICATION DISTRIBUTION

Health care providers write medication orders, pharmacists dispense medications, and nurses deliver medications to patients. A number of technologies for medication distribution have the po-

TABLE 20-5	Factors Influencing Choice of Administration Routes

Advantages	Disadvantages/Contraindications
Oral, Buccal, Sublingual Routes	
Easy and comfortable to administer, convenient, economical; may produce local or systemic effects. Rarely causes anxiety for patient.	Avoided when patient has alterations in GI function (e.g., nausea and vomiting), with reduced GI motility (after general anesthesia or bowel inflammation) and surgical resection of portion of GI tract. Gastric secretions destroy some medications. Oral administration is contraindicated in patients who are NPO and unable to swallow (e.g., patients with neuromuscular disorders, esophageal strictures, and mouth lesions). Do not give oral medications when patient has gastric suction, before certain diagnostic tests or surgery. An unconscious or confused patient is unable or unwilling to swallow or hold sublingual medication under the tongue or buccal medication in cheek. Oral medications sometimes irritate the lining of the GI tract, discolor teeth, or have an unpleasant taste.
Parenteral (Subcutaneous, Intramuscular, Intravenous, Intradermal, Epidural) Routes	
Routes provide means of administration when oral medications are contraindicated. More rapid absorption occurs than with topical or oral routes.	Risk for introducing infection, and medications are expensive. Some patients experience pain from repeated needle sticks. Subcutaneous, IM, and ID routes avoided in patients with bleeding tendencies. Risk for tissue damage with subcutaneous injections.
IV infusion provides medication delivery when patient is critically ill or long-term therapy is necessary. If peripheral perfusion is poor, IV route is preferred over injections.	IV and IM routes have higher absorption rates, thus placing patient at higher risk for reactions.
Epidural provides excellent pain control.	Limits mobility during administration. Risk for infection.
Skin	
Topical	
Topical skin applications provide primarily local effect. Route is usually painless. Limited side effects occur.	Extensive applications often require dressings that are bulky for a patient when maneuvering. Do not apply to skin if abrasions are present, unless that is the reason for order. Medications can be absorbed by person applying it if gloves are not worn.
Transdermal	
Transdermal applications provide prolonged systemic effects, with limited side effects.	Application leaves oily or pasty substance on skin and may soil clothing. Some patients have sensitivity to adhesive.
Mucous Membranes (Includes Eyes, Ears, Nose, Vaginal, Rectal, Buccal, and Sublingual Routes)	
Therapeutic effects are provided by local application to involved sites. Aqueous solutions are readily absorbed and capable of causing systemic effects.	Mucous membranes are highly sensitive to some medication concentrations. Insertion of rectal and vaginal medications often causes embarrassment.
Mucous membranes provide route of administration when oral medications are contraindicated.	Rectal suppositories are contraindicated if patients have had rectal surgery or if active rectal bleeding is present. If eardrum is ruptured, otic medications are usually contraindicated.
Inhalation	
Inhalation provides rapid relief for local respiratory problems. There is also now available an inhaled form of insulin. Route provides easy access for introduction of general anesthetic gases.	Some local agents cause serious systemic effects. If patients unable to administer inhaler correctly, medication will be ineffective. Difficult to learn for older adults and children.
Intraocular Disk	
Route is advantageous in that it does not require frequent administration like eye drops. The patient can also wear disk when sleeping or swimming. Dry eyes do not affect medication delivery.	Local reactions occur such as tearing, itching, or redness of the eyes. Patient needs to know how to insert disk into and remove from the eye. Medication is often expensive. Medication is contraindicated in patients with infections of the eye.

GI, Gastrointestinal; *NPO,* nothing by mouth; *IM,* intramuscular; *ID,* intradermal; *IV,* intravenous.

tential for reducing medication errors and ADEs. These technologies are now in numerous health care settings. The technologies include computerized physician order entry (CPOE), automated medication dispensing system (AMDS), and bar coding (Oren and others, 2003; Skibinski, 2007). AMDS often reduce the chance of medication errors (Manno, 2006).

Computerized Physician Order Entry

CPOE is a system that allows prescribers to electronically enter orders for medications, eliminating the need for written orders. With use of CPOE, there is increased accuracy and legibility of medication orders, integration of clinical decision support into the order-entry process, and optimization of prescriber, nurse, and pharmacist time (Oren and others, 2003; Rask, 2007). Decision support software, integrated into a CPOE system, allows for automatic drug allergy checks, dosage indications, and identification of potential drug interactions. When a prescriber enters an order through CPOE, the information about the order immediately transmits to the pharmacy and ultimately to the nurses' MAR without the need for written transcription. Researchers estimate that CPOE implementation at all nonrural hospitals in the United States will possibly prevent over 500,000 serious medication errors annually (Skibinski, 2007).

Distribution Systems

 Advanced / Safe Medication Administration / Using Medication Administration Systems

Institutions providing nursing care have a special area for stocking and dispensing medications. Special medication rooms, portable locked carts, computerized medication cabinets, and individual storage units next to patients' rooms are examples of storage areas used. All medications must be in a locked environment or under constant surveillance.

Unit Dose

The standard for medication distribution is the unit-dose system. The system uses AMDS or carts containing a drawer with a 24-hour supply of medications for each patient. Each drawer has a label with the name of the patient in the designated room. The unit dose is the ordered dose of medication the patient receives at one time. Each tablet or capsule is wrapped in a foil or paper container. Liquid doses come in prepackaged foil or plastic cups. At a designated time each day the pharmacist or a pharmacy technician refills the drawers in the cart with a fresh supply. Controlled substances are not in the individual patient drawer; they are in a larger locked drawer to keep them secure. A unit-dose system is designed to reduce the number of medication errors and saves steps in dispensing medications.

Automated Medication Dispensing System

Unit dose systems that use an AMDS provide computerized control of unit-dose medication dispensing (Fig. 20-3). All procedures connected to an AMDS are controlled electronically via a patient's profile. A nurse accesses a patient name and his or her drug profile order before the AMDS dispenses a medication. Each nurse has a security code allowing access to the system. In these systems the nurse selects the desired medication, dosage, and route from a list displayed on the computer screen. The system causes the drawer containing the medication to open, records it, and charges it to the patient. Frequently these systems link to computer software programs in the pharmacy that detect dosage errors and incompatible medications or send alerts regarding potential interactions and patients' medication allergies. When a CPOE system is used, medication orders transmit directly to an AMDS. There is evi-

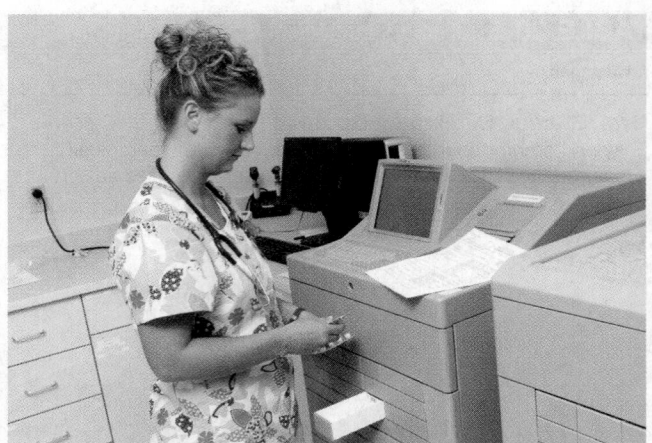

FIG. 20-3   Automated medication dispensing system.

dence of an increase in reported medication errors with use of the system. Typically there are fewer missing doses reported with AMDS (Oren and others, 2003). An AMDS is not foolproof. The system has mechanical moving parts, electronics, and software that can fail. Errors can occur with an AMDS system, including errors by pharmacists on manual order entry and cabinet loading or by nurses on the retrieval of medications.

Bar Coding

Recently steps have been taken to require bar code labels on all medications, vaccines, and over-the-counter (OTC) drugs used in hospitals (Roark, 2004). The use of electronic bar codes on medication labels and packaging has the potential to improve patient safety in a number of ways. Bar codes electronically link with a hospital's computer system. A patient's MAR entered into the computer database and encoded in the patient's wristband is accessible to a nurse through a handheld device. The device scans the patient's wristband and then displays the MAR. When administering a medication, the nurse scans the drug's bar code and the patient's medical record number on the wristband and the nurse's code on her identification badge. The computer then processes the scanned information, charts it, and updates the patient's MAR record appropriately (Roark, 2004). The use of bar codes improves accuracy of patient identification and correct medication use and improves medical record keeping (Paoletti and others, 2007). Hospitals that have point-of-care systems in which nurses verify patient and drug information at the bedside find bar coding very useful.

SYSTEMS OF MEDICATION MEASUREMENT

NSO *Safe Medication Administration Module / Lesson 3*

The proper administration of medication depends on a nurse's ability to calculate medication doses accurately and measure medications correctly. Calculation mistakes often lead to fatal errors. The prescriber and patient depend on you to check doses before administering medications. The most common medication measurement system is the metric system. The apothecary and household measurement systems are used less frequently.

Metric System

As a decimal system, the metric system is the most logically organized measurement system. Metric units are easy to convert and compute through simple multiplication and division. Each basic unit of measurement is organized into units of 10. Multiplying or dividing by 10 forms secondary units. In multiplication the decimal point moves to the right; in division the decimal moves to the left. For example:

$$10 \text{ mg} \times 10 = 100 \text{ mg}$$

$$10 \text{ mg} \div 10 = 1 \text{ mg}$$

When designating a metric dosage it is important to **never have a trailing zero** (e.g., 1.0 mg is incorrect) and **always include a zero before a decimal point** (e.g., 0.1 mL is correct). The basic units of measure in the metric system are the meter (length), the liter (volume), and the gram (weight). For medication calculations only use the volume and weight units. The following are examples of metric system abbreviations:

$$\text{Gram} = \text{g or Gm}$$

$$\text{Liter} = \text{l or L}$$

Use only lowercase letters for abbreviations for subdivisions of major units:

$$\text{Milligram} = \text{mg}$$

The one exception: Milliliter = ml or mL

A system of Latin prefixes designates subdivision of the basic units: deci- (1/10 or 0.1), centi- (1/100 or 0.01), and milli- (1/1000 or 0.001). Greek prefixes designate multiples of the basic units: deka- (10), hecto- (100), and kilo- (1000). For example: 1 gram = 1000 milligrams (mg). When writing medication dosages in metric units, prescribers and nurses use either fractions or multiples of a unit. Convert fractions to decimals:

$$500 \text{ mg or } 0.5 \text{ g, not } \tfrac{1}{2} \text{ g}$$

$$10 \text{ mL or } 0.01 \text{ L, not } \tfrac{1}{100} \text{ L}$$

Apothecary System

The apothecary system is one of the oldest measurement systems. It is conducive to errors because of its symbols and abbreviations. Many hospitals no longer permit its use. The basic units of measure in the apothecary system include weight (grains) and volume (minims, drams, and ounces). The system uses Roman numerals and fractions. The symbol "ss" is used for the fraction ½. In the apothecary system you write the abbreviation or symbol for a unit of measure before the amount or quantity. For example:

$$\text{gr 15 or gr xv}$$

Household Measurements

Household units of measure are familiar to most people. The disadvantage is their inaccuracy. Regular household utensils such as teaspoons and drinking cups vary in size. Scales to measure pints or quarts are often not well calibrated. Household measures include drops, teaspoons, tablespoons, and cups for volume, and pints and quarts for weight. When the accuracy of a medication dose is not critical (e.g., over-the-counter medications), it is safe to use household measures. Recommend the use of measuring cups or spoons used for cooking.

Solutions

Nurses use solutions of various concentrations for injections, irrigations, and infusions. A solution is a given mass of solid substance dissolved in a known volume of fluid or a given volume of liquid dissolved in a known volume of another fluid. When a solid is dissolved in a fluid, the concentration is in units of mass per units of volume (e.g., g/L or mg/mL). You can also express the concentration of a solution as a percentage. A 10% solution, for example, is 10 g of solid dissolved in 100 mL of solution. A proportion also expresses concentrations. A 1/1000 solution represents a solution containing 1 g of solid in 1000 mL of liquid or 1 mL of liquid mixed with 1000 mL of another liquid.

SAFE MEDICATION ADMINISTRATION

 Advanced / Safe Medication Administration / Ensuring the Six Rights of Medication Administration

Standards are those actions that ensure safe nursing practice. To ensure safe medication administration, nurses follow the nursing standard called the *six rights of medication administration* consistently every time they administer medications. All medication errors are linked, in some way, to an inconsistency in adhering to the six rights. The six rights of medication administration include:

1 The right medication
2 The right dose
3 The right patient
4 The right route
5 The right time
6 The right documentation

Right Medication

A medication order is required for any drug you administer to a patient. Prescribers typically write orders by hand in a patient's chart. Alternatively, some agencies use CPOE, eliminating the need for written orders. Regardless of how you receive the order, you compare the prescriber's written orders with the MAR when the medication is initially ordered. Also verify medication information whenever new MARs are written or distributed or when patients transfer from one nursing unit or health care setting to another (TJC, 2007b).

A state's nurse practice act and institutional policies define which providers, other than physicians, are able to prescribe medications. As a nurse, you need to know the proper abbreviations to use when writing and transcribing medication orders. Each organization has a list of acceptable abbreviations. The Joint Commission (2007a) has identified a list of prohibited or "dangerous" abbreviations that when used frequently lead to error. Recently a study was completed showing that abbreviation-related errors more often originate from medical staff, thus requiring nurses to carefully check all orders (Brunetti, 2007). In addition, this same study found that in nearly 40% of the errors in which abbreviations were identified as the cause of error, the exact abbreviation could not be identified. Table 20-6 includes the Institute for Safe Medication Practices' (ISMP's) list of error-prone abbreviations, in addition to The Joint Commission's prohibited abbreviations that were first effective in 2004.

Types of orders based on frequency and/or urgency of medication administration include standing or routine orders, prn orders (given only when a patient requires it), STAT orders (drug given immediately and only once), and single, one-time orders (medication ordered for specific time). Each order needs to include the patient's name, the drug ordered, dosage, route of administration, and time(s) of administration.

Even though there are hospitals that have CPOE, most institutions still use a written order system. Written orders need to be transcribed either by hand or electronically on an MAR (Fig. 20-4). A nurse or a designated unit secretary writes the prescriber's complete order on the MAR. The transcribed order includes the

TABLE 20-6	Institute for Safe Medication Practice List of Error-Prone Abbreviations

These abbreviations, symbols, and dose designations have been reported to ISMP though the USP-ISMP Medication Error Reporting Program for being frequently misinterpreted and involved in harmful medication errors. They should never be used when communicating medical information. The Joint Commission has established a National Patient Safety Goal that specifies that certain abbreviations must appear on an accredited organization's do-not-use list; those items are indicated with a double asterisk (**).

Abbreviations	Intended Meaning	Misinterpretation	Correction
μg	Microgram	Mistaken as "mg"	Use "mcg"
AD, AS, AU	Right ear, left ear, each ear	Mistaken as OD, OS, OU (right eye, left eye, each eye)	Use "right ear," "left ear," or "each ear"
OD, OS, OU	Right eye, left eye, each eye	Mistaken as AD, AS, AU (right ear, left ear, each ear)	Use "right eye," "left eye," or "each eye"
BT	Bedtime	Mistaken as "BID" (twice daily)	Use "bedtime"
cc	Cubic centimeters	Mistaken as "u" (units)	Use "mL"
D/C	Discharge or discontinue	Premature discontinuation of medication if D/C (intended to mean "discharge") has been misinterpreted as "discontinued" when followed by a list of discharge medications	Use "discharge" and "discontinue"
IJ	Injection	Mistaken as "IV" or "intrajugular"	Use "injection"
IN	Intranasal	Mistaken as "IM" or "IV"	Use "intranasal" or "NAS"
HS	Half-strength	Mistaken as bedtime	Use "half-strength"
hs	At bedtime, hour of sleep	Mistaken as half-strength	Use "bedtime"
IU**	International unit	Mistaken as IV (intravenous) or 10 (ten)	Use "units"
o.d. or OD	Once daily	Mistaken as "right eye" (OD—*oculus dexter*), leading to oral liquid medications administered in the eye	Use "daily"
OJ	Orange juice	Mistaken as OD or OS (right or left eye); drugs meant to be diluted in orange juice may be given in the eye	Use "orange juice"
Per os	By mouth, orally	The "os" can be mistaken as "left eye" (OS—*oculus sinister*)	Use "PO," "by mouth," or "orally"
q.d. or QD**	Every day	Mistaken as q.i.d., especially if the period after the "q" or the tail of the "q" is misunderstood as an "i"	Use "daily"
qhs	Nightly at bedtime	Mistaken as "qhr" or every hour	Use "nightly"
qn	Nightly or at bedtime	Mistaken as "qhr" or every hour	Use "nightly" or "at bedtime"
q.o.d. or QOD**	Every other day	Mistaken as q.d. (daily) or q.i.d. (4 times daily) if the "o" is poorly written	Use "every other day"
q1d	Daily	Mistaken as q.i.d. (4 times daily)	Use "daily"
q6PM, etc	Every evening at 6 PM	Mistaken as every 6 hours	Use "6 PM nightly" or "6 PM daily"
SC, SQ, sub q	Subcutaneous	SC mistaken as SL (sublingual); SQ mistaken as "5 every"; the "q" in "sub q" has been mistaken for "every" (e.g., a heparin dose ordered "sub q 2 hours before surgery" misunderstood as every 2 hours before surgery)	Use "subcut" or "subcutaneously"
ss	Sliding scale (insulin) or ½ (apothecary)	Mistaken as "55"	Spell out "sliding scale"; use "one-half" or "½"
SSRI	Sliding scale regular insulin	Mistaken as selective-serotonin reuptake inhibitor	Spell out "sliding scale (insulin)"
SSI	Sliding scale insulin	Mistaken as Strong Solution of Iodine (Lugol's)	Spell out "sliding scale (insulin)"
i/d	One daily	Mistaken as "tid"	Use "1 daily"
TIW or tiw	3 times a week	Mistaken as "3 times a day" or "twice a week"	Use "3 times weekly"
U or u**	Unit	Mistaken as the number 0 or 4, causing a 10-fold overdose or greater (e.g., 4U seen as 40 or 4u seen as 44); mistaken as "cc" so dose given in volume instead of units (e.g., 4u seen as 4cc)	Use "unit"

Used with permission, Institute for Safe Medication Practice (ISMP), http://www.ismp.org.
**These abbreviations are included on The Joint Commission's "minimum list" of dangerous abbreviations, acronyms, and symbols that must be included on an organization's "Do Not Use" list, effective January 1, 2004.

	Room: 3700-03	Saint Francis Medical Center

MEDICATION ADMINISTRATION RECORD

Patient: PDM, Pharmacy
Birth: 11/30/79 Admit: 01/01/00
MRN: 2000403 Acct: 900015
A Doctor: Jim Smith

Date: 01/18/09 – 01/19/09

Age: 20 y Ht: 5 ft 2 in   Wt: 125.2 lbs
Metric: Ht: 1 m 57 cm Wt: 56.79 kg

ADEs/Nondrug allergies: Latex – Zosyn – Amoxicillin – Insulins – Darvocet – Lugols soln. – Antihi +

	0800	0900	1000	1100	1200	1300	1400	1500	1600	1700	1800	1900	2000	2100	2200	2300	2400	0100	0200	0300	0400	0500	0600	0700
P00014 Bacitracin ointment AKA: Bacitracin ointment Dose: Apply STRGH: 30 gm/tube TID Topical: Right lower leg For external use only Testing			RL 10																					
P00029 Insulin/human regular AKA: Humulin R Dose: 15 units Strgh: 1 ml = 100 units AC subcut	RL 0730																							
P00030 Fexofenadine 60 mg/psuedo 120 mg AKA: Allegra–D Sr Tab Dose: 1 tab STRGH: 60/120/tab BID Oral Auto Sub: 1 Allegra–D Tab bid For Claritin–D 12 hr and 24 hr Per P&T Comm			RL 10																					
P00036 Aspirin AKA: Aspirin 325 mg Tab Dose: 2 tab 650 mg STRGH: 325 mg/tab q3–4h Oral Testing						RL 1315																		
P00039 Haloperidol tablet AKA: Haldol 0.5 mg tab Dose: 1 mg STRGH: 1 mg/tab QHS Oral																								
P00035 Zolpidem AKA: Ambien 5 mg tab Dose: 5 mg STRGH: 5/tab QHS PRN Oral MR × 1 Testing																								

Circle = Dose not given
Initials = Dose given
Deltoid = R.D., L.D.
Vastus Lateralis = R.V.L., L.V.L.
Lower Abdominal = R.L.A., L.L.A.
Anterior Gluteal = R.A.G., L.A.G.
Posterior Gluteal = R.P.G., L.P.G.

Page: 01 (continued)

0800	0900	1000	1100	1200	1300	1400	1500	1600	1700	1800	1900	2000	2100	2200	2300	2400	0100	0200	0300	0400	0500	0600	0700

Initials and signature	Initials and signature	Initials and signature
Rita Lassater RL		
Initials and signature	Initials and signature	Initials and signature
Initials and signature	Initials and signature	Initials and signature

Fig. 20-4 Medication administration record (MAR). (*Courtesy St. Francis Medical Center.*)

patient's full name; date the order is written; date the medication order expires (if applicable); medication name, dose, and frequency (time ordered); and route of administration. The transcriber makes sure the patient's room and bed number (which are usually pre-stamped on the order form) are accurate on the form. *Transcription errors are one of the most common sources of medication errors.* With unit-dose systems, only one transcription is necessary. When you transcribe an order in written form, be sure the names, dosages, symbols, and abbreviations are legible and not smudged. Always clarify an order that is not legible. When checking an order transcribed by a unit secretary, check the accuracy and legibility of every element. An RN is responsible for checking and initialing all transcribed orders against the original orders.

A verbal order is a medication or treatment order received by a nurse in the presence of the prescriber. Verbal orders are to be accepted only in emergency situations when the prescriber has no time to write the order. When a nurse takes a verbal order, he or she writes the order on the MAR and then reads back the complete order to the independent practitioner who made the order. The Joint Commission (2007b) requires the verification process. The nurse enters verbal orders into the patient's medical record by transcribing the same way as if the prescriber wrote the order. The nurse writes the name of the prescriber next to that of the nurse.

Telephone orders are medication orders given over the phone, usually after you update the prescriber about a change in a patient's condition. You transcribe a telephone order the same as a verbal order, and it also requires a read-back by the person receiving the order. In some states only RNs can take verbal and telephone orders. Institutional and state regulations require the prescriber to sign verbal and telephone orders within 24 hours. Therefore it is important to limit their use as much as possible. *Nursing students are prohibited from receiving verbal and telephone orders.*

Once you determine that information on the patient's MAR is accurate, use the MAR to prepare and administer medications. When preparing medications from bottles or containers, *compare the label of the medication container with the MAR three times:* (1) before removing the container from the supply drawer, (2) when placing the medication in an administration cup/syringe, and (3) before administering the medication to the patient. Never prepare medications from unmarked containers or containers with illegible labels (TJC, 2007b). With unit-dose prepackaged medications, check the label with the MAR when taking medications out of the medication dispensing system. Finally, verify all medications at the patient's bedside with the patient's MAR, and use at least two

identifiers before giving the patient any medications (TJC, 2007b).

Nurses administer only the medications they prepare. If an error occurs, the nurse who administers the medication is responsible for the error. If a patient questions the medication a nurse prepares, it is important not to ignore these concerns. An alert patient will know whether a medication is different from those received before. Withhold the medication until you are able to recheck the preparation against the order. If a medication order seems incorrect or inappropriate, always consult the prescriber.

Right Dose

The unit-dose system is designed to minimize errors. When nurses prepare a medication from a larger volume or strength than needed or when the prescriber orders a system of measurement different from what the pharmacist supplies, the chance of error increases. When performing medication calculations or conversions, have another qualified nurse check the calculated doses.

The Joint Commission now discourages the use of range orders for prn medications. An example of a range order is "morphine sulfate 2 to 6 mg IV push q2-4 hr prn for pain." Range orders are often unclear and have been the source of medication errors. The Joint Commission recommends that organizations develop practice guidelines that define how to implement range orders (Rich, 2002). An example of a practice guideline is "Increase the dose 50% to 100% if pain is moderate to severe."

After calculating doses, prepare the medication using standard measurement devices (e.g., graduated cups, syringes, and scaled droppers). At home, teach patients to use kitchen measuring spoons rather than teaspoons and tablespoons, which vary in volume. Key principles to observe when using measuring receptacles include:

1 Pour liquid medication into a medication cup while holding the cup at eye level so you can accurately see the desired amount. The amount of poured liquid should be even with the base of the meniscus (Fig. 20-5).

2 Pour liquid medications away from a label to ensure that liquid will not run down a label, making it difficult to read.

3 Draw liquid medication into a syringe (without a needle) slowly to prevent air bubbles from entering the syringe. Air displaces medications and leads to inaccurate measurement of doses.

At times it is necessary to administer a portion of a tablet to ensure accurate dosage. Only break tablets that the manufacturer has scored. You can request the pharmacy split medications and

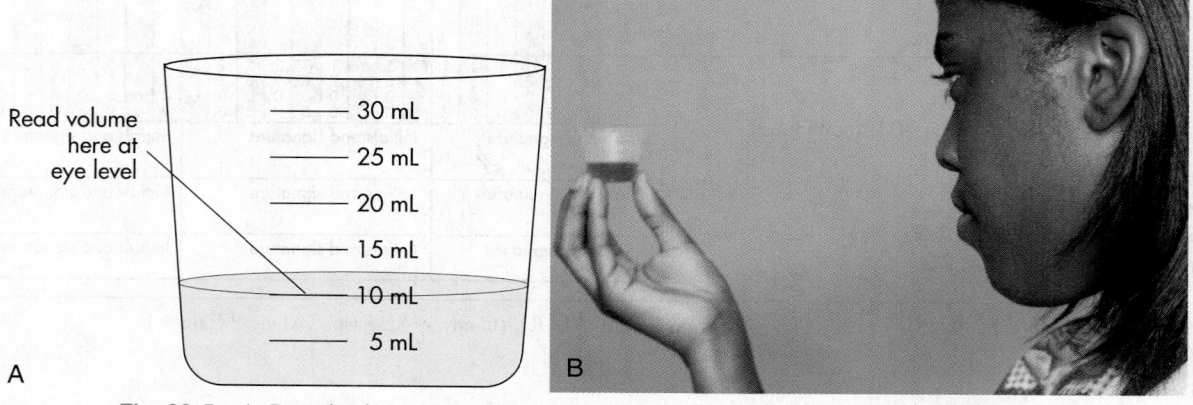

Fig. 20-5 **A,** Pour the desired volume of liquid so that base of meniscus is level with line on scale. **B,** Hold cup at eye level to confirm volume poured.

repackage with a label for the correct dose. When breaking a scored tablet, make sure the break is even. Cut a scored tablet in half by using a knife-edge or a cutting device. Discard tablets that do not break evenly. Some agencies allow a nurse to save the unadministered portion of the tablet that remains for the next dose if the remaining medication is repackaged and labeled. Verify agency policy before administering a tablet that has been opened, cut, and repackaged. Because pill splitting is particularly problematic in the home care setting, the ISMP (2006) has developed suggestions to help with this process. Nurses need to evaluate if a patient has the motor dexterity or visual acuity to split tablets. If at all possible, prescribers need to avoid ordering medications that require splitting.

Often a nurse prepares a tablet by crushing it and then mixing it in food. Always check to determine whether a medication can be crushed (see Chapter 21). Clean the crushing device completely before crushing a tablet. Remnants of previously crushed medications increase a medication's concentration or result in a patient receiving a portion of an unprescribed medication. Mix crushed medications with very small amounts of food or liquid. Do not use a patient's favorite foods or liquids because medications alter their taste and decrease the patient's desire for them. This is especially a concern for pediatric patients.

Right Patient

Medication errors often occur because one patient gets a drug intended for another patient. Therefore a key step in administering medications safely is being sure that you give the right medication to the right patient. It is difficult to remember every patient's name and face. Before giving a medication to a patient, you need to use at least two patient identifiers whenever administering medications (TJC, 2007b). Acceptable patient identifiers include the patient's name, an identification number assigned by a health care agency, or date of birth. The Joint Commission (2007a) does not require patients to state their names and other identifiers when nurses administer medications. The required identification process mandates collecting patient identifiers reliably when a patient is first admitted to a health care agency. Once identifiers are assigned to a patient (e.g., putting identifiers on an armband and placing the armband on the patient), a nurse uses the identifiers to match the patient with the patient on the MAR. Do not use the patient's room number as an identifier.

To identify a patient correctly in an acute care setting, go to the patient's bedside and compare the patient identifiers on the MAR with those on the patient's identification bracelet (Fig. 20-6). Asking patients to state their full names and identification information is a third way to verify that you are giving medications to the right patient. If an identification bracelet becomes smudged or illegible, or is missing, get a new one for the patient. In health care settings that are not acute care settings, The Joint Commission (2007a) does not require the use of armbands for identification. However, nurses still need to use a system that verifies the patient's identification with at least two identifiers before administering medications.

Right Route

The prescriber's order needs to designate a route of administration. If the route of administration is missing, or if the specified route is not the recommended route, consult the prescriber immediately. You make clinical judgments in recommending a route; for example, when a patient is nauseated, recommend the prescriber order an acetaminophen (Tylenol) suppository for pain instead of a capsule. When administering injections, use only preparations intended for parenteral use. Injection of a liquid intended for oral use produces local complications, such as sterile abscess, or fatal systemic effects. Medication companies label parenteral medication "for injectable use only."

Right Time

Nurses need to understand why a medication is ordered for a certain time of the day and whether a medication time schedule can be changed. For example, two medications are ordered, one q8h (every 8 hours) and the other 3 times per day. You are to give both medications 3 times over 24 hours. The prescriber intends for you to give the q8h medication around-the-clock to maintain therapeutic blood levels of the medication. In contrast, you need to give the other medication during the waking hours. Each agency has a recommended time schedule for medications ordered at frequent intervals. Nurses alter these recommended times if necessary or appropriate.

Prescribers often give specific instructions about when to administer a medication. A preoperative medication to be given "on call" means that you give the medication when the operating room staff members notify you that they are coming to get the patient for surgery. Give a medication ordered "after meals" within half an hour after a meal, when the patient has a full stomach. Give a STAT medication immediately.

Give priority to medications that must act at certain times For example, give insulin at a precise interval before a meal. Give antibiotics on time around-the-clock to maintain therapeutic blood levels. Give all routinely ordered medications within 60 minutes of the times ordered (30 minutes before or after the prescribed time).

Some medications require a nurse's clinical judgment in determining the proper time for administration. Administer a prn sleeping medication when the patient is ready for bed. Also use judgment when administering prn analgesics. For example, a nurse sometimes needs to obtain a STAT order from the prescriber if the

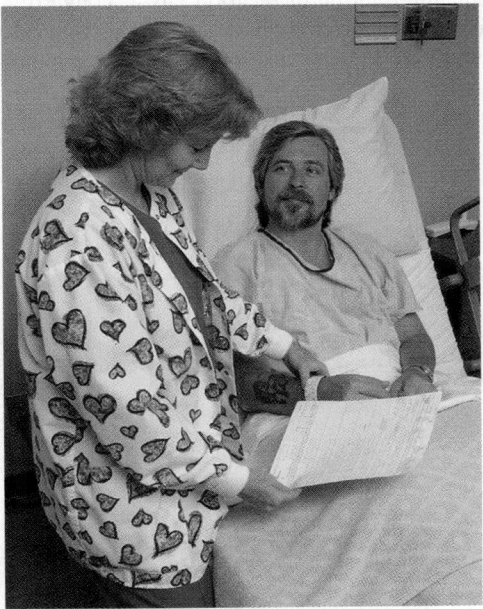

Fig. 20-6 Before administering any medications, check the patient's identification and allergy bracelets.

patient requires a medication before the prn interval has elapsed. A nurse always documents whenever the nurse calls a patient's health care provider to obtain a change in a medication order.

Before discharging patients from the hospital, evaluate their medication regimen, especially if a patient was admitted to the hospital because of a problem with medication self-administration. Patients often leave the hospital with a basic knowledge of their medications but are unable to safely self-administer medications once they return back home. Before discharge, evaluate with the prescriber whether the medications are adequate or prescribed at therapeutic levels for the patient. Help patients plan schedules based on preferred medication intervals, pharmacokinetics of the medication, and the patient's daily schedule. For patients who have difficulty remembering when to take medications, make a chart that lists the times when the patient will take each medication or prepare a special container to hold each timed dose.

Right Documentation

 Advanced / Safe Medication Administration / Documenting Medication Administration

Accurate documentation enhances medication safety. Nurses need to document appropriately before and after giving medications. Written orders and medication forms need to include the patient's name, the name of the ordered medication, and the medication dosage, route, and frequency. If any of these pieces of information is missing, contact the prescriber to verify the order. After administering a medication, record the name of the ordered medication, the time of administration, and the dosage, route, and frequency as soon as possible. After evaluating the drug's effect, document the patient's response. Accurate documentation is a way for health care providers to communicate with each other and to prevent an accidental dose from being administered to a patient.

PREPARATION OF MEDICATIONS

A nurse performs several steps before actual administration of medications: interpreting medication labels, converting measurement units within a system or between systems, and calculation of medication doses. Remember: *Medications ordered in units and mil-*

liequivalents are not convertible to metric, apothecary, or household measurements.

Interpreting Medication Labels

Medication labels include seven pieces of information: the medication trade name in large letters, the generic name in smaller letters, the form of the medication, dose, expiration date, lot number, and the manufacturer's name (Fig. 20-7). The trade name suggests the action of the medication. Always read a label carefully, uninterrupted, especially if you are required to administer only a portion of the medication made available.

Clinical Calculations

To administer medications safely, it is essential to understand basic arithmetic to calculate medication doses and mix solutions. This skill is important because medications are not always dispensed in the unit of measure in which the prescriber orders them. This occurs because medication companies package and bottle medications in standard dosages. For example, a prescriber orders 20 mg of a medication that is available only in 40-mg vials. Nurses have to convert available units of volume and weight to desired doses. Therefore be aware of equivalents in all major measurement systems, and make use of conversion tables. In addition to medication administration, nurses use volume and weight conversions in a variety of other nursing activities, including converting fluid ounces to milliliters to measure intake and output (I&O) or converting volume equivalents to calculate IV flow rates.

EVIDENCE-BASED PRACTICE TRENDS

Many medication errors occur when nurses become distracted or lose focus during medication administration. Errors also occur when nurses fail to follow standard nursing protocols and procedures related to medication administration. Nurses experience multiple interruptions and distractions in today's health care environment. Areas for medication administration preparation are highly visible locations with high levels of staff traffic (Potter and others, 2005). Nurses become interrupted while accessing dispensing systems, depositing medications into delivery containers, and confirming orders on computer screens. Nurses need systems in place to avoid distractions to help prevent medication errors. In a

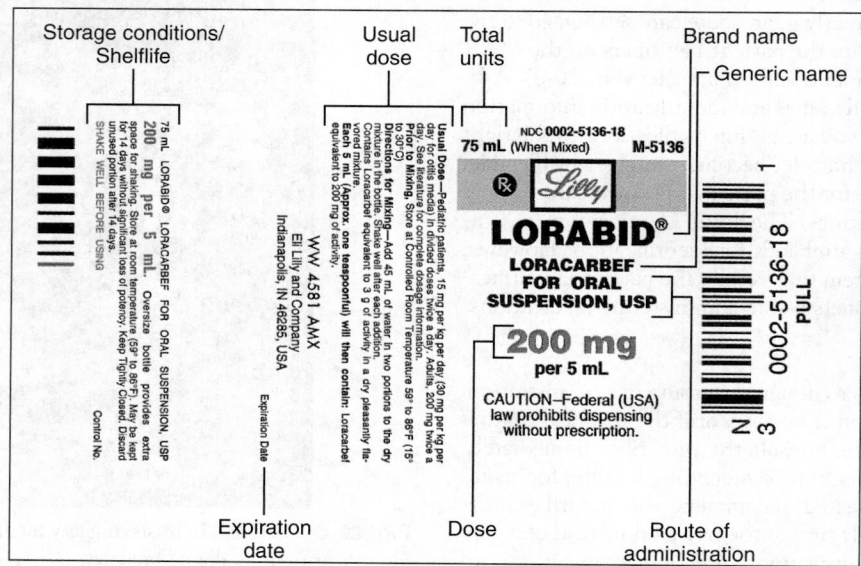

Fig. 20-7 Interpreting a medication label. (*Courtesy Eli Lilly and Co, Indianapolis, Ind.*)

research study by Pape and others (2005), researchers provided nurses techniques to help them focus on medication administration. The nurses used small checklist cards that listed the steps of medication administration. The cards were similar to checklists used by airplane pilots during the take-off and landing of airplanes. Reported medication errors decreased after 3 weeks. Then researchers posted "Do Not Disturb" signs in medication preparation areas to help remind everyone in the hospital not to disturb nurses during medication preparation. Following the interventions, nurses were better able to follow the hospital's medication administration procedure, and they perceived fewer distractions during medication administration. Findings from the study strengthen the importance of nurses consistently following protocols for medication administration to decrease medication errors. Nurses who experience fewer distractions during medication administration have fewer medication errors.

Conversions Within One System

Converting measurements within one system is relatively easy; simply divide or multiply in the metric system. For example, to change milligrams to grams, divide by 1000 or move the decimal three points to the left.

$$1000 \text{ mg} = 1 \text{ g}$$

$$350 \text{ mg} = 0.35 \text{ g}$$

To convert liters to milliliters, multiply by 1000 or move the decimal three points to the right.

$$1 \text{ L} = 1000 \text{ mL}$$

$$0.25 \text{ L} = 250 \text{ mL}$$

To convert units of measurement within the apothecary or household system, consult an equivalency table. For example, when converting fluid ounces to quarts, you know that 32 ounces is the equivalent of 1 quart. To convert 8 ounces to a quart measurement, divide 8 by 32 to get the equivalent, ¼ quart.

Conversion Between Systems

You will frequently determine the correct dose of a medication by converting weights or volumes from one system of measurement to another. For example, often you will convert metric units to equivalent household measures for use at home. To convert from one measurement system to another, use equivalent measurements. Tables of equivalent measurements are available in all health care institutions.

Before making a conversion, compare the measurement system available with that ordered. For example, a prescriber orders Robitussin 30 mL, but the patient only has tablespoons at home. To provide proper instruction to the patient, you will convert milliliters to tablespoons. By referring to an equivalency table (Table 20-7), you determine that 30 mL = 2 tablespoons. Therefore you instruct the patient to take 2 tablespoons of Robitussin.

Dose Calculations

There are many formulas used to calculate medication doses. Apply the following basic formula when preparing solid or liquid forms:

$$\frac{\text{Dose ordered}}{\text{Dose on hand}} \times \text{Amount on hand} = \text{Amount to administer}$$

The dose ordered is the amount of medication prescribed (e.g., 20 mg). The dose on hand is the dose (e.g., milligrams, milliliters, units) of medication supplied by the pharmacy. The amount on hand is the weight or volume of medication available and supplied by the pharmacy. It is on the medication label as the contents of a tablet or capsule or as the amount of medication dissolved per unit volume of liquid. The amount on hand is the basic quantity of the medication that contains the dose on hand. For solid medications the amount on hand is often one capsule; the amount of liquid on hand is often 1 mL or 1 L. The amount to administer (e.g., milliliters or milligrams) is always expressed in the same measure as the amount on hand.

Example I: The prescriber orders the patient to receive morphine sulfate 2 mg IV (dose ordered). The medication is available in a vial containing 10 mg (dose on hand) in 1 mL (amount on hand). You apply the formula as follows:

$$\frac{2 \text{ mg}}{10 \text{ mg}} \times 1 \text{ mL} = \text{Amount in milliliters to administer}$$

In this case, divide numerator and denominator by 2:

$$\frac{1}{5} \times 1 \text{ mL} = \frac{1}{5} \text{ mL to administer}$$

Syringes are calibrated only in decimals. Convert the fraction ⅕ to 0.2 to prepare the correct dose.

Example II: The prescriber orders 0.125 mg orally (PO) of digoxin. The medication is available in tablets containing 0.25 mg. You apply the formula as follows:

$$\frac{0.125 \text{ mg}}{0.250 \text{ mg}} \times 1 \text{ tablet} = \text{Number of tablets to administer}$$

The fraction $^{0.125}\!/_{0.250}$ equals ½. Therefore

$$\frac{1}{2} \times 1 \text{ tablet} = \frac{1}{2} \text{ tablet to administer}$$

Often, liquid medications come prepared in volumes greater than 1 mL. In applying the formula, be careful to use the correct concentration to avoid a medication error. Follow the next example.

Example III: The order is "erythromycin suspension 250 mg PO." The pharmacy delivers 100-mL bottles with the label stating, "5 mL contains 125 mg of erythromycin." Thus the appropriate concentration to use in this example to obtain the correct dose of medication is 125 mg in 5 mL.

$$\frac{250 \text{ mg}}{125 \text{ mg}} \times 5 \text{ mL} = \text{Volume to administer}$$

The fraction $^{250}\!/_{125}$ equals 2. Therefore

$$2 \times 5 \text{ mL} = 10 \text{ mL to administer}$$

Some agencies require a nurse to double-check calculations with another nurse before administering the medication, especially when the risk for administering the wrong medication dosage is

TABLE 20-7	Equivalents of Measurement	
Metric	**Apothecary**	**Household**
1 mL	15-16 minims (m)	15 drops (gtt)
4-5 mL	1 fluidram (fl dr)	1 teaspoon (tsp)
16 mL	4 fluidrams (fl dr)	1 tablespoon (tbsp)
30 mL	1 fluid ounce (fl oz)	2 tablespoon (tbsp)
240 mL	8 fluid ounces (fl oz)	1 cup (c)
480 mL (approx 0.5 L)	1 pint (pt)	1 pint (pt)
960 mL (1 L)	Approx 1 quart (qt)	Approx 1 quart (qt)

high (e.g., heparin or insulin). **Always** double-check calculations or confer with another nurse or health care professional if an answer to a calculation seems unreasonable.

Pediatric Doses

Calculating children's medication doses requires caution. Children metabolize medications at different rates compared with adults. Other factors that influence medication dosages in children include the difficulty in evaluating the desired effect and the hydration status of the child. In most cases the prescriber will calculate the dose for a child before ordering the medication. However, it is your responsibility to be aware of the safe dosage range for any medication administered to a child. Therefore be aware of the formulas used to calculate pediatric doses and recheck all doses before administration. Various formulas to determine appropriate medication dosages for children exist. These formulas often take the child's age, weight, body surface area, and/or the medication amount into consideration. However, the most accurate method of calculating pediatric doses uses a child's body surface area (Hockenberry and Wilson, 2007). Use a standard nomogram (e.g., the West nomogram) to estimate a child's body surface area.

Use the formula below to calculate a pediatric dose. The formula is a ratio of the child's body surface area compared with the body surface area of an average adult (1.7 square meters, or 1.7 m^2).

$$\text{Child's dose} = \frac{\text{Surface area of child}}{1.7\ m^2} \times \text{Normal adult dose}$$

For example, a prescriber orders ampicillin for a child weighing 11.4 kg. The normal adult dose for ampicillin is 250 mg. The West nomogram (Fig. 20-8) shows that a child weighing 11.4 kg has a surface area of 0.51 m^2. Using this information, calculate the appropriate child's dose.

$$\text{Child's dose} = \frac{0.51\ m^2}{1.7\ m^2} \times 250\ mg$$

The m^2 units are canceled out.

$$\text{Child's dose} = \frac{0.51}{1.7} \times 250\ mg$$

$$\frac{0.51}{1.7} = 0.3$$

$$\text{Child's dose} = 0.3 \times 250\ mg = 75\ mg$$

Older Adult Dosages

Older adults require special consideration during medication administration. The changes of aging alter pharmacokinetics (Table 20-3). As a result, nurses caring for older adults must be aware of drug dosing and alterations in drug response (Hunter and Cyr, 2006). Chronic disease is more prevalent among older adults, and multiple disease states also affect medication use and response.

A common problem for older adult patients is polypharmacy, the use of a number of different medications, prescribed or not, for one or more health problems (McKenry and others, 2006). When several medications have similar effects, polypharmacy increases the chances of medication interactions. These interactions can be mistaken as medication toxicity, an increase in disease severity, suboptimal treatment, or an unrelated event. It is important to know that the majority of undesirable drug effects resulting from polypharmacy are preventable. McKenry and others (2006) recommend that nurses make geriatric medication therapy as simple as possible. Confer with the prescriber to limit the number of medications a patient is taking. The nurse, prescriber, and pharmacist share the responsibility of reducing or

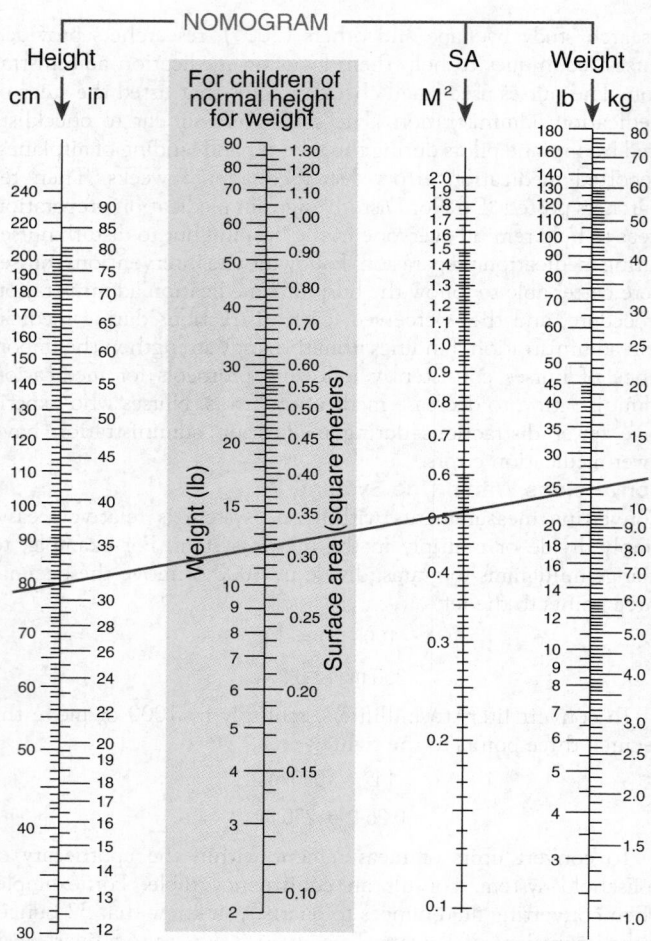

Fig. 20-8   West nomogram for estimation of surface areas in children. A straight line is drawn between height and weight. The point where the line crosses the surface area column is the estimated body surface area. (*From Behrman RE and others, editors:* Nelson textbook of pediatrics, *ed 17, Philadelphia, 2004, WB Saunders.*)

eliminating the adverse risk factors associated with various medication regimens older adults receive. Thoroughly assess the patient's health status, current medication regimen (including OTC drugs and herbal products), the reason for existing and proposed medications, and any environmental factors that influence accurate and safe medication administration by the patient and caregivers. Although there are no standardized dosages for older adults, you need to recognize physiological changes in the patient that influence dosages prescribed. Prescribers often lower recommended adult dosages to treat older adult patients. The potent medications available to treat older adults often have a narrow index between effectiveness and toxicity (McKenry and others, 2006). Box 20-4 lists medications that commonly cause problems for older adults.

NURSING PROCESS IN MEDICATION ADMINISTRATION

Always perform medication administration in a safe and orderly manner. Application of the nursing process ensures that critical thinking and clinical judgment are integrated into a patient's care.

TABLE 20-3 | Altered Pharmacokinetics in Older Adults

Absorption	↑ Gastric pH ↓ Intestinal blood flow and motility
Distribution	↓ Lean body mass ↓ Total body mass ↑ Adipose (fat) stores ↓ Total body water ↓ Serum albumin
Metabolism	↓ Liver size ↓ Liver blood flow ↓ Liver functions (microsomal enzyme activity)
Excretion	↓ Glomerular filtration rate

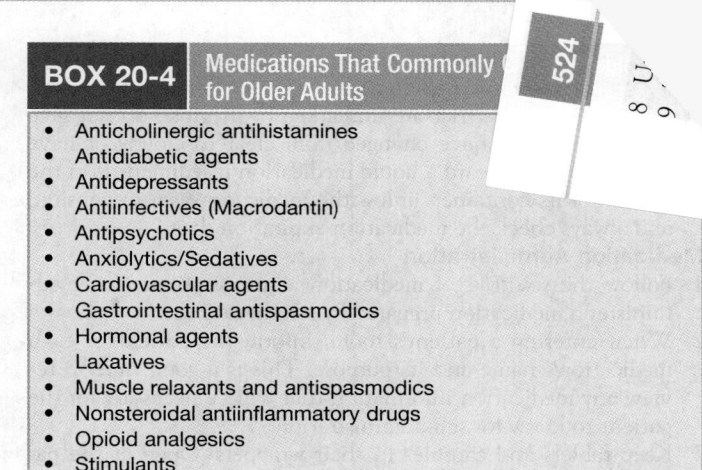

BOX 20-4 | Medications That Commonly (for Older Adults

- Anticholinergic antihistamines
- Antidiabetic agents
- Antidepressants
- Antiinfectives (Macrodantin)
- Antipsychotics
- Anxiolytics/Sedatives
- Cardiovascular agents
- Gastrointestinal antispasmodics
- Hormonal agents
- Laxatives
- Muscle relaxants and antispasmodics
- Nonsteroidal antiinflammatory drugs
- Opioid analgesics
- Stimulants

From McKenry LM and others: *Mosby's pharmacology in nursing*, ed 22, Mosby, St. Louis, 2006.

Assessment

Before administering medications, perform a patient assessment and medication review. Determine if a patient has a history of medication allergies. Ask the patient, "Are there any drugs or medicines that have given you problems?" Then assess whether patients have allergies or if they have simply experienced side effects from medications. Make sure the hospitalized patient's medical record is clearly marked with a list of allergies. Also ensure that the patient has an allergy band. *Never give a patient a medication to which he or she is known to be allergic.*

Assess the patient's physiological status. How is the patient tolerating food or liquids by mouth? Does the patient have abnormal laboratory values suggesting a change in renal or liver function? Does the patient's blood pressure or pulse rate contraindicate administration of a medication? Is the patient becoming less responsive at times, making him or her prone to aspiration of a liquid medication? These are just examples of conditions you consider when judging the appropriateness of a medication and/or the route for administration. Nursing assessment also reveals if it is necessary to withhold a prescribed medication. Report any withheld medication to the prescriber.

Assessing the patient's current medication history helps to determine the reason for the patient's presenting signs and symptoms. This is especially true in urgent situations. In clinic and medical office settings, nurses ask patients to bring a list of their current medications for review. Review of current medications allows you to also assess the patient's knowledge level, which is necessary for safe self-administration. Does the patient know each medication's dosage schedule, purpose, common side effects, and actions to take when side effects develop?

In the home, nursing assessment includes a review of the environment in which the patient self-administers medications (see Chapter 42). Are medications stored safely away from children? Are there facilities to adequately prepare the medications? Does the patient use a system to organize medications and remember dosage schedules? Is there a mechanism to dispose of biomedical equipment (e.g., needles and syringes)? Also determine the family member's or significant other's ability to assist with medication administration.

A medication review requires you to methodically consider what you know about each medication. You need to know a medication's purpose, action, normal dosage and route, time interval for action, expected side effects, and the specific reason why a patient has the medication prescribed. Nursing implications for administering each medication safely will depend on the type of medication being given (e.g., all antihypertensives should require a blood pressure measure-

ment before administration). When in doubt about medication information, check available medication references or the pharmacy.

Planning

When administering medications, meet these three basic goals:
1. The patient achieves the medication's therapeutic effect.
2. The patient experiences no complications related to the prescribed medication and the method of administration.
3. The patient and family are able to describe how to self-administer medications safely.

Implementation

Follow the principles of safe and effective medication preparation and administration for each patient.

Preadministration Activities
1. Minimize distractions during medication preparation—ask colleagues to not interrupt you, close the door of the medication room, and do not try to perform other tasks while preparing a medication.
2. Make sure you have a written order for every medication that you are responsible for administering. Ensure that a medication order has not expired. Follow institutional policy for medication order renewal.
3. Make sure that the information on the medication computer sheet or MAR corresponds exactly with the prescriber's written order and with the medication container label.
4. Read the label on the medication container, and compare it with the MAR at least three times: before removing the container from the supply drawer, when placing the medication in an administration cup/syringe, and just before administering the medication to the patient.
5. Follow guidelines described earlier for medication calculation. Remember: Take your time with all calculations, and have another nurse check any calculation.
6. Review any preadministration assessments (e.g., vital signs, review of laboratory results).
7. Use medical aseptic technique; perform hand hygiene before preparing a dose of medication. Avoid touching tablets and capsules. Use sterile technique for parenteral medications (see Chapter 8).

...e correct equipment when preparing a medication.
...o avoid common errors do not prepare medications from containers with labels that are unmarked or illegible; do not give medications that have changed from clear to cloudy or have changed color; discard a liquid medication if sediment is in the bottom of its container, unless the medication is a suspension; and always check the medication expiration date.

Medication Administration

1 Follow the *six rights* of medication administration. Never administer a medication prepared by another nurse.
2 When entering a patient's room, inform the patient of each medication's name and its purpose. This is a good time to review any medication information that will be necessary for the patient to know for self-administration.
3 Keep tablets and capsules in their wrappers. Open at the patient's bedside. This allows you to review each medication with the patient. Respect the patient's right to refuse a medication. If a patient refuses medication, never return unwrapped medication to a container; discard it according to agency policy. If the medication wrapper remains intact, return the medication to the patient's unit-dose drawer. When a patient refuses a medication, determine the reason for it, and take action. Document refusal of medications, and notify the prescriber.
4 Medications interact with certain foods or beverages. Know what is compatible. Milk and grapefruit juice are examples of liquids that alter the absorption and metabolism of medications (Hunter and Cyr, 2006). It is always safe to offer water with oral medications. In the home, make sure patients know to never take alcohol with medications. Of the more than 100 most commonly prescribed drugs, more than half contain at least one ingredient known to interact adversely with alcohol (McKenry and others, 2006).
5 Remain with the patient as the patient takes the medication. Provide assistance if necessary (e.g., for the patient who is weak and unable to administer eyedrops). Do not leave medications at a patient's bedside without a prescriber's order to do so. If such an order is written, check back with the patient to be sure the medication has been taken.

Postadministration Activities

1 After administering a medication, record the following information on the MAR or other appropriate form (e.g., nurses' notes) required by the institution:
   • Medication name
   • Dose
   • Route of administration
   • Time of administration
   • Any unexpected patient responses (see evaluation)
   • Pertinent data or assessment collected at the time of administration
   • Signature and title of nurse administering medication
2 If the patient refuses a medication, document the reason for refusal in the nurses' notes. The MAR sometimes requires you to enter a special symbol that indicates that the patient refused the medication.

Evaluation

After you administer a medication, evaluate the patient's condition and response to the medication, while considering how the medication is expected to affect the patient. You look for therapeutic effects, as well as adverse effects. If adverse effects develop, you need to recognize the clinical signs and respond quickly.

1 Monitor patient's physical response to the medication (e.g., vital signs, urine output, relief of pain).
2 Monitor patient's behavioral responses to the medication (e.g., level of anxiety, agitation, consciousness).
3 Observe injection sites for bruises, inflammation, localized pain, numbness, or bleeding.
4 Determine patient's understanding of medication therapy and ability to self-administer medication.

GENETIC AND CULTURAL FACTORS IN ADMINISTERING MEDICATIONS

Research over the last 15 years shows that there are significant differences among racial and ethnic groups in their drug metabolism rates, clinical drug responses, and adverse effects of drugs (McKenry and others, 2006). A new scientific field, pharmacogenetics, involves the study of the genetic influence on drug response that occurs from inherited metabolic defects or deficiencies. As a nurse, you cannot detect a genetic abnormality. However, you can learn to become aware of cultural differences in drug responses so as to better monitor drug therapy. Evans and McLeod (2003) report genetic variation in a number of important sites of drug action:

• *Beta-adrenergic receptor:* Site of drug action for many pulmonary drugs
• *Angiotensin-converting enzyme (ACE):* Affecting the treatment of hypertension and heart failure
• *Dopamine receptors:* Site of action of antipsychotic drugs
• *Serotonin receptors:* Site of action of antidepressants and treatments for nausea and vomiting

Culturally, a patient's values and beliefs affect medication response. A patient's level of education, prior experience with medication therapy, and the family's influence on actions significantly influence medication adherence. For example, in Japan it is not acceptable to complain about gastrointestinal problems, so it is common for patients to not report nausea, vomiting, and bowel changes related to medication use. Some cultures' use of herbal and homeopathic remedies alters response to a medication. Most practitioners do not consider ethnicity when prescribing medications at this time; however, with new scientific findings this will change.

SPECIAL HANDLING OF MEDICATIONS

Controlled Substances

Nurses are responsible for following federal and state laws regarding the administration of controlled substances or narcotics. Violations of the Controlled Substances Act are punishable by fines, imprisonment, and loss of nurse licensure. Hospitals and other health care institutions have policies for the proper storage, distribution, and disposal of narcotics. AMDSs make counting and tracking of narcotics more efficient, because these systems automatically count and record the nurse's electronic signature as the dose is dispensed. RNs investigate any discrepancies found in a narcotic count. Report any narcotics unaccounted for to the nurse manager or supervisor immediately. When administering narcotics to a patient, follows these general guidelines:

• Store all narcotics in a locked, secure cabinet. (Computerized, locked cabinets are preferred.)
• Count narcotics frequently, during the opening of narcotic drawers and/or at shift change.
• Report discrepancies in narcotic counts immediately.
• Use a special inventory record each time a narcotic is dispensed. Records are often electronic and provide an accurate ongoing

count of narcotics used and remaining, as well as information about narcotics that are wasted.

- Use the record to document the patient's name, date, time of medication administration, name of medication, dose, and signature of nurse dispensing the medication.
- If you give only part of a premeasured dose of a controlled substance, a second nurse witnesses disposal of the unused portion. Both nurses sign their names on the required form. Computerized systems record the nurses' names electronically. Do not place wasted portions in the sharps containers. Instead, dispose of medications properly following institutional policy.

REPORTING MEDICATION ERRORS

 Advanced / Safe Medication Administration / Preventing Medication Errors

Medication errors often harm patients because of inappropriate medication use. Medication errors include inaccurate prescribing, administration of the wrong medication, route, and time interval, as well as administering extra doses or failing to administer a medication. Medication errors are related to professional practice, health care product design, or procedures and systems such as product labeling and distribution. When an error occurs, the patient's safety and well-being become the top priority. The nurse assesses and examines the patient's condition and notifies the physician or prescriber of the incident as soon as possible. Once the patient is stable, the nurse reports the incident to the appropriate person in the institution (e.g., manager or supervisor).

The nurse is also responsible for preparing a written incident or occurrence report that must be filed usually within 24 hours of the incident (see Chapter 4). The report includes patient identification information; the location and time of the incident; an accurate, factual description of what occurred and what the nurse did; the patient's outcome, and the signature of the nurse involved. Brunetti (2007) recommends that any report of a medication error also include the cause of the error, a brief description of the cause (e.g., an abbreviation that was misread), and any contributing factors. The incident report is an internal audit tool and not a permanent part of the medical record. Do not refer to an incident report in the nurses' notes. This is to legally protect the health care professional and institution. Institutions use incident reports to track incident patterns and to initiate performance improvement programs as needed. Depending on the circumstances and the severity of the outcome, the nurse or institution may be responsible for reporting the incident to The Joint Commission, MedWatch (FDA's Medical Products Reporting Program), or U.S. Pharmacopeia's Medication Errors Reporting Program.

It is good risk management to report all medication errors, including mistakes that do not cause obvious or immediate harm or near misses. You should feel comfortable in reporting an error and not fear repercussions from managerial staff. Even when a patient suffers no harm from a medication error, the institution can still learn why the mistake occurred and what to do in the future to avoid similar errors. Box 20-5 lists steps to take in preventing medication errors.

PATIENT AND FAMILY TEACHING

A properly informed patient is more likely to take medications correctly than one who is unsure about the purpose of a medication and how it will affect his or her daily lifestyle. When planning education, consult with the prescriber to simplify the drug regimen as much as possible (e.g., use once-daily dosing versus multiple times when appropriate). Offer simple, clear written instructions in a large font (Schlenk and others, 2004). If your patient has a health literacy problem, realize that he or she will have difficulty. When individuals have limited literacy skills, they are unable to read complex texts, are reluctant to ask questions, have difficulty listening, and have limited mathematical skills. Health literacy skills are needed for patients to have dialogue and discussion, interpret graphics or charts, read health information, use medical equipment (e.g., syringes) for family care, and calculate timing and dose of medications (IOM, 2004).

When possible, assess a patient's reading level. There are standard literacy assessment tools (e.g., the Rapid Estimate of Adult Literacy in Medicine [REALM]) available. Begin instruction as soon as possible so that you can have several teaching sessions. It is ideal to use instructional materials written no higher than a sixth-grade reading level. When providing instruction, have the patient or family member repeat the name and use for each medication plus the dosing instructions. Have the patient demonstrate preparing and setting up a medication. Provide time to discuss problem scenarios (e.g., side effects develop or a syringe becomes contaminated) to test the patient's knowledge of what to do should something go wrong. Determine if the patient requires a compliance aid or memory cue. This is especially important in older adults. Medication dose containers, organized by the hours and days of the week, are very useful. In the event patients miss a dose of medication, they need to know how to adjust their medication schedule safely.

Evaluating the effectiveness of teaching ensures that the patient is able to administer medications in a safe manner. Have pa-

---

BOX 20-5	**Steps in Preventing Medication Errors**

- Follow the six rights of medication administration.
- If unfamiliar with a medication, check pharmacology resources.
- Be sure to read labels at least three times (comparing MAR with label): before removing the container from the supply drawer, when placing the medication in an administration cup/syringe, and just before administering the medication to the patient.
- Use at least two patient identifiers whenever administering a medication.
- Do not allow any other activity to interrupt your administration of medication to a patient.
- Double-check all calculations, and verify with another nurse.
- Do not interpret illegible handwriting; clarify with prescriber.
- Question unusually large or small doses.
- Document all medications as soon as they are given.
- When you have made an error, reflect on what went wrong; ask how you could have prevented the error.
- Evaluate the context or situation in which a medication error occurred. This helps to determine if nurses have the necessary resources for safe medication administration.
- When repeated medication errors occur within a work area, identify and analyze the factors that may have caused the errors and take corrective action.
- Attend in-service programs that focus on the medications you commonly administer.

MAR, Medication administration record.

tients describe their medication schedules, and then have a discussion that allows them to ask questions and clarify their understanding:

- Why are you taking this medication?
- How often do you take this medication?
- How much do you take?
- What side effects should you look for?
- What do you do when side effects occur?

It is often helpful to have actual medication bottles labeled with the medication name available at a teaching session. Medication bottles often have fine print and are not always easy to read, especially for the patient with impaired visual acuity. This is the time to discover visual limitations so that you can provide a larger print label.

Also evaluate the patient's sensory, motor, and cognitive functions, which, when impaired, will affect the patient's ability to safely self-administer medications. This includes the ability to open medication containers, prepare a dose in a syringe, or read a label. When you assess an impairment, include family members, friends, or home care aides in any discussion.

 ## CRITICAL THINKING EXERCISES

Justin Brown is a 72-year-old patient who visits the medicine clinic 1 month following a myocardial infarction (heart attack). He denies any chest pain since his angioplasty, which involved insertion of a stent into one of his coronary arteries. He is currently taking an antidepressant, a thyroid supplement, a fecal softener, a cardiac drug (beta-adrenergic blocker), and an antihypertensive. In addition, he takes melatonin, an herbal preparation for sleep. The physician has revised Mr. Brown's antihypertensive medication to metoprolol (Lopressor). He is now instructed to take 75 mg by mouth twice daily. Mr. Brown tells the clinic nurse that he has experienced some weakness and dizziness since he has been taking Lopressor.

1 Which of the medications taken by Mr. Brown are likely to cause problems for him because of his age?
2 What does the weakness and dizziness likely indicate?
3 What might the physician do after receiving the nurse's report of Mr. Brown's weakness and dizziness?
4 The medication order is for 75 mg of Lopressor by mouth. The medication comes in 50-mg tablets. What would be the correct amount of medication to administer?
5 As the nurse, what would be important to assess in order for Mr. Brown to take the 75-mg dose safely?

REVIEW QUESTIONS

1 An older adult patient is weak and malnourished. What should the nurse be especially watching for after administering the patient's usual medications?
   1 Signs and symptoms of drug toxicity
   2 Increased dependence on the medication
   3 Side effects of the medication
   4 An allergic reaction
2 The nurse needs to draw a serum trough level of a medication. When should the nurse obtain the blood sample?
   1 Right before the next dose of the drug is due
   2 Midpoint between the times the drug doses are given
   3 Two hours after the medication is given
   4 When the serum level is due to plateau, usually early in the morning
3 A patient has asked for a pain medication to relieve the discomfort from her abdominal incision. She has experienced nausea since this morning, after several bites of her soft-diet breakfast. She last received a dose of her ordered oral analgesic 4 hours ago. The medication, hydrocodone 10 mg PO, is ordered q4h prn. Which of the following rights of drug administration most likely will challenge the nurse caring for this patient?
   1 Right route
   2 Right patient
   3 Right dose
   4 Right time
4 A medication order is for 0.5 g PO every 12 hours. The medication is available in 250-mg tablets. How many tablets should the nurse administer?
   1 One-half tablet
   2 One tablet
   3 One and one-half tablets
   4 Two tablets
5 A patient has been having enemas until clear for an upcoming intestinal surgery. He is on several oral medications. What effect do the enemas have on the absorption of the medications?
   1 They increase the rate of excretion of the medications.
   2 They decrease the rate of excretion of the medications.
   3 They will prolong the medications' effects.
   4 It is unknown because the mechanism of medication excretion is not stated.

REFERENCES

Arnold GJ: Clinical recognition of adverse medication reactions: obstacles and opportunities for the nursing profession, *J Nurs Care Qual* 13(2):45, 1998.
Birkmeyer J and others: Leapfrog safety standards: potential benefits of universal adoption, Washington, DC, 2000, Leapfrog Group.
Burke KG: Executive summary: the state of the science on safe medication administration symposium, *J Intraven Nurs* 28(3):4, 2005.
deWit S: *Fundamental concepts and skills for nursing,* ed 2, Philadelphia, 2005, WB Saunders.
Hockenberry MJ, Wilson D: *Wong's nursing care of infants and children,* ed 8, St. Louis, 2007, Mosby.
Hughes RG, Ortiz E: Medication errors: why they happen, and how they can be prevented, *Am J Nurs* 105:79, 2005.
Hunter K, Cyr D: Pharmacotherapeutics in older adults, *J Wound Ostomy Continence Nurs* 33(6):630, 2006.
Institute of Medicine: *Report brief, to err is human: building a safer health system,* 2003, http://iom.edu/CMS/8089/5575/4117.aspx.
Institute of Medicine: *Health literacy: a prescription to end confusion,* Washington, DC, 2004, National Academies Press.
Institute for Safe Medication Practices: Preventing errors with tablet splitting, 2006, http://www.accessdata.fda.gov/scripts/cdrh/cfdocs /psn/transcript.cfm?show=54#7, accessed August 5, 2007.
Kohn LT and others, editors, Committee on Quality of Health Care in America, Institute of Medicine: *To err is human: building a safer health system,* Washington, DC, 2000, National Academies Press, Institute of Medicine.
McIntyre LJ, Courey TJ: Safe medication administration, *J Nurs Care Qual* 22(1):40, 2007.
McKenry LM and others: *Mosby's pharmacology in nursing,* ed 22, St. Louis, 2006, Mosby.
Rich DS: Ask The Joint Commission, *Hosp Pharm* 37(6):1, 2002.
Roark DC: Bar codes and drug administration, *Am J Nurs* 104(1):63, 2004.
Schlenk EA and others: Medication nonadherence among older adults: a review of strategies and interventions for improvement, *J Gerontol Nurs* 30(7):33, 2004.

The Joint Commission: *Comprehensive accreditation manual for hospitals*, Oakbrook Terrace, Ill, 2007a, The Commission.

The Joint Commission: 2008 *National patient safety goals*, Oakbrook Terrace, Ill, 2007, The Commission, http://www.jointcommission.org/PatientSafety/NationalPatientSafetyGoals/08_npsg_facts.htm, accessed August 5, 2007b.

RESEARCH REFERENCES

Brunetti L and others: The impact of abbreviations on patient safety. *Jt Comm J Qual Patient Saf* 33(9):576, 2007.

Evans WE, McLeod HL: Drug therapy: pharmacogenomics—drug disposition, drug targets, and side effects, *N Engl J Med* 348(6):538, 2003.

Fitzpatrick J and others: *Annual review of nursing research: Focus on patient safety*, New York, New York, Springer Publishing, 2006.

Manno M: Preventing adverse drug events, *Nursing* 36(3):56, 2006.

Oren E and others: Impact of emerging technologies on medication errors and adverse drug events, *Am J Health Syst Pharm* 60(14):1447, 2003.

Paoletti R and others: Using bar-code technology and medication observation methodology for safer medication administration, *Am J Health Syst Pharm* 64:536, 2007.

Pape TM and others: Innovative approaches to reducing nurses' distractions during medication administration, *J Cont Ed Nurs* 36(3):108, 2005.

Potter P and others: Understanding the cognitive work of nursing in the acute care environment, *J Nurs Adm* 35(7/8):327, 2005.

Rask K and others: Adopting national quality forum medication safe practices: Progress and barriers to hospital implementation, *J Hosp Med* 2(4):212, 2007.

Skibinski K and others: Effects of technological interventions on the safety of a medication-use system, *Am J Health Syst Pharm* 64(1):90, 2007.

Tang F and others: Nurses relate the contributing factors involved in medication errors, *J Clin Nurs* 16(3):447, 2007.

U.S. Food and Drug Administration: *MedWatch*, 2007, http://www.fda.gov/medwatch, accessed September 23, 2008.

Oral and Topical Medications

MEDIA RESOURCES

- **evolve** *learning system* http://evolve.elsevier.com/Perry/skills
  - Review Questions
  - Video Clips

- **View Video!** Mosby's Nursing Video Skills, 3.0

- **NSO** Nursing Skills Online

Mastery of content in this chapter will enable the nurse to:

- Correctly administer a medication by oral, nasogastric or other enteral tube, skin (topical), ophthalmic, otic, nasal, inhaled, vaginal, and rectal routes.
- Correctly administer medications for irrigation and instillation.
- Identify guidelines for administering oral, nasogastric or other enteral tube, and topical medications.
- Describe factors to assess before administering medications.
- Differentiate types of topical administrations that require sterile technique and those that require clean medical aseptic technique.
- Instruct patients in proper use of metered-dose inhalers (MDIs), dry powder inhaler (DPI) medications, and small-volume nebulizers.
- Identify conditions contraindicating the administration of medications by various oral and topical routes.
- Prepare a teaching plan regarding medication use for a selected patient.

The oral route is the easiest and most desirable way to administer medications. Patients usually ingest or self-administer oral medication with few problems. Certain situations often arise that contraindicate a patient's receiving medications by mouth, such as gastrointestinal alterations, the inability of the patient to swallow food or fluids, and the use of gastric suction. If an enteral tube is present, first ensure that the medications are appropriate for tube administration and that the tube is in the correct location before giving medications. In addition, some oral medication formulations cannot be crushed.

Topical medications are applied locally to skin, mucous membranes, or tissue membranes. There are a variety of methods and formulations for applying medication to the skin. Adhesive-backed medicated disks applied to the skin provide a continuous release of medication over several hours or days. Topical administration avoids puncturing the skin and decreases the risk for infection and tissue injury that may occur with injections. Rotation of application sites helps reduce the severity of localized reactions, which may occur with topically applied medications. Systemic effects from topical drugs occur if the skin is thin, if the drug concentration is high, or if contact with the skin is prolonged.

Drugs applied to membranes, such as the cornea of the eye or the rectal mucosa, are absorbed quickly because of the membrane's vascularity. Mucous and other tissue membranes differ in their sensitivity to medications. Patients commonly experience burning sensations during administration of eye and nose drops, but medications applied to vaginal or rectal mucosa are generally less irritating.

You can administer medications for topical use in the following ways:

1 *Direct application of liquid:* Eyedrops, gargling, swabbing the throat.
2 *Inserting drug into a body cavity:* Rectal or vaginal suppositories, vaginal creams, or foams.
3 *Instillation of fluid into body cavity (fluid is retained):* Ear drops, nose drops, bladder and rectal instillation.
4 *Irrigation of body cavity (fluid is not retained):* Flushing eye, ear, vagina, bladder, or rectum with medicated fluid.
5 *Spraying:* Instillation into nose or throat, or under the tongue (sublingually).
6 *Inhalation of medicated aerosol spray:* Distributes medication throughout the nasal passages and the tracheobronchial airway. There are two types of devices designed for this purpose: metered-dose inhalers (MDIs) and small-volume nebulizers.
7 *Inhalation of dry powder medication:* Distributes medication in powder form throughout the tracheobronchial airway. The device designed for this purpose is the dry powder inhaler (DPI).
8 *Direct application to skin or mucosa:* Lotion, ointment, cream, powder, foam, spray, patch, and disk.
9 *Sublingual:* Medication placed under the tongue and allowed to dissolve.
10 *Buccal:* Medication placed between the upper or lower molar teeth and cheek area and allowed to dissolve.

EVIDENCE-BASED PRACTICE TRENDS

Medication errors continue to be a problem in the clinical setting. Madegowda and others (2007) investigated medication errors during various shifts in a small rural hospital. Findings revealed an increased number of errors on the second shift (3 PM to 11 PM) and on the general medical surgical unit. The authors conclude that this type of study would be helpful for other nursing units in developing quality improvement programs to reduce medication errors.

Stetina and others (2005) studied nurses' understanding and management of medication errors. Although the nurses were familiar with the standard "rights" of medication safety, they believed that late medication administration is not always a medication error, and the nurses used their own judgment to determine when and if a medication should be given. In addition, the researchers noted that the nurses rely more heavily on computerized systems to prevent medication errors and less on systematic checking against errors in medication orders.

Patients using MDIs need to learn how to determine when the canister is empty. Severe problems result if a patient tries to use an empty medication inhaler during an acute asthma attack. Rubin and Durotoye (2005) note that patients use a variety of methods to determine whether a canister is empty, but none of the methods is reliable. Many patients do not realize that their inhaler canisters are empty and are using the inhalers long past the intended duration for the MDI. The researchers strongly recommend instructing patients in dose counting (calculating the number of puffs used per day and calculating how many days the inhaler should last). Sander and others (2006) studied how patients evaluate whether their MDIs are empty and whether they are discarding inhalers that still contain medication or using inhalers beyond the recommended number of doses. More than half of the respondents refilled their MDI prescriptions more frequently than recommended by national guidelines, and 25% of the respondents found their MDI empty during an asthma exacerbation.

Education about proper technique for using MDIs is essential. Burkhart and others (2005) studied the accuracy of children's MDI technique and whether teaching proper MDI administration would improve performance of the medication. It is crucial for nurses to reinforce MDI use with children and their family members at every visit. Both children and parents need to understand how to use MDIs and have the opportunity to practice their use before going home.

CULTURAL CONSIDERATIONS

When giving oral and topical medications to patients of different cultures, it is important to incorporate cultural practices that are appropriate to the patient. In some instances these cultural practices affect only the method of administration; they do not alter the medication's effectiveness. However, there are times when cultural preferences, such as dietary preferences, timing of medication administration, or adherence to the medication regimen, are in conflict with the medication order. It is important to carefully determine when cultural preferences are safe to integrate into the administration of oral and topical medications (Andrews and Boyle, 2007).

- Before administering any medications, assess the patient's use of herbal therapies or folk remedies. Such practices may interfere with medications.
- If the medication requires equipment, such as an MDI, nebulizer, or medication dropper, ensure that patients from different cultures clearly understand the instructions.
- Some cultural groups such as Haitians, Southeast Asians, and Sudanese have a tendency to share medications and discontinue Western medications as soon as symptoms are resolved (Kemp and Rasbridge, 2001).
- When giving oral medications to Hindus and Muslims, use the right hand, not the left (Al-Shahri, 2002). They consider the right hand clean and the left hand dirty.
- Southeast Asians believe that Western medicines are too strong, and some stop taking them once symptoms are relieved (Nowak, 2003).
  - Emphasize the importance of completing a prescribed regimen.
  - Develop patient and family awareness of dangers associated with taking medications without medical supervision.
  - Encourage patient and family to ask questions without making any value judgment.
- Obtain the patient's consent before instilling eye and ear medications or performing ear irrigations.
  - Among Africans and Southeast Asians touching the head of the patient by a nonrelative is believed to predispose loss of one's spirit and power (Mashaba, 2002).

- Assess the meaning of the illness and the healing modalities used by different cultural groups.
  - Some Latinos believe that asthma is a cold disease and prefer medications with colors symbolizing hot properties, such as orange casing for inhalers.

Skill Performance Guidelines

1. Assess patient's sensory function, including sight, hearing, touch, and physical coordination. Sensory and coordination deficits impair patient's ability to see medications, open prescription bottles, and read labels at home.
2. Patients often receive more than one oral medication at a time. Evaluate each medication for potential drug-drug or drug-food interactions. Always consult with the pharmacist when in doubt.
3. Always assess for drug allergies. If the patient reports having an allergy, ask about the type of reaction that occurred.
4. Evaluate if patient can take medication with food. In most cases, the presence of food in the stomach will delay drug absorption. Some drugs irritate the stomach lining and should always be taken with food.
5. For all medications administered, review prescriber's order for patient's name, name of drug, dosage, time of administration, and site of application.
6. For all medications administered, gather information pertinent to the drug(s) ordered: purpose, normal dosage and route, common side effects, time of onset and peak action, contraindications, and nursing implications.
7. Determine if medications require any specific nursing actions. For example, monitor the patient's apical pulse and serum drug levels before administering digoxin.
8. If patients are mentally and physically able, prepare them for discharge by instructing them in self-administration techniques. Include family members and/or caregivers if possible.
9. Check the expiration date for all medications.

SKILL 21-1 Administering Oral Medications

 Advanced / Nonparenteral Medication Administration / Administering Oral Medication

NSO *Safe Medication Administration Module / Lesson 5*

The easiest and most desirable way to administer medications is by mouth. The majority of medications are given orally. The nurse usually prepares the medications in an area designed for medication preparation or at a unit-dose cart.

Delegation Considerations

The skill of administering oral medications cannot be delegated to nursing assistive personnel (NAP). The nurse directs the NAP about:
- Potential side effects of medications and to report their occurrence.

- Informing the nurse if patient's symptoms (e.g., pain, itching) continue after the medication was given.

Equipment
- ❑ Medication cart or tray
- ❑ Disposable medication cups
- ❑ Glass of water, juice, or preferred liquid
- ❑ Drinking straw
- ❑ Pill-crushing or pillating device (*optional*)
- ❑ Paper towels
- ❑ Medication administration record (MAR)
- ❑ Clean gloves

STEP	RATIONALE

ASSESSMENT

1. Check accuracy and completeness of each MAR with prescriber's written medication order. Check patient's name, drug name and dosage, route of administration, and time for administration. Clarify incomplete or unclear orders with the prescriber before implementation.

The order sheet is the most reliable source and only legal record of drugs patient is to receive. Ensures patient receives correct medication. *This is the first check for accuracy.*

STEP	RATIONALE
2 Assess for any contraindications to patient's receiving oral medication: Is patient suffering from nausea/vomiting? Is patient diagnosed as having bowel inflammation or reduced peristalsis? Has patient had recent gastrointestinal surgery? Does patient have gastric suction? Is patient restricted to nothing by mouth (NPO)? What is patient's level of consciousness?	Gastrointestinal alterations interfere with drug absorption, distribution, and excretion. Patients with gastrointestinal suction do not receive benefit from the medication because they may be suctioned from the gastrointestinal tract before it can be absorbed. Patients with altered levels of consciousness may not be able to swallow oral medications.
3 Assess risk for aspiration (see Skill 30-3). Is patient able to swallow? Assess patient's swallow, cough, and gag reflexes. Determine patient's ability to swallow safely (Box 21-1, p. 536).	Aspiration occurs when food, fluid, or medication intended for gastrointestinal administration is inadvertently administered into the respiratory tract. Patients with altered ability to swallow are at higher risk for aspiration (Nowlin, 2006).

Critical Decision Point *Patients with neuromuscular disorders, esophageal strictures, or lesions of the mouth and those who are unresponsive or comatose and cannot swallow or patients with high risk for aspiration should not receive oral medications. Request the prescriber to order the medication by an alternative route. When contraindications to oral medications exist, or if in doubt about the patient's ability to safely swallow the medication, temporarily withhold the medication and inform the prescriber.*

STEP	RATIONALE
4 Assess patient's medical history, history of allergies, medication history, and diet history. Drug allergies should be listed on each page of the MAR and prominently displayed on patient's medical record, and patient should be wearing the facility's allergy bracelet.	These factors influence how certain drugs act. Information also reflects patient's need for medications. Medication history reveals past problems with medication administration. Assessment for drug allergies is necessary before medication administration.
5 Gather and review physical assessment findings and laboratory data that will influence drug administration, such as vital signs, and results of renal and liver function studies.	Physical examination findings or laboratory data may contraindicate drug administration. Renal and liver function status affects metabolism and excretion of medications (Lilley and others, 2007).
6 Assess patient's knowledge regarding health and medication use. Consider drug use problems such as drug tolerance, noncompliance, abuse, addiction, or dependence.	Determines patient's need for drug education. Also assists in identifying patient's adherence to drug therapy at home. If you suspect a substance abuse problem, refer patient to appropriate health care professional.
7 Assess patient's preferences for fluids.	Offering fluids during drug administration is an excellent way to increase patient's fluid intake. Fluids ease swallowing and facilitate absorption from the gastrointestinal tract. However, maintain fluid restrictions if ordered.
8 Assess whether you can administer the medication with the preferred fluid.	Some fluids interfere with absorption of the medication. For example, taking tetracyclines with milk products greatly reduces their absorption (Lilley and others, 2007).
9 After confirming order, recopy or reprint any portion of the MAR that is illegible.	Soiled or illegible MAR forms are a source of drug error.

NURSING DIAGNOSES

- Deficient knowledge regarding drug self-administration
- Health-seeking behaviors (self-care)
- Impaired swallowing
- Ineffective therapeutic regimen management
- Noncompliance regarding drug regimen
- Risk for aspiration

Individualize related factors based on patient's condition or needs.

PLANNING

1 Expected outcomes following completion of procedure:	
• Patient experiences desired medication effect within period of onset of medication.	Drug has exerted its therapeutic action.
• Patient denies any gastrointestinal discomfort or symptoms of alterations.	Oral medications irritate gastrointestinal mucosa.
• Patient explains purpose of medication and drug dose schedule.	Demonstrates understanding of drug therapy.
2 Explain procedure to patient. Be specific if patient wishes to self-administer medications.	Makes patient a participant in care and minimizes anxiety. Begins patient teaching regarding medications. Enables patient to self-administer drug if physically able.

IMPLEMENTATION

1 Prepare medications: a Perform hand hygiene.	Reduces transfer of microorganisms.

STEP	RATIONALE
b Plan medication administration to avoid interruptions during drug preparation.	Avoidance of interruptions will reduce risk for medication errors.
c Arrange medication tray and cups in medication preparation area, or move medication cart to position outside patient's room.	Organization of equipment saves time and reduces error.
d Unlock medicine drawer or cart or access the automated medication dispensing system.	Medications are safeguarded when locked in cabinet, cart, or automated dispensing system.
e Prepare medications for one patient at a time. Keep all pages of MAR for one patient together.	Prevents preparation errors.
f Select correct drug from automated medication dispensing system, unit-dose drawer, or stock supply. Compare label of medication with MAR (see illustration). Be sure to exit the automated dispensing system after removing drugs.	Reading label first time and comparing it against transcribed order reduces errors. Exiting the automated dispensing system ensures that no one else can remove medications using your identity.
g Calculate drug dose as necessary. Double-check calculation.	Double-checking reduces risk for error.
h To prepare tablets or capsules from a floor-stock bottle, pour required number into bottle cap, and transfer medication to medication cup. Do not touch medication with fingers.	Avoids waste by removing only what is needed. Avoids contamination of medications.
i If you have to break a medication to administer half the dosage, use a clean, gloved hand to break the tablet or cut with a clean pillating device (see illustration). Tablets that are to be broken in half must be prescored—containing a manufactured line that transverses the center of the tablet.	Reduces contamination of the tablet. Tablets that are not prescored cannot be broken into equal halves, and the result will be an inaccurate dose. Using a cutting device results in a more even split of the tablet (Institute for Safe Medication Practices [ISMP], 2006c).
j To prepare unit-dose tablets or capsules, place packaged tablet or capsule directly into medicine cup. (Do not remove wrapper.)	Wrapper maintains cleanliness of medications and identifies drug name and dose.

Critical Decision Point   *If preparing controlled substances (i.e., opioid), check controlled substance record for previous drug count and compare with supply available, and maintain adherence to controlled substance laws.*

k Place all tablets or capsules patient will receive in one medicine cup, except for those requiring preadministration assessments (e.g., pulse rate or blood pressure).	Keeping medications that require preadministration assessments separate from others makes it easier to withhold drugs as necessary.
l If patient has difficulty swallowing, use pill-crushing device to crush pills (see illustration). Mix ground tablet in small amount of soft food (custard or applesauce).	Large tablets are often difficult to swallow. Ground tablet mixed with palatable soft food is usually easier to swallow.

Critical Decision Point   *Not all drugs can be crushed (e.g., capsules, enteric-coated and long-acting/slow-release drugs). The coating of these drugs protects the stomach from irritation or protects the drug from destruction by stomach acids. Consult with pharmacist when in doubt (Box 21-2, p. 536).*

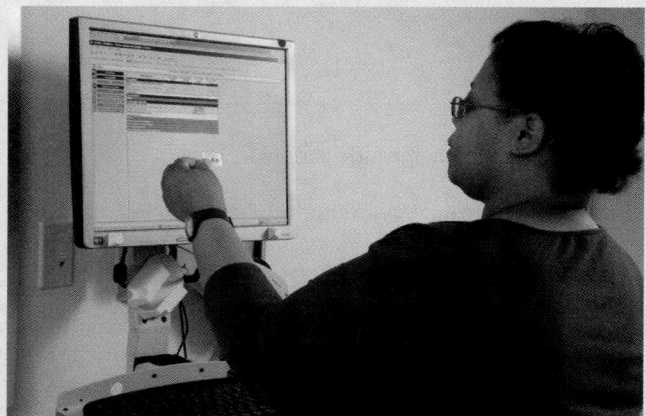

STEP 1f   The nurse checks the label of the medication with the transcribed medication order on the computerized MAR.

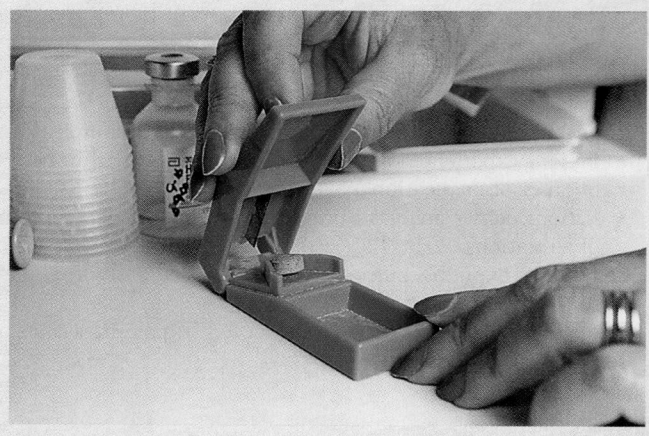

STEP 1i   Tablet is placed in a pillating device and cut in half.

STEP	RATIONALE

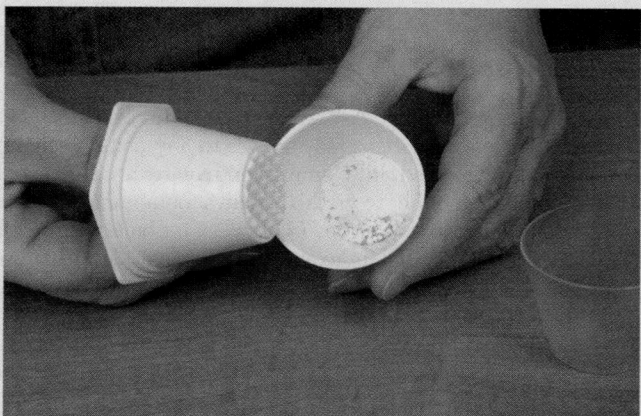

STEP 1l Crushing a tablet with a pill-crushing device.

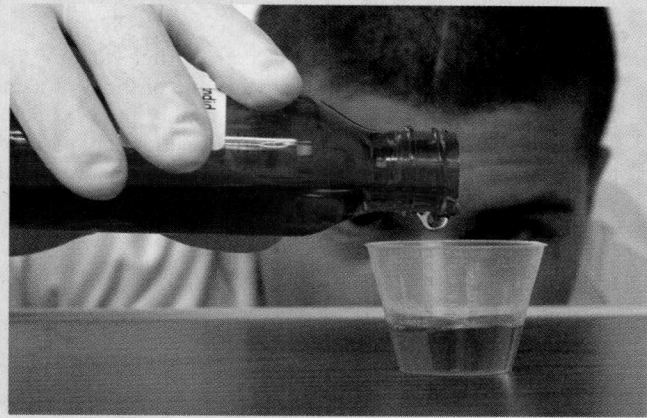

STEP 1m(3) Pour the desired volume of liquid so that base of meniscus is level with line on scale.

m Prepare liquids:

(1) Gently shake container. If medication is in a unit-dose container with the correct amount to administer, no further preparation is necessary. If medication is in a multidose bottle, remove bottle cap from container, and place cap upside down on work surface.

Shaking container ensures medication is mixed before administering. Prevents contamination of inside of cap.

(2) Hold bottle with label against palm of hand while pouring.

Prevents spilled liquid from dripping and soiling label.

(3) Hold medication cup at eye level, and fill to desired level on scale. Scale should be even with fluid level at its surface or base of meniscus, not edges (see illustration).

Ensures accuracy of measurement.

(4) Discard any excess liquid into sink. Wipe lip and neck of bottle with paper towel, and recap the bottle.

Prevents contamination of bottle's contents and prevents bottle cap from sticking.

(5) For doses of liquid medications less than 10 mL, draw liquid into a calibrated oral syringe. Do not use a hypodermic syringe or a syringe with a needle or syringe cap.

A calibrated oral syringe allows for accurate measuring of small doses of liquid medications.

Critical Decision Point *Only use syringes specifically designed for oral use when administering liquid medications. If using hypodermic syringes, the medication may be inadvertently administered parenterally, or the syringe cap or needle, if not removed from the syringe before administration, may become dislodged and accidentally aspirated when the syringe plunger is pressed (ISMP, 2001).*

n Check expiration date on all medications.

Medications used past expiration date may be inactive or harmful to patient.

o When preparing controlled substances, check controlled substance record for previous drug count and compare with supply available.

Controlled substance laws require careful monitoring of dispensed opioids and other controlled drugs.

p Compare MAR with prepared drugs, and continue.

This is the second check for accuracy.

q Return stock containers or unused unit-dose medications to shelf or drawer, and read label again.

Third check of label reduces administration errors.

r Label medicine cups and poured medications with patient's name before leaving the medication preparation area. Do not leave drugs unattended.

Ensures that the correct medications are prepared for the correct patient. Nurse is responsible for safekeeping of drugs (The Joint Commission [TJC], 2007).

STEP	RATIONALE

2 Administer medications:

  a Take medications to patient at correct time. Identify patient using two identifiers (i.e., name and birthday or name and account number, according to facility policy). Compare these identifiers with the information on patient's identification bracelet. Ask patient to state name. Check name on patient's identification bracelet. Replace any missing or faded identification bracelets.

Identification bracelets are made at time of patient's admission and are the most reliable source of identification. Ensures correct patient receives medication. Ask patient to state his or her name. A sedated or confused patient may answer to any name, including the wrong name. The Joint Commission requires at least two patient identifiers (neither to be the patient's room number) whenever administering medications (TJC, 2007). Some facilities are now using a bar code system to assist with patient identification.

  b Explain purpose of each medication and its action to patient. Allow patient to ask any questions about drugs.

Patient has right to be informed, and patient's understanding of purpose of each medication improves compliance with drug therapy.

Critical Decision Point *If patient expresses concern regarding accuracy of a medication, do not give the medication. Explore patient's concern, and verify physician's order before administering. Listening to patient's concerns may prevent a medication error.*

  c Assist patient to a seated or side-lying position if sitting is contraindicated by patient's condition.

Decreases risk for aspiration during swallowing.

  d *For tablets:* Some patients wish to hold solid medications in hand or cup before placing in mouth. Offer water or juice to help patient swallow medications.

Patient can become familiar with medications by seeing each drug. Choice of fluid promotes patient's comfort and can improve fluid intake.

  e *For orally disintegrating formulations (tablets or strips):* Remove medication from blister packet just before use. Do not push the tablet through the foil. Place medication on top of patient's tongue. Caution patient against chewing the medication.

Orally disintegrating formulations begin to dissolve when placed on the tongue. Water is not needed for these medications. Careful removal from packaging is necessary because the tablets and strips are thin and fragile (Uko-Ekpenyong, 2006).

  f *For sublingual-administered medications:* Have patient place medication under tongue and allow it to dissolve completely (see illustration). Caution patient against swallowing tablet or saliva.

Drug is absorbed through blood vessels of undersurface of tongue. If swallowed, drug is destroyed by gastric juices or so rapidly detoxified by liver that therapeutic blood levels are not attained.

  g *For buccal-administered medications:* Have patient place medication in mouth against mucous membranes until it dissolves (see illustration).

Buccal medications act locally or systemically as they are swallowed in saliva.

Critical Decision Point *Avoid administering liquids until orally disintegrating, buccal, or sublingual medication is completely dissolved.*

  h *For powdered medications:* Mix with liquids at bedside, and give to patient to drink.

When prepared in advance, powdered drugs thicken and some even harden, making swallowing difficult.

  i Caution patient against chewing or swallowing lozenges.

Drug acts through slow absorption through oral mucosa, not gastric mucosa.

  j Give effervescent powders and tablets immediately after dissolving.

Effervescence improves unpleasant taste of drug and often relieves gastrointestinal problems.

  k If patient is unable to hold medications, place medication cup to the lips and gently introduce each drug into the mouth, one at a time. Do not rush.

Administering single tablet or capsule eases swallowing and decreases risk for aspiration.

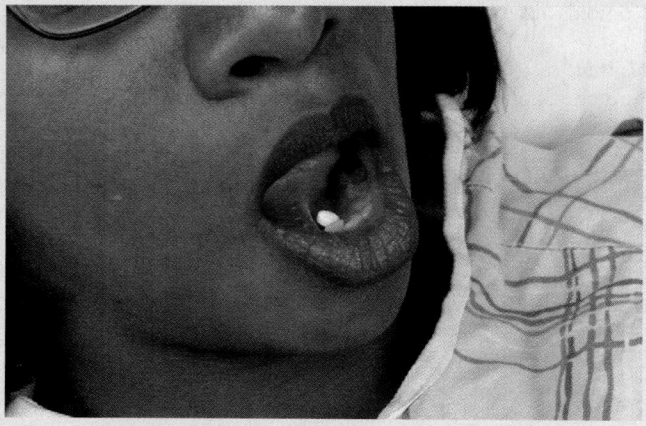

STEP 2f   Proper placement of sublingual tablet in sublingual pocket.

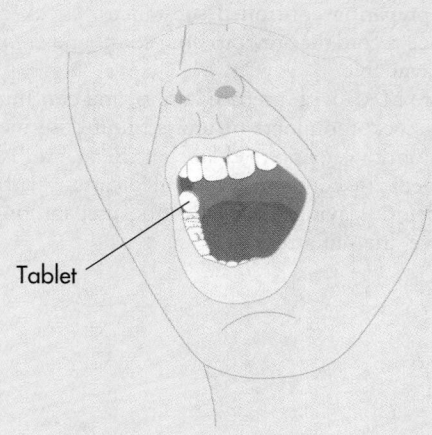

Tablet

STEP 2g   Buccal administration of a tablet.

STEP	RATIONALE

Critical Decision Point   *If tablet or capsule falls to the floor, discard it and repeat preparation. Drug is contaminated.*

l Stay until patient completely swallows each medication. Ask patient to open mouth if uncertain whether medication has been swallowed.	Nurse is responsible for ensuring that patient receives ordered dosage. If left unattended, patient may not take dose or may save drugs, causing risk to health.
m For highly acidic medications (e.g., aspirin), offer patient a nonfat snack (e.g., crackers) if not contraindicated by patient's condition.	Reduces gastric irritation. The fat content of foods may delay absorption of the medication.
n Assist patient in returning to comfortable position.	Maintains patient's comfort.
o Dispose of soiled supplies, and perform hand hygiene.	Reduces transmission of microorganisms.
3 Record administration of medication on MAR. Return MAR to appropriate file for next administration time.	Timely recording reduces medication errors. The MAR indicates when next dose is due. Failure to document medications given, or loss of MAR can lead to administration error.

EVALUATION

1 Return within an appropriate time to evaluate patient's response to medications.	Evaluates drug's therapeutic benefit and helps to detect onset of side effects or allergic reactions.
2 Ask patient or family member to identify drug name and explain purpose, action, dose schedule, and potential side effects of drug.	Determines level of knowledge gained by patient and family.

Unexpected Outcomes

1 Patient exhibits adverse effects (side effect, toxic effect, allergic reaction).

2 Patient is unable to explain drug information.

3 Patient refuses medication.

Related Interventions

- Withhold further doses.
- Assess vital signs.
- Notify prescriber and pharmacy.
- Symptoms such as urticaria, rash, pruritus, rhinitis, and wheezing may indicate an allergic reaction.

- Further assess the patient's or family member's knowledge of medications and guidelines for drug safety.
- Further instruction is necessary.

- Assess why patient is refusing medication.
- Do not force patient to take medications.
- Notify prescriber.
- Record refused medication and patient's stated reason.

Recording and Reporting

- Record actual time each drug was administered on MAR immediately after administration. Do not chart medication administration until *after* you give it to patient. If you withhold a drug, record reason in nurses' notes and follow agency's policy for noting withheld doses.
- Report adverse effects/patient response and/or withheld drugs to nurse in charge or physician. Depending on medication, immediate prescriber notification may be required.

Teaching Considerations

- Instruct patient in specific information pertaining to drug regimen (purpose, action, dose, dosage intervals, side effects, foods to avoid or take with drugs).
- All patients should learn the basic guidelines for drug safety in the home (see Skill 42-6).

Pediatric Considerations

- Liquid forms of medication are safer to swallow to avoid aspiration of small pills.
- Children will refuse bitter or distasteful oral preparations. Mix the drug with a small amount (about 1 teaspoon) of a sweet-tasting substance, such as jam, applesauce, sherbet, ice cream, or fruit pu-

ree. Do not use honey in infants because of the risk for botulism. Offer the child juice or a flavored ice pop after medication administration. Do not place medication in an essential food item, such as milk or formula; the child may refuse the food at a later time.
- Measure small amount of liquid medications using a plastic calibrated oral dosing syringe or a hollow-handled medicine spoon. Amounts less than a teaspoon are impossible to measure accurately with a molded medicine cup (Hockenberry and Wilson, 2007).

Gerontological Considerations

- Physiological changes of aging influence how oral medications are distributed, absorbed, and excreted. Common changes include loss of elasticity in oral mucosa; reduction in parotid gland secretion, causing dry mouth; delayed esophageal clearance, impaired swallowing; reduction in gastric acidity and stomach peristalsis, increased susceptibility to highly acidic drugs; reduced liver function, resulting in altered drug metabolism; and, lastly, reduced renal function and reduced colon motility, slowing drug excretion. Both altered drug metabolism and excretion may lead to drug toxicity (Ebersole and others, 2007).
- The most common adverse reactions that occur in older adults are lethargy, sedation, falls, confusion, constipation, and gastrointestinal upset.

- Administer a full glass of water (unless restricted) with medications to aid passage of the drug. Give patient time to swallow.
- Some older adults have several health problems or chronic conditions requiring the use of multiple drugs, often prescribed by different health care providers. This polypharmacy creates a high risk for drug interactions and adverse reactions (Wooten and Galavis, 2005).

Home Care Considerations
- When measuring liquid medications at home, patients should use kitchen measuring spoons, not eating utensil spoons that vary in volume.
- See Skill 41-3, Medication and Medical Device Safety, and Skill 42-6, Teaching Patients Self-Medication Administration.

BOX 21-1	Dysphagia

Dysphagia, or difficulty in swallowing, may lead to aspiration. A variety of signs and symptoms may be associated with dysphagia:
- Choking while eating or drinking, or increased congestion after eating or drinking
- Frequent need to clear the throat or need for oropharyngeal suctioning
- Unusually intense chewing or repeated swallowing of one bite of food
- Drooling or leakage of food from the mouth
- Coughing or gagging during or after meals

- Holding pockets of food in the cheeks
- Gurgling voice quality after eating
- Patient tells nurse that it feels as though food is lodged in the throat or behind the sternum, or has pain when swallowing

If swallowing difficulties are suspected or detected, notify the physician and request a referral to a speech pathologist who can perform a bedside swallow assessment. Further testing may be needed for a definitive diagnosis. Dysphagia that is not recognized or safely managed may lead to aspiration pneumonia (Nowlin, 2006).

BOX 21-2	Altering Oral Doses: Safety First

Safe Actions	Unsafe Actions
Swallow oral doses with a full glass of water to ensure that the medication reaches the stomach and to promote dissolution of the drugs.	Swallowing oral medications with small sips of water may result in the tablets becoming lodged in the esophagus. Damage to the mucosal lining may result as the medication dissolves.
Stay in an upright position after swallowing medications.	Swallowing oral medications while reclining may result in aspiration of liquid; the medication may not reach the stomach.
Allow oral disintegrating, sublingual, and buccal tablets to dissolve completely. Avoid swallowing saliva while the tablets dissolve.	Chewing these formulations will result in the destruction of the medication by gastric juices, thus reducing therapeutic effects.
Swallow enteric-coated tablets or capsules whole, without chewing, crushing, or opening them.	Crushing or chewing enteric-coated tablets or opening capsules results in reduced therapeutic effect because of destruction by acidic gastric juices. Some drugs are enteric coated to protect the stomach from irritation (McKenry and others, 2006).
Swallow sustained-release tablets or capsules whole.	Crushing or chewing sustained-release tablets may result in rapidly elevated drug levels, quickly followed by reduced levels. Steady therapeutic levels are not maintained (Lilley and others, 2007).
Sometimes patients must split tablets. If instructed to split tablets at home, use a pill splitter for accurate cutting. Do not put different strengths of split tablets in the same bottle.	Failure to split tablets as instructed will result in overdosing. Mixing different strengths of split tablets will also alter doses. Splitting tablets by hand may result in crumbled or unevenly split tablets (ISMP, 2006c).
Unless instructed to take medications with food to reduce gastric irritation, take them on an empty stomach with a full glass of water to promote absorption.	Taking irritating drugs on an empty stomach will result in gastric distress. The presence of food in the stomach delays medication absorption, thus delaying therapeutic effect.

SKILL 21-2   Administering Medications by Nasogastric or Enteral Tube

NSO   *Enteral Nutrition Module / Lesson 5*

Enteral tubes are inserted when patients cannot receive food or medications by mouth. Nasogastric feeding tubes generally are small-bore tubes that are inserted into the stomach via one of the nares. For long-term enteral feedings, a percutaneous endoscopic gastrostomy (PEG) tube or a jejunostomy tube may be surgically inserted. Do not administer medications into nasogastric tubes that are inserted for decompression.

Preferably, medications administered by enteral tubes should be in liquid form. If liquid form is not available, you will need to modify the form of the medication tablet by crushing or dissolving it. However, you cannot crush sustained-release, chewable, long-

acting, or enteric-coated tablets and capsules. Therefore do not administer these medications by enteral tubes. Consult with the hospital pharmacy when in doubt. It is essential to verify correct placement of a nasogastric tube before administering medications (see Skill 31-1).

Delegation Considerations
The skill of administering medications by nasogastric or enteric tubes cannot be delegated to NAP. The nurse directs the NAP to:
- Keep the head of the bed elevated for 15 to 30 minutes after medication administration.

- Monitor for signs of aspiration, such as coughing, choking, gagging, or drooling of liquid or moistened pills after swallowing, and inform the nurse immediately if these occur.

Equipment

❑ 60-mL syringe: catheter tip for large-bore tubes; Luer-Lok tip for small-bore tubes

❑ Gastric pH indicator strip (scale of 0.0 to 14.0)
❑ Graduated container
❑ Water
❑ Medication to be administered
❑ Pill crusher if medication in tablet form
❑ Medication administration record (MAR)
❑ Clean gloves

STEP	RATIONALE

ASSESSMENT

1. Check accuracy and completeness of each MAR with prescriber's written medication order. Check patient's name, drug name and dosage, route of administration, and time for administration.

The order sheet is the most reliable source and only legal record of drugs patient is to receive. Ensures patient receives correct medication.

2. Assess for any contraindications to patient's receiving medication enterally. Has patient been diagnosed as having bowel inflammation or reduced peristalsis? Has patient had recent gastrointestinal surgery? Does patient have gastric suction? Can the suction be temporarily turned off?

Alterations in gastrointestinal function interfere with drug distribution, absorption, and excretion. Patients with gastrointestinal suction should not receive medications via nasogastric tube because it may be suctioned from gastrointestinal tract before it can be absorbed.
This is the first check for accuracy.

Critical Decision Point *Always review patient's postoperative orders for gastric tube care. Manipulation and irrigation of tube or instillation of medication may be contraindicated.*

3. Assess patient's medical history, history of allergies, medication history, and diet history. If contraindications exist, withhold medication and inform prescriber of findings.

These factors influence how certain drugs act. Information also reflects patient's need for medications. Medication history often reveals past problems with medication administration.

4. Gather and review physical assessment and laboratory data that may influence drug administration, such as vital signs, and results of renal and liver function studies.

Physical examination or laboratory data may contraindicate drug administration. Renal and liver function status affect metabolism and excretion of medications (Lilley and others, 2007).

5. Before administration of medications verify placement of the feeding tube (see Skill 31-2).

Reduces the risk for aspiration.

NURSING DIAGNOSES

- Feeding self-care deficit
- Impaired swallowing
- Risk for aspiration

Individualize related factors based on patient's condition or needs.

PLANNING

1. Expected outcomes following completion of procedure:
   - Patient experiences desired medication effect within period of onset of medication.

   Drug has exerted its therapeutic action.

   - Patient's feeding tube remains patent after administration of medication.

   A patent enteric tube indicates passage of medication into stomach, ensuring proper absorption. If the tube becomes blocked, then administration of other medications and feedings will not be possible.

2. Explain procedure to patient, including description of medication to be instilled into enteric tube.

   Makes patient a participant in care and minimizes anxiety. Begins patient teaching regarding medications.

IMPLEMENTATION

1. Perform hand hygiene.

   Reduces transfer of microorganisms.

2. If the medication is not compatible with the feeding solution, or if patient needs to take medication on an empty stomach, stop the feeding 15 to 30 minutes before medication administration.

   Facilitates absorption of medication (Monahan and others, 2006).

3. Prepare medications for instillation into feeding tube. Check label against MAR three times (see Skill 21-1). Fill graduated container with 50 to 100 mL of tepid water.

   Adequate preparation saves nursing time. Ensures patient receives correct medication. Cold water causes gastric cramping.

Critical Decision Point *Whenever possible, use liquid medications instead of crushed tablets, but if you have to crush tablets, the tubing must be flushed before and after the medication to prevent the drug from adhering to the inside of the tube. In addition, make sure concentrated medications are thoroughly diluted. Never add crushed medications directly to the tube feeding (Monahan and others, 2006).*

STEP	RATIONALE

a Crush tablets using a pill-crushing device to grind pills into a fine powder. If a pill-crushing device is not available, place tablet between two medication cups and grind with a blunt instrument. Dissolve in at least 30 mL of warm water.

b *Capsules:* Ensure that contents of capsule (granules or gelatin) can be expressed from the covering (consult with pharmacist). Open capsule, or pierce gelcap with sterile needle, and empty contents into 30 mL of warm water. You can also dissolve gelcaps in warm water. | Ensures contents of tablets or capsules are a fine powder or solution to prevent occlusion of the tube.

4 Identify patient using two identifiers and comparing these identifiers with the information on patient's identification bracelet. Ask patient to state name. Check name on patient's identification bracelet. | Ensures correct patient receives medication. You need to use at least two patient identifiers (neither can be the patient's room number) whenever administering medications (TJC, 2007).

5 Prepare patient by placing in a high-Fowler's position (if not contraindicated by patient's medical condition). | Reduces risk for aspiration.

6 Apply clean gloves. | Reduces transfer of microorganisms.

7 If a continuous enteric tube feeding is infusing, adjust the infusion pump to hold the tube feeding. | Feeding solution should not infuse while residuals are checked or while medications are administered.

8 Check placement of feeding tube by observing gastric contents and checking pH of aspirate contents. *Gastric pH should be 4 or less* (see Skill 31-2). | Ensures proper tube placement and reduces the risk for introducing fluids into the respiratory tract (Metheny and Titler, 2001).

9 Check for gastric residual. Draw up 30 mL of air with the syringe. Connect syringe to end of feeding tube and flush with air. Then pull back slowly to aspirate gastric contents. Return aspirated contents to stomach. | Residual volume indicates if gastric emptying is delayed. Return of aspirate prevents fluid and electrolyte imbalance. Irrigation clears tubing (Lewis and others, 2007).

Critical Decision Point   *If you find a large volume of aspirate (e.g., 200 mL or more), return aspirate to patient, withhold medication, and notify patient's health care provider. Check agency policy. Some agency policies will hold the tube feeding as well. Large-volume aspirates indicate delayed gastric emptying, which contributes to gastric distention, esophageal reflux, and vomiting, all of which place patient at risk for aspiration (Lewis and others, 2007).*

10 Pinch nasogastric/enteric tube, and remove syringe. Draw up 30 mL of water in syringe. Reinsert tip of syringe into nasogastric/enteric tube, and flush tube. Pinch tube again, and remove the syringe. | Pinching tube prevents leakage or spillage of stomach contents. Flushing ensures tube is patent.

a Some nasogastric/enteric tubes are connected to continuous feeding tubing with a stopcock apparatus, such as a Lopez valve, that contains a medication port (see illustration). If present, attach the tip of the syringe to the medication port on the stopcock, and turn the "off" setting of the stopcock away from patient and toward the infusion tubing. Flush the enteric tube, then set stopcock "off" again to the medication port. Remove the syringe.

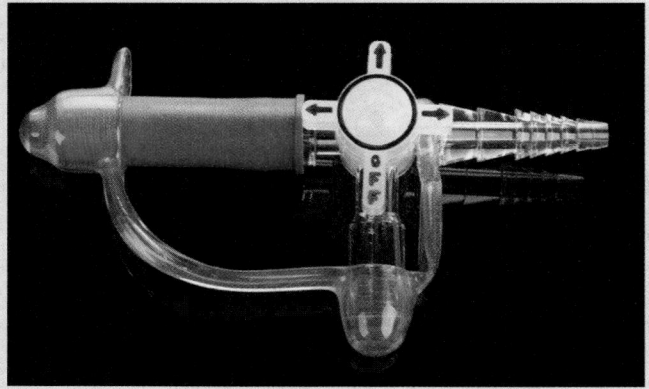

STEP 10a Lopez valve with a medication port. (*Courtesy ICU Medical, Inc, San Clemente, Calif.*)

STEP	RATIONALE
11 Remove bulb or plunger of syringe. Reinsert syringe into enteric tube (or medication port).	Removal of bulb or plunger prepares syringe for delivery of medications.
12 Administer first dose of dissolved medication by pouring into syringe.	

Critical Decision Point *If water or medication does not flow freely, raise the height of the syringe to increase the rate of flow, or try having the patient change position slightly because the end of the feeding tube may be against the gastric mucosa. If these measures do not improve the flow, a gentle push with bulb of Asepto syringe or plunger of the syringe may facilitate flow of fluid.*

STEP	RATIONALE
a If giving only one dose of medication, flush with 30 mL of water after administration.	Maintains patency of nasogastric/enteric tube.
b To administer more than one medication, give each separately, and flush between medications with 15 to 30 mL of water.	Keeping the medications separate allows for accurate identification of medication if a dose is spilled. In addition, some medications are not compatible with each other, which will cause clogging of tube (Monahan and others, 2006).
c Follow last dose of medication with 30 to 60 mL of water.	Maintains patency of nasogastric/enteric tube. Ensures passage of medication into stomach (Padula and others, 2004).
13 When a tube feeding is not being administered, clamp the proximal end of the feeding tube, and cap end of tube.	Prevents air from entering the stomach between medication doses.
14 When continuous tube feeding is being administered by an infusion pump:	
a Follow medication administration Steps 1 to 12. If the medications are not compatible with the feeding solution, then hold the feeding for an additional 30 to 60 minutes.	Allows for adequate absorption of medication, and avoids potential drug-food interaction between medication and enteral feeding.
15 Assist patient to comfortable position, but keep the head of the bed elevated for 1 hour after administering the medication.	Prevents aspiration.
16 Dispose of soiled supplies, rinse graduated container and syringe with tap water, remove and dispose of gloves, and perform hand hygiene.	Reduces transmission of microorganisms.

EVALUATION

1 Return within 30 minutes to evaluate patient's response to medications.	Monitoring patient's response helps assess drug's therapeutic benefit and helps detect onset of side effects or allergic reactions.

Unexpected Outcomes	Related Interventions
1 Patient exhibits signs of aspiration of administered medications/fluids, which include respiratory distress, changes in vital signs, or changes in oxygen saturation.	• Stop all medications/fluids through the tube. • Elevate the head of the bed, and stay with the patient. • Assess vital signs and breath sounds while another staff member notifies the patient's physician.
2 Patient does not receive medication as prescribed because of a blocked nasogastric/enteric tube.	• Requires interventions to unclog tube to ensure drug delivery (Box 21-3, p. 540).
3 Patient exhibits adverse effects (side effect, toxic effect, allergic reaction).	• Withhold further doses. • Always notify prescriber and pharmacy when patient exhibits adverse effects. • Symptoms such as urticaria, rash, pruritus, rhinitis, and wheezing indicate an allergic reaction.

Recording and Reporting

- Record in nurses' notes method used to check placement of nasogastric tube, volume of stomach aspirate, and pH of stomach aspirate. Record actual time each drug was administered on MAR immediately after administration. Do not chart medication administration until *after* it is given to patient. If you withhold a drug, record reason in nurses' notes and follow institution's policy for noting withheld doses and notifying prescriber.
- Record total amount of fluid used for medication administration on proper intake/output sheet.
- Report adverse effects/patient response to nurse in charge or physician. Depending on medication, immediate prescriber notification may be required.

Teaching Considerations

- In the home setting, provide instruction so patients/family members can administer medications safely:
  - Instruct patient or family in how to store medications and tube-feeding supplements (see Chapter 31).
  - Teach patient or family how to verify correct placement of tube before medication or tube feeding administration.
  - Demonstrate to family how to prepare medications, including crushing medications if appropriate.
  - Instruct family in the importance of consistent flushing of feeding tube following medication administration.

Pediatric Considerations

- Volumes for instillation of medications or for irrigation of nasogastric tubes may be smaller. Check agency policy (Hockenberry and Wilson, 2007).

BOX 21-3	Unclogging a Blocked Feeding Tube
<ul><li>Prevent tube from becoming blocked by flushing it with at least 30 mL of tepid water before and after administering each dose of medication, before and after checking gastric residual volumes, and every 4 to 6 hours around-the-clock.</li><li>If a tube becomes blocked, first try to irrigate it gently with tepid water.</li></ul>	<ul><li>If irrigation with water is not effective, obtain an order for a pancrelipase tablet (such as Viokase) and follow manufacturer's guidelines for irrigation of the tube. In addition, a declogging stylus may be used.</li><li>The tube may have to be removed and a new one inserted if the medication is urgent.</li></ul>

Modified from Lewis SM and others: *Medical-surgical nursing: assessment and management of clinical problems,* ed 7, St. Louis, 2007, Mosby.

SKILL 21-3 Administering Skin Applications

Advanced / Nonparenteral Medication Administration / Administering Topical Medications Applying an Estrogen Patch or Nitroglycerin Paste

NSO *Nonparenteral Medication Administration Module / Lesson 2*

Many locally applied drugs such as lotions, patches, pastes, and ointments create systemic and local effects if absorbed through the skin. To protect from accidental exposure, apply these drugs using gloves and applicators. Skin encrustations and dead tissue harbor microorganisms and block contact of medications with the affected tissues. Simply applying new medications over previously applied drugs does little to prevent infection or offer therapeutic benefit. Cleanse the skin or wound thoroughly before applying a new dose of medication. Apply each type of medication, whether an ointment, lotion, powder, or patch, in a specific way to ensure proper penetration and absorption.

Delegation Considerations

The skill of administering skin (topical) medications cannot be delegated to NAP. However, some institutions may permit NAP to apply some forms of topical agents, such as lotions, ointment, and powders, to irritated skin or for the protection of the perineum during morning or perineal care. Check agency policies. The nurse directs the NAP about:

- The correct method and site of application and the six rights of medication administration if NAP are permitted to apply topical agents.
- The expected therapeutic effects and potential side effects of medications and the importance of reporting their occurrence.

Equipment

- ☐ Clean gloves (for intact skin) or sterile gloves (for nonintact skin)
- ☐ Ordered agent (powder, cream, lotion, ointment, spray, patch)
- ☐ Cotton-tipped applicators or tongue blades (*optional*)
- ☐ Basin of warm water, washcloth, towel, nondrying soap
- ☐ Sterile dressing, tape (if needed)
- ☐ Medication administration record (MAR)

STEP	RATIONALE

ASSESSMENT

| 1 Check accuracy and completeness of each MAR with prescriber's written medication order. Check patient's name, drug name and dosage, route of administration, and time for administration. | The order sheet is the most reliable source and only legal record of drugs patient is to receive. Ensures patient receives correct medication. |

STEP	RATIONALE
2 When topical medications are applied to wounds or skin alterations, assess condition of patient's skin. If there is an open wound, apply clean gloves. First wash site thoroughly with mild, nondrying soap and warm water, rinse, and dry. Be sure to remove any previously applied medication or debris. Also remove any blood, body fluids, secretions, or excretions. Assess for symptoms of skin irritation such as pruritus or burning.	Cleansing site thoroughly promotes a proper assessment of skin surface. Assessment provides baseline to determine change in condition of skin after therapy. Application of certain topical agents can lessen or aggravate these symptoms.
3 Further inspect the condition of the skin or membranes. Do not administer topical medications to skin if integrity is altered, unless indicated.	Break in skin integrity can affect drug absorption and actions.
4 Determine whether patient has known allergy to topical agent. Ask if patient has had reaction to a cream or lotion applied to the skin. Also ask if patient has allergy to latex.	Allergic contact dermatitis is relatively common and can worsen dermatological (skin) condition. In addition, some patients may be allergic to preservatives or fragrances in topical medications. Latex allergy requires use of nonlatex gloves.
5 Determine amount of topical agent required for application by assessing affected area, reviewing prescriber's order, and reading application directions carefully (a thin, even layer is usually adequate).	An excessive amount of topical agent can cause chemical irritation of skin, negate drug's effectiveness, and/or cause adverse systemic effects, such as decreased white cell counts.
6 Assess patient's knowledge of action and purpose of medication being given and interest in treating health problem.	Reveals patient's level of understanding and whether instruction is necessary.
7 Determine if patient is physically able to apply medication by assessing fine grasp, hand strength, reach, and coordination.	Necessary if patient is to self-administer drug in the home.

NURSING DIAGNOSES

- Deficient knowledge regarding medication application
- Impaired physical mobility

- Impaired skin integrity
- Ineffective therapeutic regimen management

- Pain (acute or chronic)
- Risk for infection

Individualize related factors based on patient's condition or needs.

PLANNING

1 Expected outcomes following completion of procedure:	
• Patient is able to identify drug and describe action, purpose, dose, side effects, and schedule of medication.	Demonstrates learning.
• Patient is able to apply medication without assistance on prescribed schedule.	Demonstrates learning and compliance.
• With repeated applications, skin becomes clear, without inflammation or drainage from lesions.	Existing lesions heal and/or disappear as a result of medication's therapeutic action.
2 Prepare medications for application. Check label of medication against MAR three times (see Skill 21-1).	Ensures patient receives correct medication.
3 Identify patient using two identifiers and comparing these identifiers with the information on patient's identification bracelet. Ask patient to state name.	Ensures correct patient receives medication. You need to use at least two patient identifiers (neither can be the patient's room number) whenever administering medications (TJC, 2007).
4 Explain procedure to patient, including description of skin area you will treat.	Makes patient a participant in care and minimizes anxiety.

IMPLEMENTATION

1 Perform hand hygiene, and arrange supplies at bedside. If skin is broken (e.g., wound), use sterile gloves; otherwise apply clean gloves.	Reduces transmission of infection. Sterile gloves are used when applying agents to open noninfectious skin lesions. Topical agents are not usually premeasured in medication room. The use of gloves also prevents absorption of the medication into the nurse's skin.
2 Close room curtain or door, and position patient comfortably. Remove gown or bed linen so as to keep unaffected skin areas draped.	Provides patient privacy and easy access to area being treated. Promotes patient's comfort.
3 Apply topical agent.	
a Technique for applying creams, ointments, and oil-based lotions:	

STEP	RATIONALE
(1) Place required amount of medication in palm of gloved hand and soften by rubbing briskly between hands.	Softening of topical agent makes it easier to spread on skin.
(2) Once medication is softened, spread it evenly over skin surface, using long, even strokes that follow direction of hair growth. Do not vigorously rub skin. Apply to the thickness specified by manufacturer's instructions.	Ensures even distribution and sufficient dosage of medication. Technique prevents irritation of hair follicles.
(3) Explain to patient that skin may feel greasy after application.	Ointments often contain oils.
b Technique for applying nitroglycerin (an antianginal) ointment:	
(1) Apply desired number of inches of ointment over paper measuring guide (see illustration).	Ensures correct dose of medication. Antianginal (nitroglycerin) ointments are usually ordered in inches, or portions of an inch, and can be measured on small sheets of paper marked off in ½-inch markings. Unit-dose packages are available.

Critical Decision Point   *One package equals 1 inch; smaller amount should not be measured from this package. Use a tube to deliver amounts less than 1 inch (National Library of Medicine–National Institutes of Health, Health and Human Services, 2006).*

STEP	RATIONALE
(2) Remove previous dose paper. Fold used paper containing any residual medication with used sides together and dispose of properly. Wipe off residual medication with tissue.	Prevents overdose that can occur with multiple dose papers left in place. Proper disposal protects others from accidental exposure to medication.
(3) Apply antianginal medication to the chest area, back, upper arm, or legs. Do not apply on hairy surfaces or over scar tissue.	If patient complains of headaches, apply ointment farther from head. Application on hairy surfaces or scar tissue may interfere with absorption.
(4) Rotate site when applying nitroglycerin ointment.	Prevents skin irritation.
(5) Apply ointment to skin surface by holding edge or back of the paper measuring guide and placing ointment and wrapper directly on the skin (see illustration). Do not rub or massage ointment into skin.	Minimizes chance of ointment covering gloves and later touching nurse's hands. Medication is designed to absorb slowly over several hours; massaging increases absorption rate.
(6) Date and initial paper, and note time.	Prevents missing doses.
(7) Secure ointment and paper with a transparent dressing or strip of tape. Plastic wrap may be used as an occlusive dressing.	Prevents staining of clothing or inadvertent removal of the medication (Lilley and others, 2007).

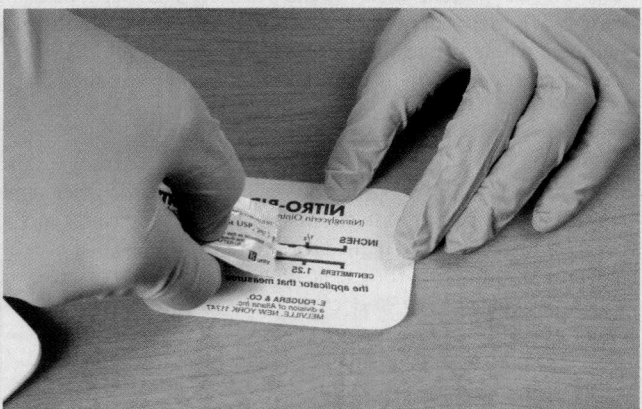

STEP 3b(1)   Ointment spread in inches over measuring guide.

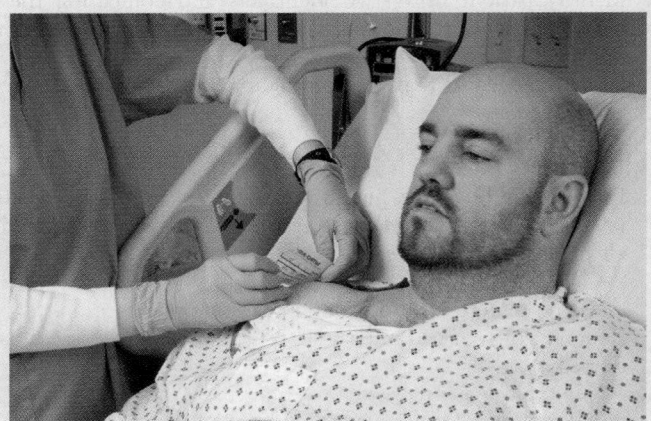

STEP 3b(5)   Nurse applies wrapper with medication to patient's skin.

STEP	RATIONALE

c   A variety of medications are available as transdermal (skin) patches (see illustration). Technique for applying a transdermal patch:

(1)   Locate and remove old patch before applying a new one. Check beneath skin folds, if necessary. Cleanse the area.

Failure to remove the old patch can result in drug overdose if a new patch is applied and the old patch remains on. Many transdermal patches are small, clear, or flesh-colored and can be easily hidden beneath skin folds. Cleansing the area removes traces of the older dose and adhesive, which may irritate the skin (McErlane, 2005).

(2)   Date and initial the outer side of the patch before applying it, and note time. Use a soft-tip or felt-tip marker pen.

Visual reminder prevents missing or extra doses. It is better to write on the patch before applying it to patient's skin. Damaging the patch with a pen will alter the delivery of the medication.

(3)   Choose a clean, dry area of the body that is free of hair. Some patches have specific instructions for the placement locations (e.g., Testoderm scrotal patches).

Increases absorption. Proper placement ensures correct delivery of drug.

Critical Decision Point   *Do not attempt to apply transdermal patches on skin that is oily, burned, broken out, cut, or irritated in any way. In addition, never apply heat, such as with a heating pad, over a transdermal patch. These actions will result in an increased rate of absorption with potentially serious adverse effects (ISMP, 2005).*

(4)   Carefully remove the patch from its protective covering. Hold the patch by the edge; do not touch the adhesive edges.

Touching only the edges ensures that the patch will adhere and that the medication dose has not changed. Removing the protective covering allows the medication to be absorbed through the skin.

(5)   Immediately apply the patch, pressing firmly with the palm of one hand for 10 seconds. Make sure it sticks well, especially around the edges. Apply overlay if provided with patch.

Sufficient pressure is necessary to ensure that the adhesive will keep the patch on the skin surface.

(6)   When the next dose is due, remove the old patch and choose a different site. Do not apply to previously used sites for at least 1 week.

Rotation of sites reduces skin irritation from medication and adhesive.

Critical Decision Point   *It is recommended that nitroglycerin transdermal patches be removed after 10 to 12 hours to allow for a nitrate-free interval and reduce the chance of tolerance to the medication. Check with patient's prescriber (Lilley and others, 2007).*

(7)   Dispose of patches by folding in half with sticky sides together. Throw the patch in the trash away from children and pets. Some agencies require the patch to be cut before disposal.

Proper disposal protects others from accidental exposure to medication (Schulmeister, 2005).

d   Technique for applying aerosolized medication (spray):

(1)   Shake container vigorously.

Mixes contents and propellant to ensure distribution of fine, even spray.

(2)   Read container's label for distance recommended to hold spray away from area (usually 15 to 30 cm [6 to 12 inches]).

Proper distance ensures fine spray hits skin surface. Holding container too close results in thin, watery distribution.

(3)   If spraying neck or upper chest, ask patient to turn face away from spray or briefly cover face with towel.

Prevents inhalation of spray.

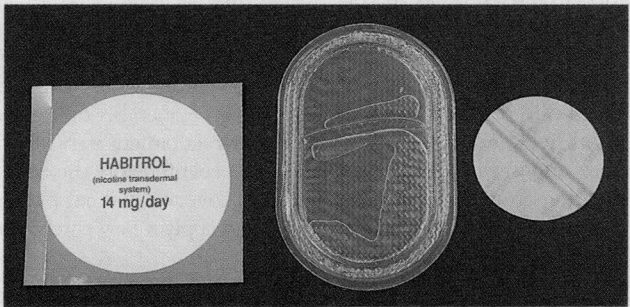

STEP 3c   Examples of transdermal (skin) patches.

STEP	RATIONALE
(4) Spray medication evenly over affected site (in some cases spray is timed for select period of seconds).	Ensures that affected area of skin is medicated.
e Technique for applying a suspension-based lotion:	
(1) Shake container vigorously.	Mixes powder throughout liquid to form well-mixed suspension.
(2) Apply small amount of lotion to small gauze dressing or pad, and apply to skin by stroking evenly in direction of hair growth.	Method of application leaves protective film of powder on skin after water base of suspension dries. Technique prevents irritation to hair follicles.
(3) Explain to patient that area will feel cool and dry.	Water evaporates to leave thin layer of powder.
f Technique for applying a powder:	
(1) Be sure skin surface is thoroughly dry.	Minimizes caking and crusting of powder.
(2) Fully spread apart any skin folds such as between toes or under axilla, and dry with a towel.	Fully exposes skin surface for application.
(3) If target area is near the face, ask patient to turn face away from powder or briefly cover face with towel.	Prevents inhalation of powder.
(4) Dust skin site lightly with dispenser so that area is covered with fine, thin layer of powder.	A thin layer of powder has slight lubricating properties to reduce friction and promote drying (Lilley and others, 2007).
(a) Cover skin area with dressing if ordered by physician.	Helps prevent agent from being rubbed off skin. Protects clothing from being stained.
4 Assist patient to comfortable position, reapply gown, and cover with bed linen as desired.	Provides for patient's sense of well-being.
5 Dispose of soiled supplies in receptacle especially designated for such articles, remove and dispose of gloves, and perform hand hygiene.	Keeps patient's environment neat and reduces transmission of infection and/or residual medication to children, pets, or others.

EVALUATION

1 Ask patient or significant other to name the medication and its action, purpose, dose, schedule, and side effects.	Evaluates learning.
2 Have patient keep a diary of doses taken.	Confirms compliance with prescribed therapy.
3 Observe patient apply lotion, ointment, or patch.	Return demonstration measures learning.
4 Inspect condition of skin between applications.	Determines if skin condition improves.

Unexpected Outcomes	Related Interventions
1 Skin site appears inflamed and edematous with blistering and oozing of fluid from lesions. These signs are indicative of subacute inflammation or eczema that can develop if skin lesions are getting worse.	• Notify prescriber; alternative therapies may be needed.
2 Patient continues to complain of pruritus and tenderness. Indicates slow or impaired healing.	• Notify prescriber; alternative therapies may be needed.
3 Patient is unable to explain information about drug or does not administer as prescribed.	• Identify possible reasons for noncompliance. • Reinstruction is necessary, or patient is unable to learn. • Offer patient or family opportunity to apply topical agent during next application and to ask questions. • Reexplore patient's health beliefs and resources.

Recording and Reporting

- Record actual time each drug was administered, type of agent applied, strength, and site of application in nurses' notes and on MAR immediately after administration. Describe condition of skin before topical agent application in nurses' notes. Do not chart medication administration until *after* it is given to patient. If you withhold a drug, record reason in nurses' notes and follow institution's policy for noting withheld doses.
- Report adverse effects/patient response and/or withheld drugs to nurse in charge or physician. Depending on medication, immediate prescriber notification may be required.
- Report any abnormalities in condition of skin to nurse in charge or physician.

Teaching Considerations

- If skin is inflamed, instruct patients to use only warm water rinse without soap for cleansing.
- When instructing patient, be sure lighting is adequate and area to be treated is well exposed. Have patient demonstrate the application technique to ensure effective therapy and compliance. Include a family member or friend if possible (Lilley and others, 2007).
- Instruct patient in how to manage a transdermal patch that begins to peel off before the next dose is due. Rather than tape the patch or cover it, instruct patient to remove the patch, clean the skin, and apply a new patch to a different area (Schulmeister, 2005).

Gerontological Considerations

- Changes in the skin of an older adult patient include increased wrinkling, dryness, flaking, and increased tendency to bruise. Be aware of these changes when applying topical medications to ensure proper application. Older skin is often more fragile and must be handled gently when applying topical medications.

Home Care Considerations

- Instruct patient to wrap applicators, used patches, and similar materials and dispose into cardboard or plastic disposable containers. Careful disposal is necessary to ensure the safety of patient, other adults, pets, and children.

SKILL 21-4   Administering Eye Medications

 Advanced / Nonparenteral Medication Administration / Administering Eye Medications

NSO *Nonparenteral Medication Administration Module / Lesson 3*

Common eye (ophthalmic) medications used by patients are drops and ointments, including over-the-counter preparations such as artificial tears and vasoconstrictors (e.g., Visine and Murine). However, many patients receive prescribed ophthalmic drugs for eye conditions such as glaucoma and infections and following cataract extraction. In addition, there is a third type of delivery system, the intraocular disk. Medications delivered by disk resemble a contact lens, but the disk is placed in the conjunctival sac, not on the cornea, and it remains in place for up to 1 week.

The eye is the most sensitive organ to which the nurse applies medications. The cornea is richly supplied with sensitive nerve fibers. Care must be taken to prevent instilling medication directly onto the cornea. The conjunctival sac is much less sensitive and thus a more appropriate site for medication instillation.

Any patient receiving topical eye medications should learn correct self-administration of the medication, especially patients with glaucoma, who must often undergo lifelong medication administration for control of their disease. Nurses can easily instruct patients while administering medications. At times it will become necessary for family members to learn how to administer eye medications. This is particularly true immediately after eye surgery, when a patient's vision is so impaired that it is difficult to assemble needed supplies and handle applicators correctly.

Delegation Considerations

The skill of administering eye medications cannot be delegated to NAP. The nurse directs the NAP about:

- Potential side effects of medications and to report their occurrence.
- The potential for temporary visual impairment after administration of eye medications.

Equipment

- ❏ Medication bottle with sterile eyedropper, ointment tube, or medicated intraocular disk
- ❏ Cotton ball or tissue
- ❏ Washbasin filled with warm water and washcloth
- ❏ Eye patch and tape (*optional*)
- ❏ Clean gloves
- ❏ Medication administration record (MAR)

STEP	RATIONALE

ASSESSMENT

STEP	RATIONALE
1 Check accuracy and completeness of each MAR with prescriber's written medication order. Check patient's name, drug name and dosage, route of administration, number of drops (if a liquid), and eye (right, left, or both) to receive medication.	Ensures patient receives correct medication.
2 Assess condition of external eye structures (you can do this just before drug instillation).	Provides baseline to later determine if local response to medications occurs. Also indicates need to clean eye before drug application.
3 Determine whether patient has any known allergies to eye medications. Also ask if patient has allergy to latex.	Protects patient from risk for allergic drug response. Latex allergy requires use of nonlatex gloves.
4 Determine whether patient has any symptoms of visual alterations.	Certain eye medications act to either lessen or increase these symptoms. Establishes baseline to recognize change in patient's condition.
5 Assess patient's level of consciousness and ability to follow directions.	If patient becomes restless or combative during procedure, a greater risk for accidental eye injury exists.
6 Assess patient's knowledge regarding drug therapy and desire to self-administer medication.	Indicates need for health teaching. Motivation influences teaching approach.
7 Assess patient's ability to manipulate and hold dropper.	Reflects patient's ability to learn to self-administer drug.

NURSING DIAGNOSES

- Deficient knowledge regarding drug and self-administration
- Disturbed sensory perception (visual)
- Health-seeking behaviors (self-care)
- Impaired physical mobility
- Pain (acute or chronic)
- Risk for injury

Individualize related factors based on patient's condition or needs.

STEP	RATIONALE

PLANNING

1 Expected outcomes following completion of procedure:
   - Patient experiences desired effect of medication.
   - Patient denies discomfort.
   - Patient experiences no side effects, and symptoms (e.g., irritation) are relieved.
   - Patient is able to discuss information about medication and technique correctly.
   - Patient demonstrates self-instillation of eyedrops.

Drug is administered correctly without injury to patient.
Drug is administered correctly without injury to patient.
Drug is distributed and absorbed properly.

Demonstrates learning.

Demonstrates learning.

2 Prepare medications for instillation. Check label of medication against MAR three times (see Skill 21-1).

Adequate preparation saves nursing time. Ensures patient receives correct medication.

3 Identify patient using two identifiers and comparing these identifiers with the information on patient's identification bracelet. Ask patient to state name.

Ensures correct patient receives medication. You need to use at least two patient identifiers (neither can be the patient's room number) whenever administering medications (TJC, 2007).

4 Explain procedure to patient.

Relieves anxiety and promotes patient participation.

IMPLEMENTATION

1 Perform hand hygiene, and arrange supplies at bedside; apply clean gloves.
   a If storing eyedrops in refrigerator, rewarm to room temperature before administering.

Reduces transmission of microorganisms; ensures a smooth, orderly procedure.
Reduces irritation to eye due to cold temperature of solution.

2 Ask patient to lie supine or sit back in chair with head slightly hyperextended.

Position provides easy access to eye for medication instillation and minimizes drainage of medication through tear duct.

Critical Decision Point   *Do not hyperextend the neck of a patient with cervical spine injury.*

3 If drainage or crusts are present along eyelid margins or inner canthus, gently wash away. Soak any crusts that are dried and difficult to remove by applying a warm, damp washcloth or cotton ball over eye for a few minutes. Always wipe clean from inner to outer canthus (see illustration).

Drainage or crusts harbor microorganisms. Soaking allows easy removal and prevents pressure from being applied directly over eye. Cleansing from inner to outer canthus avoids entrance of microorganisms into lacrimal duct (Lilley and others, 2007).

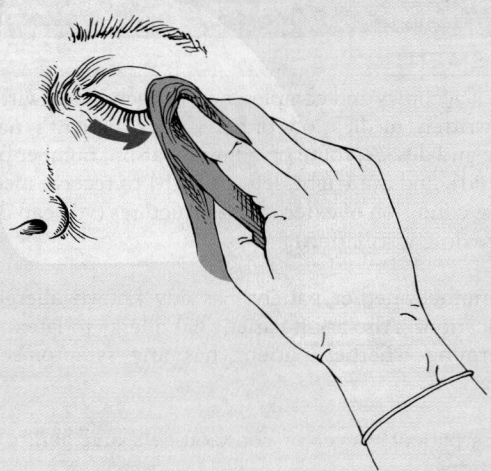

STEP 3   Cleanse eye, washing from inner to outer canthus before administering drops or ointment.

4 Ask a patient to look at ceiling, and explain steps to patient.

Action moves sensitive cornea up and away from conjunctival sac and reduces stimulation of blink reflex; explanation facilitates patient's cooperation with the procedure.

5 Instill eyedrops.
   a Hold cotton ball or clean tissue in nondominant hand on patient's cheekbone just below lower eyelid.

Cotton or tissue absorbs medication that escapes eye.

STEP	RATIONALE

b With tissue or cotton resting below lower lid, gently press downward with thumb or forefinger against bony orbit. Never press directly against patient's eyeball.

Technique exposes lower conjunctival sac. Retraction against bony orbit prevents pressure and trauma to eyeball and prevents fingers from touching eye. Pressure to the eyeball may cause damage.

c With dominant hand resting on patient's forehead, hold filled medication eyedropper approximately 1 to 2 cm (½ to ¾ inch) above conjunctival sac.

Helps prevent accidental contact of eyedropper tip with eye structures, thus reducing risk for injury to eye and transfer of infection to dropper. Ophthalmic medications are sterile.

d Drop prescribed number of medication drops into conjunctival sac (see illustration).

Conjunctival sac normally holds one or two drops. Provides even distribution of medication across eye.

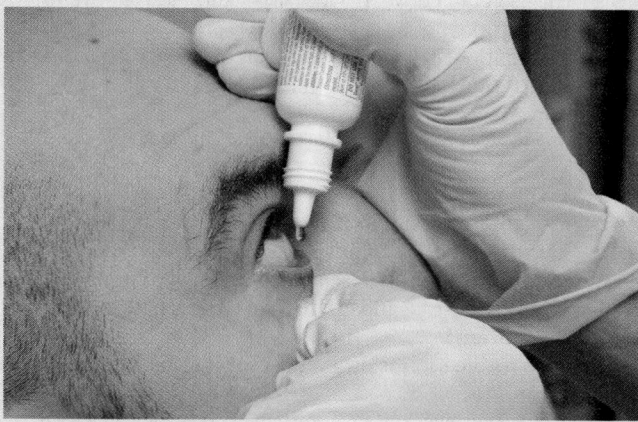

STEP 5d Hold eyedropper over the lower conjunctival sac.

e If patient blinks or closes eye, or if drops fall on outer lid margins, repeat procedure.

Therapeutic effect of drug is obtained only when drops enter conjunctival sac.

f After instilling drops, ask patient to close eye gently.

Helps to distribute medication. Squinting or squeezing of eyelids forces medication from conjunctival sac.

g When administering drugs that cause systemic effects, with a clean tissue apply gentle pressure to patient's nasolacrimal duct for 30 to 60 seconds (see illustration).

Prevents overflow of medication into nasal and pharyngeal passages. Prevents absorption into systemic circulation.

6 Instill eye ointment:

a Holding ointment applicator above lower lid margin, apply thin ribbon of ointment evenly along inner edge of lower eyelid on conjunctiva (see illustration) from the inner canthus to outer canthus.

Distributes medication evenly across eye and lid margin.

b Have patient close eye and rub lid lightly in circular motion with cotton ball, if not contraindicated.

Further distributes medication without traumatizing eye.

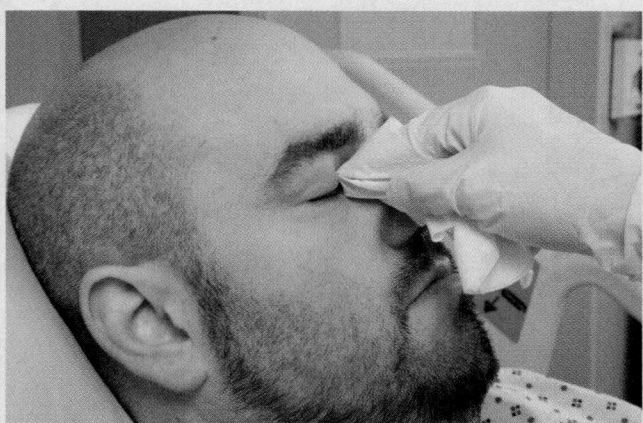

STEP 5g Apply gentle pressure against the nasolacrimal duct after giving eye medications.

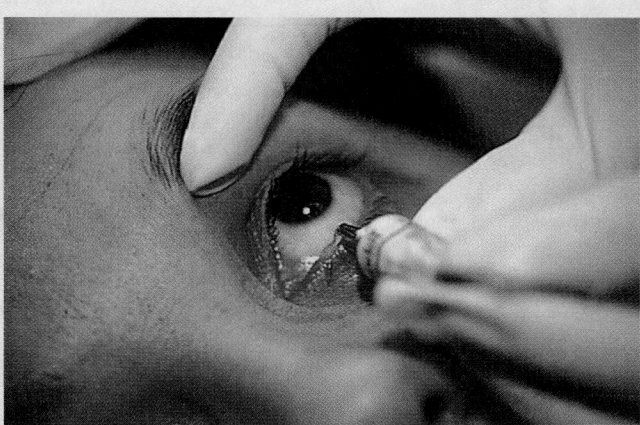

STEP 6a Nurse applies ointment along the inner edge of the lower eyelid from the inner to outer canthus.

STEP	RATIONALE

7 Insert intraocular disk

   a Open package containing the disk. Gently press your fingertip against the disk so that it adheres to your finger. (NOTE: It is sometimes necessary to moisten gloved finger with sterile saline.) Position the convex side of the disk on your fingertip.

Allows nurse to inspect disk for damage or deformity. Prepares disk for proper administration.

   b With your other hand, gently pull patient's lower eyelid away from the eye. Ask patient to look up.

Prepares conjunctival sac for receiving medicated disk.

   c Place the disk in the conjunctival sac, so that it floats on the sclera between the iris and lower eyelid (see illustration).

Ensures delivery of medication.

   d Pull patient's lower eyelid out and over the disk (see illustration).

Ensures accurate medication delivery.

Critical Decision Point *You should not be able to see the disk at this time. Repeat Step (e) if you can see the disk.*

8 Remove intraocular disk

   a Explain procedure to patient.

   b Gently pull on patient's lower eyelid to expose the disk.

   c Using your forefinger and thumb of your other hand, pinch the disk, and lift it out of the patient's eye (see illustration).

Intraocular disks may remain in place for up to 1 week (duration varies).

9 If excess medication is on eyelid, gently wipe it from inner to outer canthus.

Promotes comfort and prevents trauma to eye.

10 If patient had eye patch, apply clean one by placing it over affected eye so entire eye is covered. Tape securely without applying pressure to eye.

Clean eye patch reduces chance of infection.

11 Assist patient to comfortable position.

Provides for patient's sense of well-being.

12 Dispose of soiled supplies in proper receptacle, remove and dispose of gloves, and perform hand hygiene.

Maintains neat environment at bedside and reduces transmission of microorganisms.

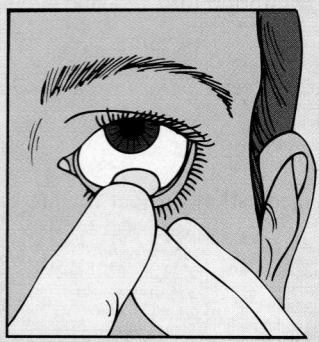

STEP 7c Place intraocular disk in the conjunctival sac between the iris and the lower eyelid.

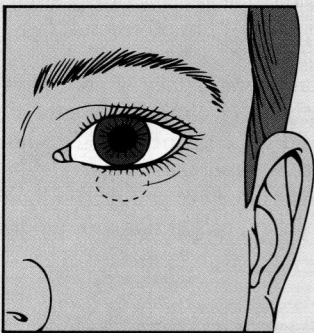

STEP 7d Gently pull the patient's lower eyelid over the disk.

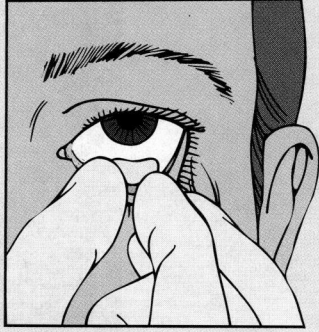

STEP 8c Carefully pinch the disk to remove it from the patient's eye.

STEP	RATIONALE

13 Patients experienced in self-instillation may be allowed to give drops under nurse's supervision (check agency policy).

EVALUATION

1 Note patient's response to instillation; ask if patient felt any discomfort.

Determines if procedure was performed correctly and safely.

2 Observe response to medication by assessing visual changes, asking if symptoms are relieved, and noting any side effects.

Evaluates effects of medication.

3 Ask patient to discuss drug's purpose, action, side effects, and technique of administration.

Determines patient's level of understanding.

4 Have patient demonstrate self-administration of next dose.

Provides feedback regarding competency with skill.

Unexpected Outcomes

1 Patient complains of burning or pain or experiences local side effects (e.g., headache, bloodshot eyes, local eye irritation). The drug concentration and the patient's sensitivity both influence the chances of side effects developing.

2 Patient experiences systemic effects from drops (e.g., increased heart rate and blood pressure from epinephrine, decreased heart rate and blood pressure from timolol).

Related Interventions

- Eyedrops may have been instilled onto the cornea, or the dropper touched the surface of the eye.
- Notify prescriber for a possible adjustment in medication type and dosage.
- Notify prescriber immediately.
- Remain with patient. Assess vital signs.
- Withhold further doses.
- Systemic absorption through tear duct can cause potentially dangerous effects.
- Ophthalmic anesthetics and antibiotics may cause the same type of adverse reactions as systemically administered drugs (e.g., anaphylaxis).

Recording and Reporting

- Record drug, concentration, number of drops, time of administration, and which eye (left, right, or both) received medication on MAR immediately after administration. Record appearance of eye in nurses' notes. Do not chart medication administration until *after* it is given to the patient. If you withhold a drug, record reason in nurses' notes and follow institution's policy for noting withheld doses.
- Report adverse effects/patient response and/or withheld drugs to nurse in charge or physician. Depending on medication, immediate prescriber notification may be required.

Teaching Considerations

- Warn patients that mydriatics will temporarily blur vision. Wearing sunglasses will reduce photophobia. If necessary, make arrangements for someone else to drive patient home from an office or clinic visit.
- Patients who receive medications that paralyze the ciliary muscles of the eye (e.g., scopolamine, Isopto-Hyoscine, atropine, Isopto Atropine, and cycloplegics) should not drive or attempt to perform any activity that requires acute vision after receiving medication.

Pediatric Considerations

- When instilling drops in an infant or young child, have parent gently restrain child's head with child in parent's lap. Be sure that child's hands do not interfere with instillation.

- Infants often clench the eyes tightly to avoid eyedrops. To administer drops in an uncooperative infant, with the head gently restrained, place the drops at the nasal corner where the lids meet. When the child opens the eye the medication will flow into the eye.
- When both eyedrops and ointment are ordered, administer the drops first, wait 3 minutes, then administer the ointment. This allows time for each medication to have an effect.
- If the eye ointment is to be given once a day, administer at bedtime because it will blur the child's vision (Hockenberry and Wilson, 2007).

Gerontological Considerations

- Before discharging older adult patient, evaluate patient's ability to perform all the necessary steps for the administration of eyedrops and ointments.

Home Care Considerations

- When using over-the-counter eyedrops, patients should not share medications with other family members. Risk for infection transmission is high. In addition, instruct patients to follow manufacturer's instructions carefully for dosing.

SKILL 21-5 Administering Ear Drops

Advanced / Nonparenteral Medication Administration / Administering Ear Drops

NSO *Nonparenteral Medication Administration Module / Lesson 4*

When administering ear (otic) medications, be aware of certain safety precautions. Internal ear structures are very sensitive to temperature extremes. Failure to instill a solution at room temperature can cause vertigo (severe dizziness) or nausea and debilitate a patient for several minutes. Although structures of the outer ear are not sterile, use sterile drops and solutions in case the eardrum is ruptured. Entrance of nonsterile solutions into the middle ear can cause serious infection. A final precaution is to avoid forcing any solution into the ear. Do not occlude the ear canal with a medicine dropper, because this can cause pressure within the canal during instillation and subsequent injury to the eardrum. If you follow these precautions, instillation of ear drops is a safe and effective therapy.

Delegation Considerations

The skill of administering ear medications cannot be delegated to NAP. The nurse directs the NAP about:

- Potential side effects of medications and to report their occurrence.
- Reporting any dizziness or light-headedness to the nurse for further assessment.

Equipment

- ❑ Medication bottle with dropper
- ❑ Cotton-tipped applicator
- ❑ Cotton ball (*optional*)
- ❑ Clean gloves (*optional*, only if patient has drainage)
- ❑ Medication administration record (MAR)

STEP	RATIONALE
ASSESSMENT	
1 Check accuracy and completion of MAR with prescriber's written medication order. Check patient's name, drug name, dosage, route of administration, number of drops to instill, ear (right, left, or both) to receive medication, and time of administration. Clarify incomplete or unclear orders with the prescriber before implementation.	Ensures patient receives correct medication.
2 Assess condition of external ear structures and canal (see Chapter 19).	Provides baseline to later determine if local response to medication occurs, whether patient's condition improves, or whether it will be necessary to clean ear before instilling medication.
3 Determine whether patient has symptoms of discomfort and/or hearing impairment.	Disorders of external ear are painful. Occlusion of external ear canal by swelling, drainage, or cerumen (earwax) can impair hearing acuity. These conditions may change after drug instillation and require ongoing monitoring.
4 Assess patient's level of consciousness and ability to follow instructions.	Patient must lie still during drug administration. Sudden movements can cause injury from ear dropper.
5 Assess patient's level of knowledge regarding drug therapy and motivation to self-administer medication.	Patient's knowledge level determines whether health teaching is required. Motivation influences teaching approach.
6 Assess patient's ability to grasp and manipulate dropper.	Determines patient's ability to self-administer drug.

NURSING DIAGNOSES

- Deficient knowledge regarding drug actions and purpose
- Disturbed sensory perception (auditory)
- Health-seeking behaviors (self-care)
- Impaired physical mobility
- Pain (acute or chronic)
- Risk for injury

Individualize related factors based on patient's condition or needs.

PLANNING

1 Expected outcomes following completion of procedure:	
• Patient denies discomfort during administration.	Procedure is performed correctly without injury to patient.
• Ear canal becomes clear, without drainage, excess cerumen, or inflammation, as medication is repeatedly instilled.	Drug action is effective.
• Patient's hearing acuity improves.	This response occurs only if hearing loss was caused by obstruction in external ear canal.
• Patient is able to explain steps for instilling ear drops and demonstrates technique for administration.	Cognitive and psychomotor learning occurs.
2 Prepare medication for instillation. Check label of medication against MAR three times (see Skill 21-1).	Adequate preparation saves nursing time. Ensures patient receives correct medication.

STEP	RATIONALE

3 Identify patient using two identifiers and comparing these identifiers with the information on patient's identification bracelet. Ask patient to state name.

Ensures correct patient receives medication. You need to use at least two patient identifiers (neither can be the patient's room number) whenever administering medications (TJC, 2007).

4 Explain each step of procedure to patient, allowing for questions.

Reduces patient anxiety; timing of instruction enhances learning.

IMPLEMENTATION

1 Perform hand hygiene, and arrange supplies at bedside. Apply clean gloves (if drainage is present).

Reduces transmission of microorganisms; helps nurse perform procedure smoothly.

2 Warm medication by running warm water over the bottle (without damaging the label directions or allowing water to get into the bottle).

Prevents nausea and vertigo that may occur if the medication is too cold.

3 Have patient assume side-lying position (if not contraindicated by patient's condition) with ear to be treated facing up, or patient may sit in chair or at the bedside. Stabilize the patient's head.

Position provides easy access to ear for instillation of medication. Ear canal is in position to receive medication. Stabilizing the head promotes safety during instillation with a dropper.

4 For adults and children older than 3 years, gently pull the pinna up and outward; in children 3 years of age or less, pull the pinna down and back (see illustrations).

Straightening of ear canal provides direct access to deeper external ear structures. Developmental differences in younger children and infants necessitate different methods of medication administration (Lilley and others, 2007).

5 If cerumen or drainage occludes outermost portion of ear canal, wipe out gently with cotton-tipped applicator (see illustration). Do not use the cotton-tipped applicator to clean the ear canal.

Cerumen and drainage harbor microorganisms and can block distribution of medication. Use of a cotton-tipped applicator to clean the ear canal may force wax inward, occluding the canal.

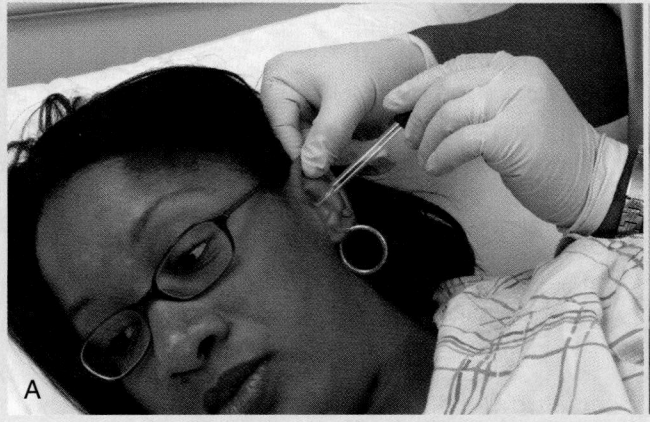

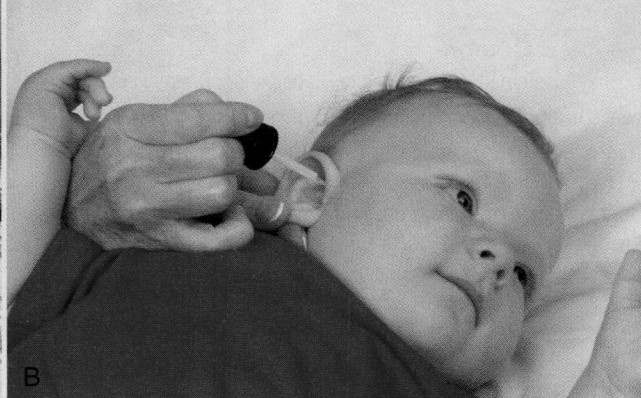

STEP 4 **A,** Pull the pinna up and outward for adults and children older than 3 years. **B,** Pull the pinna down and back for children 3 years of age or less.

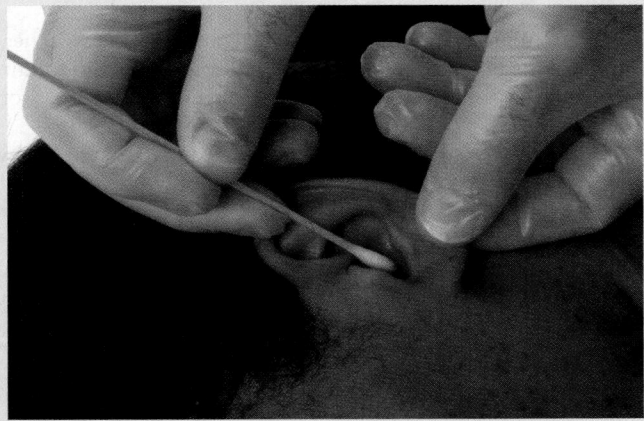

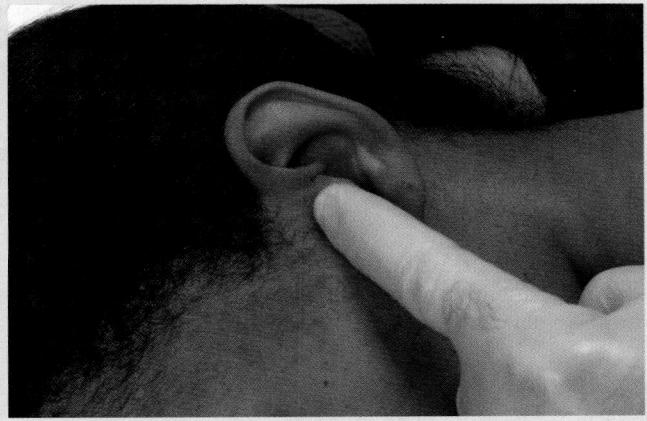

STEP 5 Always cleanse only outer canal. Do not push secretions into ear.

STEP 7 Nurse applies pressure to tragus of ear after instilling drops.

STEP	RATIONALE
6 Instill prescribed drops holding dropper 1 cm (½ inch) above ear canal (see illustrations for Step 4).	Forceful instillation of drops into occluded canal can cause injury to eardrum.
7 Ask patient to remain in side-lying position for a few minutes. Apply gentle massage or pressure to tragus of ear with finger (see illustration, p. 551).	Allows complete absorption of medication. Pressure and massage move medication inward.

Critical Decision Point *If medication is ordered for both ears, ask the patient to stay in the side-lying position for at least 10 minutes after the dose before turning to the other side.*

STEP	RATIONALE
8 At times, the prescriber orders insertion of portion of cotton ball into outermost part of canal. Do not press cotton into canal.	Inserting cotton into outer canal prevents escape of medication when patient sits or stands. Cotton should not block canal to impair hearing.
9 Remove cotton after 15 minutes.	Time period promotes drug distribution and absorption.
10 Dispose of soiled supplies, remove and dispose of gloves, and perform hand hygiene.	Reduces transmission of microorganisms.
11 Assist patient to comfortable position after drops are absorbed.	Restores comfort.

EVALUATION

1 Ask if patient feels any discomfort during instillation.	Determines if procedure is performed correctly and reveals severity of symptoms.
2 Evaluate condition of external ear between drug instillations.	Determines response to medication.
3 Evaluate patient's hearing acuity.	Hearing may change after drug administration.
4 Ask patient to explain technique for instilling ear drops and purpose of medication.	Evaluates degree of learning.
5 Have patient demonstrate self-administration of next dose.	Provides feedback regarding competency with skill.

Unexpected Outcomes	Related Interventions
1 Ear canal is inflamed, swollen, tender to palpation. Drainage is present.	• Symptoms of continuing ear infection are present; notify prescriber.
2 Patient's hearing acuity continues to be reduced.	• Obstruction within ear canal is unrelieved. Notify prescriber.
3 Cerumen is occluding ear canal.	• Wax has become impacted in the canal. Ear irrigation may be necessary to remove wax impaction.
4 Patient is unable to explain drug information and steps for drug instillation.	• Repeat instructions. Patient may be unable to learn. • Include family or caregivers when instructing.
5 Patient has difficulty self-administering ear drops.	• Reinstruction is needed. Have patient demonstrate instillation of ear drops until performed.

Recording and Reporting

- Record drug, concentration, number of drops, actual time administered, and ear (left, right, or both) into which drops instilled on MAR immediately after administration. Record condition of ear canal in nurses' notes. Do not chart medication administration until *after* it is given to patient. If you withhold a drug, record reason in nurses' notes and follow institution's policy for noting withheld doses.
- Record condition of ear canal in nurses' notes.
- Report adverse effects/patient response and/or withheld drugs to nurse in charge or physician. Depending on medication, immediate prescriber notification may be required.

Teaching Considerations

- Instruct patient in proper way to cleanse ears and to avoid use of sharp objects in ear canal.

Pediatric Considerations

- Ensure that parents and/or caregivers are aware of the proper method of administration (e.g., for children younger than 3 years gently pull the pinna of the ear downward and straight back).
- Restrain infants or young children in supine position with head turned to expose affected ear. Hold child in this position until the drug has time to be absorbed (Hockenberry and Wilson, 2007).
- Teach the signs of hearing loss and the need for frequent follow-ups to parents with children who have chronic otitis media.

Gerontological Considerations

- Some older adults experience excessive accumulation of cerumen in the ear. Have this removed before administering medication.

SKILL 21-6   Administering Nasal Instillations

Patients with nasal sinus alterations may receive drugs by spray, drops, or tampons. The most commonly administered form of nasal instillation is a decongestant spray or drops used to relieve sinus congestion and cold symptoms. Many over-the-counter nasal preparations contain sympathomimetic drugs (e.g., Afrin or Neo-Synephrine). These drugs are relatively safe when administered nasally because only small doses are needed. However, the drugs can enter the systemic circulation by way of the nasal mucosa, or by the gastrointestinal tract if an excess amount is swallowed, causing restlessness, nervousness, tremors, or insomnia in some patients. Long-term use of decongestant nasal spray can actually worsen nasal congestion because of a rebound effect. Nasal sprays are easy for a patient to self-administer.

Delegation Considerations

The skill of administering nasal medications cannot be delegated to NAP. The nurse directs the NAP about:

- Potential side effects of medications and to report their occurrence.
- Reporting any bloody nasal drainage.

Equipment

- ❑ Prepared medication with clean dropper or spray container
- ❑ Facial tissue
- ❑ Small pillow (*optional*)
- ❑ Washcloth (*optional*)
- ❑ Clean gloves
- ❑ Medication administration record (MAR)

STEP	RATIONALE
ASSESSMENT	
1 Check accuracy and completeness of each MAR with prescriber's written medication order. Check patient's name, drug name and dosage, route of administration, and time for administration.	The order sheet is the most reliable source and only legal record of drugs patient is to receive. Ensures right drug is administered.
2 For antiinfective nasal drops, determine which sinus is affected by referring to medical record.	Prescribed nasal drops often contain antibiotics for the treatment of sinus infections. Proper positioning of patients during instillation of drops is essential for medication to reach the affected sinus.
3 Assess patient's history of hypertension, heart disease, diabetes, and hyperthyroidism.	These conditions contraindicate use of decongestants that stimulate the central nervous system. Side effects of transient hypertension, tachycardia, palpitations, and headache may occur.
4 Inspect condition of nose and sinuses. Palpate sinuses for tenderness. Note type of drainage, if present.	Provides baseline to monitor effects of medication. Presence of discharge interferes with drug absorption. Clear nasal discharge indicates sinus problem. Yellow or greenish discharge indicates infection.
5 Assess patient's knowledge regarding use of nasal instillations and technique for instillation and willingness to learn self-administration.	Requires health teaching regarding use of drugs. Motivation influences teaching approach.

NURSING DIAGNOSES

- Deficient knowledge regarding drug action and purpose
- Health-seeking behaviors (self-care)
- Pain (acute or chronic)
- Risk for injury

Individualize related factors based on patient's condition or needs.

STEP	RATIONALE
PLANNING	

1 Expected outcomes following completion of procedure:
  • Patient is able to breathe with ease through nose.
  • Patient's nasal sinuses become clear, moist, pink, without drainage after repeated instillations (applies to antiinfective medications).
  • Patient is able to explain medication's purpose and administers nasal instillations correctly.
	Nasal congestion has been relieved.
	Inflammation of mucosa has been relieved.
	
	Feedback reflects patient's learning.

2 Prepare medication for instillation. Check label of solution against MAR three times (see Skill 21-1).	Adequate preparation saves nursing time. Ensures patient receives correct medication.
3 Identify patient using two identifiers and comparing these identifiers with the information on patient's identification bracelet. Ask patient to state name.	Ensures correct patient receives medication. You need to use at least two patient identifiers (neither can be the patient's room number) whenever administering medications (TJC, 2007).

STEP	RATIONALE
4 Explain procedure to patient regarding positioning and sensations to expect, such as burning or stinging of mucosa or choking sensation as medication trickles into throat.	Helps patient anticipate experience of procedure to reduce anxiety.

IMPLEMENTATION

1 Perform hand hygiene. Arrange supplies and medications at bedside. Apply clean gloves (if drainage is present).	Reduces transmission of microorganisms; ensures smooth, orderly procedure.
2 Instruct patient to clear or blow nose gently unless contraindicated (e.g., risk for increased intracranial pressure or nosebleeds).	Removes mucus and secretions that can block distribution of medication.
3 Administer nose drops	
a Assist patient to supine position.	Proper positioning provides access to specific nasal passages.
b Position head properly:	
(1) For access to posterior pharynx, tilt patient's head backward.	
(2) For access to ethmoid or sphenoid sinus, tilt head back over edge of bed, or place small pillow under patient's shoulder and tilt head back (see illustration).	
(3) For access to frontal and maxillary sinus, tilt head back over edge of bed or pillow with head turned toward side to be treated (see illustration).	Position allows medication to drain into affected sinus.
c Support patient's head with nondominant hand.	Prevents straining of neck muscles.
d Instruct patient to breathe through mouth.	Mouth breathing reduces chance of aspirating nasal drops into trachea and lungs.
e Hold dropper 1 cm (½ inch) above nares, and instill prescribed number of drops toward midline of ethmoid bone.	Avoids contamination of dropper. Instilling toward ethmoid bone facilitates distribution of medication over nasal mucosa.
f Have patient remain in supine position 5 minutes.	Prevents premature loss of medication through nares.
4 Administer nasal spray:	
a Determine number of sprays to administer. Some sprays (i.e., decongestants) are administered by one spray into each nostril. Others sprays, such as calcitonin, are administered by one single spray.	

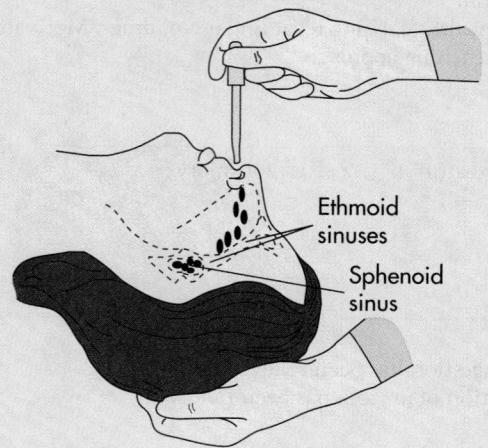

STEP 3b(2)   Position for instilling nose drops into ethmoid or sphenoid sinus.

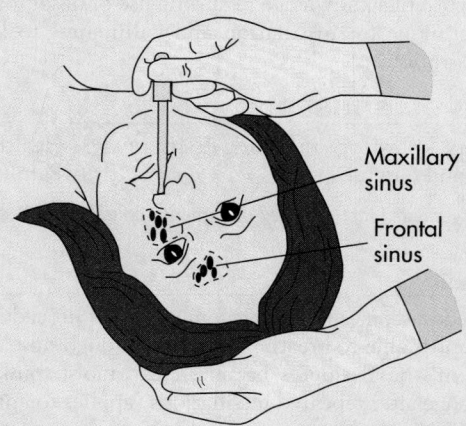

STEP 3b(3)   Position for instilling nose drops into frontal and maxillary sinus.

STEP	RATIONALE
b Position patient in upright position with head tilted slightly forward.	Proper positioning permits the medication spray to reach the nasal passages
c Insert tip of nasal spray into one nostril, and occlude the other nostril with a finger (see illustration). Point the spray tip toward the nasal turbinates and away from the nasal septum.	Allows for proper administration of medication.
d Instruct patient to inhale with mouth closed, and spray the nasal spray into the nostril.	Allows for proper administration and distribution of nasal medication as high into the nasal passages as possible.
e If a second spray is indicated, repeat Steps a to d through the other nostril.	

Critical Decision Point   *Some medications are designed for one spray per dose. Examples include calcitonin (salmon), desmopressin, and sumatriptan. It is essential to ensure that the patient understands the correct number of sprays to use per dose in order to prevent overdosing of these strong medications (ISMP, 2006a).*

5 Offer facial tissue to blot runny nose, but caution patient against blowing nose for several minutes.	Allows maximal amount of medication to be absorbed.
6 Assist patient to a comfortable position after drug is absorbed.	Restores comfort.
7 Dispose of soiled supplies, remove and dispose of gloves, and perform hand hygiene.	Maintains neat, orderly environment. Reduces spread of microorganisms.

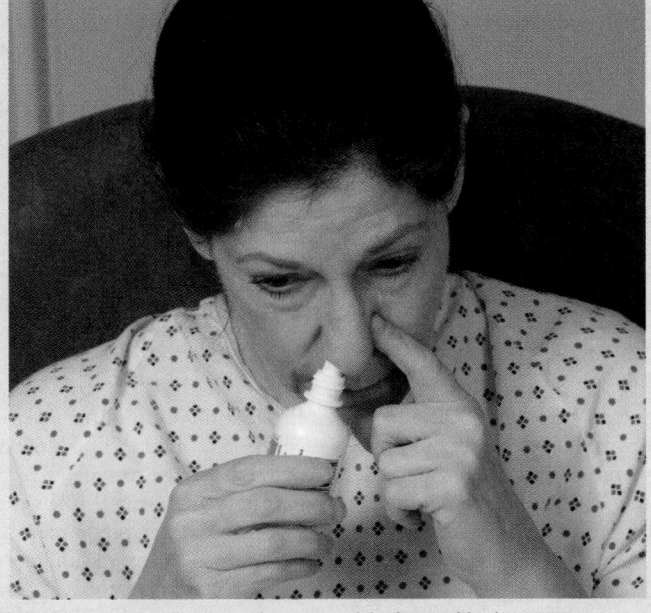

STEP 4c   Occlude the other nostril before self-administering nasal spray.

EVALUATION

1 Observe patient for onset of side effects 15 to 30 minutes after administration.	Drugs absorbed through mucosa can cause systemic reaction.
2 Ask if patient is able to breathe through nose after decongestant administration. May be necessary to have patient occlude one nostril at a time and breathe deeply.	Determines effectiveness of decongestant medication.
3 Reinspect condition of nasal passages between instillations.	Condition of mucosa reveals response to medication.
4 Ask patient to describe risks of overuse of decongestants and methods for administration.	Feedback ensures that patient can self-administer drugs properly.
5 Have patient demonstrate self-medication.	Feedback demonstrates learning.

Unexpected Outcomes	Related Interventions
1 Patient is unable to breathe easily through nasal passages. Mucosa appears swollen, and congestion is unrelieved.	• Patient may be experiencing rebound effect, or medication may not be effective. • Stop medication use, and notify prescriber. Consider alternative therapy.
2 Nasal mucosa remains inflamed and tender, with discharge from nares.	• Inflammatory or infectious process remains. Consider alternative therapy.
3 Patient complains of sinus headache. Sinuses remain congested.	• Consider alternative therapy.
4 Patient is unable to explain technique and risks of drug therapy.	• Further explanation is required. • Include family members or caregiver when possible.
5 Patient is unable to self-administer medication.	• Reinstruction is necessary. • Include family members or caregiver when possible.

Recording and Reporting

• Record medication administration on MAR immediately after administration, including drug name, concentration, number of drops; nostril into which drug was instilled; and actual time of administration. Do not chart medication administration until *after* it is given to patient. If you withhold a drug, record reason in nurses' notes and follow institution's policy for noting withheld doses.

• Report any unusual systemic effects or adverse effects/patient response and/or withheld drugs to nurse in charge or physician. Depending on medication, immediate prescriber notification may be required.

Teaching Considerations

• Instruct patients that each family member should have a different dropper or spray applicator. Instruct patients to wash or rinse applicators after each use.

• Use over-the-counter nasal sprays or nose drops for only one illness; bottles become easily contaminated with bacteria.

• Caution patients against overuse of nasal spray decongestants because they cause rebound effect, worsening of mucosal swelling. Risk increases as more drug is used.

Pediatric Considerations

• Positioning child with head extended over edge of bed or pillow facilitates smooth instillation of nasal drops. Instruct child or parent to remain in this position for at least 1 minute to ensure that drops come into contact with affected tissue.

• Infants are nose breathers, and the possible congestion caused by nasal medications may inhibit their sucking. Administer nose drops, if ordered, 20 to 30 minutes before feedings (Hockenberry and Wilson, 2007).

SKILL 21-7   Using Metered-Dose Inhalers

Advanced / Nonparenteral Medication Administration / Using a Metered-Dose Inhaler

[NSO]   *Nonparenteral Medication Administration Module / Lesson 5*

Inhaled medications are usually designed to produce local effects; for example, bronchodilators open narrowed bronchioles, and mucolytic agents liquefy thick mucous secretions. However, because these medications are absorbed rapidly through the pulmonary circulation, some have the potential for producing systemic side effects (e.g., albuterol may cause palpitations, tremors, and tachycardia).

Patients who receive drugs by inhalation frequently suffer from chronic respiratory disease. Drugs administered by inhalation provide control of airway hyperactivity or constriction. Because patients depend on these medications for disease control, they must learn about the medications and how to administer them safely. Inhalers and small-volume nebulizers (see Skill 21-9) are devices that deliver inhaled medications.

Metered-dose inhalers (MDIs) are handheld devices that disperse medications through an aerosol spray or mist to penetrate lung airways. Dry powder inhalers (DPIs) deliver inhaled medication in a fine powder formulation to the respiratory tract (see Procedural Guideline 21-1). Fig. 21-1 illustrates examples of MDIs and DPIs. The deeper passages of the respiratory tract provide a large surface area for drug absorption, and the alveolar-capillary network absorbs medication rapidly.

An MDI delivers a measured dose of the drug with each push of a canister. Approximately 5 to 10 pounds of pressure must be used to activate the aerosol. This is a problem for some older patients because hand strength diminishes with age. Because use of an MDI requires coordination during the breathing cycle, many patients spray only the back of their throats and fail to receive a full dose. The inhaler must be depressed to expel medication just as the patient inhales. This ensures the medication reaches the lower airways. Poor coordination can be solved by the use of spacer devices (AeroChamber, InspirEase) or the use of a breath-activated MDI, such as the Maxair Autoinhaler (Burkhart and others, 2005). Box 21-4 summarizes common problems in using an inhaler.

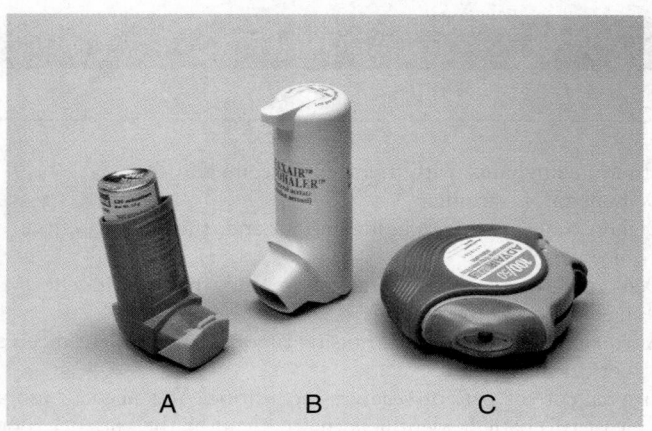

FIG 21-1 **A,** Metered-dose inhaler (MDI). **B,** Automated MDI. **C,** Dry powder inhaler (DPI).

Delegation Considerations

The skill of administering MDI medications cannot be delegated to NAP. The nurse directs the NAP about:

- Potential side effects of medications and to report their occurrence.
- Reporting paroxysmal coughing, audible wheezing, and patient's report of breathlessness or difficulty breathing.

Equipment

- ❑ Metered-dose inhaler with medication canister
- ❑ Stethoscope
- ❑ Spacer device, such as AeroChamber or InspirEase *(optional)*
- ❑ Facial tissues *(optional)*
- ❑ Washbasin or sink with warm water
- ❑ Paper towel
- ❑ Medication administration record (MAR)

BOX 21-4	Common Problems in Using an Inhaler

- *Not taking the medication as prescribed:* Taking either too much or too little.
- *Incorrect activation:* This usually occurs through pressing the canister *before* taking a breath. Both should be done simultaneously so that the drug can be carried down to the lungs with the breath.
- *Forgetting to shake the inhaler:* The drug is in a suspension, and therefore particles may settle. If the inhaler is not shaken, it may not deliver the correct dose of the drug.

- *Not waiting long enough between puffs:* The whole process should be repeated to take the second puff, otherwise an incorrect dose may be delivered, or the drug may not penetrate into the lungs.
- *Failure to clean the valve:* Particles may jam up the valve in the mouthpiece unless it is cleaned occasionally. This is a frequent cause of failure to get 200 puffs from one inhaler.
- *Failure to observe whether the inhaler is actually releasing a spray:* If it is not, this should be checked with the pharmacist.

STEP	RATIONALE

ASSESSMENT

1. Check accuracy and completeness of each MAR with prescriber's written medication order. Check patient's name, drug name and concentration, route of administration, number of inhalations, and time for administration.

The order sheet is the most reliable source and only legal record of drugs patient is to receive. Ensures patient receives correct medication.

2. Assess respiratory pattern, and auscultate breath sounds.

Establishes baseline of airway status for comparison during and after treatment.

3. Assess patient's readiness to learn: patient asks questions about medication, disease, or complications; requests education in use of inhaler; is mentally alert; participates in own care.

Affects patient's ability to understand explanations and actively participate in teaching process.

4. Assess patient's ability to learn: patient should not be fatigued, in pain, or in respiratory distress; assess level of understanding of technical vocabulary terms.

Mental or physical limitations affect patient's ability to learn and methods nurse uses for instruction.

5. Assess patient's knowledge and understanding of disease and purpose and action of prescribed medications.

Knowledge of disease is essential for patient to realistically understand use of inhaler.

6. Assess patient's ability to hold, manipulate, and depress canister and inhaler.

Any impairment of grasp or presence of hand tremors interferes with patient's ability to depress canister within inhaler. A spacer device is often necessary.

7. Assess drug schedule and number of inhalations prescribed for each dose.

Determines the type of instruction nurse provides for use of inhaler.

8. If previously instructed in self-administration of inhaled medicine, assess patient's technique in using an inhaler.

Instruction may require only simple reinforcement, depending on patient's level of dexterity.

NURSING DIAGNOSES

- Activity intolerance
- Anxiety
- Deficient knowledge regarding use of MDI

- Health-seeking behaviors (self-care)
- Impaired gas exchange
- Ineffective breathing pattern

- Ineffective therapeutic regimen management
- Risk for injury

Individualize related factors based on patient's condition or needs.

STEP	RATIONALE

PLANNING

1 Expected outcomes following completion of procedure:
   • Patient describes techniques for use of MDI.
   • Patient correctly self-administers metered dose.
   • Patient's breathing pattern improves, and airways become less restricted.
   • Patient's gas exchange is adequate.

   Ensures compliance with therapeutic regimen.
   Demonstrates learning.
   Demonstrates proper administration and therapeutic effect of medication.
   Demonstrates proper administration and therapeutic effect of medication.

2 Prepare medication for instillation. Check label on inhaler against MAR three times (see Skill 21-1).

   Adequate preparation saves nursing time. Ensures patient receives correct medication.

3 Identify patient using two identifiers and comparing these identifiers with the information on patient's identification bracelet. Ask patient to state name.

   Ensures correct patient receives medication. You need to use at least two patient identifiers (neither can be the patient's room number) whenever administering medications (TJC, 2007).

4 Explain procedure to patient. Be specific if patient wishes to self-administer drug. Explain where and how to set up in the home.

   Makes patient a participant in care and minimizes anxiety.

5 Provide adequate time for teaching session.

   Prevents interruptions. Instruction should occur when patient is receptive.

IMPLEMENTATION

1 Perform hand hygiene, and arrange equipment needed.

   Reduces transfer of microorganisms and saves time.

2 Allow patient opportunity to manipulate inhaler, canister, and spacer device. Explain and demonstrate how canister fits into inhaler.

   Patient must be familiar with how to use equipment.

Critical Decision Point *If the patient is using an MDI that is new or has not been used for several days (with or without a spacer), push a "test spray" into the air before administering the dose (Burkhart and others, 2005).*

3 Explain what metered dose is, and warn patient about overuse of inhaler, including drug side effects.

   Patient must not use inhaler excessively because of risk for serious side effects and/or tolerance developing to medications. When drug is given in recommended doses, side effects are uncommon.

4 Explain steps for administering inhaled dose of medication (demonstrate steps when possible):

   Use of simple, step-by-step explanations allows patient to ask questions at any point during procedure.

   a Remove mouthpiece cover from inhaler after MDI canister is inserted into the holder.

   b Shake inhaler well for 2 to 5 seconds (five or six shakes).

   Ensures mixing of medication in canister.

   c Hold inhaler in dominant hand.

   d Instruct patient to position inhaler in one of two ways:

   (1) Place mouthpiece in mouth with opening toward back of throat, closing lips tightly around it (see illustration).

   (2) Position the mouthpiece 2 to 4 cm (1 to 2 inches) in front of widely opened mouth (see illustration), with opening of inhaler toward back of throat. Lips should not touch the inhaler.

   Directs aerosol spray toward airway. Positioning the mouthpiece 2 to 4 cm from the mouth is the best way to deliver the medication without a spacer.

   e Have patient take a deep breath and exhale completely.

   Prepares patient's airway to receive the medication.

   f With inhaler properly positioned, have patient hold inhaler with thumb at the mouthpiece and the index finger and middle finger at the top. This is a three-point or bilateral hand position.

   Proper hand position ensures proper activation of MDI (Lilley and others, 2007).

   g Instruct patient to tilt head back slightly, inhale slowly and deeply through mouth for 3 to 5 seconds, and depress medication canister fully.

   Medication is distributed to airways during inhalation. Inhalation through mouth rather than nose draws medication more effectively into airways.

   h Have patient hold breath for approximately 10 seconds.

   Allows tiny drops of aerosol spray to reach deeper branches of airways (Burkhart and others, 2005).

STEP	RATIONALE

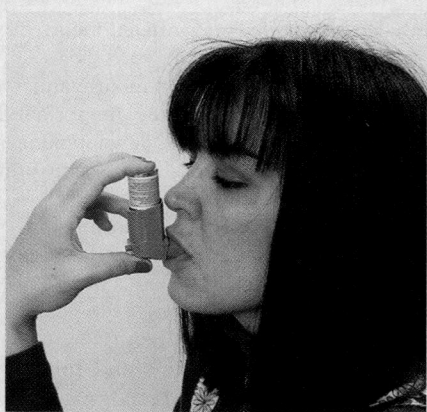

STEP 4d(1)   The patient opens lips and places inhaler mouthpiece in mouth with opening toward back of throat.

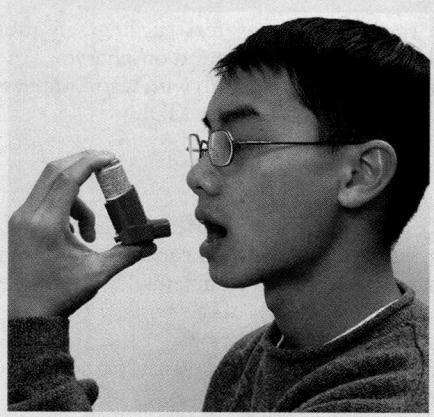

STEP 4d(2)   The patient positions the inhaler mouthpiece 2 to 4 cm (1 to 2 inches) from the widely open mouth. This is considered the best way to deliver the medication without a spacer.

i Remove the MDI from the mouth before exhaling, then exhale slowly through nose or pursed lips.

Keeps small airways open during exhalation.

5 Explain steps to administer inhaled dose of medication using a spacer device (demonstrate when possible):

a Remove mouthpiece cover from MDI and mouthpiece of spacer device.

Inhaler fits into end of spacer device.

b Shake inhaler well for 2 to 5 seconds (five or six shakes).

Ensures mixing of medication in canister.

c Insert MDI into end of spacer device.

A spacer device traps medication released from MDI; patient then inhales the drug from the device. These devices improve delivery of correct dose of inhaled medication (Capriotti, 2005).

d Place spacer device mouthpiece in mouth and close lips. Do not insert beyond raised lip on mouthpiece. Avoid covering small exhalation slots with the lips.

Medication should not escape through mouth.

e Breathe normally through spacer device mouthpiece (see illustration).

Allows patient to relax before delivering medication.

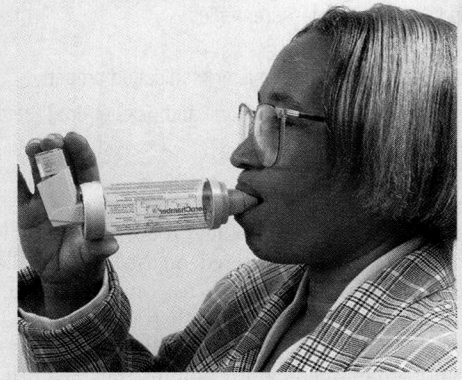

STEP 5e   Using a spacer device with an MDI.

f Depress medication canister, spraying one puff into spacer device.

The spacer device contains the fine spray and allows patient to inhale more medication.

g Breathe in slowly and fully (for 5 seconds).

Ensures particles of medication are distributed to deeper airways.

h Hold full breath for 10 seconds.

Ensures full drug distribution.

6 Instruct patient to wait 20 to 30 seconds between inhalations (if it is the same medication), or 2 to 5 minutes between inhalations if the medications are different.

Drugs must be inhaled sequentially. If bronchodilators are administered with inhaled steroids, the bronchodilators should be given first in order to dilate the airway passages for the second medication (Lilley and others, 2007).

7 Instruct patient against repeating inhalations before next scheduled dose (see Box 21-4).

Drugs are prescribed at intervals during day to provide constant drug levels and minimize side effects. Beta-adrenergic MDIs are used either on an "as needed" basis or regularly every 4 to 6 hours.

STEP	RATIONALE
8 Explain that patient may feel gagging sensation in throat caused by droplets of medication on pharynx or tongue.	Results when inhalant is sprayed and inhaled incorrectly.
9 Instruct patient to rinse mouth with warm water, then spit the water out after each use of the MDI.	Inhaled bronchodilators may cause dry mouth and taste alterations. Inhaled corticosteroids may alter the normal flora of the oral mucous membrane and cause the development of oral candidiasis. Rinsing the mouth after MDI use can prevent these problems (Lilley and others, 2007).
10 For daily cleaning, instruct patient to remove the medication canister, rinse the inhaler and cap with warm running water, and ensure the inhaler is completely dry before reuse. Do not get the valve mechanism of the canister wet.	Removes residual medication. Reduces transmission of microorganisms. Water may damage the valve mechanism of the canister (Rubin and Durotye, 2004).
11 Ask if patient has any questions.	Clarifies misconceptions or misunderstanding.
12 Perform hand hygiene, and assist patient to comfortable position.	Reduces the spread of microorganisms and promotes patient comfort.

EVALUATION

1 Have patient explain and demonstrate steps in use of inhaler.	Return demonstration provides feedback for measuring patient's learning.
2 Ask patient to explain drug schedule.	Improves likelihood of compliance with therapy.
3 Ask patient to describe side effects of medication and criteria for calling physician.	Allows patient to recognize signs of overuse and need to seek medical support when drugs are ineffective.
4 After medication administration, assess patient's respirations and breath sounds, and assess peak flow measures if ordered.	Determines status of breathing pattern and adequacy of ventilation/gas exchange.

Unexpected Outcomes
Related Interventions

Unexpected Outcomes	Related Interventions
1 Patient's respirations are rapid and shallow; breath sounds indicate wheezing.	• Reassess type of medication and/or delivery method. • Notify prescriber.
2 Patient experiences paroxysms of coughing. Aerosolized particles can irritate posterior pharynx.	• Reassess type of medication and/or delivery method. • Notify prescriber.
3 Patient needs a bronchodilator more than every 4 hours.	• Indicates respiratory problems. • Reassessment of type of medication and delivery methods needed. • Notify prescriber.
4 Patient experiences cardiac dysrhythmias (light-headedness, syncope), especially if receiving beta-adrenergics.	• Withhold all further doses of medication. Assess vital signs. • Notify prescriber for reassessment of type of medication and delivery method.
5 Patient is not able to self-administer medication properly.	• Explore alternative delivery routes or devices.
6 Patient is unable to explain technique and risks of drug therapy.	• Further teaching is necessary. • Include family members or caregivers when possible.

Recording and Reporting

- Record drug administered, dosage, route, and actual time and date each drug was administered on MAR immediately after administration. Record patient's response to the medication, including pulse, respirations, breath sounds assessed, and any adverse effects. Follow institution's policy for initials and signature. Do not chart medication administration until *after* it is given to patient.
- Document what skills you taught and patient's ability to perform them.
- Report adverse effects/patient response and/or withheld drugs to nurse in charge or physician. Depending on medication, immediate prescriber notification may be required.

Teaching Considerations

- Allow for supervised practice of the procedures. Patients may have difficulty with timing inspiration with medication dispersal without proper instruction (Lewis and others, 2007).

- Teach patient to keep track of the number of inhalations in the MDI (Box 21-5).
- Do not try to teach patient how to use an inhaler during an episode of shortness of breath. Patient's attention span will be very poor.
- Ensure that patient knows the proper sequence and spacing of medications if two different types of inhalers (i.e., bronchodilator and inhaled corticosteroid) are due to be given at the same time (Lilley and others, 2007).
- Teach patients to use small handheld peak flow meters to monitor response to therapy when inhalers are prescribed (Pruitt, 2005).
- Teach patient to rinse his or her mouth with water after the use of inhalers (Lilley and others, 2007).
- Teach patient how to clean the inhaler mouthpiece daily.

Pediatric Considerations

- Because of difficulty coordinating inhaler activation and inhalation, the use of a spacer device is recommended for young children (Burkhart and others, 2005).

- Bronchodilators are used often in children, but use with extreme caution and monitor for adverse effects such as tremors, restlessness, dizziness, gastrointestinal upset, and tachycardia (Lilley and others, 2007).
- Educate child and parent about the need to use inhaler during school hours. Help family find resources within the school or day care facility. Keep in mind that many school systems do not permit self-administration of MDIs. Follow the school's policy regarding having the MDI available for use during school hours. A physician's order may be necessary.

Gerontological Considerations
- Some older adult patients are unable to depress medication canister because of weakened grasp or are unable to coordinate actuation of the canister with inhalation. The use of a spacer device is necessary.

Home Care Considerations
- Remind patients to carry prescribed inhalers to use as immediate treatment in case of an acute asthma attack.

BOX 21-5 | Counting Doses in a Metered-Dose Inhaler

Most metered-dose inhalers (MDIs) currently do not have automatic dose counters. Patients need to keep careful track of the number of inhalations used in their MDIs. Failure to do so may result in patients using an empty inhaler during an acute exacerbation of a respiratory problem. To track doses:
- Note first day of use on a calendar.
- Note number of inhalations in the canister. Example: 200 inhalations per MDI.

- Note number of inhalations used per day. Example: 2 inhalations a day, 3 times a day, equals 6 inhalations per day.
- Divide the total number of inhalations in the canister by the number of inhalations needed per day to determine the number of days the inhaler should last. Example: 200 inhalations divided by 6 inhalations per day equals approximately 33 days of 3-times-a-day dosing.
- Mark on a calendar the date the inhaler will be empty, and obtain a refill of the inhaler a few days before this target date.

Data from Rubin DK, Durotoye L: How do patients determine that their metered dose inhaler is empty? *Chest* 126(4):1134, 2005; Capriotti T: Changes in inhaler devices for asthma and COPD, *Medsurg Nurs* 14(3):185, 2005.

PROCEDURAL GUIDELINE 21-1   Using Dry Powder Inhaled Medications

 Advanced / Nonparenteral Medication Administration / Using a Dry Powder Inhaler

Delegation Considerations
The skill of administering DPI medications cannot be delegated to NAP. The nurse directs the NAP about:
- Potential side effects of medications and to report their occurrence.
- Reporting paroxysmal coughing, audible wheezing, and patient's report of breathlessness or difficulty breathing.

Equipment
- ❑ Dry powder inhaler (see Fig. 21-1, C)
- ❑ Stethoscope
- ❑ Washbasin or sink with warm water
- ❑ Medication administration record (MAR)
- ❑ Facial tissues (*optional*)

Procedural Steps
1 Check accuracy and completeness of MAR with prescriber's written medication order. Check patient's name, drug name, drug concentration, route of administration, number of inhalations, and time for administration.
2 Assess respiratory pattern, and auscultate breath sounds.
3 Assess patient's readiness to learn: Patient asks questions about medication, disease, or complications; requests education in use of DPI; is mentally alert; participates in own care.
4 Assess patient's ability to learn: patient should not be fatigued, in pain, or in respiratory distress; assess level of understanding of technical vocabulary terms.
5 Assess patient's knowledge and understanding of disease and purpose and action of prescribed medications.
6 Determine patient's ability to hold, manipulate, and activate the dry powder inhaler.
7 If previously instructed in self-administration of inhaled medicine, assess patient's technique in using a DPI.

8 Prepare medication for instillation, check label on inhaler against MAR three times.
9 Identify patient using two identifiers and compare these identifiers with the information on patient's identification bracelet.
10 If the DPI has an external counter, note the number indicated.
11 Prepare DPI for administration. Some DPIs require loading with the medication before administration. Some DPIs simply require a rotation of a lever to load the medication. Some require insertion of a capsule; some require insertion of a disk into the inhaler device. Follow manufacturer's specific instructions.

Critical Decision Point   *DPIs do not contain propellant. The patient's inhaled breath pulls the drug into the airway. DPIs may differ as to how fast the patient should inhale the medication; consult manufacturer's specific instructions. In addition, do not shake DPI because powdered medication may spill out of the device.*

12 Have patient place lips over the mouthpiece of the DPI and inhale quickly and deeply. Remove inhaler from mouth as soon as inhalation is complete, but before exhalation. Instruct patient that he or she may not taste the powdered medication.
13 Have patient hold breath for 10 seconds, or as long as possible, then exhale. Do not exhale into the DPI.
14 After using the DPI, have patient rinse mouth with warm water, then spit out water, to reduce throat irritation and prevent oral candidiasis.
15 Return DPI to closed position, or remove loaded capsule or disk, if necessary.
16 If an external counter is present, note the number, which should be one less than the number in Step 10.
17 Assess for therapeutic effects of the medication.

SKILL 21-8 Administering Nebulized Medications

Nebulization is a process of adding medications or moisture to inspired air by mixing particles of various sizes with air. Adding moisture to the respiratory system through nebulization improves clearance of pulmonary secretions. Medications such as bronchodilators, mucolytics, and corticosteroids are often administered by nebulization.

Small-volume nebulizers provide medications in an aerosolized form that can be inhaled by a patient into the tracheobronchial tree and possibly into the bloodstream through the alveoli. As a result, systemic effects from the medications may occur.

Patients who receive drugs by inhalation frequently suffer from chronic lung disease. Drugs administered by inhalation provide control of airway hyperactivity or constriction. Because patients depend on these medications for disease control, they must learn how the drugs work and how to administer them safely.

Delegation Considerations

In many facilities, a respiratory therapist performs the skill of administering medications by nebulizer. The nurse must be aware of the type of and actions of the inhaled medication the patient is receiving.

The skill of administering medications by nebulizer cannot be delegated to NAP. The nurse directs the NAP about:
- Potential side effects of medications and to report their occurrence.
- Reporting paroxysmal coughing, ineffective breathing patterns, and other respiratory difficulties.

Equipment
- ☐ Medication ordered and diluent (if needed)
- ☐ Nebulizer bottle and tubing assembly
- ☐ Small-volume nebulizer machine (often called handheld nebulizer or simply "nebulizer")
- ☐ Pulse oximeter
- ☐ Stethoscope
- ☐ Medication administration record (MAR)

STEP	RATIONALE
ASSESSMENT	
1 Check accuracy and completion of MAR with prescriber's written medication order. Check patient's name, drug name, dosage, type and amount of diluent (if unit dose is not available), and frequency of administration.	Ensures correct drug and dosage.
2 Assess patient's medical history, history of allergies, medication and diet history.	These factors influence how certain drugs act. Information also reflects patient's need for medications.
3 Assess patient's ability to assemble, hold, and manipulate the nebulizer equipment.	Any impairment of grasp or presence of hand tremors interferes with patient's ability to use the equipment.

Critical Decision Point *Unit-dose medications do not require dilution; however, a diluent may be used along with a unit-dose medication if a different percentage of drug is desired.*

4 Assess pulse, respirations, breath sounds, pulse oximetry, and peak flow measurement (if ordered) before beginning treatment.	Establishes a baseline for comparison during and after treatment.

NURSING DIAGNOSES

- Activity intolerance
- Anxiety
- Deficient knowledge regarding use of nebulizers
- Health-seeking behaviors (self-care)
- Impaired gas exchange
- Ineffective breathing pattern
- Ineffective therapeutic regimen management
- Risk for injury

Individualize related factors based on patient's condition or needs.

PLANNING

1 Expected outcomes following completion of procedure:	
• Patient's breathing patterns are effective.	Demonstrates proper administration and therapeutic effect of medication.
• Patient's gas exchange is adequate.	Demonstrates proper administration and therapeutic effect of medication.
• Patient describes techniques for use of a nebulizer.	Increases likelihood of compliance with therapeutic regimen.
• Patient correctly self-administers medication using a nebulizer.	Demonstrates learning.
2 Prepare medication for instillation. Check label on medication against MAR three times (see Skill 21-2).	Ensures patient receives correct medication.

STEP	RATIONALE
3 Identify patient using two identifiers and comparing these identifiers with the information on patient's identification bracelet. Ask patient to state name.	Ensures correct patient receives medication. You need to use at least two patient identifiers (neither can be the patient's room number) whenever administering medications (TJC, 2007).
4 Explain procedure to patient. Be specific if patient wishes to self-administer drug.	Makes patient a participant in care and minimizes anxiety. Begins patient teaching regarding medications. Enables patient to self-administer drug if physically able and motivated.

IMPLEMENTATION

1 Perform hand hygiene, and arrange equipment needed.	Reduces transfer of microorganisms and saves time.
2 Explain the use of the nebulizer, and warn patient of possible drug side effects.	Helps to make patient more knowledgeable about treatment and medication.
3 Assemble nebulizer equipment per manufacturer's directions.	Assembly may vary slightly with different manufacturers. Proper assembly ensures safe delivery of medication.
4 Add prescribed medication and diluent (if needed) to nebulizer cup (see illustration).	Ensures proper dose and delivery of ordered medication.
5 Have patient hold mouthpiece between lips with gentle pressure (see illustration).	
a If patient is an infant, child, or fatigued adult or unable to follow instructions, use a face mask.	Use of a face mask does not require patient to remember to hold mouthpiece correctly. Correct delivery ensures sufficient deposition of medication.
b Use special adapters for patients with a tracheostomy.	Promotes greater deposition of medication in the airways.
6 Turn on the small-volume nebulizer machine, and ensure that a sufficient mist is formed.	Verifies that the equipment is working properly during delivery of medication.
7 Have patient take a deep breath, slowly, to a volume slightly greater than normal. Encourage a brief, end-inspiratory pause. Then have patient exhale passively.	Improves effectiveness of medication.
a If patient is dyspneic, encourage patient to hold every fourth or fifth breath for 5 to 10 seconds.	Maximizes effectiveness of medication.
b Remind patient to repeat the breathing pattern described in Step 7 until the drug is completely nebulized.	Maximizes effectiveness of medication.
(1) Some practitioners set a timed limit as the length of the treatment rather than waiting for the medication to completely nebulize.	
c Tap the nebulizer cup occasionally during treatment and toward the end of the treatment.	Releases droplets that are clinging to the side of the cup, thus allowing for renebulization of the solution.
d Monitor patient's pulse during procedure, especially if beta-adrenergic bronchodilators are used.	Enables nurse to observe for potential side effects of medications.
8 When medication is completely nebulized, turn off machine, and store tubing assembly per agency policy.	Proper storage reduces transfer of microorganisms.
9 Shake the nebulizer bottle, attempting to remove all remaining solution. NEVER rinse with tap water. Allow to air dry.	Tap water may contain microorganisms.

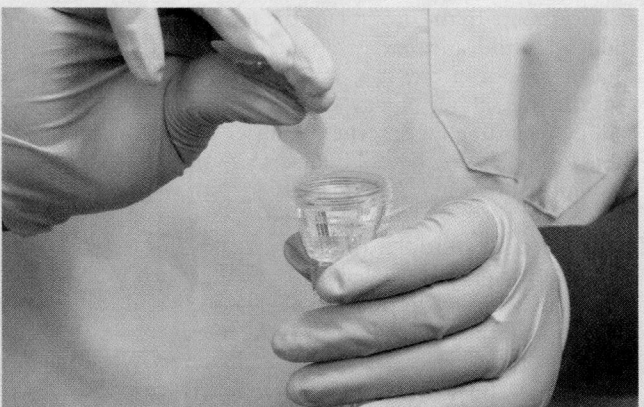

STEP 4 Add prescribed medication (and diluent, if needed) to nebulizer cup.

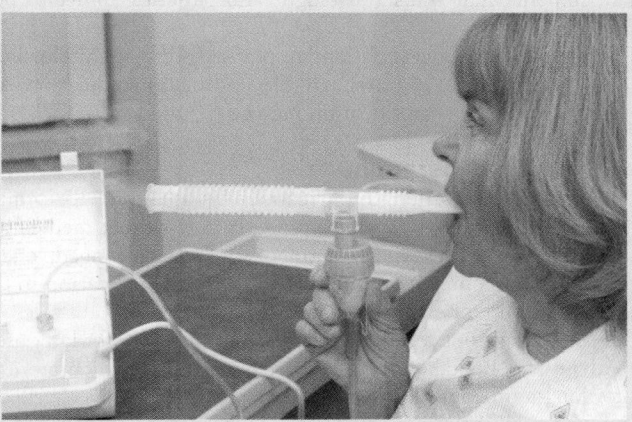

STEP 5 Nebulizer mouthpiece placed between patient's lips.

STEP	RATIONALE
10 If steroids are nebulized, instruct patient to rinse mouth and gargle with warm water after nebulizer treatment.	Removes medication residue from oral cavity and helps to prevent oral candidiasis, a possible adverse effect of inhaled steroid therapy.
11 Perform hand hygiene, and assist patient to comfortable position.	Reduces the spread of microorganisms and promotes patient comfort.

Critical Decision Point *Some respiratory medications can cause systemic effects such as restlessness, nervousness, and palpitations. Administer these medications with caution to patients with cardiac disease because of the possibility of hypertension, dysrhythmias, or coronary insufficiency. If severe bronchospasm occurs during treatment, discontinue drug immediately and notify physician.*

EVALUATION

1 Assess patient's respirations, breath sounds, cough effort, sputum production, and pulse oximetry, and assess peak flow measures if ordered.	Determines status of breathing pattern and adequacy of ventilation/gas exchange. Allows comparison with baseline data and evaluation of effectiveness of procedure.
2 Have patient explain and demonstrate steps in use of nebulizer.	Return demonstration provides feedback for measuring patient's learning.
3 Ask patient to explain drug schedule.	Improves likelihood of compliance with therapy.
4 Ask patient to describe side effects of medication and criteria for calling physician.	Allows patient to recognize signs of overuse and need to seek medical support when drugs are ineffective.

Unexpected Outcomes

Related Interventions

1 Patient's breathing pattern is ineffective; respirations are rapid and shallow; breath sounds indicate wheezing.
- Reassess type of medication and/or delivery method.
- Notify prescriber.

2 Patient experiences paroxysms of coughing. Aerosolized particles can irritate posterior pharynx.
- Reassess type of medication and/or delivery method.
- Notify prescriber.

3 Patient experiences cardiac dysrhythmias (light-headedness, syncope), especially if receiving beta-adrenergics.
- Withhold all further doses of medication. Assess vital signs.
- Notify prescriber for reassessment of type of medication and delivery method.

4 Patient may not be able to self-administer medication properly.
- Explore alternative delivery routes or devices.

5 Patient is unable to explain technique and risks of drug therapy.
- Further teaching may be required.
- Include family members or caregivers when possible.

Recording and Reporting

- Record drug administered, dosage and concentration, route, and time and date of administration on MAR immediately after administration. Record patient's response to the medication, including pulse, respirations, breath sounds, and pulse oximetry assessed. Do not chart medication administration until *after* it is given to patient. If you withhold a drug, record reason in nurses' notes and follow agency's policy for noting withheld doses.
- Document what skills you taught and patient's ability to perform them.
- Report adverse effects/patient response and/or withheld drugs to nurse in charge or physician. Depending on medication, immediate prescriber notification may be required.

Teaching Considerations

- Teach patient that length of treatment is usually 10 to 15 minutes, if equipment is working properly and correct medication and diluent are used. If treatment time is prolonged, check nebulizer or compressor function. Use all the medication in the nebulizer cup for each treatment.
- Teach patient not to store medication in nebulizer for later use.
- Advise patients taking long-acting beta-agonists, which are used for long-term control of symptoms, about possible adverse effects: nervousness, restlessness, tremor, headache, nausea, rapid or pounding heart, and dizziness. Emphasize that the drug should only be taken as ordered so that a tolerance to the drug is not developed.

- Teach patients to use small handheld peak flow meters to monitor response to therapy when inhaled drugs are prescribed (Pruitt, 2005).

Pediatric Considerations

- Use a mask for the nebulizer treatment if child is too young to hold mouthpiece correctly for the duration of the treatment (Hockenberry and Wilson, 2007).
- Instruct child to breathe normally with mouth open to provide a direct route to the airways for the medication.
- Educate child and parent about the need to use nebulizer during school or day care hours. Help family find resources within the school or day care facility. Follow the school's policy regarding having the nebulizer and medication available for use during school hours. A physician's or health care provider's order may be necessary.

Home Care Considerations

- When at home, rinse nebulizer parts after each use with clear water and air dry. In addition, clean parts daily with warm, soapy water, rinse, and allow them to dry.
- Never store nebulizer parts until totally dried. Wet equipment encourages growth of bacteria and mold. Twice weekly, patient should wash the L-shaped mouthpiece with mild dishwashing soap and warm water, rinse, and dry it well (McKenry and others, 2006) (see manufacturer's instructions).

SKILL 21-9 Administering Vaginal Instillations

NSO *Nonparenteral Medication Administration Module / Lesson 6*

Female patients can develop vaginal infections that require topical application of antiinfective agents. Vaginal medications are available in foam, jelly, cream, or suppository form. Medicated irrigations or douches can also be given. However, their excessive use can lead to vaginal irritation (Iannacchione, 2004).

Vaginal suppositories are oval shaped and come individually packaged in foil wrappers. They are larger and more oval than rectal suppositories. (Fig. 21-2 provides a comparison with rectal suppositories.) Storage in a refrigerator prevents the solid suppositories from melting. A suppository is inserted into the vagina with an applicator or a gloved hand. After insertion, body temperature causes the suppository to melt, and the medication is distributed. Foam, jellies, and creams are administered with an inserter or applicator. Patients often prefer administering their own vaginal medications, and you should give them privacy to do so. After instillation of the drug, a patient may wish to wear a perineal pad to collect excess drainage. Because vaginal medications are frequently given to treat infection, any discharge is often foul smelling. Follow good aseptic technique, and offer the patient frequent opportunities for perineal hygiene (see Skill 17-1).

Delegation Considerations

The skill of administering vaginal instillations cannot be delegated to NAP. The nurse directs the NAP about:

- Potential side effects of medications and to report their occurrence.
- Reporting any change in comfort level or new or increased vaginal discharge or bleeding to the nurse for further assessment.

Equipment

- ❑ Vaginal cream, foam, jelly, tablet, suppository, or irrigating solution
- ❑ Applicators (if needed)
- ❑ Clean gloves
- ❑ Tissues
- ❑ Towels and/or washcloths
- ❑ Perineal pad
- ❑ Drape or sheet
- ❑ Water-soluble lubricants
- ❑ Bedpan
- ❑ Irrigation or douche container (if needed)
- ❑ Medication administration record (MAR)

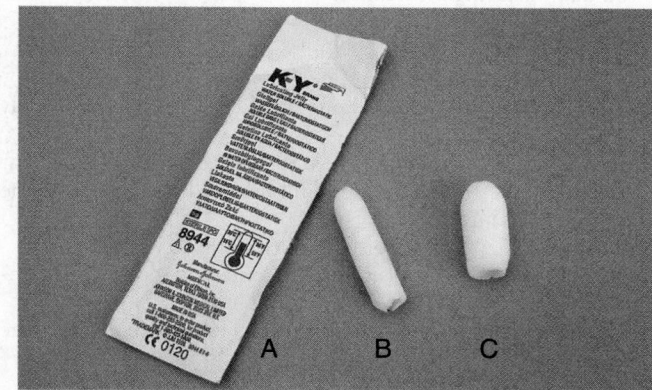

FIG 21-2 A, K-Y lubricating jelly. **B,** Rectal suppository. **C,** Vaginal suppository. Note that vaginal suppositories are larger and more oval than rectal suppositories.

STEP	RATIONALE

ASSESSMENT

1 Check accuracy and completeness of MAR with prescriber's written medication order, including patient's name, drug name, form (foam, jelly, cream, tablet, suppository, or irrigating solution), route, dosage, and time of administration.

The order sheet is the most reliable source and only legal record of drugs patient is to receive. Ensures safe and correct administration of medication.

2 Review pertinent information related to medication, including action, purpose, side effects, and nursing implications.

Allows nurse to administer drug properly and to monitor patient's response.

3 Ask if patient is experiencing any symptoms of pruritus, burning, or discomfort.

Identifies symptoms of vaginal irritation.

4 Have patient void.

Empties bladder and promotes comfort during medication insertion.

5 Assess patient's ability to manipulate applicator, suppository, or irrigation equipment and to properly position self to insert medication (may be done just before insertion).

Presence of mobility restrictions indicates need for assistance from nurse.

6 Review patient's knowledge of purpose of drug therapy and interest in self-administering medication.

Indicates need for health teaching. Understanding influences compliance with therapy.

NURSING DIAGNOSES

- Deficient knowledge regarding vaginal medication administration
- Health-seeking behaviors (self-care)
- Impaired physical mobility
- Noncompliance with drug therapy
- Pain (acute or chronic)
- Sexual dysfunction

Individualize related factors based on patient's condition or needs.

STEP	RATIONALE

PLANNING

1 Expected outcomes following completion of procedure:

- Vaginal tissues are pink and smooth. Genitalia are clear and without discharge.

- Patient denies symptoms of discomfort and expresses relief from symptoms of infection/inflammation. A small amount of discharge that is the color of medication is present.

- Patient is able to discuss information about prescribed drug.
- Patient self-administers suppository, medication, or irrigation.

2 Prepare medication for instillation. Check label on medication against MAR three times (see Skill 21-1).

3 Identify patient using two identifiers and comparing these identifiers with the information on patient's identification bracelet. Ask patient to state name.

4 Explain procedure to patient. Be specific if patient plans on self-administering medication.

Tissues take on normal characteristics.

Inflammation or infection has resolved. When suppository or cream becomes distributed, small amount may escape from the vaginal orifice.

Feedback reflects patient's learning.
Demonstrates learning.
Ensures right medication is administered.

Ensures correct patient receives medication. You need to use at least two patient identifiers (neither can be the patient's room number) whenever administering medications (TJC, 2007).

Promotes patient's understanding. Enables patient to self-administer drug if physically able.

IMPLEMENTATION

1 Close room curtain or door.

2 Perform hand hygiene, arrange supplies at bedside, and apply clean gloves.

3 Assist patient with lying in dorsal recumbent position. Patients with restricted mobility in knees or hips may lie supine with legs abducted.

4 Keep abdomen and lower extremities draped.

5 Be sure vaginal orifice is well illuminated by room light. Otherwise, position portable gooseneck lamp.

6 Inspect condition of external genitalia and vaginal canal (see Chapter 6).

7 Insert vaginal suppository:

  a Remove suppository from wrapper, and apply liberal amount of water-soluble lubricant to smooth or rounded end (see illustration). Be sure that suppository is at room temperature. Lubricate gloved index finger of dominant hand.

  b With nondominant gloved hand, gently separate labial folds in the front-to-back direction.

  c With dominant gloved hand, insert rounded end of suppository along posterior wall of vaginal canal entire length of finger (7.5 to 10 cm [3 to 4 inches]) (see illustration).

Provides privacy.
Reduces transfer of microorganisms; helps nurse perform procedure smoothly.

Position provides easy access to and good exposure of vaginal canal. Dependent position also allows suppository to completely dissolve in the vagina.

Minimizes patient's embarrassment by limiting exposure.

Proper insertion requires visualization of external genitalia if not self-administered.

Provides baseline to monitor effect of medication.

Lubrication reduces friction against mucosal surfaces during insertion. Use of petroleum jelly may leave a residue that harbors bacteria and yeast fungi.

Exposes vaginal orifice.

Proper placement of suppository ensures equal distribution of medication along walls of vaginal cavity.

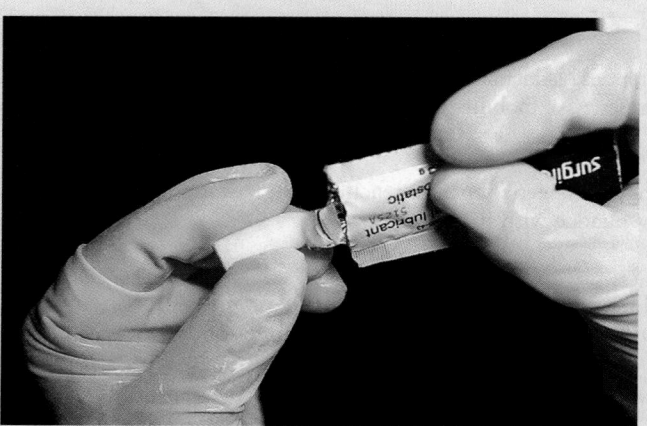

STEP 7a   Lubricate tip of suppository.

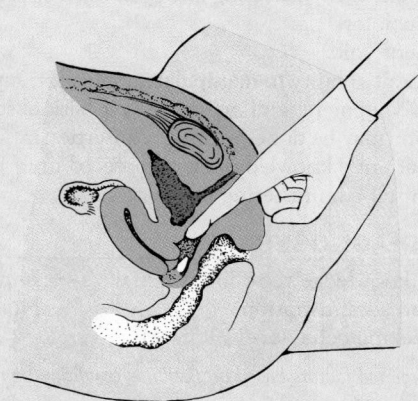

STEP 7c   Angle of vaginal suppository insertion.

STEP	RATIONALE

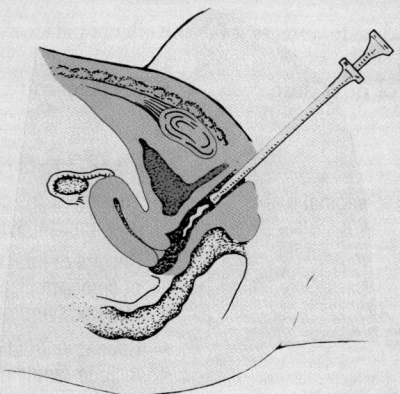

STEP 8c   Applicator inserted into vaginal canal. Plunger pushed to instill medication.

d Withdraw finger, and wipe away remaining lubricant from around orifice and labia with a tissue or cloth.	Maintains comfort.
8 Apply cream or foam:	
a Fill cream or foam applicator following package directions.	Dose is based on volume in applicator.
b With nondominant gloved hand, gently separate labial folds.	Exposes vaginal orifice.
c With dominant gloved hand, insert applicator approximately 5 to 7.5 cm (2 to 3 inches). Push applicator plunger to deposit medication into vagina (see illustration).	Allows equal distribution of medication along vaginal walls.
d Withdraw applicator, and place on paper towel. Wipe off residual cream from labia or vaginal orifice with a tissue or cloth.	Maintains patient comfort. Residual cream on applicator may contain microorganisms.
9 Administer irrigation and douche:	
a Place patient on bedpan with absorbent pad underneath.	Allows hips to be higher than shoulders and solution reaches posterior wall of vagina. Bedpan collects solution.
b Be sure fluid is at body temperature. Run fluid through container nozzle (priming the tubing).	Body temperature promotes patient comfort. Priming tubing removes air and moistens the nozzle tip.
c Gently separate labial folds, and direct nozzle toward sacrum, following the floor of the vagina.	Correct angle allows nozzle access into the vagina.
d Raise container approximately 30 to 50 cm (12 to 20 inches) above level of vagina. Insert nozzle 7 to 10 cm (3 to 4 inches). Allow solution to flow while rotating nozzle. Administer all the irrigating solution.	Rotating nozzle allows irrigation of all areas in vagina.
e Withdraw nozzle, and assist patient to a comfortable sitting position.	Remaining solution drains by gravity.
f Allow patient to remain on bedpan for a few minutes. Cleanse perineum with soap and water.	Ensures all solution drains from vagina. Provides comfort for the patient.
g Assist patient off bedpan. Dry perineal area.	
10 Instruct patient who received suppository, cream, or tablet to remain on her back for at least 10 minutes.	Allows melting and spreading of the medication throughout vaginal cavity and prevents loss through the vaginal orifice.
11 If using an applicator, wash with soap and warm water, rinse, and store for future use.	Vaginal cavity is not sterile. Soap and water assist in removal of bacteria and residual cream from applicator.
12 Offer perineal pad when patient resumes ambulation.	Provides patient comfort.
13 Discard gloves by turning them inside out, and dispose of gloves and other soiled equipment in appropriate receptacle. Perform hand hygiene.	Reduces transmission of microorganisms.

EVALUATION

1 Don clean gloves. Inspect condition of vaginal canal and external genitalia between applications. Assess vaginal discharge, if present.	Determines whether vaginal medication effectively reduced irritation or inflammation of tissues.
2 Question patient regarding continued pruritus, burning, discomfort, or discharge.	Determines whether symptoms are relieved.

STEP	RATIONALE
3 Ask patient to discuss purpose, action, and side effects of medication.	Reflects patient's understanding of drug therapy.
4 Observe patient demonstrate administration of next dose.	Reflects learning of technique.

Unexpected Outcomes	Related Interventions
1 A thick, white, patchy, curdlike discharge is clinging to vaginal walls. Vaginal walls appear bright pink or inflamed.	• Possible signs of yeast infection. Continue medication administration, and report if symptoms continue or appear to get worse.
2 Patient reports localized pruritus and burning.	• Results of infection or inflammation, but may be a possible side effect of some medications (such as miconazole). • Monitor symptoms; report if they are worse.
3 Patient is unable to discuss drug therapy correctly.	• Repeat instructions, or assess if patient is able to learn. • Include family members or caregiver when appropriate.
4 Patient is unable to self-administer medications.	• Reinstruction is necessary.

Recording and Reporting

- Record actual time each drug (or solution if vaginal instillation) was administered on MAR immediately after administration. Record appearance of vaginal canal and genitalia in nurses' notes, and report any unusual findings.
- Report to prescriber if patient states that symptoms do not disappear or that symptoms get worse.
- Report adverse effects/patient response and/or withheld drugs to nurse in charge or physician.

Teaching Considerations

- Teach patient value of and technique for regular perineal hygiene.

- Encourage patient to take *all* of the medication as prescribed, for the prescribed amount of time, to ensure effectiveness of the treatment.
- Women taking antifungal medications for the treatment of vaginal infections should abstain from sexual intercourse until the treatment is completed and the infection is resolved. Women should be told to continue to take the medication even if actively menstruating. Patients should notify the physician if symptoms persist past the treatment time period (Lilley and others, 2007).
- Many women prefer to self-administer vaginal irrigations and medications. These procedures may be self-administered while patient is sitting on the toilet. Ensure that patient is able to perform the procedure correctly.

SKILL 21-10   Administering Rectal Suppositories

 Advanced / Nonparenteral Medication Administration / Inserting a Rectal Suppository

NSO *Nonparenteral Medication Administration Module / Lesson 6*

There are a variety of rectal medications. Drugs administered rectally exert either a local effect on gastrointestinal mucosa, such as promoting defecation, or exert systemic effects, such as relieving nausea or providing analgesia. The rectal route is not as reliable as oral or parenteral routes in terms of drug absorption and distribution. However, the medications are relatively safe, because they rarely cause local irritation or side effects. Rectal medications are contraindicated in patients with rectal surgery or active rectal bleeding (Lilley and others, 2007).

Rectal suppositories differ in shape from vaginal suppositories, being thinner and bullet shaped (see Fig. 21-2, p. 565) for comparison with vaginal suppositories.) The rounded end prevents anal trauma during insertion. When the nurse administers the suppository, placing it past the internal anal sphincter and against the rectal mucosa is important. Improper placement can result in expulsion of the suppository before the medication dissolves and is absorbed into the mucosa. If a patient prefers to self-administer a suppository, give specific instructions so that the medication is deposited correctly. Do not cut the suppository into sections to divide the dosage; the active

drug may not be distributed evenly within the suppository, and the result may be an inaccurate dose (Lilley and others, 2007).

Delegation Considerations

The skill of rectal medication administration cannot be delegated to NAP. The nurse directs the NAP about:

- Expected fecal discharge or bowel movement and to report occurrence to the nurse.
- Potential side effects of medications and to report their occurrence.
- Informing nurse of any rectal discharge, pain, or bleeding.

Equipment

- ❏ Rectal suppository
- ❏ Lubricating jelly (water soluble)
- ❏ Clean gloves
- ❏ Tissue
- ❏ Drape
- ❏ Medication administration record (MAR)

STEP	RATIONALE

ASSESSMENT

1   Check accuracy and completeness of MAR with prescriber's written medication order, including patient's name, drug name, dosage, form, route, and time of administration.

The order sheet is the most reliable source and only legal record of drugs patient is to receive. Ensures safe and correct administration of medication.

2   Review pertinent information related to medication, including action, purpose, side effects, and nursing implications.

Allows nurse to administer drug properly and to monitor patient's response.

3   Review medical record for history of rectal surgery or bleeding.

Conditions contraindicate use of suppository.

Critical Decision Point   *Do not palpate patient's rectum if patient has had rectal surgery. Generally a rectal suppository is contraindicated in the presence of active rectal bleeding or diarrhea (Lilley and others, 2007).*

4   Review any presenting signs and symptoms of gastrointestinal alterations (e.g., constipation or diarrhea).

Conditions indicate use of suppository.

5   Assess patient's ability to hold suppository and to position self to insert medication.

Mobility restriction indicates need for nurse to assist with drug administration.

6   Review patient's knowledge of purpose of drug therapy and interest in self-administering suppository.

Indicates need for health teaching. Level of motivation influences teaching approach.

NURSING DIAGNOSES

- Bowel incontinence
- Constipation
- Deficient knowledge regarding suppository administration
- Health-seeking behaviors (self-care)
- Impaired physical mobility
- Pain (acute or chronic)

Individualize related factors based on patient's condition or needs.

PLANNING

1   Expected outcomes following completion of the procedure:
- Patient reports relief or reduction in symptoms for which medication is prescribed.

Drug acts effectively.

- Patient describes purpose of medication.

Feedback reflects patient's learning.

- Patient self-administers suppository.

Demonstrates learning.

2   Prepare medication for administration. Check label on medication against MAR three times (see Skill 21-1).

Ensures right medication is administered.

3   Identify patient using two identifiers and comparing these identifiers with the information on patient's identification bracelet. Ask patient to state name.

Ensures correct patient receives medication. You need to use at least two patient identifiers (neither can be the patient's room number) whenever administering medications (TJC, 2007).

4   Explain procedure to patient. Be specific if patient wishes to self-administer drug.

Promotes patient's understanding and cooperation. Enables patient to self-administer drug safely if physically able and motivated.

IMPLEMENTATION

1   Close room curtain or door.

Maintains privacy and minimizes embarrassment.

2   Perform hand hygiene, arrange supplies at bedside, and apply clean gloves.

Reduces transfer of microorganisms, helps nurse perform procedure smoothly.

3   Assist patient in assuming a left side-lying Sims' position with upper leg flexed upward.

Position exposes anus and helps patient to relax external anal sphincter. Left side-lying Sims' position lessens the likelihood of the suppository or feces being expelled.

Critical Decision Point   *If patient has mobility impairment that prevents a left side-lying Sims' position, assist patient to a left lateral position. Obtain assistance from another health care provider to help patient turn, and use pillows under patient's upper arm and leg for support and comfort.*

4   Keep patient draped with only anal area exposed.

Maintains privacy and facilitates relaxation.

5   Examine condition of anus externally, and palpate rectal walls as needed (e.g., if impaction is suspected) (see Chapter 6). Dispose of gloves by turning them inside out and placing them in proper receptacle if they become soiled.

Determines presence of active rectal bleeding. Palpation determines whether rectum is filled with feces, which interferes with suppository placement. Reduces transmission of infection.

6   Apply new pair of clean gloves (if previous gloves were soiled and discarded).

Minimizes contact with fecal material to reduce transmission of infection.

STEP	RATIONALE
7 Remove suppository from foil wrapper, and lubricate rounded end with water-soluble lubricant. Lubricate gloved index finger of dominant hand. If patient has hemorrhoids, use a liberal amount of lubricant and handle area gently.	Lubrication reduces friction as suppository enters rectal canal.
8 Ask patient to take slow deep breaths through mouth and to relax anal sphincter.	Forcing suppository through constricted sphincter causes pain.
9 Retract patient's buttocks with nondominant hand. With gloved index finger of dominant hand, insert suppository gently through anus, past internal sphincter, and against rectal wall, 10 cm (4 inches) in adults (see illustration) or 5 cm (2 inches) in infants and children.	Suppository needs to be against rectal mucosa for eventual absorption and therapeutic action.

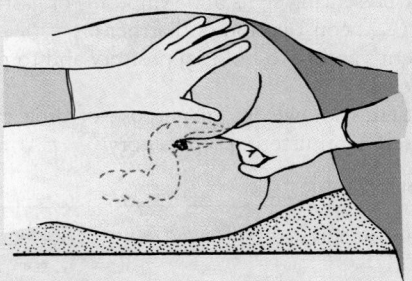

STEP 9   Insert rectal suppository past sphincter and against rectal wall.

Critical Decision Point   *Do not insert suppository into a mass of fecal material; this will reduce effectiveness of medication.*

STEP	RATIONALE
10 Withdraw finger, and wipe patient's anal area.	Provides comfort.
11 Discard soiled supplies and gloves by turning them inside out and dispose of them in appropriate receptacle. Perform hand hygiene.	Reduces transfer of microorganisms.
12 Ask patient to remain flat or on side for 5 minutes.	Prevents expulsion of suppository.
13 If suppository contains laxative or fecal softener, place call light within reach so patient can obtain assistance to reach bedpan or toilet.	Ability to call for assistance provides patient with sense of control over elimination.
14 If the suppository was given for constipation, remind patient *not* to flush the commode after the bowel movement.	Allows staff to evaluate results of the suppository.

Critical Decision Point   *Suppositories may be given through a colostomy (not ileostomy) if ordered. Use a small amount of water-soluble lubricant for insertion.*

EVALUATION

1 Return within 5 minutes to determine if suppository was expelled.	Determines if drug is properly distributed. Reinsertion may be necessary.
2 Ask if patient experienced localized anal or rectal discomfort during insertion.	Determines whether insertion of suppository was irritating.
3 Evaluate patient for relief of symptoms for which medication was prescribed (within time expected action of drug occurs).	Determines medication's effectiveness.
4 Ask patient to explain purpose of medication.	Reflects patient's understanding of drug therapy.
5 Have patient demonstrate administration of next dose of medication.	Demonstration measures learning.

Unexpected Outcomes	Related Interventions
1 Side effects of specific medication develop.	• Explore alternative therapy.
2 Symptoms previously reported are unrelieved.	• Explore alternative therapy.
3 Patient experiences decreased heart rate during rectal suppository insertion.	• Unintended vagal stimulation may occur, resulting in bradycardia in some patients. • Monitor heart rate of patient. Rectal route may not be suitable for certain cardiac conditions.
4 Patient reports rectal pain during insertion.	• Suppository may need more lubrication. • Rectal route may not be suitable; assess and notify prescriber.
5 Patient is unable to explain purpose of drug therapy.	• Reinstruction is necessary, or patient is unwilling or unable to learn.

Recording and Reporting

- Record drug administered, dosage, route, and actual time and date of administration on MAR immediately after administration. Record patient's response to medication, including any unusual reactions. Do not chart medication administration until *after* it is given to patient. If you withhold a drug, record reason in nurses' notes and follow institution's policy for noting withheld doses.
- Report adverse effects/patient response and/or withheld drugs to nurse in charge or physician. Depending on medication, immediate prescriber notification may be required.

Teaching Considerations

- Be certain that patient is aware that the foil wrapper must be removed before insertion and that the suppository is to be in-

serted rectally, not eaten (ISMP, 2006b). If patient chooses to self-administer suppositories, teach principles and techniques of infection control to prevent contact with and spread of fecal material.

Pediatric Considerations

- With children, it is often necessary to gently hold or tape the buttocks together for 5 to 10 minutes to relieve pressure on the anal sphincter until the urge to expel the suppository is gone (Hockenberry and Wilson, 2007).

Gerontological Considerations

- Older adult patients with loss of sphincter control may have difficulty with retaining suppository.

 CRITICAL THINKING EXERCISES

Mrs. Martin, a 75-year-old African-American homemaker, was in the hospital for 3 days with a diagnosis of dehydration. She has a history of hypertension, asthma, angina, and osteoarthritis in her hands. She also has an abscess on her right calf that was caused by a bug bite that became infected. One week after her discharge, the home care nurse visits Mrs. Martin to review her medications and to check her wound care. Mrs. Martin's medications include:

- Hydrochlorothiazide 25 mg every morning by mouth (PO) (diuretic)
- Diltiazem SR capsule, 60 mg twice a day PO (calcium channel blocker)
- Albuterol (Proventil) MDI 2 puffs 4 times a day (inhaled bronchodilator)
- Bacitracin topical ointment (500 units/g) applied topically to wound twice a day.
- Nitroglycerin transdermal patch (Nitro-Dur), 0.2 mg/hr, one each morning topically
- Nitrostat sublingual tablets, 400 mcg, as needed for chest pain

1. The nurse observes Mrs. Martin as she gives herself the inhaler. Mrs. Martin complains that she "just can't seem to breathe in at the same time as I press the inhaler." The nurse should take what action?
2. Mrs. Martin has a new refill of the albuterol. The canister label says that it contains 200 actuations ("puffs"). How many days will this canister of albuterol last for Mrs. Martin?
3. While inspecting Mrs. Martin's abscess, the nurse finds that there is a thick crust of old medication on the wound. Mrs. Martin explains, "I don't like to waste the medication that is already there, so I just put the new medicine on top of it all. I am sure that all that antibiotic there will help it to heal faster." How should the nurse intervene?
4. While listening to Mrs. Martin's breath sounds, the nurse notes that she has three nitroglycerin transdermal patches on her chest. What should the nurse do?
5. The nurse asks Mrs. Martin about taking the sublingual nitroglycerin tablets. Mrs. Martin explains, "Well, if I have chest pains, I sit down and chew one pill. If it doesn't work, I chew another one. Usually by the second one I am starting to feel better, but sometimes I have to chew a third pill." Explain the nurse's appropriate response.

☑ **REVIEW QUESTIONS**

1. An infant is to receive 4 mL of an antibiotic. What equipment would be most appropriate for preparation and administration?
   1. A teaspoon
   2. A plastic medication cup
   3. A syringe
   4. An oral-dosing syringe
2. A patient says he prefers to chew rather than swallow his pills. One of the medications is an extended-release tablet. Which of the following is an appropriate action in response to his request?
   1. Break the tablet into halves or quarters.
   2. Allow him to chew the tablet if he prefers.
   3. Explain why he should not chew the tablet.
   4. Use a mortar and pestle to crush the tablet.
3. A patient is to receive medications through a gastrostomy. Which nursing actions would be appropriate? Select all that apply.
   1. Verify tube placement after medications are given.
   2. Mix all crushed medications together, and give all at once.
   3. Flush tube with a minimal amount of water after giving medications.
   4. Flush tube with 30 to 60 mL of water after the last dose of medication.
   5. Check for gastric residual before giving the medications.
   6. Keep the head of the bed elevated after the medications are given.
4. An immunocompromised patient has a massive open wound that needs topical medication. Which nursing technique is most appropriate?
   1. Use clean gloves when applying the medication.
   2. Use sterile gloves when applying the medication.
   3. Previously applied medication should remain on the wound surface.
   4. Be sure to apply a thick layer of medication over the wound.
5. A patient is using transdermal patches to relieve his mild cardiac pain. Which patient statement demonstrates understanding of the use of transdermal patches?
   1. "I will apply the patch to a different area each time."
   2. "I need to leave the old patch on to make sure I receive all the medicine."
   3. "If I get a headache from this medicine, I will cut the patch in half."
   4. "It does not matter where I throw away the old patch because the medicine is gone."

REFERENCES

Andrews M, Boyle J: *Transcultural concepts in nursing care*, ed 5, Philadelphia, 2007, Lippincott.

Al-Shahri MZ: Culturally sensitive caring for Saudi patients, *J Transcult Nurs* 13(2):133, 2002.

Capriotti T: Changes in inhaler devices for asthma and COPD, *Medsurg Nurs* 14(3):185, 2005.

Ebersole P and others: *Toward healthy aging*, ed 6, St. Louis, 2007, Mosby.

Hockenberry MJ, Wilson D: *Wong's nursing care of infants and children*, ed 8, St. Louis, 2007, Mosby.

Iannacchione MA: The vagina dialogues: do you douche? *Am J Nurs* 104(1):40, 2004.

Institute for Safe Medication Practices: Hazard alert! Asphyxiation possible with syringe tip caps, *ISMP Medication Safety Alert*, August 22, 2001, http://www.ismp.org/MSAarticles/Hypodermic.html, accessed October 28, 2007.

Institute for Safe Medication Practices: New fentanyl warnings: more needed to protect patients, *ISMP Medication Safety Alert*, August 11, 2005, http://www.ismp.org/Newsletters/acutecare/articles/20050811.asp, accessed November 4, 2007.

Institute for Safe Medication Practices: One or both nostrils? *ISMP medication safety alert* 11(13), 2006a, http://www.ismp.org/Newsletters/acutecare/articles/20060629_2.asp, accessed November 4, 2007.

Institute for Safe Medication Practices: Suppository stories, *ISMP Medication Safety Alert*, 2006b, http://www.ismp.org/consumers/Suppository.asp, accessed November 4, 2007.

Institute for Safe Medication Practices: Tablet splitting: do it only if you "half" to, and then do it safely, *ISMP medication safety alert* 11(10), 2006c, http://www.ismp.org/Newsletters/acutecare/archives/ May06.asp#18, accessed October 28, 2007.

Kemp C, Rasbridge LD: Culture and the end of life: East African cultures. II. Sudanese, *J Hosp Palliat Nurs* 3(3):110, 2001.

Lewis SM and others: *Medical-surgical nursing: assessment and management of clinical problems*, ed 7, St. Louis, 2007, Mosby.

Lilley LL and others: *Pharmacology and the nursing process*, ed 5, St. Louis, 2007, Mosby.

Mashaba G: South African culturally based health-illness patterns and humanistic care practices. In Leininger M, McFarland M: *Transcultural nursing*, New York, 2002, McGraw-Hill.

McErlane K: Keeping track of the patch, *Am J Nurs* 105(6):36, 2005.

McKenry and others: *Mosby's pharmacology in nursing*, ed 22, St. Louis, 2006, Mosby.

Monahan F and others: *Phipps' medical-surgical nursing*, ed 8, St. Louis, 2006, Mosby.

National Library of Medicine-National Institutes of Health, Health and Human Services (NLM-NIHS), DailyMed: *Nitro-Bid (nitroglycerin) ointment [E. Fougera and Co.]*, 2006, http://dailymed.nlm.nih.gov/ dailymed/drugInfo.cfm?id=1351, retrieved October 27, 2007.

Nowak T: People of Vietnamese heritage. In Purnell L, Paulanka B: *Transcultural healthcare*, Philadelphia, 2003, FA Davis.

Nowlin A: The dysphagia dilemma: how you can help, *RN* 69(6):44, 2006.

Padula, CA and others: Enteral feedings: what the evidence says, *Am J Nurs* 104(7):62, 2004.

Pruitt WC: Teaching your patient to use a peak flowmeter, *Nursing* 35(3):54, 2005.

Rubin BK, Durotoye L: How do patients determine that their metered dose inhaler is empty? *Chest* 126(4):1134, 2004.

Schulmeister L: Transdermal drug patches: medicine with muscle, *Nursing* 35(1):48, 2005.

The Joint Commission: *2008 National patient safety goals, hospital program*, http://www.jointcommission.org/PatientSafety/NationalPatientSafetyGoals/08_hap_npsgs.htm, accessed October 28, 2007.

Uko-Ekpenyong G: Improving medication adherence with orally disintegrating tablets, *Nursing* 36(9):20, 2006.

Wooten J, Galavis J: Polypharmacy, *RN* 68(8):44, 2005.

RESEARCH REFERENCES

Burkhart PV and others: An evaluation of children's metered-dose inhaler technique for asthma medications, *Nurs Clin North Am* 40(1):167, 2005.

Madegowda B and others: Medication errors in a rural hospital, *Medsurg Nurs* 16(3):175, 2007.

Metheny NA, Titler MG: Assessing placement of feeding tubes, *Am J Nurs* 101(5):36, 2001.

Rubin DK, Durotoye L: How do patients determine that their metered dose inhaler is empty? *Chest* 126(4):1134, 2005.

Sander N and others: Dose counting and the use of pressurized metered-dose inhalers: running on empty, *Ann Allergy Asthma Immunol*: 97(1):34, 2006.

Stetina P and others: Managing medication errors—a qualitative study, *Medsurg Nurs* 14(3):174, 2005.

Parenteral Medications

MEDIA RESOURCES

- **evolve** learning system   http://evolve.elsevier.com/Perry/skills
  - Review Questions
  - Video Clips

- **View Video!**   Mosby's Nursing Video Skills, 3.0

- **NSO**   Nursing Skills Online

KEY TERMS

Adverse reaction
Air embolus
Allergic reaction
Ampule
Anaphylactic reaction
Aqueous
Aspirate
Blunt-tip vial access cannula
Bolus
Compatibility
Continuous subcutaneous infusion (CSQI or CSCI)
Diluent
Extravasation
Hematemesis
Hematuria
Heparin lock
Hypodermoclysis
Incompatibility
Induration

Infiltration
Infusion
Injection
Intradermal (ID) injection
Intramuscular (IM) injection
Intravenous (IV) injection
Medication administration record (MAR)
Parenteral
Phlebitis
Piggyback infusion
Saline lock
Subcutaneous injection
Tandem setup
Vial
Volume-control administration set (Volutrol)
Z-track method

OBJECTIVES

Mastery of content in this chapter will enable the nurse to:
- Correctly prepare injectable medications from a vial and an ampule.
- Identify advantages, disadvantages, and risks of administering medications by each injection route.
- Explain the importance of selecting the proper-size syringe and needle for an injection.
- Discuss factors to consider when selecting injection sites.
- Discuss ways to promote patient comfort while administering an injection.
- Correctly administer intradermal, subcutaneous, and intramuscular injections.
- Correctly add medications to intravenous fluid containers.
- Compare the risks of three different intravenous routes.
- Correctly administer an intravenous infusion by intravenous piggyback, intermittent infusion, or bolus through a hanging intravenous line or a saline lock.
- Initiate, maintain, and discontinue a continuous subcutaneous infusion.

The route of administration is the path by which a drug comes in contact with the body. *Parenteral* means taken into the body or administered in a manner other than through the digestive tract. Parenteral administration of medication instills medications into body tissues and into the circulatory system by injection. These procedures are invasive and thus pose greater risks than those associated with administering oral or topical medications. Because infections originate from a variety of sources, you must use aseptic technique (Table 22-1). The effects of parenterally administered medication reach the bloodstream either directly or by rapid absorption through the tissues. Therefore closely monitor the patient's response, be aware of potential adverse or allergic reactions, and understand the risk for infection.

You can administer parenteral medication through four different routes:

1 *Subcutaneous injection:* Injection into tissues just under the dermis of the skin
2 *Intramuscular (IM) injection:* Injection into the body of a muscle
3 *Intradermal injection:* Injection into the dermis just under the epidermis
4 *Intravenous (IV) injection or infusion:* Injection into a vein

Each type of injection requires a certain set of skills to ensure that the medication reaches the proper location. Failure to inject a medication correctly will result in complications such as an inappropriate drug response (e.g., too rapid or too slow), nerve injury with associated pain, localized bleeding, tissue necrosis, and sterile abscess.

EQUIPMENT

Administer parenteral medication by using a needle and a syringe, available in a variety of sizes. Determine the appropriate size of syringe, length and gauge of needle, volume of solution, and medication route. These decisions are based on the quantity and type of medication prescribed and the body size of the patient. Most syringes come with needleless systems or safety needles that help prevent needle-stick injuries (Fig. 22-1). There are a variety of electronic infusion pumps that deliver intravenous or continuous subcutaneous infusions. Infusion pumps ensure a constant and accurate delivery of medication.

SYRINGES

Syringes have a cylindrical barrel with a close-fitting plunger and a tip designed to fit the hub of a hypodermic needle (Fig. 22-2). Syringes are single use, disposable, and are classified as Luer-Lok or non–Luer-Lok. The design of the syringe tip influences the name. Luer-Lok syringes (Fig. 22-3, A) require special needles, which are twisted onto the tip and lock themselves in place. The design prevents the unintentional removal of the needle from the syringe. Non–Luer-Lok syringes use needles that slip onto the tip (Fig. 22-3, B to D).

Syringes come in different sizes, ranging from 0.5 to 60 mL in capacity (see Fig. 22-3). A 1- to 3-mL syringe is adequate for IM and subcutaneous injections (see Fig. 22-3, A), and rarely is a syringe larger than 5 mL used for an injection. Larger syringes are used to administer some IV medications, add medications to IV solutions, and irrigate drainage tubes. Some syringes are packaged with their needle attached, and some syringes require you to change the needle based on the viscosity of the medication, route of administration, and the size of the patient.

Some syringes have two scales along the barrel; one is divided into minims and the other into tenths of a milliliter. The tuberculin syringe (see Fig. 22-3, B) has a long, thin barrel with

TABLE 22-1	Preventing Infection During an Injection	
Principle	**Technique**
Prevent contamination of solution.	Add date, time, and initials to vials when opened. A multidose vial, properly labeled, can be used up to 30 days. Swab top of opened multidose vial with alcohol before piercing. Ampules should not sit open, and medication should be removed quickly.
Prevent needle contamination.	Avoid letting needle touch contaminated surface: outer edges of ampule or vial, outer surface of needle cap, your hands, countertop, or table surface. Avoid touching the length of the plunger or inner part of the barrel. Keep tip of syringe covered with cap or needle.
Prepare skin.	Wash skin soiled with dirt, drainage, or feces with soap and water. Use friction and a circular motion while cleaning with an antiseptic swab. Swab from center of site, and move outward in a 5-cm (2-inch) radius.
Before handling any equipment, hand hygiene is essential to reduce the transfer of microorganisms.	Perform hand hygiene for a minimum of 15 seconds.

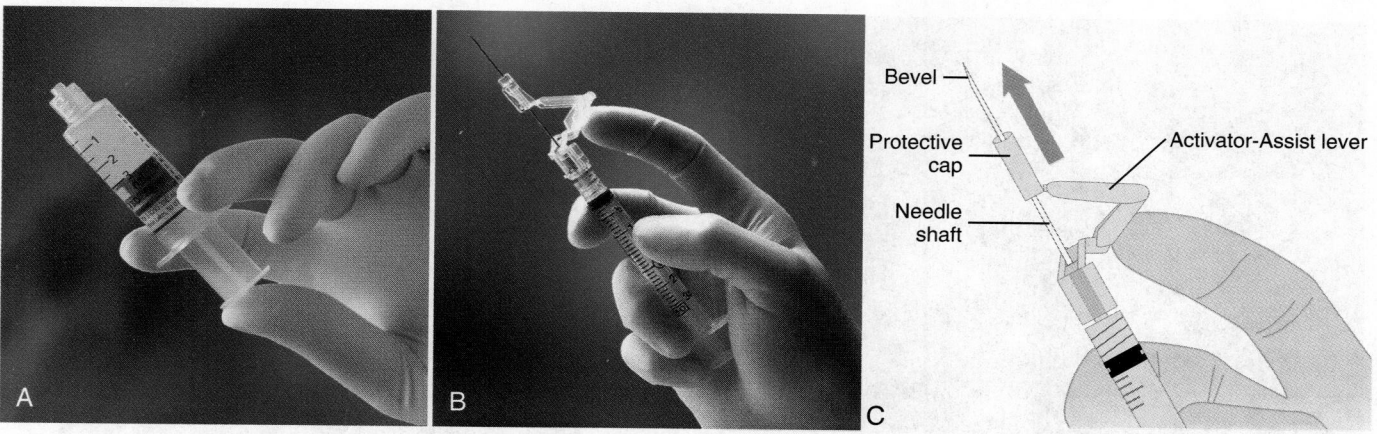

FIG 22-1 **A,** Needleless system. **B,** Safety needle system. **C,** Detail of safety needle system. (*A and B, Courtesy and © Becton, Dickinson and Company.*)

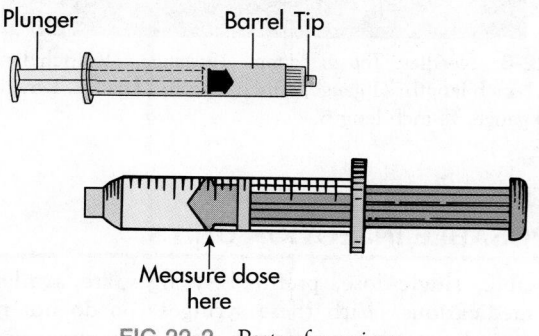

FIG 22-2 Parts of a syringe.

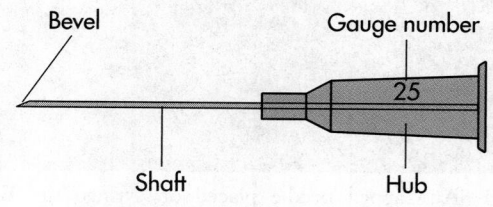

FIG 22-4 Parts of a needle.

a preattached thin needle. The syringe is calibrated in six-teenths of a minim and hundredths of a milliliter and has a capacity of 1 mL. You use tuberculin syringes to prepare small amounts of medication such as small, precise doses for infants or young children. You also use them for intradermal and subcutaneous injections.

Insulin syringes (see Fig. 22-3, *C* and *D*) hold 0.3 mL to 1 mL, come with a preattached needle that cannot be removed, and are calibrated in units. Low-dose insulin syringes (30 units per 0.3 mL or 50 units per 0.5 mL) hold 0.3 mL and 0.5 mL. People with visual problems and children diagnosed with diabetes usually use this syringe. Most insulin syringes are U-100s, designed for use with U-100–strength insulin. Each milliliter of solution contains 100 units of insulin. Before use, carefully examine the syringe to determine the measurement scale and to ensure that you use the correct syringe for preparing the ordered medication.

NEEDLES

Some needles come attached to syringes. Other needles come packaged individually to allow flexibility in selecting the right needle for a patient. Most needles are stainless steel and are disposable. The needle has three parts: the hub, which fits onto the tip of a syringe; the shaft, which connects to the hub; and the bevel,

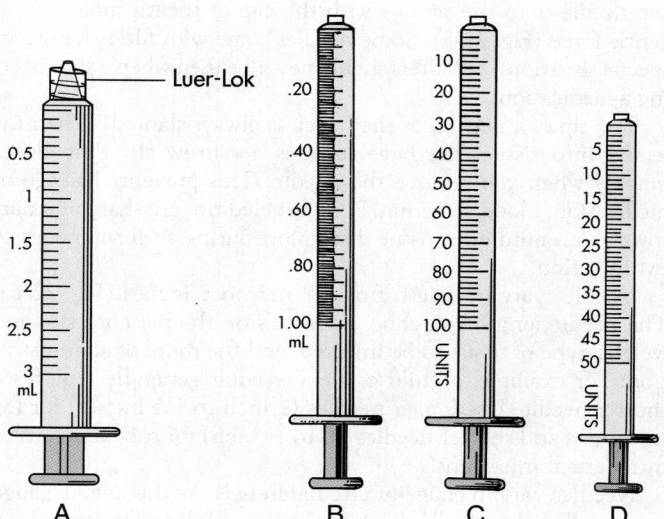

FIG 22-3 Types of syringes. **A,** Luer-Lok syringe with 3-mL capacity is marked in 0.1 (tenths). **B,** Tuberculin syringe marked in 0.01 (hundredths) for doses of less than 1 mL. **C,** Insulin syringe marked in units (100). **D,** Insulin syringe marked in units (50).

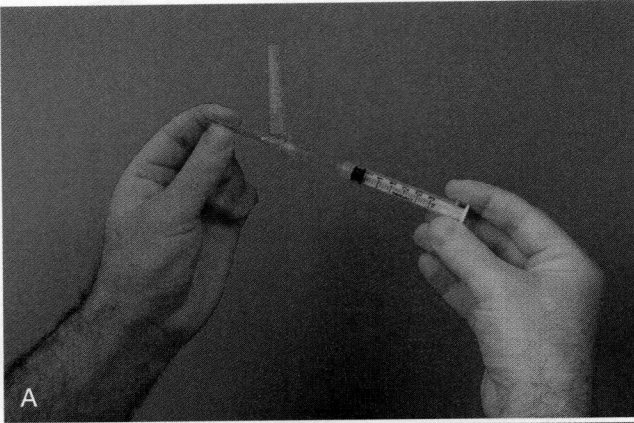

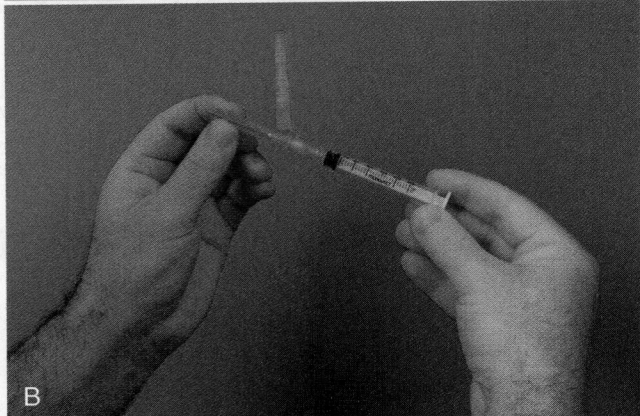

FIG 22-5 **A,** Capped needle placed on syringe tip. **B,** Needle secured.

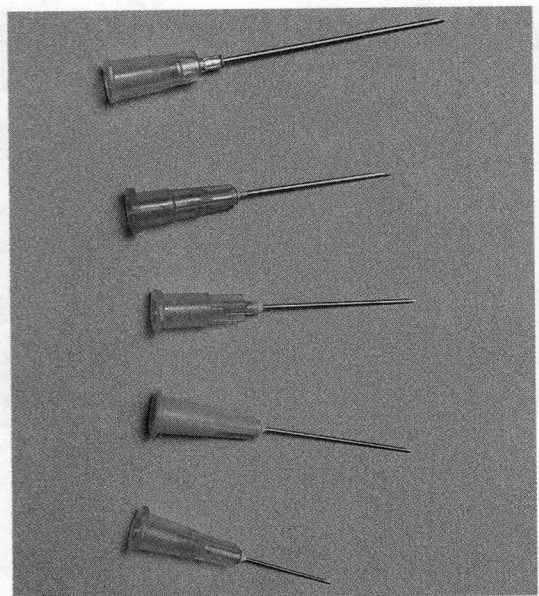

FIG 22-6 Needles. *Top to bottom:* 19 gauge, 1½-inch length; 20 gauge, 1-inch length; 21 gauge, 1-inch length; 23 gauge, 1-inch length; and 25 gauge, ⅝-inch length.

or slanted tip (Fig. 22-4). The needle hub, shaft, and bevel must remain sterile at all times. To prevent contamination, you place the needle onto the syringe with the cap or sheath intact, using gentle force (Fig. 22-5). Some needles come with filters for use in special situations, but filters should never be used when administering a medication.

The tip of a needle, or the bevel, is always slanted. When injected into tissue, the bevel creates a narrow slit that closes quickly when you remove the needle. This prevents leakage of medication, blood, or serum. Long beveled tips are sharp and narrow, which minimizes tissue discomfort during a subcutaneous or IM injection.

Needles vary in length from ⅜ inch to 3 inches (Fig. 22-6). The needle length you choose depends on the patient's size and weight, type of tissue to be injected, and the route of administration. For example, a child or slender adult generally requires a shorter needle. Use longer needles (1 inch to 1½ inches) for IM injections and shorter needles (⅜ to ⅝ inch) for subcutaneous or intradermal injections.

Needles vary in gauge or circumference. As the needle gauge gets smaller, the needle diameter becomes larger, for example, a 21-gauge needle is larger than a 25-gauge needle. The selection of a gauge depends on the viscosity of fluid you will inject or infuse.

DISPOSABLE INJECTION UNITS

Disposable, single-dose, prefilled syringes are available for some medications. With these syringes you do not need to prepare medication doses, except perhaps to expel unneeded portions of medication or air.

Prefilled unit-dose systems such as Tubex and Carpuject injection systems include reusable plastic syringe holders and disposable, prefilled, sterile, glass cartridge units (Fig. 22-7). To use a prefilled system, load the cartridge, Luer tip first, into the plastic syringe holder, then secure it following manufacturer's instructions. Check for air bubbles in the syringe. You expel air and excess medication by advancing the plunger, as with a regular syringe. You may use the glass cartridge with safety needles or needleless systems. After giving the medication, dispose of the glass cartridge safely in a puncture-proof and leak-proof container. This design reduces the risk for needle-stick injury.

PROTECTING YOURSELF FROM NEEDLE-STICK INJURY

The most frequent route of exposure to blood-borne disease for health care workers is from needle-stick injuries (American Nurses Association, 2007; Wilburn and Eijkemans, 2004). Exposure to blood-borne pathogens is one of the deadliest hazards nurses are exposed to on a daily basis. However, the implementation of safe needle devices can prevent over 81% of needle-stick injuries (American Nurses Association, 2007). The Needlestick Safety and Prevention Act is a federal law that became effective in April 2001. This federal law mandates health care facilities to use safe needle devices to reduce the frequency of needle-stick

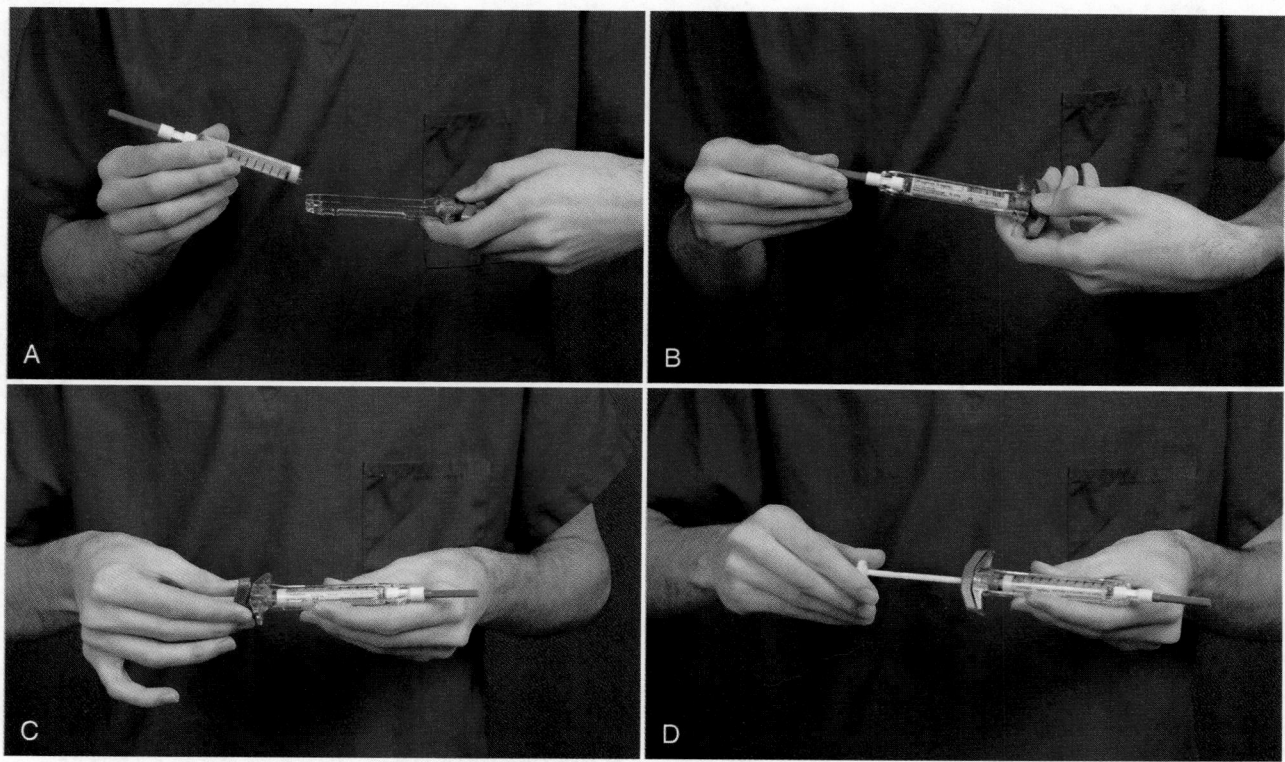

FIG 22-7 **A,** Carpuject syringe holder and prefilled sterile cartridge with needle. **B,** Assembling the Carpuject. **C,** The cartridge slides into the syringe barrel, turns, and locks at the needle end. **D,** The plunger then screws into the cartridge end.

injury (see Figure 22-1, C). One type of safe needle device is the safety syringe, which has a plastic guard or shield that slips over the needle as you withdraw it from the skin (Fig. 22-8, A and B). Another type of safety device can be found on needleless IV line connection systems (Fig. 22-8, C, D, and E). Box 22-1 (p. 579) provides recommendations for decreasing the risk for needle-stick injuries.

EVIDENCE-BASED PRACTICE TRENDS

Administering parenteral medication via IM injections is an important responsibility of the professional nurse. Complications from IM injections include abscess formation, sciatic nerve injury, local induration, erythema, persistent pain, hematoma, and bleeding (Prettyman, 2005). The choice of an injection site is based on sound clinical judgment, best evidence, and patient assessment (Small, 2004). Site selection and injection technique are important to minimizing damage to blood vessels and nerves. Nurses need to administer an IM injection only when medically necessary and ensure that every IM injection is given safely (Prettyman, 2005; World Health Organization [WHO], 2007).

Certain scientific reasons justify the need for an IM injection (Greenway and others, 2006; Nisbet, 2006; Prettyman, 2005); for example, some medications are irritating to subcutaneous tissue and can only be administered IM. Consideration of the medication's onset of action, intensity of effect, and duration also help determine the need for an IM injection. Medications that are not readily soluble provide sustained release when administered in a suspension form and given IM (Ansel and others, 2004).

Recent evidence supports avoiding the traditional dorsogluteal route in favor of the ventrogluteal site (Greenway and others, 2006; Ramtahal and others, 2006). Studies demonstrate the exact location of the sciatic nerve varies from one person to another. If a needle hits the sciatic nerve, the patient may experience permanent or partial paralysis of the involved leg. Therefore the dorsogluteal site **should not** be used as a site for IM injections (Greenway, 2006; Ramtahal and others, 2006; Small, 2004). The injection site used for IM injections is the most predictive factor associated with complications (Prettyman, 2005). To avoid these complications, assess the patient's age, medication type, medication volume, and viscosity in selecting the appropriate injection site. Appropriate technique for administering IM injections facilitates the best patient outcomes in all health care settings (Hockenberry and Wilson, 2007; Wynaden and others, 2005).

Based on the evidence, the recommendation for pediatric IM injection sites includes use of the vastus lateralis site for infants up to 12 months of age, deltoid in children 12 months and older, and ventrogluteal site for children of all ages (Cook and others, 2006; Hockenberry and Wilson, 2007). Research suggests that the ventrogluteal area is the most appropriate site for all age-groups of children (Cook and Murtagh, 2006; Schechter and others, 2007). Preferred IM injection sites for children and adolescents include the deltoid or ventrogluteal, and the preferred sites for adults are the ventrogluteal or vastus lateralis. Administer medications that are irritating or are in an oily solution in the ventrogluteal. Administer vaccines in the vastus lateralis in infants and young children and in the deltoid in older children and adults.

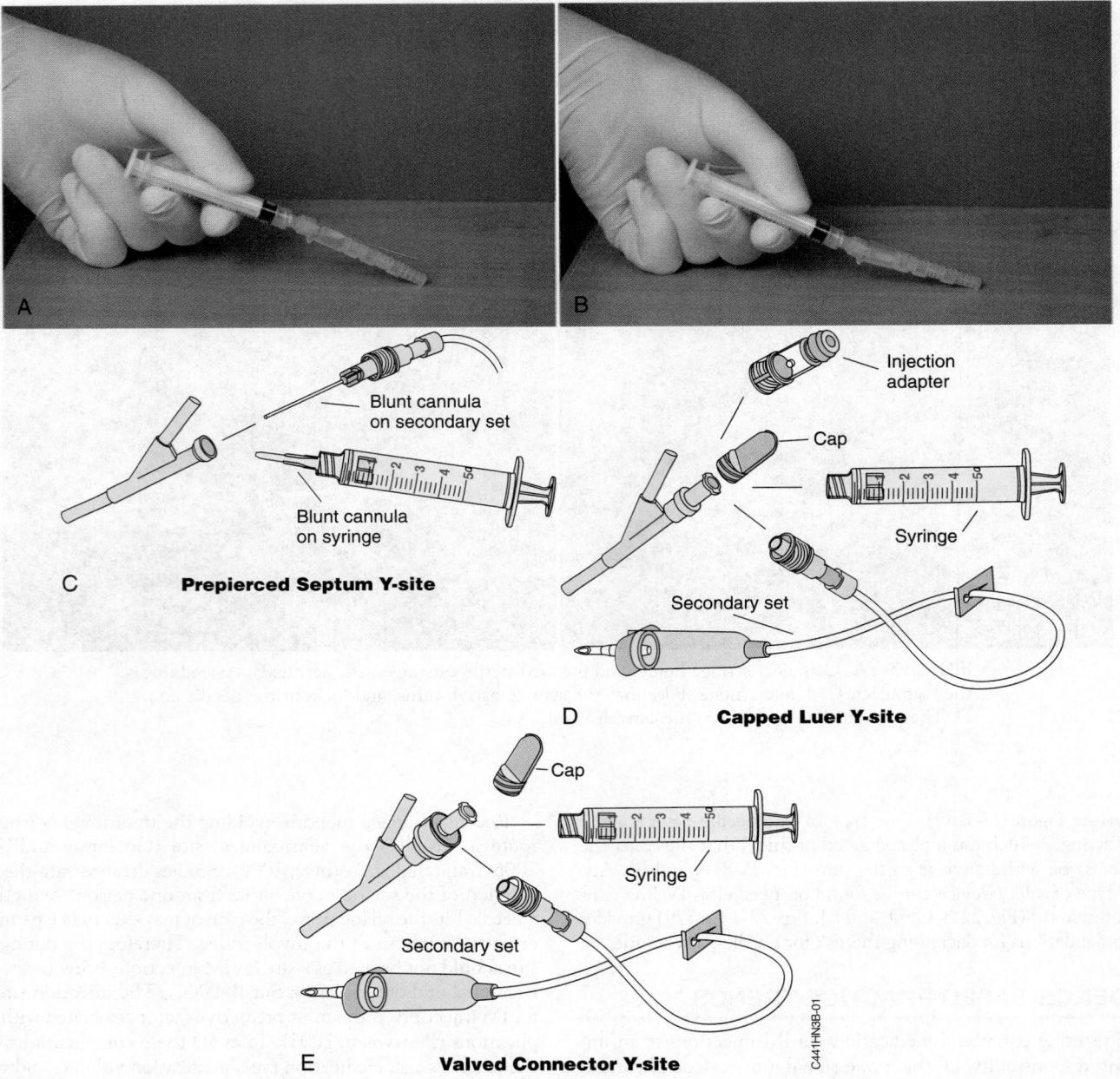

FIG 22-8 **A,** Protective syringe shown with sheath partially retracted. **B,** Sheath pulled and locked over needle. **C,** Prepierced septum Y-site. **D,** Capped Luer Y-site. **E,** Valved connector Y-site. (*C, D, and E from* Health Devices Needlestick-Prevention Device Selection Guide, *Plymouth Meeting, Pa, 2000, ECRT.*)

Administer volumes of 1 mL or less to infants and small children. As the child approaches adult size, use adult volumes of greater than 1 mL. Larger volumes require a large muscle mass (Hockenberry and Wilson, 2007). To reduce pain associated with intramuscular injections, apply manual pressure or a vapocoolant to the injection site before administering the injection, and use distraction when administering the injection (Hockenberry and Wilson, 2007; Schechter and others, 2007).

CULTURAL CONSIDERATIONS

Research shows that ethnicity, genetics, and culture influence drug response, pharmacokinetics, and pharmacodynamics, as well as patient adherence and education (Lea, 2005; Munoz and Hilgenberg, 2005). Knowledge about variations in therapeutic dose and adverse effects is essential in administering medications to different ethnic groups. Some patients experience a

---

BOX 22-1 | Recommendations for the Prevention of Needle-Stick Injuries

1 Avoid using needles when effective needleless systems or sharps with engineered sharps injury protection (SESIP) safety devices are available.
2 Do not manually recap needles.
3 Plan safe handling and disposal of needles before beginning a procedure that requires the use of a needle.
4 Immediately dispose of used needles, needleless systems, and SESIP into puncture-proof and leak-proof sharps disposal containers.
5 Maintain a sharps injury log that includes:
   A Type and brand of device involved in the incident
   B Location of the incident (e.g., department or work area)
   C Description of the incident
   D Methods to maintain privacy of employees who have experienced sharps injuries

6 Participate in educational offerings regarding blood-borne pathogens, and follow recommendations for infection prevention, including receiving the hepatitis B vaccine.
7 Report all needle-stick and sharps-related injuries immediately, according to institutional policies to ensure the receipt of appropriate follow-up care.
8 Participate in the selection and evaluation of needleless systems and devices with safety features within your place of employment whenever possible.
9 Support legislation that promotes the safe use of needles and sharps.

Data from Occupational Safety and Health Administration: Occupational exposure to blood borne pathogens, needlestick, and other sharps injuries: final rule, 29 CFR part 1910 (*Fed Regist* 66:5317, Jan 18, 2001), updated April 2007, http://www.osha.gov/pls/oshaweb/owadisp.show_document?p_id516265&p_table5FEDERAL_REGISTER.

---

therapeutic response at a lower dose than recommended and require careful monitoring. For example, Japanese and Taiwanese patients require lower doses of lithium (Munoz and Hilgenberg, 2005). You need skills in communicating with and educating diverse patient populations. If a culture values patience and modesty, make your questions specific rather than general to elicit information about adverse drug effects. The Transcultural Assessment Model considers areas of communication, space, social organization, time, environmental control, and biological variations important for teaching and education of patients (Giger and Davidhizar, 2004). Cultural assessment also yields information about dietary preferences, tobacco and alcohol use, and use of herbal remedies that affect drug action and response. Cultural context is essential in planning education for patients and families (Schim, 2007).

Skill Performance Guidelines

1 Use strict aseptic technique during all steps of medication preparation and administration.
2 To prevent contamination and maintain sterility of a syringe, avoid letting the needle touch contaminated surfaces (e.g., outer edges of ampule or vial, outer surface of needle cap, your hands, countertop, table surface). Avoid touching the length of the plunger or inner part of the barrel. Keep tip of syringe covered with cap or needle.
3 Know the volume and characteristics of the medication you will administer. Injecting too large a volume of medication can cause adverse effects, extreme pain, and local tissue damage. Avoid tracking medication through superficial tissues.
4 Identify the bony prominences and anatomical structures that outline the chosen injection sites. Correct identification of the specific muscle mass will prevent injury to major nerves and blood vessels located near the injection site.
5 Select a site that is free from irritation and infection; palpate the area for sensitivity or hardness.

6 Insert the needle at the proper angle to deliver medication into the correct tissue (Fig. 22-9).
7 Attempt to minimize the patient's discomfort when giving an injection:
   • Use sharp beveled needles in the shortest length and smallest gauge possible.
   • Change the needle if liquid medication has coated the shaft of the needle.
   • Position and flex the patient's limbs to reduce muscular tension.
   • Divert the patient's attention away from the injection procedure.
   • Spray vapocoolant on the site 15 seconds before injection, or place wrapped ice on site for a minute before injection.
   • Insert the needle smoothly and quickly. Do not hesitate, and slowly push the needle into tissue.
   • Inject the medication slowly but smoothly to reduce pain.
   • Hold the syringe steady once the needle is in the tissue to prevent tissue damage.
   • Withdraw the needle smoothly at the same angle used for insertion.
   • Gently apply an antiseptic pad (e.g., alcohol) or dry, sterile gauze pad to the site.
   • Apply gentle pressure at the injection site.
   • Rotate injection sites to prevent the formation of indurations and abscesses.
8 Use the guidelines for administering medications, including the six rights of medication administration, listed in Chapter 20, when giving parenteral medications.
9 Do not recap needles after administering injections, and dispose of all needles in an appropriate puncture-proof and leak-proof container (Occupational Safety and Health Administration [OSHA], 2006).

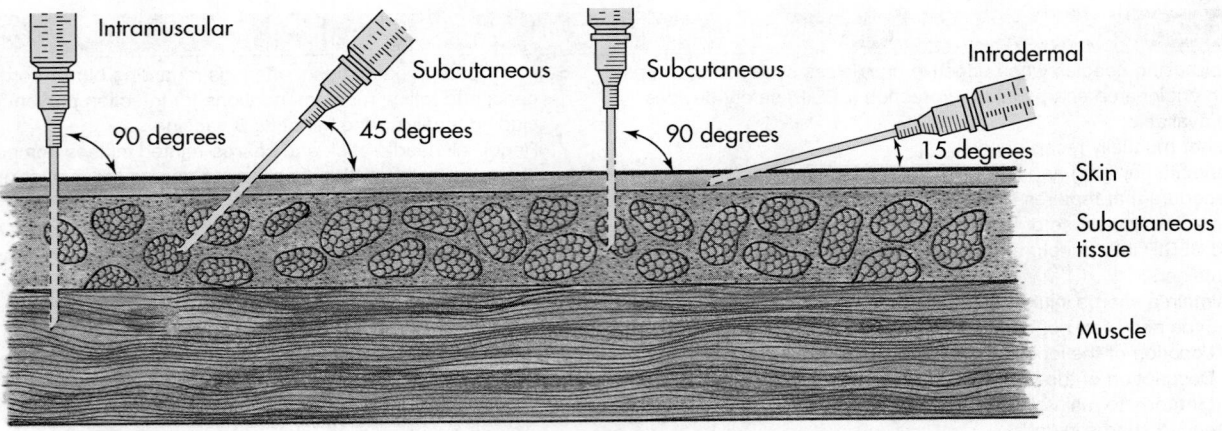

FIG 22-9 Comparison of the angles of insertion of intramuscular (90 degrees), subcutaneous (45 to 90 degrees), and intradermal (15 degrees) injections.

SKILL 22-1 Preparing Injections From Ampules and Vials

 Advanced / Injections / Preparing Injections
From Ampules
Preparing Injections From Vials

[NSO]   Injections Module/ Lesson 2

Ampules contain single doses of injectable medication in a liquid form and are available in sizes from 1 to 10 mL or more (Fig. 22-10, A). An ampule is made of glass with a constricted, prescored neck that you need to snap off to allow access to the medication. A colored ring around the neck indicates where the ampule is prescored. Aspiration of medication from the ampule is achieved with a filter needle and syringe. Filter needles prevent glass particles from being drawn into the syringe (Stein, 2006). Medication enters the syringe because pulling on the plunger creates a vacuum in the syringe barrel. Place an appropriate-size needle on the syringe after withdrawing a medication.

A vial is a single-dose or multidose container with a rubber seal at the top, protected by a metal or plastic cap (Fig. 22-10, B). Re-

move the cap when preparing the vial for use. Vials contain liquid or dry forms of medications. Medications that are unstable in solution are packaged dry. The vial label specifies the solvent or diluent used to dissolve the medication and the amount of diluent needed to prepare a desired drug concentration. Normal saline and sterile distilled water are solutions commonly used to dissolve medications.

Some vials have two chambers separated by a rubber stopper. One chamber contains the diluent solution and the other the dry medication. Before preparing the medication, you push on the upper chamber, which dislodges the rubber stopper and allows the powder and the diluent to mix. Unlike the ampule, the vial is a closed system and you inject air into the container to permit with-

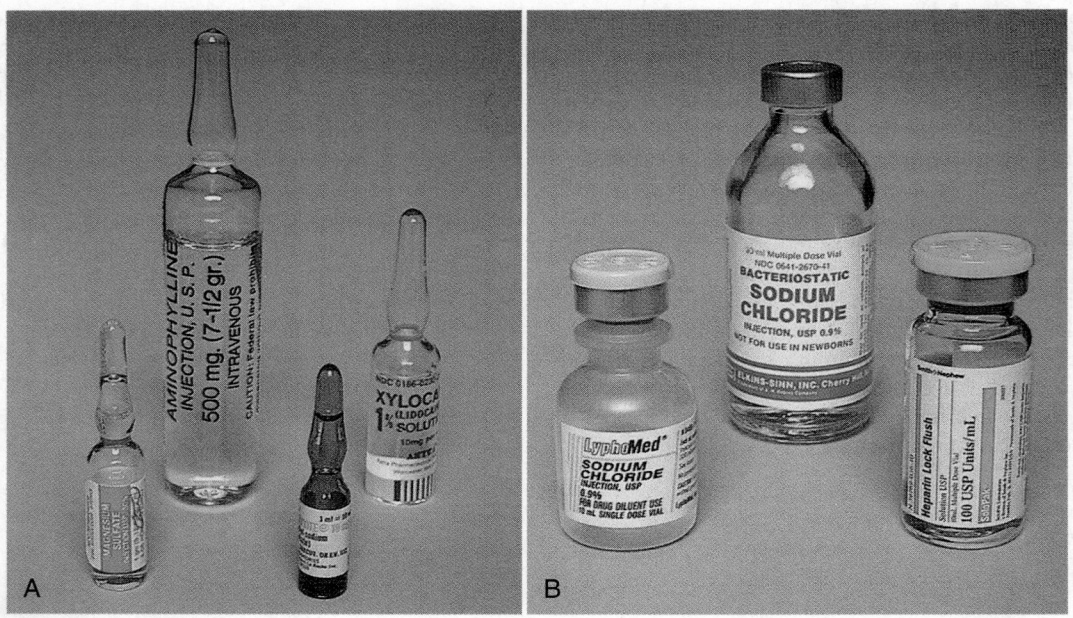

FIG 22-10 **A,** Medication in ampules. **B,** Medication in vials.

drawal of the solution. Some medications, even when in a vial, may need to be drawn up with a filter needle because of the nature of the medication. Institutional policies will indicate which drugs you need to prepare with a filter needle.

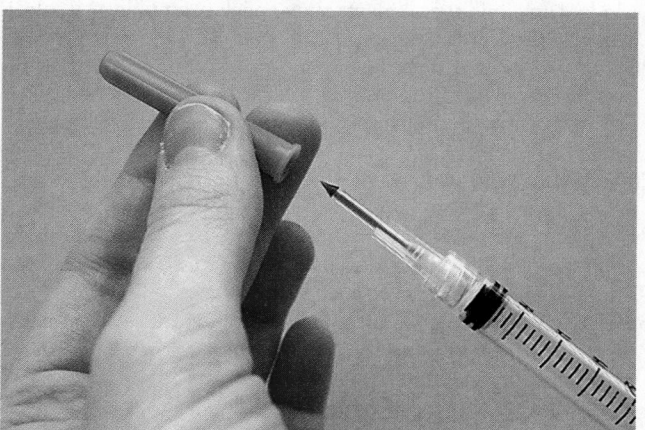

FIG 22-11 Syringe with needleless vial access adapter.

Delegation Considerations

The skill of preparing injections from ampules and vials cannot be delegated to nursing assistive personnel (NAP).

Equipment

Medication in an Ampule
❑ Syringe, needle, and filter needle
❑ Small sterile gauze pad or unopened alcohol swab

Medication in a Vial
❑ Syringe and two needles
❑ Needles:
  • Blunt-tip vial access cannula (if needleless system used) (Fig. 22-11) or needle for drawing up medication (if needed)
  • Filter needle for ampules
  • Needle for injection
❑ Small sterile gauze pad or alcohol swab
❑ Diluent (e.g., 0.9% sodium chloride or sterile water) (if indicated)

Both
❑ Medication administration record (MAR) or computer printout

STEP	RATIONALE

ASSESSMENT

1 Check accuracy and completeness of the MAR or computer printout with prescriber's written medication order. Check patient's name, medication name and dosage, route of administration, and time of administration. Recopy or re-print any portion of MAR that is difficult to read.

Helps to ensure that the six rights of medication administration are met. The order sheet is the most reliable source and legal record of the patient's medications. Ensures that patient receives the correct medication.
Illegible MARs are a source of medication errors.

2 Assess patient's medical and medication history.

Identifies need for medication.

3 Assess patient's history of allergies: Know type of allergies and normal allergic response.

Do not prepare medication if there is a known patient allergy.

4 Review medication reference information related to medication, including action, purpose, side effects, normal dose, rate of administration, time of peak onset, and nursing implications.

Allows you to administer drug properly and to monitor patient's response.

5 Assess the patient's body build, muscle size, and weight if giving subcutaneous or IM medication.

Determines type and size of syringe and needles for injection.

PLANNING

1 Expected outcomes following completion of procedure:
  • Proper dose is prepared. No air bubbles are in syringe barrel.

Ensures right dose. Air bubbles displace medication. Elimination of air ensures the accuracy of medication dose.

IMPLEMENTATION

1 Perform hand hygiene, and prepare supplies.

Reduces transmission of microorganisms.

2 Check date of expiration for medication vial or ampule.

Medication potency increases or decreases when outdated.

3 Prepare medication for one patient at a time following six rights of medication administration (see Chapter 20). Select ampule or vial from unit-dose drawer or automated dispensing system. Compare the label of the medication with the MAR.

Establishing a medication preparation routine, eliminating distractions, and double-checking the transcribed order reduce error (Pape and others, 2005; Ridge, 2007; Wolf, 2007).
This is the first check for accuracy.

STEP	RATIONALE

4   Preparing an ampule:

   a   Tap top of ampule lightly and quickly with finger until fluid moves from neck of ampule (see illustration).

Dislodges any fluid that collects above neck of ampule. All solution moves into lower chamber.

   b   Place small gauze pad or unopened alcohol swab around neck of ampule (see illustration).

Placing pad around neck of ampule protects nurse's fingers from trauma as glass tip is broken off. Do not use opened alcohol swab to wrap around top of ampule because alcohol may leak into ampule.

   c   Snap neck of ampule quickly and firmly away from hands (see illustration).

Protects nurse's fingers and face from shattering glass.

   d   Draw up medication quickly, using a filter needle long enough to reach bottom of ampule.

System is open to airborne contaminants. Ensures needle is long enough to access medication for preparation. Filter needles filter out glass fragments (Stein, 2006).

   e   Hold ampule upside down, or set it on a flat surface. Insert filter needle into center of ampule opening. Do not allow needle tip or shaft to touch rim of ampule.

Broken rim of ampule is considered contaminated. When ampule is inverted, solution dribbles out of ampule if needle tip or shaft touches rim of ampule.

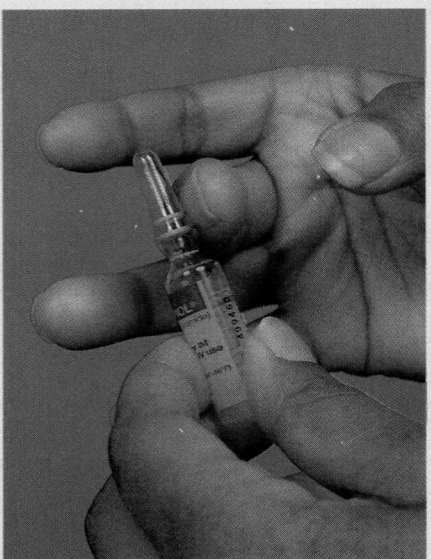

STEP 4a   Tapping moves fluid down neck.

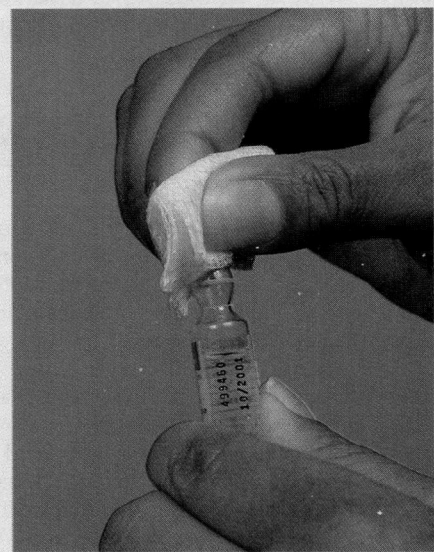

STEP 4b   Gauze pad placed around neck of ampule.

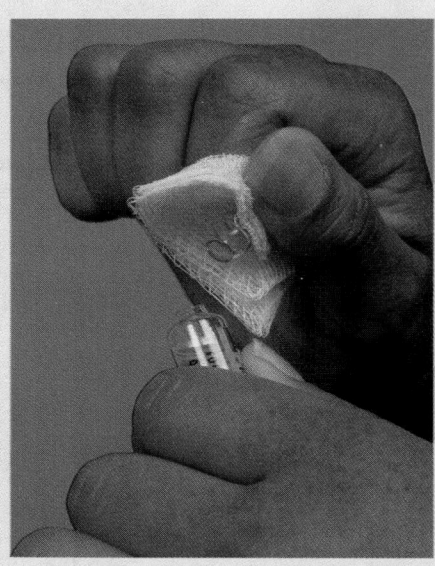

STEP 4c   Neck snapped away from hands.

STEP	RATIONALE
f Aspirate medication into syringe by gently pulling back on plunger (see illustrations).	Withdrawal of plunger creates negative pressure within syringe barrel, which pulls fluid into syringe.
g Keep needle tip under surface of liquid. Tip ampule to bring all fluid within reach of the needle.	Prevents aspiration of air bubbles.
h If air bubbles are aspirated, do not expel air into ampule.	Air pressure forces fluid out of ampule and medication will be lost.
i To expel excess air bubbles, remove needle from ampule. Hold syringe with needle pointing up. Tap side of syringe to cause bubbles to rise toward needle. Draw back slightly on plunger, and then push plunger upward to eject air. Do not eject fluid.	Withdrawing plunger too far will remove it from barrel. Holding syringe vertically allows fluid to settle in bottom of barrel. Pulling back on plunger allows fluid within needle to enter barrel so fluid is not expelled. You then expel air at top of barrel and within needle.
j If syringe contains excess fluid, use sink for disposal. Hold syringe vertically with needle tip up and slanted slightly toward sink. Slowly eject excess fluid into sink. Recheck fluid level in syringe by holding it vertically.	Safely dispenses excess medication into sink. Position of needle allows you to expel medication without it flowing down needle shaft. Rechecking fluid level ensures proper dose.
k Cover needle with its safety sheath or cap. Do not engage the sheath, or it will lock. Replace filter needle with a needleless access device or an appropriate-size needle for injection.	Minimizes needle sticks. Filter needles cannot be used for injection.
5 Preparing a vial containing a solution:	
a Remove cap covering top of unused vial to expose sterile rubber seal. If a multidose vial has been used, cap is already removed. Firmly and briskly wipe surface of rubber seal with alcohol swab, and allow it to dry.	Vial comes packaged with cap that cannot be replaced after seal removal. Not all drug manufacturers guarantee that rubber seals of unused vials are sterile. Therefore swab with alcohol before preparing medication. Allowing alcohol to dry prevents alcohol from coating needle and mixing with medication.
b Pick up syringe, and remove needle cap or cap covering needleless vial access device. Pull back on plunger to draw amount of air into syringe equivalent to volume of medication to be aspirated from vial.	Injecting air prevents buildup of negative pressure in vial when aspirating medication.

Critical Decision Point   *Some medications and institutions require that a filter needle be used when preparing medications from a vial. Check agency policy to determine if use of filter needle is indicated (Stein, 2006).*

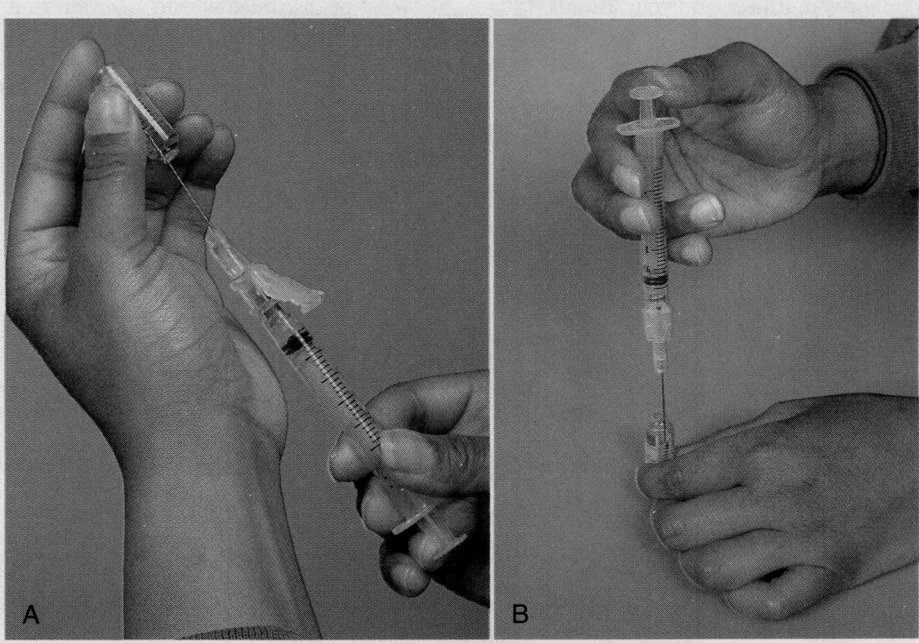

STEP 4f   A, Medication aspirated with ampule inverted. **B,** Medication aspirated with ampule on flat surface.

STEP	RATIONALE
c With vial on flat surface, firmly insert tip of needle or needleless vial access device through center of rubber seal.	Center of seal is thinner and easier to penetrate. Using firm pressure prevents dislodging rubber particles that could enter vial or needle.
d Inject air into the vial's air space, holding on to plunger. Hold plunger with firm pressure; plunger is sometimes forced backward by air pressure within vial.	Air must be injected before aspirating fluid. Injecting into vial's air space prevents formation of bubbles and inaccuracy in dose.
e Invert vial while keeping firm hold on syringe and plunger (see illustration). Hold vial between thumb and middle fingers of nondominant hand. Grasp end of syringe barrel and plunger with thumb and forefinger of dominant hand to counteract pressure in vial.	Inverting vial allows fluid to settle in lower half of container. Position of hands prevents forceful movement of plunger and permits easy manipulation of syringe.
f Keep tip of needle in the fluid while withdrawing medication.	Prevents aspiration of air.
g Allow air pressure from the vial to fill syringe gradually with medication. If necessary, pull back slightly on plunger to obtain correct amount of medication.	Positive pressure within vial forces fluid into syringe.
h When desired volume has been obtained, position needle into vial's air space; tap side of syringe barrel gently to dislodge any air bubbles. Eject any air remaining at top of syringe into vial.	Forcefully striking barrel while needle is inserted in vial may bend needle. Accumulation of air displaces medication and causes dose errors.
i Remove needle or needleless vial access device by pulling back on barrel of syringe.	Pulling plunger rather than barrel causes plunger to separate from barrel, resulting in loss of medication.
j Hold syringe at eye level, at 90-degree angle, to ensure correct volume and absence of air bubbles. Remove any remaining air by tapping barrel to dislodge any air bubbles (see illustration). Draw back slightly on plunger; then push plunger upward to eject air. Do not eject fluid. Recheck volume of medication.	Holding syringe vertically allows fluid to settle in bottom of barrel. Pulling back on plunger allows fluid within needle to enter barrel so fluid is not expelled. Air at top of barrel and within needle is then expelled.

Critical Decision Point   *When preparing medication from single-dose vial, do not assume that volume listed on label is total volume in vial. Some manufacturers provide small amount of extra liquid, expecting loss during preparation. Be sure to draw up only desired volume.*

k If medication will be injected into patient's tissue, change needle to appropriate gauge and length according to route of medication administration.	Inserting needle through a rubber stopper dulls beveled tip. New needle is sharper. Because no fluid is along shaft, needle will not track medication through tissues.
l For multidose vial, make label that includes date of mixing, concentration of drug per milliliter, and your initials.	Ensures that nurses will prepare future doses correctly. Some drugs must be discarded within a certain time frame of mixing.

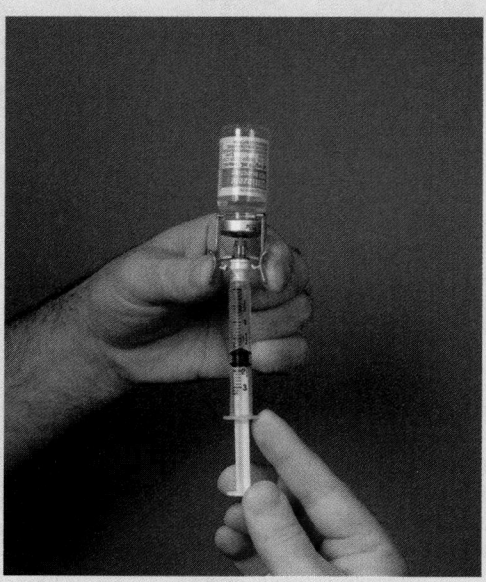

STEP 5e   Withdraw fluid with vial inverted.

STEP	RATIONALE

6 Vial containing a powder (reconstituting medications):

   a Remove cap covering vial of powdered medication and cap covering vial of proper diluent. Firmly swab both rubber seals with alcohol swab, and allow alcohol to dry.

         Not all drug manufacturers guarantee that rubber seals of unused vials are sterile. Allowing alcohol to dry prevents alcohol from coating needle and mixing with medication.

   b Draw up manufacturer's suggestion for volume of diluent into syringe following Steps 5b to j.

         Prepares diluent for injection into vial containing powdered medication.

   c Insert tip of needle or needleless access device through center of rubber seal of vial of powdered medication. Inject diluent into vial. Remove needle.

         Diluent begins to dissolve and reconstitute medication.

   d Mix medication thoroughly. Roll in palms. Do not shake.

         Ensures proper dispersal of medication throughout solution and prevents formation of air bubbles.

   e Reconstituted medication in vial is ready to be drawn into new syringe. Read label carefully to determine dose after reconstitution.

         Once you add diluent, concentration of medication (mg/mL) determines dose you give.

   f Draw up reconstituted medication into syringe following Steps 5b to l.

         Prepares medication for administration.

7 Compare MAR, computer screen, or computer printout with prepared medication and label of containers.

         This is the second check for accuracy.

8 Some institutions require that medications prepared for parenteral administration be verified by another nurse. Check institution policies before administering medication.

         Ensures accuracy of parenteral medication dose.

9 Dispose of soiled supplies. Place broken ampule and/or used vials and used needle or needleless access device in punctureproof and leak-proof container. Clean work area, and perform hand hygiene.

         Proper disposal of glass and needle prevents accidental injury to staff (OSHA, 2006).
Controls transmission of infection.

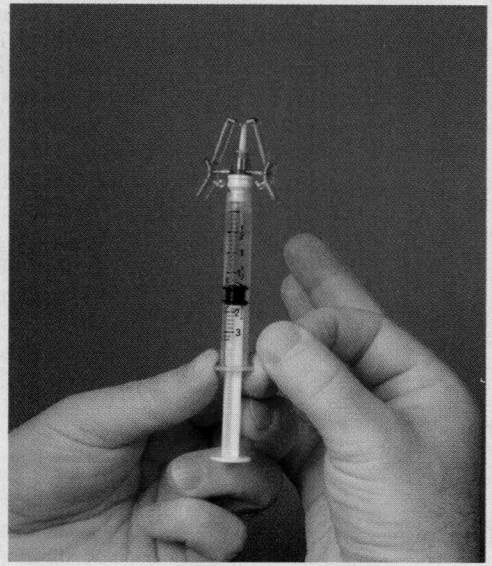

STEP 5j Hold syringe upright; tap barrel to dislodge air bubbles.

EVALUATION

1 Just before administering drug to patient, compare MAR with label of prepared drug, and compare dose in syringe with desired dose.

         Ensures that dose is accurate. *This is the third check for accuracy.*

Unexpected Outcomes	Related Interventions
1 Air bubbles remain in syringe.	• Expel air from syringe, and add medication to syringe until you prepare the correct dose.
2 Incorrect dose of medication is prepared.	• Discard prepared dose. • Prepare correct new dose.

PROCEDURAL GUIDELINE 22-1   Mixing Parenteral Medications in One Syringe

Advanced / Injections / Drawing Up More Than One Type of Insulin

There are medications that need to be mixed from two vials or from a vial and an ampule. Mixing compatible medications avoids the need to give a patient more than one injection. Most nursing units have medication compatibility charts. Compatibility charts are in drug reference guides or are posted within patient care areas. If you are uncertain about medication compatibilities, consult a pharmacist. When mixing medications, you must correctly aspirate fluid from each type of container. When using multidose vials, do not contaminate the vial's contents with medication from another vial or ampule.

When you mix medications from a vial and an ampule, you prepare medications from the vial first. Then you withdraw medication from the ampule using the same syringe and a filter needle. When mixing medications from two vials, do not contaminate one medication with another, ensure that the final dose is accurate, and maintain aseptic technique.

You need to give special consideration to the proper preparation of insulin, which comes in vials. Insulin is the hormone used to treat diabetes mellitus. Insulin is classified by rate of action, including short acting, intermediate, and long acting. A patient with diabetes sometimes requires more than one type of insulin. In addition, some patients require several injections in a day that combine two different insulin preparations to duplicate the normal pattern of a patient's insulin production.

If more than one type of insulin is required to manage the patient's diabetes, you can mix two different types of insulin into one syringe if they are compatible. This may result in a patient response to insulin that is different than the response that would occur if the insulins had been given separately. Box 22-2 (p. 588) lists recommendations from the American Diabetes Association for mixing insulins.

Delegation Considerations

The skill of mixing medications from two vials or a vial and an ampule cannot be delegated to NAP. The nurse instructs the NAP about:

❑ Potential side effects of medications and the need to report their occurrence.

Equipment

❑ Single-dose or multidose vials and ampules containing medication
❑ Syringe and two needles
❑ Needles:
   • Blunt-tip vial access cannula (if needleless system is used)
   • Filter needle if indicated
   • Needle for drawing up medication (if needed) and needle for injection
❑ Alcohol swab
❑ Puncture-proof container for disposing of syringes, needles, and glass
❑ Medication administration record (MAR) or computer printout

Procedural Steps

1   Check accuracy and completeness of the MAR or computer printout with prescriber's written medication order. Check patient's name, medication name and dosage, route of administration, and time of administration. Recopy or re-print any portion of MAR that is difficult to read.

2   Review pertinent information related to medication, including action, purpose, side effects, and nursing implications.

3   Assess the patient's body build, muscle size, and weight if giving subcutaneous or IM medication.

4   Consider medications to be mixed, compatibility of medications, and type of injection.

5   Perform hand hygiene.

6   Check medication's expiration date printed on vial or ampule.

7   Prepare medication for one patient at a time following the six rights of medication administration (see Chapter 20). Select ampule or vial from the unit-dose drawer or automated dispensing system. Compare the label of each medication with the MAR or computer printout. In the case of insulin, ensure the correct types of insulin are prepared. *This is the first check for accuracy.*

8   Mixing medications from two vials:
   a   Take syringe with needleless access device or filter needle, and aspirate volume of air equivalent to first medication dose (vial A).
   b   Inject air into vial A, making sure needle or needleless access device does not touch solution (Fig. 22-12, A).
   c   Holding on to plunger, withdraw needle or needleless access device and syringe from vial A. Aspirate air equivalent to second medication dose (vial B) into syringe.
   d   Insert needle or needleless access device into vial B, inject volume of air into vial B, and then withdraw medication from vial B into syringe (Fig. 22-12, B).
   e   Withdraw needle or needleless access device and syringe from vial B. Ensure that proper volume has been obtained.
   f   Determine on syringe scale what the combined volume of medications should measure.
   g   Insert needle or needleless access device into vial A, being careful not to push plunger and expel medication within syringe into vial. Invert vial, and carefully withdraw the desired amount of medication from vial A into syringe (Fig. 22-12, C).
   h   Withdraw needle or needleless access device, and expel any excess air from syringe. Check fluid level in syringe for proper dose. Medications are now mixed.

> **Critical Decision Point**   *If too much medication is withdrawn from second vial, discard syringe and start over. Do not push medication back into either vial.*

   i   Change needle or needleless access device for appropriate-size needle if medication is being injected. Replace filter needle with needleless system or with appropriate-size needle according to route of medication. Keep needle or needleless device capped until administration time.

9   Mixing insulin:
   a   If patient takes insulin that is cloudy, roll the bottle of insulin between the hands to resuspend the insulin preparation.
   b   Wipe off tops of both insulin vials with alcohol swab.
   c   Verify insulin dose against MAR.
   d   If mixing rapid- or short-acting insulin with intermediate- or long-acting insulin, take insulin syringe and aspirate volume of air equivalent to dose to be withdrawn from intermediate- or long-acting insulin first (see illustration). If

PROCEDURAL GUIDELINE 22-1 Mixing Parenteral Medications in One Syringe—cont'd

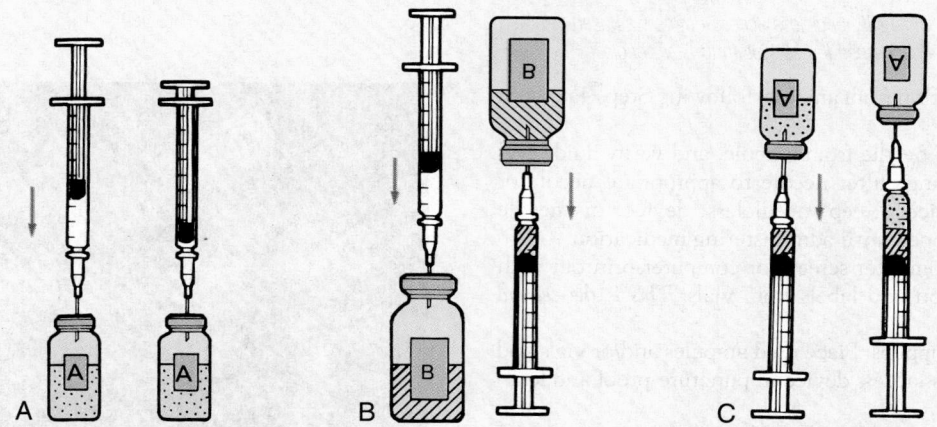

FIG 22-12 **A,** Injecting air into vial A. **B,** Injecting air into vial B and withdrawing dose. **C,** Withdrawing medication from vial A; medications are now mixed.

two intermediate- or long-acting insulins are mixed, it makes no difference which vial is prepared first.

> **Critical Decision Point** *If long-acting insulin glargine (Lantus) is ordered, note that this is a clear insulin that should not be mixed with other insulin preparations.*

e Insert needle, and inject air into vial of intermediate- or long-acting insulin. Do not let the tip of the needle touch solution.

f Remove the syringe from vial of insulin without aspirating medication.

g With the same syringe, inject air, equal to the dose of rapid- or short-acting insulin, into the vial and withdraw the correct dose into the syringe (see illustration).

h Remove the syringe from the rapid- or short-acting insulin, and remove any air bubbles to ensure accurate dose.

> **Critical Decision Point** *Some institutions require insulin doses to be verified by another nurse for accuracy. If indicated by institutional policy, have dose of clear insulin verified before proceeding with mixing of insulin at this time. Have dose verified a second time after the medications are mixed.*

i Verify short-acting insulin dosage with MAR, then show insulin prepared in syringe to another nurse to verify cor-

rect dosage of insulin was prepared. Then determine to which point on syringe scale combined units of insulin should measure by adding the number of units of both insulins together (e.g., 4 units Regular + 10 units NPH = 14 units total). Verify the combined dosage.

j Place the needle of the syringe back into the vial of intermediate- or long-acting insulin. Be careful not to push plunger and inject insulin in syringe into the vial.

k Invert the vial, and carefully withdraw the desired amount of insulin into syringe (see illustration, p. 588).

l Withdraw needle, and check fluid level in syringe. Keep needle of prepared syringe sheathed or capped until ready to administer medication.

> **Critical Decision Point** *Administer mixture of insulin within 5 minutes of preparation. Rapid- or short-acting insulin can bind with intermediate- or long-acting insulin, thus reducing the action of the more rapid-acting insulin (American Diabetes Association [ADA], 2007).*

10 Mixing medications from a vial and an ampule:

a Prepare medication from vial first, following Steps 5a to j in Skill 22-1.

b Determine on syringe scale what the combined volume of medications should measure.

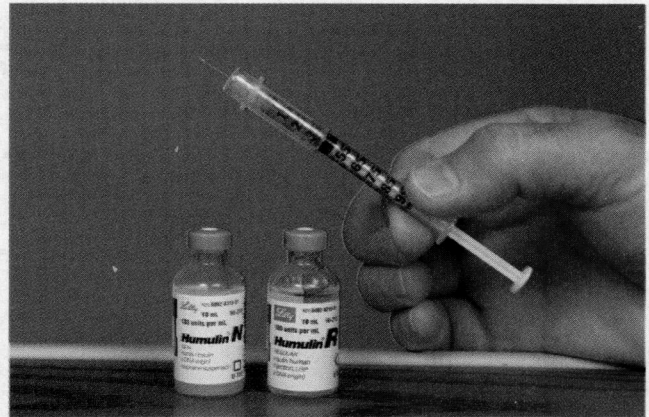

STEP 9d Vials of intermediate- or long-acting insulin and rapid- or short-acting insulin and syringe with air aspirated.

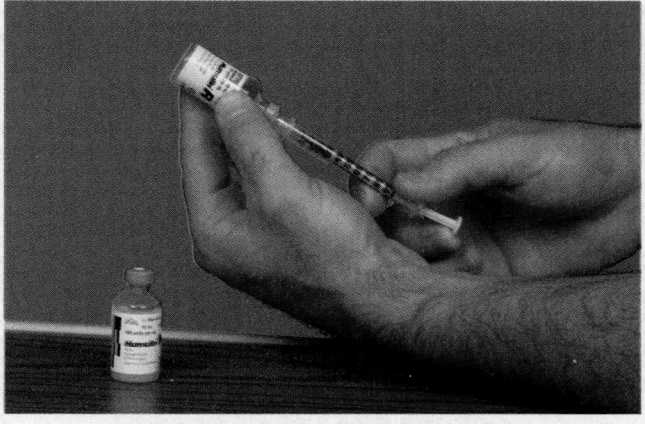

STEP 9g Withdrawal of short-acting insulin.

Continued

PROCEDURAL GUIDELINE 22-1　Mixing Parenteral Medications in One Syringe—cont'd

Critical Decision Point　*If needleless access device was used in preparing medication from vial, change needleless system to filter needle.*

 c　Prepare medication from ampule, following Steps 4a to k in Skill 22-1.

 d　Withdraw filter needle from ampule, and verify fluid level in syringe. Change filter needle to appropriate needle or needleless device. Keep needleless device or needle sheathed or capped until administering medication.

11　Compare MAR, computer screen, or computer printout with prepared medication and labels from vials. *This is the second check for accuracy.*

12　Dispose of soiled supplies. Place used ampules and/or vials and needle or needleless access device in puncture-proof and leak-proof container.

13　Clean work area, and perform hand hygiene.

14　Check syringe again carefully for total combined dose of medications.

15　*The third check for accuracy occurs at patient's bedside.*

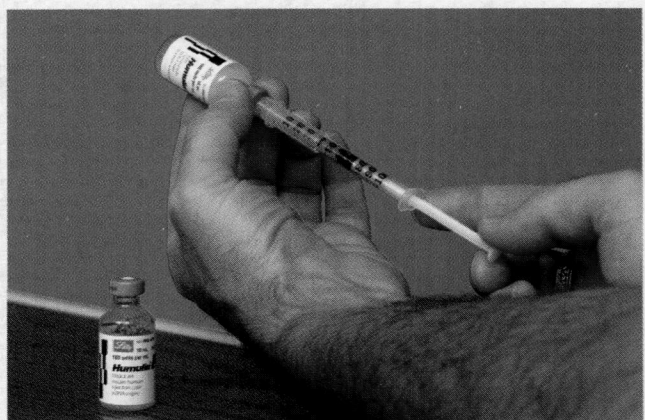

STEP 9k　Withdrawal of modified insulin.

BOX 22-2　Recommendations for Mixing Insulins

- Patients whose blood sugar levels are well controlled on a mixed-insulin dose maintain their individual routine when preparing and administering their insulin.
- Do not mix insulin with any other medications or diluents unless approved by the prescriber.
- Never mix insulin glargine (Lantus) or insulin detemir (Levemir) with any other types of insulin.

- Inject rapid-acting insulins mixed with NPH, Lente, or Ultralente insulins within 15 minutes before a meal.
- Do not mix short-acting and Lente insulins unless the patient's blood glucose levels are currently under control with this mixture.
- Do not mix phosphate-buffered insulins (e.g., NPH) with Lente insulins.

No-SS10168-TK. Copyright © 2004 *American Diabetes Care* 27:5106-5109, 2004. Reprinted with permission from the American Diabetes Association.

SKILL 22-2　Administering Intradermal Injections

 Advanced / Injections / Administering an Intradermal Injection

NSO　*Injections Module / Lesson 4*

A nurse typically gives intradermal injections for skin testing, for example, in tuberculin screening and allergy tests. Because such medications are potent, you inject them into the dermis, where blood supply is reduced and drug absorption occurs slowly. A patient may have an anaphylactic reaction if the medications enter the patient's circulation too rapidly. For patients with a history of numerous allergies, a physician may perform skin testing.

Skin testing often requires you to visually inspect the test site; therefore make sure intradermal sites are free of lesions and injuries and are relatively hairless. The inner forearm and upper back are ideal locations.

To administer an injection intradermally use a tuberculin or small syringe with a short (⅜ to ⅝ inch), fine-gauge (25 to 27) needle. The angle of insertion for an intradermal injection is 5 to 15 degrees (see Fig. 22-9). You inject only small amounts of medication (0.01 to 0.1 mL) intradermally. If a bleb does not appear, or if the site bleeds after needle withdrawal, the medication may have entered subcutaneous tissues. In this situation skin test results will not be valid.

Delegation Considerations

The skill of administering intradermal injections should not be delegated to NAP. The nurse directs the NAP about:

- Potential medication side effects and to report their occurrence to the nurse.
- Reporting any change the NAP notices in the patient's condition to the nurse.

Equipment

- ❏ 1-mL tuberculin syringe with preattached 25- or 27-gauge needle
- ❏ Small gauze pad
- ❏ Alcohol swab
- ❏ Vial or ampule of skin test solution
- ❏ Clean gloves
- ❏ Medication administration record (MAR) or computer printout
- ❏ Skin pencil (*optional*)

STEP	RATIONALE

ASSESSMENT

1 Check accuracy and completeness of the MAR or computer printout with prescriber's written medication order. Check patient's name, medication name and dosage, route of administration, and time of administration. Recopy or re-print any portion of MAR that is difficult to read.

The order sheet is the most reliable source and legal record of the patient's medications.
Ensures patient receives the correct medication.
Illegible MARs are a source of medication errors.

2 Review drug reference information about expected reaction when testing skin with specific allergen or medication and appropriate time to read site.

Type of reaction depends on patient's ability to mount a cell-mediated immune response. Knowledge of expected and adverse reactions to skin testing helps you determine what symptoms to monitor for, how frequently, and when to reassess patient.

3 Assess patient's history of allergies; know type of allergens and normal allergic reaction.

You do not administer any medication if there is a known patient allergy.

4 Assess patient's knowledge of purpose and response to skin testing.

Reveals patient teaching needs.

NURSING DIAGNOSES

- Anxiety
- Deficient knowledge regarding skin testing

- Fear

- Health-seeking behaviors regarding disease screening practices

Individualize related factors based on patient's condition or needs.

PLANNING

1 Expected outcomes following completion of procedure:
  - Patient experiences very mild burning sensation during injection but no discomfort after injection.

  Normal reaction to medication deposited in dermis.

  - Small, light-colored bleb approximately 6 mm (¼ inch) in diameter forms at site and gradually disappears. Minimal bruising may be present.

  Medication is in dermis and is eventually absorbed. Bruising is result of minor bleeding from capillaries.

  - Patient is able to identify signs of a skin reaction and their significance.

  Demonstrates learning.

IMPLEMENTATION

1 Perform hand hygiene. Prepare medication for one patient at a time following the six rights of medication administration (see Chapter 20). Compare label of the medication with the MAR or computer printout two times (see Skill 22-1) when preparing medication from ampules or vials in syringe.

Establishing a medication preparation routine, eliminating distractions, and double-checking the transcribed order reduce error (Pape and others, 2005; Ridge, 2007; Wolf, 2007). *First and second checks for accuracy ensure right medication administered.*

2 Take medication to patient at right time, and perform hand hygiene.

Ensures patient experiences effect of intradermal injection at correct time. Reduces transfer of microorganisms.

3 Close room curtain or door.

Provides privacy.

4 Verify patient's identity by using at least two patient identifiers. Compare patient's name and one other identifier, such as hospital identification number, with MAR. Ask patient to state name as a third identifier.

Complies with The Joint Commission requirements and improves medication safety. In most acute care settings, the patient's name and identification number on armband and MAR are used to identify patients (The Joint Commission [TJC], 2007).

5 Compare the label of the medication with the MAR one final time at the patient's bedside.

Comparison decreases risk for medication administration errors. *This is the third check for accuracy.*

6 Explain the procedure, and tell patient injection will cause a slight burning or stinging.

Helps minimize patient's anxiety.

7 Apply clean gloves.

Reduces transfer of organisms.

8 Select appropriate injection site. Inspect skin surface over sites for bruises, inflammation, or edema. Note lesions or discolorations of skin. Select site three to four finger widths below antecubital space and one hand width above wrist (Centers for Disease Control and Prevention [CDC], 2007). If forearm cannot be used, inspect the upper back. If necessary, use sites appropriate for subcutaneous injections (see Fig. 22-13, p. 592).

Intradermal injections sites need to be free of discoloration or hair so that you can see results of skin test and interpret them correctly (CDC, 2007).

STEP	RATIONALE
9 Assist patient to comfortable position. Have patient extend elbow and support it and forearm on flat surface.	Stabilizes injection site for easiest accessibility.
10 Cleanse site with an antiseptic swab. Apply swab at center of the site, and rotate outward in a circular direction for about 5 cm (2 inches).	Mechanical action of swab removes secretions containing microorganisms.
11 Hold swab or gauze between third and fourth fingers of nondominant hand.	Gauze or swab remains readily accessible when withdrawing needle.
12 Remove needle cap from needle by pulling it straight off.	Preventing needle touching sides of cap prevents contamination.
13 Hold syringe between thumb and forefinger of dominant hand with bevel of needle pointing up.	Smooth injection requires proper manipulation of syringe parts. With bevel up, you are less likely to deposit medication into tissues below dermis.
14 With nondominant hand, stretch skin over site with forefinger or thumb.	Needle pierces tight skin more easily.
15 With needle almost against patient's skin, insert it slowly at 5- to 15-degree angle until resistance is felt. Then advance needle through epidermis to approximately 3 mm (⅛ inch) below skin surface. Needle tip can be seen through skin (see illustration).	Ensures that needle tip is in dermis. Inaccurate results will be obtained if needle is not injected at correct angle and depth (CDC, 2007).
16 Inject medication slowly. Normally you feel resistance. If not, needle is too deep; remove and begin again.	Slow injection minimizes discomfort at site. Dermal layer is tight and does not expand easily when you inject solution.

Critical Decision Point   *It is not necessary to aspirate because dermis is relatively avascular.*

STEP	RATIONALE
17 While injecting medication, note that small bleb (approximately 6 mm [¼ inch]) resembling mosquito bite appears on skin surface (see illustration).	Bleb indicates you deposited medication in dermis.
18 After withdrawing needle apply alcohol swab or gauze gently over site.	Support of tissue around injection site minimizes discomfort during needle withdrawal. Dry gauze minimizes discomfort associated with alcohol on nonintact skin.
19 Touch lightly with gauze; even gentle pressure could displace medication. Do not massage site. Apply bandage to site if needed.	Massage damages underlying tissue. Massage of intradermal site may disperse medication into underlying tissue layers and alter test results.
20 Assist patient to comfortable position.	Gives patient sense of well-being.
21 Discard uncapped needle or needle enclosed in safety shield and attached syringe in puncture-proof and leak-proof receptacle.	Prevents injury to patients and health care personnel. Recapping needles increases risk for a needle-stick injury (Occupational Safety and Health Administration [OSHA], 2006).
22 Remove clean gloves, and perform hand hygiene.	Reduces transmission of microorganisms.
23 Stay with patient for several minutes, and observe for any allergic reactions.	Dyspnea, wheezing, and circulatory collapse are signs of severe anaphylactic reaction.

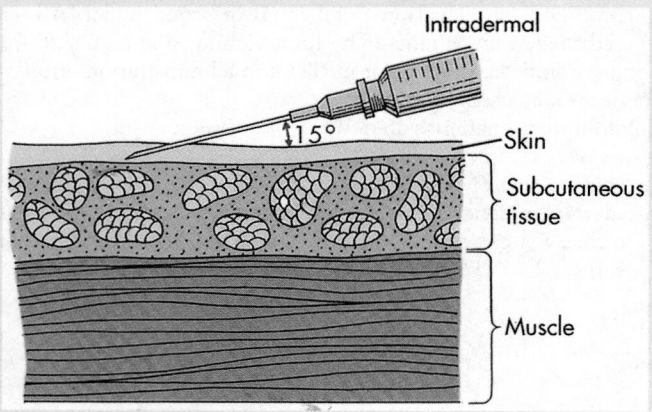

STEP 15   Intradermal needle tip inserted into dermis.

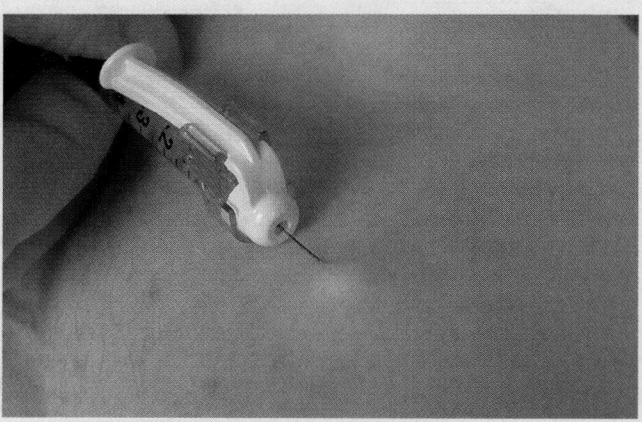

STEP 17   Injection creates small bleb.

STEP	**RATIONALE**

EVALUATION

1 Return to room in 15 to 30 minutes, and ask if patient feels any burning or stinging at injection site.

2 Ask patient to discuss implications of skin testing and signs of hypersensitivity.

3 Inspect bleb. *Optional:* Use skin pencil, and draw circle around perimeter of injection site. Read tuberculin (TB) test at 48 to 72 hours. Positive TB reaction is indicated by induration (hard, dense, raised area) of skin around injection site of:
- 15 mm or more in patients with no known risk factors for TB
- 10 mm or more in patients who are recent immigrants; injection drug users; residents and employees of high-risk settings; patients with certain chronic illnesses; children less than 4 years of age; and infants, children, and adolescents exposed to high-risk adults
- 5 mm or more in patients who are human immunodeficiency virus (HIV) positive, have fibrotic changes on chest x-ray film consistent with previous TB infection, have had organ transplants, or are immunosuppressed (CDC, 2007)

Rationale column:

Continued discomfort could indicate injury to underlying tissues.

Patient's ability to recognize signs of skin testing helps to ensure timely reporting of results.

Degree of reaction will vary based on patient condition.

Site must be read at various intervals to determine test results. Pencil marks make site easy to find. You determine the results of skin testing at various times, based on the type of medication used or the type of skin testing completed. Manufacturer's directions determine when to read the test results.

Unexpected Outcomes	Related Interventions
1 Raised, reddened, or hard zone (induration) forms around intradermal test site.	• Notify patient's health care provider. • Document sensitivity to injected allergen or positive test if tuberculin skin testing was completed.
2 Allergic reaction develops within minutes.	• Notify patient's health care provider. • Follow institutional policy or guidelines for appropriate response to allergic reactions (e.g., administration of antihistamine such as diphenhydramine [Benadryl] or epinephrine). • Add allergy information to patient's record.
3 Patient is unable to explain purpose or signs of skin testing.	• Provide further teaching. • Recognize patient is unable to learn at this time.

Recording and Reporting
- Immediately after administration, record amount and type of testing substance, site, time and date given on MAR. Correctly sign MAR according to institutional policy.
- Record area of intradermal injection and appearance of skin in your notes.
- Report any undesirable effects from medication to patient's health care provider, and document adverse effects according to institutional policy.
- Record adverse effects according to institutional policy.

Teaching Considerations
- Instruct patient not to squeeze medication out of injection site.
- Teach patients that negative skin tests may not rule out allergies, especially when low concentrations of medication are used.
- Patient should wear medical identification band listing all allergies.

- Caution patient not to wash off pencil markings around injection site.
- Explain to patient how to observe for skin reactions.

Pediatric Considerations
- Only administer amounts up to 0.1 mL intradermally to children (Hockenberry and Wilson, 2007).
- Children who are exposed to persons with confirmed or suspected infectious TB should be tested for TB immediately following exposure (Hockenberry and Wilson, 2007).
- Children who are exposed to high-risk individuals (e.g., HIV-infected, homeless, incarcerated) should be tested for TB every 2 to 3 years (Seleckman, 2006).

Gerontological Considerations
- The older adult has skin that is less elastic and must be held taut to ensure the intradermal injection is administered correctly.

SKILL 22-3   Administering Subcutaneous Injections

 Advanced / Injections / Administering a Subcutaneous Injection   NSO *Injections Module / Lesson 3*

Subcutaneous injections involve depositing medication into the loose connective tissue underlying the dermis. Because subcutaneous tissue is not as richly supplied with blood vessels as muscles are, medications are absorbed more slowly than with IM injections. Physical exercise or application of hot or cold compresses, which influences the rate of drug absorption, affects local blood flow to tissues. Any condition that impairs blood flow is a contraindication for subcutaneous injections.

You give subcutaneous medications in small doses of 0.5 to 1 mL. They are isotonic, nonirritating, nonviscous, and water soluble. Examples of subcutaneous medications include epinephrine, insulin, allergy medications, narcotics, and heparin. Because subcutaneous tissue contains pain receptors, the patient often experiences some discomfort.

The best subcutaneous injection sites include the outer aspect of the upper arms, the abdomen from below the costal margins to the iliac crests, and the anterior aspects of the thighs (Fig. 22-13). These areas are easily accessible, and are large enough to allow rotating multiple injections within each anatomical location.

Choose an injection site that is free of skin lesions, bony prominences, and large underlying muscles or nerves. Site rotation prevents the formation of lipohypertrophy or lipoatrophy in the skin. The patient's body weight and amount of adipose tissue indicate the depth of the subcutaneous layer. Therefore base the needle length and angle of needle insertion on the patient's weight and estimate of subcutaneous tissue. Generally a 25-gauge ⅝-inch needle inserted at a 45-degree angle (Fig. 22-14) or a ½-inch needle inserted at a 90-degree angle deposits medications into the subcutaneous tissue of a normal-size patient. A child usually requires a 26- to 30-gauge ½-inch needle inserted at a 90-degree angle (Hockenberry and Wilson, 2007). If the patient is obese, pinch the tissue and use a needle long enough to insert through the fatty tissue at the base of the skinfold. Thin patients sometimes have insufficient tissue for injections. Therefore the upper abdomen is the best injection site for patients with little peripheral subcutaneous tissue. To ensure a subcutaneous medication reaches subcutaneous tissue, use the following rule to determine the angle of injection: If you can grasp 5 cm (2 inches) of tissue, insert the needle at a 90-degree angle; if you can grasp 2.5 cm (1 inch) of tissue, insert the needle at a 45-degree angle (Rushing, 2004). Aspiration after an injection, including heparin and insulin, is not necessary. Piercing a blood vessel and causing a hematoma formation is rare (ADA, 2007; Annersten and Willman, 2005).

Injection pens are a new technology that patients can use to self-administer medications (e.g., epinephrine, insulin, or interferon) using the subcutaneous route (Fig. 22-15). This offers a convenient delivery method using prefilled, disposable cartridges. A patient pinches the skin, inserts the needle, and injects a predetermined medication dose. Teaching is essential to ensure patients use the correct injection technique and deliver the correct dose of medication. The disadvantages to this technology include increased risk for needle-stick injury, lack of knowledge and skill in administration technique, and inappropriate storage of device (Moshang, 2005; Pellissier and others, 2006; Shih-Wen, 2007).

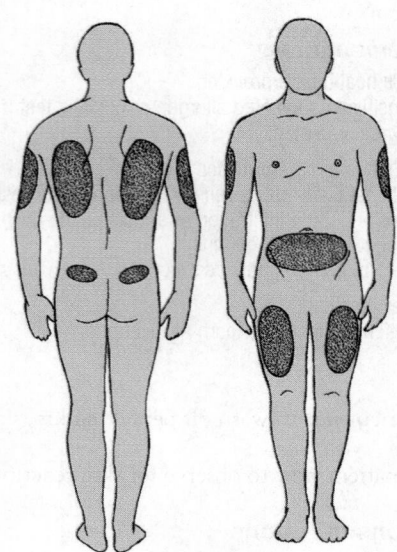

FIG 22-13   Common sites for subcutaneous injections.

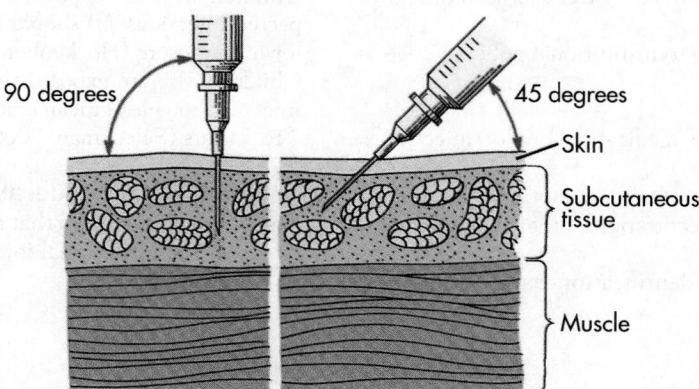

FIG 22-14   Subcutaneous injection. Angle and needle length depend on the thickness of skinfold.

SPECIAL CONSIDERATIONS FOR ADMINISTRATION OF INSULIN

 Advanced / Injections / Preparing Insulin

Insulin is the hormone used to treat diabetes mellitus. Patients often receive a combination of different types of insulin to control their blood glucose levels. Although inhaled insulin (Exubera) has been approved for use, most patients manage type 1 diabetes with insulin injections (Appel and Wright, 2007). Injection site rotation is no longer necessary because newer human insulins carry a lower risk for hypertrophy. Patients choose one anatomical area (e.g., the abdomen) and systematically rotate sites within that region, which maintains consistent insulin absorption from day to day. Absorption rates of insulin vary based on the injection site. Insulin is most quickly absorbed in the abdomen, followed by the arms, thighs, and buttocks (Ridge, 2007).

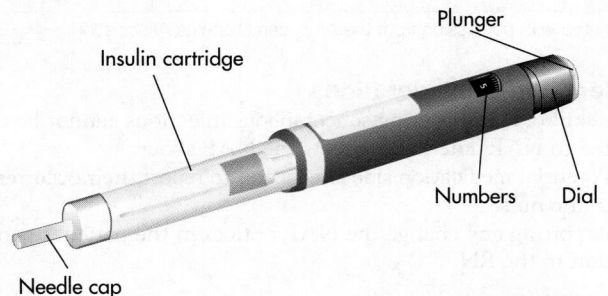

FIG 22-15 Injection pen. (*From Lewis and others*, Medical-surgical nursing: assessment and management of clinical problems, *ed 7*, St. Louis, 2007, Mosby.)

The timing of injections is critical to correct insulin administration. When planning insulin injection times, determine the current blood glucose level and when the patient will eat. Knowing the peak action and duration of the insulin protocol is essential when developing an effective diabetes management plan. Table 22-2 compares a variety of insulin preparations. Box 22-3 provides general guidelines for insulin administration.

SPECIAL CONSIDERATIONS FOR ADMINISTRATION OF HEPARIN

Heparin therapy provides therapeutic anticoagulation to reduce the risk for thrombus formation by suppressing clot formation. Therefore patients receiving heparin are at risk for bleeding, including bleeding gums, hematemesis, hematuria, or melena. Results from coagulation blood tests (e.g., activated partial thromboplastin time [aPTT] and partial thromboplastin time [PTT]) allow you to monitor the desired therapeutic range for IV heparin therapy.

Before administering heparin, assess for preexisting conditions that contraindicate the use of heparin, including threatened abortion, cerebral or aortic aneurysm, cerebrovascular hemorrhage, severe hypertension, blood dyscrasias, and recent ophthalmic surgery or neurosurgery. In addition, assess for conditions in which increased risk for hemorrhage is present: recent childbirth, severe diabetes, severe renal disease, liver disease, severe trauma, vasculitis, and active ulcers or lesions of the gastrointestinal (GI), genitourinary (GU), or respiratory tract. Obtain information about the patient's current medication regimen, including use of over-the-counter (OTC) and herbal medications (e.g., garlic, ginger, ginkgo, horse chestnut, or feverfew), for possible interaction with heparin. Other medications that interact with heparin include aspirin, nonsteroidal antiinflammatory drugs

TABLE 22-2	Comparison of Insulin Preparations		
Insulin Type	**Onset (Hours)**	**Peak Effect**	**Duration of Action**
Rapid-Acting (Clear)			
Insulin lispro (Humalog)	15 min	60-90 min	3-5 hr
Insulin aspart (NovoLog)	15 min	60-90 min	3-5 hr
Short-Acting (Clear)			
Regular human insulin* (e.g., Humulin R, Novolin R)	30-60 min	2-3 hrs	3-6 hr
Intermediate-Acting (Cloudy)			
NPH (Humulin N)	2-4 hr	4-10 hr	10-16 hr
NPH (Novolin N)	2-4 hr	4-10 hr	10-16 hr
Combination Insulins (Cloudy)			
Humulin 70/30 (70% NPH, 30% Regular)	30 min	2-12 hr	24 hr
Novolin 70/30 (70% NPH, 30% Regular)			
Humulin 50/50 (50% NPH, 50% Regular)	15 min	1 hr	24 hr
Humalog 75/25 (75% lispro protamine suspension/25% lispro)			
Long-Acting (Clear)			
Insulin detemir (Levemir) [†]	1-2 hr	No pronounced peak	24+ hr
Insulin glargine (Lantus) [†]	1-2 hr	No pronounced peak	24+ hr

Modified from McKenry LM and others: *Mosby's pharmacology in nursing*, ed 22, St. Louis, 2006, Mosby.
*Regular insulin is the only insulin for intravenous use; intravenously, the onset of action is within 10 to 30 minutes, peak effect within 20 to 30 minutes, and duration of action within 30 minutes to 1 hour.
[†]*Cannot* be mixed with other insulins.

BOX 22-3 | General Guidelines for Insulin Administration

- Store vials of insulin in the refrigerator. Keep vials of insulin currently in use at room temperature to reduce irritation at the injection site. Do not inject cold insulin.
- Inspect insulin vials before each use for changes in appearance (e.g., clumping, frosting, precipitation, change in clarity or color) as this indicates a loss in potency.
- Do not interchange insulin types unless approved by the patient's prescriber.
- The usual recommended interval between injection of short-acting insulin and a meal is 30 minutes.
- Preferred injection sites include the upper arm, anterior and lateral aspects of the thigh, buttocks, and abdomen, avoiding a 2-inch radius around the navel. Base site selection on anticipated rate of absorption. Insulin absorbs quickest in the abdomen, followed by the arms, thighs, and buttocks.
- Have the patient self-administer insulin whenever possible. Consider the child's developmental level when determining the appropriate age for self-administration. Generally, children begin self-administration of insulin by adolescence.

- Patients who use insulin need to self-monitor their blood sugars whenever possible.
- Various changes in patient status may require a different insulin dose. Information about blood glucose levels helps patients adjust their insulin dosage during times of illness or stress.
- All patients who take insulin should carry at least 15 g carbohydrate (e.g., 4 ounces juice, 8 ounces milk) to be eaten or taken in liquid form in the event of a hypoglycemic reaction. Monitor blood glucose levels.
- Teach significant others how to administer insulin and glucagon for situations in which the patient is unable to self-administer insulin or is unable to ingest oral carbohydrates during hypoglycemic reactions.

No-SS10168-TK. Copyright © 2004 *American Diabetes Care* 27:5106-5109, 2004. Reprinted with permission from the American Diabetes Association.

(NSAIDs), cephalosporins, antithyroid agents, probenecid, and thrombolytics.

You administer heparin subcutaneously or intravenously. Low-molecular-weight (LMW) heparins (e.g., enoxaparin) are more effective than heparin in some patients. The anticoagulant effects are more predictable (McKenry and others, 2006). LMW heparins have a longer half-life and require less laboratory monitoring but are expensive. These medications often come from the manufacturer in a prepared syringe (see manufacturer's guidelines). To minimize the pain and bruising associated with LMW heparin, it is given subcutaneously on the right or left side of the abdomen, at least 2 inches away from the umbilicus; this area is commonly referred to as a patient's "love handles" (Aventis, 2008). LMW heparin requires no dietary monitoring, and it has fewer hemorrhagic complications (Cranwell-Bruce, 2007).

Delegation Considerations

The skill of administering subcutaneous injections cannot be delegated to NAP. The nurse directs the NAP about:

- Potential medication side effects and to report their occurrence to the nurse.
- Reporting any change the NAP notices in the patient's condition to the RN.

Equipment

- ❑ Syringe (1 to 3 mL)
- ❑ Needle (25 to 27 gauge, ⅜ to ⅝ inch)
- ❑ Small gauze pad *(optional)*
- ❑ Alcohol swab
- ❑ Medication vial or ampule
- ❑ Clean gloves
- ❑ Medication administration record (MAR) or computer printout

STEP	RATIONALE

ASSESSMENT

1 Check accuracy and completeness of the MAR or computer printout with prescriber's written medication order. Check patient's name, medication name and dosage, route of administration, and time of administration. Recopy or re-print any portion of MAR that is difficult to read.

The order sheet is the most reliable source and legal record of the patient's medications.
Ensures patient receives the correct medication.
Illegible MARs are a source of medication errors.

2 Assess patient's medical and medication history.

Identifies need for medication.

3 Review medication reference information related to medication, including action, purpose, side effects, normal dose, rate of administration, time of peak onset, and nursing implications.

Knowledge of medication allows you to give medication safely and monitor patient's response to therapy.

4 Assess patient's history of allergies; know type of allergens, and normal allergic reaction.

Certain substances have similar compositions; it may harm patients to give a medication if there is a known allergy.

5 Observe patient's previous verbal and nonverbal responses toward injection.

Injections are sometimes painful. Anticipating patient's anxiety allows you to use distraction to reduce pain awareness.

6 Assess for contraindication to subcutaneous injections. Assess for factors such as circulatory shock or reduced local tissue perfusion.

Reduced tissue perfusion interferes with drug absorption and distribution.

7 Assess patient's symptoms before initiating medication therapy.

Provides information to evaluate desired effect of medication.

STEP	RATIONALE
8 Assess adequacy of patient's adipose tissue.	Physiological changes of aging or patient illness influences the amount of subcutaneous tissue a patient possesses. This influences methods for administering injections.
9 Assess patient's knowledge regarding medication to be received.	Poses implications for patient education.

NURSING DIAGNOSES

- Acute pain
- Anxiety

- Deficient knowledge regarding medication administration or drug therapy

- Fear
- Ineffective health maintenance

Individualize related factors based on patient's condition or needs.

PLANNING

1 Expected outcomes following completion of procedure:	
• Patient experiences no pain or mild burning at injection site.	Medications may cause minor tissue irritation.
• Patient achieves desired effect of medication with no signs of allergies or undesired effects.	Medication administered without patient injury.
• Patient explains purpose, dosage, and effects of medication.	Demonstrates learning.

IMPLEMENTATION

1 Perform hand hygiene. Prepare medication for one patient at a time following the six rights of medication administration (see Chapter 20). Compare label of the medication with the MAR or computer printout two times (see Skill 22-1) when removing ampules or vial from storage area and after preparing medication in syringe.	Establishing a medication preparation routine, eliminating distractions, and double-checking the transcribed order reduce error (Pape and others, 2005; Ridge, 2007; Wolf, 2007). *First and second checks ensure right medication is administered.*
2 Take medication to patient at right time, and perform hand hygiene.	Ensures patient experiences effect of injection at correct time. Reduces transfer of microorganisms.
3 Close room curtain or door.	Provides privacy.
4 Verify patient's identity by using at least two patient identifiers. Compare patient's name and one other identifier, such as hospital identification number, with MAR. Ask patient to state name as a third identifier.	Complies with The Joint Commission requirements to improve medication safety. In most acute care settings, the patient's name and identification number on armband and MAR are used to identify patients (TJC, 2007).
5 Compare the label of the medication with the MAR one final time at the patient's bedside.	Comparison decreases risk for medication administration errors. *This is the third check for accuracy.*
6 Explain the procedure, and tell patient injection will cause a slight burning or stinging.	Helps minimize patient's anxiety.
7 Apply clean gloves.	Reduces transfer of microorganisms.
8 Keep sheet or gown draped over body parts not requiring exposure.	Respects patient dignity during injection.
9 Select appropriate site for injection. Inspect skin surface over sites for bruises, inflammation, or edema.	Injection sites are free of abnormalities that interfere with drug absorption. Sites used repeatedly become hardened from lipohypertrophy (increased growth in fatty tissue). Do not use an area that is bruised or has signs associated with infection.
NOTE:	
• When administering heparin, use abdominal injection sites.	Anticoagulant causes local bleeding and bruising when injected into areas such as arms and legs.
• When administering LMW heparin, choose a site on the right or left side of the abdomen, at least 2 inches away from the umbilicus.	Injecting LMW heparin on the side of the abdomen will help decrease pain and bruising at the injection site (Aventis, 2008).
• When administering insulin, rotate the injection site within the same anatomical area (e.g., the abdomen) and systematically rotate sites within that area.	Rotating insulin sites within the same anatomical area helps maintain consistency in insulin absorption from day to day (ADA, 2004b).

Critical Decision Point   *Applying ice to the injection site for 1 minute before the injection may decrease the patient's perception of pain (Hockenberry and Wilson, 2007).*

10 Palpate for masses or tenderness. Be sure needle is correct size by grasping skinfold at site with thumb and forefinger. Measure fold from top to bottom. Make sure needle is one-half length of fold.	Subcutaneous injections can mistakenly be given into muscle, especially in the abdomen and thigh sites. Appropriate size of needle ensures that medication is injected into the subcutaneous tissue (Prettyman, 2005).

STEP	RATIONALE

11 Assist patient into comfortable position. Have patient relax arm, leg, or abdomen, depending on site selection.

Relaxation of site minimizes discomfort.

> **Critical Decision Point**   *Pain during insulin injections may be decreased by injecting room temperature insulin, allowing alcohol to dry before injecting insulin, relaxing muscles around the injection site, and injecting the needle quickly (ADA, 2007).*

12 Relocate injection site using anatomical landmarks.

Injection into correct anatomical site prevents injury to nerves, bone, and blood vessels.

13 Cleanse site with antiseptic swab. Apply swab at center of site, and rotate outward in circular direction for about 5 cm (2 inches) (see illustration).

Mechanical action of swab removes secretions containing microorganisms.

14 Hold swab or gauze between third and fourth fingers of nondominant hand.

Swab or gauze remains readily accessible withdrawing needle.

15 Remove needle cap by pulling it straight off.

Preventing needle touching sides of cap prevents contamination.

16 Hold syringe between thumb and forefinger of dominant hand, hold as dart, palm down (see illustration).

Quick, smooth injection requires proper manipulation of syringe parts.

17 Administer injection:

  a For average-size patient, pinch skin with nondominant hand.

Pinching skin elevates subcutaneous tissue and desensitizes area.

  b Inject needle quickly and firmly at 45- to 90-degree angle. Then release skin, if pinched. *Option:* When using injection pen or giving heparin, continue to pinch skin while injecting medicine.

Quick, firm insertion minimizes discomfort. (Injecting medication into compressed tissue irritates nerve fibers). Correct angle prevents accidental injection into muscle.

  c For obese patient, pinch skin at site and inject needle at 90-degree angle below tissue fold.

Obese patients have fatty layer of tissue above subcutaneous layer (Zaybak, 2007).

  d After needle enters site, grasp lower end of syringe barrel with nondominant hand to stabilize it. Move dominant hand to end of plunger, and slowly inject medication over 30 seconds (Zaybak and Khorshid, 2006) (see illustration). Avoid moving syringe. *Option:* While continuing to pinch skin, use dominant hand to inject medicine and release skin after injection.

Movement of syringe may displace needle and cause discomfort. Slow injection of medication minimizes discomfort.

> **Critical Decision Point**   *Aspiration after injecting a subcutaneous medication is not necessary. Piercing a blood vessel in a subcutaneous injection is very rare (Prettyman, 2005). Aspiration after injecting heparin and insulin is not recommended (ADA, 2004b).*

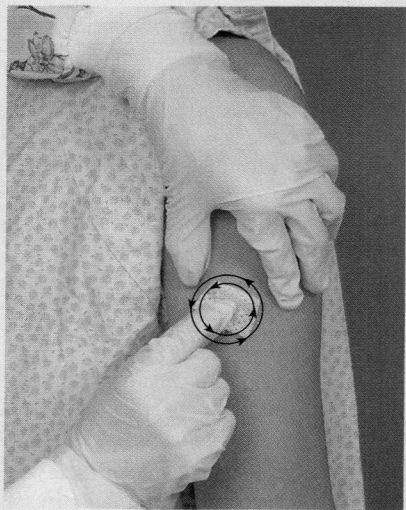

STEP 13   Cleansing site with circular motion.

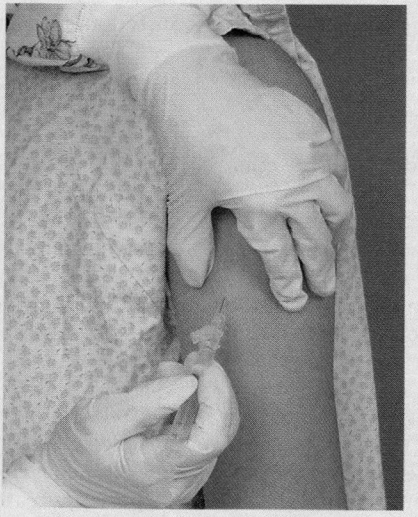

STEP 16   Holding syringe as if grasping a dart.

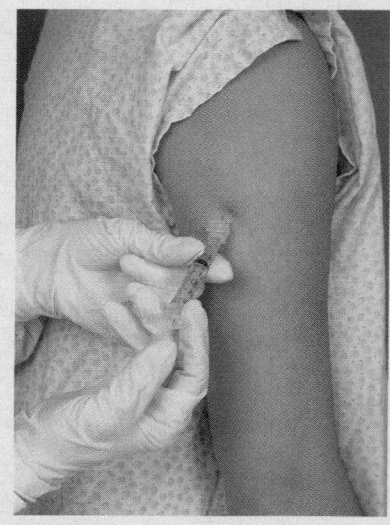

STEP 17(d)   Inject medication slowly.

STEP	RATIONALE

e Withdraw needle quickly while placing antiseptic swab or gauze gently over site.

Supporting tissues around injection site minimizes discomfort during needle withdrawal. Dry gauze may minimize patient discomfort associated with alcohol on nonintact skin.

18 Apply gentle pressure to site. *Do not massage site.* (If heparin is given, hold alcohol swab or gauze to site for 30 to 60 seconds.)

Aids absorption. Massage can damage underlying tissue. Time interval prevents bleeding at site.

19 Assist patient to comfortable position.

Gives patient a sense of well-being.

20 Discard uncapped needle or needle enclosed in safety shield (see illustrations) and attached syringe into a puncture-proof and leak-proof receptacle.

Prevents injury to patients and health care personnel. Recapping needles increases risk for a needle-stick injury (OSHA, 2006).

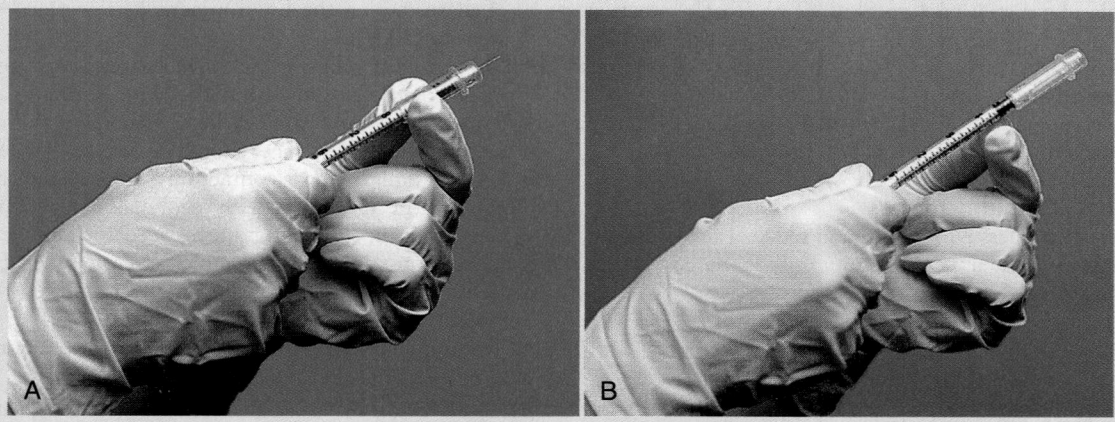

STEP 20   Needle with plastic guard to prevent needle sticks. **A,** Position of guard before injection. **B,** After injection the guard locks in place, covering the needle.

21 Remove clean gloves, and perform hand hygiene.

Reduces transmission of microorganisms.

22 Stay with patient for several minutes, and observe for any allergic reactions.

Dyspnea, wheezing, and circulatory collapse are signs of severe anaphylactic reaction.

EVALUATION

1 Return to room in 15 to 30 minutes, and ask if patient feels any acute pain, burning, numbness, or tingling at injection site.

Continued discomfort may indicate injury to underlying bones or nerves.

2 Inspect site, noting bruising or induration.

Bruising or induration indicates complication associated with injection. Provide warm compress to site.

3 Observe patient's response to medication at times that correlate with the medication's onset, peak, and duration.

Adverse effects of parenteral medications develop rapidly. Evaluate effect of medication based on the onset, peak, and duration of action.

4 Ask patient to explain purpose and effects of medication.

Evaluates patient's understanding of information taught.

Unexpected Outcomes	Related Interventions
1 Patient complains of localized pain, numbness, tingling, or burning at injection site.	• Assess injection site; may indicate potential injury to nerve or tissues. • Notify patient's health care provider, and do not reuse site.
2 Patient displays adverse reaction with signs of urticaria, eczema, pruritus, wheezing, and dyspnea.	• Monitor patient's heart rate, respirations, blood pressure, and temperature. • Follow institutional policy or guidelines for appropriate response to allergic reactions (e.g., administration of antihistamine such as diphenhydramine [Benadryl] or epinephrine), and notify patient's health care provider immediately. • Add allergy information to patient's record.
3 Hypertrophy of skin develops from repeated injection.	• Do not use site for future injections. • Instruct patient not to use site for 6 months.

Recording and Reporting

- Immediately after administration, record medication, dose, route, site, time, and date given on MAR. Correctly sign MAR according to institutional policy.
- Record patient's response to medication.
- Report any undesirable effects from medication to patient's health care provider, and document adverse effects in record.

Teaching Considerations

- Instruct patient to wear medical identification bracelet indicating important medical information, including bleeding tendencies, illnesses (e.g., diabetes) and allergies.
- Patients who require daily injections will need to learn techniques of self-administration (see Skill 42-6). Teach injection techniques to a family member or a significant other.

Pediatric Considerations

- Only administer amounts up to 0.5 mL subcutaneously to small children (Hockenberry and Wilson, 2007).

Gerontological Considerations

- Aging patients have less elastic skin and reduced subcutaneous skinfold thickness. The upper abdominal site is the best site to use when the patient has little subcutaneous tissue.

Home Care Considerations

- Improper disposal of used needles and sharps in the home setting poses a health risk to the public and waste workers. Several options for safe sharps disposal at home exist, including allowing patients to transport their own sharps containers from home to collection sites (e.g., doctor's office, a hospital, or a pharmacy); mailing their used syringes to a collection site (mailback programs); syringe exchange programs; or special devices that destroy the needle on the syringe, rendering it safe for disposal. If the patient cannot implement any of these options, have patient dispose of needles and other sharps in a hard plastic or metal container with a tightly sealed lid (e.g., empty detergent bottle or coffee can). Pamphlets for safe home disposal of sharps are on the Environmental Protection Agency (EPA) website (2007).
- Most insulin preparations have bacteriostatic properties that inhibit bacterial growth on the skin. Therefore patients with diabetes may reuse their syringes at home if they can safely recap the needles. Syringes should be discarded when the needles become dull, bent, or contact any surface other than the skin. Wiping the needle off with alcohol is not recommended, because the silicon coating on the needle is removed, making injections more painful. Immunocompromised patients and patients with poor personal hygiene, acute illness, or open hand wounds should not reuse syringes (ADA, 2007).
- Teach injection techniques that minimize patient discomfort.

SKILL 22-4   Administering Intramuscular Injections

 Advanced / Injections / Administering an Intramuscular Injection

NSO *Injections Module / Lesson 5*

The IM injection route deposits medication into deep muscle tissue, which has a rich blood supply, allowing medication to absorb faster than by the subcutaneous route. However, there is an increased risk for injecting drugs directly into blood vessels. Any factor that interferes with local tissue blood flow affects the rate and extent of drug absorption.

An IM injection requires a longer and larger-gauge needle to penetrate deep muscle tissue (see Fig. 22-9). The viscosity of the medication, injection site, patient's weight and amount of adipose tissue influence needle size selection. An obese patient requires a needle over 1½ inches, whereas a thinner patient only requires a ½- to 1-inch needle (Zaybak and Khorshid, 2007). Recommendations for needle length in average-size children include use of a

1-inch needle for infants, 1- to 1¼-inch needle in toddlers, and 1½- to 2-inch needle in older children. Based on the evidence, the recommendation for pediatric IM injection sites includes use of the anterolateral thigh for infants up to 12 months of age, deltoid in children 12 months and older, and ventrogluteal site for children of all ages (Cook and Murtagh, 2006; Hockenberry and Wilson, 2007).

Needle gauge is determined by the medication to be administered. Immunizations and parenteral medications in aqueous solutions should be administered with a 20- to 25-gauge needle. Medications that are viscous or in oil-based solution are administered with an 18- to 25-gauge needle. For children, a small-gauge needle (25- to 30-gauge) is used unless the medication is viscous.

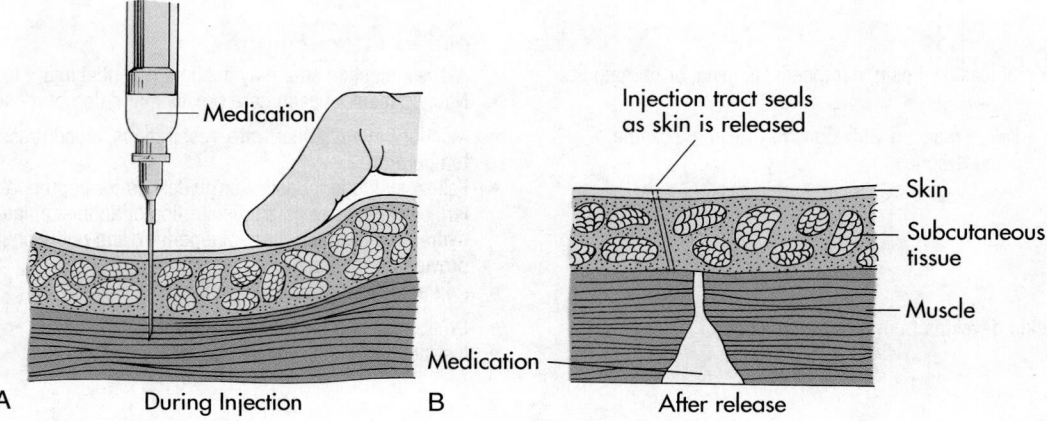

FIG 22-16   **A,** Pulling on overlying skin during IM injection moves tissue to prevent later tracking. **B,** The Z-track left after injection prevents the deposit of medication through sensitive tissue.

Administer IM injections so that the needle is perpendicular to the patient's body and as close to a 90-degree angle as possible (Cook and others, 2007). Intramuscular injection sites should also be rotated to decrease the risk for hypertrophy. Emaciated or atrophied muscles absorb medication poorly, so avoid their use when possible.

Muscle is less sensitive to irritating and viscous medication. A normal, well-developed adult can safely tolerate 2 to 5 mL of medication in larger muscles such as the ventrogluteal (Prettyman, 2005). However, clinically it is unusual to administer over 3 mL of medication in a single injection because the body does not absorb it well. Older adults and thin patients often tolerate only 2 mL in a single injection. The muscles of older infants and small children can tolerate 1 mL of medication in a single site. Larger muscles are often able to tolerate a maximum volume of 2 mL of medication (Hockenberry and Wilson, 2007).

The Z-track method is recommended for IM injections. The Z-track technique, pulling the skin laterally before injection, prevents leakage of medication into subcutaneous tissue, seals medication in the muscle, and minimizes irritation (Pullen, 2005). To use the Z-track method, apply the appropriate-size needle to the syringe, and select an IM site, preferably in a large, deep muscle, such as the ventrogluteal. Pull the overlying skin and subcutaneous tissues approximately 2.5 to 3.5 cm (1 to 1½ inches) laterally to the side with the ulnar side of the nondominant hand. Hold the skin in this position until you have administered the injection. After cleansing the site, inject the needle deeply into the muscle. If there is no blood return on aspiration, slowly inject the medication. Keep the needle inserted for 10 seconds to allow the medication to disperse evenly. Then release the skin after withdrawing the needle. This leaves a zigzag path that seals the needle track wherever tissue planes slide across each other (Fig. 22-16). The medication is sealed in the muscle tissue.

INJECTION SITES

When selecting an IM site, determine that the site is free of pain, infection, necrosis, bruising, and abrasions. Also consider the location of underlying bones, nerves, and blood vessels and the volume of medication you will administer. Because of the sciatic nerve location, the dorsogluteal muscle is not recommended as an injection site. If a needle hits the sciatic nerve, the patient may experience partial or permanent paralysis of the leg (Cook and Murtagh, 2006; Ramtahal and others, 2007; Small, 2004).

VENTROGLUTEAL SITE

The ventrogluteal site involves the gluteus medius and minimus and is a safe injection site for adults and children (Greenway, 2006; Hockenberry and Wilson, 2007). Research has shown that injuries such as fibrosis, nerve damage, abscess, local induration, hematoma, tissue necrosis, muscle contraction, gangrene, and pain are associated with all the common IM sites except the ventrogluteal site (Cook and Murtagh, 2006; Prettyman, 2005).

To locate the ventrogluteal site, place the heel of the hand over the greater trochanter of the patient's hip with the wrist almost perpendicular to the femur. Use the right hand for the left hip, and the left hand for the right hip. Point the thumb toward the patient's groin, the index finger points to the anterior superior iliac spine, and extend the middle finger back along the iliac crest toward the buttock. The index finger, the middle finger, and the iliac crest form a V-shaped triangle. The injection site is the center of the triangle (Fig. 22-17). To relax this site, patients lie on their side or back, flexing the knee and hip.

VASTUS LATERALIS MUSCLE

The vastus lateralis muscle is another injection site used in adults and is the preferred site for administration of biologicals (e.g., immunizations) to infants, toddlers, and children (Hockenberry and Wilson, 2007). The muscle is thick and well developed and is located on the anterior lateral aspect of the thigh. It extends in an adult, from a handbreadth above the knee to a handbreadth below the greater trochanter of the femur (Fig. 22-18). Use the middle third of the muscle for injection. The width of the muscle usually extends from the midline of the thigh to the midline of the thigh's outer side. With young children or cachectic patients, it helps to grasp the body of the muscle during injection to be sure that the medication is deposited in muscle tissue. To help relax the muscle, ask the patient to lie flat with the knee slightly flexed and foot externally rotated or assume a sitting position.

DELTOID MUSCLE

Although the deltoid site is easily accessible, the muscle is not well developed in many adults. There is potential for injury because the axillary, radial, brachial, and ulnar nerves and the brachial artery lie within

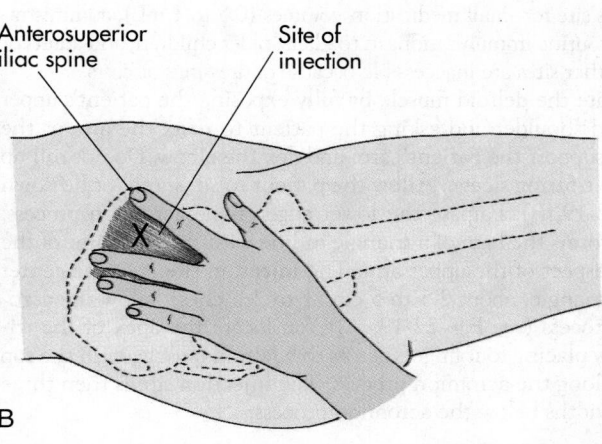

FIG 22-17   A, Injection at the ventrogluteal site avoids major nerves and blood vessels. **B,** Anatomical view of ventrogluteal injection site.

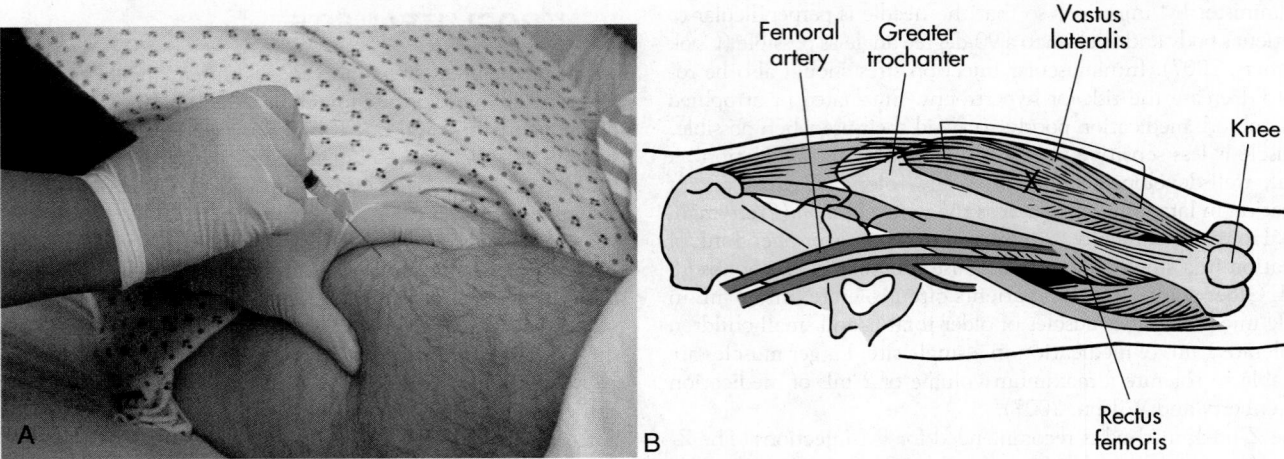

FIG 22-18 **A,** Giving IM injection in vastus lateralis site. **B,** Landmarks for vastus lateralis site.

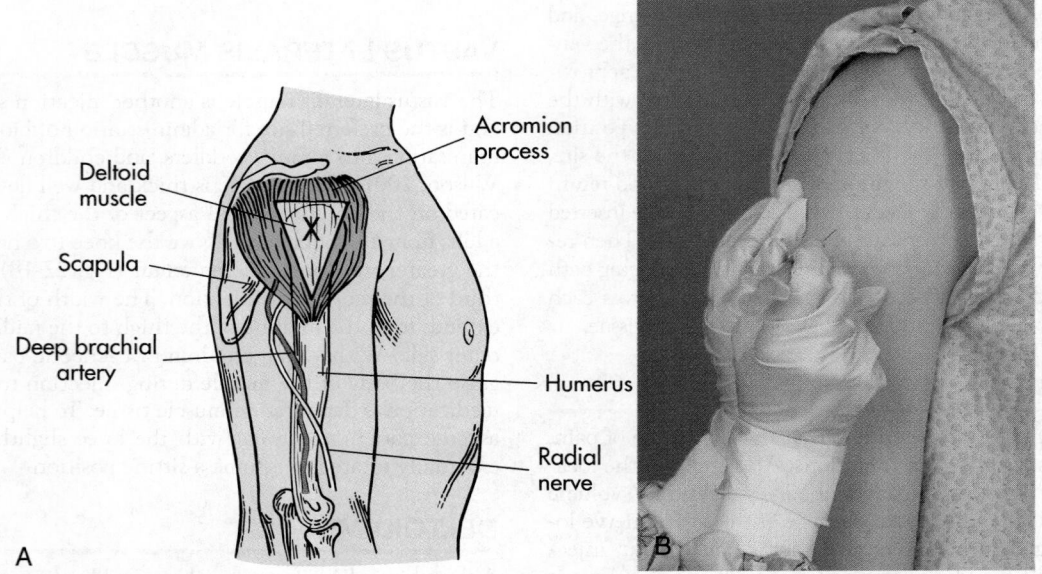

FIG 22-19 **A,** Landmarks for deltoid site. **B,** Giving IM injection in deltoid site.

the upper arm under the triceps and along the humerus (Fig. 22-19, A). Use this site for small medication volumes (0.5 to 1 mL), administration of routine immunizations in toddlers, older children, and adults or when other sites are inaccessible because of dressings or casts.

Locate the deltoid muscle by fully exposing the patient's upper arm and shoulder and asking the patient to relax the arm at the side or support the patient's arm and flex the elbow. Do not roll up any tight-fitting sleeve. Allow the patient to sit, stand, or lie down (Fig. 22-19, B). Palpate the lower edge of the acromion process, which forms the base of a triangle in line with the midpoint of the lateral aspect of the upper arm. The injection site is in the center of the triangle, about 2.5 to 5 cm (1 to 2 inches) below the acromion process (see Fig. 22-19, A). You locate the apex of the triangle by placing four fingers across the deltoid muscle, with the top finger along the acromion process. The injection site is then three finger widths below the acromion process.

Delegation Considerations
The skill of administering subcutaneous injections cannot be delegated to NAP. The nurse directs the NAP about:

- Potential medication side effects and to report their occurrence to the nurse.
- Reporting any change the NAP notices in the patient's condition to the RN.

Equipment
❑ Proper-size syringe and needle:
  - 2 to 3 mL for adult
  - 0.5 to 1 mL for infants and small children
❑ Needle length corresponds to site of injection, age of patient, and body size according to the following guidelines:
  - Infants and children: 1 inch
  - Vastus lateralis (adults): ½ to 2 inches
  - Deltoid (adults): ½ to 1½ inches
  - Ventrogluteal (adults): ½ to 2 inches
❑ Alcohol swab
❑ Small gauze pad
❑ Vial or ampule of medication
❑ Clean gloves
❑ Medication administration record (MAR) or computer printout

STEP	RATIONALE

ASSESSMENT

1 Check accuracy and completeness of the MAR or computer printout with prescriber's written medication order. Check patient's name, medication name and dosage, route of administration, and time of administration. Recopy or re-print any portion of MAR that is difficult to read.

> The order sheet is the most reliable source and legal record of the patient's medications.
> Ensures patient receives the correct medication.
> Illegible MARs are a source of medication errors.

2 Assess patient's medical and medication history.

> Identifies need for medication.

3 Review medication reference information related to medication, including action, purpose, side effects, normal dose, rate of administration, time of peak onset, and nursing implications.

> Knowledge of medication allows you to give medication safely and monitor patient's response to therapy.

4 Assess patient's history of allergies, type of allergens, and normal allergic reaction.

> Certain substances have similar compositions; it may harm patients to give a medication if there is a known allergy.

5 Observe patient's previous verbal and nonverbal responses toward injections.

> Injections are sometimes painful. Anticipating patient's anxiety allows you to use distraction to reduce pain awareness.

6 Assess for contraindications for IM injections. Assess for factors such as muscle atrophy, reduced blood flow, or circulatory shock.

> Atrophied muscle absorbs medication poorly. Factors interfering with blood flow to muscles impair drug absorption (McKenry and others, 2006).

7 Assess patient's symptoms before initiating medication therapy.

> Provides information for nurse to evaluate the desired effects of medication.

Critical Decision Point *Because of the documented adverse effects of IM injections, other routes of medication injection are preferred. Consider contacting health care provider for alternative route of medication administration (Prettyman, 2005; WHO, 2007).*

8 Assess patient's knowledge regarding medication to be received.

> Poses implications for patient education.

NURSING DIAGNOSES

- Acute pain
- Anxiety
- Deficient knowledge regarding medication administration or drug therapy
- Fear

Individualize related factors based on patient's condition or needs.

PLANNING

1 Expected outcomes following completion of procedure:
- Patient experiences no pain or mild burning at injection site.

> Medications may cause minor tissue irritation.

- Patient achieves desired effect of medication with no signs of allergies or undesired effects.

> Medication administered without patient injury.

- Patient explains purpose, dosage, and effects of medication.

> Demonstrates learning.

IMPLEMENTATION

1 Perform hand hygiene. Prepare medication for one patient at a time following the six rights of medication administration (see Chapter 20). Compare label of the medication with the MAR or computer printout two times (see Skill 22-1) when using ampules or vials from storage area and after drawing up medication in syringe.

> Establishing a medication preparation routine, eliminating distractions, and double-checking the transcribed order reduce error (Pape and others, 2005; Ridge, 2007; Wolf, 2007). *First and second checks for accuracy ensures right medication is administered.*

2 Take medication to patient at right time, and perform hand hygiene.

> Ensures patient experiences effect of injection at correct time.
> Reduces transfer of microorganisms.

3 Close room curtain or door.

> Provides privacy.

4 Verify patient's identity by using at least two patient identifiers. Compare patient's name and one other identifier, such as hospital identification number, with MAR. Ask patient to state name as a third identifier.

> Complies with The Joint Commission requirements to improve medication safety. In most acute care settings, the patient's name and identification number on armband and MAR are used to identify patients (TJC, 2007).

5 Compare the label of the medication with the MAR one final time at the patient's bedside.

> Comparison decreases risk for medication administration errors. *This is the third check for accuracy.*

6 Explain the procedure, and tell patient injection will cause a slight burning or stinging.

> Helps minimize patient's anxiety.

7 Apply clean gloves.

> Reduces transfer of microorganisms.

STEP	RATIONALE
8 Keep sheet or gown draped over body parts not requiring exposure.	Respects patient's dignity while exposing injection site.
9 Select appropriate site for injection. Inspect skin surface over sites for bruises, inflammation, or edema.	Injection sites are free of abnormalities that interfere with drug absorption. Sites used repeatedly become hardened from lipohypertrophy (increased growth in fatty tissue). Do not use an area that is bruised or has signs associated with infection.
10 Note integrity and size of muscle, and palpate for tenderness or hardness. Avoid these areas. If patient receives frequent injections, rotate sites.	The ventrogluteal site is preferred injection site for adults and children, including infants receiving irritating or viscous solutions (Cook and Murtagh, 2006; Hockenberry and Wilson, 2007; Small, 2004).
11 Assist patient to comfortable position. Position patient depending on chosen site (e.g., sit, lie flat, on side, or prone).	Reduces strain on muscle and minimizes injection discomfort.

Critical Decision Point   *Ensure that medical condition (e.g., circulatory shock) does not contraindicate patient's position for injection.*

STEP	RATIONALE
12 Relocate injection site using anatomical landmarks.	Injection into correct anatomical site prevents injury to nerves, bone, and blood vessels.
13 Cleanse site with antiseptic swab. Apply swab at center of site, and rotate outward in circular direction for about 5 cm (2 inches).	Mechanical action of swab removes secretions containing microorganisms.
Optional: Use a vapocoolant spray (e.g., ethyl chloride) just before injection.	Decreases pain at injection site.
14 Hold swab or gauze between third and fourth fingers of nondominant hand.	Swab or gauze remains readily accessible for use when withdrawing needle.
15 Remove needle cap by pulling it straight off.	Preventing needle from touching sides of cap prevents contamination.
16 Hold syringe between thumb and forefinger of dominant hand; hold as dart, palm down.	Quick, smooth injection requires proper manipulation of syringe parts.
17 Administer injection.	
a Position ulnar side of nondominant hand just below site and pull skin laterally approximately 2.5 to 3.5 cm. Hold position until medication is injected. With dominant hand, inject needle quickly at 90-degree angle into muscle.	Z-track creates zigzag path through tissues that seals the needle track to avoid tracking medication. A quick dartlike injection reduces discomfort. Z-track injections can be used for all IM injections (Pullen, 2005).
b *Optional:* If patient's muscle mass is small, grasp body of muscle between thumb and forefingers.	Ensures that the medication reaches the muscle mass (Cook and others, 2007; Hockenberry and Wilson, 2007).
c After needle pierces skin, use thumb and forefinger of nondominant hand to hold syringe barrel while still pulling on skin. Move dominant hand to end of plunger. Avoid moving syringe.	Stabilizes syringe. Smooth manipulation of syringe reduces discomfort from needle movement. Skin remains pulled until after medication is injected to ensure Z-track administration.
d Pull back on plunger 5 to 10 seconds. If no blood appears, inject medication slowly at a rate of 1 mL/10 sec.	Aspiration of blood into syringe indicates possible placement into a vein. Slow injection reduces pain and tissue trauma.

Critical Decision Point   *If blood appears in syringe, remove needle, dispose of medication and syringe properly, and prepare another dose of medication for injection.*

STEP	RATIONALE
e Wait 10 seconds, then smoothly and steadily withdraw needle, release skin, and apply alcohol swab or gauze gently over site.	Allows time for medication to absorb into muscle before syringe is removed. Dry gauze minimizes discomfort associated with alcohol on nonintact skin.
18 Apply gentle pressure to site. Do not massage site. Apply bandage if needed.	Massage damages underlying tissue.
19 Assist patient to comfortable position.	Gives patient sense of well-being.
20 Discard uncapped needle or needle enclosed in safety shield and attached syringe into a puncture-proof and leak-proof receptacle.	Prevents injury to patients and health care personnel. Recapping needles increases risk for a needle-stick injury (OSHA, 2006).
21 Remove clean gloves, and perform hand hygiene.	Reduces transmission of microorganisms.

STEP	RATIONALE
22 Stay with patient for several minutes, and observe for any allergic reactions.	Dyspnea, wheezing, and circulatory collapse are signs of severe anaphylactic reaction.

EVALUATION

1 Return to room in 15 to 30 minutes, and ask if patient feels any acute pain, burning, numbness, or tingling at injection site.	Continued discomfort may indicate injury to underlying bones or nerves.
2 Inspect site; note any bruising or induration.	Bruising or induration indicates complication associated with injection. Document findings, and notify health care provider. Apply warm compress to site.
3 Observe patient's response to medication at times that correlate with the medication's onset, peak, and duration.	Intramuscular medications are absorbed rapidly. Adverse effects of parenteral medications develop rapidly. Evaluate effect of medication based on the medication's onset, peak, and duration of actions.
4 Ask patient to explain purpose and effects of medication.	Evaluates patient's understanding of information taught.

Unexpected Outcomes	Related Interventions
1 Patient complains of localized pain or continued burning at injection site, indicating potential injury to nerve or vessels.	• Assess injection site. • Notify patient's health care provider.
2 During injection, blood is aspirated.	• Immediately stop injection, and remove needle. • Prepare new syringe of medication for administration.
3 Patient displays adverse reaction with signs of urticaria, eczema, pruritus, wheezing, and dyspnea.	• Follow institutional policy or guidelines for appropriate response to allergic reactions (e.g., administration of antihistamine such as diphenhydramine [Benadryl] or epinephrine). • Notify patient's health care provider immediately. • Add allergy information to patient's record.

Recording and Reporting

- Immediately after administration, record medication, dose, route, site, time, and date given on MAR. Correctly sign MAR according to institutional policy.
- Record patient's response to medication.
- Report any undesirable effects from medication, to patient's health care provider, and document adverse effects in record.

Teaching Considerations

- Patients who require regular injections (e.g., vitamin B_{12}) will need to learn techniques of self-administration. Teach a family member or significant other injection techniques and the importance of rotating sites to decrease the risk for hypertrophy.
- Instruct patient and family member or significant other to observe injection sites for complications and to immediately report complications to a health care provider.
- Instruct patient and family member or significant other to observe for effectiveness of medication and adverse reactions and report ineffectiveness of medication and adverse reactions to the health care provider.
- Have patient perform several return demonstrations of medication preparation to validate learning has taken place.

Pediatric Considerations

- Children can be very anxious or fearful of needles. Assistance with proper positioning and holding of the child is

sometimes necessary. Distraction, such as blowing bubbles and pressure at the injection site before giving the injection, can help alleviate the child's anxiety (Schechter and others, 2007).

- If possible, apply EMLA cream on injection site at least 2½ hours before IM injection or use a vapocoolant spray (e.g., ethyl chloride) just before injection to decrease pain (Hockenberry and Wilson, 2007).

Gerontological Considerations

- Older patients may have decreased muscle mass, which reduces drug absorption from IM injections. In addition, older adults may have loss of muscle tone and strength that impairs mobility, placing them at high risk for falls from guarding an injection site (Prettyman, 2005).

Home Care Considerations

- Self-administration of an IM injection is difficult, especially in the vastus lateralis. Teach a significant other to identify and administer injections in this site.
- Instruct adult patients who require frequent injections to apply EMLA cream to the injection site before administration.
- Patients will need instruction in safe disposal of syringes and needles (see Skill 22-3, Home Care Considerations).
- See Skill 42-1 for information about modifying safety risks in the home.

SKILL 22-5   Adding Medications to Intravenous Fluid Containers

Advanced / Intravenous Medication Administration / Adding Medications to Intravenous Fluid Containers

NSO   *IV Medication Administration Module / Lessons 1 and 4*

Nurses administer IV medication by direct injection into a vein or through a large volume IV infusion. IV medication enters the bloodstream directly, producing a rapid response. It is essential to observe patients closely for symptoms of adverse reactions. Avoid errors in administration by verifying the dose calculation, rate of administration, and drug preparation. Follow the six rights of safe drug administration, know the desired action and potential side effects of each medication, and document the medication according to agency policy. If the medication has an antidote or antagonist, have it available during medication administration. Some medications require assessment of vital signs before, during, and after the IV infusion.

Mixing medications in large volumes of fluids is the safest and easiest method of administration. For adults, medications are diluted in large volumes of 500 to 1000 mL of compatible IV fluids, such as normal saline or lactated Ringer's solution. Although nurses mixed medications commonly in the past, this practice is no longer supported on a routine basis (TJC, 2008; UPA, 2006). Safety risks include inaccurate calculations and nonaseptic preparation. Preparation of IV medications in IV fluids is now usually done by a manufacturer or pharmacist. Nurses should add medications to IV fluid containers only in emergent situations. Vitamins and potassium chloride are two types of medications commonly added to IV fluids. Never add high-alert medications (e.g., heparin, dopamine, nitroglycerin, or potassium). Verify any medications you add to IV fluids with another nurse. Do not add IV medications to IV bags that are already hanging. Add medications only to new IV fluid containers.

Some parenteral medications are alkaline and irritating to muscle and subcutaneous tissue, so administering them via the IV route minimizes discomfort. Administer IV medications by the following methods:

1 As a mixture within large volumes of IV fluids
2 By piggyback infusion of a solution containing the prescribed medication and a small volume of IV fluid through an adjoining container or existing IV line (see Skill 22-6)

3 By a volume-control device, in which a small container, holding 50 to 150 mL of fluid, is attached below the primary infusion bag (see Skill 22-6)
4 By electronic infusion devices (see Skill 22-6)
5 By injection of a bolus or small volume of medication through an existing IV infusion line or intermittent venous access (heparin or saline lock) (see Skill 22-7)

In all methods, the patient has either an existing IV infusion line or an IV site (heparin or saline lock) that is accessed at prescribed intervals for infusion. In most agencies, policies and procedures identify the medications that nurses can administer intravenously.

Delegation Considerations
The skill of adding medications to IV fluid containers cannot be delegated to NAP. The nurse directs the NAP about:
- Potential medication actions and side effects of the medications and to report their occurrence to the nurse.
- Reporting any change the NAP notices in the patient's condition to the nurse.
- Reporting any patient complaints of moisture or discomfort around IV insertion site to the nurse.

Equipment
- ❑ Vial or ampule of prescribed medication
- ❑ Syringe of appropriate size (1 to 20 mL)
- ❑ Sterile needle (19 to 21 gauge, 1 to 1½ inch) with special filters, only if needleless syringe not available
- ❑ Correct diluent if indicated (e.g., sterile water, 0.9% sodium chloride)
- ❑ Sterile IV fluid container (bag or bottle, 25 to 1000 mL in volume)
- ❑ Alcohol or antiseptic swab
- ❑ Label to attach to IV bag or bottle
- ❑ Medication administration record (MAR) or computer printout

STEP	RATIONALE

ASSESSMENT

1 Check accuracy and completeness of each MAR or computer printout with prescriber's written medication order. Check patient's name, medication name, dosage, route of administration, and time for administration. Recopy or re-print any portion of MAR that is difficult to read.

The order sheet is the most reliable source and only legal record of medications patient is to receive.
Ensures patient receives the correct medications.
Illegible MARs are a source of medication errors.

2 Assess patient's medical and medication history.
3 Review medication reference information including action, purpose, side effects, normal dose, rate of administration, time of peak onset, and nursing implications.

Identifies need for medication
Allows nurse to give medication safely and to monitor patient's response to therapy.

4 When adding more than one medication to IV solution, assess for compatibility of medications. Check institutional reference for drug compatibility list.

Some medications are incompatible when mixed together. Chemical reactions that occur result in clouding or crystallization of IV fluids.

5 Assess patient's systemic fluid balance, as reflected by skin hydration and turgor, body weight, pulse, and blood pressure.

In continuous IV infusions there is danger that fluids may infuse too rapidly, causing circulatory overload, especially in older adults and children (Hockenberry and Wilson, 2007; Rosenthal, 2007).

6 Assess patient's history of medication allergies; know type of allergens and normal allergic reaction.

IV administration of medications may cause rapid response. Allergic response is immediate.

7 Assess patient's symptoms before initiating medication therapy.

Provides information to evaluate the desired effects of medication.

8 Perform hand hygiene.

Reduces transfer of microorganisms

STEP	RATIONALE
9 Assess IV insertion site for signs of infiltration or phlebitis (see Chapter 28). Assess patency of existing IV infusion line.	An intact, properly functioning site ensures that medication is given safely. Presence of complication will require IV to be restarted.
10 Assess patient's understanding of purpose of medication therapy.	Poses implications for patient education.

NURSING DIAGNOSES

- Deficient knowledge regarding medication therapy
- Risk for imbalanced fluid volume

Individualize related factors based on patient's condition or needs.

PLANNING

1 Expected outcomes following completion of this procedure:
   - Patient experiences no medication side effects or adverse reactions.
   - Patient develops no signs or symptoms of fluid volume excess.
   - IV site is free of swelling, inflammation, or pain.
   - Patient explains purpose and side effects of medication.

Medication prepared and administered safely with therapeutic effect achieved.
IV rate is correctly maintained.
IV fluid was delivered without infusion site complications.
Demonstrates learning.

IMPLEMENTATION

STEP	RATIONALE
1 Perform hand hygiene. Prepare medication for one patient at a time following the six rights of medication administration (see Chapter 20). Compare label of the medication with the MAR or computer printout two times (see Skill 22-1) when removing ampules or vials from storage area and after drawing up medication in syringe.	Ensures correct medication is given to patient. Establishing a medication preparation routine, eliminating distractions, and double-checking the transcribed order reduce error (Pape and others, 2005; Ridge, 2007; Wolf, 2007). *First and second checks for accuracy ensure right medication is administered.*
2 Add medication to new container (usually done in medication room or at medication cart):	Reduces transfer of microorganisms.
a *Solution in a bag:* Locate medication injection port on plastic IV solution bag. Port has small rubber stopper at end. Do not select port for IV tubing insertion or air vent.	Medication injection port on plastic IV bag is self-sealing to prevent introduction of microorganisms after repeated use.
b *Solution in bottles:* Locate injection site on IV solution bottle, which is often covered by a metal or plastic cap.	Accidental injection of medication through main tubing port or air vent alters pressure within bottle and cause fluid leaks through air vent. Cap seals bottle to maintain its sterility.
c Wipe off port or injection site with alcohol or antiseptic swab (see illustration).	Reduces risk for introducing microorganisms into bag during needle insertion.
d Remove needle cap from syringe, and insert needleless cannula needle of syringe through center of injection port or site; inject medication (see illustration).	Insertion of needle into sides of port or site may produce a leak, which leads to fluid contamination.

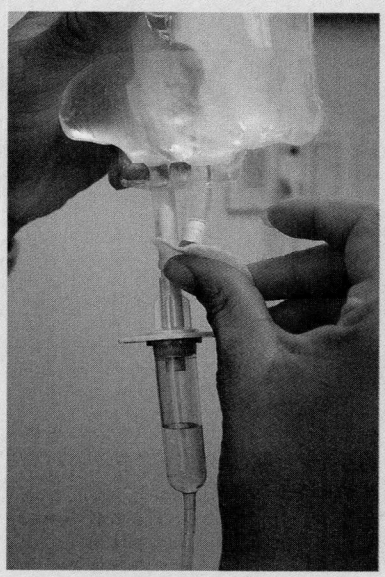

STEP 2c Injection port cleansed with alcohol.

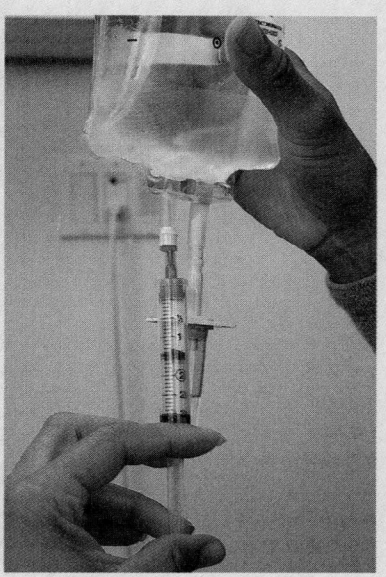

STEP 2d Medication injected through port.

STEP	RATIONALE
e Withdraw syringe from bag or bottle.	Withdrawal of syringe allows injection port to self-seal, preventing introduction of microorganisms.
f Mix medication and IV solution by holding bag or bottle and turning it gently end to end.	Allows even distribution of medication.
g Discard uncapped needle or engaged sheet over needle and syringe into a puncture-proof and leak-proof container.	Prevents injury to patient and health care personnel.
h Complete medication label with name and dose of medication, date, time, and your initials. Stick it on bottle or bag (see illustration). *Optional* (check institution's policy): Apply a flow strip that identifies the time the solution was hung and intervals indicating fluid levels.	Label is easily read during infusion of solution and informs other nurses and health care providers of contents of bag or bottle.

Critical Decision Point   *Do not use felt-tip markers on plastic surfaces. The ink will penetrate the plastic and leach into the IV solution.*

i If new tubing is required, spike bag or bottle with IV tubing; prime IV tubing (see Chapter 28).	Follows standards for changing IV tubing (Infusion Nurses Society [INS], 2006).
j Bring assembled items to patient's bedside at correct time, and perform hand hygiene.	Organization reduces errors. Hand hygiene reduces transfer of microorganisms.
k Verify patient's identity by using at least two patient identifiers. Compare patient's name and one other identifier, such as hospital identification number, with MAR. Ask patient to state name as a third identifier.	Complies with The Joint Commission requirements to improve medication safety. In most acute care settings, the patient's name and identification number on armband and MAR are used to identify patients (TJC, 2007).
l Compare label on IV bag with the MAR a final time.	Final comparison of medication label with the MAR reduces risk for medication errors. *This is the third check for accuracy.*
m Prepare patient by explaining the procedure and that there should be no discomfort during the medication infusion. Tell patient to report any symptoms of discomfort.	Most IV medications do not cause pain or discomfort when properly diluted and administered. Pain at IV insertion site may be early indication of infiltration.

Critical Decision Point   *Potassium chloride is irritating to veins. Some medications such as potassium chloride cause adverse reactions, including cardiac dysrhythmias. Always infuse these medications on an IV pump. Institutional guidelines and policies will identify which medications to administer on an IV pump.*

n Connect bag with new infusion tubing to IV site, or spike bag with existing tubing. Regulate infusion at prescribed rate (see Chapter 31).	Prevents rapid infusion of fluid and medication.

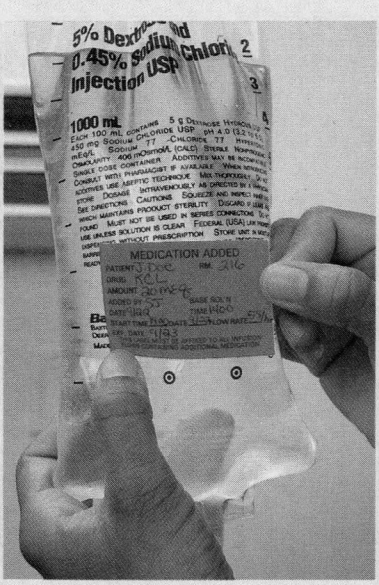

STEP 2h   Label affixed to IV bag.

STEP	RATIONALE

Critical Decision Point   *Because there is no way to know exactly how much IV fluid is in an existing hanging IV container, there is no way to determine the exact concentration of the medication in the IV solution. Therefore it is highly recommended that you add medications to new IV fluid containers only.*

o Regulate infusion at ordered rate.	Prevents rapid infusion of fluid and medication.
3 Discard uncapped needle or needle enclosed in safety shield and syringe into a puncture-proof and leak-proof receptacle. Properly dispose of equipment and supplies.	Proper disposal of needle prevents injury to nurse and patient. Capping of needles increases risk for needle-stick injuries (OSHA, 2006).
4 Perform hand hygiene.	Reduces transmission of microorganisms.

EVALUATION

1 Observe patient for signs or symptoms of medication reaction.	IV medications can cause rapid responses.
2 Observe for signs and symptoms of fluid volume excess.	Rapid uncontrolled infusion causes circulatory overload.
3 Return to patient's room at regular intervals to assess IV insertion site and rate of infusion.	Time may cause an IV site to become infiltrated, or cannulas move out of position. Flow rate may change according to patient's position or volume remaining in container.
4 Observe IV site for signs or symptoms of IV infiltration or phlebitis.	Infiltrated medications can injure tissue. Phlebitis indicates need to restart IV.
5 Have patient explain purpose and effects of medication therapy.	Demonstrates learning.

Unexpected Outcomes	Related Interventions
1 Patient has adverse or allergic reaction to medication.	• Stop medication infusion immediately. • Follow institutional policy or guidelines for appropriate response to allergic reaction (e.g., administration of antihistamine such as diphenhydramine [Benadryl] or epinephrine) and reporting of adverse medication reactions. • Notify patient's health care provider of adverse effects immediately. • Add allergy information to patient record.
2 Patient develops signs of fluid volume excess (e.g., abnormal breath sounds [crackles], blood pressure changes, jugular venous distention, shortness of breath, intake greater than output).	• Assess patient for circulatory compromise. • Stop IV infusion, or reduce rate to maintain IV site access for emergency. • Notify patient's health care provider of fluid excess immediately.
3 IV site becomes swollen, warm, reddened, and tender to touch, indicating phlebitis (see Chapter 28).	• Stop IV infusion and discontinue IV. • Treat IV site as indicated by institutional policy. • Insert new IV catheter if therapy continues.
4 IV site becomes cool, pale, and swollen, indicating infiltration (see Chapter 28).	• Stop IV infusion and discontinue IV. • Determine how much damage the IV medication can produce in subcutaneous tissue. • Provide IV extravasation care (e.g., injecting phentolamine [Regitine] around the IV infiltration site) as indicated by institutional policy, or use a medication reference, or consult pharmacist to determine appropriate follow-up care.

Recording and Reporting

- Record IV solution, medication added, and infusion rate on appropriate form (Fig. 22-20).
- Report any adverse effects to patient's health care provider, and document adverse effects according to institutional policy.

Pediatric Considerations

- IV bags that hold no more than 250 to 500 mL of fluid, a graded Buretrol, and an infusion pump are used to regulate fluids and prevent fluid overload (Hockenberry and Wilson, 2007).

Gerontological Considerations

- Altered pharmacokinetics of medications and the effects of polypharmacy place older adults at risk for medication toxicity.

Carefully monitor the response of older adults to IV medication therapy (Hadaway, 2006; McKenry and others, 2006).

- Older adults are at risk for developing fluid volume overload and require careful assessment for signs of overload and heart failure (e.g., intake greater than output, peripheral edema, shortness of breath).

Home Care Considerations

- Patients or their caregivers can discard IV tubing with their regular garbage.

<u>BARNES</u>

B15

PARENTERAL FLUID

4838 rev 9/90

Check if infusion device in use

Amt.	Type of Fluid	Product # or Medication Added	Date/ Hr. Start	Init.	Date/ Hr. Comp.	Init.	Amt. Rec'd	I.V. Site Appearance	√	IV Site Care Date/Hr.	Tubing Change Date/Hr.	Init.
1 L	D₅NS	20 meq KCl	1-16 / 0800	PN	1/16 / 1530	PN	1 L	ⓇANTECUBITAL, NO REDNESS, TENDERNESS s̄ INFILTRATION	√			
500 mL	D₅NS		1-16 / 1000	RN			400 mL	ⓁFOREARM – NO REDNESS, TENDERNESS s̄ INFILTRATION				
1 L	D₅NS	20 meq KCl	1-16 / 1530	CS				ⓇANTECUBITAL TENDERNESS AT SITE NO REDNESS	√		1-16 / 1530	CS

FIG 22-20 Example of documentation form for parenteral fluids.

SKILL 22-6 Administering Intravenous Medications by Piggyback, Intermittent Infusion Sets, and Miniinfusion Pumps

*Advanced / Intravenous Medication Administration /
Administering Medication by Intravenous Piggyback
Administering Medication by Miniinfusion Pump*

NSO *IV Medication Administration Module / Lesson 2*

One method of administering IV medications uses small volumes (25 to 250 mL) of compatible IV fluids infused over a desired period of time. This method reduces the risk for rapid dose infusion and provides independence for the patient. Patients must have an established IV line that is kept patent by intermittent flushes of normal saline. You can administer intermittent infusion of medication with any of the following methods:

1 *Piggyback:* A piggyback is a small (25 to 250 mL) IV bag or bottle connected to a short tubing line that connects to the *upper* Y-port of a primary infusion line (Fig. 22-21) or to an intermittent venous access. The piggyback tubing is a microdrip or macrodrip system (see Chapter 28). The set is called a "piggyback" because the small bag or bottle is set *higher* than the primary infusion bag or bottle. In the piggyback setup the main line does not infuse when a compatible piggybacked medication is infusing. The port of the primary IV line contains a back-check valve that automatically stops the flow of the primary infusion once the piggyback infusion flows. After the piggyback solution infuses and the solution within the tubing falls below the level of the primary infusion drip chamber, the back-check valve opens and the primary infusion starts to flow again.

2 *Tandem:* A tandem setup is a small (25 to 250 mL) IV bag or bottle connected to a short tubing line to the *lower* Y-port of a primary infusion line or to an intermittent venous access. You place the tandem set at the same height as the primary infusion bag or bottle. In the tandem setup the tandem and the main line infuse simultaneously. Monitor the tandem setup closely. If the tandem setup is not immediately clamped when the medication is infused, the IV solution from the primary line will back up into the tandem line.

3 *Volume-control administration:* Volume-control administration sets (e.g., Volutrol, Buretrol, Pediatrol) are small (50 to 150 mL) containers that attach just below the primary infusion bag or bottle. The set is attached and filled in a manner similar to that used with a regular IV infusion. However, the priming filling of the set is different, depending on the type of filter (floating valve or membrane) within the set. Follow package directions for priming sets.

4 *Miniinfusion pump:* The miniinfusion pump is battery operated and delivers medication in very small amounts of fluid (5 to 60 mL) within controlled infusion times using standard syringes (Fig. 22-22).

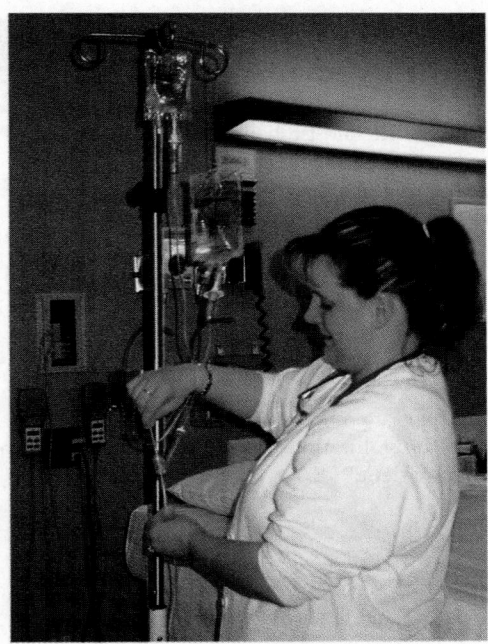

FIG 22-21 Piggyback infusion set.

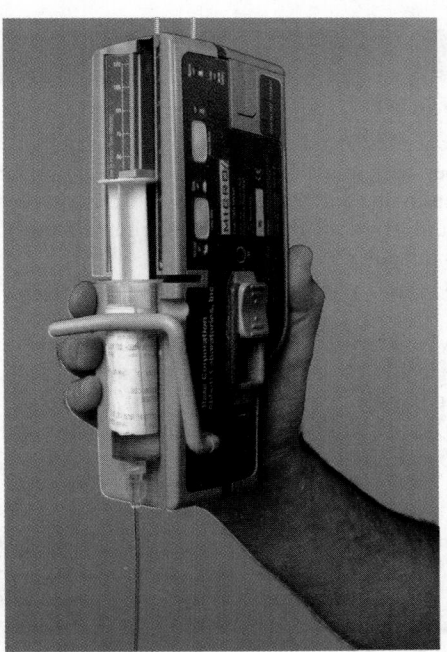

FIG 22-22 Miniinfusion pump.

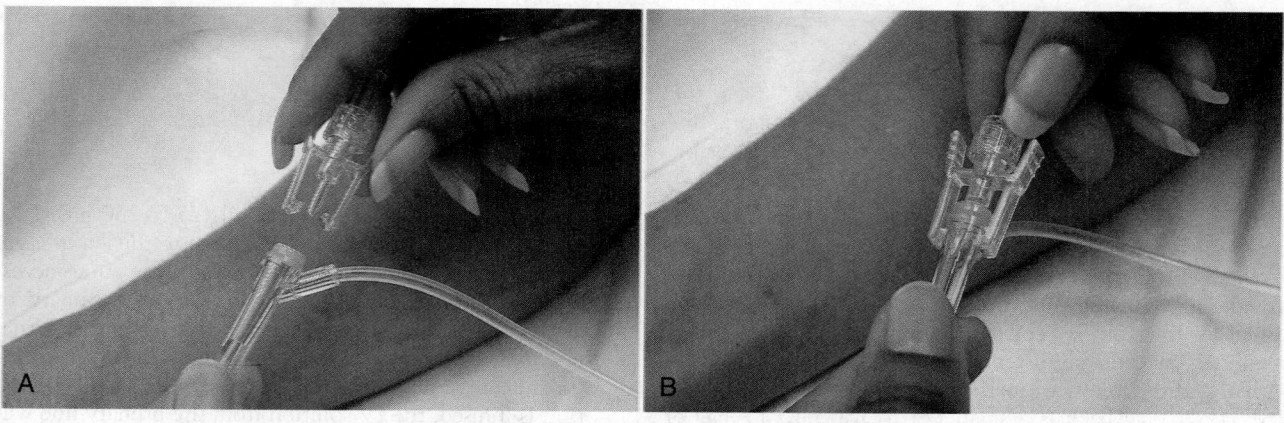

FIG 22-23   **A,** Needleless lever lock cannula system. **B,** Blunt-ended cannula inserts into port and locks.

NEEDLE SAFETY

The Needle Safety and Prevention Act of 2001 mandates that health care institutions use safe needle devices and manufactured needleless systems (Fig. 22-23) to reduce needle-stick injury. Systems with catheter ports or Y-connector sites are designed to contain a needle housed in a protective covering. Needleless infusion lines allow a direct connection with the IV line via a recessed connection port or a blunt-ended cannula or shielded-needle device, eliminating the risk for exposure to an IV needle (OSHA, 2006).

Delegation Considerations

The skill of administering IV medications by piggyback, intermittent infusion sets, and miniinfusion pumps cannot be delegated to NAP. The nurse directs the NAP about:

• Potential medication side effects and to report their occurrence to the nurse.
• Reporting patient's report of any discomfort at infusion site to the nurse.
• Reporting any change in the patient's condition or vital signs to the nurse.

Equipment
❑ Adhesive tape *(optional)*
❑ Antiseptic swab
❑ IV pole or rack
❑ Medication administration record (MAR) or computer printout
Piggyback, Tandem, or Miniinfusion Pump
❑ Medication prepared in 50- to 250-mL labeled infusion bag or syringe
❑ Short microdrip or macrodrip IV tubing set for piggyback (preferably with needleless system attached)
❑ Needleless device or stopcocks, preferred if available
❑ Needles (21 or 23 gauge, **only** if stopcocks or other needleless systems are not available)
❑ Miniinfusion pump and tubing
Volume-Control Administration Set
❑ Volutrol, Buretrol, or Pediatrol
❑ Infusion tubing (may have needleless system attachment)
❑ Syringe (1 to 20 mL)
❑ Vial or ampule of ordered medication

STEP	RATIONALE

ASSESSMENT

1 Check accuracy and completeness of each MAR or computer printout with prescriber's original medication order. Check patient's name and medication name, dosage, route, and time for administration. Recopy or re-print any portion of MAR that is difficult to read.	The order sheet is the most reliable source and only legal record of medications patient is to receive. Ensures patient receives the correct medications. Illegible MARs are a source of medication errors.
2 Assess patient's medical and medication history.	Indicates type of appropriate IV solution to be used and patient's need for medication.
3 Review medication reference information, including action, purpose, side effects, normal dose, time of peak onset, and nursing implications.	Allows nurse to give medication safely and to monitor patient's response to therapy.
4 Assess compatibility of medication with existing IV solution.	Medications that are incompatible with IV solutions result in clouding or crystallization of solution in the IV tubing, which could harm patient.

Critical Decision Point   *Never administer IV medications through tubing that is infusing blood, blood products, or parenteral nutrition solutions.*

5 Assess patency of patient's existing IV infusion line or saline lock (see Chapter 28).	For medication to reach venous circulation effectively, IV line must be patent and fluids must infuse easily.

STEP	RATIONALE

Critical Decision Point   *If the patient's IV site is saline locked, cleanse the port with alcohol, and assess the patency of the IV line by flushing it with 2 to 3 mL of sterile 0.9% sodium chloride.*

STEP	RATIONALE
6 Perform hand hygiene.	Reduces transmission of microorganisms.
7 Assess IV insertion site for signs of infiltration or phlebitis: redness, pallor, swelling, and tenderness on palpation.	Confirmation of placement of IV needle or catheter and integrity of surrounding tissues ensures that medication is administered safely.
8 Assess patient's history of drug allergies; know type of allergens and normal allergic reaction.	Effects of medications can develop rapidly after IV infusion. Be aware of patients at risk.
9 Assess patient's symptoms before initiating medication therapy.	Provides information to evaluate the desired effects of medication.
10 Assess patient's understanding of purpose of medication therapy.	Poses implications for patient education.

NURSING DIAGNOSES

- Deficient knowledge regarding medication therapy
- Risk for imbalanced fluid volume
- Risk for ineffective health maintenance

Individualize related factors based on patient's condition or needs.

PLANNING

1 Expected outcomes following completion of procedure:	
• Patient experiences no adverse reactions.	Medication was given safely with desired therapeutic effect.
• Medication infuses within desired time frame.	IV line remains patent.
• Patient's IV site remains intact without signs of swelling or inflammation or symptoms of tenderness at site.	Fluid infuses into vein, not tissues.
• Patient is able to explain medication purposes, action, side effects, and dosage.	Demonstrates learning.

IMPLEMENTATION

1 Perform hand hygiene. Prepare medication for one patient at a time following the six rights of medication administration (see Chapter 20). Compare label of the medication with the MAR or computer printout two times (see Skill 22-1) when removing ampules, vials, or infusion bags from storage area for medication preparation.	Ensures correct medication is given to patient. Establishing a medication preparation routine, eliminating distractions, and double-checking the transcribed order reduce error (Pape and others, 2005; Ridge, 2007; Wolf, 2007). *First and second checks for accuracy ensure right medication is administered.*
2 Assemble medication and supplies at bedside.	Organizes procedure.
3 Give medication to patient at right time, and perform hand hygiene.	Ensures patient will experience medication effects at right time. Reduces risk for transmission of organisms.
4 Verify patient's identity by using at least two patient identifiers. Compare patient's name and one other identifier, such as hospital identification number, with MAR. Ask patient to state name as a third identifier.	Complies with The Joint Commission requirements to improve medication safety. In most acute care settings, the patient's name and identification number on armband and MAR are used to identify patients (TJC, 2007).
5 Explain purpose of medication and side effects to patient, and explain that medication will be given through existing IV line. Encourage patient to report symptoms of discomfort at site.	Keeps patient informed of procedures and therapies. Patients who verbalize pain at the IV site help detect IV infiltrations early, lessening damage to surrounding tissues.
6 Compare label on IV bag or syringe with the MAR a final time.	Final comparison of medication label with the MAR reduces risk for medication errors. *This is the third check for accuracy.*
7 Administer infusion:	
a Piggyback or tandem infusion:	
(1) Connect infusion tubing to medication bag (see Chapter 28). Allow solution to fill tubing by opening regulator flow clamp. Once tubing is full, close clamp, and cap end of tubing.	Infusion tubing needs to be filled with solution and free of air bubbles to prevent air embolus.

STEP	RATIONALE

Optional: Saline lock: Attach appropriate IV tubing, and administer the medication via piggyback, miniinfusion, or volume-control administration set. When the infusion is completed, disconnect the tubing, cleanse the port with alcohol, and flush the IV line with 2 to 3 mL sterile 0.9% sodium chloride. Maintain sterility of IV tubing between intermittent infusions.

   (2) Hang piggyback medication bag above level of primary fluid bag (see illustration). (Use hook to lower main bag.) Hang tandem infusion at same level as primary fluid bag.

Height of fluid bag affects rate of flow to patient.

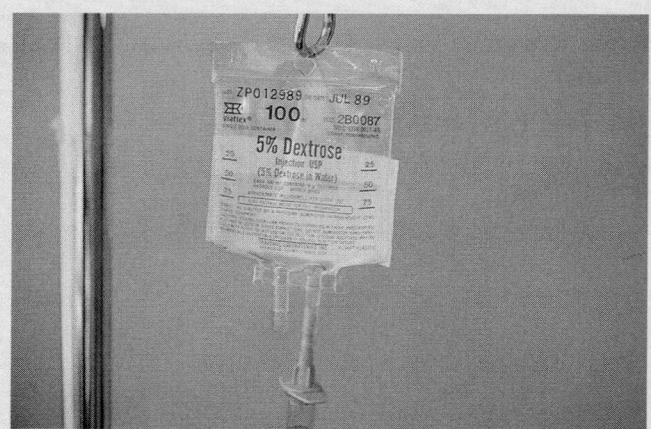

STEP 7a(2)   Small-volume minibag for piggyback infusion.

   (3) Connect tubing of piggyback or tandem to appropriate connector on primary infusion line:

      (a) *Needleless system:* Wipe off needleless port on main IV line, and insert tip of piggyback or tandem infusion tubing.

Needleless connections prevent accidental needle-stick injuries (OSHA, 2006).
Establishes route for IV medication to enter main IV line.
Stopcock eliminates need for needle.

      (b) *Stopcock:* Wipe off stopcock port with alcohol swab, and connect tubing. Turn stopcock to open position.

      (c) *Tubing port:* Connect sterile needle to end of piggyback infusion tubing, remove cap, cleanse injection port on main IV line, and insert needle through center of port. Secure by taping connection.

Use this step *only* if needleless system is not available.
Prevents introduction of microorganisms during needle insertion.

   (4) Regulate flow rate of medication solution by adjusting regulator clamp or IV pump infusion rate. (Infusion times vary, so refer to medication reference or institutional policy for safe flow rate).

Provides slow, safe, intermittent infusion of medication and maintains therapeutic blood levels.

   (5) After medication has infused, check flow rate of primary infusion. The primary infusion automatically restarts after the piggyback solution is completed. If using a stopcock, turn stopcock to the off position. If a tandem setup is used, turn off tandem tubing and adjust flow rate of primary infusion.

Back-check valve on piggyback prevents flow of primary infusion until medication infuses. The tandem and primary infusions flow together until the tandem set empties. Checking flow rate ensures proper administration of IV fluids.

   (6) Regulate main infusion line to ordered rate, if necessary.

Infusion of medication sometimes interferes with main line infusion rate.

   (7) Leave IV piggyback or tandem bag and tubing in place for future drug administration, or discard in puncture-proof and leak-proof container.

Establishment of secondary line produces route for microorganisms to enter main line. Repeated changes in tubing increase risk for infection transmission (check institutional policy).

STEP	RATIONALE

b **Volume-control administration set (e.g., Volutrol):**

(1) Fill Volutrol with desired amount of IV fluid (50 to 100 mL) by opening clamp between Volutrol and main IV bag (see illustration).

IV medication is diluted with small fluid volume and reduces risk for rapid infusion.

(2) Close clamp, and check to be sure clamp on air vent Volutrol chamber is open.

Prevents additional leakage of fluid into Volutrol. Air vent allows fluid in Volutrol to exit at regulated rate.

(3) Clean injection port on top of Volutrol with antiseptic swab.

Prevents introduction of microorganisms during needle insertion.

(4) Remove needle cap, and insert needleless syringe tip through port, then inject medication (see illustrations). Gently rotate Volutrol between hands.

Rotating mixes medication with solution in Volutrol to ensure equal distribution.

(5) Regulate IV infusion rate to allow medication to infuse in time recommended by institutional policy, a pharmacist, or a medication reference manual.

For optimal therapeutic effect, medication should infuse in prescribed time interval.

(6) Label Volutrol with name of medication, dosage, total volume including diluent, and time of administration.

Alerts nurses to medication being infused. Prevents other medications from being added to Volutrol.

(7) Dispose of uncapped needle or needle enclosed in safety shield and syringe in puncture-proof and leak-proof container. Discard supplies in appropriate container. Perform hand hygiene.

Prevents accidental needle sticks (OSHA, 2006).
Reduces transmission of microorganisms.

c **Miniinfuser administration:**

(1) Connect prefilled syringe to miniinfusion tubing.

Special tubing designed to fit syringe delivers medication to main IV line.

(2) Carefully apply pressure to syringe plunger, allowing tubing to fill with medication.

Ensures tubing is free of air bubbles to prevent air embolus.

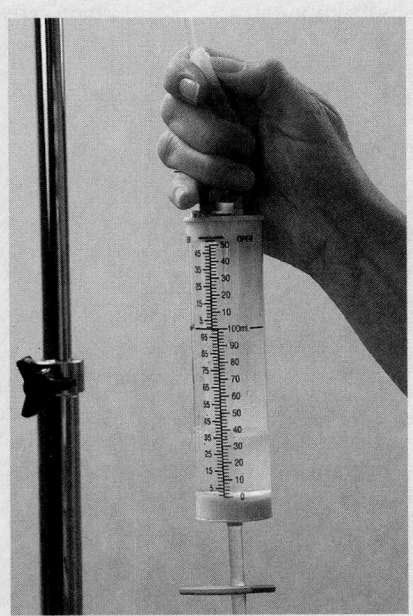

STEP 7b(1) Filling volume-control administration device.

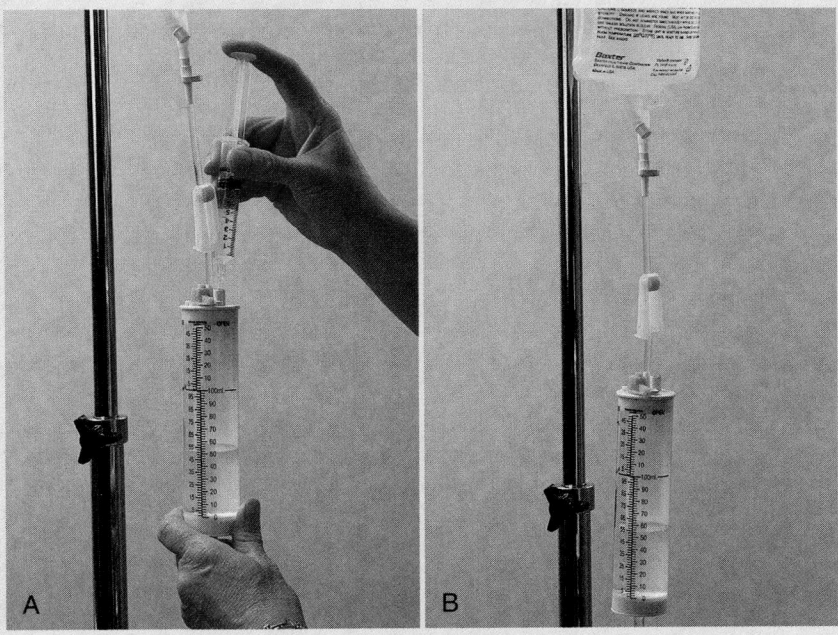

STEP 7b(4) **A,** Medication injected into device. **B,** Prepared device.

STEP	RATIONALE
(3) Place syringe into miniinfusion pump (follow product directions). Be sure syringe is secured (see illustration).	Secure placement is needed for proper medication administration.

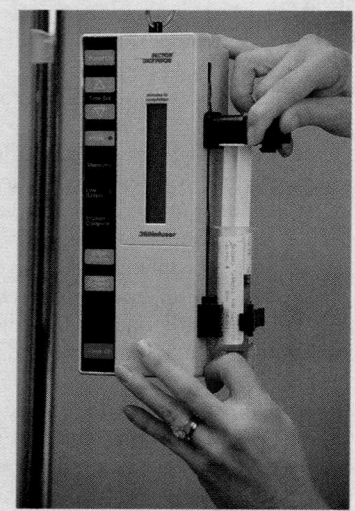

STEP 7c(3)   Ensure syringe is secure after placing it into miniinfusion pump.

STEP	RATIONALE
(4) Connect miniinfusion tubing to main IV line:	Establishes route for IV medication to enter main IV line.
(a) *Needleless system:* Wipe off needleless port on main IV line, and insert tip of miniinfusion tubing.	Needleless connections reduce risk for accidental needle-stick injuries (OSHA, 2006).
(b) *Stopcock:* Wipe off stopcock port with alcohol swab, and connect tubing. Turn stopcock to open position.	Stopcock reduces risk for accidental needle-stick injuries.
(c) *Tubing port:* Connect sterile needle to miniinfusion tubing, remove cap, cleanse injection port on main IV line or saline lock, and insert needle through center of port. Secure by taping connection.	Use this method *only* if needleless system is not available. Cleansing reduces transmission of microorganisms. Prevents introduction of microorganisms during needle insertion.
(5) Hang infusion pump with syringe on IV pole alongside main IV bag. Set pump to deliver medication within time recommended by institutional policy, a pharmacist, or a medication reference manual. Press button on pump to begin infusion.	Pump automatically delivers medication at safe, constant rate based on volume in syringe.
(6) After medication has infused, check flow rate on primary infusion. The infusion normally continues to flow while medication infuses. Regulate main infusion line to ordered rate as needed. (NOTE: If using a stopcock, turn off miniinfusion line.)	Maintains patent primary IV fluids.
d Dispose of supplies in puncture-proof and leak-proof container.	Prevents accidental needle sticks (OSHA, 2006).
e Perform hand hygiene.	Reduces transmission of microorganisms.

EVALUATION

1 Observe patient for signs or symptoms of adverse reaction.	IV medications act rapidly.
2 During the infusion, periodically check infusion rate and condition of IV site.	IV must remain patent for proper drug administration. Infiltration of IV site necessitates discontinuing infusion.
3 Ask patient to explain purpose and side effects of medication.	Evaluates patient's understanding of instruction.

Unexpected Outcomes	Related Interventions
1 Patient has adverse or allergic reaction to medication.	• Stop medication infusion immediately. • Follow institutional policy or guidelines for appropriate response to allergic reaction (e.g., administration of antihistamine such as diphenhydramine [Benadryl] or epinephrine) and reporting of adverse medication reactions. • Notify patient's health care provider of adverse effects immediately. • Add allergy information to patient record per agency policy.
2 Medication does not infuse over established time frame.	• Determine reason (e.g., flow rate calculated incorrectly, IV needle position, site infiltration). • Resolve problem, and resume infusion.
3 IV site becomes swollen, warm, reddened, and tender to touch, indicating phlebitis (see Chapter 28).	• Stop IV infusion and discontinue IV. • Treat IV site as indicated by institutional policy. • Insert new IV catheter if therapy continues.
4 IV site becomes cool, pale, and swollen, indicating infiltration (see Chapter 28).	• Stop IV infusion and discontinue IV. • Determine how harmful IV medication is to subcutaneous tissue. • Provide IV extravasation care (e.g., injecting phentolamine [Regitine] around the IV infiltration site) as indicated by institutional policy, or use a medication reference, or consult pharmacist to determine appropriate follow-up care. • Insert new IV catheter if therapy continues.

Recording and Reporting

- Immediately record medication, dose, route, and time administered on MAR or computer printout.
- Record volume of fluid in medication bag or Volutrol on intake and output (I&O) form.
- Report any adverse reactions to patient's health care provider.

Teaching Considerations

- Review all IV medications with the patient and significant others, including why the patient is receiving the medication and potential adverse effects, including allergic responses.
- Teach the patient and/or significant others not to alter the ordered rate of infusion without consulting the prescriber. IV medications need to be infused at a specified rate to achieve their desired effect and to avoid adverse effects.
- Teach the patient and/or significant others to report any adverse effects immediately.

Pediatric Considerations

- Infants and young children are more vulnerable to alterations in fluid balance, and do not adjust quickly to changes in fluid balance. Therefore, to assess fluid balance, monitor I&O

carefully when infusing IV medications (Hockenberry and Wilson, 2007).

Gerontological Considerations

- Altered pharmacokinetics of medications and the effects of polypharmacy place older adults at risk for medication toxicity. Carefully monitor the response of older adults to IV medication therapy (Hadaway, 2006; McKenry and others, 2006).
- Older adults are at risk for developing fluid volume overload and require careful assessment for signs of overload and heart failure (e.g., intake greater than output, peripheral edema, shortness of breath).

Home Care Considerations

- Patients or significant others who administer IV medications at home require education about the steps of medication administration. The patient or significant other needs to perform several return demonstrations of IV medication administration before performing this skill independently. In addition, patients and significant others need to know signs of IV medication administration complications, such as phlebitis and infiltration, and what to do for any problems.

SKILL 22-7 Administering Medications by Intravenous Bolus

Advanced / Intravenous Medication Administration / Administering Medication by Intravenous Bolus

NSO *IV Medication Administration Module / Lesson 4*

An IV bolus involves introducing a concentrated dose of a medication directly into the systemic circulation via a vein. An IV bolus or "push" usually requires small volumes of fluid, which is an advantage for patients who are at risk for fluid overload. Institutional policy dictates which medications to give by IV push. There are advantages and disadvantages to administering IV push medications (Box 22-4).

The IV bolus is a dangerous method to administer medications because it allows no time to correct errors. Therefore be very careful in calculating the correct amount of the medication to give. In addition, a bolus may cause direct irritation to the lining of blood vessels, so always confirm placement of the IV catheter or needle. Never give an IV bolus if the insertion site appears puffy, edematous, or reddened or if the IV fluids do not flow at the ordered rate. Accidental injection of some medications into tissues surrounding a vein can cause pain, sloughing of tissues, and abscesses.

Administering an IV push medication too quickly can cause serious negative patient outcomes, including death. The Institute for Safe Medication Practices (2007) has identified the following three strategies to reduce harm from rapid IV push medications:

- Make sure information regarding rate of administration of IV push medication is readily available.
- Use less concentrated solutions whenever possible.
- Avoid using terms in orders such as *IV push*, *IVP*, or *IV bolus* with medications that should be administered over 1 minute or longer. Use more descriptive terms such as *IV over 5 minutes*.

You need to verify the rate of administration of IV push medication using institutional guidelines or a medication reference manual. Review the amount of medication the patient will receive each minute, the recommended concentration, and rate of administration. For example, if a patient is to receive 6 mL of a medication over 3 minutes, give 2 mL of the IV bolus medication every minute. Understand the purpose of the medication and any potential adverse reactions related to the rate and route of administration.

Delegation Considerations

The skill of administering intravenous medications by intravenous bolus cannot be delegated to NAP. The nurse directs the NAP about:

- Potential medication side effects or reactions and to report their occurrence to the nurse.
- Reporting patient's discomfort at infusion site to the nurse.
- Obtaining any required vital signs and reporting them to the nurse.

Equipment

- ❑ Watch with second hand
- ❑ Clean gloves
- ❑ Antiseptic swab
- ❑ Medication in vial or ampule
- ❑ Syringe
- ❑ Needleless device or sterile needle (21 to 25 gauge)
- ❑ IV push (IV lock): vial of appropriate flush solution (saline most common, but heparin may be used; if heparin is used, most common concentration is 10 to 100 units/mL; check agency policy)
- ❑ Medication administration record (MAR) or computer printout

BOX 22-4	Advantages and Disadvantages of the Intravenous Push Method

Advantages

- Rapid onset of medication effects, which is useful in patients experiencing critical or emergent health problems.
- Medications can be prepared quickly and given over a shorter time than by IV piggyback.
- Doses of short-acting medications can be titrated based on a patient's needs and responses to the drug therapy. This is important for infants, children, and older patients.
- Method provides a more accurate dose of medication delivered because no medication is left in IV tubing (Rosenthal, 2007).

Disadvantages

- *Not all medications can be delivered IV push.*
- Higher risk for infusion reactions; some are mild to severe, because the medication action peaks quickly.
- When giving medication quickly (e.g., less than 1 minute), there is very little opportunity to stop the injection if an adverse reaction occurs.
- There is increased risk for infiltration and phlebitis, especially if a highly concentrated medication, a small peripheral vein, or a short venous access device is used.
- Hypersensitivity reaction can cause an immediate or delayed systemic reaction to a medication, requiring supportive measures (Hadaway, 2006).

STEP	RATIONALE

ASSESSMENT

1 Check accuracy and completeness of each MAR or computer printout with prescriber's original medication order. Check patient's name and medication name, dosage, route, and time for administration. Recopy or re-print any portion of MAR that is difficult to read.

The order sheet is the most reliable source and only legal record of medications patient will receive.

Ensures patient receives the correct medications.

Illegible MARs are a source of medication errors.

Critical Decision Point *Some IV medications can only be given IV push safely when the patient is being continuously monitored for dysrhythmias, blood pressure changes, or other adverse effects. Therefore you can push some medications only in specific areas within a health care agency (e.g., critical care unit). Confirm institutional guidelines regarding requirements for special monitoring.*

STEP	RATIONALE
2 Review medication reference information, including action, purpose, side effects, normal dose, time of peak onset, how slowly to give the medication, and nursing implications, such as the need to dilute the medication or administer it through a filter.	Allows for safe medication administration and ability to monitor patient's response to therapy.
3 If pushing medication through an existing IV line, determine compatibility of medication with IV fluids and any additives within IV solution.	IV medication is not always compatible with IV solution and/or additives.
4 Perform hand hygiene. Assess condition of IV or saline (heparin) lock insertion site for signs of infiltration or phlebitis.	Do not administer medication if site is edematous or inflamed.
5 Assess patency of patient's existing IV infusion line or saline lock (see Chapter 28).	For medication to reach venous circulation effectively, IV line must be patent, and fluids must infuse easily.
6 Check patient's medical history and medication allergies.	IV bolus delivers medication rapidly. Adverse reactions could prove fatal.
7 Check date of expiration for medication vial or ampule.	Medication potency may increase or decrease when medication is outdated.
8 Assess patient's symptoms before initiating medication therapy.	Provides information to evaluate the desired effects of medication.
9 Assess patient's understanding of purpose of drug therapy.	Poses implication for education.

NURSING DIAGNOSES

- Acute pain
- Deficient knowledge regarding medication therapy

Individualize related factors based on patient's condition or needs.

PLANNING

1 Expected outcomes following completion of procedure:	
• Patient experiences no medication side effects or adverse reactions.	Medication administered safely with desired therapeutic effect achieved.
• IV site remains clear, without swelling.	Medication infuses without complications to IV site and surrounding tissues.
• Patient explains purpose and side effects of medication.	Demonstrates learning.

Critical Decision Point *Some IV medications require dilution before administration. If giving a small amount of medication (e.g., less than 1 mL), dilute medication in 5 to 10 mL of 0.9% sodium chloride or sterile water so that the medication does not collect in the "dead spaces" (e.g., Y-site injection port, IV cap) of the IV delivery system.*

IMPLEMENTATION

1 Perform hand hygiene. Prepare medication for one patient at a time following the six rights of medication administration (see Chapter 20). Compare label of the medication with the MAR or computer printout two times (see Skill 22-1) when removing ampules or vials from storage and after drawing up medication in syringes.	Ensures correct medication is given to patient. Establishing a medication preparation routine, eliminating distractions, and double-checking the transcribed order reduce error (Pape and others, 2005; Ridge, 2007; Wolf, 2007). *First and second checks for accuracy ensures right medication is administered.*
2 Take medication to patient at right time, and perform hand hygiene.	Ensures patient will experience medication effects at right time. Reduces risk for transmission of organisms.
3 Verify patient's identity by using at least two patient identifiers. Compare patient's name and one other identifier, such as hospital identification number, with MAR. Ask patient to state name as a third identifier.	Complies with The Joint Commission requirements to improve medication safety. In most acute care settings, the patient's name and identification number on armband and MAR are used to identify patients (TJC, 2007).
4 Compare label of the medication with the MAR a final time.	Final comparison of medication label with the MAR reduces risk for medication errors. *This is the third check for accuracy.*
5 Explain purpose of medication and side effects to patient, and explain that medication will be given through existing IV line. Encourage patient to report symptoms of discomfort at site.	Keeps patient informed of procedures and therapies. Patients who verbalize pain at the IV site help detect IV infiltrations early, lessening damage to surrounding tissues.
6 Apply clean gloves.	Reduces transmission of microorganisms and reduces risk for blood exposure (OSHA, 2006).
7 Intravenous push (existing line):	
a Select injection port of IV tubing closest to patient. Whenever possible, use a stopcock or other needleless component.	Follows provisions of the Needle Safety and Prevention Act of 2001 (OSHA, 2006).

STEP	RATIONALE
b Clean injection port with antiseptic swab. Allow to dry.	Prevents introduction of microorganisms during needle insertion.
c Connect syringe to IV line: Insert needleless tip of syringe containing drug through center of port (see illustration).	Prevents introduction of microorganisms. Prevents damage to port diaphragm and possible leakage from site.
d Occlude IV line by pinching tubing just above injection port (see illustration). Pull back gently on syringe's plunger to aspirate for blood return.	Final check ensures that medication is being delivered into bloodstream.

Critical Decision Point   *In some cases, especially with a smaller gauge IV needle, blood return is not always aspirated, even if IV is patent. If IV site does not show signs of infiltration, and IV fluid is infusing without difficulty, proceed with IV push.*

e Release tubing, and inject medication within amount of time recommended by institutional policy, pharmacist, or medication reference manual. Use a watch to time administrations (see illustration). IV line may be pinched while pushing medication and released when not pushing medication. Allow IV fluids to infuse when not pushing medication.	Ensures safe medication infusion. Rapid injection of IV drug can be fatal. Allowing IV fluids to infuse while pushing IV drug will enable medication to be delivered to patient at prescribed rate.
f After injecting medication, withdraw syringe, and recheck IV fluid infusion rate.	Injection of bolus may alter rate of fluid infusion. Rapid fluid infusion can cause circulatory fluid overload.

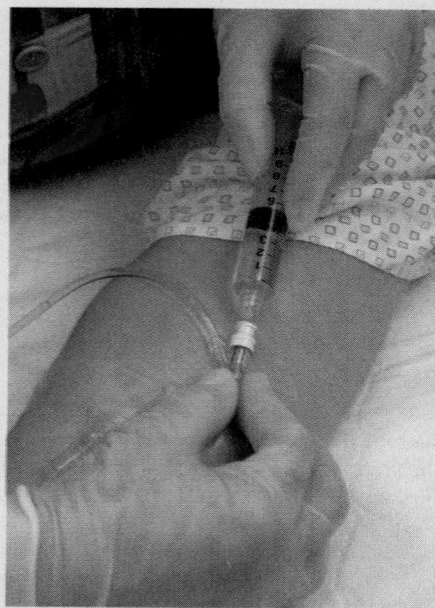

STEP 7c   Connecting syringe to IV line with needleless blunt cannula tip.

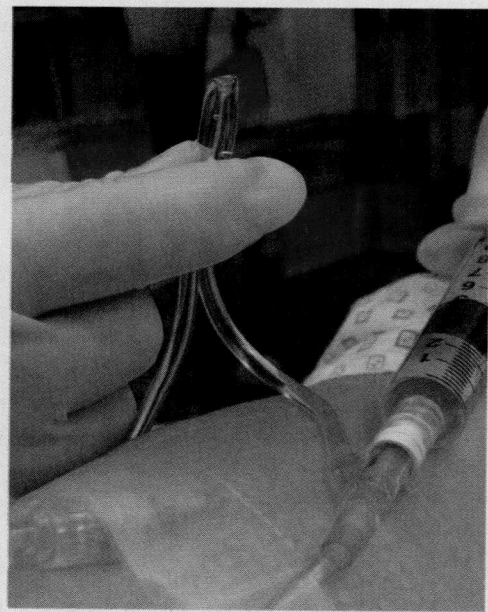

STEP 7d   Occluding IV tubing above injection port.

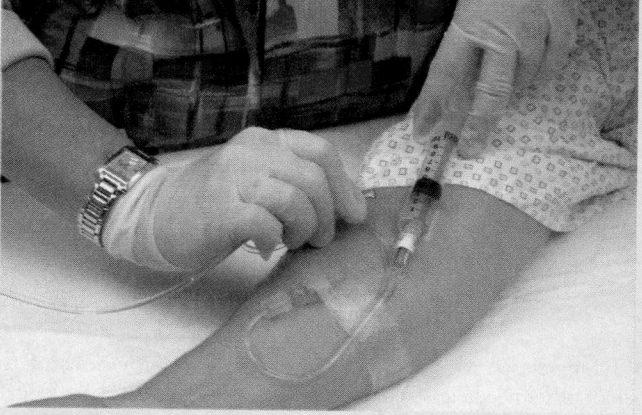

STEP 7e   Using a watch to time an IV push medication.

STEP	RATIONALE

8 Intravenous push (intravenous lock):
  a Prepare flush solutions according to institutional policy.
    (1) *Saline flush method (preferred method):* Prepare two syringes filled with 2 to 3 mL of 0.9% sodium chloride. | Normal saline is effective in keeping IV locks patent and is compatible with a wide range of medications (Fujita and others, 2006).
    (2) *Heparin flush method (traditional method):*
      (a) Prepare one syringe with ordered amount of heparin flush solution.
      (b) Prepare two syringes with 2 to 3 mL of 0.9% sodium chloride.
  b Administer medication:
    (1) Clean lock's injection port with antiseptic swab. | Prevents introduction of microorganisms during needle insertion.
    (2) Insert syringe with 0.9% sodium chloride through injection port of IV lock (see illustrations).
    (3) Pull back gently on syringe plunger, and check for blood return. | Indicates if needle or catheter is in vein.
    (4) Flush IV site with 0.9% sodium chloride by pushing slowly on plunger. | Clears needle and reservoir of blood. Flushing without difficulty indicates patent IV.

Critical Decision Point   *Carefully observe the area of skin above the IV catheter. Note any puffiness or swelling as the IV site is flushed, which could indicate infiltration into the vein, requiring removal of catheter.*

    (5) Remove saline-filled syringe.
    (6) Clean lock's injection port with antiseptic swab. | Prevents transmission of microorganisms.
    (7) Insert syringe containing prepared medication through injection port of IV lock. | Allows administration of medication.
    (8) Inject medication within amount of time recommended by institutional policy, pharmacist, or medication reference manual. Use a watch to time administration. | Many medication errors are associated with IV pushes being administered too quickly. Following guidelines for IV push rates promotes patient safety (Nicholas and Agius, 2005).
    (9) After administering medication, withdraw syringe.
    (10) Clean lock's injection site with antiseptic swab. | Prevents transmission of microorganisms.
    (11) Flush injection port.
      (a) Attach syringe with 0.9% sodium chloride, and inject normal saline flush at the same rate the medication was delivered. | Flushing IV line with saline prevents occlusion of IV access device and ensures all medication delivered. Flushing IV site at same rate as medication ensures that any medication remaining within IV needle is delivered at the correct rate.
      (b) *Heparin flush option for use with central lines:* After instilling saline, attach syringe containing heparin flush. Inject heparin slowly, and then remove syringe. | Maintains patency of central line by inhibiting clot formation. *SASH method:* Saline, Administration of medication, Saline, Heparin (Guthrie and others, 2007).
9 Dispose of uncapped needles or needle engaged in safety shield and syringes in puncture-proof and leak-proof container. | Prevents accidental needle-stick injuries and follows Centers for Disease Control and Prevention (CDC) guidelines for disposal of sharps (OSHA, 2006).
10 Remove clean gloves, and perform hand hygiene. | Reduces transmission of microorganisms.

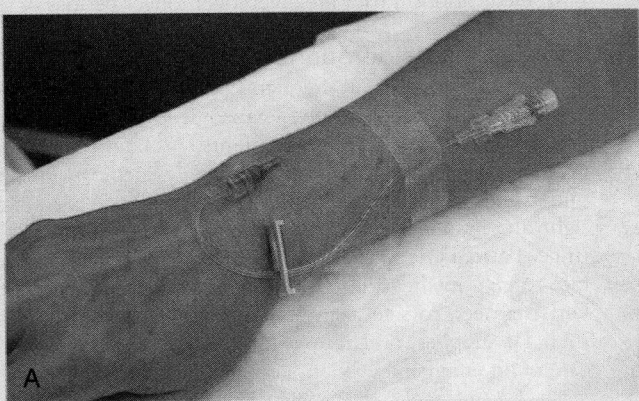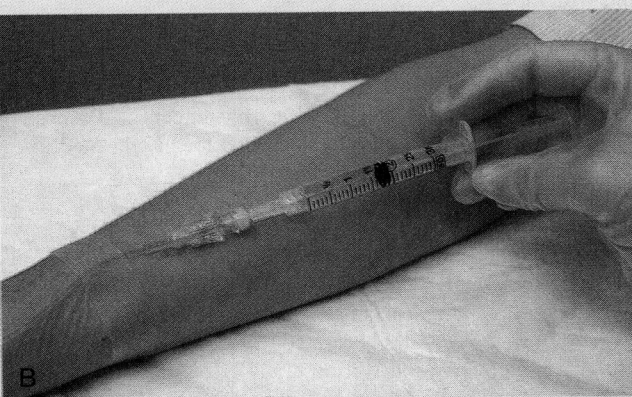

STEP 8b(2)   **A,** Intravenous catheter with saline lock adapter. **B,** Syringe inserted into injection port.

STEP	RATIONALE

EVALUATION

1 Observe patient closely for adverse reactions during administration and for several minutes thereafter.

IV medications act rapidly.

2 Observe IV site during injection for sudden swelling and for 48 hours after IV push.

Swelling indicates infiltration into tissues surrounding vein. Signs of infiltration may not occur for 48 hours (Hadaway, 2006).

3 Assess patient's status after giving medication to evaluate the effectiveness of the medication.

Some IV bolus medications can cause rapid changes in the patient's physiological status. Some medications require careful monitoring and assessment and possibly future laboratory testing (e.g., vasopressors and antiarrhythmics require blood pressure and heart rate monitoring, and heparin requires laboratory studies after administration to determine therapeutic levels).

4 Ask patient to explain medication's purpose and side effects.

Evaluates learning.

Unexpected Outcomes

1 Patient develops adverse reaction to medication.

Related Interventions

- Stop delivering medication immediately, and follow institutional policy or guidelines for appropriate response to allergic reaction (e.g., administration of antihistamine such as diphenhydramine [Benadryl] or epinephrine) and reporting of adverse drug reactions.
- Notify patient's health care provider of adverse effects immediately.
- Add allergy information to patient's record.

2 IV medication is incompatible with IV fluids (e.g., IV fluid becomes cloudy).

- Stop the IV fluids, and clamp the IV line.
- Flush the IV with 10 mL of 0.9% sodium chloride or sterile water.
- Give the IV bolus over the appropriate amount of time.
- Flush with another 10 mL of 0.9% sodium chloride or sterile water at the same rate as the medication was administered.
- Restart the IV fluids at the prescribed rate.
- If unable to stop IV infusion, start a new IV site (see Chapter 28), and administer medication using the IV push (IV lock) method.

3 IV site becomes cool, pale, and swollen, indicating signs of infiltration (see Chapter 28).

- Stop IV infusion immediately, or discontinue access device.
- Determine how much damage the IV medication can produce in subcutaneous tissue.
- Provide IV extravasation care (e.g., injecting phentolamine [Regitine] around the IV infiltration site) as indicated by institutional policy, or use a medication reference, or consult pharmacist to determine appropriate follow-up care.
- Restart new IV site if therapy continues.

4 Patient is unable to explain medication information.

- Provide patient with additional information, or patient is unable to learn at this time.

Recording and Reporting

- Immediately record medication administration, including medication name, dose, route, and time.
- Report any adverse reactions to patient's health care provider. Patient's response sometimes indicates need for additional medical therapy.
- Record patient's medication response in nurses' notes.

Teaching Considerations

- Teach patient and/or significant other that effects of IV push medications occur rapidly. Explain reasons for giving medication slowly, and teach signs of adverse effects.

Pediatric Considerations

- The therapeutic dosage of IV push medications for infants and children is often small and difficult to accurately prepare, even with a tuberculin syringe. You need to infuse these medications slowly and in small volumes because of the risk for fluid volume overload (Hockenberry and Wilson, 2007). To maintain pediatric patient safety, carefully follow institutional policies when administering medications via IV bolus (Rosenthal, 2007).

Gerontological Considerations

- The central nervous system and cardiovascular system are most affected by the aging process. To reduce the risk for adverse effects of IV push medications, smaller dosages are often prescribed (McKenry and others, 2006). Older patients may tolerate IV push medications if they are given over longer periods of time.

Home Care Considerations

- IV push medications are frequently given in the home setting. Nurses, pharmacists, and physicians need to collaborate closely in the care of these patients. Patients and families who are independently responsible for managing IV medications need to understand all aspects of administration safety. Adequate eyesight and manual dexterity are necessary to manipulate the syringe. Patients need to understand their venous access device, rate to give medications, and how to flush their access device. Patients need to safely store their medications and dispose of their IV supplies, and they should know whom to contact in case of an emergency (Nicholas and Agius, 2005).

SKILL 22-8 Administering Continuous Subcutaneous Infusions

The continuous subcutaneous infusion (CSQI or CSCI) route of medication administration is an alternative to IV, IM, or subcutaneous injections. The CSQI route is for continuous administration of selected medications (e.g., opioids or insulin). The route is also effective with medications to stop preterm labor (e.g., terbutaline) and to treat pulmonary hypertension (e.g., trepostrenil sodium). One factor that determines the infusion rate of CSQI is the rate of medication absorption. Most patients can absorb 2 to 5 mL/hr of medication (Owens, 2005; Pasero and McCaffery, 2005).

Many settings use CSQI because it enables patients to manage their illness and/or pain without the risks and expenses involved with IV medication administration. When used for home pain management, this route is relatively easy for patients and families to learn and understand. CSQI improves oncological and postoperative pain control in different patients, including infants, children, and adults (Morton, 2007; Owens, 2005; Pasero and McCaffery, 2005). Box 22-5 summarizes benefits associated with the use of CSQI for pain management.

Patients with diabetes who are using CSQI for management of blood glucose levels receive intense diabetes self-management education from qualified diabetes educators and insulin pump trainers. The newest system integrates an insulin pump with real-time continuous glucose monitoring (Fig. 22-24) (MedTronic MiniMed, 2007). Patients with diabetes who are using insulin pumps generally require 25% less insulin because insulin is absorbed and used more efficiently (Webb, 2006). Box 22-6 lists criteria to use when selecting insulin pumps for patient use.

| BOX 22-5 | Benefits Associated With Pain Management Delivered by Continuous Subcutaneous Infusion |

- Can be used in patients with poor venous access.
- Provides pain relief to patients who are unable to tolerate oral pain medications.
- Allows patients greater mobility.
- Onset of action takes about 20 minutes.
- Provides better pain control than IM injections.
- Costs are almost half of those associated with IV infusions.

Modified from Wurhman and others: Authorized and unauthorized dosing of analgesic infusion pumps, *Pain Manag Nurs* 8(1):4, 2007.

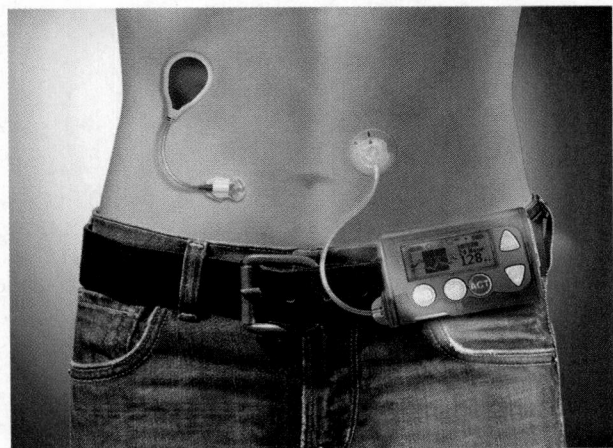

FIG 22-24 MiniMed Paradigm Real-Time Insulin Pump and Continuous Glucose Monitoring System. (*Courtesy MedTronic, Inc., Northridge, Calif.*)

The procedure to initiate and discontinue CSQI therapy is similar regardless of the type of medication being delivered. However, nursing assessment and interventions vary depending on the type of medication administered. For example, if the medication is for diabetes glucose management, you evaluate the patient's blood glucose levels and episodes of hypoglycemia or hyperglycemia (Weissberg-Benchell and others, 2007).

Use a small-gauge (25 to 27) winged butterfly IV needle or special commercially prepared Teflon cannula to deliver medications through CSQI. Although Teflon cannulas are generally more expensive, they tend to be more comfortable for the patient and have lower rates of complications than winged IV needles. They are associated with fewer needle-stick injuries (Abbas, 2005). You base the choice of needle type on institutional guidelines or patient preference. Use the needle with the shortest length and the smallest gauge necessary to establish and maintain the infusion.

Use the same anatomical sites for subcutaneous injections (see Fig. 22-13) and the upper chest. Site selection depends on the patient's activity level and the type of medication delivered. For example, pain medications given to ambulatory patients are best delivered in the upper chest, which allows the patient to move freely. Insulin is absorbed most consistently in the abdomen, thus a site in the abdomen away from the waistline is the preferred administration site. Always avoid sites where the tubing of the pump could be disturbed. Sites should be free from irritation and away from bony prominences and the waistline. Rotate sites at least every 72 hours or whenever complications such as leaking occur (INS, 2006; MedTronic MiniMed, 2007).

The CSQI route requires a computerized pump with safety features, including lockout intervals and warning alarms. A variety of medication pumps are currently available. Ideally, medication pumps are individualized based on the medication being delivered and the patient's needs. You also need to consider the availability and cost of the pump and its supplies. When possible, have patients select the pump that fits their individual and home needs and is easiest to use.

| BOX 22-6 | Selection Criteria for Patients Using Insulin Pumps |

- Possesses strong motivation and commitment to use diabetes management skills
- Requires or desires improved control of blood glucose levels
- Requires greater flexibility than allowed by traditional insulin injection schedules
- Is willing to participate in a formal diabetes education program
- Possesses strong critical thinking and problem-solving skills
- Accepts responsibilities associated with the self-management of diabetes
- Is able to perform self–blood glucose monitoring and to operate the insulin pump
- Displays evidence of effective coping patterns
- Has support systems available
- Secures financial resources to cover costs associated with CSQI

Data from American Diabetes Association: Continuous subcutaneous insulin infusion, *Diabetes Care* 27(suppl 1):S110, 2004; Retnakarn R, Zinman B: Continuous subcutaneous insulin infusion versus multiple daily injections, *Diabetes Care* 28:763, 2005.
CSQI, Continuous subcutaneous infusion.

Delegation Considerations

The skill of administering continuous subcutaneous medications cannot be delegated to NAP. The nurse directs the NAP about:

- Potential medication side effects or reactions and to report their occurrence to the nurse.
- Reporting complications (e.g., leaking, redness, discomfort) at the insertion site to the nurse.
- Obtaining any required vital signs and reporting them to the nurse.

Equipment

Initiation of CSQI

❑ Clean gloves
❑ Alcohol swab

❑ Antibacterial skin preparation, such as chlorhexidine
❑ Small (25 to 27) gauge winged IV catheter with attached tubing or CSQI designed catheter (e.g., Sof-Set)
❑ Infusion pump
❑ Occlusive, transparent dressing
❑ Tape
❑ Medication in appropriate syringe or container
❑ Medication administration record (MAR) or computer printout

Discontinuing CSQI

❑ Clean gloves
❑ Small, sterile gauze dressing
❑ Tape or adhesive bandage
❑ Alcohol swab and chlorhexidine (optional)

STEP	RATIONALE

ASSESSMENT

1. Check accuracy and completeness of each MAR or computer printout with prescriber's original medication order. Check patient's name and medication name, dosage, route, and time for administration. Recopy or re-print any portion of MAR that is difficult to read.

The order sheet is the most reliable source and only legal record of medications patient will receive.
Ensures patient receives the correct medications.
Illegible MARs are a source of medication errors.

2. Review medication reference information, including action, purpose, side effects, normal dose, time of peak onset, how slowly to give the medication, and nursing implications, such as the need to dilute the medication or administer it through a filter.

Allows for safe medication administration and ability to monitor patient's response to therapy.

3. Assess patient's medical and medication history.

Indicates patient's need for medication.

4. Assess patient's history of allergies; know type of allergens and normal allergic reaction.

Certain substances have similar compositions; it may harm patients to give a medication if there is a known allergy.

5. Assess patient's previous verbal and nonverbal response to needle insertion.

Injections are sometimes painful. Anticipating patient's anxiety allows you to use distraction to reduce pain awareness.

6. Assess for contraindications to CSQI (e.g., thrombocytopenia or reduced local tissue perfusion).

Reduced tissue perfusion interferes with medication absorption and distribution.

7. Assess adequacy of patient's adipose tissue to determine appropriate site.

Physiological changes of aging or patient illness influence the amount of subcutaneous tissue, which affects choice of catheter insertion site.

8. Assess patient's knowledge regarding medication to be received and use of the medication pump.

Information poses implications for patient education.

9. Assess patient's symptoms before initiating medication therapy. Determine severity of pain (if using analgesia), or measure blood glucose level (if using insulin).

Provides information to evaluate desired effects of CSQI medication.

NURSING DIAGNOSES

- Anxiety
- Deficient knowledge regarding CSQI therapy
- Fear
- Ineffective health maintenance
- Pain (acute, chronic)
- Risk for infection
- Risk for injury

Individualize related factors based on patient's condition or needs.

PLANNING

1. Expected outcomes following completion of procedure:
   - Needle insertion site remains free from infection.

   Risk for infection at needle insertion site is a potential complication of CSQI therapy (Abbas, 2005).

   - Patient achieves desired effect of medication with no signs of adverse reactions.

   Medication is delivered safely with desired therapeutic effect achieved.

   - Patient explains purpose, dosage, and effects of medication and verbalizes understanding of CSQI therapy.

   Demonstrates learning.

IMPLEMENTATION

1. Review manufacturer's directions.

Ensures proper use of equipment.

STEP	RATIONALE
2 Perform hand hygiene. Prepare medication for one patient at a time following the six rights of medication administration (see Chapter 20). Check dose on prefilled syringe. Compare label of the medication with the MAR or computer printout two times (see Skill 22-1) when removing prefilled syringe from storage area and after preparing to prime tubing.	Ensures correct medication is given to patient. Establishing a medication preparation routine, eliminating distractions, and double-checking the transcribed order reduce error (Pape and others; Ridge, 2007; Wolf, 2007). *First and second checks for accuracy ensure right medication is administered.*
3 Prime tubing with medication, being careful not to lose any medication. Obtain and program medication administration pump.	Ensures that medication dose administered is accurate.
4 Take medication to patient at right time, and perform hand hygiene. Place syringe in pump.	Ensures patient will experience medication effects at right time. Reduces risk for transmission of organisms.
5 Verify patient's identity by using at least two patient identifiers. Compare patient's name and one other identifier, such as hospital identification number, with MAR. Ask patient to state name as a third identifier.	Complies with The Joint Commission requirements and improves medication safety. In most acute care settings, the patient's name and identification number on armband and MAR are used to identify patients (TJC, 2007).
6 Compare label of the medication with the MAR a final time.	Final comparison of medication label with the MAR reduces risk for medication errors. *This is the third check for accuracy.*
7 Explain steps of procedure, and tell patient that needle insertion will cause slight burning or stinging.	Keeps patient informed of procedures and therapies.
8 Position patient, drape, and provide for privacy.	Respects patient's dignity.
9 Initiate CSQI:	
a Assist patient to comfortable position.	Eases pain associated with insertion of needle.
b Select appropriate injection site. Most common sites used are subclavicular, abdomen, upper arms, or thighs.	Site must be free from irritation and not over bony prominences.
c Apply clean gloves.	Reduces transmission of microorganisms and reduces risk for blood exposure (OSHA, 2006).
d Cleanse injection site with alcohol using a circular motion, followed by antiseptic, using straight cleansing strokes. Allow both agents to dry.	Reduces risk for infection at insertion site.
e Hold needle in dominant hand, and remove needle guard.	Prepares needle for insertion.
f Gently pinch or lift up skin with nondominant hand.	Ensures needle will enter subcutaneous tissue.
g Gently and firmly insert needle at a 45- to 90-degree angle (see illustration). Some prepackaged needles (e.g., Sof-Set, Sub-Q-Set) are inserted at a 90-degree angle. These needles are shorter than butterfly needles. Refer to manufacturer's directions.	Decreases pain related to insertion of needle.
h Release skinfold, and apply tape over "wings" of needle.	Secures needle.

Critical Decision Point   *Some cannulas have a sharp needle covered with a plastic catheter. In this case, remove the needle and leave the plastic catheter in the skin.*

i Place occlusive, transparent dressing over insertion site (see illustration).	Protects site from infection and allows you to assess site during medication infusion.

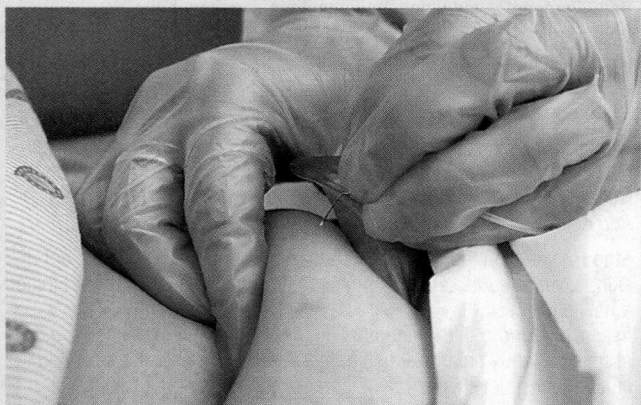

STEP 9g   Insertion of butterfly needle into subcutaneous tissue of abdomen.

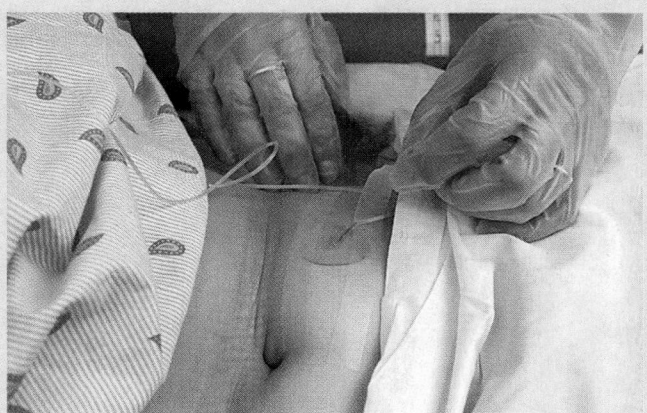

STEP 9i   Placement of transparent dressing over insertion site.

STEP	RATIONALE
j Attach tubing from needle to tubing from infusion pump, and turn pump on.	Allows you to administer medication.
k Dispose of any sharps in appropriate leak-proof, puncture-proof container. Discard used supplies, and perform hand hygiene.	Prevents accidental needle-stick injuries and follows CDC guidelines for disposal of sharps (OSHA, 2006).
l Assess site before leaving patient, and instruct patient to inform you if site becomes red or begins to leak.	Initiate a new site with a new needle whenever erythema or leaking occurs. If the site is free from complications, rotate the needle every 3 to 5 days (INS, 2006).
10 Discontinue CSQI:	
a Verify order, and establish alternative method for medication administration if applicable.	If medication will be required after discontinuing CSQI, a different medication and/or route is often necessary to continue to manage patient's illness or pain.
b Stop infusion pump.	Prevents medication from spilling.
c Perform hand hygiene, and apply clean gloves.	Follows CDC recommendations to prevent accidental exposure to blood and body fluids (OSHA, 2006).
d Remove dressing without dislodging or removing the needle.	Exposes needle.

Critical Decision Point   *If site is infected or if included in institutional guidelines, cleanse site with alcohol and antiseptic. Apply triple antibiotic cream to site if it is excoriated (abraded).*

STEP	RATIONALE
e Remove tape from the wings of needle, and pull needle out at the same angle it was inserted.	Minimizes patient discomfort.
f Apply gentle pressure at site until no fluid leaks out of skin.	Dressing will adhere to site if skin remains dry.
g Apply small sterile gauze dressing or adhesive bandage to site.	Prevents bacterial entry into puncture site.
11 Dispose of uncapped needles and syringes in puncture-proof and leak-proof container.	Prevents accidental needle-stick injuries and follows CDC guidelines for disposal of sharps (OSHA, 2006).
12 Remove gloves, and perform hand hygiene.	Reduces transmission of microorganisms.

EVALUATION

1 Evaluate patient's response to medication.	Determines effect of therapy. Decreased or absent response to medication may indicate patient is not receiving medication into subcutaneous tissue (e.g., pump malfunction, medication leaking at site).
2 Assess site at least every 4 hours for redness, pain, drainage, or swelling.	Indicates infection at insertion site.
3 Ask patient to verbalize understanding of medication and CSQI therapy.	Demonstrates learning.

Unexpected Outcomes

1   Patient complains of localized pain or burning at needle's insertion site, or site appears red, swollen, or is leaking, indicating potential infection or needle dislodgment.

2   Patient displays signs of allergic reaction to medication.

3   CSQI becomes dislodged.

Related Interventions

- Remove needle, and place new needle in a different site.
- Continue to monitor original site for signs of infection, and notify health care provider if you suspect infection.
- Stop delivering medication immediately, and follow institutional policy or guidelines for appropriate response to allergic reaction (e.g., administration of antihistamine such as diphenhydramine [Benadryl] or epinephrine) and reporting of adverse drug reactions.
- Notify patient's health care provider of adverse effects immediately.
- Add allergy information to medical record.
- Stop the infusion, apply pressure at the site until no fluid leaks out of skin, cover site with a gauze dressing or adhesive bandage, and initiate a new site.
- Assess patient to determine effects of not receiving medication (e.g., assess patient's pain level using age-appropriate pain scale, obtain blood glucose level).

Recording and Reporting

- After initiating CSQI, immediately chart medication, dose, route, site, time, date, and type of medication pump in patient's medical record.
- If medication is an opioid, follow institutional policy to document waste.
- Record patient's response to medication and appearance of site every 4 hours or according to institutional policy in nurses' notes.
- Report any adverse effects from medication or infection at insertion site to patient's health care provider, and document according to institutional policy. Patient's condition often indicates need for additional medical therapy.

Teaching Considerations

- Instruct patient to wear medical alert bracelet along with medical information, including disease (e.g., diabetes) and allergies, and a contact phone number for the pump manufacturer for technical support.
- Instruct patients to carry back-up batteries and extra medication if they are going to be away from home.
- Patients receiving insulin require intensive diabetes management education (Box 22-7).
- Never immerse pumps in water or expose them to x-rays or magnetic resonance imaging.

Pediatric Considerations

- CSQI improves glycemic control in children and adolescents. There is a decreased rate of severe hypoglycemia, catheter-site infection, and weight gain (Mack-Fogg and others, 2005; Nimri and others, 2006). Parents experience higher levels of confidence and independence in diabetes management with appropriate education and guidance (Weissberg-Benchell and others, 2007).
- Insulin pumps offer more flexibility with adolescents (Cook and Plotnick, 2005). You can place the responsibility of diabetes management on the child. Extensive child and family education is necessary to ensure effective diabetes management using CSQI (Hockenberry and Wilson, 2007).

Gerontological Considerations

- CSQI delivers isotonic IV solutions to dehydrated older adults, known as hypodermoclysis therapy. This method of providing hydration avoids the need to transfer the patient from home or long-term care facility to an acute care hospital. Fluids should infuse slowly (e.g., 30 mL/hr) during the first hour of therapy. If the patient remains comfortable, you can increase the rate of infusion. Usually infusion rates do not exceed 80 mL/hr. Hypodermoclysis provides an easy-to-use, safe, and cost-effective alternative to intravenous hydration for older adults (Walsh, 2005).

Home Care Considerations

- Patients in the home using CSQI need a responsible caregiver, if available. Educate the patient, family, and/or significant others about the desired effect of the medication, side effects and adverse effects of the medication, operation of the pump, how to evaluate the effectiveness of the medication, when and how to assess and rotate injection sites, and when to call a health care provider for problems. Patients need to know where and how to obtain and dispose of all required supplies.
- Patients managing CSQI at home may use an antibacterial soap (e.g., Hibiclens, pHisoHex) instead of alcohol and chlorhexidine to cleanse insertion site.

BOX 22-7   Education Topics for Patients Receiving Insulin With Continuous Subcutaneous Infusion

- Blood glucose monitoring
- Meal planning and food choices
- Incorporating exercise into daily routine
- How to program and use the insulin pump
- Illness guidelines and management
- Management of hypoglycemia

- Prevention and management of hyperglycemia
- Prevention of infection, especially at infusion site
- Problem-solving and decision-making skills
- Special considerations and precautions (e.g., what to do with pump when showering and sleeping)

Modified from Dalton M and others: Safety issues: use of continuous subcutaneous insulin infusion pumps (CSII) in hospitalized patients, *Hosp Pharm* 41(10):956, 2006.

 CRITICAL THINKING EXERCISES

You are assigned to care for a patient newly diagnosed with thrombophlebitis of the left calf. The patient is placed on bed rest, and the physician has ordered heparin 5000 units to be given subcutaneously every 8 hours to prevent further clot formation. You have just received the order and are getting ready to start this medication.

1 What information do you need to know about the medication before you prepare it?
2 What information do you need to know about the patient before you administer the heparin?
3 The heparin arrives on the unit in a multiple-dose vial. What will you do with this vial before administering the medication?
4 You assess the patient and find that she weighs 100 kg (220 pounds). Your drug calculation has determined that you will administer 1 mL of heparin. What size syringe and needle will you use to administer her injection? What site will you choose to administer the medication?
5 In addition to the subcutaneous heparin, the physician has ordered morphine sulfate 1 mg IV push every 6 hours as needed. What do you assess before you give the morphine?

 REVIEW QUESTIONS

1 The nurse needs to reconstitute a medication for an intramuscular injection and can choose the concentration of medication that would be best for his patient. What action by the nurse indicates he has done the procedure appropriately?
 1 The nurse shakes the vial after the fluid is injected into the vial to mix it well.
 2 The nurse determines the amount of prepared medication and concentration needed before adding the diluent.
 3 The powder is injected slowly into the vial of diluent.
 4 The nurse evaluates the medication's concentration after the diluent and powder are mixed.
2 The nurse is going to mix two medications in one syringe with one medication from a multidose vial and the other from an ampule. Which sequence of preparation is correct?
 1 The nurse withdraws the medication from the vial first.
 2 The nurse prepares the medication from the ampule first.
 3 The nurse draws all the medication out of both the ampule and the vial.
 4 The nurse inserts air into the ampule first.

3   An average-size 30-year-old woman is to have an intramuscular injection in the ventrogluteal site. Which needle is appropriate for administering the aqueous-based medication?
  1   26 gauge, ⅝ inch
  2   22 gauge, 1½ inch
  3   25 gauge, 1 inch
  4   20 gauge, 1½ inch

4   While the nurse is giving an intravenous (IV) infusion of a piggyback medication, the patient's IV site becomes cool, pale, and swollen. Upon assessing these symptoms, the nurse should take which action?
  1   Stop the current IV infusion and change to another site.
  2   Slow down the rate of the IV infusion.
  3   Flush the IV line with normal saline.
  4   Retape the IV catheter to decrease the pressure.

5   The nurse is getting ready to administer an IV push medication. What is the most important action for the nurse to take before administering the IV push medication?
  1   Assess the condition of the IV insertion site.
  2   Stop the maintenance of IV fluids.
  3   Dilute the medication to decrease irritation.
  4   Ensure that the correct-size filter needle is applied to the syringe

REFERENCES

American Diabetes Association: Continuous subcutaneous insulin infusion, *Diabetes Care* 27(suppl 1):S110, 2004a.

American Diabetes Association: Insulin administration: position statement, *Diabetes Care* 27(suppl 1):S106, 2004b.

American Diabetes Association: Standards of medical care in diabetes—2007, *Diabetes Care* 30(suppl 1):S4, 2007.

American Nurses Association: *2007 study of injectable medication errors,* http://www.nursingworld.org/coeh/resources/ANA_InviroSurveyFacts061507.pdf, accessed July 23, 2007.

Ansel H and others: *Pharmaceutical dosage forms and drug delivery systems,* ed 8, Philadelphia, 2004, Lea & Febiger.

Appel S, Wright M: Teach your patient to administer: inhaled insulin, *Nursing* 37(1):49, 2007.

Aventis: *Lovenox (enoxaparin sodium injection),* http://www.lovenox.com/, updated February 2008, accessed July 2007.

Centers for Disease Control and Prevention: *Mantoux tuberculin skin test facilitator guide,* 2007, http://www.cdc.gov/tb/pubs/Mantoux/part1.htm, retrieved July 28, 2007.

Cranwell-Bruce L: Anticoagulation therapy: reinforcing patient education, *Medsurg Nurs* 16(1):55, 2007.

Dalton M and others: Safety issues: use of continuous subcutaneous insulin infusion pumps (CSII) in hospitalized patients, *Hosp Pharm* 41(10):956, 2006.

Environmental Protection Agency: *Disposal of medical sharps,* 2007, http://www.epa.gov/epaoswer/other/medical/disposal.htm, retrieved July 29, 2007.

Fujita T and others: Normal saline flushing for maintenance of peripheral intravenous sites, *J Clin Nurs* 15(1):103, 2006.

Giger JN, Davidhizar RE: *Transcultural nursing: assessment and intervention,* ed 4, St. Louis, 2004, Mosby.

Greenway K and others: using the ventrogluteal site for intramuscular injections, *Learn Disabil Pract* 9(8):34, 2006.

Guthrie D and others: I.V. rounds: what you need to know about PICCs, *Nursing* 37(9):14, 2007.

Hadaway L: Practical considerations in administering intravenous medications, *J Neurosci Nurs* 38(2):119, 2006.

Hockenberry MJ, Wilson D: *Wong's nursing care of infants and children,* ed 7, St. Louis, 2007, Mosby.

Infusion Nurses Society: Infusion nursing standards of practice, *J Intraven Nurs* 29(1S), 2006.

Institute for Safe Medication Practices: *How fast is too fast for IV push medications?* 2007 Practices, http://www.ismp.org/newsletters/acutecare/articles/20030515.asp, accessed August 3, 2007.

Lea D: Tailoring drug therapy with pharmacogenetics, *Nursing* 35(40):22, 2005.

McKenry LM and others: *Mosby's pharmacology in nursing* ed 22, St. Louis, 2006, Mosby.

MedTronic MiniMed: *Pump infusion set overview,* 2007, http://www.minimed.com/products/insulinpumps, accessed August 3, 2007.

Morton N: Management of postoperative pain in children, *Arch Dis Child* 92:14, 2007.

Moshang J: Making a point about insulin pens, *Nursing* 35(2):46, 2005.

Munoz C, Hilgenberg C: Ethnopharmacology, *Am J Nurs* 105(8):40, 2005.

Nicholas P, Agius C: Toward safer IV medication administration: the narrow safety margins of many IV medications make this route particularly dangerous, *Am J Nurs* 105(3):25, 2005.

Nisbet AL: Intramuscular gluteal injections in the increasingly obese population: retrospective study, *Br Med J* 333(7542):637, 2006.

Occupational Safety and Health Administration: Occupational exposure to blood borne pathogens, needlestick, and other sharps injuries: final rule, CFR 29, part 1910 (*Fed Regist* 66:5317, Jan 18, 2001), updated April 2006, http://www.osha.gov/SLTC/bloodbornepathogens/index.html.

Occupational Safety and Health Administration: Occupational exposure to blood borne pathogens, needlestick, and other sharps injuries: final rule, 29 CFR part 1910 (*Fed Regist* 66:5317, Jan 18, 2001), updated April 2007, http://www.osha.gov/pls/oshaweb/owadisp.show_document?p_id=16265&p_table=FEDERAL_REGISTER.

Owens D: Interdisciplinary team consult—continuous subcutaneous infusions, *J Hosp Palliat Nurs* 7(6):310, 2005.

Pape T and others: Innovative approaches to reducing nurses' distractions during medication administration, *J Contin Educ Nurs* 36(3):108, 2005.

Pasero C, McCaffery M: Authorized and unauthorized use of PCA pumps, *Am J Nurs* 105(7):30, 2005.

Prettyman J: Subcutaneous or intramuscular? Confronting a parenteral administration dilemma, *Medsurg Nurs* 14(2):93, 2005.

Pullen R: Administering medication by the Z-track method, *Nursing* 35(7):24, 2005.

Ramtahal J and others: Sciatic nerve injury following intramuscular injection: a care report and review of the literature, *J Neurosci Nurs* 38(4):239, 2006.

Retnakarn R, Zinman B: Continuous subcutaneous insulin infusion versus multiple daily injections, *Diabetes Care* 28:763, 2005.

Ridge R: Boosting insulin safety, *Nursing* 37(2):14, 2007.

Rosenthal K: Avoiding common perils of drug administration, *Nursing* 37(4):20, 2007.

Rushing J: How to administer a subcutaneous injection, *Nursing* 34(6):32, 2004.

Schechter NL and others: Pain reduction during pediatric immunizations: evidence-based review and recommendations, *Pediatrics* 119(5):1184, 2007.

Schim S: Culturally congruent care, *J Transcult Nurs* 18(2):103, 2007.

Selekman J: Changes in the screening for tuberculosis in children, *Pediatr Nurs* 32(1):73, 2006.

Small S: Preventing sciatic nerve injury from intramuscular injections: literature review, *J Adv Nurs* 47(3):287, 2004.

Stein H: Glass ampules and filter needles: an example of implementing the sixth 'R' in medication administration, *Medsurg Nurs* 15(5):290, 2006.

The Joint Commission: *2008 National patient safety goals hospital program,* http://www.jointcommission.org, accessed July 2007.

Walsh G: Hypodermoclysis: an alternate method for rehydration in long-term care, *J Infus Nurs* 28(2):123, 2005.

Webb K: Use of insulin pumps for diabetes management, *Medsurg Nurs* 15(2):61, 2006.

Wilburn S, Eijkemans G: Preventing needlestick injuries among healthcare workers: A WHO-ICN collaboration, *Int J Occup Environ Health* 10:451, 2004.

Wolf Z: Pursuing safe medication use and the promise of technology, *Medsurg Nurs* 16(2):92, 2007.

World Health Organization: *Injection safety,* 2007, http://www.who.int/injection_safety/WHOGuidPrinciplesInjEquipFinal.pdf, accessed July 19, 2007.

Wurhman E and others: Authorized and unauthorized dosing of analgesic infusion pumps, *Pain Manag Nurs* 8(1):4, 2007.

RESEARCH REFERENCES

Abbas S: The use of metal or plastic needles in continuous subcutaneous infusion in a hospice setting, *Am J Hosp Palliat Care* 22(2):134, 2005.

Annersten R, Willman A: Performing subcutaneous injections: a literature review, *Worldviews Evid Based Nurs* 2(3):122, 2005.

Cook D, Plotnick L: Care of children and adolescents with type I diabetes, *Diabetes Care* 28(1):186, 2005.

Cook I, Murtagh J: Ventrogluteal area—a suitable site for intramuscular vaccination of infants and toddlers, *Vaccine* 24(13):2403, 2006.

Cook I and others: Definition of needle length required for intramuscular deltoid injection in elderly adults: an ultrasonographic study, *Vaccine* 24(7):937, 2007.

Mack-Fogg J and others: Continuous subcutaneous insulin infusion in toddlers and children with type 1 diabetes is safe and effective, *Pediatr Diabetes* 6(1):17, 2005.

Nimri R and others: Insulin pump therapy in youth with type 1 diabetes: a retrospective paired study, *Pediatrics* 117(6):2126, 2006.

Pellissier G and others: Risk of needlestick injuries by injection pens, *J Hosp Infect* 63(1):60, 2006.

Shih-Wen H: Evaluating the results of teaching epinephrine auto-injector use in an allergy clinic, *Pediatr Asthma Allergy Immunol* 20(1):19, 2007.

Weissberg-Benchell J and others: The use of continuous subcutaneous insulin infusion (CSII): parental and professional perceptions of self-care master and autonomy in children and adolescents, *J Pediatr Psychol* 32(7):1, 2007.

Wynaden D and others: Establishing best practice guidelines for administration of intramuscular injections in the adult: a systematic review of the literature, *Contemp Nurse* 20(2):268, 2005.

Zaybak A and others: Does obesity prevent the needle from reaching muscle in intramuscular injections, *J Adv Nurs* 58(6):552, 2007.

Zaybak A, Khorshid L: A study on the effect of the duration of subcutaneous heparin injection on bruising and pain, *J Clin Nurs* 15(11):1365, 2006.

23

Oxygen Therapy

MEDIA RESOURCES

- **evolve** learning system   http://evolve.elsevier.com/Perry/skills

  - Review Questions
  - Video Clips

-  Mosby's Nursing Video Skills, 3.0

OBJECTIVES

Mastery of content in this chapter will enable the nurse to:
- Discuss indications for oxygen therapy.
- Discuss methods for administering oxygen therapy.
- Demonstrate applying a nasal cannula and an oxygen mask.
- Demonstrate administering oxygen therapy to a patient with an artificial airway.
- Demonstrate proper peak expiratory flow rate measurements (PEFR).
- Demonstrate proper use of incentive spirometry.
- Demonstrate use of noninvasive ventilation using continuous positive airway pressure (CPAP) or bilevel positive airway pressure (BiPAP).
- Demonstrate care of the patient receiving mechanical ventilation.

Oxygen therapy is the administration of supplemental oxygen (O_2) to a patient to prevent or treat hypoxia. Hypoxia is a condition in which there is insufficient oxygen to meet the metabolic demands of the tissues and cells. Hypoxia results from hypoxemia, a deficiency of arterial blood oxygen. Hemoglobin is the carrier of respiratory gases, oxygen, and carbon dioxide (CO_2). It combines with a gas to carry it to and from the cells. Decreased hemoglobin levels reduce the amount of oxygen transported to the cells and carbon dioxide transported away from the cells. Hemoglobin levels and acid-base status directly affect oxygenation. Acidemia increases the ability of hemoglobin to release oxygen to the tissues. Alkalemia decreases the ability of hemoglobin to release oxygen to the tissues.

Various diseases require the use of oxygen therapy, for example, pneumonia. Pneumonia results in impaired gas exchange because of fluid and secretions in the lung, which decrease the diffusion of oxygen from the lungs to the arterial blood supply. Some patients with chronic bronchitis, a form of chronic obstructive pulmonary disease (COPD), have normal arterial oxygen levels during the day but have oxygen desaturation, a reduction in the arterial oxygen level, during sleep. Frequently these patients require daytime and nocturnal oxygen therapy to prevent hypoxemia (Langenhof and Fichter, 2005).

Patients with COPD are at risk for retaining carbon dioxide and developing carbon dioxide narcosis induced by administration of high levels of oxygen. Normally the chemoreceptors monitor carbon dioxide levels. In the individual with healthy lungs, the chemoreceptors are sensitive to small changes in carbon dioxide levels and effectively regulate ventilation. When the carbon dioxide level rises to a certain level, the person inhales air. In patients with COPD who retain carbon dioxide, the chemoreceptors are not sensitive to small changes in carbon dioxide and regulate ventilation poorly. In these patients it is the change in the oxygen level that stimulates changes in ventilation. When you administer high levels of oxygen, this extinguishes the stimulus to breathe.

Patients with cardiovascular disease, such as left ventricular failure, are not always able to supply oxygen to the tissues because of decreased cardiac output. Supplemental oxygen helps decrease the work of the left ventricle and increase oxygen delivery to the tissues.

The nursing assessment of a patient requiring supplemental oxygen therapy sometimes reveals findings associated with hypoxia (Box 23-1). Presenting symptoms depend on the patient's age, level of health, present disease process, and the presence of chronic illnesses. Anxiety, confusion, and restlessness are early signs of hypoxia (Carbery, 2008).

Initially blood pressure is elevated. If hypoxia remains uncorrected, hypotension develops. Respiratory rate and depth increase. As hypoxia worsens, the patient's activity tolerance decreases, vital signs worsen, and the patient's level of consciousness decreases.

Cyanosis, a bluish discoloration of the skin and mucous membranes, is a late sign of hypoxia. Vasoconstriction of the peripheral blood vessels or decreased oxyhemoglobin causes cyanosis. Cyanosis is present in patients who have decreased level of oxyhemoglobin, are very cold, or have decreased peripheral circulation because of vascular disease. Never assume a lack of cyanosis means adequate oxygenation. Cyanosis caused by hypoxia is observed in the oral mucosa, the conjunctiva of the eye, and around the lips, known as circumoral cyanosis.

OXYGEN SYSTEMS

Oxygen therapy is inexpensive, widely available, and used in a variety of settings. Patients with decreased tissue oxygenation benefit from controlled oxygen administration. Long-term oxygen treatment is one of the few interventions that improve survival in COPD (O'Reilly and Bailey, 2007). Treat oxygen therapy as a medication. It has dangerous side effects, such as atelectasis or oxygen toxicity or carbon dioxide retention in certain patients with COPD (O'Reilly and Bailey, 2007). As with any drug, continuously monitor the dosage or concentration of oxygen. Routinely check the health care provider's orders to verify that the patient is receiving the prescribed oxygen concentration. The six rights of medication administration also pertain to oxygen administration (see Chapter 20).

Selection of the type of oxygen delivery system depends on the level of oxygen support the patient needs, based on the severity of the hypoxia and the disease process. Consider other factors, such as the patient's age, level of health and orientation level, the presence of an artificial airway, whether the setting is in the hospital or the home, the type of home environment, and the type of support and care given after discharge. Common oxygen delivery systems include nasal cannula; face mask, or noninvasive ventilation (NIV); and mechanical ventilation.

Oxygen is available in a number of systems. In a hospital or institutional setting oxygen is available in a bulk liquid oxygen system designed to store the oxygen at a precise and safe temperature and

---

| **BOX 23-1** | **Assessment of Signs and Symptoms Associated With Hypoxia** |

- Apprehension, anxiety, behavioral changes
- Decreased level of consciousness, confusion, drowsiness, altered concentration
- Increased pulse rate
- Increased rate and depth of respiration or irregular respiratory patterns
- Decreased lung sounds, adventitious lung sounds (e.g., crackles, wheezes)
- Elevated blood pressure evolving to decreased blood pressure

- Pulse oximetry (SpO_2) less than 90%
- Dyspnea
- Use of accessory muscles of respiration, rib retractions
- Cardiac dysrhythmias
- Pallor, cyanosis
- Increased fatigue
- Dizziness
- Clubbing of nails resulting from prolonged, chronic hypoxia

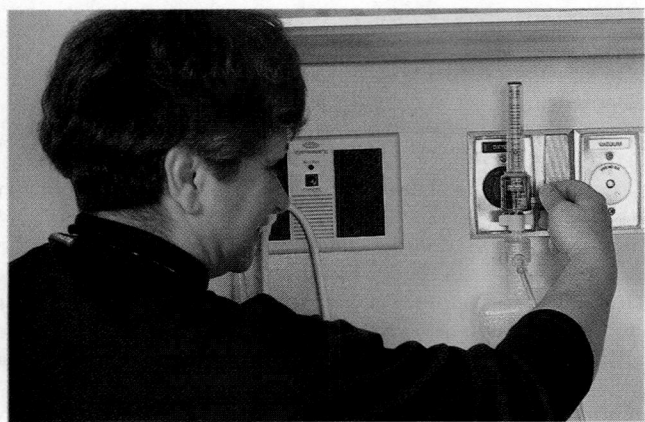

FIG 23-1   Flowmeter attached to oxygen source.

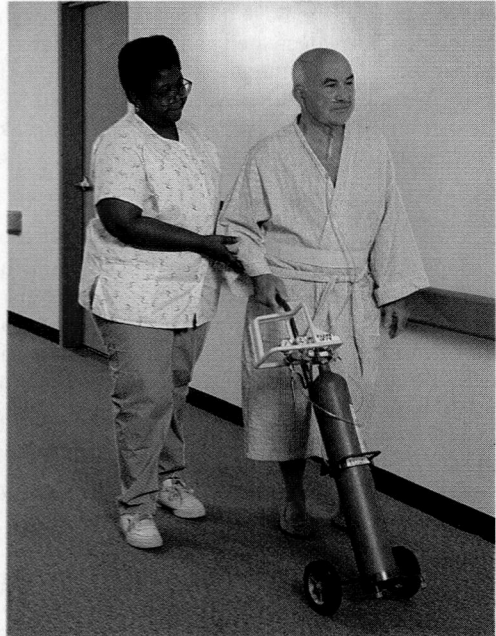

FIG 23-2   Smaller E tank for portability.

deliver it as a gas through wall outlets in a patient's room. An oxygen flowmeter regulates the flow rate in liters per minute (Fig. 23-1).

Oxygen is available as a liquid, which is lighter and more convenient for patients. It is also available as compressed gas in various-size cylinders and exists as a nonliquid gas stored at a precise temperature under high pressure and measured as pounds per square inch (psi). Oxygen cylinders used in hospital and institutional care settings include large cylinders and smaller E cylinders (Fig. 23-2). In addition, still smaller, easily transported cylinders are available for use in the home. Patients using home oxygen also use concentrators, some of which are portable.

EVIDENCE-BASED PRACTICE TRENDS

Oxygen remains one of the most effective therapeutic agents available (Langenhof and Fichter, 2005). Although this therapy benefits hypoxemic patients with pulmonary problems and those with acute exacerbations of COPD, it also relieves pulmonary vasoconstriction and right-sided heart workload and decreases myocardial ischemia. As a result, cardiac output improves. In addition, there is evidence that improved oxygen delivery to the lungs enhances pulmonary defenses

and assists mucociliary transport and mucous clearing (O'Reilly and Bailey, 2007).

Current long-term oxygen therapy reduces mortality risk in patients with COPD and severe arterial hypoxemia (O'Reilly and Bailey, 2007). In addition, long-term oxygen improves quality of life, functional status, and activity tolerance (Ram and Wedzicha, 2007).

A major concern in the administration of oxygen therapy to patients with acute exacerbations of COPD is resultant elevations in carbon dioxide levels (hypercarbia) and increased risk for respiratory failure. Administration of oxygen, even at low levels of 24% to 28%, will possibly result in hypercarbia; thus you need to administer oxygen with caution (Kuebler, 2008).

CULTURAL CONSIDERATIONS

Orient patients and family members to the oxygen setup and precautions they need to observe. Patients and visitors with limited English proficiency are not able to understand signs posted in the room. Safely accommodate valued practices of cultural groups when using oxygen. For example, Indian, Thai, and Chinese patients sometimes burn incense, which does not have a flame, to promote healing of ill members (Galanti, 2004). When oxygen is used in the home, designate areas where patient can safely burn incense, and encourage family members to bring the ashes to the bedside. Jewish patients light candles during Sabbath and accept use of battery-operated candles while in the hospital (Spector, 2008). Collaborate with family members and religious leaders on how to accommodate these practices during illness and recovery.

Skill Performance Guidelines

1   Know the patient's normal range of vital signs and pulse oximetry (SpO_2) values. Hypoxia affects a patient's vital signs and pulse oximetry values.
2   Review the patient's medical history. It is important to be aware of the patient with COPD who retains carbon dioxide. High inspired oxygen concentrations result in severe side effects such as respiratory depression and oxygen toxicity.
3   Be aware of environmental conditions. Patients with chronic respiratory diseases have difficulty maintaining optimal oxygen levels in polluted environments. If a patient is to receive home oxygen therapy, complete an environmental assessment to determine respiratory hazards in the home, such as the use of gas stoves or kerosene space heaters or the presence of smokers in the home.
4   Document the patient's smoking history. Smoking damages the lungs' mucociliary clearance mechanism and paralyzes the ciliary action, resulting in a decreased ability to clear mucus from the airways. Chronic bronchitis is caused primarily by smoking and results in pooling of mucus in the airways, creating an environment for the development of infections. Long-term chronic bronchitis ultimately results in hypoxia.
5   Know the patient's most recent hemoglobin values and past and current arterial blood gas (ABG) values.
6   Oxygen is a medication. Increasing the oxygen liter flow rate for shortness of breath is similar to doubling heart, asthma, or other medications.
7   Provide education to the patient and family about home oxygen therapy so that the patient and family understand proper use of the equipment. Safety measures for oxygen use are very important (Box 23-2).

BOX 23-2 | Oxygen Safety Guidelines

- Remind patients that oxygen is a medication and is not adjusted without a physician's order.
- In the home setting place an "Oxygen in Use" sign on the door of the residence.
- Keep oxygen delivery systems 10 feet from any open flames in the home.
- Oxygen supports combustion; however, it will not explode.
- No smoking is allowed on the premises.
- When using oxygen cylinders, secure them so that they will not fall over. Store oxygen cylinders upright, chained, or in appropriate holders.

- Determine that all electrical equipment in the room is functioning correctly and is properly grounded (see Chapter 13). An electrical spark in the presence of oxygen will result in a serious fire.
- Avoid using items that create a spark (e.g., electric razor) with a nasal cannula in use; electrical or mechanical toy in oxygen tent; objects of synthetic fabrics that cause static electricity.
- Check the oxygen level of portable tanks before transporting a patient to ensure that there is enough oxygen in the tank.

SKILL 23-1 Applying a Nasal Cannula or Oxygen Mask

 Intermediate / Respiratory Care and Suctioning / Applying a Nasal Cannula or Face Mask

NASAL CANNULA

A nasal cannula is a simple, effective, comfortable device for delivering oxygen to a patient (Fig. 23-3). It allows the patient to breathe through the mouth or nose, is available for all age-groups, and is adequate for short-term or long-term use. Cannulas are inexpensive, disposable, and easily accepted by most patients. The two tips of the cannula, about 1.5 cm (½ inch) long, protrude from the center of a disposable tube and are inserted into the nostrils. Oxygen is delivered via the cannula at a flow rate from 1 to 6 L/min. Higher flow rates dry airway mucosa and do not increase the inspired oxygen concentration (FIO_2). You do not use humidification for rates less than 4 L/min. At flow rates greater than 4 L/min, humidification helps prevent drying of nasal and oral mucous membranes. You can estimate approximate FIO_2 by the flow rate (Table 23-1). The delivered oxygen percentage will vary, depending on the rate and depth of the patient's breathing.

OXYGEN MASK

The simple face mask (Fig. 23-4) is for short-term oxygen therapy. It fits loosely and delivers oxygen concentrations from 30% to 60%. The mask is contraindicated for patients with carbon dioxide retention because it will make the retention worse. The percentage

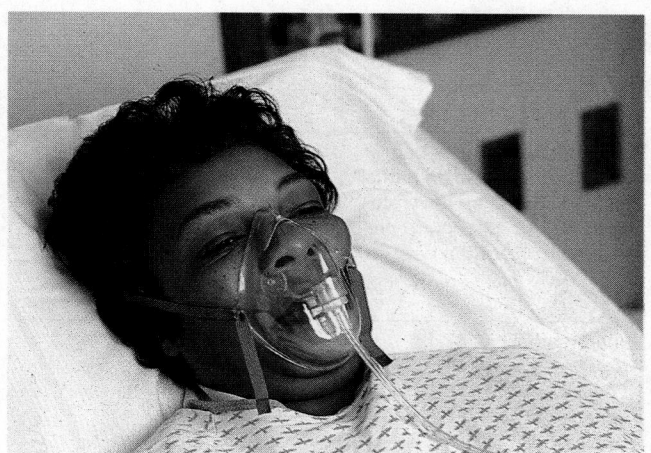

FIG 23-4 Simple face mask.

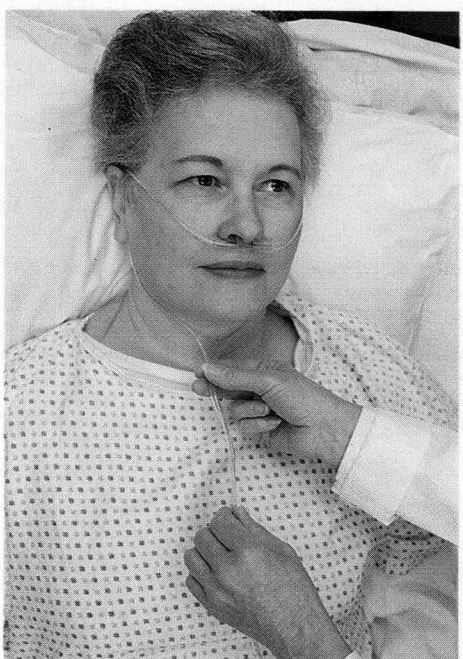

FIG 23-3 Nasal cannula is useful for low oxygen concentration (2 L/min) for patients with chronic lung disease.

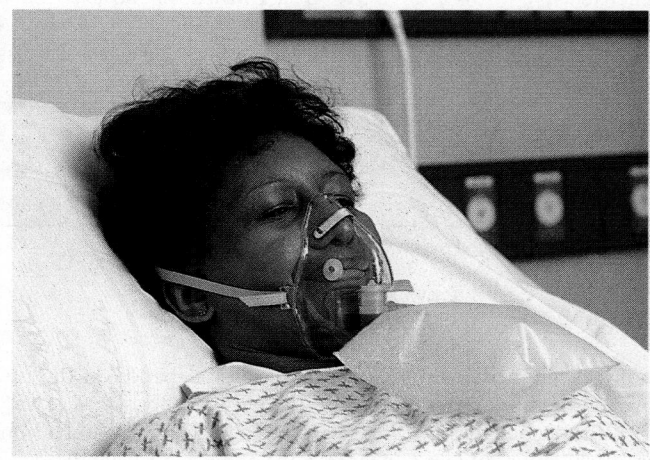

FIG 23-5 Plastic face mask with reservoir bag.

TABLE 23-1 | Oxygen Delivery Systems

Delivery System	FiO$_2$ Delivered	Advantages	Disadvantages
Nasal cannula	1 L/min: 24% 2 L/min: 28% 3 L/min: 32% 4 L/min: 36% 5 L/min: 40% 6 L/min: 44%	Safe and simple. Easily tolerated. Delivers low concentrations while allowing the patient to eat, speak, and drink. Does not impede eating or talking. Inexpensive, disposable.	Unable to use with nasal obstruction. Drying to mucous membranes. Can dislodge easily. May cause skin irritation or breakdown. Patient's breathing pattern will affect exact FiO$_2$.
OXYMIZER	1-15 L/min: 24%-60%	Higher concentrations without mask. Releases O$_2$ only on inhalation. Conserves O$_2$, increased portability. Does not require humidification.	Nasal reservoir may interfere with drinking from cup. May be cosmetically unappealing. Potential reservoir membrane failure. Patient's breathing pattern will affect exact FiO$_2$.
Simple face mask	5-6 L/min: 40% 6-7 L/min: 50% 7-8 L/min: 60% >8 L/min: 60%	Can assist in providing humidified O$_2$.	Exact FiO$_2$ level is difficult to estimate. Requires high FiO$_2$ levels to prevent rebreathing of CO$_2$. Patient inhales room air through the side holes in the mask.
Venturi mask	4 L/min: 24%-28% 8 L/min: 35%-40% 12 L/min: 50%-60%	Controls the amount of specified oxygen concentration. Delivers percentage of FiO$_2$ from 24% to 60%. Does not dry mucous membranes. Delivers humidity with oxygen concentration.	Hot and confining, increased levels of humidification may irritate skin. A specific flow rate is necessary to deliver a specific FiO$_2$, and the FiO$_2$ can be decreased if the mask does not fit properly. Interferes with eating and talking.
Partial nonrebreather—bag should always remain partially inflated. Therefore flow rate must be high enough to prevent collapse of the bag.	6 L/min: 60% 7 L/min: 70% 8 L/min: 80% 9 L/min: 90% 10 L/min: 95%	Delivers increased FiO$_2$. It is useful for patients requiring a high concentration of O$_2$ (e.g., asthma, multiple trauma). Easily humidifies O$_2$. Does not dry mucous membranes.	No inspiratory valve, so exhaled air mixes with inspired air. Hot and confining, may irritate skin, tight seal necessary. Interferes with eating and talking. Bag may twist or kink.
Nonrebreather	6-15 L/min: 60%-100%	Valve closes during expiration, so exhaled air does not enter reservoir and mix with inhaled air. Delivers highest possible FiO$_2$ without intubation. Does not dry mucous membranes.	Requires tight seal, difficult to maintain and uncomfortable. May irritate skin. Bag should not totally deflate.
Face tent	8-12 L/min: 28%-100%	Alternative to aerosol mask. Provides high humidity with O$_2$.	Difficult to keep in place, and the FiO$_2$ cannot be controlled.
Oxygen hood—usually pediatric use	5-8 L/min: 28%-40% 8-12 L/min: 49%-85%	Provides warmed humidified oxygen at a specific temperature.	Flow rate of less than 5 L/min may lead to CO$_2$ narcosis.
Oxygen tent—usually pediatric use	10-15 L/min: up to 50%	Provides humidified O$_2$ and can provide a cool environment to control body temperature.	Can be isolating for the child because every time the tent is opened the O$_2$ and humidity levels change.

FiO$_2$, Fraction of inspired oxygen concentration.

of oxygen delivered with a simple face mask depends on the liter flow and depth of respirations (see Table 23-1).

A plastic face mask with a reservoir bag (Fig. 23-5) and a Venturi mask deliver higher concentrations of oxygen. When used as a nonrebreather, the plastic face mask with a reservoir bag delivers 60% to 100% oxygen at appropriate flow rates (see Table 23-1). This oxygen mask maintains a high-concentration oxygen supply in the reservoir bag. Frequently inspect the bag to make sure it is inflated. If it is deflated, the patient breathes in large amounts of exhaled carbon dioxide.

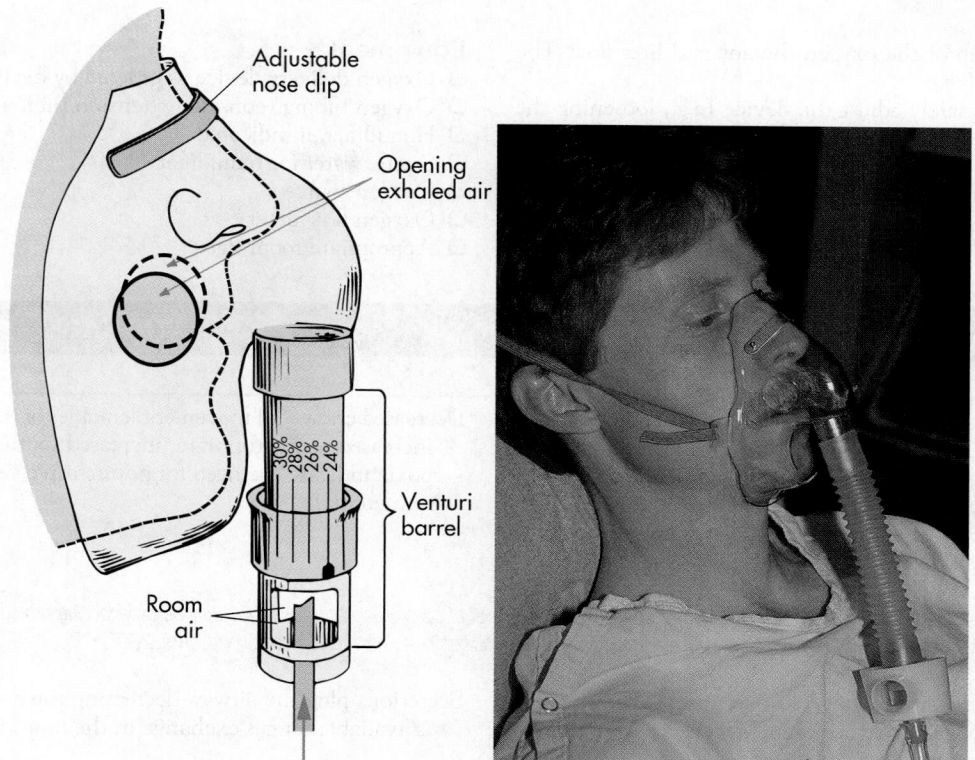

Adjustable
nose clip

Opening
exhaled air

Venturi
barrel

30%
28%
26%
24%

Room
air

FIG 23-6   Venturi mask.

A Venturi mask is a cone-shaped device with entrainment ports of various sizes at the base of the mask (Fig. 23-6). The entrainment ports adjust to permit regulation of FiO_2 from 24% to 60%. This mask is useful because it delivers a more precise concentration of oxygen to the patient (see Table 23-1).

The face tent is a shieldlike device that fits under the patient's chin and sweeps around the face (Fig. 23-7). It is used primarily for humidification and for oxygen only when the patient cannot or will not tolerate a tight-fitting mask. Because it is so close to the patient's face, there is no way to estimate how much oxygen is delivered to the patient.

Oxygen hoods and tents are commonly used in the pediatric setting. These devices are able to provide high concentrations of humidified oxygen. This is particularly useful in the child with airway inflammation, epiglottitis (croup), or other respiratory tract infections.

Delegation Considerations

The skill of applying a nasal cannula or oxygen mask can be delegated to nursing assistive personnel (NAP). The nurse is responsible for assessing the patient's respiratory system, response to oxy-

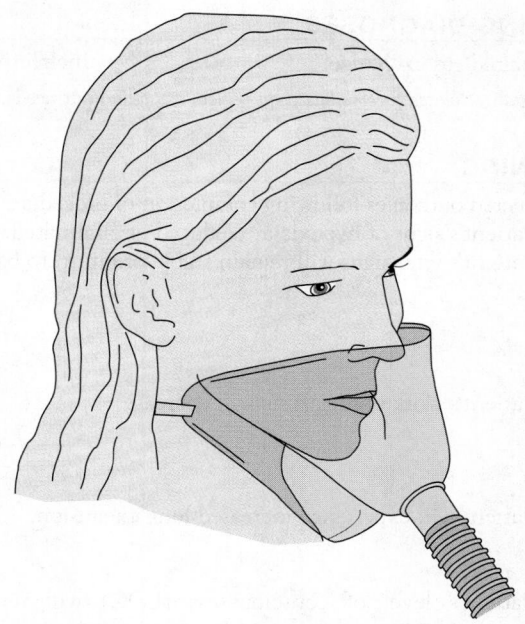

FIG 23-7   Face tent for oxygen delivery.

gen therapy, and setup of the oxygen therapy and liter flow. The nurse directs the NAP by:

- Informing how to safely adjust the device (e.g., loosening the strap on oxygen cannula or mask).
- Instructing to inform the nurse immediately about any vital sign changes; skin irritation from the cannula, mask, or straps; or patient complaints of pain or breathlessness.

Equipment
❑ Oxygen delivery device as ordered by health care provider
❑ Oxygen tubing (consider extension tubing)
❑ Humidifier, if indicated
❑ Sterile water for humidifier
❑ Oxygen source
❑ Oxygen flowmeter
❑ Appropriate room signs

STEP	RATIONALE

ASSESSMENT

1. Assess patient's respiratory status, including symmetry of chest wall expansion, chest wall abnormalities (e.g., kyphosis), temporary conditions (such as pregnancy, trauma) affecting ventilation, respiratory rate and depth, sputum production, and lung sounds (see Chapter 6) and for signs and symptoms associated with hypoxia (see Box 23-1).

Decreased chest wall movement, crackles or decreased lung sounds, increased respiratory rate, increased sputum production, or hypoxia indicate the need for noninvasive ventilation to improve oxygenation.

Critical Decision Point   *Patients with sudden changes in their vital signs, level of consciousness, or behavior may be experiencing profound hypoxia. Patients who demonstrate subtle changes over time may have worsening of a chronic or existing condition or a new medical condition (Jarvis, 2006).*

2. Observe for patent airway, and remove airway secretions by having patient cough and expectorate mucous or by suctioning (see Chapter 25).

Secretions plug the airway, decreasing the amount of oxygen that is available for gas exchange in the lungs.

3. If available, note patient's most recent ABG results or SpO_2 value.

Objectively documents the patient's pH, arterial oxygen, arterial carbon dioxide, or arterial oxygen saturation.

4. Review patient's medical record for the medical order for oxygen, noting delivery method, flow rate, and duration of oxygen therapy.

Ensures safe and accurate oxygen administration. Safe oxygen delivery includes the six rights of medication administration (see Chapter 20).

NURSING DIAGNOSES

- Impaired gas exchange
- Ineffective airway clearance
- Ineffective breathing pattern

Individualize related factors based on patient's condition or needs.

PLANNING

1. Expected outcomes following completion of procedure:
   - Patient's signs of hypoxia are reduced or eliminated.
   - Patient's vital signs will remain stable or return to baseline.

Patient demonstrates improved oxygenation.

When there is no underlying cardiovascular disease, patients adapt to decreased oxygen levels by increasing pulse and blood pressure. This is a short-term adaptive response. Once the signs of hypoxia are reduced or controlled, the patient's vital signs usually return to normal.

   - Patient's work of breathing will decrease.

Pulmonary conditions such as pneumonia or asthma cause varying degrees of airway narrowing. With improved oxygenation, the patient's airways are open, and the work of breathing decreases.

   - Patient will experience increased lung expansion.

Improved oxygenation assists in resolving collapsed and constricted airways, improves the work of breathing, and thus improves lung expansion.

   - Patient's level of consciousness (LOC) will return to baseline.

Improvement in oxygenation relieves hypoxia and improves the patient's mental status.

   - Arterial blood gas values or SpO_2 will return to normal or baseline.

Documents physiological response to oxygen therapy.

   - Patient's nares and nasal mucosa remain intact.

Oxygen cannula applied correctly.

2. Explain the procedure to patient and family.

Increases compliance and cooperation of the patient and family.

STEP	**RATIONALE**

IMPLEMENTATION

1 Perform hand hygiene.

2 Attach oxygen delivery device (e.g., cannula, mask) to oxygen tubing, and attach to humidified oxygen source adjusted to prescribed flow rate (see Fig. 23-1).

3 Position tips of cannula properly in nares, and adjust elastic headband or plastic slide on cannula or face mask so that a snug comfortable fit is achieved (see Figs. 23-3 and 23-4).

4 Maintain sufficient slack on oxygen tubing, and secure to patient's clothes.

5 Observe for proper function of oxygen delivery device:

   a *Nasal cannula:* Cannula is positioned properly in the nares.

   b *Reservoir nasal cannula OXYMIZER:* Fit as for nasal cannula. Reservoir is positioned under patient's nose or worn as a pendant.

   c *Nonrebreathing mask:* Apply mask over patient's mouth and nose to form a tight seal. The valves on the mask close, so exhaled air does not enter reservoir bag.

   d *Partial rebreathing mask (see Fig. 23-5):* Apply mask over patient's mouth and nose to form a tight seal. Ensure that the bag remains partially inflated.

   e *Venturi mask (see Fig. 23-6):* Apply mask over patient's mouth and nose to form a tight seal. Select appropriate flow rate (see Table 23-1).

   f *Face tent (see Fig. 23-7):* Apply tent under patient's chin and over the mouth and nose. It will be loose, and a mist is always present.

6 Verify setting on flowmeter and oxygen source for proper setup and prescribed flow rate.

7 Check cannula/mask every 8 hours. Keep humidification container filled at all times.

8 Perform hand hygiene.

Rationale (Step 1): Reduces transmission of microorganisms.

Rationale (Step 2): Humidity prevents drying of nasal and oral mucous membranes and airway secretions. Ensures correct O_2 delivery.

Rationale (Step 3): Directs flow of oxygen into patient's upper respiratory tract. Patient is more likely to keep device in place if it fits comfortably.

Rationale (Step 4): Allows patient to turn head without causing mask to shift position or dislodge nasal cannula.

Rationale (Step 5): Ensures patency of delivery device and accuracy of prescribed oxygen flow rate.

Rationale (a): Provides prescribed oxygen rate and reduces pressure on tips of nares.

Rationale (b): Delivers higher flow of oxygen than cannula without changing to a mask, which is claustrophobic for some patients. Delivers a 2:1 ratio (e.g., 6 L/min nasal cannula is approximately equivalent to 3.5 L/min with OXYMIZER device).

Rationale (c): Does not allow exhaled air to be rebreathed. Valves on mask side ports permit exhalation but close during inhalation to prevent inhaling room air.

Rationale (d): Allows the exhaled air to mix with the inhaled air. Ports on the side of the mask permit most of the expired air to escape; however, the bag remains partially inflated.

Rationale (e): Reduces carbon dioxide buildup.

Rationale (f): Excellent source of humidification; however, you cannot control oxygen concentrations.

Rationale (Step 6): Ensures delivery of prescribed oxygen therapy in conjunction with the specific cannula/mask.

Rationale (Step 7): Ensures patency of cannula and oxygen flow. Oxygen is a dry gas; when oxygen is administered via any route, you must add humidification so that patient inhales humidified oxygen (Woodrow, 2007).

Rationale (Step 8): Reduces transmission of microorganisms.

EVALUATION

1 Monitor patient's response to changes in the oxygen flow rate with pulse oximetry. NOTE: Monitor ABGs when ordered; however, obtaining ABG measurement is an invasive procedure and ABGs are not frequently measured.

2 Observe for decreased anxiety, improved LOC and cognitive abilities, decreased fatigue, absence of dizziness, decreased respiratory rate, improved color, improved oxygen saturation, and return to patient's baseline vital signs.

3 Assess adequacy of oxygen flow each shift.

4 Observe patient's external ears, bridge of nose, nares, and nasal mucous membranes for evidence of skin breakdown.

Rationale (1): Continual monitoring with pulse oximetry is required for patients on oxygen therapy. Base changes in supplemental oxygen on individual patient's oxygen saturation levels.

Rationale (2): Evaluates patient's response to supplemental oxygen. As the patient's oxygen level improves, physical signs and symptoms improve.

Rationale (3): Ensures patency of the oxygen delivery device.

Rationale (4): Oxygen therapy sometimes causes drying of nasal mucosa. The delivery device can cause skin breakdown where the device comes in contact with the face, neck, and ears.

Unexpected Outcomes	Related Interventions
1 Patient experiences skin irritation or breakdown (e.g., at ears, bridge of nose, nares, other pressure areas), drying of nasal and oral mucosa, sinus pain, or epistaxis.	• Increase humidification to oxygen delivery system. • Provide appropriate skin care.
2 Patient experiences continued hypoxia.	• Obtain health care provider's orders for follow-up pulse oximetry monitoring or ABG determinations. • Notify the physician or health care provider. • Consider measures to improve airway patency, coughing techniques, and oropharyngeal or orotracheal suctioning.
3 Patient experiences nasal and upper airway mucosa	• If oxygen flow rate is greater than 4 L/min, determine the need for humidification. • Assess the patient's fluid status, and increase fluids if appropriate. • Provide frequent oral care. • Obtain physician or health care provider order for use of sterile nasal saline intermittently.

Recording and Reporting

- Record the respiratory assessment findings; method of oxygen delivery, flow rate, patient's response; any adverse reactions or side effects; change in health care provider's orders.
- Report any unexpected outcome to health care provider or nurse in charge.

Teaching Considerations

- If oxygen therapy continues after discharge, teach the patient and family the importance of and rationale for oxygen therapy, how to use the oxygen delivery device, how to contact the supplier of medical equipment, and when to contact the health care provider.
- Discuss safety precautions for oxygen use (see Box 23-2) with the patient and family.
- Discuss signs of oxygen toxicity and carbon dioxide retention (e.g., confusion, headache, decreased LOC, somnolence, carbon dioxide narcosis, respiratory arrest) that the patient needs to report to the health care provider.

Pediatric Considerations

- Some infants and small children are able to tolerate a nasal cannula. Secure the prongs of the cannula with Dermiclear tape or strips of transparent dressing over the child's cheek.
- Typically infants receive oxygen therapy via an oxygen hood. Place the hood over the patient's head (sometimes over the shoulders of a small infant). Sufficient room must exist between the curve of the hood and the patient's neck to allow carbon dioxide to escape.
- Inspect toys placed in the tent for safety and suitability. Any source of sparks (e.g., from mechanical or electrical toys) is a potential fire hazard (Hockenberry and Wilson, 2007).

- Provide comfort and reassurance to the child. Make sure the child is able to see someone nearby (Hockenberry and Wilson, 2007).

Gerontological Considerations

- Because of the fragility of older adults' skin and mucous membranes, offer oral hygiene and skin care more frequently. Water-based gels, such as Aquagel, are useful but will also dry quickly and need more frequent application (Woodrow, 2007).
- Older adults often have a reduced oxygen-carrying capacity if they have a decreased hemoglobin level as a result of poor nutrition or other underlying illnesses.

Home Care Considerations

- Obtain appropriate referrals to determine if the patient meets the standards for third-party reimbursement (e.g., PaO_2 55 mm Hg or less during sleep or exercise). If patients have dependent edema, pulmonary hypertension, or hematocrit greater than 56%, they are eligible with a PaO_2 of 56 to 59 mm Hg (O'Reilly and Bailey, 2007).
- Oxygen tubing in the home setting is available in lengths of 15 m (50 feet).
- Provide information about a reliable oxygen therapy equipment vender within the community to determine if patient and family are able to use a home-fill system with an oxygen concentrator, which provides patient opportunity to fill portable canister as needed (Stegmaier, 2005).
- Consider using oxygen-conserving devices (e.g., OXYMIZER) that administer oxygen during inhalation. These reduce the use and cost of long-term oxygen therapy.

SKILL 23-2   Administering Oxygen Therapy to a Patient With an Artificial Airway

Patients with an artificial airway require constant humidification to the airway (see Chapter 25). An artificial airway bypasses the normal filtering and humidification process of the nose and mouth. The two devices that supply humidified gas to an artificial airway are a T tube and a tracheostomy collar.

The T tube, also called a Briggs adaptor, is a T-shaped device with a 15-mm (⅗-inch) connection that connects an oxygen source to an artificial airway such as an endotracheal (ET) tube or tracheostomy (Fig. 23-8). The recommended flow rate is 10 L/min with a nebulizer set to the appropriate FiO_2.

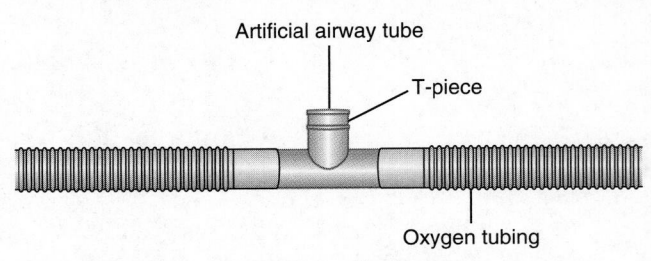

FIG 23-8   T tube.

A tracheostomy collar is a curved device with an adjustable strap that fits around a patient's neck (Fig. 23-9). There are two ports: an exhalation port that remains patent at all times and the port that connects to the oxygen source with large-bore tubing. The flow rate is set at 10 L/min with a nebulizer set to the appropriate F_IO_2 that provides humidification to the lower airways via the tracheostomy tube opening.

Delegation Considerations

The skill of administering oxygen therapy to a patient with an artificial airway cannot be delegated to NAP. The nurse is responsible for assessing the patient's respiratory system, response to oxygen therapy, and setup of the oxygen therapy device and flow rate. The nurse directs the NAP by:

- Informing about patient-specific variations for application of the T tube or tracheostomy collar (e.g., methods to avoid pressure or pulling on the artificial airway, methods for handling accumulated secretions in devices).
- Informing to immediately report to the nurse unexpected outcomes, such as increase in anxiety, change in vital signs, and increased secretions, associated with the oxygen delivery device.

Equipment

- ❑ T tube or tracheostomy collar
- ❑ Large-bore oxygen tubing
- ❑ Nebulizer

- ❑ Sterile water for nebulizer
- ❑ Oxygen or gas source
- ❑ Clean gloves
- ❑ Goggles (if splash risk exists)
- ❑ Flowmeter

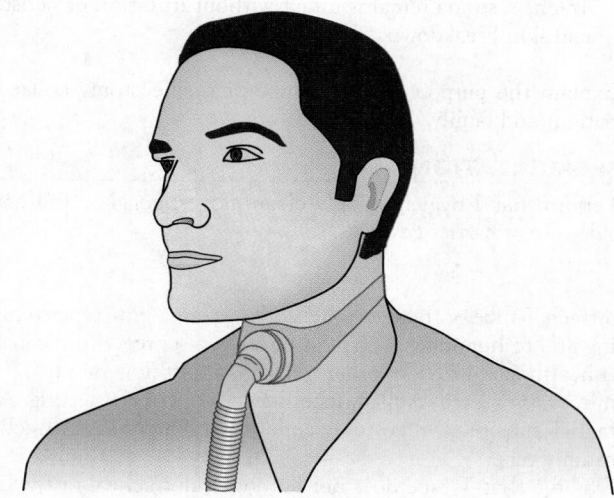

FIG. 23-9   Tracheostomy collar.

STEP	RATIONALE

ASSESSMENT

1. Assess patient's respiratory status, including symmetry of chest wall expansion, respiratory rate and depth, sputum production, and lung sounds (see Chapter 6), and assess for signs and symptoms associated with hypoxia (see Box 23-1). | Decreased chest wall movement, crackles or decreased lung sounds, increased respiratory rate, increased sputum production, or signs of hypoxia indicate worsening respiratory status and the need for other therapies.

2. Observe for patent airway, and remove airway secretions by having patient cough and by suctioning (see Chapter 25). | Secretions plug the airway, decreasing the amount of oxygen available for gas exchange in the lung. Secretions also occlude the T tube or tracheostomy collar, impeding oxygen delivery to the patient.

3. Monitor pulse oximetry (SpO_2), and if available, note patient's most recent ABG results. | Objectively documents the patient's pH, arterial oxygen, arterial carbon dioxide or arterial oxygen saturation.

4. Review patient's medical record for the medical order for oxygen, noting delivery method, flow rate, and duration of oxygen therapy. | Ensures safe and accurate oxygen administration.

NURSING DIAGNOSES

- Impaired gas exchange   • Ineffective airway clearance   • Ineffective breathing pattern

Individualize related factors based on patient's condition or needs.

PLANNING

1. Expected outcomes following completion of procedure:
   - Signs of hypoxia are reduced or eliminated. | Patient experiences improved oxygenation.
   - Patient's vital signs will return to baseline. | When there is no underlying cardiovascular disease, patients adapt to decreased oxygen levels by increasing pulse and blood pressure. This is a short-term adaptive response. Once the signs of hypoxia are reduced or controlled, the patient's vital signs usually return to normal.
   - Patient's work of breathing will decrease. | With improved oxygenation, tissue oxygen demand is met and the work of breathing decreases.
   - Patient will experience increased lung expansion. | Improved oxygenation assists in resolving collapsed and constricted airways, improves work of breathing, and thus improves lung expansion.

STEP	RATIONALE
• Patient's LOC will return to baseline.	Improvement in oxygenation relieves hypoxia and improves the patient's mental status.
• ABG values or arterial oxygen saturation will return to normal or baseline.	Documents physiological response to oxygen therapy.
• Tracheal stoma remains intact without irritation or peristomal skin breakdown.	Tension on the tracheal stoma from the oxygen therapy equipment has the potential to cause pressure on the stoma and surrounding skin.
2 Explain the purpose of the T tube or tracheostomy collar to patient and family.	Explanation decreases patient's anxiety and reduces oxygen consumption.

IMPLEMENTATION

1 Perform hand hygiene, apply clean gloves, goggles, and consider use of barrier gown.	Reduces transmission of microorganisms by preventing contact with pulmonary secretions. Patients with excessive secretions or forceful productive coughs place the caregiver at risk for splash contact.
2 Attach T tube or tracheostomy collar to large-bore oxygen tubing and to humidified room air or oxygen source, if indicated.	Provides supplemental humidification to avoid drying of the airway.
3 If health care provider orders oxygen, adjust flow rate to 10 L/min or as ordered. Adjust nebulizer to proper FiO$_2$ setting. Attach T tube or tracheostomy collar to endotracheal or tracheostomy tube.	Flow rate ensures humidification; nebulizer regulates FiO$_2$.
4 Observe that T tube does not pull on endotracheal or tracheostomy tube. Observe for secretions within T tube or tracheostomy collar, and suction as necessary (see Chapter 25).	Pulling effect increases patient's discomfort and causes pressure to side of patient's mouth or tracheal stoma. Maintains patent airway.
5 Observe oxygen tubing frequently for accumulation of fluid. If fluid is present, drain tube away from patient, and discard fluid in proper receptacle.	Excess water is medium for bacterial growth. Draining contaminated water into proper receptacle prevents contamination of entire humidifying unit.
6 Set up suction equipment at patient's bedside.	Some patients experience increased airway secretions resulting from humidification.
7 Remove gloves and goggles; perform hand hygiene.	Reduces transmission of microorganisms.

EVALUATION

1 Monitor patient's response to changes in the oxygen flow rate with pulse oximetry.	Monitoring with pulse oximetry allows for noninvasive, cost-effective trending of the patient's arterial oxygen saturation and pulse rate.
2 Observe the position of the oxygen delivery device to ensure that it is not pulling on the artificial airway.	Pulling on the artificial airway results in damage to the oral cavity or stoma.
3 Monitor ABG levels or observe pulse oximetry.	Documents patient's level of oxygenation.

Unexpected Outcomes	Related Interventions
1 Patient experiences tracheal stoma irritation; thick, tenacious secretions; pressure areas on neck or near stoma site.	• Implement measures to maintain skin integrity (see Chapter 18). • Increase frequency of airway care. • Suction secretions from artificial airway and lungs as indicated.
2 Patient experiences continued hypoxia.	• Determine if the cause of the continued hypoxia is the oxygen delivery device, plugging of the airway, the oxygen flow rate, or a new clinical problem. • Notify physician or health care provider of continued or worsening hypoxia.

Recording and Reporting

• Record the respiratory assessment findings; method of oxygen delivery, flow rate, condition of tracheal stoma, patient's response; any adverse reactions or side effects; change in health care provider's orders.
• Report any unexpected outcome to physician or nurse in charge.

Teaching Considerations

• See Teaching Considerations for Skill 23-1.

Home Care Considerations

• Some patients with an artificial airway who are at home have a permanent tracheostomy, as well as a T tube or a tracheostomy collar. The patient or caregiver needs to be physically able to perform tracheostomy care and suctioning techniques (see Chapter 25).

SKILL 23-3 Using Incentive Spirometry

Incentive spirometry assists the patient in deep breathing. An incentive spirometer (IS) is most often used following abdominal or thoracic surgery to help reduce the incidence of postoperative pulmonary atelectasis. The use of incentive spirometry is especially important in patients with underlying pulmonary diseases because of their risk for postoperative pneumonia. Studies demonstrate that although postoperative deep breathing and coughing are as effective as incentive spirometry, the use of an IS in combination with coughing and other methods for lung expansion (e.g., chest physiotherapy and intermittent positive pressure) lowers rates of postoperative pneumonia (Lawrence and others, 2006).

Incentive spirometry provides visual feedback to patients about the depth of their breaths. The two types of spirometers are flow oriented and volume oriented. Flow-oriented incentive spirometry devices have one or more plastic chambers with freely movable, colored balls. As a patient inhales slowly, the balls are elevated to a premarked area (Fig. 23-10). The patient's goal is to keep the balls elevated for as long as possible to ensure maximal sustained inhalation, not to snap the balls to the top of the chamber with a rapid, very brief, low-volume breath. Even if a very slow inspiration does not elevate the balls, this pattern helps the patient improve lung expansion. The advantage of a flow-oriented IS is the slow, steady expansion of the lung.

Volume-oriented devices use a bellows that a patient must raise to a predetermined volume by inhaling slowly (Fig. 23-11). An achievement light or counter provides feedback to the patient. Some devices have a marker that moves up as a patient inhales. The advantage of the volume-oriented IS is that a patient can achieve a known inspiratory volume and can measure it with each breath.

Incentive spirometry encourages patients to breathe deeply and achieve their normal inspiratory capacity. Before surgery it is helpful to determine a patient's baseline inspiratory capacity. An inspiratory volume half to three quarters of baseline is an acceptable postoperative volume. Patients benefiting from incentive spirometry include those using it preoperatively, especially before abdominal, cardiac, or orthopedic surgery; patients with a history of smoking, pneumonia, or chronic respiratory disease; and patients with atelectasis (Lawrence and others, 2006).

Delegation Considerations
The skill of using incentive spirometry can be delegated to NAP. The nurse is responsible for patient assessment, monitoring, and evaluating the patient response. The nurse directs the NAP by:
- Informing about the patient's target goal for spirometry.
- Informing to immediately notify the nurse about any unexpected outcomes, such as chest pain, excessive sputum production, and fever.

Equipment
❑ Flow-oriented IS or volume-oriented IS

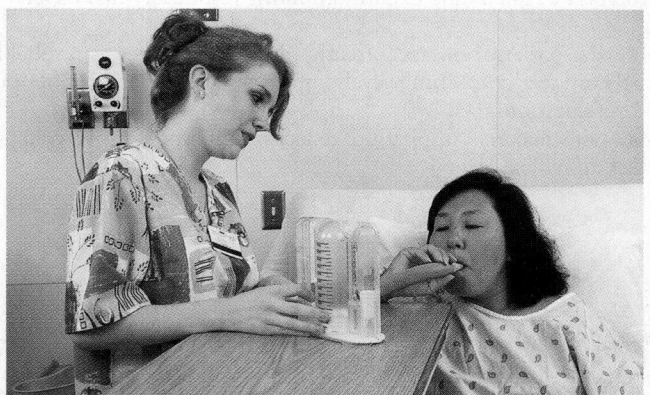

FIG 23-10   Flow-oriented incentive spirometer.

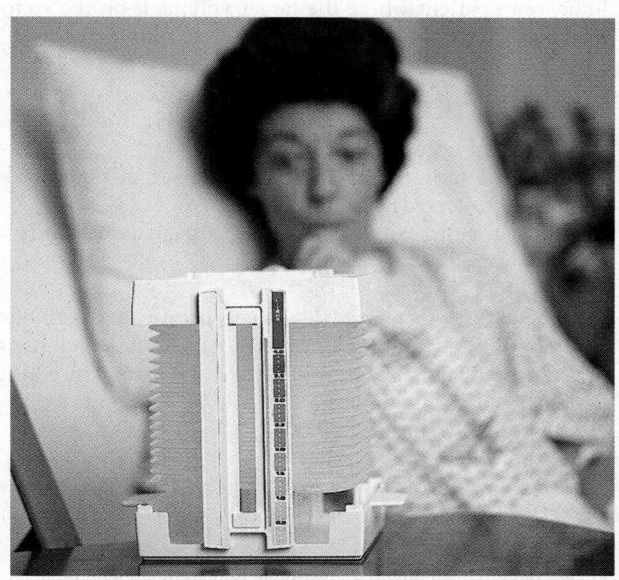

FIG 23-11   Volume-oriented incentive spirometer.

STEP	RATIONALE

ASSESSMENT

1 Identify patients who will benefit from incentive spirometry, especially those who have existing pulmonary disease, are overweight, or have other debilitating chronic illnesses (Lawrence and others, 2006; Ruse and Molyneux, 2006).

Alerts health care personnel to those patients at risk for respiratory complications during illness or postoperatively.

2 Assess patient for confusion, malnutrition, cognitive impairment, and decreased necessary motor skills.

Determines risks for having difficulty with incentive spirometry.

Critical Decision Point   *Incentive spirometry is usually contraindicated in patients with flail chest. These patients require other respiratory maneuvers to correct asymmetrical chest wall motion.*

STEP	RATIONALE
3 Assess patient's respiratory status, including symmetry of chest wall expansion, respiratory rate and depth, sputum production, and lung sounds (see Chapter 6).	Decreased chest wall movement, crackles or decreased lung sounds, increased respiratory rate, or increased sputum production can indicate a need for incentive spirometry to improve lung expansion.
4 Assess level of pain.	Pain decreases effective incentive spirometry because the patient restricts chest expansion and at times coughing.
5 Review the health care provider's order for incentive spirometry.	Health care institutions frequently require a medical order for incentive spirometry in order to receive third-party reimbursement for the spirometer.

NURSING DIAGNOSES

• Impaired gas exchange	• Ineffective airway clearance	• Ineffective breathing pattern

Individualize related factors based on patient's condition or needs.

PLANNING

1 Expected outcomes following completion of procedure:	
• Patient will demonstrate correct use of the IS.	Demonstrates learning.
• Patient achieves target volume and number of repetitions per hour.	Demonstrates increased lung expansion.
• Patient has improved breath sounds.	Incentive spirometry assists the patient in deep breathing and managing airway secretions.
2 Explain the procedure to patient and family.	Understanding the purpose of incentive spirometry and its proper use will improve compliance with use.
3 Indicate to patient where the target volume is on the spirometer. NOTE: If possible, demonstrate use of spirometer.	Encourages patients to "do better" with each breath and to meet or exceed the target volume. When patients have a visual target, they can gauge their improvement.

IMPLEMENTATION

1 Perform hand hygiene.	Reduces transmission of microorganisms.
2 Position patient in the most erect position (e.g., high-Fowler's position, if tolerated) (Pruitt, 2006).	Promotes optimal lung expansion during respiratory maneuver.
3 Instruct patient to exhale completely through mouth and place lips tightly around the mouthpiece.	Showing patient how to correctly place mouthpiece is a reliable technique for teaching psychomotor skill and enables patient to ask questions.
4 Instruct patient to take a slow, deep breath and maintain a constant flow, like pulling through a straw. When patient cannot inhale any more, patient has reached maximal inspiration. Patient needs to hold breath for at least 3 seconds and then exhale normally (Pruitt, 2006).	Maintains maximal inspiration; reduces risk for progressive collapse of individual alveoli.

Critical Decision Point   *Some patients with COPD are able to hold their breath for only 2 to 3 seconds. Encourage patients to do their best and to try to extend the duration of breath holding. Allow patients to rest between IS breaths to prevent hyperventilation and fatigue.*

5 Have patient repeat the maneuver, encouraging patient to reach the prescribed goal.	Ensures correct use of the spirometer and patient's understanding of use.
6 Remind patient to perform IS exercises 5 to 10 times followed with controlled coughing every hour while awake or as directed by health care provider. Keep IS device within patient's reach.	Repeated use of IS improves lung expansion and promotes clearing of airways, especially in patients with underlying lung disease (Lawrence and others, 2006). Atelectasis can start within an hour post anesthesia (Pruitt, 2006). Using controlled cough techniques reduces the risk for coughing spasms.
7 Perform hand hygiene.	Reduces transmission of microorganisms.

EVALUATION

1 Observe patient's ability to use incentive spirometry by return demonstration.	Determines patient's ability to perform breathing exercise correctly.

STEP	RATIONALE
2 Assess if the patient is able to achieve the target volume or frequency.	Measures compliance with therapy and lung expansion.
3 Auscultate chest during respiratory cycle.	Documents lung expansion, identifies any abnormal lung sounds, and determines if airways are clear.

Unexpected Outcomes

1 Patient is unable to achieve incentive spirometry target volume.

Related Interventions

- Encourage patient to attempt incentive spirometry more frequently followed by rest periods.
- Teach cough-control exercises.
- Teach patient how to splint and protect incision sites during deep breathing.

2 Patient has decreased lung expansion and/or abnormal breath sounds.

- Teach patient cough-control exercises.
- Provide assistance with suctioning if patients cannot effectively cough up their secretions.

Recording and Reporting

- Record the lung sounds before and after incentive spirometry, the frequency of use, the volumes achieved, and any adverse effects.
- Report any changes in respiratory assessment or patient's inability to use IS to health care provider.

Teaching Considerations

- Do not let patient use the device if patient cannot understand or demonstrate proper use.
- Teach patient to examine sputum for consistency, amount, and color changes.

Pediatric Considerations

- Incentive spirometry is not typically used in pediatrics except for school-age children; a pediatric patient needs the fine motor skills and ability to follow instructions to effectively use IS (Hockenberry and Wilson, 2007).
- Allowing a child to play with and try out the IS assists in decreasing the child's anxiety and encourages participation in care.

- Use games or bubbles and balloons to encourage small children to take deep breaths. These activities will help achieve the same goals as incentive spirometry in some children.

Gerontological Considerations

- Older adults with chronic illnesses or arthritis have difficulty coordinating the use of the IS. They will require additional time to demonstrate the procedure (Meiner and Lueckenotte, 2006).
- COPD, common in the older adult population, is an important patient-related risk factor; in addition, heart failure, cigarette use, obesity, obstructive sleep apnea, and decreased cognitive status are also risks for developing postoperative pulmonary complications. Using IS preoperatively and postoperatively has the potential to reduce these risks.
- Weakened respiratory muscles and decreased elastic recoil properties of the lungs affect a patient's ability to cough and deep breathe. Therefore it takes an older adult longer to achieve the target volume (Ruse and Molyneux, 2005).

SKILL 23-4   Care of a Patient Receiving Noninvasive Ventilation

Intermediate / Respiratory Care and Suctioning / Ensuring Oxygen Safety / Maintaining an Airway

Noninvasive ventilation (NIV) maintains positive airway pressure and improves alveolar ventilation without the need for an artificial airway. In addition, this mechanical ventilation alternative reduces and reverses atelectasis, improves oxygenation, reduces pulmonary edema, and improves cardiac function (Frace, 2008). Continuous positive airway pressure (CPAP) keeps the terminal airways (alveoli) partially inflated, reducing the risk for atelectasis; and if atelectasis has occurred, positive pressure assists in reinflation. Because the alveoli remain partially inflated, there is continued exchange of respiratory gases, and as a result the patient's oxygenation improves (Jarvis, 2006). In a cardiac patient, NIV reduces pulmonary edema because the increased alveolar pressure forces interstitial fluid out of the lungs and back into the pulmonary circulation. In patients with altered cardiac function secondary to sleep apnea, NIV provides improved myocardial oxygenation and function.

In selected patients, such as those with postpolio syndrome and other neuromuscular diseases, congestive heart failure, sleep disorders, and pulmonary diseases, NIV is often the treatment of choice in supporting ventilation without the hazards associated with endotracheal intubation (Frace, 2008). In addition, there is a reduced risk for pneumonia, gastric aspiration, and ventilator dependency when using NIV.

NIV delivers both inspiratory positive airway pressure (IPAP) and an expiratory positive airway pressure (EPAP) (Jarvis, 2006). Thus NIV has the option of providing CPAP or bilevel positive airway pressure (BiPAP). For most patients it is recommended to try CPAP initially. If this delivery mechanism is not effective, then BiPAP is tried.

CPAP maintains a set positive airway pressure, measured by centimeters of water (cm H_2O) throughout the patient's inspiratory and expiratory breathing cycles (Fig. 23-12). A CPAP of 5 cm H_2O provides 5 cm of pressure during inspiration and expiration. It is very beneficial in patients who retain carbon dioxide, such as with obstructive sleep apnea (OSA) or acute exacerbations of COPD (Balami, 2006). CPAP keeps the airway open and prevents upper airway collapse. As a result of CPAP therapy a patient breathes more normally, sleeps better, and has markedly reduced snoring. In OSA the upper airway collapses during sleep and prevents normal airflow. When the airflow is interrupted, there is a drop in the patient's oxygen saturation and frequent awakenings occur. The usual CPAP pressure is 4 to 10 cm H_2O (Frace, 2008). However, there are disadvantages to this device (Table 23-2).

BiPAP is delivered via face mask, so some patients find it uncomfortable and noisy (see Table 23-2). BiPAP works by providing assistance during inspiration and preventing airway closure during expiration. BiPAP uses two modes of pressure: one for inspiration and one for expiration. The health care provider designates the pressure during inspiration. BiPAP generates a preset positive pressure support, during inspiration, which increases the patient's tidal volume and ultimately alveolar ventilation. This inspiratory pressure support ends when the patient initiates the expiratory phase. As a result, there is an increase in the functional residual capacity (the amount of air remaining in the lungs at the end of expiration), reduced airway closure, reexpansion of atelectatic areas, and improved oxygenation. During expiration BiPAP delivers sufficient expiratory pressure to keep the airways open (Frace, 2008).

For patients who have measurable changes with flow of their airways, such as patients with asthma, peak expiratory flow rates (PEFRs) measurements are useful. The PEFR is the maximum flow that a patient forces out during one quick exhalation and is measured in liters. These measurements provide an objective indicator of the patient's current status or the effectiveness of treatment (see Procedural Guideline 23-1, p. 645). The National Institutes of Health (NIH) has developed a peak flow zone system organized in a "traffic light" pattern to assist patients with their peak flow meter changes (see http://www.nhlbi.nih.gov).

The goals for NIV include improved oxygenation, decreased carbon dioxide retention, improved sleep, enhanced quality of

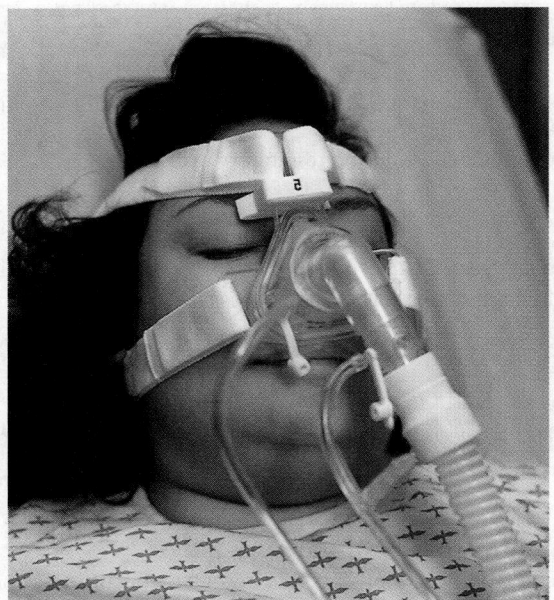

FIG 23-12 Mask suitable for continuous positive airway pressure (CPAP).

life, reduced morbidity, improved physical and physiological function, and cost-effectiveness (Balami, 2006; Frace, 2008). Patients and families who are candidates for NIV are prepared for discharge by a multidisciplinary team including representatives of nursing, medicine, dietary service, social service, the home care nurse, and the home care durable medical equipment company.

Delegation Considerations

The skill of caring for a patient receiving noninvasive ventilation cannot be delegated to NAP. The nurse directs the NAP by:

- Informing about the need to immediately report to the nurse any changes in patient's pulse, blood pressure, respiratory rate, oxygen saturation, mental status, or skin color.

TABLE 23-2	Problems Associated With Continuous Positive Airway Pressure (CPAP) and Bilevel Positive Airway Pressure (BiPAP)
Problem	**Cause**
Discomfort	Tight-fitting mask that fits over patient's nose. Oxygen flow rate causes dry mucous membranes.
Psychosocial	Difficult for relationship with sleep partner. Possible sensations of claustrophobia.
Risks to skin integrity	Tight fit of the mask causes diaphoresis, pressure, and increased risk for skin breakdown. Patients need to remove the mask to relieve pressure.
Hypercapnia	Although CPAP improves alveolar function, which increases carbon dioxide clearance from the blood, it also causes air trapping. In some patients this causes a rise in carbon dioxide levels. Initially, you need to monitor the patient's ABG levels.
Gastric distention	CPAP/BiPAP forces more air into the stomach, which causes distention and discomfort.
Noise	Some patients find the older machines very noisy, not only interfering with sleep but also leisure activities, such as watching TV or listening to music.

Data from Frace M: Noninvasive ventilation: CPAP and BiPAP on the medical-surgical unit, *Med-Surg Matters* 17(3):12, 2008; Jarvis H: Exploring the evidence base of the use of non-invasive ventilation, *Br J Nurs* 15:756, 2006.
ABG, Arterial blood gas.

- Instructing on how to modify care, such as how long the mask can be removed, oral care, or any special skin care needs.
- Informing about the prescribed settings on the NIV equipment and notifying nurse of any change in settings or patient comfort.

Equipment

(NOTE: When device is used in the home, the home care equipment vendor provides the equipment.)

❑ Nasal mask/full face mask (with quick-release straps), or nasal pillows

❑ Oxygen source and tubing
❑ CPAP/BiPAP per health care provider order
❑ Humidification source, if needed
❑ Pressure generator (in institutional health care settings the patient's room may have a pressure source)
❑ Delivery tubing
❑ Pulse oximetry
❑ Clean gloves
❑ Gown, mask, and goggles (if splash risk exists)

STEP	RATIONALE
ASSESSMENT	
1 Assess patient's respiratory status, including symmetry of chest wall expansion, respiratory rate and depth, oxygen saturation, sputum production, and lung sounds (see Chapter 6). When possible, ask patient about dyspnea, and observe for signs and symptoms associated with hypoxia (see Box 23-1).	Decreased chest wall movement, crackles or decreased lung sounds, increased respiratory rate, increased sputum production, or signs of worsening hypoxia indicate a need for mechanical ventilation or changes in the current ventilator settings to improve oxygenation.
2 Observe patient's skin over the bridge of nose, around the external ears, back of the head.	The mask can place pressure on the skin and increase the risk for skin breakdown.
3 Observe patient's ability to clear and remove airway secretions.	Secretions plug the airway, decreasing the amount of oxygen that is available for gas exchange in the lung.
4 Obtain pulse oximetry results, and when available, note patient's most recent ABG results.	Objectively documents patient's pH, arterial oxygen, arterial carbon dioxide, or arterial oxygen saturation.
5 Obtain vital signs and pulse oximetry before initiation of therapy.	Provides baseline data to compare desired or untoward vital sign changes resulting from the therapy.

Critical Decision Point *NIV is contraindicated in cardiac or respiratory arrest, nonrespiratory organ failure, facial surgery or trauma, inability to protect the airway and/or high risk for aspiration, and inability to clear secretions (Nava and Cerianna, 2004).*

6 Review patient's medical record for the medical order for CPAP/BiPAP and appropriate settings.	Health care provider's order is necessary for this therapy.

NURSING DIAGNOSES

- Activity intolerance
- Impaired gas exchange
- Sleep deprivation

Individualize related factors based on patient's condition or needs.

PLANNING

1 Expected outcomes following completion of procedure:	
• Patient will have increased lung expansion.	Patient experiences improved oxygenation.
• Patient will maintain ABG levels or oxygen saturation within normal range or at baseline.	NIV delivered appropriately based on patient assessment data.

Critical Decision Point *When first initiating CPAP/BiPAP, it is important to monitor ABG levels in addition to pulse oximetry, especially in patients with COPD, pulmonary edema, or acute respiratory failure. You do this to observe for carbon dioxide retention (Jarvis, 2006; Nava and Cerianna, 2004).*

• Patient experiences reduction in feelings of dyspnea and work of breathing.	In patients with acute conditions there is usually an improvement in dyspnea within 30 to 60 minutes (Balami, 2006; Woodrow, 2003b). Patients with chronic pulmonary diseases often require nocturnal CPAP/BiPAP indefinitely to achieve long-term benefits.
• Patient's vital signs and respiratory assessment parameters improve.	Reduced pulse and respiratory rate, improved mental status, improved skin color, and decreased use of accessory and abdominal muscles occurs because patient's work of breathing decreases as the level of oxygenation improves (Frace, 2008).
2 Explain to patient and family the purpose and reasons for CPAP/BiPAP.	Helps reduce the sense of claustrophobia from the mask. In addition, information reduces anxiety and increases cooperation and compliance with the therapy.

STEP	RATIONALE

IMPLEMENTATION

1 Perform hand hygiene; apply clean gloves and goggles. Apply mask, gown, and goggles if secretions are projectile.

Reduces transmission of microorganisms and exposure to pulmonary secretions.

2 Determine correct mask size. Masking charts are supplied to determine the correct size (S, M, L, XL). **NOTE: It is imperative that the mask have quick-release straps.**

Mask should fit snugly over patient's nose (CPAP) or nose and/or mouth (BiPAP) to create a tight seal for delivering positive pressure. In the case of an emergency (e.g., vomiting, respiratory arrest) quick-release straps allow the mask to be quickly removed. This system also allows patient to remove the mask quickly as needed (Frace, 2008).

3 Connect CPAP/BiPAP device delivery tubing to pressure generator.

Ensures patient is receiving proper NIV as ordered.

4 Connect patient to pulse oximetry.

It is important to continually monitor patient's level of oxygenation when initiating NIV (Jarvis, 2006).

5 Set CPAP/BiPAP initial settings:

These settings allow the health care team to determine initial patient response.

a CPAP: 4 to 8 cm H_2O

CPAP provides single positive pressure throughout the breathing cycle, which helps to keep the alveoli open at end-expiration.

b BiPAP:
   Inspiratory pressure usually set at 10 to 15 cm H_2O
   Expiratory pressure usually set at 4 to 10 cm H_2O (Frace, 2008)

BiPAP supplies pressures at both inhalation and exhalation. The inhalation pressure is set according to health care provider's order and helps to prevent airway closure. The expiratory pressure is set according to health care provider's order and assists in keeping the alveoli open at end-expiration (Frace, 2008).

6 Perform frequent skin assessment to determine the presence of pressure, skin irritation, or skin breakdown.

A mask that is too tight increases the risk for skin breakdown over the bridge of the nose (Jarvis, 2006).

7 Dispose of supplies as appropriate, and perform hand hygiene.

Reduces transmission of microorganisms.

EVALUATION

1 Observe for decreased anxiety; improved LOC and cognitive abilities; decreased fatigue; absence of dizziness; decreased pulse, regular rhythm; decreased respiratory rate and work of breathing; return to normal blood pressure; improved color (Jarvis, 2006).

Determines patient's response to NIV. As hypoxia and hypercapnia are reduced or corrected, the patient's physical assessment parameters improve.

2 Monitor ABG levels—observe pulse oximetry.

Documents patient's level of oxygenation. When first initiating NIV, especially in patients with underlying COPD, it is important to obtain ABG levels after the first hour and every 2 to 6 hours during the first day because these patients may retain carbon dioxide.

3 Observe skin integrity over the bridge of the patient's nose.

A mask that is too tight causes skin breakdown, and frequent skin assessment is necessary.

4 If NIV is planned for use in the home, observe and monitor patient and family's ability to manipulate device and face mask.

Determines patient's ability to perform self-care and adhere to CPAP/BiPAP plan. The success of noninvasive ventilation depends largely on patient acceptance and adherence (Nava and Cerianna, 2004).

Unexpected Outcomes	Related Interventions
1 Patient experiences hypoxia.	• Notify physician or health care provider. • Reassess patient. • Determine correct settings and integrity of NIV.
2 Patient experiences hypercapnia.	• Notify physician or health care provider. • Reassess patient. • Determine correct settings and integrity of NIV.
3 Patient states a sense of smothering or claustrophobia.	• Explain system to patient again. • Demonstrate use of quick-release straps. • Have patient demonstrate use of quick-release straps.

Recording and Reporting

- Record respiratory assessment findings, CPAP/BiPAP settings, vital signs and pulse oximetry, patient response, patient teaching outcomes.
- Report to charge nurse or health care provider: Sudden change in patient's respiratory status and any decline in ABG levels or pulse oximetry values.

Teaching Considerations

- Teach the patient and family the best hours to use the machine (e.g., bedtime, watching TV); usually the patient receives 6 to 8 hours of continual CPAP/BiPAP.
- Teach the patient and family how to apply the mask, connect it to the machine, and how to add oxygen if ordered.
- Instruct family to bring the machine, along with a list of correct settings, to the hospital any time the patient is admitted.

- When patients require home NIV, instruct in complete care of the CPAP/BiPAP system. Skills include assembling the system, cleaning the system, and daily equipment maintenance.

Home Care Considerations

- The durable medical equipment provider, the home care nurse, and the primary care nurse develop a teaching plan to ensure that patient and family have working knowledge of the system before discharge.
- Instruct patient and primary caregiver in what to do in case of respiratory distress or power failure.
- Notify appropriate power company so that in the event of a power outage, the home is on priority for restoring power.

PROCEDURAL GUIDELINE 23-1   Use of a Peak Flow Meter

Delegation Considerations

Assessment of a patient's condition cannot be delegated. The skill of follow-up peak expiratory flow rate measurements (PEFR) can be delegated to NAP.

Equipment

Peak flow meter, patient diary/action plan, if appropriate.

1. Instruct patient about the purpose and rationale.
2. Patient should be standing. If patient cannot stand, assist patient to high-Fowler's position.
3. Slide the mouthpiece into base of the numbered scale to zero position.
4. Instruct patient to take a deep breath.
5. Have patient place meter mouthpiece in the mouth and close lips, making a firm seal.
6. Have patient blow out as hard and fast as possible through the mouth only in one single breath.

7. Repeat maneuver two additional times, with the highest number recorded in the chart or patient's diary.
8. If patient is to record PEFR at home, have patient demonstrate PEFR technique independently and assess ability to record PEFR accurately on chart using "traffic light" pattern. Green zone (80% to 100% of personal best number) indicates that no asthma symptoms are present. Yellow zone (50% to 80% of personal best number) signals caution. Red zone (less than 50% of personal best number) signals a medical alert and patient should call health care provider immediately (Zoidus, 2005).
9. Help patient implement an appropriate action plan as prescribed by health care provider.
10. Instruct patient to clean unit weekly, following manufacturer's instructions.

SKILL 23-5   Care of a Patient on a Mechanical Ventilator

 Intermediate / Respiratory Care and Suctioning / Suctioning an Artificial Airway

Patients requiring mechanical ventilation need support for ventilation and/or oxygenation. Clinical problems such as respiratory failure, exacerbation of chronic obstructive lung disease, spinal cord trauma, respiratory muscle paralysis, and pneumonia require mechanical ventilation support. Patients receiving mechanical ventilation are most often in an intensive care unit.

There are two types of mechanical ventilation: positive pressure and negative pressure. Positive-pressure ventilation is the usual method of ventilation that delivers a positive pressure to inflate the lungs. There are multiple complications associated with positive-pressure ventilation: decreased cardiac output, aspiration, tension pneumothorax (see Chapter 25), bronchospasm, laryngeal trauma, sinusitis, and ventilator-associated pneumonia. In addition, as the length of time needed for mechanical ventilation increases, there is an increased risk for failure to wean from the ventilator (Carbery, 2008). Be alert for these side effects. An artificial airway, such as an ET or tracheostomy tube, is necessary (see Chapter 25).

Negative-pressure ventilation is a noninvasive, negative-pressure ventilation technique that is used for patients with primary neuromuscular illnesses that interfere with normal respiratory muscle function, such as multiple sclerosis and muscular dystrophy. You fit the patient with a poncho or shell that is connected to the ventilator. Air is removed from between the patient's chest wall and the interior wall of the poncho or shell, causing the patient to inhale. A patient using negative-pressure ventilation does not need an artificial airway.

This skill described in this chapter focuses on positive-pressure mechanical ventilation frequently used in acute, subacute, and in some selective home care settings. There are many types of positive-pressure mechanical ventilators available for acute care use. Mechanical ventilators are available in pressure-cycled and volume-cycled machines. Pressure-cycled ventilation delivers a specified pressure to the patient, achieving a tidal volume, or amount of air, in milliliters per breath (Fig. 23-13). Volume-cycled ventilation delivers a specified tidal volume. Volume-cycled ventilators are most often used in the clinical setting. Patients using pressure-cycled ventilators are at higher risk for development of pneumothorax, hypotension, and decreased cardiac output as a result of the ventilator's achieving the prescribed pressure without regard for

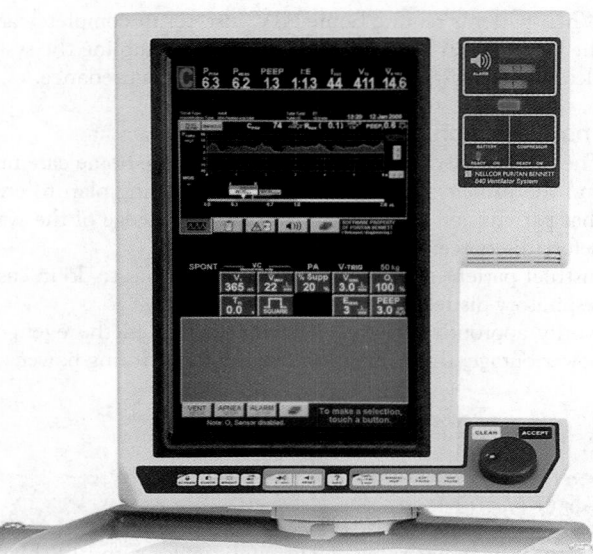

FIG 23-13 840 Series Ventilator System. *(Reprinted by permission from Nellcor Puritan Bennet LLC, Boulder, Colo, Part of Covidien.)*

lung compliance. Volume-cycled ventilators achieve tidal volume with preset pressure limits and are more sensitive to lung compliance. Time-cycled ventilators provide an inspiratory phase until a preset time is reached. This often results in varying tidal volumes.

MODES OF VENTILATION

There are many different modes of mechanical ventilation to support different conditions and physiological processes. Mechanical ventilation controls or assists the patient's respirations when the patient is unable to maintain adequate gas exchange because of respiratory or ventilatory failure (Table 23-3). The ventilator takes over the physical work of moving air into and out of the lungs, but it does not replace or alter the physiological function of the lung. Mechanical ventilation maintains or improves ventilation, oxygenation, and breathing pattern. Patients with impaired ventilation have low oxygen level (hypoxia), retain carbon dioxide (hypercapnia), and have difficulty breathing. Invasive mechanical ventilation requires an artificial airway (see Chapter 25).

It is important that patients remain on mechanical ventilation only as long as necessary. When patients wean from the ventilator,

TABLE 23-3	Overview of Mechanical Ventilation	
Types	**Description**	**Nursing Considerations**
Continuous positive airway pressure (CPAP)	Applies positive pressure during entire respiratory cycle.	Used for patients who breathe spontaneously but have hypoxemic respiratory failure; useful during weaning.
Positive end-expiratory pressure (PEEP)	Applies positive pressure during expiration.	Used for treating hypoxemic respiratory failure.
Volume-cycled	Delivers a preset volume to patient; peak inspiratory pressure varies.	Use in short-term ventilation and with ventilator weaning
Pressure-cycled	Delivers volume to patient until a preset pressure is reached; tidal volume varies.	Useful when excessive inspiratory pressures could damage lungs, as in neonates; tidal volume varies with airway resistance and lung compliance.
High-Frequency		
High-frequency jet ventilation (HFJV)	Delivers gas rapidly under low pressure via special injector cannula. Delivers 100-200 breaths per minute with tidal volume of 50-400 mL.	Patient on any mode of high-frequency ventilation requires continuous sedation and neuromuscular blocking agent administration.
High-frequency oscillatory ventilation (HFOV)	Delivers over 200 breaths per minute or 900-3000 vibrations, with tidal volume of 50-80 mL, airway pressures controlled.	Most common of high-frequency types: maintains alveolar ventilation with low airway pressure; useful for treating esophageal or bronchopleural fistulas or pneumothorax; helps avert barotraumas in high-risk patients if used early in treatment.
High-frequency positive-pressure ventilation (HFPPV).	Delivers 60-100 breaths per minute, with tidal volume of 3-6 mL/kg.	Tidal volume is less than the normal 8-10 mL/kg (Manno, 2005).
Mode of Use		
Control	Fully regulates ventilation in patient with paralysis or in arrest. Delivers set tidal volume at prescribed rate, using predetermined inspiratory and expiratory times.	Some patients require sedation to reduce competition with ventilator.
Assist	Patient initiates inspiration and receives preset tidal volume that augments ventilatory effort.	
Assist-control	Patient initiates breathing, but backup control delivers a preset number of breaths at a set volume.	
Synchronized intermittent mandatory ventilation (SIMV)	Ventilator delivers set number of breaths as specified volume. Some patients breathe spontaneously between SIMV breaths at volumes differing from those set on the machine.	Requires frequent monitoring during weaning from mechanical ventilation.

the goal is to avoid reintubation within 24 to 48 hours. Caring for the patient on mechanical ventilation and weaning from mechanical ventilation requires an interdisciplinary collaboration. Nursing care includes provision of emotional support, prevention of complications (e.g., pneumothorax, atelectasis, decreased cardiac output, pulmonary barotraumas, stress ulcer, or infection), promotion of optimal respiratory gas exchange, and monitoring for equipment failure.

ALARMS AND SETTINGS

The mechanical ventilator has a number of settings to adjust the amount of oxygen delivered, the amount of tidal volume, the time for inspiration and expiration, and the pressure at which each breath is delivered. The tidal volume, the amount of air per breath, is usually set by the patient's ideal body weight (5 to 7 mL/kg). If the patient has a restrictive lung disease, such as pulmonary fibrosis, or a flail chest or recent thoracic surgery, the tidal volumes are usually set lower.

The respiratory rate is usually set at 10 to 16 breaths per minute. Initially the FiO_2 is usually set at 100% and is quickly reduced to less than 40% based on patient ABG levels. The goal of providing oxygenation is to maintain a PaO_2 of ≥60 mm Hg using an FiO_2 of 40% or less. Table 23-4 lists the ventilator parameters you need to become familiar with to care for a patient on mechanical ventilation.

There are several alarms on the ventilator to ensure patient safety. Each ventilator is a little different; however, the basic alarms are similar. Alarms common to all ventilators include high-pressure, low-pressure, low-exhaled volume, and oxygen alarms (Table 23-5). You need to know how to respond to the ventilator alarms and what nursing actions are required to preserve the pa-

tient's respiratory status. The two most frequent alarms are the high-pressure and low-pressure alarms. The high-pressure alarm is usually set at 10 to 15 cm greater than the peak airway pressure. When this alarm sounds, it indicates the ventilator has met resistance to delivering the tidal volume and requires more pressure to inflate the lungs. Some patients have coughed during the inspiratory cycle; some need suctioning or have changed position. More acute problems that require immediate nursing intervention include the development of a pneumothorax or displacement of the ET or tracheostomy tube. The low-pressure alarm sounds when the ventilator has no resistance to inflating the lung. The patient may be disconnected from the ventilator, or a leak has developed in the ventilator circuit.

HOME MECHANICAL VENTILATION

The patient on mechanical ventilation can be successfully managed in the home. Neuromuscular disease such as amyotrophic lateral sclerosis (ALS), muscular dystrophy, brain and spinal cord diseases, chest wall disease, central hypoventilation syndrome, and advanced COPD are a few of the diseases that can be managed at home on mechanical ventilators. Many factors determine if a patient and family are candidates for home ventilation. Assessment criteria include the desire of the patient and family, the patient's acceptance of ventilator dependence, the patient's and family's ability to understand and perform daily care procedures, the home environment, personal resources, monetary resources, and resources and technologies for support in the community.

The goals of long-term ventilator care include extension of life, enhancement of the quality of life, provision of an environment that enhances individual potential, reduction of morbidity, improvement of physical and physiological function, and cost-

TABLE 23-4	Ventilator Parameters	
Parameter	**Definition**	**Ventilator Setting**
Tidal volume (V_T)	Amount of air inspired and expired with each breath	5-8 mL/kg of ideal body weight (patients with nonrestrictive pulmonary diseases) (Manno, 2005).
Respiratory rate (R or RR)	Number of breaths delivered per minute	Usual rate is 10-16 breaths per/min. However, the rate can be set 4-20 breaths per/min with the lower rates used during weaning (Manno, 2005).
Fraction of inspired oxygen (FiO_2)	Amount of oxygen the patient receives	Ideally less than 40% to maintain PaO_2 >60 mm Hg and SpO_2 >90% (Manno, 2005).
Positive end-expiratory pressure (PEEP) (see also Table 23-3)	Positive pressure applied at end-expiration to improve oxygenation	3-5 cm H_2O may be used to approximate physiological PEEP.* May require higher levels (>5 cm H_2O) in respiratory failure (e.g., acute respiratory disease syndrome).
Sigh	Larger than normal breath to provide hyperinflation; helps prevent atelectasis	Usually twice the tidal volume breath; about 10-15 mL/kg. Rate is usually set at 10-15 times per hour.
Sensitivity	Determines the inspiratory effort required to trigger the ventilator	Set to respond to an inspired volume of <1% of the patient's tidal volume.
Peak airway pressure	The maximal pressure level required to deliver the desired tidal volume	<40 cm H_2O. Normally set 1:1, 1:2, or 1:3.
I:E ratio	Comparison of inspiratory (I) to expiratory (E) time	Example: inspiration 2 seconds, expiration 4 seconds, then I:E = 1:2 to 1:1.5 (Manno, 2005).
Exhaled minute ventilation (V_E)	Measures the exhaled minute ventilations in liters	Alarm set at 15% greater than patient's average V_E.

*Some clinicians believe that the endotracheal tube with inflated cuff creates a closed system with the ventilator and does not require 3-5 cm of PEEP.

TABLE 23-5 Troubleshooting Mechanical Ventilation

Ventilator Alarm	Possible Causes	Nursing Interventions
Sudden increase in peak airway pressure (high-pressure alarm)	Coughing Airway plugging Changes in patient position Pneumothorax Incorrect ET tube position Kinked ventilator circuit Excessive water in ventilator circuit	Clear secretions by suctioning. Reposition patient. Assess breath sounds and chest wall movement. Verify placement of ET tube. Assess breath sounds. Verify centimeter level of ET tube. Check circuit; unkink tubing. Drain ventilator tubing.
Gradual increase in peak airway pressure	Decreasing lung compliance Exacerbation of acute process	Evaluate breath sounds; suction. Check for reversible causes: airway plugging, bronchospasm.
Sudden decrease in peak airway pressure (low-pressure alarm)	Patient disconnected from ventilator Leak in ventilator circuit	Check for disconnection. Evaluate circuit connections; tighten loose connections.
Change in minute ventilation or tidal volume	Leak in ET cuff	Check cuff seal.
Decrease	Airway secretions System leak Increased respiratory rate	Suction excessive secretions. Check circuit connections. Evaluate respiratory rate.
Increase	Hypoxia	Evaluate for signs of hypoxia. Evaluate need to obtain ABG sample or monitor pulse oximetry.
Change in respiratory rate	Patient anxiety Increased metabolic demand Hypoxia	Reassure patient. Evaluate body temperature, heart rate, and rhythm. Monitor pulse oximetry and obtain ABG levels.

ET, Endotracheal; *ABG,* arterial blood gas.

effectiveness. Patients and families who are candidates for home mechanical ventilation are prepared for discharge by a multidisciplinary team including representatives of nursing, medicine, dietary service, social service, the home care nurse, and the home care durable medical equipment company. The nurse in the hospital needs to be familiar with the home ventilator to assist the patient with discharge planning and education.

Delegation Considerations
The skill of caring for a patient on a mechanical ventilator cannot be delegated to NAP. The nurse directs the NAP by:
- Informing to immediately report to the nurse any change in the patient's respiratory status or patient indication of breathlessness, oxygen saturation, or vital signs.
- Informing to immediately inform the nurse if any of the ventilator's alarms sound.

Equipment
- ☐ Appropriate mechanical ventilator
- ☐ Oxygen source
- ☐ Pulse oximetry (SpO_2) probe and monitor
- ☐ Capnography ($EtCO_2$) window and monitor
- ☐ Stethoscope
- ☐ 10-mL syringe
- ☐ Oral airway/bite block
- ☐ Manual resuscitation bag (bag-valve-mask) with oxygen connecting tubing and flowmeter
- ☐ Clean gloves
- ☐ Goggles (if splash risk exists)
- ☐ Suction equipment at bedside (in-line/individual catheters)
- ☐ Chlorhexidine solution and toothbrush for oral care
- ☐ Method for patient communication
- ☐ Ventilator flow sheet to document ventilator changes and settings

STEP	RATIONALE

ASSESSMENT

1 Assess patient's LOC and ability to cooperate with mechanical ventilation and the need for special positioning, such as head of bed at 30 degrees or the need for selected prone position.

2 Assess patient's need for administering sedation (check agency policy).

Determines patient's ability to cooperate and understand aspects of care. Anxious and combative patients may require sedation to tolerate mechanical ventilation.

Sedation is sometimes used in mechanically ventilated patients to reduce respiratory efforts, decrease oxygen demand, and improve ABG levels and oxygen saturation levels.

Critical Decision Point *When patients on mechanical ventilation become excessively anxious, combative, or try to override the ventilator, sedation is often used. Check agency policy for the specific indications for sedation and the specific protocol for administering and monitoring sedation levels for these patients.*

STEP	RATIONALE
3 Assess patient's respiratory status, including symmetry of chest wall expansion, respiratory rate and depth, sputum production, and lung sounds (see Chapter 6), and assess for signs and symptoms associated with hypoxia (see Box 23-1).	Decreased chest wall movement, crackles or decreased lung sounds, increased respiratory rate, increased sputum production, or signs of worsening hypoxia indicates a need for mechanical ventilation or changes in the current ventilator settings to improve oxygenation.
4 Check ventilator, EtCO$_2$ (if available), SpO$_2$, and ventilator and cardiac alarms at the beginning of each shift and periodically throughout care, and compare with health care provider's orders.	Verifies that the ventilator settings are as ordered by the health care provider.
5 Verify placement of artificial airway through auscultation of lung sounds and verification of distal tip marking on endotracheal tube. Determine that tube is securely placed (see Chapter 25).	Prevents migration of the tube into the right or left bronchus and accidental extubation.
a Auscultate over trachea for presence of air leak. When an air leak is present, you will hear the movement of air over the trachea.	Cuff of artificial airway needs to be inflated to create a seal in order for positive-pressure ventilation to occur.
b Using minimal occlusive pressure, check inflation of cuff of artificial airway (see Chapter 25).	

Critical Decision Point   *When patients have a chest x-ray examination, also verify placement of the artificial airway.*

6 Observe for patent airway, and remove airway secretions by suctioning (see Chapter 25).	Secretions plug the airway, decreasing the amount of oxygen that is available for gas exchange in the lung. Secretions also occlude the **T** tube or tracheostomy collar, impeding oxygen delivery to the patient.
7 If available, note patient's most recent ABG results or SpO$_2$. Determine if any factors have changed during mechanical ventilation.	Objectively documents the patient's pH, arterial oxygen, arterial carbon dioxide, or arterial oxygen saturation.
8 Determine a method for communication with patient. If possible, review previous communication techniques with patient and family.	Patients with an artificial airway and mechanical ventilation cannot communicate verbally. In addition, some of these patients are too weak to use a note pad to communicate their needs. Therefore assessing for and determining communication needs before instituting mechanical ventilation is ideal. However, each time the patient has a new caregiver, assess communication preferences.
9 Review patient's medical record for the medical order for mechanical ventilation, noting mode of ventilation, respiratory rate, oxygen setting, and tidal volume.	Mechanical ventilation and changes in the ventilator settings require a health care provider's order.

NURSING DIAGNOSES

- Dysfunctional ventilatory weaning response
- Impaired gas exchange
- Impaired spontaneous ventilation
- Impaired verbal communication
- Ineffective airway clearance
- Ineffective breathing pattern
- Risk for infection

Individualize related factors based on patient's condition or needs.

PLANNING

1 Expected outcomes following completion of procedure:	
• Patient will have improved lung expansion.	As patient's lungs and lung mechanics improve, patient's lung expansion increases.
• Patient will maintain ABG levels and oxygen saturation within normal range or at patient baseline.	Verifies that the ventilator settings are effective in improving or maintaining patient's level of oxygenation.
• Patient's vital signs and respiratory assessment parameters improve.	Reduced pulse and respiratory rate, improved mental status, improved skin color, and decreased use of accessory and abdominal muscles occurs because patient's work of breathing decreases as the level of oxygenation improves (Carbery, 2008).
• Patient experiences reduction in feelings of dyspnea and work of breathing.	As the pulmonary problem resolves, the patient's perceptions of dyspnea and the actual work of breathing decline (Twibell and others, 2003).

STEP	RATIONALE
• Patient uses communication board, paper and pencil, or computer to state needs.	Appropriate communication system matches patient's abilities.
2 Explain the ventilator system to the patient and family, and be sure to include the purpose of and reasons for initiation of mechanical ventilation.	Helps patient to express fears and wishes. Plays a role in the weaning process (Manno, 2005).
3 Position patient with the head of bed elevated at least 30 degrees.	Positioning of patients with the head of bed at 30 degrees or higher significantly reduces gastric reflux, thereby decreasing the risk for ventilator-associated pneumonia (VAP) (American Association of Critical-Care Nurses [AACN], 2004).

IMPLEMENTATION

1 Perform hand hygiene; apply clean gloves and goggles. Apply mask, gown, and goggles if secretions are projectile.	Reduces transmission of microorganisms and exposure to pulmonary secretions.
2 Attach mechanical ventilator to ET or tracheostomy tube. Observe for proper functioning of mechanical ventilator.	Connects the artificial airway to the ventilator and ensures closed system, which enables the ventilator to exert appropriate pressure or volume to meet patient's oxygen demands.

Critical Decision Point *The mechanical ventilator requires programming of accurate settings before attaching to the patient. This is most often the responsibility of the respiratory therapist; however, it is usually a collaborative responsibility of the nurse.*

3 Verify that the ET or tracheostomy tube is properly positioned during an inspiratory and expiratory cycle by listening to both lungs and assessing chest wall symmetry.	Properly placed artificial airway will ensure that both lungs are equally ventilated. Improper airway placement will lead to unilateral lung ventilation.
4 Observe patient for synchronization with mechanical ventilation and response to therapy.	Ensures patient is comfortable using ventilator and has not experienced any adverse hemodynamic effects.
5 Monitor heart rate, blood pressure, respiratory rate, and cardiac rhythm.	Implementation of mechanical ventilation will result in decreased venous return and associated hemodynamic changes.
6 Note and mark the level of the ET tube at the lips or nares (see Chapter 25).	Provides a baseline for depth of tube placement. Endotracheal tube must be placed through the vocal cords into the trachea. Ensures that the tube is not too close to carina or in the right mainstem bronchus.
7 Set up suction equipment, including oral suctioning as well (see Chapter 25).	Need to provide airway care and suctioning as needed of ET or tracheostomy tube to prevent plugging of the airway and to reduce the risk for infection.
8 Position patient to promote best oxygenation and ventilation. This position can be high-Fowler's, lateral, or even prone. Monitor SpO_2 levels during and after positioning.	Positioning affects oxygenation and ventilation. SpO_2 will drop during a position change and recover once the patient is completely positioned. In other patients, a change in position (e.g., high-Fowler's to lateral) will result in a sustained drop in SpO_2, thus indicating that the patient in unable to tolerate that particular position at that time.
9 Collaborate with the health care provider frequently about the status of the patient, the response to therapy, and ongoing monitoring.	Assesses oxygenation status and continued need for mechanical ventilation.
a Monitor SpO_2 continuously.	Provides the ability to continually assess oxygenation levels.
b Monitor $EtCO_2$ continually and with serial ABG levels to detect possible overventilation or inadequate alveolar ventilation.	Overventilation causes respiratory alkalosis from decreased carbon dioxide. Inadequate alveolar ventilation causes respiratory acidosis from increased carbon dioxide retention (Carbery, 2008; Manno, 2005).
c Obtain ABG levels with changes in patient's condition or ventilator changes.	Provides more accurate measure of oxygen saturation and partial pressures of oxygen and carbon dioxide.
10 Do hourly safety checks on patient and ventilator system:	
a Make sure patient can reach call light.	Provides mechanism for patient to contact health care personnel.
b Check the security of all ventilator connections; make sure alarms are all turned on, including both high- and low-pressure alarms and volume alarms.	Ensures continuous safe and proper functioning of the ventilator system. Enables you to identify and correct problems in a timely manner.

STEP	RATIONALE
c Verify that all ventilator settings are correct and correspond to health care provider's orders (Manno, 2005).	Maintains integrity of the system and ensures that all settings are consistent with health care provider's orders.
d Check and refill humidifier as needed. Check corrugated tubing for condensation; drain and appropriately discard liquid.	Ensures continuous humidification. Condensation that returns to humidifier can cause possible bacterial contamination.
e When present, observe temperature gauges on the panel of the mechanical ventilator, making sure that gas is delivered at the correct temperature. Desired ranges of inspired gas are between 89.6° F (32° C) and 98.6° F (37° C).	The temperature of inspired gas will artificially alter the patient's body temperature.
11 Perform mouth care at least 4 times per 24 hours (see Chapter 17). Use a toothbrush and solution such as chlorhexidine, which is effective in reducing oral bacteria and the risk for ventilator-associated pneumonia (Munro and Grap, 2006).	Ventilator-associated pneumonia is common, and it is associated with microaspiration of oropharyngeal secretions. Frequent mouth care reduces patient's risk for ventilator-associated pneumonia. Oral care at least 4 times per 24 hours helps reduce the risk for pneumonias (AACN, 2006; Berry and others, 2007; Grap and others, 2004; Munro and others, 2006).
12 Perform nursing activities to prevent hazards of immobility (e.g., assist patient with changing position, assist with range-of-joint motion, encourage independence and activity as tolerated by the patient).	Maintaining activity avoids complications associated with decreased mobility, such as pressure ulcers, pneumonia, deep vein thrombosis (DVT), and activity intolerance. Patients receiving mechanical ventilation need assistance with activity.
13 Keep patient informed on progress and plan for weaning from the mechanical ventilator.	Apprehension and anxiety occur when the patient is not properly informed about progress, changes in care, or changes in ventilator setting. Patients need information, as well as emotional support, to successfully tolerate and wean from mechanical ventilation (Carbery, 2008).
14 Remove gloves and goggles; perform hand hygiene.	Reduces transmission of microorganisms and exposure to pulmonary secretions.

EVALUATION

1 Reassess and monitor patient's response to mechanical ventilation every 2 to 4 hours.	Patients requiring mechanical ventilation have unstable physiological status. It is important to perform key focused evaluating measures frequently as the patient's condition warrants.
a *Neurological assessment:* LOC, orientation, sleepiness, changes in anxiety	
b *Pulmonary assessment:* Lung sounds, airway clearance, work of breathing, breathing pattern, rate of respirations, SpO_2, $EtCO_2$	
c *Cardiovascular assessment:* Vital signs, heart rhythm, heart sounds, lower extremity edema	
2 Observe pulse oximetry, and monitor ABG levels.	Documents patient's level of oxygenation and ventilation.
3 Observe integrity of patient ventilator system.	Ensures adequate delivery of mechanical ventilation.
4 Observe and evaluate effectiveness of the communication methods:	Communication, or lack of it, will increase the patient's frustration, sense of powerlessness, and confusion during mechanical ventilation and the weaning process (Carbery, 2008).
a Ask patient if needs and concerns are addressed.	
b Observe for signs of frustration (e.g., patient shaking head in irritation, crying, withdrawal).	
c Observe patient/family and health care personnel use communication methods.	

Unexpected Outcomes	Related Interventions
1 Patient experiences stiff, noncompliant lung; alveolar edema; pulmonary congestion; chest pain; intraalveolar hemorrhage; substernal chest pain; pneumothorax; continued decrease in blood pressure related to use of positive pressure.	• Notify health care provider. • Remain with patient. • Conduct a complete cardiac and pulmonary assessment.
2 Patient experiences hypoxia, hypercapnia.	• Notify health care provider. • Assess patient. • Assess integrity of ventilator system. • Expect ventilator change (increase positive end-expiratory pressure [PEEP] levels).
3 Patient experiences self-extubation.	• Maintain patent airway. • Provide oxygen. • Assess patient's respiratory status and level of oxygenation and ventilation. • Notify health care provider.
4 Patient experiences tension pneumothorax, as evidenced by sudden respiratory distress: air hunger, distended neck veins, tracheal/mediastinal shift, hypotension, and tachycardia.	• Remain with patient, and remove patient from ventilator and ventilate with bag-valve-mask (see Chapter 27). • Notify health care provider. • Ask nursing assistive personnel to obtain chest tube insertion kit. • Ask additional personnel to obtain patient's vital signs.
5 Pressure alarm sounds.	• Assess for airway obstruction (e.g., secretions, patient biting on endotracheal tube). • Remove obstruction (e.g., ET suctioning, inserting oral airway/bite block).
6 Low-volume alarm sounds.	• Assess integrity of the ventilator tubing, and reconnect if disconnected. • Check for airway displacement (e.g., extubation). • Assess integrity of the airway cuff (e.g., deflate and reinflate, and determine if seal is present) (see Chapter 25). • Remain with patient, and remove patient from ventilator and ventilate with bag-valve-mask.

Recording and Reporting

• Record in progress notes: respiratory assessment findings; mode of mechanical ventilation, oxygen level, actual patient tidal volume, actual patient respiratory rate, peak airway pressure, patient's response to mechanical ventilation, level of the ET, any adverse reactions or side effects.

• Report to nurse in charge or health care provider: sudden change in patient's respiratory status, ventilator-associated problems.

Teaching Considerations

• Teach patient and family about the rationale for mechanical ventilation.

• Teach patient and family about the alarms and what they mean.

• Teach patient and family alternative communication techniques to reduce frustration and fear.

Pediatric Considerations

• There are increasing numbers of children on home mechanical ventilation. For this reason it is important to include the parent in the child's care as appropriate. Parents also need to be prepared that when a readmission to a hospital occurs, due to the chronic nature of the illness, the child may not be readmitted to an intensive care unit, but rather may remain on the general medical or surgical area.

• Once the child is stable on the mechanical ventilator, promote normal or near-normal activities as the child's condition warrants (e.g., promote play, resume school activities, encourage mobility).

Gerontological Considerations

• Presence of underlying chronic illnesses increase patient's risk for longer intensive care, hospital stays.

• Older adults are usually not able to tolerate the usual sedative, antianxiety medications ordered. The prescribed dose is based on patient's baseline kidney and liver functions (Balami, 2006; Smetana, 2003).

Home Care Considerations

• Patients requiring home mechanical ventilation need to learn complete care of the mechanical ventilator system, suctioning, and artificial airway care. Skills include assembling the ventilator circuit, cleaning the circuit, and daily equipment maintenance.

• Use a checklist for ensuring consistency of care for a patient on a ventilator.

• Evaluate the following areas during each visit: oxygen flow, alarm system, inspiratory pressure, high-pressure alarm, tidal volume setting, humidifier, respiratory rate, tubing, temperature, resuscitation bag, tracheostomy care, breath sounds, suctioning, and tubing changes.

• The durable medical equipment provider, the home care nurse, and the primary care nurse develop a teaching plan to ensure that patient and family have a complete working knowledge of the ventilator before discharge.

• Instruct patient and primary caregiver in what to do in case of respiratory distress or power failure. Check to determine availability of emergency batteries.

• Instruct family in use of the bag-valve-mask (see Chapter 27).

• Patients who require long-term mechanical ventilation are sometimes transferred to a chronic ventilator facility or a long-term ventilator dependency floor within the hospital. The purpose of such a transfer is to aggressively rehabilitate the patient through physical therapy, occupational therapy, and speech therapy. The overall goal is to effectively wean patient from the mechanical ventilator.

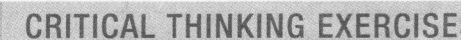

CRITICAL THINKING EXERCISES

You are caring for newly admitted Mr. Landon, who has a history of COPD that is well controlled. However, 2 weeks ago he developed an upper respiratory tract infection; he was treated with antibiotics. He completed his full course of antibiotics, but his symptoms continued. He has a 4-day history of high fever greater than 102.8° F, fatigue, productive coughing, worsening dyspnea, and decreased activity tolerance. His physician does a complete examination, orders a chest x-ray examination, and obtains a sputum specimen. Preliminary chest x-ray results indicate right lower lobe pneumonia. Mr. Landon is admitted to a general medicine floor for treatment with intravenous (IV) antibiotics, supplemental oxygen, and pulmonary hygiene measures.

1   You observe him and notice that he is fatigued, has difficulty speaking, and in general looks very uncomfortable. You decide to do a focused assessment. What systems will you assess, and what information will you obtain? State your rationale for choosing these systems.

2   Mr. Landon is started on oxygen therapy via nasal cannula at 2 L/min. What is the approximate FiO_2 level, and what are the hazards for oxygen therapy in this patient?

3   Mr. Landon continues to remove the cannula because of discomfort at the nares and ears from the device. What are the causes of this discomfort? What are your interventions to reduce the discomfort?

4   One of the nurses suggests a partial rebreather mask for Mr. Landon's oxygen therapy. You do not think this is a good idea, and the rationale for your decision is:
  A   Increased inspired oxygen percentage
  B   Decreased carbon dioxide retention
  C   Decreased oxygen percentage
  D   Increased carbon dioxide retention

5   As the day progresses, Mr. Landon is getting more breathless and fatigued. He is unable to clear his secretions effectively and needs nasotracheal suctioning. His level of consciousness is declining; he is difficult to arouse and at times appears confused and continually takes off his nasal cannula. His pulse oximetry value is 85%; ABG levels show slight acidemia with CO_2 retention. The physicians want to try Mr. Landon on BiPAP in the hope of avoiding intubation and mechanical ventilation.
  a   What concerns do you have with Mr. Landon's confusion and initiation of BiPAP? What are your interventions?
  b   The physician orders hourly ABG measurements and continuous pulse oximetry. What is the rationale?

6   As you continue to assess Mr. Landon, what assessment parameters indicate a worsening status?
  A   Increased respiratory rate, decreased oxygen saturation, decreased carbon dioxide level, sleepiness
  B   Increased respiratory rate, decreased oxygen saturation, increased carbon dioxide level, sleepiness
  C   Decreased respiratory rate, increased oxygen saturation, decreased carbon dioxide level, alertness
  D   Increased respiratory rate, increased oxygen saturation, decreased carbon dioxide level, alertness

REVIEW QUESTIONS

1   A patient arrives on the nursing unit because of a sudden onset of dyspnea. Which assessment data would the nurse expect to find?
  1   A respiratory rate of 24 breaths per minute
  2   Cyanosis
  3   Clubbing of the fingers
  4   A regular breathing pattern

2   A patient with an oxygen mask with a reservoir bag is seen while making initial rounds. What problem might the patient experience if the reservoir bag becomes deflated?
  1   Elevated oxygen levels
  2   Elevated carbon dioxide levels
  3   Drying of the nasal mucous membranes
  4   A decrease in the number of respirations

3   A patient with a tracheostomy tube and humidification collar also has an underlying diagnosis of chronic obstructive pulmonary disease. The nurse hears a bubbling sound on approaching the patient, although the patient is lying calmly and quietly. What is the appropriate action for the nurse to take?
  1   Suction the patient's tracheostomy tube.
  2   Liquefy the patient's pulmonary secretions.
  3   Check the oxygen tubing for fluid accumulation.
  4   Elevate the patient's head slightly to improve oxygenation.

4   The use of noninvasive ventilation (CPAP or BiPAP) has the potential to cause carbon dioxide retention in selected patients. Patients with which of the underlying diagnoses are at greatest risk for carbon dioxide retention? Those with an underlying dignosis of:
  1   Congestive heart failure
  2   Pulmonary fibrosis
  3   Chronic obstructive pulmonary disease
  4   Pulmonary edema

5   The low-pressure alarm has sounded on a patient's ventilator. The nurse would check to see which of the following situations has occurred. The patient may:
  1   Have a leak in the ventilator circuit
  2   Have just coughed during the inspiratory cycle
  3   Need his or her airway suctioned
  4   Have changed his or her position

REFERENCES

Berry A and others: Systematic literature review of oral hygiene practices for intensive care patients receiving mechanical ventilation, *Am J Crit Care* 16(6):552, 2007.

Carbery C: Basic concepts in mechanical ventilation, *Journal of Perioperative Practice* 18(3):106, 2008.

Frace M: Non-invasive ventilation: CPAP and BiPAP on the medical-surgical unit, *Med-Surg Matters*, 17(3):12, 2008.

Galanti GA: *Caring of patients from different cultures*, ed 3, Philadelphia, 2004, University of Pennsylvania Press.

Hockenberry MJ, Wilson D: *Wong's clinical manual of pediatric nursing*, ed 7, St. Louis, 2007, Mosby.

Kuebler K and others: Differentiating chronic obstructive pulmonary disease from asthma, *Journal of the American Academy of Nurse Practitioners*, 20(9):445, 2008.

Manno MS: Managing mechanical ventilation, *Nursing* 35(12):36, 2005.

Meiner SE, Lueckenotte AG: *Gerontologic nursing,* ed 3, St. Louis, 2006, Mosby.

Nava S, Ceriana P: Causes of failure of noninvasive mechanical ventilation, *Respir Care* 49(3):295, 2004.

O'Reilly P, Bailey W: Long-term continuous oxygen treatment in chronic obstructive pulmonary disease: proper use, benefits and unresolved issues, *Curr Opin Pulm Med* 12:120, 2007.

Pruitt B: Help your patient combat atelectasis, *Nursing* 36(5):64, 2006.

Ruse C and Molyneux A: Management and implications of chronic obstructive pulmonary disease (COPD) for older patients, *Rev Clin Gerontol* 15:91, 2006.

Spector R: *Cultural diversity in health and illness,* Upper Saddle River, NJ, 2008, Prentice Hall.

Stegmaier J: Emerging technology in home respiratory care, *AARC Times,* September 23, 2005.

Woodrow MA: Caring for patients receiving oxygen therapy, *Nursing Older Adults* 19(1):31, 2007.

Zoidus J: Peak flow monitoring for asthma, *J Respir Care Pract,* Currant Communications, December 2005, http://www.rtmagazine.com/articles.asp, accessed September 14, 2008.

RESEARCH REFERENCES

American Association of Critical-Care Nurses: *Practice alert—ventilator associated pneumonia,* Mission Viejo, Calif, 2004, The Association.

American Association of Critical-Care Nurses: *Practice alert—oral care in the critically ill,* Mission Viejo, Calif, 2006, The Association.

Balami JS: Non-invasive ventilation for respiratory failure due to acute exacerbations of chronic obstructive disease in older patients, *Age and ageing* 35(1):75, 2006.

Frace M: Noninvasive ventilation: CPAP and BiPAP on the medical-surgical unit, *Med-Surg Matters* 17(3):12, 2008.

Grap MJ and others: Duration of action of a single, early oral application of chlorhexidine on oral microbial flora in mechanically ventilated patients: a pilot study, *Heart Lung* 33(2):83, 2004.

Jarvis H: Exploring the evidence base of the use of non-invasive ventilation, *Br J Nurs* 15: 756, 2006.

Langenhof S, Fichter J: Comparison of two demand oxygen delivery devices for administration of oxygen in COPD, *Chest* 128:2082, 2005.

Lawrence VA and others: Strategies to reduce postoperative pulmonary complications after noncardiothoracic surgery: systematic review for the American College of Physicians, *Ann Intern Med* 144:596, 2006.

Munro CL, Grap MJ: Oral health and care in the intensive care unit: state of the science, *Am J Crit Care* 13(1):25, 2006.

Munro CL and others: Oral health status and development of ventilator associated pneumonia: a descriptive study, *Am J Crit Care* 15(5):453, 2006.

Ram FSF, Wedzicha JA: Ambulatory oxygen for chronic obstructive pulmonary disease, *The Cochrane Database Syst Rev* 2:2007.

Ruse CE, Molyneux AWP: Management and implications of chronic obstructive pulmonary disease (COPD) for older adults, *Rev Clin Gerontol* 15:91, 2005.

Smetana GW and others: Preoperative pulmonary risk stratification for noncardiothoracic surgery: systematic review for the American College of Physicians, *Ann Intern Med* 144:581, 2006.

Performing Chest Physiotherapy

KEY TERMS

Chest
  physiotherapy
  (CPT)
Mucociliary
transport

Percussion
Postural drainage
  (PD)
Shaking
Vibration

MEDIA RESOURCES

- **evolve** http://evolve.elsevier.com/Perry/skills
  learning system

  - Review Questions

OBJECTIVES

Mastery of content in this chapter will enable the nurse to:
- Assess the need to perform chest physiotherapy (CPT) maneuvers.
- Determine the need to modify or discontinue CPT maneuvers, including contraindications and individual variations.
- Explain how to prepare a patient and family for the performance of each CPT maneuver.
- Perform the outlined CPT maneuvers, including standard and modified versions.
- Describe expected and unexpected outcomes of each CPT maneuver.
- Describe discharge teaching and planning related to the use of each CPT maneuver in the home setting.

Chest physiotherapy (CPT) consists of physical chest wall maneuvers such as percussion, vibration and shaking, postural drainage (PD), and cough. Percussion is a rhythmical force that a caregiver provides by clapping cupped hands against a patient's thorax. Percussion assists in loosening retained secretions from the airway. Vibration and shaking move secretions from small distal airways into larger central airways. The caregiver contracts all muscles in the upper extremities and causes vibration while applying pressure to a patient's chest wall. Shaking is a stronger bouncing maneuver supplying a concurrent, compressive force to the chest wall.

Postural drainage requires positioning a patient so that the position of the lung segment to be drained allows gravity to have its greatest effect (Denehy and Berney, 2006; Oermann and others, 2000). After CPT moves secretions into the large central airways, secretions are removed through coughing or suctioning. Cough occurs when the patient takes a deep breath, closing the glottis to build up a back pressure, and then forcefully exhaling. During the expiratory phase of a cough, the airways are compressed, causing the airway to narrow. Airway narrowing and forced exhalation increase the force of airflow in the large central airways, and mucus moves up and out of the trachea. CPT and coughing maneuvers assist with airway clearance of mucus in patients with retained tracheobronchial secretions (van der Schans and others, 2000).

Secretions accumulate in the airways of patients with bronchitis, asthma, cystic fibrosis (CF), pneumonia, and bronchiectasis. Surgical patients in the postoperative period sometimes have excess secretions because of the effects of anesthesia and ineffective coughing because of incision pain. Mucous plugs, atelectasis, and lobular collapse occur when secretions accumulate in the airway.

CPT is often used in combination with other therapies, including antibiotics, bronchodilators, mucolytic agents, and systemic hydration. These therapies along with CPT reduce mucus production and promote airway clearance. The goals of these therapies are (1) to clear the airways of excessive secretions in order to reduce the work of breathing and (2) to improve the patient's ability to cough up secretions.

In the normal lung the mucociliary transport system clears the airways of excessive mucus and inhaled particles. This system lines the internal lumen of the entire tracheobronchial tree and consists of a thin layer of mucus that is constantly being propelled toward the larynx by cells that have hairlike projections called cilia. Inhaled particles are trapped on the mucus, and the cilia act as a conveyor belt to sweep the mucus toward the throat, where it is swallowed or removed by coughing. Airways normally remain clear, and mucus is constantly being cleared almost as fast as it is made. Normal mucus remains thin, white, and watery. When disease causes excessive sputum production, therapeutic interventions help natural airway clearance mechanisms (cough and mucociliary transport) clear the airways of obstructing mucus.

In various disease states, mucus clearance slows down or the cilia are overwhelmed by production of large quantities of mucus. The lung no longer clears the mucus as fast as it is produced. Secretions stagnate in the airways, change color, and become thick and sticky. The cilia cannot remove large amounts of thick mucus from the lungs. In addition, many people with lung disease cannot cough effectively to clear airways. Therefore it is important to use other maneuvers to aid in clearing excess lung secretions and provide adequate hydration.

Help the patient maintain adequate hydration. Fluids help to thin the oral secretions so they are easily coughed up and expectorated after CPT. Unless contraindicated by other disease states, such as congestive heart failure or renal failure, provide fluids throughout the day to assist in making mucus thin and watery. During an acute pulmonary illness, it often takes three or four CPT treatments per day and 2 L or more of fluid a day to clear and thin secretions.

EVIDENCE-BASED PRACTICE TRENDS

CPT is effective in selected patients, such as those with cystic fibrosis or bronchiectasis (McCool and Rosen, 2006). Newer studies compare the effectiveness of newer airway clearance methods (oscillating positive expiratory pressure devices, such as the Acapella device [see Procedural Guideline 24-1, p. 664], high-frequency chest wall oscillators, and intrapulmonary compression ventilators) with standard manual CPT (Main and others, 2005; Marks, 2007; Varekojis and others, 2003). These studies demonstrate that CPT and the newer devices are safe and effective modalities for the clearance of airway secretions in a variety of adult and pediatric lung diseases (Patterson and others, 2005). More severely impaired patients with cystic fibrosis have better oxygenation during CPT if it is administered in conjunction with noninvasive ventilation (Holland and others, 2003). Although there are few studies on the effectiveness of CPT in the adult with chronic obstructive pulmonary disease (COPD) and pneumonia, CPT does assists in clearing some airway secretions in these patients (McCool and Rosen, 2006).

The use of mechanical devices often improves patient satisfaction and adherence with CPT (Oermann and others, 2000, 2001; Patterson and others, 2005; Varekojis and others, 2003). With the mechanical devices there is a greater degree of patient use, because they are often self-administered (Oermann and others, 2000; Patterson and others, 2005). In addition, these devices are easy to use and do not cause any discomfort.

CULTURAL CONSIDERATIONS

The skills in this chapter include a great deal of patient touching. Asian and Muslim cultures consider it very poor taste to touch in public. Health care providers need to be sensitive to these cultural concerns and provide for gender-congruent health care providers (Galanti, 2004). In addition, the skills of physical therapy sometimes involve a gentle percussion or shaking of a patient's rib cage. Patients and families from cultures where violence is an everyday occurrence need detailed information about the procedure so they do not misunderstand the intent and objective of CPT. In these situations it is important to establish a solid relationship with the patient and explain what type of touching is involved, what the patient may feel during the treatment, and provide an opportunity for the patient to temporarily stop and rest during the procedure.

Skill Performance Guidelines

Plan a patient's care and subsequent selection of CPT skills based on specific assessment findings. The following guidelines help guide physical assessment and subsequent decision making:

1 Know the patient's normal range of vital signs. Conditions such as atelectasis and pneumonia requiring CPT can affect a patient's vital signs. The degree of change is related to the level of hypoxia, overall cardiopulmonary status, and tolerance to the procedure.

2 Know the patient's present medications. Some medications, particularly diuretics and antihypertensives, cause fluid and hemodynamic changes. These changes affect the patient's tolerance of the positional changes. Steroid medications, age, and malnutrition increase the patient's risk for pathological rib fractures and often contraindicate rib shaking.

3 Know the patient's medical and surgical history. Certain conditions, such as increased intracranial pressure, spinal cord injuries, abdominal aneurysm resection, bone metastases, or severe osteoporosis, contraindicate the positional changes of postural drainage (Box 24-1). Thoracic trauma contraindicates percussion, vibration, and shaking.

4 Know the patient's level of cognitive function. Alteration in mental status often makes it difficult or impossible for the patient to cough and expectorate secretions. Participation in controlled cough techniques requires the patient to understand and to follow instructions. If the patient cannot cough and clear secretions, be prepared to suction out the airway secretions (see Chapter 25).

5 Assess the patient's exercise tolerance. CPT maneuvers are exhausting. When the patient is not used to physical activity, initial tolerance of the maneuvers decreases. However, with gradual increases in activity and planned CPT, the patient's tolerance improves.

| **BOX 24-1** | **Contraindications for Postural Drainage** |

- Increased intracranial pressure
- Head and neck injury until stabilized
- Active hemorrhage with hemodynamic instability
- Recent spinal surgery (e.g., laminectomy) or acute spinal injury
- Active hemoptysis
- Empyema
- Bronchopleural fistula
- Pulmonary edema associated with congestive heart failure
- Large pleural effusions
- Pulmonary embolism
- Aged, confused, or anxious patients who are unable to tolerate position change
- Rib fracture, with or without flail chest
- Surgical wound or healing tissue

Trendelenburg's Position Is Contraindicated for the Following:

- Uncontrolled hypertension
- Distended abdomen
- Esophageal surgery
- Recent gross hemoptysis
- Uncontrolled airway at risk for aspiration

Modified from AARC clinical practice guideline: postural drainage therapy, *Respir Care* 36(12):1418, 1991.

SKILL 24-1 Performing Postural Drainage

Postural drainage achieves gravitational clearance of airway secretions from specific bronchial segments by using several different body positions. Each position drains a specific corresponding section of the tracheobronchial tree, from either the upper, middle, or lower lung field, into the trachea. Coughing or suctioning helps remove secretions from the trachea. Fig. 24-1 shows the anatomy of the upper, middle, and lower lobe bronchi. The images in Table 24-1 show the bronchial lobes and the corresponding body postures for drainage of each.

Clinicians select areas for drainage based on (1) knowledge of the patient's condition and disease process, (2) physical assessment of the chest, (3) chest x-ray examination results, and (4) the extent of the pathological condition and lobe involvement based on the physical examination and chest x-ray findings.

Delegation Considerations

The skill of chest physiotherapy can be delegated to appropriately trained nursing assistive personnel (NAP) in special situations. It is the nurse's responsibility to assess the patient, review laboratory and x-ray examination results, and determine that the patient is stable and able to tolerate the procedure. The nurse directs the NAP to:

- Be alert for the patient's tolerance of procedure, such as comfort level and changes in breathing pattern, and to immediately report changes to the nurse.
- Use specific patient precautions related to disease or treatment.

- Avoid specific positioning restrictions or problems unique to the patient.

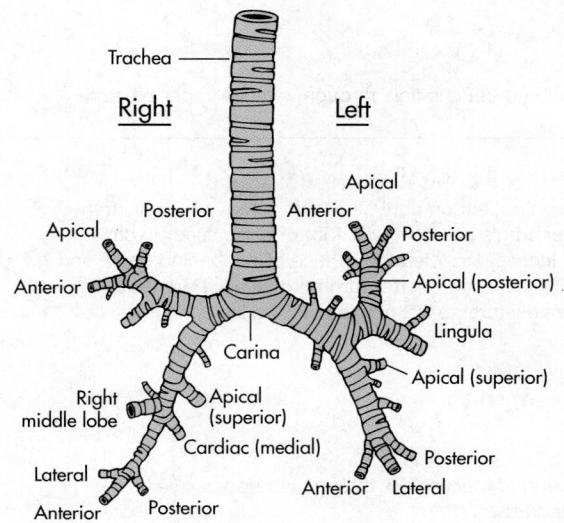

FIG 24-1 Tracheobronchial tree. *(Modified from Frownfelter DL, Dean E: Principles and practice of cardiopulmonary therapy, ed 3, St. Louis, 1996, Mosby.)*

TABLE 24-1 | Positions and Procedures for Drainage, Percussion, Vibration, and Shaking

Area and Procedure	Anatomical Area	Position of Patient
Left and Right Upper Lobe Anterior Apical Bronchi Position patient in chair, or high-Fowler's, leaning back. Percuss and vibrate with heel of hands at shoulders and fingers over collarbones (clavicles) in front; do both sides at same time. Note body posture and arm position of nurse. Nurse's back is kept straight, and elbows and knees are slightly flexed.	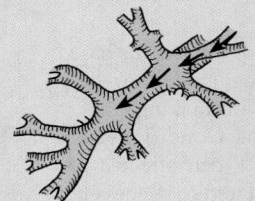	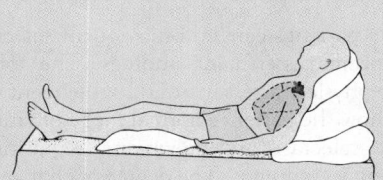 Anterior apical segments
Direction of mucus flow through upper lobe anterior apical bronchi.	Position hands for chest physiotherapy over left and right upper lobe anterior apical bronchi.	
Left and Right Upper Lobe Posterior Apical Bronchi Position patient in chair, leaning forward on pillow or table. Percuss and vibrate with hands on either side of upper spine. Do both sides at same time.	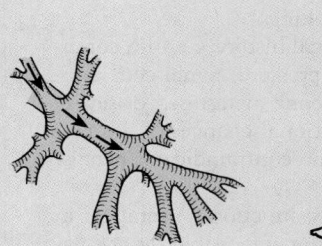	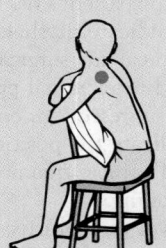 Posterior apical segments
Direction of mucus flow through upper lobe posterior apical bronchi.	Position hands for chest physiotherapy over left and right upper lobe posterior apical bronchi.	
Right and Left Anterior Upper Lobe Bronchi Position patient flat on back with small pillow under knees. Percuss and vibrate just below clavicle on either side of sternum.	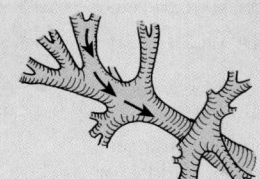	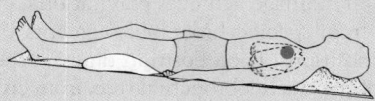 Left and right anterior upper lobe segments
Direction of mucus flow through anterior upper bronchi.	Position hands for chest physiotherapy over right and left anterior upper lobe bronchi.	
Left Upper Lobe Lingular Bronchus Position patient on right side with arm overhead in Trendelenburg's position, with foot of bed raised 30 cm (12 inches), as tolerated.* Place pillow behind back, and roll patient one-quarter turn onto pillow. Percuss and vibrate lateral to left nipple below axilla.	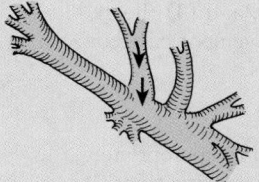	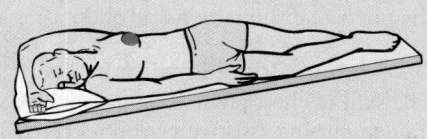 Left upper lobe lingular segment
Direction of mucus flow through left upper lobe lingular bronchus.	Position hands for chest physiotherapy over left upper lobe lingular bronchus.	

*In adult settings Trendelenburg's position is not used as frequently. Verify use with agency policy and health care provider's order.

| **TABLE 24-1** | Positions and Procedures for Drainage, Percussion, Vibration, and Shaking—cont'd |

Area and Procedure	Anatomical Area	Position of Patient

Right Middle Lobe Bronchus

Position patient on left side or abdomen. Place pillow behind back, and roll patient one-quarter turn onto pillow. Percuss and vibrate to right nipple below axilla.

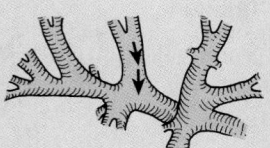 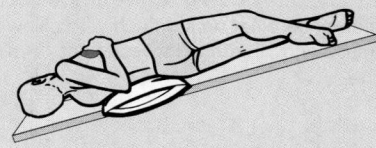

Right middle lobe segment

Direction of mucus flow through right middle lobe bronchus.

Position hands for chest physiotherapy over right middle lobe bronchus.

Left and Right Anterior Lower Lobe Bronchi

Position patient on back, with foot of bed elevated 45 to 50 cm (18 to 20 inches). Have knees bent on pillow. Percuss and vibrate over lower anterior ribs on both sides.

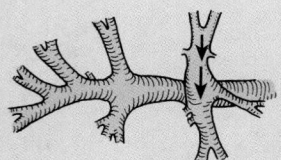 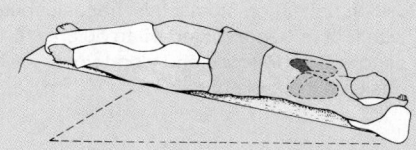

Left and right anterior lower lobe segments

Direction of mucus flow through anterior lower lobe bronchi.

Position hands for chest physiotherapy over left and right anterior lower lobe bronchi.

Right Lower Lobe Lateral Bronchus

Position patient on abdomen in Trendelenburg's position with foot of bed raised 45 to 50 cm (18 to 20 inches), as tolerated. Percuss and vibrate on left and right side of chest below shoulder blades (scapulas) posterior to midaxillary line.

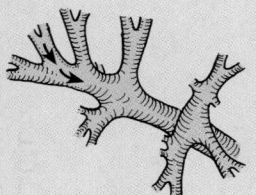 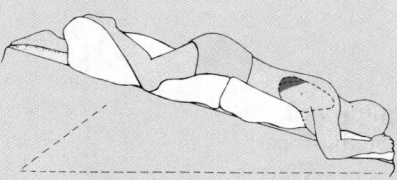

Left and right lower lateral lobe segments

Direction of mucus flow through right lower lobe lateral bronchus.

Positions hands for chest physiotherapy over right lower lobe lateral bronchus.

Left Lower Lobe Lateral Bronchus

Position patient on right side in Trendelenburg's position with foot of bed raised 45 to 50 cm (18 to 20 inches), as tolerated. Percuss and vibrate on left side of chest below scapulas posterior to midaxillary line.

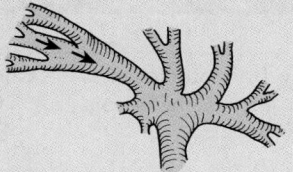 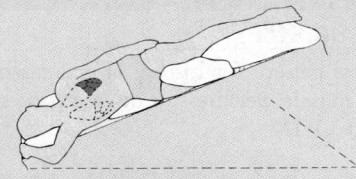

Left lower lobe lateral segment

Direction of mucus flow through left lower lobe lateral bronchus.

Position hands for chest physiotherapy over left lower lobe lateral bronchus.

Continued

TABLE 24-1	Positions and Procedures for Drainage, Percussion, Vibration, and Shaking—cont'd	
Area and Procedure	**Anatomical Area**	**Position of Patient**
Right and Left Lower Lobe Superior Bronchi Position patient flat on stomach with pillow under stomach. Percuss and vibrate below scapulas on either side of spine.	Right and left lower lobe superior segments	
Direction of mucus flow through lower lobe superior bronchi.	Position hands for chest physiotherapy over right and left lower superior bronchi.	
Right and Left Posterior Basal Bronchi Position patient on stomach in Trendelenburg's position with foot of bed elevated 45 to 50 cm (18 to 20 inches), as tolerated. Percuss and vibrate over lower posterior ribs on either side of spine.	Right and left posterior segments	
Direction of mucus flow through posterior basal bronchi.	Position hands for chest physiotherapy over right and left posterior lower lobe bronchi.	

Equipment
- ❑ Stethoscope
- ❑ Pulse oximeter
- ❑ Trendelenburg's hospital bed or tilt table, more common in pediatric agencies
- ❑ Water in pitcher and glass
- ❑ Chair (for draining upper lobes)

- ❑ One to four pillows
- ❑ Tissues and paper bag
- ❑ Clear graduated screw-top container
- ❑ Clean gloves (if there is a risk for exposure to patient's respiratory secretions)
- ❑ Suction equipment (if patient unable to cough and clear own secretions)

STEP	RATIONALE
ASSESSMENT	
1 Assess patient for history of decreased level of consciousness and muscle weakness or disease processes, such as pneumonia and COPD.	Conditions that pose risk for impaired airway clearance will require CPT.

Critical Decision Point   *If the use of Trendelenburg's position or other postures causes severe hypertension, severe hypoxemia, or severe shortness of breath, therapy is contraindicated (see Box 24-1).*

| 2 Review medical record, and assess patient for signs and symptoms, including x-ray film changes consistent with atelectasis, lobar collapse pneumonia, or bronchiectasis; ineffective coughing; thick, sticky, tenacious, and discolored secretions that are difficult to cough up; and abnormal breath sounds, such as wheezing and rhonchi. | Indicates need to perform postural drainage. X-ray film data and signs and symptoms indicate accumulation of pulmonary secretions and ineffective airway clearance. |

STEP	RATIONALE
3 Review chest x-ray examination reports, and auscultate over all lung fields decreased breath sounds, crackles, wheezes, and rhonchi. Palpate the chest wall over all lung fields to assess for increased or decreased fremitus and asymmetrical chest wall expansion.	Findings identify bronchial segments needing drainage. Areas of lung congestion and postures for drainage will vary, depending on disease process, patient condition, and clinical problems. Areas in need of postural drainage usually are easily identified by the presence of early inspiratory crackles and palpable crepitus.
4 Assess vital signs and pulse oximetry.	Provides baseline to evaluate patient's response to therapy.
5 Determine patient's understanding of and ability to perform home postural drainage.	Identifies potential areas for instruction. Home care CPT is indicated in patients with chronic inability to clear lung secretions adequately, such as those with cystic fibrosis, chronic bronchitis, asthma, or bronchiectasis.

NURSING DIAGNOSES

- Deficient knowledge regarding postural drainage and airway clearance
- Impaired gas exchange
- Ineffective airway clearance
- Ineffective breathing pattern

Individualize related factors based on patient's condition or needs.

PLANNING

1 Expected outcomes following completion of procedure:	
• Lung sounds improve or become clear.	Airways are clear of retained secretions.
• Sputum is more easily coughed and expectorated or suctioned out.	CPT provides a mechanical stimulus to loosen secretions from the wall of the airway, and thus secretions are easier to expectorate.
• Secretions appear more normal in color and consistency.	Result of increased hydration and in resolving infection.
• Dyspnea decreases.	As secretions are removed, patient exchange of respiratory gases improves, and dyspnea gradually declines.
• Chest x-ray film shows improvements: lobar collapse and atelectasis are decreased or eliminated.	CPT improves atelectasis and facilitates the removal of secretions from the airways. As a result there is visual improvement on chest x-ray film.
2 Prepare patient for procedure:	
a Explain purpose and rationale for procedure. Explain positioning, sensations, how long it will take, and any discomforts or side effects.	Helps promote cooperation. Well-prepared patient is usually more relaxed and comfortable, which is essential for effective drainage.
b Encourage high fluid intake program unless contraindicated by other diseases and if physician approves. Maintain record of fluid intake and output.	Fluids thin secretions and make them easier to cough up. Patients need close monitoring and encouragement when first starting high fluid intake program.
c Plan treatments so they do not overlap with meals or tube feeding. Avoid postural drainage 1 to 2 hours before a meal or 1 to 2 hours after meals or bolus tube feedings. Stop all continuous gastric tube feedings for 30 to 45 minutes before postural drainage. Check for residual feeding in patient's stomach; if greater than 100 mL, hold treatment.	Performing postural drainage when patient's stomach is empty helps avoid gastric reflux or vomiting and aspiration of stomach contents.
d Schedule treatments at appropriate times during day (e.g., coordinate with any bronchodilator therapy, which is usually administered 20 minutes before CPT).	Scheduling of CPT avoids conflict with other interventions and/or diagnostic testing.

Critical Decision Point *If patient is receiving inhaled bronchodilator, nebulizers, or aerosol treatment, postural drainage is done 20 minutes after such therapy.*

e Have patient remove any tight or restrictive clothing.	Helps patient relax and promotes deep breathing.

IMPLEMENTATION

1 Close room door or pull curtains around patient's head. Perform hand hygiene, and apply gloves as indicated.	Maintains privacy. Reduces transmission of microorganisms.
2 Select congested areas for draining based on assessment of all lung fields, clinical data, and chest x-ray data.	Individualized treatment helps relieve specific areas of congestion identified during patient assessment.

STEP	RATIONALE
3 Position patient to drain congested areas; first area selected usually varies from patient to patient. (Refer to Table 24-1 for positioning to drain upper, middle, and lower lobe bronchi.) Help patient assume position as needed. Teach patient correct posture and arm and leg positioning. Place pillows for support and comfort. Drape patient appropriately.	Proper patient positioning promotes drainage of pulmonary secretions.
4 Have patient maintain posture for 10 to 15 minutes.	In adults, draining each area takes time.
5 During 10 to 15 minutes of drainage in selected postures, perform chest percussion and vibration and shaking (see Procedural Guideline 24-2, p. 665) over affected lung region. Table 24-1 shows all postures and hand placement for percussion and vibration and shaking.	Provides mechanical forces to help move airway secretions.
6 After 10 to 15 minutes of drainage in first posture, have patient sit up and cough. If indicated, save expectorated secretions in a clear container. If patient cannot cough, suctioning is necessary.	Any secretions moved to the central airways are removed by cough or suctioning before placing patient into next drainage position. Coughing is most effective when patient is sitting up and leaning forward.

Critical Decision Point *Sometimes patients experience transient dyspnea and fatigue because of airway irritation and bronchospasm from the secretions. These patients often benefit from an oscillating or vibrating device, such as an Acapella device (see Procedural Guideline 24-1). Dyspnea and bronchospasm usually subside after secretions are removed.*

7 Have patient rest briefly if necessary.	Short rest periods between postures help prevent fatigue and increase tolerance for the therapy.
8 Have patient take sips of water.	Keeping mouth moist aids in expectoration of secretions.
9 Repeat Steps 3 to 8 until all congested areas selected are drained. Make sure each treatment does not exceed 30 to 60 minutes.	Postural drainage is used only to drain areas involved and is based on individual assessment.
10 Offer or assist patient with oral hygiene.	Promotes comfort and reduces bad breath.
11 Perform hand hygiene.	Reduces transmission of microorganisms.

EVALUATION

1 Auscultate lung fields.	Clearance of secretions usually relieves gurgling, early inspiratory crackles, and palpable crepitus.
2 Inspect character and amount of sputum.	Determines if secretions are adequately thinned.
3 Review diagnostic reports, including sputum collections/cultures, chest x-ray films, and blood gas levels.	Provides objective data on improvements in lung function.
4 Obtain vital signs, pulse oximetry.	Procedure can result in dysrhythmias and decreases in oxygen saturation in some patients.

Unexpected Outcomes

1 Patient experiences severe dyspnea, bronchospasm, hypoxemia, hypercarbia, and/or is unable to tolerate treatment.

2 Little to no secretions are obtained, and there is no improvement in chest assessment or chest x-ray examination results.

Related Interventions

- Identify patients at risk such as (1) those with severe lung disease who have high $PaCO_2$ levels and/or who require high concentrations of oxygen and (2) those who are severely debilitated with altered mental status.
- Discontinue, modify, or shorten treatments.
- Administer bronchodilator or nebulizer therapy 20 minutes before CPT.
- Notify health care provider.
- Suction and ventilate with bag-valve-mask as needed, and closely monitor arterial blood gas (ABG) levels, oxygen saturation, and vital signs.

- Initially, increase treatments, and encourage and teach coughing exercises (sometimes there is a lack of secretions, or they are too thick for the patient to cough up).
- Consult health care provider because patient may need sputum culture, change in antibiotics, mucolytics, or a bronchoscopy to remove thick mucous plugs.
- Increases hydration.

Unexpected Outcomes	Related Interventions
3 Hemoptysis occurs, or patient develops acute hypotension, severe chest pain, vomiting, aspiration, and/or dysrhythmias.	• Stop therapy, place patient in high-Fowler's position, and obtain vital signs. • Notify health care provider. • Remain calm, stay with patient, call for help, and keep patient comfortable, calm, warm, and quiet. • If patient vomits or aspirates, suction airway and place patient on his or her side.
4 Patient has difficulty tolerating treatment, and/or family is unable to learn technique for home use.	• Modify treatments by shortening duration or eliminating techniques that cause discomfort. • Consider trial use of chest vest because patients usually tolerate it well. These vests are also self-applied, so patient can use it independently at home. • Use an oscillating or vibrating airway clearance mechanism, such as an Acapella device (see Procedural Guideline 24-1) in conjunction with postural drainage.

Recording and Reporting

- Record pretherapy and posttherapy assessment of chest and chest x-ray findings; frequency and duration of treatment; postures used and bronchial segments drained; cough effectiveness; need for suctioning; color, amount, and consistency of sputum; hemoptysis or other unexpected outcomes; and patient's tolerance and reactions.
- If patient and family receive instruction in home care, chart instructions given, understanding of therapy, demonstration of skill, patient acceptance of home care, barriers to learning and implementation, and referrals for home care or rehabilitation.

Teaching Considerations

- Best times for treatments are (1) in the morning before breakfast, when patient can clear secretions that accumulate overnight, and (2) about 1 hour before bedtime, so that lungs are clear before sleeping and patient has time after treatment to cough up any mobilized secretions. Frequency depends on need and patient's tolerance and varies from once daily to every 2 to 4 hours in an acute situation.
- Instruct patient's family or primary caregiver in recognizing when the patient's respiratory status requires breathing exercises or postural drainage.
- Teach patient and significant others how to assume postures at home. Some postures need modification to meet patient needs. For example if the patient is very short of breath, place the patient in a supine, side-lying semi-Fowler's or side-lying Trendelenburg's position to drain lateral lower lobes.

Pediatric Considerations

- In a child with cystic fibrosis, chest physiotherapy is a cornerstone therapy and is usually performed at least twice daily, on rising in the morning and in the evening (Hockenberry and others, 2007). Many CF patients use the chest vest when at home so they are independent.
- Chest physiotherapy is not recommended during acute exacerbations of asthma.

Gerontological Considerations

- Take extra care and assessment when using postural drainage in older adults. Change positions more slowly, and closely assess for any changes in oxygen saturation or vital signs with position changes.
- Older adults with chronic cardiac and pulmonary conditions do not always tolerate a supine or side-lying position for CPT. In these positions patients experience decline in forced vital capacity (FVC) and subsequent decline in oxygen saturation (Manning and others, 1999).

Home Care Considerations

- If specialized home or outpatient follow-up is needed, refer patient to pulmonary nurse specialist, pulmonary rehabilitation team, or home care personnel.
- Obtain foam wedge or multiple pillows for correct positioning (Rice, 2000).
- In the home setting Trendelenburg's position is achieved in several ways. Select the most comfortable and practical method that best suits patient (note that this is more common for the pediatric patient). Purchase a slant board or make one out of old door or tabletop and pad the surface with foam or blankets; elevate patient's hips with a stack of old newspapers and pillows or foam wedge (these props are often uncomfortable and often flatten out because of patient's body weight); or place a wedge or stack of papers under bed board.

PROCEDURAL GUIDELINE 24-1 Using an Acapella Device

The Acapella device is one of many airway clearance devices aimed at assisting patients with cystic fibrosis, COPD, and other lung diseases to easily remove secretions from their airways (Marks and others, 2004). These airway clearance devices are easy to use, and patients are able to perform airway clearance interventions independently (Volsko and others, 2003). The Acapella is a hand-held airway clearance device (Fig. 24-2). It provides positive expiratory pressure (PEP) with oral airway oscillations. Positive expiratory pressure stabilizes airways and improves aeration of the distal lung areas. During exhalation, pressure from the airways is transmitted to the Acapella device, which helps mucus dislodge from the airway walls and as a result prevents airway collapse, accelerates expiratory flow, and moves mucus toward the trachea (Marks, 2007).

This device combines resistive features of positive expiratory pressure and vibration to mobilize airway secretions. Patients with chronic conditions, such as cystic fibrosis, appear to receive the greatest benefit from this type of treatment (Holland and others, 2003; Marks, 2007) (see Box 24-1).

Delegation Considerations

The skill of using an Acapella device can be delegated to appropriately trained NAP. The nurse is responsible for determining respiratory assessment and that the procedure is appropriate and that the patient is able to tolerate the procedure and for evaluating the patient's response to the procedure. The nurse directs the NAP to:

- Be alert for the patient's tolerance of procedure, such as comfort level and changes in breathing pattern, and to immediately report changes to the nurse.
- Use specific patient precautions related to disease or treatment.
- Use any positioning restrictions or problems unique to the patient.

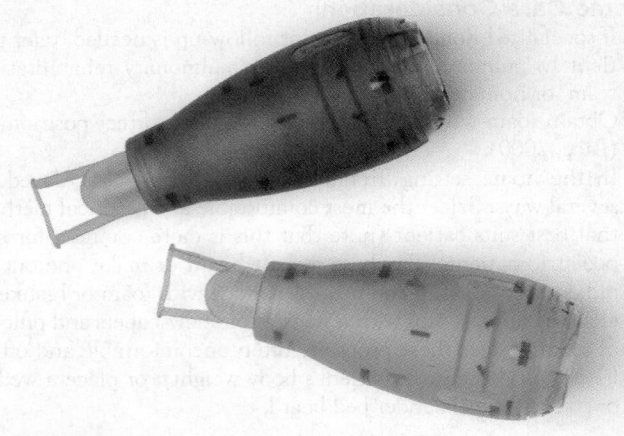

FIG 24-2 Acapella device. (*Used with permission, Smithsmedical.com.*)

Equipment

- ❏ Stethoscope
- ❏ Pulse oximeter
- ❏ Water and glass
- ❏ Chair
- ❏ Tissues and paper bag
- ❏ Clear graduated screw-top container
- ❏ Suction equipment (if patient unable to cough and clear own secretions)
- ❏ Acapella device (see Fig. 24-2)
- ❏ Clean gloves (*optional*)
- ❏ Patient education materials

Procedural Steps

1 Verify the need for a physician's order per agency's policy.
2 Assess respirations, and auscultate lung sounds for signs and symptoms indicating the need for this treatment.
3 Assess patient and family understanding of the device and procedure, and explain and clarify procedure as needed.
4 Prepare Acapella device; initial setting: turn Acapella frequency adjustment dial counterclockwise to lowest resistance setting. As patient improves or is more proficient, adjust the proper resistance level upward by turning the dial clockwise. This initial setting helps patient to adjust to the device.

Critical Decision Point *Determine if aerosol drug therapy is ordered. If so, attach a nebulizer to the end of the Acapella valve.*

5 Instruct patient to (Fink and Mahlmeister, 2002):
   a Sit comfortably.
   b Take in a breath that is larger than normal, but not to fill lungs completely. Instruct patient to inhale to about 75% of inspiratory capacity (Marks, 2007).
   c Place mouthpiece into the mouth, maintaining a tight seal.
   d Hold breath for 2 to 3 seconds.
   e Try not to cough and to exhale slowly for 3 to 4 seconds through the device while it vibrates.

Critical Decision Point *If patient cannot maintain an exhalation for this length of time, adjust the dial clockwise. Clockwise adjustment increases the resistance of the vibrating opening, which will allow the patient to exhale at a lower flow rate.*

   f Repeat cycle for 5 to 10 breaths as tolerated.
   g Remove mouthpiece and perform one to two forceful exhalations and "huffs" coughs (Marks, 2007).
   h Repeat Steps a through g as ordered.
6 Auscultate lung fields.
7 Obtain vital signs, pulse oximetry.
8 Inspect color, character, and amount of sputum.
9 Assist patient with oral hygiene.
10 Review Unexpected Outcomes for Skill 24-1.

PROCEDURAL GUIDELINE 24-2   Performing Percussion, Vibration, and Shaking

During postural drainage a nurse, respiratory therapist, or trained family member sometimes uses physical maneuvers, such as percussion, vibration, and shaking, on the rib cage over lung tissue. The techniques are used on specific parts of the rib cage over each affected lung region. Normally the mucociliary escalator and cough transport can effectively clear airway secretions. However, when the patient's ability to clear the airways is reduced, the techniques of percussion, vibration, and shaking are combined with postural drainage.

Percussion involves clapping the chest wall with cupped hands. If done correctly, it painlessly sets up vibrations in the chest to dislodge retained secretions. Vibration is a sustained contraction of the upper extremities of the caregiver. Vibration produces a downward vibrating pressure, done only during exhalation, with the flat part of the palm over the area. Shaking is a more vigorous downward rocking motion on the rib cage done with the flat part of the hand during exhalation. These last two maneuvers are performed as the patient exhales through pursed lips. They augment the natural movement of the rib cage during exhalation and assist with secretion clearance. The clavicles, breast tissue, sternum, spine, waist, and abdomen are never used for percussion and vibration. Perform percussion, vibration, and shaking only over the ribs.

Delegation Considerations

The skill of performing percussion, vibration, and shaking can be delegated to NAP. The nurse is responsible for the respiratory assessment and review of the patient's chest x-ray film to determine that the patient is stable, which areas of the lungs are affected, and specific positions for the patient to assume. The nurse directs the NAP to:

- Be alert for the patient's tolerance of the procedure, to monitor vital signs, and be alert to any patient precautions related to disease or treatment
- Report any problems with tolerance of the procedure, pain, dyspnea, or changes in vital signs.

Equipment

- ❑ Stethoscope
- ❑ Hospital bed (tilt table placed in Trendelenburg's position, optional, check agency policy)
- ❑ Chair (for upper lobes)
- ❑ One to four pillows
- ❑ Water pitcher and glass
- ❑ Tissues and paper bag
- ❑ Clear graduated screw-top container
- ❑ Mechanical vibrator or percussor (*optional*)
- ❑ Single layer of clothing
- ❑ Clean gloves (if there is a risk for exposure to patient's respiratory secretions)
- ❑ Suction equipment (*optional*)

Procedural Steps

1. Assess breathing pattern, including muscles used for breathing, respiratory rate and depth, extent of excursion, and chest wall movement.
2. Assess patient, and review medical record for signs and symptoms and conditions that indicate need to perform these skills (see Skill 24-1, Assessment).

Critical Decision Point   *Percussion, vibration, and shaking are contraindicated with rib fracture, fracture of other rib cage structures such as clavicle or sternum, pain, severe dyspnea, and severe osteoporosis. Thin, frail patients with osteoporosis are most susceptible to injury and are taught other secretion control measures (e.g., forceful coughing, humidification).*

3. Identify and assess area of rib cage over affected bronchial segment for pain, tenderness, abnormal configuration, abnormal excursion or chest wall movement during breathing, and muscle tension.
4. Determine patient's understanding, and assess patient's ability to cooperate with therapy, both in hospital and at home.
5. Explain procedure in detail: patient's positioning, sensations, how it will be done, how long it will take, and any discomforts or side effects.
6. Help patient to relax and deep breathe during procedure. Have patient practice exhaling slowly through pursed lips while relaxing chest wall muscles. Instruct patient to blow out using abdominal muscles, not rib cage muscles.
7. Perform hand hygiene, and apply clean gloves as appropriate.
8. Elevate bed to comfortable working height, and stand close to bed with arms directly in front and knees slightly bent.
9. Position patient in appropriate drainage position (see Skill 24-1, Implementation, Steps 1 to 3); assess and identify lung region for percussion and vibration (see Table 24-1).
10. Perform percussion for 3 to 5 minutes in each position as tolerated. Begin percussion on appropriate part of chest wall over draining area (see Table 24-1). Always ask if patient is experiencing any discomfort, such as undue pressure or stinging of the skin.
    a. Place hands side by side on chest wall over area to be drained. Cup hands with fingers and thumbs held tightly together. Make sure that entire outer portion of hand makes contact with chest wall to avoid air leaks (see Table 24-1).
    b. When clapping, most of arm movement comes from the elbow and wrist joints. Clapping is often done for 5 minutes without stopping or 2 to 3 minutes, alternating with vibration and shaking.
    c. Alternately clap chest with cupped hands to create rhythmic popping sound resembling galloping horse. Perform clapping at moderate or fast speed; whichever is most comfortable and effective.

Continued

PROCEDURAL GUIDELINE 24-2   Performing Percussion, Vibration, and Shaking—cont'd

11 Perform chest wall vibration and shaking over each affected area (see Table 24-1). Vibrations are usually done in sets of three followed by coughing so that any loosened secretions are expectorated.

   a Place hands over area, and have patient take slow, deep breath through nose.

   b Gently resist chest wall as it rises during inhalation.

   c Have patient hold breath and then exhale through pursed lips, while contracting abdominal muscles and relaxing chest wall muscles. Chest wall relaxes and falls.

   d While patient is exhaling, gently push down and vibrate with flat part of hand.

   e Repeat vibration three times, and then have patient cascade cough by taking deep breath and doing series of small coughs until end of breath. Instruct patient not to inhale between coughs. Vibrate chest wall as patient coughs. When applying pressure to ribs, always follow natural movement of rib cage. Allow patient to sit up and cough as needed.

   f Monitor patient's tolerance of vibration and ability to relax chest wall and breathe properly as instructed.

12 Perform shaking with vibration:

   a Place flat part of hand over area, and have patient inhale slowly through nose.

   b During inhalation, apply light pressure on ribs and stretch skin so it is tight.

   c Have patient hold breath for 2 seconds.

   d As patient exhales, increase pressure. Maintain pressure while applying intermittent rocking motion on ribs. Pressure is directed toward following natural expiratory rib cage movement.

   e Instruct patient to exhale through pursed lips and relax chest wall muscles as much as possible.

   f Repeat shaking three times, have patient inhale deeply, and then do rib shaking during cascade cough.

13 Perform a total of three or four sets of three vibrations and shaking and coughing in each posture as tolerated. Strength and frequency of vibration and shaking will vary. Vibration requires all muscles in arm and shoulder to contract and tremble. Shaking requires applying controlled pressure from shoulders and back while slightly leaning on chest; rocking motion is created by flexing and extending elbows using triceps.

14 Suction if patient is unable to cough up mucus (see Chapter 25).

15 Assist patient with oral hygiene.

16 Remove gloves, and perform hand hygiene.

17 If long-term therapy is needed, teach patient and significant others the procedure for home use. If they cannot learn or use, refer for outpatient or home care follow-up.

18 Auscultate lung fields.

19 Obtain vital signs, pulse oximetry.

20 Inspect color, character, and amount of sputum.

CRITICAL THINKING EXERCISES

Mr. Meyersohn is a 29-year-old college student with a history of cystic fibrosis. He was admitted to the hospital 3 days ago for pneumonia. He has a fever to 38.8° C and bilateral lower lobe pneumonia and lobar collapse of his right middle lobe.

1 Chest physiotherapy was ordered. What positions would you use?
2 Based on the chest x-ray findings, what would you expect to find on physical examination of the chest, and what additional signs and symptoms would you expect to see?
3 After 24 hours of aggressive CPT a chest x-ray examination was repeated. It showed improvement with good expansion of the right middle lobe and improved aeration of the lower lobes. Were the improvements in the x-ray examination a result of the CPT? What other clinical improvement would you expect?
4 What would you document regarding the CPT and clinical assessment?

 ## REVIEW QUESTIONS

1 A patient was hospitalized with respiratory failure due to exacerbation of severe emphysema and bronchiectasis. Chest x-ray examination revealed good lung expansion except for left lower lobe collapse. In which position should you place the patient for the ordered chest physiotherapy?
   1 Right side-lying Trendelenburg's
   2 Left side-lying Trendelenburg's
   3 Right side-lying flat
   4 Right side-lying Trendelenburg's with one-quarter turn back onto a pillow
2 A patient was admitted with recurrence of bilateral upper lobe lung abscesses due to tuberculosis. Chest computed tomography examination showed fluid- and air-filled abscesses in bilateral upper lobes anteriorly. How should you position the patient to drain these areas?
   1 Sitting up in a chair and leaning backward onto a pillow
   2 Sitting up in a chair and leaning forward onto a pillow or table
   3 Lying on back flat in bed
   4 Lying prone with bed flat
3 A patient needing chest physiotherapy finished his lunch at 1 PM. When is the soonest he should receive postural drainage?
   1 An hour from now
   2 At 2 PM
   3 Before his next snack
   4 Right after dinner
4 A frail older adult patient needs chest physiotherapy because during assessment retained respiratory secretions were auscultated. What approach would be most appropriate to help this patient get rid of these secretions?
   1 Encourage him to increase his oral fluid intake.
   2 Teach the patient how to forcefully cough.
   3 Perform postural drainage on the affected lobes.
   4 Use vibration and shaking over the affected lobes.

5 A patient experiences severe dyspnea and hemoptysis during a session of chest physiotherapy. After stopping the CPT, what is the initial appropriate nursing intervention?
   1 Notify the physician.
   2 Administer a bronchodilator to ease the dyspnea.
   3 Assess the patient.
   4 Elevate the head of the patient's bed.

REFERENCES

AARC clinical practice guideline: postural drainage therapy, *Respir Care* 36(12):1418, 1991.
Fink JB, Mahlmeister MJ: High frequency oscillation of the airway and chest wall, *Respir Care* 47(7):797, 2002.
Frownfelter DL, Dean E: *Principles and practice of cardiopulmonary therapy*, ed 3, St. Louis, 1996, Mosby.
Galanti GA: *Caring for patients from different cultures*, ed 3, Philadelphia, 2004, University of Pennsylvania Press.
Hockenberry MJ, Wilson D: *Wong's nursing care of infants and children*, ed 8, St. Louis, 2007, Mosby.
Manning F and others: Effects of side lying on lung function in older individuals, *Phys Ther* 79(5):456, 1999.
Marks JH: Airway clearance devices in cystic fibrosis, *Paediatr Respir Rev* 8:17, 2007
Rice R: *Manual of home health nursing procedures*, ed 2, St. Louis, 2000, Mosby.
Volsko TA and others: Performance comparison of two oscillating positive expiratory pressure devices: Acapella versus Flutter, *Respir Care* 48(2):124, 2003.

RESEARCH REFERENCES

Denehy L, Berney S: Physiotherapy in the intensive care unit, *Phys Ther Rev* 11:49, 2006.
Holland AE and others: Non-invasive ventilation assists chest physiotherapy in adults with acute exacerbations of cystic fibrosis, *Thorax* 58:880, 2003.
Main E and others: Conventional chest physiotherapy compared to other airway clearance techniques for cystic fibrosis, *Cochrane Database Syst Rev* (1): CD002011, 2005.
Marks JH and others: Pulmonary function and sputum production in patients with cystic fibrosis: a pilot study comparing the PercussiveTech HF device and standard chest physiotherapy, *Chest* 125:1507, 2004.
McCool FD, Rosen MJ: Nonpharmacologic airway clearance therapies—ACCP evidence-based clinical practice guidelines, *Chest* 129:205S, 2006.
Oermann CM and others: Validation of an instrument measuring patient satisfaction with chest physiotherapy techniques in cystic fibrosis, *Chest* 118:92, 2000.
Oermann CM and others: Comparison of high-frequency chest wall oscillation and oscillating positive expiratory pressure in the home management of cystic fibrosis: a pilot study, *Pediatr Pulmonol* 32:372, 2001.
Patterson JE and others: Airway clearance in bronchiectasis: a randomized crossover trial of active cycle of breathing techniques versus Acapella, *Respiration* 72:239, 2005.
van der Schans C and others: Chest physiotherapy compared to no chest physiotherapy for cystic fibrosis, *Cochrane Database Syst Rev* 2000(2):CD001401, DOI:10.1002/14651858.CD001401.
Varekojis SM and others: A comparison of the therapeutic effectiveness of and preference for postural drainage and percussion, intrapulmonary percussive ventilation, and high-frequency chest wall compression in hospitalized cystic fibrosis patients, *Respir Care* 48(1):24, 2003.

KEY TERMS

Artificial airway
Atelectasis
Bronchospasm
Closed system
  suction catheter
Endotracheal (ET)
  tube
Hypercapnia
Hypoxemia
Hypoxia
Intubation

Laryngospasm
Obturator
Outer and inner
  cannula
Respiratory
  distress
Suction
Suction catheter
Tracheostomy
Yankauer suction

SKILLS AND PROCEDURES

MEDIA RESOURCES

- **evolve** *learning system* http://evolve.elsevier.com/Perry/skills
  - Review Questions
  - Video Clips

- **View Video!** Mosby's Nursing Video Skills, 3.0

- **NSO** Nursing Skills Online

OBJECTIVES

Mastery of content in this chapter will enable the nurse to:
- Identify guidelines used in managing the airway.
- Describe the methods for airway management.
- Discuss the indications for airway suctioning.
- Discuss the indications for tracheostomy care.
- Provide oropharyngeal suctioning.
- Provide airway suctioning.
- Provide endotracheal care.
- Provide tracheostomy tube care.
- Inflate the cuff on an endotracheal or tracheostomy tube.
- Change a tracheostomy tube.

Airway management involves maintaining the patency of the nose, upper airway, trachea, and lower airway of the respiratory system. Many courses of action are available to promote an open or patent airway, which has the potential to become obstructed by mucus, mechanical obstruction (i.e., soft tissue in upper airway), or a foreign body. These actions do not always require a physician's order. Consult the physician if there are any concerns about the appropriateness of the intervention or when an airway obstruction is present, even when treatment relieves the obstruction. Hydration, positioning, nutrition, chest therapy airway clearance techniques, mucous clearance device therapy, deep breathing, coughing, humidity, and aerosol therapy are noninvasive techniques that are helpful in maintaining a patent airway.

When a patient is unable to clear airway secretions with coughing, chest physiotherapy, or other noninvasive techniques, more invasive measures, such as suctioning, are needed. These additional measures directed at maintaining a patent airway are necessary, especially in a weak, confused, or critically ill patient. This chapter focuses on nonemergent, invasive techniques to maintain airway patency, including artificial airways.

EVIDENCE-BASED PRACTICE TRENDS

Preoxygenation and deep breathing, sometimes referred to as hyperventilation, assist in reducing suction-induced hypoxemia (Demir and Dramali, 2005). Preoxygenation provides a patient with a short-term increase in supplemental oxygen, such as increasing oxygen flow rate on a nasal cannula or oxygen mask, increasing the percent of inspired oxygen of breaths delivered by the mechanical ventilator, or increasing oxygen flow rates to artificial airways. Not every patient requires preoxygenation unless he or she is hypoxemic before suctioning. Hyperinflation is the process of providing 100% oxygen to a patient before airway suctioning (Pruitt, 2005).

Following suctioning, return a patient's oxygen level to presuctioning levels to avoid increased risk for oxygen toxicity. In addition, there is also a risk for absorption atelectasis from prolonged administration of high concentrations of oxygen and increased carbon dioxide retention in patients with chronic obstructive lung diseases (Demir and Dramali, 2005).

The practice of normal saline instillation (NSI) into artificial airways to improve secretion removal is inconclusive. Clinical studies comparing the results of suctioning using NSI with those of standard suctioning do not show any clinical or significant results (Celik and Kanan, 2006). A review of the literature indicates that suctioning with or without isotonic normal saline (INS) produces similar amounts of secretions and significant decreases in oxygen saturation. In addition, these studies show increases in heart rate for 4 to 5 minutes after suctioning with INS as opposed to dry suctioning. The review also indicates that the level of a patient's dyspnea after suctioning with or without INS was not significantly different. Last, the review notes that the use of INS with suctioning has the potential to increase ventilator-associated pneumonia because INS can dislodge bacteria from the upper airway to the lower portions of the airway (Celik and Kanan, 2006; Grap and Munro, 2004).

Psychosocial consequences of airway suctioning often occur. Patients who remember the suctioning report it as painful, suffocating, or stressful. Patients recalled some of the physiological results of suctioning, such as sleep disturbances, tachycardia, confusion, shortness of breath, and dizziness (Lindgren and Ames, 2005).

CULTURAL CONSIDERATIONS

Communication is vital. Artificial airways alter patients' ability to communicate. Patients, especially those from other cultures, feel frightened, frustrated, and vulnerable. In addition, measures used to maintain airway patency are new and frightening. Assess the meaning of oropharyngeal suctioning to the patient and family members. Explain anticipated effects such as gagging and tearing, which are very distressing to family members. Many Vietnamese believe that objects entering the body cause illness, so some may interpret suctioning as introducing illness to the patient (Edmonds and Brady, 2003). A balance between positive and negative forces, or the yin and yang, are important components of Vietnamese culture and must be maintained for optimal health.

Provide culturally congruent explanations of the purpose and therapeutic effects of the procedure. Whenever possible, demonstrate suctioning techniques and encourage patient and family members to participate. If available, a professional interpreter is a valuable asset for explanation of procedures, especially those that are invasive and need to be repeated multiple times, such as suctioning and tracheostomy tube care. If an interpreter is not available, have a family or community member explain invasive procedures such as insertion of endotracheal tube or tracheostomy. Encourage family members at the bedside to provide support for a patient who has limited English proficiency. Collaborate with the family in providing alternative means of communication for the patient. Provide educational materials to the patient and family in their native language for maximal understanding.

Skill Performance Guidelines

1 Know the patient's normal range of vital signs and oxygen saturation levels. Baseline vital signs serve as a means to identify individual abnormalities and to recognize the onset of worsening of an illness.

2 Know the patient's medical history. Smoking alters normal mucociliary clearance. Certain disorders such as chronic obstructive pulmonary disease (COPD), asthma, cystic fibrosis, pneumonia, thoracic surgery, chest trauma, and abdominal surgery place the patient at increased risk for an obstructed airway.

3 Identify conditions that increase the patient's risk for aspiration of gastric contents into the lung, resulting in airway obstruction. These include the presence of enteral feeding tubes or other nasal or oral gastric tubes, a decreased level of consciousness, and a decreased swallowing ability.

4 Determine if the patient has a history of nasal problems, such as nasal trauma, nasal polyps, deviated nasal septum, or chronic sinusitis. Allergy problems causing mucosal swelling

narrow nasal passages, which affect your ability to easily pass a suction catheter.

5 Review the patient's respiratory assessments. Review the patient's condition from the past 12 or 24 hours. These are relative baseline measurements that assist in distinguishing between gradual and acute changes in the patient's status.

6 Perform a systematic respiratory assessment of upper and lower airways, including identifying respiratory rate, respiratory pattern, respiratory muscles used, breath sounds, ability to cough effectively, integrity of the rib cage, and the characteristics of sputum production.

7 Determine the type and frequency of intervention, based on assessment findings. Care that is appropriate for one day or shift can change, resulting in an increase or decrease in frequency of care or alterations in the type of intervention.

8 Identify and become familiar with the use of equipment available at the institution. Many types of artificial airways, suction catheters, and suction machines are available. Knowing how to operate the equipment before using it will benefit both you and the patient.

9 Test all equipment before use. Have adequate supplies on hand at the bedside. Equipment must work properly to provide safe nursing care. Determine that the suction machine is generating adequate negative suction pressure (Table 25-1) and that there are suction catheters and appropriate equipment at the bedside.

TABLE 25-1	Vacuum Pressure Settings for Suctioning
Age	**Pressure Setting**
Preterm infants	60-80 mm Hg
Infants	80-100 mm Hg
Children	100-120 mm Hg
Adults	100-150 mm Hg

Data from *AARC clinical practice guidelines: nasotracheal suctioning—2004 revision and update,* 2004, http://www.rcjournal.com/cpgs/pdf/09.04.1080. pdf, accessed September 13, 2007.

10 Know the patient's home care plan. Absence or interruption of certain therapies such as bronchodilators places the patient at risk for an obstructed airway during the hospitalization or after discharge from the hospital.

11 Know the side effects of medications and other therapies. Some medications such as beta-adrenergic blockers have the side effect of bronchospasm. An adverse effect of opioids and sedatives is respiratory depression. Similarly, too much oxygen reduces the drive to breathe in patients with chronic hypercapnia (elevated arterial carbon dioxide tension). Some position changes affect the patient adversely. For example, in patients with impaired spinal cord innervations of the respiratory muscles, supine positions place the diaphragm at a mechanical disadvantage and increase the risk for aspiration.

SKILL 25-1 Oropharyngeal Suctioning

 Intermediate / Respiratory Care and Suctioning / Performing Oropharyngeal Suctioning

NSO *Airway Management Module / Lesson 3*

A Yankauer, or tonsillar tip, suction device is used for oropharyngeal suctioning (Fig. 25-1). A Yankauer suction catheter is made of rigid, minimally flexible plastic. The tip of this suction catheter usually has one large and several small eyelets through which the mucus enters with application of negative pressure. The Yankauer suction catheter is angled to facilitate removal of pharyngeal secretions through the mouth. This catheter is used instead of a standard suction catheter when oral secretions are extremely copious and thick because it can handle large volumes of secretions better than a standard suction catheter. The Yankauer suction catheter is not used to suction the nares because of its size.

The Yankauer suction device is useful in the removal of secretions from the mouth in patients after oral and maxillofacial surgery, trauma to the mouth, or neurovascular injury and cerebrovascular accident causing hemiparesis and drooling or impaired swallowing. Patients with artificial airways and impaired swallowing require use of the Yankauer suction device to provide oral hygiene.

Delegation Considerations
The skill of performing oropharyngeal (Yankauer) suctioning can be delegated to nursing assistive personnel (NAP). Do not routinely delegate this skill for patients with oral or neck surgery in the immediate postoperative period. The nurse is responsible for assessing the patient's respiratory status. The nurse directs the NAP about:

- Appropriate suction limits for oropharyngeal suctioning for the particular patient, for example, the appropriate suction pressure, expected frequency of suctioning, and the expected color and volume of secretions.
- The risks of applying excessive or inadequate suction pressure.
- Avoiding mouth sutures, applying suction against sensitive tissues, and dislodging tubes in the patient's nose or mouth.
- Avoiding stimulation of the gag reflex.

Equipment
- ❑ Towel, cloth, or disposable paper drape
- ❑ Clean gloves
- ❑ Yankauer or tonsillar tip suction catheter
- ❑ Mask, goggles, or face shield
- ❑ Disposable cup or nonsterile basin
- ❑ Tap water or normal saline (about 100 mL)
- ❑ Suction equipment
- ❑ Connecting tubing (6 feet)
- ❑ Oral airway (if indicated)
- ❑ Washcloth (if indicated)
- ❑ Pulse oximeter

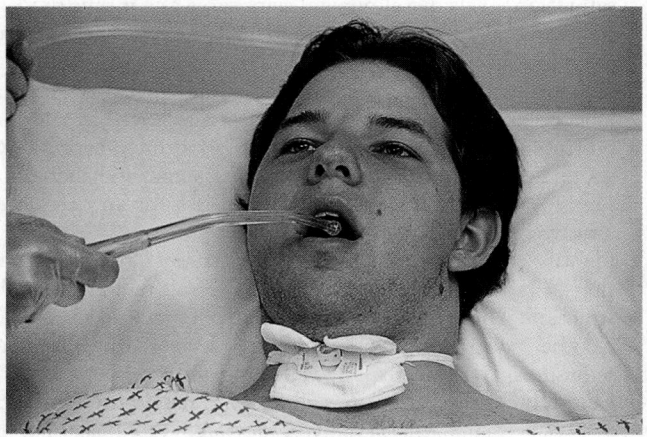

FIG 25-1 Oropharyngeal suctioning.

STEP	RATIONALE

ASSESSMENT

1 Assess signs and symptoms of upper airway obstruction requiring oropharyngeal suctioning: gurgling on inspiration or expiration, restlessness, obvious excessive oral secretions, drooling, gastric secretions or vomitus in mouth, or coughing without clearing secretions from upper airway.

Physical signs and symptoms result from pooling of secretions in upper airway. Worsening secretions may result in total airway obstruction and hypoxia. The risk for aspiration of gastric contents and airway obstruction is increased in patients with vomiting, delayed gastric emptying, impaired esophageal sphincter control, hiatal hernia, impaired cough, impaired swallowing, or impaired gag reflex.

2 Assess for signs and symptoms associated with hypoxia (low oxygen utilization at the cellular or tissue level), hypoxemia (low oxygen tension in the blood), or hypercapnia (elevated carbon dioxide tension in the blood) and associated symptoms of apprehension, anxiety, decreased ability to concentrate, lethargy, decreased level of consciousness (especially acute), increased fatigue and dizziness, behavioral changes (especially irritability and restlessness), increased pulse rate, increased rate of breathing, decreased depth of breathing, elevated blood pressure, cardiac dysrhythmias, pallor, cyanosis, dyspnea, and use of accessory muscles for breathing (Considine, 2005).

Suctioning of airways is indicated with alterations in oxygenation associated with secretion accumulation.

3 Obtain patient's oxygen saturation level via pulse oximetry (SpO_2) (see Chapter 5). Keep oximeter in place.

Provides an objective baseline measure of the oxygen saturation and provides an early objective indication of worsening oxygenation status.

4 Determine patient's knowledge about use of suction catheter.

Reveals need for patient instruction.

5 Identify risk factors for airway obstruction such as impaired cough or gag reflex, weakened respiratory muscles, impaired swallowing, and decreased level of consciousness, as well as patient's inability to manipulate and use the catheter device.

Risk factors prevent patient from protecting the airway from aspiration or from clearing secretions safely. Physical factors such as impaired mobility of the upper extremities prevent patient from using the catheter to help control oral secretions.

6 Auscultate for presence of adventitious sounds.

Determines if lower airway secretions are present (see Skill 25-2).

NURSING DIAGNOSES

- Deficient knowledge regarding airway clearance techniques and devices
- Impaired gas exchange
- Impaired swallowing
- Ineffective airway clearance
- Ineffective breathing pattern
- Risk for aspiration
- Risk for infection

Individualize related factors based on patient's condition or needs.

PLANNING

1 Expected outcomes following completion of procedure:
- Upper airway (oral pharynx) is cleared of secretions.
- No gurgling sounds are heard in patient's pharynx on inspiration and expiration.
- Drooling is diminished or absent.

- Vomitus or gastric secretions are absent from mouth.

- SpO_2 improves or remains the same.

Suctioning is effective.

Presence of secretions in large upper airway produces noisy respirations.

Excessive drooling indicates that patient is unable to handle oral secretions.

Gastric secretions retained in oral cavity increase patient's risk for aspiration pneumonia.

Removal of secretions helps to improve oxygen saturation level.

Critical Decision Point *In patients with chronic pulmonary disease, the SpO_2 value may remain the same after suctioning.*

2 Explain to patient how the procedure helps clear airway secretions and relieves some breathing problems. Explain that coughing, gagging, or (less commonly) sneezing is normal and lasts only a few seconds. Encourage patient to cough out secretions during procedure. Practice coughing if able. Show patient how to splint surgical incisions, if necessary.

Gagging or coughing occurs when the posterior pharynx is deeply suctioned or as a result of excess secretions. Coughing secretions out of lower airway or posterior pharynx decreases the amount of suctioning required. Splinting reduces abdominal incision discomfort during coughing or gagging.

3 Position patient (usually semi-Fowler's or sitting upright). Place towel, cloth, or paper drape across patient's neck and chest.

Promotes patient comfort and removal of airway secretions. Towel protects patient's gown and bed linen from contamination by secretions.

STEP	RATIONALE

IMPLEMENTATION

1 Perform hand hygiene, and apply clean gloves. Apply mask or face shield if splashing is likely.

Reduces transmission of microorganisms.

2 Fill cup or basin with approximately 100 mL of water or normal saline.

Aids in cleansing catheter after suctioning.

3 Connect one end of connecting tubing to suction machine and other to Yankauer suction catheter. Turn on suction equipment, set vacuum regulator to appropriate setting (see manufacturer's instructions).

Prepares suction apparatus. Elevated pressure settings increase risk for trauma to the oral mucosa.

4 Check that equipment is functioning properly by suctioning small amount of water or normal saline from cup or basin.

Ensures equipment function and lubricates catheter.

5 Remove patient's oxygen mask, if present. Nasal cannula may remain in place. Keep oxygen mask near patient's face.

Allows access to mouth. Reduces chance of hypoxia.

Critical Decision Point   *Be prepared to quickly reapply supplemental oxygen if SpO$_2$ value falls below 90% or respiratory distress develops during or at the end of suctioning (Considine, 2005; Pease, 2006).*

6 Insert catheter into mouth along gum line to pharynx. Move catheter around mouth until secretions have cleared. Encourage patient to cough. Replace oxygen mask.

Movement of catheter prevents the suction tip from invaginating oral mucosal surfaces and causing trauma. Coughing moves secretions from lower airway into mouth and upper airway.

7 Rinse catheter with water in cup or basin until connecting tubing is cleared of secretions. Turn off suction. Wash face if secretions are present on patient's skin.

Rinses catheter and reduces probability of transmission of microorganisms. Clean suction tubing enhances delivery of set suction pressure. Prevents skin breakdown.

8 Observe respiratory status. Repeat procedure, if indicated. May need to use standard suction catheter to reach into trachea if respiratory status not improved (see Skill 25-2).

Directs nurse to continue or cease intervention or to choose another intervention.

9 Remove towel, cloth, or disposable drape, and place in trash or in laundry if soiled. Reposition patient; Sims' position encourages drainage and should be used if patient has decreased level of consciousness.

Reduces transmission of microorganisms.
Facilitates drainage of oral secretions.

10 Discard remainder of water into appropriate receptacle. Rinse basin in warm soapy water, and dry with paper towels. Discard disposable cup into appropriate receptacle. Place catheter in clean, dry area.

Reduces transmission of microorganisms and maintains medical asepsis. Moist environment encourages microorganism growth.

Critical Decision Point   *Keep catheter in nonairtight container such as brown paper or plastic bag attached to bed rail or in suction canister area. Do not store the catheter where it will come in contact with secretions or excretions, which promote bacterial growth.*

11 Remove gloves and mask or face shield, and dispose of in appropriate receptacle. Perform hand hygiene.

Reduces transmission of microorganisms to other patients and equipment.

12 Position patient, and provide oral hygiene as needed.

Promotes patient's comfort.

EVALUATION

1 Compare assessment findings before and after procedure.

Identifies physiological response to the suction procedure.

2 Auscultate chest and airways for adventitious sounds.

Presence of lower airway adventitious sounds suggests a need for lower airway suctioning.

3 Obtain postsuction SpO$_2$ measure.

Provides objective postsuction data to compare with baseline and is another objective measure of the effectiveness of the suction procedure (AARC, 2004).

4 Observe patient or family perform Yankauer suctioning.

Demonstrates learning.

Unexpected Outcomes

1 Worsening respiratory distress.

2 Return of bloody secretions.

Related Interventions

- Suction further or implement nasal or tracheal suctioning.
- Evaluate need for other means to protect airway (e.g., oral intubation, oral airway, positioning).
- Provide supplemental oxygen.
- Notify physician.

- Assess oral cavity for trauma or lesions.
- Reduce the amount of suction pressure used.
- Observe catheter tip for nicks, which cause mucosal trauma.
- Increase frequency of oral hygiene.

Recording and Reporting

- Record the amount, consistency, color, and odor of secretions and the patient's response to the procedure; document presuction and postsuction cardiopulmonary assessment.
- Record instruction to caregivers and ability to correctly perform procedure.

Teaching Considerations

- Instruct family or caregiver not to allow catheter to fall to the floor.
- Provide information regarding signs and symptoms of worsening respiratory status.
- Assess knowledge level of patient and family caregiver to determine amount of instruction required and frequency of home health visits necessary to reach goals.

Pediatric Considerations

- Maintain healthy infant in supine position (American Academy of Pediatrics, 2005).
- Position infants with breathing problems or excessive vomitus in prone position (Hockenberry and Wilson, 2007; Pease, 2006).
- Airways of infants and children are smaller than those of an adult; even small amounts of mucus cause airway obstruction.

- Use bulb syringe. Compress syringe before insertion to prevent forcing secretions into infant's bronchi (Hockenberry and Wilson, 2007). If more forceful suctioning is necessary, use mechanical suction.

Gerontological Considerations

- Some patients with dysphagia benefit from oral suctioning before, during, and after meals.
- Oral mucosa in older adults is fragile, and a lower suction pressure is needed.
- Older adults are prone to aspiration of oral secretions because of decreased cough and gag reflexes (Meiner and Lueckenotte, 2006).

Long-Term and Home Care Considerations

- In the long-term care or home setting, make sure patient knows to clean and disinfect or change the secretion collection container every 24 hours according to home care or institutional protocol. Many institutions seal and dispose of the entire disposable secretion collection canister as biohazardous material.
- Assess home for the presence of respiratory irritants, including cigarette smoke, dust, pollen, animal dander, mold, and chemicals.

SKILL 25-2 Airway Suctioning

 Intermediate / Respiratory Care and Suctioning / Suctioning an Artificial Airway

NSO *Airway Management Module / Lessons 1, 5, and 6*

The major differences between oropharyngeal and tracheal airway suctioning are the depth suctioned, sterile procedure, and the potential for complications. Oropharyngeal suctioning only removes secretions from the back of the throat. Tracheal airway suctioning extends into the lower airway. Suctioning is necessary to remove respiratory secretions and maintain optimum ventilation and oxygenation in patients who are unable to independently remove these secretions (Demir and Dramali, 2005). Assess the patient to determine frequency and depth of suctioning. Some patients require suctioning every hour or two, whereas others need suctioning only once or twice a day (Considine, 2005).

If the secretions are only in the nose and mouth, then only the pharynx requires suctioning, although in most instances you will suction both the pharynx and the trachea. Suction secretions from the pharynx as often as necessary. Secretions that are not removed are more likely to be aspirated into the lungs, increasing the risk for infection and respiratory failure.

The suctioning procedure has many risks associated with it. The most serious relate to hypoxemia, which often results in cardiac dysrhythmias; laryngeal spasm; bradycardia, which is associated with stimulation of the vagus nerve; and nasal trauma and bleeding, which can develop from trauma of the suction catheter (Demir and Dramali, 2005).

NASOPHARYNGEAL AND NASOTRACHEAL SUCTIONING

 Intermediate / Respiratory Care and Suctioning / Performing Nasotracheal Suctioning

NSO *Airway Management Module / Lesson 4*

Nasopharyngeal and nasotracheal suctioning assist in maintaining a patent airway by removing secretions from the pharynx or throat and the trachea. This type of suctioning is used when oral suctioning with a Yankauer device is ineffective or inappropriate or when the lower airway requires removal of secretions. It involves inserting a small rubber or soft plastic tube into the nares to the pharynx or trachea and then applying negative pressure to withdraw mucus.

ARTIFICIAL AIRWAY SUCTIONING

Endotracheal (ET) tubes and tracheostomy ("trach") tubes (TTs) are artificial airways inserted to relieve airway obstruction, provide a route for mechanical ventilation, permit easy access for secretion removal, and protect the airway from gross aspiration in patients with impaired cough or gag reflexes (Fig. 25-2).

Endotracheal Tubes

NSO *Airway Management Module / Lesson 7*

Endotracheal intubation is a procedure performed by a physician or specially trained personnel (e.g., certified registered nurse anesthesiologist, respiratory therapist, or rescue personnel). An ET tube is inserted through the nares (nasal ET tube) or the mouth (oral ET tube) past the epiglottis and vocal cords into the trachea (Fig. 25-2, A).

The length of time that an ET tube remains in place is somewhat controversial; however, in most cases after 2 to 4 weeks a tracheostomy tube is inserted (Lindgren and Ames, 2005). ET tubes are usually made of plastic or rubber (Fig. 25-2, B). Adult sizes of ET tubes have a cuff molded onto the tube to (1) prevent the aspiration of oral secretions or gastric contents into the lung and/or (2) obstruct the escape of air from mechanical ventilator breaths through the upper airway.

Tracheostomy Tubes

Although ET tubes are temporary, a tracheostomy tube can be temporary or permanent depending on the patient's condition. A tracheostomy tube is inserted directly into the trachea through a small incision made in the patient's neck. Tracheostomy tubes are made of several different materials, including various polyvinyl chloride–based or silicone-based plastics and stainless steel or metallic compounds. Metal tracheostomy tubes are thermal sensitive and must be protected from extreme heat and cold to prevent tissue injury in the patient. Most metal and plastic tracheostomy tubes contain an inner cannula that is temporarily withdrawn for cleaning airway-occluding mucus without removing the entire tracheostomy tube (see Skill 25-4) (Roman, 2005; St. John and Malen, 2004).

A cuff on a tracheostomy tube serves the same purpose as one on an ET tube. Cuffs are made of a balloonlike inflatable plastic; usually you manually inflate them with air (see Skill 25-5). Plastic-covered foam cuffs are self–air inflating if the inflation port is left open to the atmosphere (St. John and Malen, 2004).

Some institutions use a closed suction catheter system or in-line suction catheter device to assist in minimizing infections, especially in critically ill or immunosuppressed patients (Grap and Munro, 2004; Pruitt, 2005). Use of a closed system catheter (in-line) allows quicker lower airway suctioning without applying gloves or a mask and does not interrupt ventilation and oxygenation in critically ill patients (see Procedural Guideline 25-1, p. 682). With a closed system method the patient's artificial airway is not disconnected from the mechanical ventilator (Mohan and Bollineni, 2007; Pruitt, 2005).

Delegation Considerations

The skills of nasotracheal suctioning and suctioning a new artificial airway cannot be delegated to NAP. When the patient has an established tracheostomy and you determine the patient is stable, you can delegate suctioning a tracheostomy. The nurse directs the NAP about:

- Any unique modifications of the skill, such as the need for supplemental oxygen or the use of a clean versus sterile suction technique.

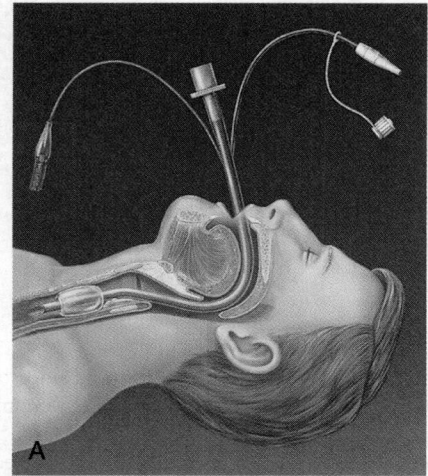

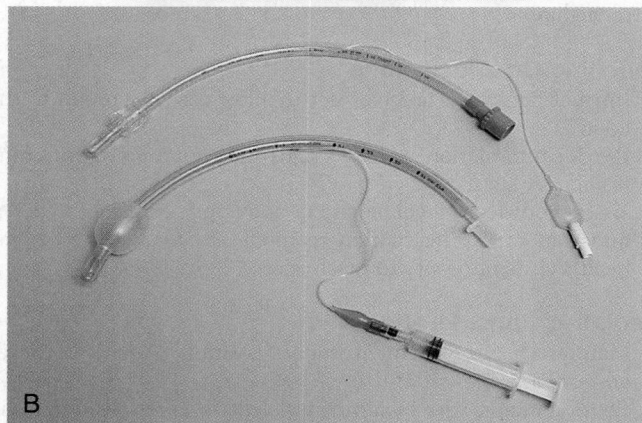

FIG 25-2 **A,** Endotracheal (ET) tube with inflated cuff. **B,** ET tubes with uninflated and inflated cuffs and syringe for inflation.

- Appropriate suction limits for suctioning tracheostomy tube and risks of applying excessive or inadequate suction pressure.
- Signs and symptoms of hypoxemia, such as change in patient's respiratory status, confusion, and restlessness, and to report these signs immediately to the nurse.
- Reporting any change in secretion quality, quantity, and color.

Equipment

- ❏ Appropriate-size suction catheter (smallest diameter that will remove secretions effectively) (Table 25-2)
- ❏ Nasal or oral airway (if indicated)
- ❏ Two sterile gloves or one sterile and one clean glove
- ❏ Clean towel or paper drape
- ❏ Suction machine/source
- ❏ Mask, goggles, or face shield
- ❏ Connecting tubing (6 feet)
- ❏ Small Y-adapter (if catheter does not have a suction control port)
- ❏ Water-soluble lubricant
- ❏ Sterile basin
- ❏ Sterile normal saline solution or water, about 100 mL
- ❏ Pulse oximeter and stethoscope

TABLE 25-2 | Equipment Guidelines* for Intubation and Suctioning

Equipment	Infant (Premature Infant to 1 Year)	Small Child (2-5 Years)	School-Age Child (6-12 Years)	Adolescent to Adult
Airway size:				
Oral	00-2	2-3	3-4	4-5
Nasal (French)	5-8	10-20	20-25	25-36
Handheld resuscitator size	Child	Child	Child/adult	Adult
Mask size	Premature infant/child	Child	Small adult	Adult
Laryngoscope blade size	0-1 (straight)	2 (straight)	2-3 (straight or curved)	4-5 (straight or curved)
Endotracheal tube size (mm)	2.5-4.0	4.0-5.0	5.0-6.5	7.0-9.0
Tracheostomy tube: Jackson size	000-1	1-2	3-4	4-10
Inner diameter (mm)	2.5-3.5	3.5-4.0	4.5-5.0	5.0-9.0
Suction catheter size (French)[†]	5-6	6-8	8-10	10-16

Data from St. John RE: Airway management, *Crit Care Nurse* 19(4):79, 1999.
*These guidelines should be used as an estimate only: actual sizes depend on the size and individual needs of the patient.
[†]Catheter outer diameter should not exceed half the internal diameter of the tube.

STEP	RATIONALE

ASSESSMENT

1 Assess signs and symptoms of upper and lower airway obstruction requiring nasal, tracheal, or nasopharyngeal suctioning, including wheezes, crackles, or gurgling on inspiration or expiration; restlessness; ineffective coughing; unilateral, segmental, or lobar absent or diminished breath sounds (absent in patients with pneumonectomy or lobectomy); tachypnea; hypertension or hypotension; cyanosis; decreased level of consciousness, especially acute; or excess nasal secretions, drooling, or gastric secretions or vomitus in mouth (Considine, 2005).

Physical signs and symptoms result from decreased oxygen to tissues, as well as pooling of secretions in upper and lower airways. Assessment is necessary before and following the suction procedure (AARC, 2004; Demir and Dramali, 2005).

2 Determine the presence of apprehension, anxiety, decreased ability to concentrate, lethargy, decreased level of consciousness (especially acute), increased fatigue, dizziness, behavioral changes (especially irritability), decreased oxygen saturation (using pulse oximetry), increased pulse rate, increased rate of breathing, decreased depth of breathing, elevated blood pressure, cardiac dysrhythmias, pallor, cyanosis, dyspnea, or use of accessory muscles.

Signs and symptoms indicate hypoxia (low oxygen at the cellular or tissue level), hypoxemia (low oxygen tension in the blood), or hypercapnia (elevated carbon dioxide tension in the blood). Anxiety and pain consume oxygen and in turn worsen the signs of hypoxia (Considine, 2005). Patients with conditions such as acute respiratory distress syndrome, pulmonary edema, and congestive heart failure are at particular risk.

3 Assess for risk factors for upper or lower airway obstruction, including obstructive lung disease; pulmonary infections; impaired mobility; sedation; decreased level of consciousness; seizures; presence of feeding tube; decreased gag or cough reflex; and decreased swallowing ability.

Presence of these risk factors sometimes impairs the patient's ability to clear secretions from the airway, increases risk for retaining secretions, and necessitates nasopharyngeal or nasotracheal suctioning

4 Assess for additional factors that anatomically influence upper or lower airway function: recent surgery; head, chest, or neck tumors, facial or nasal trauma; and neuromuscular diseases.

Abnormal anatomy impairs normal drainage of secretions. For example, nasal swelling, deviated septum, or facial fractures impair nasal drainage. Tumors in or around the lower airway impair secretion removal by occluding or externally compressing the lumen of the airway.

5 Assess factors that affect volume and consistency of secretions.
  a Fluid balance

Thickened or copious secretions increase risk for airway obstruction.
Fluid overload increases amount of secretions. Dehydration promotes thicker secretions.

  b Lack of humidity

The environment influences secretion formation and gas exchange, necessitating airway suctioning when the patient cannot clear secretions effectively.

  c Infection (e.g., pneumonia)

Patients with respiratory infections are prone to increased secretions that are thicker and sometimes more difficult to expectorate.

  d Allergies, sinus drainage

Increases volume of secretions in pharynx.

STEP	RATIONALE
6 Identify contraindications to **nasotracheal** suctioning (AARC, 2004): 　a Facial or neck trauma/surgery 　b Bleeding disorders 　c Nasal bleeding 　d Epiglottitis or croup 　e Laryngospasm 　f Irritable airway 　g Gastric surgery with high anastomosis	These conditions are contraindications because the passage of a catheter through the nasal route causes additional trauma, increases nasal bleeding, or causes severe bleeding in the presence of bleeding disorders. In the presence of epiglottitis, croup, laryngospasm, or irritable airway, the entrance of a suction catheter via the nasal route causes intractable coughing, hypoxemia, and severe bronchospasm; this may necessitate emergency intubation or tracheostomy.
7 Examine sputum microbiology data.	Certain bacteria are easier to transmit or require isolation because of virulence or antibiotic resistance.
8 Assess patient's understanding of procedure.	Reveals need for patient instruction and encourages cooperation.

NURSING DIAGNOSES

- Deficient knowledge regarding airway clearance techniques and devices
- Fatigue
- Impaired gas exchange

- Impaired spontaneous ventilation
- Impaired swallowing
- Ineffective airway clearance
- Ineffective breathing pattern

- Risk for aspiration
- Risk for infection

Individualize related factors based on patient's condition or needs.

PLANNING

1 Expected outcomes following completion of procedure: 　• Lower and upper airways demonstrate absent or diminished adventitious sounds and gurgles, crackles, wheezes, and gurgles on inspiration and expiration; return of absent or diminished breath sounds.	Airways are cleared of secretions.
• Normalization of heart rate, blood pressure, respiratory rate and effort, and pulse oximetry readings.	When airway secretions are removed and oxygenation improves, the patient's vital signs, pulse oximetry readings, and respiratory assessment findings improve (Considine, 2005; Lindgren and Ames, 2005).
• Absence of drooling, gastric secretions, or vomitus in mouth, and nasal secretions.	Secretions retained in oral cavity increase patient's risk for pneumonia.
• Patient verbalizes easier breathing, if able.	Patent airway reduces work of breathing.
2 Explain to patient how procedure will help clear airway and relieve breathing problems. Explain that temporary coughing, sneezing, gagging, or shortness of breath is normal during the procedure. Encourage patient to cough out secretions. Practice coughing, if able. Splint surgical incisions, if necessary.	Encourages cooperation and minimizes risks, anxiety, and pain of procedure.
3 Explain importance of and encourage coughing during procedure.	Facilitates secretion removal and reduces frequency and duration of future suctioning.
4 Assist patient with assuming position comfortable for nurse and patient (usually semi-Fowler's or sitting upright with head hyperextended, unless contraindicated).	Reduces stimulation of gag reflex, promotes patient comfort and secretion drainage, and prevents aspiration and nurse strain. Hyperextension facilitates insertion of catheter into trachea.
5 Place pulse oximeter on patient's finger. Take reading and leave oximeter in place. Place towel across patient's chest, if needed.	Provides baseline SpO_2 value to determine patient's response to suctioning. Reduces transmission of microorganisms by protecting gown from secretions.

IMPLEMENTATION

1 Perform hand hygiene, and apply mask, goggles, or face shield if splashing is likely.	Reduces transmission of microorganisms.
2 Connect one end of connecting tubing to suction machine, and place other end in convenient location near patient. Turn suction device on, and set vacuum regulator to appropriate negative pressure (see Table 25-1).	Excessive negative pressure damages nasal pharyngeal and tracheal mucosa and induces greater hypoxia.
3 If indicated, increase supplemental oxygen therapy to 100% or as ordered by physician. Encourage patient to deep breathe.	Hyperoxygenation provides some protection from suction-induced decline in oxygenation. Hyperoxygenation is most effective in the presence of hyperinflation, such as encouraging the patient to deep breathe or increasing ventilator tidal volume settings (Demir and Dramali, 2005).

STEP	RATIONALE

4   Prepare suction catheter.

   a   One-time-use catheter

      (1)   Using aseptic technique, open suction kit or catheter. If sterile drape is available, place it across patient's chest or on the over-bed table. Do not allow the suction catheter to touch any nonsterile surfaces.

Prepares catheter, maintains asepsis and reduces transmission of microorganisms. Provides sterile surface on which to lay catheter between passes.

      (2)   Unwrap or open sterile basin, and place on bedside table. Be careful not to touch inside of basin. Fill with about 100 mL sterile normal saline solution or water (see illustration).

Saline or water is used to clean tubing after each suction pass.

      (3)   Open lubricant. Squeeze small amount onto open sterile catheter package without touching package. NOTE: Lubricant is not necessary for artificial airway suctioning.

Prepares lubricant while maintaining sterility. Using water-soluble lubricant helps avoid lipoid aspiration pneumonia. Excessive lubricant occludes catheter.

   b   Closed (in-line) suction catheter: see Procedural Guideline 25-1, p. 682.

5   Apply sterile glove to each hand, or apply nonsterile glove to nondominant hand and sterile glove to dominant hand.

Reduces transmission of microorganisms and maintains sterility of suction catheter.

6   Pick up suction catheter with dominant hand without touching nonsterile surfaces. Pick up connecting tubing with nondominant hand. Secure catheter to tubing (see illustration).

Maintains catheter sterility. Connects catheter to suction.

7   Check that equipment is functioning properly by suctioning small amount of normal saline solution from basin.

Ensures equipment function. Lubricates internal catheter and tubing.

8   Suction airway:

   a   Nasopharyngeal and nasotracheal suctioning:

      (1)   Lightly coat distal 6 to 8 cm (2 to 3 inches) of catheter with water-soluble lubricant.

Lubricates catheter for easier insertion.

      (2)   Remove oxygen delivery device, if applicable, with nondominant hand. Without applying suction and using dominant thumb and forefinger, gently but quickly insert catheter into nares. Then instruct patient to deep breathe and insert the catheter following natural course of the nares. Slightly slant the catheter downward or through mouth. Do not force through nares (see illustration).

Application of suction pressure while introducing catheter into trachea increases risk for damage to mucosa and increases risk for hypoxia because of removal of entrained oxygen present in airways. Passing catheter during inhalation improves likelihood of entering trachea.

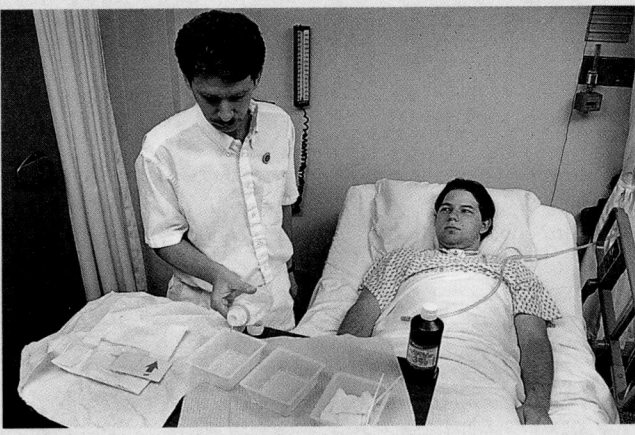

STEP 4a(2)   Pouring sterile saline into tray.

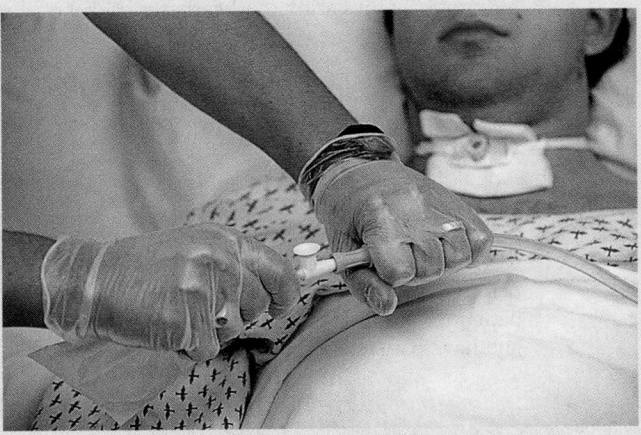

STEP 6   Attaching catheter to suction.

STEP	RATIONALE

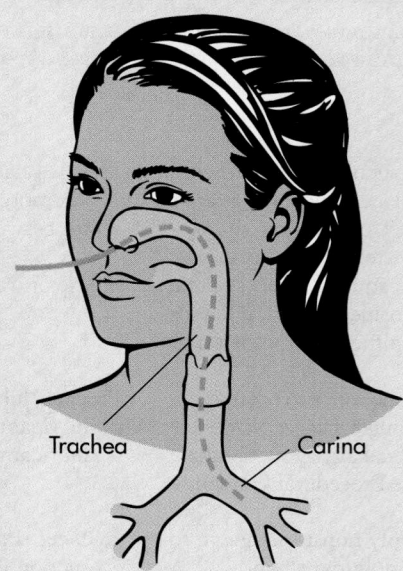

Trachea   Carina

STEP 8a(2) Pathway for nasotracheal catheter progression.

(a) Nasopharyngeal suctioning (without applying suction): In adults, insert catheter about 16 cm (6 inches); in older children, 8 to 12 cm (3 to 5 inches); in infants and young children, 4 to 8 cm (2 to 3 inches). Rule of thumb is to insert catheter distance from tip of nose (or mouth) to angle of mandible.

Ensures that catheter tip reaches pharynx for suctioning.

(b) Nasotracheal suctioning (without applying suction): In adults, insert catheter about 20 cm; in older children about 16 to 20 cm (6 to 8 inches); and in young children and infants, 8 to 14 cm (3 to 5½ inches).

Ensures that catheter tip reaches trachea.

Critical Decision Point   *When there is difficulty passing the catheter, ask patient to cough or say "ahh," or try to advance the catheter during inspiration. Both measures assist in opening the glottis to permit passage of the catheter into the trachea.*

(3) Positioning: In some instances turning patient's head to right helps you suction left mainstem bronchus; turning head to left helps you suction right mainstem bronchus. If you feel resistance after insertion of catheter for maximum recommended distance, catheter has probably hit carina. Pull catheter back 1 to 2 cm before applying suction.

Turning the patient's head to the side elevates the bronchial passage on the opposite side.

Critical Decision Point   *Use the nasal approach, and perform tracheal suctioning before pharyngeal suctioning whenever possible. The mouth and pharynx contain more bacteria than the trachea does. If copious oral secretions are present before beginning the procedure, suction mouth with oral suction device first.*

(4) Apply intermittent suction for 10 to 15 seconds (AARC, 2004; Pruitt, 2005) by placing and releasing nondominant thumb over vent of catheter and slowly withdrawing catheter while rotating it back and forth between dominant thumb and forefinger. Encourage patient to cough. Replace oxygen device, if applicable, and have patient deep breathe.

Intermittent suction and rotation of catheter prevents injury to mucosa. If catheter "grabs" mucosa, remove thumb to release suction. Suctioning longer than 15 seconds causes cardiopulmonary compromise, usually from hypoxemia or vagal overload.

Critical Decision Point   *Monitor patient's vital signs and oxygen saturation using pulse oximetry throughout suction procedure. If the patient's pulse drops more than 20 beats per minute or increases more than 40 beats per minute, or if pulse oximetry falls below 90% or 5% from baseline, cease suctioning (Lindgren and Ames, 2005).*

STEP	RATIONALE

(5) Rinse catheter and connecting tubing with normal saline or water until cleared.

Secretions that remain in suction catheter or connecting tubing decrease suctioning efficiency.

(6) Assess for need to repeat suctioning procedure. Do not perform more than two passes with the catheter. Observe for alterations in cardiopulmonary status. When possible, allow adequate time (at least 1 minute) between suction passes for ventilation and oxygenation (AARC, 2004). Encourage patient to deep breathe and cough.

Suctioning can induce hypoxemia, dysrhythmias, laryngospasm, and bronchospasm. Deep breathing ventilates and reoxygenates alveoli. Repeated passes clear the airway of excessive secretions but can also remove oxygen and may induce laryngospasm.

b Artificial airway suctioning:

(1) Hyperinflate and/or hyperoxygenate patient before suctioning, using manual resuscitation bag-valve device connected to oxygen source or sigh mechanism on mechanical ventilator. Some mechanical ventilators have a button that when pushed delivers 100% oxygen for a few minutes and then resets to the previous value.

Hyperinflation decreases the risk for atelectasis caused by negative pressure of suctioning (Demir and Dramali, 2005). Preoxygenation converts large proportion of resident lung gas to 100% oxygen to offset amount used in metabolic consumption while ventilation or oxygenation is interurupted, as well as to offset volume lost during suctioning (Bourgault and others, 2006).

Critical Decision Point   *Suctioning can cause elevations in intracranial pressure (ICP) in patients with head injuries. Reduce this risk by presuction hyperventilation, which results in hypocarbia, which in turn induces vasoconstriction. Vasoconstriction reduces the potential for an increase in ICP. Limit suctioning to two times with each suctioning procedure (Considine, 2005; Demir and Dramali, 2005).*

---

(2) If patient is receiving mechanical ventilation, open swivel adapter, or if necessary remove oxygen or humidity delivery device with nondominant hand.

Exposes artificial airway.

(3) Without applying suction, gently but quickly insert catheter using dominant thumb and forefinger into artificial airway (it is best to try to time catheter insertion into the artificial airway with inspiration) until you meet resistance or patient coughs, then pull back 1 cm (½ inch).

Application of suction pressure while introducing catheter into trachea increases risk for damage to tracheal mucosa, as well as increased hypoxia related to removal of entrained oxygen present in airways. Pulling back stimulates cough and removes catheter from mucosal wall so that catheter is not resting against tracheal mucosa during suctioning.

Critical Decision Point   *If unable to insert catheter past the end of the ET tube, the catheter is probably caught in the Murphy eye (i.e., side hole at the distal end of the ET tube that allows for collateral airflow in the event of tracheal mainstem intubation) (Lindgren and Ames, 2005). If this happens, rotate the catheter to reposition it away from the Murphy eye, or withdraw it slightly and reinsert with the next inhalation. Usually the catheter meets resistance at the carina. One indication that the catheter is at the carina is acute onset of coughing, because the carina contains many cough receptors. Pull the catheter back 1 cm (½ inch).*

---

(4) Apply intermittent suction by placing and releasing nondominant thumb over vent of catheter; slowly withdraw catheter while rotating it back and forth between dominant thumb and forefinger (see illustration). Encourage patient to cough. Watch for respiratory distress.

Intermittent suction and rotation of catheter prevent injury to tracheal mucosal lining. If catheter "grabs" mucosa, remove thumb to release suction.

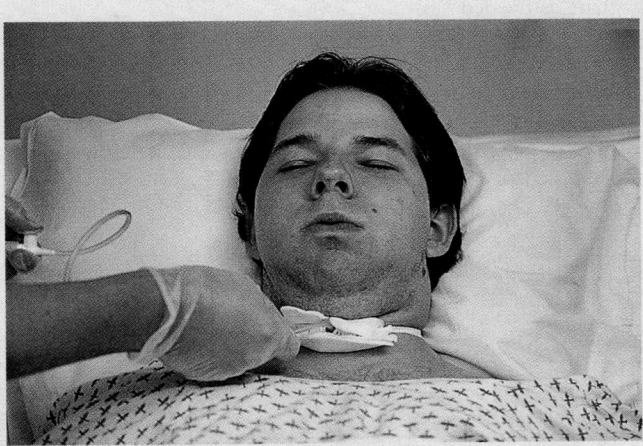

STEP 8b(4) Suctioning tracheostomy.

STEP	RATIONALE

Critical Decision Point *If patient develops respiratory distress during the suction procedure, immediately withdraw catheter and supply additional oxygen and breaths as needed. In an emergency administer oxygen directly through the catheter. Disconnect suction, and attach oxygen at prescribed flow rate through the catheter.*

STEP	RATIONALE
(5) If patient is receiving mechanical ventilation, close swivel adapter, or replace oxygen delivery device.	Reestablishes artificial airway.
(6) Encourage patient to deep breathe, if able. Some patients respond well to several manual breaths from the mechanical ventilator or bag-valve device.	Reoxygenates and reexpands alveoli. Suctioning causes hypoxemia and atelectasis.
(7) Rinse catheter and connecting tubing with normal saline until clear. Use continuous suction.	Removes catheter secretions. Secretions left in tubing decrease suctioning efficiency and provide environment for microorganism growth.
(8) Assess patient's cardiopulmonary status for secretion clearance. Repeat Steps (1) through (7) once or twice more to clear secretions. Allow adequate time (at least 1 full minute) between suction passes.	Suctioning can induce dysrhythmias, hypoxia, and bronchospasm and impair cerebral circulation or adversely affect hemodynamic stability (Demir and Dramali, 2005; Lindgren and Ames, 2005).
(9) When pharynx and trachea are sufficiently cleared of secretions, perform oropharyngeal suctioning to clear mouth of secretions. Do not suction nose again after suctioning mouth.	Removes upper airway secretions. More microorganisms are generally present in mouth. Upper airway is considered "clean" and lower airway is considered "sterile." Therefore you can use the same catheter to suction from sterile to clean areas (e.g., tracheal suctioning to oropharyngeal suctioning) but not from clean to sterile areas.
9 When you have completed suctioning, disconnect catheter from connecting tubing. Roll catheter around fingers of dominant hand. Pull glove off inside out so that catheter remains coiled in glove. Pull off other glove over first glove in same way to seal in contaminants. Discard in appropriate receptacle. Turn off suction device.	Reduces transmission of microorganisms.
10 Remove towel, place in laundry or appropriate receptacle, and reposition patient. (Apply clean gloves to continue personal care.)	Reduces transmission of microorganisms. Promotes comfort.
11 If indicated, readjust oxygen to original level because patient's blood oxygen level should have returned to baseline.	Prevents absorption atelectasis and oxygen toxicity while allowing patient time to reoxygenate blood.
12 Discard remainder of normal saline into appropriate receptacle. If basin is disposable, discard into appropriate receptacle. If basin is reusable, rinse it out, and place it in soiled utility room.	Reduces transmission of microorganisms.
13 Remove face shield, and discard into appropriate receptacle. Perform hand hygiene.	Reduces transmission of microorganisms.
14 Place unopened suction kit on suction machine table or at head of bed.	Provides immediate access to suction catheter for next procedure.
15 Assist patient to a comfortable position, and provide oral hygiene as needed.	

EVALUATION

1 Compare patient's respiratory assessments and SpO$_2$ values before and after suctioning.	Identifies physiological effects of suction procedure to restore airway patency.
2 Ask patient if breathing is easier and if congestion is decreased.	Provides subjective confirmation that suctioning procedure has relieved airway.
3 Observe character of airway secretions.	Provides data to document presence or absence of respiratory tract infection or thickened secretions.

STEP	RATIONALE

Unexpected Outcomes

Related Interventions

1 Worsening respiratory status.

- Limit length of suctioning.
- Determine need for more frequent suctioning, possibly of shorter duration.
- Determine need for supplemental oxygen. Supply oxygen between suctioning passes.
- Notify physician.

2 Return of bloody secretions.

- Determine amount of suction pressure used. May need to be decreased.
- Ensure suction completed correctly using intermittent suction and catheter rotation.
- Evaluate suctioning frequency.
- Provide more frequent oral hygiene.

3 Unable to pass suction catheter through nares at first attempt.

- Try other nares or oral route.
- Increase lubrication of catheter.
- Insert nasal airway, especially if suctioning through patient nares frequently.
- If obstruction is mucus, apply suction to relieve obstruction, but do not apply suction to mucosa. If you think obstruction is a blood clot, consult with physician.

4 Paroxysms of coughing.

- Administer supplemental oxygen.
- Allow patient to rest between passes of suction catheter.
- Consult with physician regarding need for inhaled bronchodilators or topical anesthetics.

5 No secretions obtained.

- Evaluate patient's fluid status.
- Assess for signs of infection.
- Determine need for chest physiotherapy (see Chapter 24).
- Assess adequacy of humidification on oxygen delivery device.

Recording and Reporting

- Record the amount, consistency, color, and odor of secretions, route of suctioning, and patient's response to suctioning. Document patient's presuctioning and postsuctioning cardiopulmonary status.

Teaching Considerations

- Instruct patient that coughing increases during the procedure.
- Explain why supplemental oxygen is given before and after suctioning, if indicated.

Pediatric Considerations

- Small-diameter suction catheters required in pediatrics should be half the diameter of the child's tracheostomy tube (Hockenberry and Wilson, 2007).
- Because of small diameter of suction catheter, thick secretions are often more difficult to remove.
- Make sure distance suctioned is not greater than 0.5 cm beyond the tip of the artificial airway. To determine distance, place catheter near a sample artificial airway (Hockenberry and Wilson, 2007).
- Infant airways have less cartilage and may collapse easily, especially in premature infants or those with reactive airways.
- Suctioning should not last beyond 5 seconds (Hockenberry and Wilson, 2007).

Gerontological Considerations

- Older adults have lost some properties of elastic recoil and gas exchange.
- Capillaries of older adults are often fragile, predisposing patient to bleeding problems.
- Some older patients have coronary artery disease, which places them at increased risk for cardiopulmonary compromise. In addition, some older adults take antiplatelet and/or anticoagulant medications such as aspirin or warfarin (Coumadin) for the prevention of coronary or cerebral artery occlusion.

Home Care Considerations

- Although most patients with airway clearance problems at home have a tracheostomy, some also require nasal pharyngeal suctioning. Catheters are often used for a 24-hour period and then cleaned and disinfected; or catheters are cleaned with soapy water after each use and discarded after 24 hours.
- In the home, instruct the patient to clean and disinfect or change the secretion collection container every 24 hours according to home care or institutional protocol.
- In the home setting, stress the importance of brief intervals of applying suction pressure. Instruct those performing suctioning to hold their breath during the application of negative suction pressure to help them remember to not suction too long.

PROCEDURAL GUIDELINE 25-1   Closed (In-Line) Suction Catheter

[NSO] *Airway Management Module / Lesson 6*

Delegation Considerations

The skill of airway suction with a closed (in-line) suction catheter cannot be routinely delegated to NAP. In special situations, such as suctioning a permanent tracheostomy, this procedure may be delegated to NAP. The nurse is responsible for cardiopulmonary assessment and evaluation of patient. The nurse directs the NAP about:

- Any individualized aspects of patient care that pertain to suctioning (e.g., position, duration of suction, pressure settings).
- Expected quality, quantity, and color of secretions and to inform the nurse immediately if there are changes.
- Patient's anticipated response to suction and to immediately report to the nurse changes in vital signs, complaints of pain, shortness of breath, confusion, or increased restlessness.

Equipment

- ❏ Closed system or in-line suction catheter
- ❏ Suction machine
- ❏ 6 feet of connecting tubing
- ❏ Two clean gloves *(optional)*
- ❏ Mask, goggles, or face shield
- ❏ Pulse oximeter and stethoscope

Procedural Steps

1 Perform assessment as in Skill 25-2 (p. 673).
2 Explain the procedure to the patient and the importance of coughing during the suctioning procedure.
3 Assist patient with assuming a position of comfort for both patient and nurse, usually semi- or high-Fowler's position. Place towel across the patient's chest.
4 Perform hand hygiene, apply face shield and gloves, and attach suction.
 a In many institutions a respiratory therapist attaches the catheter to the mechanical ventilator circuit. If catheter is not already in place, open suction catheter package using aseptic technique, attach closed suction catheter to ventilator circuit by removing swivel adapter and placing closed suction catheter apparatus on ET or tracheostomy tube, and connect Y on mechanical ventilator circuit to closed suction catheter with flex tubing (see illustrations).
 b Connect one end of connecting tubing to suction machine, and connect other to the end of a closed system or in-line suction catheter, if not already done. Turn suction device on, and set vacuum regulator to appropriate negative pressure. Many closed system suction catheters re-

quire slightly higher suction pressures; consult manufacturer's guidelines (Lindgren and Ames, 2005).
5 Hyperinflate and/or hyperoxygenate patient with bag-valve device or manual breathing mechanism on mechanical ventilator according to institution protocol and clinical status (usually 100% oxygen).
6 Unlock suction control mechanism if required by manufacturer. Open saline port, and attach saline syringe or vial.
7 Pick up suction catheter enclosed in plastic sleeve with dominant hand.

Critical Decision Point   *The use of normal saline instillation with closed in-line suction catheters may not be appropriate for all patients and needs further investigation. Normal saline instillation in conjunction with endotracheal tube suctioning may lead to the dispersion of microorganisms into the lower respiratory tract (Celik and Kanan, 2006).*

8 Insert catheter; use a repeating maneuver of pushing catheter and sliding (or pulling) plastic sleeve back between thumb and forefinger until resistance is felt or patient coughs.
9 Encourage patient to cough, and apply suction by squeezing on suction control mechanism while withdrawing catheter. It is difficult to apply intermittent pulses of suction and nearly impossible to rotate the catheter compared with a standard catheter. Be sure to withdraw catheter completely into plastic sheath so it does not obstruct airflow (AARC, 2004).
10 Reassess cardiopulmonary status, including pulse oximetry, to determine need for subsequent suctioning or complications. Repeat Steps 5 to 9 one more time to clear secretions. Allow adequate time (at least 1 full minute) between suction passes for ventilation and reoxygenation (AARC, 2004).
11 When airway is clear, withdraw catheter completely into sheath. Be sure that colored indicator line on catheter is visible in the sheath. Squeeze vial or push syringe while applying suction to rinse inner lumen of catheter. Use at least 5 to 10 mL of saline to rinse the catheter until it is clear of retained secretions, which can cause bacterial growth and increase the risk for infection (AARC, 2004). Lock suction mechanism, if applicable, and turn off suction.
12 If patient requires oral or nasal suctioning, perform Skill 25-1 or 25-2 with separate standard suction catheter.
13 Reposition patient.
14 Remove gloves and face shield and discard into appropriate receptacle, and perform hand hygiene.
15 Compare patient's respiratory assessments before and after suctioning, and observe airway secretions.

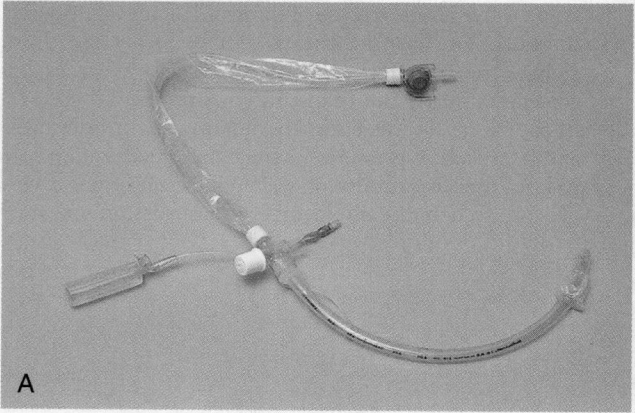
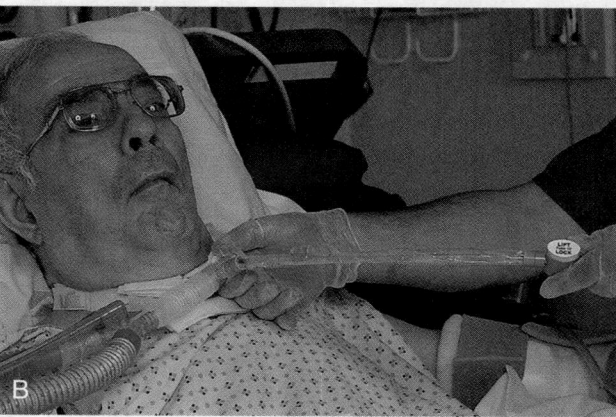

STEP 4a   A, Closed system suction catheter attached to endotracheal tube. **B,** Suctioning tracheostomy with closed system suction catheter.

SKILL 25-3   Endotracheal Tube Care

NSO *Airway Management Module / Lesson 7*

Endotracheal (ET) tubes are used as short-term artificial airways to administer mechanical ventilation, relieve upper airway obstruction, protect against aspiration, and clear secretions. Routine care maintains correct position of the tube and good hygiene (Lindgren and Ames, 2005).

After insertion of an ET tube, the cuff is inflated. Preventing cuff-related problems is a critical component of nursing care and depends on securing the tube and inflating the cuff properly. In many institutions these functions are shared by nursing and respiratory therapy staff. Allowing an ET tube to slip lower into the airway can prevent ventilation of a lung, usually the left lung (and sometimes the right upper lobe also). Allowing an ET tube to slide too far up the tracheobronchial tree can allow air to escape through or damage the vocal cords. Properly securing the ET tube prevents incidental extubation from coughing or pulling on the tube. Additional risks of movement of an artificial airway are tracheal stenosis, tracheomalacia, erosion of the innominate artery, and tracheoesophageal fistula, particularly when the cuff is overinflated. Risks for each of these complications are reduced with proper nursing care (Considine, 2005).

After the tube is inserted and secured and the cuff is inflated (see Skill 25-5), the chief concern of the nurse is to maintain patency of the ET tube. In patients who cannot clear their secretions, patency is achieved primarily through periodic suctioning of the artificial airway.

EVIDENCE-BASED PRACTICE TRENDS

Ventilator-associated pneumonia (VAP) occurs in 10% to 65% of ventilated patients, causes 90% of nosocomial infections in ventilated patients, and causes an increase in hospital length of stay and mortality. VAP is defined as developing after 48 hours following intubation. Best practice guidelines indicate the following interventions are advantageous in preventing VAP:

1 Elevating the head of the bed at 30 to 40 degrees to prevent aspiration.
2 Changing patient position every 30 minutes to decrease risk for atelectasis and pulmonary infections.

3 Providing oral care with a toothbrush every 8 hours to remove dental plaque organisms. Toothettes are not adequate to clean the dental plaque, but they may be used between brushing for comfort.
4 Maintaining the endotracheal cuff pressures at 20 cm H_2O to decrease movement of secretions to the lower airways.
5 Carefully monitoring patient for aspiration when enteral feedings are infusing (Abbott and others, 2006; Grap and Munro, 2004; Tolentino-DelosReyes and others, 2007).

Delegation Considerations

This skill of performing endotracheal tube care cannot be delegated to NAP. NAP may assist the nurse with endotracheal tube care. The nurse directs the NAP to:

- Immediately report any signs of respiratory problems or increased airway secretions.
- Immediately report if the ET tube appears to have moved or become obstructed or dislodged.
- Immediately report changes in patient's mood, level of consciousness, irritability, vital signs, or decreased pulse oximetry value.

Equipment

- ❑ Towel
- ❑ Endotracheal and oropharyngeal suction equipment
- ❑ 1- or 1½-inch-wide adhesive or waterproof tape (do not use paper or silk tape) or commercial ET tube holder and mouthguard (follow manufacturer's instructions for securing)
- ❑ Clean gloves (two pairs)
- ❑ Adhesive remover swab or acetone on cotton ball
- ❑ Nonalcohol mouthwash or toothpaste
- ❑ Toothbrush, toothette, and shaving supplies
- ❑ One wet and one soapy washcloth or paper towels
- ❑ Clean 2 × 2 inch gauze
- ❑ Tincture of benzoin, liquid adhesive, or skin prep pads
- ❑ Tongue blade (*optional*)
- ❑ Mask, goggles, face shield, if indicated
- ❑ Stethoscope

STEP	RATIONALE

ASSESSMENT

1 Auscultate lungs and observe respiratory rate and depth.

2 Observe for soiled or loose tape; pressure sore on nares, lips, or corner of mouth; excess nasal or oral secretions; patient moving tube with tongue, biting tube or tongue; tube repositioned by physician or other specially trained personnel; foul-smelling mouth.

3 Observe for factors that increase risk for complications from ET tube: type and size of tube, movement of tube up and down trachea (in and out), duration of tube placement, cuff overinflation or underinflation, presence of facial trauma, malnutrition, and neck or thoracic radiation.

Provides baseline measure of ventilation.

Presence of ET tube impairs ability of patient to swallow oral secretions. Patient is at increased risk for development of pressure areas from impaired circulation as tube is pulled or pressed against nasal or oral mucosa.

Nasal tube cannot be rotated from side to side like oral tube. Pressure sores are more likely. Tube moving up and down trachea predisposes patient to develop tracheoesophageal fistula or tracheomalacia. The tube can become dislodged from the lower airway (incidental extubation), or it can enter mainstem bronchus. Cuff underinflation increases risk for aspiration, whereas cuff overinflation may cause ischemia or necrosis of tracheal tissue from obstruction of capillary bed. Patient can "tongue" oral tube easily and dislodge it. Longer duration of intubation is associated with increased risk for lower airway complications, as in facial trauma. Tissue is more prone to breakdown in presence of malnutrition and radiation.

STEP	RATIONALE
4 Determine proper ET tube depth as noted by centimeters at lip or gum line. This line is marked on the tube and recorded in the patient's record at time of intubation.	Ensures that tube is a proper depth to adequately ventilate both lungs and that the tube is not too high, which causes vocal cord damage, or too low, which results in right mainstem intubation, in which only the right lung is ventilated.
5 Assess patient's knowledge of procedure.	Encourages cooperation, minimizes risks and anxiety. Identifies teaching needs.

NURSING DIAGNOSES

- Deficient knowledge regarding airway clearance techniques and devices
- Fatigue
- Impaired gas exchange

- Impaired skin integrity
- Impaired spontaneous ventilation
- Impaired swallowing
- Ineffective airway clearance

- Ineffective breathing pattern
- Risk for aspiration
- Risk for infection

Individualize related factors based on patient's condition or needs.

PLANNING

1 Expected outcomes following completion of procedure:	
• ET tube remains in correct position in patient's trachea.	Complications of lower airway and vocal cord trauma prevented.
• Patient's skin around mouth and oral mucous membranes does not have pressure areas or other injury from biting: tube is repositioned on opposite side of mouth or center of mouth at least every 24 to 48 hours according to institution protocol (oral ET tube only). Oral airway, if used, is cleaned and reinserted to prevent biting of tongue or inner cheeks.	ET tube does not place undue pressure against corners of mouth, causing pressure area. Patient is not able to bite inner cheeks or tongue.
• ET tube is resecured at proper depth as evidenced by the following: clean tape is firmly secured to cheeks, upper lip, or top of nose and tube only; depth of tube is same as when started or as ordered (same centimeter marking at gums or lips); bilateral breath sounds are equal.	ET tube care prevents movement of tube out of airway or into mainstem bronchus. Position of the tube should be at the level of the gums or lips. This is generally at 23 cm for men and 21 cm for women (Vollman, 2006).
2 Obtain assistance from available staff in this procedure.	Reduces risk for incidental extubation of ET tube.
3 Explain procedure and patient's participation, including importance of the following: not biting or moving ET tube with tongue; trying not to cough when tape is off ET tube; keeping hands down and not pulling on tubing; removal of tape from face can be uncomfortable.	Reduces anxiety, encourages cooperation, and reduces risks.
4 Assist patient with assuming position comfortable for both nurse and patient (usually supine or semi-Fowler's).	Promotes patient comfort; prevents nurse muscle strain.
5 Place towel across chest.	Reduces transmission of organisms and protects patient's gown and bed linen from contamination.

IMPLEMENTATION

1 Perform hand hygiene. Apply mask, goggles, or face shield if indicated.	Reduces transmission of microorganisms.
2 Administer endotracheal, nasopharyngeal, or oropharyngeal suction (see Skills 25-1 and 25-2).	Removes secretions. Diminishes patient's need to cough during procedure.
3 Connect oral suction catheter to suction source.	Prepares patient for oropharyngeal suctioning.
4 Prepare method to secure ET tube.	
a *Tape method:* Cut a piece of tape long enough to go completely around patient's head from naris to naris plus 6 inches: adult, 30 to 60 cm (1 to 2 feet). Lay tape adhesive-side up on bedside table. Cut and lay 8 to 15 cm (3 to 6 inches) of second piece of tape, adhesive sides together, in center of the long strip to prevent tape from sticking to hair. Smaller strip of tape should cover area between ears around back of head.	Preparing tape ahead allows you to have one hand positioned on ET tube throughout procedure. Adhesive tape needs to encircle head below ears with sufficient tape left to wrap around tube.

STEP	RATIONALE
b *Commercially available ET tube holder:* Open package per manufacturer's instructions. Set device aside with the head guard in place and the Velcro strips open.	Commercial devices are latex free, fast, and convenient. These devices avoid the need for tape and the resultant skin breakdown and are easily applied in the presence of facial hair.
5 Apply clean gloves. Instruct helper to apply pair of gloves and hold ET tube firmly at patient's lips or nares. Note the number marking on the ET tube at the gumline or lips.	Reduces transmission of microorganisms. Maintains proper tube position and prevents incidental extubation.

Critical Decision Point *Do not allow helper to hold the tube away from the lips or nares. Doing so allows too much "play" in the tube and increases the risk for tube movement and accidental extubation. Never let go of the ET tube because the tube could become dislodged.*

STEP	RATIONALE
6 Remove old tape or device.	Provides nurse with access to skin under tape for assessment and hygiene. Reduces transmission of microorganisms.
a *Tape:* Carefully remove tape from ET tube and patient's face. If tape is difficult to remove, moisten with (soapy) wet washcloth, water, or adhesive tape remover. Discard tape in appropriate receptacle if nearby.	
b *Commercially available device:* Remove Velcro strips from ET tube, and remove ET tube holder from patient.	The Velcro adhesive strips hold the ET tube in place and provide a marker to measure distance to patient's lips or gums. These devices all permit access to patient's mouth and lips for ease in oropharyngeal suctioning and oral hygiene.
7 Remove any secretions or adhesive from patient's face.	Promotes hygiene. Adhesive causes damage to skin. Prevents poor adhesion of new tape.
a Use adhesive remover swab to remove excess adhesive left on face after tape removal. Wash adhesive remover from face.	
8 Remove oral airway or bite block, if present, and place on towel.	Provides access to and complete observation of patient's oral cavity.

Critical Decision Point *Do not remove oral airway if patient is actively biting ET tube. Wait until tape is partially or completely secured to ET tube.*

STEP	RATIONALE
9 Clean mouth, gums, and teeth opposite ET tube with non–alcohol-based mouthwash solution and toothpaste on toothbrush or toothette. Brush teeth thoroughly. Administer oropharyngeal suctioning with Yankauer suction catheter during brushing and rinsing.	Promotes hygiene and reduces risk for infection to teeth and gums. Alcohol-based mouthwashes dry oral mucosa (Lewis and others, 2007). Suctioning removes pooled sescretions.
10 *Oral ET tube only:* Remembering "cm" ET tube marking at the level of the gums or lips, with help of assistant move ET tube to opposite side or center of mouth. Do not change tube depth (Vollman, 2006).	Prevents formation of pressure sores at sides of patient's mouth. Ensures correct position of tube. Measuring the tube at the lip line can be distorted due to edema, trauma, or disease process (Vollman, 2006).
11 Repeat oral cleaning as in Step 9 on opposite side of mouth.	Removes secretions from mouth and oral pharynx.
12 Clean face and neck with soapy washcloth, rinse, and dry. Shave male patient as necessary (see Chapter 17).	Moisture and beard growth prevent adhesive tape adherence.
13 Pour small amount of skin protectant or liquid adhesive on clean 2 × 2 inch gauze, and dot on upper lip (oral ET tube) or across nose (nasal ET tube) and cheeks to ear. Allow to dry completely.	Protects skin from tape burns and makes more adherent.

STEP	RATIONALE

14 Secure ET tube.
  a Tape method:
  (1) Slip tape under patient's head and neck, adhesive side up. Take care not to twist tape or catch hair. Do not allow tape to stick to itself. It helps to gently stick tape to tongue blade, which serves as a guide. Then slide tongue blade under patient's neck. Center tape so that double-faced tape extends around back of neck from ear to ear.

Positions tape to secure ET tube in proper position.

  (2) On one side of face, secure tape from ear to nares (nasal ET tube) or over lip to ET tube (oral ET tube). Tear remaining tape in half lengthwise, forming two pieces that are ½ to ¾ inch wide. Secure bottom half of tape across upper lip (oral ET tube) or across top of nose (nasal ET tube) to opposite ear (see illustration A). Wrap top half of tape around tube and up from bottom (see illustration B). Tape should encircle tube at least two times for security.

Secures tape to face. Using top tape to wrap prevents downward drag on ET tube.

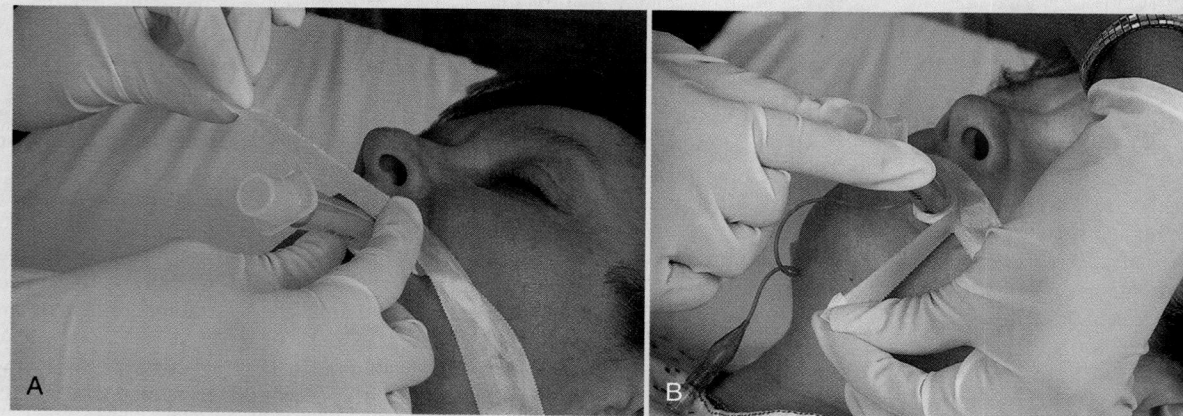

STEP 14a(2)   **A,** Securing bottom half of tape across patient's upper lip. **B,** Securing top half of tape around tube.

STEP	**RATIONALE**
(3) Gently pull other side of tape firmly to pick up slack, and secure to opposite side of face and ET tube the same as the first piece (see illustration). NOTE: ET tube is secured. Assistant can release hold. (You may want assistant to help reinsert oral airway.)	Secures tape to face and tube. ET tube should be at same depth at the lips or gum line. Check earlier assessment for verification of tube depth in centimeters.
b Commercially available device:	
(1) Thread ET tube through the opening designed to secure the ET tube. Be sure that the pilot balloon is accessible.	Commercially available holders have a slit in the front of the holder designed to secure the ET tube.
(2) Place strips of ET holder under the patient at the occipital region of the head.	
(3) Verify that the ET tube is at the established depth using the lip or gum line marker as a guide.	Ensures that the ET tube remains at the correct depth as determined during assessment.
(4) Attach the Velcro strips at the base of the patient's head. Leave 1 cm (½ inch) slack in the strips (see illustration).	
(5) Verify that tube is secure, it does not move forward from the patient's mouth or backward down into the patient's throat, and there are no pressure areas on the oral mucosa or the occipital region of the head.	The tube must be secure so that the position of the tube remains at the correct depth. The tube can be secured without being tight and causing pressure.
15 Remove and clean oral airway in warm soapy water, and rinse well. A half hydrogen peroxide and half normal saline solution aids in removal of crusted secretions. A mouthwash rinse will freshen patient's mouth. Shake excess water from oral airway. Be sure to rinse hydrogen peroxide mixture from the airway.	Promotes hygiene. Reduces transmission of microorganisms.
16 Reinsert oral airway without pushing tongue into oropharynx, and secure with tape (see Chapter 27).	Prevents patient from biting ET tube and allows access for oropharyngeal suctioning.
17 Discard soiled items in appropriate receptacle. Remove towel, and place in laundry.	Reduces transmission of microorganisms.
18 Reposition patient.	Promotes comfort.
19 Remove gloves and mask, goggles, or face shield, discard in receptacle, and perform hand hygiene. Assistant is also to remove gloves and perform hand hygiene before leaving patient's room. Place clean items (e.g., tincture of benzoin, mouthwash, excess swabs) in place of storage.	Reduces transmission of microorganisms. Ensures contaminated gloves and hands do not touch clean items.

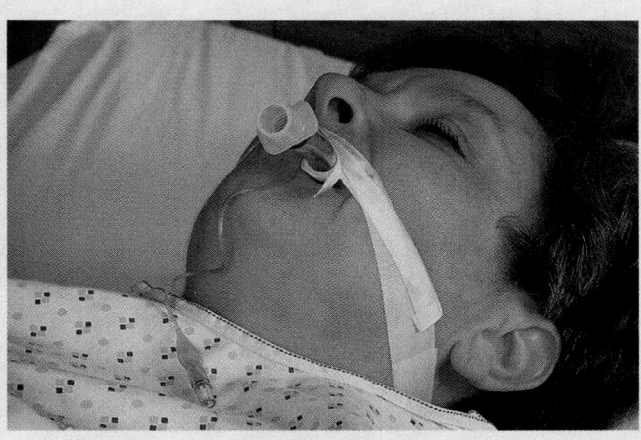

STEP 14a(3) Tape securing endotracheal tube.

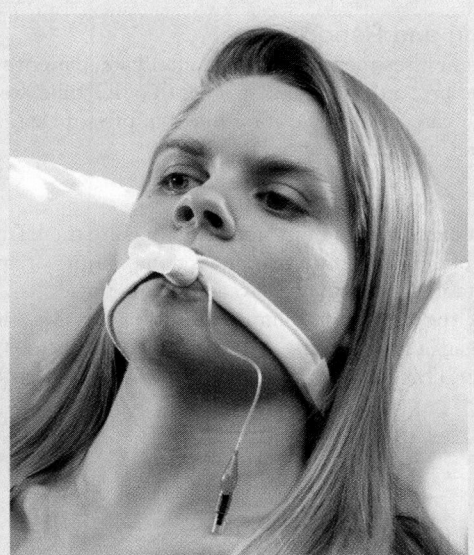

STEP 14b(4) Endotracheal tube holder in place with pilot balloon accessible and Velcro strips secured. (*Courtesy Dale Medical Products, Plainesville, Mass.*)

STEP	RATIONALE

EVALUATION

1 Compare respiratory assessments before and after ET tube care.	Identifies any changes in presence and quality of breath sounds after procedure.
2 Observe depth and position of ET tube according to physician recommendation.	Position of ET tube should not be altered.
3 Assess security of tape by gently tugging at tube.	Tape should remain attached to face. Patient may cough.
4 Assess skin around mouth and oral mucous membranes for intactness and pressure areas.	Tape should not tear skin. Pressure areas should be absent.

Unexpected Outcomes	Related Interventions
1 Unexpected extubation.	• Remain with patient. • Call for assistance. • Assist respirations with bag-valve-mask as needed. • Assess patient for airway patency, spontaneous breathing, and vital signs • Prepare for reintubation.
2 Movement of ET tube.	• Repeat taping or securing procedure. • In very active patients without facial injury who are at risk for self-extubation, consider applying a second piece of tape around the back of the head.
3 Unequal breath sounds.	• Suction patient. • Evaluate ET tube for proper depth before and after ET tube care. If ET tube is deeper or shallower, reposition tube only if allowed by institution and nurse has received appropriate instructions. • Notify physician, who may order chest x-ray film to verify placement, and then reposition ET tube.
4 Pressure areas from tube.	• Increase frequency of ET tube care. • Apply antimicrobial ointment per institutional protocol. • Align oxygen and humidity supply tubing so that they do not pull ET tube, creating pressure areas. • Monitor for infection. If skin tear is present on cheeks or over nose or upper lip, apply protective barrier such as stoma adhesive patch or hydrocolloid dressing, and apply tape to this.
5 Air escaping around tube (see Skill 25-5).	• Verify correct position of tube. If tube position is correct, assess proper cuff inflation. If tube position is incorrect, reposition according to protocol or notify physician (see Skill 25-5).

Recording and Reporting

• Document assessments before and after care, patient's tolerance of procedure, ordered and actual depth of ET tube, frequency of ET tube care, integrity of oral mucosa, pressure sore care, and frequency and extent of ET tube care.

Teaching Considerations

• Instruct patient and family not to manipulate the ET tube, tape, or ET tube holder. If the patient is complaining or appears uncomfortable, instruct family to ask for the nurse.
• Instruct the patient and family to inform the nurse if the tube causes gagging. The nurse will perform interventions to reduce gagging. This may include repositioning of the tube and/or sedation.

Pediatric Considerations

• Neonatal and pediatric procedures for securing ET tubes and suctioning airways vary (Hockenberry and Wilson, 2007).
• Infant skin is more prone to tearing when removing tape (Hockenberry and Wilson, 2007).
• Because of infants' delicate skin, you will not always use skin preparation before securing ET tube. ET tube holders are best used in this population.

Gerontological Considerations

• Older adult skin is more prone to tearing when removing tape.
• Older adults with tendency toward inadequate nutrition are more prone to complications (e.g., infection, breakdown of oral mucosa).

SKILL 25-4 Tracheostomy Care

Intermediate Skills / Respiratory Care and Suctioning / Providing Tracheostomy Care

NSO *Airway Management Module / Lesson 8*

A tracheostomy is placed in patients who require long-term airway management due to airway obstruction, airway clearance needs, and long-term intubation (St. John and Malen, 2004). Some patients with a tracheostomy tube are able to cough secretions out of the tracheostomy tube completely, whereas others are only able to cough secretions up into the tracheostomy tube.

A tracheostomy tube has a flange that fits against the patient's neck, an outer cannula or primary airway, a removable inner cannula for cleansing, and an inflatable cuff that surrounds the outer cannula (Fig. 25-3, A). An inflation tube and valve connect to the cuff for inflation. The pilot balloon expands and contracts on inflation and deflation. An inflated cuff keeps the tube stable within the trachea.

A comprehensive plan includes properly securing the tube, inflating the cuff to an appropriate pressure, maintaining patency by suctioning, and encouraging communication and oral hygiene. A tracheostomy tube can cause development of granulation tissue on the vocal cords, epiglottis, or trachea secondary to inappropriate cuff inflation. (See additional material related to cuff inflation in Skill 25-5.)

The intubated patient is unable to speak because placement of the ET and tracheostomy tube prevents normal airflow over and vibration of the vocal cords. When caring for an intubated patient, use verbal and nonverbal communication skills to communicate. Alphabet charts, pen and paper, slates or chalkboards, or magnetic pen doodle boards are some common communication tools. Place a cap or speaking valve over the tracheostomy tube, which allows the patient to speak (St. John and Malen, 2004; Wilson, 2005).

One type of tracheostomy tube is fenestrated, which means that the outer cannula has precut openings (Fig. 25-3, B). When the inner cannula is removed and the cuff is deflated, patients can speak. A speech pathologist must evaluate patients for aspiration risk before cuff deflation and inner cannula removal (Roman, 2005; St. John and Malen, 2004).

Delegation Considerations

The skill of performing tracheostomy care is not routinely delegated to NAP. In some settings, patients who have well-established tracheostomy tubes may have the care delegated to NAP. The nurse is responsible for assessing the patient and evaluating for proper artificial airway care. The nurse directs the NAP to:

- Immediately report any changes in the patient's respiratory status, level of consciousness, confusion, restlessness or irritability, or change in level of comfort.
- Immediately report any dislodgment or excessive movement of the tracheostomy tube.
- Immediately report abnormal color of tracheal stoma and drainage.

Equipment

- ❑ Bedside table
- ❑ Towel
- ❑ Tracheostomy suction supplies (see Skill 25-2)
- ❑ Sterile tracheostomy care kit, if available (be sure to collect supplies listed that are not available in kit), or two sterile 4 × 4 inch gauze pads
  - Sterile cotton-tipped applicators
  - Sterile tracheostomy dressing (precut and sewn surgical dressing)
  - Sterile basin
  - Normal saline
  - Small sterile brush (or disposable inner cannula)
  - Roll of twill tape, tracheostomy ties, or tracheostomy holder
  - Scissors
- ❑ Clean gloves (two)
- ❑ Mask, goggles, or face shield

Tracheostomy tie strings

Flange

Outer cannula

15-mm adapter

Cuff

Inflation tube

Hollow inner cannula

Pilot balloon

Obturator

A One-way valve   Rounded tip

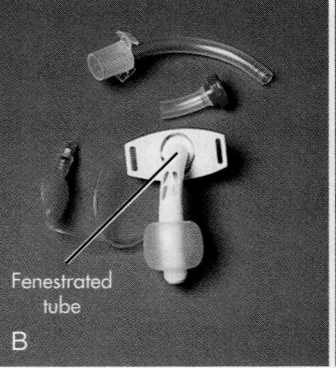

Fenestrated tube

B

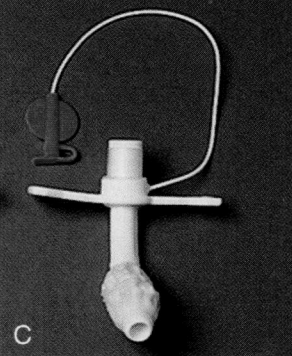

C

FIG 25-3 **A,** Parts of a tracheostomy tube. **B,** Fenestrated tracheostomy tube with cuff, inner cannula, decannulation plug, and pilot balloon. **C,** Tracheostomy tube with foam cuff and obturator. (*From Lewis SL and others,* Medical-surgical nursing: assessment and management of clinical problems, *ed 7, St. Louis, 2007, Mosby.*)

STEP	RATIONALE

ASSESSMENT

1   Observe for signs and symptoms of need to perform tracheostomy care: excess peristomal secretions, excess intratracheal secretions, soiled or damp tracheostomy ties, soiled or damp tracheostomy dressing, diminished airflow through tracheostomy tube, or signs and symptoms of airway obstruction requiring suctioning (see Skill 25-2).

Signs and symptoms are related to presence of secretions at stoma site or within tracheostomy tube. Fig. 25-3 shows a partially inflated cuff on an outer cannula, a syringe used for cuff inflation, and an obturator that is used to insert outer cannula.

2   Assess patient's hydration status, humidity delivered to airway, status of existing infection, patient's nutritional status, and ability to cough.

Determines factors that affect amount and consistency of secretions in the tracheostomy and patient's ability to clear airway.

3   Assess patient's understanding of and ability to perform own tracheostomy care.

Allows nurse to identify potential need for instruction.

4   Check when tracheostomy care was last performed.

Tracheostomy care is provided at least every 8 hours and more often if indicated (e.g., increased airway secretions, infection [airway or stoma], increased secretions around stoma) (Roman, 2005; Wilson, 2005).

NURSING DIAGNOSES

- Deficient knowledge regarding airway clearance techniques and devices
- Impaired gas exchange
- Impaired spontaneous ventilation
- Impaired swallowing
- Ineffective airway clearance
- Ineffective breathing pattern
- Risk for aspiration
- Risk for impaired skin integrity
- Risk for infection

Individualize related factors based on patient's condition or needs.

PLANNING

1   Expected outcomes following completion of procedure:
- Inner cannula and outer cannula of tracheostomy tube are free of secretions; ties are clean, secured snugly, and tied in double square knot.

Tracheostomy tube is patent and secure. Tracheostomy tube that is clear and free of secretions optimizes the amount of oxygen delivered to patient and limits risk for infection from retained secretions.

- Stoma site is pink, does not bleed, and is free of secretions.

Indicates absence of infection at stoma site. Dry, intact tracheostomy stoma reduces risk for subsequent systemic infection.

2   Have another nurse or family member assist in this procedure.

Prevents accidental extubation of tracheostomy tube (Roman, 2005).

3   Explain procedure and patient's participation.

Encourages cooperation, minimizes risks, and reduces anxiety.

4   Assist patient to position comfortable for both nurse and patient (usually supine or semi-Fowler's).

Promotes patient comfort and prevents nurse muscle strain.

5   Place towel across patient's chest.

Reduces transmission of microorganisms.

IMPLEMENTATION

1   Perform hand hygiene, and apply gloves and face shield if applicable.

Reduces transmission of microorganisms.

2   Suction tracheostomy (see Skill 25-2). Before removing gloves, remove soiled tracheostomy dressing, and discard in glove with coiled catheter.

Removes secretions to avoid occluding outer cannula while inner cannula is removed. Reduces need for patient to cough.

3   While patient is replenishing oxygen stores, prepare equipment on bedside table.

Prepares equipment and allows for smooth, organized completion of tracheostomy care.

   a   Open sterile tracheostomy kit. Open two 4 × 4 inch gauze packages using aseptic technique, and pour normal saline on one package. Leave second package dry. Open two cotton-tipped swab packages, and pour normal saline on one package. Do not recap normal saline.

   b   Open sterile tracheostomy dressing package.

   c   Unwrap sterile basin, and pour about 0.5 to 2 cm (½ to 1 inch) of normal saline into it.

   d   Open small sterile brush package, and place aseptically into sterile basin.

STEP	RATIONALE

e Prepare length of twill tape long enough to go around patient's neck two times, about 60 to 75 cm (25 to 30 inches) for an adult. Cut ends on diagonal. Lay aside in dry area.

Cutting ends of tie on diagonal aids in inserting tie through eyelet.

f If using commercially available tracheostomy tube holder, open package according to manufacturer's directions.

4 Apply sterile gloves. Keep dominant hand sterile throughout procedure.

Reduces transmission of microorganisms.

5 Hyperoxygenate the patient, if the patient has oxygen saturation levels below 92% (Demir and Dramali, 2005). Apply oxygen source loosely over tracheostomy if patient desaturates during procedure.

Helps to reduce the amount of desaturation.

Critical Decision Point *For tracheostomy tube with no inner cannula or Kistner button, continue with Step 8.*

6 Care of tracheostomy with inner cannula:

a While touching only the outer aspect of the tube, unlock and remove the inner cannula with nondominant hand. Drop inner cannula into normal saline basin.

Removes inner cannula for cleaning. Normal saline loosens secretions from inner cannula.

b Replace tracheostomy collar, T tube, or ventilator oxygen source over outer cannula (NOTE: Do not attach T tube and ventilator oxygen devices to all outer cannulas when the inner cannula is removed.)

Maintains supply of oxygen to patient as needed.

c To prevent oxygen desaturation in affected patients, quickly pick up inner cannula, and use small brush to remove secretions inside and outside inner cannula (see illustration).

Tracheostomy brush provides mechanical force to remove thick or dried secretions.

d Hold inner cannula over basin, and rinse with normal saline, using nondominant hand to pour normal saline.

Removes secretions and normal saline from inner cannula.

e Replace inner cannula (see illustration), and secure "locking" mechanism. Reapply ventilator after hyperventilating the patient if needed.

Secures inner cannula and reestablishes oxygen supply.

7 Tracheostomy with disposable inner cannula:

a Remove new cannula from manufacturer's packaging.

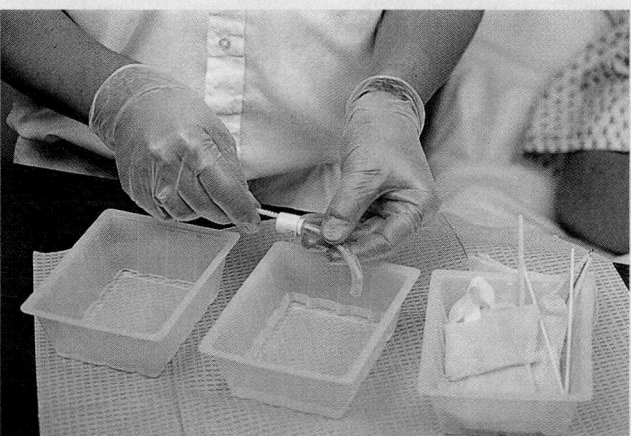

STEP 6c Cleansing the tracheostomy inner cannula.

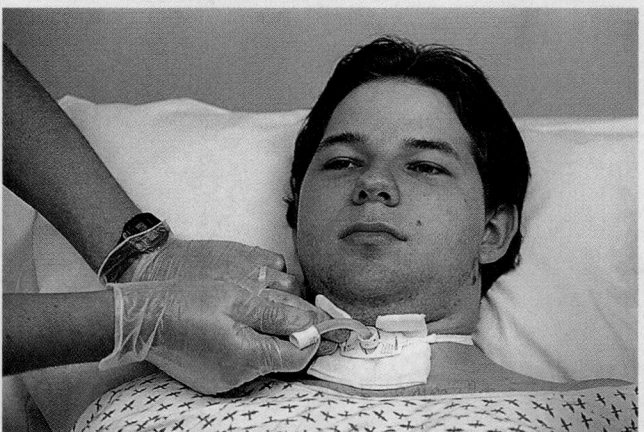

STEP 6e Reinserting the inner cannula.

STEP	RATIONALE

b While touching only the outer aspect of the tube, withdraw inner cannula, and replace with new cannula. Lock into position.

c Dispose of contaminated cannula in appropriate receptacle, and apply ventilator.

8 Using normal saline–saturated cotton-tipped swabs and 4 × 4 inch gauze, clean exposed outer cannula surfaces and stoma under faceplate extending 5 to 10 cm (2 to 4 inches) in all directions from stoma (see illustration). Clean in circular motion from stoma site outward using dominant hand to handle sterile supplies.

Aseptically removes secretions from stoma site. Moving in outward circle pulls mucus and other contaminants from stoma to periphery.

9 Using dry 4 × 4 inch gauze, pat lightly at skin and exposed outer cannula surfaces.

Dry surfaces prohibit formation of moist environment for microorganism growth and skin excoriation.

10 Secure tracheostomy.

a Tracheostomy tie method:

(1) Instruct assistant, if available, to apply gloves and securely hold tracheostomy tube in place. With assistant holding tracheostomy tube, cut old ties.

Promotes hygiene and reduces transmission of microorganisms. Secures tracheostomy tube to prevent incidental extubation.

Critical Decision Point   *Assistant must not release hold on tracheostomy tube until new ties are firmly tied. If working without an assistant, do not cut old ties until new ties are in place and securely tied (Roman, 2005; St. John and Malen, 2004).*

(2) Take prepared tie and insert one end of tie through faceplate eyelet, and pull ends even (see illustration).

(3) Slide both ends of tie behind the head and around neck to other eyelet, and insert one tie through second eyelet.

(4) Pull snugly.

Secures tracheostomy tube.

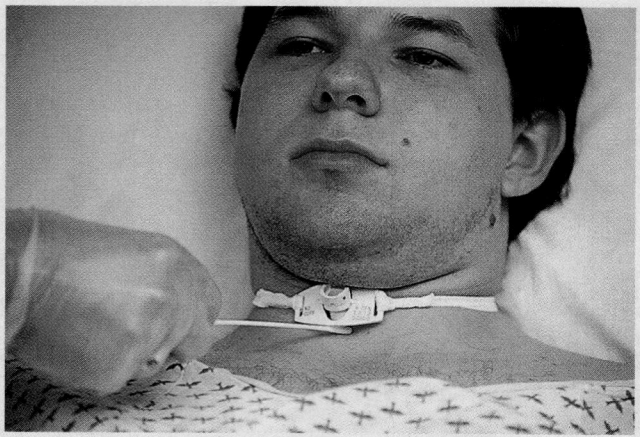

STEP 8   Cleansing around the stoma.

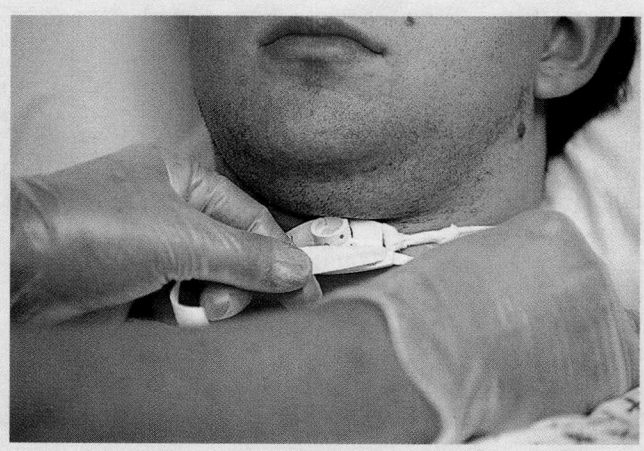

STEP 10a(2)   Replacing tracheostomy ties. Do not remove old tracheostomy ties until new ones are secure.

STEP	RATIONALE
(5) Tie ends securely in double square knot, allowing space for only one loose or two snug finger widths in tie (see illustration).	One finger width of slack prevents ties from being too tight when tracheostomy dressing is in place and also prevents movement of tracheostomy tube into lower airway.
(6) Insert fresh tracheostomy dressing under clean ties and faceplate (see illustration).	Absorbs drainage. Dressing prevents pressure on clavicle heads.
b Tracheostomy tube holder method:	
(1) While wearing gloves, maintain a secure hold on the tracheostomy tube. This can be done with an assistant or, when an assistant is not available, leave the old tracheostomy tube holder in place until the new device is secure.	Prevents incidental dislodgement of tube.
(2) Align strap under patient's neck. Be sure that the Velcro attachments are on either side of the tracheostomy tube.	
(3) Place narrow end of the ties under and through the faceplate eyelets. Pull ends even, and secure with the Velcro closures.	
(4) Verify that there is space for only one loose or two snug finger widths under neck strap (see illustration).	
11 Position patient comfortably, and assess respiratory status.	Promotes comfort. Some patients require post–tracheostomy care suctioning.
12 Replace any oxygen delivery sources.	
13 Remove gloves and face shield, and discard in appropriate receptacle.	Reduces transmission of microorganisms.

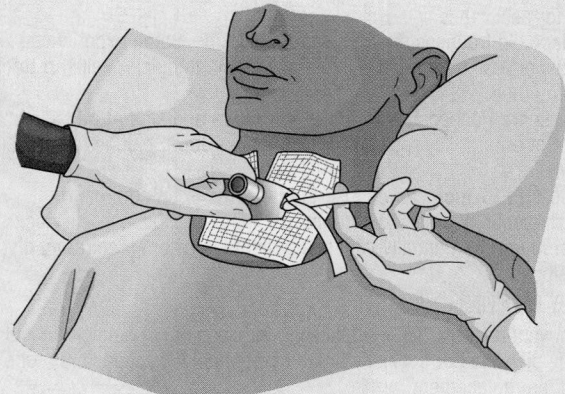

STEP 10a(5)   Tracheostomy ties properly placed. (*From Sorrentino SA:* Mosby's textbook for nursing assistants, *ed 6, St. Louis, 2004, Mosby.*)

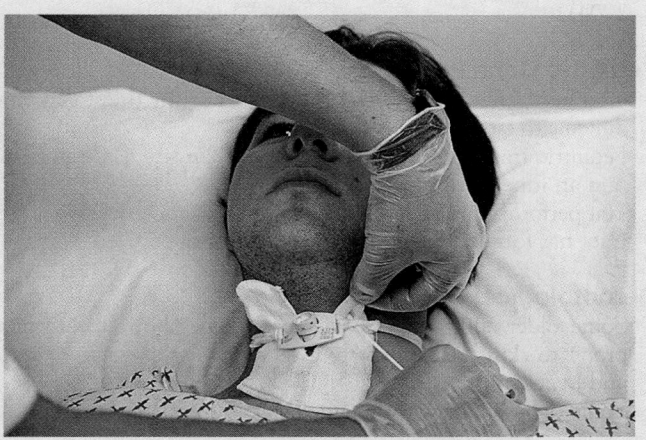

STEP 10a(6)   Applying tracheostomy dressing.

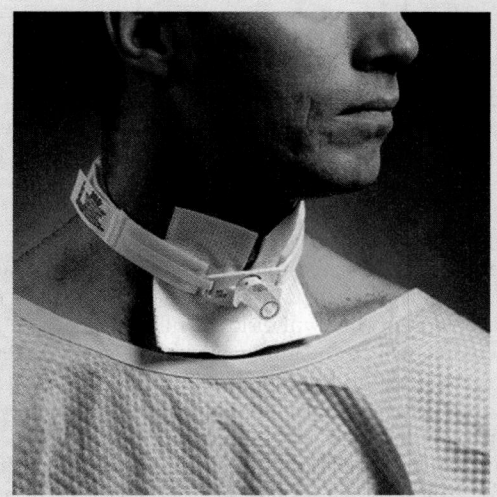

STEP 10b(4)   Tracheostomy tube holder in place. (*Courtesy Dale Medical Products, Plainesville, Mass.*)

STEP	RATIONALE
14 Replace cap on normal saline bottles. Store reusable liquids and unused supplies in appropriate place.	Once opened, normal saline is considered free of bacteria for 24 hours.
15 Perform hand hygiene.	Reduces transmission of microorganisms among patients.

EVALUATION

1 Compare assessments before and after tracheostomy care.	Determines effectiveness of tracheostomy care.
2 Assess fit of new tracheostomy ties and ask patient if tube feels comfortable.	Tracheostomy ties are uncomfortable and place patient at risk for injury when they are too loose or too tight.
3 Inspect inner and outer cannulas for secretions.	Presence of secretions on cannulas indicates the need for more vigorous tracheostomy care.
4 Assess stoma for signs of infection or skin breakdown.	Broken skin places patient at risk for infection. Stoma infection necessitates change in tracheostomy skin care plan.

Unexpected Outcomes	Related Interventions
1 Excessively loose or tight tracheostomy ties/tracheostomy holder.	• Adjust ties, or apply new ties/tracheostomy holder.
2 Inflammation of the tracheostomy stoma.	• Increase frequency of tracheostomy care.
	• Apply topical antibacterial solution, and allow it to dry and provide bacterial barrier.
	• Apply hydrocolloid or transparent dressing just under stoma to protect skin from breakdown. Consult with skin care specialist.
3 Pressure area around tracheostomy tube.	• Increase frequency of tracheostomy care, and keep dressing under faceplate at all times.
	• Consider using double dressing or applying hydrocolloid or stoma adhesive dressing around stoma.
4 Accidental decannulation.	• Call for assistance.
	• Replace old tracheostomy tube with new tube. Some experienced nurses or respiratory therapists may be able to quickly reinsert tracheostomy tube.
	• Keep spare tracheostomy tube of same size and kind at bedside in event of emergency replacement (Roman, 2005; St. John and Malen, 2004).
	• Same-size ET tube can be inserted in stoma in an emergency.
	• Insert suction catheter to confirm that the new tube is in the trachea.
	• Be prepared to manually ventilate patients in whom respiratory distress develops.
	• Notify physician.
5 Respiratory distress from mucus plug in cannula.	• Remove inner cannula, if applicable, for cleaning, or suction cannula.
	• Notify physician or specially trained personnel if tracheostomy tube requires replacement.

Recording and Reporting

• Record respiratory assessments before and after care, the type and size of tracheostomy tube, frequency and extent of care, patient tolerance of procedure, and special care in event of unexpected outcomes.

Teaching Considerations

• Different types of tracheostomy tubes have different faceplates. Some are rigid, others are not. Instruct caregivers not to lift up rigid faceplates or they will dislodge tube.
• Some commercial tracheostomy tube holders require removal of excess tie material to fit properly.
• If you anticipate long-term placement of tracheostomy, plan to teach patient and family tracheostomy care.
• Patients with new tracheostomy frequently have bloody secretions for 2 to 3 days after procedure and for 24 hours after each tracheostomy tube change (Roman, 2005; St. John and Malen, 2004).

Pediatric Considerations

• Children generally have shorter necks, making the stoma more difficult to clean.
• Pediatric tracheostomy tubes (smaller than size 4) do not contain an inner cannula.
• You perform routine tracheostomy tube changes weekly after a tract has formed (Hockenberry and Wilson, 2007).

Gerontological Considerations

• Some older adults may have more fragile skin and are more prone to skin breakdown from secretions or pressure (Meiner and Lueckenotte, 2006).
• Some older adults with impaired nutrition do not heal well.

SKILL 25-5   Inflating the Cuff on an Endotracheal or Tracheostomy Tube

The goals of correctly inflating the cuff on an artificial airway are to promote lung inflation for mechanical ventilation, to prevent aspiration of gastric contents, and at the same time to allow drainage of secretions that accumulate between the epiglottis and the cuff (Box 25-1). The amount of air inserted in a cuff is based on several factors; the two most important factors are the size of the patient's trachea and the external diameter of the artificial airway. If two patients of approximately the same size are intubated—one with a size 6 and one with a size 8—the patient with the larger tube (size 8) will require less air in the cuff. This is because the larger tube occludes more of the airway than the smaller tube does. If the cuff pressures are too high, permanent damage to the tracheal mucosa occurs (Roman, 2005; St. John and Malen, 2004). Maintain cuff pressures between 20 and 25 mm Hg or less (Roman, 2005).

No recommendation exists on a preferred method for cuff inflation. The minimal leak technique and the minimal occlusive technique are both acceptable methods (Roman, 2005; St. John and Malen, 2004) (Table 25-3).

Delegation Considerations

The skill of inflating the cuff on an endotracheal or tracheostomy tube cannot be delegated to NAP. However, you can delegate other aspects of care to NAP. Direct the NAP to:
- Immediately report any change in vital signs, respiratory status, confusion, restlessness, or discomfort.
- Immediately report any indication of the artificial airway moving or appearing loose.

Equipment

- ❑ Endotracheal/tracheostomy suction equipment (see Skill 25-2)
- ❑ Stethoscope
- ❑ 5- or 10-mL syringe
- ❑ Alcohol wipe
- ❑ Mask, goggles, face shield, if indicated
- ❑ Clean gloves, if indicated

BOX 25-1	Indications for Cuff Inflation

Mechanical Ventilation
- Continuous airway pressure
- Positive end-expiratory pressure (PEEP)
- Inability to meet ventilatory requirements with cuff down
- Inability to meet oxygen requirements with cuff down

Risk for Aspirating Gastric Contents
- Feeding tube, especially large bore, in stomach
- Gastroesophageal reflux disease
- Hiatal hernia
- During and after meals
- Impaired gastric emptying
- Decreased gag reflex
- Impaired swallowing

TABLE 25-3	Endotracheal and Tracheostomy Cuff Inflation Methods	
Inflation Method	**Procedure**	
Minimal occlusive technique	1	Place stethoscope over patient's trachea. Inject air into the cuff until no airflow is auscultated over the trachea during the peak inflation pressure of a positive pressure breath.
	2	Record the cuff volume.
Minimal leak technique	1	Inject air into the cuff until the air leak around the cuff is eliminated.
	2	Remove a small amount of air from the cuff until a slight leak occurs (50 to 100 mL tidal volume decrease) at peak inflation pressure during a positive pressure breath.
	3	Record the cuff volume.

From St. John RE, Malen J: Contemporary issues in adult tracheostomy management, *Crit Care Nurs Clin North Am* 16:413, 2004.

STEP	RATIONALE

ASSESSMENT

1 Observe for signs and symptoms of need to adjust cuff inflation, including gurgling on expiration, decreased exhaled tidal volume (mechanically ventilated patient), spasmodic coughing, tense test balloon on tube, flaccid test balloon on tube, and unexpected phonation.

Partially deflated cuff allows secretions to enter trachea and permits vocalization. High cuff pressure can result in necrosis, tracheomalacia, or tracheoesophageal fistula. Overinflated cuff may cause patient to cough (Roman, 2005; St. John and Malen, 2004).

2 If patient is to be discharged with a cuffed tracheostomy tube, determine family caregiver's understanding of and ability to perform procedure.

Identifies teaching needs.

NURSING DIAGNOSES

- Deficient knowledge regarding airway clearance techniques and devices
- Impaired gas exchange

- Impaired spontaneous ventilation
- Impaired swallowing
- Ineffective airway clearance

- Ineffective breathing pattern
- Risk for aspiration
- Risk for infection

Individualize related factors based on patient's condition or needs.

STEP	RATIONALE

PLANNING

1 Expected outcomes following completion of procedure:
   • Mechanically ventilated patient receives prescribed tidal volume.
   • Minimal leak is auscultated at end of inspiration.

   Proper inflation of cuff ensures patient receives tidal volume.

   Allows drainage of secretions during inhalation when airway is at widest but prevents gross aspiration during exhalation when airway is narrower. Prevents continuous contact of tracheal mucosa with cuff.

   • No evidence of excessive phonation, aspiration of gastric or mouth contents, tracheoesophageal fistula, or tracheomalacia is present.

   Proper level of cuff inflation is consistently maintained. Aspiration and phonation occur when cuff is underinflated. Tracheoesophageal fistula and tracheomalacia occur when the cuff is overinflated (Roman, 2005; St. John and Malen, 2004).

2 Explain procedure and how patient can participate. Explain that some coughing during procedure is normal.

   Encourages cooperation, minimizes risks, and reduces anxiety.

3 Assist patient to position comfortable for nurse and patient (usually semi-Fowler's).

   Promotes patient comfort, prevents nurse muscle strain, and facilitates drainage.

IMPLEMENTATION

1 Perform hand hygiene. Apply gloves and face shield, if indicated.

   Reduces transmission of microorganisms.

2 Suction secretions through ET or tracheostomy tube and also mouth.

   Ensures patent airway and facilitates hearing airflow with stethoscope. Prevents aspiration of oral secretions during cuff deflation.

3 Connect syringe to pilot balloon.

   Allows immediate access to equipment for adjusting cuff pressure.

4 Place stethoscope in sternal notch or above tracheostomy tube, and listen for minimal amount of air leak at end of inspiration (see illustration).

   Assesses proper cuff inflation.

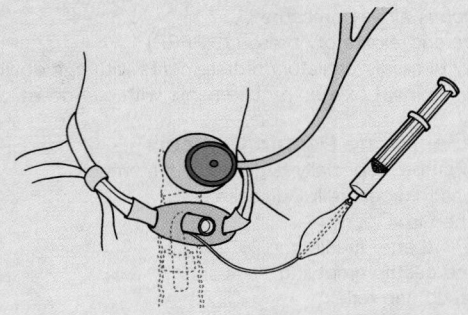

STEP 4 Inflating cuff on tracheostomy while listening with stethoscope.

5 If you do not hear an air leak, remove all air from cuff.

   Releases excessive cuff pressure, which reduces capillary blood flow and increases risk for tissue necrosis.

6 Inflate cuff according to agency policy (see Table 25-3).

   Inflates cuff to minimal leak. If air leak is audible with ear, air leak is too large. If you do not hear an air leak, cuff is overinflated.

7 If you hear excessive air leak, slowly add air as in Step 6.

   Air leak may prevent adequate lung expansion and increase risk for aspiration.

8 Remove stethoscope, and wipe diaphragm with alcohol wipe.

   Reduces transmission of microorganisms.

9 Remove syringe, and discard into appropriate receptacle or store per policy. Do not leave attached to pilot balloon valve.

   Reduces transmission of microorganisms.

10 Reposition patient.

   Promotes comfort.

11 Remove gloves and face shield. Discard into appropriate receptacle. Perform hand hygiene.

   Reduces transmission of microorganisms.

EVALUATION

1 Compare respiratory assessments before and after cuff care.

   Determines effectiveness of cuff care procedure.

2 Observe exhaled tidal volume from mechanical ventilator. Exhaled tidal volume should be not less than 50 mL of delivered tidal volume.

   Ensures appropriate ventilation of lungs.

3 Auscultate for audible air leak.

   Air leak should be heard only with stethoscope.

4 Observe for excessive phonation, presence of gastric secretions in airway secretions, or tracheoesophageal fistula.

   Occurs with inadequate or excessive cuff inflation.

Unexpected Outcomes

1 Cuff pressure is excessive.

2 Excessive volume is required to inflate cuff.

3 Excessive air leak is present.

4 Cuff requires increased amounts of air to maintain minimal leak.

Related Interventions

- Remove air from cuff.
- Reinflate with appropriate minimal leak technique.
- Notify physician.
- Patient may need insertion of larger tube.
- Reposition patient or tubing.
- Reinflate cuff if needed.
- Prepare for insertion of new tube by physician or trained personnel if cuff ruptures.
- Prepare to manually ventilate patient if needed.
- Reassess position of tube.
- Cuff of ET tube is sometimes higher in trachea (where airway is wider) than previously.
- Withdraw all air from cuff so pilot balloon is completely deflated (flat).
- Remove syringe from pilot balloon. Watch to see if air reenters pilot balloon (cuff). If so, there is leak in cuff, and tube requires replacement.
- Fill cuff appropriately.

Recording and Reporting

- Document presence of minimal leak at end of inspiration, volume of air injected into cuff, secretions obtained when suctioning, frequency of cuff care, patient tolerance of procedures and safe cuff pressure levels.

Pediatric Considerations

- Pediatric tracheostomy tubes do not have cuffs.
- Neonatal and many pediatric ET tubes do not contain cuffs.

? CRITICAL THINKING EXERCISES

You are assigned to care for Mrs. Karlowski, a 55-year-old bank manager. The only information you are given is that she has a history of chronic lung disease; a 1-week history of upper respiratory symptoms with shortness of breath; and a 2-day history of increasing fever, cough, malaise, nausea, and worsening shortness of breath.

1 Mrs. Karlowski complains of secretions in her mouth. She feels that she can cough up the pulmonary secretions, but the secretions still remain in her mouth, and they make her nauseous. What intervention would you select to assist her in clearing oral secretions? Explain your choice.
   A Yankauer suctioning
   B Nasotracheal suctioning
   C Orotracheal suctioning

2 As the day progresses, Mrs. Karlowski is becoming more fatigued, pulmonary crackles are worsening, and the sputum is thicker and progressively more difficult to clear. The patient has an intravenous (IV) line and humidified source of oxygen present. However, coughing, deep breathing, and chest physical therapy are not efficient in maintaining a clear airway. As you, the charge nurse, and the physician discuss this patient, what type of airway measures do you anticipate? Explain your choice.
   A Yankauer suctioning
   B Nasotracheal suctioning
   C Orotracheal suctioning

3 When you are performing airway management interventions, the risk for health-care associated pneumonia is always present. What can you do to reduce this risk when using a suction technique to clear tracheal secretions? Select all that apply. Explain your choice(s).
   A Perform hand hygiene.
   B Use sterile suction technique.
   C Use clean suction technique.
   D Use humidified oxygen.
   E All of the above.

4 While suctioning Mrs. Karlowski, you observe that the returned sputum is thicker and is brown tinged. This is very different from earlier sputum. What action would you take? Select all that apply. Explain your choice(s).
   A Notify physician or nurse in charge.
   B Decrease humidification.
   C Increase fluids.
   D Obtain artificial airway.
   E Obtain sputum specimen.

✓ REVIEW QUESTIONS

1 A patient hospitalized for acute pneumonia has a 10-year history of chronic lung disease and cannot clear her respiratory secretions from the upper airway even with coughing. Which suctioning intervention is appropriate?
   1 Oropharyngeal
   2 Nasopharyngeal
   3 Endotracheal
   4 Tracheal

2 A patient needs both the trachea and the oral pharynx suctioned. In what order should the nurse suction these areas and why? Select all correct answers.
   1 Suction the oral cavity last.
   2 Suction the oral cavity first.
   3 Suction nasotracheally first.
   4 Suction nasotracheally last.

3 Secretions within an airway affect a patient's ability to oxygenate. What assessment data would the nurse expect as a result of these secretions?
   1 A decreased airway size would raise the respiratory rate.
   2 A decreased airway size would decrease the respiratory rate.
   3 An increased airway size would raise the respiratory rate.
   4 An increased airway size would decrease the respiratory rate.

4 The nurse is caring for a patient with an artificial airway whose pulse oximeter reading drops from 90% to 85%. What is the priority action?
 1 Check for the presence of a pulse.
 2 Assess for an adequate blood pressure.
 3 Check for a patent airway.
 4 Check the connections of the oxygen supply.

5 A patient with an endotracheal tube has unequal breath sounds, even after being suctioned and repositioned. What nursing intervention is indicated at this time?
 1 Notify the physician.
 2 Call for help.
 3 Suction the airway.
 4 Reposition the patient's endotracheal tube deeper.

REFERENCES

AARC clinical practice guidelines: nasotracheal suctioning—2004 revision and update, 2004, http://www.rcjournal.com/cpgs/pdf/09.04.1080.pdf, accessed September 13, 2007.

American Academy of Pediatrics: The changing concept of sudden infant death syndrome: diagnostic coding shifts, controversies regarding the sleeping environment, and new variables to consider in reducing risk, Pediatrics 116(5):1245, 2005.

Celik S, Kanan N: A current conflict: use of isotonic sodium chloride solution on endotracheal suctioning in critically ill patients, Dimens Crit Care Nurs 25(1):11, 2006.

Considine J: The role of nurses in preventing adverse events related to respiratory dysfunction: literature review, J Adv Nurs 49(6):624, 2005.

Edmonds V, Brady P: Healthcare for Vietnamese immigrants, J Multicult Nurs Health, 2, 2003, http://findarticles.com/p/articles/mi_qa3919/is_200307/ai_n9271299, accessed September 13, 2007.

Grap M, Munro C: Preventing ventilator-associated pneumonia: evidence-based care, Crit Care Nurs Clin North Am 16:349, 2004.

Hockenberry MJ, Wilson D: Wong's nursing care of infants and children, ed 8, St. Louis, 2007, Mosby.

Lewis SL and others: Medical-surgical nursing: assessment and management of clinical problems, ed 7, St. Louis, 2007, Mosby.

Lindgren V, Ames N: Caring for patients on mechanical ventilation: what research indicates is best practice, Am J Nurs 105(5):50, 2005.

Meiner SE, Lueckenotte AG: Gerontologic nursing, ed 3, St. Louis, 2006, Mosby.

Mohan A, Bollineni S: Closed system suctioning: why is the debate still open? Indian J Med Sci 61(4):177, 2007.

Pease P: Oxygen administration: is practice based on evidence? Paediatr Nurs 18(8):14, 2006

Pruitt B: Clear the air with closed suctioning, Nursing 35(7):44, 2005.

Roman M: Tracheostomy tubes, Medsurg Nurs 14(2):143, 2005.

Sorrentino SA: Mosby's textbook for nursing assistants, ed 6, St. Louis, 2004, Mosby.

St. John RE: Airway management, Crit Care Nurse 19(4):79, 1999.

St. John RE, Malen J: Contemporary issues in adult tracheostomy management, Crit Care Nurs Clin North Am 16:413, 2004.

Vollman, K: Ask the experts, Crit Care Nurse 26(4):53, 2006.

Wilson M: Tracheostomy management, Paediatr Nurs 17(3):38, 2005.

RESEARCH REFERENCES

Abbott C and others: Adoption of a ventilator-associated pneumonia clinical practice guideline, Worldviews Evid Based Nurs 3(4):139, 2006.

Bourgault AM and others: Effects of endotracheal tube suctioning on arterial oxygen tension and heart rate variability, Biol Res Nurs 7:268, 2006.

Demir F, Dramali A: Requirement for 100% oxygen before and after closed suction, J Adv Nurs 51(3): 245, 2005.

Jongerden I and others: Open and closed endotracheal suction systems in mechanically ventilated intensive care patients: a meta-analysis, Crit Care Med 35(1):260, 2007.

Tolentino-DelosReyes and others: Evidence-based practice: use of ventilator bundle to prevent ventilator-associated pneumonia, Amer J Crit Care 16(1):20, 2007.

Closed Chest Drainage Systems

MEDIA RESOURCES

- **evolve** *learning system* http://evolve.elsevier.com/Perry/skills
  - Review Questions
  - Video Clips

- **NSO** Nursing Skills Online

KEY TERMS

Air leak
Atmospheric pressure
Chest tube
Hemothorax
Intrapleural pressure
Mediastinal shift
Negative pressure
Parietal pleura
Pneumothorax
Positive pressure
Subcutaneous emphysema
Tension pneumothorax
Tidaling
Visceral pleura

OBJECTIVES

Mastery of content in this chapter will enable the nurse to:

- Explain the physiology of normal respiration.
- List three common sites for chest tube placement.
- List three conditions requiring chest tube insertion.
- Describe closed chest drainage systems: water-seal and waterless systems.
- Describe principles and mechanisms of chest tube suction.
- Describe methods of troubleshooting chest tube systems.
- Discuss the nursing principles in caring for patients with chest tubes.
- Describe autotransfusion.

The chest cavity is a closed structure bound by muscle, bone, connective tissue, vascular structures, and the diaphragm. This cavity has three distinct sections, each sealed from the others: one section for each lung and a third section for the mediastinum, which surrounds structures such as the heart, esophagus, trachea, and great vessels.

The lungs are covered with a membrane called the visceral pleura. The interior chest wall is lined with a membrane called the parietal pleura (Fig. 26-1). The potential space between the visceral and parietal pleura is called the pleural space and is filled with approximately 4 mL of lubricating fluid to help the pleura slide during respiration. A negative intrapleural pressure is needed to expand the lungs. During inspiration the intercostal muscles pull outward and the diaphragm contracts and pulls downward, thereby increasing the size of the chest cavity. As a result there is an increase in the amount of negative pressure (vacuum effect) being exerted in the intrapleural space.

During inspiration increased negative pressure pulls the lungs against the expanded chest cavity, increasing their size. The expanding lungs cause the intrapulmonic (alveoli) pressure to fall lower than atmospheric pressure, thus increasing the negative pressure within the lungs. This change in pressure causes air to rush into the lungs until the intrapulmonic pressure is equal to the pressure in the atmosphere. When the chest cavity stops expanding and the lungs are full of air, the respiratory muscles and diaphragm relax and return the chest cavity to its resting stage. Expiration (exhalation) is a passive process that results from relaxation of the inspiratory muscles that decrease the space in the chest cavity.

Trauma, disease, or surgery can result in air, blood, or fluid leaking into the intrapleural space, creating a positive pressure that collapses lung tissue. Small leaks (24% or less) are sometimes absorbed spontaneously and may not require a chest tube. The usual intervention for larger leaks is a chest tube to remove air and fluid from the pleural space, prevent air or fluid from reentering the pleural space, and reestablish normal intrapleural and intrapulmonary pressures.

The amount of pleural fluid is small and contains 1 to 2 g of protein per 100 mL. The protein content maintains the hydrostatic-osmotic pressure and regulates the balance of pleural fluid. Pleural fluid originates in the pleural capillaries, interstitial spaces, intrathoracic lymphatic vessels, intrathoracic blood vessels, or peritoneal cavity (Light, 2007). Factors causing an increase in protein content and/or an increase in fluid entry or a decrease in fluid exit cause an accumulation of pleural fluid (Allibone, 2006). This is called a pleural effusion, and it is classified as either transudate or exudate effusion.

Transudate effusions are usually bilateral and occur from a variety of conditions, such as congestive heart failure, hepatic disease, or nephrotic syndrome. An exudate effusion is usually unilateral, and the fluid is high in protein. It is the result of many clinical conditions, such as cancer, infection, pancreatitis, connective tissue disease (e.g., rheumatoid arthritis), or collagen vascular diseases. When a pleural effusion is present, the patient usually needs

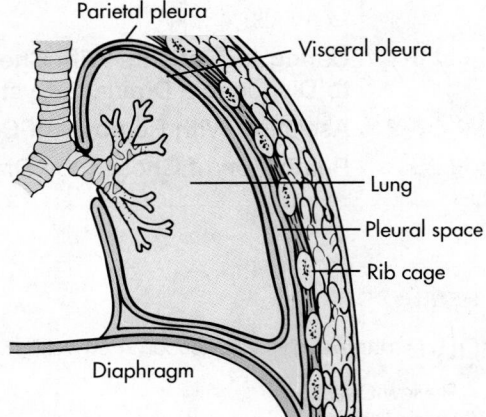

FIG 26-1   Partial structures of the lungs.

a diagnostic thoracentesis and pleural fluid analysis to determine the cause of the exudate (see Chapter 44). Patients usually need one or more chest tubes to promote drainage of the excess fluid and lung expansion (Allibone, 2006).

A pneumothorax is a collapse of the lung caused by a collection of air in the pleural space. The loss of negative intrapleural pressure causes the lung to collapse. There are a variety of mechanisms that cause a pneumothorax. A traumatic pneumothorax develops as a result of penetrating chest trauma, such as a stabbing or the chest striking the steering wheel in an automobile accident. A spontaneous or primary pneumothorax sometimes occurs from the rupture of a small bleb (blister) on the surface of the lung or from an invasive procedure, such as insertion of a subclavian intravenous (IV) line. Secondary pneumothorax occurs because of underlying disease, such as emphysema. A patient with a pneumothorax usually feels pain because atmospheric air irritates the parietal pleura. The pain may be sharp and pleuritic. Dyspnea is common and worsens as the size of the pneumothorax increases.

A tension pneumothorax occurs from rupture in the pleura when air accumulates in the pleural space more rapidly than it is removed. It is a life-threatening situation. The pleural space functions as a one-way valve, causing an increase in the amount of air and pressure. If left untreated, the lung on the affected side collapses, the mediastinum shifts to the opposite (unaffected side), and venous return and subsequent cardiac output decrease. The patient has sudden chest pain, a fall in blood pressure, and tachycardia, and cardiopulmonary arrest can occur. The patient usually experiences acute pleuritic pain, diaphoresis, and dry cough (Allibone, 2003). Patients with chest trauma, fractured ribs, invasive thoracic bedside procedures (such as insertion of central lines), and those on high-pressure mechanical ventilation are at risk for tension pneumothorax (Leigh-Smith and Harris, 2005).

A hemothorax is a collapse of the lung caused by an accumulation of blood and fluid in the pleural cavity between the chest wall

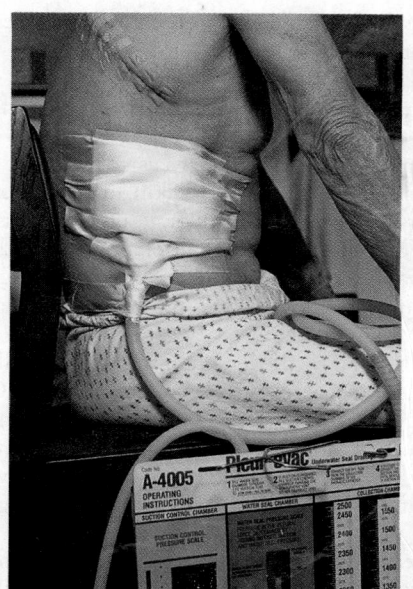

FIG 26-2 Pleural chest tube in place following thoracic surgery.

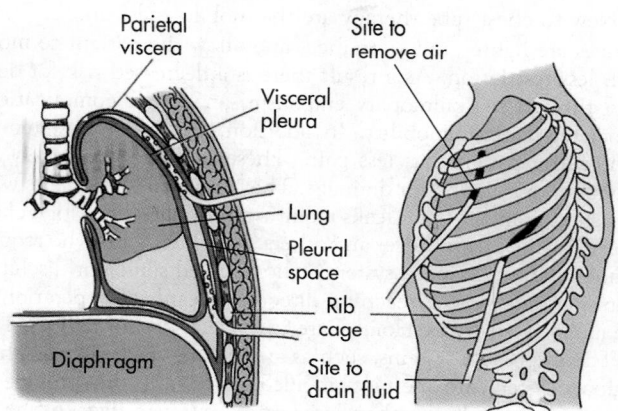

FIG 26-3 Diagram of sites for chest tube placement.

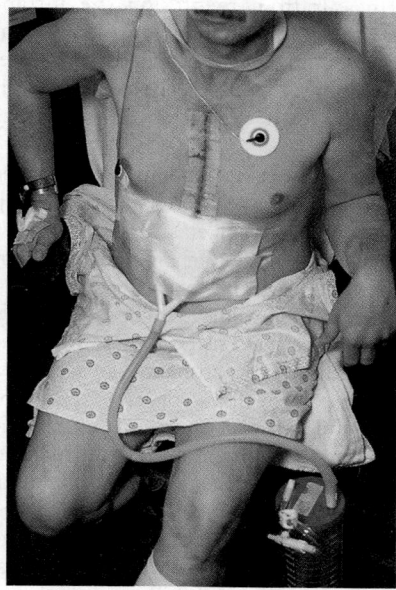

FIG 26-4 Mediastinal chest tube.

and the lung, usually as a result of trauma. It produces a counterpressure and prevents the full expansion of the lung. A hemothorax is also caused by rupture of small blood vessels from inflammatory processes, such as pneumonia or tuberculosis. In addition to pain and dyspnea, signs and symptoms of shock can develop if blood loss is severe.

Chest tube insertion is the treatment for most types of pneumothorax and postoperative chest surgery or trauma. A chest tube is a large catheter inserted through the thorax to remove fluid, blood, and/or air. There are a variety of chest tubes on the market. Small-bore chest tubes (12 to 20 Fr) are sufficient to remove air, and large-bore (24 to 32 Fr) tubes are needed to remove fluid and blood. In some settings the traditional reusable glass three-bottle system is still used. The newest system available is the mobile chest drain, which allows the patient to move about with less restriction (Carroll, 2005). Regardless of the system used, the principles of patient management are the same (Rieger and others, 2007). A pleural chest tube (Fig. 26-2) is inserted when air or fluid enters the pleural space, compromising oxygenation or ventilation (e.g., chest trauma, open chest surgery, or a large pleural leak). A closed chest drainage system with or without suction is attached to the chest tube to promote drainage of air and fluid. Lung reexpansion occurs as the fluid or air is removed from the pleural space.

The location of the chest tube indicates the type of drainage expected. Apical (second or third intercostal space) and anterior chest tube placement promotes removal of air. Because air rises, these chest tubes are placed high, allowing evacuation of air from the intrapleural space and lung reexpansion (Fig. 26-3). The air is discharged into the atmosphere, and there is little or no drainage in the collection chamber.

Chest tubes placed low (usually in the fifth or sixth intercostal space) and posterior or lateral drain fluid (see Fig. 26-3). Fluid in the intrapleural space is affected by gravity and localizes in the lower portion of the lung cavity. Tubes placed in these positions drain blood and fluid. Frequently applying suction assists this drainage. Fluid drainage is expected after open chest surgery and with some chest trauma.

A mediastinal chest tube is placed in the mediastinum, just below the sternum (Fig. 26-4), and is connected to a drainage system. This tube drains blood or fluid, preventing its accumulation around the heart. A mediastinal tube is commonly used after open heart surgery.

Occasionally, in emergency situations and for some small pneumothoraces, a catheter is inserted through the chest wall, and a rubber flutter one-way valve (e.g., a Heimlich valve) is attached to the catheter (Carroll, 2005). As the patient exhales, the positive pressure generated by the air leaving the chest enters the tubing, causing the valve to open so the air is released. During inspiration, the tube collapses on itself, preventing air from reentering the chest (Carroll, 2005). No drainage chamber is used with this device, and therefore it is not used when patients need fluid drained, such as from a hemothorax or a pleural effusion.

New smaller "pigtail catheters" are also used and are less traumatic than the large-bore tubes. In addition, if they occlude, the health care provider can irrigate them using sterile water. However, because these tubes are small, the size of the tube lumen does not promote drainage of blood, and they are not used for chest trauma (Lewis and others, 2008).

New to chest tube therapy are the mobile chest drains. These devices are lighter, self-contained, and allow the patient to move with less restriction. As a result there is a decreased risk for deep vein thrombosis, pulmonary embolism, and other complications associated with immobility. In addition, because the system is lighter, the patient has less pain. These mobile systems rely on gravity or dry suction for drainage. They are ideal for patients with persistent drainage or air leaks requiring prolonged need for a chest tube (Carroll, 2005; Rieger and others, 2007). Patients who require a mobile chest drainage system at home need sufficient discharge planning and patient teaching directed toward safe operation of the mobile system (see Home Care Considerations for Skill 26-1).

The disposable systems, such as an Atrium or Pleur-Evac chest drainage system, are one-piece molded plastic units that provide for a single- or multiple-chamber closed drainage system (Fig. 26-5).

A single chamber system allows air from a pneumothorax to bubble out of the water seal and escape through the air outlet while preventing air from reentering the intrapleural space. This system is not recommended for the evacuation of fluid because drainage would raise the level of the water-seal liquid. An increased height of fluid in the water seal increases the resistance to drainage on expiration and eventually stops the drainage entirely.

A two- or three-chamber system drains both a hemothorax and a pneumothorax effectively. The two-chamber system permits liquid to flow into the collection chamber, and air flows into the water-seal chamber. A three-chamber system promotes the drainage of fluid and air with controlled suction. In both systems the first chamber provides a compartment for fluid or blood drainage and a second compartment for either a water seal or a one-way valve. In the three-chamber system, the third compartment is for suction control, which may or may not be used. The disposable units appear to be the system of choice because they are cost-effective and some facilitate autotransfusion, a common practice in open heart surgeries. Knowledge of the basics of chest tube management and troubleshooting maneuvers reduces the patient's risk for complications.

Water-seal or the newer waterless chest drainage systems are also used. Researchers are trying to determine which system is most effective. Marshall and others (2002) compare the two systems in patients who had lung resection surgery. They conclude that placing chest tubes on water seal for a brief period following surgery decreases the duration of air leak and length of time needed for the chest tube. Multiple-chamber, water-seal, and waterless systems are presented in this text.

EVIDENCE-BASED PRACTICE TRENDS

There continues to be controversy as to whether to "strip" or "milk" a chest tube. Stripping or milking a chest tube is a process used to clear a tube of clots. Milking or stripping is the manual compression of a chest tube in an attempt to move the chest tube drainage toward the collection device. Stripping causes a dangerous increase in intrathoracic pressure that causes damage to the lung tissue. Milking is achieved by gently squeezing and releasing the drainage tube along the length of the tubing. Milking does not alter the intrathoracic pressure as much as stripping (Coughlin and Parchinsky, 2006). However, this technique is used only in selected situations, such as following thoracic surgery when chest tube drainage has multiple clots. Milking is never routinely done and usually requires a health care provider's order or agency written protocol.

When chest tube occlusions are due to clotting, the literature is contradictory regarding interventions. Chest tube milking or stripping is usually contraindicated because the techniques do not improve catheter patency (Coughlin and Parchinsky, 2006). Ideally, the tube is changed if a blockage is detected (Allibone, 2003). However, in some select situations, such as with early postoperative chest surgeries, it may be necessary to clear the tube of blood clots. In these situations milking of the chest tube is done by experienced nurses who are following specific agency guidelines. The danger of stripping or milking the chest tube is a sudden rise in intrathoracic pressures, which increases the risk lung injury or injures the surgical area. However, a nonfunctional chest tube may cause a more severe problem, and gently milking the chest tube may be the only option (Coughlin and Parchinsky, 2006).

Careful management of chest tube drainage prevents the need to milk chest tubes. Institute nursing interventions to maintain tube patency. Avoid dependent loops of the drainage tube, or when these loops cannot be avoided, such as when the patient is sitting, lift and clear the tube every 15 minutes (Roman and Mercado, 2006). In addition, it is important to tailor the length of the drainage tube to the patient. The length of the tubing is long enough to allow the patient to move, but not so long that dependent loops hang down the side of the bed. If the tubing is coiled, looped, or clotted, the drainage is impeded and can result in a tension pneumothorax (Allibone, 2003; Roman and Mercado, 2006).

▋ Skill Performance Guidelines

1   Document patient's baseline vital signs, oxygen saturation, lung sounds, and respiratory status. Changes in the vital signs or respiratory status often indicate a malfunction of the chest drainage system.

2   Observe the water seal for intermittent bubbling from its **U** tube or a rise and fall of fluid that is synchronous with respirations. (For example, in a non–mechanically ventilated patient the fluid rises during inspiration, and the fluid level falls during expiration. When a patient is on a mechanical ventilator, the opposite occurs.)

   a   Constant bubbling in the water seal or a sudden, unexpected stoppage of water-seal activity is considered abnormal and requires immediate attention.

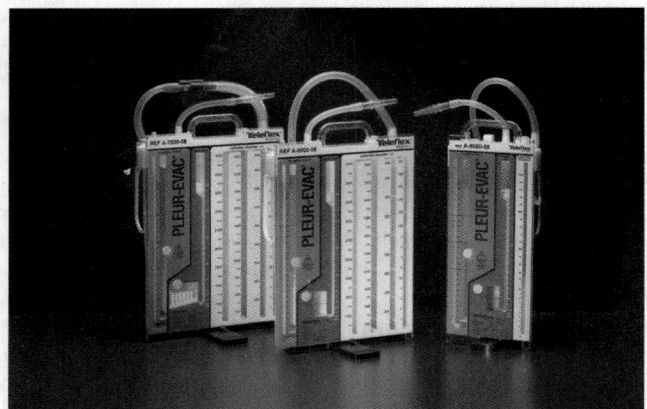

FIG 26-5 Disposable chest drainage systems. (*Pleur-Evac images courtesy Teleflex Medical, Research Triangle Park, NC.*)

b Unexpected stoppage of activity may indicate a blockage. In these situations immediate attention and correction are indicated. After 2 to 3 days, tidaling or bubbling on expiration is expected to stop, indicating that the lung has reexpanded.

3 In the waterless system look for a rise and fall of fluid in the diagnostic air-leak indicator synchronous with respirations. Constant left-to-right bubbling (when facing the indicator) or violent rocking is considered abnormal and may indicate an air leak.

4 Know the amount of expected chest tube drainage.

a A sudden decrease in the amount of chest tube drainage can indicate a possible clot or obstruction in the chest tube.

b A sudden increase of more than 70 mL of drainage can indicate fresh bleeding from the thorax.

c Drainage from a pneumothorax is generally limited. Any fluid buildup is caused by chest tube insertion trauma. The chest tubes promote the removal of air from the intrapleural space.

5 Know the expected color of the drainage. Drainage from recent open chest surgery is initially bright red and gradually becomes serous as the postoperative course continues. Blood-tinged fluid usually indicates malignancy, pulmonary infarction, or severe inflammation (Allibone, 2006). Frank blood indicates a hemothorax. Pus indicates an empyema, which is a collection of pus in the pleural cavity, and the drainage is pus colored (Coote and Kaye, 2005).

6 In the water system, observe for constant, gentle bubbling in the suction control chamber when it is connected to suction. In the waterless system, a designated amount of suction is maintained by setting the suction source and dialing the prescribed suction level in the float ball column.

7 Assess both types of systems for air leaks. If an air leak exists, determine whether the air leak is in the patient (patient-centered air leak) or in the chest tube system (system-centered air leak). Remember that continuous bubbling in the water-seal chamber with an absence of bubbles in the suction control chamber indicates that there is a leak in the system (Roman and Mercado, 2006). Ensure that all tubing connections are tight.

8 Note the color and amount of chest tube drainage on a regular basis (e.g., every hour initially and then every 4 hours). Make a mark to indicate the fluid level on the side of the drainage collection chamber at the end of the shift. Note the drainage amount as output.

SKILL 26-1 Caring for Patients With Chest Tubes Connected to Disposable Drainage Systems

NSO *Chest Tubes Module / Lessons 1 and 3*

There are two types of commercial drainage systems: the water-seal and the waterless systems.

WATER-SEAL SYSTEMS

NSO *Chest Tube Module / Lesson 2*

Two-Chamber Water-Seal System

On expiration, fluid or air is forced out of the intrapleural space. Suction pulls air or fluid through the chest tube into the drainage collection chamber. On entering the drainage collection chamber, this fluid or air displaces the air present in the chamber by pushing it through the water seal and out of the system into the atmosphere. The water-seal chamber is left open to air in order to drain. If the tubing is clamped, there is no mechanism for air to vent. To maintain the water-seal system, the chest tube system must remain upright. When it is tipped or overturned, the water seal is disrupted.

Three-Chamber Water-Seal System

If suction is used, the three-chamber water-seal system (Fig. 26-6) is set up with the suction control chamber added. A prescribed amount of sterile fluid (e.g., 20 cm of water) is poured into the suction control chamber, which is then attached to a suction source by tubing. The amount of sterile water added depends on the manufacturer's recommendations. The chamber is filled to the set volume for the prescribed amount of suction. Sterile water is added several times a day because of evaporation. As the fluid level decreases, the amount of suction also declines. The wall or portable suction device is turned up until the water in the suction control bottle exhibits a continuous, gentle bubbling. This provides the prescribed amount of suction (negative pressure).

If the suction source delivers more negative pressure than the suction control chamber water level allows, there is no danger because atmospheric air is pulled into the suction control chamber through an inlet, causing the excess suction to dissipate. The extra air pulled into the chamber causes vigorous bubbling. If this occurs, lower the suction source setting to reduce noise and evaporation of the fluid. The absence of bubbling indicates that no suction is being exerted into the system. Raise the suction setting to restore gentle bubbling.

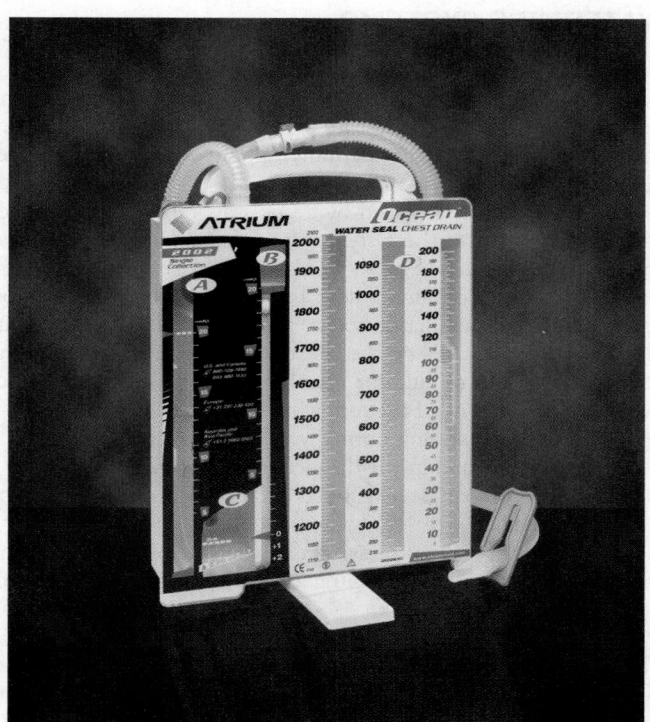

FIG 26-6 Disposable waterless chest drainage system with suction.

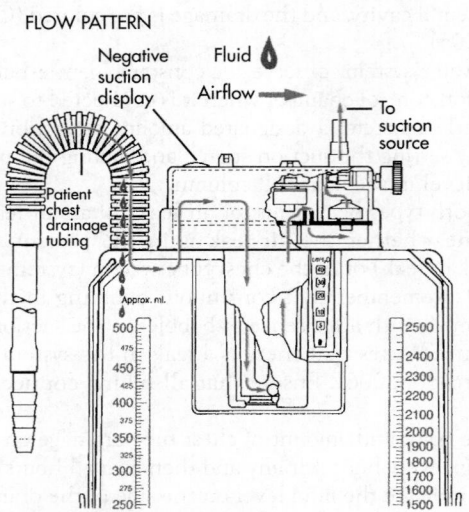

FIG 26-7   Disposable waterless chest drainage system with suction.

The middle chamber of a traditional chest drainage system is the water seal. The main purpose of the water seal is to allow air to exit from the pleural space on exhalation and prevent air from entering the pleural cavity or mediastinum on inhalation. When the appropriate amount of sterile water is added, a 2-cm water seal is established. To maintain effective water seal the chest drainage unit must remain upright and you must monitor the water level in the water-seal chamber to check for evaporation. Bubbling in the water-seal chamber indicates an air leak.

WATERLESS SYSTEMS

Two-Chamber Waterless System

The principles of the waterless system are similar to those of the water-seal system except that fluid is not required for setup. Because water is not used, accidentally tipping over the system does not compromise the patient's condition.

The water seal is replaced by a one-way valve (Fig. 26-7) located near the top of the system. Most of the container serves as the drainage chamber. The suction chamber does not depend on water. Instead, it contains a float ball, which is set by a suction control dial after the suction source is turned on. A diagnostic air-leak indicator is located on the face of the unit. It does require the addition of 15 mL of fluid for visualization. The indicator's function is to identify one of the following:

1 The lung is expanding normally. This is indicated by a gentle tidaling of the fluid in the diagnostic indicator.
2 The lung is probably reexpanded if after 2 or 3 days the tidaling has stopped.
3 There is an air leak in the system if, when facing the system, the observer sees the fluid bubbling left to right. Locate and correct the source of the air leak.

Three-Chamber Waterless System

When suction is ordered, attach the suction chamber port to the suction source by tubing, turn the suction on, and set the float ball to the prescribed setting. If the float ball does not rise to the pre-

scribed level, increase the suction source setting until it does. The system is now functioning with suction.

There are usually two suction settings: one at either the suction control chamber or the float ball setting and the other at the suction source. The chamber or float ball setting is a safety factor to reduce the possibility that the intrapleural tissues receive too much suction, causing injury.

Dry Suction System

Dry suction control systems provide many advantages (Fig. 26-8). Higher suction pressure levels are achieved, set up is easy, and the lack of continuous bubbling provides for quiet operation. There is no fluid to evaporate, which decreases the amount of suction necessary. A self-compensating regulator controls dry suction units. A dial is set to the prescribed suction control setting. These units are preset to −20 cm of water pressure, but they are adjustable from −10 to −40 cm of water pressure. However, the dry suction control systems do require sterile water in the water-seal chamber.

Delegation Considerations

The skill of caring for a patient with a chest tube connected to a disposable drainage system cannot be delegated to nursing assistive personnel (NAP). However, NAP may assist with other aspects of the patient's care, such as monitoring vital signs. The nurse directs the NAP about:

- Proper positioning of the patient with chest tubes to facilitate chest tube drainage and optimal functioning of the system
- How to ambulate and transfer patient with chest drainage
- Immediately informing the nurse of any changes in vital signs, chest pain, or sudden shortness of breath, or excessive bubbling in water-seal chamber
- Immediately informing the nurse if there is disconnection of system, change in type and amount of drainage, sudden bleeding, or sudden cessation of bubbling

EQUIPMENT

- ❑ Disposable chest drainage system as ordered
- ❑ Suction source and setup (wall canister or portable)
  - *Water suction system:* Add sterile water or normal saline (NS) solution to cover the lower 2.5 cm (1 inch) of water-seal U tube, sterile water or NS to pour into the suction control chamber if suction is to be used (see manufacturer's directions)
  - *Waterless system:* Add vial of 30 mL injectable sodium chloride or water, 20-mL syringe, 21-gauge needle, and antiseptic swab
- ❑ Clean gloves
- ❑ Sterile gauze sponges
- ❑ Local anesthetic, if this is not an emergent procedure
- ❑ Chest tube tray (all items are sterile): Knife handle (1), chest tube clamp, small sponge forceps, needle holder, knife blade No. 10, 3-0 silk sutures, tray liner (sterile field), curved 8-inch Kelly clamps (2), 4 × 4 inch sponges (10), suture scissors, hand towels (3), sterile gloves
- ❑ Dressings: Petrolatum gauze, split chest-tube dressings, several 4 × 4 inch gauze dressings, large gauze dressings (2), and 4-inch tape or elastic bandage (Elastoplast)
- ❑ Head cover
- ❑ Face mask/face shield
- ❑ Sterile gloves
- ❑ Rubber-tipped hemostats for each chest tube (2)
- ❑ 1-inch adhesive tape for taping connections
- ❑ Stethoscope, sphygmomanometer, and pulse oximeter

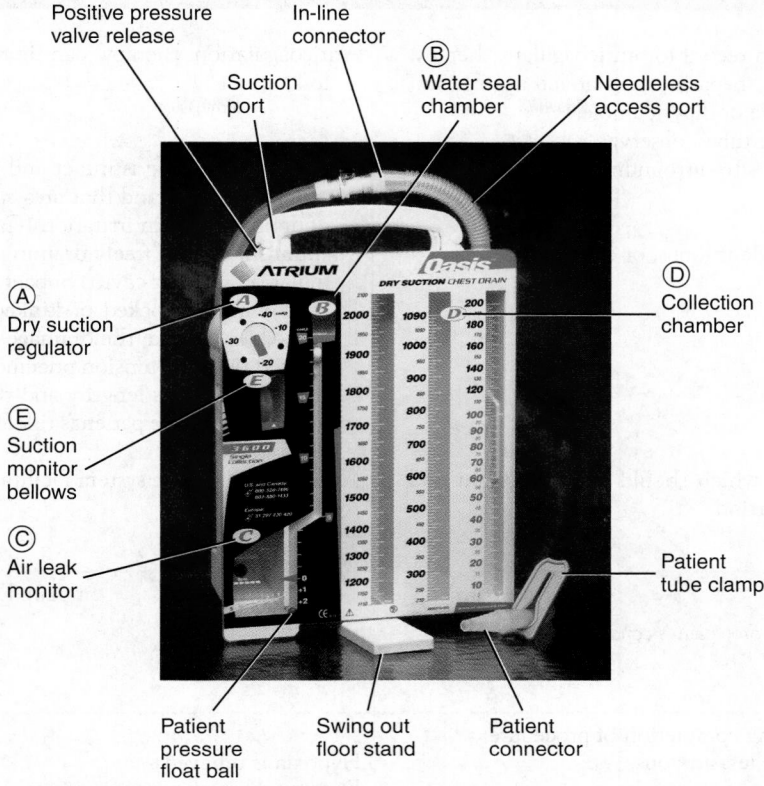

FIG 26-8   Dry suction chest drainage system. (*Courtesy Atrium Medical Corp.*)

STEP	RATIONALE

ASSESSMENT

1 Obtain baseline and serial vital signs, oxygen saturation (SpO_2), and level of orientation.

Baseline vital signs are essential for any invasive procedure. Patients requiring chest tube insertion frequently have respiratory distress. Changes in vital signs and level of orientation may indicate decreased levels of oxygen and/or hypoxia.

2 Know patient's current hemoglobin and hematocrit levels.

Provides measure reflecting blood loss and subsequent levels of oxygenation.

3 Assess pulmonary status:

Patients in need of chest tubes have impaired oxygenation and ventilation.

a Signs and symptoms of increased respiratory distress: Displaced trachea, decreased breath sounds over the affected and nonaffected lungs, marked cyanosis, asymmetrical chest movements.

The degree of the signs and symptoms associated with respiratory distress is related to the size of the pneumothorax, hemothorax, or preexisting illness of the patient.

b Assess for sharp, stabbing chest pain or chest pain on inspiration, hypotension, and tachycardia (Carroll, 2002). If possible, ask patient to rate level of comfort on a scale of 0 to 10.

Sharp stabbing chest pain with or without decreased blood pressure and increased heart rate may indicate a tension pneumothorax. The presence of a pneumothorax or hemothorax is painful, frequently causing sharp inspiratory pain. In addition, there is discomfort associated with the presence of a chest tube, not just with the insertion of the tube. As a result of this discomfort, patients tend to not cough or change position in an effort to minimize this pain (Milgrom and others, 2004).

4 Assess patient for known allergies. Ask patients if they have had a problem with medications, latex, or anything applied to the skin.

Povidone-iodine or chlorhexidine are antiseptic solutions used to cleanse the skin during tube insertion (Coughlin and Parchinsky, 2006). Lidocaine is a local anesthetic administered to reduce pain. The chest tube will be held in place with tape. Iodine, lidocaine, and tape are common allergens.

STEP	RATIONALE
5 Review patient's medication record for anticoagulant therapy, including aspirin, warfarin, heparin, or platelet aggregation inhibitors such as ticlopidine or dipyridamole.	Anticoagulation therapy can increase procedure-related blood loss.
6 For patients who have chest tubes, observe:	
a Chest tube dressing and site surrounding tube insertion	Ensures that dressing is intact and occlusive seal remains without air or fluid leaks and that area surrounding insertion site is free of drainage or skin irritation (Carroll, 2002).
b Tubing for kinks, dependent loops, or clots	Maintains a patent, freely draining system, preventing fluid accumulation in chest cavity. Subcutaneous emphysema can occur if the tubing is blocked or kinked. When the tubing is coiled, looped, or clotted, the drainage is impeded, and there is an increased risk for a tension pneumothorax or surgical emphysema. If the drainage is lengthy and the chest tube remains in place for some time, the patient's risk for infection increases (Allibone, 2003).
c Chest drainage system, which should remain upright and below level of tube insertion	An upright drainage system facilitates drainage and maintains the water seal.

NURSING DIAGNOSES

- Anxiety
- Acute pain
- Impaired gas exchange

Individualize related factors based on patient's condition or needs.

PLANNING

1 Expected outcomes following completion of procedure:	
• Patient is oriented and is less anxious.	Hypoxia is relieved.
• Vital signs are stable.	Decreased hypoxia improves vital sign measures.
• Patient reports no chest pain.	Reexpansion of the lung reduces chest pain.
• Breath sounds are auscultated in all lobes. Lung expansion is symmetrical, SpO$_2$ is stable or improved, and respirations are nonlabored.	Reexpansion of the lung promotes normal respirations.
• Chest tube remains in place, and chest drainage system remains airtight.	Indicates correct placement and patency of the chest tube drainage system.
• Gentle tidaling (fluctuations or rocking) is evident in water seal or diagnostic indicator.	Indicates system is functioning normally. Reflects changes in intrapleural pressure.
2 Check agency policy, and determine whether informed consent is needed.	In nonemergent situations most institutions require informed, written permission for chest tube insertion.
3 Review health care provider's role and responsibilities for chest tube placement (Table 26-1, p. 712). **The nursing responsibilities and interventions are detailed in the steps of this skill.**	Helps differentiate health care provider and nurse roles so that the nurse can function more effectively.
4 Explain procedure to patient.	Reduces anxiety and promotes patient cooperation.
5 Perform hand hygiene.	Reduces transmission of microorganisms.
6 Set up the prescribed drainage system. NOTE: *Open the system when health care provider is ready to insert chest tube.*	Premature opening of the sterile chest drainage system increases risk for contamination of sterile equipment.
a Prepare a water-seal drainage system (check manufacturer's guidelines):	System permits displaced air to pass into the atmosphere.
(1) Obtain chest drainage system. Remove wrappers, and prepare to set up the system.	Maintains sterility of the system. The system is packaged for use in sterile operating room conditions.
(2) While maintaining sterility of the drainage tubing, stand the system upright, and add sterile water or normal saline to the appropriate compartments.	Reduces possibility of contamination.
(a) *For a two-chamber system (without suction):* Add 2 cm sterile water to the water-seal chamber (second chamber), which is enough to submerge the water-seal tube and create a one-way valve (Roman and Mercado, 2006).	The water seal creates a one-way valve allowing fluid and air to drain from the patient's chest and not return (Roman and Mercado, 2006).

STEP	RATIONALE
(b) *For a three-chamber system (with suction):* Add 2 cm sterile water to the water-seal chamber (middle chamber). Add amount of sterile solution prescribed by health care provider to the suction control (third chamber), usually 20 cm water pressure (8 inches). Connect tubing from suction control chamber to suction source. (Tailor length of drainage tube to patient.) (See illustration.)	The amount of fluid in the suction control chamber governs the suction's intensity, not the amount of suction delivered from an outside suction source, such as a portable or wall suction unit (Roman and Mercado, 2006). For example, 20 cm of water is approximately −20 cm of water pressure.

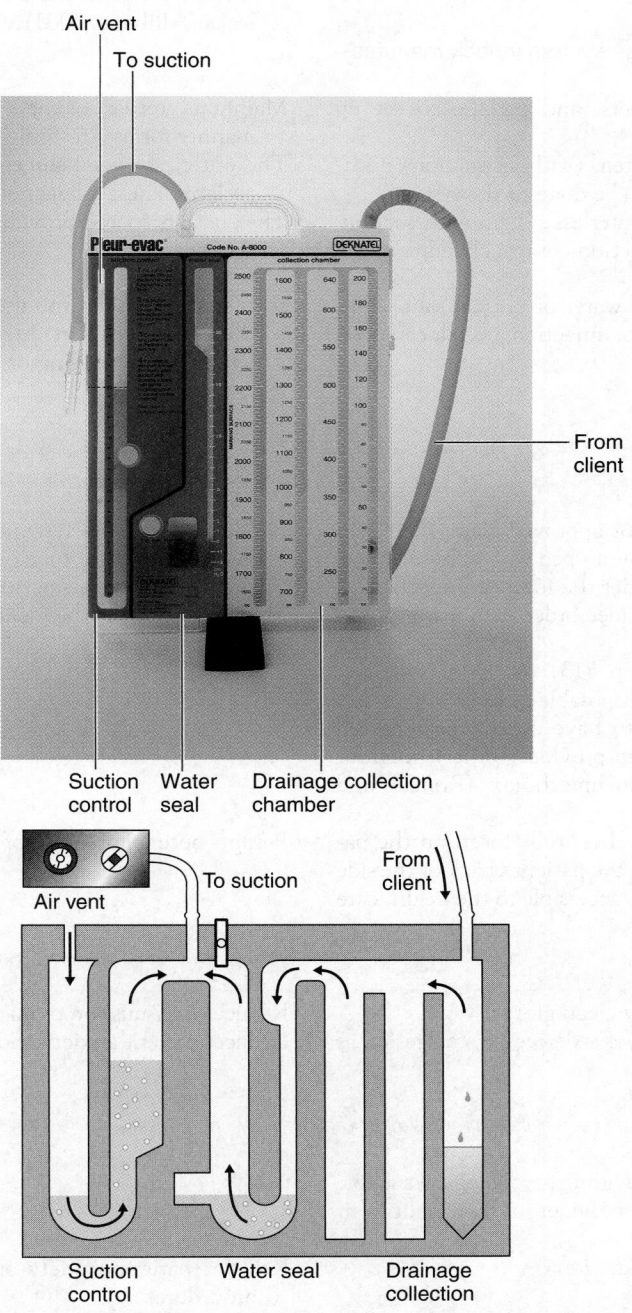

STEP 6a(2)(b)   *Top,* The Pleur-Evac drainage system, a commercial three-chamber chest drainage device. *Bottom,* Schematic of the drainage device.

STEP	RATIONALE
(c) *For a dry suction system:* Fill the water-seal chamber with 2 cm sterile water. Adjust the suction control dial to the prescribed level of suction; suction ranges from –10 to –40 cm of water pressure. The suction control chamber vent is never occluded when suction is used. NOTE: *On a dry suction system, DO NOT obstruct the positive pressure relief valve. This allows air to escape.*	The automatic control valve on the dry suction control device adjusts to changes in patient air leaks and fluctuation in suction source and vacuum to deliver the prescribe amount of suction (Roman and Mercado, 2006). Provides a safety factor of releasing excess negative pressure into the atmosphere through the suction control vent. Too little suction prevents lung reexpansion and increases patient's risk for infection, atelectasis, and tension pneumothorax. Too much suction damages the lung tissue and perpetuates existing air leaks (Allibone, 2003).
b Prepare a waterless drainage system (check manufacturer's guidelines):	
(1) Remove sterile wrappers, and prepare to set up equipment.	Maintains sterility of the system. The system is packaged in this manner for use in sterile operating room conditions.
(2) For a two-chamber system (without suction) nothing is added or needs to be done to the system.	The waterless two-chamber system is ready for connecting to the patient's chest tube after opening the wrappers.
(3) For a three-chamber waterless system with suction, connect tubing from suction control chamber to the suction source.	The suction source provides additional negative pressure to the system.
(4) Instill 15 mL of sterile water or normal saline into the diagnostic indicator injection port located on top of the system.	Instillation of water into the injection port enables observation of the rise and fall in the diagnostic air-leak window. Constant left-to-right bubbling or rocking is abnormal and may indicate an air leak.

Critical Decision Point   *This step is not necessary for mediastinal drainage because there will be no tidaling. Also, in an emergency it is not necessary because the system does not require water for setup.*

STEP	RATIONALE
7 Provide two shodded hemostats or approved clamps for each chest tube, attached to top of patient's bed with adhesive tape. Chest tubes are clamped only under the following specific circumstances per health care provider order or nursing policy and procedure:	Shodded hemostats have a covering to prevent hemostat from penetrating chest tube once changed. The application of these shodded hemostats or other clamps to a chest tube prevents air from reentering the pleural space (Allibone, 2003).
a To assess air leak (Table 26-2, p. 713)	
b To quickly empty or change disposable systems	
c To assess if patient is ready to have chest tube removed (which is done by health care provider's order); monitor the patient for recurrent pneumothorax (Roman and Mercado, 2006)	
8 Position the patient: During the chest tube insertion the patient will need to be positioned so the patient's back or the side in which the tube will be placed is accessible to the health care provider.	Permits optimal drainage of fluid and/or air.

IMPLEMENTATION

1 Perform hand hygiene, and apply clean gloves.	Reduces transmission of microorganisms.
2 Administer premedication, such as sedatives or analgesics, as ordered.	Reduces patient anxiety and pain during procedure.

Critical Decision Point   *During procedure carefully monitor patient for changes in level of sedation.*

3 Assist health care provider in providing psychological support to the patient. (See health care provider's responsibilities in Table 26-1, p. 712.)	
a Reinforce preprocedure explanation.	Reduces patient anxiety and assists in efficient completion of procedure.
b Coach and support patient throughout procedure.	

STEP	RATIONALE
4 Show local anesthetic to health care provider.	Allows health care provider to read label of drug before administering it to patient.
5 Hold anesthetic solution bottle upside down with label facing health care provider. Health care provider will withdraw solution and inject into patient's skin.	Allows health care provider to withdraw solution properly while maintaining surgical asepsis.
a Health care provider places chest tube. (A standard procedure is detailed in Table 26-1, p. 712.)	
6 Help health care provider attach drainage tube to chest tube.	Connects drainage system and suction (if ordered) to the chest tube.
7 After the chest tube is inserted, secure connection between chest tube and chest drainage system with waterproof adhesive tape. Tape all connections in a double spiral fashion with 1-inch adhesive tape; be sure not to totally obliterate view of drainage. (NOTE: Taping of the chest tube is usually done by the health care provider at time of tube placement; check agency policy.) Then:	Secures chest tube to drainage system and reduces risk for air leak causing breaks in airtight system.
a Check systems for proper functioning:	
(1) Clamp the drainage tubing that will connect the patient to the system.	Provides a chance to ensure an airtight system before connecting it to the patient. Allows correction or replacement of system if it is defective before connecting it to the patient.
(2) Connect tubing from the float ball chamber to the suction source.	NOTE: Bubbling will be seen at first because there is air in the tubing and system initially. This usually stops after a few minutes unless there are other sources of air entering the system.
(3) Turn on the suction to the prescribed level.	

Critical Decision Point *If bubbling continues, check connections and locate source of the air leak, as described in Table 26-2 (p. 713).*

STEP	RATIONALE
b Check chest tube placement with x-ray film.	Verifies chest tube placement.
8 Turn off suction source, and unclamp drainage tubing before connecting patient to the system.	Having the patient connected to suction when it is being inserted has the potential to damage pleural tissues from sudden increase in negative pressure. The suction source is turned on again after the patient is connected to the three-chamber system.
9 Check patency of air vents in system:	
a Confirm that water-seal vent is not occluded.	Permits the displaced air to pass into the atmosphere.
b Confirm that suction control chamber vent is not occluded when suction is used.	Provides safety factor of releasing excess negative pressure into the atmosphere.
c Confirm that valves are unobstructed.	Provides safety factor of releasing excess negative pressure.
NOTE: Waterless systems have relief valves without caps. For dry suction systems, the positive pressure relief valve must remain unobstructed.	
10 Lay excess tubing horizontally on mattress next to patient. Secure with a rubber band and safety pin or the system's clamp.	Prevents excess tubing from hanging over the edge of the mattress in a dependent loop. Drainage collected in the loop can occlude the drainage system, which predisposes patient to a tension pneumothorax (Roman and Mercado, 2006).
11 Adjust tubing to hang in a straight line from the chest tube to the drainage chamber.	Promotes drainage and prevents fluid or blood from accumulating in the pleural cavity.

Critical Decision Point *Frequent gentle lifting of sections of the drain allows gravity to assist blood and other viscous material to move to the drainage bottle. Patients with recent chest surgery or trauma need to have the chest drain lifted based on assessment of the amount of drainage; some patients might need chest tube drains lifted every 5 to 10 minutes until drainage volume decreases (Lehwaldt and Timmins, 2005). However, when coiled or dependent looping of tubing is unavoidable, the tubing is lifted every 15 minutes at a minimum to promote drainage (Allibone, 2003).*

Critical Decision Point *Check institutional policy before stripping or milking chest tubes (see Evidence-Based Practice section). This practice is being discontinued at most institutions because it is believed that stripping the tube greatly increases intrathoracic pressure, which damages the pleural tissue and causes or worsens an existing pneumothorax. However, even though the literature is contradictory, milking may be done in selected patients (e.g., fresh postoperative thoracic surgery in presence of multiple clots). The rationale for this selective use of stripping or milking is that the presence of clotted tube drainage causes decreased rate of reexpansion and increases risk for tension pneumothorax (Allibone, 2003). In these selected cases the benefits outweigh the risks.*

STEP	RATIONALE
12 Gently lift sections of the postoperative mediastinal chest tubes. Observe drainage for clots or debris in the tubing.	Maintains tubing in dependent position and facilitates drainage (Roman and Mercado, 2006).
13 After the tube is placed, assist patient to a comfortable position:	Reduces patient anxiety and promotes cooperation.
a Semi-Fowler's to high-Fowler's position to evacuate air (pneumothorax)	Air rises to the highest point in the chest. Pneumothorax tubes are usually placed on the anterior aspect at the mid-clavicular line, second or third intercostal space (Allibone, 2003).
b High-Fowler's position to drain fluid (hemothorax, pleural effusion)	Permits optimal drainage of fluid. Posterior tubes are placed on the mid-axillary line, fifth or sixth intercostal space.
14 Remove gloves, and dispose of used soiled equipment.	Prevents accidents involving contaminated equipment.
15 Perform hand hygiene.	Reduces spread of microorganisms.

EVALUATION

1 Monitor vital signs, oxygen saturation, and insertion site every 15 minutes for the first 2 hours.	Provides immediate information about procedure-related complications such as respiratory distress and leakage.
2 Monitor chest tube drainage:	
a Assessment after chest tube insertion is done every 15 minutes for the first 2 hours. This assessment interval then changes *on the basis of patient's status*. Mark the time and level of drainage on the calibrated write-on strip periodically.	Permits timely and efficient account of the amount of drainage from the chest tube. Drainage is marked at specified periods of time and documented in the nurses' notes and intake and output (I&O) sheet. Ensures early detection of complications.
b Observe type and amount of fluid drainage: Note color and amount of drainage, patient's vital signs, and skin color. Look at the fluid in the collection tubing, not just the fluid in the collection chamber. Is the drainage bright red, dark red, or pink? Is it opaque, or can you see through it?	
c *Expected drainage in the adult:* Less than 50 to 200 mL/hr immediately after surgery in a mediastinal chest tube. Approximately 500 mL in the first 24 hours.	Dark-red drainage is expected only during the immediate postoperative period. This drainage turns serous over time.
d *Expected drainage in the adult:* Between 100 and 300 mL of fluid may drain from a pleural tube during the first 3 hours after insertion. The 24-hour rate is 500 to 1000 mL. Drainage is grossly bloody during the first several hours after surgery and then changes to serous. Remember that a sudden gush of drainage may be retained (dark) blood and not active (bright red) bleeding. This increased drainage can result from patient position changes.	Reexpansion of the lungs forces drainage into the tube. Coughing can also cause large gushes of drainage or air. Acute bleeding indicates hemorrhage.

Critical Decision Point   *If drainage suddenly increases, is bright red, or there is more than 100 mL/hr of bloody drainage (except for the first 3 hours postoperatively), the nurse notifies the health care provider, remains with the patient, and assesses vital signs and cardiopulmonary status.*

3 Evaluate patient for decreased respiratory distress and chest pain, breath sounds over affected lung area, and change in oxygen saturation.	Increase in respiratory distress and/or chest pain, decrease in breath sounds over the affected and nonaffected lungs, marked cyanosis, asymmetrical chest movements, presence of subcutaneous emphysema around tube insertion site or neck, hypotension, tachycardia, and/or mediastinal shift are critical and indicate a severe change in patient status, such as excessive blood loss or tension pneumothorax (Allibone, 2003; Roman and others, 2003). Notify health care provider immediately.
4 Ask patient to rate level of comfort on a scale of 0 to 10.	Indicates need for analgesia. Patient with chest tube discomfort hesitates to take deep breaths and as a result is at risk for pneumonia and atelectasis.
5 Observe the drainage system:	
a Inspect chest tube dressing and drainage.	Ensures that dressing is occlusive.

Critical Decision Point   *Check the dressing carefully. It can come loose from the skin, although this may not be readily apparent.*

b Inspect tubing for kinks and dependent loops.	Straight and coiled drainage tube positions are optimal for pleural drainage. However, when dependent loop is unavoidable, periodic lifting and draining of the tube will also promote pleural drainage (Allibone, 2003; Lehwaldt and Timmons, 2005).

STEP	RATIONALE
c The chest drainage system remains upright and below level of tube insertion. Note presence of clots or debris in tubing.	Maintains proper functioning, facilitates drainage, and maintains the water seal.

Critical Decision Point *Monitor the position of the system relative to the chest tube carefully, especially during patient transport.*

STEP	RATIONALE
d Inspect water seal for fluctuations with patient's inspiration and expiration.	
(1) *Waterless system:* Diagnostic indicator for fluctuations with patient's inspirations and expirations.	In the non–mechanically ventilated patient, fluid rises in the water seal or diagnostic indicator with inspiration and falls with expiration. The opposite occurs in the patient who is mechanically ventilated. This indicates that the system is functioning properly (Lewis and others, 2008).
(2) *Water-seal system:* Bubbling in the water-seal chamber (see Table 26-2, p. 713).	When system is initially connected to the patient, bubbles are expected from the chamber. These are from air that was present in the system and in the patient's intrapleural space. After a short time the bubbling stops. Fluid continues to fluctuate in the water seal on inspiration and expiration until the lung is reexpanded or the system becomes occluded.
(3) *Water-seal system:* Bubbling in the suction control chamber (when suction is being used) (see Table 26-2, p. 713).	Suction control chamber has constant, gentle bubbling. Tubing to the suction source remains free of obstruction, and the suction source is turned to the appropriate setting.
e *Waterless system:* Bubbling in diagnostic indicator.	Mechanism to observe for the presence of tidaling. Character of drainage indicates if normal or if infection or hemorrhage is developing.
f *Waterless system:* The suction control (float ball) indicates the amount of suction the patient's intrapleural space is receiving.	The suction float ball dictates the amount of suction in the system. The float ball allows no more suction than dictated by its setting. If the suction source is set too low, the suction float ball cannot reach the prescribed setting. In this case the suction is increased for the float ball to reach the prescribed setting.
6 After first 2 hours, assess patient's physical and psychological status at least every 4 hours or according to agency policy.	Detects early signs and symptoms of complications: *Apprehension:* Increase in patient anxiety, restlessness, and inability to concentrate *Respiratory distress:* Alteration in rate and/or depth of respirations, difficulty breathing, and breath sounds *Subcutaneous emphysema:* Air that is being trapped in the subcutaneous tissue

Unexpected Outcomes	Related Interventions
1 Air leak unrelated to patient's respirations occurs.	• Locate source (see Table 26-2, p. 713). • Notify health care provider.
2 There is no chest tube drainage.	• Observe for kink in chest drainage system. • Observe for possible clot in chest drainage system. • Observe for mediastinal shift or respiratory distress (medical emergency). • Notify health care provider.
3 Chest tube is dislodged.	• Immediately apply pressure over chest tube insertion site. • Have assistant apply occlusive gauze dressing, and tape three sides. • Notify health care provider.
4 Substantial increase in bright red drainage occurs.	• Obtain vital signs. • Monitor drainage. • Assess patient's cardiopulmonary status. • Notify health care provider.
5 Continuous bubbling is seen in water-sealed chamber, indicating leak between patient and water seal.	• Tighten loose connections. • Check agency policy, and if instructed, cross-clamp chest tube closer to patient's chest. If bubbling stops, air leak is inside patient's thorax or at chest tube insertion site. • Unclamp chest tube. • Reinforce dressing. • Notify health care provider.

Recording and Reporting

- Record level of patient comfort, baseline vital signs, including oxygen saturation. If postoperative patient, record vital signs and oxygen saturation every 15 minutes for at least 2 hours postoperatively. Record chest drainage output hourly for at least 2 hours, and then record as patient status indicates. Document time, type, and amount of drainage. Record integrity of chest suction system (e.g., record the amount of bubbling in the water-seal suction control chamber, level of suction, intactness of system).
- Report patient response to chest tube insertion or continuation, noting level of comfort, drainage, and intactness of the system.

Teaching Considerations

- Instruct patient and family regarding proper functioning of chest tube and drainage system.
- Instruct patient to immediately report any changes in chest comfort.

Pediatric Considerations

- If possible, using pictures and special dolls, familiarize child and family with equipment before inserting chest drainage system (Hockenberry and Wilson, 2007).
- Allow child to play with equipment and special dolls before inserting chest drainage system.
- Chest tube drainage greater than 3 mL/kg/hr for more than 2 consecutive hours is excessive and may indicate postoperative hemorrhage (Hockenberry and Wilson, 2007).

Gerontological Considerations

- Fragility of the older adult's skin requires special care and planning for management of chest tube dressing. Frequently assess surrounding skin for signs of skin breakdown (Meiner and Lueckenotte, 2006).

Home Care Considerations

- Patients with chronic conditions (e.g., uncomplicated pneumothorax, effusions, empyema) that require long-term chest tube may be discharged with smaller mobile drains (Carroll, 2002, 2005).
- Instruct patient in how to ambulate and remain active with a mobile chest tube drainage system.
- Instruct patient and caregivers in when to contact health care professionals regarding changes in the drainage system (e.g., chest pain, breathlessness, change in color or amount of drainage, leakage on the dressing around the chest tube).
- Provide patient and caregiver information specific to the type of drain, and when possible have patient demonstrate proper maintenance of the mobile drainage system. Most of these systems do not have a suction control chamber and use a mechanical one-way valve instead of a water-seal chamber. For example, if a one-way flutter valve is used, the arrow on the housing must always point away from the patient. Otherwise there is a risk for air trapping and a recurrent pneumothorax. The Pneumostat and Express Mini mobile devices have built-in collection chambers, and the Express Mini uses dry suction set at -20 cm H_2O (Carroll, 2005).

TABLE 26-1	Physician's or Advanced Practice Nurse's Role in Chest Tube Placement
Role	**Purpose**
Explain purpose, procedure, and possible complications to the patient, and have patient sign consent form.	Provides informed consent.
Have pain medication available to administer before or immediately after chest tube insertion as appropriate according to patient's condition.	Analgesia improves patient comfort throughout the procedure and assists patient in taking appropriate deep breaths to promote lung reexpansion and drainage of fluid in the pleural space.
Perform hand hygiene. Cleanse chest wall with antiseptic.	Reduces transmission of microorganisms.
Apply mask and gloves.	Maintains surgical asepsis.
Drape area of chest tube insertion with sterile towels.	Maintains surgical asepsis.
Inject local anesthetic, and allow time to take effect.	Decreases pain during procedure.
Make a small incision over the rib space where tube is to be inserted. Thread a clamped chest tube through the incision. Health care provider clamps chest tube until system is connected to water seal.	Inserts chest tube into the intrapleural space. Clamping prevents entry of atmospheric air into the chest and worsening of the pneumothorax.
Suture chest tube in place, if suturing is policy or health care provider preference.	Secures chest tube in place.
Cover the chest tube insertion site with sterile 4 × 4 inch gauze and large dressing to form an occlusive dressing supported with an elastic bandage (Elastoplast). Sterile petrolatum gauze is used around the tube.	Holds chest tube in place and occludes site around chest tube. Helps stabilize chest tube and holds dressing tightly in place. Sterile petrolatum gauze helps prevent air leak.
Water-Seal System	
Remove connector cover from patient's end of chest drainage tubing with sterile technique. Secure drainage tubing to the chest tube and drainage system.	Health care provider is responsible for making certain that the system is set up properly, the proper amount of water is in the water seal, the dressing is secure, and the chest tube is securely connected to the drainage system.

TABLE 26-1	Physician's or Advanced Practice Nurse's Role in Chest Tube Placement—cont'd

Water-Seal Suction

Connect system to suction, or supervise a nurse connecting it to suction, if suction is to be used.	The health care provider is responsible for determining and checking the amount of fluid that is to be added to the suction control chamber and prescribing the suction setting.

Waterless System

Remove connector cover from patient's end of chest drainage tubing with sterile technique. Secure drainage tubing to the chest tube and drainage system.	Health care provider is responsible for making certain that the system is set up properly and the chest tube is securely connected to the drainage system.

Waterless Suction

Turn on suction source. Set float ball level to prescribed setting.	Health care provider is responsible for prescribing level of float ball and prescribing the suction setting.
The health care provider or nurse adds sterile water or normal saline to diagnostic indicator.	Allows quick assurance that the system is functioning properly. Connects chest tube to drainage.
Unclamp the chest tube.	Verifies correct chest tube placement.
In both systems the health care provider orders and reviews chest x-ray studies.	

TABLE 26-2	Troubleshooting With Chest Tubes

Assessment	Intervention
Air leak can occur at insertion site, connection between tube and drainage, or within drainage device itself. Determine when the air leak occurs during respiratory cycle (e.g. inspiration or expiration). Continuous bubbling is noted in water-seal chamber, and water seal indicates a leak during the inspiratory and expiratory phases (Cerfolio, 2005).	Check all connections between the chest tube and drainage system. Locate leak by clamping tube at different intervals along the tube. Leaks are corrected when constant bubbling stops. If present on chest drainage system, such as the Sahara S 1100a Pleur-Evac, observe the air leak meter to determine the size of the leak.
Assess for location of leak by clamping chest tube with two rubber-shod or toothless clamps close to the chest wall. If bubbling stops, air leak is inside patient's thorax or at chest insertion site.	Unclamp tube, reinforce chest dressing, and notify health care provider immediately. Leaving chest tube clamped can cause collapse of lung, mediastinal shift, and eventual collapse of other lung from buildup of air pressure within the pleural cavity.
If bubbling continues with the clamps near the chest wall, gradually move one clamp at a time down drainage tubing away from patient and toward suction control chamber. When bubbling stops, leak is in section of tubing or connection between the clamps.	Replace tubing, or secure connection and release clamps.
If bubbling still continues, this indicates the leak is in the drainage system.	Change the drainage system. Make sure chest tubes are patent: remove clamps, eliminate kinks, or eliminate occlusion.
Assess for tension pneumothorax; indicated by: • Severe respiratory distress • Low oxygen saturation • Chest pain • Absence of breath sounds on affected side • Tracheal shift to unaffected side • Hypotension and signs of shock • Tachycardia	Obstructed chest tubes trap air in intrapleural space when air leak originates within the thorax. Notify health care provider immediately, and prepare for another chest tube insertion. A one-way flutter (Heimlich) valve or large-gauge needle may be used for short-term emergency release of pressure in the intrapleural space. Have emergency equipment, oxygen, and code cart available because condition is life threatening.
Water-seal tube is no longer submerged in sterile fluid due to evaporation.	Add sterile water to water-seal chamber until distal tip is 2 cm under surface level.

SKILL 26-2 Assisting With Removal of Chest Tubes

NSO *Chest Tubes Module / Lesson 4*

Actual removal of a chest tube is the function of health care providers and advanced practice nurses (APNs). If nurses are to remove a chest tube, this procedure is part of the agency's policy and procedure standards. This skill details nursing responsibilities and health care provider action for chest tube removal.

Prepare the patient for chest tube removal by (1) assessing the need for preremoval analgesia and obtaining the required medication orders and (2) instructing the patient about the process and what will be requested of the patient (Freisner and others, 2006; Milgrom and others, 2004). During removal of the chest tube, it is important to instruct the patient to take a deep breath and hold it until the tube is removed. This maneuver prevents air from being sucked into the chest as the tube is pulled out and an occlusive dressing is applied.

Delegation Considerations

The skill of assisting with removal of chest tubes cannot be delegated to NAP. However, following chest tube removal certain aspects of care can be delegated. The nurse directs the NAP to:

- Immediately report to the nurse any patient sensations of shortness of breath, increased chest pain, dizziness, or increased anxiety.
- Report to the nurse any drainage or an occlusive dressing.

Equipment

- ❏ Suture set
- ❏ Sterile scissors
- ❏ Sterile forceps
- ❏ Clean gloves
- ❏ Sterile gloves
- ❏ Face mask/face shield
- ❏ Prepared sterile dressing: petrolatum-impregnated gauze, 4 × 4 inch gauze dressings, and large dressings
- ❏ 4-inch adhesive tape or elastic bandage (Elastoplast) cut into strips
- ❏ Stethoscope, sphygmomanometer, pulse oximeter

STEP	RATIONALE

ASSESSMENT

1 Assess status of patient's lung reexpansion:	
a Provide health care provider with results of chest x-ray film.	Reveals position of lung tissue in chest cavity and whether sufficient lung reexpansion has occurred.
b Note trend in water-seal fluctuation over last 24 hours. Determine if bubbling is present.	Pleura of the expanded lung seals the holes on the internal tip of the chest tube, halting fluctuation in the water seal. A halt in fluctuation for 24 hours indicates lung is expanded. When bubbling is present, this usually indicates that the lung has not fully expanded.
c Confirm that drainage has decreased to less than 50 mL/day.	Pleural drainage was removed, allowing the lung to reexpand.
d Percuss lung for resonance.	Normal resonance occurs with reexpansion.
e Auscultate lung sounds.	Normal breath sounds are heard bilaterally with reexpansion.
2 Assess patient's level of comfort using a 0 to 10 scale, and determine when the last analgesic medication was given.	Presence of chest tubes is painful, and patient frequently requires analgesic medication. It is important to note the last dose of the medication. Chest tube removal is painful, and additional analgesia or breathing exercises may be necessary (Allibone, 2003; Freisner and others, 2006).
3 Determine patient's understanding of the chest tube removal procedure.	Assists in determining what the patient needs to know about the procedure and assists in reducing anxiety.
4 Clamp chest tube before removal as ordered by the health care provider. Assess for changes in vital signs, oxygen saturation, chest pain, apprehension, and symptoms of tension pneumothorax.	Health care provider orders tube clamping before removal to assess patient's tolerance (Roman and Mercado, 2006).

Critical Decision Point *If the patient develops respiratory distress when the tube is clamped, assess the patient, unclamp the tube, reestablish suction, and immediately notify health care provider (Roman and Mercado, 2006).*

NURSING DIAGNOSES

- Acute pain
- Anxiety
- Risk for impaired gas exchange

Individualize related factors based on patient's condition or needs.

STEP	RATIONALE

PLANNING

1 Expected outcomes following completion of procedure:
   • Lung reexpansion is maintained.
   • Patient does not experience discomfort.
   • Spontaneous healing of chest tube insertion site occurs after removal of tube without infection or other complications.
2 Explain procedure to patient.
3 Verify analgesia orders before chest tube removal.

Source of air or fluid loss is sealed or has healed.
Pain management is achieved.
Large nonporous occlusive dressing at puncture site promotes uncomplicated healing.
Reduces anxiety and promotes patient cooperation.
Anticipatory management of pain related to chest tube removal reduces patient's anxiety and assists patient in taking the required deep breath. After procedure, the patient will be able to deep breathe and cough and move more effectively (Milgrom and others, 2004).

IMPLEMENTATION

1 Administer prescribed medication for pain relief about 30 minutes before procedure.

Reduces discomfort and relaxes patient. Medication reaches peak effect at time of tube removal. Patients do report sensations ranging from pain to pulling when the chest tube is removed (Allibone, 2003; Milgrom and others, 2004).

2 Perform hand hygiene, and apply gloves and face shield if needed.

Reduces transmission of microorganisms.

3 Assist patient in sitting on edge of bed or lying supine or on the side without chest tubes.

Health care provider prescribes patient's position to facilitate tube removal.

4 Health care provider or APN prepares an occlusive dressing of petrolatum-impregnated gauze on a pressure dressing and sets it aside on a sterile field, and applies sterile gloves.

Essential to prepare in advance for quick application to the wound on tube withdrawal.

5 Support patient physically and emotionally while health care provider or APN removes dressing and clips sutures.

Patients state that when they know the tube is being pulled, they can mentally prepare themselves for the procedure. Support from the health care team reduces anxiety and promotes cooperation.

6 Health care provider or APN asks the patient to take a deep breath and hold it or exhale completely and hold it.

Prevents air from being sucked into the chest as the tube is removed (Roman and Mercado, 2006). A complication associated with removal of chest tubes is recurrent pneumothorax, which results from atmospheric air reentering the pleural cavity. This occurs when the patient inhales during tube removal (Allibone, 2003).

7 Health care provider or APN quickly pulls out the chest tube and tightens and ties purse string suture if present. After which the patient is instructed to breathe normally.

This forms an airtight seal and prevents entry of air through the chest wound. Sutures aid in skin closure.

8 Aseptically apply sterile occlusive dressing over the wound, and firmly secure it in position with elastic bandage (Elastoplast) or wide tape.

Keeps wound aseptic. Prevents entry of air into the chest. Wound closure occurs spontaneously.

9 Assist patient to a comfortable position.

Assists in patient's return to a comfortable status. Patients report that proper positioning and rest following chest tube removal assists in relief of procedure-related sensations of pain and pulling (Milgrom and others, 2004).

10 Remove used equipment from bedside. Place it in appropriate area for medical waste products.

Prevents spread of microorganisms.

11 Remove gloves, and perform hand hygiene.

Reduces transmission of microorganisms.

EVALUATION

1 Auscutate lung sounds. Palpate over lung where tube was inserted, and observe patient for subcutaneous emphysema. Evaluate for respiratory distress immediately after tube removal and during the first few hours after removal.

Provides for early notification of health care provider if adverse symptoms occur. Chest tubes may need reinsertion. Subcutaneous emphysema results from the entrance of air into the subcutaneous space. It is painful, and as a result, patients may not take full lung expansion.

Critical Decision Point   *If air is heard escaping from the chest tube site, reinforce the occlusive dressing and immediately notify health care provider.*

STEP	RATIONALE
2 Evaluate patient's vital signs, oxygen saturation, pulmonary status, and psychological status.	Detects early signs and symptoms of complications.
3 Review chest x-ray film.	Identifies early signs of incomplete lung expansion.
4 Ask about the patient's level of pain or comfort. Observe for nonverbal cues of pain, and assess level of discomfort on a scale of 0 to 10.	Indicates that the wound did not close well. Determines patient's tolerance of procedure.
5 Check chest dressing for drainage and patency. When changing dressing, note wound for signs of healing.	Ensures occlusion and proper healing of chest wound.

Unexpected Outcomes

1   Dyspnea, labored respirations

Related Interventions

- Potential recurrence of pneumothorax, hemothorax, or effusion.
- Notify health care provider, obtain vital signs and oxygen saturation, and remain with patient.
- Prepare for possible chest tube reinsertion.

Recording and Reporting

- Record removal of tube, amount of drainage in the collection bottle, appearance of wound and dressing, and patient's response. Patient's response also includes vital signs and respiratory assessment.
- Report patient's response to chest tube removal to next shift.

Teaching Considerations

- Instruct patient and family to immediately report signs of chest pain, shortness of breath, or sensations of chest discomfort.

Pediatric Considerations

- Pediatric patients usually require analgesia (e.g., morphine sulfate 0.1 mg/kg in combination with midazolam [Versed]) before the chest tube removal (Hockenberry and Wilson, 2007).
- EMLA (locally applied anesthetic patch) placed under the occlusive dressing at the chest tube insertion site 1 hour before tube removal reduces pain of procedure. However, child may still feel the "pulling" sensation of tube removal (Hockenberry and Wilson, 2007).

SKILL 26-3   Reinfusion of Chest Tube Drainage

Reinfusion of chest tube drainage into the patient's circulatory system is widely used because the public has become aware of the risks associated with blood transfusions. When reinfusion is linked with chest drainage, it is a relatively risk-free, inexpensive, and easy method of replacing mediastinal blood previously lost during emergencies and open heart or thoracic surgery. Patients requiring this skill must also have an IV line in place (see Chapter 31). Reinfusion is contraindicated in patients with coagulation disorders; pericardial, mediastinal, or systemic infections; pulmonary infections; malignant neoplasms; contaminated thoracoabdominal cavities; or intraoperative thoracic or mediastinal cavity use of topical thrombin, microfibrillar hemostatic agents, or povidone-iodine gels or solutions (Atrium, 2004).

Delegation Considerations

The skill of reinfusion of chest tube drainage cannot be delegated to NAP. The nurse directs the NAP to:

- Immediately inform nurse of changes in patient's vital signs or SpO$_2$ levels.
- Immediately inform nurse about increased drainage from mediastinal tube.
- Immediately inform nurse about decreased drainage from mediastinal tube.

Equipment

- ❏ Adult/pediatric single-use chest drainage and autotransfusion unit (Fig. 26-9)
- ❏ *Optional:* Continuous autotransfusion system (ATS) with a blood-compatible infusion pump (check agency policy)

- ❏ Microaggregate blood filter (40-μm filter, see manufacturer's instructions)
- ❏ Nonvented blood-compatible IV administration set
- ❏ Infusion pump (see manufacturer's instructions)
- ❏ Replacement bag
- ❏ Gown, clean gloves, and mask as needed

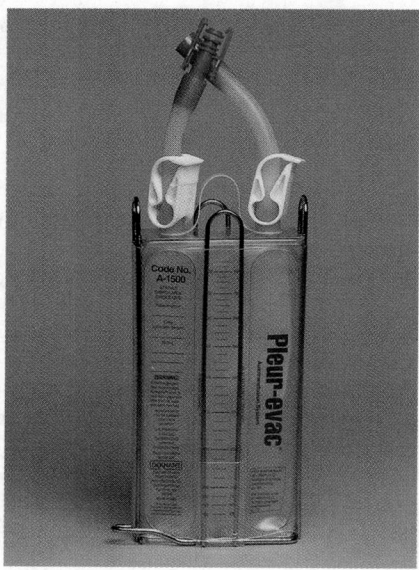

FIG 26-9   Example of autotransfusion unit.

STEP	RATIONALE

ASSESSMENT

1 See Assessment for Skill 26-1.
2 Determine presence of active bleeding, at least 50 to 100 mL/hr through mediastinal tube. — Indicates the need for possible reinfusion of mediastinal tube drainage.

> **Critical Decision Point** *Collected blood never remains in the chest drain or ATS blood bag for more than 6 hours before autotransfusion (Atrium, 2004).*

3 Assess IV site (see Chapter 28); note size of IV catheter. — Determines presence of adequate and patent IV site for the administration of blood products (e.g., 18-gauge angiocatheter).
4 Obtain baseline laboratory data (e.g., hemoglobin and hematocrit). — Provides data to measure the effectiveness of the reinfusion of chest drainage on the patient's circulating blood volume.

NURSING DIAGNOSES

- Decreased cardiac output
- Ineffective peripheral tissue perfusion
- Risk for infection

Individualize related factors based on patient's condition or needs.

PLANNING

1 Expected outcomes following completion of procedure:
- Vital signs, hematocrit, and hemoglobin will stabilize. — Reinfusion reduces significant blood loss associated with closed chest drainage.
- The drainage system will function correctly, and the lung will reexpand in 48 to 72 hours. — Negative pressure will have been reestablished in the intrapleural space.
- The IV line will remain patent. — A patent IV is necessary for reinfusion of cleansed mediastinal tube drainage.

2 Explain procedure to patient. — Reduces anxiety and promotes patient cooperation.

IMPLEMENTATION

1 System setup
  a Set up the ATS according to technique that maintains the sterility of the unit and following the three steps printed on the front of the unit. — Contamination of the unit provides a ready source of infection to patient.
  b Make certain all connections are tight and all clamps are open. — Tight connections ensure an airtight system, and open clamps allow chest drainage to enter the ATS bag.
  c A 200-μm double-sided mesh filter is located in the ATS bag to filter the drainage. — Filtering the drainage removes extraneous materials and microemboli.
  d The ATS collection bag has a capacity of 1000 mL marked in increments of 25 mL and an area for marking times and amounts. — *Expected drainage in the adult:* Less than 50 to 200 mL/hr immediately after surgery in a mediastinal chest tube. Approximately 500 mL in the first 24 hours. Dark-red drainage is expected only during the immediate postoperative period. This drainage turns serous over time.

> **Critical Decision Point** *Continuous ATS is prescribed following cardiac surgery. This is a closed system with a specific infusion pump and IV circuit. This system requires specific education and is used in selected situations (Atrium, 2004). Check agency policy.*

2 Perform hand hygiene, and apply gloves. — Reduces transmission of microorganisms.
3 Prepare chest drainage for reinfusion:
  a Following manufacturer's directions, open a replacement bag, and close the two white clamps. — Contamination of the unit provides a ready source of contamination to the patient. The closed clamps maintain a closed system during replacement.
  b Use the high-negativity relief valve to reduce excessive negativity. — This eases the removal of the initial collection bag from the metal support stand.
  c Bag transfer:
     (1) Close clamp on chest drainage tubing. — Prevents air from entering the chest cavity through the tube and collapsing the lung.
     (2) Close the clamps on the top of the initial ATS collection bag. — Maintains a closed system for the reinfusion, preventing contamination of the blood.
     (3) Connect the chest drainage tube to the new ATS bag. — Establishes a new autotransfusion system.
     (4) Make certain that all connections are tight. — Ensures an airtight system.
     (5) Open all clamps on chest drainage tube and replacement bag. — Reestablishes an autotransfusion collection system.

STEP	RATIONALE
d Connect the connectors on top of the initial collection bag, and remove it by lifting it from the side hook and then from the foot hook.	Maintains a closed system within the bag and removes it for use in autotransfusion.
e Secure the replacement bag by connecting the foot hook, replacing the metal frame into the side hook of the chest drainage unit, and pushing down to secure the frame onto the hook.	Provides safe attachment of the replacement bag to the chest drainage unit.
f Place the thumbs on the top of the metal frame, and push up with the fingers to slide the bag out; remove the replacement bag.	
4 Reinfuse chest drainage:	
a Use a new microaggregate filter to reinfuse each autotransfusion bag.	Prevents the infusion of microemboli and provides maximal filtration for each bag.
b Access the bag by inverting it and spiking the bag through the spike port with the microaggregate filter and twisting.	Connects the autotransfusion bag to the transfusion tubing.
c With the bag upside down, gently squeeze the bag to remove the air, and prime the filter with blood.	Gentle pressure is used to prevent hemolysis.
d Hang the bag on an IV pole, and continue to prime the tubing until all air is gone. Clamp the tubing, attach it to the patient's IV access, and adjust the clamp to deliver the reinfusion at the appropriate rate.	Removes all air from the transfusion tubing. Reinfusion delivered either by gravity, application of a blood cuff (not to exceed 150 mm Hg pressure), or a blood-compatible IV pump (see Chapter 28).
e If ordered, anticoagulants (Anticoagulant Citrate Dextrose Solution-A or Citrate Phosphate Dextrose Solution, USP) are added to the reinfusion through the self-sealing port in the autotransfusion connector.	Prevents clotting in the autotransfusion. Reversing heparin with protamine to preoperative levels or collection of nonheparinized blood following emergency chest trauma may require a citrate anticoagulant (Atrium, 2004).
f Monitor patient's vital signs and SpO$_2$ according to patient condition and agency policy. For some patients this may be as frequent as every 15 minutes; for other patients it may be every hour.	Patients who require autotransfusion usually have complex physiological needs, and their vital signs change quite rapidly. Consistent, frequent monitoring allows for timely identification of changes and initiation of appropriate interventions to restore physiological stability.
5 Discontinue autotransfusion:	
a Clamp the chest drainage tube, and connect it directly to the chest drainage unit with the red and blue connectors.	Prevents air from entering the chest cavity through the tube and collapsing the lung.
b Open the chest drainage tube clamp.	All drainage will be collected directly in the drainage unit and appropriately discarded.
6 Discard used supplies, and perform hand hygiene.	Reduces transmission of microorganisms.

EVALUATION

1 Monitor vital signs, hematocrit, and hemoglobin.	Helps determine the effects of the treatment.
2 Monitor chest drainage system and patient's lung sounds.	Helps determine the proper functioning of the system and its effectiveness.
3 Evaluate the IV infusion site for infiltration and phlebitis.	A patent IV infusion site is maintained.

Unexpected Outcomes	Related Interventions
1 Chest tube is displaced.	• Immediately apply pressure over chest tube insertion site. • Have assistant apply sterile petrolatum-impregnated occlusive dressing. • Notify health care provider.
2 Patient has dyspnea, chest pain, and labored respirations.	• Verify that chest tube is patent and draining. • Obtain vital signs. • Notify health care provider.
3 Patient has signs of infection, fever, and chills.	• Obtain wound cultures as ordered. • Obtain vital signs.

Recording and Reporting

- Record drainage and reinfusion with times and amounts of each. Describe condition of IV infusion site.
- Report unusual findings and patient responses to nurse in charge or health care provider.

Teaching Considerations

- Prepare patient and family for the procedure so they will understand when the patient's blood from the previous mediastinal drainage is reinfused. Patients and their families may have had this instruction preoperatively and need reinforcement. Patients who have had emergent thoracic surgery will need more in-depth and frequent information.

CRITICAL THINKING EXERCISES

Mr. Robert is in his first postoperative day following open heart surgery. He has pleural and mediastinal chest tubes to drainage. His last vital signs were blood pressure (BP), 110/64 mm Hg; pulse, 126 beats per minute; respirations on mechanical ventilator, 16 breaths per minute; SpO₂, 90%; temperature, 99.0° F (rectally). The last hourly chest tube drainage was 75 mL from the pleural tube and 100 mL from the mediastinal tube.

1 Why is it important to check vital signs, check for air leaks, and note the amount of chest drainage every 15 to 30 minutes for at least 2 hours after he returns from surgery?

2 Mr. Robert's chest tube drainage ranged from 75 to 100 mL from both chest tubes over the last 3 hours. What measures do you take to maintain chest tube patency?

3 It is now 12 hours after surgery, and Mr. Robert is transferred from bed to chair. Immediately following this transfer you note drainage of 50 mL of dark red fluid. What are your actions?

4 Mr. Robert is discharged to the step-down area. His chest tube is out. Your assessment of this patient noted that the dressing over the puncture site was occlusive and without visible drainage. Vital signs were stable; patient was free of pain and sitting in a chair. The nursing assistive personnel tell you he is "breathing funny." You immediately reassess Mr. Robert and find your patient is in respiratory distress. His vital signs are BP, 90/60 mm Hg; pulse, 120 beats per minute; respirations, 32 breaths per minute; and SpO₂, 82%. Mr. Robert complains of severe chest pain and is pale. What are your actions?

 REVIEW QUESTIONS

1 The nurse is caring for a patient with a new chest tube. The patient is anxious and fearful of taking pain medications because he knows he needs to be active, take deep breaths, and cough. He feels that taking pain medications will make him sleepy. The nurse's actions include:
   1 Telling him that the medication will not make him sleepy
   2 Explaining that by controlling pain he will be able to be active and cough well
   3 Notifying his physician
   4 Giving him the medication anyway

2 A postoperative thoracotomy patient complains of increased sharp chest pain. The nurse's assessment reveals an increased respiratory rate, increased pulse rate, and increased anxiety. When assessing the chest tube system, the nurse notes the water-seal chamber of the collection tubing is empty. The patient's chest pain is due to:
   1 Improper function of the chest tube system
   2 Improved pneumothorax
   3 Tension pneumothorax
   4 Incisional pain

3 Patients with chest tubes that assist in the removal of bloody drainage from the chest cavity have many care priorities. Two important priorities related to management of the chest tube system include:
   1 Monitoring chest tube drainage and maintaining chest tube patency
   2 Monitoring chest tube drainage and promoting activity
   3 Promoting airway clearance and maintaining chest tube patency
   4 Promoting activity and airway clearance

4 Patients who have a pneumothorax have which type of chest tubes?
   1 Pleural tubes placed in the second or third intercostal space
   2 Pleural tubes placed in the fifth or sixth intercostal space
   3 Pleural tubes placed laterally
   4 Pleural tubes placed posteriorly

5 The nurse is caring for a patient with a chest tube to treat a pneumothorax. His tube and occlusive dressing become dislodged. The nurse's immediate action is to:
   1 Call for help and take vital signs
   2 Take vital signs and perform a pulmonary assessment
   3 Place an occlusive dressing over chest tube site and take vital signs
   4 Notify the physician and prepare to insert a new chest tube

REFERENCES

Allibone L: Nursing management of chest drains, *Nurs Stand* 17(22):45, 2003.
Allibone L: Assessment and management of patients with pleural effusions, *Nurs Stand* 20(22):55, 2006.
Atrium: *Managing chest drainage-autotransfusion*, Hudson, NH, 2004, Atrium, Welcome to Atrium, last accessed August 2007.
Carroll P: A guide to mobile chest drains, *RN* 65(5):56, 2002.
Carroll P: Keeping up with mobile chest drains, *RN* 68(10):27, 2005.
Hockenberry MJ and Wilson D: *Nursing care of infants and children*, ed 8, St. Louis, 2007, Mosby.
Leigh-Smith S, Harris T: Tension pneumothorax—time for a re-think, *Emerg Med J* 22(8):8, 2005.
Lewis ML and others: *Medical-surgical nursing: assessment and management of clinical problems*, ed 7, St. Louis, 2008, Mosby.
Light LW: *Pleural diseases*, ed 5, Philadelphia, Lippincott Williams & Wilkins, 2007.
Meiner S, Lueckenotte AG: *Gerontologic nursing*, ed 3, St. Louis, 2006, Mosby.
Rieger KM and others: Postoperative outpatient chest tube management: initial experience with a new portable system, *Ann Thorac Surg* 84:630, 2007.
Roman M, Mercado D: Review of chest tube use, *Medsurg Nurs* 15(1):41, 2006.
Roman M and others: Primary spontaneous pneumothorax, *Medsurg Nurs* 12(3):161, 2003.
The Joint Commission: *2008 National Patient Safety Goals Hospital Program*, http://www.jointcommission,org,accessed August 2007, 2007, Oakbrook Terrace, IL, The Commission.

RESEARCH REFERENCES

Cerfolio RJ: Recent advances in the treatment of air leaks, *Curr Opin Pulm Med* 11:319, 2005
Coote N, Kay E: Surgical versus non-surgical management of pleural empyema, *Cochrane Database Syst Rev* 2005(4):CD001956, DOI:10.1002/14651858.CD001956.pub2.
Coughlin AM, Parchinsky C: Go with the flow of chest tube therapy, *Nursing* 36(3):36, 2006.
Freisner SA and others: Comparison of two pain-management strategies during chest tube removal: relaxation exercise with opioids and opioids alone, *Heart Lung* 35:269, 2006.
Lehwaldt D, Timmins F: Nurses' knowledge of chest drain care: an exploratory descriptive study, *Nurs Crit Care* 10(4):192, 2005.
Marshall MB and others. Suction vs water seal after pulmonary resection: a randomized prospective study, *Chest* 121(3):831, 2002.
Milgrom LB and others: Pain levels experienced with activities after cardiac surgery, *Am J Crit Care* 13(2):116, 2004.

KEY TERMS

Advance directive
Automated external defibrillator (AED)
Bag-mask device
Cardiopulmonary resuscitation (CPR)
Code event
Do not resuscitate (DNR)
Dysrhythmia
Endotracheal intubation
Manual defibrillator
Oral airway

MEDIA RESOURCES

- **evolve** learning system   http://evolve.elsevier.com/Perry/skills
  - Review Questions

OBJECTIVES

Mastery of content in this chapter will enable the nurse to:

- Discuss indications for oral airway insertion.
- Identify need for automated external defibrillator (AED) application and indications for use.

- State indications for cardiopulmonary resuscitation (CPR).
- Discuss code management.
- State the end points for CPR.
- Demonstrate in a laboratory or clinical situation: insertion of an oral airway, use of an AED, and performance of CPR.

Life is dependent on the adequacy of oxygen transport to the body's tissues. Oxygen transport depends on the health of the respiratory and cardiovascular systems that power three mechanisms: ventilation, diffusion, and perfusion. Ventilation is the movement of oxygen and carbon dioxide into and out of the lungs. Diffusion is the movement of oxygen and carbon dioxide into and out of cells and tissues. The final mechanism to ensure oxygen delivery is perfusion or blood flow to the tissues. Anytime one or more of these three mechanisms fail, a cardiopulmonary arrest may occur.

Cardiopulmonary arrests are emergency situations that you must be prepared to handle at any time. During an arrest, ventilation and/or perfusion becomes limited. Respiratory arrest, or cessation of ventilation, results in the absence of oxygen delivery to the alveoli. Causes of a respiratory arrest include airway obstruction, cardiopulmonary illnesses, traumatic injury, or exposure to toxic substances. Early intervention in a respiratory arrest usually prevents a cardiac arrest.

Cardiac arrest is the cessation of circulating blood flow, which halts oxygen delivery to the tissues. Many cardiac arrests are caused by irregular heart rhythms known as dysrhythmias. The causes of dysrhythmias may include electrolyte disturbances (potassium, magnesium, or calcium), heart damage, and certain prescribed or recreational medications. Dysrhythmia causes symptoms that vary in severity from minor to lethal. Lethal dysrhythmias include ventricular tachycardia (VT) and ventricular fibrillation (VF) and require electrical shock for treatment. Early defibrillation or shock may quickly return the heart to normal without further deterioration of the patient's status. The majority of arrests involve the collapse of both the respiratory and cardiovascular systems. This is defined as a cardiopulmonary arrest. Unless otherwise indicated within a patient's advance directive or a do-not-resuscitate (DNR) physician's order, all patients receive cardiopulmonary resuscitation (CPR) in the event of an arrest.

A resuscitation attempt is approached in a systematic and organized fashion to ensure the most expeditious care. Within most hospitals this arrest situation is referred to as a "code" (e.g., "code blue," "code 7"). Each institution has a specific code or signal to summon immediate assistance in the event of a cardiac and/or respiratory arrest. The goal is to provide resuscitation in a timely manner to restore cardiopulmonary function and avoid poor neurological outcomes or death. Most nurses and nursing students are required to be certified in basic life support measures. Two specific skills utilized during basic life support are inserting an oral airway and use of an automated external defibrillator (AED). This chapter covers both of these skills, as well as organizational skills used during a resuscitation or code event.

EVIDENCE-BASED PRACTICE TRENDS

The Committee on Emergency Cardiac Care (American Heart Association [AHA], 2005) reviews and conducts research on cardiac arrest treatment and outcomes and has created guidelines for both initial care (basic life support, or BLS) and ongoing measures (advanced cardiovascular life support, or ACLS) (Field, 2006). These guidelines are evidence based.

Overall survival rates following cardiopulmonary arrests are dismal. Mortality statistics from the largest of the recent studies reveal overall survival rates of 6.4% after out-of-hospital arrest and 17.5% after in-hospital arrest (Cooper and others, 2006). It appears that quality CPR and ACLS can make a difference in outcomes regardless of the underlying disease state. Recent studies quantify the quality of chest compressions for both in- and out-of-hospital arrests (Abella and others, 2005; Berg, 2003; Wik and others, 2005). Results demonstrate that chest compressions are frequently too shallow, frequently interrupted, and withheld in 48% of pulseless resuscitation time. During interruptions, a patient does not receive cerebral and coronary perfusion. This directly contributes to the poor survival rates listed above. The 2005 American Heart Association (AHA) resuscitation guidelines recommend performing chest compressions at a rate of 100 per minute, with few and very brief interruptions for ventilation, pulse checks, intubation, and defibrillation.

The Joint Commission set a standard for hospitals to improve recognition and response to changes in a patient's condition in an effort to reduce the number of preventable deaths. The 2008 National Patient Safety Goal 16A from The Joint Commission states, "The organization (should) select a suitable method that enables health care staff members to directly request additional assistance from a specially trained individual(s) when the patient's condition appears to be worsening." Many hospitals have initiated the use of rapid response teams as their method of choice. The team members and criteria for activation vary, but the team's goal is to provide early intervention to stabilize or transport the patient to the intensive care unit (ICU), thereby reducing the number of non-ICU arrests. Effectiveness of these teams is still being assessed, but the initial case reports are positive (Institute for Healthcare Improvement, 2008).

Immediate bystander CPR and defibrillation within 3 to 5 minutes of collapse have resulted in survival rates of 41% to 75% for victims of witnessed VF arrest in airports, casinos, and first-responder programs with police officers (Bunch and others, 2005). Data suggest that every minute a patient remains in an untreated shockable rhythm, the likelihood of survival is reduced by 7% to 10% (Field, 2006). Because of these statistics, many hospitals and large public areas are providing the tools needed for the first 3 to 5 minutes of an arrest, including AEDs. AEDs are very user friendly and provide an automated analysis of the heart's rhythm and recommendation for electrical shock.

The 2005 AHA guidelines recommend postresuscitation cooling in certain circumstances to help preserve neurological function (Hazinski and others, 2006). Widespread cerebral ischemia and edema due to brain injury after an arrest can clearly exacerbate the degree of permanent neurological damage (Kozik, 2007). Lowering the body temperature to 33° C (91.4° F) improves the neurological recovery of out-of-hospital, post–ventricular fibrillation arrest victims (Bernard and others, 2002; Hypothermia After

Cardiac Arrest Study Group, 2002). Many hospitals have developed protocols for using external cooling techniques and intravascular cooling devices.

Advance directives (ADs) are documents that inform the health care professional (HCP) of a patient's wishes regarding the extent of resuscitation measures. Nurses, because of their unique relationship with patients and the associated high level of trust, are in an ideal position to initiate discussion of advance directives. The American Nurses Association (ANA) *Position Statement: Nursing Care and Do-Not-Resuscitate (DNR) Decision* (2003) states that the DNR decision should be directed by what the informed patient wants or would have wanted. This demands that communication regarding end-of-life issues occurs between all involved parties (patient, HCPs, and family members; the latter as defined by the patient) and that appropriate DNR orders be written before a life-threatening crisis occurs. Many hospitals have resources to assist a patient/family with this issue. Health care providers may consult with pastoral care, social services, and/or hospital-based ethics committees to assist patients and their families.

Many hospitals now allow family members/significant others to remain in the patient's room during resuscitative efforts and invasive procedures. Evaluation of these programs, pioneered by critical care and emergency nurses, confirms a remarkable level of approval and gratitude by participating family members (Emergency Nurses Association, 2005; MacLean and others, 2003). These evaluations note significant reduction in posttraumatic stress and self-reports of a greater sense of resolution and fulfillment among witnesses of resuscitative efforts compared with nonwitnesses. Make provisions for a designated professional to accompany family members during the event to answer questions, explain, and offer emotional support. In addition, the accompanying professional can observe for signs of acute discomfort in the family members and end the observation. Although few hospitals have written policies and guidelines to support this practice, many critical care and emergency nurses have allowed family to be present during a patient's resuscitation.

CULTURAL CONSIDERATIONS

Whenever a patient requires resuscitation, their family is also a prime nursing concern. When caring for patients from diverse cultures and religions, consider the individual's meaning and interpretation of life support and resuscitation. There are many interventions you can perform to assist the family during emergency situations, such as the following:

- Use a professional language interpreter to explain the patient's status to the family.
- Use cultural and religious support personnel to facilitate understanding of the events by family members. Accommodate patient's religious and cultural practices.

- Be prepared to handle large numbers of visitors who may remain at the bedside to provide support for the family and/or pray for the patient. Collaborate with the family decision maker and leader to plan rotating visits at the bedside. Designate a waiting area to accommodate the group. Assign a contact person from the unit to interact with the patient's family and visitors. Promote cultural understanding by staff (Emergency Nurses Association, 2003).
- Consult religious leaders and family decision maker regarding measures to be taken in the event of an emergency.
- Initiate discussions about advance directives, DNR status, and organ donation with the guidance of the religious leader and consent of the family decision maker. Include in the discussion a representative of the organ procurement organization working with your hospital.
- Be aware that autopsy and organ donation may be refused by persons from certain cultures.

The following cultural considerations may affect a patient's approach to resuscitation or death. Orthodox Jews bury all body fluids with the body. In the event of a death, tubes with fluids, dressings, bloody sheets, etc. go with the body. Some African Americans will not readily accept advance directives because of their distrust of the health care system. Buddhists and Hindus generally believe that life is determined by one's karma or deeds in a previous life. Muslims believe in predestination of life by Allah. Collectivistic groups (e.g., Asians or Hispanics) tend to make decisions together rather than use individual decision making (Doorenbos, 2003). Some Sudanese families rely on community elders to make decisions.

Although individuals may be part of a specific cultural or religious group, an individual may not follow all aspects of that culture or religion. Therefore it is essential that you consider each individual's interpretation and wishes to ensure the right of self-determination.

Skill Performance Guidelines

1 Know the patient's baseline vital signs, noting any irregularities in cardiac rhythm. Dysrhythmias can precipitate a cardiopulmonary arrest. Cardiovascular conditions that place the patient at risk for dysrhythmias include coronary artery disease, myocardial infarction, open heart surgeries, acid-base imbalances, and toxicities.

2 Know the patient's most recent serum electrolyte values. Electrolyte imbalances (e.g., those involving potassium, magnesium, and calcium) can precipitate cardiopulmonary arrest.

3 When a patient has been exposed to a chemical or drug, attempt to determine the type and amount of the substance involved. Certain chemicals, such as ethanol, tranquilizers, and depressants, depress the respiratory center and can result in a respiratory arrest. Overdoses of some drugs can cause ventricular dysrhythmias and cardiopulmonary arrest.

SKILL 27-1   Inserting an Oral Airway

An oral airway is a semicircular, minimally flexible, curved piece of hard plastic (Fig. 27-1). When inserted, it extends from just outside the lips, over the tongue, and to the pharynx (Fig. 27-2). Oral airways enable you to suction through a central core or along the side of the airway and maintain airway patency in the unconscious patient.

Oral airways vary in length and width. Pediatric sizes are 000, 00, 0, 1, 2, and 3. School-age children are usually size 3. Adult sizes are 4 through 6 or small, medium, and large. Choose the size of an oral airway based on the patient's age and the width and length of the patient's mouth. Size is correct if, when the flange is held paral-

lel to the front teeth with the airway against the patient's cheek, the end of the curve reaches the angle of the jaw. Table 27-1 provides general size guidelines for choosing an oral airway for children.

Delegation Considerations

The skill of inserting an oral airway cannot be delegated to nursing assistive personnel (NAP). The nurse directs the NAP to:

- Immediately report to the nurse changes in vital signs or patient's color.

Equipment

- ❑ Appropriate-size oral airway
- ❑ Clean gloves
- ❑ Tissues or washcloths
- ❑ Suction equipment, if indicated
- ❑ Nonallergenic tape *(optional)*
- ❑ Face shield for the nurse, if there is a potential for splattering oral contents
- ❑ Tongue blade

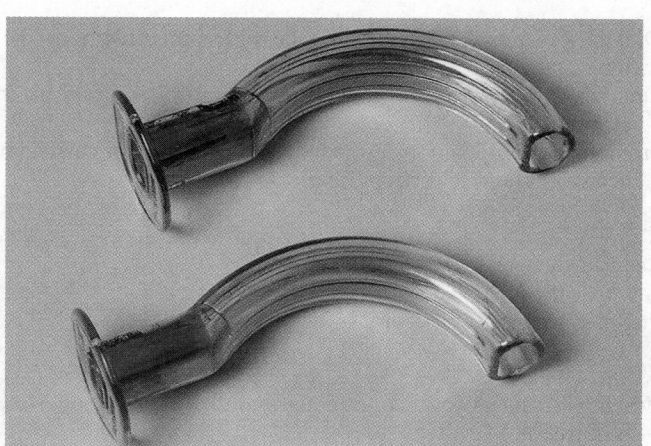

FIG 27-1   Oral airways.

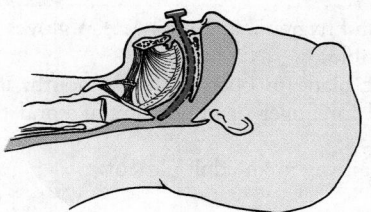

FIG 27-2   Placement of oral airway.

TABLE 27-1	Oral Airway Guidelines for Size* by Age		
Size	**Age**	**Size**	**Age**
30-34 mm or size 000	Premature neonates	80 mm or size 3	6 to 18 yr
40 mm or size 00	Newborn	90 mm or size 4	Adult medium
50 mm or size 0	Newborn to 1 yr	100 mm or size 5	Adult large
60 mm or size 1	1 to 2 yr	110 mm or size 6	Adult extra large
70 mm or size 2	2 to 6 yr		

*Measure from the corner of the mouth to the angle of the jaw just below the ear for size estimation.

STEP	RATIONALE

ASSESSMENT

1   Identify need to insert oral airway. Signs and symptoms include upper airway gurgling with breathing, absence of gag reflex, increased oral secretions, excessive drooling, grinding teeth, clenched teeth, biting of orotracheal or gastric tubes, labored respirations, and increased respiratory rate.

These conditions place patient at risk for obstruction of the upper airway. Use oral airways only in unconscious patients. Oral airways may stimulate vomiting or laryngospasm if inserted in a semiconscious or conscious patient.

2   Determine factors that normally influence upper airway functioning, such as age (children have a proportionally larger tongue) and the presence of a nasal or oral airway or drainage tubes (swallowing is more difficult with tubes in place).

Allows nurse to accurately assess need for oral airway placement. Patients at greater risk for upper airway obstruction are infants, children, and adults with upper airway congestion, loss of consciousness, seizure disorders, neuromuscular diseases, increased oral secretions, or facial trauma.

3   Assess for presence of gag reflex; gently place tongue blade on back of patient's tongue.

Provides guide as to when oral airway can be safely removed in a postoperative patient.

Critical Decision Point   *Never insert an oral airway in a conscious patient or a patient with recent oral trauma, oral surgery, or loose teeth. Never force an airway into place.*

STEP	RATIONALE
4 Assess family's knowledge of procedure.	Identifies learning needs of family. Patient will be unconscious.

NURSING DIAGNOSES

- Impaired gas exchange
- Ineffective airway clearance
- Ineffective breathing pattern
- Risk for aspiration
- Risk for infection

Individualize related factors based on patient's condition or needs.

PLANNING

1 Expected outcomes following completion of procedure:	
• Patient's respiratory status improves, as evidenced by easier respirations with normal rate, easier removal of secretions, and lack of gurgling noise in throat with respirations.	Airway is clear of secretions.
• Patient is not able to grind teeth or bite tubes.	Oral airway prevents tooth contact with other teeth or with tubes.
• Patient's tongue does not obstruct airway, making it easer to bag-mask ventilate the patient.	Oral airway keeps tongue in correct position to maintain patent airway.
2 Position patient; semi-Fowler's position is preferred.	Promotes patient comfort, provides easy access to oral cavity, and decreases the work of breathing.

IMPLEMENTATION

1 Perform hand hygiene, and apply clean gloves and face shield (when possible).	Reduces transmission of microorganisms.
2 Use tongue blade to open patient's mouth; if necessary, use thumb and forefinger of nondominant hand to pry jaws and teeth apart.	Provides access to oral cavity.
3 Insert oral airway in an adult patient:	When inserting airway, take care not to push patient's tongue into pharynx.
a Hold oral airway with curved end up, insert distal end until airway reaches back of throat, then turn airway over 180 degrees and follow natural curve of tongue. You can also hold airway sideways, insert halfway, and then rotate airway 90 degrees while gliding it over natural curvature of tongue. Make sure outer flange is just outside patient's lips.	Prevents displacement of patient's tongue into posterior oropharynx.

Critical Decision Point   *In a pediatric patient, DO NOT rotate the oral airway on insertion because the airway tip will damage the soft palate.*

4 Suction secretions, as needed.	Removes secretions; maintains patent airway.
5 Reassess patient's respiratory status.	Directs nurse to initiate intervention.
6 Clean patient's face with soft tissue or washcloth.	Promotes hygiene.
7 Discard tissue into appropriate receptacle, place washcloth in dirty or soiled linen bag, remove gloves and face shield, and discard in appropriate receptacle; perform hand hygiene.	Reduces transmission of microorganisms.
8 Administer mouth care frequently.	Increases patient comfort and removes debris. It also provides moisture to oral mucosal tissues.

Critical Decision Point   *Do not use lemon glycerin swabs for oral care because they are drying to mucosal tissues and promote bacterial growth. Oral airway will need to be removed, cleaned or discarded, and replaced in patients with excessive oral secretions. Frequent suctioning of the oral cavity may be required. Oral airways are not a long-term solution. They can cause significant lip and tongue erosion.*

EVALUATION

1 Observe patient's respiratory status, and compare respiratory assessments before and after insertion of oral airway.	Identifies patient's response to insertion of airway.
2 Assess that airway is patent and that patient's tongue does not obstruct airway.	Ensures a route for oxygen delivery to patient.
3 If patient pushes airway out with tongue or coughs, reassess need for the oral airway.	Patient's ability to clear their own airway may have returned.

Unexpected Outcomes	Related Interventions
1 Patient continually coughs and gags when airway is inserted.	• Do not continue inserting airway if patient begins to gag. Stimulation of gag reflex can cause vomiting and aspiration. • Remove oral airway, and position patient on side. • Reassess need for artifical airway.
2 Airway obstruction not relieved.	• Obtain immediate assistance. • Reinsert airway. • Assess for other causes of obstruction.
3 Patient pushes airway out of place or out of mouth.	• Reinsert airway again, and secure. • Reassess patient's need for oral airway.
4 Nurse is unable to insert oral airway in patient; patient is combative, or nurse is unable to pry mouth open.	• Obtain assistance. • Reassess patient's need for oral airway. • Provide sedation, as ordered.

Recording and Reporting

- Record in nurses' notes and/or patient progress notes: assessment findings while inserting oral airway; size of oral airway; other interventions performed at same time, especially positioning, suctioning; and patient's response to procedure.
- Report presence of respiratory distress, vomiting, or pain.

Pediatric Considerations

- Oral airways are seldom used in treatment of airway obstruction in children and infants. Due to narrowness of child's airway, oral airways are often more occlusive than beneficial. Because of the low frequency of use, competency validation may be required before health care professional is allowed to perform pediatric oral airway insertion.
- For infants and children the preferred method for inserting airway is with tip pointing downward, over the tongue (Hockenberry and Wilson, 2007).

Gerontological Considerations

- Be sure patient does not have dentures in place before attempting an oral airway insertion.

SKILL 27-2 Use of an Automated External Defibrillator

The advantage of an AED is that laypersons or health care providers trained in basic life support, who have less training than ACLS personnel, can defibrillate. AEDs eliminate the need for training in rhythm interpretation and make early defibrillation practical and achievable. The AED is a defibrillator that incorporates a rhythm analysis system. The device attaches to a patient by two adhesive pads and connecting cables. The technology of the AED is available in several different devices. Most AEDs are stand-alone boxes with very simple three-step function (Fig. 27-3) and verbal prompts to guide the responder. All AEDs offer automated rhythm analysis, whereby the rhythm is compared to thousands of other rhythms stored in the AED's computer software. Upon rhythm identification, some AEDs will automatically provide the electrical shock after a verbal warning (fully automated). Other AEDs will recommend a shock, if needed, and then prompt the responder to press the shock button.

Delegation Considerations

Basic life support certification provides hands-on training with an AED for laypersons, NAP, and licensed health care professionals. Most hospitals using AEDs have given the authority to use an AED to all CPR-certified personnel, including NAP. Refer to the specific hospital policies for use of the AED.

Equipment

☐ Automated external defibrillator
☐ Pair of AED adhesive pads

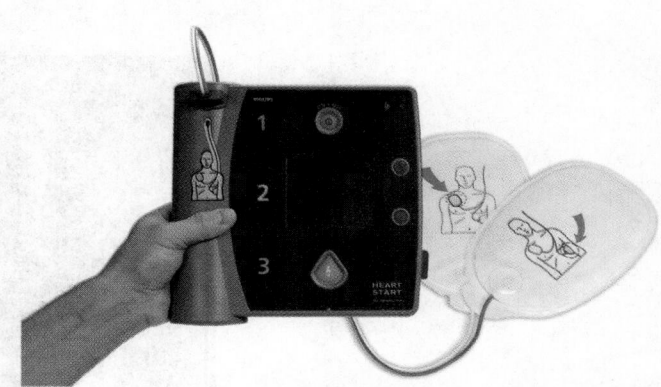

FIG 27-3 Automated external defibrillator device. (*Courtesy Philips Medical Systems.*)

STEP	RATIONALE

ASSESSMENT

1 Establish a person's unresponsiveness, and call for help. (In a community setting have someone call 9-1-1.)	This information assists in determining if the individual is unresponsive rather than asleep, intoxicated, hearing impaired, or postictal. Rapid response by qualified professionals ensures ongoing resusciation support.
2 Establish absence of respirations and the lack of circulation: no pulse, no respirations, no movement.	

STEP	RATIONALE

Critical Decision Point *An AED should be applied only to a patient who is unconscious, not breathing, and pulseless. For children younger than 8 years old, AED pads designed for children should be used. If child pads are not available, use adult AED pads (AHA, 2005).*

NURSING DIAGNOSES

- Decreased cardiac output
- Impaired spontaneous ventilation
- Ineffective breathing pattern
- Ineffective tissue perfusion

Individualize related factors based on patient's condition or needs.

PLANNING

1 Expected outcomes following completion of procedure:	
• Patient's cardiac rhythm is converted back to stable rhythm.	Defibrillation provides the electrical shock to convert a lethal dysrhythmia.
• Patient regains pulse and respirations.	CPR and defibrillation were successful.
2 Within a hospital activate the code team in accordance with hospital policy and procedure.	First available person to bring the resuscitation cart and AED.

IMPLEMENTATION

1 Deliver two breaths using a mouth-to-mouth with barrier device or mouth-to-mask device or bag-mask device. Watch for chest rise and fall.	In a hospital setting where protected methods of artificial ventilation are available, mouth-to-mouth without a barrier device is not recommended because of the risk for microbial contamination.
2 Start chest compressions, and continue until AED is attached to patient and the device's verbal prompt advises you, "Do NOT touch the patient."	To minimize the interruption time of chest compressions, continue CPR while the AED is being applied and turned on.
3 Place AED next to the patient near the chest or head (see illustration).	Ensures easy access to device.

Critical Decision Point *If the AED is immediately available, attach AED to patient as soon as possible. The faster defibrillation is delivered, the better the survival rate.*

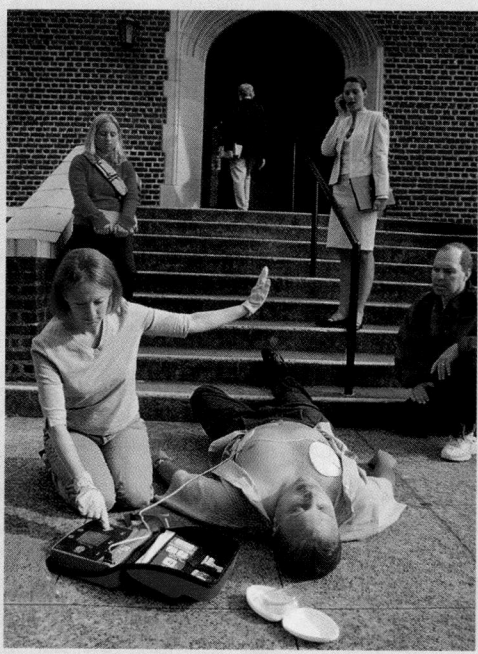

Step 3   Placement of AED pads with device next to patient.
(Courtesy Philips Medical Systems.)

STEP	RATIONALE

4 Turn on the power (see illustration).

Turning on the power will begin the verbal prompts to guide you through the next steps.

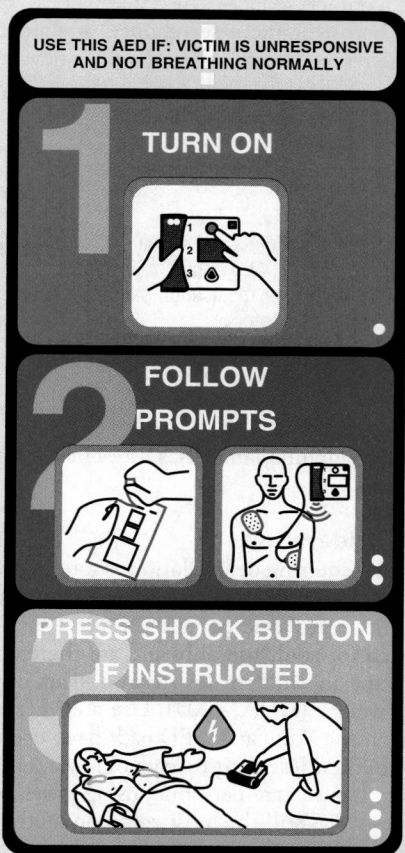

USE THIS AED IF: VICTIM IS UNRESPONSIVE AND NOT BREATHING NORMALLY

1 TURN ON

2 FOLLOW PROMPTS

3 PRESS SHOCK BUTTON IF INSTRUCTED

STEP 4 Power panel with AED prompts. (*Courtesy Philips Medical Systems.*)

5 Attach the device. Place the first AED pad on the upper right sternal border directly below the clavicle. Place the second AED pad lateral to the left nipple with the top of the pad a few inches below the axilla (see illustration for Step 4). Ensure that the cables are connected to the AED. Do not attach pads to a wet surface, over a medication patch, or over a pacemaker or implanted defibrillator. Patients with large amounts of chest hair may require shaving to obtain adequate pad contact.

Alternative placement of the AED pads is not recommended. The fastest application technique is the one mentioned. AEDs analyze most heart rhythms using lead II. If the AED pads are placed as directed, the patient's heart rhythm will be analyzed in lead II.

Wet surfaces, implanted defibrillators, and medication patches reduce the effectiveness of the defibrillation attempt and result in complications.

6 Do NOT touch the patient when the AED prompts you to not touch the patient. Direct rescuers and bystanders to avoid touching the patient by announcing "Clear!" Allow the AED to analyze the rhythm. Some devices will require that an analysis button be pressed. The AED will take approximately 5 to 15 seconds to analyze the rhythm.

Each brand of AED is different, so familiarity with the model is important.

Not touching the patient when directed prevents artifact errors, avoids all movement during analysis (Field, 2006), and prevents shock from being delivered to bystanders.

7 Before pressing the shock button, announce loudly to clear the victim, and perform a visual check to ensure that no one is in contact with victim.

Clearing the patient ensures safety for those involved in rescue efforts.

8 Immediately begin chest compression after the shock, and continue for 2 minutes.

Continues cardiac perfusion.

9 After 2 minutes of CPR, the AED will prompt you not to touch the patient and will resume analysis of the patient's rhythm. This cycle will continue until the patient regains a pulse or until the physician determines death.

STEP	RATIONALE

EVALUATION

1 Inspect the pad adhesion to chest wall. If the pads are not in good contact with chest wall, remove the AED pads and apply a new set. Attach new set of pads to the AED.

Poor pad-skin contact reduces the effectiveness of the shock, causes skin burns, or increases chance of shocking those involved in the rescue efforts. Always apply a new set of pads. Do NOT reuse.

2 Continue resuscitative efforts until the patient regains pulse or until the physician determines death.

Unexpected Outcomes

1 Patient's heart rhythm does not convert into a stable rhythm with pulse after defibrillation.

2 Patient's skin has burns under AED pads.

Related Interventions

- Assess pad contact on patient's chest wall.
- Do not touch patient during AED's rhythm analysis.
- Avoid placing AED pads over medication patches, pacemaker, or implantable defibrillator generators.
- Assess AED pad contact on the chest.
- Ensure the chest is dry before applying pads to chest.

Recording and Reporting

- Immediately report arrest via the hospital-wide communication system, indicating exact location of victim.
- Cardiopulmonary arrest requires precise documentation. Most hospitals use a form designed specifically for in-hospital arrests.
- Record in nurses' notes or on designated CPR worksheet: onset of arrest, time and number of AED shocks (you will not know the exact energy level used by the AED), time and energy level of manual defibrillations, medications given, procedures performed, cardiac rhythm, use of CPR, and the patient's response.

Teaching Considerations

- If patient is at risk for cardiopulmonary arrest, instruct the family or caregivers in CPR or encourage them to obtain certification through an instructor from the hospital, American Red Cross, or AHA.
- Patient and family should keep emergency numbers taped to the phone or consider programming them into speed dial function on both home and mobile phones. Stress the use of 9-1-1.

- It is extremely helpful if family has list of medications patient is presently taking.

Pediatric Considerations

- Cardiac arrest requiring defibrillation is rare in children. If you must consider defibrillation, lower energy requirements are necessary in the pediatric population. Most AEDs are specifically designed for adult use only and are therefore not recommended for use in children less than 8 years old or less than 25 kg body weight (AHA, 2005). Use an AED on a pediatric patient only if the AED and AED pads have been specially designed for children less than 8 years old. Manual defibrillation performed by health care personnel using lower energy settings (2 to 4 joules/kg) is still the most common method of pediatric defibrillation (AHA, 2005).

Home Care Considerations

- AEDs are available for use in the community and home setting.

SKILL 27-3   Code Management

All who respond to cardiopulmonary arrests should follow a simple, standardized, easy-to-remember approach. The ACLS provider course (AHA, 2005) teaches the primary and secondary survey approach to arrest situations. The memory aid A-B-C-D describes two sets of actions for each of four steps. With each step the responder performs an assessment and then, if the assessment so indicates, a management intervention. Initially a code is managed by the first responder performing the basic skills of CPR, which includes the primary survey of A (airway), B (breathing), C (circulation), and D (early defibrillation). Interventions must be continued until the code team arrives. The initial process also includes notification of the hospital's resuscitation or code team. The team usually includes a physician, critical care nurse, respiratory care personnel, anesthesia provider, and ancillary support. Most code team members have been educated in ACLS and performance of the secondary survey of A (airway intubation), B (confirmation of airway and ventilation), C (rhythm analysis of cardiac rhythm), and D (differential diagnosis of the cause). Both surveys must be continually used to reassess and manage the patient as appropriate throughout the code situation.

An early primary survey of ABCD is crucial for a favorable patient outcome. Without oxygen delivery, brain damage can begin within 4 minutes of arrest; brain damage almost always occurs at 6 minutes, and brain death is certain at 10 minutes (AHA, 2005). The ability of a non–ACLS-certified nurse to initiate resuscitative efforts can prevent lethal dysrhythmias such as ventricular fibrillation from deteriorating to asystole (absence of cardiac electrical activity) and provide a chance for the heart to return to its normal rhythm. Table 27-2 summarizes a few basic cardiac arrhythmias. Early CPR and defibrillation delivered within the primary ABCD survey optimizes heart and brain function, leading to improved survivability. Equipment may be readily available at the bedside or in a designated area of the hospital unit. It is the nurse's responsibility to know how to use this equipment and to know its location and the contents of the resuscitation or crash cart (Fig. 27-4).

As stated earlier in this chapter, CPR certification is required of most nurses and nursing students. Therefore CPR will not be covered in detail within this chapter. Table 27-3 (p. 731) summarizes a few points regarding CPR skills, including differences in adult, child, and infant techniques.

Delegation Considerations

NAP who are certified in basic life support techniques by the AHA or the American Red Cross can perform the basic skills of CPR. Hospitals differ in how the skill of defibrillation is delegated. In most hospitals, CPR-certified NAP or nurses can use the AED to perform defibrillation. In situations in which the AED is unavailable, a manual defibrillator is used. Most hospitals reserve the skill of manual defibrillation for licensed personnel who are ACLS certified or have received competency validation to perform manual defibrillation. All others skills required in the code situation will require physician-directed interventions performed by nurses, respiratory therapists, and other physicians.

Equipment

❏ Crash cart or resuscitation cart (see Fig. 27-4): Most carts have the following equipment:
- Clean gloves, gown, protective eyewear
- Oxygen source
- Pocket mask or CPR mask
- Bag-mask device or resuscitation bag
- Laryngoscope handle, straight and curved blades
- Endotracheal (ET) tubes, various sizes (5 to 9 mm for adults; 0 to 4 mm for pediatrics)
- Tape or commercial ET tube holder
- Backboard
- AED and/or manual defibrillator with AED/defibrillator pads
- Intravenous (IV) needles (sizes for adults and pediatrics)
- Central venous catheter (CVC) kit
- IV tubing and fluids (normal saline and 5% dextrose in water [D_5W])
- Syringes
- Laboratory specimen tubes
- Arterial blood gas kit
- Code medications
- ACLS guidelines or algorithms

❏ Suction source and suction equipment if not with crash cart
❏ Documentation form

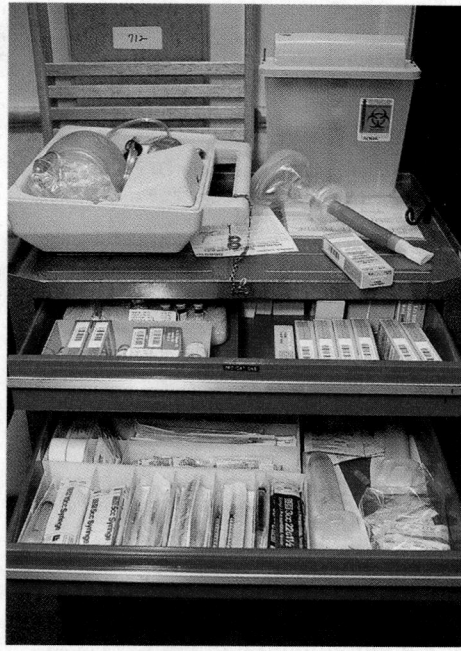

FIG 27-4 Emergency resuscitation cart.

TABLE 27-2	Common Basic Cardiac Dysrhythmias
Rhythm Characteristics and Etiology	**Clinical Significance and Management**

Sinus Tachycardia

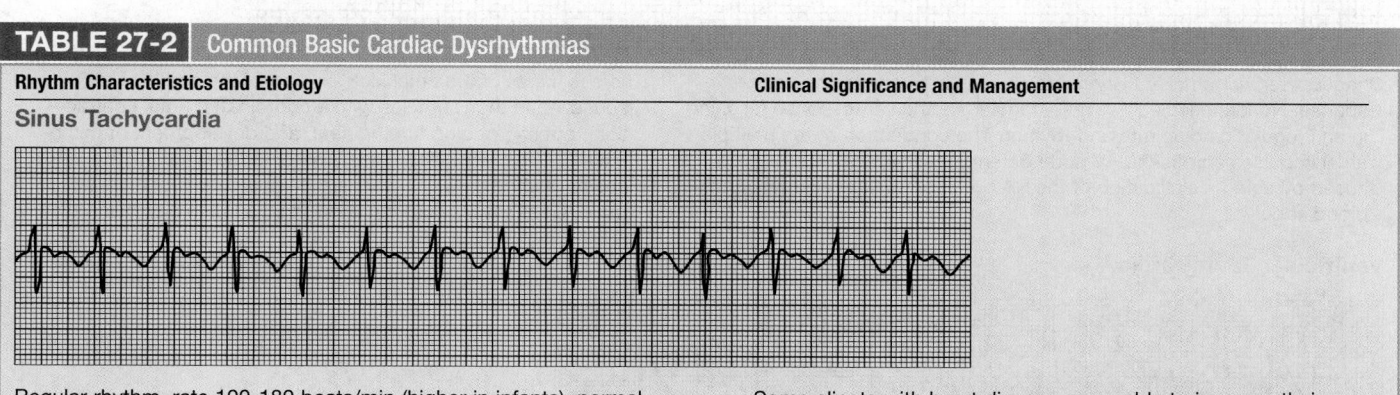

Rhythm Characteristics and Etiology	Clinical Significance and Management
Regular rhythm, rate 100-180 beats/min (higher in infants), normal P wave, normal QRS complex Rate increase is often normal response to exercise, emotion, or stressors such as pain, fever, pump failure, hyperthyroidism, and certain drugs (e.g., caffeine, nitrates, epinephrine, nicotine)	Some clients with heart disease are unable to increase their heart rate to meet increased oxygen demands. Correct underlying factors; discontinue drugs producing the side effect

Continued

TABLE 27-2 | Common Basic Cardiac Dysrhythmias—cont'd

Rhythm Characteristics and Etiology	**Clinical Significance and Management**

Sinus Bradycardia

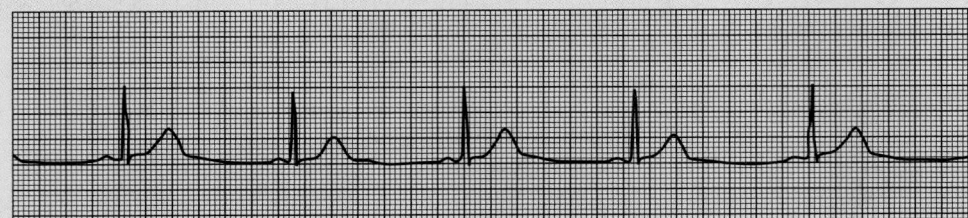

Regular rhythm, rate less than 60 beats/min, normal P wave, normal PR interval, normal QRS complex

Rate decrease is a normal response to sleep or in well-conditioned athlete; diminished blood flow to SA node, vagal stimulation, hypothyroidism, increased intracranial pressure, or pharmacological agents (e.g., digoxin, propranolol, quinidine, procainamide) sometimes cause abnormal drops in rate

No clinical significance unless associated with signs and symptoms of reduced cardiac output such as dizziness or syncope or presence of chest pain

Bradycardia with hypotension and decreased cardiac output is treated with atropine; a pacemaker is sometimes necessary

Atrial Fibrillation (A-fib)

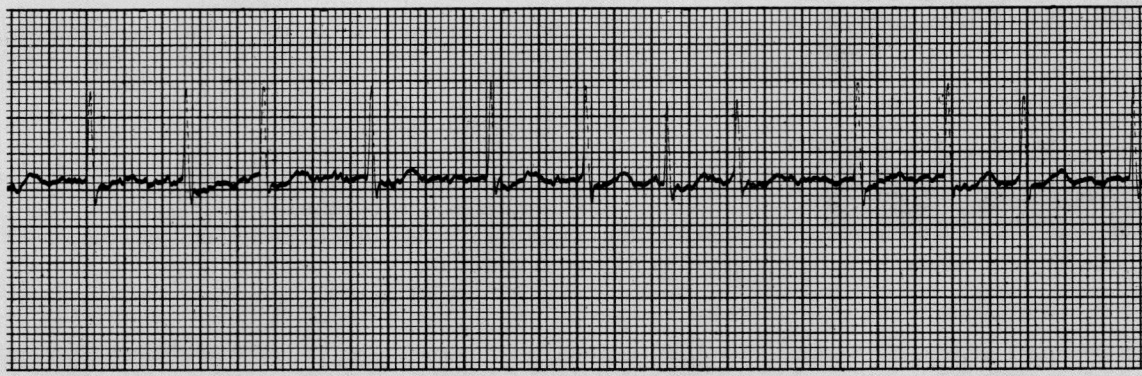

Chaotic, irregular atrial activity resulting in an irregular ventricular response. No identifiable P waves. Irregular ventricular response resulting in an irregular cardiac rate and rhythm. The conduction of the multiple atrial impulses across the AV node determines the rate.

Caused by aging, calcification of the SA node, or changes in myocardial blood supply

There is a loss of the atrial kick (portion of the cardiac output squeezed in the ventricles with a coordinated atrial contraction), pooling of blood in the atria, and development of microemboli. The client often complains of fatigue, a fluttering in the chest, or shortness of breath if the ventricular response is rapid. Commonly occurring dysrhythmia in the aging and older adult

Ventricular Tachycardia

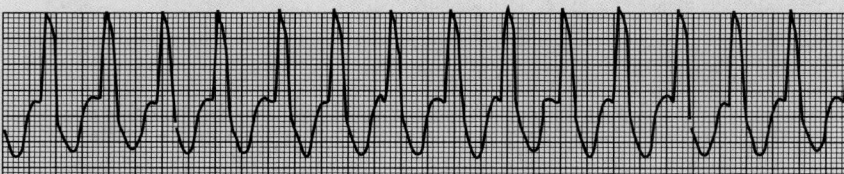

Rhythm slightly irregular, rate 100-200 beats/min, P wave absent, PR interval absent, QRS complex wide and bizarre, >0.12 second

Caused by changes in the normal pacemaker of the heart such as decrease in blood flow, ischemia, or embolus

Results in decreased cardiac output due to decreased ventricular filling time; often leads to severe hypotension and loss of pulse and consciousness

If refractory to defibrillation, amiodarone 300 mg IV followed by an additional 150 mg IV in 3-5 minutes (American Heart Association [AHA], 2005a)

TABLE 27-2	Common Basic Cardiac Dysrhythmias—cont'd

Rhythm Characteristics and Etiology	Clinical Significance and Management

Ventricular Fibrillation

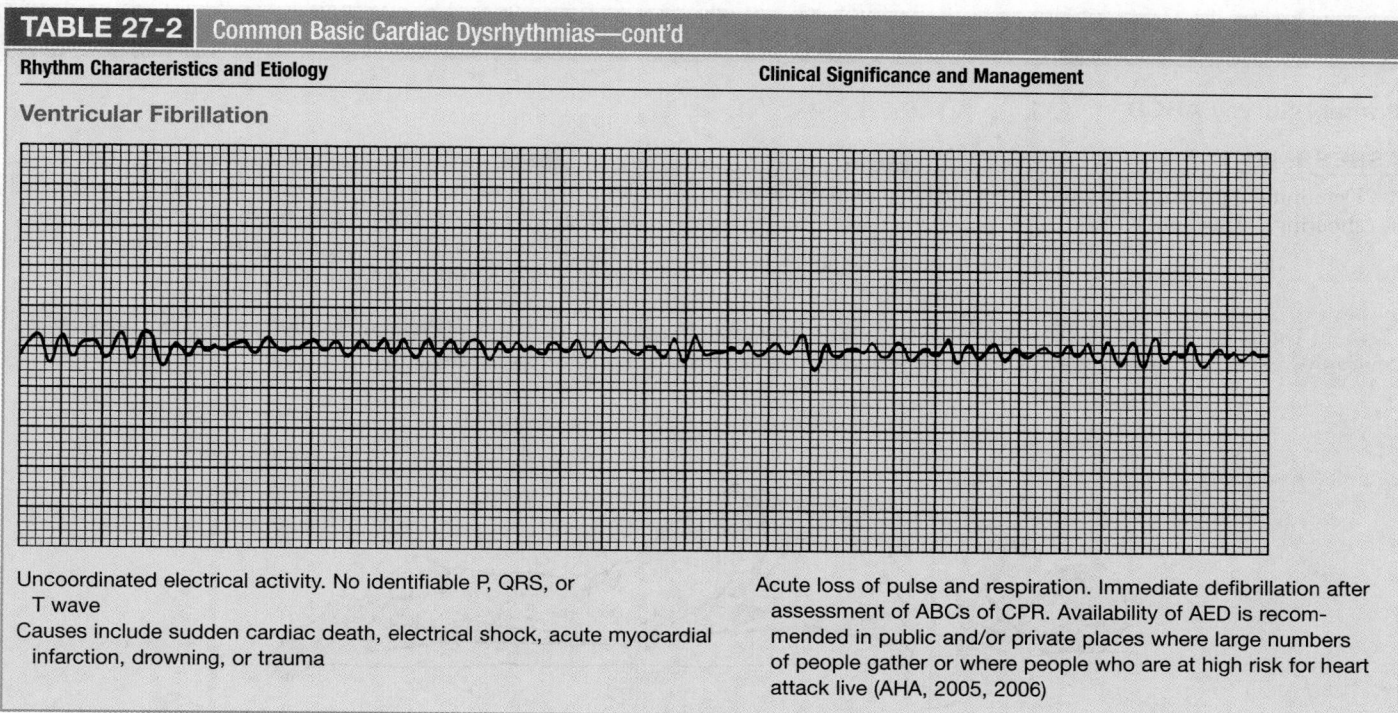

Uncoordinated electrical activity. No identifiable P, QRS, or T wave Causes include sudden cardiac death, electrical shock, acute myocardial infarction, drowning, or trauma	Acute loss of pulse and respiration. Immediate defibrillation after assessment of ABCs of CPR. Availability of AED is recommended in public and/or private places where large numbers of people gather or where people who are at high risk for heart attack live (AHA, 2005, 2006)

Modified from Canobbio MM: *Cardiovascular disorders*, St. Louis, 1990, Mosby. *SA,* Sinoatrial; *AV,* atrioventricular; *AED,* automated external defibrillator.

TABLE 27-3	Adult, Child, and Infant CPR Techniques for Health Care Providers

Technique	Adult	Child (1-8 Years Old)	Infant
Airway	Head tilt–chin lift (HCP-suspected trauma, use jaw thrust)	Head tilt–chin lift (HCP-suspected trauma, use jaw thrust)	Head tilt–chin lift (HCP-suspected trauma, use jaw thrust)
Initial breathing	2 breaths at 1 sec per breath	2 effective breaths at 1 sec per breath	2 effective breaths at 1 sec per breath
HCP: Rescue breathing without chest compressions	10-12 breaths/min (approximately 1 breath every 5 seconds)	12-20 breaths/min (approximately 1 breath every 3-5 seconds)	12-20 breaths/min
HCP: Rescue breaths for CPR with advanced airway (endotracheal tube/tracheotomy)	8-10 breaths/min	8-10 breaths/min	8-10 breaths/min
Foreign body airway obstruction	Abdominal thrusts	Abdominal thrusts	Five back blows and five chest thrusts
Chest compressions	Lower half of sternum, between nipples Heel of one hand, other hand on top 1½-2 in *One or two rescuers:* 30 compressions, 2 breaths (30:2) 100 compressions/min	Lower half of sternum, between nipples Heel of one hand only or as for adults Approximately one-third to one-half depth of chest *One rescuer:* 30 compressions, 2 breaths (30:2) *Two rescuers (HCPs):* 15 compressions, 2 breaths (15:2) 100 compressions/min	Just below nipple line (lower half of sternum) Two fingers, two thumbs (encircling hands) Approximately one-third to one-half depth of chest *One rescuer:* 30 compressions, 2 breaths (30:2) *Two rescuers (HCPs):* 15 compressions, 2 breaths (15:2) 100 compressions/min

Data from American Heart Association guidelines for cardiopulmonary resuscitation and emergency cardiovascular care, *Circulation* 112:IV-1, 2005.
CPR, Cardiopulmonary resuscitation; *HCP,* health care provider.

STEP	RATIONALE

Primary Survey ABCD

ASSESSMENT

1 Determine if patient is unconscious by shaking the patient and shouting, "Are you OK?"

Confirms that patient is unresponsive as opposed to intoxicated, sleeping, or hearing impaired. Unconsciousness can also be caused by substance abuse, hypoglycemia, toxicities, seizures, trauma, ketoacidosis, and shock.

Critical Decision Point *If unresponsive person has adequate respirations and pulse, remain until further assistance is present. Place victim in a lateral recovery position (see illustration). Continue to determine presence of respirations and pulse because a recurrent arrest may develop.*

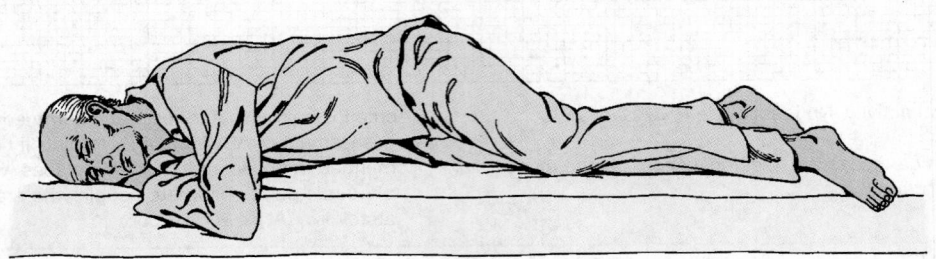

STEP 1 Recovery position.

NURSING DIAGNOSES

- Decreased cardiac output
- Impaired gas exchange
- Impaired spontaneous ventilation
- Ineffective breathing pattern
- Ineffective tissue perfusion

Individualize related factors based on patient's condition or needs.

PLANNING

1 Expected outcomes following completion of procedure:
   - Patient regains pulse and respirations.
   - Physician may terminate CPR.
   - Provide postresuscitation care:
     - Transport to ICU.
     - Continue ongoing care in the ICU.
     - Postmortem care.

CPR was successful.

2 Immediately activate the hospital's code team or emergency medical services (EMS). Tell co-workers to bring AED (if available) and crash cart to bedside.

Ensures timely application of defibrillation, CPR, and ACLS to the arrest victim.

IMPLEMENTATION

Primary Survey ABC

1 Primary survey: A (AIRWAY)
   a Apply clean gloves and face shield.

   Reduces transmission of microorganisms.

   b Open airway using:
      (1) Head tilt–chin lift (no trauma) (see illustration) *or*

   Determine if patient has spontaneous respirations. The tongue is the most common cause of blocked airway in an unresponsive patient.

      (2) Jaw thrust (cervical trauma is suspected) (see illustration)

   Consider spinal cord injury in patients with trauma. In these situations a rescuer must use jaw-thrust maneuver. Prevention of head extension and neck movement is very important to prevent paralysis or spinal cord injury. Apply a rigid cervical collar as soon as possible to reduce cervical spine motion.

STEP	RATIONALE

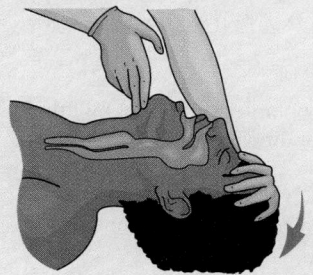

STEP 1b(1)   Head tilt-chin lift. (*From Sorrentino S: Mosby's text-book for nursing assistants, ed 7, St. Louis, 2008, Mosby.*)

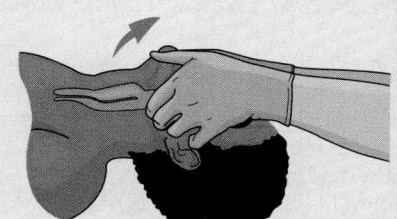

STEP 1b(2)   Jaw thrust without head tilt.

2 Primary survey: B (BREATHING)
   a Give two breaths to the patient using one of these methods:
      (1) Mouth-to-mouth using a barrier device.
      (2) Mouth-to-mask using a pocket mask or CPR mask (see illustration).
      (3) Bag-mask device (see illustrations). If available, attach bag-mask device or mouth-to-mask device to supplemental oxygen supply.

Form an airtight seal to prevent air from escaping.

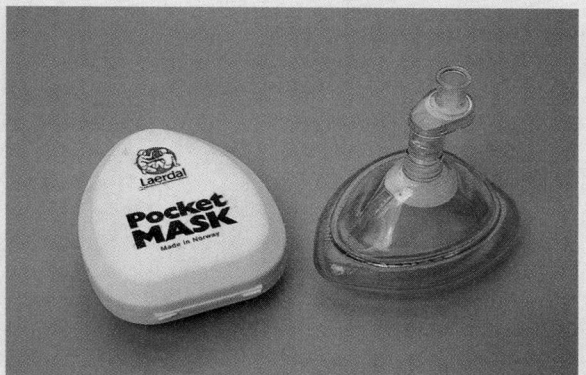

STEP 2a(2)   Pocket mask.

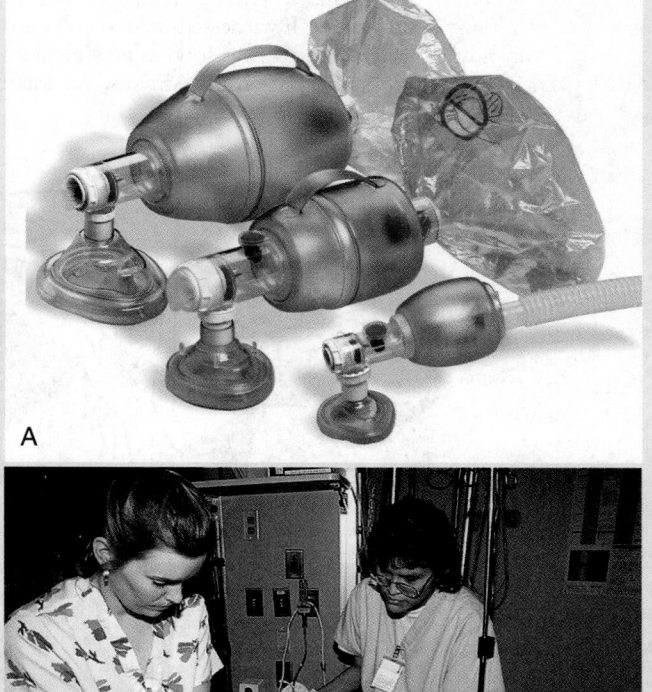

STEP 2a(3)   **A,** Bag-mask device. (*Courtesy Ambu USA.*) **B,** Two-rescuer breathing with bag-mask device.

STEP	RATIONALE

Critical Decision Point   *Give breaths with only enough force to make the chest rise. In a hospital setting where protected methods of artificial ventilation are available, mouth-to-mouth without a barrier device is not recommended because of the risk for microbial contamination.*

b If the patient cannot be ventilated, insert oral airway (see Skill 27-1).

Maintains tongue on anterior floor of mouth and prevents obstruction of posterior airway by tongue.

c Give two initial breaths at 1 second per breath, watching for chest rise and fall.

d Suction secretions if necessary.

Suctioning clears airway obstruction.

3 Primary survey: C (CIRCULATION)

a Check carotid pulse on an adult or child. Check for brachial or femoral pulse in an infant. Palpate for no more than 10 seconds (AHA, 2005).

Carotid pulse is the easiest to locate in adults and children. Femoral pulse may also be palpated in a child or infant. The neck of an infant is usually short, so the carotid pulse is difficult to locate.

b Place victim on hard surface such as floor, ground, or backboard. Victim must be flat. Logroll victim to flat, supine position using spine precautions if trauma is suspected.

External compression of heart is facilitated. Heart is compressed between sternum and spinal vertebrae, which must be on hard and firm surface. Do NOT delay the start of CPR. Positioning the patient on a hard surface may take more than one or two rescuers. You may need to wait to safely move the patient. Place the backboard or position the patient as soon as appropriate assistance is present.

c If pulse is absent, begin chest compressions until AED is applied, ACLS team arrives, or the patient starts to move. Continue chest compression at 100/min at a ratio of 30 compressions to 2 breaths until the AED is applied and the verbal prompt instructs you to clear the patient.

Early CPR and early defibrillation are the hallmarks of successful resuscitation. Specific hand position, compression depth, and ratio are different for adults, children, and infants to avoid injury to the heart, lung, or liver (see illustrations and Table 27-3).

(1) *Children:* Use AED after five cycles of CPR (out of hospital). Use pediatric AED system if available. If not, use adult system. If witnessed sudden collapse or in-hospital arrest, use AED as soon as possible.

(2) *Infant:* No recommendation for AED use for infants less than 1 year of age.

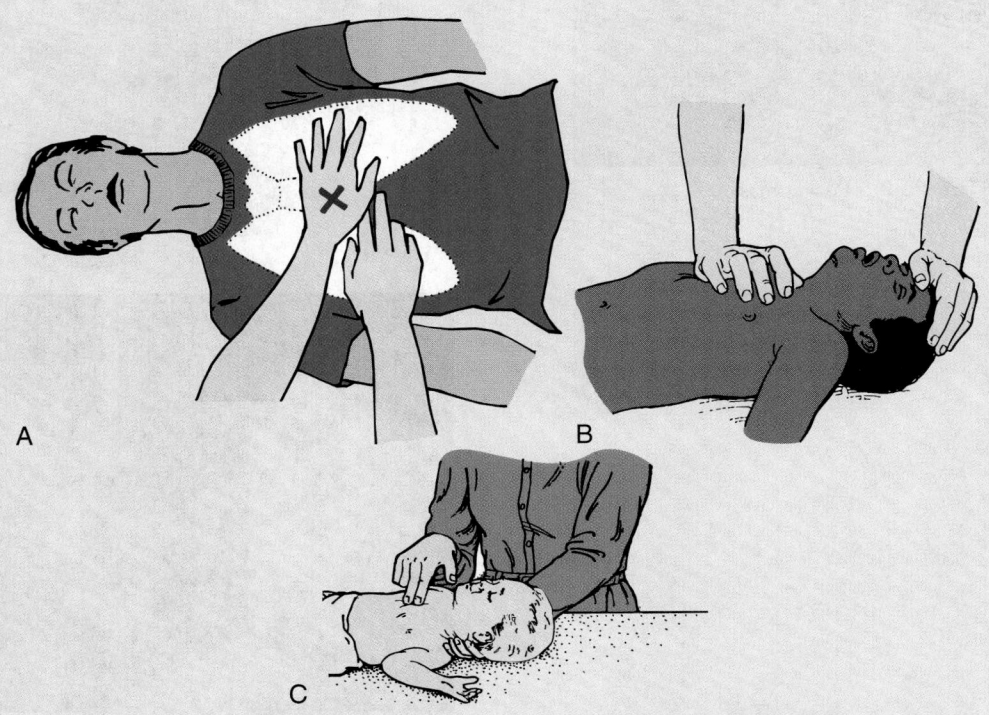

STEP 3c   **A,** Proper hand position—adult. **B,** Proper hand position—child. **C,** Proper hand position—infant.

STEP	RATIONALE
d When instructed by the AED verbal prompt, stop compressions for AED rhythm analysis.	For accurate AED analysis, patient movement must be limited.
(1) If the AED advises a shock, do NOT touch the patient, and press the shock button when prompted.	ACLS guidelines specify 2 minutes of CPR immediately following one shock to provide blood flow and perfusion before attempting another shock (AHA, 2005).
e Resume CPR for 2 minutes immediately after the shock or if the AED advises NO Shock. The AED will prompt you to clear patient in 2 minutes to analyze the patient's rhythm and provide a shock/no shock prompt. Repeat Steps 3c to 3e.	
f If no AED available, continue cycles of 30 compressions to 2 breaths until the ACLS providers take over or the victim starts to move.	

Critical Decision Point *When performing adult CPR, ensure fingers are off the ribs and the lowermost part of the xiphoid process. This minimizes the chance of rib fracture that could result in punctured lung or liver laceration, which will further compromise cardiopulmonary status.*

Secondary Survey ABCD

STEP	RATIONALE
1 Upon arrival of sufficient personnel, delegate tasks as appropriate while a core group continues with resuscitation efforts:	Delegation of duties is essential to meet the critical needs of the patient and his or her family in a timely matter.
• Code leader/physician directs the resuscitation efforts, gives orders. The code leader should be the voice of authority in the room, positioned at the foot of the bed.	
• Airway expert and/or respiratory care will manage the advanced airway at the head of the bed.	
• Bedside nurse will be involved with medication administration, vital signs, assisting with procedures.	
• Crash cart nurse to get medications and supplies from the crash cart to hand off to code team members.	
• Recorder to document the events of the code	
• Small team of CPR-certified staff to switch every 2 minutes when performing chest compressions.	After 2 minutes, a rescuer's ability to maintain quality chest compression declines (Abella, 2005). Frequent rotation of chest compressors will help to maintain quality.
• Staff to bring patient's chart to the bedside or refer to the patient's electronic chart for latest data and to clarify code status and allergies.	
• Pastoral care, social work, or other nurses to communicate with family.	
• Staff to remain with and support family that may remain at the patient's bedside.	
• Staff to assist the victim's roommate or visitors away from the code scene.	
• Staff to remove excess furniture or equipment from the room.	
• Give code leader brief verbal report of events just before code, vital signs, medical diagnosis, and code interventions performed before the code team's arrival.	This information is critical to the selection of appropriate treatment for the patient.
2 Secondary survey: A (INTUBATE AIRWAY)	
a If respirations are absent, assist the code team with endotracheal intubation.	Intubation provides a secure airway and facilitates pulmonary ventilation (Field, 2006).
(1) Have available laryngoscope handle, curved and straight blades, ET tubes, stylet, suction, and tape or ET tube holder. Ensure that the light source on the laryngoscope is functional.	Light is necessary on the laryngoscope to visualize the vocal cords and intubate the trachea. Batteries may need to be changed.

STEP	RATIONALE

3 Secondary survey: B (CONFIRMATION OF AIRWAY AND VENTILATION)

   a Assist in confirmation of endotracheal tube placement by auscultating epigastric area for lack of breath sounds and then the lungs for bilateral breath sounds. Intubation personnel usually perform secondary confirmation by using a carbon dioxide detector.

   b Ventilate using a bag-mask device upon intubation at a rate of 8 to 10 breaths/min.

Tracheal tube placement in the esophagus does not provide ventilation of the lungs.

Chest x-ray film is usually obtained after patient has been stabilized to confirm placement of endotracheal tube and central venous catheters.

Avoid hyperventilation. The increased intrathoracic pressure due to incomplete exhalation results in reduced cardiac output (Field, 2006).

4 Secondary survey: C (ANALYSIS OF CARDIAC RHYTHM)

   a Attach manual defibrillator/monitor to patient using electrocardiogram (ECG) electrodes; Quick-Look paddles with gel pads or "hands-off" defibrillation pads/cable will also provide visualization of the heart rhythm (see illustration).

Quick-Look paddle placement on the chest immediately reveals the patient's heart rhythm. AED pads often are compatible with the hands-off defibrillator cable. This also offers a very fast approach to connecting to the manual defibrillator. "Hands-off" pads or cable allows defibrillation without coming into contact directly with the patient during shock delivery. Not all manual defibrillators have this function.

   b If cardiac rhythm is shockable, assist code team with manual defibrillation.

     (1) Place paddles or pads on patient's chest wall. ACLS-certified personnel will charge defibrillator to appropriate energy and discharge the device after announcing "Clear!"

Manual defibrillation is performed only by trained licensed personnel.

Good skin to paddle/pad contact ensures appropriate discharge of current and decreases chance of skin burns (Field, 2006).

   c Establish IV access with the largest possible IV catheter, and begin infusion of 0.9% normal saline or lactated Ringer's solution.

     (1) If you cannot obtain peripheral IV access, physicians may pursue central venous or intraosseous access.

Provides a route for rapid drug administration, access for blood samples, and fluid administration. Physiological saline is isotonic.

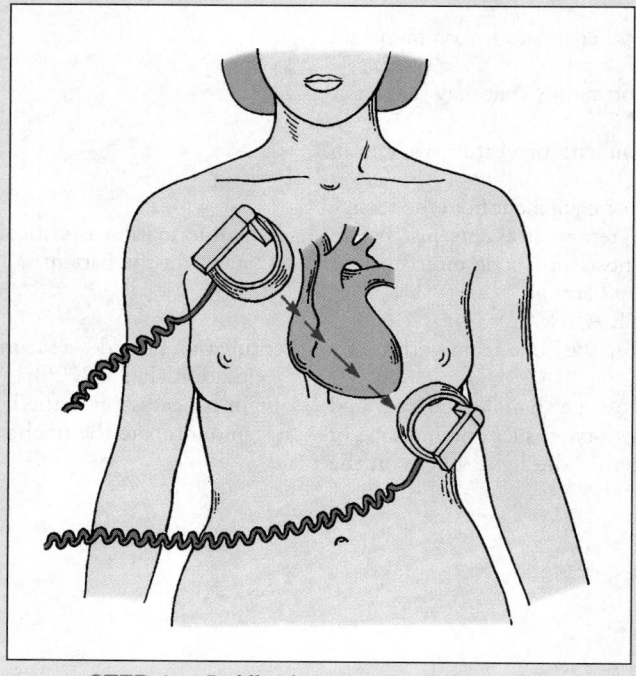

STEP 4a Paddle placement for defibrillation.

STEP	RATIONALE
d Assist with procedures as needed.	Much of the equipment needed for special procedures during a code is on the crash cart. Knowledge of the crash cart contents is very helpful in the code to provide personnel with the appropriate equipment.
5 Secondary survey: D (DIFFERENTIAL DIAGNOSIS) a Assist physician with differential diagnosis.	Physician will need laboratory/diagnostic testing or further procedures to help identify the cause of the arrest.

EVALUATION

1 Reassess the primary and secondary surveys (ABCDs) throughout the code event.	This will keep the process organized and address the immediate needs of the patient.
2 Palpate carotid pulse at least every 5 minutes after first minute of CPR.	Documents adequacy of external cardiac compressions.
3 Observe for spontaneous return of respirations or heart rate.	
4 Ensure that interruptions in CPR are minimized.	Interruptions are associated with reduced coronary artery perfusion pressure and lower mean coronary perfusion pressure (Berg and others, 2003).

Unexpected Outcomes	Related Interventions
1 Patient develops skeletal injury, such as fractured ribs or sternum, or internal organ injury, such as lacerated lung or liver, as a result of chest compressions.	• Obtain appropriate diagnostic tests to document injuries. • Assess patient's postarrest breathing for symmetry and pain. • Observe for intrathoracic or intraabdominal bleeding. • Observe for distending abdomen.
2 Patient's CPR is unsuccessful.	• Contact chaplain services. • Contact social worker. • Complete postmortem care on patient. • Provide for privacy for patient's family to say their good-byes to patient.
3 Rescuer is unassisted, tires, and is unable to continue.	• Obtain assistance.

Recording and Reporting

- Immediately report arrest, indicating exact location of victim.
- In hospital setting, follow hospital policy. In community setting, activate the emergency response system.
- Cardiopulmonary arrest requires precise documentation. Most hospitals use a form designed specifically for in-hospital arrests.
- Record in nurses' notes or on designated CPR worksheet: onset of arrest, time and number of AED shocks (you will not know the exact energy level used by the AED), time and energy level of manual defibrillations, medications given, procedures performed, cardiac rhythm, use of CPR, and the patient's response.

Teaching Considerations

- If patient is at risk for cardiopulmonary arrest, instruct the family or caregivers in CPR or encourage them to obtain certification through an instructor from the hospital, American Red Cross, or AHA.
- Patient and family should keep emergency numbers taped to the phone or consider programming them into speed dial function on both home and mobile phones. Stress the use of 9-1-1.

- It is extremely helpful if family has list of medications patient is presently taking.

Pediatric Considerations

- All persons involved in administering CPR must understand different breathing/compression ratios, hand (fingers) placement, and depth of compression in children and infants compared with adults.
- Infants and children experience respiratory arrest much more frequently than full cardiopulmonary arrest.
- Quick reference, color-coded guides are frequently utilized in pediatric codes to quickly determine appropriate drug doses and equipment sizes.

Gerontological Considerations

- In older adults, compressions often result in rib or cartilage fractures. You should continue cardiopulmonary resuscitation.
- Remove loose-fitting dentures to avoid obstructing the airway. If dentures fit securely, leave them in to provide a tight seal when providing ventilations.

Home Care Considerations

- In the community and long-term care settings, patients may have implanted cardioverter defibrillators (ICDs) and/or pacemakers. For these patients, families need to know how to administer CPR and the specific capabilities of the patient's ICD/pacemaker. Placement of defibrillator or AED pads/paddles may need to be altered to avoid placement directly on top of an ICD or pacemaker generator. Remove medication patches from chest.
- Soft surfaces such as a mattress, car seat, or grassy surface decrease efficiency of external cardiac compressions.

Long-Term Care Considerations

- It is important for patients and their families to clarify the patient's code status upon entering a long-term care environment. Patients need to detail their wishes regarding resuscitative care in an advance directive or other legal document. Families must also understand that a copy of the patient's advance directive should accompany the patient upon transfer to another health care facility if necessary. Families may consider keeping a copy of this document to take with them to the health care facility if their family member is transferred.

CRITICAL THINKING EXERCISES

You are the charge nurse for night shift on a general medical floor. On your rounds you find your patient, Ethel Waters, lying unresponsive on the floor of the bathroom. She is 85 years old and was admitted with heart failure. An AED is available down the hall.

1 What should you do first? Explain your choice.
   A Apply AED.
   B Call for help.
   C Check for a pulse.
   D Open airway and provide two breaths.
2 You look, listen, and feel for Mrs. Waters' breathing. No breathing is detected. You open her airway and deliver two breaths. Which of the following is the *least* desired method to provide artificial ventilations/breaths? Explain your choice.
   A Mouth-to-mouth
   B Mouth-to-mouth with barrier device
   C Mouth-to-mask
   D Bag-mask device
3 After you successfully ventilate Mrs. Waters, your co-worker arrives with the AED. What is your next step? Explain your choice.
   A Check for a pulse.
   B Start chest compressions.
   C Apply the AED.
   D Continue with 8 to 10 breaths per minute.
4 Your co-worker has started chest compressions on Mrs. Waters. Under which of the following circumstances should you interrupt performance of the chest compressions? Explain your choice.
   A Arrival of the code team
   B AED advises, "Do NOT touch the patient."
   C Initiation of bag-mask ventilation
   D IV insertion
5 The code team has arrived to continue resuscitation attempts on Mrs. Waters. What activities will be involved in the code team's work? How can you participate?

REVIEW QUESTIONS

1 A nurse is reviewing the procedure for insertion of an oropharyngeal airway. Which of the following is true about an oral airway?
   1 It eliminates the need to position the head of the unconscious patient.
   2 It eliminates the possibility of an upper airway obstruction.
   3 It needs to be inserted even when a patient has had recent oral trauma.
   4 It may stimulate vomiting or laryngospasm if inserted in the semiconscious patient.
2 A visitor suffers a cardiac arrest, and resuscitation is begun. The nurse would be correct doing CPR and operating an AED if which sequence was followed?
   1 Call for help, check for a pulse, attach the AED, open the airway, provide two breaths if needed, then turn on the AED.
   2 Wait for the AED, then open the airway, provide two breaths if needed, check for a pulse, and if no pulse, attach the AED.
   3 Call for help, get the AED, open the airway, provide two breaths if needed, check for a pulse, continue compressions if no pulse is present, attach the AED.
   4 Provide two breaths, check for a pulse, call for the AED, provide chest compressions until the AED arrives, attach the AED.
3 The airway needs to be established in a suspected trauma victim. Which technique would the nurse use to open the airway in this patient?
   1 Head tilt
   2 Chin lift
   3 Jaw thrust
   4 Lateral lying position
4 The nurse is participating in a code on an adult and are awaiting the AED to be applied. At what rate should the compressions and breaths be delivered?
   1 60 chest compressions per minute at a ratio of 30 compressions to 2 breaths
   2 60 chest compressions per minute at a ratio of 15 compressions to 2 breaths
   3 80 chest compressions per minute at a ratio of 15 compressions to 2 breaths
   4 100 chest compressions per minute at a ratio of 30 compressions to 2 breaths
5 The nurse is involved in resuscitating a patient. The AED has just delivered a shock. What should be done after the shock has been delivered if no pulse is present?
   1 Continue CPR for another minute until the AED recharges.
   2 Start an IV of normal saline with a large-size IV catheter.
   3 Reposition the patient's head for better respiratory effort.
   4 Continue CPR for 2 minutes before attempting another shock.

REFERENCES

Abella BS and others: Quality of cardiopulmonary resuscitation during in-hospital cardiac arrest, JAMA 293:305, 2005.

American Heart Association guidelines for cardiopulmonary resuscitation and emergency cardiovascular care, *Circulation* 112:IV-1, 2005.

American Heart Association: Community lay rescuer automated external defibrillator programs, *Circulation* 113:1260, 2006.

American Nurses Association: *Position statement: nursing care and do-not-resuscitate (DNR) decision,* Washington DC, 2003, The Association.

Cooper JA and others: Cardiopulmonary resuscitation: history, current practice and future direction, *Circulation* 114:2839, 2006.

Doorenbos AZ: The use of advance directives in a population of Asian Indian Hindus, *J Transcult Nurs* 14(1):17, 2003.

Emergency Nurses Association position statement: diversity in emergency care, Des Plaines, Ill, 2003, The Association.

Emergency Nurses Association position statement: family presence at the bedside during invasive procedures and cardiopulmonary resuscitation, Des Plaines, Ill, 2005, The Association.

Field JM, editor: *Advanced cardiovascular life support (ACLS) provider manual,* Dallas, 2006, American Heart Association.

Hazinski MF and others: Major changes in the 2005 AHA guidelines on CPR and ECC: Reaching the tipping point for change, *Circulation* 112(24, suppl):IV206, 2006.

Hockenberry MJ, Wilson D: *Wong's nursing care of infants and children,* ed 8, St. Louis, 2007, Mosby.

Institute for Healthcare Improvement: Establish a rapid response team, 2008, http://www.ihi.org/IHI/Topics/CriticalCare/IntensiveCare/Change/EstablishaRapidResponseTeam.htm.

The Joint Commission: *2009 National Patient Safety Goals,* http://www.jointcommission.org/PatientSafety/NationalPatientSafetyGoals/08_hap_npsgs.htm, accessed 2008.

Kozik TM: Induced hypothermia for patients with cardiac arrest: role of a clinical nurse specialist, *Crit Care Nurse* 27(5):36, 2007.

Nolan JP and others: Therapeutic hypothermia after cardiac arrest: an advisory statement by the Advanced Life Support Task Force of the International Liaison Committee on Resuscitation, *Circulation* 108:118, 2003.

Sorrentino S: *Mosby's textbook for nursing assistants,* ed 7, St. Louis, 2008, Mosby.

RESEARCH REFERENCES

Berg RA and others: Automated external defibrillation versus manual defibrillation for prolonged ventricular fibrillation: lethal delays of chest compressions before and after countershocks, *Ann Emerg Med* 42:458, 2003.

Bernard SA and others: Treatment of comatose survivors of out-of-hospital cardiac arrest with induced hypothermia, *N Engl J Med* 346:557, 2002.

Bunch TJ and others: Outcomes after ventricular fibrillation out-of-hospital cardiac arrest: expanding the chain of survival, *Mayo Clin Proc* 80:774, 2005.

Hypothermia After Cardiac Arrest Study Group: Mild therapeutic hypothermia to improve the neurological outcome after cardiac arrest, *N Engl J Med* 346:549, 2002.

MacLean S and others: Family presence during cardiopulmonary resuscitation and invasive procedures: practices of critical care and emergency nurses, *Am J Crit Care* 12:246, 2003.

Wik L and others: Quality of cardiopulmonary resuscitation during out-of-hospital cardiac arrest, *JAMA* 293:299, 2005.

Intravenous and Vascular Access Therapy

MEDIA RESOURCES

- **evolve**   http://evolve.elsevier.com/Perry/skills
  - Review Questions
  - Video Clips

- Mosby's Nursing Video Skills, 3.0

- NSO   Nursing Skills Online

OBJECTIVES

Mastery of content in this chapter will enable the nurse to:

- Discuss patient conditions requiring intravenous (IV) therapy.
- Explain how to prepare a patient and family for IV therapy.
- Discuss complications of IV therapy.
- Identify individualized outcomes for patients requiring IV therapy.
- Explain techniques for preventing transmission of infection for

a patient receiving IV therapy.
- Demonstrate initiation of IV therapy, regulation of IV flow rate, changing of IV solutions, changing of IV tubing, changing of IV dressings, and discontinuing a peripheral IV.
- Identify common types of central vascular access devices (CVADs) and describe their care and maintenance.
- Identify the educational needs of patients with CVADs.

One way to replace fluid and electrolytes is through the infusion of fluids directly into the bloodstream rather than via the digestive system. The use of intravenous (IV) therapy for a patient with an alteration in fluid and electrolyte balance is standard in nursing practice. Parenteral replacement includes IV fluid and electrolyte (crystalloids) therapy, blood and blood component (colloids) administration (see Chapter 29), total parenteral nutrition (TPN), and peripheral parenteral nutrition (PPN) (see Chapter 32). The goal of IV therapy is to maintain or prevent fluid and electrolyte imbalances without any complications associated with the delivery of IV medications and fluids (Burke, 2005). Evidence-based practice guides the safe, efficient, quality care necessary to provide infusion therapy. Follow the six rights of medication and IV fluid administration: right drug/solution, right dose/concentration, right patient, right route, right date/time, and right documentation (Hodgson and Kizor, 2006). This includes knowledge of the correct solution and equipment and how to initiate an infusion, regulate infusion rate, care for and maintain the system, identify and correct problems, and discontinue the infusion. To safely and correctly

provide infusion therapy, you need astute clinical management and specialized IV therapy skills in addition to your knowledge and professional accountability.

INTRAVENOUS SOLUTIONS

Many prepared IV solutions are available for use (Table 28-1). Intravenous solutions fall into the following categories: isotonic, hypotonic, and hypertonic. Isotonic fluids have the same osmolality as body fluids and are used most often to replace extracellular volume (e.g., prolonged vomiting). Isotonic fluids effectively mimic the body's fluid loss in the absence of an electrolyte imbalance. Hypotonic solutions are those that have an effective osmolality less than that of body fluids. Hypertonic solutions are those that have an effective osmolality greater than body fluids. The patient's specific fluid and electrolyte imbalance guides the need for hypotonic or hypertonic solutions.

Administer all IV fluids carefully, especially hypertonic solutions, because these solutions pull fluid into the vascular space by osmosis,

TABLE 28-1 | Intravenous Solutions

Solution	Concentration	Other Names
Dextrose in Water Solutions		
Dextrose 5% in water*	Isotonic	D_5W
Dextrose 10% in water	Hypertonic	$D_{10}W$
Dextrose 50% in water	Hypertonic	$D_{50}W$
Saline Solutions		
0.45% sodium chloride (half normal saline)	Hypotonic	½ NS 0.45% NS
0.33% sodium chloride (one-third normal saline)	Hypotonic	⅓ NS
0.9% sodium chloride† (normal saline)	Isotonic	NS 0.9% NS 0.9% NaCl
3%-5% sodium chloride	Hypertonic	3%-5% NS 3%-5% NaCl
Dextrose in Saline Solutions		
Dextrose 5% in 0.9% sodium chloride	Hypertonic	$D_5$0.9% NaCl $D_5$0.9% NS D_5NS
Dextrose 5% in 0.45% NaCl sodium chloride	Hypertonic	$D_5$0.45% NaCl $D_5$0.45% NS D_5½ NS
Multiple Electrolyte Solutions		
Lactated Ringer's‡	Isotonic	LR
Dextrose 5% in Lactated Ringer's	Hypertonic	D_5LR

*Dextrose is quickly metabolized, leaving free water to be distributed evenly in all fluid compartments (Heitz and Horne, 2005).
†Although it is isotonic because the total concentration of electrolytes equals plasma concentration, it contains 154 mEq of both sodium and chloride, which is a higher concentration of these electrolytes than is found in the plasma, which can cause fluid volume excess (Heitz and Horne, 2005).
‡Contains sodium, potassium, calcium, chloride, and lactate.

resulting in an increased vascular volume that will possibly result in pulmonary edema. This is common in high-risk patients with cardiac or renal disease. A patient's serum electrolyte values and fluid volume balance will determine the appropriate type and amount of IV solution.

Certain additives, most commonly vitamins and potassium chloride (KCl), are frequently added to IV solutions. Some IV fluids arrive from the manufacturer with potassium already added to decrease the chance of medication error. If this is unavailable, the pharmacy prepares the IV admixture. You add potassium to IV solutions only after there is verification of a patient's adequate urine output to reduce the risk for hyperkalemia. During IV therapy, monitor the patient's laboratory values and assess for fluid and electrolyte balance. *Under no circumstances should you give potassium chloride by IV push. A direct IV infusion of KCl may be fatal.* Before adding additives to an IV, obtain a health care provider's order that includes the required additives, for example, Bag 1: 1000 mL D$_5$½ NS with 20 mEq KCl at 100 mL/hr.

INTRAVENOUS CATHETERS

Peripheral venous catheters are made of polymers, such as polyurethane, silicone, or polyethylene. Commonly used over-the-needle catheters (ONCs) comprise a metal stylet, which you will use to pierce the skin, and a Teflon, polyurethane, or silicone catheter, which is threaded into a vein and remains there for the infusion of fluid. These flexible catheters do not dislodge from the vein as easily as stainless steel needles. Steel-winged devices (butterfly needles) are for limited, short-term situations because of vein trauma and complications (e.g., infiltration and phlebitis). An 18- to 24-gauge flexible catheter is used for adults, whereas a 22- to 24-gauge catheter is used for children and or any patient with small or fragile veins.

The Needlestick Safety and Prevention Act, enacted in 2001, requires health care facilities to use effective and safer medical devices to reduce the risk for needle-stick and sharp injuries. Common needle-stick injuries include recapping needles, assembling or accessing IV tubing devices with needles, disposing of contaminated sharps, and using alternative methods to cover used needles. IV catheters and steel-winged catheters are devices commonly associated with a high risk for injuries. There are safer medical devices such as sliding sheaths that cover used needles, retracting needles, and needleless systems. There are currently three types of needleless systems available: prepierced septum/blunt catheter, Luer-activated device (LAD), and pressure-activated safety valve device. To help prevent accidental injury, do not recap needles, but place them directly in puncture-proof containers, referred to as sharps containers. Safety standards now recommend the use of needleless devices that eliminate the use of needles altogether. Needleless devices use protective covers and valvelike systems and come in a variety of needle, catheter, and tubing products.

EVIDENCE-BASED PRACTICE TRENDS

Established standards for routine replacement of peripheral IV catheters and IV administration sets recommend a maximum of 72 hours to reduce IV fluid contamination and prevention of catheter site complications (Ahlqvist and others, 2006; Centers for Disease Control and Prevention [CDC], 2002; Eggimann, 2007; Infusion Nurses Society [INS], 2006). Prevention of complications such as bloodstream infection, infiltration, and phlebitis are important and require regular replacement of IV administration sets and rotation of peripheral catheter sites. Advanced catheter materials such as polyurethane are more biocompatible and are associated with less traumatic insertions, more blood vessel preservation, and increased cost savings (Occupational Safety and Health Administration [OSHA], 2006).

The Needlestick Safety and Prevention Act was enacted to prevent risks related to inadvertent injuries with vascular access devices (VADs) and sharps (Deacon, 2004; OSHA, 2006). VADs and ancillary sharps such as Huber access needles are available with safety features, and health care facilities usually require their use (INS, 2006). Research suggests that a dedicated, nurse-driven IV team that implements the most current technologies, maintains IV therapy knowledge and aseptic technique, and incorporates the current standards and guidelines will improve patient outcomes and reduce complications (Ean and others, 2006; Eggimann, 2007; Richardson, 2007).

CULTURAL CONSIDERATIONS

Current standards of nursing and evidence-based practice dictate the need for culturally competent practices in health care settings. These standards promote an environment and plan of care that is inclusive of cultural and other forms of diversity. Communication and education are essential components of positive therapeutic outcomes with diverse populations. Educate patients and caregivers regarding their IV therapy with attention to cultural and linguistic sensitivity. Education includes clear and concise terms for all aspects of IV therapy and individualized training that includes self-care practices (INS, 2006; Pearson and others, 2007).

Skill Performance Guidelines

1 Know the patient's baseline vital signs before initiating IV therapy. Fluid and electrolyte imbalances affect vital signs. Dehydration sometimes produces hypotension and tachycardia. Fluid overload results in hypertension and bounding pulses. Alterations in serum potassium results in an irregular pulse.

2 The proportion of total body water to body mass changes from infancy to older adult years.

3 Know the patient's weight. Body size affects total body water. Fat contains no water; the overweight patient has proportionately less body water.

4 Know the patient's medical history, current medications, and therapies. Medications affect fluid and electrolyte balance (e.g., diuretics or steroids). Determine the patient's previous experience with IV therapy.

5 Beware of prolonged environmental conditions that affect the patient's fluid status (e.g., exposure to hot, humid weather) leading to fluid and electrolyte imbalances, particularly in the infant, older adult, and the chronically ill.

6 Know if the patient is right- or left-handed. For comfort and mobility, place an IV in the nondominant arm.

7 Ensure that an IV system is intact, and there is no evidence of phlebitis or infiltration. An intact system ensures that you have maintained sterility and that no fluid or medication has been lost.

8 Note the date of the last IV administration set and dressing change (Box 28-1).

9 Maintain sterility of a patent IV system using the INS standards (see Box 28-1).

10 Know the standard precautions for infection control and the Occupational Safety and Health Administration (OSHA) standards for occupational exposure to blood-borne pathogens (Box 28-2).

BOX 28-1	INS Standards to Decrease Intravascular Infection Related to Intravenous Therapy

- Palpate catheter insertion site for tenderness daily through the intact dressing.
- Directly inspect a catheter site if patient develops tenderness at site, fever without obvious source, or symptoms of local or bloodstream infection.
- Perform hand hygiene before and after palpating, inserting, replacing, or dressing any intravascular device.
- Cleanse skin site before venipuncture with an appropriate single-use antiseptic solution.
- Allow site to air-dry before proceeding with procedure.
- Do not palpate insertion site after skin has been cleansed with single-use antiseptic solution.
- Use catheter stabilization device that allows visual inspection of access site.
- Gauze dressings that cover a catheter site must be changed every 48 hours.
- Intravenous tubing administration sets can remain sterile for 72 hours. Do not change more often than 72-hour intervals unless clinically indicated.
- Replace tubing used to administer blood, blood products, or lipid emulsions within 24 hours of initiating infusion.
- After being added to an administration set, change parenteral medications and fluids every 24 hours.
- Replace dressing over peripheral venous catheters when replacing catheter or when dressing becomes damp, loosened, or soiled.
- Clean injection ports with single-use antiseptic solution before accessing system.
- Replace short, peripheral venous catheters and rotate sites every 72 hours or immediately when complications appear.
- There is no recommendation for the frequency of replacement of a peripherally inserted central catheter (PICC).

Modified from Infusion Nurses Society: Infusion nursing standards of practice, *J Intraven Nurs* 29(suppl 1):S1, 2006.
INS, Infusion Nurses Society. *IV,* Intravenous; *OSHA,* Occupational Safety and Health Administration.

BOX 28-2	Standards for Reducing Occupational Exposure to Blood-Borne Pathogens

1 Gloves are necessary when there is a reasonable expectation that the employee may contact blood; for example, during vascular access procedures or while changing IV administration sets.
2 Immediately place contaminated needles, needleless devices, and other sharps in puncture-resistant, leak-proof containers properly labeled as a biohazard; when the containers are full, seal and dispose of them properly.
3 Do not bend, shear, recap, or remove contaminated needles from the syringe after use.
4 OSHA requires reports of needle-stick injuries, and the health care agency must provide medical evaluation and follow-up.
5 Hepatitis B vaccination should be made available to all employees who have occupational exposure.
6 Training and education about exposure prevention and use of protective equipment must be offered to high-risk workers who initiate IV therapy.
7 Each facility must have an infection control plan, including methods to reduce health care worker's exposure to biohazardous wastes.
8 Facilities must have engineering and work practice controls to eliminate or minimize employee exposure. Controls may include sharps disposal containers and self-sheathing needles.

Modified from Occupational Safety and Health Administration: Occupational exposure to blood borne pathogens, needlestick, and other sharps injuries: final rule, CFR 29, part 1910 (*Fed Regist* 66:5317, Jan 18, 2001), updated April 2006, http://www.osha.gov/SLTC/bloodbornepathogens/index.html.

SKILL 28-1 Initiating Intravenous Therapy

 Advanced / Intravenous Fluid Therapy Administration / Preparing an Infusion Site
Performing Venipuncture and Initiating an Infusion

NSO *IV Fluid Administration Module / Lessons 1 and 2*

The goal of IV fluid administration is correction or prevention of fluid and electrolyte disturbances in patients. For example, a patient who is NPO (nothing by mouth) after surgery routinely receives IV fluid replacement to prevent fluid and electrolyte imbalances. Another reason for IV access is to administer intermittent or emergency medication. IV administration often occurs through the use of an injection port (e.g., saline lock), which is an IV catheter attached to an injection cap to maintain a closed system. Sometimes you use a short piece of extension tubing. Flush the saline lock with 0.9% sodium chloride solution (see agency protocol) or after each administration of medication to maintain patency of the IV catheter (see Chapter 22). Peripherally placed catheters are for short-term use (e.g., fluid restoration postoperatively and short-term antibiotic administration). Central venous access devices (CVADs), which include nontunneled and tunneled catheters, peripherally inserted central catheters (PICC), and implanted ports are for long-term use. These devices are more effective than peripherally placed catheters for administering medications and solutions that are irritating to veins. Increased use of CVADs requires education in the care of these devices.

Delegation Considerations
The skill of initiating peripheral intravenous therapy cannot be delegated to nursing assistive personnel (NAP). Delegation to licensed practical nurses (LPNs) varies by state Nurse Practice Act. The nurse directs the NAP to:
- Inform the nurse if the patient complains of burning, bleeding, swelling, or coolness at the catheter insertion site.
- Inform the nurse if the patient's IV dressing becomes wet.
- Inform the nurse if the solution of fluid in the IV bag is low or the electronic infusion device (EID) alarm is sounding.

Equipment
- ❑ Correct IV solution
- ❑ Proper IV safety access device for venipuncture (will vary with patient's body size and reason for IV fluid administration). In an adult a peripheral 22-gauge cannula is appropriate for fluid maintenance (Rosenthal, 2005). Use a steel-winged infusion set only for short-term therapy (INS, 2006).
- ❑ IV start kit (available in some agencies): may contain a sterile drape to place under the patient's arm, tourniquet, cleansing and antiseptic preparations, dressings, and a small roll of sterile tape

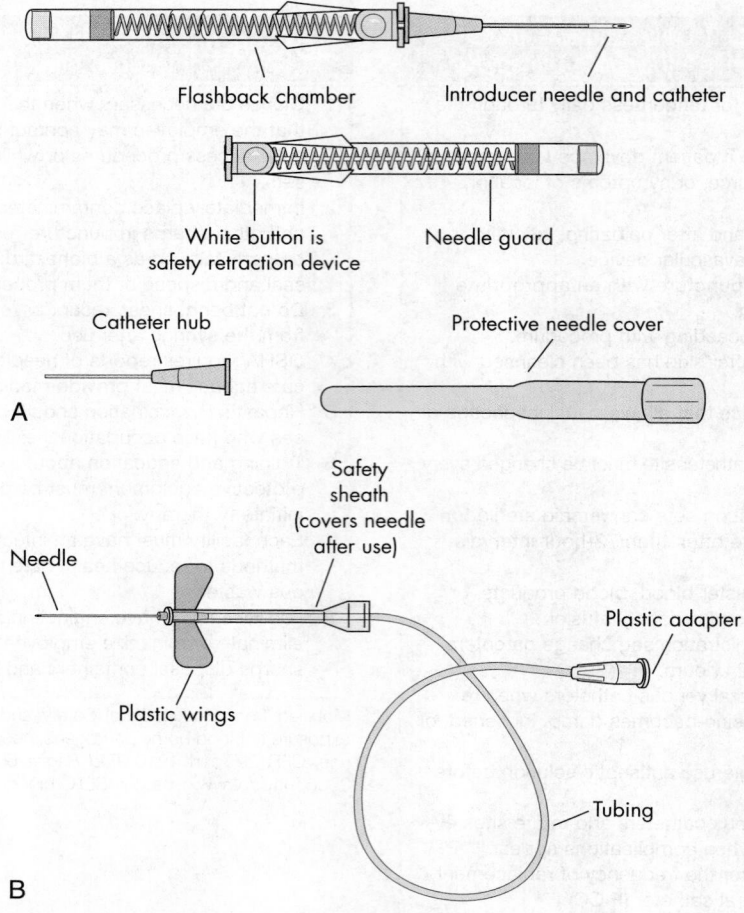

FIG 28-1 Intravenous access device options. **A,** Over-the-needle catheter (ONC) device. **B,** Steel butterfly needle.

❑ Local anesthetic (e.g., intradermal lidocaine, topical transdermal anesthetic, vapocoolant)

For IV Fluid Infusion

❑ Administration set (choice depends on type of solution and rate of administration; infants and children, patients with cardiac and renal disease, and certain medications require microdrip tubing, which provides 60 gtt/mL)

❑ 0.22-mm filter (if required by agency policy or if particulate matter is likely; size appropriate to type of solution)

❑ Extension tubing

❑ Antiseptic swabs or sticks (i.e., chlorhexidine gluconate, providine-iodine, or alcohol) (INS, 2006)

❑ Clean gloves

❑ Protective equipment: goggles, mask (optional, check agency policy)

❑ Tourniquet (Determine type of tourniquet based on patient assessment, e.g., blood pressure cuff [older adult], rubber band [infants]. Tourniquets are a source of contamination; use a single-use product.)

❑ Nonallergenic tape and sterile tape

❑ Towel (to place under patient's hand or arm)

❑ IV pole, rolling or ceiling mounted

❑ Special patient gown with snaps at shoulder seams (makes removal with IV tubing easier), if available

❑ Needle disposal container (also called sharps container)

❑ IV site protection device (*optional*)

For Heparin or Normal Saline Lock

❑ Injection cap (also called IV plug, prn adapter)

❑ IV loop or short piece of extension tubing, if necessary

❑ Syringe filled with 1 to 3 mL of 0.9% sodium chloride or heparin flush (10 units/mL as ordered)

Transparent Dressing Only

❑ Transparent dressing

Gauze Dressing Only

❑ 2 × 2 or 4 × 4 inch sterile gauze sponge

❑ Sterile tape

STEP	RATIONALE

ASSESSMENT

1   Review accuracy and completeness of health care provider's order for type and amount of IV fluid, medication additives, infusion rate, and length of therapy. Follow six rights of medication administration (see Chapter 20).

Before implementing this procedure, an order from a health care provider to initiate a peripheral VAD and administration of an IV solution is needed. Ensures safe and correct administration of IV therapy.

STEP	RATIONALE

Critical Decision Point   *In most medical facilities, health care providers do not write an order to "initiate peripheral access" or "perform venipuncture." The statement "Start IV" may be written followed by the exact IV therapy order. The order to perform the venipuncture is implied. If the order is confusing or in question, clarify with the health care provider before proceeding.*

STEP	RATIONALE
2 Assess for clinical factors/conditions that will respond to or be affected by IV fluid administration:	Provides baseline to determine effect IV fluids have on patient's fluid and electrolyte balance.
a Peripheral edema—rate severity by assessing pitting over bony prominences: 1+, indicating barely detectable edema, to 4+ indicating deep, persistent pitting (see Chapter 6).	Indicates expanded interstitial volume. This is usually most evident in dependent areas (i.e., feet and ankles). Fluid overload will worsen edema.
b Body weight.	Daily weights document fluid retention or loss. Change in body weight of 1 kg corresponds to 1 L of fluid retention or loss (Heitz and Horne, 2005).
c Dry skin and mucous membranes.	Suggests fluid volume deficit (FVD).
d Distended neck veins.	Suggests fluid volume excess (FVE).
e Blood pressure changes.	Elevated blood pressure may indicate FVE due to increase in stroke volume. Decreased blood pressure may indicate FVD due to a decrease in stroke volume.
f Irregular pulse rhythm; increased pulse rate.	Rhythm changes may occur with potassium, calcium, and/or magnesium abnormalities; rate change may occur with FVD.
g Auscultation of crackles or rhonchi in lungs.	May signal fluid buildup in the lungs due to FVE.
h Poor skin turgor (after pinching, skin fails to return to normal position within 3 seconds).	With FVD, the pinched skin stays elevated for several seconds. This is called "tenting."

Critical Decision Point   *Tenting is a less reliable indicator for older adults because their skin has lost elasticity naturally due to aging (Meiner and Lueckenotte, 2006).*

STEP	RATIONALE
i Anorexia, nausea, and vomiting.	Occurs with acute FVD or FVE.
j Thirst.	Symptomatic of FVD.
k Decreased urine output.	During dehydration, kidney attempts to restore fluid balance by reducing urine production. Average daily adult urine output is 1500 mL; urine output of less than 400 mL/24 hr (oliguria) signals the retention of metabolic wastes (Heitz and Horne, 2005).
l Behavioral changes (e.g., restlessness, confusion).	Occurs with FVD or acid-base imbalance.
m Decreased capillary refill.	Indicates poor tissue perfusion.
3 Assess patient's previous or perceived experience with IV therapy and arm placement preference.	Determines level of emotional support and instruction needed. If hypersensitive to venipunctures, a local anesthetic may be indicated.
4 Obtain information from drug reference books or pharmacist about composition of IV fluids, purposes of administration, potential incompatibilities, and possible side effects. Include information about the most appropriate type of catheter to use for administration.	Allows detection of an inadvisable IV fluid order and helps to determine priority assessments.
5 Determine if patient is to undergo any planned surgeries or procedures.	Allows anticipation and placement of appropriate VAD and size for fluid infusion and to avoid placement in an area that will interfere with medical procedures.
6 Assess for the following risk factors: child or older adult; presence of heart failure or renal failure, skin lesions, infection, low platelet count; or receiving anticoagulants.	Older adults develop fluid imbalances more rapidly because they have a proportionately larger extracellular fluid volume, persons with heart failure cannot adapt to sudden increases in vascular volume, and persons with renal failure cannot eliminate excess extracellular fluid. Skin lesions or infection influence choice of access site. Low platelet count or use of anticoagulants increases patient's risk for bleeding from VAD and affects venous integrity, increasing the risk for seepage of blood from puncture site during venipuncture attempt.
7 Assess laboratory data and patient's history of allergies, especially to iodine, adhesive, or latex.	Reveals information that affects insertion of devices, such as fluid volume deficit or allergy.
8 Assess patient's understanding of purpose of IV therapy.	Poses implications for patient education.

NURSING DIAGNOSES

- Anxiety
- Deficient knowledge regarding IV therapy
- Risk for deficient fluid volume
- Risk for imbalanced fluid volume
- Risk for infection

Individualize related factors based on patient's condition or needs.

STEP	RATIONALE

PLANNING

1   Expected outcomes following completion of procedure:
   • Fluid and electrolyte balance returns to normal.
   • Vital signs are stable and within normal limits for patient.

   • No swelling, pallor, pain, inflammation, or infiltration is present at venipuncture site.
   • IV line is patent, and infusion is delivered at ordered rate.
   • Patient is able to explain purpose and risks of IV therapy.

Indicates fluid and electrolyte imbalance is resolved.
Demonstrates circulatory system's response to fluid and electrolyte replacement.
Ensures catheter is in vein without evidence of complications.

Ensures instillation of IV fluids without obstruction.
Demonstrates learning.

IMPLEMENTATION

1   Instruct patient about the rationale for IV, fluids, and medications, procedure for initiating an IV, and signs and symptoms of complications.

Provides patient with information about procedure and promotes compliance.

2   Assist patient to comfortable sitting or supine position. Position yourself level with patient. Provide adequate lighting.

Promotes comfort and relaxation of patient. Provides proper body mechanics for nurse. Aids in successful vein location.

3   Verify patient's identity by using at least two patient identifiers. Compare patient's name and one other identifier, such as hospital identification number, with medication administration record (MAR). Ask patient to state name as a third identifier.

Complies with The Joint Commission requirements and improves patient safety. In most acute care settings, patient's name and identification number on armband and MAR are used to identify patients (The Joint Commission [TJC], 2007).

4   Perform hand hygiene. Organize equipment on clean, clutter-free bedside stand or over-bed table.

Reduces transmission of infection and risk for accidents.

5   Change patient's gown to the more easily removed gown with snaps at the shoulder, if available.

Use of a special IV gown makes it easier to safely remove the gown once you have inserted the IV.

6   Open sterile packages using sterile aseptic technique (see Chapter 8).

Maintains sterility of equipment and reduces spread of microorganisms.

7   Prepare IV infusion tubing and solution.

   a   Check IV solution, using six rights of medication administration (see Chapter 20). Be sure prescribed additives, such as potassium and vitamins, have been added. Check solution for color, clarity, and expiration date. Check bag for leaks. This is easier if you do it before reaching the bedside.

IV solutions are medications and need to be carefully checked to reduce risk for error. Do not use solutions that are discolored, contain particles, or are expired. Do not use leaky bags because they present an opportunity for infection.

   b   Open infusion set, maintaining sterility of both tubing ends. Many sets allow for priming of tubing without removal of end cap. EID pumps sometimes have a special dedicated administration set.

Prevents touch contamination, which allows microorganisms to enter infusion equipment and bloodstream.

   c   Place roller clamp (see illustration) about 2 to 5 cm (1 to 2 inches) below drip chamber, and move roller clamp to "off" position (see illustration).

Close proximity of roller clamp to drip chamber allows more accurate regulation of flow rate. Moving clamp to "off" prevents accidental spillage of IV fluid on patient, nurse, bed, or floor.

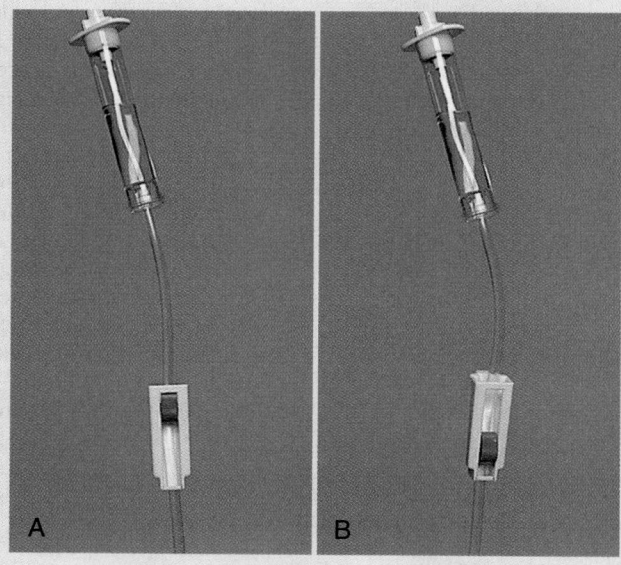

STEP 7c   **A,** Roller clamp in open position. **B,** Roller clamp in closed position.

STEP	**RATIONALE**
d Remove protective sheath over IV tubing port on plastic IV solution bag (see illustration) or top of bottle.	Provides access for insertion of infusion tubing into solution.
e Insert infusion set into fluid bag or bottle. Remove protector cap from tubing insertion spike, not touching spike, and insert spike into tubing port of IV container (see illustration). Cleanse rubber stopper on glass bottled solution with single-use antiseptic, and insert spike into black rubber stopper of IV bottle.	Flat surface on the top of bottled solution may contain contaminants, whereas opening to plastic bag is recessed. Prevents contamination of bottled solution during insertion of spike.

Critical Decision Point   *Do not touch spike because it is sterile. If contamination occurs (e.g., spike is accidentally dropped on the floor), then discard that IV tubing, and obtain a new one.*

f Prime infusion tubing by filling with IV solution: Compress drip chamber and release, allowing it to fill one-third to one-half full (see illustration).	Ensures tubing is clear of air before connection with VAD. Creates suction effect; fluid enters drip chamber to prevent air from entering tubing.
g Remove protector cap on end of tubing (you can prime some tubing without removal), and slowly open roller clamp to allow fluid to travel from drip chamber through tubing to needle adapter. Return roller clamp to "off" position after priming tubing (filled with IV fluid).	Slow fill of tubing decreases turbulence and chance of bubble formation. Removes air from tubing and permits tubing to fill with solution. Closing the clamp prevents accidental loss of fluid.
h Be certain tubing is clear of air and air bubbles. To remove small air bubbles, firmly tap IV tubing where air bubbles are located. Check entire length of tubing to ensure that all air bubbles are removed (see illustration). If using multiple-port tubing, turn port upside down, and tap to fill and remove air.	Large air bubbles act as emboli.

Critical Decision Point   *You may add extension tubing to IV tubing to allow for more length, which will enable patient to move more freely while still keeping IV line stable.*

i Replace cap protector on end of infusion tubing.	Maintains system sterility.
8 *Option:* Saline lock (capped catheter)	
a If you need a loop or short extension tubing because of awkward VAD placement, use sterile technique to connect extension to the IV tubing.	Used when continuous infusions are not needed.
b Swab injection cap with antiseptic swab. Insert syringe with 1 to 3 mL saline or heparin flush solution, and inject through the injection cap into the loop or short extension tubing.	Removes air from tubing and prevents air from being introduced into the vein.

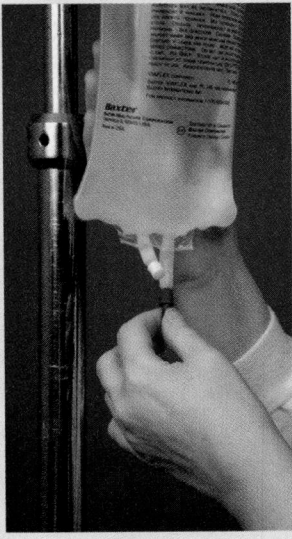

STEP 7d Removing protective sheath from IV bag port.

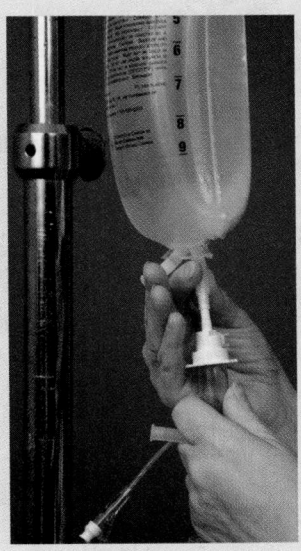

STEP 7e Inserting spike into IV bag.

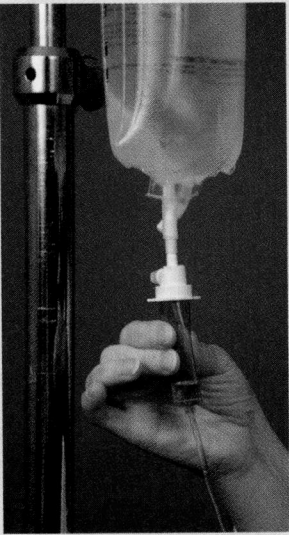

STEP 7f Squeezing drip chamber to fill with fluid.

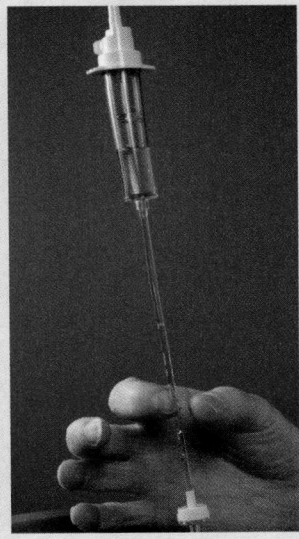

STEP 7h Removing air bubbles from tubing.

STEP	RATIONALE

9 Apply clean gloves. Wear eye protection and mask (see agency policy) if splash or spray of blood is possible.

Reduces transmission of microorganisms. Decreases exposure to human immunodeficiency virus (HIV), hepatitis, and other blood-borne organisms (CDC, 2006; INS, 2006). Prevents spraying blood from contacting your mucous membranes.

10 Identify accessible vein for VAD. Apply tourniquet around arm above antecubital fossa 10 to 15 cm (or 4 to 6 inches) above the proposed insertion site (see illustration). Do not apply tourniquet too tightly to avoid injury or bruising the skin. Check for presence of radial pulse. Apply tourniquet on top of a thin layer of clothing such as a gown sleeve. Sometimes it is necessary to remove tourniquet and move lower down arm. *Option*: Apply blood pressure cuff instead of tourniquet. Inflate to a level just below patient's normal diastolic pressure (less than 50 mm Hg). Maintain inflation at that pressure until you have completed venipuncture.

Tourniquet slows down venous return but should not occlude arterial flow. If you cannot find a vein in the hand or lower arm, move up to the antecubital fossa.

Use of blood pressure cuff reduces trauma to underlying skin and tissues.

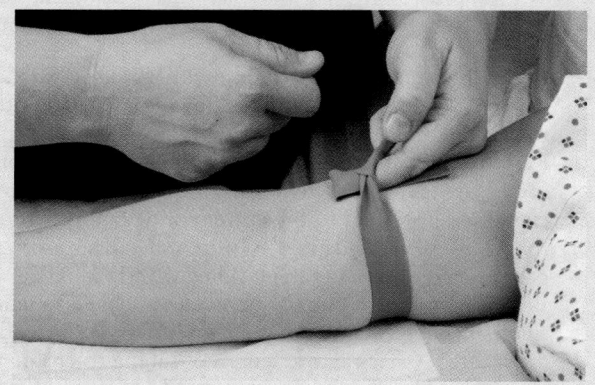

STEP 10   Tourniquet placed on arm for initial vein selection.

11 Vein distention.
 a Select well-dilated vein. Other methods to foster venous distention include:
 (1) Stroking the extremity from distal to proximal below the proposed venipuncture site.
 (2) Applying warmth to the extremity for several minutes, for example, with a warm washcloth.

Increases the volume of blood in the vein at the venipuncture site.
Promotes venous filling.

Increases blood supply and fosters venous dilation.

Critical Decision Point   *Gloves are not necessary to locate vein but must be applied before preparing the site.*

12 Vein selection. Select the vein for VAD insertion (see illustration). Veins found on the dorsal and ventral surfaces of upper extremities (e.g., cephalic, basilic, and median veins) are preferred in adults.

Ensures adequate vein that is easier to puncture with needle and less likely to rupture.

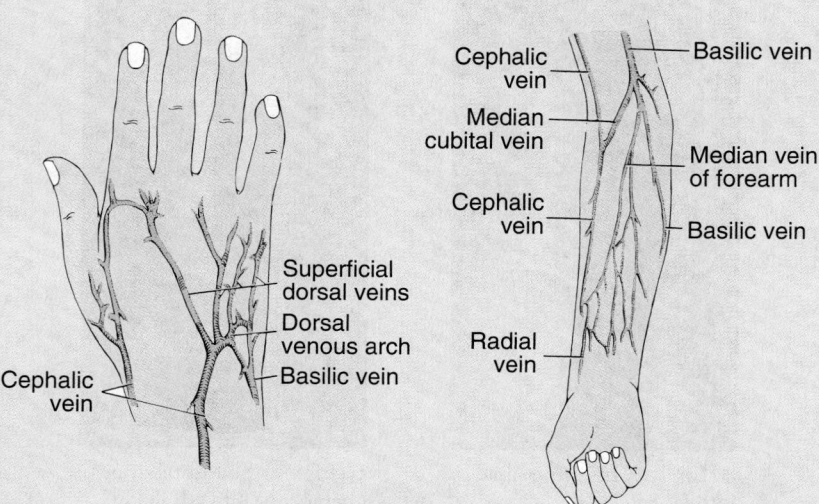

STEP 12   Cephalic, basilic, and median cubital veins are best for IV placement in adults.

STEP	RATIONALE
a Use the most distal site in the nondominant arm, if possible. Clip arm hair with scissors if necessary.	You perform venipuncture distal to proximal, which increases the availability of other sites for future IV therapy. Hair impedes venipuncture or adherence of dressing.

Critical Decision Point *Do not shave area with a razor. Shaving causes microabrasions and predisposes patient to infection (INS, 2006).*

STEP	RATIONALE
b Avoid areas affected by:	
(1) Pain, infection, or wound	Indicates inflammation.
(2) Previous cerebrovascular accident (CVA), paralysis, or mastectomy	Increases risk for complications such as infection, lymphedema, or vessel damage.
c Select a vein large enough for VAD.	Prevents interruption of venous flow while allowing adequate blood flow around the catheter.
d Choose a site that will not interfere with patient's activities of daily living (ADLs) or planned procedures.	Keeps patient as mobile as possible.
e With the index finger, palpate the vein by pressing downward. Note the resilient, soft, bouncy feeling while releasing the pressure (see illustration).	Fingertip is more sensitive and is better to assess vein condition.
f If possible, place extremity in dependent position.	Permits venous dilation and visibility.

Critical Decision Point *Vigorous friction and multiple tapping of the veins, especially in older adults, causes hematoma and/or venous constriction.*

STEP	RATIONALE
g Avoid sites distal to previous venipuncture site, veins in the antecubital fossa or inner wrist, sclerosed or hardened veins, infiltrate site or phlebotic vessels, bruised areas, and areas of venous valves.	Such sites cause infiltration of newly placed VAD and excessive vessel damage. Antecubital fossa area is used for blood draws; also limits mobility (Otto, 2005).
h Avoid fragile dorsal veins in older adult patients and vessels in an extremity with compromised circulation (e.g., in cases of mastectomy, dialysis graft, or paralysis).	Venous alterations increase risk for complications (e.g., infiltration and decreased catheter dwell time).
13 Release tourniquet temporarily and carefully. *Option:* At this point of the procedure there is the option of applying a local anesthetic to site. Monitor patient for allergic reaction.	Restores blood flow and prevents venospasm when preparing for venipuncture. Most patients prefer a local anesthetic (Earhart and others, 2007).
14 Apply clean gloves if not done in Step 9.	Reduces transmission of microorganisms.
15 Place adapter end of infusion tubing or extension/injection cap for saline lock nearby on sterile gauze or sterile towel.	Permits smooth, quick connection of infusion to VAD once vein is accessed.

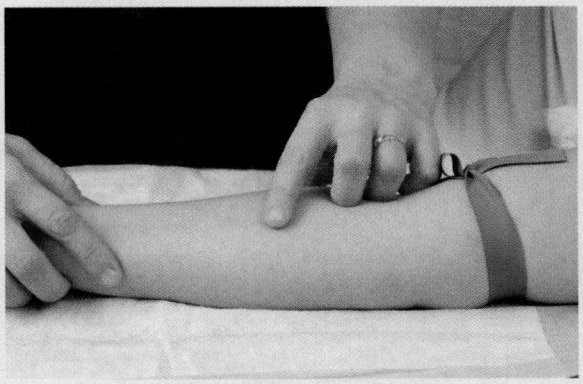

STEP 12e Palpate vein.

STEP	RATIONALE

16 If area of insertion appears to need cleansing, use soap and water first, then dry. Then use antiseptic swab to cleanse insertion site, working in a horizontal plane with first swab, vertical plane with second swab, and a circular motion, moving outward with third swab (see illustration). Allow to dry completely. Refrain from touching the cleansed site unless using sterile technique.

Mechanical friction in this pattern allows penetration of the antiseptic solution into the cracks and fissures of the epidermal layer of the skin (INS, 2006). Allowing antiseptic solutions to air-dry completely, effectively reduces microbial counts (INS, 2006). Drying allows time for maximum microbicidal activity of agents (Hadaway, 2006). Chlorhexidine 2% preparation is preferred (INS, 2006).

Touching cleansed area introduces microorganisms from your finger to site. If this happens, prepare the site again.

17 Reapply tourniquet 10 to 15 cm (4 to 6 inches) above anticipated insertion site. Check presence of distal pulse.

Diminished arterial flow prevents venous filling. The pressure of the tourniquet causes the vein to dilate.

18 Perform venipuncture. Anchor vein below site by placing thumb over vein and gently stretching the skin against the direction of insertion 4 to 5 cm (1½ to 2 inches) distal to the site (see illustration). Warn patient of a sharp, quick stick.

Stabilizes vein for needle insertion. Places VAD parallel to vein.

a *ONC with safety device:* Insert with the bevel up at 10- to 30-degree angle slightly distal to actual site of venipuncture in the direction of the vein (see illustration).

Places needle at a 10- to 30-degree angle to the vein. When vein is punctured, risk for puncturing posterior vein wall is reduced. Superficial veins require a smaller angle. Deeper veins require a greater angle.

b *Winged needle:* Hold needle at 10- to 30-degree angle with bevel up, slightly distal to actual site of venipuncture.

Critical Decision Point   *Use each VAD only once for each insertion attempt.*

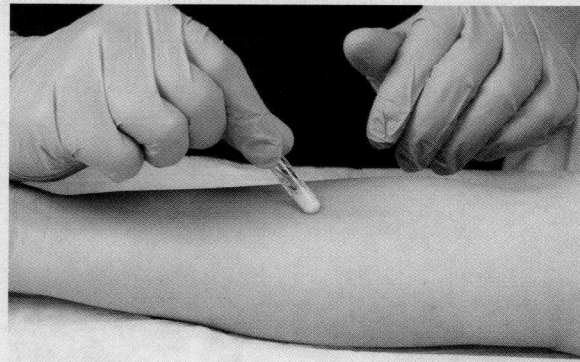

STEP 16   Cleanse site with chlorhexidine.

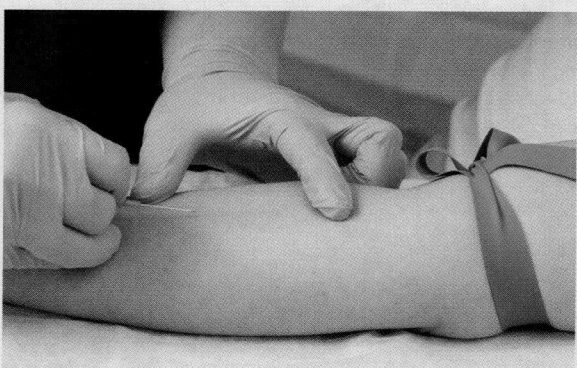

STEP 18   Stabilize vein below insertion site.

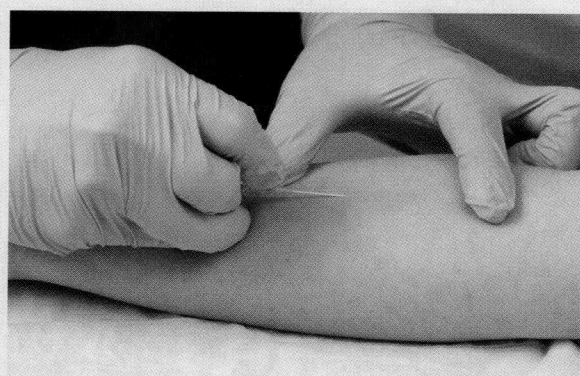

STEP 18a   Puncture skin with catheter at 10- to 30-degree angle.

STEP	**RATIONALE**
19 Observe for blood return through flashback chamber of catheter or tubing of winged catheter, indicating that bevel of needle has entered vein (see illustration A). Lower catheter/winged needle until almost flush with skin. Advance catheter/needle approximately ¼ inch into vein, and then loosen stylet if using ONC. Continue to hold skin taut while stabilizing the needle, and advance catheter off the needle to thread just the catheter into vein until hub is almost at insertion site (see illustration B). *Do not reinsert the stylet once it is loosened.* Advance the catheter while the safety device automatically retracts the stylet. (Note: Techniques for retracting stylet will vary with each IV device.) Advance winged cannula until hub rests at venipuncture site. Place needle/stylet directly into sharps container. Follow manufacturer's guidelines for specific safety catheter use.	Increased venous pressure from tourniquet increases backflow of blood into catheter or tubing. Allows for full penetration of the vein wall, placement of the catheter in the vein's inner lumen, and advancement of the catheter off the stylet. Reduces risk for introduction of microorganisms along catheter. Advancing the entire stylet into the vein may penetrate the wall of the vein, resulting in a hematoma. Reinsertion of stylet causes catheter shearing in the vein and potential catheter embolization.

Critical Decision Point   *A single nurse should not make more than two attempts at initiating IV access (INS, 2006). In that case, the nurse should have another nurse attempt the insertion.*

20 Stabilize catheter with one hand, and release tourniquet or blood pressure cuff with other. Apply gentle but firm pressure with middle finger of nondominant hand 3 cm (1¼ inches) above the insertion site. Keep catheter stable with index finger.	Permits venous flow, reduces backflow of blood, and allows connection with administration set with minimal blood loss.

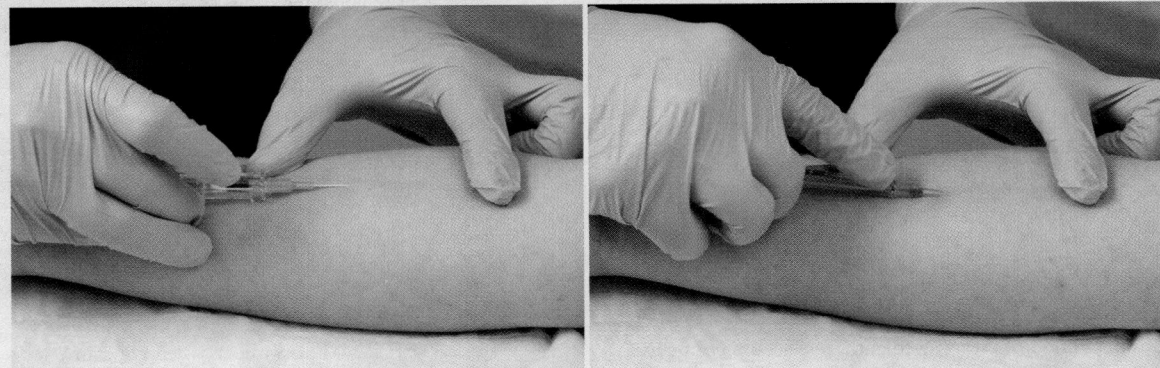

STEP 19   **A,** Observe for blood return in flashback chamber. **B,** Advance catheter into vein until hub is near insertion site.

STEP	RATIONALE
21 Quickly connect end of the prepared saline lock or the continuous infusion tubing set to end of catheter (see illustration). Do not touch point of entry of connection. Secure connection.	Prompt connection of infusion set maintains patency of vein and prevents risk for exposure to blood. Maintains sterility.
22 Flush injection cap of saline lock (see illustration), or begin infusion by slowly opening the slide clamp or adjusting the roller clamp of the IV tubing.	Initiates flow of fluid through IV catheter, preventing clotting of device.
23 Secure catheter (procedures differ; follow agency policy).	
a *Manufactured catheter stabilization device*: Wipe selected area with single-use skin protectant, and allow to dry. Slide device under catheter hub, and center hub over device. Holding catheter in place, peel off half of liner, press to adhere to skin. Repeat on other side. Holding catheter in place, pull tab out from center of device to create opening, insert catheter into slit. This frames the IV site (see illustration). Cover insertion site with a transparent or sterile gauze dressing.	The manufactured catheter stabilization device is a sterile, adhesive pad that holds the catheter in place and reduces the risk for infection and needle-stick injuries and improves patient outcomes (INS, 2006; Rosenthal, 2007).
b *Transparent dressing*: Secure catheter with nondominant hand while preparing to apply dressing.	Prevents accidental dislodgment of catheter.
c *Sterile gauze dressing*: Place narrow piece (½ inch) of sterile tape over catheter hub (see illustration). If sterile tape is not available, apply nonsterile tape around catheter hub or stabilization device. Place tape only on the catheter, *never* over the insertion site. Secure site to allow easy visual inspection. Avoid applying tape or gauze around arm.	Use only sterile tape under a sterile dressing to prevent site contamination. Prevents back-and-forth motion, which will irritate the vein and introduce microorganisms on the skin into the vein. Wrapping anything around the arm prevents visualization of the insertion site.
24 Observe site for swelling.	Swelling indicates infiltration, and the catheter would need to be removed.

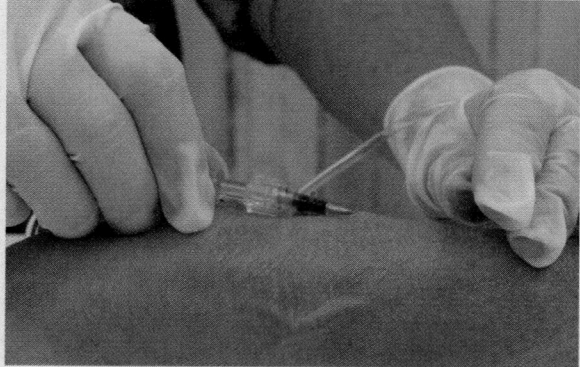

STEP 21 Connect end of IV tubing to catheter. Secure connection.

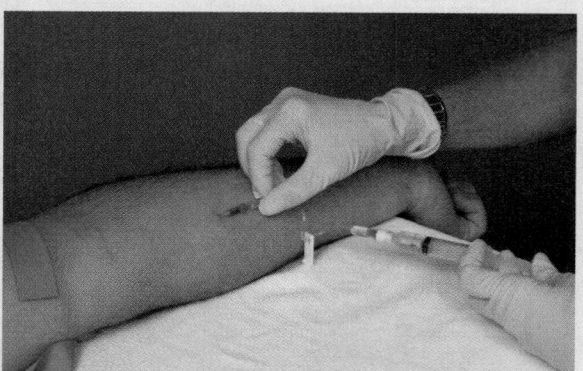

STEP 22 Flush injection cap of saline lock.

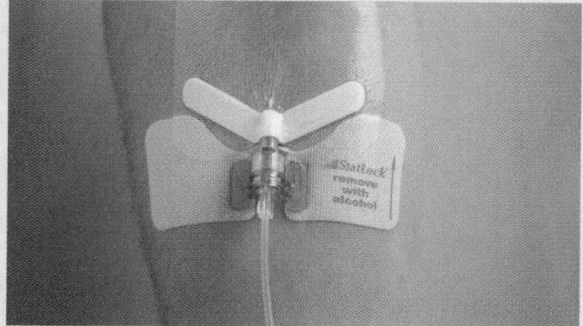

STEP 23a Catheter stabilization device in place. (*Courtesy C.R. Bard, Inc.*)

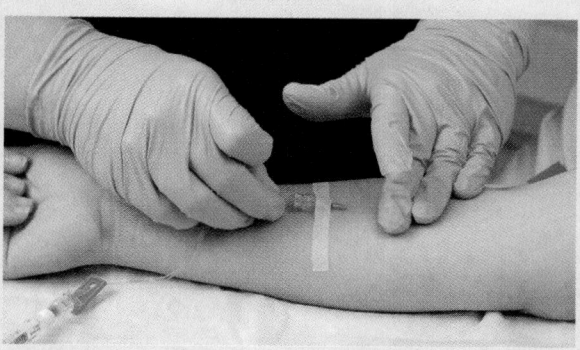

STEP 23c Tape over catheter hub.

STEP	RATIONALE

Critical Decision Point   *Be sure to calculate rate so as not to infuse IV solution too rapidly or too slowly.*

25 Apply sterile dressing over site.

  a Transparent dressing:

    (1) Carefully remove adherent backing. Apply one edge of dressing, and then gently smooth remaining dressing over IV site, leaving connection between IV tubing and catheter hub uncovered. Remove outer covering, and smooth dressing gently over site (see illustration).

Occlusive dressing protects site from bacterial contamination. Connection between administration set and hub needs to be uncovered to facilitate changing the tubing if necessary.

    (2) Take a 1-inch piece of tape, and place it over extension or administration set tubing (see illustration). Do not apply tape on top of transparent dressing.

Removal of tape from a transparent dressing will possibly cause accidental removal of the catheter.
Tape on top of a transparent dressing prevents moisture from being carried away from the skin.

  b Sterile gauze dressing:

    (1) Place 2 × 2 inch gauze pad over insertion site and catheter hub. Secure all edges with tape. Do not cover connection between IV tubing and catheter hub (see illustration).

    (2) Fold a 2 × 2 inch gauze in half, and cover with a 1 inch–wide tape extending about an inch from each side. Place under the tubing/catheter hub junction (see illustration).

Tape on top of gauze makes it easier to access hub/tubing junction. Gauze pad elevates hub off skin to prevent pressure area.

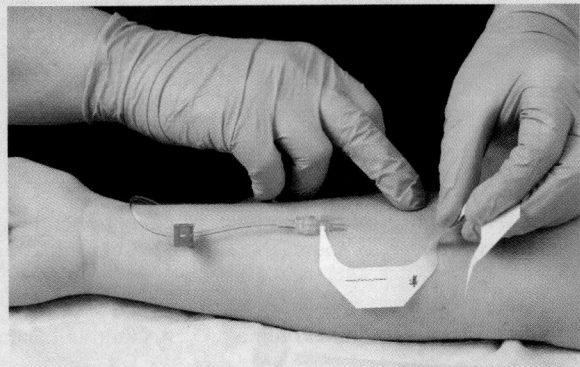

STEP 25a(1)   Apply transparent dressing.

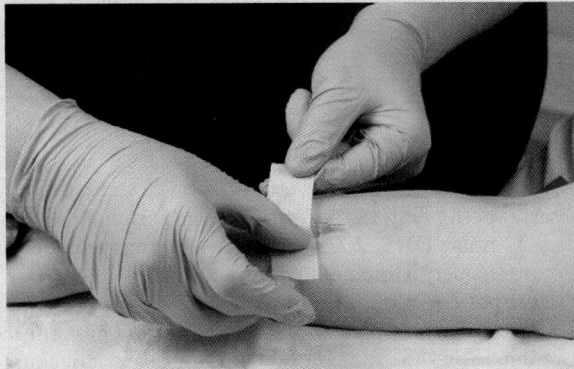

STEP 25a(2)   Place tape over administration set tubing.

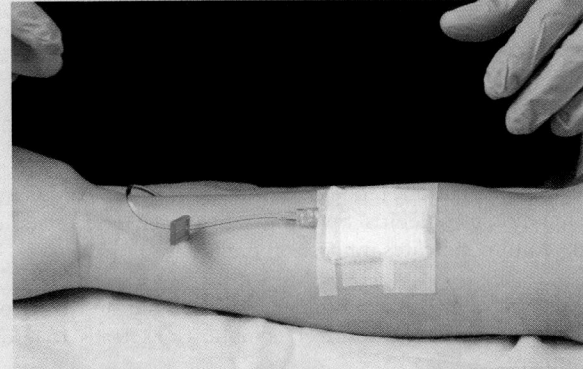

STEP 25b(1)   Place 2 × 2 inch gauze over insertion site and catheter hub.

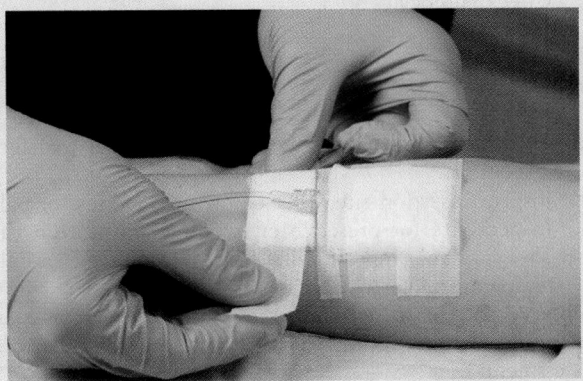

STEP 25b(2)   Apply 2 × 2 inch gauze dressing under tubing junction.

STEP	RATIONALE
26 Curl a loop of tubing alongside the arm, and then place a second piece of tape directly over the tubing and secure (see illustration).	Securing loop of tubing reduces risk for dislodging catheter if the IV tubing is pulled (i.e., the loop comes apart before the catheter dislodges).
27 For IV fluid administration, recheck flow rate and correct drops per minute (see Skill 28-2), and connect to EID as per agency policy.	Manipulation of catheter during dressing application alters flow rate. Maintains correct rate of flow for IV solution. Flow fluctuates, so it must be checked at intervals for accuracy.
28 Label dressing per agency policy. Include date and time of IV insertion, VAD gauge size and length, and your initials (see illustration).	Provides immediate access to data as to when IV was inserted and when to change dressing and rotate site.
29 Dispose of used stylet or other sharps in appropriate sharps container. Discard supplies. Remove gloves, and perform hand hygiene.	Reduces transmission of microorganisms, prevents accidental needle-stick injuries, and follows CDC guidelines for disposal of sharps (OSHA, 2006).
30 Instruct patient in how to move or turn without dislodging VAD.	Prevents accidental dislodgment of catheter.

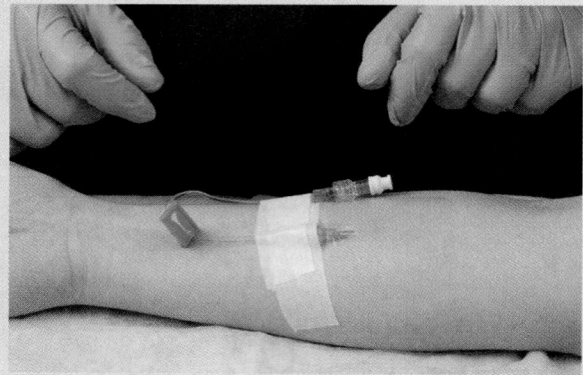

STEP 26   Loop and secure tubing.

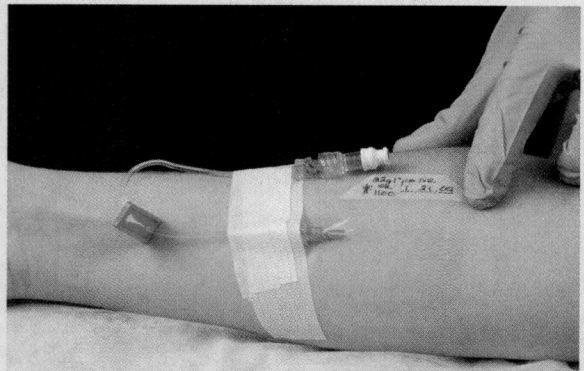

STEP 28   Label IV dressing.

EVALUATION

1 Observe peripheral IV access. Change peripheral IV access every 72 hours (INS, 2006) or per health care provider orders or more frequently if complications occur.	Incidences of complications are higher when peripheral IV remains in a vein over 72 hours (INS, 2006; Rosenthal, 2007).
2 Observe patient every 1 to 2 hours:	
a Check if correct amount of IV solution has infused by comparing time tape on IV container or by checking EID record.	Correct administration of fluid volume prevents fluid imbalance.
b Count drip rate (if gravity drip), or check rate on infusion pump.	Accurate monitoring of drip rate further ensures correct volume administration.
c Check patency of VAD.	Flow rate will be slowed or stopped.

Critical Decision Point   *If IV is positional, fluid will run less slowly or stop depending on position of patient's arm. Instruct patient to position arm to maintain flow; if this continues, you may have to restart IV.*

d Observe patient during palpation of vessel for signs of discomfort.	Tenderness is an early sign of phlebitis.
e Inspect insertion site, note color (e.g., redness or pallor). Inspect site for presence of swelling, infiltration (Table 28-2, p. 756), and phlebitis (Table 28-3, p. 756). Palpate temperature of skin above dressing.	Redness, inflammation, tenderness, and warmth indicate vein inflammation or phlebitis. Swelling above insertion site and cool temperature indicates infiltration of fluid into tissues.
3 Observe patient to determine response to therapy (e.g., intake and output [I&O], weights, vital signs, postprocedure assessments).	IV fluids and additives maintain or restore fluid and electrolyte balance. Early recognition of complications leads to prompt treatment.

Unexpected Outcomes

1. FVD as manifested by decreased urine output, dry mucous membranes, decreased capillary refill, a disparity in central and peripheral pulses, tachycardia, hypotension, shock.

2. FVE as manifested by crackles in the lungs, shortness of breath, edema.

3. Electrolyte imbalances indicated by abnormal serum electrolyte levels, changes in mental status, alterations in neuromuscular function, cardiac arrhythmias, and changes in vital signs.

4. Infiltration as indicated by swelling and possible pitting edema, pallor, coolness, pain at insertion site, possible decrease in flow rate (see Table 28-2, p. 756).

5. Phlebitis is indicated by pain, increased skin temperature, erythema along path of vein.

6. Bleeding occurs at venipuncture site.

Related Interventions

- Notify health care provider.
- Requires readjustment of infusion rate.

- Reduce IV flow rate if symptoms appear.
- Notify health care provider.

- Notify health care provider.
- Adjust additives in IV or type of IV fluid per order.

- Stop infusion, and discontinue IV (see Procedural Guideline 28-1, p. 770).
- Elevate affected extremity.
- Restart new IV if continued therapy is necessary.
- Document degree of infiltration and nursing intervention (see Table 28-2).

- Stop infusion, and discontinue IV (see Procedural Guideline 28-1).
- Restart new IV if continued therapy is necessary.
- Place moist warm compress over area of phlebitis.
- Document degree of phlebitis and nursing interventions per agency policy and procedure (see Table 28-3, p. 756).

- Verify that system is intact, and place a dressing over site or change dressing. NOTE: If using gauze dressing, remove it to accurately assess insertion site.
- Restart new IV if bleeding from site does not stop or if IV is dislodged.

Recording and Reporting

- Record in nurses' notes number of attempts and sites of insertion; precise description of insertion site (e.g., cephalic vein on dorsal surface of right lower arm, 2.5 cm above wrist); flow rate; size and type, length, and brand of catheter; and time infusion started. Use an infusion therapy flow sheet when available.
- If using an EID, document type and rate of infusion and device identification number.
- Record patient's status, IV fluid, amount infused, and integrity and patency of system according to agency policy.
- Report to oncoming nursing staff: type of fluid, flow rate, status of VAD, amount of fluid remaining in present solution, expected time to hang subsequent IV container, and patient condition.
- Report to health care provider adverse reactions such as pulmonary congestion, shock, or thrombophlebitis.

Teaching Considerations

- Instruct patient in signs and symptoms of infiltration, phlebitis, and inflammation. Patient will report early onset to nurse.
- Instruct patient to inform nurse or NAP if flow slows or stops or if patient sees blood in the tubing or on the dressing.
- Instruct patient in how to ambulate with IV pole or stand.
- Instruct patient to protect IV when performing hygiene activities.

Pediatric Considerations

- Perform venipuncture in a neutral space to allow the child's room to be a safe place.
- Pediatric veins are very fragile. Avoid sites that are easily moved or bumped. Use transparent site protectors to cover area.
- In addition to the usual venipuncture sites, use the veins in the scalp or the foot in infants.
- Use local anesthesia cream before venipuncture to lessen needle-related pain (check agency policy).
- Allow older children to select IV site to increase cooperation so they feel they have some control over their treatment.
- Most IV infusions in pediatric patients require a 22- to 24-gauge catheter.

- Avoid using chlorhexidine as a prepping agent in infants less than 1000 g; this is associated with dermatitis (INS, 2006).
- Employ distraction techniques such as blowing bubbles for nonpharmacological pain control.
- To maintain safety in positioning, have extra help when starting an IV on a child. Use therapeutic hugging, usually in a sitting position, to provide close contact (Rosenthal, 2005). NAP can help with positioning. Allow parents to stay with their child to help them cope with the procedure.
- When child requires long-term IV access, use a PICC, Broviac catheter, or implanted port to access larger veins (see Skill 28-6).
- Choose age-appropriate activities compatible with the maintenance of the IV infusion to maintain normal growth and development.

Gerontological Considerations

- Gerontological veins are very fragile; there is less subcutaneous support tissue, and there is thinning of the skin (Hadaway, 2006). Avoid sites that are easily moved or bumped. Sometimes dorsal metacarpal veins are not the best choice. Use a commercial protective device to protect site (Fig. 28-2, p. 756).
- In older patients, use the smallest gauge possible. For example, a 22-gauge needle is adequate for fluid and medication therapy; use a 24-gauge in frail, older adults. Smaller-gauge catheters are less traumatizing to the vein but still allow blood flow to provide increased hemodilution of the IV fluids or medications.
- If possible, avoid the back of the older adult's hand or the dominant arm for venipuncture because use of these sites interferes with the older adult's independence.
- Minimize pressure from tourniquets, or avoid them if possible. Apply a blood pressure cuff upside-down for effective compression (Rosenthal, 2005).
- As older adults lose subcutaneous tissue, the veins lose stability and roll away from the needle. To stabilize the vein, pull the skin taut and toward you with your nondominant hand and anchor the vein with your thumb.

- Reduce the angle of insertion (e.g., 5 to 15 degrees on insertion) to accommodate more superficial veins (Coulter, 2004; Rosenthal, 2005).
- Use mesh dressing or securement device on fragile skin (Coulter, 2004).
- Some older adults do not complain of pain at the insertion site. A large amount of fluid may infiltrate before a patient experiences discomfort.

Home Care Considerations

- Ensure that the patient is able and willing to self-administer IV therapy or that there is a reliable caregiver to provide IV therapy care at home.
- Ensure that all sharps and equipment contaminated by blood are disposed of in puncture-resistant containers with lids. Some suppliers will provide sharps containers for needle disposal. Teach patient and family to dispose of any open and sheathed needles into sharps container. Store all sharps containers in safe area away from children (see Chapter 42).
- Instruct patient and primary caregiver about procedures of IV therapy, including hand hygiene and aseptic technique while handling syringes and other supplies.
- Teach patient and primary caregiver to protect IV site during hand hygiene or during bathing to avoid getting it wet. If using an EID, unplug around water. For showering, protect the IV site and dressing from getting wet by covering completely with plastic.
- Instruct patient to wear clothes that avoid pressure on IV site.
- Teach primary caregiver to apply pressure with sterile gauze if catheter falls out and, if patient is on anticoagulant therapy, to tape several pieces of sterile gauze in place for at least 20 minutes with pressure or until bleeding stops.

- Teach patient about activity restrictions, for example, avoiding strenuous exercise of the arm with the IV.

Long-Term Care Considerations

- If a patient is highly active or disturbs IV, a securement device is recommended to prevent dislodgment of the catheter. Ensure that securement device does not restrict patient's movement or impair circulation.

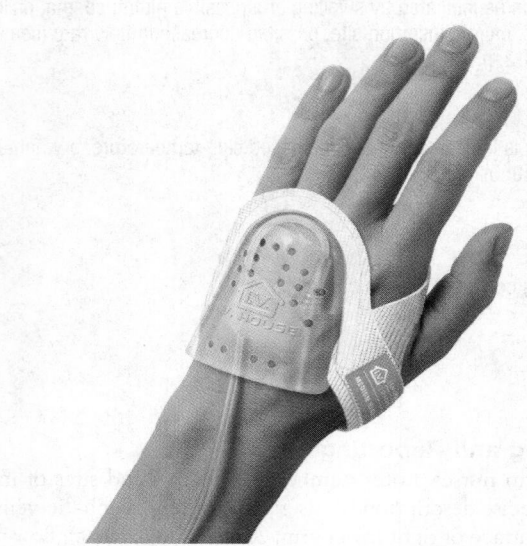

FIG 28-2 I.V. House Protective Device. (*Courtesy I.V. House.*)

TABLE 28-2	Infiltration Scale
Grade	**Clinical Criteria**
0	No symptoms
1	Skin blanched Edema, <1 inch in any direction Cool to touch With or without pain
2	Skin blanched Edema 1-6 inches in any direction Cool to touch With or without pain
3	Skin blanched, translucent Gross edema >6 inches in any direction Cool to touch Mild-moderate pain Possible numbness
4	Skin blanched, translucent Skin tight, leaking Skin discolored, bruised, swollen Gross edema >6 inches in any direction Deep pitting tissue edema Circulatory impairment Moderate to severe pain Infiltration of any amount of blood product, irritant, or vesicant

From Infusion Nurses Society: Infusion nursing standards of practice, *J Intraven Nurs* 29(1S):S60, 2006.

TABLE 28-3	Phlebitis Scale
Grade	**Clinical Criteria**
0	No symptoms
1	Erythema at access site with or without pain
2	Pain at access site with erythema and/or edema
3	Pain at access site with erythema and/or edema Streak formation Palpable venous cord
4	Pain at access site with erythema and/or edema Streak formation Palpable venous cord >1 inch in length Purulent drainage

From Infusion Nurses Society: Infusion nursing standards of practice, *J Intraven Nurs* 29(1S):S59, 2006.

SKILL 28-2   Regulating Intravenous Flow Rate

 Advanced / Management of Intravenous Fluid Therapy / Regulating an Intravenous Infusion

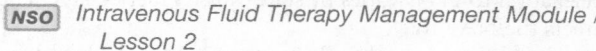 *Intravenous Fluid Therapy Management Module / Lesson 2*

After initiating the IV infusion and ensuring the line is patent, regulate the rate of infusion according to the health care provider's order. Accurate infusion rates are essential in the delivery of fluids and medications. Appropriate regulation of fluid rates reduces complications (e.g., phlebitis, infiltration, fluid overload, or clotting of the IV device) associated with IV therapy. Changes in patient position, flexion of the IV site extremity, and occlusion of the IV device influence infusion rates. Vasospasm of the vein, venous trauma, or manipulation of device also affects infusion rates. A patient will achieve therapeutic outcomes and fewer complications when the IV system and flow rate are assessed systematically.

There are a variety of methods for calculating infusion rates. The minimal rate used to keep a vein patent is about 10 to 15 mL/hr. Infusion devices maintain correct flow rates, maintain catheter patency, and prevent an unexpected bolus of IV infusion. Many infusion devices provide a record of the volume of fluid infused over a period of time.

An EID delivers a measured amount of fluid over a period of time (e.g., 100 mL/hr) using positive pressure. Infusion pumps are necessary for patients requiring low hourly rates, at risk for volume overload, with impaired renal clearance, or receiving medications or fluids that require a specific hourly volume. EIDs use an electronic sensor and an alarm that signals if the pressure in the system changes and the desired flow rate alters. For example, when an infiltration occurs in the subcutaneous tissue or a patient's position obstructs intravenous flow, pressure builds up and the alarm sounds. An infiltration is sometimes extensive before a positive-pressure EID alarm responds. Frequent inspection and palpation of the IV site ensures timely detection of an infiltration.

Nonelectronic infusion devices, such as an IV controller, deliver small fluid volumes with the aid of gravity. Patient and mechanical factors (e.g., height of the IV fluid container, IV tubing size, or fluid viscosity) affect an IV gravity controller. IV controllers cannot overcome increased resistance in the IV system, so an IV controller detects infiltrations more quickly than by an EID. An example of a volume-control device is a calibrated chamber placed between the IV container and the insertion spike and drip chamber of the administration set (Fig. 28-3). You place a small volume of IV fluid in the chamber and regulate it for administration. The advantage of this system is that only the smaller volume of fluid infuses if the rate of the IV is inadvertently increased. Volume-control devices are beneficial when administering fluids to neonates, very young children, and older adults. With either type of device, the patient requires consistent monitoring to verify the accurate infusion of the IV solution and to detect and prevent complications.

There is a new generation of IV infusion safety systems that reduce medication administration errors. Known as smart pumps, they are designed to be a final step in preventing errors that relate directly to administration of IV medications (Fig. 28-4) (Bates, 2007). They have built-in software programmed from health care pharmacy databases with unit-specific profiles. The pump has an audible and visual alert when the pump setting does not match the medication administration guidelines, assisting in preventing infusion errors. Each pump has the potential to use add-on syringe pumps, permit multiple infusions, and administer patient-controlled analgesia. The potential reduction in serious medication errors and the improved patient outcomes have prompted many organizations to implement this technology (Cohen, 2007; TJC, 2007).

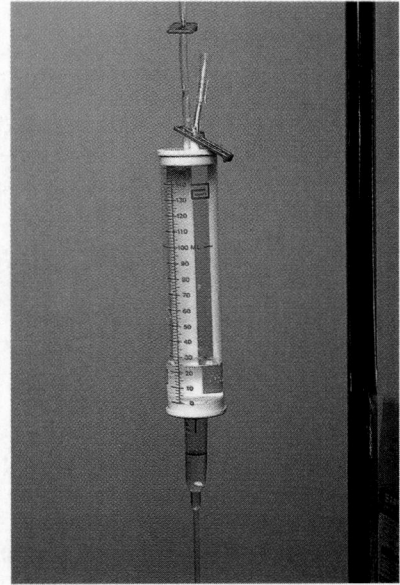

FIG 28-3   Volume-control device.

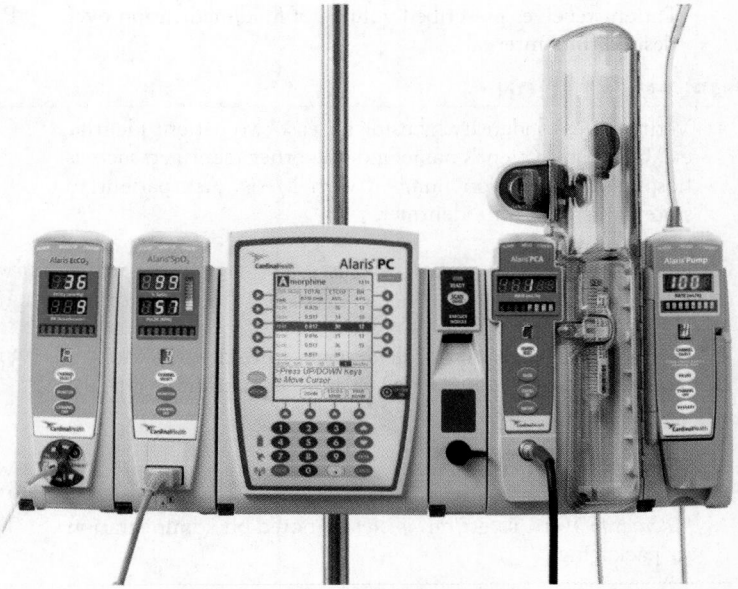

FIG 28-4   Smart pump. (*Photo courtesy Cardinal Health, Dublin, Ohio.*)

Delegation Considerations

The skill of regulating intravenous flow rate cannot be delegated to NAP. Delegation to LPNs varies by state Nurse Practice Act. The nurse directs the NAP to:

- Inform the nurse when the electronic infusion device alarm signals.
- Inform the nurse when the fluid container is almost empty.
- Report any patient complaints of any discomfort at the IV site.

Equipment

- ☐ Watch with second hand
- ☐ Calculator, paper, and pencil
- ☐ Tape
- ☐ Label
- ☐ IV flow-control device: EID (optional), volume-control device (*optional*)

STEP	RATIONALE

ASSESSMENT

1 Review accuracy and completeness of health care provider's order in patient's medical record for patient name and correct solution: type, volume, additives, rate, and duration of IV therapy. Follow the six rights of drug administration (see Chapter 20).	Ensures that correct IV fluid is administered (Ketchum and others, 2005).
2 Perform hand hygiene.	Prevents transmission of microorganisms.
3 Assess patient's knowledge of how positioning of IV site affects flow rate.	Fosters patient participation in maintaining most effective position of arm with IV equipment. Nurse is responsible for positioning of control clamp or setting infusion device rate.
4 Inspect IV site, verify patency, and verify with patient how site feels (e.g., determine if there is pain, burning, or tenderness at site).	Pain or burning is an early indication of phlebitis. Includes patient in decision making.
5 Observe for patency of VAD and IV tubing.	For fluid to infuse at proper rate, IV tubing and VAD must be free of kinks, knots, and clots.
6 Identify patient risk for fluid imbalance (e.g., neonate, history of cardiac or renal disease, electrolyte imbalance).	Volume control needs to be strict. Guides choice of infusion device.

NURSING DIAGNOSES

- Deficient fluid volume
- Excess fluid volume
- Risk for imbalanced fluid volume

Individualize related factors based on patient's condition or needs.

PLANNING

1 Expected outcomes following completion of procedure:	
• Serum electrolyte levels remain within normal limits.	IV fluid assists in maintaining fluid and electrolyte levels.
• Patient receives prescribed volume of fluid/medication over desired time interval.	Patient will achieve therapeutic outcomes.

IMPLEMENTATION

1 Verify patient's identity by using at least two patient identifiers. Compare patient's name and one other identifier, such as hospital identification number, with MAR. Ask patient to state name as a third identifier.	Complies with The Joint Commission requirements and improves medication safety. In most acute care settings, patient's name and identification number on armband and MAR are used to identify patients (TJC, 2007).

Critical Decision Point *It is common for health care providers to write an abbreviated IV order such as: "D5W with 20 mEq KCl 125 mL/hr continuous." This order implies that the IV should be maintained at this rate until order has been written for IV to be discontinued.*

2 Have paper and pencil or calculator to calculate flow rate.	Use mathematical calculations to obtain correct rate.
3 Know calibration (drop factor) in drops per milliliter (gtt/mL) of infusion set used by agency:	
Microdrip: 60 gtt/mL	Microdrip tubing universally delivers 60 gtt/mL. Used when small or very precise volumes are to be infused.
Macrodrip: 10 to 15 gtt/mL is clearly noted on administration set packaging.	There are different commercial parenteral administration sets for macrodrip tubing. Used when large volumes or fast rates are necessary. Know the drip factor for the tubing being used.

STEP	RATIONALE
4 Determine how long each liter of fluid should run. Calculate milliliters per hour (hourly rate) by dividing volume by hours: $$mL/hr = \frac{total\ infusion\ (mL)}{hours\ of\ infusion}$$ 1000 mL/8 hr = 125 mL/hr or if 3 L is ordered for 24 hours: 3000 mL/24 hr = 125 mL/hr	Provides even infusion of fluid over prescribed hourly rate.
5 Select one of the following formulas to calculate minute flow rate (drops per minute) based on drop factor of infusion set: a mL/hr/60 min = mL/min Drop factor × mL/min = drops/min Or b mL/hr × drop factor/60 min = drops/min Use the following formula to calculate minute flow rate for bag 1:1000 mL with 20 mEq KCI @ 125 mL/hr. *Microdrip:* 125 mL/hr × 60 gtt/mL = 7500 gtt/hr 7500 gtt ÷ 60 minutes = 125 gtt/min *Macrodrip:* 125 mL/hr ×15 gtt/mL = 1875 gtt/hr 1875 gtt ÷ 60 minutes = 31-32 gtt/min	Once you determine the hourly rate, these formulas compute correct flow rate. When using microdrip, milliliters per hour (mL/hr) always equals drops per minute (gtt/min). Multiply volume by drop factor, and divide the product by time (in minutes).
6 Confirm hourly infusion rate, and place marked adhesive tape or commercial fluid indicator tape on existing IV container next to volume markings. Document each IV fluid bag sequentially, and note type of fluid, patient's name, infusion span, and expected start and end time of infusion.	Provides a visual scale to assess progress of hourly infusion. Use time tapes for all IV infusions, including those on EIDs. NOTE: Some patient's receive secondary infusions that affect the visual time tape scale.

Critical Decision Point   *On IV bags made of polyvinylchloride (PVC) avoid drawing directly with felt-tip pens or permanent markers because the ink could contaminate the solution (Hadaway and Millam, 2005).*

STEP	RATIONALE
7 *For gravity infusions:* Confirm hourly rate and minute rate based on drop factor of infusion set. Microdrip infusion set has a drop factor of 60 gtt/mL. Regular drip or macrodrip infusion set used in this example has drop factor of 15 gtt/mL. Using formula (see Implementation, Step 5), calculate flow rate.	Calculates minute flow rate for regulation of infusion.
8 Regulate flow rate by counting drops in drip chamber for 1 minute by watch, then adjust roller clamp to increase or decrease rate of infusion.	Regulates flow to prescribed rate.
9 *For use of EID for infusion:* Follow manufacturer's guidelines for setup of EID. a Consult manufacturer's directions for setup of the infusion. If using a gravity controller, ensure that IV container is 36 inches above IV site.	IV controller works by gravity. Heights of 36 to 48 inches will overcome venous pressure and other resistance from tubing and catheter (INS, 2006).

STEP	RATIONALE
b Insert IV tubing into chamber of control mechanism (see manufacturer's directions) (see illustration).	Most electronic infusion pumps use positive pressure to infuse. Infusion pumps propel fluid through tubing by compressing and milking the IV tubing.
c Turn on power button, select required drops per minute or volume per hour, close door to control chamber, and press start button (see illustration).	

Critical Decision Point   *An anti–free flow safeguard (preventing bolus infusion in the event of machine malfunction or when tubing removed from machine) is an important element of an electronic infusion device and is required. Always check manufacturer's recommendations for specific device features.*

d Open drip regulator completely while EID is in use.	Ensures that pump freely regulates infusion rate.
e Monitor infusion rate and IV site for complications according to agency policy. Use watch to verify rate of infusion, even when using EID.	Infusion controllers or pumps are not perfect and do not replace frequent, accurate nursing evaluation. EIDs continue to infuse IV fluids after a complication has begun.
f Assess patency of system when alarm signals.	Alarm indicates some blockage in the system. Empty solution container, tubing kinks, closed clamp, infiltration, clotted catheter, air in the tubing, and/or low battery will all trigger the EID alarm.
10 *For a smart pump* (see Fig. 28-4): a Place pump module into the computer. b Insert the IV tubing into the pump module, and close the door. c Computer screen will require the patient unit to be entered.	Manufacturer's guidelines and health care facility programming automatically configure the computer to the specific unit (e.g., obstetrics, critical care).
d From the list on the screen, choose the medication and concentration. e Program the dose and infusion rate ordered. If the entered order matches the database, the pump will begin the infusion. f Follow manufacturer's directions for programming.	The pump checks the programming against the medication database.
g If the programming does not match the database, a visual and audible alarm sounds.	Prevents medication and infusion errors.
h If an alarm sounds, the pump will automatically turn off. You must reprogram it within the facility's database.	Prevents medication and infusion errors.
i Reconfirm that the medication is infusing at the ordered rate.	The pump maintains a log of all alarms, including time, date, medication, medication concentration, rate, and any actions.
11 *For a volume-control device:* a Place volume-control device between IV container and insertion spike of infusion set using aseptic technique (see Fig. 28-3).	Delivers small fluid volumes, but needs refilling as volume becomes low. Reduces risk for sudden fluid infusion.
b Place no more than 2 hours allotment of fluid into device by opening clamp between IV bag and device.	Allows for a continuous infusion of fluid if you do not return in exactly 60 minutes to refill volume. If infusion rate accidentally increases, patient receives only a 2-hour allotment of fluid.

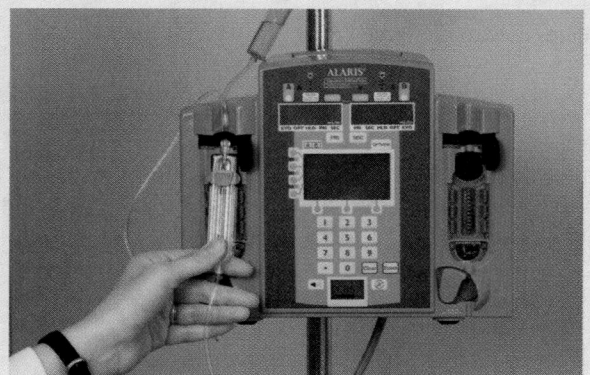

STEP 9b   Insert IV tubing into chamber of control mechanism.

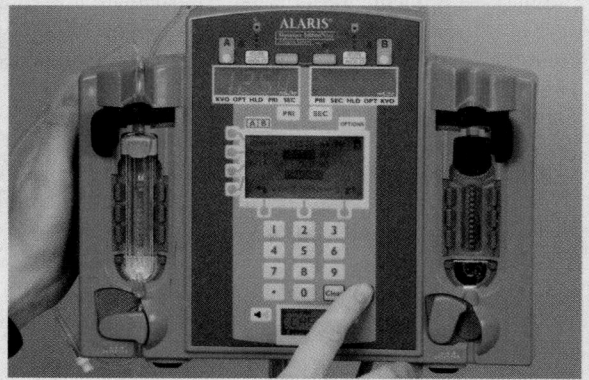

STEP 9c   Select rate and volume to be infused, and press start button.

STEP	RATIONALE
c Assess system at least hourly; add fluid to volume-control device. Regulate flow rate.	Maintains patency of system and patient monitoring.
12 Instruct patient in the purpose of the alarms, to avoid raising hand or arm that affects flow rate, and to avoid touching the control clamp.	Information allows patient to protect IV site and informs patient about rationale for not altering control rate.

EVALUATION

1 Monitor IV infusion at least every hour, noting volume of IV fluid infused and rate.	Ensures correct volume infuses over prescribed time period.
2 Observe patient for signs of overhydration or dehydration to determine response to therapy and restoration of fluid and electrolyte balance.	Signs and symptoms of dehydration or overhydration warrant changing rate of fluid infused.
3 Evaluate for signs of complications related to IV flow rate: infiltration, inflammation at site, occluded VAD, kink or knot in infusion tubing.	Prevents complications that decrease or stop flow rate.

Unexpected Outcomes	Related Interventions
1 Sudden infusion of large volume of solution occurs with patient having symptoms of dyspnea, crackles in the lung, and increased urine output, indicating fluid overload.	• Slow infusion to keep vein open (KVO) rate, and notify health care provider immediately. • Place patient in high-Fowler's position. • Anticipate new IV orders. • Administer diuretics if ordered.
2 IV fluid container empties with subsequent loss of IV line patency.	• Discontinue present IV, and restart new VAD.
3 The IV infusion is slower than ordered.	• Check for positional change that affects rate, height of IV container, kinking of tubing or obstruction. • Check VAD site for complications. • Consult health care provider for new order to provide necessary fluid volume.

Recording and Reporting

- Record rate of infusion in drops per minute or milliliters per hour, in nurses' notes or on parenteral fluid form according to agency policy.
- Immediately record in nurses' notes any new IV fluid rates.
- Document use of any EID or controlling device and identification number on that device.
- At change of shift or when leaving on break, report rate of and volume left in infusion to nurse in charge or next nurse assigned to care for patient.

Teaching Considerations

- Instruct patient to contact staff if a complication develops.
- Patient using an EID should know its preset rate and the significance of alarms.
- Teach patient about factors affecting flow rate, to protect IV site, and importance of not altering rate control.

Pediatric Considerations

- Consider physiological differences in children, particularly focusing on total body weight (85% to 90% water). Dehydration is a common cause of fluid and electrolyte imbalance; assessment of fluid needs includes meter square weight or caloric method (Phillips, 2005).
- Infusion pumps (especially syringe pumps) are almost always used in pediatrics because they infuse very small amounts of fluids and accurately provide the prescribed volume of IV solution.
- Use only small-volume containers for infusions (250 mL for children younger than 12 months, 500 mL for older children)

(Hockenberry and Wilson, 2007). Microdrip tubing is recommended for children.

Gerontological Considerations

- Renal changes in older adults reduce the kidney's ability to concentrate and dilute urine in response to water or salt excess. Combined with cardiac deficiencies and decreased blood flow to organs, an older patient balances between dehydration and fluid overload. Use an EID and microdrip tubing to administer fluids. Monitor electrolyte levels, blood urea nitrogen (BUN), creatinine, urine output, and daily weight.
- Some older patients easily develop cerebral edema from rapid dextrose infusions. Older patients with impaired renal function often develop hypernatremia from normal saline infusions.

Home Care Considerations

- Ensure that patient is able and willing to operate an infusion pump and administer IV therapy. If patient is unable to provide self-care, be sure that a reliable caregiver is available in the home.
- Ensure proper EID function before use with patient.
- Teach patient and primary caregiver what EID alarms mean, methods to troubleshoot them, and how to disconnect the tubing from the EID pump in the event of a pump failure.
- Provide patient with a contact phone number that patient can access 24 hours a day for problems.
- If using gravity infusion, teach patient and primary caregiver to time drops per minute using watch with second hand.
- Ensure that patient's electrical outlets are properly grounded.

SKILL 28-3 Changing Intravenous Solutions

Advanced / Management of Intravenous Fluid Therapy / Changing Intravenous Tubing and Fluids

NSO *Intravenous Fluid Therapy Management Module / Lesson 3*

Patients receiving IV therapy over time require periodic changes of IV solutions. IV containers include plastic bags and glass bottles. A nurse will change a container when there is an order for a new solution or when it becomes time to change an empty container for a full container. It becomes clinically appropriate to change a solution depending on a patient's fluid and electrolyte balance and goals of therapy. The Centers for Disease Control and Prevention (CDC) (2002) does not have a recommendation for hang time of IV fluids, but the Infusion Nurses Society (INS) recommends changing the container within 24 hours after adding an administration set (INS, 2006). Fluid containers on ambulatory infusion devices may remain longer than 24 hours if you use aseptic technique, the system remains closed without injection ports or add-on tubing, and the medication is stable for a longer time period (Depledge, 2006; INS, 2006). It is important to organize tasks and follow proper technique, so you can complete this procedure in time before the solution container is empty and to prevent clot formation in the catheter.

Delegation Considerations
The skill of changing an intravenous solution cannot be delegated to NAP. Delegation to LPNs varies by state Nurse Practice Act. The nurse directs the NAP to:
• Inform the nurse when an IV container is near completion.
• Report any cloudiness or precipitate in the IV solution.

Equipment
❑ IV solution as ordered by health care provider
❑ Time tape

STEP	RATIONALE
ASSESSMENT	
1 Review accuracy and completeness of health care provider's order in patient's medical record for patient name and correct solution: type, volume, additives, rate, and duration of IV therapy. Follow the six rights of drug administration (see Chapter 20).	Ensures that correct IV fluid is administered (Ketchum and others, 2005).
2 Note date and time when IV tubing and solution were last changed.	INS recommends a hang time no longer than 24 hours after addition of an administration set to ensure sterility of solutions in bag or bottle (INS, 2006). Administration sets need to be changed every 72 hours (INS, 2006).
3 Determine the compatibility of all IV fluids and additives by consulting appropriate literature or the pharmacy.	Incompatibilities cause physical, chemical, and therapeutic patient changes.
4 Determine patient's understanding of the need for continued IV therapy.	Reveals need for patient education.
5 Assess patency of current VAD site by carefully adjusting the roller clamp to observe an increase in flow rate and then regulate back to prescribed rate. *Lowering IV container below level of IV site for presence of blood return (retrograde) is an unreliable indicator of patency.*	New IV access site is necessary if IV is not patent.
6 Assess IV insertion site for swelling, coolness to touch, or tenderness around site.	Indicates infiltration.
7 Assess IV tubing for puncture, contamination, or occlusions.	Indicates need for tubing change.

NURSING DIAGNOSES

• Deficient fluid volume • Deficient knowledge related to purpose for IV therapy • Risk for imbalanced fluid volume
  • Risk for infection

Individualize related factors based on patient's condition or needs.

PLANNING

1 Expected outcomes following completion of procedure:	
• IV solution is correct.	Patient receives fluids ordered for condition.
• IV line remains patent.	Ensures infusion of fluid into intravascular space.
• Patient and family can explain purpose of IV solution change.	Demonstrates learning.

IMPLEMENTATION

1 Collect equipment. Have next solution prepared at least 1 hour before needed. If solution is prepared in pharmacy, ensure that it has been delivered to patient care unit. Allow solution to warm to room temperature if it has been refrigerated. Check that solution is correct and properly labeled. Check solution expiration date.	Adequate planning reduces risk for clot formation in vein caused by empty IV container. Checking that solution is correct prevents medication error.

STEP	RATIONALE
2 Verify patient's identity by using at least two patient identifiers. Compare patient's name and one other identifier, such as hospital identification number, with MAR. Ask patient to state name as a third identifier.	Complies with The Joint Commission requirements and improves medication safety. In most acute care settings, patient's name and identification number on armband and MAR are used to identify patients (TJC, 2007).
3 Prepare to change solution when about 50 mL of fluid remains in container. Be sure drip chamber is half full.	Prevents air from entering tubing and vein from clotting from lack of flow.
4 Change administration set tubing with fluid container when possible (see Skill 28-4).	Decreases number of times system is open and maintains sterility.
5 Prepare patient and family by explaining the procedure, its purpose, and what is expected of patient.	Decreases anxiety and promotes cooperation.
6 Perform hand hygiene.	Reduces transmission of microorganisms.
7 Prepare new solution for changing. If using plastic bag, remove protective cover from IV tubing port. If using glass bottle, remove metal cap and metal and rubber disks.	Permits quick, smooth, and organized change from old to new solution.
8 Position roller clamp on existing solution to stop flow rate. Remove tubing from EID (if used). Then remove old IV fluid container from IV pole. Hold container with tubing port pointing upward.	Prevents solution remaining in drip chamber from emptying while changing solutions. Prevents solution from spilling.
9 Quickly remove spike from old solution container and, without touching tip, insert spike into new container.	Reduces risk for solution in drip chamber becoming empty and maintains sterility.

Critical Decision Point *If spike is contaminated, you will need a new IV tubing set. You can use sterile IV tubing for 72 hours unless compromised.*

STEP	RATIONALE
10 Hang new container of solution on IV pole.	Gravity assists with delivery of fluid into drip chamber.
11 Check for air in tubing. If bubbles form, remove them by closing roller clamp, stretching tubing downward, and tapping tubing with finger (bubbles rise in fluid to drip chamber) (see illustration). For a larger amount of air, swab port below the air and allow to dry, insert needleless syringe into the port and aspirate the air into the syringe. Reduce air in tubing by priming slowly instead of allowing a wide-open flow.	Reduces risk for air entering tubing. Use of an air-eliminating filter also reduces risk.
12 Make sure drip chamber is one-third to one-half full. If the drip chamber is too full, pinch off tubing below drip chamber, invert container, squeeze drip chamber (see illustration), release, and turn the solution container upright, and unpinch the tubing.	Reduces risk for air entering tubing. If chamber is completely filled, you cannot observe or regulate drip rate.

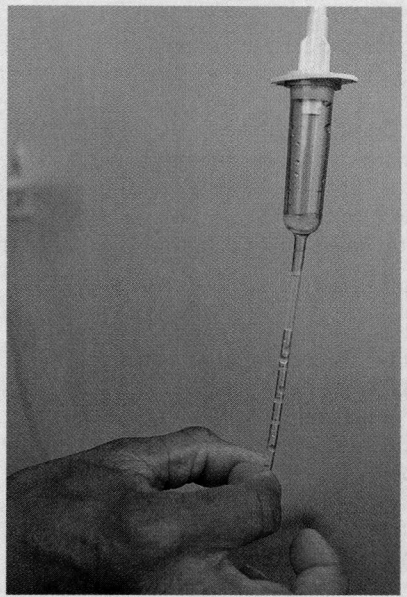

STEP 11   Tap tubing to cause air bubbles to rise up to drip chamber.

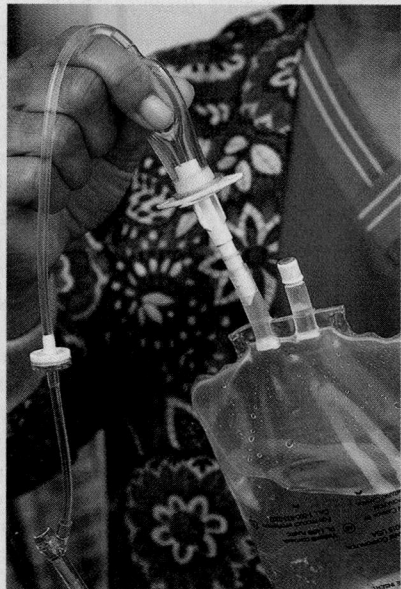

STEP 12   Squeeze drip chamber to fill with fluid. Be sure to leave chamber one-third to one-half full.eter into vein.

STEP	RATIONALE
13 Regulate flow to ordered rate using either the roller clamp on the tubing or programming EID.	Maintains measures to restore fluid balance and deliver IV fluid as ordered.
14 Place time label on the side of container, and label with the time hung, the time of completion, and appropriate intervals. If using plastic bags, mark only on the label and not the container.	Provides a visual comparison of volume infused compared with prescribed rate of infusion. Ink on container sometimes leaks into plastic bags.

EVALUATION

1 Evaluate flow rate hourly, and observe connection site for leaking.	Ensures proper fluid administration.
2 Observe patient for signs of FVD or FVE to determine response to IV therapy.	Provides ongoing evaluation of patient's fluid and electrolyte status.
3 Check IV system for patency.	Prevents improper fluid infusion.

Unexpected Outcomes	Related Interventions
1 Flow of IV fluid is decreased or absent.	• Assess IV system for patency • Reregulate drip rate. • Assess IV site for complications.
2 Flow rate is incorrect; patient receives too little or too much fluid.	• Readjust infusion rate to ordered rate. • Evaluate patient for adverse effects of infusion. • Determine and correct the cause of incorrect flow rate (e.g., change in position, tubing kink). • Use EID when accurate flow rate is critical. • Notify health care provider.

Recording and Reporting

- Record amount and type of fluid infused and amount and type of fluid started according to agency policy.
- Record solution and tubing change on patient's record. Use parenteral (IV) therapy flow sheet, if available.

Teaching Considerations

- Inform patient of new solution, additives, flow rate, and potential side effects.

Home Care Considerations

- Instruct patient and primary caregiver in how to perform an IV solution change. Observe them performing procedure.

SKILL 28-4 Changing Infusion Tubing

 Advanced / Management of Intravenous Fluid Therapy / Changing Intravenous Tubing and Fluids

NSO *Intravenous Fluid Therapy Management Module / Lesson 3*

An important component of patient care is maintaining the integrity of an IV to prevent infection through the conscientious use of infection control principles (Hindley, 2004). Intravenous tubing administration sets remain sterile for 72 hours (CDC, 2002; INS, 2006), thus the Centers for Disease Control and Prevention (2002) recommends changing tubing no more frequently than every 72 hours. The INS (2006) recommends 72-hour intervals for continuous tubing changes, adding that more frequent changes may occur if the tubing has been compromised or contaminated. You change primary intermittent sets every 24 hours because the IV system becomes interrupted, which increases the risk for contamination (INS, 2006). In addition, administration set changes need to coincide with peripheral IV site rotation. The exception is tubing containing blood, blood products, and lipid emulsions, which often requires more frequent tubing changes (e.g., every 24 hours) because they are more likely to promote bacterial growth (see agency policy). Whenever possible, schedule tubing changes when it is time to hang a new IV container (see Skill 28-1). To prevent entry of bacteria into the bloodstream, maintain sterility during tubing and solution changes. Situations arise when you change the tubing without hanging a new bag. Such situations include accidental puncture of the tubing or after infusion of blood or a blood product.

Delegation Considerations

The skill of changing infusion tubing cannot be delegated to NAP. Delegation to LPNs varies by state Nurse Practice Act. The nurse directs the NAP to:

- Report to the nurse any leakage from or around the IV tubing.

Equipment

- ☐ Clean gloves
- ☐ 0.22-μm filter and extension

Continuous IV Infusion

- ☐ Microdrip or macrodrip infusion tubing, as appropriate
- ☐ 0.22-μm filter and extension tubing (if necessary)
- ☐ Tubing label
- ☐ Antiseptic swab (2% chlorhexidine)

Intermittent Saline Lock

- ☐ 5-mL syringe filled with preservative-free normal saline
- ☐ Loop or short extension tubing (if necessary), injection cap or prn adapter
- ☐ Antiseptic swab

STEP	RATIONALE

ASSESSMENT

1 Note date and time when IV tubing was last changed. Agency policy will indicate frequency of routine change for IV administration sets and saline/heparin locks.

CDC (2002) and INS (2006) recommend tubing change no more often than 72-hour intervals or whenever tubing has been compromised or contaminated. Change primary intermittent tubing sets every 24 hours (INS, 2006).

2 Assess tubing for puncture, contamination, or occlusion that requires immediate change.

Compromised tubing results in fluid leakage and bacterial contamination.

3 Determine patient's understanding of the need for continued IV therapy.

Reveals need for patient instruction.

NURSING DIAGNOSIS

- Deficient knowledge related to purpose for IV therapy
- Risk for infection

Individualize related factors based on patient's condition or needs.

PLANNING

1 Expected outcomes following completion of procedure:
- Patient's IV site will be free from infection, redness, swelling, pain, or exudate.

Sterile IV tubing prevents microbial growth.

- Patient will experience no leakage of solution from or around IV tubing.

Intact system decreases risk for microbial contamination.

- Patient's IV tubing will be patent.

Brief interruption of IV infusion will not result in thrombus formation.

- Patient and family will explain the procedure, purpose, and what is expected of patient.

Demonstrates learning.

IMPLEMENTATION

1 Verify patient's identity by using at least two patient identifiers. Compare patient's name and one other identifier, such as hospital identification number, with MAR. Ask patient to state name as a third identifier.

Complies with The Joint Commission requirements and improves patient safety. In most acute care settings, patient's name and identification number on armband and MAR are used to identify patients (TJC, 2007).

2 Prepare patient and family by explaining the procedure, its purpose, and what is expected of patient.

Decreases anxiety, promotes cooperation, and prevents sudden movement of extremity, which could dislodge IV catheter.

3 Coordinate tubing changes with bag changes when possible.

Decreases number of times system is open.

4 Perform hand hygiene.

Reduces transmission of microorganisms.

5 Open new infusion set, and connect add-on pieces (e.g., filters, extension tubing). Keep protective coverings over infusion spike and distal adapter. Secure all connections.

Securing connections reduces the risk later of air emboli, hemorrhage, and infection. Protective covers reduce entrance of microorganisms.

6 Apply clean gloves.

Reduces transmission of microorganisms. Infections related to IV therapy are most often caused by catheter hub contamination; use careful technique throughout the tubing change (CDC, 2006; INS, 2006).

7 If cannula hub is not visible, remove IV dressing (see Skill 29-5). Do not remove tape securing cannula to skin.

Cannula hub must be visible to provide smooth transition when removing old and inserting new tubing.

8 Prepare infusion tubing with new bag. Refer to Skill 28-1, Steps 7c to 7i.

9 Prepare infusion tubing with existing continuous IV infusion
   a Move roller clamp on new IV tubing to "off" position.

Prevents fluid spillage.

   b Slow rate of infusion to existing IV by regulating roller clamp on old tubing to KVO rate.
   c Compress and fill drip chamber of old tubing.

Ensures fluid chamber remains full until new tubing is changed.

   d Invert container and remove old tubing. Keep spike sterile and upright. *Optional:* Tape old drip chamber to IV pole without contaminating spike.

Fluid in drip chamber will continue to run and maintain catheter patency.

   e Place insertion spike of new tubing into solution container. Hang solution bag on IV pole, compress and release drip chamber on new tubing, and fill drip chamber one-third to one-half full.

Permits flow of fluid from solution into new infusion tubing.

STEP	RATIONALE

f   Slowly open roller clamp, remove protective cap from adapter (if necessary), and flush new tubing with solution. Stop infusion and replace cap. Place end of adapter near patient's IV site.

Removes air from tubing and replaces it with IV solution. Equipment is positioned for a quick connection of new tubing.

g   Turn roller clamp on old tubing to "off" position.

Prevents fluid spillage.

10 Prepare tubing with intermittent saline lock

a   If a loop or short extension tubing is needed, use sterile technique to connect the new injection cap to the new loop or tubing.

b   Swab injection cap with antiseptic swab. Insert syringe with 1 to 3 mL of saline solution, and inject through the injection cap into the loop of the extension tubing.

Maintains patency of catheter. Volume of saline solution should not exceed 30 mL in a 24-hour period (INS, 2006).

11 Reestablish infusion

a   Gently disconnect old tubing from extension tubing (or from IV catheter), and quickly insert adapter of new tubing or saline lock into tubing connection (or IV catheter hub) (see illustrations).

Allows smooth transition from old to new tubing, minimizing time system is open.

b   For continuous infusion, open roller clamp on new tubing, allowing solution to run rapidly for 30 to 60 seconds, and then regulate drip rate using roller clamp or electronic infusion device (see illustration).

Ensures catheter patency and prevents occlusion.

c   Attach a piece of tape or preprinted label with date and time of tubing change onto tubing below the drip chamber.

Provides reference to determine next time for tubing change.

d   Form a loop of tubing, and secure it to patient's arm with a strip of tape.

Avoids accidental pulling against site and stabilizes catheter.

12 Remove and discard old IV tubing. If necessary, apply new dressing (see Skill 28-5). Remove and dispose of gloves. Perform hand hygiene.

Reduces transmission of microorganisms.

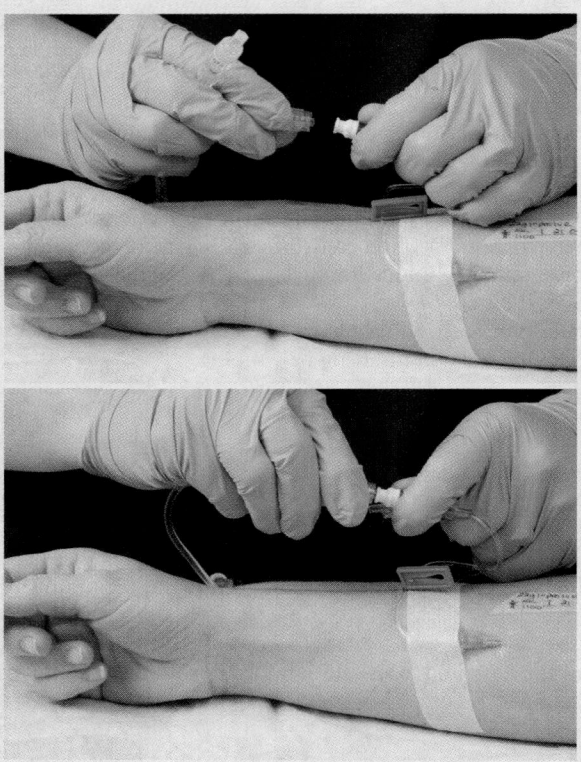

STEP 11a   **A,** Disconnect old tubing. **B,** Insert adapter of new tubing.

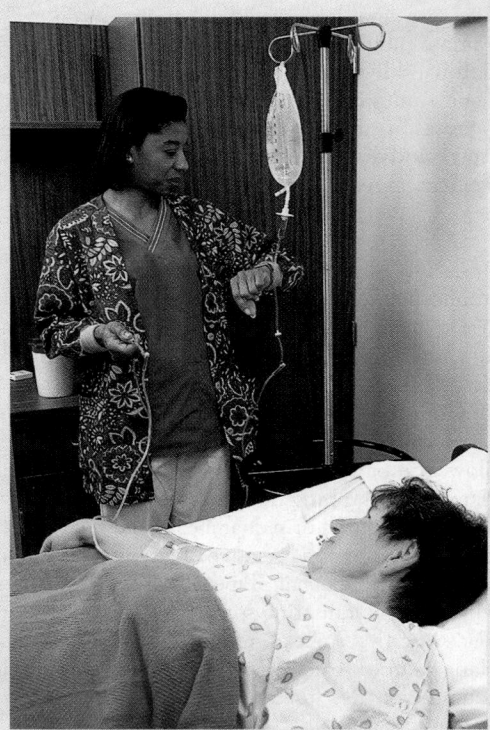

STEP 11b   Regulate flow of IV.

Unexpected Outcomes

1 Decreased rate or obstructed flow indicates decreased or absent flow of IV fluid.

Related Interventions

- Assess IV infusion system for patency by opening roller clamp, slide clamps, and check for kinks in tubing.
- Recalibrate drip rate.
- Assess patient for complaints of pain or discomfort at IV site.

Recording and Reporting

- Record tubing change, type of solution, volume, and rate of infusion on patient's record. Use a special IV therapy flow sheet for parenteral fluids.
- Mark a piece of tape or preprinted label with date and time of tubing change, and attach to tubing below the level of drip chamber.

Teaching Considerations

- Instruct patient to notify nurse if fluid leaks from or around IV site or tubing or if tubing separates from catheter.

Home Care Considerations

- Instruct patient or primary caregiver in procedure for performing a sterile IV tubing change.
- Ensure that patient is able and willing to perform tubing change and maintain IV access site or that there is a reliable person at home to provide this IV therapy care.

SKILL 28-5   Changing a Peripheral Intravenous Dressing

 Advanced / Management of Intravenous Fluid Therapy / Changing Intravenous Dressings

| NSO | *Intravenous Fluid Therapy Management Module / Lesson 4*

Peripheral IV catheters and infusion therapy are frequently associated with complications such as local or systemic infections, phlebitis, and infiltration. Diligent IV site care and management helps prevent or minimize complications (Eggimann, 2007). The skin insertion site is the most common source of colonization and infection for IV catheters (Hadaway, 2005). Therefore you need to securely apply catheter dressings and change dressings when wet, soiled, or loosened. You stabilize peripheral IV catheters with a manufactured stabilization device, sterile tapes, or surgical strips and cover with a transparent semipermeable dressing or sterile gauze (INS, 2006; Smith, 2007). You change a transparent dressing during catheter site rotation and immediately if integrity of the dressing is compromised. Change gauze dressings every 48 hours and immediately if integrity is compromised. When using gauze under a transparent dressing, it is considered a gauze dressing and should be changed every 48 hours (INS, 2006).

- Report to the nurse if a patient complains of moistness or loosening of an IV dressing.
- Protect the IV dressing during hygiene and ADLs.

Equipment

- ☐ Antiseptic swabs (2% chlorhexidine)
- ☐ Adhesive remover *(optional)*
- ☐ Skin protectant swab
- ☐ Clean gloves
- ☐ Strips of nonallergenic tape
- ☐ Commercially available IV site protection *(optional)*

For Transparent Dressing
- ☐ Sterile transparent semipermeable dressing

For Gauze Dressing
- ☐ Sterile 2 × 2 or 4 × 4 inch gauze pad

Delegation Considerations

The skill of changing a peripheral intravenous dressing cannot be delegated to NAP. The nurse directs the NAP to:

STEP	RATIONALE

ASSESSMENT

1 Determine when dressing was last changed. Many institutions require dressing label to include date and time dressing applied, size and type of VAD, and date the VAD was inserted.

Provides information regarding length of time that present dressing has been in place. In addition, you are able to plan for dressing change.

2 Perform hand hygiene. Observe present dressing for moisture and intactness. Determine if moisture is from site leakage or from external source.

Moisture is medium for bacterial growth and renders dressing contaminated. Nonadhering dressing increases risk for bacterial contamination to venipuncture site or displacement of IV catheter.

3 Observe IV system for proper functioning or complications (e.g., current flow rate, tubing, or catheter kinks). Palpate the catheter site through the intact dressing for complaints of tenderness, pain, or burning. (NOTE: Apply clean gloves if a gauze dressing is moist.)

Unexplained decrease in flow rate indicates problems with VAD placement and patency. Pain is associated with phlebitis and infiltration.

4 Monitor body temperature.

Elevated temperature is possibly related to infection at VAD site.

5 Assess patient's understanding of the need for continued IV infusion.

Reveals need for patient instruction.

NURSING DIAGNOSES

- Acute pain
- Risk for infection

Individualize related factors based on patient's condition or needs.

STEP	RATIONALE

PLANNING

1 Expected outcomes following completion of procedure:
   • IV insertion site will remain free of infection, redness, swelling, tenderness, or exudate.
   • Patient and family can explain procedure and purpose of VAD dressing change.

Proper care maintains IV site.

Demonstrates learning.

IMPLEMENTATION

1 Explain procedure and purpose to patient and family. Explain that patient will need to hold affected extremity still. Explain how long procedure will take.

Decreases anxiety, promotes cooperation, and gives patient time frame around which to plan personal activities.

2 Perform hand hygiene. Collect equipment. Apply clean gloves.

Reduces transmission of microorganisms. Infections related to IV therapy are most often caused by catheter hub contamination, so you need to use careful technique throughout the dressing change (CDC, 2006; INS, 2006).

3 Verify patient's identity by using at least two patient identifiers. Compare patient's name and one other identifier, such as hospital identification number, with MAR. Ask patient to state name as a third identifier.

Complies with The Joint Commission requirements and improves patient safety. In most acute care settings, patient's name and identification number on armband and MAR are used to identify patients (TJC, 2007).

4 Remove tape from old dressing one layer at a time by pulling toward the insertion site, leaving tape that secures VAD to skin intact. Be cautious if IV tubing becomes tangled between two layers of dressing. Remove transparent semipermeable dressing by pulling up one corner and pulling the side laterally while holding the catheter hub (see illustration). Repeat on other side. When removing transparent dressing, hold catheter hub and tubing with nondominant hand.

Prevents accidental displacement of VAD.

5 Observe insertion site for signs and/or symptoms of infection: tenderness, redness, swelling, and exudate. If complication exists or if ordered by health care provider, discontinue infusion (see Procedural Guideline 28-1, p. 770).

Presence of infection or complication indicates need to remove VAD at current site.

6 Prepare new tape strips for use. If IV is infusing properly, gently remove tape securing VAD. Stabilize VAD with one finger. Use adhesive remover to cleanse skin and remove adhesive residue, if needed.

Exposes venipuncture site. Stabilization prevents accidental displacement of VAD. Adhesive residue decreases ability of new tape to adhere securely to skin.

Critical Decision Point   *Keep one finger over catheter at all times until tape or dressing secures placement. If patient is restless or uncooperative, it is helpful to have another staff member assist with procedure.*

7 While stabilizing IV, cleanse insertion site with antiseptic swab using friction in a horizontal plane, then a vertical plane, followed by a circular motion, moving from the insertion site outward (see illustration). Allow antiseptic solution to dry completely.

Mechanical friction in this pattern allows penetration of the antiseptic solution into the epidermal layer of the skin (Hadaway and Milam, 2005).

Allowing antiseptic solutions to air-dry completely effectively reduces microbial counts (INS, 2006).

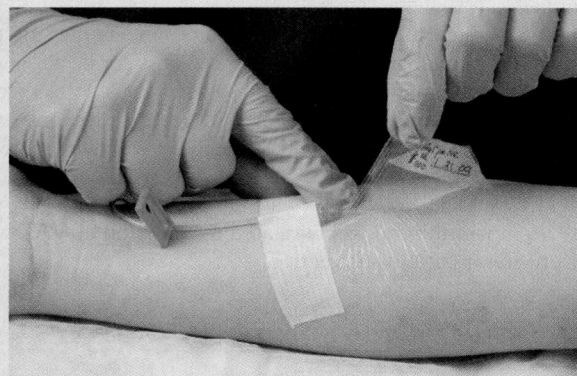

STEP 4   Remove transparent dressing by pulling side laterally.

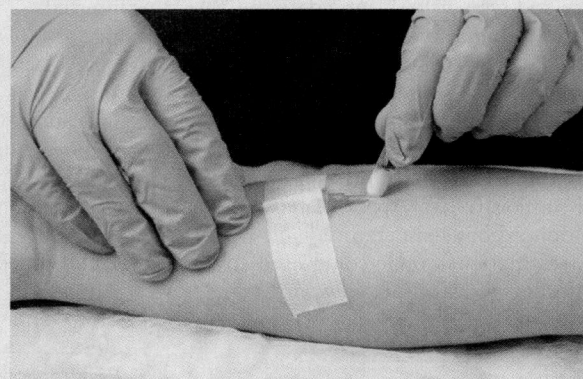

STEP 7   Cleanse peripheral insertion site with antiseptic swab.

STEP	**RATIONALE**
8 *Optional:* Apply skin protectant solution (e.g., Skin Prep, No Sting Barrier Film) to the area where you will apply the tape or dressing. Allow to dry.	Coats the skin with protective solution to maintain skin integrity, prevents irritation from the adhesive, and promotes adhesion of the dressing.
9 While securing catheter, apply sterile dressing over site (procedures differ; follow agency policy).	
a *Manufactured catheter stabilization device:* Apply catheter stabilization device as directed in Skill 28-1, Step 23a.	The manufactured catheter stabilization device is a sterile, adhesive pad that holds the catheter in place and reduces the risk for infection and needle-stick injuries and improves patient outcomes (INS, 2006; Rosenthal, 2007).
b *Transparent dressing:* Apply transparent dressing as directed in Skill 28-1, Step 23b.	Prevents accidental dislodgment of catheter. Occlusive dressing protects site from bacterial contamination. Connection between administration set and hub needs to be uncovered to facilitate changing the tubing if necessary.
c *Sterile gauze dressing:* Apply sterile gauze dressing as directed in Skill 28-1, Step 23c.	Only use sterile tape under a sterile dressing to prevent site contamination. Prevents back-and-forth motion, which will irritate the vein and introduce microorganisms on the skin into the vein. Tape on top of gauze makes it easier to access hub/tubing junction. Gauze pad elevates hub off skin to prevent pressure area. Securing loop of tubing reduces risk for dislodging catheter if the IV tubing is pulled (i.e., the loop will come apart before the catheter dislodges).

Critical Decision Point   *Because Band-Aids are not occlusive and nonsterile tape increases the risk for insertion site infection, do not use either over catheter insertion points.*

STEP	**RATIONALE**
10 Remove and discard gloves.	Prevents transmission of microorganisms.
11 *Optional:* Apply site protection device (e.g., I.V. House Protective Device).	Reduces the risk for phlebitis and infiltration from mechanical motion.
12 Anchor IV tubing with additional pieces of tape if necessary. When using transparent dressing, avoid placing tape over dressing.	Prevents accidental displacement of VAD.
13 Label dressing per agency policy. Information on label includes date and time of IV insertion, VAD gauge size and length, and your initials.	Communicates type of device and time interval for dressing change and site rotation.
14 Discard equipment, and perform hand hygiene.	Reduces transmission of microorganisms.

EVALUATION

1 Observe function, patency of IV system, and flow rate after changing dressing.	Validates that IV is patent and functioning correctly. Manipulation of catheter and tubing will affect rate of infusion.
2 Inspect condition of VAD site, noting color. Palpate for skin temperature, edema, and tenderness.	Complications such as phlebitis and infiltration require removal of VAD and insertion of new VAD at another site.
3 Monitor patient's body temperature.	Elevated temperature indicates an infection that is possibly associated with contamination of the venipuncture site.

Unexpected Outcomes	**Related Interventions**
1 VAD is infiltrated, as evidenced by decreased flow rate or edema, pallor, or decreased temperature around insertion site.	• Stop infusion, and remove VAD (see Procedural Guideline 28-1). • Restart new VAD in other extremity or above previous insertion site, if continued therapy is necessary. • Elevate affected extremity.
2 Phlebitis is present, as evidenced by erythema and tenderness along vein pathway.	• Stop infusion, and remove VAD (see Procedural Guideline 28-1). • Restart new VAD in other extremity if continued therapy is necessary. • Apply warm moist compress to affected site (see Chapter 39) until resolved.
3 VAD is accidentally removed.	• Restart VAD if continued therapy needed.
4 Patient has an elevated temperature.	• Notify health care provider. • Prepare to obtain blood culture or culture of IV site to evaluate source of infection.
5 Insertion site is red and/or edematous and/or painful and/or has presence of exudate, indicating infection at venipuncture site.	• Notify health care provider. Culture of catheter tip and/or exudate will probably be ordered. (Confirm before removal of IV.) • Remove VAD (see Procedural Guideline 28-1). • Antibiotic therapy may be ordered. (Do not begin until blood cultures obtained, if ordered.)

Recording and Reporting

- Record time peripheral dressing was changed, reason for change, type of dressing material used, patency of system, and description of venipuncture site.
- Report to nurse in charge or oncoming nursing shift that dressing was changed and any significant information about integrity of system.
- Report to health care provider and document any complications.

Teaching Considerations

- Instruct patient to notify nurse if skin under dressing or tape becomes reddened, itches, or burns or if dressing becomes compromised.

Pediatric Considerations

- Pediatric patients are not always able to fully understand explanations. Presence of parent or security toy during procedure will help to decrease fear and increase cooperation. Perform procedure on patient's toy or doll first.
- Assistance is necessary to keep patient still and protect IV catheter from dislodgment.

Gerontological Considerations

- Some older adults have fragile skin, so prevent skin tears by minimizing the use of tape directly on the skin and applying skin protectant before applying tape.

Home Care Considerations

- Instruct patient and caregiver about the signs and symptoms of infiltration and phlebitis and therapies to implement for complications.
- Ensure that there is a reliable caregiver or person at home to provide this IV therapy care.
- Instruct patient and caregiver in whom to notify if IV dressing becomes compromised.

PROCEDURAL GUIDELINE 28-1 Discontinuing Peripheral Intravenous Access

 Advanced / Intravenous Fluid Therapy Administration / Discontinuing Intravenous Therapy

[NSO] *Intravenous Fluid Administration Module / Lesson 4*

You discontinue a peripheral intravenous line when the prescribed length of therapy is completed or a complication occurs (e.g., phlebitis, infiltration, or catheter occlusion). The technique for discontinuing a peripheral IV line follows infection control guidelines to minimize the chance of the patient's acquiring an infection. When discontinuing a peripheral IV line, catheter tips can break off, causing an embolus, an emergency situation.

Delegation Considerations

The skill of discontinuing a peripheral intravenous line cannot be delegated to NAP. Delegation to LPNs varies by state Nurse Practice Act. The nurse directs the NAP to:

- Report to the nurse any bleeding after the catheter has been removed.

Equipment

- ❑ Clean gloves
- ❑ Sterile 2 × 2 or 4 × 4 inch gauze sponge
- ❑ Antiseptic swab
- ❑ Tape

Procedural Steps

1. Observe existing IV site for signs and symptoms of infection, infiltration, or phlebitis.
2. Review accuracy and completeness of health care provider's order for discontinuation of IV therapy.
3. Assess patient's understanding of the need for IV to be discontinued.
4. Verify patient's identity by using at least two patient identifiers. Compare patient's name and one other identifier, such as hospital identification number, with MAR. Ask patient to state name as a third identifier.
5. Explain procedure to patient, describing sensation (burning) the patient will feel when you remove catheter. Explain that the patient needs to hold affected extremity still. Also explain how long procedure will take (about 5 minutes).
6. Turn IV tubing roller clamp to "off" position, or turn EID off and then turn roller clamp to "off" position.
7. Perform hand hygiene. Apply clean gloves.
8. Remove IV site dressing and stabilizing IV device (see Skill 28-5). Then remove the tape securing catheter.

> **Critical Decision Point** *Never use scissors to remove the tape or dressing because you may accidentally cut the catheter.*

9. Hold catheter, and clean site with antimicrobial swab. Allow to dry completely.
10. Place clean sterile gauze above site and withdraw catheter, using a slow, steady motion. Keep the hub parallel to the skin (see illustration).

> **Critical Decision Point** *Do not raise or lift catheter before it is completely out of the vein to avoid trauma or hematoma formation.*

11. Apply pressure to site for 2 to 3 minutes, using a dry, sterile gauze pad. Secure with tape. NOTE: Apply pressure for 5 to 10 minutes if patient is on anticoagulants.
12. Inspect catheter for intactness after removal; note tip integrity and length.
13. Apply clean folded gauze dressing over insertion site, and secure with tape.
14. Discard used supplies, remove gloves, and perform hand hygiene.
15. Observe site for evidence of bleeding.
16. Observe site for redness, pain, drainage, or swelling.

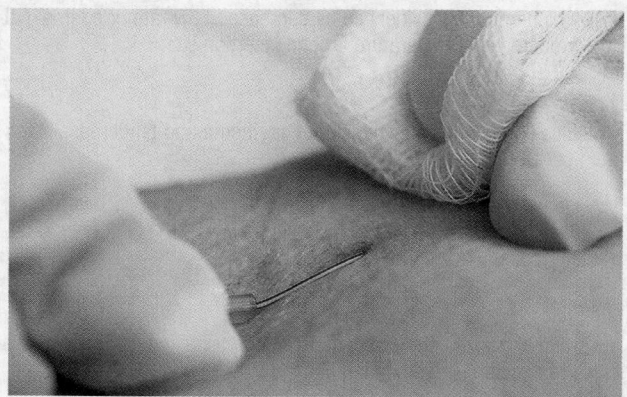

STEP 10 IV catheter is removed slowly, keeping catheter parallel to vein.

SKILL 28-6 Insertion and Care of Central Venous Access Devices

Long-term IV therapy (including parenteral nutrition) can be achieved with the use of medically inserted central venous access devices (CVADs) for administration of medications and solutions. The use of this type of vascular access depends on the length of infusion therapy, the type of medications and osmolarity of solutions needed, and the patient's current health status. CVADs are used in the home, hospital, and long-term care for patients who require supplemental nutrition (see Chapter 32), blood and blood products (see Chapter 29), continuous fluids, medications, hemodynamic monitoring, and blood sampling. These devices minimize peripheral IV therapy complications by reducing the need for frequent venipuncture and multiple IV lines. Use of peripheral IV therapy increases the risk for patients to develop infection, vein sclerosis, phlebitis, and infiltration.

The need for safe and convenient IV therapy has led to the development of vascular access devices designed for long-term access to the venous or arterial systems. Physicians or credentialed advanced practice nurses place these devices into the central venous system. The nurse's role is to assist the health care provider in placing a CVAD. Attention to asepsis and positioning, reassuring the patient during the procedure, and ensuring that the right equipment is available are critical to the success of the insertion. There are four types of CVAD: nontunneled percutaneous central venous catheters, tunneled central venous catheters, peripherally inserted central catheter (PICC), and implanted subcutaneous ports. A PICC is inserted through a larger arm vein (e.g., cephalic or basilic vein) and advanced until the tip enters the central venous system in the lower third of the superior vena cava (INS, 2006). Other CVADs enter chest and neck sites, which are preferred because they are immobile areas and blood flows through large veins at a rapid rate. The catheters are made of silicone or polyurethane materials and may be coated with heparin, antibiotics, or chlorhexidine. CVADs are inserted and threaded into the superior vena cava just above the right atrium and require radiological confirmation of accurate placement. You must be able to maintain the integrity and educate patients about the care and maintenance of CVADs for the duration of their use.

PICCs provide alternative IV access when the patient requires intermediate-length venous access (longer than 7 days to several months). PICCs can be single lumen or multilumen, vary in size from 16 to 24 gauge, and vary in length from 40 to 65 cm (16 to 26 inches). The length is chosen based on the distance from the patient's proposed insertion site to the superior vena cava. The tip placement requires x-ray confirmation to use (Trerotola and others, 2007). PICCs can be used to infuse IV fluids, parenteral nutrition, blood and blood products, and medications such as antibiotics.

Nontunneled percutaneous central venous catheters are inserted directly through the skin and into the internal or external jugular (Fig. 28-5), subclavian, or femoral veins. The tip of the catheter rests in the superior vena cava. These catheters are usually 15 to 20 cm in length (6 to 8 inches) and have one to four lumens. You choose the catheter based on the type and the manufacturer's recommendations, the length of therapy, and the condition/functionality of the catheter. These catheters are used for shorter placements (e.g., 5 to 10 days).

Tunneled central venous catheters are surgically inserted through a tunnel into subcutaneous tissue, usually between the clavicle and nipple (Fig. 28-6), into the internal jugular or subclavian vein, with the catheter tip resting in the distal end of the superior vena cava (Fig. 28-7). The subcutaneous tunnel allows the catheter to remain in place for months to years. The catheter is

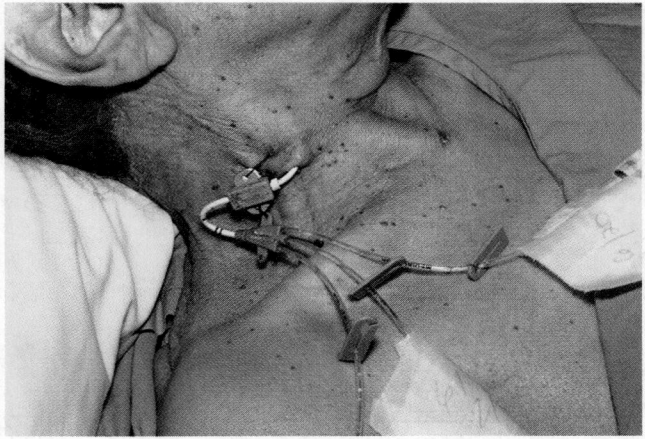

FIG 28-5 Triple-lumen CVAD placed in jugular vein.

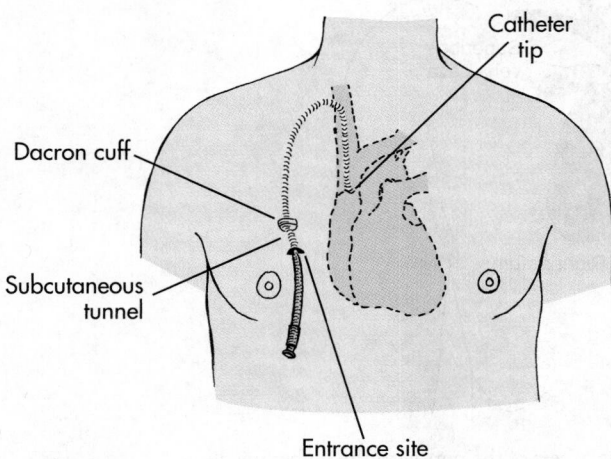

FIG 28-6 Small-gauge tunneled catheter is in place, threaded into superior vena cava.

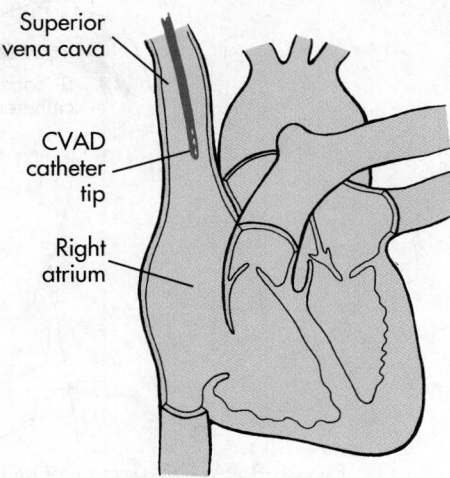

FIG 28-7 Catheter tip from CVAD lies in superior vena cava.

held in place with a Dacron cuff that provides long-term catheter stabilization by creating scar formation that seals the tract and creates an antimicrobial barrier between the skin and the venous system. The catheters are available in different sizes, lengths, and number of lumens depending on manufacturer (e.g., Hickman, Broviac, Groshong).

Subcutaneous implanted ports consist of a portal body, a central septum, a reservoir, and a catheter (Fig. 28-8, A). Single or dual septal ports are available. The infusion port is surgically implanted in a subcutaneous pocket in the chest, arm, forearm, or abdominal wall, and the catheter is inserted into a large vein and threaded into the superior vena cava (Fig. 28-8, B). The port is easy to palpate to determine placement. Specially designed noncoring Huber needles (straight or with 90-degree angles) are inserted through the skin into a self-sealing injection port (Fig. 28-8, C). Implanted infusion ports are used for long-term and complex IV therapy. When not in use, no external catheter is present, and the port manufacturers recommend the port be heparinized every 4 weeks to maintain patency. No other care is required for an unused port.

Primary complications associated with CVADs are usually related to infection caused by contamination of the catheter from the skin of the patient or from the health care worker (Hamilton, 2006; Richardson, 2007). Care of CVADs requires knowledge of the purpose and function of the devices and prevention of complications. Patients with CVADs require health education and teaching about asepsis and skin care.

Delegation Considerations

The skill of caring for a central vascular access device in an acute care setting cannot be delegated to NAP. Delegation to LPNs varies by state Nurse Practice Act. The nurse directs the NAP to:

- Report the following immediately: patient's dressing becomes damp or soiled, catheter line appears to be pulled out farther than original insertion position, IV line becomes disconnected, patient has a fever, patient complains of pain at the site.
- Assist with positioning patient during insertion.

Equipment
Insertion and Dressing Care
- ☐ Hair clippers
- ☐ Subclavian insertion tray *or* the following:
  - ☐ Caps
  - ☐ Sterile gowns
  - ☐ Sterile drapes
  - ☐ Masks and protective eyewear
- ☐ Nonsterile gloves

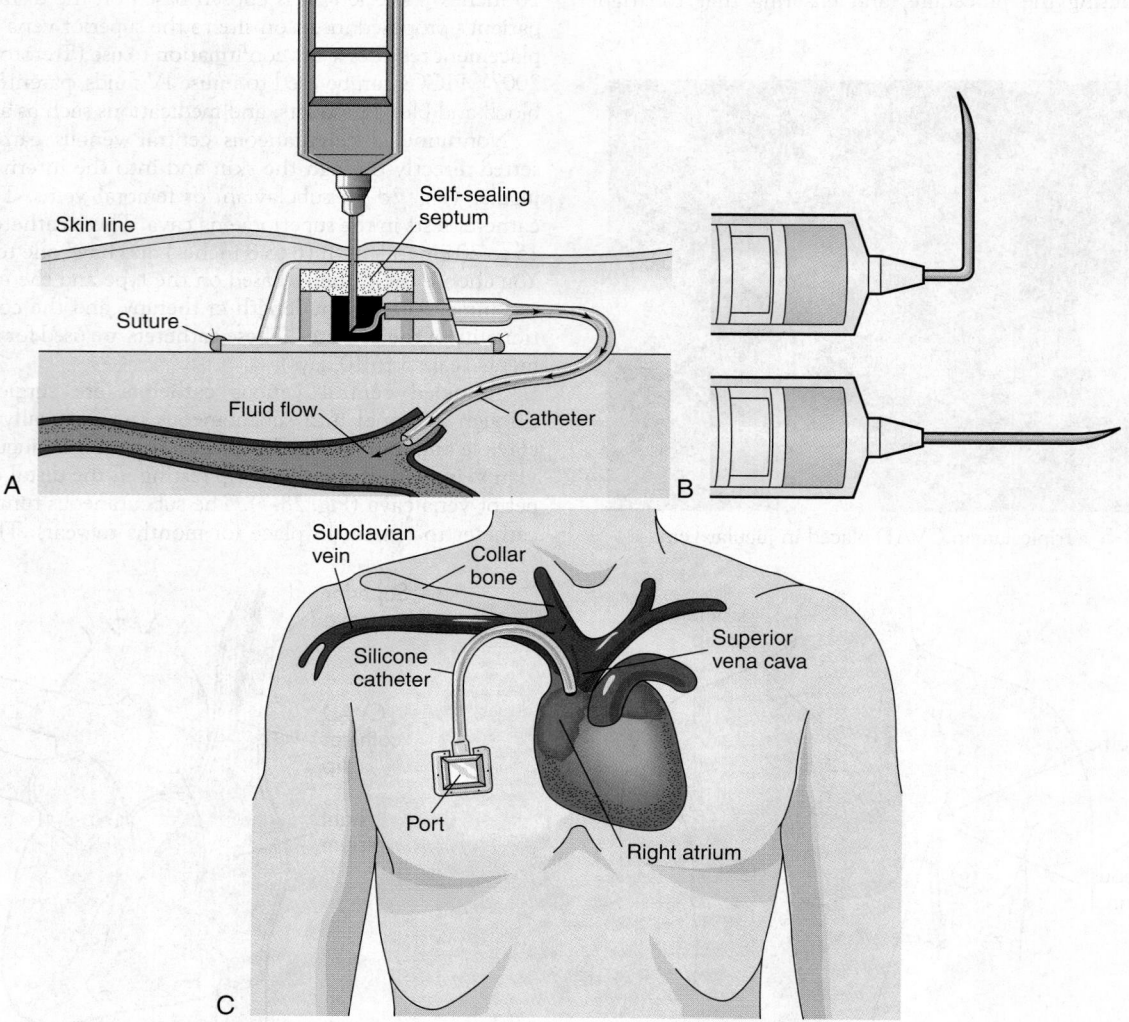

FIG 28-8   **A,** Cross section of implantable port showing access of the port with the Huber needle. **B,** Two Huber needles used to enter implanted port. The 90-degree needle is used for top-entry ports for continuous infusion. **C,** Implanted port and catheter.

❑ Sterile gloves (powder free)
❑ Gauze pads
❑ Surgical towels
❑ Antimicrobial solutions: chlorhexidine gluconate, 70% alcohol, iodophor solution, as single agents or in combination
❑ 1% lidocaine (Xylocaine)
❑ Central line catheter kit
❑ Sterile drapes
❑ 5-mL syringe
❑ Bath blanket or towel and protective pad
❑ 500-mL bottle of 5% dextrose in water
❑ Transparent dressing or gauze dressing for catheter insertion site
❑ Tape
❑ IV infusion pump
❑ Tincture of benzoin (optional)

Site Care and Dressing Change
❑ Clean gloves, mask
❑ Sterile gloves
❑ Antimicrobial swabs (e.g., 2% chlorhexidine, alcohol, iodophor solution; see agency policy)
❑ Transparent gauze dressing or tape
❑ Label
❑ Catheter stabilization device with sterile tape or sterile surgical strips (if not sutured) for PICC or nontunneled catheters

Blood Sampling
❑ Clean gloves
❑ Antimicrobial swabs (e.g., 2% chlorhexidine, alcohol)
❑ 5-mL Luer-Lok syringes
❑ 10-mL Luer-Lok syringes

❑ Vacutainer system (see agency policy)
❑ 3-mL syringe with heparin flush (100 units/mL)
❑ Preservative-free saline flush
❑ Blood tubes, including waste tubes, labels
❑ Needleless injection cap
❑ Access syringe (5 mL or 10 mL—see agency policy)
❑ 10-mL syringe with 5 to 10 mL saline flush
❑ 10-mL syringe with 3 mL heparin flush (100 units/mL)
❑ Clean gloves
❑ Sterile needleless access

Changing the Injection Cap
❑ Clean gloves
❑ Antimicrobial swabs (e.g., 2% chlorhexidine, 70% alcohol, iodophor solution)
❑ Injection cap(s)
❑ 10-mL syringe with 10 mL normal saline flush

Flushing a Positive Pressure Device
❑ Clean gloves
❑ Alcohol swabs
❑ Positive pressure injection cap
❑ 10-mL prefilled saline syringe

Discontinuation of a Nontunneled Catheter or PICC
❑ Central venous access device dressing change kit
❑ Tape
❑ Antimicrobial solutions: 70% alcohol, 2% chlorhexidine-based preparation, or iodophor solution
❑ Suture removal kit (if sutures are in place)
❑ Goggles, gown, mask, and clean gloves

STEP	RATIONALE

ASSESSMENT

1 Review accuracy and completeness of health care provider's order for insertion of CVAD for size and type. Assess treatment schedule: times for administration of IV fluids, medications, blood products, nutrition, and blood sampling. Follow six rights of medication administration (see Chapter 20). Be prepared to witness when physician obtains written informed consent from patient.

Identifies patient's need for vascular access, evaluate response to therapy, and determine education needs. Insertion of central catheter requires informed consent (INS, 2006). Physician may request a certain type or size of catheter.

2 Assess patient's hydration status: skin turgor, texture, and fluid intake and output.

Provides a baseline. Also, dehydration is a depletion of fluid volume and makes insertion of a central vein catheter more difficult.

3 Assess patient for any surgical procedures of the upper chest or anatomical irregularities.

Previous surgical procedures or central venous catheterizations indicates that you should not use a particular site. Scoliosis or other spine deformities make positioning difficult.

4 Inspect condition of skin overlying supraclavicular and infraclavicular area.

Certain skin conditions in which skin integrity is broken contraindicate catheter insertion.

5 Assess patient for allergy to iodine, lidocaine, latex, or medications in a parenteral nutrition solution (see Chapter 32).

Medications, solutions used during catheter insertion, and use of gloves will cause serious allergic response.

6 Assess CVAD placement site for skin integrity and signs of infection (i.e., redness, swelling, tenderness, exudate, bleeding).

Patients requiring long-term IV therapy often have conditions placing them at risk for alterations in skin integrity and immune function. CVAD site is an insult to skin integrity and provides access for pathogens through the skin as well as pathogens to migrate from the catheter.

7 When CVAD is in place, assess the type of device. Review manufacturer's directions concerning the catheter and maintenance.

Care and management depends on type and size of catheter or port, number of lumens, purpose of therapy.

STEP	RATIONALE
8 Assess need to use existing CVAD for blood sampling.	Scheduling blood sampling minimizes number of times health care providers enter CVAD system and allows for timely collection of specimens. Risk for infection increases with multiple entries into vascular system, especially in immunocompromised patients.

Critical Decision Point *In most situations, you can run several tests from one blood tube sample (e.g., potassium, calcium, and magnesium). Always draw blood cultures first. Always anticipate the need for a blood test (e.g., blood cultures if a patient has developed an elevated temperature). If your next task is to draw blood for electrolyte results, you will eliminate reaccessing the CVAD at a later time by asking the health care provider if blood cultures need to be drawn. Consultation with laboratory services will provide specific instructions.*

STEP	RATIONALE
9 Assess for proper function of existing CVAD before therapy: integrity of catheter, septum port (if used), ability to irrigate or infuse fluid, ability to aspirate blood.	Ensures proper function of CVAD without complications.
10 Assess if any lumens require flushing or site needs dressing change by referring to medical record, nurses' notes, agency policies, and manufacturer's recommended guidelines for use.	Provides guidelines for maintaining catheter patency and preventing infection.
11 Assess patient's reaction to CVAD and knowledge of purpose, care, and maintenance. For long-term use, ask patient to discuss steps in care and to perform procedure (e.g., catheter site cleansing or dressing change).	Determines patient's level of understanding. Provides opportunity to educate patient for home care of CVAD.
12 Assess patient's understanding of need for inserting/discontinuing CVAD.	Promotes cooperation with procedures.

NURSING DIAGNOSES

- Deficient fluid volume
- Deficient knowledge regarding use of CVAD
- Excess fluid volume
- Impaired skin integrity
- Risk for infection
- Risk for injury

Individualize related factors based on patient's condition or needs.

PLANNING

STEP	RATIONALE
1 Expected outcomes following completion of procedure:	
• Insertion occurs without complication.	Placement of a central vein catheter carries risks.
• Placement of catheter tip is in the superior vena cava.	Confirmation of placement relies on x-ray examination.
• CVAD site is intact and with no evidence of clotting, local inflammation, phlebitis, systemic infection, venous thrombosis, air embolus, extravasation (medication leaks into tissues around site), or catheter migration.	Catheter is patent, properly placed, and without evidence of complications.
• Fluids, medications, blood products, parenteral nutrition (see Chapter 32) infuse without difficulty.	Catheter remains patent.
• Patient and family are able to explain the purpose of CVAD therapy and perform dressing changes and skin care.	Demonstrates that patient and family have an understanding and competency in caring for CVAD.

IMPLEMENTATION

STEP	RATIONALE
1 Explain procedure and purpose to patient and family. Instruct patient not to move during procedure.	Decreases anxiety and promotes cooperation.
2 Verify patient's identity by using at least two patient identifiers. Compare patient's name and one other identifier, such as hospital identification number, with MAR. Ask patient to state name as a third identifier.	Complies with The Joint Commission requirements and improves patient safety. In most acute care settings, patient's name and identification number on armband and MAR are used to identify patients (TJC, 2007).
3 **Catheter insertion:**	
a Physician, with assistance of nurse, positions patient flat in bed, lying supine. Place rolled towel or bath blanket between patient's scapulas, and place protective pad under shoulder area.	Opens angle between clavicle and first rib; dilates veins to facilitate eventual catheter insertion.
b If necessary, use scissors or electric clippers to remove any hair around insertion site.	Transient microorganisms reside in body hair. Clippers do not cause microabrasions, which harbor microorganisms (INS, 2006).

STEP	RATIONALE
c Physician applies cap, mask, and eyewear and performs surgical hand scrub. Applies surgical gown and powder-free sterile gloves.	Maximum barrier precautions needed when inserting central venous catheter (INS, 2006).
d Nurse puts on cap (optional), mask, and eyewear. Performs hand hygiene. (Check agency policy because some institutions require strict precautions.)	Appropriate barrier precautions necessary for nurse to assist in positioning and comforting patient, obtaining additional supplies as needed, regulating IV flow rate once line is inserted.
e Physician opens central vein kit and adds any sterile equipment to kit for use during insertion (see Chapter 8).	Maintains sterile field.
f Nurse saturates 4 × 4 inch gauze pads with preferred antimicrobial antiseptic. Physician applies antiseptics either as a combination solution or in a series (INS, 2006): Alcohol is usually first, followed by chlorhexidine. Alcohol should not be applied after the application of iodophor solution. Physician scrubs area using circular motion from shoulder to ear to chin to nipple for approximately 1 minute.	Alcohol cleans and defats skin. Antiseptics remove resident and transient bacteria.
g Physician cleans same area for 1 minute using antimicrobial swabs (chlorhexidine or iodophor).	Removes surface skin bacteria.
h Allow antimicrobial solution to air-dry completely.	Ensures maximum antimicrobial effect (INS, 2006).
i Physician removes sterile gloves and applies new pair of sterile gloves.	Gloves become contaminated from surface bacteria picked up in solution.
j Physician uses large sterile drape and sterile towels to create a sterile field. Physician finds anatomical landmarks and places fenestrated drape appropriately.	Provides sterile work space for catheter insertion. Patients whose catheters were placed using a mask, cap, sterile gloves, gown, and large drape had lower colonization rate of bacteria than patients whose catheters were placed using sterile gloves and a small drape (Richardson, 2007).
k Physician arranges equipment in kit in preparation for catheter insertion.	Ensures smooth, orderly procedure.
l Nurse sets up IV bag, fills tubing, and covers end of tubing with a sterile cap (see Skill 28-1).	IV tubing is ready to be connected to IV catheter.
m Nurse places patient on right side in 10-degree Trendelenburg's position without a rolled towel and turns patient's head away from site of insertion.	Presence of a rolled towel does not improve filling of subclavian vein. With head down, below heart, position without towel promotes maximal filling and distention with an increase in the diameter of the subclavicular vein (Biemans and others, 2007). A 10-degree tilt effectively achieves increase in diameter of vein (Clenaghan and others, 2005).

Critical Decision Point *Trendelenburg's position is contraindicated in patients with head injuries, increased intracranial pressure, certain respiratory conditions, and spinal cord injuries.*

n Nurse wipes off top of 1% lidocaine bottle with alcohol swabs and holds bottle upside down. *Optional:* Topical transdermal anesthetic agents can be applied before insertion.	Removes surface bacteria; allows physician to withdraw lidocaine while maintaining asepsis. Lidocaine has the potential for creating allergic reaction and tissue damage.
o Physician injects needle into bottle and withdraws approximately 3 to 4 mL lidocaine. Physician injects needle into site for subclavian puncture and anesthetizes venipuncture site, waiting 1 to 2 minutes for effect to take place.	Minimizes discomfort patient feels during venipuncture.

Critical Decision Point *Just before time of insertion, ask patient to hold breath and strain. This is a Valsalva maneuver, which increases central venous pressure in order to prevent entry of air into the catheter. The Valsalva maneuver is the preferred method, although breath holding and humming may be a necessary option in uncooperative patients (Lewin and others, 2007). In addition, if patient is unable to perform maneuvers, compress patient's abdomen gently.*

STEP	RATIONALE
p Physician inserts IV catheter into subclavian vein. Usually physician does this by locating the vein with a large-bore cannula, removing the needle from the cannula, threading a wire into the cannula and vein, removing the cannula over the wire, and threading the central vein catheter over the wire to the appropriate location (Seldinger technique) (Varon and Nyman, 2007).	Large vein is selected because it will be less irritated by hypertonic solutions or medications.
q Physician determines patency of line by withdrawing blood with 5-mL syringe. When blood return is evident and catheter placement is appropriate, physician connects IV tubing to IV catheter. Nurse should confirm tubing connection.	Connecting IV solution prevents air from entering venous system. Tubing misconnections involving central IV catheters have led to patient injury and death (TJC, 2006).
r Infusion of fluid into the catheter does not begin until the location of the catheter tip is confirmed by x-ray film (see agency policy).	Prevents accidental infusion of fluid into chest cavity.
s Physician applies catheter securement device (e.g., manufactured stabilization device, sterile tape, or surgical Steri-Strips) to secure central venous catheter in place.	Suturing catheter to skin at insertion site increases risk for infection. Catheter securement devices are noninvasive and preferred for preventing catheter dislodgment (INS, 2006).
t Physician removes sterile drapes and completes procedure.	Occurs only if physician is not applying occlusive dressing to IV site.
u Physician orders chest film.	X-ray film of the central catheter's tip location is the method recommended to confirm location of catheter tip (INS, 2006).
v Nurse adjusts IV infusion to prescribed rate and connects to electronic infusion pump once chest x-ray study is obtained.	Central line cannulations increase risk for pneumothorax (entrance of air into pleural space). Chest x-ray examination verifies absence of pneumothorax and confirms location of IV catheter before fluids are administered at a rapid flow.
4 Insertion site care and dressing change:	
a Position patient in comfortable position with head slightly elevated.	Provides access to patient. Infusion port requires palpation.
b *Gauze dressing:* Provide insertion site care every 48 hours and as needed. *Transparent dressings:* Provide insertion site care every 7 days and as needed.	Insertion sites require regular inspection for early detection of infection and complications. An intact transparent dressing may remain in place without increasing the risk for infection (INS, 2006).
c Perform hand hygiene, and apply mask.	Reduces transfer of microorganisms, prevents spread of airborne microorganisms over CVAD insertion site.
d Apply clean gloves. Remove old dressing by lifting and removing tape in the direction of the catheter insertion. Discard in appropriate biohazard container.	Stabilizes catheter as you remove dressing.
e Remove catheter stabilization device if used. Must be removed with alcohol.	Allows clear visualization of insertion site and surrounding skin (INS, 2006).

Critical Decision Point   *If sutures are used for initial catheter stabilization and become loosened or are no longer intact, alternative stabilization measures should be used (INS, 2006). Recent recommendations include use of a stabilization device because of the increased risk for infection when the catheter is sutured (Dougherty, 2007).*

f Inspect catheter, insertion site, and surrounding skin.	Insertion site requires regular inspection for complications.
g Remove and discard clean gloves, perform hand hygiene; open CVAD dressing kit using sterile technique, and **apply sterile gloves**.	Sterile technique is required to apply new dressing.

STEP	RATIONALE

h Using antiseptic swab, cleanse catheter and site, working in a horizontal plane with first swab, vertical plane with second swab, and a circular motion, moving outward with third swab (see illustration). Allow to dry completely.

Allowing antiseptic solutions to air-dry completely effectively reduces microbial counts (INS, 2006). Drying allows time for maximum microbicidal activity of agents (Hadaway, 2006). Chlorhexidine 2% preparations are preferred (INS, 2006).

i Apply skin protectant to entire area. Allow to dry completely so that skin is not tacky.

Skin protectant is used to protect irritated or fragile skin from the dressing. It must be used if a catheter stabilization device is used.

j Apply new catheter stabilization device per manufacturer's instructions if the catheter is not sutured in place (see illustration).

Provides catheter stability to minimize dislodgment.

k Apply sterile, transparent semipermeable dressing or gauze dressing over insertion site (see Skill 28-5).

Transparent dressing allows for clear visualization of catheter site between dressing changes.

l Apply label with date, time, and your initials.

Provides information about next dressing change.

m Dispose of soiled supplies and used equipment. Remove gloves, and perform hand hygiene.

Reduces transmission of microorganisms.

5 **Blood sampling:**

a Perform hand hygiene.

Reduces transmission of microorganisms.

b Apply clean gloves.

Prevents transfer of body fluids.

c Turn off any infusion for at least 1 minute before drawing blood. NOTE: If you cannot stop infusion, draw blood from a peripheral vein.

Prevents interruption of critical fluid therapy.

d If sampling through an injection cap, cleanse injection cap with alcohol, and allow to dry completely. Use proximal (red or brown) lumen to draw blood if device has more than one lumen.

Maximizes bactericidal effectiveness of antiseptic swab.
The proximal (red or brown) lumen typically is the largest-gauge lumen.

e Flush catheter with 5 to 10 mL 0.9% sodium chloride (check agency policy). Do not flush before drawing blood for blood cultures.

Determines catheter patency and clears IV.
Blood that has been sitting in the catheter is needed for blood cultures.

f If sampling through the catheter hub, clamp the catheter, remove end of IV tubing or injection cap from the catheter hub. Attach a 10-mL syringe with 10 mL of 0.9% normal saline, unclamp the catheter, and flush per agency policy.

Prevents air from entering system.

g Slowly aspirate 5 mL blood from catheter. Discard syringe in biohazard container. *Optional*: Use Vacutainer device to draw one red-top blood tube for discard. **NOTE: Check agency policy for use of Vacutainers with central lines.**

Initial sample clears catheter of fluid and medication before blood is drawn.
Vacutainer system reduces risk for blood exposure.

Critical Decision Point   *If blood cultures have been ordered, do not discard any blood. Use initial specimen for blood cultures.*

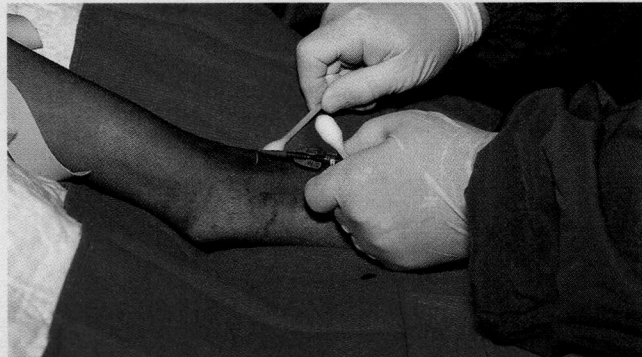

STEP 4h   Cleanse central venous access device site.

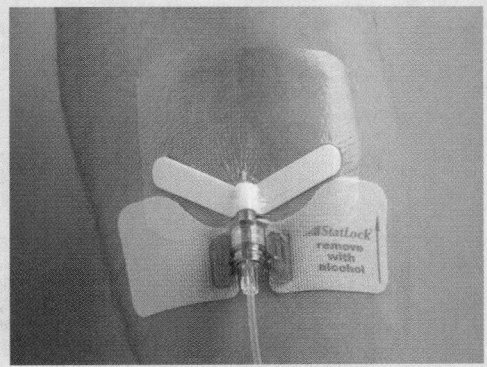

STEP 4j   CVAD in stabilization device. (*Photo courtesy Bard Medical.*)

STEP	RATIONALE
h Cleanse injection cap with antiseptic swab, and allow to dry completely. Attach or insert appropriate size syringe, and withdraw blood required for specimen. Clamp catheter. If available, obtain specimens with Vacutainer system. If using syringes, transfer blood using a transfer vacuum device (see illustration). Dispose of syringe or Vacutainer in biohazard container.	You can draw multiple blood specimens at a one time and place them in different laboratory tubes. Consult laboratory manual for correct amount of blood and tube needed for ordered tests. If coagulation specimens are ordered, check laboratory policy for amount of blood discard and volume needed.
i Swab injection cap with antiseptic swab and insert 10-mL syringe of 0.9% sodium chloride. Unclamp catheter, and slowly flush. Reclamp catheter using positive pressure on plunger (follow manufacturer's guidelines when flushing during the last 0.5 mL of solution through an injection cap). **NOTE:** Some injection caps create positive pressure, and the catheter should not be clamped until the syringe is removed. Other caps need to use positive pressure flush and clamp.	Reduces risk for catheter clotting after procedure.
j Flush catheter port with syringe containing heparin solution (check agency policy).	Heparin flush volume and concentration varies by agency and type of catheter. Flush Groshong catheters with 0.9% sodium chloride only.

Critical Decision Point *Always use a 10-mL syringe on central lines to minimize pressure during injection.*

k Remove syringe. Attach IV tubing, and resume infusion or place new injection cap.	Maintains sterile seal to catheter.

Critical Decision Point *There are new positive pressure devices for CVADs that allow blood drawing and fluid administration without removing caps from system.*

l Dispose of soiled equipment and used supplies. Remove gloves, and perform hand hygiene.	Reduces transmission of microorganisms.
6 **Changing injection cap:**	
a Determine if injection caps should be changed.	Injection caps are usually changed when removed for IV fluid administration, if integrity is compromised, or if they have been accessed beyond manufacturer's directions.
b Prepare new injection cap(s): (1) Remove cap from package, and cleanse septum with alcohol using friction.	

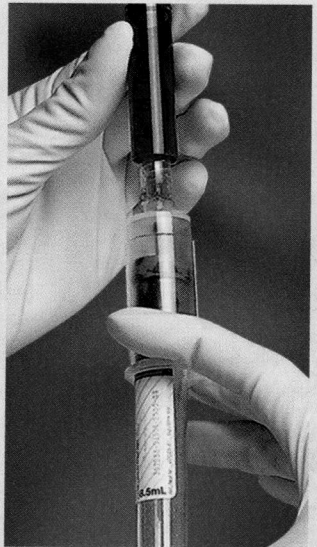

STEP 5h Blood specimen transfer device. *(Courtesy and © Becton Dickinson, and Company.)*

STEP	RATIONALE
(2) Keep the protective cap on the tip of the injection cap.	Maintains sterility.
(3) Prime the injection cap by flushing with 0.9% normal saline through cap until fluid is seen in the protective cap. Keep syringe attached.	Removes air from the system.
c Clamp catheter lumens one at a time by using slide or squeeze clamp.	Prevents air from entering system when opened. Patient can also perform Valsalva maneuver during cap changes.
d Remove old injection caps using aseptic technique.	Routine injection cap changes decrease catheter infections
e Cleanse catheter hub with antiseptic swab. Connect new injection cap(s) on catheter hub.	Allowing antiseptic solutions to air-dry completely effectively reduces microbial counts (INS, 2006). Drying allows time for maximum microbicidal activity of agents (Hadaway, 2006).
f Flush catheter with 10-mL syringe of 0.9% sodium chloride, or attach new IV tubing and begin infusion.	Prevents clot formation.
g Dispose of all soiled supplies and used equipment. Remove gloves, and perform hand hygiene.	Reduces spread of microorganisms.
7 Flushing a positive pressure device:	
a Perform hand hygiene, and apply clean gloves.	Reduces transmission of microorganisms.
b Prepare positive pressure device by attaching prefilled saline syringe. Prime through the device, and leave syringe attached.	Maintains sterility of device.
c Vigorously cleanse the cap-catheter junction with alcohol swab for 5 to 10 seconds.	
d Clamp catheter. Remove needleless cap and discard.	
e Connect the positive pressure device, unclamp the catheter, and flush through with saline as ordered.	Do not add extension tubing, which negates positive pressure action of the valve.
f Do **not** reclamp catheter.	Reclamping negates the positive pressure action of the valve.
g Dispose of all soiled supplies and used equipment. Remove gloves, and perform hand hygiene.	Reduces spread of microorganisms.
8 Discontinuing nontunneled catheters or PICCs:	
a Verify physician's order to discontinue line. Check agency policy because most require physician to discontinue CVAD. In some settings critical care nurses are certified for removal of line.	Verifies appropriateness of procedure. Only a competent health care professional can remove a CVAD.
b If IV fluids or medications are to continue, prepare to convert them to a peripheral IV before CVAD discontinuation.	Prevents interruption of IV medication/fluid therapy.
c Perform hand hygiene.	Prevents transmission of microorganisms
d Turn off IV fluids infusing through the central line.	Prevents fluid loss during CVAD removal.
e Place moisture-proof pad under site.	Minimizes soiling of bed linen.
f Apply gown, mask, goggles, and clean gloves.	Prevents transmission of microorganisms and nurse's exposure to blood-borne pathogens.
g Gently remove CVAD dressing. Discard in biohazard container. Inspect catheter and insertion site.	Prevents skin tears. Provides information about catheter and site before removal. Disposal prevents transmission of microorganisms.
h Remove gloves, perform hand hygiene, and apply new pair of clean gloves.	Prevents transfer of organisms on soiled dressing to catheter insertion site.
i Cleanse CVAD site using combination antiseptic or chlorhexidine swabs (check agency policy). Begin at insertion site and move outward in a circular motion or, with chlorhexidine only, use a back-and-forth scrub method. Allow to dry completely.	Removes microorganisms from skin surrounding insertion site. Allowing antiseptic solutions to air-dry completely effectively reduces microbial counts (INS, 2006).
j If catheter securement device is present, carefully disconnect catheter from device and remove device with alcohol. If sutures are present, remove clean gloves and open suture removal kit.	Alcohol aids in removal of securement device.
k To remove sutures, apply sterile gloves. With nondominant hand, grasp suture with forceps. Using dominant hand, carefully cut suture with sterile scissors, avoid damaging skin or catheter. Lift suture out and discard. Continue until all sutures are removed.	Technique prevents pulling contaminated end of suture through patient's skin.

STEP	RATIONALE
l Position patient in 10-degree Trendelenburg's position.	Position promotes venous filling and prevents air embolus during catheter removal.
m Using nondominant hand, apply sterile 4 × 4 inch gauze to site. Instruct patient to take a deep breath and hold it as you withdraw catheter.	Valsalva maneuver reduces the risk for air embolus by decreasing negative pressure in respiratory system.
n With dominant hand, remove catheter in a smooth, continuous motion an inch at a time. Note any resistance while removing the catheter. Inspect catheter for intactness, especially along tip. Keeping fingers near insertion site, immediately apply pressure to site and continue to hold for 5 minutes or until bleeding stops.	Gentle removal of catheter prevents stretching and breaking of the catheter. Damaged catheter may break off and leave a piece of catheter in patient's arm. Direct pressure reduces risk for bleeding and hematoma formation.

Critical Decision Point   *It is often necessary to apply pressure longer if patient is receiving anticoagulation therapy or has prolonged clotting times.*

STEP	RATIONALE
o Apply antiseptic ointment to exit site (*optional:* see agency policy). Apply sterile occlusive dressing such as transparent dressing or sterile gauze to site. Change dressing every 24 hours until healed.	Reduces chance of bacterial growth at old insertion site. Inspection of catheter removal site for bleeding and infection until healed is necessary (INS, 2006).
p Label dressing with date, time and your initials.	Identifies date of catheter removal and need for dressing change.
q Inspect catheter integrity, and discard in biohazard container.	If catheter tip is broken or compromised, place in container and label for possible follow-up.
NOTE: Some protocols recommend sending catheter tip for routine culture.	
r Return patient to comfortable position. Be sure peripheral IV is infusing at correct rate.	Maintains IV fluid therapy
s Dispose of soiled supplies; remove gloves and personal protective equipment. Perform hand hygiene.	Reduces transmission of microorganisms.

EVALUATION

1 Observe patient for shortness of breath, pain in the chest or shoulder after CVAD insertion. Auscultate for breath sounds.	Pain, shortness of breath, and absent breath sounds indicate complication of pneumothorax.
2 Observe patient for bleeding or swelling at the insertion site and occlusiveness of dressing.	Symptoms indicate infiltration of IV fluids into subcutaneous tissues or damage to vessel lumen. Dressing must remain occlusive to protect against entrance of microorganisms.
3 Monitor I&O every 4 hours for fluid balance, and monitor laboratory values for electrolyte balance as indicated.	Assesses patient's circulatory system and indicates fluid volume excess or deficit.
4 Routinely assess vital signs of patient, noting changes symptomatic of infection.	Catheter-related sepsis causes fever, chills, flushed skin, tachycardia.
5 Observe catheter insertion site or port exit when sites are exposed for erythema, warmth, tenderness, edema or drainage.	Continual monitoring for signs of inflammation or infection is essential.
6 Observe all catheter connection points periodically.	An intact system prevents accidental blood loss or entrance of air.
7 Inspect condition of catheter and connection tubing every 8 hours for leaks or tears, secure connections, kinks or obstructions, correct solution, or cracked hubs.	Break in integrity of system predisposes patient to hemorrhage or air embolus.
8 Observe for clot formation in catheter, air embolism, extravasation during infusions, and catheter migration.	Early detection of complications improves patient outcomes.
9 Consult x-ray examination reports for catheter placement.	A routine chest x-ray examination will locate position of catheter tip.
10 Evaluate ability of patient and family to provide care and maintain catheter or infusion port through discussion and return demonstrations of dressing changes and skin care. Determine need for restrictions on daily activities.	Measures patient's ability to care for self and any additional learning needs.

Unexpected Outcomes	Related Interventions
For catheter complications, see Table 28-4.	
1 Patient or family member is unable to explain or perform CVAD care.	• Indicates need for home care referral or additional instruction.

| TABLE 28-4 | Complications of Vascular Access Devices | | |

Complication	Assessment	Prevention	Intervention
Catheter damage, breakage	Every shift, observe for pinholes, leaks, tears. Assess for drainage from site after flushing.	Follow proper clamping procedure. Avoid sharp objects near the catheter. Use needleless system device. Use only 5- to 10-mL syringe for flushing. Never flush against resistance.	Clamp the catheter near insertion site and place sterile gauze over break or hole until repaired. Use permanent repair kit, if available. Remove catheter.
Occlusion: thrombus, precipitation, malposition	Assess insertion site and sutures. Assess for blood return. Assess for ability to infuse fluid. Assess equipment. If port, reaccess and verify Huber needle placement. Assess with syringe directly on catheter. Assess for discomfort or pain in shoulder, neck, ear, or arm at insertion site. Assess for neck or shoulder edema.	Follow routine flushing with positive pressure and/or use positive pressure valve injection cap. Secure with catheter stabilization device to prevent tension on CVAD. Administer low-dose oral anticoagulant therapy. Do not flush against resistance. Flush between medications. Flush vigorously after viscous solutions. Avoid mixing incompatible drugs. Avoid kinking catheter.	Reposition patient. Have patient cough and deep breathe. Raise patient's arm overhead. Obtain venogram if ordered. Administer thrombolytics if ordered. Remove catheter (CVAD requires order). Obtain x-ray film as ordered. If precipitate, try hydrochloric acid or ethanol solution per orders. Do not use a 1-mL syringe to instill saline because pressure exceeds 200 psi.
Infection and sepsis: exit site, tunnel, thrombus, port pocket	Assess exit site for redness, drainage, edema, or tenderness. Assess for signs of systemic infection. Monitor laboratory findings.	Use aseptic technique. Prevent contamination of catheter hub. Adhere to dressing change technique. Apply transparent semipermeable dressing over exit site.	Obtain blood cultures first, from peripheral and CVAD if ordered. Administer antibiotic therapy as ordered. Remove catheter (CVAD requires order). Administer thrombolytic agent if ordered. Replace catheter.
Dislodgment	Assess length of catheter daily. Inform patient of possible catheter dislodgment. Identify edema at exit site or drainage. Palpate exit site and tunnel for coiling (catheter can feel cordlike underneath the skin). Assess for distended neck veins.	Loop and tape the catheter securely. Use catheter stabilization device and transparent semipermeable dressing. Avoid pulling on CVAD. Avoid manipulating catheter by hand. Protect site with soft outer cover.	Insert new catheter. Secure with catheter stabilization device. Teach patient not to manipulate catheter.
Catheter migration (e.g., length of catheter moved from original position), pinch-off syndrome (e.g., compression of catheter between the clavicle and the first rib), port separation or catheter fracture (e.g., internal fracture or separation of catheter)	Assess for patient complaints of gurgling sounds. Assess for change in patency of catheter by evaluating change in flow rate, local irritation, swelling, occlusion, tenderness, pain, inability to aspirate fluid and/or blood. Pain at site when flushed or symptoms of embolus. Obtain x-ray examination. Assess edema of arm and hand on side of insertion. Assess for distended neck veins. Assess for inability to infuse fluids. Assess length of catheter daily.	Avoid trauma. Avoid placement near site of local infection, scarring, or skin disorder.	Reposition under fluoroscopy as ordered. Remove catheter as ordered. Stop all fluid administration.

TABLE 28-4 | Complications of Vascular Access Devices—contd

Complication	Assessment	Prevention	Intervention
Skin erosion (e.g., mechanical loss of skin tissue), hematomas (e.g., local collection of blood), cuff extrusion (e.g., tissue at edges of insertion site separate), scar tissue formation over port	Assess for loss of viable tissue over septum site. Assess for separation of exit site edges. Assess for drainage at exit site. Assess for redness. Assess for edema, contusions. Note if tunneled catheter is exposed.	Maintain nutritional status. Avoid pressure or trauma. Rotate with each port access. Do not reinsert a Huber needle in the same "hole" of a previous insertion. This creates a permanent hole in the septum.	Remove CVAD as ordered. Improve nutrition. Provide appropriate skin care.
Infiltration, extravasation	Assess for erythema. Assess for edema. Assess for spongy feeling. Assess for swelling around the IV site and at the termination of the catheter tip. Assess for labored breathing. Assess for aspiration of fluid and/or blood. Assess for complaints of pain. Assess for no free-flow IV drip.	Immediately, stop vesicant administration. Administer antidote or therapeutic medications to maintain tissue integrity according to protocol.	Apply cold/warm compresses according to specific vesicant protocol. Provide emotional support. Obtain x-ray film if ordered. Use antidotes per protocol. Discontinue IV fluids.
Pneumothorax, hemothorax, air emboli, hydrothorax	Assess for subcutaneous emphysema by inspecting and palpating skin around insertion site and along arm. Inspection may reveal edema where the air is located, and the air may travel if the skin is loose. Palpation reveals a crackling sensation such as popping plastic bubble wrap. Assess for chest pain. Assess for dyspnea, apnea, hypoxia, tachycardia, hypotension, nausea, confusion.	Use injection cap on distal end when not in use. Do not leave catheter open to air.	Administer oxygen as ordered. Elevate feet. Aspirate air, fluid. If air emboli suspected, place patient on left side with head down. Remove catheter as ordered. Assist with insertion of chest tubes as ordered.
Incorrect placement	Assess for cardiac dysrhythmias. Assess for hypotension. Assess for neck distention. Assess for narrow pulse pressure. Assess for inadequate blood withdrawal. Assess for retrograde flow of blood (the flow of blood back into the tubing usually caused by decreased pressure gradient between the venous system and the access device unit [e.g., IV infusion, heparin lock]).	Obtain x-ray examination after placement. Reposition catheter as warranted.	Stop all fluid administration until placement is confirmed. Discontinue catheter (requires order). Obtain x-ray and electrocardiogram (for PICC and CVAD). Administer support medications as ordered.

CVAD, Central venous access device; *CVC,* central venous catheter; *IV,* intravenous; *PICC,* peripherally inserted central catheter.

Recording and Reporting
- Immediately notify health care provider of signs and symptoms of any complications.
- Document catheter site care in nurses' notes: size of catheter, change of injection caps, appearance of site, condition and type of securement device, date and time of dressing change.
- Document in nurses' notes condition of exit site or port insertion site, including skin integrity, signs of infection, placement, integrity, and functionality of catheter.
- Document in nurses' notes catheter removal: patient position, appearance of site, integrity of catheter after removal, dressing applied, patient's tolerance of procedure, and presence/absence of bleeding from site every 15 minutes for 1 hour.
- Document in nurses' notes blood draw: date, time, sample drawn.
- Document in nurses' notes unexpected outcomes, health care provider notification, interventions, and patient response to treatment.

Teaching Considerations
- Instruct patient to report discomfort around the site; discomfort in arms, shoulders, or side of the neck; or any shortness of breath.
- Discuss and provide written emergency measures and telephone numbers of health care personnel to be used in case of catheter damage, displacement, swelling, redness, or leakage at insertion site; occlusion of port or catheter; temperature above 100° F; and shaking chills.
- Provide written instruction for dressing changes, inspection of insertion site, irrigations, and tubing changes.
- Arrange for instruction and return demonstration of skills by patient or caregiver.
- Have patient or caregiver maintain a list of caregivers and telephone numbers (e.g., physician, nurse, social worker, pharmacist, dietitian).

Pediatric Considerations
- The use of chlorhexidine gluconate in infants weighing less than 1000 g has been associated with contact dermatitis. For neonates, alcohol is not recommended for site care (INS, 2006).
- Central vein catheters that are of a smaller diameter and shorter length are available for children and infants.
- Take care to secure infant catheters in a manner that does not allow them to twist. Small-diameter catheters are fragile, and twisting them will cause them to tear.
- Amount and dosage of flush solution (heparin/saline) varies with age and size. Record volume of blood draws on intake and output record.
- In neonates, PICCs have a reduced risk for infections compared with umbilical venous catheters.

Gerontological Considerations
- Some older adults have difficulty with lying flat in bed, and a modification of the totally supine position during CVAD insertion is often necessary. Positioning on the right side in Trendelenburg's position is preferred (Biemans and others, 2007).

Home Care Considerations
- Initiate early referral for discharge planning to social service, counselor, or home care coordinator for assessment of resources.
- Provide patient with written list of providers for supplies and equipment.
- Instruct patient or caregiver in flushing technique, site care and dressing change, and emergency interventions.
- Instruct patient and caregiver in adaptations of hospital procedures that they can make at home (e.g., good hand hygiene instead of sterile gloves).
- Ongoing assessment by the home care provider is essential in the early detection of complications and preservation of CVADs.
- Assess home environment, and determine suitable area for dressing changes, avoiding areas where contaminants are potential hazards.
- Provide appropriate information about home disposal of soiled dressings and equipment (see Chapter 42).

☒ CRITICAL THINKING EXERCISES

A patient is admitted from the emergency department to the medical unit with a diagnosis of pneumonia and dehydration. The health care provider has ordered 1000 mL $D_5\frac{1}{2}NS$ at 100 mL/hr to be started in the right hand on admission. The patient has an IV running in her left antecubital fossa that shows evidence of inadequate flow rate, and the patient complains of discomfort at the site.

1 Using a microdrip tubing, what would be the correct drip rate for this IV? Using a 15 gtt/mL macrodrip tubing, what would be the correct drip rate for this IV?
2 When you obtain the IV fluids for the patient, what steps are necessary before you initiate the IV?
3 What assessments and interventions are required for the existing IV in the left arm?
4 Discuss the information to document after discontinuing the left antecubital IV.
5 The IV has been started and is infusing by EID. What teaching considerations should you share with the patient?

☑ REVIEW QUESTIONS

1 A patient is receiving a liter of D_5 LR every 12 hours using an administration set with a drop factor of 15 gtt/mL. At what rate should the nurse set this infusion?
   1 10 gtt/min
   2 21 gtt/min
   3 33 gtt/min
   4 83 gtt/min
2 A patient had his IV catheter inserted 48 hours ago to receive antibiotic therapy. During assessment of his IV site the nurse observes redness and tenderness on palpation. The nurse documents that the IV was discontinued and restarted because of which complication of IV therapy?
   1 Clotting of the IV catheter
   2 Infiltration
   3 Phlebitis
   4 Puncturing of the opposite side of the vein

3   A patient just had a PICC placed in his right antecubital site. When reading the x-ray report verifying correct placement of the catheter, the nurse knows the tip of the PICC is located correctly if it is in which vessel?

  1   The inferior vena cava
  2   The basilic vein
  3   The cephalic vein
  4   The superior vena cava

4   An obese patient who had a right mastectomy several years ago has better veins in her right hand but is left handed. Where should the nurse place the IV catheter?

  1   In her right hand
  2   In her left lower arm
  3   Wherever the patient wants
  4   In her right antecubital site

5   The physician discontinued a patient's anticoagulant therapy. What nursing intervention is most appropriate after the nurse removes the IV catheter from his hand?

  1   Apply pressure to the IV site for 5 minutes.
  2   Convert the catheter to an intermittent heparin lock for 24 hours.
  3   Encourage the patient to keep his hand elevated for 10 minutes.
  4   Use a warm compress at the site for several minutes.

REFERENCES

Bates D: Preventing medication errors: a summary, *Am J Health Syst Pharm* 64(S9): S3, 2007.

Burke KG: Executive summary: the state of the science on safe medication administration symposium, *J Infus Nurs* 28(2):87, 2005.

Centers for Disease Control and Prevention: Guidelines for the prevention of intravascular catheter-related infections, *MMWR Morb Mortal Wkly Rep* 51(No. RR-10):1, 2002.

Cohen M: Only as smart as the user, *Nursing* 37(7):12, 2007.

Coulter K: Older adult patient. In Macklin D, Chernecky C: *Real world nursing survival guide IV therapy,* St. Louis, 2004, Saunders.

Depledge J and others: Developing a strategic approach for IV therapy in the community, *Br J Community Nurs* 11(11): 462, 2006.

Dougherty L: *Central venous access devices: care and management,* Malden, Mass, 2007, Wiley.

Earhart A and others: Assessing pediatric patients for vascular access and sedation, *J Infus Nurs* 30(4):226, 2007.

Hadaway LC: IV rounds: skin flora: unwanted dead or alive, *Nursing* 35(7):20, 2005.

Hadaway LC: Practical considerations in administering intravenous medications, *J Neurosci Nurs* 38(2):119, 2006.

Hadaway M, Milam D: On the road to successful IV starts, *Nursing* 35(suppl):22, 2005.

Hamilton H: Complications associated with venous access devices: part I, *Nurs Stand* 20(26):43, 2006.

Heitz UE, Horne MM: *Pocket guide to fluid, electrolyte, and acid-base balance,* ed 5, St. Louis, 2005, Mosby.

Hindley G: Infection control in peripheral cannulae, *Nurs Stand* 18(27):39, 2004.

Hockenberry MJ, Wilson D: *Wong's nursing care of infants and children,* ed 8, St. Louis, 2007, Mosby.

Hodgson B, Kizor R: *Saunders nursing drug handbook 2006,* St. Louis, 2006, Elsevier.

Infusion Nurses Society: Infusion nursing standards of practice, *J Intraven Nurs* 29(suppl 1):S1, 2006.

Ketchum K and others: Medication reconciliation, *Am J Nurs* 105(11):78, 2005.

Meiner S, Lueckenotte A: *Gerontologic nursing,* ed 3, St. Louis, 2006, Mosby.

Occupational Safety and Health Administration: Occupational exposure to blood borne pathogens, needlestick, and other sharps injuries: final rule, CFR 29, part 1910 (*Fed Regist* 66:5317, Jan 18, 2001), updated April 2006, http://www.osha.gov/SLTC/bloodbornepathogens/index.html.

Otto S: *Pocket guide to infusion therapy,* ed 5, St. Louis, 2005, Mosby.

Phillips D: *Manual of IV therapeutics,* ed 4, Philadelphia, 2005, FA Davis.

Richardson D: Vascular access nursing—standards of care, and strategies in the prevention of infection: a primer on central venous catheters, *J Assoc Vasc Access* 12(1):19, 2007.

Rosenthal K: Tailor your IV insertion techniques for special populations, *Nursing* 35(5):37, 2005.

Rosenthal K: Safer sharps in clinical practice—has federal legislation been effective in protecting healthcare workers? *US Infect Dis* 1:40, 2007.

Smith B: New standards for improving peripheral IV catheter securement, *Nursing* 37(3):72, 2007.

The Joint Commission: Maximizing the benefits of smart pump technology: addressing potential error proactively, *Joint Commission Perspect Patient Safety* 7(6):7, 2007.

The Joint Commission: Tubing misconnections: a persistent and potentially deadly problem, *Sentinel Event Alert* 3b, April 3, 2006.

The Joint Commission: *2009 National patient safety goals hospital program,* Oakbrook Terrace, Ill, 2008, The Commission, http://www.jointcommission.org, accessed October 2008.

RESEARCH REFERENCES

Ahlqvist M and others: Handling of peripheral intravenous cannulae: effects of evidence-based clinical guidelines, *J Clin Nurs* 15(11):1354, 2006.

Biemans JM and others: Optimal patient position for catheterisation of the subclavian vein: in the Trendelenburg position without a rolled towel between the shoulder blades, *Ned Tijdschr Geneeskd* 151(4):243, 2007.

Clenaghan S and others: Relationship between Trendelenburg tilt and internal jugular vein diameter, *Emerg Med J* 22(12):867, 2005.

Deacon VL: The Safe Medical Device Act and its impact on clinical practice, *J Infus Nurs* 27(1):31, 2004.

Ean R and others: A nurse-driven peripherally inserted central catheter team exhibits excellence through teamwork, *J Assoc Vasc Access* 11(3):135, 2006.

Eggimann P: Prevention of intravascular catheter infection, *Curr Opin Infect Dis* 20(4):360, 2007.

Lewin M and others: Humming is as effective as Valsalva's maneuver and Trendelenburg's position for ultrasonic visualization of the jugular venous system and common femoral veins, *Ann Emerg Med* 50(1):73, 2007.

Pearson A and others: Systematic review on embracing cultural diversity for developing and sustaining a healthy work environment in healthcare, *Int J Evid Based Healthc* 5:54, 2007.

Trerotola S and others: Analysis of tip malposition and correction in peripherally inserted central catheters placed at bedside by a dedicated nursing team, *J Vasc Intervent Radiol* 18(4):513, 2007.

Varon J, Nyman U: Sven-Ivar Seldinger: the revolution of radiology and acute intravascular access, *Resuscitation* 75(1):7.

Blood Transfusions

MEDIA RESOURCES

- **evolve** http://evolve.elsevier.com/Perry/skills
  learning system
  - Review Questions
  - Video Clips

KEY TERMS

Agglutinate

Allogeneic

Anemia

Autologous
transfusion

Autotransfusion

Blood group

Blood transfusion

Blood type

Hemolysis

Reinfusion

Thrombocytopenia

Transfusion
reaction

Transfusion-related
acute lung injury
(TRALI)

OBJECTIVES

Mastery of content in this chapter will enable the nurse to:
- Discuss indications for blood therapy.
- Describe various transfusion reactions.
- Demonstrate the following skills on selected patients: initiating blood therapy, implementing autotransfusion, and monitoring for adverse reactions to transfusion.

Transfusion therapy or blood replacement is the intravenous (IV) administration of whole blood, its components, or plasma-derived product for therapeutic purposes. The average adult has about 5 L of blood. Transfusions are used to restore intravascular volume with whole blood or albumin, to restore oxygen-carrying capacity of blood with red blood cells, and to provide clotting factors and/or platelets. Specified components are withdrawn from a unit of whole blood. The most common method of blood transfusion is allogeneic blood, or blood donated from someone else. Despite precautions, transfusion therapy carries risks. Compatibility of the patient and the donor is essential. Human-related errors (e.g., improper labeling or completion of requisition) that may lead to the administration of incompatible transfusions can occur in every step of the process. In addition, incompatibility and/or disease transmission is also a possibility. Comprehensive screening and testing reduce these occurrences considerably. There are currently new blood products in use to reduce patients' risk for transfusion reactions. These modified blood products include washed, irradiated, or leukocyte-poor blood.

In autologous transfusion, or autotransfusion, the donor is the patient. The obvious advantage to autologous transfusions is increased patient safety with the elimination of incompatibility reactions, but it also conserves blood supply, especially if the patient has a rare blood type (Kirschman, 2004). Human errors and infectious disease contamination and transmission remain potential risks. Autologous donation occurs preoperatively for a planned surgery, perioperatively (during a surgical procedure), or postoperatively. Sometimes a patient who is scheduled for a surgical procedure that involves a large volume of blood loss will elect to supply a unit of blood in the event of a needed transfusion (Kirschman, 2007). Donations are not recommended within 72 hours of surgery to avoid hemodynamic compromise. Like allogeneic blood, autologous units are tested for disease and pathogen transmissions. A unit of RBCs can be stored for 4 weeks, or if frozen, for several years (American Association of Blood Banks [AABB], 2005). Accurate identification of the patient and blood unit is vital with preoperative donation (Scarlet, 2006).

Blood for an autologous transfusion can also be salvaged perioperatively or intraoperatively (during a surgical procedure) using a machine that washes and filters the blood to remove anticoagulants and activated clotting factors before reinfusion into the patient's circulation (AABB, 2005). The reinfused blood from perioperative blood salvage contains more viable red blood cells than does stored blood, its pH is normal, and there is a higher level of 2,3-diphospho-glycerate (2,3-DPG, a chemical that increases the oxygen-carrying capacity of hemoglobin).

A patient's blood can also be salvaged postoperatively. The patient's blood is removed through tubes from the site of bleeding and filtered before reinfusion. An anticoagulant, such as heparin, acid citrate dextrose, or citrate phosphate dextrose (CPD) helps prevent clotting (AABB, 2005). Salvaged blood must be reinfused within 6 hours of the beginning of collection. If more than 50% of the patient's total blood volume is reinfused, replacement of clotting factors is necessary.

Although transfusions require a health care provider's order, you will assess the patient before, during, and after a transfusion. You need to understand the rationale for transfusion of any component given, the expected outcomes, and any possible unexpected outcomes so that you will immediately recognize any adverse effects of the therapy and implement appropriate action.

ABO SYSTEM

There are three blood typing systems, ABO, Rh, and HLA typing, used to ensure a close match between transfused products and the recipient's blood. The presence or absence of specific antigens on the surface of red blood cells determines blood type in the ABO system. When the type A antigen is present, the blood group is called type A. When the type B antigen is present, the blood group is type B. When both A and B antigens are present, the blood group is type AB, and when neither A nor B antigens are present, the blood group is type O (Table 29-1).

Antibodies that react against the A and B antigens are naturally present in the plasma of people whose red blood cells do not carry the antigen. These antibodies (agglutinins) react against the foreign antigens (agglutinogens). Incompatible red blood cells agglutinate (clump together) and result in a life-threatening hemolytic transfusion reaction. People with type A blood have anti-B antibodies; people with type B blood have anti-A antibodies. People with type AB blood have neither antibody and can receive all blood types. People with type O blood have both A and B antibodies and can receive only type O blood.

Rh SYSTEM

Although six common types of Rh antigen may be present on the surface of red blood cells, the type D antigen is widely prevalent and is most likely to elicit an immune response. It is the presence or absence of the D antigen that determines a person's Rh type. A person with the D antigen is Rh positive, and a person without the D antigen is Rh negative. Unlike the ABO antigens, there are no naturally occurring antibodies to the Rh (D) antigen. A person with Rh-negative blood must first be exposed to Rh-positive blood before any Rh antibodies are formed. A person with Rh-negative blood who is exposed to a large amount (200 mL or more) of Rh-positive blood will develop enough antibodies to mount a severe transfusion reaction with repeat exposure. These antibodies take up to 2 weeks to form. Therefore, in the case of massive transfusion as used in trauma situations, Rh-positive blood may be used for a person with Rh-negative blood without adverse effect, provided that the person has not been previously exposed to Rh-positive blood.

An Rh-negative mother previously exposed to Rh antigen can transfer Rh antibodies across the placenta to an Rh-positive fetus. This can result in severe fetal hemolysis, the breakdown of red blood cells, with resultant anemia and jaundice, and is often fatal to the infant.

EVIDENCE-BASED PRACTICE TRENDS

Safety and risk management are key factors in transfusion therapy. ABO incompatibility is one of the most serious errors with transfu-

TABLE 29-1 | ABO System

Patient Blood Type (Rh Factor)	Red Blood Cell Antigen	Transfuse With Type A	Transfuse With Type B	Transfuse With Type AB	Transfuse With Type O	Transfusion Options
A (+)	A	Yes	No	No	Yes	A+, A– O+, O–
A (–)	A	Yes	No	No	Yes	A–, O–
B (+)	B	No	Yes	No	Yes	B+, B– O+, O–
B (–)	B	No	Yes	No	Yes	B–, O–
AB (+)	AB	Yes	Yes	Yes	Yes	A+, A– B+, B– O+, O– Universal recipient
AB (–)	AB	Yes	Yes	Yes	Yes	A– B– O–
O (+)	None	No	No	No	Yes	O+, O–
O (–)	None	No	No	No	Yes	O– Universal donor

sions and usually has fatal outcomes (Gray and others, 2007). It most often involves misidentification of the patient or the unit of blood or mislabeling the pre-transfusion blood sample (Dzik, 2007). Almost all fatal hemolytic transfusion reactions occur as a result of human error.

Bar code technology helps prevent errors in the identification process between the patient and the compatible blood unit (Carayon and others, 2007). Systems designed to improve identification processes demonstrate improved practice; however, a barrier warning label on blood units to remind staff to compare the patient's identification band with the blood unit before removal of the label is ineffective (Murphy and others, 2007). Better error-prevention systems are needed to avoid human-related errors (Koshy, 2005; Seiden and Barach, 2006). Radiofrequency transponder microchips used to standardize and document key steps in the blood collection and confirmation of the recipient–blood unit matching at the bedside demonstrates safety benefits (Roark and Miguel, 2006; Sandler and others, 2007). Results from a national audit indicate that the most important error contributing to "wrong blood" is the failure of bedside check of the patient/blood identity (Parris and Grant-Casey, 2007). Compliance with standards, policies, and education is essential to maintain patient safety and reduce potential errors (Gray and others, 2005).

Advanced technological laboratory screening procedures are other trends ensuring safe transfusion. Screening identifies and thereby reduces pathogen transmission. Better assessment of blood and plasma cell integrity are available to avoid loss of blood component function (Thiele and others, 2007). Blood alternative therapies with pharmacological developments such as colloids, crystalloids, erythropoietin, antifibrinolytics, and hematinics reduce the risks associated with transfusing human blood (Kirschman, 2007). Research concerning a hemoglobin substitute is ongoing. Autologous transfusion and cell salvaging reduces blood loss and the need for allogeneic transfusions postoperatively without compromising patient outcomes (Murphy and others, 2007). Blood conservation involves transfusion-free surgery and mechanical options aimed at limiting blood loss (Jabbour and others, 2005; Kirschman, 2007).

CULTURAL CONSIDERATIONS

When administering blood products, you need to consider a patient's cultural beliefs and the acceptance of blood therapy. Some religions do not allow blood transfusions. For example, members of Jehovah's Witness do not allow blood transfusions or organ donation if it involves blood exchange (Jabbour and others, 2005). It is helpful to consult a religious leader when caring for patients in need of blood therapy. Be familiar with the organizational policies and procedures to follow when patients refuse blood transfusion, and inform the physician of a patient's decision.

 Skill Performance Guidelines

1 Review hospital or agency policy and procedure regarding administration of blood or blood products. These are designed to ensure safe administration of blood products.
2 Know the patient's normal range of vital signs and medical history, including allergies and previous transfusion reactions. Administration of blood products increases intravascular volume and may elevate a patient's blood pressure. Sometimes this is one of the desired effects of therapy. However, some patients cannot tolerate the volume load of a blood transfusion and develop fluid volume excess, leading to markedly elevated blood pressure, tachycardia, pulmonary edema, or cardiac failure.
3 Monitor and document the patient's temperature and vital signs immediately before initiation of therapy and closely during blood therapy as well. Policies differ among institutions regarding timing of vital sign monitoring during blood transfusions. An elevation in temperature or heart rate is one of the first signs that a person is having an adverse reaction to a transfusion. Some patients also experience marked hypotension if a severe reaction occurs (Table 29-2).
4 Understand the indications and the goal of the transfusion therapy. This will allow you to assist the physician or health care provider in evaluating the outcome and assessing the need for any further therapy.

5 Assess the patient's most recent serum electrolyte values. When blood is stored, there is continual destruction of red blood cells, which releases potassium from the cells into the plasma. If blood is transfused rapidly, there may be transient hyperkalemia before the potassium is reabsorbed. Blood that is preserved with CPD contains a high concentration of citrate ions. The excess citrate may combine with the ionized calcium in the recipient's blood, resulting in transient low ionized calcium levels. Al-though ionized calcium deficiency resulting from blood transfusions is rare, it is more likely to occur in young children, older adults, or patients with osteoporosis.

6 Patients receiving multiple transfusions need to be assessed for iron overload.

7 Verify the patient's understanding of the procedure and its rationale. This helps to alleviate any anxiety the patient has over receiving blood products.

TABLE 29-2 | Transfusions Reactions

Reaction	Mechanism	Onset	Signs and Symptoms	Prevention	Nursing Intervention
Acute hemolytic transfusion reaction	ABO, Rh incompatibility; causes intravascular destruction of transfused RBCs as antibodies in recipient's plasma attach to antigens on donor RBCs.	Within 15 min of transfusion initiation	Severe pain in kidney area and chest; increased temperature (up to 105° F), increased heart rate; sensation of heat and pain along vein receiving blood; chills, low back pain, headache, nausea, chest or back pain, chest tightness, dyspnea, bronchospasm, anxiety, hypotension, vascular collapse, disseminated intravascular coagulation, possibly death	Carefully identify patient and blood sample obtained for blood typing and compatibility screening. When blood released from blood bank, match with patient information. Follow agency's verification procedures at bedside before transfusion.	Stop transfusion. Remove blood product and tubing. Maintain IV access. Notify health care provider. Monitor vital signs at least every 15 min. Administer ordered therapy to correct arterial blood pressure and coagulopathy. Insert Foley catheter. Monitor intake and output hourly. Assess for shock. Dialysis may be required. Obtain blood and urine samples, and send to laboratory with unused portion of unit of blood. Document reaction according to agency policy.
Delayed hemolytic transfusion reaction	Immune response mounted by recipient against non-ABO donor antigens; usually the result of destruction of transfused RBCs by alloantibodies not detected during the crossmatch.	2-14 days	Unexplained fever, unexplained decrease in Hgb/Hct, increased bilirubin levels, jaundice	Careful crossmatching of donor and recipient blood. Potential to be missed because it may occur several days after transfusion.	Monitor laboratory values for anemia. (Recognition is important because subsequent transfusions may cause an acute hemolytic reaction.) If detected, notify physician and blood bank. Most delayed hemolytic reactions require no treatment.
Febrile, nonhemolytic	Accompanies less than 1% of transfusions; possible sensitivity of recipient to the leukocytes or platelets in donor's blood.	30 min after initiation to 6 hr after completion of transfusion	Fever greater than 1° C above baseline, flushing, chills, headache, muscle pain; occurs most frequently in immunosuppressed patients	Use leukocyte-reduced blood products in patients who have experienced febrile nonhemolytic reactions in the past.	Stop transfusion. Administer antipyretics as ordered. Monitor temperature every 4 hr.
Allergic reaction (mild to moderate)	Caused by recipient allergy to a plasma protein in donor's blood.	During transfusion to 1 hr after transfusion	Local erythema, hives and urticaria, itching or pruritus	May administer antihistamines before transfusion if prescribed.	Stop transfusion. Notify health care provider and blood bank. Administer antihistamines as ordered. Monitor and document vital signs every 15 min. Transfusion may be restarted if fever, dyspnea, and wheezing are not present.

TABLE 29-2 | Transfusions Reactions—cont'd

Reaction	Mechanism	Onset	Signs and Symptoms	Prevention	Nursing Intervention
Allergic reaction (severe)	Caused by recipient allergy to a donor antigen (usually IgA). Agglutination of RBCs obstructing capillaries and blocking blood flow, causing symptoms to all major organ systems.	Within 5-15 min of initiation of transfusion	Coughing, nausea, vomiting, respiratory distress, wheezing, hypotension, loss of consciousness, possible cardiac arrest	Transfusion of saline-washed or leukocyte-depleted RBCs.	This is a life-threatening reaction. Stop transfusion. Maintain IV access. Notify health care provider and blood bank. Administer antihistamines, corticosteroids, epinephrine, and antipyretics as ordered. Measure and document vital signs until stable. Initiate cardiopulmonary resuscitation if necessary.
Graft-versus-host disease	Donor lymphocytes are destroyed by recipient's immune system. In immunocompromised patients, the donor lymphocytes are identified as foreign; however, the patient's immune system is not capable of destroying, and, in turn, the patient's lymphocytes are destroyed.	Days to weeks	Skin rash, fever, jaundice due to liver dysfunction, bone marrow suppression	Administer irradiated blood and/or leukocyte-depleted RBC products as prescribed.	Administer methotrexate, corticosteroids as ordered.
Circulatory overload	Occurs with transfusion of excessive volume or excessively rapid rate; can lead to pulmonary edema.	Anytime during or within 1-2 hr after transfusion	Dyspnea, cough, crackles at lung bases, tachypnea, headache, hypertension, tachycardia, increased central venous pressure, distended neck veins	Administer blood or component at prescribed rate, usually no greater than 2-4 mL/kg/hr; pay particular attention to rate and volume in older adults, young children, and patients with cardiac and renal disorders. Administer PRBCs instead of whole blood. Minimize amount of saline infused with transfusion.	Slow or stop transfusion as ordered. Elevate patient's head. Notify health care provider. Administer diuretics as ordered.
Infectious disease transmission	Microorganism contamination of infused product.	During transfusion to 2 hr after transfusion	High fever, chills, abdominal cramping, vomiting, diarrhea, profound hypotension, flushed skin, back pain	Proper care of blood or blood product from time of procurement through end of administration. Complete transfusion within 4 hr.	Stop transfusion. Remove blood product and tubing. Maintain IV access. Notify health care provider. Monitor and document vital signs. Obtain samples for blood culture and Gram stain from recipient. Administer IV fluids, broad-spectrum antimicrobials, vasopressors, and steroids as ordered.
Iron overload	Iron from donated blood binds to protein and is not eliminated.	May occur with multiple transfusions or with chronic transfusion therapy	Cardiac dysfunction, SOB, arrhythmias, congestive heart disorder, increased serum transferrin, increased liver enzymes, jaundice	Chelation, phlebotomy, monitor serum Fe levels.	Monitor patient for CHF, cardiac disorder, liver disorder, serum transferrin.

Data from Otto SE: *Mosby's pocket guide to infusion therapy,* ed 5, St. Louis, 2005, Mosby; American Association of Blood Banks: *Technical manual,* ed 15, Bethesda, Md, 2005, The Association.

CHF, Congestive heart failure; *Hct,* hematocrit; *Hgb,* hemoglobin; *IV,* intravenous; *PRBCs,* packed red blood cells; *RBC,* red blood cell; *SOB,* shortness of breath.

SKILL 29-1 Initiating Blood Therapy

Clinical indications differ among blood products (Table 29-3). The patient's medical condition determines which blood component is indicated. A physician's or health care provider's order is required for the administration of a blood product. You are responsible for understanding which components are appropriate in various situations. You must ensure that a blood sample has been collected and sent to the laboratory within 72 hours for typing and compatibility screening. The blood sample collector must be meticulous when labeling the patient's identification information on the blood tube. This is the first step in the prevention of error.

Blood is stored in a refrigerated environment. In emergency situations, rapid transfusion of cold blood may lead to dysrhythmias and a reduction of core temperature. Sometimes a blood warmer machine is used for large transfusions of greater than 50 mL/kg/hr or patients with cold agglutinins (Ackley and others, 2008). Heating blood products in a microwave or with hot water is dangerous and may destroy blood cells.

Delegation Considerations

The skill of initiating blood therapy cannot be delegated to nursing assistive personnel (NAP). After the transfusion has been started

TABLE 29-3 | Blood and Blood Component Products*

Blood Product and Source	Volume and Infusion Time	Able to Transmit HIV/HBV	ABO/Rh Testing Needed	Actions/Uses
Whole blood—single donor: allogeneic or autologous	300-550 mL Within 4 hr	Yes	Yes—Must be ABO identical; Rh—Yes	Replaces red cell mass and plasma volume; expected to raise hemoglobin 1 g/100 mL and hematocrit by 3% in nonhemorrhaging adult.
Packed RBCs—single donor: allogeneic or autologous	250-350 mL Within 4 hr	Yes	Yes/Yes	Preferred method of replacing red blood cell mass; expected to raise Hgb/Hct level same as whole blood.
Leukocyte-poor RBCs—single donor: allogeneic or directed	200-250 mL Within 4 hr	Yes	Yes/Yes	Replaces RBCs while preventing febrile, nonhemolytic transfusion reactions; reduces risk for CMV† transmission.
Irradiated RBCs—single donor: allogeneic or directed	250-350 mL Within 4 hr	Yes	Yes/Yes	Replaces RBCs while preventing transfusion-associated graft-versus-host disease; used in immunodeficient patients (any blood component can be irradiated).
Fresh frozen plasma—single donor	200-250 mL Infuse within 24 hr of thawing Within 4 hr	Yes	Yes/No	Replaces plasma without RBCs or platelets; contains most coagulation factors and complement; used in the control of bleeding where replacement of coagulation factors is needed (e.g., DIC, TTP).
Cryoprecipitate—multiple donors, pooled	5-20 mL/unit; 1 unit/10 kg body weight 1-2 mL/min Infuse within 6 hr of thawing or 4 hr of pooling	Yes	No/No	Replaces factors VIII, XIII, von Willebrand's factor, and fibrinogen.
Platelets—multiple/random donor, pooled	40-70 mL/unit; 1 unit/10 kg body weight Within 6 hr of pooling	Yes	Yes/Yes	Used in patients with thrombocytopenia. Certain microaggregate filters are not to be used with platelets—check manufacturer's instructions.
Platelets—single donor	200-500 mL Within 4 hr	Yes	Yes/Yes	Single-donor platelets are most useful in immunologically refractory patients when given as HLA matched with recipient. Each unit expected to raise platelet count by 5000-10,000/mL in a 70-kg patient.
Colloid components—albumin 5% pooled	250-500 mL 1-10 mL/min	No	No/No	Oncotically equivalent to plasma; used to treat hypoproteinemia in burns and hypoalbuminemia in shock and ARDs; used to support blood pressure in dialysis and acute liver failure.
Colloid components—albumin 25% pooled	50-100 mL 0.2-0.4 mL/min	No	No/No	Increased circulating blood volume by increasing intravascular oncotic pressure.

Data from Miller Y and others: *Practice guidelines for blood transfusion: a compilation from recent peer-reviewed literature*, ed 2, 2007, http://www.redcross.org/services/biomed/profess/pgbtscreen.pdf, accessed September 3, 2007; McKenry L and others: *Mosby's pharmacology in nursing*, ed 22, St. Louis, 2006, Mosby.
*Other, less commonly used blood components include factors VIII and IX concentrates, granulocytes, immunoglobulin, and saline-washed RBCs.
ARD, Acute respiratory disease; *CMV*, cytomegalovirus; *DIC*, disseminated intravascular coagulation; *HBV*, hepatitis B virus, *Hct*, hematocrit; *Hgb*, hemoglobin; *HIV*, human immunodeficiency virus; *HLA*, human leukocyte antigen; *RBC*, red blood cell; *TTP*, thrombotic thrombocytopenic purpura.

and the patient is stable, monitoring of a patient by NAP does not relieve you of the responsibility and accountability to continue to assess the patient during the transfusion. The nurse directs the NAP about:

- Frequency of vital sign monitoring.
- Reviewing what to observe, such as complaints of shortness of breath, hives, and/or chills, and reporting this information to the nurse.
- Obtaining blood components from the blood bank (if agency allows).
- Assisting in the verification procedure before the initiation of blood therapy (if agency allows). (Many facilities require two licensed professionals to verify blood units.)

Equipment
❑ Y-type blood administration set (in-line filter)

❑ 250-mL bag 0.9% NaCl (normal saline) IV solution
❑ Antiseptic wipes
❑ Clean gloves
❑ Tape
❑ Vital sign equipment: thermometer, blood pressure cuff, and stethoscope
❑ Signed transfusion consent form

Optional Equipment
❑ Rapid infusion pump
❑ Electronic infusion device (EID) (Verify pump can be used to deliver blood and blood products)
❑ Leukocyte-depleting filter
❑ Blood warmer
❑ Pressure bag
❑ Pulse oximeter

STEP	RATIONALE

ASSESSMENT

1 Verify physician's or health care provider's order for blood component transfusion with date, time of transfusion, duration, and any pretransfusion or posttransfusion medications you will administer.

A physician's or health care provider's order must be present before transfusing a blood product. Verifying order helps to ensure that appropriate blood component will be administered (Davis and others, 2006). Premedications such as an antihistamine or antipyretic may be ordered especially if patient demonstrated previous transfusion sensitivity.

2 Obtain patient's transfusion history, and note known allergies, including previous transfusion reactions. Verify that the type and crossmatch have been completed within 72 hours of transfusion.

Identifies patient's prior response(s) to transfusion of blood components. If patient has experienced a reaction in the past, anticipate a similar reaction, and be prepared to rapidly intervene.

3 Verify that IV cannula is patent and without complications such as infiltration or phlebitis. In emergency situations that require rapid transfusions, a large-gauge cannula is preferred; however, transfusions for therapeutic indications may be infused with cannulas ranging from 20 to 24 gauge (INS, 2006). If it is necessary to initiate venous access, do so before obtaining blood from blood bank.

Patent IV ensures that transfusion will be initiated and infused within established time guidelines. The gauge of the IV cannula should be appropriate for accommodating the infusion of blood and/or blood components (Infusion Nurses Society [INS], 2006). Large-gauge cannulas (18 or 20 gauge) promote rapid flow of blood components. Use of smaller cannula gauges, such as 24 gauge, often require the blood bank to divide the unit so that each half can be infused within the allotted time or require pressure-assisted devices.

4 Check that patient has properly completed and signed transfusion consent before retrieving blood.

Most agencies require patients to sign consent forms before receiving blood component therapy because of the inherent risks.

5 Know indication for blood product to be transfused (e.g., packed red blood cells [PRBCs] for a patient with a low hematocrit level from gastrointestinal bleeding or surgery blood loss).

Allows you to anticipate patient's response to therapy.

6 Obtain and record pretransfusion vital signs, including temperature, immediately before initiation of transfusion. If patient is febrile (temperature greater than 100°F [37.8°C]), notify physician or health care provider before initiating transfusion.

Change from baseline vital signs during infusion will alert nurse to a potential transfusion reaction or adverse effect of therapy.

7 Assess patient's need for IV fluids or medications while transfusion is infusing.

If IV medications need to be administered during the transfusion, a second IV site is necessary because the blood may cause incompatibilities (INS, 2006).

8 Assess patient's understanding of procedure and rationale.

Clarifying patient's need for and associated benefits of therapy will alleviate some of the anxiety patient may have.

NURSING DIAGNOSES

• Activity intolerance	• Deficient fluid volume	• Excess fluid volume
• Decreased cardiac output	• Deficient knowledge regarding purpose and risks of blood transfusions	• Ineffective peripheral tissue perfusion

Individualize related factors based on patient's condition or needs.

STEP	RATIONALE

PLANNING

1 Expected outcomes following completion of the procedure:
- Patient will verbalize understanding of rationale for therapy.

    Indicates patient's understanding and ability to make an informed decision for consent.

- Patient experiences improved activity tolerance.

    Oxygenation is improved.

- Mucous membranes are pink, and patient has brisk capillary refill.

    Tissue perfusion is improved.

- Patient's cardiac output returns to baseline.

    Intravascular volume is restored.

- Patient's systolic blood pressure improves, and urine output is 0.5 to 1 mL/kg/hr.

    Parameters reflect optimal fluid status and adequate renal blood flow.

- Patient's laboratory values will reflect improvement in targeted areas (hematocrit, coagulation values, platelet count).

    Components in blood are reflected in improved targeted laboratory values such as complete blood count [CBC], red blood cell count, hemoglobin [Hgb], hematocrit [Hct], platelet count, and/or coagulation values.

2 Explain procedure to patient and family.

    Promotes patient's cooperation and ability to report complications.

IMPLEMENTATION

1 Preadministration protocol:

a Obtain blood component from blood bank following agency protocol (see illustration). Blood transfusion must be initiated within 30 minutes after release from laboratory or blood bank (INS, 2006).

    Timely acquisition ensures product is safe to administer. Agency protocol usually encompasses safeguards to ensure quality control throughout transfusion process.

b Check appearance of blood product for leaks, bubbles, clots, or purplish color.

    Do not transfuse blood if integrity is compromised. Air bubbles, clots, or discoloration indicate bacterial contamination or inadequate anticoagulation of the stored component and are contraindications for transfusion of that product (Gray and others, 2005). Blood serves as a medium for bacterial growth.

c Verbally compare and correctly verify patient and blood product. Blood is double-checked with another person considered qualified by your agency (e.g., registered nurse [RN], licensed practical nurse [LPN], patient care technician) before initiating transfusion.

    Strict adherence to verification procedures before administration of blood or blood components reduces risk for administering the wrong blood to patient. Clerical errors are the cause of most hemolytic transfusion reactions (AABB, 2005; Parris and Grant-Casey, 2007).

    Some facilities require each individual to check separately to prevent one relying on another (see illustration).

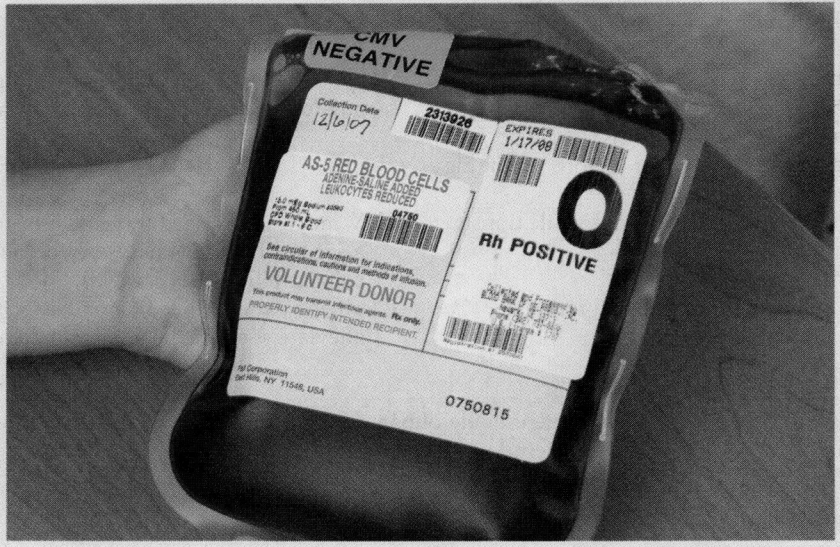

STEP 1a   Unit of blood with label.

STEP	RATIONALE
(1) Transfusion record number and patient's identification number match.	Prevents accidental administration of wrong component.
(2) Patient's name is correct on all documents. Check patient's identification number and date of birth on identification band and patient record.	
(3) Check unit number on blood container with blood bank form to ensure they are the same.	
(4) Blood type matches on transfusion record and blood bag. Verify that component received from blood bank is the same component physician or health care provider ordered (e.g., packed red cells, platelets) (see illustration).	Ensures patient receives correct therapy. One of the most common causes of the patient's receiving the incorrect transfusion is obtaining the wrong blood component from the blood bank (Gray and others, 2005).
(5) Check that patient's blood type and Rh type are compatible with donor blood type and Rh type (e.g., Patient A+: Donor A+ or 0+).	Verifies accurate donor blood type and compatibility.
(6) Check expiration date and time on unit of blood.	Never use expired blood, because the cell components deteriorate and may contain excess citrate ions (Gray and others, 2005).
(7) Check patient's first and last names by having patient state name, if able. Identify patient using at least two identifiers. When you notice a discrepancy during verification procedure, do not administer the product. Notify blood bank and appropriate personnel as indicated by agency policy. Return blood to blood bank until discrepancy resolved.	At least two identifiers are required to administer blood (The Joint Commission, 2008).
(8) At the point of initiation, check the patient identification information with the blood unit label information (see illustration). Do not administer blood to a patient without an identification bracelet (see illustration).	Serves as the last point of patient and blood confirmation and is the most important step in the verification process (Stainsby and others, 2006).
(9) Both individuals verifying the patient and unit identification record verification process as directed by agency policy.	Documentation is the legal medical record.
d Review purpose of the transfusion, and ask patient to report any changes he or she may feel during the transfusion.	Signs and symptoms of transfusion reactions include chills, low back pain, shortness of breath, rash, hives, or itching (Scarlet, 2006). Prompt notification aids in early intervention.
e Empty urine drainage collection container, or have patient void.	If a transfusion reaction occurs, a urine specimen containing urine produced after initiation of the transfusion will be sent to the laboratory.

Critical Decision Point *Initiate the blood transfusion within 30 minutes from time of release from blood bank. If you cannot do this because the patient is in the bathroom or the health care provider has to be notified of an elevated temperature, immediately return the blood to the blood bank, and retrieve it when you can administer it.*

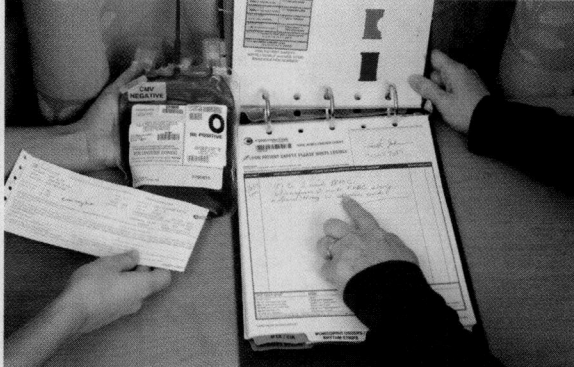

STEP 1c(4) Two clinicians verifying blood type with physician order.

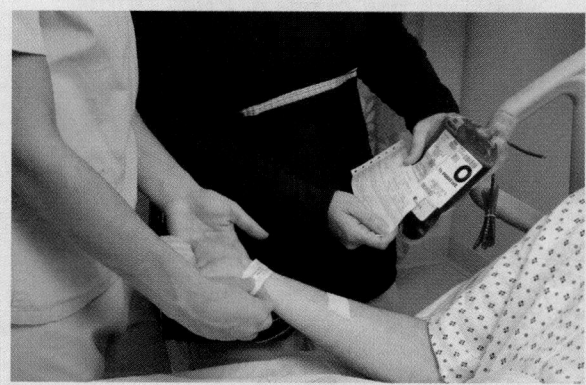

STEP 1c(8) Two clinicians verifying identification of patient and blood product.

STEP	RATIONALE

2 Administration:

a Perform hand hygiene, and apply clean gloves and appropriate attire.

Using standard precautions reduces risk for transmission of microorganisms.

Critical Decision Point *Standard blood administration set is for single unit use and must be changed when unit completed or after 4 hours. If multiple units are ordered, use a blood administration multiset (INS, 2006).*

b Open Y-tubing blood administration set.

Y-tubing facilitates maintenance of IV access in case a patient will need more than 1 unit of blood. Both a unit of blood and a container of normal saline are connected to the system.

c Set all clamp(s) to "off" position.

Setting clamps to "off" position prevents accidental spilling and wasting of product.

d Spike 0.9% normal saline IV bag with one of Y-tubing spikes. Hang the bag on an IV pole, and prime tubing. Open the upper clamp on normal saline side of tubing, and squeeze the drip chamber until fluid covers the filter and one-third to one-half of the drip chamber (see illustration).

Primes tubing with fluid to eliminate air in Y-tubing. Closing the clamp prevents spillage and waste of fluid.

e Maintain clamp on blood product side of Y-tubing in off position. Open common tubing clamp to finish priming the tubing to the distal end of tubing connector. Close tubing clamp when tubing is filled with saline. All three tubing clamps should be closed. Maintain protective sterile cap on tubing connector.

This will completely prime the tubing with saline, and the IV line is ready to be connected to the patient's vascular access device (VAD). Some patient conditions (e.g., sodium restriction, potential fluid overload) contraindicate the infusion of normal saline, and it is necessary to connect the blood component to prime the common tubing.

f Prepare blood component for administration. Gently agitate blood unit bag. Remove protective covering from access port. Spike blood component unit with other Y connection. Close normal saline clamp above filter and open clamp above filter to blood unit, and prime tubing with blood. Blood will flow into the drip chamber (see illustration). Tap the filter chamber to ensure residual air is removed. Allow saline in tubing to flow into receptacle, being careful to ensure any blood spillage is contained in blood precaution container.

Gentle agitation suspends the red blood cells in the anticoagulant. A protective barrier drape may be used to catch any potential blood spillage. The tubing is primed with the blood unit and ready for transfusion into the patient.

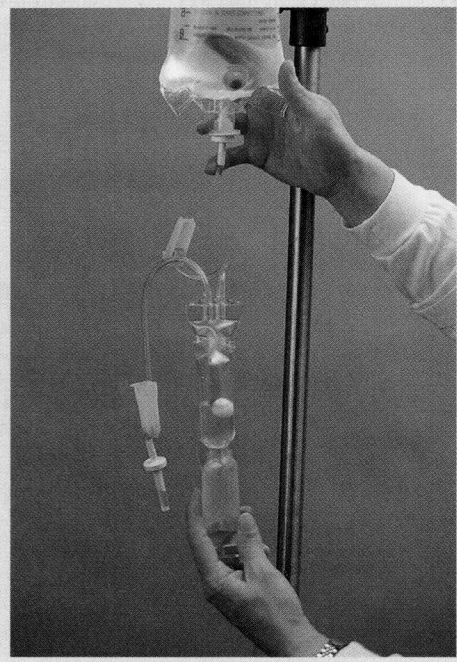

STEP 2d Blood administration set primed with normal saline.

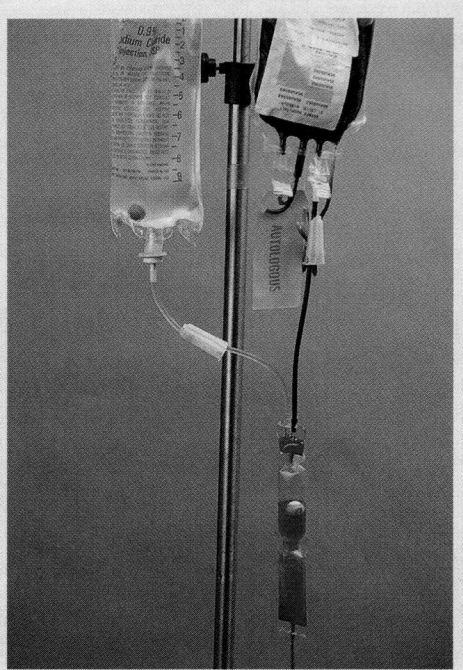

STEP 2f Unit of blood connected to Y-tubing setup.

STEP	RATIONALE

Critical Decision Point *Normal saline is compatible with blood products, unlike solutions that contain dextrose, which causes coagulation of donor blood.*

g Maintaining asepsis, attach primed tubing to patient's VAD. Open common tubing clamp, and regulate blood infusion to allow only 2 mL/min to infuse in the initial 15 minutes.

This initiates infusion of blood product into patient's vein.

h Remain with patient during the first 15 minutes of a transfusion. Initial flow rate during this time should be 2 mL/min, or 20 gtt/min (using macrodrip of 10 gtt/mL).

Most transfusion reactions occur within the first 15 minutes of a transfusion (Rosenthal, 2004). Infusing a small amount of blood component initially minimizes the volume of blood to which the patient is exposed, thereby minimizing the severity of a reaction.

Critical Decision Point *If signs of a transfusion reaction occur, stop the transfusion, start normal saline with new primed tubing directly to the VAD at keep vein open (KVO) rate, and notify the health care provider immediately. (Refer to Skill 29-2 for signs and symptoms of a transfusion reaction.)*

i Monitor patient's vital signs at 5 minutes, 15 minutes, and every 30 minutes until 1 hour after transfusion (AABB, 2005) or per agency policy.

Frequent monitoring of vital signs will help to quickly alert you to a transfusion reaction (Parris and Grant-Casey, 2007).

j If there is no transfusion reaction, regulate rate of transfusion according to health care provider's orders. Check the drop factor for the blood tubing.

Maintaining the prescribed rate of flow decreases risk for fluid volume excess while restoring vascular volume. Drop factor for most blood tubing is 10 gtt/mL.

Critical Decision Point *Do not let a unit of blood hang for more than 4 hours because of the danger of bacterial growth. Administration sets should be changed every 12 hours or after 4 units to reduce bacterial contamination (Ackley, 2008). Never store blood in a facility's refrigerator.*

Critical Decision Point *Never inject medication into the same IV line with a blood component because of the risk for contaminating the blood product with pathogens and the possibility of incompatibility. A separate IV access must be maintained if the patient requires IV infusion (total parenteral nutrition [TPN], pain control) during the transfusion.*

k After blood has infused, clear IV line with 0.9% normal saline, and discard blood bag according to agency policy. When consecutive units are ordered, maintain IV patency with 0.9% saline at keep open rate and retrieve subsequent unit for administration.

Infusing IV saline solution infuses remainder of blood in IV tubing and keeps IV line patent for supportive measures in case of a transfusion reaction (INS, 2006).

l Appropriately dispose of all supplies. Remove gloves, and perform hand hygiene.

Standard precautions during a transfusion reduce transmission of microorganisms.

EVALUATION

1 Monitor IV site and status of infusion each time vital signs are taken.

Detects presence of infiltration or phlebitis and verifies continuous and safe infusion of blood product.

2 Observe for any changes in vital signs and for chills, flushing, itching, dyspnea, rash, or other signs of transfusion reaction.

Compare presenting signs and symptoms to baseline assessment of patient before transfusion. These are early signs of a transfusion reaction (see Table 29-2).

3 Observe patient, and assess laboratory values to determine response to administration of blood component

This aids in determining whether goals of therapy have been reached or if further blood component therapy will be required.

Unexpected Outcomes	Related Interventions
1 Patient displays signs and symptoms of a transfusion reaction, which occurs when donor blood is incompatible with recipient's blood or when recipient has sensitivity to a plasma protein in the transfused (donor's) blood.	• Stop transfusion immediately. • Connect normal saline–primed tubing at VAD hub to prevent any subsequent blood from infusing from tubing. • Disconnect blood tubing at VAD hub, and cap distal end with sterile connector to maintain sterile system. • Keep vein open with slow infusion of normal saline at 10 to 12 gtt/min to ensure venous patency and maintain venous access for medication or to resume transfusion. It is important to regulate flow rate to minimize administration of excess IV fluid, especially in patients who are prone to fluid overload such as patients with cardiac and renal disorders, pediatric patients, and older adults. Notify health care provider. • See Table 29-2 for interventions.
2 Patient develops infiltration or phlebitis at venipuncture site.	• Remove IV, and insert new VAD at different site. Restart the product if remainder can be infused within 4 hours of initiation of transfusion. • Institute nursing measures to reduce discomfort at infiltrated or infected site.
3 Rate of infusion slows in the absence of infiltration.	• Verify IV catheter is patent and all clamps are open. Gently flush IV line with normal saline, or use a pressure bag or EID that permits blood transfusion to increase flow rate of product.
4 Fluid overload occurs, and/or patient exhibits difficulty breathing or has crackles on auscultation.	• Slow or stop transfusion, elevate head of bed, and inform physician of physical findings. KVO venous access. • Administer diuretics, morphine, and/or oxygen as ordered by physician. • Continue frequent assessments, and closely monitor vital signs, intake and output.
5 Patient displays signs and symptoms associated with decreased cardiac output: hypotension, tachycardia, cold skin, decreased urine output.	• Ensure that transfusion is infusing at ordered rate, so that rate of volume replacement is sufficient. • If blood loss is too rapid, allogeneic transfusion may be necessary.

Recording and Reporting

• Record pretransfusion medications, vital signs, and location and condition of IV system.
• Record type and volume of blood component, blood unit/donor/recipient identification, compatibility, and expiration date according to agency policy, along with patient's response to therapy. Document on transfusion record nurses' notes, medication administration record, flow sheet, and/or intake and output sheet, depending on agency policy.
• Report signs and symptoms of a transfusion reaction immediately to the health care provider.
• Record amount of blood received by autotransfusion and patient's response to therapy.
• Report to health care provider any intratransfusion/posttransfusion deterioration in cardiac, pulmonary, and/or renal status.
• Record volume of normal saline and blood component infused.
• Record vital signs before, during, and after transfusion.

Teaching Considerations

• Instruct patient regarding rationale for transfusion and anticipated amount of time for completion of transfusion.
• Discuss with patient and family the rationale for frequent vital sign monitoring throughout transfusion.
• Inform patient and family to notify nurse if the patient experiences itching, swelling, dizziness, dyspnea, low back pain, and/or chest pain, because these may be indicative of a transfusion reaction.
• Instruct patient to inform nurse if pain, swelling, or redness occurs at IV site, because these are indicative of infiltration.

Pediatric Considerations

• Infuse the first 50 mL or 20% of volume (whichever is smaller) of a blood transfusion very slowly in a pediatric patient, 5 mL/min for the first 15 minutes. Nurse should stay with the child during this time frame (Hockenberry and Wilson, 2007).
• Smaller portions of blood are often available for use with pediatric patients (AABB, 2008).
• A 27-, 26-, or 24-gauge cannula can be used to infuse packed red cells without significant hemolysis (Hockenberry and Wilson, 2007). The use of a small-gauge cannula often requires positive pressure through an infusion pump when the blood will not infuse by gravity alone.

Gerontological Considerations

• Some older adults have decreased cardiac function, thus requiring a slower infusion time. Half units may be obtained if a patient is unable to tolerate the volume in a whole unit of blood or blood component.
• In older adults at risk for circulatory overload, regulate flow rate at 1 mL/kg/hr.

Home and Long-Term Care Considerations

• Patients who have had prior transfusion reactions, acute angina, or congestive heart failure are not good candidates for home transfusion.
• Initiate the transfusion as soon as possible after component is obtained from blood bank. Transport blood in an insulated container with coolant to maintain temperature.
• Nursing personnel must be present during the entire transfusion process and for 30 to 60 minutes after transfusion.

- When blood sample is obtained for blood typing and cross-matching, identification band should be attached to patient, with full name and identification number used by laboratory. This provides clear identification of patient when blood component transfusion is initiated.
- Before transfusion initiation, confirmation with patient identification and blood unit is imperative to avoid error.

- Instruct patient and caregiver regarding signs and symptoms of a delayed hemolytic transfusion reaction (unexplained fever, decrease in hemoglobin and hematocrit levels 2 to 14 days after transfusion), so that they can report them and receive treatment if necessary.
- Return the container, empty bags, and tubing to the home care agency after completion of the transfusion.

SKILL 29-2   Monitoring for Adverse Reactions to Transfusion

Adverse reactions may occur anytime during transfusion of blood products. Life-threatening reactions usually occur within the first 15 minutes of transfusion. Remain with the patient during this time to monitor physiological responses.

A hemolytic reaction is a systemic response to the administration of a blood product that is incompatible with that of the recipient, contains allergens to which the recipient is sensitive or allergic, or is contaminated with pathogens. Some patients who have a history of frequent transfusion may require premedication with diphenhydramine (Benadryl) to combat acquired sensitivities.

Several types of adverse reactions may result from a blood transfusion (see Table 29-2). Currently each blood unit undergoes extensive serological testing, thereby minimizing the risk for patients' acquiring a blood-borne disease. Symptoms that indicate an adverse reaction range from fever, chills, and skin rash to hypotension and cardiac arrest. Some patients also experience a delayed transfusion reaction, which sometimes does not occur for days or

weeks after the transfusion. Other possible adverse outcomes that result from transfusion therapy include transmission of diseases, circulatory overload, and transfusion-related acute lung injury (TRALI), characterized by noncardiogenic pulmonary edema with an onset within 6 hours of transfusion (Knippen, 2006). The most fatal risk for transfusion-associated death is the erroneous transfusion of ABO-incompatible allogeneic units (Stainsby and others, 2006). Agencies must report fatalities that occur as the result of a transfusion reaction to the Food and Drug Administration.

Delegation Considerations

The skill of monitoring for adverse blood transfusion reactions cannot be delegated to NAP. The nurse is responsible and accountable for patient assessment and monitoring and evaluating for blood transfusion reactions. The nurse directs the NAP about:
- Vital sign monitoring.
- The signs and symptoms of a transfusion reaction patient may exhibit and to immediately report these to the nurse.

STEP	RATIONALE

ASSESSMENT

1 Observe for fever with or without chills.

Fever indicates onset of an acute hemolytic reaction, febrile nonhemolytic reaction, or bacterial sepsis.

2 Assess patient for tachycardia and/or tachypnea and dyspnea.

Indicates acute hemolytic reaction or circulatory overload. In the case of circulatory overload, a cough may accompany these symptoms.

3 Observe patient for hives or skin rash, including assessment of the trunk and back.

These are early indications of an allergic reaction, anaphylaxis, or graft-versus-host disease, which occurs after transfusion.

4 Observe patient for flushing.

Flushing is sometimes present in an acute hemolytic reaction or a febrile nonhemolytic reaction. Sometimes localized flushing presents with an allergic reaction.

5 Observe patient for gastrointestinal symptoms.

Nausea and vomiting is present in acute hemolytic transfusion reactions, anaphylactic reactions, or sepsis. Diarrhea is sometimes present in graft-versus-host disease or sepsis.

6 Observe patient for a fall in blood pressure.

Hypotension is indicative of an acute hemolytic reaction, anaphylaxis, or sepsis.

Critical Decision Point   Report sepsis and other infections due to blood transfusion to the blood bank and the agency's infection control department, which will then communicate the information to the state health department and the Centers for Disease Control and Prevention.

7 Observe the patient for wheezing, chest pain, and possible cardiac arrest.

These are all indications of an anaphylactic reaction.

8 Be alert to patient complaints of headache or muscle pain in the presence of a fever.

Both indicate a febrile nonhemolytic reaction.

9 Monitor patient for disseminated intravascular coagulation, renal failure, and hemoglobinemia/hemoglobinuria by reviewing laboratory test results.

All are late signs of an acute hemolytic reaction.

STEP	RATIONALE
10 Auscultate patient's lungs, and monitor central venous pressure (CVP), if possible.	Crackles in bases of lungs and a rising CVP are indications of circulatory overload.
11 Observe patient for jaundice and increased liver enzyme levels, indicating liver damage, and decreased red blood cells, white blood cells, and platelets, indicating bone marrow suppression.	These are indicative of graft-versus-host disease and would occur following transfusion.
12 Monitor patient's laboratory values (e.g., CBC, Hgb, Hct) for anemia refractory to transfusion therapy.	This could signify a delayed hemolytic reaction.
13 In patients receiving massive transfusions, observe patient for mild hypothermia, cardiac dysrhythmias, hypotension, hypocalcemia, and hemochromatosis (iron overload).	Cold blood products affect the cardiac conduction system, resulting in ventricular dysrhythmias. Other cardiac dysrhythmias, hypotension, and tingling indicate hypocalcemia, which occurs when citrate (used as a preservative for some blood products) combines with patient's calcium. Iron overload may occur after 10 transfusions and presents with shortness of breath, cardiac dysrhythmias, chest pain, and elevated liver enzyme levels. It is usually seen in patients who require chronic transfusions.

NURSING DIAGNOSES

- Acute pain
- Anxiety
- Decreased cardiac output
- Excess fluid volume
- Hyperthermia
- Hypothermia
- Impaired gas exchange
- Risk for infection

Individualize related factors based on patient's condition or needs.

PLANNING

1 Expected outcomes following completion of the procedure:	
• Patient will have pink mucous membranes and brisk capillary refill.	Tissue perfusion is improved.
• Patient's cardiac output will return to baseline.	Intravascular volume is restored.
• Patient will maintain core body temperature of 97° to 99° F.	Helps to confirm absence of transfusion reaction, infection, and sepsis.
• Patient will have urine output of 0.5 to 1 mL/kg/hr.	Reflects optimal fluid status.
• Patient will maintain stable blood pressure.	Intravascular volume is restored. Absence of transfusion reaction.
• Patient will maintain oxygen saturation of greater than 95%.	Improved tissue perfusion.
• Patient will be comfortable and calm.	Absence of transfusion reaction. Appropriate nursing measures applied to keep patient at ease.
2 Explain treatment of a reaction to patient and family.	Calms anxiety and helps patient/family anticipate nurse's actions.

IMPLEMENTATION

1 Interventions in the event of a transfusion reaction:	
a Stop the transfusion.	Severity of reaction is related to amount of component infused and the cause of reaction. It is imperative to prevent any more blood from infusing into the patient.
b Remove blood and tubing containing blood product, and replace them with new saline bag and tubing (see Chapter 28), except as noted below, in the case of mild allergic reaction.	Prevents additional blood in tubing from being infused.
c Maintain patent IV line using 0.9% normal saline.	Normal saline tubing should be connected at the cannula hub to prevent additional blood from being infused. Medications and fluids may need to be administered for certain reactions.
d Obtain and document vital signs. Remain with the patient for continuous monitoring and assessment.	Vital signs serve as an objective measure of patient condition. The patient's condition can rapidly deteriorate. The patient should not be left alone.
e Notify physician or health care provider.	Transfusion reactions require immediate medical intervention. Follow protocol for emergency interventions for anaphylactic reactions. In the event of a mild allergic reaction, stop transfusion and administer antihistamine per order. Transfusion may then be restarted per health care provider's order.

STEP	RATIONALE
f Notify blood bank.	Blood bank will have a procedure to follow when notified of a transfusion reaction.
g Obtain blood samples (if needed) from extremity opposite the extremity receiving transfusion. Check agency policy regarding number and type of tubes to be used.	Typically, one tube of blood will be crossmatched to pretransfusion sample to ensure that correct blood was given to recipient, and the blood will be checked for antibodies to determine the type of reaction. A second blood sample will be checked for free hemoglobin in the serum, indicating hemolysis, and a bilirubin level should be obtained.
h Return remainder of blood component and attached blood tubing to the blood bank according to agency policy. (Blood will not usually need to be returned in the case of circulatory overload.)	A sample of this blood will be crossmatched to patient's pretransfusion and posttransfusion samples to determine if error in crossmatching occurred.
i Monitor and document patient's vital signs every 15 minutes or more frequently if needed.	Maintains ongoing assessment of health care provider's cardiopulmonary status.
j Administer prescribed medications according to type and severity of transfusion reaction.	Follow medical protocol or physician's orders.
(1) Epinephrine	Stimulates sympathetic nervous system to relieve respiratory distress and combat vasodilation in anaphylaxis.
(2) Antihistamine	Parenteral antihistamine diminishes some aspects of allergic response by blocking histamine receptors. May also be ordered before transfusion in some cases.
(3) Antibiotics	Administered when bacterial contamination/sepsis is suspected.
(4) Antipyretics/analgesics	Administered to relieve fever and discomfort in acute hemolytic reactions, febrile nonhemolytic reactions, graft-versus-host disease, and bacterial sepsis.
(5) Diuretics/morphine	May be administered in circulatory overload to reduce intravascular volume and decrease vascular tone.
(6) Corticosteroids	Stabilizes cell membranes, decreasing histamine release. Administered in severe allergic reactions.
(7) IV fluids	Rapid administration of IV fluids helps to counteract some of symptoms of anaphylactic shock.
k In the event of cardiac arrest, initiate cardiopulmonary resuscitation (see Chapter 27).	Anaphylaxis can quickly lead to cardiopulmonary arrest. Prompt resuscitation may prevent further complications.
l Obtain first voided urine sample, and send to laboratory. You may need to insert a catheter to obtain the urine (see Chapter 33).	Hemoglobinuria occurs with acute hemolytic reactions. Degree of damage to kidneys is influenced by pH of urine and rate of urinary excretion. Attempts will be made to initiate diuresis and alkalinize the urine. If kidney damage is severe, dialysis may be required.
m Complete transfusion reaction report.	Documentation is part of the medical record.

EVALUATION

1 Observe patient, and conduct necessary nursing measures to determine response to end of transfusion or institute measures to reduce transfusion reaction.	Provides continued monitoring of patient's cardiopulmonary status and physiological response.

Unexpected Outcomes

1 Patient's physiological status worsens.

Related Interventions

• Appropriate interventions depend on the nature of crisis. Table 29-2 provides general guidelines.

Recording and Reporting

• Document patient's response to transfusion in nurses' notes/transfusion form or agency form.
• Immediately report presence of transfusion reaction and patient's physical assessment findings to nurse in charge and health care provider.
• Record exact time of transfusion reaction, assessment findings, and nursing and medical actions taken.

Teaching Considerations

• Teach patients and caregivers signs and symptoms of transfusion reactions and steps to take if they occur.

Pediatric Considerations

• Irradiated red blood cells and platelets are preferable in children under 6 years of age because of their immature immune systems and to avoid graft-versus-host disease.

Gerontological Considerations

• Administer blood components cautiously to older adults, considering both rate and amount of infusion, because they are at risk for developing circulatory overload.

Home and Long-Term Care Considerations

• Certain adverse outcomes (development of hepatitis) or transfusion reactions (delayed hemolysis) occur days to weeks after patient has received transfusion and may become evident in the home setting. It is important that patient, family, and home care workers are aware of signs and symptoms of these adverse occurrences, and steps to be taken should they occur.

CRITICAL THINKING EXERCISES

Catherine Cooper is a 68-year-old white woman scheduled for a total knee replacement of the right knee in 6 weeks. She has a history of previous injury from years of playing tennis and basketball. She states that she is concerned about the possibility of receiving a blood transfusion. She has read stories of people contracting diseases and viruses, and her friends have told her about someone who became very ill and distressed from a transfusion.

1 You are conducting Ms. Cooper's preoperative planning. How should you respond to her concerns?

2 Ms. Cooper decided to donate a unit of blood before her operation in the event that she needed transfusion therapy postoperatively. She comments to you that she is so glad she does not have to worry about anything going wrong with receiving her blood. What information does she require to ensure that the donation of blood will be successful?

3 Following type and cross, it is determined that Mrs. Cooper has AB+ blood. What type of blood can she recieve? What type of antigens does she carry on her red blood cells?

4 Describe your responsibilities associated with initiation and monitoring of the transfusion.

5 The physician orders another transfusion of red blood cells. Because Ms. Cooper had only 1 unit of autologous blood, she consents to a unit of allogeneic blood. Within 15 minutes of the blood initiation, Ms. Cooper complains of itching. What actions should you take?

☑ REVIEW QUESTIONS

1 The nurse is preparing a blood transfusion infusion set. Which solution should be used to prime the tubing?
   1 0.45% sodium chloride (½NS)
   2 Dextrose 5% in 0.45% sodium chloride (D_5½NS)
   3 0.9% sodium chloride (normal saline)
   4 Dextrose 5% in 0.9% sodium chloride (D_5NS)

2 A patient with A− blood type needs a blood transfusion. Which blood types are appropriate for him to receive?
   1 A+ or A−
   2 A− or O+
   3 A− or O−
   4 A+ or AB−

3 A patient is to receive blood that has been stored for quite a period of time. What recent laboratory value should the nurse check before administering the unit?
   1 Sodium
   2 Hematocrit
   3 Hemoglobin
   4 Potassium

4 A patient is to receive a blood transfusion. Which nursing action has the greatest impact on reducing a potential transfusion reaction?
   1 Administering an antihistamine 15 minutes before the transfusion
   2 Comparing the patient's identification bracelet with the blood bag label number
   3 Ensuring that the patient knows what his or her blood type is
   4 Obtaining the patient's previous transfusion history

5 A patient receiving a blood transfusion begins having signs and symptoms of a transfusion reaction. Other than stopping the transfusion and assessing vital signs, what else should the nurse do?
   1 Hang a new infusion setup with D_5W to maintain an access for medications.
   2 Finish infusing the blood remaining in the tubing, then flush the tubing with the normal saline hanging on the Y-tubing.
   3 Keep the existing tubing patent with a dextrose solution in case diphenhydramine is needed.
   4 Hang a new infusion setup with normal saline to maintain an IV access.

REFERENCES

Ackley B and others: *Evidence-based nursing care guidelines,* St. Louis, 2008, Mosby.

American Association of Blood Banks: *Technical manual,* ed 15, Bethesda, Md, 2005, The Association.

American Association of Blood Banks: *AABB guidelines and standards for blood banks and transfusion services,* ed 25, Bethesda, Md, 2008, The Association.

Davis K and others: Transfusing safely: a 2006 guide for nurses, *Aust Nurs J* 13(6):38, 006.

Dzik WH: New technology for transfusion safety, *Br J Haematol* 136(2):181, 2007.

Gray A and others: Improving blood transfusion: a patient-centered approach, *Nurs Stand* 19(26):38, 2005.

Gray A and others: Safe transfusion of blood and blood components, *Nurs Stand* 21(51):40, 2007.

Hockenberry MJ, Wilson D: *Wong's nursing care of infants and children,* ed 8, St. Louis, 2007, Mosby.

Infusion Nurses Society: Infusion nursing standards of practice, *J Infus Nurs* 29(suppl 1):S1, 2006.

Kirschman RA: Finding alternatives to blood transfusion, *Holist Nurs Pract* 18(6):177, 2004.

Kirschman RA: Finding alternatives to blood transfusion, *Nursing* 34(6):58, 2007.

Knippen MA: Transfusion-related acute lung injury: a rare but potentially lethal result of allogeneic blood transfusion, TRALI resembles acute respiratory distress syndrome. Early intervention can save lives, *Am J Nurs* 106(6):61, 2006.

Koshy R: Navigating the information technology highway: computer solutions to reduce errors and enhance patient safety, *Transfusion* 45(suppl):189S, 2005.

McKenry L and others: *Mosby's pharmacology in nursing,* ed 22, St. Louis, 2006, Mosby.

Otto SE: *Mosby's pocket guide to intravenous therapy,* ed 5, St. Louis, 2005, Mosby.

http://www.redcross.org/services/biomed/profess/pgbtscreen.pdf, accessed September 3, 2007.

Roark DC, Miguel K: RFID: bar coding's replacement? *Nurs Manage* 37(2):28, 2006

Rosenthal K: Avoiding bad blood: key steps to safe transfusions, *Nursing Made Incredibly Easy* 2(5):20, 2004.

Scarlet C: Anaphylaxis, *J Infus Nurs* 29(1):39, 2006.

Stainsby D and others: Serious hazards of transfusion: a decade of hemovigilance in the UK, *Transfus Med Rev* 20(4):273, 2006.

The Joint Commission: *Accreditation program: critical access hospital,* National Patient Safety Goals, 2009, http://www.jointcommission.org/patientsafety/nationalpatientsafetygoals/09.

RESEARCH REFERENCES

Carayon P and others: Evaluation of nurse interaction with bar code medication administration technology in the work environment, *J Patient Safety* 3(1):34, 2007.

Jabbour N and others: Transfusion-free techniques in pediatric live donor liver transplantation, *J Pediatr Gastroenterol* 40(4):521, 2005.

Murphy MF and others: Prevention of bedside errors in transfusion medicine (PROBE-TM) study: a cluster-randomized, matched-paired clinical areas trial of a simple intervention to reduce errors in the pretransfusion bedside check, *Transfusion* 47(5):771, 2007.

Parris E, Grant-Casey J: Promoting safer blood transfusion practice in hospital, *Nurs Stand* 21(41):35, 2007.

Sandler SG and others: Radiofrequency identification technology can standardize and document blood collections and transfusions, *Transfusion* 47(5):763, 2007.

Seiden SC, Barach P: Wrong-side/wrong-site, wrong-procedure, and wrong-patient adverse events: are they preventable? *Arch Surg* 141(9):931, 2006.

Thiele T and others: Proteomics of blood-based therapeutics: a promising tool for quality assurance in transfusion medicine, *Biodrugs* 21(3):179, 2007.

Oral Nutrition

MEDIA RESOURCES

- 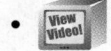 http://evolve.elsevier.com/Perry/skills
  - Review Questions
  - Video Clips

- View Video! Mosby's Nursing Video Skills, 3.0

OBJECTIVES

Mastery of content in this chapter will enable the nurse to:
- Perform accurate nutritional screening.
- Identify and refer patients for nutritional assessment to a registered dietitian.
- Assess a patient's ability to swallow.
- Identify risk factors for aspiration related to dysphagia.
- Evaluate a patient's tolerance of oral nutrition.
- Identify appropriate meals for a patient to receive.
- Demonstrate how to properly feed a patient who cannot self-feed.

Nutrition is a basic component of health that affects a patient's rate of recovery from illness, surgery, or extensive procedures. When a patient is unable to obtain adequate oral nutrition, nutritional status becomes compromised. A nurse's role includes performing nutritional screening to assess a patient's risk status for malnutrition, assessing and assisting an adult patient with feeding, and identifying patients at risk for aspiration during oral feeding.

SCREENING FOR NUTRITIONAL RISK

The prevalence of disease-related malnutrition is high across all types of medical specialties and health care settings (Stratton and Elia, 2007). Routine identification of malnutrition with screening of patients in health care settings is a requirement of many accrediting organizations. Nutritional screening is the process of identifying patient characteristics associated with nutritional problems and risk factors for malnutrition (American Society for Parenteral and Enteral Nutrition [ASPEN], 2007; Hammond and others, 2007). It is the first step in the nutritional assessment process. As a nurse, you learn to conduct an initial nutritional screening. Your findings determine the need for consultation with a registered dietitian (RD). Nutritional risk is the potential to become malnourished because of primary factors such as inadequate intake or secondary factors such as disease. Box 30-1 provides a list of risk factors for nutritional problems (Grodner and others, 2007). An effective nutritional screening is simple, uses readily available data or data that are easy to obtain, includes data relevant to nutritional status, leads to interventions, and is cost-effective. The Malnutrition Universal Screening Tool (MUST) (Fig. 30-1) is an example of an evidence-based, easy-to-use screening tool for all adults (Elia, 2003).

Nutritional screening identifies patients at risk for nutritional problems. But remember, no single objective measure alone is an effective predictor of nutritional risk. Nurses work with RDs to complete more comprehensive nutritional assessments. An RD is a food and nutrition expert who has met the minimum academic and professional requirements to qualify for the credential RD (American Dietetic Association, 2008). In a comprehensive nutritional assessment, RDs use data collected from several different sources to assess patients' nutritional needs, often using the ABCD approach: **A**nthropometrics, **B**iochemical tests, **C**linical observations, and **D**iet evaluation.

The Joint Commission (TJC) (2007) standards require the identification of patients who are nutritionally at risk by means of an initial screening mechanism. This screening must be completed within 24 hours of admission to a hospital, within 14 days of admission to a long-term care facility, or within a facility-defined period of time in ambulatory care and home care settings. Patients who are identified as being at risk need to have a nutritional assessment completed by an RD. Collaborating with the RD, you then design, implement, and periodically reevaluate the multidisciplinary nutritional plan of care based on individual patient needs. The Joint Commission also requires education and training of patients regarding nutritional intervention, modified diets, and oral health.

Nutrition Screening Initiative

The aging of America has increased the prevalence of age-related chronic disease. Disease-specific nutritional screening and intervention are fundamental to the management of many chronic diseases. The Nutrition Screening Initiative (NSI) (1997) was a multidisciplinary endeavor led by the American Academy of Family Physicians and the American Dietetic Association. Disciplines represented include nutrition, dentistry, pharmacology, mental health, managed care, home care, and community social services. The NSI's goal is to incorporate nutritional screening and intervention into the nation's health care delivery system for older Americans (American Academy of Family Physicians, 2003). One tool designed as a result of the NSI to identify older adults at nutritional risk is the "DETERMINE Your Nutritional Health Checklist" (Fig. 30-2, p. 806). This 10-item questionnaire is a self-report instrument that a patient completes and brings to his or her physician's office. Referrals to an appropriate health care professional are made based on the outcomes of each individual patient's form.

Global Assessment

The Mini Nutritional Assessment (MNA) (Fig. 30-3, p. 808), developed by Guigoz with Nestlé Nutritional Corporation, is an assessment tool used by health care providers to identify geriatric patients (over 65 years of age) at risk for malnutrition. The 18-item tool includes questions for screening or assessment. The screening includes questions related to change in oral intake, weight loss, mobility, stress, and body mass index (BMI). A score of less than

Text continued on p. 809

BOX 30-1 | Risk Factors for Potential Nutritional Problems

- Clear- or full-liquid diets for more than 3 days without nutrient supplementation or inappropriate or insufficient nutrient supplementation
- Intravenous feeding (dextrose or saline) or NPO for more than 3 days without supplementation
- Low intakes of prescribed diet or tube feedings
- Weight 20% above or 10% below desirable body weight (accounting for edema)
- Pregnancy weight gain deviating from normal patterns
- Diagnoses that increase nutritional needs or decrease nutrient intake (or both): cancer, malabsorption, diarrhea, hyperthyroidism, excessive inflammation, postoperative status, hemorrhage, infected or draining wounds, burns, infection, major trauma
- Chronic use of drugs, especially alcohol, that affect nutritional intake
- Alterations in chewing, swallowing, appetite, taste, and smell
- Body temperature consistently above 37° C (98.6° F) for more than 2 days
- Hematocrit: <43% in men, <37% in women; hemoglobin <14 g/dL in men, <12 g/dL in women
- Absolute decrease in lymphocyte count (<1500 cells/mm³)
- Elevated (>250 mg/dL) or decreased (<130 mg/dL) total plasma cholesterol
- Serum albumin <3 g/dL in patients without renal or liver disease, generalized dermatitis, overhydration

Modified from Grodner M and others: *Foundations and clinical applications of nutrition: a nursing approach,* ed 4, St. Louis, 2007, Mosby.
NPO, Nothing by mouth.

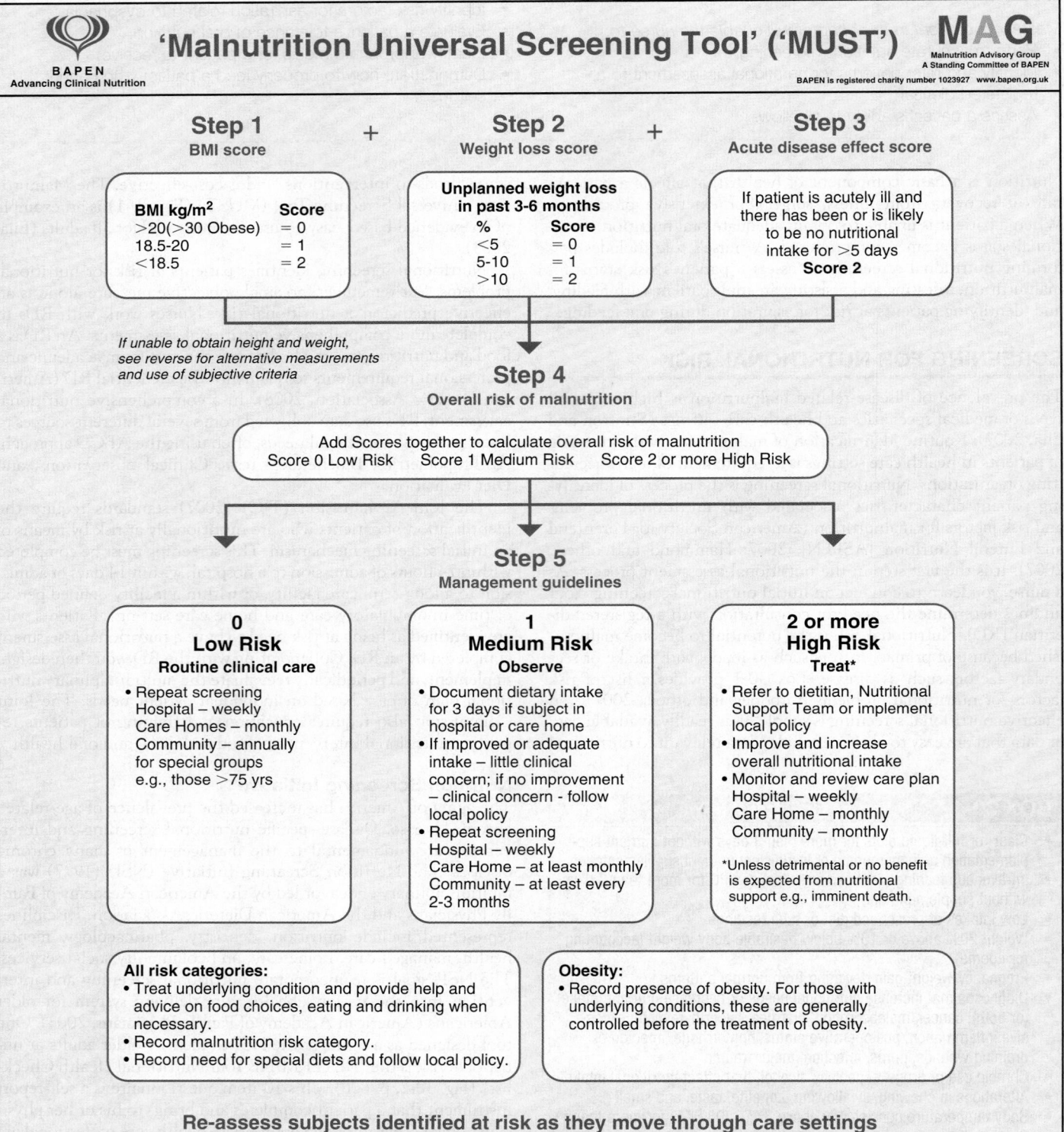

FIG 30-1   The Malnutrition Universal Screening Tool (MUST). *(Courtesy BAPEN.)*

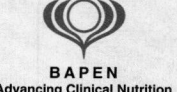

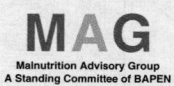

'Malnutrition Universal Screening Tool' ('MUST')

BAPEN
Advancing Clinical Nutrition

Malnutrition Advisory Group
A Standing Committee of BAPEN
BAPEN is registered charity number 1023927   www.bapen.org.uk

Alternative measurements and considerations

Step 1: BMI (body mass index)

If height cannot be measured
- Use recently documented or self-reported height (if reliable and realistic).
- If the subject does not know or is unable to report their height, use one of the alternative measurements to estimate height (ulna, knee height or demispan).

If height and weight cannot be obtained
- Use mid upper arm circumference (MUAC) measurement to estimate BMI category.

Step 2: Recent unplanned weight loss

If recent weight loss cannot be calculated, use self-reported weight loss (if reliable and realistic).

Subjective criteria

If height, weight or BMI cannot be obtained, the following criteria which relate to them can assist your professional judgement of the subject's nutritional risk.

1. BMI
- Clinical impression – thin, acceptable weight, overweight. Obvious wasting (very thin) and obesity (very overweight) can also be noted.

2. Unplanned weight loss
- Clothes and/or jewelry have become loose fitting (weight loss).
- History of decreased food intake, reduced appetite or swallowing problems over 3-6 months and underlying disease or psycho-social/physical disabilities likely to cause weight loss.

3. Acute disease effect
- No nutritional intake or likelihood of no intake for more than 5 days.

FIG 30-1, cont'd

The Warning Signs of poor nutritional health are often overlooked. Use this checklist to find out if you or someone you know is at nutritional risk.

Read the statements below. Circle the number in the yes column for those that apply to you or someone you know. For each yes answer, score the number in the box. Total your nutritional score.

DETERMINE YOUR NUTRITIONAL HEALTH

	YES
I have an illness or condition that made me change the kind and/or amount of food I eat.	2
I eat fewer than 2 meals per day.	3
I eat few fruits or vegetables, or milk products.	2
I have 3 or more drinks of beer, liquor or wine almost every day.	2
I have tooth or mouth problems that make it hard for me to eat.	2
I don't always have enough money to buy the food I need.	4
I eat alone most of the time.	1
I take 3 or more different prescribed or over-the-counter drugs a day.	1
Without wanting to, I have lost or gained 10 pounds in the last 6 months.	2
I am not always physically able to shop, cook and/or feed myself.	2
	TOTAL

Total Your Nutritional Score. If it's —

0-2   **Good!** Recheck your nutritional score in 6 months.

3-5   **You are at moderate nutritional risk.** See what can be done to improve your eating habits and lifestyle. Your office on aging, senior nutrition program, senior citizens center or health department can help. Recheck your nutritional score in 3 months.

6 or more   **You are at high nutritional risk.** Bring this checklist the next time you see your doctor, dietitian or other qualified health or social service professional. Talk with them about any problems you may have. Ask for help to improve your nutritional health.

These materials developed and distributed by the Nutrition Screening Initiative, a project of:

 AMERICAN ACADEMY OF FAMILY PHYSICIANS

 THE AMERICAN DIETETIC ASSOCIATION

 NATIONAL COUNCIL ON THE AGING

Remember that warning signs suggest risk, but do not represent diagnosis of any condition. Turn the page to learn more about the Warning Signs of poor nutritional health.

FIG 30-2   Tool for nutritional screening of older adults.

The Nutrition Checklist is based on the Warning Signs described below. Use the word <u>DETERMINE</u> to remind you of the Warning Signs.

DISEASE

Any disease, illness or chronic condition which causes you to change the way you eat, or makes it hard for you to eat, puts your nutritional health at risk. Four out of five adults have chronic diseases that are affected by diet. Confusion or memory loss that keeps getting worse is estimated to affect one out of five or more of older adults. This can make it hard to remember what, when or if you've eaten. Feeling sad or depressed, which happens to about one in eight older adults, can cause big changes in appetite, digestion, energy level, weight and well-being.

EATING POORLY

Eating too little and eating too much both lead to poor health. Eating the same foods day after day or not eating fruit, vegetables, and milk products daily will also cause poor nutritional health. One in five adults skip meals daily. Only 13% of adults eat the minimum amount of fruit and vegetables needed. One in four older adults drink too much alcohol. Many health problems become worse if you drink more than one or two alcoholic beverages per day.

TOOTH LOSS/ MOUTH PAIN

A healthy mouth, teeth and gums are needed to eat. Missing, loose or rotten teeth or dentures which don't fit well or cause mouth sores make it hard to eat.

ECONOMIC HARDSHIP

As many as 40% of older Americans have incomes of less than $6,000 per year. Having less--or choosing to spend less--than $25-30 per week for food makes it very hard to get the foods you need to stay healthy.

REDUCED SOCIAL CONTACT

One-third of all older people live alone. Being with people daily has a positive effect on morale, well-being and eating.

MULTIPLE MEDICINES

Many older Americans must take medicines for health problems. Almost half of older Americans take multiple medicines daily. Growing old may change the way we respond to drugs. The more medicines you take, the greater the chance for side effects such as increased or decreased appetite, change in taste, constipation, weakness, drowsiness, diarrhea, nausea, and others. Vitamins or minerals when taken in large doses act like drugs and can cause harm. Alert your doctor to everything you take.

INVOLUNTARY WEIGHT LOSS/GAIN

Losing or gaining a lot of weight when you are not trying to do so is an important warning sign that must not be ignored. Being overweight or underweight also increases your chance of poor health.

NEEDS ASSISTANCE IN SELF CARE

Although most older people are able to eat, one of every five have trouble walking, shopping, and buying and cooking food, especially as they get older.

ELDER YEARS ABOVE AGE 80

Most older people lead full and productive lives. But as age increases, risk of frailty and health problems increase. Checking your nutritional health regularly makes good sense.

The Nutrition Screening Initiative, 2626 Pennsylvania Avenue, NW, Suite 301, Washington, DC 20037

© The Nutrition Screening Initiative is funded in part by a grant from Ross Laboratories, a division of Abbott Laboratories.

A5944(1.00)/DECEMBER 1995

FIG 30-2, cont'd For legend see opposite page.

Mini Nutritional Assessment
MNA®

Last name: _____   First name: _____   Sex: _____   Date: _____

Age: _____   Weight, kg: _____   Height, cm: _____   I.D. Number: _____

Complete the screen by filling in the boxes with the appropriate numbers.
Add the numbers for the screen. If score is 11 or less, continue with the assessment to gain a Malnutrition Indicator Score.

Screening

A Has food intake declined over the past 3 months due to loss of appetite, digestive problems, chewing or swallowing difficulties?
0 = severe loss of appetite
1 = moderate loss of appetite
2 = no loss of appetite

B Weight loss during the last 3 months
0 = weight loss greater than 3 kg (6.6 lbs)
1 = does not know
2 = weight loss between 1 and 3 kg (2.2 and 6.6 lbs)
3 = no weight loss

C Mobility
0 = bed or chair bound
1 = able to get out of bed/chair but does not go out
2 = goes out

D Has suffered psychological stress or acute disease in the past 3 months
0 = yes   2 = no

E Neuropsychological problems
0 = severe dementia or depression
1 = mild dementia
2 = no psychological problems

F Body Mass Index (BMI) (weight in kg)/(height in m)^2
0 = BMI less than 19
1 = BMI 19 to less than 21
2 = BMI 21 to less than 23
3 = BMI 23 or greater

Screening score (subtotal max. 14 points)

12 points or greater Normal–not at risk–no need to complete assessment
11 points or below   Possible malnutrition–continue assessment

Assessment

G Lives independently (not in a nursing home or hospital)
0 = no   1 = yes

H Takes more than 3 prescription drugs per day
0 = yes   1 = no

I Pressure sores or skin ulcers
0 = yes   1 = no

J How many full meals does the patient eat daily?
0 = 1 meal
1 = 2 meals
2 = 3 meals

K Selected consumption markers for protein intake
• At least one serving of dairy products (milk, cheese, yogurt) per day?   yes ☐   no ☐
• Two or more servings of legumes or eggs per week?   yes ☐   no ☐
• Meat, fish or poultry every day   yes ☐   no ☐
0.0 = if 0 or 1 yes
0.5 = if 2 yes
1.0 = if 3 yes

L Consumes two or more servings of fruits or vegetables per day?
0 = no   1 = yes

M How much fluid (water, juice, coffee, tea, milk...) is consumed per day?
0.0 = less than 3 cups
0.5 = 3 to 5 cups
1.0 = more than 5 cups

N Mode of feeding
0 = unable to eat without assistance
1 = self-fed with some difficulty
2 = self-fed without any problem

O Self view of nutritional status
0 = views self as being malnourished
1 = is uncertain of nutritional state
2 = views self as having no nutritional problem

P In comparison with other people of the same age, how does the patient consider his/her health status?
0.0 = not as good
0.5 = does not know
1.0 = as good
2.0 = better

Q Mid-arm circumference (MAC) in cm
0.0 = MAC less than 21
0.5 = MAC 21 to 22
1.0 = MAC 22 or greater

R Calf circumference (CC) in cm
0 = CC less than 31   1 = CC 31 or greater

Assessment (max. 16 points)

Screening score

Total Assessment (max. 30 points)

Malnutrition Indicator Score
17 to 23.5 points   at risk of malnutrition

Less than 17 points   malnourished

Ref.: Vellas B, Villars H, Abellan G, et al. Overview of the MNA® - Its History and Challenges. J Nutr Health Aging 2006;10:456–465.

Rubenstein LZ, Harker JO, Salva A, Guigoz Y, Vellas B. Screening for Undernutrition in Geriatric Practice Developing the Short-Form Mini Nutritional Assessment (MNA-SF). J Geront 2001;56A: M366–377.

Guigoz Y. The Mini-Nutritional Assessment (MNA®) Review of the Literature – What does it tell us? J Nutr Health Aging 2006;10:466–487.

FIG 30-3   The Nestlé Mini Nutritional Assessment tool used to assess the nutritional status of geriatric patients. (Courtesy Nestlé Nutrition Institute.)

11 in the screening component suggests malnutrition and the need to complete the remainder of the form. The assessment component includes arm and calf circumference, specific questions related to eating habits, and questions related to medical history. A total score (0 to 30 points) provides a subjective judgment of protein energy malnutrition (PEM). A score of less than 17 points denotes malnutrition; a score of 17 to 23.5 indicates risk for malnutrition (DiMaria and Gaenter, 2008; Nestlé Clinical Nutrition, 2003).

Nutritional Assessment by a Registered Dietitian

Dietitians work closely with nursing personnel to provide comprehensive nutritional care. The care provided by a registered dietitian (RD) is medical nutrition therapy (MNT), defined as "nutritional diagnostic, therapy, and counseling services for the purpose of disease management which are furnished by a registered dietitian or nutrition professional" (Lacey and Pritchett, 2004). In 2003 the American Dietetic Association published the Nutrition Care Process (NCP) and model. The process provides structure for the provision of nutritional care to all patients and provides a framework for an RD to think critically and make decisions regarding medical nutrition therapy (Lacey and Pritchett, 2004). There are four steps to the process: nutrition assessment, nutrition diagnosis, nutrition intervention, and nutrition monitoring and evaluation (Lacey and Pritchett 2004). The nutritional assessment is a comprehensive evaluation of a patient's nutritional status, performed by an RD. The assessment includes medical, social, nutritional, and medication history; physical examination; anthropometric measurements; and laboratory data. The nutritional assessment builds on information collected from the nutritional screening (Hammond and others, 2007). The goal of the assessment is to develop an effective nutritional plan of care that addresses problems identified from the assessment and screening. The RD makes a nutritional diagnosis from the assessment. A nutritional diagnosis is a label that describes "an actual occurrence, risk for, or potential for developing a nutritional problem that dietetics professionals are responsible for treating independently" (Lacey and Pritchett, 2004). The nutritional intervention is the activity intended to address that problem. You then monitor and evaluate the effects of this intervention, making changes as necessary.

FOUNDATIONS OF NUTRITION

Several agencies and organizations in the United States regularly publish and update dietary guidelines. The guidelines change as nutritional researchers discover new knowledge. In 2005 the U.S. Department of Agriculture (USDA) revised the food guide pyramid, MyPyramid (Fig. 30-4), as a part of the Food Guidance System. The pyramid better educates the American public on healthy eating for weight maintenance and health promotion. Recommendations in MyPyramid are consistent with recommendations to control obesity and diabetes mellitus, heart disease and stroke, hypertension, cancer, and osteoporosis (Krebs-Smith and Kris-Etherton, 2007).

EVIDENCE-BASED PRACTICE TRENDS

Patients who are hospitalized or reside in long-term care settings often receive special diets to maintain oral intake when patients have gastrointestinal (GI) limitations or alterations (Table 30-1). When these diets are not supplemented with nutrients, patients are at risk for malnutrition. Oral nutritional supplements (ONS) are ready-made, multinutrient liquid supplements that are energy dense and contain both macronutrients (protein, carbohydrate, and fat) and micronutrients (vitamins, minerals, and trace elements) (Stratton and Elia, 2007). Current evidence suggests that ONS are more effective than diet alone in the treatment of certain patient groups, including postoperative patients (Baldwin and others, 2003; Stratton and others, 2006). Research shows that mortality rates are significantly lower in patients receiving ONS versus patients who are unsupplemented (Stratton and others, 2003). Studies involving GI surgical patients show lower rates of postoperative complications, retention of skeletal muscle strength, and improved physical and mental health in patients receiving supplementation compared with those on routine hospital diets. There are improvements resulting from ONS in older adults and cancer patients. Evidence shows that liquid supplements do not suppress appetite and food intake substantially, making supplementation an effective treatment for patients with poor appetite (Stratton and Elia, 2007). The use of ONS effectively improves total energy and nutritional intake in most patient groups.

TABLE 30-1	**Types of Therapeutic Diets**
Diet	**Description**
Clear liquid	Foods that are clear and liquid at room or body temperature (e.g., water, clear fruit juice, Jello, Popsicles). Prevents dehydration and minimizes colon contents, thereby resting the colon. Ordered for patients immediately postoperatively or for patients being prepared for GI procedures. Is inadequate in regard to protein, fat, or energy sources. Should not be used for more than 24 hours. Caution should be exercised in regard to amount of caffeine patients receive on clear liquids.
Full liquid	Consists of foods that are liquid at room temperature. Provides oral nourishment for patients who have difficulty chewing or swallowing solid foods. Offers more variety than clear liquids (e.g., milk products, orange and tomato juice), and ONS can be used to supply adequate amounts of nutrients. Diet can cause problems for patients who are lactose intolerant. Many patients do not tolerate fat or lactose following surgery.
Mechanical or dental—soft	Consists of chopped, ground, mashed, or pureed foods for patients who have problems with chewing or swallowing. Consistency can be varied according to patient's own ability to chew or swallow. Small amounts of liquids added to foods help reach an appropriate consistency. Liquids that are added should complement the food and not conceal food's original flavor. Butter, margarine, and honey can be added to increase caloric density.
Diet as tolerated	Used for patients who do not require dietary restrictions or modifications. Hospitals offer self-select menus for patients.
Special	Prescribed specifically for patient's medical condition (e.g., diabetic diet, lactose intolerant diet, renal diet).

GI, Gastrointestinal; *ONS*, oral nutritional supplements.

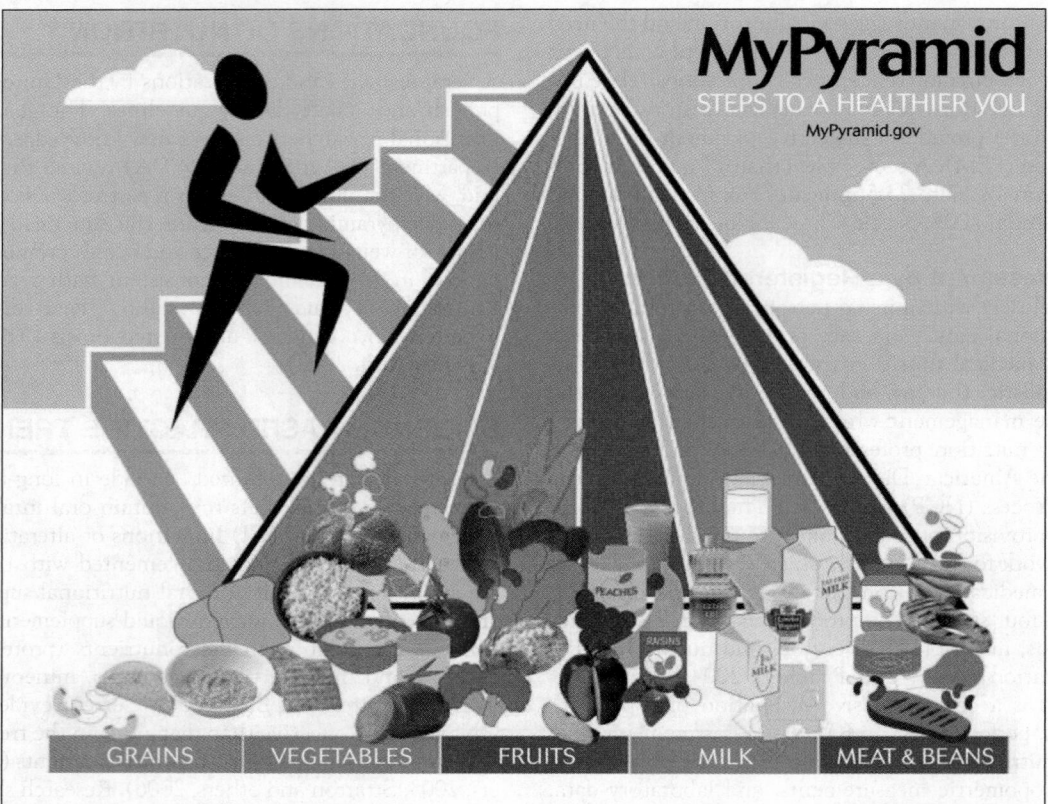

MyPyramid.gov
STEPS TO A HEALTHIER YOU

FIG 30-4 Food Guide Pyramid for adults. (*From U.S. Department of Agriculture, Center for Nutrition Policy and Promotion, April 2005, http://www.MyPyramid.gov.*)

CULTURAL CONSIDERATIONS

It is important to assess the meaning of food and food preferences for a patient and family. Foods are often associated with caring and love, as well as health promotion, maintenance, and restoration. For example:

- Asians achieve a balance between yin and yang through dietary practices (Kitayama and others, 2007).
- Among Koreans, mothers consume seaweed soup postpartum to cleanse the blood, promote lactation, and restore yang because postpartum is a predominantly yin state.
- Asians, Hispanics, Eastern Europeans, and Africans believe in the hot and cold theory of health and illness. Foods are classified as cold or hot based on their characteristics, independent of the temperature at which they are served. There is no universal agreement across cultures on which foods are hot or cold.
- African Americans and Mexicans have large extended family networks. Eating food prepared by family members or loved ones can meet nutritional needs and serve as an expression of love.

Determine the nutritional practices of the patient and family. Collect information on the types of foods and beverages that are generally given for different types of conditions. For example, some pregnant Hispanic and African American women have specific cravings and believe they need to eat starch or red clay to promote the baby's health. Some African Americans also believe that certain foods build blood, thereby preventing anemia. When providing nutritional care to patients of diverse cultures and religions:

- Avoid making value judgments about their practices.
- Understand food practices, and collaborate to develop healthy alternatives.
- Assess religious and cultural influences on nutritional practices.
  - Buddhists and Hindus are generally vegetarians because of their respect for life and belief in transmigration of the soul.
  - Vegetarians and vegans will prefer meat substitutes.
  - Hindus generally avoid eating beef, but some eat chicken and lamb.
  - Muslims eat *halal* foods and avoid those that are classified as *haram* (pork, alcohol).
  - Orthodox Jews generally eat kosher foods and avoid serving meat and dairy at the same time, eat fish with fins and scales, eat animals that chew their cud, and eat nonpredatory birds.
  - Muslims fast all day, including food and water, during the month of Ramadan. They eat before dawn and during evenings.
  - Some Hindus fast to obtain blessing from their gods.
- Accommodate food patterns of the culture.
  - Assess which ingredient or food content you need to reduce. For example, a Chinese patient on a low-sodium diet needs to use low-sodium soy sauce and avoid shrimp paste and oyster sauce.
  - Counsel diabetic Puerto Ricans to use exchanges within the cultural dietary pattern. Rice, beans, corn, potatoes, and plantains all belong to the same carbohydrate food group.
  - Most Southeast Asians, Jews, and African Americans are lactose intolerant.
  - Allow family members to prepare food for the patient by teaching them how to accommodate the prescribed modification. Note that not all groups will be able to read food labels.
  - Use an interpreter to provide culture-specific teaching. Instruct family members in how to store and heat the food they bring for the patient (Kitayama and others, 2007).

Skill Performance Guidelines

1. Be aware of signs and symptoms of malnutrition, and identify those patients at risk (see Table 30-2).
2. Use a systematic and organized approach when obtaining a nutritional assessment.
3. Be aware of patients' social history, cultural preferences, and economic factors. Some patients will be interested in healthy nutritional practices but are unable to implement them (e.g., no refrigeration at home, lack of money to buy food or infant formula). Each of these factors, alone and in combination, affects a patient's nutritional status and ability to follow a therapeutic diet.
4. Review the patient's medical history for diseases, medications, and medical problems that influence nutritional status. Some patients with medical problems or nonfunctioning GI tracts cannot be treated with oral nutrition. Enteral or parenteral therapies are sometimes necessary.

TABLE 30-2 | Components of Physical Examination for Nutritional Screening

Body Area	Signs and Symptoms of Nutritional Risk	Nutritional Implications
Hair	Dull, shedding, easily pluckable	Generalized protein calorie malnutrition
Face	Malar pigmentation (dark skin over cheeks and under eyes)	Niacin, B vitamins
	Bitemporal wasting	Malnutrition
	Nasolabial seborrhea	Niacin, riboflavin, vitamin B_6 deficiency
	Edematous	Protein deficiency
	Moon face	Corticosteroid impact
	Pallor	Inadequate Fe^{++}, undernutrition
Eyes	Pale eye membranes	Inadequate Fe^{++}
Lips	Cheilosis (red/swelling) Angular fissures	Inadequate niacin, vitamin B_6, riboflavin, Fe^{++}
Gingiva	Spongy, bleeding, abnormal redness	Inadequate vitamin C
Tongue	Glossitis (red, raw, fissured)	Inadequate folate, niacin, riboflavin, Fe^{++}, vitamin B_6, vitamin B_{12}
	Pale, atrophic, smooth/slick (filiform papillary atrophy)	Inadequate Fe^{++}, vitamin B_{12}, niacin, folate
	Magenta	Inadequate riboflavin
Nails	Spoon shaped, brittle, ridged	Inadequate Fe^{++}
Back	Bony prominences along shoulder girdle	Malnutrition

5 Verify that the type of feeding ordered is what has been provided to the patient at the proper temperature. Knowledge of the different types of oral therapeutic diets will help you properly plan and recommend food choices to meet patient needs.

6 Promote factors that improve a patient's appetite, such as encouraging the patient to select foods; providing small, frequent meals; and arranging pleasant and comfortable surroundings.

7 An organized approach when feeding a patient of any age helps the patient feel more at ease, and appetite increases in a relaxed atmosphere.

8 Be aware of the psychological effects on an adult patient who cannot self-feed. Feeding in a timely, well-paced, and understanding manner that allows maximal patient independence lessens the negative aspects of being fed by someone else. Instruct family members to provide a relaxed, social atmosphere when feeding the patient and to allow the patient to be as independent in feeding as possible.

9 Encourage patients and family members to keep menus from the hospital meal tray to use as a guide for preparing meals at home.

SKILL 30-1   Performing Nutritional Assessment

There are four basic components of a nutritional assessment: (1) patient history (medical, psychological, and social); (2) dietary history; (3) physical examination and anthropometric measurements; and (4) biochemical parameters (Grodner and others, 2007; Lacey and Pritchett, 2004). Elements of the patient history, such as appetite, psychosocial factors affecting intake, economics, and cultural issues, give background to factors influencing current nutritional status. Collect the history by reviewing the patient's medical record or by direct interview. The medical history indicates medications, surgery, and coexisting medical conditions compromising nutrition. The psychological history includes screening for depression, alcohol abuse, or abnormal psychiatric behavior leading to decreased food intake. A social history gives important insight into poverty, avoidance of specific food groups, and food customs influencing nutritional education. Assessment of dietary intake by eating habits will sometimes indicate food practices or avoidance of food groups that impair nutritional status. A physical examination reveals signs and symptoms of impaired nutrition. Finally, biochemical parameters offer information on immune function and protein status.

Assessment of nutritional status is an essential part of patient care. This assessment involves the verification of data and the analysis of all data to establish a database to form nursing judgments. Interpreting the data in a meaningful and relevant way allows nursing diagnoses to be identified that provide direction for nursing care. Therefore the steps of performing a nutritional assessment include delegation, assessment, nursing diagnoses, and evaluation.

PHYSICAL EXAMINATION

Physical examination is an important component of a thorough nutritional screening. Table 30-2 lists the body systems to assess and some of the external characteristics of malnutrition.

ANTHROPOMETRICS

Anthropometrics are measures of height; weight; head, arm, muscle circumferences; and skinfold thickness. Nurses typically measure height and weight. Registered dietitians more typically measure circumferences and skinfold thickness. Height and weight are useful in determining the nutritional status of both children and adults. The height and weight of a child is plotted on a growth chart and evaluated against standards based on the normal U.S. population. This information is essential to tracking the growth of children over time, which reflects nutritional adequacy. Measure height directly or indirectly (see Chapter 6). The direct measurement of height involves a measuring rod, and the individual must be able to stand or lie flat. This is sometimes impossible because of a patient's condition, so indirect methods, such as recumbent length, arm span, or knee height estimate height.

Body weight is a simple, gross estimate of body composition. It is one of the most important measurements in assessing nutritional status and for predicting energy expenditure (Grodner and others, 2007). You gather weight information in several ways, including usual body weight (UBW), ideal body weight (IBW), actual body weight (ABW), and BMI. A thorough nutritional assessment usually requires the collection of all of these weight measures. The change in a patient's weight over time is an inexpensive and relatively accurate method of predicting nutritional status. The magnitude and direction of weight change are more meaningful than standardized weight references when dealing with sick or debilitated patients (Grodner and others, 2007). Percent of weight change is a useful nutrition index.

$$\text{\% Weight change} = \frac{(\text{Usual weight} - \text{Actual weight})}{\text{Usual weight}} \times 100$$

Table 30-3 summarizes weight changes that indicate nutritional status. BMI provides a definition for adiposity by measuring weight corrected for height. The easiest way to calculate BMI is to refer to a standard BMI chart (Fig. 30-5). Box 30-2 lists BMI by degree of adiposity. BMI alone is not a perfect predictor of overweight or obesity. Use clinical judgment when evaluating muscular patients such as body builders or those patients with large amounts of edema or ascites because these physiological states will lead to false overestimation of the degree of fatness (Expert Panel on the Identification, 2000).

BIOCHEMICAL INDICES

Biochemical indices help to determine the effects of nutritional factors or of medical conditions on the health status of patients (Grodner and others, 2007). There is no single test available for evaluating short-term response to medical nutritional therapy. Use laboratory tests along with other assessment measures. Laboratory tests conducted over time will give more accurate information than a single test. The most important biochemical measures are visceral protein status and immune function. Tests of serum albumin and prealbumin measure visceral protein. Total lymphocyte count (TLC) measures immune function.

Normal serum albumin values are within 3.5 to 5.0 g/dL. For nutritional analysis, values between 2.8 and 3.5 g/dL indicate compromised protein status (Grodner and others, 2007). Albumin is a useful test for monitoring long-term nutrition changes because

Body Mass Index (BMI)

BMI	Weight in pounds													
Height	120	130	140	150	160	170	180	190	200	210	220	230	240	250
4'6	29	31	34	36	39	41	43	46	48	52	43	46	48	60
4'8	27	29	31	34	36	38	40	43	45	47	49	52	54	56
4'10	25	27	29	31	34	36	38	40	42	44	46	48	50	52
5'0	23	25	27	29	31	33	35	37	39	41	43	45	47	49
5'2	22	24	26	27	29	31	33	35	37	38	40	42	44	46
5'4	21	22	24	26	28	29	31	33	34	36	38	40	41	43
5'6	19	21	23	24	26	27	29	31	32	34	36	37	39	40
5'8	18	20	21	23	24	26	27	29	30	32	34	35	37	38
5'10	17	19	20	22	23	24	26	27	29	30	32	33	35	36
6'0	16	18	19	20	22	23	24	26	27	28	30	31	33	34
6'2	15	17	18	19	21	22	23	24	26	27	28	30	31	32
6'4	15	16	17	18	20	21	22	23	24	26	27	28	29	30
6'6	14	15	16	17	19	20	21	22	23	24	25	27	28	29
6'8	13	14	15	17	18	19	20	21	22	23	24	25	26	28

KEY

Obese (30+)
Overweight (25–29)
Healthy weight (Below 25)

FIG 30-5 Body mass index grid. (From Expert Panel on Identification, Evaluation, and Treatment of Overweight and Obesity in Adults: *The practical guide to identification, evaluation, and treatment of overweight and obesity in adults,* Bethesda, MD, 2000, National Institutes of Health.)

TABLE 30-3	Weight Change as an Indicator of Nutritional Status	
% Weight Change	**Time Period**	**Nutritional Status**
1-2	1 week	Moderate weight loss
>2	1 week	Severe weight loss
5	1 month	Moderate weight loss
>5	1 month	Severe weight loss

From Grodner M and others: *Foundations and clinical applications of nutrition: a nursing approach,* ed 3, St. Louis, 2004, Mosby.

BOX 30-2 Body Mass Index

To calculate BMI:

$$BMI = Weight\ (kg)/Height\ (m)^2$$

OR

$$BMI = \frac{Weight\ (lb)}{Height\ (inches) \times Height\ (inches)} \times 703$$

Classification of BMI in Adults

Degree of Adiposity	BMI
Underweight	$<18.5\ kg/m^2$
Normal Weight	$18.5\text{-}24.9\ kg/m^2$
Overweight	$25\text{-}29.9\ kg/m^2$
Obesity (Class 1)	$30\text{-}34.9\ kg/m^2$
Obesity (Class 2)	$35\text{-}39.9\ kg/m^2$
Extreme Obesity (Class 3)	$\geq40\ kg/m^2$

From Expert Panel on the Identification, Evaluation, and Treatment of Overweight and Obesity in Adults: *The practical guide: identification, evaluation, and treatment of overweight and obesity in adults,* Bethesda, Md, 2000, National Institutes of Health.
BMI, Body mass index.

normal values may still be found among patients who are malnourished. In addition, patients who are dehydrated or have received infusions of albumin, fresh frozen plasma, or whole blood serum albumin will have levels that appear normal. Prealbumin normally ranges from 20 to 50 mg/dL. The test is useful in monitoring short-term changes in visceral protein (Grodner and others, 2007). It has a short half-life of 2 days. A patient has compromised protein status when levels are between 10 and 15 g/dL.

TLC is a useful measure of immune function. A normal TLC is greater than 1500 cells/mm^3. You must assess a measure of TLC along with other diagnostic indicators. A count of less than 1500/mm^3 indicates possible immunocompromise associated with protein-energy malnutrition (Grodner and others, 2007). However, abnormally low TLCs are also associated with severe stress, corticosteroid therapy, renal failure, and cancer. High TLCs indicate infections, leukemia, myeloma, cancer, and adrenal insufficiency.

Delegation Considerations

The skill of interpreting nutritional assessment cannot be delegated to nursing assistive personnel (NAP). However, measurement of a patient's height and weight can be delegated. The nurse directs the NAP to:

- Recalibrate a scale before measuring a patient's weight.
- Measure patient's weight after voiding.
- Measure a recumbent height if patient is not capable of weight bearing.

Equipment

- ❑ Tongue blade, stethoscope, penlight (for physical assessment)
- ❑ Scale
- ❑ Assessment sheet and pen or computerized assessment form

STEP	RATIONALE

ASSESSMENT

1. Ask patient to report usual body weight, noting recent changes in the last month. Emphasize the importance of an accurate estimate.

   Women tend to underestimate their weight more than men, and for both sexes the extent of underreporting increases as actual weight increases (Grodner and others, 2007).

2. Obtain complete and thorough nursing history (see Chapter 6), including social, economic, and psychological factors affecting nutrition.

   Allows you to identify those patients who are at nutritional risk or are at risk for developing nutrient deficiencies.

3. Perform physical assessment (see Chapter 6), including condition of skin, hair, nails, oral mucosa, and eyes.

   Provides data on patient's nutritional status.

4. Review results of relevant laboratory tests.

   Test data provide clues about nutritional status.

5. Determine the medications and other dietary supplements patient is taking (over-the-counter and prescribed).

   Certain medications inhibit or increase the action of other medications. Also, some medications (e.g., coumarin anticoagulants) and nutrients (e.g., foods rich in vitamin K, dark green vegetables) interact to decrease medication function. Nutrients such as mineral oil laxatives impair nutrient use. Be aware of common drug-drug and drug-nutrient interactions.

6. Measure actual weight:

   a. Have patient void. Be sure patient is in hospital gown; try to weigh at the same time of day, each day.

   Improves accuracy of actual weight for comparison over time.

   b. Calibrate scale. Help patient to standing position, and be sure patient is free of restrictive clothing.

   Ensures accurate measurement. Prevents risk for fall when patient stands.

   c. Have patient stand on scale, or if patient is unable to stand, use chair, bed, or sling type of scale. Instruct patient to remain still, and record weight at nearest 0.1 kg or 0.25 pound.

   An accurate weight is a useful index of patient's nutritional well-being.

7. Measure actual height:

   a. Assist patient to standing position; have patient stand erect with weight equally distributed on both feet.

   Balance is necessary for patient to stand erect.

   b. Instruct patient to let arms hang free at the sides with palms facing the thighs.

   Prevents movement of shoulders, which will result in inaccurate measurement.

   c. Have patient look straight ahead, take a deep breath, and hold position while bringing horizontal bar firmly on top of head. Measure to nearest 0.1 cm or ⅛ inch.

   Steady position ensures accurate measurement. Make sure your eyes are level with the bar to read measurement.

8. Calculate IBW:

   a. Calculate via standard height and weight chart. IBW range for normal is 10% above and 10% below IBW.

   Use IBW to compare with patient's actual weight in determining if patient is at risk for nutritional alteration.

   b. Use the following formulas to calculate IBW:
   Male: 106 lb (48.1 kg) for the first 5 feet, then add 6 lb per additional inch (2.7 kg per 2.5 cm).
   Female: 100 lb (45.4 kg) for the first 5 feet, then add 5 lb per additional inch (2.25 kg per 2.5 cm).

STEP	RATIONALE
9 Calculate BMI:	Assesses patient's adiposity (obesity) against national standards.
Wt (kg)/Ht (m)^2	
a Divide weight in pounds by 2.2.	Converts pounds into kilograms.
b Multiply height in inches by 2.54, and divide result by 100.	Converts height to meters.
c Multiply height in meters by itself.	Computes square meters.
d Divide weight in kilograms by square of height in meters.	Computes BMI.
10 Assess patient's diet history, including current diet, food choices/preferences, appetite, explanations for any restrictions, food allergies, and food intolerances.	Allows for assessment of factors affecting diet adequacy and appetite.
11 Have patient provide 24-hour diet recall. Ask patient to report all foods and beverages consumed over past 24 hours.	Screens patient's compliance with dietary recommendations or reported diet pattern.
12 Determine patient's ability to manipulate eating utensils and self-feed.	Difficulty in self-feeding creates significant risk for malnutrition (Ebersole and others, 2008).
13 Explain to patient that nutritional assessment is complete.	Allows time for patient to ask questions about assessment.
14 Report diet restrictions and preferences to food and nutrition department.	Ensures an inpatient or resident will receive appropriate diet.

NURSING DIAGNOSES

- Deficient knowledge regarding nutritional intake
- Feeding self-care deficit
- Imbalanced nutrition: more than body requirements
- Risk for aspiration
- Risk for deficient fluid volume

Individualize related factors based on patient's condition or needs.

EVALUATION

1 Review history and physical findings. Note abnormal findings or areas of concern.	Completeness of data obtained from history and physical findings permits prompt identification of risk for malnutrition and need for nutritional interventions.
2 Compare patient's weight for height with ideal weight. Compare BMI with recommended BMI for height.	Significant weight fluctuations or weight outside of normal range indicates nutritional risk.
3 Compare normal laboratory test levels with patient's levels.	Abnormal values, when considered with other nutritional parameters, indicate malnutrition.

Unexpected Outcomes	Related Interventions
1 Body weight is below or above usual body weight and/or ideal body weight.	• Check weight daily while in acute care, then weekly after discharge. Assess for change over time. Report changes to RD or health care provider.
	• Document significant changes in intake, especially if patient is at risk for malnutrition.
	• If patient has experienced an unintentional weight loss, consult the RD for medical nutrition therapy.
	• The RD will conduct a nutritional assessment, calculate patient's caloric needs (calories per kilogram), determine amount of protein patient requires, determine route of nutrition (enteral versus parenteral) (see Chapters 31 and 32).
2 Laboratory test results are not within normal limits.	• Inform health care provider.
	• Obtain serial laboratory parameters as ordered by physician or dietitian.

Recording and Reporting

- Record results on nutritional screening form, making referral to the RD and documenting any significant differences from the norm.

Pediatric Considerations

- Anthropometric data include measurement of length, weight, and head circumference in children. Compare these measurements with standard growth charts to determine percentiles. The most commonly used growth charts are from the National Center for Health Statistics (Hockenberry and Wilson, 2007). These charts now include BMI for age and weight for stature percentiles.

Gerontological Considerations

- The "normal" anthropometric standards are based on a healthy middle-age population. However, there are methods of compar-ing anthropometric measurements over time for older adults (Meiner and Lueckenotte, 2006).

Long-Term Care Considerations

- Protein-calorie malnutrition (PCM) is prevalent among newly admitted older adult nursing home residents. Malnutrition risk factors on the Minimum Data Set (MDS) that were significant predictors for PCM included weight loss, leaves 25% or more of food uneaten at most meals, psychiatric/mood diagnoses, and deteriorated ability to participate in activities of daily living. In contrast, residents who used fingerfoods, verbal cueing, and were on therapeutic diets were more likely to have a normal BMI (Ebersole, 2008).

SKILL 30-2 Assisting an Adult Patient With Oral Nutrition

 Basic / Nutrition and Fluids / Assisting With Meals

Hospitalized patients receive a number of different oral diets (see Table 30-1). You can modify a regular diet in two ways: quantita-tively or qualitatively (Grodner and others, 2004). Qualitative di-ets include modifications in consistency, texture, or nutrients, such as clear or full liquid. Quantitative diets include modifications in number or size of meals served or amounts of specific nutrients, such as six small feedings or kcalorie diets. You can supplement any diet with oral nutrition supplements. As the nurse, you are respon-sible for preparing a patient and offering the type of assistance necessary so that the patient can successfully eat a full meal.

Assisting adults with oral nutrition requires time, patience, knowledge, and understanding. Most people eat without assis-tance. However, with illness, trauma, or altered oral integrity, some patients are physically unable to eat independently. Physical im-pairments that limit self-feeding, altered dentition, improper fit-ting dentures, oral lesions or infections, or diseases causing im-paired digestion limit the types and consistencies of foods tolerated. Hemiplegia, fractured arm, quadriplegia, debilitating illness, or generalized weakness limits self-feeding ability and appetite. The presence of intravenous (IV) catheters or tubing, dressings, and bandages limits the mobility needed for self-feeding as well. In ad-dition, some older adults tire quickly and need assistance even though they can eat independently. An adult who needs help to eat needs compassion and understanding. Use common sense when feeding the adult, and provide a socially meaningful mealtime experience.

Delegation Considerations

The skill of assisting a patient with oral nutrition can be delegated to NAP. The nurse directs the NAP by:

- Explaining any specific swallowing strategies/techniques unique to the patient.
- Reviewing when to stop feeding and report immediately to the nurse incidences of coughing, gagging, or difficulty swallowing.

Equipment

- ❑ Stethoscope
- ❑ Two-handled cup with lid
- ❑ Plate with plate guard
- ❑ Utensils with splints
- ❑ Utensils with enlarged handles
- ❑ Towels
- ❑ Tongue blade

STEP	RATIONALE

ASSESSMENT

1 Assess if patient passes flatus and is without nausea. Auscultate bowel sounds.	Determines if GI tract is functioning normally. Your awareness of specific diet order ensures patient gets an appropriate meal tray.
2 Review physician's or health care provider's diet order.	Awareness of specific diet order ensures patient gets appropriate meal tray.
3 Assess patient's ability to swallow. In patients with neurologi-cal condition, assess cranial nerves V, VII, IX, and X. Place a tongue blade on the back of patient's tongue to assess gag reflex.	Some patients (those who have neurological diseases or are handi-capped) have reduced gag reflex and/or dysphagia, increasing risk for aspiration. Change in consistency of diet (thickened liquids, pureed, soft), swallow training, or alternative means of nutrition is often necessary and requires a speech therapist or RD.
4 If patient wears dentures, check to ensure they fit well and are clean.	Ensures patient is able to chew food and swallow more normally.
5 Assess patient's level of energy.	Patients eat better when well rested.

STEP	RATIONALE
6 Determine to what extent patient is able to self-feed. Assess physical motor skills, level of consciousness, visual acuity and peripheral vision, and mood.	Patients with any level of independence should not be totally fed by hospital staff. Thorough understanding of patient's physical and cognitive limitations alerts you to type of assistance patient needs.
7 Assess patient's appetite, tolerance of foods, recent fluid intake, cultural and religious preferences, and food likes and dislikes.	Provides baseline of food and fluid intake. Allows you to prepare patient appropriately, determine time and pacing of feeding, and offer foods that patient will likely eat.

NURSING DIAGNOSES

- Disturbed sensory perception (gustatory)
- Feeding self-care deficit
- Impaired swallowing
- Risk for aspiration
- Risk for deficient fluid volume

Individualize related factors based on patient's condition or needs.

PLANNING

1 Expected outcomes following completion of procedure:	
• Patient denies any biting, chewing, or swallowing problem or food intolerances.	Patient tolerates diet.
• Patient's weight is maintained or changes according to the nutritional care plan.	Nutritional intake meets daily needs.
• Patient completes meal.	Prescribed dietary intake consumed.
• Patient is able to feed self independently.	Assistance successfully promotes self-feeding.
2 Collaborate with dietitian in adapting quality or quantity of meals. For example, if patient is on a pureed diet, make foods more attractive by pureeing each item separately. Use a cake decorating tool to enhance the appearance of pureed meals, or use molds to shape foods.	Improves likelihood that patient will be interested in eating and meal is more appealing in appearance.
3 Prepare patient's room for mealtime:	
a Perform hand hygiene. Clear over-bed table.	
b Set up chair for patient and for yourself. Help patient to comfortable sitting position in chair, or place bed in high-Fowler's position. If patient is unable to sit, turn patient on side with the head of the bed elevated. Conditions such as pressure ulcer, traction, or spinal surgery prevent positioning with head elevated.	Upright position assists patient with keeping food toward front of mouth before swallowing, reducing aspiration.
4 Prepare patient for meal:	
a Assist patient with elimination needs.	Increases patient's comfort and enjoyment of meal, which helps increase patient's nutritional intake.
b Help patient perform hand hygiene.	Reduces spread of microorganisms.
c Assist patient with mouth care. Patients with dysphagia or dry mouth often benefit from toothbrushing or clear water rinsing.	Moist and clean oral mucosa and teeth improve taste and increase appetite.
d Patients with stomatitis (inflammation of oral mucosa) benefit from rinsing with a solution containing hydrogen peroxide, warm saline, sodium bicarbonate, or a combination of all agents. Consult with physician regarding an oral analgesic (e.g., lidocaine 2% viscous) (Munro and others, 2006).	Some patients avoid foods because of pain from oral infections or lesions.
e Help patient to put in dentures and put on eyeglasses or insert contact lenses if used. Check that dentures fit properly.	Enhances patient's ability to bite, chew, and swallow as well as see food. Ill-fitting dentures inhibit normal chewing and pose a safety risk.

STEP	RATIONALE

f Obtain special devices and needed supplies to facilitate feeding (two-handled cup with lid, plate with plate guard, utensils with splints, utensils with enlarged handles, towels) before meal (see illustration).

Ensures organized, unhurried atmosphere.

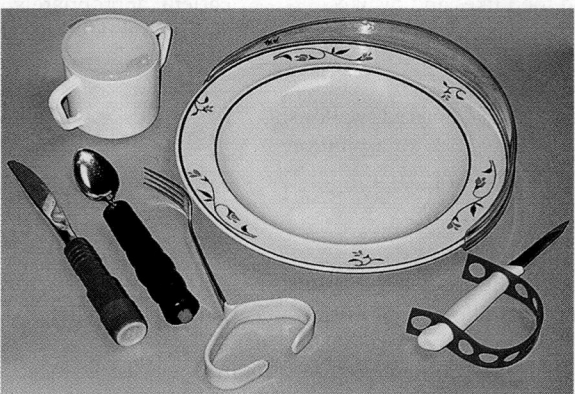

STEP 4f   Mealtime equipment. *Clockwise from upper left:* Two-handled cup with lid, plate with plate guard, utensils with splints, and utensils with enlarged handles.

IMPLEMENTATION

1 Prepare patient's tray:
   a Perform hand hygiene before preparing patient's tray.
   b Assess tray for completeness and correct diet.
   c Prepare tray to meet patient's needs: open cartons, remove lids, cut food, and season food after asking patient's preferences.
   d If patient is able to eat independently, stop here. Return after 10 to 20 minutes.
2 Assist patient who cannot eat independently:
   a Put yourself in a comfortable position.

   b Ask in what order patient would like to eat, and cut food into bite-size pieces.
   c It is helpful for disoriented, visually impaired, or easily fatigued patients to have food identified by location on plate as if the plate were a clock (see illustration).
   d Feed patient in a manner that facilitates chewing and swallowing.
      (1) *Older adult:* Feed small amounts at a time, observing biting, chewing, swallowing, and fatigue. Be sure between bites that patient has swallowed food.

Reduces spread of microorganisms.
Prevents ingestion of incorrect or incomplete meal.
Patients with cognitive, visual, or physical impairments do not always have the ability to prepare tray for eating.

Determines how well patient is tolerating diet.

Sitting or standing close to patient during feeding promotes psychologically comforting and caring environment, which often increases appetite. It is important to be comfortable when feeding a patient, so as not to rush him or her through the meal.
Allows patient more independence and control. Small pieces are easier to chew and minimize risk for aspiration.
Assists in patient's ability to locate food items.

Decreased saliva production impairs swallowing. Aspiration results because of a decreased or absent gag reflex and relaxation of the lower esophageal sphincter. Chewing and sitting up for feeding accelerates the onset of fatigue. Frequent rests are helpful (Ebersole and others, 2008).

Critical Decision Point   *If you suspect patient is aspirating, stop feeding immediately and suction airway.*

STEP	RATIONALE

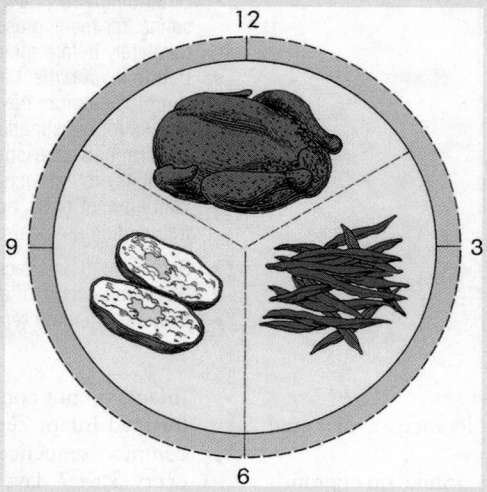

STEP 2c   Clock setup to prepare food on a plate for the visually impaired patient.

(2) *Neurologically impaired patient:* Feed small amounts at a time, and assess for ability to chew, manipulate tongue to form a bolus, and swallow. Give small amounts of thin liquids (soup, beverages), and assess for swallowing.	Some patients with limited tongue strength and control are unable to move bolus to back of mouth for swallowing. Checking for "pocketed" food in mouth prevents aspiration.

Critical Decision Point   *Patients with dysphagia who aspirate thin liquids often benefit from liquids thickened with commercial thickening products or from change in consistency of diet.*

(3) *Patient with cancer:* Check for food aversions before and during the meal.	May have strong, abnormal sense of taste and smell as side effect of medications.
e Provide fluids as requested. Do not allow patient to drink all liquids at beginning of meal.	Assists with swallowing. Prevents patient from filling up on liquids.
f Talk with patient during meal.	Meal should be a pleasant event. Conversation promotes socialization. Involve family if possible.
g Use meal as an opportunity to educate patient (e.g., topics related to nutrition, postoperative exercises, discharge plans).	Education can occur whenever nurse and patient are together.
h Assist patient with hand hygiene and performing mouth care.	Mouth care after meals helps prevent dental caries.
i Help patient to resting position, leave head elevated 45 degrees for 30 minutes after meal.	Patient may feel tired after full meal. Elevation of head reduces risk for aspiration.
j Return patient's tray to appropriate place, and perform hand hygiene.	Reduces spread of microorganisms.

EVALUATION

1 Observe patient's ability to swallow.	Determines if patient develops dysphagia and becomes prone to aspiration.
2 Weigh patient daily (if nutrition has been inadequate).	Gradual weight gain reflects improved nutritional status.
3 Determine patient's tolerance to diet.	Overfeeding causes nausea and vomiting. Underfeeding leaves patient feeling hungry.
4 Monitor patient's fluid intake, and note amount of food eaten from tray.	Helps to determine whether patient's nutritional and fluid needs are being met.
5 Observe patient's ability to feed self.	Determines if patient is gaining independence in feeding.

Unexpected Outcomes	Related Interventions
1 Patient is unable to eat entire meal.	• Determine why patient is unable to finish meal (e.g., inadequate personnel for feeding assistance, ingestion of large volume of liquids immediately before meal, food preferences). • Determine if patient is in pain, nauseated, or uncomfortable. Manage symptoms before next feeding. • Assess for constipation. • Perform oral assessment; provide oral care as needed • If inability to eat meal is a repeated problem, consult with RD. • Wait an hour or so, and offer a snack from food service. Also offer more frequent small meals.
2 Patient chokes on food.	• Suction food and secretions from mouth and airway. • If choking occurs often, contact physician or health care provider. • Make appropriate referrals (e.g., speech therapy).

Recording and Reporting

- Document in patient's chart: patient's tolerance of diet and amount eaten.
- If patient is on calorie counts, record caloric intake on appropriate form; if evaluating intake and output, record fluid intake on appropriate form.
- If patient is receiving oral nutritional supplements (e.g., Ensure, Boost), record the amount taken and communicate patient tolerance (likes or dislikes, supplements to fill or replace meals) to the health care team.
- Report any swallowing difficulties, food dislikes, refusal to eat to nurse in charge.

Teaching Considerations

- Discuss dietary concerns of the patient's illness. Explain why specific foods are not included in a meal or why only limited amounts are allowed (Grodner and others, 2007).
- Instruct patient and family to maintain a balanced diet and to monitor intake of fluids and percent or amount of meals and snacks consumed. If intake falls below 75% for any length of time, refer the patient to an RD for medical nutrition therapy.
- Teach family members techniques to safely assist patient in feeding. Have family encourage patient to do as much as possible in feeding self.

Pediatric Considerations

- Human milk is the most desirable complete diet for infants during the first 6 months. Infants who are breast- or bottle-fed do not require additional fluids, especially water or juice, during the first 4 months of life. Excessive intake of water causes water intoxication, failure to thrive, and hyponatremia. Typically, infants do not consume solid foods until 6 months of age. Iron-fortified infant cereal is usually the first solid food to offer. A common sequence for introducing solid food is one new food every 5 to 7 days. Strained fruits followed by vegetables, and finally meats is the usual pattern (Hockenberry and others, 2007).
- Do not mix solid foods in a bottle and feed through a nipple with a larger hole (Hockenberry and Wilson, 2007).

Gerontological Considerations

- Some older adult patients have diminished appetite because of loss of taste and smell and decreased number of taste buds.
- Interactions between nutrients and medications affect taste of foods or metabolism, absorption, digestion, or excretion of drugs.

Home Care Considerations

- Assess financial resources of patient and family to determine if they are able to purchase proper foods for patient.
- Help patient and family to identify ways to make meals in the home pleasant and enjoyable experiences.

Long-Term Care Considerations

- Meals are part of a resident's social interaction with other residents and staff, and, as a result, residents rarely eat meals in their rooms. Meals in long-term care settings are often in a social dining program, where residents eat in a dining room and food is served as in a restaurant; family dining, in which residents serve themselves from a common serving bowl; or in an assistive dining program, in which residents can receive assistance with meals.

SKILL 30-3   Aspiration Precautions

 Basic / Nutrition and Fluids / Taking Aspirations Precautions

Aspiration is the inhalation of oropharyngeal secretions into the lower respiratory tract. Secretions build up in the back of the oropharynx as a result of gastroesophageal reflux or dysphagia (impairment in swallowing). When pathogenic bacteria colonize the secretions, the risk for aspiration pneumonia is high. Aspiration pneumonia can be a fatal complication, particularly in older adults. Dysphagia is a symptom or complication of a number of conditions (Box 30-3), particularly that of stroke. Dysphagia after a stroke is very common and is a marker of a patient's poor prognosis, increasing the risks for pneumonia, malnutrition, persistent disability, prolonged hospital stay, and death (Martino and others, 2005). Cerebral, cerebellar, or brain stem strokes impair swallowing in a number of ways. Cerebral lesions interrupt voluntary control of chewing and movement of food down the esophagus (White and others, 2008). Lesions of the cerebral cortex impair facial, lip, and tongue motor control (Martino and others, 2005). Impairments in cognitive function such as concentration or selective attention also affect swallowing. Because stroke is common in older adults, age-related swallowing further adds to stroke-related dysphagia.

In some patients, aspiration from dysphagia occurs silently. This means that a patient will aspirate without any outward signs of swallowing difficulty. Conditions associated with silent aspiration include local weakness/incoordination of the pharyngeal muscles, reduced laryngopharyngeal sensation, impaired ability to reflexively cough, and low levels of neurotransmitters (e.g., substance P and dopamine) (Ramsey and others, 2005).

Characteristics of dysphagia that are most predictive of aspiration risk include the following (Nowlin, 2006):
- A wet voice
- Weak voluntary cough
- Coughing or choking on food
- Prolonged swallow
- Combination of the above

Additional characteristics of dysphagia are a voice change after swallowing; abnormal lip closure and tongue movement; hoarse voice; slow, weak, imprecise, or uncoordinated speech; abnormal gag; abnormal volitional cough; delayed oral and pharyngeal transit; incomplete oral clearance; regurgitation; pharyngeal pooling; and inability to speak consistently.

NUTRITIONAL IMPLICATIONS OF DYSPHAGIA

Dysphagia often causes a decrease in food intake, which then results in malnutrition. Nutritional status changes as indicated by changes in skinfold thickness and albumin level are apparent in patients with dysphagia. In most instances this is due to difficulty in consuming an adequate volume of solids or liquids. Dietary intake may be affected for long periods of time, and the malnutrition that occurs is secondary to insufficient protein, calorie, and micronutrient intake (Ebersole and others, 2008). This significantly impedes a patient's recovery from illness.

DYSPHAGIA SCREENING

Dysphagia is typically identified by using one of three types of diagnostic techniques. An initial bedside swallow assessment is a cursory examination that you can administer with basic clinical swallowing training. If you suspect dysphagia, an extensively trained swallowing technician (e.g., speech pathologist) will conduct a more thorough test. The comprehensive testing involves assessment of cranial nerves and swallowing trials using a variety of texture-modified liquids and solids. The third diagnostic technique is use of videofluoroscopy. A patient assumes a sitting position and swallows radiopaque materials of different liquid and food textures. The videofluoroscope shows swallow physiology.

Nurses and RDs initially screen for dysphagia in patients believed to be at risk. There are many dysphagia screening tools with similar characteristics (Fig. 30-6). The Registered Dietitian Dysphagia Screening Tool, designed by Brody and others, uses medical record review, patient questioning, and observation of a meal. The screening tool includes observation of a patient at a meal for change in voice quality, posture and head control, percentage of meal consumed, eating time, drooling of liquids and solids, cough during/after a swallow, facial or tongue weakness, difficulty with secretions, pocketing, and presence of voluntary and dry cough (Brody and others, 2002). All dysphagia screening tools assess holding food in mouth, leakage from mouth, coughing, choking, breathlessness, and quality of voice after swallowing (Runions and others, 2004).

BOX 30-3	Causes of Dysphagia

Neurogenic	**Obstructive**
Stroke	Benign peptic stricture
Cerebral palsy	Lower esophageal ring
Guillain-Barré syndrome	Candidiasis
Multiple sclerosis	Head and neck cancer
Amyotrophic lateral sclerosis (Lou Gehrig disease)	Inflammatory masses
Diabetic neuropathy	Trauma/surgical resection
Parkinson's disease	Anterior mediastinal masses
	Cervical spondylosis
Myogenic	
Myasthenia gravis	**Other**
Aging	Gastrointestinal or esophageal resection
Muscular dystrophy	Rheumatological disorders
Polymyositis	Connective tissue disorders
	Vagotomy

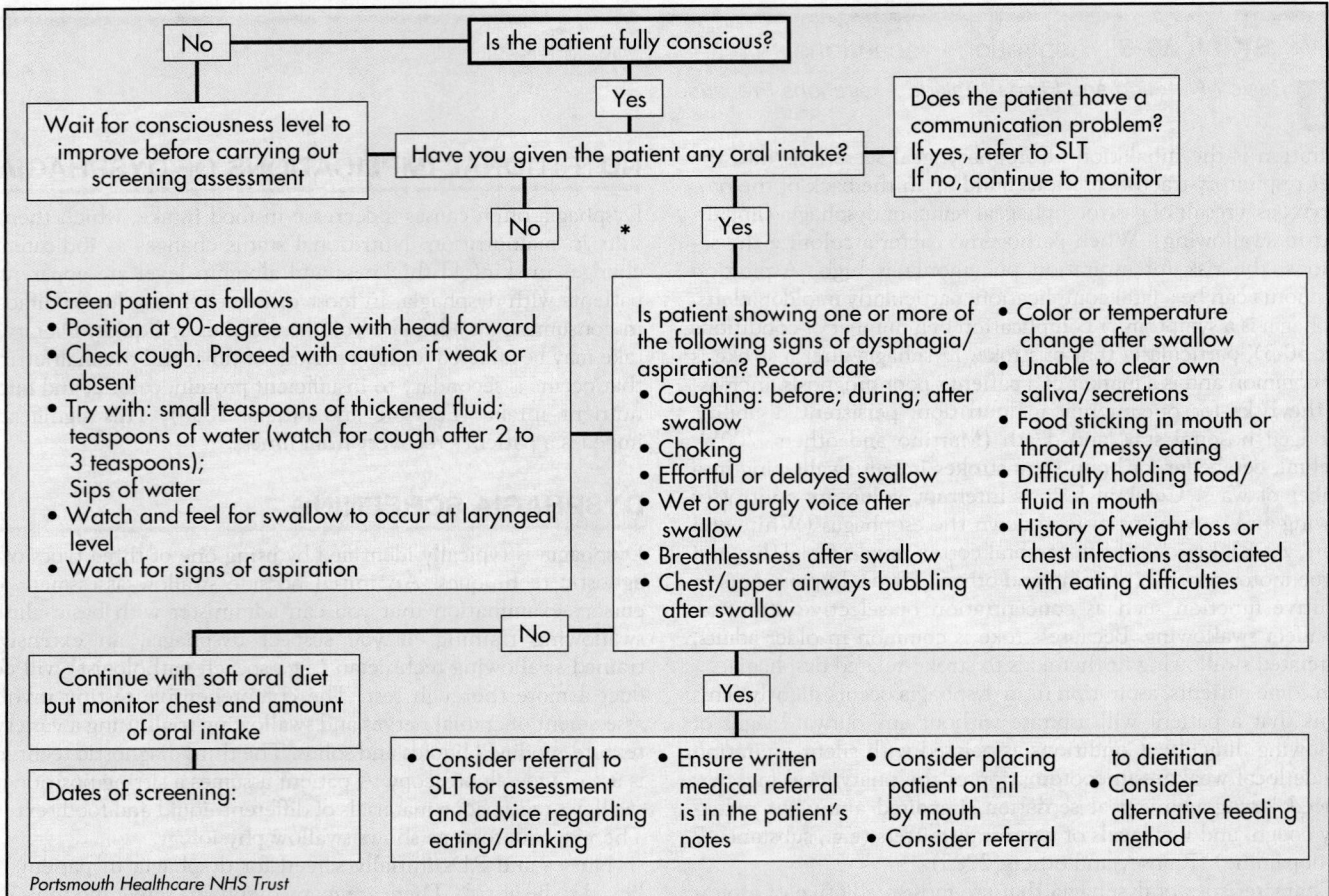

FIG 30-6 Screening assessment for dysphagic patients. *SLT*, Speech, language therapist. (*From Dangerfield L, Sullivan R: Screening for and managing dysphagia after stroke, Nurs Times 95[19]:44, 1999.*)

When assessing patients during a meal, use caution. It is important to first assess the patient's consciousness level, posture, ability to cooperate, and gross oral motor function (Metheny, 2007). After you determine that a patient is safe, test the patient with sips of water while observing for coughing or respiratory distress, voice changes, and laryngeal movement. Offer a small glass of water if the sip is cleared safely. Then, offer those without difficulties in swallowing a larger volume of water, yogurt, and normal foods, again under constant monitoring. Patients who continue to have no problems then need to receive a normal diet, with monitoring of oral intake and respiratory status for 48 hours (Ramsey and others, 2003).

When a patient has difficulty swallowing, referral for a more comprehensive examination is necessary (Box 30-4). The assessment includes observation of the patient eating a range of food textures and consistencies, resulting in a comprehensive description of the phases of swallowing and a judgment of degree of dysfunction and aspiration risk (Metheny, 2007; White and others, 2008). A speech-language pathologist performs the assessment. Clinical assessment focuses on oral-motor and oral-sensory function, protective reflexes, and respiratory status. Treatment recommendations include alterations in the consistencies of foods and the use of swallowing therapies.

DYSPHAGIA TREATMENT

There is no one clear approach to prevent aspiration in patients. Metheny (2007) and White and others (2008) reviewed the evidence on research studies involving interventions for preventing aspiration pneumonia in older adults. Positioning changes, dietary interventions, oral hygiene, pharmacological therapies, and electrical stimulation have all been tested. The benefit of these therapies is inconclusive. However, Skill 30-3 includes approaches used by researchers to minimize aspiration. A priority is the initiation of safe oral nutrition and hydration. Changes in food and/or liquid consistencies, elimination of oral intake, and initiation of tube feeding are common diet modifications. Liquid or pureed foods are sometimes the only consistency tolerated by patients with mechanical disorders that cause dysphagia, but this is not always the most appropriate choice for individuals with oropharyngeal dysphagia. Patients with oropharyngeal dysphagia have more success with semisolid consistencies that are easy to chew. Foods with increased viscosity, such as the thickness of pudding, have to be thickened with a commercial thickener to decrease transit time and allow for protection of the airway (White and others, 2008). Maintain nothing by mouth (NPO) status if aspiration is present.

BOX 30-4	Criteria for Dysphagia Referral

Before referral:

If the answer is yes to either of the following two questions, the referral at this time is not appropriate.

- Is the patient unconscious or drowsy?
- Is the patient unable to sit in an upright position for a reasonable length of time?

Please consider the next two questions before making the referral:

- Is the patient near the end of life?
- Does the patient have an esophageal problem that will require surgical intervention?

When observing the patient or giving mouth care, look for the following:

- Open mouth (weak lip closure)
- Drooling liquids or solids
- Poor oral hygiene/thrush

- Facial weakness
- Tongue weakness
- Difficulty with secretions
- Slurred, indistinct speech
- Change in voice quality
- Poor posture or head control
- Weak involuntary cough
- Delayed cough (up to 2 minutes after swallow)
- General frailty
- Confusion/dementia
- No spontaneous swallowing movements

If any of the above is present, the patient may have swallowing problems and may need referral to a speech-language pathologist.

In October 2002 the American Dietetic Association published the National Dysphagia Diet Task Force's (NDDTF's) National Dysphagia Diet (2002). The diet comprises four levels: Dysphagia Puree, Dysphagia Mechanically Altered, Dysphagia Advanced, and Regular. There are also four levels of liquid consistencies: thin liquids (low viscosity), nectarlike liquids (medium viscosity), honeylike liquids (viscosity of honey), and spoon-thick liquids (viscosity of pudding) (Table 30-4).

Delegation Considerations

The assessment of patient's risk for aspiration and determination of positioning cannot be delegated to NAP. However, NAP may feed patients after receiving instruction in aspiration precautions. The nurse directs the NAP to:

- Report to the nurse in charge, as soon as possible, any onset of coughing, gagging, a wet voice, or pocketing of food.

Equipment

- ❑ Chair or electric bed (to allow patient to sit upright)
- ❑ Thickening agents as needed (rice, cereal, yogurt, gelatin, commercial thickening agent)
- ❑ Tongue blade
- ❑ Oral hygiene supplies (see Chapter 17)
- ❑ Pulse oximeter
- ❑ Penlight
- ❑ Suction equipment

TABLE 30-4	Stages of National Dysphagia Diet	
Stage	**Description**	**Examples**
Dysphagia Puree	Uniform Pureed Cohesive Puddinglike texture	Smooth hot cereals cooked to a "pudding" consistency Mashed potatoes Pureed meat Pureed pasta or rice Pureed vegetable Yogurt
Dysphagia Mechanically Altered	Moist Soft textured Easily forms a bolus	Cooked cereals Dry cereals moistened with milk Canned fruit (excluding pineapple) Moist ground meat Well-cooked noodles in sauce/gravy Well-cooked, diced vegetables
Dysphagia Advanced	Regular foods (with the exception of very hard, sticky, or crunchy foods)	Moist breads (with butter, jelly, etc.) Well-moistened cereals Peeled soft fruits (peach, plum, kiwi) Tender, thin-sliced meats Baked potato (without skin) Tender, cooked vegetables
Regular	All foods	No restrictions

STEP	RATIONALE

ASSESSMENT

1 Perform a nutritional assessment (see Skill 30-1).

Patients with aspiration from dysphagia alter their eating patterns or choose foods that do not provide adequate nutrition (White and others, 2008).

2 Assess patients who are at increased risk for aspiration for signs and symptoms of dysphagia (see Box 30-4). Use a dysphagia screening tool if available.

Some patients show symptoms of poor lip and tongue control. Patients at risk include those who have neurological or neuromuscular diseases and those who have had trauma to or surgical procedures of the oral cavity or throat.

3 Observe patient during mealtime for signs of dysphagia. Allow patient to attempt to feed self. Note at end of meal if patient fatigues, has wet voice, or coughs after attempting to swallow (White and others, 2008).

Detects abnormal eating patterns such as frequent clearing of throat, coughing after swallowing, prolonged eating time. Fatigue increases risk for aspiration.

STEP	RATIONALE
4 Ask patient about any trouble with chewing or swallowing various textures of food.	Be alert for coughing, dyspnea, or drooling that suggest difficulty handling food, especially thin liquids.
5 Report signs and symptoms of dysphagia to the health care provider.	Some patients need to have an assessment performed by a radiologist or speech-language pathologist (White and others, 2008).
6 Place an identification on patient's chart or Kardex indicating that dysphagia/aspiration risk is present. *Option:* Some facilities use different-colored meal trays to signify patients at risk for aspiration.	Identifying patient as dysphagic reduces risk for his or her receiving oral nutrients without supervision (Nowlin, 2006).

NURSING DIAGNOSES

- Disturbed sensory perception (gustatory)   • Impaired swallowing   • Risk for aspiration

Individualize related factors based on patient's condition or needs.

PLANNING

1 Expected outcomes following completion of procedure:	
• Patient will not exhibit signs or symptoms of aspiration.	Interventions for preventing aspiration are successful.
• Patient maintains stable weight.	Patient is able to maintain oral intake.

IMPLEMENTATION

STEP	RATIONALE
1 Perform hand hygiene.	Prevents transmission of microorganisms.
2 Provide thorough oral hygiene, including brushing of tongue, before meal.	Tongue coating is associated with accumulation of bacterial cells in the saliva and aspiration pneumonia, especially in patients without dentures (Abe and others, 2007).
3 Apply pulse oximeter to patient's finger.	Studies have suggested that oxygen desaturation and hypoxia occur with aspiration (White and others, 2008).
4 Position patient upright in bed or sitting at a 90-degree angle in a chair (Loeb and others, 2003).	Position aims to prevent gastric reflux and reduces occurrence of aspiration.
5 Using penlight and tongue blade, gently inspect mouth for pockets of food.	Pockets of food in the mouth indicate difficulty swallowing.
6 Have patient assume a chin-tuck position. Begin by having patient try sips of water. Monitor for swallowing and respiratory difficulties continuously. If patient tolerates water, offer a larger volume of water, then different consistencies of foods and liquids.	Chin-tuck or chin-down position helps reduce aspiration (Huang and others, 2006). Introducing liquids and foods of different textures assesses patient's ability to swallow safely. Gradual increase in types and textures, coupled with constant monitoring, ensures patient is able to eat safely (White and others, 2008).
7 Add thickener to thin liquids to create the consistency of mashed potatoes.	Thin liquids can be easily aspirated (White and others, 2008).
8 Place ½ to 1 teaspoon of food on unaffected side of mouth, allowing utensils to touch the mouth or tongue.	Provides a tactile cue to begin eating.
9 Provide verbal cueing while feeding. Remind patient to chew and think about swallowing.	Keeps patient focused on swallowing and minimizes distractions (Metheny, 2007).
10 Observe for coughing, choking, gagging, and drooling; suction airway as necessary.	Indicates dysphagia and risk for aspiration.
11 During feeding do not rush a patient. Allow time for adequate chewing and swallowing.	Ensures oral cavity is empty between swallows.
12 Ask patient to remain sitting upright for at least 30 to 60 minutes after the meal.	Reduces the risk for gastroesophageal reflux, which causes aspiration (Ebersole and others, 2008; Nowlin, 2006).
13 Help patient to perform hand hygiene and mouth care.	Mouth care after meals helps prevent dental caries.
14 Return patient's tray to appropriate place, and perform hand hygiene.	Reduces spread of microorganisms.

EVALUATION

STEP	RATIONALE
1 Observe patient's ability to ingest foods of various textures and thicknesses.	Indicates whether aspiration risk is increased with thin liquids.
2 Monitor patient's food and fluid intake.	Some patients avoid certain types and textures of food that are difficult to swallow.
3 Monitor pulse oximetry readings.	The occurrence of desaturation indicates aspiration.
4 Weigh patient weekly.	Determines if weight is stable and reflects adequate caloric level.

Unexpected Outcomes

1 Patient coughs, gags, complains of food "stuck in throat," or has pockets of food in mouth.

2 Patient avoids certain textures of food.
3 Patient experiences weight loss.

Related Interventions

- Patient may require a swallowing evaluation by a licensed speech pathologist or videofluoroscopy.
- Consider consultation with a speech therapist for swallowing exercises and techniques to improve swallowing and reduce risk for aspiration.
- Notify physician of any symptoms that occurred during meal and which foods caused the symptoms.
- Change consistency and texture of food (see Table 30-4).
- Consult with dietitian on increasing frequency of meals or providing oral nutritional supplements.

Recording and Reporting

- Document in patient's chart: patient's tolerance of liquids and food textures, amount of assistance required, position during meal, absence or presence of any symptoms of dysphagia, fluid intake, and amount eaten.
- Report any coughing, gagging, choking, or swallowing difficulties to nurse in charge or health care provider.

Teaching Considerations

- Instruct family caregivers in ways to position patient and the signs and symptoms of aspiration to observe (Huang and others, 2006).
- Consider language barriers when instructing patient and family (Riquelme, 2007).

- For high-risk patients, have an oral suction device available for family caregivers to use.

Gerontological Considerations

- The risk for aspiration pneumonia is higher in older adults because of an increased incidence of dysphagia and gastroesophageal reflux. Older adults with stroke and Parkinson's disease and individuals with dementia are particularly at risk (Ebersole and others, 2008; White and others, 2008).
- Malnutrition occurs rapidly in older adults with dysphagia. Enteral feedings are sometimes necessary, but there is still a risk for aspiration (Ebersole and others, 2008).

CRITICAL THINKING EXERCISES

Mr. Jasper is a 73-year-old patient who has been in a retirement center for 3 months. His daughter visits frequently and usually tries to help him eat during scheduled mealtimes in the dining room. Mr. Jasper has a history of type 2 diabetes, and 4 months ago he had a stroke involving the right cerebral cortex. The stroke has caused a partial left-sided paralysis. Mr. Jasper is left handed. He currently weighs 140 pounds and is 6 feet tall. His daughter has asked to talk with the nurse in charge about her father's eating habits. For the last 2 weeks the daughter has noticed that her father has been served food prepared pureed.

1 By determining Mr. Jasper's BMI, how would you rate his nutritional status?
2 Given Mr. Jasper's history, what factors would place him at risk for not eating adequately? Explain in detail.
3 What could be done to improve Mr. Jasper's calorie intake?
4 What suggestions might you give Mr. Jasper's daughter to help prevent Mr. Jasper from aspirating when he is eating?

REVIEW QUESTIONS

1 An older adult patient is admitted to the hospital, where the mini nutritional assessment (MNA) is done and a score of 19 is obtained. What priority measure should be included in this patient's care?
 1 Observation of potential interactions between drugs and foods consumed
 2 Having the registered dietitian talk with the patient about what foods could be eaten more easily
 3 Weighing this patient every day at the same time and on the same scale

 4 An assessment of what the patient knows about sources of essential nutrients
2 A nurse is providing a nutrition education program at a senior day care center and is explaining the Nutrition Screening Initiative. What key point needs to be included in this presentation about this program?
 1 It is a federally funded program aimed at identifying older adults at nutritional risk.
 2 It is a state funded program aimed at identifying adults at nutritional risk.
 3 It is a nutritional screening program aimed at early intervention for those lacking food.
 4 It is a voluntary program aimed at early identification of nutritional risk in high-risk populations.
3 A 60-year-old vegetarian has been admitted to rule out a stroke. While doing the patient's physical assessment, the nurse notes a beefy red, fissured tongue. Which health problems may be present?
 1 The patient has glossitis and a possible vitamin B_{12} deficiency.
 2 The patient has decreased saliva production and an iron deficiency.
 3 The patient has a vitamin C deficiency and a low albumin level.
 4 The patient has a caloric deficit, causing loss of bone minerals.
4 A patient is unable to eat more than a quarter of any meal because of pain and nausea. What would be the most important measure for the nurse to take at this time?
 1 Encourage the patient to eat small amounts several times during the day.
 2 Ask the patient what foods and beverages cause the least amount of nausea.
 3 Record a chronology of what the patient has been eating for the past 2 days.
 4 Talk with the physician about strategies to decrease the pain and nausea.

5   A patient has been admitted with the diagnosis of transient weakness including a diminished gag reflex. The patient has a regular diet ordered. What is the most appropriate nursing action?

1   Keep the patient NPO until the physician can assess the patient.

2   Allow the patient to eat as long as a family member is at the bedside.

3   Elevate the head of the patient's bed while allowing the patient to drink clear liquids.

4   Change the diet order to full liquids to see how the patient tolerates the fluids.

REFERENCES

American Academy of Family Physicians: *About the Nutrition Screening Initiative (website)*, 2003, American Academy of Family Physicians, http://www.aafp.org/x16082.xml, accessed December 30, 2003.

American Society for Parenteral and Enteral Nutrition: *The science and practice of nutrition support: a case-based core curriculum*, Dubuque, Iowa, 2007, Kendall Hunt.

Brody R: Newark Beth Israel Medical Center nutrition screening, and re-assessment policy and procedure, Newark, NJ, 2002, Newark Beth Israel Medical Center.

Ebersole P and others: *Toward healthy aging*, ed 7, St. Louis, 2008, Mosby.

Elia M: The "Must" report: nutritional screening of adults: a multidisciplinary responsibility—development and use of the Malnutrition Universal Screening Tool (MUST) for adults, Redditch, 2003, BAPEN.

Expert Panel on the Identification, Evaluation, and Treatment of Overweight and Obesity in Adults: *The practical guide: identification, evaluation, and treatment of overweight and obesity in adults*, Bethesda, Md, 2000, National Institutes of Health.

Grodner M and others: *Foundations and clinical applications of nutrition: a nursing approach*, ed 4, St. Louis, 2007, Mosby.

Hammond K and others: Dietary and clinical assessment. In *Krause's food nutrition and diet therapy*, Philadelphia, 2007, Saunders, http://www.aafp.org/PreBuilt/NSI_DETERMINE.pdf.

Hockenberry MJ and Wilson D: *Wong's nursing care of infants and children*, ed 8, St. Louis, 2007, Mosby.

Krebs-Smith SM, Kris-Etherton P: How does MyPyramid compare to other population-based recommendations for controlling chronic disease? *J Am Diet Assoc* 107(5):830, 2007.

Lacey K, Pritchett E: Nutrition care process and model: ADA adopts road map to quality care and outcomes management, *J Am Diet Assoc* 103(8):1061, 2004.

Meiner S and Lueckenotte AG: *Gerontologic nursing*, ed 3, St. Louis, 2006, Mosby.

Metheny N: Preventing aspiration in older adults with dysphagia, *Medsurg Nurs* 16(4):271, 2007.

Munro C and others: Oral health measurements in nursing research: state of the science, *Biol Res Nurs* 8(1):35, 2006.

National Dysphagia Diet Task Force: *National Dysphagia Diet: standardization for optimal care*, Chicago, 2002, American Dietetic Association.

Nestlé Clinical Nutrition: *MNA—Mini Nutritional Assessment*, 2003, Nestlé Nutrition, http://www.mna-elderly.com/, accessed December 31, 2003.

Nowlin A: The dysphagia dilemma: how you can help, *RN* 69(6):44, 2006.

Nutrition Screening Initiative: DETERMINE Your Nutritional Health questionnaire, Washington, DC, 1997, American Academy of Family Physicians.

Perry L: Screening swallowing function of patients with acute stroke. I. Identification, implementation, and initial evaluation of a screening tool for use by nurses, *J Clin Nurs* 10:463, 2001a.

Riquelme L: The role of cultural competence in providing services to persons with dysphagia, *Top Geriatr Rehab* 23(3):228, 2007.

Runions S and others: Practice on acute stroke unit after implementation of a decision-making algorithm for dietary management of dysphagia, *J Neurosci Nurs* 36(4):200, 2004.

The Joint Commission: *2007 Comprehensive accreditation manual for hospitals: the official handbook*, Oakbrook Terrace, Ill, 2007, The Commission.

White G and others: Dysphagia: causes, assessment, treatment, and management, *Geriatrics* 63(5):15, 2008.

RESEARCH REFERENCES

Abe S and others: Tongue-coating as risk indicator for aspiration pneumonia in edentate elderly, *Arch Gerontol Geriatr*, epub ahead of print Oct 1, 2007.

Adams CR: Lessons learned from urban Latinas with Type 2 diabetes mellitus, *J Transcult Nurs* 14(3):255, 2003.

Baldwin C and others: *Dietary advice for illness-related malnutrition in adults (Cochrane Review)*, Oxford, 2003, Update Software.

Huang and others: Training in swallowing prevents aspiration pneumonia in stroke patients with dysphagia. *J Int Med Res* 34(3):303, 2006.

Loeb M and others: Interventions to prevent aspiration pneumonia in older adults: a systematic review, *J Am Geriatr Soc* 51(7):1018, 2003.

Martino R and others: Dysphagia after stroke: incidence, diagnosis, and pulmonary complications, *Stroke* 36(12): 2756, 2005.

Ng WQ, Neill J: Evidence for early oral feeding of patients after elective open colorectal surgery: a literature review, *J Clin Nurs* 15(6):696. 2006.

Perry L, McLaren S: Eating difficulties after stroke, *J Adv Nurs* 43(4):360, 2003.

Ramsey D and others: Early assessments of dysphagia and aspiration risk in acute stroke patients, *Stroke* 34(5):1252, 2003.

Ramsey D and others: Silent aspiration: what do we know? *Dysphagia* 20(3):218, 2005.

Schmid A and others: Recording the nutrient intake of nursing home residents by food weighing method and measuring the physical activity, *J Nutr Health Aging* 7(5):294, 2003.

Stratton R, Elia M: Who benefits from nutritional support: what is the evidence? *Eur J Gastroenterol Hepatol* 19(5):353, 2007.

Stratton RJ and others: *Disease-related malnutrition: an evidence based approach to treatment*, Oxford, 2003, CABI Publishing.

Stratton RJ and others: Food snacks or liquid oral nutritional supplements as a first line treatment for malnutrition in post-operative patients? *Proc Nutr Soc* 65:4a, 2006.

Enteral Nutrition

KEY TERMS

Enteral nutrition

Gastrostomy feeding tube

Jejunostomy feeding tube

Nasogastric (NG) feeding tube

Pulmonary aspiration

Residual volume

MEDIA RESOURCES

- **evolve** http://evolve.elsevier.com/Perry/skills
  learning system
  - Review Questions
  - Video Clips

- **View Video!** Mosby's Nursing Video Skills, 3.0

- **NSO** Nursing Skills Online

Mastery of content in this chapter will enable the nurse to:
- Assess the patient who is to receive enteral tube feedings.
- Demonstrate ability to correctly insert a small-bore feeding tube.
- Discuss the rationale for methods to determine nasogastric or nasoenteric feeding tube placement.

- Discuss the risk for pulmonary complications during the insertion and maintenance of a feeding tube.
- Demonstrate the appropriate technique for irrigating a feeding tube.
- Demonstrate three appropriate techniques for administering enteral formulas.
- Evaluate the patient's tolerance of enteral feeding.

Enteral nutrition, commonly called tube feeding, is the administration of nutrients through the gastrointestinal tract (GI) when a patient cannot ingest, chew, or swallow but can digest and absorb nutrients. The selection of tube type and placement depends on the patient's needs. Nasogastric (NG) or nasoenteric feeding is usually done for short periods of time, usually less than 30 days. A nurse passes these tubes through the nose or mouth with the end terminating in either the stomach or small bowel. Patients with long-term needs or who have no easy access to the GI tract through the nose or mouth or have other contraindications for this type of access, are in need of more-invasive access to the GI tract. These types of tubes include gastrostomy and jejunostomy tubes. There are several different methods for placement of these tubes, including endoscopy, radiological placement, and surgery. The tubes are used in a similar way; placement depends on factors related to the patient and the institution. The main complication related to feeding tubes is pulmonary aspiration with possible lung compromise. Other complications include misplaced tubes, infection, diarrhea, tube clogging, and tube dislodgment.

The nurse, dietitian, and physician collaborate to select an enteral feeding formula based on the patient's protein and calorie requirements and digestive ability. Formulas in the United States are sterile and lactose free. Disease-specific formulas are available, but research does not always support their efficacy (Worthington and Reyen, 2004a).

EVIDENCE-BASED PRACTICE TRENDS

Patients who are unable to consume adequate nutrients for short periods of time receive enteral nutrition. Nasoenteric tubes are contraindicated in patients with facial trauma, prolonged bleeding, and upper GI blockage, as with solid cancer. Once a tube is safely placed into the GI tract (esophagus), the next step is to attempt to place the tube into the stomach, and if possible, beyond the pylorus into the small bowel (Fig. 31-1). Tubes placed into the small bowel in this manner are thought to reduce the incidence of pulmonary aspiration of stomach contents, because the tube goes beyond the natural sphincters controlling reflux. However, researchers do not agree on this point (Baskin, 2006; de Aguilar-Nascimento, 2007), and tubes are reported to migrate back into the stomach.

The main complication related to nasogastric tube insertion is inadvertent pulmonary intubation. Researchers find that the incidence of this complication is as high as 5%, and it is often found in patients without adequate gag reflex (Worthington, 2004c). Patients at highest risk for pulmonary aspiration are often in need of a gastrostomy tube. Complications related to long-term placement of NG tubes include otitis media, sinusitis, nasal septum erosion, and patient discomfort. Patients needing tube feeding for a longer period (more than 30 days) are candidates for a more permanent solution, such as gastrostomy or jejunostomy tube (Worthington, 2004c).

Pulmonary aspiration is a common complication related to tube feedings. Pulmonary aspiration occurs when gastric contents enter the tracheobronchial passages. Preventive measures have been studied, but incidence of aspiration remains high, and patients with altered mental status are at highest risk. The use of gastric and intestinal pH measurements have been shown to differentiate tube placement, with the stomach having a lower pH than the intestines (Metheny, 2006). This helps to ensure the tube is beyond the pylorus, theoretically reducing the risk for aspiration. Carbon dioxide (CO_2) sensors are helpful in determining tube placement between the stomach and the lung. A small plastic piece with an imbedded yellow sensor is attached to the end of the feeding tube; the sensor changes color when carbon dioxide is present (Roberts and others, 2007). Investigators show that this reduces the incidence of inadvertent pulmonary placement. Head of bed elevation to a minimum of 30 degrees is a simple method to keep the risk for aspiration at a minimum. The nurse is instrumental in achieving this goal.

Current evidence-based practice indicates the most reliable method of feeding tube verification is chest radiograph (Rauen and others, 2008). Other methods, described above, are helpful before and after radiological confirmation is determined. Tolerance of tube feedings is usually determined by syringe aspiration of gastric contents. Researchers do not agree on an exact amount of gastric residual volume to indicate formula (feeding) tolerance. NG tubes used for feeding range in size from 8 Fr to 12 Fr. This small size makes aspiration of gastric contents difficult, and frequent aspiration may lead to clogged feeding tubes, another complication. Tube feedings are stopped if the patient has high gastric residual (more than 200 mL). Researchers agree that gastric aspiration should be used in conjunction with the patient's clinical condition before feedings are stopped (Metheny, 2006). Studies of enteral nutrition show that the best outcomes occur when an interdisciplinary team, including a nurse, a physician, a dietitian, and a pharmacist (nutrition support team), directs care (Cirgin Ellitt, 2006; Metheny, 2006; Rauen, 2008).

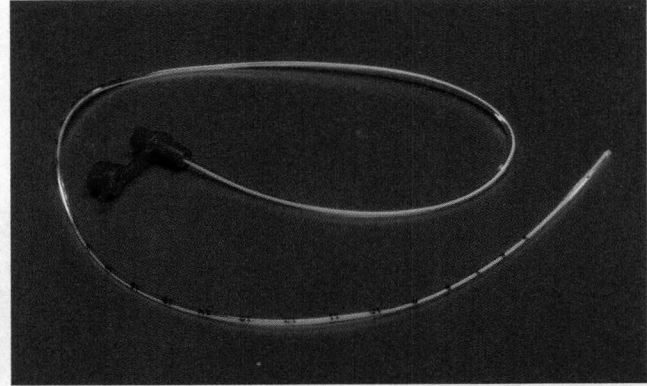

FIG 31-1   Small-bore feeding tube. (*Courtesy Kendall Brands, Mansfield, Mass.*)

CULTURAL CONSIDERATIONS

There are patients who have ethical as well as cultural concerns about artificial feedings. Patients with a living will or other advance directive may specifically refuse the use of artificial feeding by tube. This decision must be honored. Family members are not always willing to consent to this therapy whether or not an advance directive exists. Be sensitive to patients and families with strong opinions about this subject (Worthington, 2004c).

Food is an important part of life in most cultures. Many social, religious, and cultural events include food, and patients with tube feedings may participate in these events. Preparation for discharge is a good time to discuss this with caregivers, especially if a patient is going home or to another facility where group interaction is possible. If oral intake is not contraindicated, the tube-fed patient may be able to partake in some of the "real" food. This intervention may aid in the patient's well-being.

 Skill Performance Guidelines

1 Know the purpose of the feeding and the appropriate type of tube.
2 Know the psychological implications associated with the insertion and use of a feeding tube. The patient and family/significant other will need reassurance and encouragement throughout the insertion procedure.
3 Be aware of safety measures to prevent pulmonary aspiration of gastric contents and accidental dislodgment by the patient.
4 Consider the patient's medications and their route of delivery. Not all oral medications are safe to give by nasoenteric tube. Consult with physician and pharmacist, if necessary.
5 Hold tube feedings when a patient needs to travel for procedures or other therapy.

SKILL 31-1   Inserting a Nasogastric or Nasoenteric Feeding Tube

 Intermediate / Enteral Nutrition / Inserting a Nasogastric Tube

[NSO] *Enteral Nutrition Module / Lessons 1 and 2*

Throughout this chapter, feeding tubes are referred to as NG tubes or feeding tubes. Not all NG tubes are considered feeding tubes or used as feeding tubes. The composition of some NG tubes is polyvinylchloride, rendering a stiff plastic tube. These are usually used to evacuate stomach contents or for gastric decompression (see Chapter 34). They are not designed to use long term. These larger, stiffer tubes may increase pulmonary aspiration of stomach contents.

Tubes used specifically for feeding are composed of either silicone or polyurethane. They are softer and more flexible, and patients report that they are more comfortable. These tubes are more difficult to insert. Some tubes are weighted, and research shows that weighted tubes are superior to nonweighted tubes. Tubes are generally coated with a hydrophilic substance that is activated when exposed to water, making it slippery and easier to insert. A nurse activates the substance immediately before insertion by simply flushing the tube inside and out with water. Wire stylets are included with some tubes, but not all. Stylets are thought to improve insertion success but have also been implicated as increased risk for nasopulmonary intubation. You can pass a feeding tube without the use of a stylet. Nurses often pass feeding tubes through the mouth, especially in critical care when the patient is also intubated for respiratory support.

Placement of a feeding tube requires a physician's order. Patients with facial injuries or craniofacial surgery are not candidates for a nasogastric feeding tube. When facial trauma or recent maxillofacial surgery is present, there is a risk for improper placement of the tube, such as in the brain. Any type of nasogastric tube should be placed under fluoroscopy.

Delegation Considerations

The skill of feeding tube insertion cannot be delegated to nursing assistive personnel (NAP). However, NAP may assist with patient positioning during tube insertion.

Equipment

❑ Nasogastric or nasoenteric tube (8 to 12 Fr) with or without stylet (see Fig. 31-1)
❑ 60-mL catheter-tip Luer-Lok syringe
❑ Stethoscope
❑ Hypoallergenic tape, semipermeable (transparent) dressing, or tube fixation device
❑ Tincture of benzoin or other skin barrier protectant
❑ pH indicator strip (scale 0.0 to 14.0)
❑ Cup of water and straw (for patients able to swallow)
❑ Emesis basin
❑ Towel
❑ Facial tissues
❑ Clean gloves
❑ Suction equipment in case of aspiration
❑ Penlight to check placement in nasopharynx
❑ Tongue blade

STEP	RATIONALE

ASSESSMENT

1 Verify health care provider's order for type of tube and enteric feeding schedule.	A health care provider's order is needed to intubate patient with a feeding tube.
2 Assess patient's weight for height, hydration status, electrolyte balance, and organ function. Consult with nutrition support team or registered dietitian on need for enteral feedings.	Determines appropriate formula and method of administration.
3 Have patient close each nostril alternately and breathe. Examine each naris for patency and skin breakdown.	Sometimes nares are obstructed or irritated, or septal defect or facial fractures are present.
4 Review patient's medical history (e.g., for nasal problems, nosebleeds, facial trauma, nasal surgery, deviated septum, anticoagulant therapy, coagulopathy).	History of these problems may require nurse to consult with health care provider to change route of nutritional support.

STEP	RATIONALE

5 Assess patient's mental status, and assess for a gag reflex and ability to swallow.

Alert patient is better able to cooperate with procedure. If vomiting should occur, an alert patient can usually expectorate vomitus, which can help to reduce the risk for aspiration.

Critical Decision Point   *Feeding tubes may be inserted in patients with altered or decreased level of consciousness, but risk for inadvertent respiratory placement is increased if there is an impaired gag reflex (Roberts and others, 2007).*

6 Auscultate abdomen for bowel sounds.

Absence of bowel sounds may indicate decreased or absent peristalsis, contraindicating feedings.

7 Determine if the health care provider wants a prokinetic agent administered before the placement of tube.

Prokinetic agents, such as metoclopramide, given *before* tube placement help advance the tube into the intestine (Metheny, 2006).

NURSING DIAGNOSES

- Imbalanced nutrition: less than body requirements
- Readiness for enhanced nutrition
- Risk for aspiration

Individualize related factors based on patient's condition or needs.

PLANNING

1 Expected outcomes following completion of procedure:
  - Verification that tube is in stomach or intestine.
  - Feeding tube will remain patent.
  - Patient has no respiratory distress (e.g., increased respiratory rate, coughing, poor color) or signs of discomfort or nasal trauma.

2 Explain procedure to patient, including sensations that will be felt during insertion.

3 Explain to patient how to communicate during intubation by raising index finger to indicate gagging or discomfort.

Correct placement (Metheny, 2006).
Proper irrigation is achieved (Reising and Neal, 2005).
Tube correctly placed causes no interference with airway; tube correctly secured minimizes irritation to nares.

Increases patient's cooperation with intubation procedure and helps lessen anxiety.
It is important for patient to have a way of communicating to alleviate stress.

IMPLEMENTATION

1 Perform hand hygiene.

2 Position patient in high-Fowler's position, unless contraindicated. If patient is comatose, place in semi-Fowler's position with head propped forward using a pillow. If necessary, have an assistant help with positioning of confused or comatose patients. If patient is forced to lie supine, place in reverse Trendelenburg's position.

3 Determine length of tube to be inserted, and mark location with tape or indelible ink.
  a Measure distance from tip of nose to earlobe to xiphoid process of sternum (see illustration).

Reduces transmission of microorganisms.
Reduces risk for pulmonary aspiration in event patient should vomit (Metheny, 2006). Head propped assists with closure of airway and passage of the tube into the esophagus.

Length approximates distance from nose to stomach in 98% of patients.

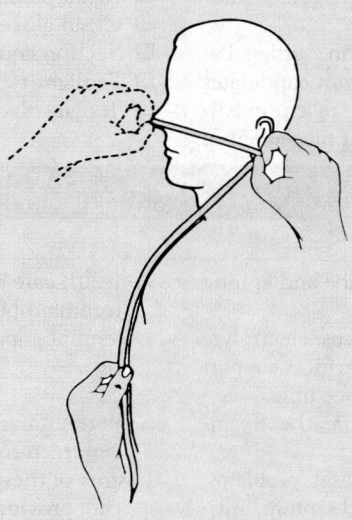

STEP 3a   Determine length of tube to be inserted.

STEP	RATIONALE

Critical Decision Point   *Tip of tube must reach stomach. Measure distance from tip of nose to earlobe to xyphoid process of sternum.*

4   Prepare nasogastric or nasoenteric tube for intubation. NOTE: Do not use plastic tubes.

   a   Perform hand hygiene.   Reduces spread of microorganisms.

   b   Inject 10 mL of water from 30-mL or larger Luer-Lok catheter-tip syringe into the tube.   Activates lubrication of tube for easier passage and ensures tube is patent. Aids in insertion.

   c   If using stylet, make certain the stylet is securely positioned against tube tip and that both Luer-Lok connections are snugly fit.   Promotes smooth passage of tube into GI tract. Improperly positioned stylet can induce serious trauma.

5   Cut hypoallergenic tape 10 cm (4 inches) long, or prepare membrane dressing or other securing device.   To be used to secure tubing after insertion.

6   Apply clean gloves.   Reduces transmission of microorganisms.

7   *Option:* Dip tube with surface lubricant into glass of room-temperature water, or apply water-soluble lubricant (see manufacturer's directions).   Activates lubricant to facilitate passage of tube into naris and GI tract.

8   Hand the alert patient a cup of water with straw (if able to swallow).   Patient will be asked to swallow water to facilitate tube passage.

9   Explain the step, and gently insert tube through nostril to back of throat (posterior nasopharynx). This may cause patient to gag. Aim back and down toward ear.   Natural contours facilitate passage of tube into GI tract.

10   Have patient flex head toward chest after tube has passed through nasopharynx.   Closes off glottis and reduces risk for tube entering trachea.

11   Encourage patient to swallow by giving small sips of water or ice chips. Advance tube as patient swallows. Rotate tube 180 degrees while inserting.   Swallowing facilitates passage of tube past oropharynx.

12   Emphasize need to mouth breathe and swallow during the procedure.   Helps facilitate passage of tube and alleviates patient's fears during the procedure.

13   When tip of tube reaches the carina (approximately 25 cm [10 inches] in the adult), stop and listen for air exchange from the distal portion of the tube.   Air may indicate that tube is in the respiratory tract; remove and start over (Baskin, 2006). Never use this step for tube verification.

14   Advance tube each time patient swallows until desired length has been passed (see illustration).   Reduces discomfort and trauma to patient.

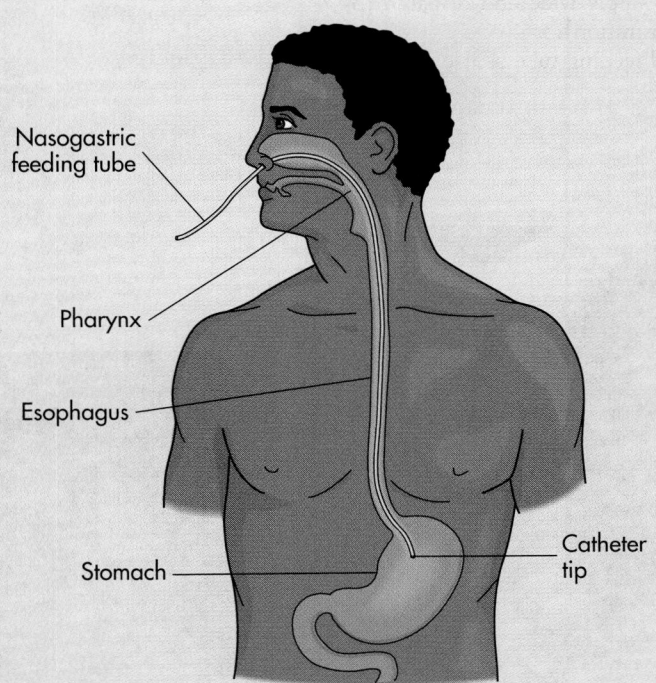

Nasogastric feeding tube

Pharynx

Esophagus

Stomach

Catheter tip

STEP 14   NG feeding tube inserted through nose and esophagus into stomach.

STEP	RATIONALE

Critical Decision Point *Do not force tube. If you meet resistance or if patient starts to cough, choke, or become cyanotic, stop advancing the tube, pull tube back, and start over.*

15 Check for position of tube in back of throat with penlight and tongue blade.	Tube may be coiled, kinked, or entering trachea.
16 Temporarily anchor tube to the nose with a small piece of tape.	Movement of the tube stimulates gagging. Assesses general position before anchoring tube more securely.
17 Check placement of tube by aspirating stomach contents (see Skill 31-2).	Proper tube position is essential before initiating feeding.

Critical Decision Point *Insufflation of air into tube while auscultating abdomen is not a reliable means to determine position of feeding tube tip (Rauen, 2008).*

18 Anchor tube to nose: After you obtain gastric aspirates, attach tube to patient's nose, avoiding pressure on nares. Mark exit site with indelible ink. Select one of the following options for anchoring:	A properly secured tube allows the patient more mobility and prevents trauma to nasal mucosa.
a Apply tape:	Prevents pulling of tube. May require frequent change if tape becomes soiled.
(1) Apply tincture of benzoin or other skin adhesive on tip of patient's nose, and allow it to become "tacky."	Helps tape adhere better. Protects skin.
(2) Remove gloves and split one end of tape lengthwise 5 cm (2 inches).	
(3) Place the intact end of tape over bridge of patient's nose. Wrap each of the 5-cm strips in opposite directions around tube as it exits nose (see illustration).	Secures tube firmly.
b Apply membrane dressing or tube fixation device:	Permits longer securement without need to change dressing.
(1) Membrane dressing: Apply tincture of benzoin or other skin protector to patient's cheek and area of tube to be secured.	
(2) Place tube against patient's cheek, and secure tube with membrane dressing, out of patient's line of vision.	Decreases risk for patient's inadvertent extubation.
(3) Tube fixation device: Apply wide end of patch to bridge of nose (see illustration).	
(4) Slip connector around feeding tube as it exits nose (see illustration).	

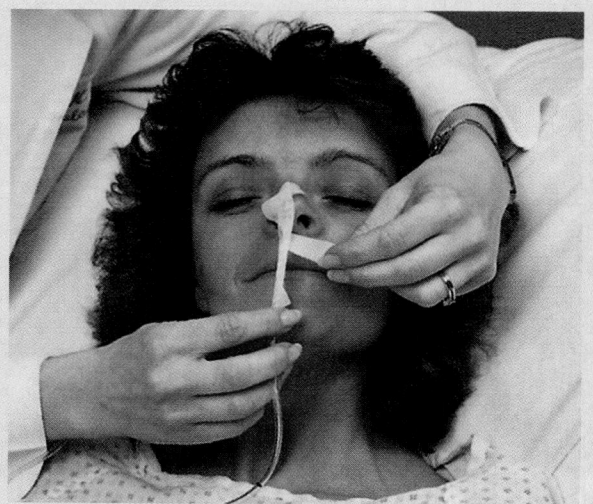

STEP 18a(3) Wrapping tape to anchor nasoenteral tube.

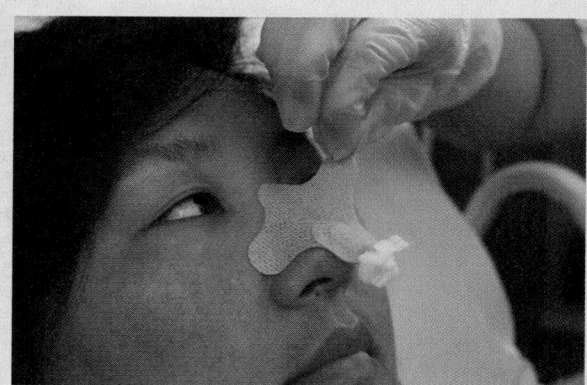

STEP 18b(3) Applying tube fixation patch to bridge of nose.

STEP	RATIONALE

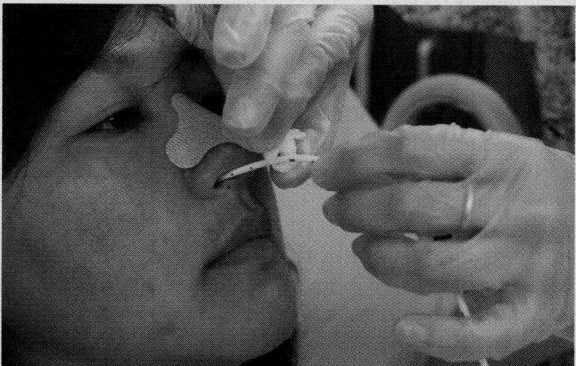

STEP 18b(4) Slip connector around feeding tube.

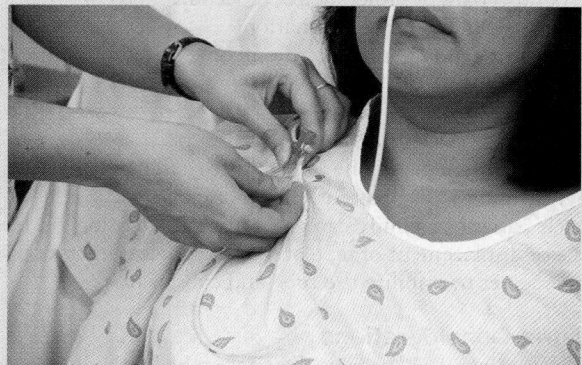

STEP 19 Fastening feeding tube to patient's gown.

19 Fasten end of NG tube to patient's gown using a clip (see illustration) or piece of tape. Do not use safety pins to pin the tube to the patient's gown.

Reduces traction on the naris if tube moves.
Safety pins become unfastened and cause injury to the patient.

20 Assist patient to a comfortable position.

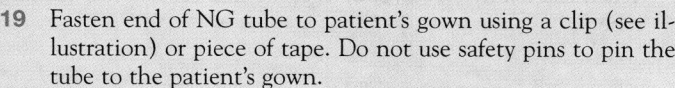

Critical Decision Point *Leave stylet in place (if used) until correct position is verified by x-ray film. Never attempt to reinsert a partially or fully removed stylet while feeding tube is in place. This can cause perforation of the tube and injure the patient.*

21 Obtain x-ray film of chest/abdomen.

X-ray examination is the most accurate method to determine feeding tube placement (Rauen, 2008).

22 Apply clean gloves and administer oral hygiene (see Chapter 17). Cleanse tubing at nostril with washcloth dampened in mild soap and water.

Promotes patient comfort and integrity of oral mucous membranes.

23 Remove gloves, dispose of equipment, and perform hand hygiene.

Reduces transmission of microorganisms.

EVALUATION

1 Observe patient to determine response to intubation. Have the patient speak. Check vital signs and oxygen saturation.

A patient who is comfortable, able to speak without difficulty, and has normal oxygen saturation is likely to have a correctly placed tube.

2 Confirm x-ray results.

Proper position is essential before initiating feedings.

3 Remove the stylet (if used) after x-ray verification of correct placement.

4 Routinely assess location of external exit site marking on the tube, as well as color and pH of fluid withdrawn from the tube.

Reveals if end of tube has changed position. However, it is possible that the tube can change position inside the GI tract with no external evidence of the change.

Unexpected Outcomes

1 Placement of the tube into the respiratory tract. This may not be discovered until the x-ray report. A small-bore tube can enter the airway without causing obvious respiratory symptoms, particularly in a semiconscious or unconscious patient.

2 Aspiration of stomach contents into respiratory tract (immediate response) in the alert patient, evidenced by coughing, dyspnea, cyanosis, or decreases in oxygen saturation values during the procedure.

3 Aspiration of stomach contents into respiratory tract (delayed response or small-volume aspiration), evidenced by auscultation of crackles or wheezes, dyspnea, or fever.

4 Clogging of feeding tube.

5 Nasal mucosa becomes inflamed, tender, and/or eroded.

Related Interventions

- Remove the tube, and report the incident to the health care provider.
- Obtain order for reinsertion.

- Position the patient on side to protect the airway.
- Suction the patient nasotracheally or orotracheally to try to remove aspirated substance (see Chapter 25).
- Report the event immediately to the health care provider.

- Report change in patient condition to the health care provider; if there has not been a recent chest x-ray film, suggest ordering one.
- Prepare for possible initiation of antibiotics.

- Irrigate tube (see Skill 31-3).

- Retape the tube in a different position to relieve pressure on mucosa.
- If the tube has been in the same site for an extended period, consider reinsertion of the tube in the opposite naris (health care provider's order required).

Recording and Reporting

- Record and report type and size of tube placed, location of distal tip of tube, patient's tolerance of procedure, and confirmation of tube position by x-ray examination.
- Report any type of unexpected outcome and the interventions performed.

Teaching Considerations

- Instruct patient or family caregiver to offer oral hygiene frequently and to keep patient's lips lubricated.
- Teach patient or family caregiver to report tension on feeding tube or displacement of tape or fixation device; instruct patient or caregiver to stabilize the tube and call for help.

Pediatric Considerations

- *Premature infant and neonate:* Estimate tube length by measuring from the nose or mouth to the earlobe then to the xiphoid process (Axelrod and others, 2006).
- *Older child:* Estimate tube length by either (1) measuring from the nose to the bottom of the earlobe then to the lower end of the xiphoid process or (2) measuring from the nose to the earlobe then to a point midway between the xiphoid process and the umbilicus (Axelrod and others, 2006).
- In infant, observe for vagal stimulation during insertion of feeding tube, resulting in decreased heart rate.

Gerontological Considerations

- Ensure adequate lubrication of tube to decrease discomfort for the older adult, because of the potential for decreased oral or nasopharyngeal secretions.

Home Care Considerations

- Assess the patient or primary caregiver's ability to maintain tube for a feeding program.
- Assess the environmental safety and sanitation of patient's home to determine potential for infection or injury.
- Teach patient or primary caregiver how to assess tube placement (see Skill 31-2).
- Teach the family caregiver correct method for securing feeding tube.

SKILL 31-2 Verifying Feeding Tube Placement

NSO *Enteral Nutrition Module / Lesson 3*

Nurses insert small-bore feeding tubes nasally or orally into the stomach for either intermittent or continuous feedings. Nurses also insert the tubes into the small intestine (duodenum or proximal jejunum) for continuous feedings. Large-bore tubes are not suitable for small bowel feedings. Intermittent feedings are boluses administered over a short time period; therefore they are only given into the stomach, because it is a natural reservoir for fluid (ASPEN, 2007).

It is possible for the tip of a feeding tube to move into a different location (from the stomach to the intestine or from the intestine into the stomach) without any external evidence that the tube has moved. The risk for aspiration of regurgitated gastric contents into the respiratory tract increases when the tip of the tube accidentally dislocates upward into the esophagus.

Following initial x-ray verification that a tube is positioned in the desired site (either the stomach or small intestine), you are responsible for ensuring that the tube has remained in the intended position before administering formula or medications through the tube. Therefore you must verify tube position every 4 to 6 hours and as needed (Metheny, 2006). Because it is not practical to do radiographic checks at this frequency, other methods of determining placement have been investigated. Certain characteristics of fluid aspirated from feeding tubes are helpful in assessing placement of the tube. Color may differentiate gastric from intestinal placement. Because most intestinal aspirates are stained by bile to a distinct yellow color, and most gastric aspirates are not, the difference can often distinguish the sites (Fig. 31-2) (Rauen and others, 2008). The pH of an aspirate offers valuable data as well in assessing placement of a feeding tube (Metheny, 2006). Bedside testing of pH using pH paper covering a range from 0 to 14 is sufficient for this purpose; a properly obtained pH value of 0 to 4 is a good indication of gastric placement (Metheny, 2006).

Delegation Considerations

The verification of tube placement is the responsibility of the nurse and may not be delegated to NAP. The nurse directs the NAP to:

- Immediately inform the nurse if patient's respirations change or patient complains of shortness of breath, coughing, or choking.
- Immediately inform the nurse if the patient vomits or the NAP notices vomitus in patient's mouth during oral hygiene.
- Immediately inform the nurse if nasal skin irritation is present.
- Immediately inform the nurse if displacement of the feeding tube occurs.

Equipment

- ❑ 60-mL Luer-Lok catheter-tip syringe
- ❑ Stethoscope
- ❑ Clean gloves
- ❑ pH indicator strip (scale of 0.0 to 14.0)
- ❑ Small medication cup

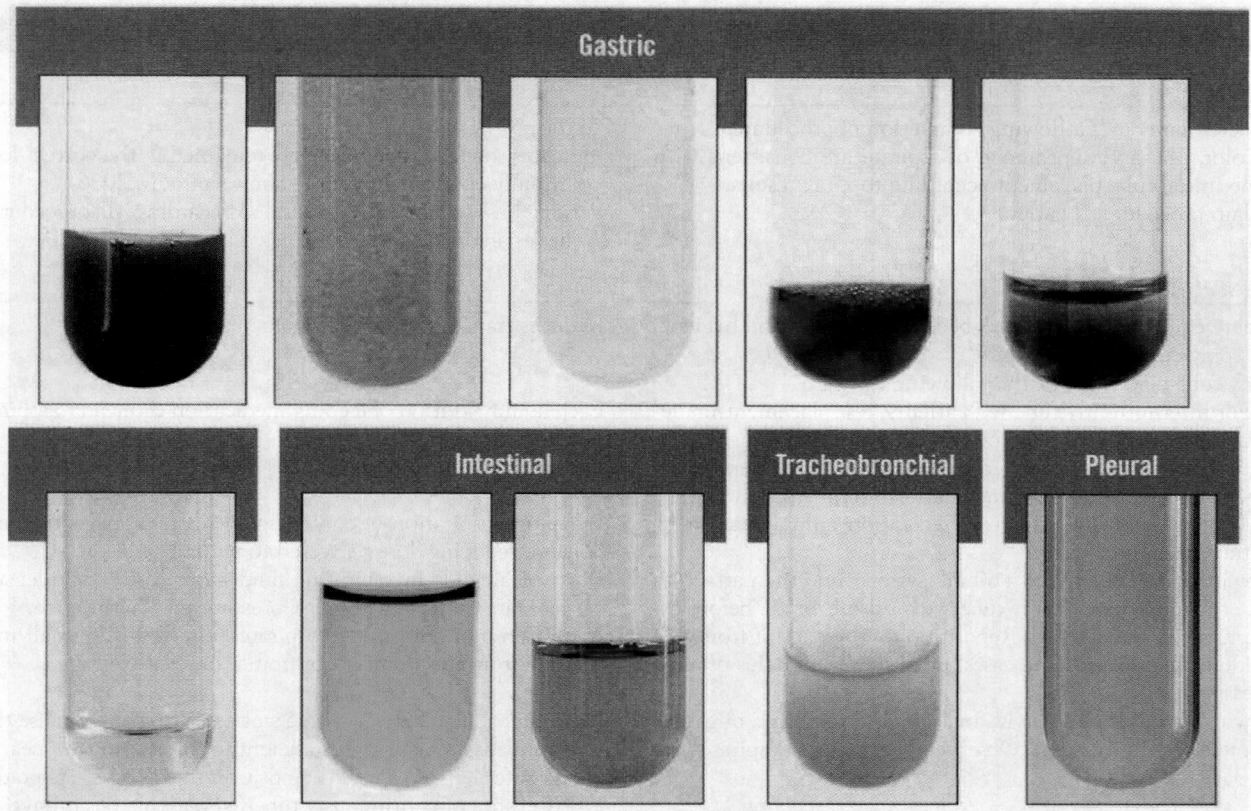

FIG 31-2 Typical color of aspirates from stomach, intestine, and airway. (*Used with permission from Metheny NA and others: pH, color, and feeding tubes*, RN 61:25, 1998.)

STEP	RATIONALE

ASSESSMENT

1 Be aware of policy and procedures for frequency and method of checking tube placement in your facility.	Maintains quality of patient care. Some facilities allow an auscultation method. Verifying tube placement by air insufflation has been proven to be an unreliable method (Rauen, 2008). Make sure x-ray confirmation was obtained at the time of placement.
2 Identify signs and symptoms of inadvertent respiratory migration of feeding tube: coughing, choking, or cyanosis.	Signs and symptoms indicate accidental migration of feeding tube into the airway. However, their absence does not ensure that respiratory migration has not occurred, especially in a patient with altered level of consciousness and/or altered gag and cough reflexes.

3 Identify conditions that increase the risk for spontaneous tube dislocation:
  a Retching/vomiting
  b Nasotracheal suction
  c Severe bouts of coughing.
	Feeding tubes may become dislocated by increases in intraabdominal pressure or coughing.

4 Observe the external portion of the tube for movement of the ink mark away from the mouth or naris (see Skill 31-1).	Increased external length of a tube indicates that the distal tip is no longer in the correct position.
5 Review patient's medication record for a gastric acid inhibitor (e.g., cimetidine, ranitidine, famotidine, nizatidine) or a proton pump inhibitor (e.g., omeprazole).	H_2 receptor antagonists reduce volume of gastric acid secretion and the acid content of secretions, thus causing the pH value to be higher, that is, more basic (Metheny, 2006).
6 Review patient's record for history of prior tube displacement.	Patients are at increased risk for repeated tube displacement.

NURSING DIAGNOSES

- Impaired gas exchange
- Risk for aspiration

Individualize related factors based on patient's condition or needs.

STEP	RATIONALE

PLANNING

1 Expected outcomes following completion of procedure:
   - Color, pH, and appearance of aspirate are consistent with the initial tube placement according to x-ray results.
2 Explain procedure to patient.

Indicates that the tube has likely remained in the correct location, initially confirmed by x-ray film (Metheny, 2006).

Patient has a right to be informed regarding all procedures. Relieves anxiety.

IMPLEMENTATION

1 Prepare equipment at patient's bedside, perform hand hygiene, and apply clean gloves.

Reduces transmission of microorganisms.

2 Verify tube placement at the following times:
   a For intermittently tube-fed patients, test placement immediately before each feeding and before medications.
   b For continuously tube-fed patients, test placement every 4 to 6 hours and before medication administration.
   c Wait at least 1 hour after medication administration by tube or mouth.

Each administration of feeding/medication can lead to aspiration if the tube is displaced.

Determines if tube migration has occurred.

Premature aspiration of contents will remove unabsorbed medication, reducing dose delivered to patient.

3 Draw up 30 mL of air into a 60-mL syringe, and then attach to end of feeding tube. Flush tube with 30 mL of air before attempting to aspirate fluid. Repositioning the patient from side to side is helpful. In some cases, more than one bolus of air is necessary.

Burst of air aids in aspirating fluid more easily. Smaller syringes generate unnecessarily high pressures inside the tube.

It is often more difficult to aspirate fluid from the small intestine than from the stomach, or from a smaller size tube.

4 Draw back on syringe slowly, and obtain 5 to 10 mL of gastric aspirate (see illustration). Observe appearance of aspirate (see Fig. 31-2).

Drawing back quickly or with a smaller syringe may cause the tube to collapse. Quantity is sufficient for pH testing. Appearance of aspirate helps to assess the position of the tube. Aspirates from NG tubes of continuously tube-fed patients often have appearance of curdled enteral formula. Gastric aspirates from intermittently tube-fed patients are not typically bile stained (unless intestinal fluid has refluxed into the stomach).

5 Gently mix aspirate in syringe. Expel a few drops into a clean medicine cup. Measure pH of aspirated GI contents by dipping the pH strip into the fluid or by applying a few drops of the fluid to the strip. Compare the color of the strip with the color on the chart (see illustration) provided by the manufacturer (Metheny, 2006).
   a Gastric fluid from patient who has fasted for at least 4 hours usually has pH range of 1 to 4.

Mixing ensures equal distribution of contents for testing. Most-accurate readings of gastric pH levels are provided by pH paper covering a minimal range of range from 0 to 14 (Metheny, 2006).

Range of 0 to 4 is a reliable indicator of stomach placement, especially when a gastric acid inhibitor is not being used.

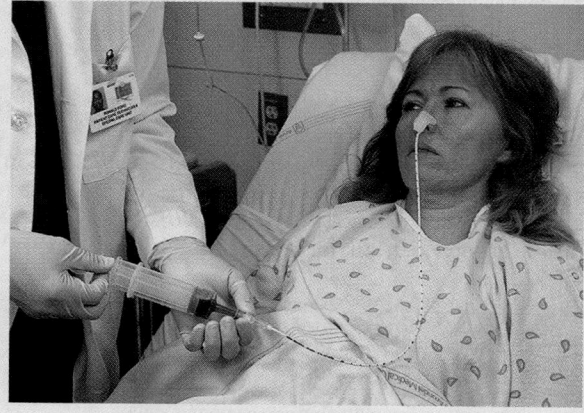

STEP 4   Obtaining gastric aspirate.

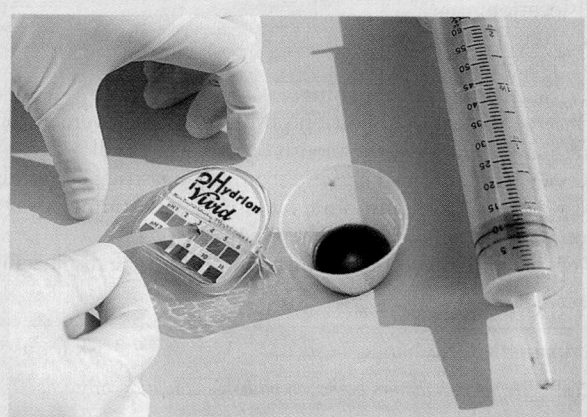

STEP 5   Compare color on test strip with color on pH chart.

STEP	RATIONALE
b Fluid from tube in small intestine of fasting patient usually has pH greater than 6.	Intestinal contents are more basic than stomach contents (Metheny, 2006).
c Patient with continuous tube feeding may have pH of 5 or higher.	Formulas contain solutions that are basic.
d The pH of pleural fluid from the tracheobronchial tree is generally greater than 6.	

Critical Decision Point *Auscultation of an air bolus is no longer considered a reliable or safe method for verification of tube position.*

STEP	RATIONALE
6 If after repeated attempts it is not possible to aspirate fluid from a tube that was confirmed by x-ray examination to be in desired position, and if (1) there are no risk factors for tube dislocation, (2) tube has remained in original taped position, and (3) patient is not experiencing respiratory distress, assume tube is correctly placed (Roberts and others, 2007).	It is reasonable to assume tube is correctly placed. When abdominal x-ray films are obtained for clinical reasons, you can take advantage of reports to monitor tube location.
7 Irrigate tube (see Skill 31-3).	Keeps tube patent.
8 Remove and dispose of gloves and supplies. Perform hand hygiene.	Reduces transmission of microorganisms.

EVALUATION

1 Observe patient for respiratory distress: persistent gagging, paroxysms of coughing, respiratory patterns (e.g., rate and depth) that are inconsistent with baseline measures.	Feeding enters airways.
2 Verify that color, pH, and appearance of aspirate are consistent with the initial tube placement according to x-ray results.	Indicates that the tip of the tube is likely to be positioned in the same place as it was following x-ray confirmation.

Unexpected Outcomes

1 Red or brown coloring (coffee grounds appearance) of fluid aspirated from a feeding tube indicates new blood or old blood, respectively, in the GI tract.

2 Patient develops severe respiratory distress (e.g., dyspnea, decreased oxygen saturation, increased pulse rate) as a result of aspiration or tube displacement into the lung.

3 Abdomen becomes distended.

Related Interventions

- If the color is not related to medications recently administered, notify the health care provider.

- Notify health care provider.
- Stop any enteral feedings.
- Obtain chest x-ray film as ordered.

- Notify health care provider.
- Stop enteral feedings.

Recording and Reporting
- Record and report pH and appearance of aspirate.

Teaching Considerations
- Instruct patient to not pull or alter position of nasoenteral tube.

Pediatric Considerations
- Decrease the amount of air insufflated according to the size of the patient (e.g., an infant may only need 1 mL of air, a small child 5 mL) before aspiration of gastric secretions.

Home Care Considerations
- Instruct patient or primary caregiver not to proceed with feedings or medication administration via the tube if there is any doubt as to proper placement of tube.

SKILL 31-3 Irrigating a Feeding Tube

Adequacy of nutritional support is essential in patient care, and for this reason feeding tubes must remain patent. Routine irrigation of a feeding tube maintains its patency. All types of feeding tubes require routine irrigation. Question the patency of a tube when you are unable to instill air or fluid through the tube.

There are other types of feeding tubes besides those inserted by nurses at the bedside. When patients cannot tolerate nasally or orally placed tubes, there are other options. See Procedural Guideline 31-1 (p. 846) for descriptions of gastrostomy and jejunostomy tubes. Both of these tubes require routine irrigation.

Delegation Considerations
The skill of irrigating a feeding tube cannot be delegated to NAP. The nurse directs the NAP to:
- Report when a continuous tube feeding stops infusing.

Equipment
- ❑ 60-mL Luer-Lok or catheter-tip syringe
- ❑ Water
- ❑ Towel
- ❑ Clean gloves

STEP	RATIONALE

ASSESSMENT

1 Inspect the volume, color, and character of gastric aspirates (if obtainable).

Thick secretions and a reduced volume of secretions indicate need to irrigate tube. Excess volume of secretions (more than 200 mL) indicates delayed gastric emptying.

2 Assess bowel sounds. Note ease with which tube feeding infuses through tubing.

Failure of formula to infuse as desired may indicate developing obstruction.

3 Monitor volume of tube-feeding formula administered during a shift, and compare with ordered amount.

Indicates whether sufficient volume of feeding is infusing.

4 Refer to agency policies regarding routine irrigation (usually every 4 to 12 hours) (Reising and others, 2005).

Determines frequency of irrigations.

NURSING DIAGNOSES

• Deficient fluid volume
• Excess fluid volume
• Imbalanced nutrition: less than body requirements

Individualize related factors based on patient's condition or needs.

PLANNING

1 Expected outcomes following completion of procedure:
  • Feeding tube remains patent.

Irrigation fluid clears inner lumen of feeding tube of accumulated solids and secretions.

  • Patient receives prescribed caloric intake.

Feeding infuses without interruption.

2 Explain procedure to patient.

Decreases patient anxiety.

3 Position patient in high-Fowler's (if tolerated) or semi-Fowler's position.

Reduces risk for aspiration during irrigation.

IMPLEMENTATION

1 Perform hand hygiene, prepare equipment at patient's bedside, and apply clean gloves.

Reduces transmission of microorganisms.
Ensures an organized approach to irrigation.

2 Verify tube placement (see Skill 31-2) if fluid can be aspirated.

With tip of tube correctly placed in stomach, irrigation will not increase risk for aspiration.

3 Draw up 30 mL of water in a syringe (see illustration). Do not use irrigation fluids from multidose bottles that are used on other patients. Patient should have personal bottle of solution.

This amount of solution will flush length of tube. Prevents contamination of fluids.

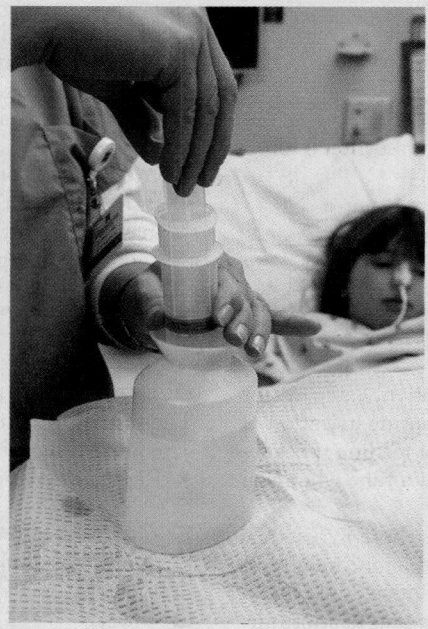

STEP 3   Draw up 30 mL of water into syringe.

STEP	RATIONALE
4 Change irrigation bottle every 24 hours.	Ensures sterile solution.
5 Position patient in semi-Fowler's position.	A slightly upright position helps prevent reflux.
6 Kink feeding tube while disconnecting it from feeding-bag tubing or while removing plug at end of tube (see illustration).	Prevents leakage of gastric secretions.
7 Insert tip of syringe into end of feeding tube. Release kink, and slowly instill irrigating solution (see illustration).	Infusion of fluid clears tubing.
8 If unable to instill fluid, reposition patient on left side, and try again.	Tip of tube may be against stomach wall. Changing patient's position may move tip away from stomach wall.
9 When water has been instilled, remove syringe. Reinstitute tube feeding, or administer medication as ordered. Irrigate before, between, and after the final medication (before feedings are reinstituted).	Tubing is clear and patent. Certain formulas have properties that predispose to tube clogging. Irrigation prevents mixing of medications in the tube, which may cause clogging. Flushes medications completely through the tube so medications do not mix with formula.
10 Remove and discard gloves; dispose of supplies. Perform hand hygiene.	Reduces transmission of microorganisms.

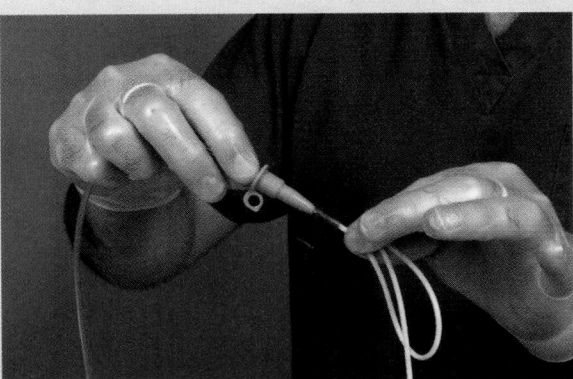

STEP 6   Kink tubing while unplugging feeding tube.

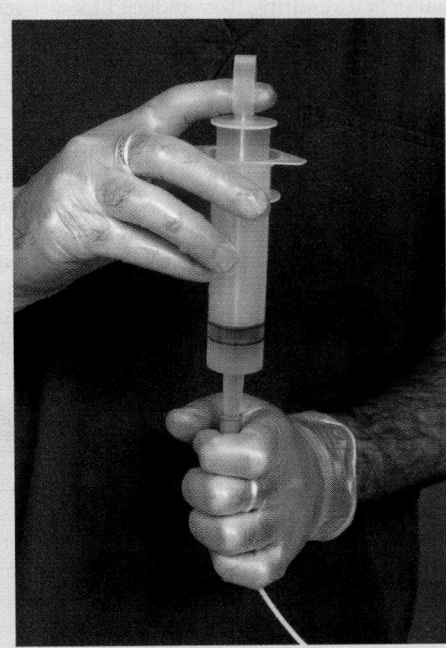

STEP 7   Irrigate feeding tube.

EVALUATION

1 Observe ease with which tube feeding instills through tubing.

A successfully irrigated tube is patent, allowing for free flow of solution.

Unexpected Outcomes

1 Tube cannot be irrigated and remains obstructed.

2 Fluid and electrolyte imbalances occur. Insufficient irrigation can cause water deficiency; excessive irrigations can cause fluid volume excess.

Related Interventions

• Reattempt irrigation; if unsuccessful, notify the health care provider. Tube may need to be removed and a new tube placed.

• Notify the health care provider of abnormal electrolyte levels or imbalanced intake and output.

Recording and Reporting

• Record time of irrigation, amount and type of fluid instilled.
• Report if tubing has become clogged.

Pediatric Considerations

• Irrigation of a tube requires a smaller volume of solution in children: 1 or 2 mL for small tubes to 5 to 15 mL or more for large ones (Axelrod and others, 2006).

SKILL 31-4   Administering Enteral Nutrition: Nasoenteric, Gasotrostomy, or Jejunostomy Tube

Intermediate / Enteral Nutrition / Providing Enteral Feedings

NSO   *Enteral Nutrition Module / Lesson 4*

Gastric feedings are the most common type of enteral nutrition, allowing tube-feeding formulas to enter the stomach and then pass more gradually through the intestinal tract to ensure absorption. Small bowel feeding occurs beyond the pyloric sphincter of the stomach, which theoretically reduces the risk for aspiration, provided that feedings do not reflux back into the stomach. Administer small bowel feedings continuously to prevent "dumping" syndrome (diarrhea).

The general indications for enteral feeding include the following:

1 Patients who cannot eat because of surgery, injury, or disease process (e.g., patients who are comatose, receiving mechanical ventilation, recovering from oral, head, and neck surgeries; patients with certain GI disorders).

2 Nutritional deficit resulting from reduced food ingestion, even when patients are physically capable of eating (e.g., confused patients, patients with head injury).

3 Patients with impaired swallowing or gag reflex (e.g., patients who have had a stroke).

Inadequate delivery of nutrients, potentially leading to malnutrition or electrolyte disturbances, sometimes occurs because of frequent interruptions in feeding (Worthington and Reyen, 2006). Administration of enteral nutrition is often delayed until after bowel sounds can be auscultated in patients. Researchers find it is safe to begin feedings before bowel sounds return, especially in patients with jejunostomy tubes, but this is not without risk. Take care to balance the benefits and risks by assessing for patient tolerance of early enteral feeding (Flesher and others, 2005).

Delegation Considerations

The skill of administration of nasoenteric tube feeding can be delegated to NAP. (Refer to agency policy.) However, a registered nurse (RN) or licensed practical nurse (LPN) must first verify tube placement and patency. The nurse directs the NAP to:

- Elevate head of bed to a minimum of 30 degrees or sit the patient up in bed or a chair.
- Infuse the feeding slowly.
- Report any difficulty infusing the feeding or any discomfort voiced by the patient.
- Report any gagging, paroxysms of coughing, or choking.

Equipment

- ❑ Disposable feeding bag, tubing, and formula or ready-to-hang system
- ❑ 30-mL or larger Luer-Lok or catheter-tip syringe
- ❑ Stethoscope
- ❑ Infusion pump (required for continuous feedings): Use pump designed for tube feedings
- ❑ pH indicator strip (scale 0.0 to 14.0)
- ❑ Prescribed enteral feeding
- ❑ Clean gloves
- ❑ Equipment to obtain blood glucose level by finger stick, if ordered

STEP	RATIONALE

ASSESSMENT

1 Assess patient's need for enteral tube feedings: decreased level of consiousness, a nutritional deficit, head or neck surgery, facial trauma, or impaired swallowing, and consult with nutrition support team or health care provider.	Identify patients who need tube feedings before they become nutritionally depleted.
2 Assess patient for food allergies.	Prevents patient from developing localized or systemic allergic responses to feeding.
3 Auscultate for bowel sounds before feeding.	Absent bowel sounds indicate decreased ability of GI tract to digest or absorb nutrients.
4 Obtain baseline weight, and review laboratory values (e.g., electrolytes, capillary blood glucose measurement). Assess patient for fluid volume excess or deficit, electrolyte abnormalities, and metabolic abnormalities (e.g., hyperglycemia).	Enteral feedings should restore or maintain a patient's nutritional status. Measures provide objective data and baseline to determine selection of formula and measure effectiveness of feedings.
5 Verify health care provider's order for formula, rate, route, and frequency.	Ensures correct formula will be administered in appropriate volume.

NURSING DIAGNOSES

- Imbalanced nutrition: less than body requirements
- Impaired swallowing
- Readiness for enhanced nutrition
- Risk for aspiration

Individualize related factors based on patient's condition or needs.

PLANNING

1 Expected outcomes following completion of procedure: • Patient experiences slow increase in weight. • Patient has no sign of respiratory distress.	Indicates that patient's nutritional status is maintained or improved. Feeding tube does not enter airway, and patient does not aspirate feeding.

STEP	RATIONALE
• Patient has no fluid or electrolyte imbalance.	Ordered schedule of feedings administered on time.
• Patient has no abdominal cramping.	Feeding administered without gastric distention.
2 Explain procedure to patient.	Decreases patient anxiety.

IMPLEMENTATION

STEP	RATIONALE
1 Perform hand hygiene.	Reduces transmission of microorganisms.
2 Prepare feeding container to administer formula:	
a Check expiration date on formula and integrity of container.	Ensures GI tolerance of formula. Prevents leakage of tube feeding.
b Have tube feeding formula at room temperature.	Cold formula causes gastric cramping and discomfort because the liquid is not warmed by mouth and esophagus.
c Connect tubing of administration set to container, or prepare ready-to-hang container. Use aseptic technique, and avoid handling the feeding system. If you need to handle the system, apply clean gloves.	The feeding system, including the bag, connections, and tubing, must be free of contamination to prevent bacterial growth (Mathus-Vliegen and others, 2006; Neely and others, 2006; Padula and others, 2004).
d Shake formula container well, and fill feeding container bag with formula (see illustration). Open roller clamp on tubing, and fill tubing (prime tubing) with formula. Close roller clamp, and cap end of tubing. Hang bag on feeding pump pole.	Filling the tubing with formula prevents excess air from entering GI tract once infusion begins.
3 For intermittent feeding have a syringe ready and be sure formula is at room temperature.	Cold formula causes gastric cramping.
4 Place patient in high-Fowler's position, or elevate head of bed at least 30 degrees. For patient forced to remain supine, place in reverse Trendelenburg's position.	Elevated head helps prevent aspiration.
5 If not applied earlier, apply gloves.	Reduces transmission of microorganisms.
6 Verify tube placement (see Skill 31-2). Attach syringe and aspirate 5 to 10 mL of gastric secretions. Observe appearance of aspirate, and note pH measure.	Gastric fluid for a patient who has fasted for 4 hours usually has a pH of 1 to 4. Continuous tube feedings elevates pH (Metheny, 2006).
a Nasoenteric (see Skill 31-2)	
b Gastrostomy tube: Attach syringe and aspirate 5 to 10 mL of gastric secretions, observe aspirate appearance, and check pH.	
c Jejunostomy tube: Aspirate intestinal secretions, observe aspirate appearance, and check pH.	Presence of intestinal fluid indicates that the end of the tube is in the small intestine.

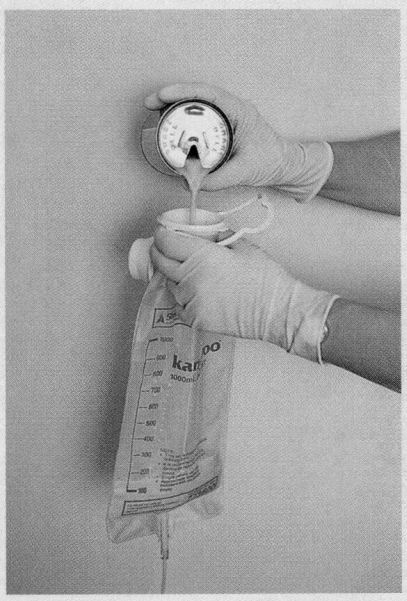

STEP 2d Pour formula into feeding container.

STEP	RATIONALE

7 Check gastric residual volume before each feeding for intermittent feedings, every 4 to 6 hours for continuous feedings (Metheny, 2006).

Intestinal residual is very small (≤10 mL); if residual volume is greater than 10 mL, displacement of the tube into the stomach may have occurred.

   a Draw up 30 mL air into syringe and connect to feeding tube.

   b Inject the air and then pull back slowly, and aspirate the total amount of gastric contents (see illustration).

   c Return aspirated contents to stomach unless volume exceeds 200 mL (check agency policy).

8 Flush with 30 mL water.

9 Initiate feeding:

   a Intermittent feeding:

     (1) Pinch proximal end of feeding tube, and remove cap.

Prevents excessive air from entering patient's stomach and leakage of gastric contents.

     (2) Attach end of administration set tubing to end of feeding tube. Label administration set as "Tube feeding only" (The Joint Commission, 2006). (NOTE: Some manufacturers now provide feeding tubes labeled "for feeding only.")

Prevents inadvertent administration of formula into intravenous access.

     (3) Set rate by adjusting roller clamp on tubing or placing on a feeding pump. Allow bag to empty gradually over 30 to 60 minutes (see illustration). Label bag with tube-feeding type, strength, and amount. Include date, time, and initials.

Gradual emptying of tube feeding by gravity from feeding bag reduces risk for abdominal discomfort, vomiting, or diarrhea induced by bolus or too-rapid infusion of tube feedings.

     (4) Change bag every 24 hours.

Decreases risk for bacterial colonization.

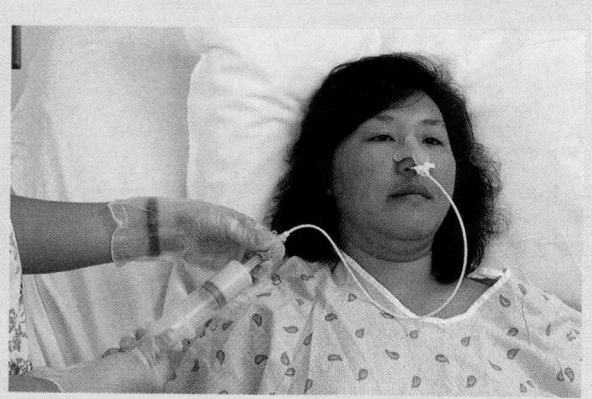

STEP 7b   Check for gastric residual volume.

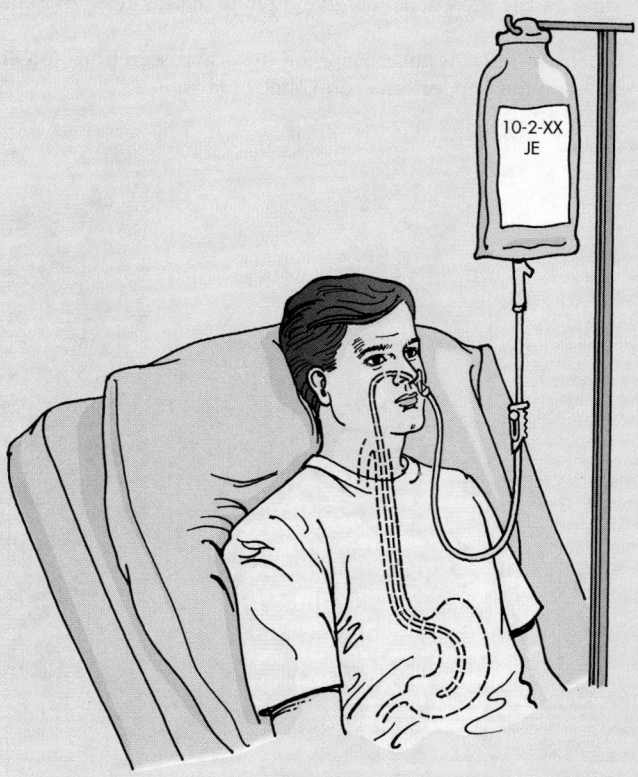

STEP 9a(3)   Administer intermittent feeding.

STEP	RATIONALE

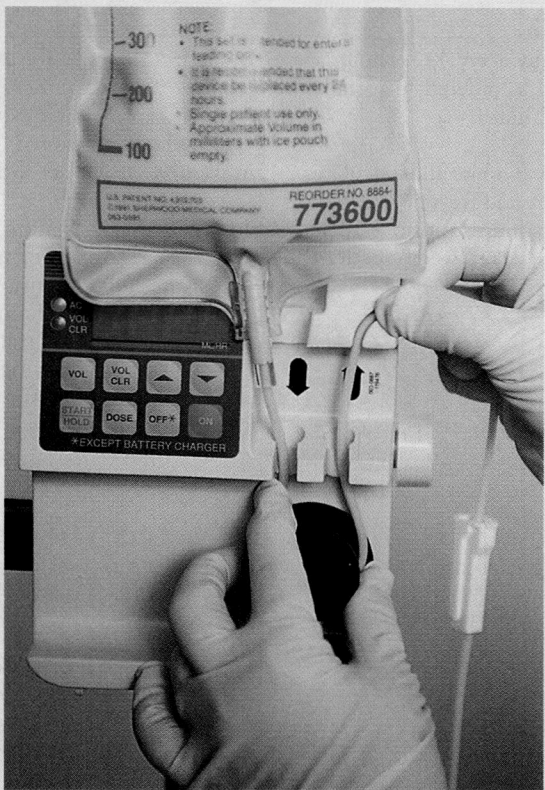

STEP 9b(2)   Connect tubing through infusion pump.

b Continuous drip method:

(1) Connect distal end of administration set tubing to proximal end of feeding tube as in Steps 9a(1) and 9a(2).

(2) Connect tubing through tube feeding pump, open roller clamp on tubing, set rate on pump, and turn on (see illustration).

Continuous feeding method is designed to deliver prescribed hourly rate of feeding. This method reduces risk for abdominal discomfort.

Delivers continuous feeding at a steady rate and pressure. Feeding pump alarms for increased resistance.

Critical Decision Point   *Maximum hang time for formula is 8 hours in an open system, 24 hours in closed, ready-to-hang system (if it remains closed). Refer to manufacturer's guidelines.*

Critical Decision Point   *Use pumps designated for tube feeding (not intravenous fluids).*

10 Advance rate of concentration of tube feeding gradually (Box 31-1).

Helps to prevent diarrhea and gastric intolerance to formula.

11 Following intermittent infusion or at end of continuous infusion, flush feeding tube with 30 mL of water. Repeat every 4 to 6 hours (check agency policy) (see Skill 31-3).

Provides patient with source of water to help maintain fluid and electrolyte balance. Clears tubing of formula.

12 When patient is receiving intermittent tube feeding, cap or clamp the proximal end of the feeding tube.

Prevents air from entering stomach between feedings.

13 Rinse bag and tubing with warm water whenever feedings are interrupted. Use a new administration set every 24 hours.

Rinsing bag and tubing with warm water clears old tube feedings and reduces bacterial growth.

14 Dispose of supplies, and perform hand hygiene.

Reduces transmission of microorganisms.

STEP	RATIONALE

EVALUATION

1 Measure residual volume per policy, usually every 4 to 6 hours.

Evaluates tolerance of tube feeding.

2 Monitor finger-stick blood glucose level as ordered, especially in patients at risk (e.g., diabetes, renal failure).

Requires physician's order. Alerts nurse to patient's tolerance of enteral nutrition. Requires physician to revise rate or type of formula administered.

3 Monitor intake and output at least every 8 hours and calculate daily totals every 24 hours (Worthington and Reyen, 2004b).

Intake and output are indications of fluid balance or fluid volume excess or deficit.

4 Weigh patient daily until maximum administration rate is reached and maintained for 24 hours, then weigh patient 3 times per week.

Slow weight gain is indicator of improved nutritional status; however, sudden gain of more than 2 pounds in 24 hours usually indicates fluid retention.

5 Monitor laboratory values.

Determines correct administration of formula rate and strength.

6 Observe patient's respiratory status.

Change in respiratory status indicates aspiration of tube feeding.

7 Observe patient's level of comfort.

Reduced gastric emptying leads to abdominal discomfort.

8 Auscultate bowel sounds.

Evaluates status of gastric peristalsis.

9 For tubes placed through the abdominal wall, inspect site for signs of impaired skin integrity.

Enteral tubes often cause pressure and excoriation at the insertion site.

Unexpected Outcomes

1 The feeding tube becomes clogged. Frequent aspiration of gastric contents and frequent administration of medications without adequate flushing increases clogging of feeding tubes (Reising and Neal, 2005).

2 Gastric residual volume exceeds 200 mL (see agency policy).

3 Patient aspirates formula.

4 Patient develops large amount of diarrhea (more than three loose stools in 24 hours). Many formulas have no fiber, so stools will always be loose.

5 Patient develops nausea and vomiting, which may indicate gastric ileus.

6 Aspirated fluid has foul odor or unusual appearance.

7 Skin around gastrostomy or jejunostomy site breaks down.

Related Interventions

- Attempt to flush the tube with water.
- Special products are available for unclogging feeding tubes; do not use soda and juice.
- Hold feeding.
- Maintain patient in semi-Fowler's position.
- Recheck residual in 1 hour.
- Notify health care provider.
- See Related Interventions following Skill 31-1.
- Notify health care provider, and meet with dietitian to determine need to change formula to provide fiber.
- Consider other causes (e.g., bacterial contamination of the feeding) (Worthington and Reyen, 2004b).
- Provide skin care.
- Determine if patient is receiving medications (e.g., containing sorbitol) that induce diarrhea (Worthington and Reyen, 2004b).
- Withhold tube feeding, and notify health care provider.
- Be sure tubing is patent; aspirate for residual.
- Notify health care provider, and document findings.
- Do not return aspirated material of unusual odor or appearance without first consulting physician.
- Institute skin care.
- Use pressure relief measures around tube.
- Provide wound care (see Chapter 38).

Recording and Reporting
- Record and report amount and type of feeding, patient's response to tube feeding, patency of tube, condition of skin at tube site if placed in abdominal wall.
- Record volume of formula and any additional water on intake and output form.
- Report type of feeding, status of feeding tube, patient's tolerance, and adverse outcomes.

Teaching Considerations
- Teach patient and caregiver that, if tolerated, patient should remain upright for 1 hour after feedings.
- Instruct patient or caregiver that patient may express feelings of fullness, increased gas, belching, or diarrhea.
- Teach patient or primary caregiver how to determine correct placement of feeding tube.

Pediatric Considerations
- Intermittent feeding is preferred in infants because of possible perforation of the stomach, nasal airway obstruction, ulceration, and irritation to mucous membranes with continuous feedings. When giving intermittent feedings to a small child, administration usually takes 20 to 30 minutes, or as long as it takes to bottle-feed the child. Hold the infant, and offer a pacifier during the feeding to simulate a more natural bottle-feeding experience (Axelrod and others, 2006).
- Temporary small-bore NG tubes are often placed in infants just before each feeding and removed afterward.

- For a neonate, an excessive residual volume is more than 20% of the ordered amount. For an older child, an excessive residual volume is greater than 50% of the ordered amount.
- For pediatric patients receiving continuous feedings, assess the residual volume with routine vitals signs, at minimum at least every 4 hours (Axelrod and others, 2006).

Gerontological Considerations
- Some older adults are more susceptible to hyperglycemia related to glucose intolerance from diabetes or other factors.
- Some older adults have decreased gastric emptying so that formula remains in the stomach longer than for younger patients. Gastric residual checks are of special importance in patients with impaired cognition to decrease the risk for aspiration during gastric feeding.

Home Care Considerations
- Instruct primary caregiver and/or patient to monitor intake and output using household measuring devices.
- Ask patient or care provider about any symptoms or discomfort during enteral feedings. Reinforce instruction to contact nurse if symptoms of discomfort occur.
- Teach patient or primary caregiver how to do skin care around the gastrostomy or jejunostomy tube and signs and symptoms of infection at insertion site.

PROCEDURAL GUIDELINE 31-1   Care of a Gastrostomy or Jejunostomy Tube

When patients cannot tolerate nasoenteral feeding tubes or require permanent enteral feeding or when nasoenteral feeding tubes interfere with rehabilitation, other options may be selected. One such option is a gastric feeding tube. Gastric feedings permit the delivery of nutrients directly to the stomach. Gastric feedings via a gastrostomy feeding tube are relatively safe to administer, provided the patient has normal gastric emptying. A physician inserts a gastrostomy tube in the operating room (called open, Stamm, or Janeway gastrostomy), during endoscopy (called percutaneous endoscopic gastrostomy, or PEG), or by radiology. A tube, generally greater than 16 Fr size, is placed in the stomach and exits through an incision in the upper left quadrant of the abdomen, where an external bumper holds it in place (Fig. 31-3).

Jejunostomy tubes, like gastrostomy tubes, can be inserted during surgery, endoscopy, or radiology. Endoscopic insertion of a jejunostomy tube may be done through a PEG tube. After insertion of the PEG tube, the percutaneous endoscopic jejunostomy (PEJ) tube is passed through the PEG and advanced into the jejunum (Fig. 31-4). A Y connector attached to a jejunostomy tube caps the PEG tube and closes the system. A Y connector labels a gastrostomy tube and designates a jejunostomy tube for feeding. Know whether a tube is gastric or jejunal or both. Patients with upper airway or upper GI cancers often use the gastric port of a tube for decompression while using the jejunal port for feeding.

Delegation Considerations

Care of a gastrostomy or jejunostomy tube feeding cannot be delegated to NAP. The nurse directs the NAP to:

- Inform the nurse of any patient complaints of discomfort at the insertion site.
- Inform the nurse of any drainage on the insertion site dressing.

Equipment

- ❑ Normal saline, dated and initialed container at patient's bedside
- ❑ 4 × 4 inch gauze
- ❑ Prepared drain-gauze dressing
- ❑ Tape
- ❑ Clean gloves

Procedural Steps

1. Determine whether exit site is left open to air or if a dressing is indicated. Check health care provider's order or verify agency policy.
2. Perform hand hygiene and apply clean gloves.
3. Remove old dressing and discard in appropriate container.
4. Assess exit site for evidence of excoriation, drainage, infection, or bleeding.
5. Cleanse skin around site with warm water and mild soap using 4 × 4 inch gauzes (Vukson, 2008).
6. Rotate external bumper 90 degrees (see Fig. 31-4).
7. Dry site completely.
8. Apply thin layer of protective skin barrier to exit site if indicated (e.g., site excoriated).
9. If dressing is ordered, place drain-gauze dressing over external bar. NOTE: Do not place dressing under external bar; this can cause gastric tissue erosion or internal abdominal wall pressure.
10. Secure dressing with tape.
11. Place date, time, and initials on new dressing.
12. Remove gloves and dispose of supplies. Perform hand hygiene.
13. Document in nurse' notes appearance of exit site, drainage noted, and dressing application.
14. Report to health care provider any exit site complications.

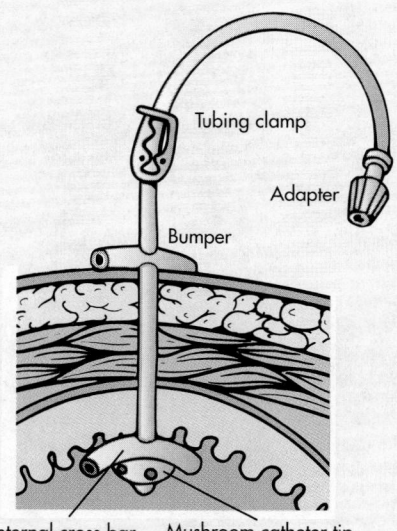

FIG 31-3   Placement of PEG tube into stomach.

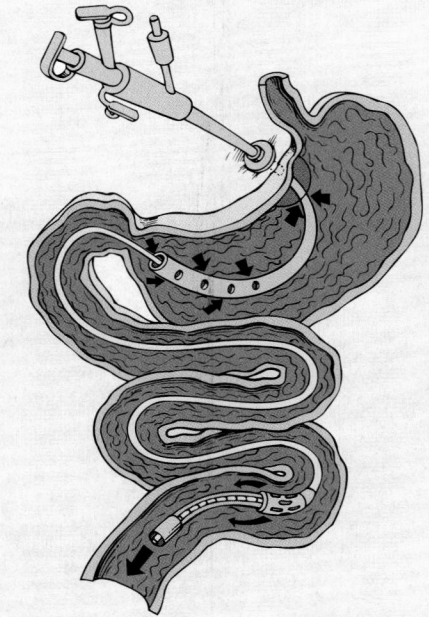

FIG 31-4   Endoscopic insertion of jejunostomy tube.

CRITICAL THINKING EXERCISES

Eugene Meeks is a 72-year-old patient admitted to the acute stroke unit following a cerebral hemorrhage. As a result of his stroke, Mr. Meeks has left-sided paralysis and is sometimes not responsive to verbal commands. He recognizes his family and at times has spoken a few words. The nutrition support team has recommended that he have a small-bore feeding tube inserted for nutritional support. A continuous tube-feeding formula has been ordered.

1 Before inserting the feeding tube, what assessments would be appropriate to determine Mr. Meeks' risk for aspiration?

2 As you prepare to insert the feeding tube, what steps of the procedure do you anticipate will be difficult for Mr. Meeks?

3 Twenty-four hours after Mr. Meeks' feeding tube was inserted, the nurse on day shift has difficulty aspirating any stomach contents from the tube. What is a common cause of tube clogging?

4 Mr. Meeks has been receiving enteral nutrition for 3 days. To ensure that the tip of the feeding tube remains in his stomach, the nurse aspirates stomach contents and measures the pH. What will be the likely pH and appearance of the aspirate?

REVIEW QUESTIONS

1 A patient has a small-bore nasal feeding tube that was just inserted. What is the most important fact that should be documented before the instillation of any type of fluids?
  1 Radiographic confirmation of nonrespiratory placement
  2 Confirmation that the tube is in the stomach
  3 Confirmation that the tube is in the intestine
  4 The type and location of the feeding tube placement

2 A patient has been receiving enteral nutrition for the last 48 hours and is also receiving an H_2 blocker. The nurse checks placement of the small-bore nasal feeding tube and obtain 80 mL of curdled cream–colored fluid with a pH of 6. Based on these findings, where is the tip of the tube most likely positioned?
  1 In the respiratory tract
  2 In the stomach
  3 In the intestine
  4 In the esophagus

3 As a result of a motor vehicle accident, a patient has had multiple facial fractures and suffered a stroke. Based on these facts, what route is the safest and most likely route for feeding tube placement?
  1 Nasoenteric
  2 Gastrostomy tube
  3 Jejunostomy tube
  4 PEG

4 What is the most important intervention the nurse can perform to prevent nosocomial infections associated with enteral nutrition?
  1 Inserting nasogastric tubes using sterile technique
  2 Performing frequent hand hygiene
  3 Wearing clean gloves when handling the feeding system
  4 Changing the feeding bags and liquid on time

REFERENCES

ASPEN: American Society for Parenteral and Enteral Nutrition: Guidelines for the use of parenteral and enteral nutrition in adult and pediatric patients, *JPEN J Parenter Enteral Nutr* 26(suppl):1SA, 2002.

Axelrod D and others: Pediatric enteral nutrition, *JPEN J Parenter Enteral Nutr* 29(suppl):S21, 2006.

Baskin WN: Acute complications associated with bedside placement of feeding tubes, *Nutr Clin Pract* 21:40, 2006.

de Aguilar-Nascimento JE, Kudsk KA: Clinical cost of feeding tube placement *JPEN J Parenter Enteral Nutr* 31:269, 2007.

Flesher ME and others: Assessing the metabolic and clinical consequences of early enteral feeding in the malnourished patient, *JPEN J Parenter Enteral Nutr* 29:108, 2005.

Mathus-Vliegen EMH and others: Analysis of bacterial contamination in an enteral feeding system *JPEN J Parenter Enteral Nutr* 29:519, 2006.

Metheny NA: Preventing respiratory complications of tube-feeding: evidence-based practice, *Am J Crit Care* 15:360, 2006.

Reising DL, Neal RS: Enteral tube flushing, *Am J Nurs* 105:58, 2005.

Roberts S and others: Devices and techniques for bedside enteral feeding tube placement, *Nutr Clin Pract* 22:412, 2007.

The Joint Commission: Tubing misconnections: a persistent and potentially deadly occurrence, *Sentinel Event Alert,* issue 36, April 3, 2006.

Worthington PH, Reyen L: Equipment and formulas for enteral nutrition. In Worthington PH, editor: *Practical aspects of nutrition support,* Philadelphia, 2004a, Elsevier.

Worthington PH, Reyen L: Initiating and managing enteral nutrition. In Worthington PH, editor: *Practical aspects of nutrition support,* Philadelphia, 2004b, Elsevier.

Worthington PH, Reyen L: Selecting candidates and delivery methods for enteral nutrition. In Worthington PH, editor: *Practical aspects of nutrition support,* Philadelphia, 2004c, Elsevier.

RESEARCH REFERENCES

ASPEN: Standards of practice for nutrition support nurses, *Nutr Clin Pract* 22:458, 2007.

Cirgin Ellett ML: Important facts about intestinal feeding tube placement, *Gastroenterol Nurs* 29(2):112, 2006.

Gottschlich M, editor: The A.S.P.E.N. *nutrition support core curriculum: a case-based approach—the adult patient,* Silver Spring, Md, 2007, ASPEN.

Rauen C and others: Seven evidence-based practice habits: putting some sacred cows out to pasture, *Crit Care Nurs* 28(2):98, 2008.

Vukson K: G-tubes and skin care, *Gastroenterol Nurs* 31(4):305, 2000.

Worthington PH, editor: *Practical aspects of nutrition support,* Philadelphia, 2004, Elsevier.

32

Parenteral Nutrition

MEDIA RESOURCES

- 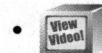 http://evolve.elsevier.com/Perry/skills
  - Review Questions
  - Video Clips

- Mosby's Nursing Video Skills, 3.0

OBJECTIVES

Mastery of content in this chapter will enable the nurse to:
- Identify patients who are candidates for parenteral nutrition.
- Discuss risks associated with parenteral nutrition.
- Describe factors influencing selection of appropriate sites for administering parenteral nutrition.
- Identify measures used to prevent complications of central parenteral nutrition.
- Demonstrate appropriate nursing care for the patient receiving parenteral nutrition.

Parenteral nutrition (PN) is a specialized form of nutritional support in which nutrients are given intravenously. When infused into a large-diameter vein, such as the superior vena cava (Fig. 32-1), PN is often called central parenteral nutrition (CPN) or total parenteral nutrition (TPN). You administer it to patients to reduce catabolism (the breakdown of protein) and to maintain nitrogen balance. In situations in which partial or complete intestinal failure has occurred and oral nutrition or enteral tube feeding is not possible, PN is the therapy of choice (Stratton and Elia, 2007) (Box 32-1). When a patient's gastrointestinal (GI) tract is functional, clinicians assess patients and choose the best method of delivering nutritional needs, which may include enteral feeding (see Chapter 31), parenteral feeding, or a combination of both. The ultimate goal is to resume use of the GI tract through enteral or oral feedings as soon as possible (American Dietetic Association, 2008; American Society for Parenteral and Enteral Nutrition [ASPEN], 2002).

In most patients, you administer PN for a few days or weeks, although a small number of patients require long-term PN (Stratton and Elia, 2007). The use of PN in the perioperative patient is controversial, and although benefits are more likely in the severely malnourished, evidence has shown little effect of PN in preventing mortality (Peter and others, 2005). Parenteral nutrition creates risks (Table 32-1). It has been associated with catheter-related bloodstream infections, noninfective complications such as pneumothorax, and increased hospital length of stay (Krein and others, 2007; Peter and others, 2005).

Patients with short-term nutritional needs often receive intravenous (IV) solutions of 5% dextrose via a peripheral vein in combination with amino acids and lipids. A solution of 10% dextrose can be administered, but it is the highest osmolarity that can be given peripherally. Peripheral solutions are not as calorically dense as PN solutions and therefore provide a temporary therapy when patients have high caloric needs. Parenteral nutrition, with greater than 10% dextrose (hypertonic solution), requires a central venous access device that delivers PN into a high-flow central vein, such as the superior vena cava. PN solutions are usually hyperosmolar, and thus you have to administer them into a large-diameter vein to prevent sclerosis of vein tissue. Examples of central venous access devices include central venous catheters, peripherally inserted central catheters (PICCs), and implanted infusion ports. Chapter 28 offers details on the insertion and care of central venous access devices. The ideal device used for PN is durable, reliable, and user friendly, because many patients receiving PN will continue to receive nutritional therapy in the home or long-term care setting.

Nurses collaborate with nutritional support teams and physicians in the administration of PN and in monitoring patients' nutritional status. Larger institutions have nutritional support teams, which consist of registered dietitians, physicians, pharmacists, and clinical nurse specialists. In order for PN to be used safely, you must closely monitor administration of PN. Special care is necessary to maintain patients' blood glucose levels in the normal range (Forbes, 2007). Higher glucose levels in patients are often associated with cardiovascular events, general infection, systemic sepsis, acute renal failure, and death. It is important to assess and identify patients at risk for malnutrition. The first sign of a developing problem is a pattern of a decline in oral food intake and reduced appetite. Patients' laboratory values may indicate a decline in albumin, prealbumin, and total protein levels. Frequently you will be the first to identify risk factors, such as progressive weight loss, restricted or limited fluid intake, intolerance to enteral feedings, increased energy need (burns, sepsis, and trauma), or being NPO (nothing by mouth) for 3 or more days. The assessment provides information for consulting with the nutritional support team and physician in an effort to initiate appropriate PN.

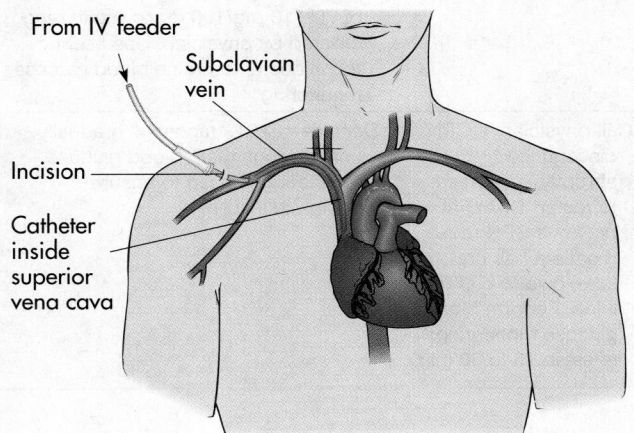

FIG 32-1 Placement of central venous catheter inserted into subclavian vein. (*Courtesy Rolin Graphics.*)

From IV feeder
Subclavian vein
Incision
Catheter inside superior vena cava

BOX 32-1	Indications for Parenteral Nutrition

Nonfunctional GI Tract
- Massive small bowel resection/GI surgery/massive GI bleed
- Paralytic ileus
- Intestinal obstruction
- Short bowel syndrome
- Trauma to abdomen, head, or neck
- Severe malabsorption
- Intolerance to enteral feeding
- Chemotherapy, radiation therapy, bone marrow transplantation

Extended Bowel Rest
- Enterocutaneous fistula
- Inflammatory bowel disease exacerbation
- Severe diarrhea
- Moderate to severe pancreatitis

Preoperative TPN
- Preoperative bowel rest
- Treatment for comorbid severe malnutrition in patients with nonfunctional GI tracts
- Severely catabolic patients when GI tract nonusable for more than 4 to 5 days

GI, Gastrointestinal; *TPN,* total parenteral nutrition.

TABLE 32-1 | Complications of Central Parenteral Nutrition

Problem	Cause	Symptoms	Immediate Action	Prevention
Pneumothorax	Tip of catheter enters pleural space during insertion, causing lung to collapse.	Sudden chest pain, difficult breathing, decreased breath sounds, cessation of normal chest movement on the affected side, tachycardia.	Remove central catheter. Administer oxygen via nasal cannula. Insert chest tube to remove air under water seal drainage or a dry one-way valve system.	Medical personnel should be properly trained to insert central catheters. Researchers suggest use of ultrasound when placing central venous catheters (de Jonge, 2007). Catheter should be properly secured to prevent migration, movement.
Air embolism	IV tubing disconnected; part of catheter system open or removed without being clamped.	Sudden respiratory distress; decreased oxygen saturation levels, shortness of breath, coughing, chest pain, decreased blood pressure.	Clamp catheter; position patient in left Trendelenburg's position; call physician; administer oxygen as needed.	Make sure all catheter connections are secure; clamp catheter when not in use. Never use a stopcock with a CVC. Instruct patient in Valsalva's maneuver for tubing changes.
Localized infection (exit site or tunnel)	Poor aseptic technique in removal of skin flora during site preparation and dressing care.	*Exit site:* Erythema, tenderness, induration or purulence within 2 cm of skin at exit site. *Tunnel:* Same as above but extends beyond 2 cm from exit site.	Call physician. *Exit:* Warm compress, daily site care, oral antibiotics. *Tunnel:* Remove catheter.	Provide catheter site care using aseptic technique; include cleansing of site, application of new stabilization device, and application of sterile dressing (INS, 2006). Change transparent dressings every 7 days, gauze dressings every 48 hours (INS, 2006). Change dressing if damp, loosened, soiled, or when inspection of site is necessary (INS, 2006). Cleanse site with chlorhexidine or povidone-iodine a minimum of 3 to 5 min. Routine use of antibiotic ointment not recommended (INS, 2006).
Catheter-related sepsis or bacteremia	Catheter hub contamination; contamination of infusate; spread of bacteria through bloodstream from distant site.	*Systemic:* Isolation of same microorganism from blood culture and catheter segment, with patient showing fever, chills, malaise, elevated white blood cell count.	*Systemic:* Antibiotics intravenously, remove catheter.	Use full sterile-barrier precautions during catheter insertion and dressing change. Use antibiotic-impregnated catheters. Do not disconnect tubing unnecessarily. Replace intravenous tubing and filter every 72 hours for standard PN (INS, 2006).
Hyperglycemia	Patient receiving CPN too quickly; too little insulin in solution.	Excessive thirst, urination, blood glucose >160 mg/100 dL, confusion.	Call physician; may need to slow infusion rate (physician order).	Review medical history for glucose intolerance or diabetes; keep rate as ordered, never increase CPN to "catch up." Maintain blood glucose in range of 70-110 mg/100 dL or within range ordered by physician. Use aseptic technique and routine blood glucose monitoring.
Hypoglycemia	CPN abruptly discontinued; too much insulin.	Patient is shaky, dizzy, nervous, anxious, senses hunger, blood glucose level <80 mg/100 dL.	Call physician; if CPN discontinued abruptly, may need to restart $D_{10}NS$ at previous CPN rate. If patient has oral intake, give ½ cup fruit juice. Perform blood glucose monitoring; retest in 15 to 30 min.	Decrease CPN, "tapering" gradually until discontinued; blood glucose monitoring is used to ensure adequate insulin.

CPN, central parenteral nutrition; *CVC,* central venous catheter; *IV,* Intravenous.

TABLE 32-2	Factors in Determining Vascular Access Device Selection for Parenteral Nutrition		
Patient Factors	**Device Characteristics**	**Therapeutic Factors**	**Duration of Therapy**
Physiological			
Condition of veins	Design of device	Numbers of lumens.	Type of disease or condition being
Hypercoagulability state	Low risk for infection (e.g.,	Durability.	treated (e.g., long-term metastatic
Diabetes	antibacterial coatings)	Characteristics of solutions or	disease vs. short-term bowel
Skin disorders		emulsions.	inflammation).
Previous surgery involving		Dextrose concentration >10%	PICCs can be placed for duration
thorax or vascular system		requires central vein access.	of 1 year.
Known allergies to catheter		Solution with osmolarity	Implanted ports may remain in
materials		>600 mOsm/L requires central	place for life of need or until por-
		vein access.	tal head does not hold needle.
Functional			Manufacturers recommend up to
Poor vision			1500 needle sticks with 20-gauge
Altered dexterity			needle can be used to access
Developmental disabilities			port.
Frailty			Hickman or Broviac catheter remains
			in place for life of need unless cath-
Psychological			eter becomes clotted or infected or
Needle phobia			there is breakdown of catheter
Body image impairment			material.
Previous experience with			Triple-lumen subclavian catheters
vascular access device			used only for duration of acute
Fear of therapy-related			care.
complications			
Social Support			
Care provider availability			
Financial resources			

PICC, Peripherally inserted central catheter.

Nurses play a role in the selection of the best vascular access site for PN administration (Table 32-2). Chapter 28 includes the skill for the insertion of a central venous access device. Selection of an ideal vascular access device depends on patient factors, device characteristics, therapeutic issues, and duration of therapy. For example, implanted ports and PICCs require the highest level of manual dexterity for home care patients to manage and manipulate dressings and tubing.

CULTURAL CONSIDERATIONS

Parenteral nutrition is a form of nutrition and thus poses problems for members of ethnic groups who restrict intake of certain types of foods. Consider the following guidelines:
- Accommodate religious and cultural beliefs of patient by making sure that you do not add prohibited substances to the parenteral solution. For example, avoid animal-based products when the patient is a strict vegetarian.
- Consult religious leaders about continuous feedings during fasting periods such as Ramadan. Although the sick usually are not required to observe these fasting periods, many devout Muslims will insist on fasting during Ramadan.
- Reinforce teaching on any technological devices such as an infusion pump, because patients from different cultures may be overwhelmed with unfamiliar information and may not remember the rationale for such devices.

EVIDENCE-BASED PRACTICE TRENDS

Home parenteral nutrition (HPN) is a life-sustaining therapy for many disease states. However, patients report alterations in their physical, psychological, and social functions that have a negative effect on their perceived quality of life (QOL). In a literature review of studies examining QOL in patients receiving HPN, Winkler (2005) reports that QOL is worse in HPN patients compared with healthy populations. QOL is poor in patients receiving HPN because of the occurrence of depression, sleep disturbance, frequent urination, fear of therapy-related complications, and the inability to eat. In addition, patients and family members find that the technical aspects of HPN administration interfere with routine daily activities. Despite study findings, it is difficult to determine whether the HPN alone or the impact of the patient's disease affects QOL (Winkler, 2005). Nonetheless, carefully consider the psychological and social effects HPN has on your patients (Kelly, 2008).

Parenteral nutrition is associated with a significant increase in the incidence of catheter-related infections (Peter and others, 2005). Pathogens are able to easily access the bloodstream via a venous access device. Researchers believe that the increased risk for infection is associated in part with poor blood glucose control and resultant hyperglycemia, creating an environment for microorganism growth. There are multiple strategies for reducing catheter-related infection, including better blood glucose control, use of sterile barrier precautions during insertion of central lines, timely replacement of IV tubing and add-on devices, application of IV site dressings, and reduction in tubing access openings.

Skill Performance Guidelines

1 Meet with the nutritional support team and physician to determine when to use peripheral vein access instead of central vein access. Patients who require short-term nutrition support, for whom central access placement is contraindicated or not reasonable, who have adequate peripheral access, and who can tolerate larger volumes of fluid are candidates for peripheral PN.

2 Know the complications associated with PN, including metabolic disturbances, fluid imbalance, technical management of catheter system, and infections.

3 Monitor the patient's vital signs, electrolyte levels, triglyceride levels, weight, and fluid status, and compare baseline with treatment values. Some patients who receive PN have rapid changes in these values.

4 Know the patient's recent temperature range. Patients with peripheral or central IV lines are susceptible to septicemia; an elevated temperature is an early indicator of a bacterial infection.

5 Routinely assess the site of a central venous access device for signs of infection.

6 Use strict aseptic technique in the care and maintenance of central venous catheters and PICC devices.

SKILL 32-1   Administering Central Parenteral Nutrition

 Advanced / Parenteral Nutrition / Providing Total Parenteral Nutrition

Administration of CPN requires the use of strict aseptic technique and application of critical thinking. Because of the composition of CPN fluids, patients can experience metabolic and fluid balance changes quickly. In addition, the clinical condition of patients receiving CPN is usually poor, especially when patients have alterations in host defenses, severe underlying illnesses, and extremes of age. You will need to anticipate changes in the patient's condition that signal developing complications. Similarly, you need to use good judgment to maintain the IV system and to ensure it is functioning properly.

Parenteral nutrition includes mixtures of carbohydrates (10% to 70% dextrose solution), amino acids (protein/nitrogen), fats (fatty acids), electrolytes, vitamins, and trace elements (e.g., zinc, copper, manganese, and chromium). Higher concentrations of dextrose solutions are used when a patient's fluids need to be restricted, whereas lower concentrations help control hyperglycemia (Grodner and others, 2007). Dextrose solutions mixed with amino acids and other nutrients form the final solution.

Lipids provide supplemental kilocalories and prevent essential fatty acid deficiencies. You can administer these emulsions through a separate peripheral line, through a central line by a Y connector tubing (see Chapter 22), or as an admixture to the PN solution. The addition of lipid emulsion to the PN solution is called a 3:1, 3-in-1, or total nutrition admixture (TNA). The advantage to a 3:1 mixture is that it allows lipid infusion over 24 hours, decreasing carbon dioxide production and reducing liver accumulation of fat from long-term glucose use (Grodner and others, 2007). The essential fatty acid present in lipid emulsion is linoleic acid. This acid cannot be made from other fats in human metabolism and therefore must be supplied. Linoleic acid is an omega-6 fatty acid. A patient with linoleic acid deficiency is immunosuppressed and thus at risk for infection. A nutritional regimen without adequate fatty acids leads to essential fatty acid deficiency (EFAD), characterized by dry scaly skin, sparse hair growth, impaired wound healing, decreased resistance to stress, increased susceptibility to respiratory tract infections, anemia, thrombocytopenia, and liver function abnormalities.

Although 3:1 admixtures are common, many institutions use 2:1 admixtures without lipids. The rationale is the potential problem of stability of the lipids when mixed with amino acids and dextrose. When administering fat (lipid) emulsions via piggyback infusion, add the solution below the infusion filter and insert it in the port nearest to the venipuncture site, because the fat particles are large and cannot pass through the infusion filter without breaking down. Not all patients should receive fat emulsion. Fat emulsions are contraindicated in patients who have a disturbance of normal fat metabolism.

Delegation Considerations

Caring for patients receiving central parenteral nutrition cannot be delegated to nursing assistive personnel (NAP). The nurse directs the NAP to:

- Immediately report to the nurse when the infusion pump alarm sounds and when the patient complains of a moist or leaking dressing/tubing.
- Perform blood glucose monitoring and report the results.

Equipment

- ❏ IV infusion tubing with Luer-Lok tip
- ❏ CPN solution (IV)
- ❏ IV filter (1.2-μm filter for three-in-one solutions or lipids, containing a membrane that is particulate retentive and air eliminating) (Infusion Nurses Society [INS], 2006)
- ❏ IV infusion pump
- ❏ Bedside glucose monitoring kit
- ❏ Adhesive tape or tubing label
- ❏ Clean gloves

ASSESSMENT

1 Assess indications of and risks for protein-calorie malnutrition: weight loss from baseline or ideal, muscle atrophy/weakness, edema, lethargy, failure to wean from ventilatory support, chronic illness, and nothing by mouth for more than 6 days. Confer with nutritional support team.

Clinical indications for parenteral nutrition.

2 Inspect condition of central vein access site for presence of inflammation, edema, and tenderness. Inspect tubing of access device for patency and kinking.

Identifies early signs of infection, infiltration, or disruption in system integrity. Development of complication contraindicates infusion of fluids and indicates need to establish new IV site.

STEP	RATIONALE
3 Assess levels of serum albumin, total protein, transferrin, pre-albumin, and triglycerides, and check blood glucose level by finger stick (see Chapter 43).	Provides baseline for measuring patient's nutritional status and tolerance to high concentration of glucose infusion.
4 Assess patient's medical history for factors influenced by CPN administration: electrolyte levels; renal, heart, and hepatic function. Assess for history of allergies.	Some patients require that CPN therapy be adapted by composition or volume (requires physician order) based on medical history. CPN includes constituents (e.g., medications) to which patient may be allergic.
5 Assess vital signs, auscultate patient's lung sounds, and measure weight.	Provides baseline for monitoring patient's response to fluid infusion and nutrients. Crackles in lungs are early indication of fluid volume excess.
6 Consult with physician and dietitian on calculation of calorie, protein, and fluid requirements for patient.	Provides multidisciplinary plan for patient's nutritional support.
7 Verify physician's order for nutrients, minerals, vitamins, trace elements, electrolytes, and added medications as well as flow rate. Check for compatibility of added medications.	Physician must order CPN, and it is often ordered daily in the hospital setting after review of laboratory values. In the home setting, orders may be obtained less frequently (e.g., weekly). Pharmacies that prepare parenteral solutions will check medication compatibility.

NURSING DIAGNOSES

• Excess fluid volume	• Imbalanced nutrition: less than body requirements	• Risk for infection

Individualize related factors based on patient's condition or needs.

PLANNING

1 Expected outcomes following completion of procedure:	
• Patient's ideal weight gain is usually between 1 and 3 lb (0.5 to 1.5 kg) per week.	Weight is an indicator of patient's nutritional status and determines fluid volume. Weight gain greater than 1 lb/day (0.5 kg) indicates fluid retention.
• Serum glucose levels are less than 150 mg/dL or maintained between 80 and 110 mg/dL. Check physician's order for desired glucose range.	High blood glucose levels have been associated with CPN complications and death (Forbes, 2007). Medical protocols will vary by institution as to the desired blood glucose range.
• Central venous access device is patent, and site is free of pain, swelling, redness, or inflammation.	Ensures that CPN is infusing into the vein rather than into surrounding tissues and that there are no signs of an access device infection.
• Patient is afebrile.	Absence of systemic infection.
2 Explain purposes of CPN.	Promotes understanding and reduces anxiety.
3 If CPN solution is refrigerated, remove from refrigeration 1 hour before infusion.	Solution should be at room temperature for administration (INS, 2006).

IMPLEMENTATION

1 Perform hand hygiene, and apply clean gloves.	Reduces transmission of microorganisms.
2 Compare label of CPN bag with medication administration record (MAR) or computer printout; check for correct additives and solution expiration date. Also check patient's name.	Prevents medication error.
3 Inspect PN solution for particulate matter or, if it is a 3:1 solution, inspect emulsion for a cream layer or separation of fat into a layer. If there is a thin layer of aggregated fat droplets about 1 to 2 cm in thickness, invert bag back and forth gently to mix.	Deterioration of a three-in-one solution results in breakdown of the emulsion.

Critical Decision Point   *Do not use PN solution if it has coalesced (thick, dense layer of fat droplets at surface, appearing 10 cm in thickness) or oiled out (fat droplets separate from solution and appear as a clear layer at surface). Notify the pharmacy, and request a new solution (Driscoll and Baron, 2000).*

4 Identify patient. Use at least two patient identifiers. Compare patient's name and one other identifier (e.g., hospital identification number) on MAR, computer printout, or computer screen with information on patient's identification bracelet.	Ensures correct patient receives correct IV solution. Complies with The Joint Commission (TJC) (2007) requirements and improves medication and patient safety.

STEP	RATIONALE

5   Attach appropriate filter to IV tubing. Prime tubing with PN solution, making sure no air bubbles remain, and turn off flow with roller clamp (see Chapter 28). Connect end of tubing to appropriate port of central catheter, and label port. Open roller clamp to rate that maintains patency of line.

Air introduced into central circulation can result in an air embolus, a fatal complication. Labeling of high-risk catheters prevents connection with an inappropriate tube or catheter (TJC, 2006).

6   Place IV tubing into IV infusion pump, open roller clamp completely, and regulate flow rate on pump as ordered (see Chapter 28) (see illustration). In some institutions the infusion rate is immediately set at the ordered rate. In other institutions an initial rate of 40 to 60 mL/hr is established, and the rate is gradually increased until patient's nutritional needs are supplied (refer to agency policy).

CPN flow rates are ordered to meet patient's metabolic and electrolyte needs. Maintaining rates prevents electrolyte imbalances.

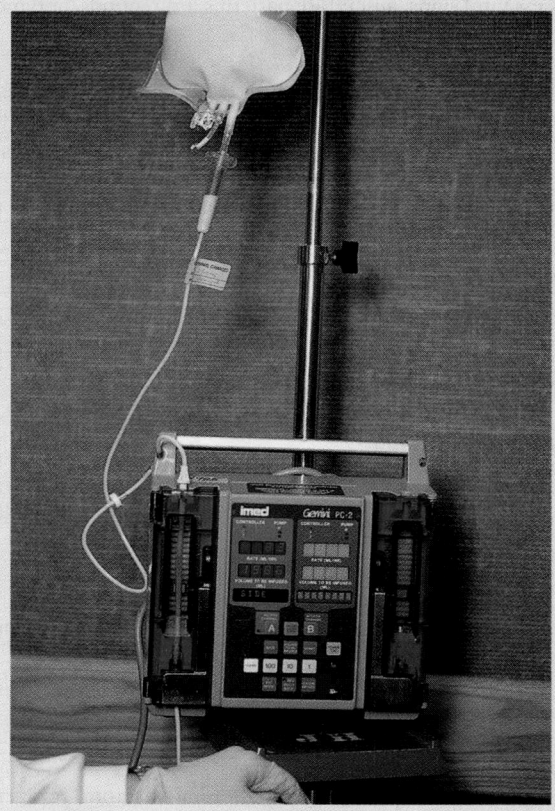

STEP 6   Parenteral nutrition solution infusing via infusion pump.

Critical Decision Point   *Increase rate of infusion gradually to prevent metabolic and electrolyte abnormalities (ASPEN, 2001). CPN is hyperosmolar, and patients usually tolerate it when it is increased incrementally. Do not abruptly discontinue CPN, because this will lead to hypoglycemia. If discontinued suddenly, hang infusion of 5% dextrose in water at same infusion rate. PN solution including lipids should be infused within 24 hours (INS, 2006).*

---

7   Infuse all IV medications or blood through an alternative IV line. Do not obtain blood samples or central venous pressure readings through same lumen or port used for CPN.

Prevents drug incompatibility. Prevents occlusion of central line and reduces risk for transmission of infection.

8   Do not interrupt CPN infusion (e.g., during showers, transport to procedure, blood transfusion), and be sure that rate does not exceed ordered rate.

Maintains continuous infusion of nutrients, prevents hypoglycemic reaction. Never attempt to catch up on a delayed infusion.

9   Change infusing tubing and filter using strict aseptic technique. Change IV administration sets for PN every 72 hours, for 3:1 and fat emulsions every 24 hours, and immediately upon suspected contamination (INS, 2006).

Prevents development of catheter-related bacteremia.

10 Discard used supplies, and perform hand hygiene.

Reduces transmission of infection.

EVALUATION

1   Monitor flow rate routinely, at least hourly.
2   Monitor fluid intake every 8 hours.

Too rapid or too slow infusion could result in metabolic disturbances.
Prevents fluid imbalance from too slow or too rapid infusion.

STEP	RATIONALE
3 Obtain daily weights or weights as ordered.	Routine measurement of weights will reflect a gain/loss resulting either from caloric intake or fluid retention. Gradual weight gain indicates adequate tolerance
4 Assess for fluid retention; palpate skin of extremities, auscultate lung sounds.	Weight gain in excess of 1 lb/day, dependent edema, lung crackles, and intake greater than output per each 24-hour period indicate fluid retention.
5 Monitor patient's glucose level every 6 hours or as ordered, and monitor other laboratory parameters daily or as ordered.	Maintenance of normal electrolyte levels, satisfactory fluid balance, acceptable serum glucose levels, and improvement in serum proteins indicates adequate tolerance to CPN.
6 Inspect central venous access site.	Determines IV patency and absence of infection, infiltration, or phlebitis.
7 Monitor for fever, elevated white blood cell count and malaise.	Signs of systemic infection.

Unexpected Outcomes	Related Interventions
1 There is redness, swelling, and tenderness around the venous access site, indicating possible exit site infection.	• Notify physician. • Apply warm compress, and initiate daily site care as ordered. • Systemic antibiotic therapy may begin.
2 Patient develops fever, malaise, and chills, indicating systemic infection.	• Check exit site for signs of infection. • Notify physician, and consult about the need to obtain cultures of exit site or blood. • Systemic antibiotic therapy may begin.
3 Infusion stops flowing or flows at a rate slower than ordered.	• Venous access device is possibly occluded with fibrin or particulate matter. Report occlusion to the physician. • If the device is a surgically placed device or PICC (see Chapter 28), a thrombolytic agent may be ordered.
4 Patient experiences weight gain greater than 1 lb/day. Taut skin turgor is also present. Crackles auscultated over lung fields.	• Notify physician. • Anticipate need to reduce IV infusion rate.
5 Serum glucose level is greater than 150 mg/dL or target set by physician. Indicates intolerance to glucose load in the CPN solution.	• Document possible need for addition of insulin to the CPN, modification of CPN solution, or sliding-scale insulin coverage.
6 Serum electrolyte levels are out of normal range.	• Indicates movement of electrolytes in response to infusion of fluids and glucose. May need to adjust the electrolyte levels in the solution.

Recording and Reporting

- Record condition of central venous access device, rate and type of infusion, catheter lumen used for infusion, intake and output (I&O) every 8 hours, blood glucose levels, vital signs, and weights.
- If signs of infection, occlusion, fluid retention, or infiltration occur, notify the physician.

Teaching Considerations

- Instruct patient and family in the purpose and goals of CPN. Keep them informed about daily care of central line.

Pediatric Considerations

- Consider children's developmental needs when they are on long-term CPN. Perform regular assessments of development to determine child's progress. Implement interventions to encourage expected milestones (Hockenberry and others, 2007).

Gerontological Considerations

- Some older adults have impaired ability to manage higher fluid volumes or are at risk for an increased incidence of hyperglycemia.

Home Care Considerations

- Patients requiring long-term PN benefit from a referral to a home nutrition therapy team.
- Patients receiving home PN usually have a tunneled catheter inserted into the subclavian vein (Fig. 32-2) inserted to reduce

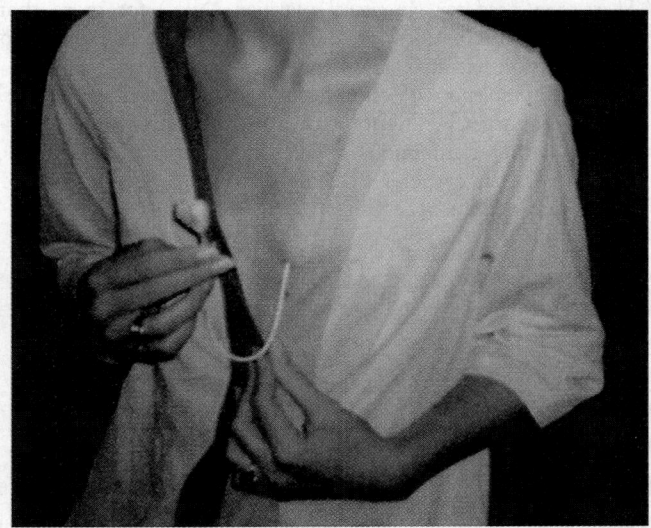

FIG 32-2 Tunneled catheter used for home central parenteral nutrition. (*From Morgan SL, Weinsier RL: Fundamentals of clinical nutrition, ed 2, St. Louis, 1998, Mosby.*)

the possibility of infection. Patients or family members need to learn to perform catheter site care, dressing changes, and techniques for adding and removing parenteral nutrition solutions.

- Some patients will receive home PN at night during sleep (cyclic total parenteral nutrition) to allow the freedom to leave home or work during the day. If the GI tract is functional, patient will receive PN only selected nights per week to supplement oral intake (Grodner and others, 2007).

- Teach patient and primary caregiver to monitor patient's weight, calorie count, I&O, and serum glucose level.
- Teach patient and primary caregiver about actions to take in case of emergency or unexpected outcomes.
- Observe patient and primary caregiver perform procedure in hospital before discharge.

SKILL 32-2 Adiminstering Peripheral Parenteral Nutrition With Lipid (Fat) Emulsion

Advanced / Parenteral Nutrition / Providing Lipid Infusion

When there is a need for short-term nutrition support, peripheral parenteral nutrition (PPN) is an option. It is used infrequently because most practitioners prefer only CPN. The administration of PN via peripheral veins requires the use of lower concentrations of dextrose and amino acids to lower tonicity and lessen the risk for vein damage (Table 32-3). Typically, 2 L of PPN consisting of 10% dextrose and 10% amino acids supplemented by 500 mL of 1% IV fat emulsion provides 2000 kcal/day. PPN is usually administered with fat emulsion. PPN is difficult to maintain because of frequent episodes of phlebitis in superficial arm veins and infiltrations of solutions into subcutaneous tissue. Therefore the final dextrose concentration must be no greater than 10%, because the peripheral vein will sclerose at higher concentrations. Solutions of lower concentration make it difficult to supply adequate calories and amino acids through a peripheral vein.

Commercial lipid emulsions are formulations of safflower oil, soybean oil, or a combination of the two, with glycerol added for isotonicity and egg phospholipids added as an emulsifier (Grodner and others, 2007). A lipid emulsion must be administered through vented IV tubing. An emulsion is administered as a primary IV or it is piggybacked. This skill describes a piggyback administration. Administration sets used for fat emulsions are changed every 24 hours and immediately upon suspected contamination. In addition, an administration set used for parenteral nutrition that has had a fat emulsion piggybacked is changed every 24 hours (INS, 2006). The administration set must have a Luer-Lok design.

Indications for PPN include the following:

1 *Short-term need for parenteral nutrition:* NPO for more than 5 days but anticipation that the patient will tolerate enteral or oral nutrition within 7 days.

2 *History of problems with central vein access or inability to establish central vein access:* Patients with a history of multiple central venous catheter infections or occlusions have increased risks associated with catheter placement. Multiple catheter placements may deplete access sites.

3 *Adequate peripheral access:* Despite its lower osmolality, PPN tends to cause phlebitis and often requires frequent changes in the access location.

4 *Ability to tolerate larger volumes of fluid:* Because of the lower concentration of dextrose in PPN, a larger volume of fluid is required to attain adequate calories. Some patients with impaired renal or cardiac function do not tolerate PPN.

5 *Ability to tolerate lipid emulsions:* Lipid is the most calorically dense nutrient, and PPN without lipid does not provide adequate calories unless very large volumes of fluid are provided. One liter of 10% dextrose provides only 340 kcal. Five hundred milliliters of 10% lipid provides 550 kcal.

Delegation Considerations

The skill of caring for a patient receiving peripheral parenteral nutrition with lipid emulsion cannot be delegated to NAP. The nurse directs the NAP to:

- Report patient complaint of burning or pain at insertion site or signs (see p. 858) of lipid intolerance.
- Report to nurse infusion pump alarms or moist IV site dressing.

Equipment

- ❑ PPN solution
- ❑ Lipid emulsion in glass container
- ❑ IV tubing for PPN with 0.2-μm filter for amino acid/dextrose solution
- ❑ Nonphthalate vented IV tubing infusion set for fat emulsion
- ❑ Needleless cannula
- ❑ Bedside glucose monitoring kit
- ❑ Antimicrobial swab
- ❑ Infusion pump
- ❑ Clean gloves

TABLE 32-3	Comparison of Central Parenteral Nutrition and Peripheral Parenteral Nutrition	
	Central Parenteral Nutrition	**Peripheral Parenteral Nutrition**
Osmolality	>600 mOsm	<600 mOsm
Route of administration	Central venous catheter	Small peripheral vein
Usual daily caloric intake	2000 to 4000	700 to 2000
Fat emulsion	Minor caloric source; provides essential fatty acid	Major caloric source; provides essential fatty acid
Objectives	Weight maintenance; weight gain	Weight maintenance
Duration of therapy	6 days or longer	7 to 10 days (INS, 2006)

STEP	RATIONALE

ASSESSMENT

1   Assess patient for potential lipid intolerance. Assess serum triglyceride level. Obtain a serum triglyceride level before initiation of fat therapy (baseline) and 6 hours after fat has infused.

Determines patient's ability to metabolize lipid.

2   Select or initiate appropriate functional IV site (18-gauge catheter) to administer PPN and lipid emulsion. Assess its patency and function (see Chapter 28).

Large-gauge catheter ensures more efficient flow of infusion.

3   Check physician's order against MAR for volume of fat emulsion and PPN solution.

Physician must order fat emulsions and PPN.

4   Check administration time for fat emulsion.

Fat emulsions cause adverse symptoms if infused too rapidly as a separate infusion. The infusion time is normally at least 4 hours. Fat emulsions should hang no longer than 10 hours as a separate infusion.

5   Use care in locating fat emulsion from supply area. Read label of solution.

Lipid emulsions are white and opaque; thus make sure to avoid confusing enteral formula with parenteral lipids.

6   Assess blood glucose level by finger stick (see Chapter 43).

Provides baseline to determine tolerance to glucose infusion.

NURSING DIAGNOSES

• Imbalanced nutrition: less than body requirements   • Risk for infection

Individualize related factors based on patient's condition or needs.

PLANNING

1   Expected outcomes following completion of procedure:
    • Triglyceride level is stable.

Indicates physical tolerance to fat.

    • Venipuncture site is free of phlebitis, pain, swelling, redness, and inflammation.

Ensures proper administration and monitoring of PPN with lipids.

    • Patient does not show signs of systemic infection (e.g., elevated temperature).

Temperature is an indication of possible systemic infection related to parenteral nutrition.

    • Patient does not show signs of side effects to lipids

Monitoring of infusion requires observation for allergic response to infusion.

2   Explain purposes of PPN and fat emulsion.

Promotes understanding and reduces anxiety.

3   Place patient in a comfortable position for IV insertion or initiation of the infusion.

When patients are comfortable, they tolerate procedures more readily.

4   If PPN solution is refrigerated, remove from refrigeration 1 hour before infusion.

Solution should be at room temperature for administration (INS, 2006).

IMPLEMENTATION

1   Perform hand hygiene, and apply clean gloves.

Reduces transmission of microorganisms.

2   Compare label of PPN bag and lipid emulsion bottle with MAR or computer printout; check for correct additives and solution expiration date. Also check patient's name.

Prevents medication error.

3   Examine the lipid solution for separation of emulsion into layers or fat globules or presence of froth.

Do not administer if these elements appear.

4   Identify patient. Use at least two patient identifiers. Compare patient's name and one other identifier (e.g., hospital identification number) on MAR, computer printout, or computer screen with information on patient's identification bracelet.

Ensures correct patient receives correct intravenous solution. Complies with The Joint Commission (2007) requirements and improves medication and patient safety.

5   Measure patient's vital signs.

Provides a baseline assessment. Immediate allergic reaction can develop once infusion begins.

6   Prepare IV tubing for PPN solution (see Skill 28-3); run solution through tubing to remove excess air. Add sterile capped needle, or place sterile cap on end of tubing. Turn roller clamp to "off" position. Follow the same procedure with the separate infusion set for the lipid infusion.

To prevent air from entering vascular system, you must clear all tubing.

STEP	RATIONALE
7 Connect the PPN solution to patient's functional peripheral IV (see Skill 22-6). Gently disconnect old PPN tubing from IV site, then insert adapter of new PPN infusion tubing. Open roller clamp on new tubing. Allow solution to run to ensure tubing is patent, then regulate IV drip rate using electronic infusion pump.	Prevents disruption of existing IV and ensures patent infusion. Pump will deliver infusion at prescribed rate.
8 Clean the needleless peripheral line tubing injection port with antimicrobial swab. (*Optional:* Use stopcock.)	Removes surface organisms at injection site and prevents organisms from entering blood system.
9 Insert needleless valve at end of fat emulsion infusion tubing into injection port of main IV, closest to patient but below the infusion filter on the main parenteral nutrition line. *Optional:* Connect at stopcock. Be sure lipid solution is at least 30 inches above IV site. Label tubing.	Fat emulsions cannot infuse through a 0.2-μm IV filter—the emulsion would separate. Refer to agency policy; if larger, 1.2-μm filter is used, lipids may be infused above filter (INS, 2006). Labeling of high-risk catheters prevents connection with an inappropriate tube or catheter (TJC, 2006). Height of solution prevents backup into main infusion tubing.
10 Open roller clamp completely on fat emulsion infusion, and then check flow rate on infusion pump.	Initial slow infusion allows you to observe for allergic response.
11 Infuse lipids initially at 1 mL/min for adults and 0.1 mL/min for child for first 15 to 30 minutes, then increase rate as ordered.	Up to 2.5 g fat per kilogram per day may be infused, but fat emulsion should not exceed 60% of total calories. Recommended daily fat percentage is 30% or less of total calories.
12 Begin PPN at ordered rate—10% fat emulsions are infused over at least 4 hours, and 20% fats are infused over at least 6 hours. All lipids can hang for 10 hours as a separate infusion.	The rate of PPN administration does not need to be gradually increased. The lower concentration of dextrose allows most patients to tolerate the full administration rate without difficulty.
13 Discard supplies, and perform hand hygiene.	Reduces transmission of microorganisms.

EVALUATION

1 Monitor flow rate routinely hourly, or more frequently if necessary.	Too rapid or too slow infusion could result in metabolic disturbances.
2 Measure vital signs and patient's general comfort level every 10 minutes for first 30 minutes.	Monitors patient for fat emulsion intolerance.
3 Monitor patient's laboratory values (e.g., triglycerides, liver function tests) daily, and perform blood glucose monitoring as ordered. Measure serum lipids 4 hours after discontinuing infusion.	Provides objective data to measure the response to therapy (e.g., liver's ability to metabolize lipids). Measurement of lipids too soon after an infusion will yield incorrect blood values.
4 Monitor temperature every 4 hours, and regularly inspect venipuncture site for signs of phlebitis or infiltration.	Determines onset of fever, a complication of intolerance to fat emulsion or sepsis. Determines integrity of IV system.
5 Assess patient's weight, I&O, condition of peripheral extremities (for edema), and breath sounds.	Weight gain, I&O imbalance, peripheral edema, and crackles in lungs indicate fluid retention.

Unexpected Outcomes

1 There is intolerance to fat emulsion, as evidenced by increased triglyceride levels, increased temperature (3° to 4° F), chills, flushing, headache, nausea and vomiting, diaphoresis, muscle ache, chest and back pain, dyspnea, pressure over the eyes, vertigo.

2 See Unexpected Outcomes and Related Interventions for Skill 32-1.

Related Interventions

- Confer with physician, and determine if fat emulsion should be discontinued.

Recording and Reporting

- Record condition of IV site, type of solutions, rate and status of infusion, catheter lumen used for infusion, I&O every 8 hours, blood glucose levels, vital signs, and weights in nurses' notes or appropriate flow sheets.
- Record any adverse reactions in nurses' notes.
- If signs of fat intolerance, infection, occlusion, fluid retention, or infiltration occur, notify the physician.

Teaching Considerations

- PPN administration rarely occurs in the home. However, if patient is discharged home, instruct patient and primary care-

giver to monitor patient's weight, calorie count, I&O, and IV site.

Pediatric Considerations

- See Skill 32-1.

Gerontological Considerations

- Some older adults have lipid intolerance.

Home Care Considerations

- See Skill 32-1.

CRITICAL THINKING EXERCISES

Mr. Giles is a 43-year-old patient admitted to the hospital with a severe exacerbation of Crohn's disease. He has lost 10 lb in the last 3 weeks and has suffered recurrent abdominal pain, cramping, and loose stools. He is unable to tolerate food orally, becoming easily nauseated. The patient is to receive bowel rest and nutritional support with CPN. The physician has inserted a central line for 3:1 parenteral nutrition (PN) therapy.

1 Identify four physical parameters that can change quickly and should thus be part of your baseline assessment before initiating PN.

2 Explain why a patient receiving PN will have an initial blood glucose measurement.

3 On the third day after central line insertion, the patient develops a fever and shows little energy, preferring to stay in bed. What might the fever indicate, and what is its source?

4 Two days after beginning PN infusion, Mr. Giles has experienced a 5-lb weight gain. He comments, "This stuff is great—I am gaining back some of the weight I lost." What would be your response? What would you include in a nursing assessment?

 REVIEW QUESTIONS

1 A patient is being switched from a standard IV solution to parenteral nutrition. What should the nurse tell the patient about the reason a large-diameter vein needs to be used for the infusion? Select all that apply.
　1 The fluid is very hyperosmolar.
　2 The fluid cannot flow through smaller veins.
　3 Peripheral veins become very irritated because of the content of the fluid.
　4 Because the patient will have the infusion for a long time, this way he will have use of both of his hands without an IV in them.

2 A patient is receiving an infusion of lipids through his central line. What symptoms might suggest that the patient is experiencing lipid intolerance?
　1 Elevated temperature, chills, nausea, and chest pain
　2 Respiratory distress, shortness of breath, chest pain, and decreased blood pressure
　3 Increased temperature, chills, malaise, and elevated white blood cell count
　4 Nausea and vomiting, and bleeding and swelling at the insertion site

3 A patient is receiving a 3:1 parenteral nutrition infusion. How often should the IV infusion tubing be changed?
　1 Once a week
　2 Every 24 hours
　3 Every 72 hours
　4 After each solution is administered

REFERENCES

American Dietetic Association: Nutritional care process model, part I: the 2008 update, *J Am Dietetic Assoc* 108(7):1113, 2008.

American Society for Parenteral and Enteral Nutrition: Standards of practice: nutrition support nurses, *Nutr Clin Pract* 16(1):56, 2001.

American Society for Parenteral and Enteral Nutrition: Guidelines for the use of parenteral and enteral nutrition in adult and pediatric patients, *JPEN J Parenter Enteral Nutr* 26(suppl 1):1SA, 2002.

de Jonge E: Placement of central venous catheters and patient safety, *Ned Tijdschr Geneeskd* 151(4):226, 2007.

Driscoll DF, Baron MN: Physiochemical stability of two types of intravenous lipid emulsions as total nutrient admixture, *JPEN J Parenter Enteral Nutr* 24(1):15, 2000.

Grodner M and others: *Foundations and clinical applications of nutrition*, ed 4, St. Louis, 2007, Mosby.

Hockenberry MJ and others: *Wong's nursing care of infants and children*, ed 8, St. Louis, 2007, Mosby.

Infusion Nurses Society: Infusion nursing standards of practice, *J Intraven Nurs* 29(suppl 1):S1, 2006.

Krein SL and others: Use of central venous catheter-related bloodstream infection prevention practices by US hospitals, *Mayo Clinic Proc* 82(6):672, 2007

Kelly L: The care of vascular access devices in community care, *Br J Community Nurs* 13(5):198, 2008

Stratton R, Elia M: Who benefits from nutritional support: what is the evidence? *Eur J Gastroenterol Hepatol* 19(5):353, 2007.

The Joint Commission: Tubing misconnections—a persistent and potentially deadly occurrence, *Sentinel Event Alert*, issue 36, April 3, 2006.

The Joint Commission: *2008 National patient safety goals hospital program*, Oakbrook Terrace, Ill, 2007, The Joint Commission, http://www.jointcommission.org, accessed July 2007.

RESEARCH REFERENCES

Forbes A: Parenteral nutrition. *Curr Opin Gastroenterol* 23(2):183, 2007.

O'Grady NP and others: Guidelines for the prevention of intravascular catheter-related infections, *MMWR Morb Mortal Wkly Rep* 51(RR-10):1, 2002.

Peter JV and others: A metaanalysis of treatment outcomes of early enteral versus early parenteral nutrition in hospitalized patients, *Crit Care Med* 33(1):213, 2005.

Winkler MF: Quality of life in adult home parenteral nutrition patients, *JPEN J Parenter Enteral Nutr* 29(3):162, 2005.

MEDIA RESOURCES

- evolve   http://evolve.elsevier.com/Perry/skills
  learning system

- View Video!   Review Questions Video Clips

- NSO   Nursing Skills Online

OBJECTIVES

Mastery of content in this chapter will enable the nurse to:

- Identify factors that alter normal voiding.
- Identify factors that increase risk for urinary infection.
- Discuss relationship between fluid balance and urinary elimination.
- Describe devices used to promote urinary elimination.

- Perform the following skills: place and remove urinal, insert urinary catheter, care for an indwelling urinary catheter, measure a bladder scan, obtain a residual urine, irrigate a catheter, remove a retention catheter, apply a condom catheter, care for a suprapubic catheter, and administer intermittent peritoneal and continuous ambulatory peritoneal dialysis.

Urinary elimination is normally a private process managed independently by a patient depending on age and developmental stage. Some patients need psychological support while adjusting to alterations in urinary elimination secondary to changes in their functional status and/or physiological status. Functional and physiological alterations limit a patient's ability for self-care and ability to manage urinary elimination independently. In addition, physiological alterations often require medical or surgical treatment, for example, an acutely ill patient may require urinary catheterization for close monitoring of urine output. You need to have an understanding of the skills and procedures used for patients with alterations in urinary elimination in order to intervene in a competent manner.

EVIDENCE-BASED PRACTICE TRENDS

Urinary catheterization is a common procedure in all health care settings. It is an invasive procedure that commonly results in catheter-associated urinary tract infections (CAUTIs). Nine percent of patients in hospitals acquire a health care associated infection and UTIs account for 35% of them (Hart 2008). CAUTI is associated with prolonged hospitalization and mortality (Toughill, 2005).

Nazarko (2008) stresses that decreasing the risk for CAUTI starts by avoiding unnecessary use of indwelling catheters and removing the catheters as soon as medically indicated. Older adult patients (older than 70 years) with limited functional ability are often catheterized to facilitate their care rather than for medical indications (Holroyd and others, 2007). The results of the study suggest that nonmedical use of indwelling catheters in older adults may result in longer hospital stays and greater risk for death secondary to development of urinary tract infection (UTI) and entrance of bacteria into the bloodstream (bacteremia or urosepsis).

Duration of catheter use, female gender, and age over 60 are some of the most important risk factors for developing UTI and gram-negative urosepsis (Pinto and Matteucci, 2008). The risk for CAUTI increases by number of days that a catheter remains in place (Nazarko, 2008). The timing of catheter removal involves a balance between avoiding infection (early removal) and avoiding the incidence of treatment-related voiding dysfunction, that is, difficulty urinating after having an indwelling catheter in place (later removal) (Fernandez and Griffiths, 2006).

Urinary catheters vary in composition and design. Limited evidenced-based research exists related to the most effective design and composition that will lower UTI risk (Gray, 2006b). Biofilm, the adherence of microorganisms to the catheter surface, leads to CAUTI. Research related to catheter composition focuses on altering the catheter surface to slow biofilm development (Trautner and others, 2005). Some newer modifications in catheter materials include indwelling catheters and intermittent-use catheters that are impregnated internally and on the outer surface with antibacterial agents such as silver oxide and nitrofurazone. These agents release slowly and are absorbed locally in the urethra. After a thorough review of the scientific literature, Saint and others (2008) conclude that short-term use of coated indwelling catheters reduces the risk for CAUTI. An intermittent catheter designed to decrease the potential for contamination is a touchless catheter. This catheter is covered by a sheath, which allows the patient to avoid touching the catheter during self-insertion, decreasing contamination risk (Hudson and Murahata, 2005).

Although not all catheterizations are unnecessary, many can be avoided by using noninvasive alternatives. For example, a frequent intervention for patients with urinary retention is to evaluate the amount of urine in the bladder using catheterization. However, you can evaluate bladder urine volume without invasive instrumentation by use of a bladder scanner or ultrasonography. When you determine urine volume is normal, catheterization may not be needed (Chen and others, 2005). Use of the bladder scan is time efficient as well; catheterization may take three to eight times the amount of time when compared to ultrasonography for measuring bladder volume (Teng and others, 2005). Experimental studies related to bladder scanner use are ongoing.

Nurses reduce the risk for CAUTI by being patient advocates. Take an active role in suggesting alternatives to catheterization use and monitoring duration of treatment. The incidence of CAUTI significantly decreases when nurses give the prescriber daily reminders to remove unnecessary catheters and suggest the use of alternative noninvasive treatments to manage urinary elimination (Holroyd and others, 2007; Nazarko, 2008).

CULTURAL CONSIDERATIONS

Consider the patient's cultural heritage in order to provide for urinary elimination in a compassionate and competent manner. The potential exposure of perineal structures during elimination care has implications for members of those cultures who hold specific beliefs about female modesty and gender-appropriate care. Use the following guidelines when caring for patients with gender-specific needs:

- Provide for gender-congruent care for cultures emphasizing separate gender roles and female modesty such as African, Hispanic, Asian, Islamic, Arabic, Hindu, Jewish Orthodox, and Amish cultures.
- Allow presence of a family member at the bedside if requested by the patient.
- Provide privacy through adequate draping and use of bedside screens.
- Prevent entrance of the opposite sex into the patient's room during the procedure.
- Use a professional, nonjudgmental manner when viewing scarring or constriction of perineal tissues indicating female circumcision. You may need to use a smaller catheter to catheterize the patient. However, if there is extensive scarring, you may not be able to insert a catheter into the urethral meatus, and the patient may need a suprapubic catheter placed (Reyners, 2004).
- Use an interpreter if needed.

- Certain cultures have meticulous hygiene practices. For example, Hindus and Muslims designate the left hand to perform unclean procedures such as catheterization. For these patients:
  - Perform hand hygiene before touching the patient, and use your right hand.
  - Use the left hand to handle the urinal and/or urinary secretions.
  - Do not place the urinal or soiled bed linens on top of the bedside table or surface used for praying or eating.
  - Provide the patient with the equipment and supplies for cleansing after elimination (Lawrence and Rozmus, 2001).

Skill Performance Guidelines

1 Consider the patient's functional status, mobility, and cognitive and psychological function, and determine how that will influence access to toileting facilities and ability to participate in self-care related to urinary elimination.

2 Know the patient's normal pattern of urination. Teach the patient not to ignore the urge to void. Assist by responding readily to the patient's request to use a bedpan, urinal, bathroom, or commode. Offer the patient the opportunity to void after meals, at regular intervals throughout the day, and before bedtime. Patients taking diuretic medications should receive them early in the morning so they do not need to void during the night.

3 Know the patient's normal range of vital signs. Abnormal fluid and electrolyte balances affect the amount of circulating blood volume (Table 33-1).

4 Know the signs of dehydration and fluid overload (see Table 33-1). Start measurement of intake and output (I&O) when there is an actual or anticipated change in fluid balance (see Chapter 6). If oral intake is not at least 1500 mL/day, develop a plan of care with the patient to increase fluids. Some patients with urinary problems hesitate to take fluids in fear of incontinence and/or increased urinary frequency. Explain the importance of fluid intake in maintaining urinary health.

5 Know the average output range for a patient. Adult urinary output averages 1000 to 2400 mL in 24 hours. An hourly output of less than 30 mL/hr for 2 hours is cause for further evaluation. Minimum average hourly output is 30 mL.

6 Weigh the patient to determine fluid status (see Chapter 6). Weigh with the same scale, at the same time of day, and with comparable articles of clothing, including bed linen if bed weights are necessary.

7 Consider the patient's age when assessing micturition (voiding) habits. Toilet training and enuresis are concerns for the toddler and preschooler. Older adults often experience disease or physiological changes that predispose them to incontinence, or the inability to control urination.

8 Assess the patient's most recent serum electrolyte measurements. Abnormal values reflect alterations in fluid balance that can lead to deterioration in patients' health.

9 Provide for the patient's privacy and comfort. A physically or psychologically uncomfortable patient may be unable to relax the external urethral sphincter and therefore may not be able to urinate or completely empty the bladder. Offer the patient a warm bedpan, assist the patient into a normal voiding position (standing for a man, squatting for a woman), or reduce pain by administering a prescribed analgesic before helping the patient walk to the bathroom. Distraction measures, such as turning on a sink faucet so the patient can hear water running, help the patient to void.

10 Identify conditions that weaken abdominal or pelvic muscles such as multiple abdominal or gynecological surgeries or pregnancies. Teach patients exercises to strengthen weak abdominal or pelvic floor muscles to increase the ability of the bladder to contract and to promote better control of the external urethral sphincter.

TABLE 33-1	Signs of Fluid Volume Deficit (FVD) and Fluid Volume Excess (FVE)
Eyes	*FVD:* Sunken eyes, dry conjunctivae, decreased or absence of tearing *FVE:* Periorbital edema, blurred vision, papilledema
Mouth	*FVD:* Sticky, dry mucous membrane; dry, cracked lips; decreased saliva; increased viscosity of saliva; furrowed, shrunken tongue *FVE:* Excessive salivation
Skin	*FVD:* Increased skin temperature; dry, scaly skin; poor turgor *FVE:* Edema, anasarca
Cardiovascular	*FVD:* Increased pulse rate, weak pulse, hypotension, decreased pulse volume/pressure, decreased capillary filling, increased hematocrit, flat neck veins *FVE:* Bounding pulse rate, blood pressure normal with or without orthostatic changes, third heart sound (S_3), distended neck veins
Gastrointestinal	*FVD:* Sunken abdomen *FVD* or *FVE:* Vomiting, diarrhea, abdominal cramps
Renal	*FVD:* Oliguria or anuria, urine specific gravity increased (normal, 1.010 to 1.030) *FVE:* Decreased urine specific gravity, diuresis (if kidneys are normal)

PROCEDURAL GUIDELINE 33-1 Assisting a Patient in Using a Urinal

Basic Skills / Elimination Assistance / Assisting With a Urinal

Bed rest or mobility restrictions interfere with a patient's ability to assume the normal position for emptying the bladder. If a patient cannot walk to the toilet facilities, a male patient may stand at the bedside and void into a urinal (Fig. 33-1). A female patient may use a bedside commode or a female urinal. If a male is unable to stand at the bedside or a female is unable to get out of bed, you will need to assist him or her in using the urinal in bed. The female urinal includes a container with a circular open top with a defined top rim portion. It is designed to come in close contact with the genitalia, which allows urine to flow into the container and not around or below the rim.

Delegation Considerations

The skill of assisting a patient in using a urinal can be delegated to nursing assistive personnel (NAP). The nurse directs the NAP about:

- The amount of functional assistance a patient requires to use a urinal.
- Reporting the following: changes in color, amount or odor of the patient's urine, and any incontinence episodes.
- Explaining the procedure to the patient and family to promote understanding and participation in care.

Equipment

- ❑ Urinal
- ❑ Clean gloves
- ❑ Graduated cylinder (used for measuring volume if urinal is not marked)
- ❑ Supplies for diagnostic urine tests and specimen collection (see Chapter 43)

Procedural Steps

1. Assess patient's normal urinary elimination habits.
2. Identify any periods of incontinence.
3. Assess for distended bladder by palpating above symphysis pubis.
4. Assess patient's functional status, including knowledge regarding urinal use.
5. Perform hand hygiene, and apply clean gloves.
6. Provide privacy by closing bedside curtain or room door.

7. Assist patient into appropriate position: *for a male patient:* on side, back, sitting with head of bed elevated, or in the standing position; *for a female patient:* lying supine.

Critical Decision Point *Always determine mobility status before having a patient stand to void, and assess for orthostatic hypotension if the patient has been on prolonged bed rest.*

8. If possible, the male patient should hold urinal and position penis in urinal. If patient is unable to position penis completely within urinal, provide needed assistance. Hold or assist in holding urinal in place. Make sure to keep the opening of the urinal higher than the base to prevent spilling the urine.
9. Assist the female patient by holding the female urinal upright.
10. Remove urinal after the patient has finished voiding. Assist patient, if able, to wash and dry penis or genitalia.
11. Measure urine, and record output on I&O record, if needed.
12. Observe characteristics of urine, empty and cleanse urinal, and return it to patient for future use.
13. Assist patient, as needed, to perform hand hygiene.
14. Remove and dispose of gloves; perform hand hygiene.

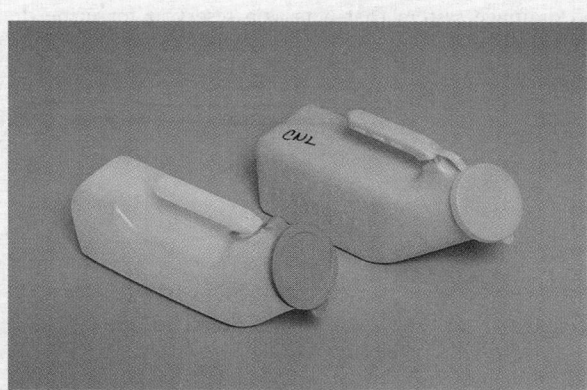

FIG 33-1 Types of male urinals.

SKILL 33-1   Inserting a Straight or Indwelling Urinary Catheter

 Intermediate / Urinary Catheter Management /
Inserting an Indwelling Catheter in a Female Patient
Inserting an Indwelling Catheter in a Male Patient
Performing Intermittent Straight Catheterization

NSO *Urinary Catheterization Module / Lessons 1 and 2*

Urinary catheters are flexible tubes inserted into the urinary bladder (Fig. 33-2). Most commonly, you will insert either a straight or an indwelling (Foley) catheter. Patients can learn how to insert straight catheters. A straight, or intermittent catheter, is a single-lumen catheter inserted into the bladder through the urethra only to empty the bladder, and then it is removed. Use this type of catheter on either a one-time basis, for example, to determine the amount of residual urine in the bladder (see Procedural Guideline 33-2), or intermittently, when the patient cannot urinate related to a urinary obstruction or neurological disorder such as a spinal cord injury. Patients use clean insertion technique in the home setting. When the patient is in an acute care or long-term care setting, sterile insertion technique is required because of the high risk for nosocomial infections (Nazarko, 2008). Patients who require self-catheterization have a variety of options in catheter products. There is a single catheter, which is prepackaged in a sterile saline solution that serves as a lubricant (called a hydrophilic catheter). In addition, self-contained systems are available, consisting of a catheter prepackaged in sterile saline with a preconnected drainage bag.

An indwelling or Foley catheter is inserted into the urethra and is usually preconnected or connected after catheterization to a closed drainage system that acts as a reservoir for urine drained

from the bladder. A Foley catheter has a separate lumen used to inflate a balloon so the catheter remains in the bladder for short- or long-term use. Indications for an indwelling catheter include (1) the presence of stage III and IV pressure ulcers (see Chapter 18) that cannot heal because of continual incontinence, (2) when accurate measurement of urinary output in critically ill patients is needed, (3) relief of urinary obstruction, and (4) postoperatively (e.g., spinal anesthesia, bladder surgery) (Gray, 2006a; Nazarko, 2008; Senese and others, 2006a).

Delegation Considerations

The skill of inserting a straight or indwelling catheter cannot be delegated. However, in some settings, for example, long-term care setting, these skills may be delegated (see agency policy). The nurse evaluates possible alternatives to catheter use and assesses the need for catheterization. The nurse directs the NAP to:

- Assist with patient positioning, focus lighting for the procedure, maintain privacy, empty urine from collection bag, and assist with perineal care.
- Report postprocedure patient discomfort or fever to the nurse.
- Report abnormal color, odor, and amount of urine in drainage bag to the nurse.

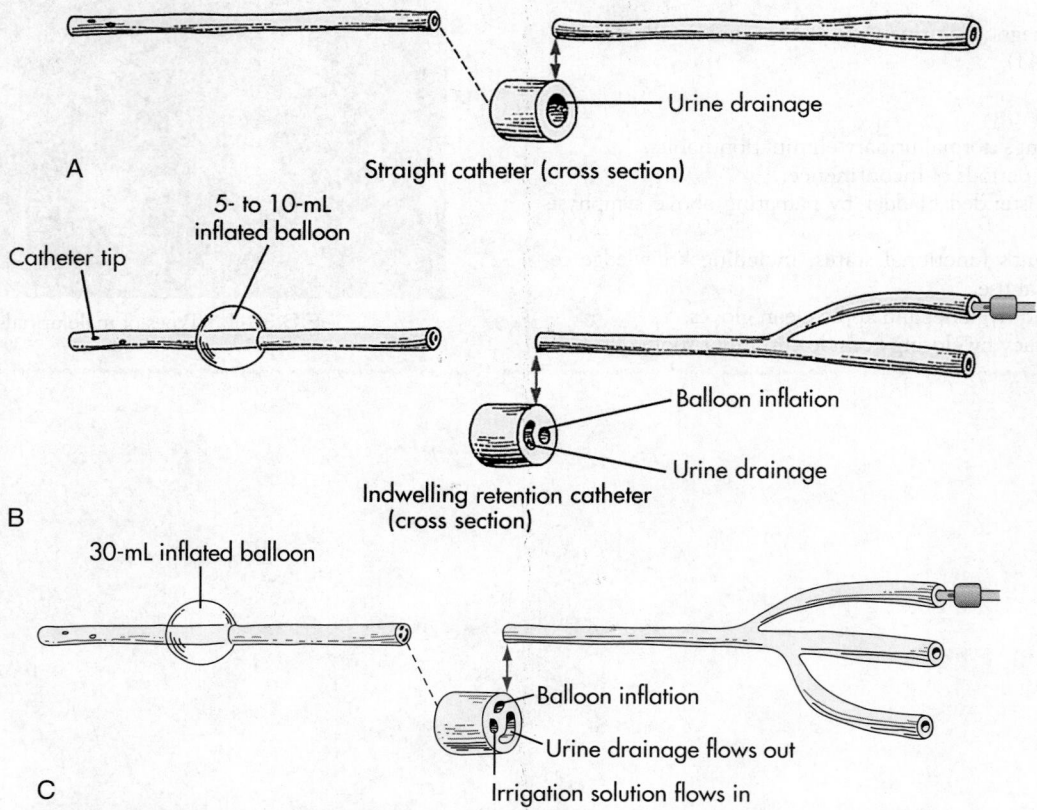

FIG 33-2 **A,** Straight catheter (cross section). **B,** Indwelling retention catheter (cross section). **C,** Triple lumen catheter for continuous closed irrigation (cross section).

Equipment

- ❏ Bladder scanner (if available)
- ❏ Catheter kit (Fig. 33-3) containing the following sterile items:
  - Proper-size urinary catheter with drainage tubing and collection bag, which are usually connected (indwelling catheter only)
  - Sterile gloves (extra pair optional)
  - Waterproof drapes (one fenestrated—has an opening in the center of drape)
  - Lubricant
  - Antiseptic cleansing agent (povidone-iodine) or alternative such as Hibiclens or Shur-Clens)
  - Cotton balls or sterile antiseptic swabs
  - Forceps
  - Prefilled syringe with sterile water (to inflate balloon of indwelling catheter only)
  - Specimen container
- ❏ Sterile drainage tubing and collection bag (if not included in the kit)
- ❏ Multipurpose Velcro tube holder or nonallergenic/paper tape
- ❏ Bath blanket
- ❏ Waterproof absorbent pad

- ❏ Clean gloves, basin with warm water, soap, washcloth, and towel for perineal care
- ❏ Additional lighting as needed (such as a flashlight or procedure light)

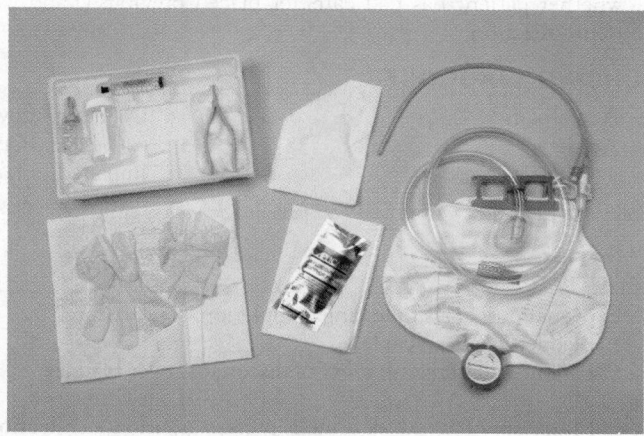

FIG 33-3 Indwelling catheterization kit (includes drainage device, specimen cup, sterile drapes, sterile gloves, indwelling catheter, cleansing solution, sterile saline, sterile cotton balls, forceps, and lubricant).

STEP	RATIONALE

ASSESSMENT

1 Review patient's medical record, including prescriber's order and nurses' notes. When appropriate, determine previous catheterization, including catheter size.	Data explains purpose of inserting catheter, such as preparation for surgery, urinary irrigations, collection of sterile urine specimen, or measurement of residual urine.
2 Assess status of patient:	
a Ask patient when was time of last urination. Check I&O flow sheet.	Determines time of last voiding or potential for bladder fullness.
b Level of awareness or developmental stage	Reveals patient's ability to cooperate during procedure, level of explanation needed, and ability to perform self-catheterization.
c Mobility and physical limitations	Determines how you will position patient.
d Gender and age	Determines catheter size: 5 to 6 Fr is generally for an infant; 8 to 10 Fr with 3-mL balloon is generally for children; 14 to 16 Fr is indicated for adult women; 12 Fr may be considered for young girls. Men often need a slightly larger size, so a 16 to 18 Fr may be used. The prescriber may order a larger size.
e Allergies	Procedure risks exposure to allergens associated with antiseptic, tape, latex, and lubricant. Povidone-iodine (Betadine) allergies are common; if client is unaware of allergy, ask if allergic to shellfish.

Critical Decision Point   *Large catheters (greater than 16 Fr) can distend the urethra and permanently damage the urethra and bladder neck, as well as cause bladder spasms and leaking around the catheter (Hart, 2008). Use the smallest size catheter possible to minimize trauma and promote adequate drainage of the periurethral glands. This will decrease the risk for infection (Hart, 2008; Senese and others, 2006a).*

3 Assess bladder for fullness (distended bladder is palpable above symphysis pubis) or use a bladder scanner (if available) (see Procedural Guideline 33-2, p. 880).	Full bladder with inability to void indicates need to insert catheter. A bladder scan noninvasively determines the amount of urine in the bladder.
4 Perform hand hygiene, apply clean gloves, and assess for perineal anatomical landmarks, erythema, drainage, and odor. Remove gloves and perform hand hygiene.	Determines condition of perineum.
5 Review medical record for any pathological condition that will impair passage of catheter (e.g., enlarged prostate gland in men).	Obstruction prevents passage of catheter through urethra into bladder.

STEP	RATIONALE
6 Assess patient's knowledge of the purpose of catheterization, whether patient has had catheter placed previously, and patient's reaction.	Reveals need for patient instruction and/or support.

NURSING DIAGNOSES

- Acute pain
- Anxiety

- Deficient knowledge regarding need for catheterization
- Impaired urinary elimination

- Risk for infection
- Urinary retention

Individualize related factors based on patient's condition or needs.

PLANNING

STEP	RATIONALE
1 Expected outcomes following completion of procedure:	
• Bladder is not palpable.	Removal of urine from bladder relieves sensation of fullness.
• Patient will verbalize relief of discomfort over bladder.	Patent catheter system keeps bladder empty and patient comfortable.
• Minimum of 30 mL of urine is present in urinary collection bag every hour (see Chapter 6).	Verifies presence of catheter in bladder, catheter patency, and adequate perfusion to kidneys.
• Patient verbalizes minimal pain during procedure.	Correct insertion technique minimizes localized trauma to urethra.
• Patient verbalizes the purpose and expectations about the procedure.	Promotes cooperation.
2 Explain procedure to patient.	Promotes cooperation.
3 Arrange for extra personnel to assist as necessary.	Some clients are unable to independently assume positioning for the procedure.

IMPLEMENTATION

STEP	RATIONALE
1 Perform hand hygiene.	Reduces transmission of microorganisms.
2 Close curtain or door.	Provides privacy and reduces embarrassment to patient, thus promoting relaxation.
3 Raise bed to appropriate working height. Facing patient, stand on left side of bed if right-handed and on right side if left-handed. If side rails in use, raise side rail on opposite side of bed and lower side rail on working side.	Successful catheter insertion requires a comfortable position with all equipment easily accessible. Use of side rails in this manner promotes patient safety.
4 Place waterproof pad under patient.	Prevents soiling of bed linen.

Critical Decision Point *Obtain assistance to position and to support weak, frail, or confused patients.*

STEP	RATIONALE
5 Position patient:	
a Female patient:	
(1) Assist to dorsal recumbent position (supine with knees flexed). Ask patient to relax thighs to externally rotate the hip joints.	Provides good visualization of perineal structures. This position is optimal because it minimizes the risk for contamination by fecal material (Cochran, 2007).
(2) Position female patient in side-lying (Sims') position with upper leg flexed at knee and hip if unable to be supine. Take extra precautions to cover rectal area with drape during procedure to reduce chance of cross contamination. Support patient with pillows if necessary to maintain position.	Use this alternative position if patient cannot abduct leg at hip joint (e.g., if patient has arthritic joints). In addition, this position is often more comfortable for patient.
b Male patient:	
(1) Assist to supine or sitting position with thighs slightly abducted.	Comfortable position for patient that aids in visualization of penis.
6 Drape patient:	Avoids unnecessary exposure of body parts and maintains patient's comfort.
a Female patient:	
(1) Drape with bath blanket. Place blanket diamond fashion over patient, with one corner at patient's neck, side corners over each arm and side, and last corner over perineum (see illustration).	Keeps legs and lower abdomen covered as nurse exposes perineum during procedure.

STEP	RATIONALE

   b Male patient:

     (1) Drape upper trunk with bath blanket, and cover lower extremities with bed sheet, exposing only genitalia.

Keeps legs and lower abdomen covered as nurse exposes genitalia during procedure.

7 Wearing clean gloves, wash perineal area with soap and water as needed; dry (see Chapter 17). Locate urinary meatus in female patients while performing perineal hygiene. Have NAP hold alternative light source to illuminate perineum as needed. Remove and discard gloves; perform hand hygiene.

Washing ensures area is not contaminated before catheter insertion (Leaver, 2007). It is sometimes difficult to see the urinary meatus of a female patient due to individual anatomical differences (Senese and others, 2006a). Additional direct lighting illuminates the perineum.

8 Open outer wrapping of either an indwelling Foley catheterization kit or intermittent catheterization kit by tearing package on paper-lined edge of plastic wrap. Place inner wrapped box on easily accessible, clean bedside table or set it in between patient's legs. Patient's size and positioning will dictate exact placement. Place empty package (outer plastic wrap) near end of bed and use for waste disposal.

Provides easy access to supplies during catheter insertion. Maintains aseptic technique during procedure.

This method works best with flexible, average-size patients.

9 Open sterile wrap covering box containing catheter supplies: Using sterile technique (see Chapter 8), fold back each flap of the sterile package one at a time, with the last flap opened toward patient.

The tray is now open and sitting on its own sterile field (see illustration, Step 6a(1)).

   a The supplies in an intermittent catheterization tray are contained in a sterile receptacle that can be used for urine collection.

Sequence of supplies will vary. Use supplies in order of use to prevent contamination of underlying supplies.

   b The supplies in an indwelling catheter box are arranged in sequence of use.

10 Apply waterproof sterile drape (when packed as first item in tray):

   Option: Sterile gloves may be packed as first item (see Step 11).

   a Female patient:

     (1) Remove the square sterile drape from the tray, touching the edges (1-inch border) only. Do not touch any other item in the kit (see Chapter 8).

Keeps drape and items sterile.

     (2) Maintain sterility of drape, and let it unfold after removing from tray. Fold top edge of drape (2.5 to 5 cm [1 to 2 inches]) away from patient to form cuff over both hands.

     (3) Have patient lift hips (if patient is unable to lift hips, get assistance).

     (4) Place sterile drape with the plastic (shiny) side down under the patient's buttocks (see illustration).

Creates a sterile field over which nurse will work during catheterization.

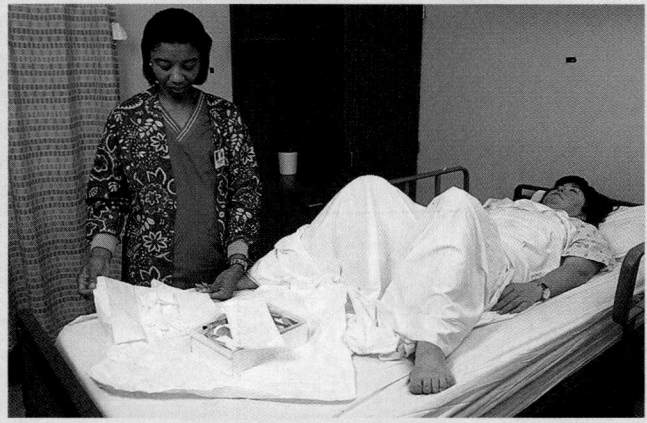

STEP 6a(1) Patient draped and in dorsal recumbent position with tray open on sterile field.

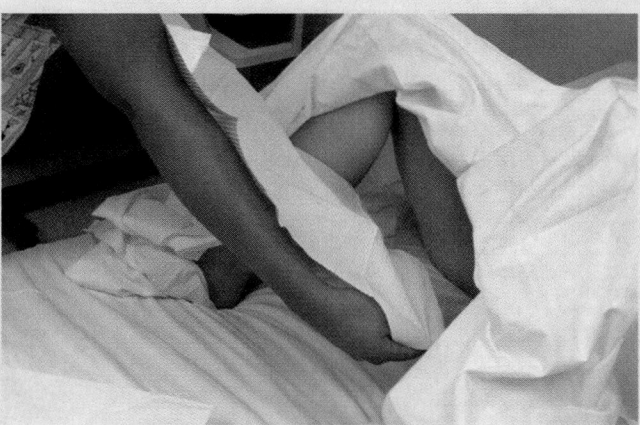

STEP 10a(4) Place sterile drape under buttocks as patient lifts hips slightly off bed.

STEP	RATIONALE
(5) Apply sterile gloves, and proceed to Step 12. **b Male patient:** (1) Use of square sterile drape is optional; you may apply a fenestrated drape instead (see Step 12). Remove and unfold as with female (see Step 10a). Apply drape over thighs just below penis (instead of under buttocks as in female).	Creates sterile field.
11 Apply sterile gloves. (When packed as first item in tray, apply and then place square drape [see Step 10].)	Nurse will apply drapes either with or without sterile gloves, depending on sequence of packaging.
12 Applying fenestrated drape: **a Female patient:** (1) Pick up fenestrated sterile drape out of tray. Allow it to unfold without touching a nonsterile surface. Form cuff from edges to protect sterile gloves. Apply drape over perineum, exposing labia and being sure not to touch contaminated surface (see illustration).	Creates sterile field around perineum with opening that allows nurse to manipulate perineum.
b Male patient: (1) Apply fenestrated drape over thighs and below penis without completely opening drape. Use this technique when you choose not to apply square sterile drape. (2) Pick up fenestrated sterile drape, allow it to unfold without touching a nonsterile surface. Form cuff from edges to protect sterile gloves; drape it over penis with fenestrated slit resting over penis (see illustration).	Either a square or a fenestrated drape may be used with the male patient to create a sterile field.
13 Move tray/box on sterile field closer to patient. In the case of a female patient, the sterile wrap under tray/box and drape under patient form a continuous field.	Prevents nurse from reaching over nonsterile area when manipulating sterile catheter.
a Organize remaining items on sterile field. *Indwelling catheter:* Take top tray out of box, and place it on sterile field. (Sterile catheter and drainage bag are under the top tray in the box). Make sure clamp on drainage port of bag is closed. If drainage bag is preconnected to the catheter, leave the bag on the sterile field until the catheter is inserted. If drainage bag is not connected to catheter, open package containing sterile collection bag and drainage tubing. Keep cover on tip of drainage tubing until ready to connect to catheter.	Maintains principles of surgical asepsis and organizes work area. Keeping cover on tip of the sterile drainage tubing prevents contamination.

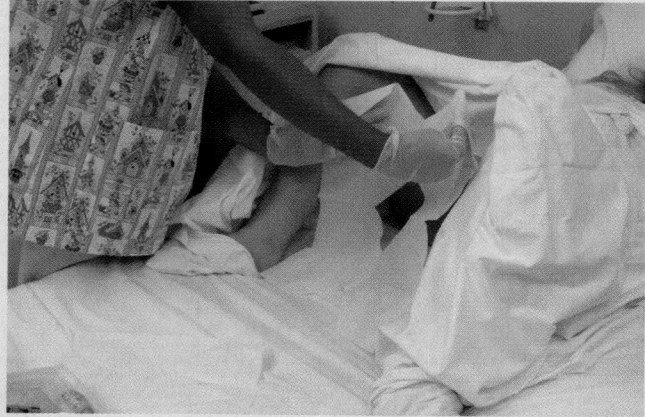

STEP 12a(1)   Place sterile fenestrated drape (with opening in center) over female's perineum with labia exposed.

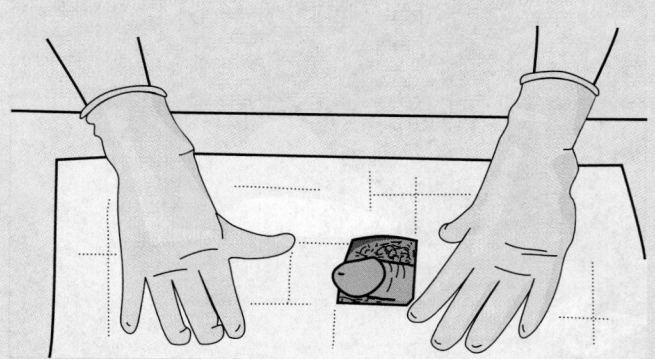

STEP 12b(2)   Draping male with fenestrated drape.

STEP	RATIONALE
b Intermittent catheter: There will be no drainage bag in container or specimen container.	
c Loosen lid on sterile specimen container if urine specimen required. Otherwise, discard into waste disposal bag.	Makes container accessible to receive urine from catheter if specimen is needed.
d Open package of sterile antiseptic solution. Pour solution over sterile cotton balls (see illustration). NOTE: Sometimes there are sterile antiseptic swabs instead of solution. If swabs are available, open package with "stick" ends up for access.	
e Open packet containing lubricant. NOTE: Lubricant is sometimes in a prefilled syringe. If in a prefilled syringe, remove protective cap. Spread lubricant into sterile tray.	Prepares lubricant for catheter.
14 Remove plastic covering from catheter (usually on indwelling catheter only). Take care to coil length of catheter in palm.	Prevents contamination of catheter.

Critical Decision Point   *Testing the balloon by injecting fluid from the prefilled sterile water syringe into the balloon port is no longer a common practice. Testing the balloon may stretch the balloon and lead to damage, causing increased trauma on insertion (check manufacturer's instruction).*

STEP	RATIONALE
15 Place length of catheter in lubricant: Lubricate catheter 2.5 to 5 cm (1 to 2 inches) for women and 12.5 to 17.5 cm (5 to 7 inches) for men (see illustration).	Lubricating catheter will minimize urethral trauma and discomfort when inserting catheter.
16 Cleanse urethral meatus:	
a Female patient:	
(1) With nondominant hand, fully expose urethral meatus by spreading labia. Have NAP use flashlight if unable to visualize meatus with available lighting. Maintain position of nondominant hand throughout procedure.	Optimal visualization of urethral meatus is possible. Fully spreading labia prevents contamination of urethral meatus during cleansing.

Critical Decision Point   *If unable to visualize urethra, place one finger of sterile gloved hand inside the vagina and apply gentle pressure upward to support and straighten the urethra. This may open the urethral meatus, creating better visualization. Insert the catheter just above the finger and below the clitoris (Senese and others, 2006b). Ensure that the patient understands what you are doing. This hand is now considered contaminated.*

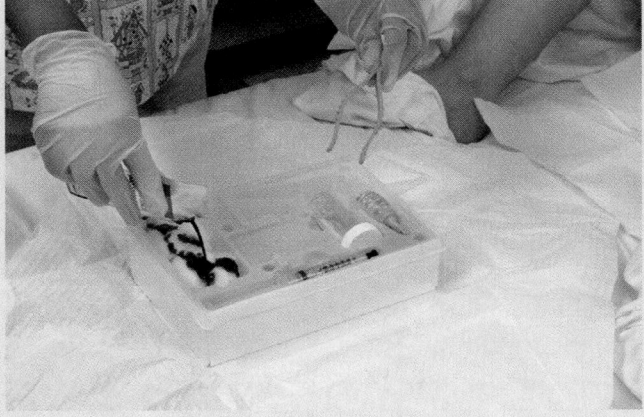

STEP 13d   Pouring antiseptic solution over cotton balls.

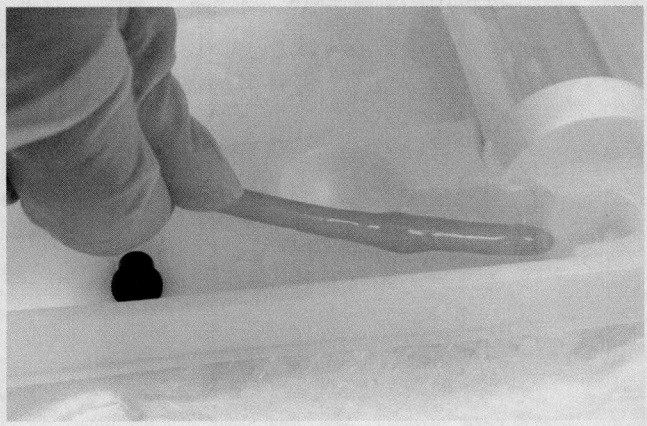

STEP 15   Lubricating catheter.

STEP	RATIONALE
(2) Using forceps in sterile dominant hand, pick up cotton ball saturated with antiseptic solution or antiseptic swab stick, and clean perineal area, wiping front to back from clitoris toward anus. Use a new cotton ball or swab for each area you cleanse: wipe the far labial fold, the near labial fold, and directly over center of urethral meatus (see illustration).	Cleansing reduces number of microorganisms at urethral meatus. Follows principles of medical asepsis (see Chapter 7). Dominant gloved hand remains sterile.

Critical Decision Point *Closure of labia during cleansing requires that the cleaning procedure be repeated because the area is now contaminated.*

STEP	RATIONALE
b Male patient:	
(1) If patient is not circumcised, retract foreskin with nondominant hand.	Exposes urethral meatus.
(a) Grasp penis at shaft just below glans.	
(b) Gently spread urethral meatus so opening is more visible. Keep nondominant hand in this position throughout procedure.	Accidental release of foreskin or dropping of penis during cleansing requires repeating the process because area becomes contaminated.
(2) With dominant hand, pick up antiseptic-soaked cotton ball with forceps or swab stick, and clean penis. Move cotton ball or swab in circular motion from urethral meatus down to base of glans. Repeat cleansing three more times, using clean cotton ball/ stick each time (see illustration).	Reduces number of microorganisms at urethral meatus. Follows principles of medical aseptic technique (see Chapter 7). Dominant gloved hand remains sterile.
17 Pick up catheter with gloved dominant hand, holding catheter 7.5 to 10 cm (3 to 4 inches) inches from catheter tip. Hold end of catheter loosely coiled in palm of dominant hand.	Hold catheter near tip because it allows easier manipulation during insertion into urethral meatus. Prevents distal end from striking contaminated surface.

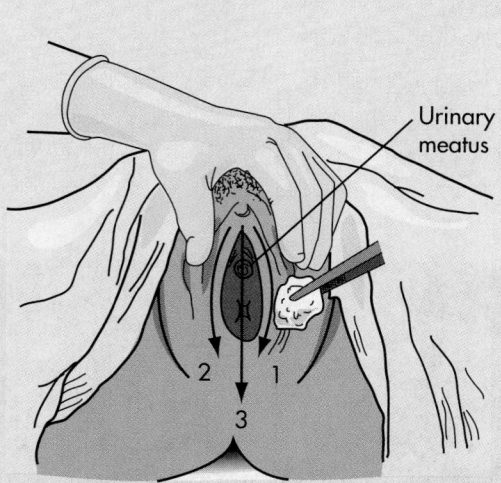

STEP 16a(2) Cleansing female perineum.

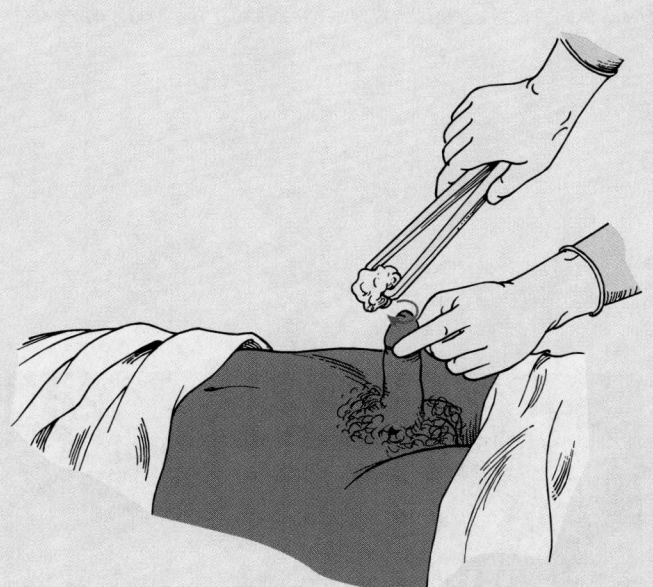

STEP 16b(2) Cleansing male urinary meatus.

STEP	RATIONALE

18 Insert catheter:

a Female patient:

(1) Ask patient to bear down gently as if to void, and slowly insert catheter through urethral meatus (see illustration).

Relaxation of external sphincter aids in insertion of catheter.

(2) Advance catheter a total of 5 to 7.5 cm (2 to 3 inches) in adult or until urine flows out catheter's end. As soon as urine appears, advance catheter another 2.5 to 5 cm (1 to 2 inches). Do not force against resistance.

Female urethra is short. Appearance of urine indicates that catheter tip is in bladder or lower urethra. Advancement of catheter ensures that the inflation balloon is in the bladder and not the urethra (Senese and others, 2006b).

Critical Decision Point   *If no urine appears, catheter may be in vagina. If misplaced, leave catheter in vagina as landmark indicating where not to insert, and insert another sterile catheter.*

(3) Release labia, and hold catheter securely with non-dominant hand. **Proceed to Step 20 for balloon inflation (indwelling Foley only).**

Bladder or sphincter contraction will cause accidental expulsion of catheter.

b Male patient:

(1) Lift penis to position perpendicular to patient's body, and apply light traction (see illustration).

Straightens urethral canal to ease catheter insertion.

(2) Ask patient to bear down as if to void, and slowly insert catheter through urethral meatus.

Relaxation of external sphincter aids in insertion of catheter.

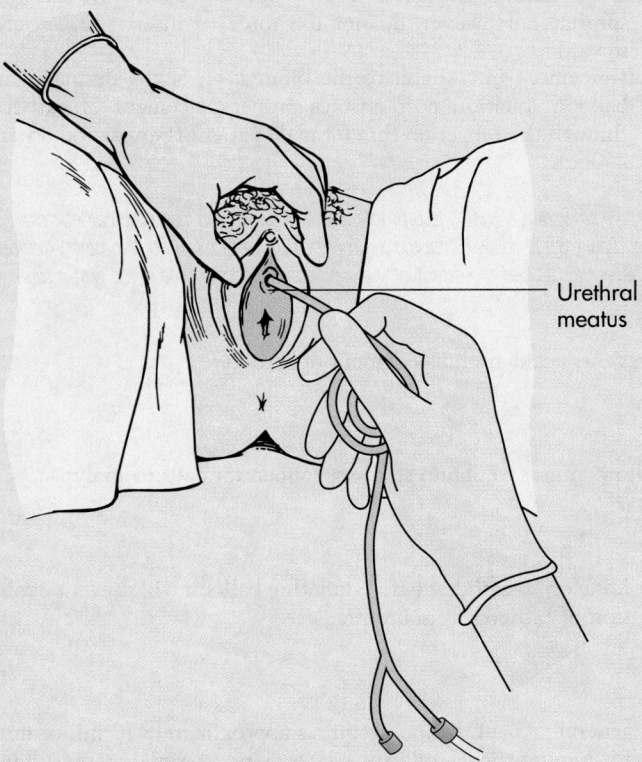

Urethral meatus

STEP 18a(1)   Inserting the catheter.

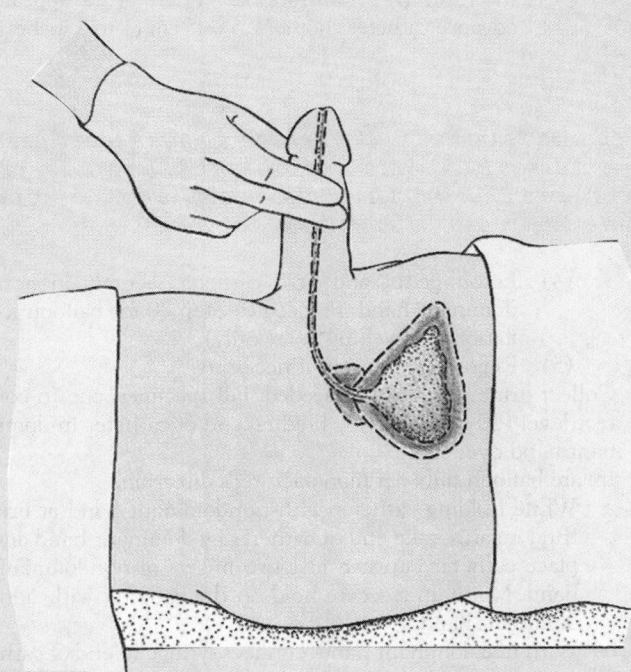

STEP 18b(1)   Hold penis perpendicular to body for catheter insertion.

STEP	RATIONALE

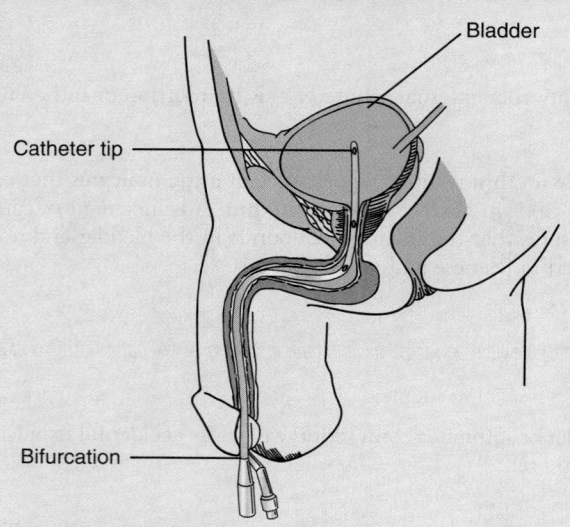

STEP 18b(3)   Male anatomy with correct catheter insertion to the bifurcation of the drainage and balloon inflation port.

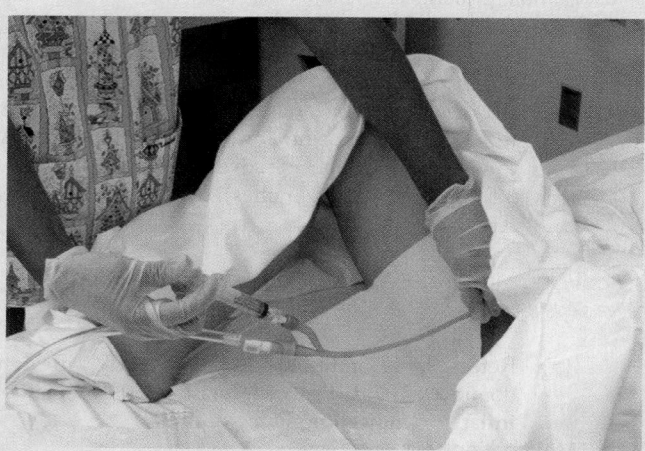

STEP 20b   Hold catheter in place with nondominant hand while inflating balloon.

(3) In the adult, advance catheter 17 to 22.5 cm (7 to 9 inches) or until urine flows out catheter end. If you meet resistance, do not attempt forceful catheter insertion (see illustration). When urine appears, advance catheter another 2.5 to 5 cm (1 to 2 inches).	There is natural resistance as the catheter enters the external sphincter. However, do not use force to insert the catheter inward. Advancement of catheter to the bifurcation of the drainage and balloon inflation port ensures proper placement of catheter through the longer urethra for male patient (Senese and others, 2006c).

Critical Decision Point   *If there is resistance to catheter insertion, have the patient take slow, deep breaths to promote relaxation while you insert the catheter slowly (Senese and others, 2006c). Another technique is to rest your arm against the patient's leg and ask him to relax. When the leg muscles begin to relax, continue the insertion process (Senese, 2004).* NOTE: *If there is persistent resistance to insertion, the patient may have an enlarged prostate. Notify the prescriber; a coudé catheter, with a slightly curved end, may be needed to facilitate insertion (Senese, 2004).*

(4) Lower penis, and hold catheter securely in nondominant hand. Proceed to Step 20 for balloon inflation (indwelling Foley only).	Prevents accidental dislodgment of catheter.
(5) Reposition foreskin if necessary.	
19 Collect urine specimen as needed. Fill specimen cup to correct level (20 to 30 mL) by holding end of catheter in dominant hand over cup.	Allows nurses to obtain sterile specimen for culture analysis.
20 Inflate balloon fully per manufacturer's direction.	
a While holding catheter with nondominant hand at urethral meatus, take end of catheter by dominant hand and place catheter between first two fingers of nondominant hand. Maintain a secure hold on the catheter with nondominant hand.	Holding on to catheter before inflating balloon will prevent expulsion of catheter from urethra.
b With free dominant hand, connect syringe to end of catheter at inflation valve and slowly inject total amount of solution (see illustration). Follow manufacturer's instructions regarding amount of fluid used for balloon inflation.	In general, a 5-mL balloon requires approximately 10 mL of fluid for symmetrical inflation. If patient complains of sudden pain, aspirate solution, and advance catheter further.

STEP	RATIONALE

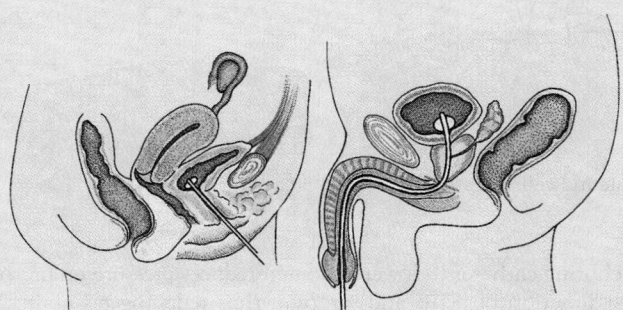

STEP 20c   Placement of inflated balloon in bladder.

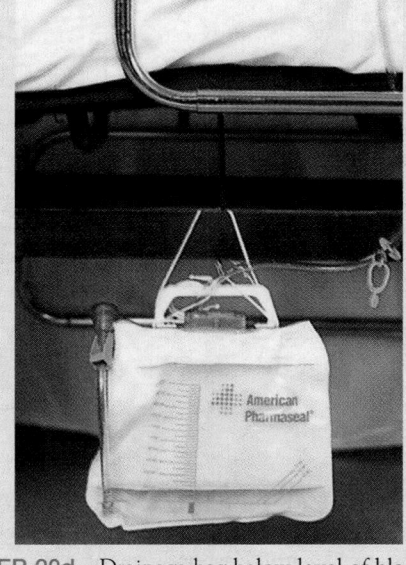

STEP 20d   Drainage bag below level of bladder.

c   After inflating balloon, pull *gently* on the catheter tubing until resistance is felt (see illustration).

Ensures that catheter tip is anchored.

Critical Decision Point   *If resistance occurs when inflating balloon or the patient verbalizes or shows nonverbal signs of pain, the balloon may not be entirely within the bladder. Stop inflation; allow fluid to flow back into syringe, and advance the catheter a little more before reattempting to inflate.*

d   Connect drainage tubing to retention catheter if it is not already preconnected. Place drainage bag below level of bladder (see illustration); do not place bag on side rails of bed.

Ensures proper drainage by gravity. Placement on side rails increases risk for tension applied to catheter, and bag can be raised above level of bladder.

21   Allow bladder to empty fully unless institution policy restricts maximal volume of urine drained with each catheterization (about 500 to 1000 mL).

Relieves bladder distention. There is no definitive evidence regarding whether there is benefit in limiting maximal volume drained.

22   Anchor catheter:

a   **Female patient:**

(1)   Secure catheter tubing to inner thigh with strip of nonallergenic tape (use paper tape if allergic to silk tape), or use a commercial multipurpose tube holder with a Velcro strap, if available. Allow for slack so movement of thigh does not create tension on catheter (see illustration). Clip drainage tubing to edge of mattress.

Securing the catheter will minimize the accidental dislodgment of the catheter (Gray, 2006a).

Also minimizes the risk for bleeding, trauma, meatal necrosis, and bladder spasms from pressure and traction (Senese and others, 2006a).

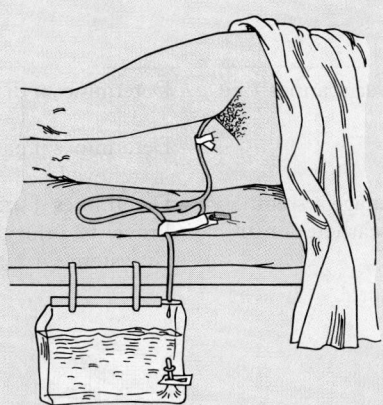

STEP 22a(1)   Securing the female indwelling catheter.

STEP	RATIONALE

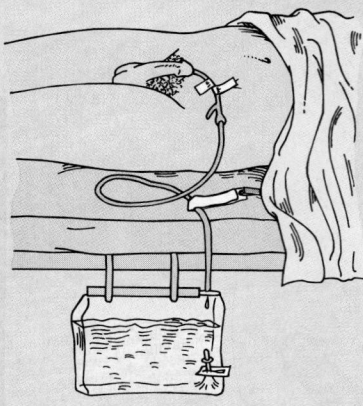

STEP 22b(1)   Securing the male indwelling catheter.

b   Male patient:
   (1)   Secure catheter tubing to top of thigh or lower abdomen (with penis directed toward chest). Allow slack in catheter so movement does not create tension on catheter (see illustration). Clip drainage tubing to edge of mattress.

Anchoring catheter to lower abdomen reduces pressure on urethra at junction of penis and scrotum, thus reducing possibility of tissue injury in this area (Senese and others, 2006a).

23   Be sure there are no obstructions in tubing. Coil excess tubing on bed, and fasten it to bottom sheet with clip from kit or with rubber band and safety pin.

Obstructions will prevent free flow of urine, leading to bladder retention.

24   Assist patient to comfortable position. Perform catheter care routinely and when secretions build up in perineum (see Skill 33-2).

25   Dispose of used equipment in appropriate receptacles. Remove gloves, and perform hand hygiene.

26   **For straight or intermittent catheter:** Follow Steps 1 to 18. Note the differences identified between an indwelling and straight catheter.

   a   Once catheter is in bladder, allow urine to drain out of end of catheter into sterile urine receptacle. Do not release hold on catheter.

The aim is to drain bladder fully without removing catheter too early.

   b   Collect urine specimen if needed by placing end of catheter over specimen container. Collect 20 to 30 mL of urine.

Urine will be used to test for microorganism growth.

   c   Withdraw catheter slowly and smoothly, while gently palpating over patient's bladder with nonsterile hand.

Allows for complete emptying of bladder.

   d   Place urine in receptacle in graduated cylinder to measure. Remember to record amount in sterile specimen container as well.

Determines urinary output.

   e   Complete Steps 24 and 25.

EVALUATION

1   Palpate bladder for distention, or apply bladder scanner (see Procedural Guideline 33-2, p. 880)

Determines if distention is relieved.

2   Ask patient to describe level of comfort.

Determines if patient's sensation of discomfort or fullness has been relieved.

3   Observe character and amount of urine in drainage system.

Determines if urine is flowing adequately.

4   Determine that there is no urine leaking from catheter or tubing connections.

Prevents injury to patient's skin and ensures a closed sterile system.

Unexpected Outcomes

1   Absence of urine in catheter drainage bag.
    Female: Catheter may be in vaginal opening.
    Male: Catheter may not be advanced far enough through prostatic urethra.

2   Bladder discomfort persists despite catheter patency, indicating urethral or bladder spasm.

3   More than 500 to 1000 mL of urine drains from the catheter.

Related Interventions

• Urine should drain freely. If not, further assess catheter placement and patient's hydration status.
• Assess the patient for discomfort, and check intake record. Immediately notify the prescriber if no urine is present within 1 hour of catheterization.
• Prescriber may order medication for relief.

• Check institution policy before beginning catheterization; some agencies restrict maximal amount of urine that can be drained at one time. This amount may vary from 500 to 1000 mL.
• Notify the prescriber.

Recording and Reporting

• Report and record type and size of catheter inserted, amount of fluid used to inflate balloon, characteristics of urine, amount of urine, reasons for catheterization, specimen collection, and, if appropriate, patient's response to procedure and teaching topics.
• Initiate I&O records (see Chapter 6).

Teaching Considerations

• Explain how the patient can cooperate and/or participate during the procedure.
• Explain to patient that burning and/or pressure sensation during catheter insertion is normal.
• Instruct patient how to position the catheter tubing while in bed. In the side-lying position facing the catheter, the tubing should drape over the thigh. In the side-lying position facing away from the catheter, the tubing should extend between the legs.
• Explain care of the catheter and drainage system. Adequate fluid intake is necessary to keep the urine dilute and to prevent catheter encrustations and subsequent blockage.

Pediatric Considerations

• For an infant or young child, explain procedures to parent. When explaining the procedure to the child, consider the developmental level of the child and adapt explanation as needed (Hockenberry and Wilson, 2007).
• Children and adolescents will experience some discomfort during catheterization. Assistance and gentle holding is sometimes necessary, especially in younger child. Most children prefer to have the parents remain with them during procedure. Ask adolescents if they would like a parent to remain with them.

• Catheterization in infants and children is easier when you use an adequate amount of lubricant that contains 2% lidocaine (Hockenberry and Wilson, 2007).

Gerontological Considerations

• A patient with a catheter is especially vulnerable to UTI. The frail older adult who is physically compromised runs the additional risk for developing urosepsis. Therefore use indwelling catheters only in select circumstances.
• Ensuring adequate oral fluid intake of 2000 mL/day and assisting the older adult with toileting on a regular timed basis will help bladder retraining and minimize the need for excessive catheterization.
• Attached equipment, such as a catheter, often makes ambulation more difficult, increasing the risks associated with decreased mobility.

Home Care Considerations

• Patients who routinely switch from large drainage bags at night to leg bags during the day have an increased risk for CAUTI.
• Instruct the patient to maintain a closed catheter system whenever possible. If the patient changes from a leg bag to a large drainage bag, instruct in the importance of hand washing and cleaning the connection ports with alcohol before changing bags (Senese and others, 2006a).
• Teach the patient with an indwelling catheter daily care of collection bags. New guidelines include using a commercial household bleach solution diluted in a 1:10 ratio with tap water. Rinse bags twice and agitate with water. Then fill the bag with 150 mL of **diluted** bleach solution (include tubing and drainage port) and agitate. Patient needs to wear gloves and avoid eye contact with solution (Senese and others, 2006a).

SKILL 33-2   Care and Removal of an Indwelling Catheter

 Intermediate / Urinary Catheter Management /
Removing an Indwelling Catheter

NSO *Urinary Catheterization Module / Lesson 5*

Bacterial growth is common where the catheter enters the urethral meatus in both men and women. Perform catheter care each shift as part of routine perineal care, after bowel incontinence, or if secretions build around the urinary meatus. Removal of a retention catheter requires the use of clean technique. You deflate the retention balloon before removal. If the retention catheter balloon remains even partially inflated, its removal will result in trauma and subsequent swelling of the urethral meatus. Always remove an indwelling catheter as soon as possible after insertion because of risk for catheter-associated urinary tract infection (CAUTI). Catheterization results in more than 1 million CAUTIs each year in the United States (Pinto and Matteucci, 2008).

A common practice before removing an indwelling catheter has been to intermittently clamp and release the catheter. The rationale for this includes an attempt to promote bladder tone and to stimulate normal filling and emptying of the bladder. However, there is no clear evidence supporting this procedure and its effectiveness. Therefore clamping indwelling catheters before removal is not a recommended clinical practice guideline (Griffiths and Fernandez, 2007).

Delegation Considerations
The skill of performing routine catheter care and removing a catheter can be delegated to NAP. (Refer to agency policy.) The nurse directs the NAP to:
- Report characteristics of the urine output from the catheter, including color, odor, and amount.
- Report the condition of the patient's perineum (color, discharge, contamination from fecal incontinence).
- Check size of balloon and size of syringe needed to deflate balloon and to report if balloon does not deflate and/or if there is bleeding or excessive burning.
- Measure first voiding and report time and amount voided.

Equipment
For Each Procedure
☐ Clean gloves (needed for care and removal)

☐ Waterproof pad
☐ Bath blanket
For Catheter Care
☐ Soap, washcloth, towel, and basin filled with warm water
☐ Cotton balls or large swabs (*optional*)
For Removing a Catheter
☐ 10-mL or larger syringe without needle—information on balloon size (mL) is printed directly on balloon inflation valve (Fig. 33-4)
☐ Correctly labeled sterile specimen container
☐ Alcohol or other disinfectant swab
☐ Washcloth and warm water to perform perineal care after removal
☐ Graduated cylinder
☐ Available urinal for patients, bedside commode or urine output commode pan for female patients for urine collection use after catheter is removed

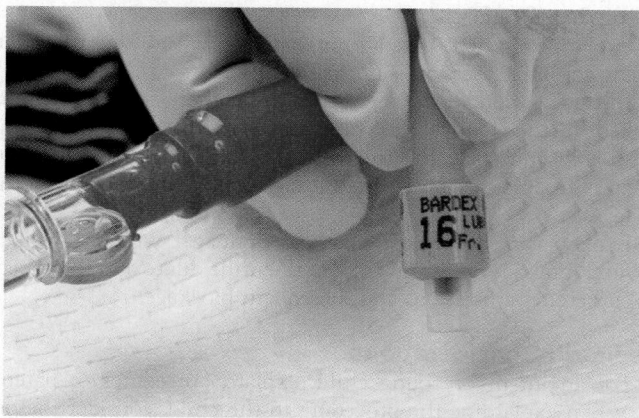

FIG 33-4   Size of balloon printed on catheter inflation valve.

STEP	RATIONALE

ASSESSMENT

1   Catheter care:
   a   Observe urinary output and urine characteristics.

Encrustation, the formation of hard deposits around the tip and inside of the drainage lumen of the catheter, leads to blockage of the drainage lumen and causes urinary retention (Hukins, 2005).

   b   Assess for history or presence of bowel incontinence.

Accumulation of fecal material irriates perineal tissue and acts as a source of bacterial growth.

   c   Assess patient's knowledge of catheter care.

Patients who perform own catheter care may be unsure of touching the catheter. Assess patient's ability and knowledge in order to provide instruction as needed (Leaver, 2007).

   d   Observe any discharge or redness around urethral meatus.

Indicates inflammatory process and possible infection.

2   Catheter removal:
   a   Assess need for catheter removal. Determine how long catheter has been in place. Check agency policy to determine time frame for Foley catheter change. Check medical record for order to remove, or obtain order as needed.

The duration of catheterization is an important risk factor for development of nosocomial UTI and gram-negative urosepsis (Hart, 2008).

STEP	RATIONALE
b Determine size of catheter inflation balloon by looking at balloon inflation valve.	Determines amount of water to remove from balloon.
c Observe any discharge or redness around urethral meatus.	Indicates inflammatory process and possible infection. Provides information for perineal care after catheter removal.

NURSING DIAGNOSES

- Impaired urinary elimination
- Risk for infection

Individualize related factors based on patient's condition or needs.

PLANNING

1 Expected outcomes following completion of procedure:	
• Urethral meatus is free of secretions and irritation.	Hygiene maintained.
• Patient will verbalize feeling of comfort after procedure is completed.	Cleansing relieves local discomfort.
• After removal of the catheter, the patient voids without discomfort within 6 to 8 hours.	Indicates return of voluntary bladder function without urinary retention.
2 Explain the procedure to the patient. Offer opportunity to perform self-hygiene care to client.	Reduces anxiety and promotes cooperation. Self-care helps to reduce patient's embarrassment.

IMPLEMENTATION

1 Close curtain, or close door.	Provides privacy and reduces embarrassment to patient, thus promoting relaxation.
2 Perform hand hygiene.	Reduces transmission of microorganisms.
3 Raise bed to appropriate working height. If side rails are raised, lower side rail on working side.	Promotes use of proper body mechanics.
4 Organize equipment for perineal care or removal of catheter.	Increases efficiency of procedure.
5 Position patient, and cover with bath blanket, exposing only perineal area (see Skill 33-1).	Reduces patient's embarrassment. Ensures easy access to perineal tissues.
a Female in dorsal recumbent position.	
b Male in supine position.	
6 Place waterproof pad under patient and drape bath blanket on patient so only perineal area is exposed.	Prevents unnecessary exposure.
7 Apply clean gloves.	
8 Remove anchor device and free tubing.	
9 With nondominant hand:	
a *Female:* Gently retract labia to fully expose urethral meatus and catheter insertion site. Maintain position of hand throughout procedure.	Provides full visualization of urethral meatus. Full retraction of labia prevents contamination of meatus during cleaning.
b *Male:* Retract foreskin, if not circumcised, and hold penis at shaft just below glans, maintaining position throughout procedure.	Retraction of foreskin provides full visualization of urethral meatus.

Critical Decision Point   *Accidental closing of labia or dropping of penis during cleansing requires procedure to be repeated.*

10 Assess urethral meatus and surrounding tissues for inflammation, swelling, and discharge, and ask patient if burning or discomfort is present.	Determines condition of perineum and the frequency and type of ongoing care required.
11 Provide routine perineal care with soap and water (see Chapter 17). Application of topical antimicrobial agents is no longer recommended.	Perineal care with soap and water is sufficient to keep the area clean (Leaver, 2007). The application of topical antimicrobial products is not effective in reducing meatal bacterial flora and reducing risk for UTI. Do not include them as a part of routine catheter care (Gray, 2004; Leaver, 2007).

STEP	RATIONALE

12 Clease catheter

   a While stabilizing catheter with dominant hand and using a clean washcloth, soap, and water, cleanse the catheter in circular motion along its length for about 10 cm (4 inches) (see illustration). Start cleansing where the catheter enters the meatus and down toward the drainage tubing. Make sure to remove all traces of soap. For male clients: Reduce or reposition the foreskin after care.

Reduces presence of secretions or drainage on outside catheter surface.

   d Replace, as necessary, the adhesive tape (remove any adhesive residue from skin) or multipurpose tube holder that anchors catheter to patient's leg or abdomen (see Skill 33-1, Step 22).

   c Avoid placing tension on the catheter.

Tension causes urethral trauma.

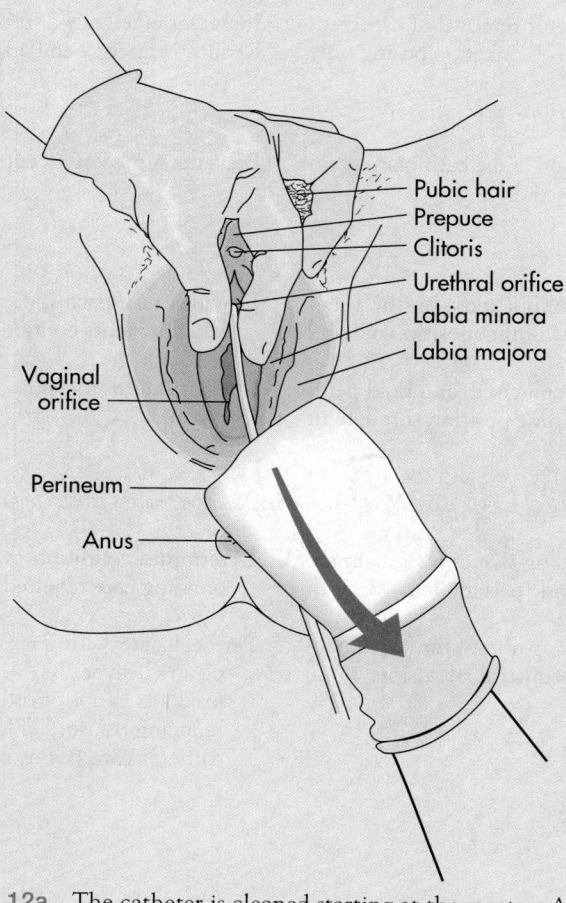

STEP 12a The catheter is cleaned starting at the meatus. About 4 inches of the catheter is cleaned.

STEP	RATIONALE
13 Catheter removal: Follow Steps 1 to 5 before catheter removal.	

a Place waterproof pad:
    (1) Between female's thighs (if in supine position)
    (2) Over male's thighs
	Prevents soiling of bed linen.

b Obtain sterile urine specimen if required (see Chapter 43).	Determines if bacteria are present in urine.
c Remove adhesive tape or Velcro tube holder used to secure and anchor catheter.	Allows for positioning of catheter for removal.
d Insert hub of syringe into inflation valve (balloon port). Allow sterile water to return into syringe by gravity until the plunger stops moving and the amount instilled is removed.	Many manufacturers recommend that fluid return to syringe by gravity. Manual aspiration leads to increased discomfort when removing catheter, resulting in the development of creases or ridges in balloon. A balloon that is not completely deflated will cause discomfort and trauma to urethral wall, which will result in bleeding as the catheter is removed.
e Pull catheter out slowly and gently while wrapping contaminated catheter in waterproof pad. Unhook collection bag and drainage tubing from bed.	Slow and gentle removal prevents possible trauma caused by deflated balloon deformation and accumulated encrustation.

Critical Decision Point   *Catheter should slide out very easily. Do not use force. If you note any resistance, repeat Step 13d) to remove any remaining fluid in inflation port. Notify prescriber.*

STEP	RATIONALE
f Reposition patient as necessary. Cleanse perineum. Lower level of bed, and position side rails accordingly.	Promotes patient comfort and safety.
g Empty, measure, and record urine present in drainage bag.	Records urinary output.
14 Dispose of all contaminated supplies in appropriate receptacle, remove gloves, and perform hand hygiene.	Reduces transmission of microorganisms.

EVALUATION

1 Inspect the condition of the urethra and surrounding tissue, and ask patient about discomfort.	Determines if area is cleansed properly and/or if patient has any irritation.
2 Observe time the patient urinates, and measure the urine; assess urine characteristics.	Urinary retention is a common occurrence after removal of an indwelling Foley catheter (Griffiths and Fernandez, 2007).
3 Evaluate patient for dysuria, small frequent voidings, or bleeding during urination.	UTI can develop after catheter removal.

Unexpected Outcomes	Related Interventions
1 Urethral or perineal irritation is present.	• Observe for leaking from around catheter; catheter may need replacement. • Make sure (if not removed) catheter is anchored and secured appropriately.
2 Patient has fever and/or urine is malodorous, small frequent voidings, or bleeding or burning occurs with urination after catheter removed.	• Monitor vital signs and urine. • Report findings to prescriber because any of these symptoms/signs indicate a UTI.
3 Patient is unable to void after catheter removal or voids in small, frequent amounts.	• Assess for bladder distention. • Assist to a normal position for voiding. • Provide privacy. • Perform bladder ultrasound (see Procedural Guideline 33-2) to assess for residual urine. Notify prescriber if residual volume is greater than 150 mL. Catheterization may be indicated (Stevens, 2005). • If patient unable to void within 6 to 8 hours of catheter removal, notify prescriber.
4 Water from inflation balloon does not return into syringe.	• Reposition patient, and ensure that catheter is not kinked. • Remove syringe, attach new syringe, and allow for passive emptying. • Attempt to empty balloon by gently pulling back on syringe.

Recording and Reporting
- Record times for catheter care in the nursing care plan.
- Record in nurses' notes time of catheter care, removal of catheter and condition of urethral meatus, condition of catheter, and character and amount of urine.
- Record urine emptied from drainage bag on I&O form.

Teaching Considerations
- Unless contraindicated, patients with a catheter should drink at least 2000 mL of fluid per day to promote continuous flushing of the bladder, preventing sediment from collecting in the catheter tubing.
- Instruct patient to hold collection bag below the level of the bladder when ambulating.
- Instruct patient not to disconnect the catheter from the collection tubing and bag.

Pediatric Considerations
- Do not force catheter out of bladder if you meet resistance. When excessive tubing has been inserted in bladder, there have been occurrences of knotting of the tube (Hockenberry and others, 2007).

Gerontological Considerations
- Some older adult patients exhibit atypical signs and symptoms of UTI. Although you should look for the usual symptoms of dysuria, urgency, frequency, odor, and hematuria, they may not be present. Also assess for less specific signs such as fever and/or mental status changes, including agitation, lethargy, and confusion.

Home Care Considerations
- Assess patient and primary caregiver for ability and motivation to participate in routine catheter care.
- Silicone catheters are a better choice for a patient in the home or in a long-term care facility, where catheterization occurs for longer periods of time, because the silicone is less likely to become encrusted. Encrustation harbors microorganisms and increases irritation.

PROCEDURAL GUIDELINE 33-2   Bladder Scan and Catheterization to Determine Residual Urine

Residual urine, also referred to as postvoid residual (PVR), is the volume of urine in the bladder after a normal voiding. PVR occurs if the patient has urinary retention or cannot empty the bladder completely. You can use a portable noninvasive bladder ultrasound device (bladder scanner) or the technique of straight/intermittent catheterization to assess PVR.

A bladder scanner is a cost-effective and accurate alternative to intermittent catheterization (Altschuler and Diaz, 2006; Stevens, 2005) used in determining the amount of urine retained in the bladder. The bladder scanner is noninvasive, so there is no risk for nosocomial UTI and possible trauma associated with urinary catheterization. It provides accurate determination of a patient's bladder volume (Altschuler and Diaz, 2006) by first creating an ultrasound image of the patient's bladder and then calculating the urine volume in the bladder (Patraca, 2005). A scanner is also helpful to assess the patient for bladder distention related to the inability to urinate secondary to medical conditions such as spinal cord injuries (Altschuler and Diaz, 2006). The scanner also determines bladder volume when the patient's urinary output from an indwelling catheter (see Skill 33-2) decreases because of a possible obstruction to urine flow (Stevens, 2005). A printed copy of the results is available from most scanners. A PVR of less than 50 mL is normal. Two or more PVR determinations greater than 150 mL are associated with the development of UTI and indicate the need for catheterization (Stevens, 2005).

Bladder scanners are not readily available for nurses to use in all clinical settings, and straight/intermittent catheterization is often the only means to determine bladder urine volume. Regardless of the method used to determine PVR, assess the amount of urine left in the bladder within 10 to 15 minutes after the patient voids (Altschuler and Diaz, 2006). Instruct the patient not to void again before the measurement.

Delegation Considerations
The skill of bladder scan and catheterization for residual urine can be delegated in some settings (see agency policy). However, the nurse is responsible for reviewing I&O trends and assessing for possible bladder distention. The nurse directs the NAP to:

- Accurately measure urine output 10 to 15 minutes before using bladder scanner or before catheterizing the patient for residual.
- Report and record residual urine volume obtained by bladder scanner or by catheterization.
- Follow manufacturer's recommendations for use of bladder scanner, if device is available for use.

Equipment
- ❏ Bladder scanner (follow manufacturer's instructions for use)
- ❏ Ultrasound gel
- ❏ A urethral catheterization tray for straight/intermittent catheterization will contain a single-use catheter and the following:
  - Sterile gloves (extra pair optional)
  - Waterproof drapes (one fenestrated drape)
  - Lubricant
  - Antiseptic cleansing agent (povidone-iodine)
  - Cotton balls (or sterile antiseptic swabs)
  - Forceps
  - Specimen container
- ❏ Bath blanket
- ❏ Waterproof absorbent pad
- ❏ Clean gloves, basin with warm water, soap, washcloth, and towel
- ❏ Appropriate additional lighting as needed (such as a flashlight or procedure light)
- ❏ *Alternative:* Antiseptic solution such as Hibiclens or Shur-Clens (if allergic to povidone iodine)

Procedural Steps
1 Review I&O record to determine urine output trends.
2 Palpate and percuss over the patient's suprapubic area for a signs of a distended bladder. (Distended bladder feels like a mass above the symphysis pubis, and there will be dullness on percussion.)
3 Review prescriber's order to determine how often to assess residual urine.
4 Assess patient's knowledge regarding urinary retention and purpose of checking residual urine volume by bladder scanner or intermittent/straight catheterization.

PROCEDURAL GUIDELINE 33-2 Bladder Scan and Catheterization to Determine Residual Urine—cont'd

5 Check time of last void; measure amount voided.
6 You will use the bladder scanner (if available) or catheterize patient within 10 to 15 minutes of urinating.

> **Critical Decision Point** *Remind ambulatory patients to let nurse or NAP know immediately after urinating. Also, remind the patient to save urine for measurement.*

7 Use bladder scanner to assess PVR:
   a Assist patient to a supine position with head elevated on a pillow.
   b Expose the patient's lower abdomen.
   c Turn on the scanner by pressing the On/Off button and then the Scan button to turn on the scanning screen.
   d Press the Gender button to select the Male or Female setting.
      (1) Use the Female option only for female patients who have not had the uterus removed (hysterectomy).
      (2) Use the Male setting when scanning female patients who **have had** the uterus removed.
   e Wipe the scan head with an alcohol pad.
   f Palpate the patient's symphysis pubis (pubic bone), and apply a generous amount of transmission/conductivity gel (2 tablespoons) or a bladder scan gel pad midline on abdomen about 2.5 to 4 cm (1 to 1.5 inches) above symphysis pubis.
   g Place the scan head on the gel with the directional icon toward the patient's head, and direct it toward the bladder (see illustration). If you do not apply the gel, the scan will be inaccurate.
   h Apply light pressure, and keep the scan head steady to prevent inaccurate readings. NOTE: For most patients,

pointing the scan head slightly downward toward the coccyx gives an accurate view of the bladder (Patraca, 2005). Press and release the scan button.

> **Critical Decision Point** *Scan to the side, above, or below any scars or dressing if present on area being scanned.*

   i Verify aim (check manufacturer's directions for details). You will hear a beep when the scan is finished. Press and hold the Done button to display the volume measurement (see illustration). Results may be printed.
8 Straight or intermittent catheterization to assess for PVR:
   a Perform hand hygiene.
   b Proceed as for inserting straight/intermittent catheter (see Skill 33-1).
   c Slowly remove the catheter to ensure complete urine drainage from the bladder.
   d Discard contaminated supplies, remove gloves, perform hand hygiene.
   e Report and record amount of urine voided, amount obtained from catheterization, and the patient's response.

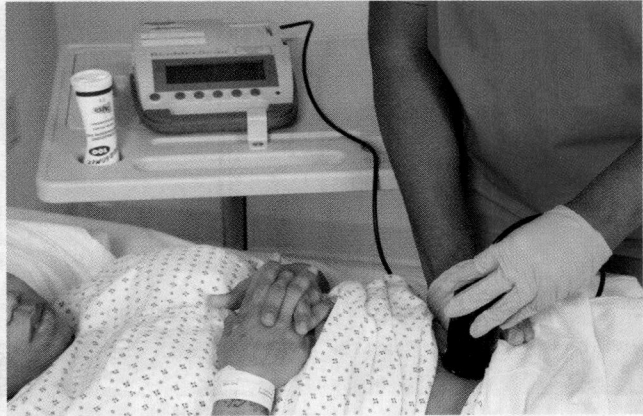

STEP 7g Placement of bladder scan head.

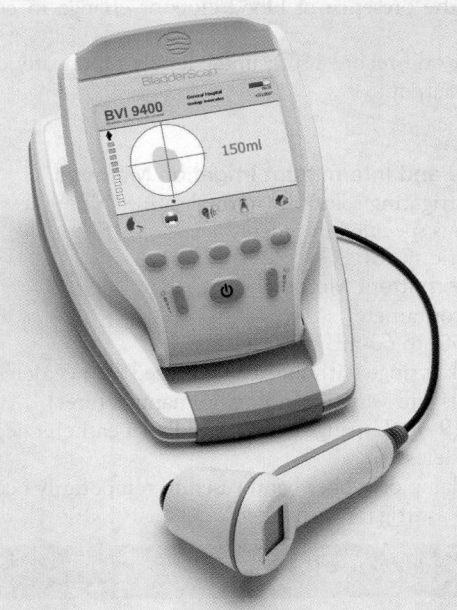

STEP 7i Bladder scan reading. (*Courtesy Verathon, Inc.*)

SKILL 33-3   Performing Catheter Irrigation

Intermediate / Urinary Catheter Management / Irrigating a Urinary Catheter

The purpose of catheter irrigation is to maintain catheter patency. Two types of irrigation techniques, closed and open, are available. Closed bladder irrigation provides intermittent or continuous irrigation of the catheter without disrupting the sterile connection between the catheter and drainage system. This technique limits the risk for UTI (Gray, 2004). An example is continuous bladder irrigation (CBI), which involves the continuous infusion of a sterile solution into the bladder, usually via a triple-lumen indwelling (Foley) catheter (Fig. 33-5). This procedure often follows genitourinary surgery to prevent occlusion of the catheter by small blood clots and mucous fragments.

You should not disconnect a urinary catheter and drainage system unless the catheter is being irrigated using the intermittent open technique. Disconnect the catheter from the drainage tubing to perform intermittent irrigation. Use strict aseptic technique to minimize contamination and risk for subsequent development of a UTI.

Delegation Considerations

The skill of catheter irrigation cannot be delegated to NAP. The nurse directs the NAP to:

- Inform the nurse about patient complaints of pain or discomfort and leakage of urine around catheter.
- Report the presence of blood clots or change in color of the urine.
- Monitor and record I&O; immediately report any decrease in urinary output.

Equipment

For Closed and Intermittent Irrigation Methods

❏ Sterile irrigating solution (normal saline [NS] unless another solution is specified in order)
❏ Antiseptic swabs

Closed Intermittent Method

❏ Sterile container
❏ Sterile 30- to 60-mL irrigation syringe
❏ Luer-Lok syringe without needle is used for needleless access port (this will vary depending on manufacturer)
❏ Sterile 19- to 22-gauge 1-inch needle (if catheter access port is *not* needleless)
❏ Screw clamp or rubber band (used to temporarily occlude catheter as irrigant is instilled)

Closed Continuous Method

❏ Bag of sterile irrigating solution
❏ Intravenous (IV) pole
❏ Irrigation tubing with clamp (with or without Y connector) (clamp regulates irrigation flow rate; Y connector allows IV bags to be connected to tubing)

Open Intermittent Method

❏ Disposable sterile irrigation kit including the following:
  - 60-mL piston type of syringe
  - Sterile collection basin
  - Sterile waterproof drape
  - Sterile solution container
  - Sterile catheter plug
  - Clean or sterile gloves
  - Nonallergenic/paper tape or Velcro tube holder

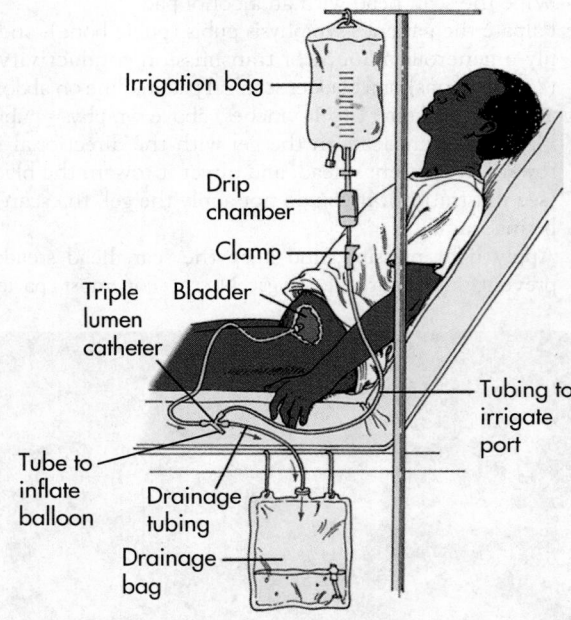

FIG 33-5   Closed continuous bladder irrigation.

STEP	RATIONALE

ASSESSMENT

1 Check patient's record to determine:
   a Purpose for bladder irrigation
   b Prescriber's order for type and amount of irrigant (e.g., sterile saline, or a medicated solution) and frequency of irrigation, and type of irrigation: continuous or intermittent.

   c Type of catheter used (see Fig. 33-2)
     (NOTE: Appropriate catheter is usually inserted during the original catheterization.
     (1) Single lumen (single use for open irrigation)

Order is required to initiate therapy. Ensures that correct medication or solution and amount is administered. Frequency of irrigation is based on need of patient (e.g., patient who has just had prostate gland surgery may require continuous irrigations for 24 hours). Knowledge of type of irrigation allows nurse to select appropriate equipment.

Directs the nurse to the type of irrigation.

STEP	RATIONALE
(2) Double lumen (one lumen to inflate the balloon, one to allow urinary drainage)	
(3) Triple lumen (one lumen to inflate balloon, one to allow urinary drainage, and one to instill irrigation solution)	
2 Assess the following:	
a Color of urine and presence of mucus, clots, or sediment	Indicates bleeding and if tissue debris is present. Determines need for increasing irrigation flow rate with continuous irrigations, and frequency of intermittent irrigations.
b Palpate bladder.	Determines presence of bladder distention.
c Existing closed continuous irrigation system: CBI	
(1) Assess ongoing urinary output and amount of irrigating solution infused.	Fluid draining from the bladder should be in excess of amount of continuous irrigating solution infused. If outflow is less than inflow, catheter may be obstructed by clots or the tubing may be kinked (Lewis and others, 2007).

<table>
<tr><td>Critical Decision Point   If urinary flow has stopped and you cannot reestablish patency of catheter by manual irrigation, stop the CBI and notify the prescriber.</td></tr>
</table>

STEP	RATIONALE
(2) Note amount of fluid remaining in existing irrigating solution container.	Allows nurse to anticipate hanging of new bag of irrigation solution.
3 Review I&O record.	Determines baseline for prior urinary output measures. Patients with CBI should have I&O measurements taken.
4 Assess patient for presence of abdominal pain or spasms, a sensation of bladder fullness, or urine leaking from around catheter.	These symptoms indicate blockage of catheter and need for irrigation (Cutts, 2005).
5 Assess patient's knowledge regarding purpose of performing any type of catheter irrigation.	Reveals need for patient instruction.

NURSING DIAGNOSES

- Acute pain
- Deficient knowledge regarding the need for bladder irrigation
- Impaired urinary elimination
- Risk for infection

Individualize related factors based on patient's condition or needs.

PLANNING

STEP	RATIONALE
1 Expected outcomes following completion of this procedure:	
• With CBI: output is greater than volume of irrigating solution used.	Indicates patency of drainage system. Patency allows drainage of urine and irrigating solution.
• Absence of bladder pain or discomfort.	Bladder empties, avoiding irritation and spasm.
• Absence of fever; lower abdominal pain, cloudy or foul-smelling urine.	Signs of UTI are not present.
• Patient can explain purpose of procedure and what to expect.	Helps patient relax and promotes cooperation.
2 Explain procedure to patient.	Reduces anxiety and promotes cooperation.

IMPLEMENTATION

STEP	RATIONALE
1 Perform hand hygiene.	Reduces transmission of microorganisms.
2 Provide privacy: Pull curtains around bed, and fold back covers to expose catheter junction where it connects to drainage tubing. Cover patient's chest with bath blanket.	Promotes patient's self-esteem; shows respect for patient while exposing only area nurse must see.
3 Position patient in supine position, and remove tape or Velcro tube holder that is anchoring catheter to patient. Be careful not to pull on catheter.	Allows for patient comfort. Removing tape enables nurse to manipulate catheter.
4 Organize appropriate supplies according to type of irrigation prescribed.	
5 Closed intermittent irrigation:	
a Pour prescribed sterile irrigating solution in sterile container.	
b Apply clean gloves.	Reduces risk for exposure to body fluids.

STEP	RATIONALE
c Draw prescribed amount of sterile irrigating solution into syringe using aseptic technique (usually 30 to 50 mL). Place sterile cap on tip of needleless syringe. Attach capped, sterile needle on end of syringe (if needleless system not used).	Ensures sterility of irrigating fluid.
d Clamp catheter tubing below soft injection port with screw clamp. Alternatively, fold catheter tubing onto itself, and secure with rubber band.	Occluding catheter tubing below the point of injection allows irrigating solution to enter catheter to clear obstruction.
e Using a circular motion, cleanse catheter port with antiseptic swab (this same port is used for specimen collections).	Reduces transmission of infection.
f Insert tip of needleless syringe using twisting motion into irrigation port. (See manufacturer's instructions for possible variation.) *Alternative:* Insert needle tip through port at 30-degree angle.	Designated port must be used for irrigation. Ensures needle tip enters lumen of catheter and that needle does not puncture tubing.
g Inject solution into catheter tubing port using slow, even pressure.	Gentle instillation of irrigating solution minimizes trauma to the bladder mucosa.
h Withdraw syringe, and remove clamp or rubber band, allowing solution to drain into urinary drainage bag. (Clamp tubing temporarily to allow instilled fluid to remain in bladder, especially if irrigant is medicated as per prescriber's order).	Allows drainage to flow via gravity.
6 Closed continuous irrigation:	
a Apply clean gloves.	Reduces transmission of microorganisms.
b Close clamp on tubing, and hang bag of irrigating solution on IV pole. Use aseptic technique to insert (spike) tip of sterile irrigation tubing into bag containing irrigation solution (see illustration). Fill drip chamber half full by squeezing the chamber.	Reduces transmission of microorganisms. Air in tubing may cause bladder spasms.
c Open clamp, and allow solution to flow through tubing, keeping end of tubing sterile; close clamp, and recap end of tubing.	Priming the tubing with fluid prevents introduction of air into bladder.
d Use aseptic technique to connect tubing securely to drainage port of **Y** connector on double/triple lumen catheter.	Reduces transmission of microorganisms.

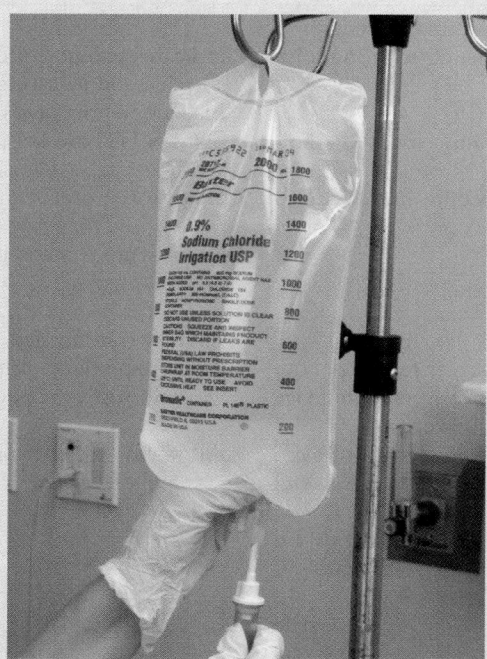

STEP 6b   Spiking a bag of sterile irrigation solution for continuous bladder irrigation.

STEP	RATIONALE
e Adjust clamp on irrigation tubing to begin flow of solution into bladder; be sure clamp on catheter drainage tubing is open, and check volume of drainage in drainage bag (see Fig. 33-5).	Discomfort, bladder distention, and possible injury may occur if outward flow of irrigant and urine is prevented. Irrigating solution is infused at a rate to keep the urine either a light pink or colorless (Lewis and others, 2007).
7 Open intermittent irrigation: a Apply clean or sterile gloves.	Irrigation is a sterile procedure, but only parts of the system in contact with the inside of the catheter must remain sterile. This includes the tip of the syringe, end of the catheter, end of the catheter tubing, and irrigant.
b Open sterile irrigation tray; establish sterile field (see Chapter 8), and pour required amount of sterile solution into sterile solution container.	Adheres to principles of surgical asepsis.
c Position sterile waterproof drape under catheter.	Maintains sterile field.
d Aspirate prescribed amount of sterile solution into irrigating syringe (usually 30 mL). Place syringe in sterile solution container until ready to use.	Prepares irrigant for instillation into catheter. Maintains sterility of irrigating syringe.
e Move sterile collection basin close to patient's thigh.	Prevents soiling of bed linen and prevents reaching over sterile area.
f Cleanse connection point between catheter and tubing with antiseptic wipe before disconnecting.	Reduces transmission of microorganisms.
g Disconnect catheter from drainage tubing, allowing urine to flow into sterile collection basin; cover open end of drainage tubing with sterile protective cap, and position tubing on sterile waterproof drape.	Maintains sterility of inner aspect of catheter lumen and drainage tubing; reduces potential of introducing pathogens into bladder.
h Insert tip of syringe into lumen of catheter, and gently instill solution (see illustration).	Gentle instillation of irrigating solution minimizes trauma to the bladder mucosa.

Critical Decision Point   *Do not force irrigation fluid into catheter. Catheter may be occluded and needs to be changed.*

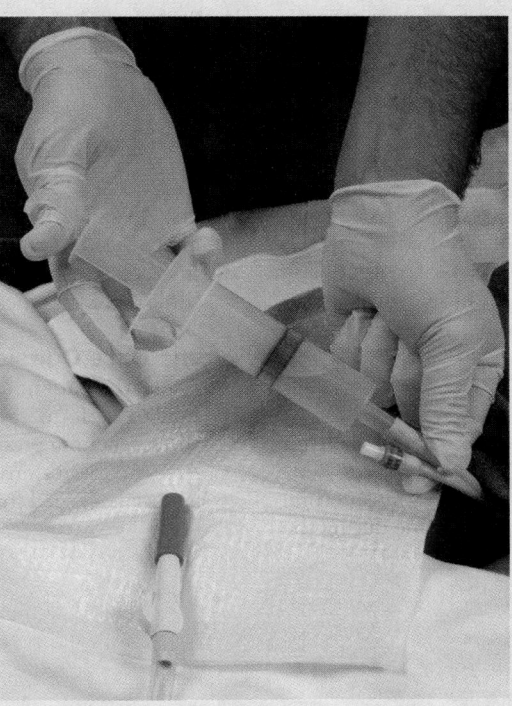

STEP 7h   Irrigation of catheter using open intermittent technique.

STEP	RATIONALE
i Remove syringe, lower catheter, and allow solution to drain into basin. Drainage solution amount should be equal to or greater than amount instilled. Repeat, instilling solution and draining several times until drainage is clear of clots and sediment.	Allows drainage to flow by gravity. Provides for adequate flushing of catheter.
j If solution does not return, have patient turn onto side facing nurse; if changing position does not help, reinsert syringe and gently aspirate solution.	Change in position may move tip of catheter in bladder, increasing likelihood that fluid instilled will flow out.
k After irrigation is complete, remove protector cap from urinary drainage tubing adapter, cleanse adapter with alcohol swab, and reinsert adapter into lumen of catheter.	Reestablishes closed urinary drainage system.
8 Anchor catheter to patient's leg or thigh with tape or Velcro multipurpose tube holder.	Prevents trauma to urethral tissue.
9 Assist patient into comfortable position.	Promotes relaxation and rest.
10 Lower bed to lowest position, and position side rails accordingly.	Promotes patient safety.
11 Dispose of contaminated supplies in appropriate receptacles. Secure catheter tubing with tape or Velcro tube holder. Remove gloves, and perform hand hygiene.	Reduces spread of microorganisms.

EVALUATION

1 Calculate fluid used to irrigate bladder and catheter, and subtract from volume drained.	Determines accurate urinary output.
2 Assess characteristics of output: viscosity, color, and presence of clots.	Data serve as baseline to judge response to therapy.
3 Observe for catheter patency.	Ensures bladder emptying freely.
4 Observe patient for signs of pain and fever.	Evaluates for presence of infection.
5 Observe urine to determine clarity, and odor.	Determines presence of UTI.

Unexpected Outcomes	Related Interventions
1 Irrigating solution does not return (intermittent irrigation) or is not flowing at prescribed rate (CBI).	• Examine tubing for clots, sediment, and kinks. • Notify prescriber if irrigant does not flow freely from the bladder, the patient complains of pain, or bladder distention occurs.
2 Signs of fever, cloudy urine, malodorous urine are present, indicating infection.	• Notify prescriber. • Monitor vital signs and character of urine.
3 Increase in bladder spasms occurs when performing intermittent irrigation, indicating blockage of catheter with foreign object (e.g., blood clot).	• Notify prescriber if large clots or sediment returns with the irrigating solution or if spasms increase or are unrelieved. • Prescriber may change irrigation method to continuous closed irrigation.

Recording and Reporting

- Record irrigation method, amount of solution used as irrigant, amount returned as drainage, characteristics of output, and urine output of drainage in nurses' notes and I&O sheet.
- Report catheter occlusion, sudden bleeding, infection, or increased pain to prescriber.

Teaching Considerations

- Instruct patient and primary caregiver to observe urine daily for changes in color, presence of mucus or blood, and odor.
- Inform patients that bleeding is common after transurethral prostatectomy and to expect bright red–tinged urine during the first 48 hours postoperatively, followed by urine ranging from pink-tinged to clear by the fifth postoperative day.
- Instruct patient to maintain adequate oral intake of 2 L/day (unless contraindicated).

Home Care Considerations

- Assess the patient and primary caregiver for ability and motivation to perform catheter irrigation. Use return demonstration when teaching procedure.
- Assess patient's environment for appropriate storage space for materials needed for procedure.

SKILL 33-4   Applying a Condom Catheter

 Basic / Elimination Assistance / Applying a Condom Catheter

NSO *Urinary Catheterization Module / Lesson 3*

A condom catheter, also referred to as an external catheter or penile sheath, is a noninvasive alternative for management of male urinary incontinence. Because it is noninvasive, there is a decreased risk for UTI (Saint and others, 2006). The device is a soft, flexible, condom-like sheath that fits over the penis (Fig. 33-6) and connects to either a small collection bag that attaches to the leg with a strap or a standard urinary collection bag that hangs on the bed frame below the level of the bladder. Most condom catheters are made of a soft silicone material to aid in reducing friction and are clear, allowing for ease of skin inspection. However, latex devices are still available; they often require removal to inspect the penile shaft and cause allergic reactions. Condoms come in different styles and sizes, so use the measuring guide supplied by the manufacturer for correct appli-

cation. Applying a condom catheter is often a nurse-initiated procedure, but a prescriber's order may be required.

Delegation Considerations
The skill of applying a condom catheter can be delegated to NAP depending on agency policy. However, the nurse determines the need for a continence device and if the patient has a latex allergy and assesses if the patient's penile shaft is free from redness, breakdown, or swelling before application of device. The nurse directs the NAP to:
- Follow the manufacturer's directions for applying the condom catheter and securing device.
- Monitor urine output and record I&O if applicable.
- Immediately report any redness, swelling, or breakdown of glans or penile shaft found during perineal care.

Equipment
- ❑ Condom catheter kit (condom sheath of appropriate size, securing device, skin preparation if prescribed [i.e., Hollister and 3M products])
- ❑ NOTE: Method to secure condom varies. Some condoms are self-adhering (the internal lining of the sheath is coated with adhesive). Other types require application of a double-sided self-adhesive strip or brush-on adhesive directly to the penis, whereas others may require an external securing device such as a reusable Velcro or foam strap or flexible self-adhesive tape to keep it in place.
- ❑ Urinary collection bag with drainage tubing or leg bag
- ❑ Basin with warm water and soap
- ❑ Towels and washcloth(s)
- ❑ Bath blanket
- ❑ Clean gloves
- ❑ Scissors, hair guard, or paper towel

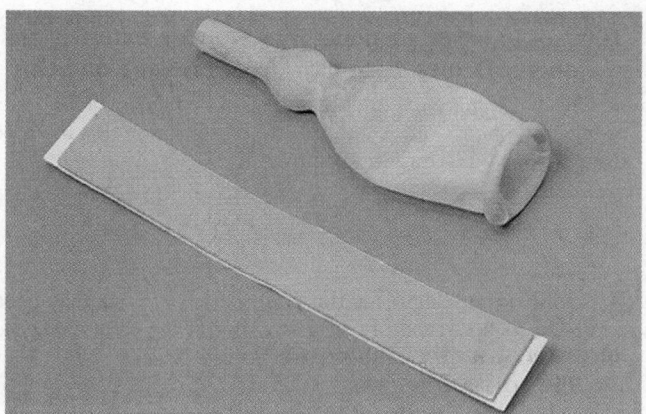

FIG 33-6   Condom catheter.

STEP	RATIONALE

ASSESSMENT

1 Assess urinary pattern, including patient's ability to empty bladder effectively, and degree of urinary continence.	Incontinent patients are at risk for skin breakdown and thus candidates for a condom catheter.
2 Assess condition of penis. Use the manufacturer's measuring guide to measure the diameter of penis in a flaccid state. The penile shaft should be at least 2 cm in length to ensure successful application.	Provides baseline to compare changes in condition of skin after condom catheter application. Measurement of the penile shaft aids in determining appropriate catheter size.
3 Assess patient's knowledge of the purpose of a condom catheter and functional ability to self-apply the device.	Reveals need for patient instruction.

NURSING DIAGNOSES

• Deficient knowledge regarding application of condom catheter	• Functional urinary incontinence • Risk for impaired skin integrity	• Toileting self-care deficit • Total urinary incontinence

Individualize related factors based on patient's condition or needs.

PLANNING

1 Expected outcomes following completion of procedure: • Patient is continent with condom catheter intact. • Glans and penile shaft are free of skin irritation or breakdown.	Catheter is secure. Catheter applied correctly.

STEP	RATIONALE
• Patient explains the purpose of the procedure and what to expect.	Helps to minimize anxiety and promotes cooperation.
2 Explain procedure to patient.	Reduces anxiety and promotes cooperation.

IMPLEMENTATION

1 Perform hand hygiene.	Reduces transmission of microorganisms.
2 Provide privacy by closing room door or bedside curtain.	Reduces embarrassment to patient.
3 Raise bed to appropriate working height. Lower side rail on working side.	Promotes use of good body mechanics.
4 Prepare urinary drainage collection bag and tubing. Clamp off drainage bag port. Secure collection bag to bed frame; bring drainage tubing up through side rails onto bed. *Optional:* Prepare leg bag for connection to condom.	Provides easy access to drainage equipment after applying condom catheter.
5 Assist patient into supine position or sitting position. Place bath blanket over upper torso. Fold sheets so that only penis is exposed.	Promotes comfort; draping prevents unnecessary exposure of body parts.
6 Apply clean gloves. Provide perineal care with soap and water (see Chapter 17), and dry thoroughly before applying device. If patient is uncircumcised, return foreskin to normal position.	Perineal care assists in removing secretions and any adhesive if previously used. Perineal care minimizes skin irritation and promotes adhesion of the new sheath (Pomfret, 2006).
7 *Optional:* Apply skin protectant film or barrier wipes used in stomal care to penis, if prescribed. Do not use barrier creams. Allow protectant to dry before applying condom.	Avoid barrier creams because they prevent the sheath from adhering to the penile shaft (Pomfret, 2005).
8 Clip hair at base of penis as necessary before application of condom sheath. Do not shave the pubic area. As an alternative to trimming pubic hair, place a hair guard, if provided by the manufacturer, over the penis before applying the device. Remove once sheath is intact. If a hair guard is not available, tear a hole in a paper towel, place it over the penis and remove following fitting of the sheath.	Pubic hair may adhere to condom and be pulled during application or removal of condom. Do not shave hair because this increases the risk for skin irritation (Pomfret, 2006).
9 Apply sheath. Ensure that it is the appropriate size to fit the patient's penis. With nondominant hand, grasp penis along shaft. With dominant hand, hold condom sheath at tip of penis and smoothly roll sheath onto penis. Allow 2.5 to 5 cm (1 to 2 inches) of space between tip of glans penis and end of condom catheter (see illustration).	If the sheath is too small for the size of the penis, it may cause constriction and tissue breakdown. If too large, it can cause urine leakage or can slip off penis (Potter, 2007).
10 Apply appropriate securing device and sheath according to manufacturer's directions. For example, a two-piece sheath system requires the application of an adhesive strip (securing device) before placing the external device over the penile shaft.	Use of an adhesive strip not designed for sheath application may be inflexible and impede circulation to penis (Pomfret, 2006).
a Spiral wrap the penile shaft with strip of supplied elastic adhesive. Do not overlap strip (see illustration).	Using the spiral wrap technique allows the supplied elastic adhesive to expand so blood flow to penis is not compromised.
b For one-piece sheath systems (self-adhesive catheters): apply catheter as in Steps 8 and 9, then apply gentle pressure on penile shaft for 10 to 15 seconds to secure catheter.	Secures catheter.

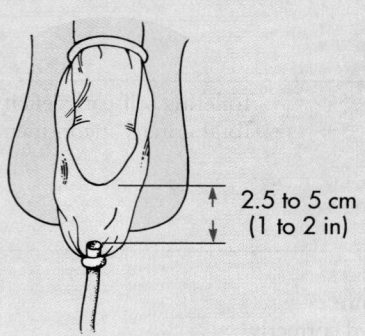

STEP 9 Distance between end of penis and tip of condom.

2.5 to 5 cm (1 to 2 in)

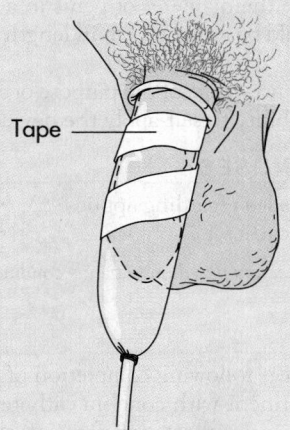

Tape

STEP 10a Tape applied in spiral fashion.

STEP	RATIONALE

11 Connect drainage tubing to end of condom catheter. Be sure condom is not twisted. Connect external catheter to large-volume bag or leg bag (see illustration).

Twisted condom prevents urine from draining into collection bag, causing skin irritation and weakening and deterioration of the adhesive, which cause sheath to come off (Pomfret, 2006).

12 Place excess coiling of tubing on bed, and secure to bottom sheet.

Prevents looping of tubing and promotes free drainage of urine.

13 Place patient in safe, comfortable position. Lower bed, and place side rails up as required.

Promotes safety and comfort.

14 Dispose of contaminated supplies, remove gloves, and perform hand hygiene.

Reduces spread of microorganisms.

15 Remove and reapply daily following the above steps unless an extended-wear device is used.

Critical Decision Point   *The best time to remove a penile sheath is during perineal hygiene. Wash the penis with warm, soapy water, and then gently roll the sheath and adhesive off the penile shaft.*

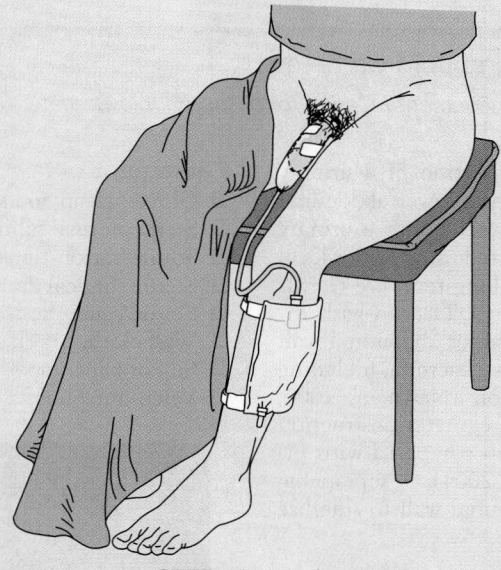

STEP 11   Leg bag.

EVALUATION

1 Observe urinary drainage.

2 Inspect penis with condom catheter in place within 30 minutes after application. Assess for swelling and discoloration, and ask patient if there is any discomfort.

Twisted condom will prevent urine from draining into collection bag.
Determines if condom is applied too tightly, impeding circulation to penis.

3 Remove and change condom. Inspect skin on penile shaft for signs of breakdown or irritation at least daily when performing perineal care and before reapplying condom.

Changing the external catheter will decrease the chance of infection (Newman, 2004).

Unexpected Outcomes	Related Interventions
1 Skin around penis is reddened and excoriated.	• Check for latex allergy, allergy to skin preparation or adhesive device. • Remove condom, and notify prescriber. • Do not reapply until penis and surrounding tissue are free from irritation. Ensure that condom is not twisted and urine flow is unobstructed after reapplication.
2 Penile swelling or discoloration occurs.	• Remove external catheter. • Notify prescriber. • Reassess current condom size. See manufacturer's size chart.
3 Condom does not stay on.	• Reassess current condom size. See manufacturer's size chart. • Observe whether outlet is kinked and urine is pooling at tip of condom. • Assess need for another brand of external catheter (i.e., one that is self-adhesive).

Recording and Reporting

- Report and record: condom application; condition of penis, skin, and scrotum; and voiding pattern.
- Monitor I&O.

Teaching Considerations

- Teach patient to keep condom and catheter kink free and positioned below the level of the bladder.
- Teach patient with leg bag to assess leg straps periodically for tightness and loosen as necessary.
- Teach patient that a collection bag that fills completely will put unnecessary tension on the catheter and lead to problems keeping the catheter intact. Patient should empty bag regularly.

Pediatric Considerations

- Condom catheters are uncommon in children. When used in adolescents, take precautions to minimize child's embarrassment.

Gerontological Considerations

- Condom catheters are not recommended in patients with chronic urinary obstruction such as benign prostatic hypertrophy.
- Evaluate patients diagnosed with neuropathy before applying condom catheter.

Home Care Considerations

- Teach patient and caregivers appropriate assessments to make and to report any signs of skin irritation or difficulty with device remaining intact.
- Teach patient the advantage of using a large-volume drainage bag at bedtime.
- Patient may need to make modifications in clothing in order to accommodate tubing and drainage device.
- Be sure patient and caregiver understand correct procedure for applying external catheter. The product manufacturer often offers training and information related to the device free of charge (Pomfret, 2005).

SKILL 33-5   Care of a Suprapubic Catheter

 Intermediate / Urinary Catheter Management / Caring for a Suprapubic Catheter

Suprapubic catheterization involves the insertion of a urinary catheter directly into the bladder through the lower abdominal wall (Fig. 33-7). Urine drains from the catheter into a urinary drainage bag. Suprapubic catheters are inserted using either local or general anesthetic and are for short- or long-term use (Lewis and others, 2007). There is a lower risk for UTI than with indwelling urethral catheters because the anterior abdominal wall normally has a lower density of gram-negative bacteria, including *Escherichia coli* than the periurethral region (Newman, 2004; Niël-Weise and others, 2004). In addition, catheter obstruction is less likely with suprapubic catheters when compared with indwelling catheters (Niël-Weise and others, 2004). A suprapubic catheter is commonly sutured to the abdominal wall to stabilize the catheter.

Delegation Considerations

The skill of care for a newly established suprapubic catheter cannot be delegated to NAP; however, care of an established suprapubic catheter may be delegated. (Refer to agency policy.) The nurse directs the NAP to:

- Report patient's discomfort related to the suprapubic catheter, change in amount and character of urine, or increased temperature.
- Empty drainage bag and document urinary output on I&O record.
- Report any signs of redness or drainage when performing site care of an established suprapubic catheter.

Equipment

- ☐ Gloves, clean and sterile
- ☐ Sterile normal saline solution
- ☐ Sterile cotton-tipped applicators
- ☐ Sterile surgical drainage sponge (split gauze)
- ☐ Sterile gauze dressing
- ☐ Washcloth, towel, soap, and water
- ☐ Silk or paper tape
- ☐ Velcro tube holder (*optional*)

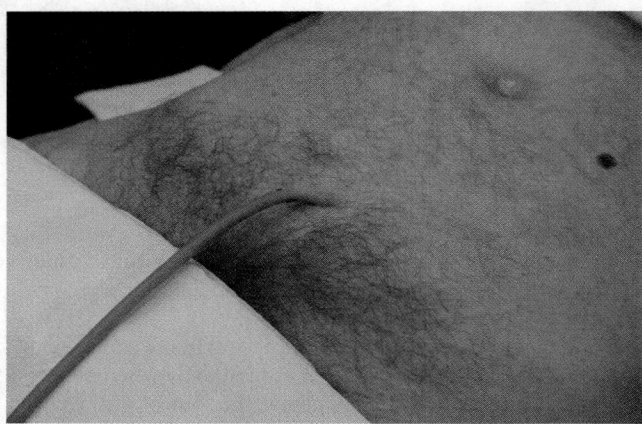

FIG 33-7   Suprapubic catheter without a dressing.

STEP	RATIONALE

ASSESSMENT

1 Assess urine in drainage bag for amount, clarity, color, odor, and sediment.	Abnormal findings indicate potential complications such as UTI, decreased urinary output, and blockage.
2 Observe dressing for drainage and intactness.	Drainage indicates potential complication such as infection. Dressing may become nonocclusive because of tape choice or drainage.
3 Assess catheter insertion site for signs of inflammation such as redness, swelling, and discharge. Ask patient if there is any pain at site; if so, have patient rate on scale of 0 to 10.	If insertion is new, slight inflammation may be expected as part of wound healing. Provides baseline to determine change following procedure.

STEP	RATIONALE
4 Assess for fever.	Increased temperature may indicate infection.
5 Assess patient's knowledge of purpose of catheter and its care.	Determines level of instruction required.

NURSING DIAGNOSES

- Acute pain
- Deficient knowledge regarding care of suprapubic catheter

- Impaired skin integrity
- Impaired urinary elimination

- Risk for infection

Individualize related factors based on patient's condition or needs.

PLANNING

1 Expected outcomes following completion of procedure:	
• Patient will deny pain or discomfort at insertion site and over bladder.	Patent catheter system keeps bladder empty and patient comfortable.
• Minimum of 30 mL of urine is present in urinary collection bag every hour.	Verifies that catheter is patent. Catheters often become blocked by clots, sediment, or position of catheter in bladder (Rushing, 2007).
• Urine remains clear without foul odor.	Removal of retained urine reduces medium for bacterial growth.
• Catheter exit site remains dry, clean, and intact.	Indicates absence of infection and irritation of skin.
• Patient remains afebrile.	Indicates that no infection is developing.
• Patient can explain the purpose and expected outcome.	Helps to minimize anxiety.
2 Explain procedure to patient.	Reduces anxiety and promotes cooperation.

IMPLEMENTATION

1 Perform hand hygiene.	Reduces transmission of infection.
2 Close curtain or room door.	Provides privacy and reduces embarrassment to patient, thus promoting relaxation.
3 Site care of the newly inserted suprapubic catheter:	
a Prepare supplies in the same manner as for applying a dry dressing (see Chapter 39).	The catheter site is surgically made and therefore is treated similarly to other incisions.
b Apply clean gloves, and remove existing dressing. Note type and presence of drainage. Remove gloves, perform hand hygiene, and put on sterile gloves.	Provides baseline for condition of suprapubic wound. Reduces transmission of microorganisms.
c Use nondominant sterile gloved hand, without creating tension, to hold catheter erect while cleaning. Use the sterile cotton-tipped applicators moistened with sterile normal saline to clean site. Using a circular motion, start closest to the catheter and continue in outward widening circles for approximately 5 cm (2 inches) (see illustration).	Follows principle of sterile technique to move from area of least contamination to most. Cleanses microorganisms that could migrate to site.
d Use a sterile gauze pad, moistened with sterile normal saline, to gently clean the base of the catheter, moving up and away from site of insertion. Do not pull catheter.	Removes microorganisms that reside on any drainage that adheres to tubing.
e With dominant sterile gloved hand, apply sterile split gauze (drainage sponge) around catheter and tape in place.	

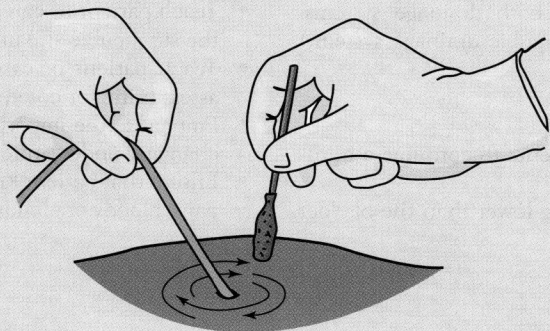

STEP 3c Cleansing around suprapubic catheter in a circular pattern.

STEP	RATIONALE
4 Site care of an established suprapubic catheter: **a** Apply clean gloves. Using warm water and soap, cleanse exit site gently with washcloth. Cleanse using a circular motion starting at the exit site and going outward. Dry completely. Remove gloves; perform hand hygiene.	A clean and dry suprapubic insertion site requires general hygienic measures; dressing is not necessary if drainage is not present (Robinson, 2005a).
5 Loop the catheter on the patient's abdomen, and secure catheter to abdomen with tape to reduce tension on insertion site.	Unsecured catheters lead to enlargement of the stomal tract, leakage, and need for larger-diameter catheters.
6 Check bag and tubing placement. Use Velcro tube holder to secure catheter drainage tubing.	
7 Coil excess tubing on bed, and fasten it to bottom sheet with clip from kit or with rubber band and safety pin.	Promotes gravity drainage and prevents kinks in tubing.

EVALUATION

1 Ask patient to rate pain or discomfort from suprapubic catheter on a scale of 0 to 10.	Determines if bladder is draining and patient is free of infection.
2 Observe patient's urine for sediment, odor, or discoloration.	Possible signs of infection when present.
3 Inspect dressing at least every shift.	Drainage may indicate infection.
4 Monitor for signs of infection: elevated white blood cell count, positive urine culture results, or elevated temperature.	Indicates systemic infection from UTI.
5 Observe catheter insertion site for erythema, edema, discharge, tenderness.	

Unexpected Outcomes	Related Interventions
1 Urinary output decreases; patient experiences lower abdominal pain.	• Check to see if the catheter bag tubing is kinked or patient is lying on tubing. • Change patient's position to see if urine output increases. • Notify the prescriber when possible occlusion is present. Do not irrigate catheter without a prescriber's order.
2 Patient develops symptoms of UTI.	• Encourage fluids to at least 2 L/day, unless contraindicated. • Monitor I&O. • Assess temperature. • Notify prescriber.
3 Dislodgment of suprapubic catheter occurs.	• Cover site with a sterile dressing. • Notify prescriber immediately. • Prescriber or specially trained nurses will need to replace catheter (Rackley and Vasavada, 2006).
4 Skin surrounding catheter exit site becomes excoriated.	• Notify prescriber. • Consult with wound care nurses for use of barrier cream or skin protectant. • Change dressing (if used) more frequently to keep site dry.

Recording and Reporting

- Report and record wound assessment, type of dressing change, and tolerance of patient to dressing.
- Some patients have both an indwelling and a suprapubic catheter after gynecological or bladder surgery. Assess and record urine characteristics and output for both drainage systems. (Most urine will drain from the suprapubic drainage system.) Record both outputs.

Teaching Considerations

- If not contraindicated, encourage patients to consume a minimum of 2000 mL of fluids daily.
- Teach patient to keep the drainage bag lower than the bladder and to keep tubing free of kinks.

- Inform patients with both suprapubic and indwelling catheters that they will have the indwelling urinary catheter removed first, usually between the second and fourth postoperative day.

Home Care Considerations

- Teach patient or caregiver how to clean and apply a dressing to the suprapubic site until clean and dry.
- Teach patient or caregiver how to empty a catheter bag and assess urine for color, odor, clarity, and amount.
- Emphasize the importance of maintaining personal hygiene and changing undergarments at least twice a day (Robinson, 2005a).
- Ensure that patient knows to report immediately any abdominal pain, bloody or cloudy urine, or urine leaking from the insertion site.

When the kidneys are diseased and unable to maintain fluid and electrolyte balance and excrete waste products from the blood, peritoneal dialysis (PD) is a treatment option (Lewis and others, 2007). A major advantage of PD is that patients can perform this procedure in the home setting. Peritoneal drainage in the home setting includes intermittent peritoneal dialysis (IPD) or continuous ambulatory peritoneal dialysis (CAPD).

A PD cycle or exchange includes three phases of inflow (fill), dwell (equilibration), and drain (Lewis and others, 2007). Each phase varies in length, and the number of exchanges depends upon an individualized prescription based on the patient's kidney function. During the inflow phase, a prescribed amount of sterile, warmed hypertonic solution (dialysate) infuses into the peritoneal cavity via a surgically placed soft silicone or polyurethane catheter (Fig. 33-8). The Tenckhoff catheter is the most commonly used PD catheter (Ash, 2006). After infusing the dialysate, an inflow clamp is closed. This starts the dwell phase where the processes of osmosis and diffusion occur between the patient's blood and the body's natural filter known as the semipermeable peritoneal membrane. During this time, excess fluid, electrolytes, and waste products cross over the patient's peritoneal membrane into the dialysate. The used dialysis solution (effluent) drains from the peritoneal cavity in the final phase, removing fluid and excess electrolytes as well as waste products.

PD is either a temporary or permanent therapy depending on degree of kidney function. It can be performed manually, or it can be automated (APD) and performed via a machine referred to as a cycler. The PD cycler delivers the dialysate and times and controls each exchange, usually while the patient sleeps (Fig. 33-9). Refer to Table 33-2, p. 895 for the most common types of PD.

Peritonitis (inflammation of the peritoneal membrane) is a serious complication of PD commonly caused by improper aseptic technique causing contamination of the dialysate and infusion set (Zeigler, 2004). It also results from a catheter exit site infection that progresses inwardly to involve the peritoneum (Lewis and others, 2007). Peritonitis often results in decreased peritoneal membrane function and subsequent removal of the dialysis access (Kelman and Watson, 2006).

Delegation Considerations

The skill of peritoneal and continuous ambulatory dialysis cannot be delegated to NAP. The nurse directs the NAP to:

- Monitor and immediately report any changes in vital signs.
- Obtain and record the patient's weight as prescribed.
- Immediately report any change in patient's condition such as presence of abdominal pain and difficulty breathing.
- Provide routine comfort measures throughout the procedure such as repositioning and elevating the head of the bed.

Equipment

- ❑ Prescribed bags of warmed dialysate solution at 37° C (98.6° F). (see agency policy and procedure for warming dialysate; dry heat [warming pad] or an incubator warming device)
- ❑ Sterile PD administration set (administration sets vary depending on agency and manufacturer)
- ❑ Povidone-iodine swabs (antimicrobial agent)
- ❑ Masks, sterile gloves, and goggles
- ❑ IV pole
- ❑ Label for any medications added to dialysate solution
- ❑ Connector tubing (continuous ambulatory peritoneal dialysis [CAPD] patients may not need)
- ❑ Sign for placement on closed door: "Dialysis in progress: Do not enter"

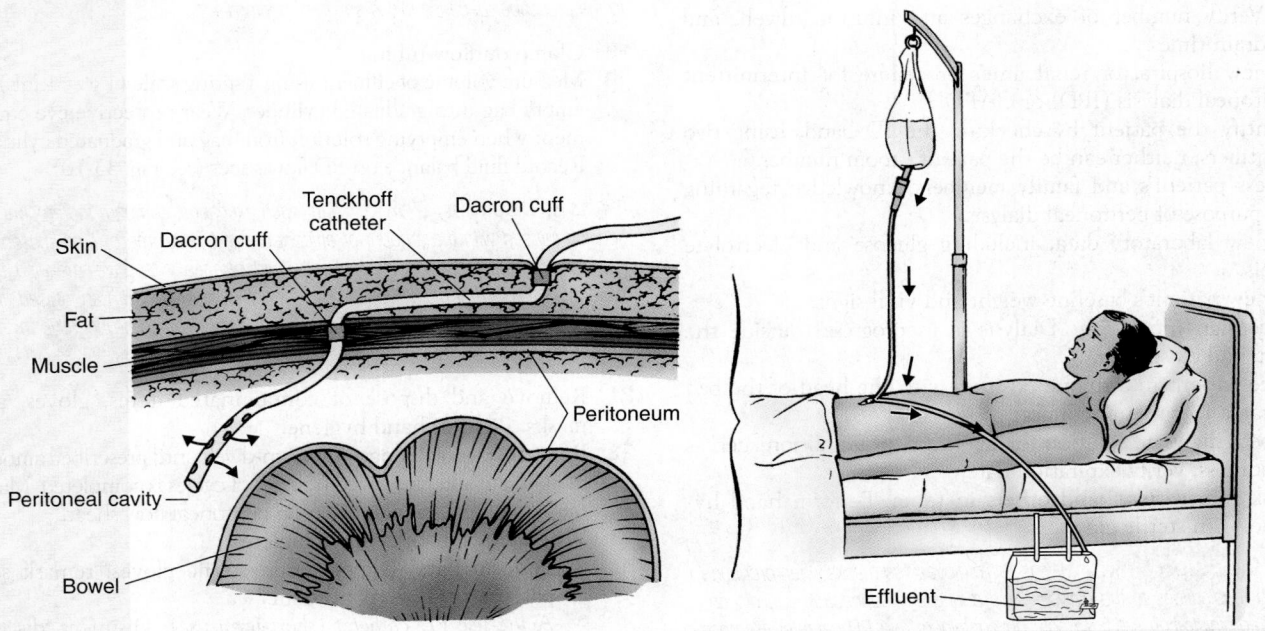

FIG 33-8 Manual peritoneal dialysis via an implanted abdominal catheter (Tenckhoff catheter). (*Modified from Lewis SM and others*: Medical-surgical nursing: assessment and management of clinical problems, *ed 4, St. Louis, 2000, Mosby.*)

Continued

PROCEDURAL GUIDELINE 33-3 Peritoneal Dialysis and Continuous Ambulatory Peritoneal Dialysis—cont'd

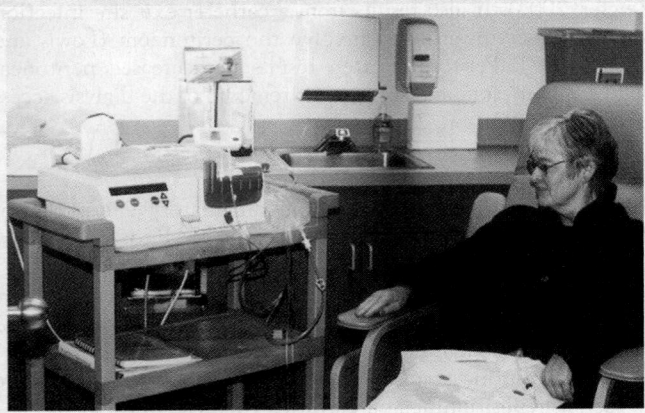

FIG 33-9 Automated peritoneal dialysis cycler, which can be used while the patient is sleeping or for hospitalized patients who require frequent exchanges.

❑ Spring scale or graduated cylinder
❑ Needleless syringe
❑ Peritoneal dialysis flow sheet (Fig. 33-10)

Supplies for Changing the Catheter Site Dressing
❑ Clean gloves, sterile gloves, masks
❑ Povidone-iodine solution or soap and water according to agency policy and procedure
❑ Precut sterile 2 × 2 inch sterile gauze pads or transparent occlusive dressing (see agency policy)
❑ "Do Not Enter" sign for the door

Procedural Steps
1 Review prescriber's orders:
   a Verify dialysis solution and the medications added to solution (added by pharmacy).
   b Verify number of exchanges and infusion, dwell, and drain times.
2 Review hospital or renal unit's procedure for intermittent peritoneal dialysis (IPD) or CAPD.
3 Identify the patient by checking the ID band, using two identifiers; neither can be the patient's room number.
4 Assess patient's and family members' knowledge regarding the purpose of peritoneal dialysis.
5 Review laboratory data, including glucose and electrolyte levels.
6 Review patient's baseline weight and vital signs.
7 Place sign indicating "Dialysis is in progress" outside the door, and close door.
8 Place patient in a supine position with the head of the bed elevated to patient's comfort.
9 Inspect dialysate solution for signs of contamination such as cloudiness; verify expiration date.
10 Mask self, patient, and others in room. Perform hand hygiene. Don sterile gloves.

Critical Decision Point *Wear sterile gloves and masks when preparing and adding medications to the dialysate and during any connection and disconnection of administration set from solution containers and PD catheter. Remove sterile gloves and masks only when system is closed.*

11 Pharmacy will usually add prescribed medications to dialysate solution bag before you receive it. If the situations calls for you to add medications (e.g., heparin, insulin, antibiotics) to dialysate bag, check institutional policy and follow the six rights of medication administration (see Chapter 20). Disinfect top of medication vial and medication port on dialysate bag with a povidone-iodine swab for 5 minutes. Draw up additive into needleless syringe, and inject medication into port on bag. Add medications immediately before the inflow phase.

12 Hang two warmed dialysate bags on IV pole, and attach to inflow tubing by spiking bags exactly as regular IV solution bags (see Chapter 28). Hanging two bags at once promotes timely, organized exchanges and maintains the integrity of the system. Prime tubing with dialysate solution before connecting to PD catheter.

13 Disinfect PD catheter cap and end of catheter with antimicrobial solution; remove cap, and disinfect adapter; connect tubing, maintaining asepsis. (With the CAPD system, you can use a Y connector that attaches on one side to the dialysate and on the other side to the drainage bag. Attach the Y connector aseptically.) Hang drainage bag on bed frame below patient.

14 Open clamp on first dialysate bag, and open clamp on patient line. Infuse solution over prescribed time (usually 2 L/10 to 15 min).

15 Clamp inflow tubing for **prescribed** dwell time (IPD: usually 30 minutes; CAPD: 3 to 5 hours).

16 Have CAPD patient fold tubing and infusion bag on abdomen, which can be concealed by clothing, and use same bag and tubing for drain cycle.

17 Replace empty dialysate bag with a third warmed bag of solution.

18 Unclamp outflow tubing, and drain for **prescribed time** (usually for 20 minutes). Evaluate drainage (effluent) for clarity and color.

Critical Decision Point *Immediately report cloudy peritoneal effluent to the prescriber because this is a sign of peritonitis.*

19 Clamp outflow tubing.
20 Measure volume of effluent using a spring scale (1 g = 1 mL), or empty bag into graduated cylinder. Wear protective eye equipment when emptying solution from bag and graduated cylinder. Record fluid balance on PD flow sheet (see Fig. 33-10).

Critical Decision Point *After each exchange, compare the amount of solution infused with the amount of effluent drained. If volume of fluid infused is more than amount drained, the patient's fluid balance is positive, meaning the patient is retaining the fluid. Conversely, if more fluid is drained than infused, the fluid balance is negative. The cumulative fluid balance should be negative for the patient receiving PD.*

21 Remove and dispose of contaminated items, gloves, and masks. Perform hand hygiene.
22 Repeat cycles of drainage-infusion-dwell until prescribed amount of dialysate and prescribed number of cycles is completed. Maintain ongoing documentation on peritoneal flow sheet.
23 When all exchanges are complete:
   a Perform hand hygiene; don sterile gloves; remask self, patient, and others in room.
   b *Acute-use PD catheter (short-term use):* Disinfect, disconnect connections, and discard tubing. Disinfect catheter rim, and securely place sterile cap on end.
   c *Chronic-use PD catheter (long-term use):* See guidelines made specifically for catheter.

PROCEDURAL GUIDELINE 33-3 Peritoneal Dialysis and Continuous Ambulatory Peritoneal Dialysis—cont'd

d *PD dressing change:*

(1) Place "Do Not Enter" sign on door, and close door.

(2) Place mask on self and patient.

(3) Perform hand hygiene; put on clean gloves.

(4) Expose patient's abdomen only.

(5) Assess catheter exit site for redness, swelling, and drainage.

(6) Remove old dressing, if applicable.

(7) Observe for signs of infection such as redness, swelling, and drainage.

(8) Remove clean gloves.

(9) Set up sterile field. Apply sterile gloves. Open sterile dressing packages, and place on field.

(10) Cleanse around the catheter insertion site with the antimicrobial-soaked sterile gauze pad (or solution designated by agency policy). Cleanse the skin around the insertion site using a circular motion, moving from the inside and cleansing outward. Pat area dry with sterile gauze pad.

(11) Apply split sterile gauze and tape edges of gauze pads, or leave open to air.

(12) Perform hand hygiene, remove masks and gloves; dispose of contaminated supplies according to agency policy.

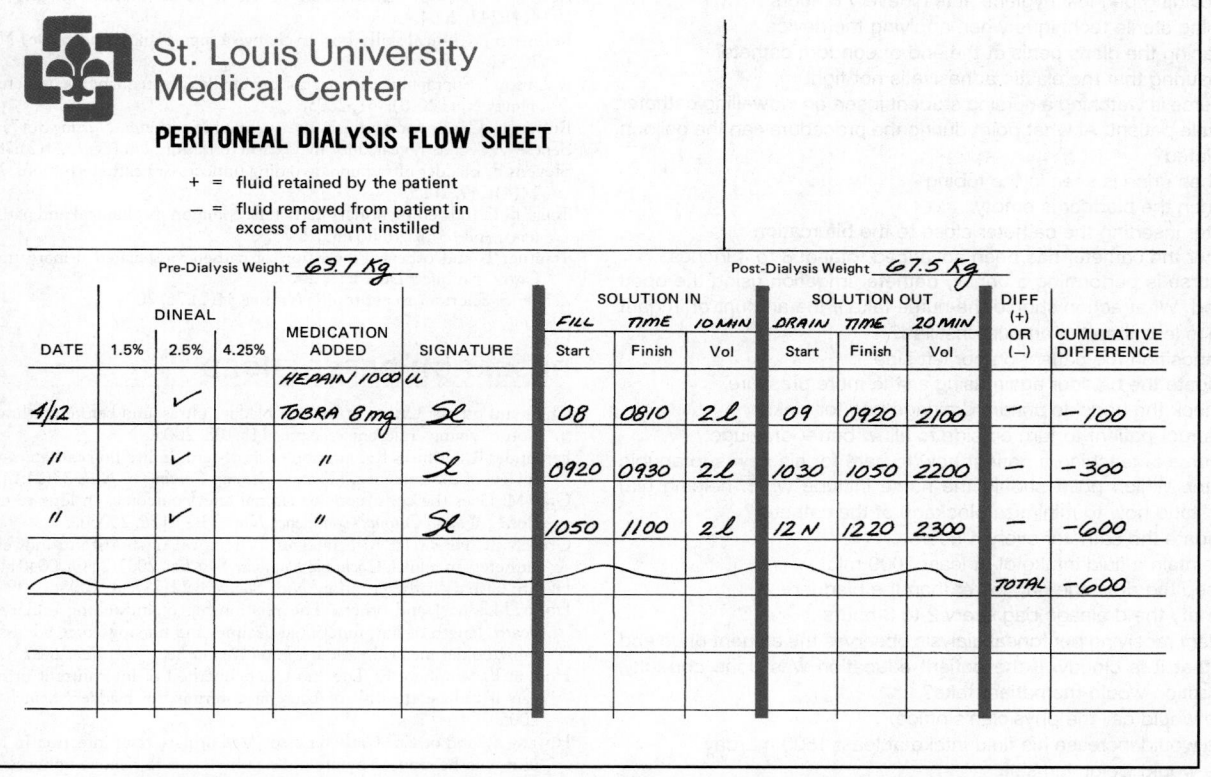

FIG 33-10   Peritoneal dialysis flow sheet. (*Courtesy Saint Louis University Medical Center, St. Louis.*)

TABLE 33-2 | Methods of Peritoneal Dialysis

Type	Description
Continuous ambulatory peritoneal dialysis (CAPD)	Manual: Three to five exchanges daily; last bag of solution remains in abdomen overnight.
Continuous cycling peritoneal dialysis (CCPD)	Cycler machine changes solution 3-5 times or more overnight; last bag of solution remains in abdomen during daytime.
Intermittent peritoneal dialysis (IPD)	Manual or automated; connected for about 10 hours, with cycle changing every 30-60 minutes; abdomen left "dry" between sessions.

CRITICAL THINKING EXERCISES

You are caring for an 80-year-old Muslim woman with a history of urinary retention. An order has been written for an intermittent catheterization for a PVR with possible indwelling catheter insertion. The clinical unit recently acquired a bladder scanner.

1 What assessments would be pertinent for this patient?
2 Explain assessment of PVR for patients with urinary retention.
3 What action would be most appropriate before catheterizing this patient? Give the rationale for your answer.
4 Explain what teaching would be appropriate before assessing PVR.

REVIEW QUESTIONS

1 An older adult patient is having a condom catheter applied for the first time. What is the most important action when caring for a patient with a condom catheter?
    1 Providing perineal hygiene at least every 8 hours
    2 Using sterile technique when applying the device
    3 Placing the glans penis at the end of condom catheter
    4 Ensuring that the elastic adhesive is not tight
2 The nurse is watching a nursing student insert an indwelling catheter in a male patient. At what point during the procedure can the balloon be inflated?
    1 When urine is seen in the tubing
    2 When the bladder is empty
    3 After inserting the catheter close to the bifurcation
    4 After the catheter has been advanced total of 3 to 4 inches
3 The nurse is performing a urinary catheter irrigation using the open method. What action should the nurse take if the amount of irrigant return is less than the amount instilled?
    1 Reposition the patient on her left side.
    2 Irrigate the bladder again using a little more pressure.
    3 Check the bedside urinary drainage bag for kinks.
    4 Instruct patient to turn on side to allow better drainage.
4 The nurse is teaching a patient how to care for his new suprapubic catheter. Which point should the nurse include when helping him understand how to minimize blockage of the catheter?
    1 Irrigate the catheter every 4 hours.
    2 Maintain a fluid intake of at least 2000 mL.
    3 Keep the drainage bag lower than the bladder.
    4 Empty the drainage bag every 2 to 3 hours.
5 A patient receiving peritoneal dialysis observes the effluent drain and sees that it is cloudy. If the patient education was done correctly, what action would the patient take?
    1 He would call the physician's office.
    2 He would increase his fluid intake at least 1500 mL/day
    3 He would weigh himself.
    4 He would change the dressing over the catheter insertion site.

REFERENCES

Altschuler V, Diaz L: Clinical "how to": bladder ultrasound, *Medsurg Nurs* 15(5):317, 2006.

Ash S: Chronic peritoneal dialysis catheters: challenges and design solutions, *Int J Artif Organs* 29(1):85, 2006.

Cochran S: Care of the indwelling urinary catheter: is it evidenced based? *J Wound Ostomy Continence Nurs* 34(3):282, 2007.

Cutts B: Developing and implementing a new bladder irrigation chart, *Nurs Stand* 20(8):48, 2005.

Emr K, Ryan R: Best practices for indwelling catheter in the home setting, *Home Heath Care Nurs* 22(12):820, 2004.

Gray M: What nursing interventions reduce the risk of symptomatic urinary tract infection in the patient with an indwelling catheter? *J Wound Ostomy Continence Nurs* 31(1):3, 2004.

Gray M: Expert review: best practices in managing the indwelling catheter, *Perspectives* 25(1):1, 2006a.

Hockenberry MJ and Wilson D: *Wong's nursing care of infants and children*, ed 8, St. Louis, 2007, Elsevier.

Kelman K, Watson D: Preventing and managing complications of peritoneal dialysis, *Nephrol Nurse* 33(6):647, 2006.

Leaver R: The evidence for urethral meatal cleansing, *Nurs Stand* 21(41):39, 2007.

Lewis and others: *Medical surgical nursing: assessment and management of clinical problems*, ed 4, St. Louis, 2000, Elsevier.

Lewis and others: *Medical surgical nursing: assessment and management of clinical problems*, ed 7, St. Louis, 2007, Elsevier.

Newman D: Incontinence products and devices for the elderly, *Urol Nurs* 24(4):316, 2004.

Patraca K: Measure bladder volume without catheterization, *Nursing* 35(4):46, 2005.

Pomfret I: Managing urinary incontinence with penile sheaths, *Nurs Residential Care* 7(9):403, 2005.

Pomfret I: Penile sheaths: a guide to selection and fitting, *Nurs Residential Care* 20(1):14, 2006.

Potter J: Male urinary incontinence—could penile sheaths be the answer, *J Comm Nurs eJournal*, 2007, http://www.jcn.co.uk/printFriend.asp?Article, accessed July 15, 2007.

Rackley R, Vasavada S: Incontinence, urinary: nonsurgical therapies, *EMedicine eJournal*, 2006, http://www.emedicine.com/med/topic3085.htm, accessed September 9, 2007.

Reyners M: Health consequences of female genital mutilation, *Rev Gynecol Pract* 4(4):242, 2004.

Robinson J: Clinical skills: how to change a suprapubic catheter, *Br J Nurs* 14(1):30, 2005a.

Robinson J: Suprapubic catheterization: challenges in changing catheters, *Br J Community Nurs* 20(8):461, 2005b.

Rushing J: Caring for your patient's suprapubic catheter, *Nursing* 36(7): 22, 2007.

Senese V: Secrets revealed for male catheterization, *Urol Nurs* 24(2):78, 2004.

Stevens E: Bladder ultrasound: avoiding unnecessary catheterizations, *Medsurg Nurs* 14(4):249, 2005.

Toughill E: Indwelling urinary catheters: common mechanical and pathogenic problems, *Am J Nurs* 105(5):35, 2005.

Trautner B and others: Prevention of catheter-associated urinary tract infection, *Curr Opin Infect Dis* 18:37, 2005.

Zeigler S: Shortcut to peritonitis *Nursing* 34(7):76, 2004.

RESEARCH REFERENCES

Chen and others: Utility of bedside bladder ultrasound before urethral catheterization in young children, *Pediatrics* 115:108, 2005.

Fernandez R, Griffiths R: Duration of short-term indwelling catheters—a systematic review of the evidence, *J Wound Ostomy Continence Nurs* 33(2):145, 2006.

Gray M: Does the construction material affect outcomes in long-term catheterization? *J Wound Ostomy Continence Nurs* 33(2):116, 2006b.

Griffiths R, Fernandez R: Strategies for removal of short-term indwelling urethral catheters in adults, *Cochrane Database Syst Rev* 2007(2):CD004011.

Hart S: Urinary catheterization, *Nurs Standard* 22(27):44, 2008.

Holroyd-Leduc J and others: The relationship of indwelling urinary catheters to death, length of stay, functional decline, and nursing home admission in hospitalized older medical patients, *J Am Geriatr Soc* 55(2):227, 2007.

Hudson E, Murahata R: The "no touch" method of intermittent urinary catheter: can it reduce the risk of bacteria entering the bladder? *Spinal Cord* 43:611, 2005.

Huyang W and others: Catheter associated urinary tract infection in intensive care units can be reduced by prompting physicians to remove unnecessary catheters, *Infect Control Hosp Epidemiol* 25(11):974, 2004.

Nazarko L: Reducing the risk of catheter-related urinary tract infection, *Br J Nurs* 17(16):1002, 2008.

Niël-Weise B, van den Broek P: Urinary catheter policies for long-term bladder drainage, *Cochrane Database Syst Rev* 2005(1):CD004201.

Pinto S and Matteucci R: Urinary catheter use and prevention of infection: evidence-based care sheet, Glendale, Calif, 2008, CINAHL Information Systems.

Saint S and others: Condom versus indwelling urinary catheters: a randomized trial, *J Am Geriat Soc* 54:1055, 2006.

Saint S and others: Prevention of nosocomial urinary tract infections, Agency for Healthcare Research and Quality, 2008, http://www.ahrg.gov/clinic/ptsafety/chap15a.htm.

Senese V and others: SUNA clinical practice guidelines: care of the patient with an indwelling catheter, *Urol Nurs* 26(1):80, 2006a.

Senese V and others: SUNA clinical practice guidelines: female urethral catheterization, *Urol Nurs* 26(4):314, 2006b.

Senese V and others: SUNA clinical practice guidelines: male urethral catheterization, *Urol Nurs* 26(4):315, 2006c.

Teng C and others: Application of portable ultrasound scanners in the measurement of post-void residual urine, *J Nurs Res* 13(3):216, 2005.

Bowel Elimination and Gastric Intubation

34

MEDIA RESOURCES

-  http://evolve.elsevier.com/Perry/skills

- **View Video!** Review Questions Video Clips

- **NSO** Nursing Skills Online

KEY TERMS

Cathartic
Cleansing enema
Constipation
Decompression
Defecation
Enema
Fracture pan
Hemorrhoids
Impaction

Medicated enema
Obstipation
Occult blood
Oil-retention
  enema
Zassi Bowel
  Management
  System

OBJECTIVES

Mastery of content in this chapter will enable the nurse to:

- Describe factors that promote and impede normal bowel elimination.
- Discuss methods to relieve constipation or impaction.
- Describe precautions to follow in administering an enema.
- Describe approaches for managing a patient's comfort during nasogastric tube insertion.
- Implement the following skills: assisting a patient in using a bedpan, digital removal of stool, enema administration, and insertion of a nasogastric tube.

Regular elimination of bowel waste products is essential for normal body functioning. Because bowel function depends on the balance of several factors, physical and psychological, elimination patterns and habits vary among individuals. When patients' functional status changes or they become ill at home or in a health care setting, they may not be able to maintain normal elimination habits. Then they require assistance, such as the use of a bedpan or enema administration. It is important for you to always show respect for a patient's privacy, provide necessary comfort measures, and attend to the patient's emotional needs when performing required skills.

To manage patients' elimination problems, you need to understand normal elimination and factors that promote, impede, or cause alterations, such as constipation, diarrhea, and fecal incontinence and perform interventions to minimize discomfort with elimination.

Assist immobilized patients with elimination by helping them on and off bedpans. Collect stool specimens, and properly handle them (see Chapter 43). If a patient is constipated, you will likely administer enemas or digitally remove impacted stool (Kyle and Prynn, 2004). When patients undergo surgery or experience an alteration in gastrointestinal (GI) peristalsis, the insertion of a nasogastric (NG) tube often becomes necessary.

EVIDENCE-BASED PRACTICE TRENDS

Constipation is a symptom, not a disease (Box 34-1). The signs of constipation usually include infrequent bowel movements (less than every 3 days), difficulty in evacuating feces, inability to defecate, and hard feces (Wilson, 2005a). When intestinal motility slows, the body absorbs additional fecal water content. The passage of dry, hard stools occurs when little water remains to soften and lubricate the stool.

There are interventions for the control of constipation. Initially changes in lifestyle, such as increased dietary fiber, increased fluids, moderate exercise, and elimination of laxative use (Bosshard and others, 2004). Also, use the following stepwise levels of interventions. Bulk-forming laxatives (e.g., psyllium [Metamucil] or methylcellulose [Citrucel]) are safe, add bulk to the fecal material, and are used in combination with a saline laxative (e.g., magnesium hydroxide [Milk of Magnesia]) or osmotic laxative (e.g., lactulose [Chronulac]). The patient should increase water intake to enhance the effectiveness of bulk-forming laxatives. If constipation continues, stimulant laxatives (e.g., bisacodyl [Dulcolax] or senna [Senokot]) usually provide relief. Avoid emollient laxatives, such as mineral oil, because they are associated with lipoid aspiration pneumonia (Lehne, 2007).

Fecal incontinence is the patient's inability to control the passage of feces and gas. Management of fecal incontinence requires a complete understanding of the causes. The presence of diarrhea is frequently associated with the incontinence episodes. Continual seepage of diarrhea may also occur with an impaction, and a digital rectal examination can verify its presence. Diarrhea is often due to diet or antibiotic use, which alters the normal flora in the GI tract (Centers for Disease Control and Prevention [CDC], 2005; Todd, 2006). Control diarrhea by supplementing course bran rather than refined fiber to slow intestinal transit time and to increase the bulk of the fecal contents (Fletcher, 2005). Treatment for controlling diarrhea encourage a more formed stool, and thus the frequency of incontinence declines. However, avoid treatments that slow intestinal transit when a patient has organism-related diarrhea (e.g., *Clostridium difficile* or food-borne pathogen) (CDC, 2005; Todd, 2006). Management strategies for fecal incontinence are diverse. One strategy to manage diarrhea is the Zassi Bowel Management System, which diverts feces away from wounds so that you can administer rectal medications and irrigations. This system is an intrarectal catheter that has a retention cuff, intraluminal balloon, three pilot balloons, anchor straps, and a port for sampling stool (Benoit and Watts, 2007) (Fig. 34-1).

CULTURAL CONSIDERATIONS

Modify nursing interventions when caring for patients from other cultural and ethnic groups to meet their elimination needs. Consider the following approaches:

- Provide gender-congruent care for patients from cultures that emphasize separate gender roles and female modesty, such as African, Hispanic, Asian, Islamic, Arabic, Hindu, Jewish Orthodox, and Amish cultures. In some cultures it is not appropriate for male nurses to provide pericare for females.
- Provide for culturally sensitive hygiene needs:
  - Certain cultures, such as Hindus and Muslims, have distinct hygienic practices, which designate the left hand to perform unclean procedures such as bowel elimination (Lawrence and Rozmus, 2001).
  - Use the right hand to first touch the patient, then use the left hand to handle the bedpan and to assist the patient in cleansing after bowel movement.

| **BOX 34-1** | Common Causes of Constipation |

- Irregular bowel habits and ignoring the urge to defecate.
- Chronic illnesses (e.g., Parkinson's disease, multiple sclerosis, rheumatoid arthritis, chronic bowel diseases, depression, eating disorders) (Wilson, Part I, 2005).
- Low-fiber diet high in animal fats (e.g., meats, dairy products, eggs), refined sugars (rich desserts), and low fluid intake slows peristalsis (Wilson, Part I, 2005).
- Lengthy bed rest or lack of regular exercise.
- Laxative misuse (Wilson, Part II, 2005).
- Older adults experience slowed peristalsis, loss of abdominal muscle elasticity, and reduced intestinal mucus secretion. Older adults often eat low-fiber foods (Stanley and others, 2005).
- Neurological conditions that block nerve impulses to the colon (e.g., spinal cord injury, tumor).
- Organic illnesses such as hypothyroidism, hypocalcemia, or hypokalemia (Wilson, Part I, 2005).
- Colonic action slowed by medications such as anticholinergics, antispasmodics, anticonvulsants, antidepressants, antihistamines, antihypertensives, antiparkinsonism drugs, bile acid sequestrants, diuretics, antacids, iron supplements, calcium supplements, opioids (Wilson, Part I, 2005).

- Promote patient's understanding of the procedure.
  - Use an interpreter if needed.
  - Repeat explanations because patient's anxiety about the loss of privacy poses distraction.

Skill Performance Guidelines

1 Determine patient's normal pattern of bowel elimination, and accommodate that pattern while the patient is in a health care setting. Determine the time the patient normally has a bowel movement and the amount of assistance needed.

2 Provide privacy to reduce patient's embarrassment. Encourage patient to use the bathroom when able.

3 Be aware of foods that promote normal peristaltic movement, including high-fiber foods such as raw fruit, whole grains, and green leafy vegetables. Make sure these are consistent with the patient's prescribed diet. Immobilized patients need to receive foods that promote peristalsis but not those that adversely affect bowel routine.

4 Unless contraindicated, encourage patient to drink six to eight glasses of water per day. Warm fluids are effective in increasing peristalsis.

5 Encourage patients to be as active as physically possible to promote peristalsis.

6 Promote comfort when patient uses the bedpan.

7 Be aware of side effects of medications patients receive. Some drugs impair normal elimination pattern by causing constipation or diarrhea. General anesthetic agents used during surgery cause temporary cessation of peristalsis and increase the risk for constipation.

8 Consider developmental changes that affect bowel functioning throughout the life span. For example, an older adult who becomes less active and has decreased muscle tone and changes in eating patterns has a higher risk for experiencing constipation.

9 When handling fecal matter, always use standard precautions.

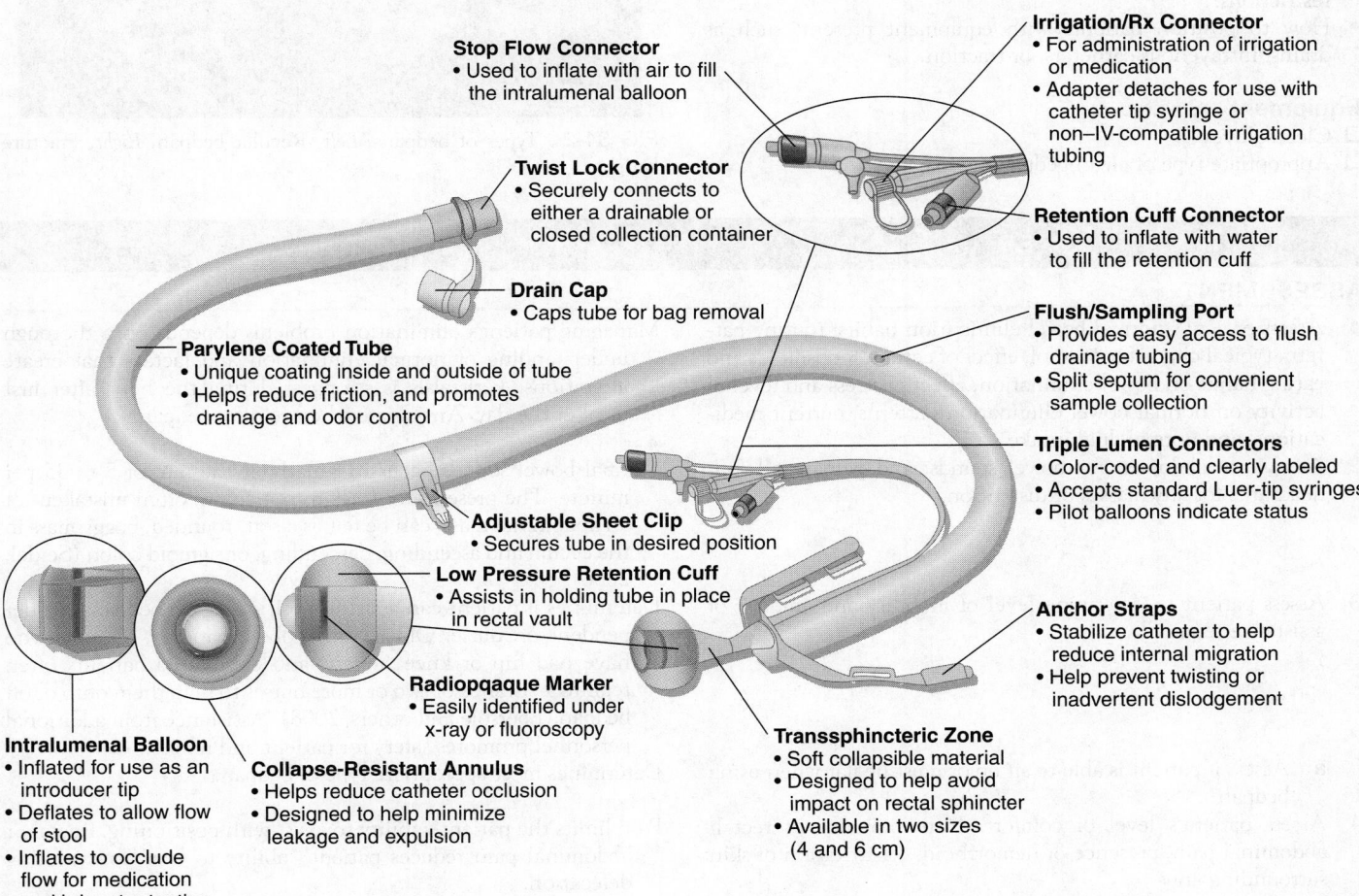

Stop Flow Connector
• Used to inflate with air to fill the intralumenal balloon

Twist Lock Connector
• Securely connects to either a drainable or closed collection container

Drain Cap
• Caps tube for bag removal

Parylene Coated Tube
• Unique coating inside and outside of tube
• Helps reduce friction, and promotes drainage and odor control

Adjustable Sheet Clip
• Secures tube in desired position

Low Pressure Retention Cuff
• Assists in holding tube in place in rectal vault

Intralumenal Balloon
• Inflated for use as an introducer tip
• Deflates to allow flow of stool
• Inflates to occlude flow for medication and irrigant retention

Collapse-Resistant Annulus
• Helps reduce catheter occlusion
• Designed to help minimize leakage and expulsion

Radiopqaque Marker
• Easily identified under x-ray or fluoroscopy

Irrigation/Rx Connector
• For administration of irrigation or medication
• Adapter detaches for use with catheter tip syringe or non–IV-compatible irrigation tubing

Retention Cuff Connector
• Used to inflate with water to fill the retention cuff

Flush/Sampling Port
• Provides easy access to flush drainage tubing
• Split septum for convenient sample collection

Triple Lumen Connectors
• Color-coded and clearly labeled
• Accepts standard Luer-tip syringes
• Pilot balloons indicate status

Anchor Straps
• Stabilize catheter to help reduce internal migration
• Help prevent twisting or inadvertent dislodgement

Transsphincteric Zone
• Soft collapsible material
• Designed to help avoid impact on rectal sphincter
• Available in two sizes (4 and 6 cm)

FIG 34-1 Zassi Bowel Management System. (*Courtesy Hollister Incorporated, Libertyville, Ill.*)

SKILL 34-1 Assisting a Patient in Using a Bedpan

Basic / Elimination Assistance / Assisting With a Bedpan

A patient restricted to bed must use a bedpan for defecation. Women use bedpans to pass urine and feces, whereas men use bedpans for defecation and urinals for urination. Sitting on a bedpan is uncomfortable. Help the patient assume a position similar to the natural squatting position.

Two types of bedpans are available (Fig. 34-2). The regular bedpan, made of metal or hard plastic, has a curved, smooth upper end and a tapered lower end. The pan is approximately 5 cm (2 inches) deep. A fracture pan, designed for patients with body or leg casts or patients restricted from raising their hips (e.g., following total joint replacement), has a shallow end approximately 1.3 cm (½ inch) deep that slips easily under a patient. The open end of the regular pan fits just under the upper thighs and the back of the pan fits under the patient's buttocks toward the sacrum. For the fracture pan, the handle is just under the thighs and the smaller portion is toward the buttocks.

Delegation Considerations

The skill of assisting a patient onto a bedpan can be delegated to nursing assistive personnel (NAP). The nurse directs the NAP about:

- The proper way to position patients who have mobility restrictions.
- How to position patients with equipment present, such as drains, intravenous catheters, or traction.

Equipment

- ❑ Clean gloves
- ❑ Appropriate type of clean bedpan
- ❑ Bedpan cover
- ❑ Toilet tissue and powder
- ❑ Specimen container (if necessary), plastic bag, clearly labeled with date, patient's name, and identification number
- ❑ Basin, washcloths, towels, and soap
- ❑ Waterproof, absorbent pads
- ❑ Clean drawsheet (optional)

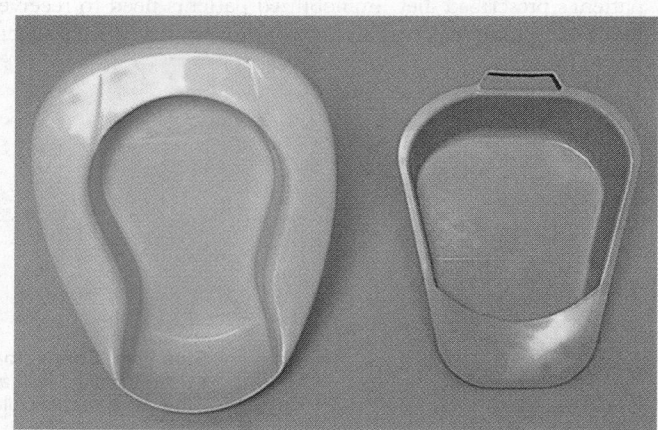

FIG 34-2 Types of bedpans. *Left,* Regular bedpan. *Right,* Fracture bedpan.

STEP	RATIONALE

ASSESSMENT

1 Assess patient's normal bowel elimination habits: routine pattern, typical character of stool, effect of certain foods/fluids and eating habits on bowel elimination, effect of stress and level of activity on normal bowel elimination patterns, current medications, and normal fluid intake.

Managing patient's elimination problems depends on a thorough understanding of normal elimination and factors that create alterations. Peristalsis is strongest during the hour after first meal of the day. Anticipate when to offer bedpan.

2 Auscultate abdomen for bowel sounds, and palpate all four quadrants for any masses or distention.

Normal bowel sounds occur irregularly at the rate of 5 to 35 per minute. The presence of feces in the colon, often mistaken for an abdominal mass, can be felt as a soft, rounded, boggy mass in the cecum and ascending, descending, or sigmoid colon (Seidel, 2006).

3 Assess patient to determine level of mobility and amount of assistance required.

Determines if patient can assist in positioning on bedpan or if dependent on nurse. Older adults, obese patients, patients who have had hip or knee surgery, and debilitated patients often require assistance of two or more nurses to help them onto or off bedpan (Ebersole and others, 2008). Assistance from additional personnel promotes safety for patient and nurses.

   a Assess if patient is able to sit up or must lie flat when using bedpan.

Determines most appropriate type of bedpan.

4 Assess patient's level of comfort. Note presence of rectal/abdominal pain, presence of hemorrhoids, or irritation of skin surrounding anus.

Pain limits the patient's ability to assist with positioning. Rectal or abdominal pain reduces patient's ability to bear down during defecation.

5 Determine need for stool specimen.

Provides opportunity to obtain specimen container before placing patient on bedpan.

STEP	RATIONALE

NURSING DIAGNOSES

- Acute pain
- Bowel incontinence
- Chronic pain
- Diarrhea
- Impaired physical mobility
- Perceived constipation
- Risk for constipation
- Toileting self-care deficit

Individualize related factors based on patient's condition or needs.

PLANNING

1 Expected outcomes following completion of procedure:
  - Perianal skin is clean and intact.
  - Patient eliminates without pain or discomfort.

2 Explain procedure to patient, including self-help tips, such as how to use a trapeze, how to move hips, etc.

3 Obtain assistance from additional nursing personnel as warranted.

Intact perianal skin.
Patient is positioned comfortably on bedpan.
Promotes independence, reduces anxiety, and helps patient to assist during procedure.
Adequate personnel resources minimize muscle strain for patient and nurse. Reduce patient's discomfort.

IMPLEMENTATION

1 Perform hand hygiene, and apply gloves.
2 Provide privacy by closing curtains around bed or door of room.
3 Place metal bedpan under warm, running water for few seconds, then dry. Be careful that pan is not too hot. Apply powder to surface of bedpan *(optional)*.

4 Put side rail in up position on opposite side of bed.

5 Raise bed horizontally according to nurse's height.

6 Have patient assume supine position.

Reduces transmission of microorganisms.
Reduces embarrassment and promotes bowel elimination.
Metal bedpans are very cold. Warm pan helps patient to relax anal sphincter. Powder reduces friction of pan against skin.

Protects patient from falling out of bed. Patient can use side rail to grasp onto and assist self in moving about in bed and onto the bedpan.
Promotes use of good body mechanics and minimizes muscle strain for nurse and patient.
Position eases eventual pan placement.

Critical Decision Point *Observe for the presence of drains, dressings, IV fluids, and traction. These devices make it difficult for a patient to assist with the procedure. You will likely need more personnel to assist in placing the patient on a bedpan.*

7 Place patient who is mobile in bed and can assist with procedure on bedpan:
  a Raise head of bed patient's head 30 to 60 degrees.

  b Remove upper bed linens so they are out of the way, but do not expose patient.
  c Instruct patient in how to flex knees and lift hips upward.

  d Place hand closest to the patient's head palm up under patient's sacrum to assist lifting. Ask patient to bend knees. As the patient raises hips, use other hand to slip bedpan under patient (see illustrations). Be sure open rim of bedpan is facing toward foot of bed. Do not force pan under patient's hips. (*Optional:* Have patient use overhead trapeze frame to raise hips.)

Prevents hyperextension of back and provides support to upper torso when patient raises hips. Sitting position promotes defecation.
Prevents embarrassment to patient; demonstrates respect for patient's sense of dignity.
If the legs, upper torso, and arms are supporting body weight, then little effort should be required of patient.
Positions the bedpan high under buttocks so feces enters pan. Incorrect placement of bedpan causes discomfort for patient and spillage of contents. Forcing bedpan under patient increases the risk for friction injury to underlying skin and tissues. Powder helps to slide the pan under the patient without friction.

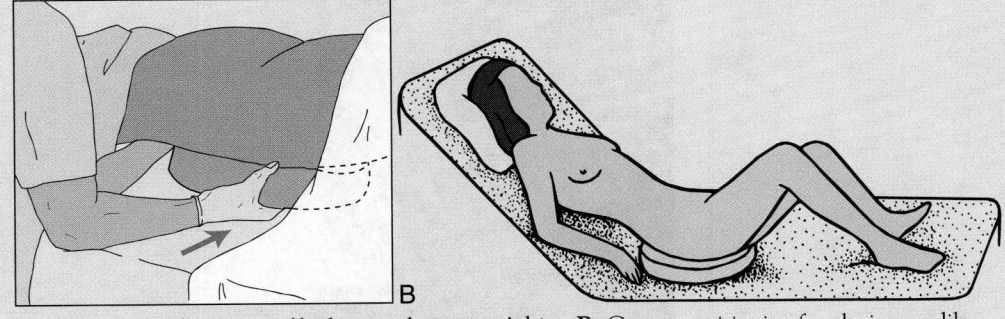

STEP 7d **A,** Placement of bedpan under patient's hips. **B,** Correct positioning for placing mobile patient on bedpan.

STEP	RATIONALE
e *Optional:* If using a fracture pan, raise hips and slip it under patient (see illustration).	Patient requires less maneuvering.
8 Place patient who is immobile or has restrictions in mobility on bedpan:	
a Put head of the bed flat (if tolerated by medical condition).	Assists patient for whom it is unsafe to exert effort when lifting hips, who must remain flat, or who is unable to lift hips, to roll onto bedpan.
b Remove top linens as necessary to turn patient while minimizing exposure.	Prevents embarrassment to patient; demonstrates respect for patient's sense of dignity.
c Assist patient with rolling onto side away from you and toward side rail. Place bedpan firmly against patient's buttocks and down into mattress. Be sure that open rim of bedpan is facing toward foot of bed (see illustrations).	Incorrect placement causes discomfort to patient and spillage of contents.

Critical Decision Point *If patient has had total hip replacement, make sure the abduction pillow placed between the legs to prevent dislocation of the new joint remain in place. Use a fracture pan.*

STEP	RATIONALE
d Keep one hand against bedpan, place other around far hip of patient. Ask patient to roll back onto bedpan, flat in bed. Do not force the pan under the patient.	Using minimal exertion, this places patient squarely on pan. Avoid forcing bedpan under patient to decreases risk for friction injury to underlying skin and tissues.
e Raise patient's head 30 to 60 degrees to a comfortable level, unless contraindicated.	Patient assumes sitting position unless condition necessitates maintaining flat position. Sitting position promotes defecation. Flat position can cause back strain.
f Raise knee gatch (unless contraindicated), or ask patient to bend the knees.	Relieves stress on back.
9 Ensure patient comfort. Cover patient for warmth. Place small pillow or rolled towel under lumbar curve of back.	Provides added comfort. Pain reduces or eliminates urge to defecate, which will result in bowel elimination problems.
10 Have call bell and toilet tissue within reach for patient.	Promotes safety by preventing patient from reaching over edge of bed for objects out of reach.
11 Ensure that bed is in lowest position and raise upper side rails.	Promotes patient safety and enables the patient to reposition the pan as needed.
12 Remove and discard gloves, and perform hand hygiene.	Reduces transmission of microorganisms.
13 Allow patient to be alone, but monitor status and respond promptly to call signal so as to remove bedpan in timely manner.	Reassures patient. Removing bedpan in a timely manner prevents pressure ulcers.
14 Perform hand hygiene, and apply new pair of gloves.	Reduces transmission of microorganisms.
15 Place patient's bedside chair close to working side of bed.	Provides area to place bedpan and contents on chair after removal from patient to prevent accidental spilling of full bedpan on bed surface.

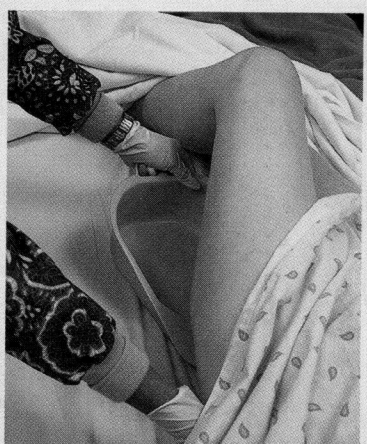

STEP 7e   Patient lifts hips as fracture pan is positioned.

STEP	RATIONALE

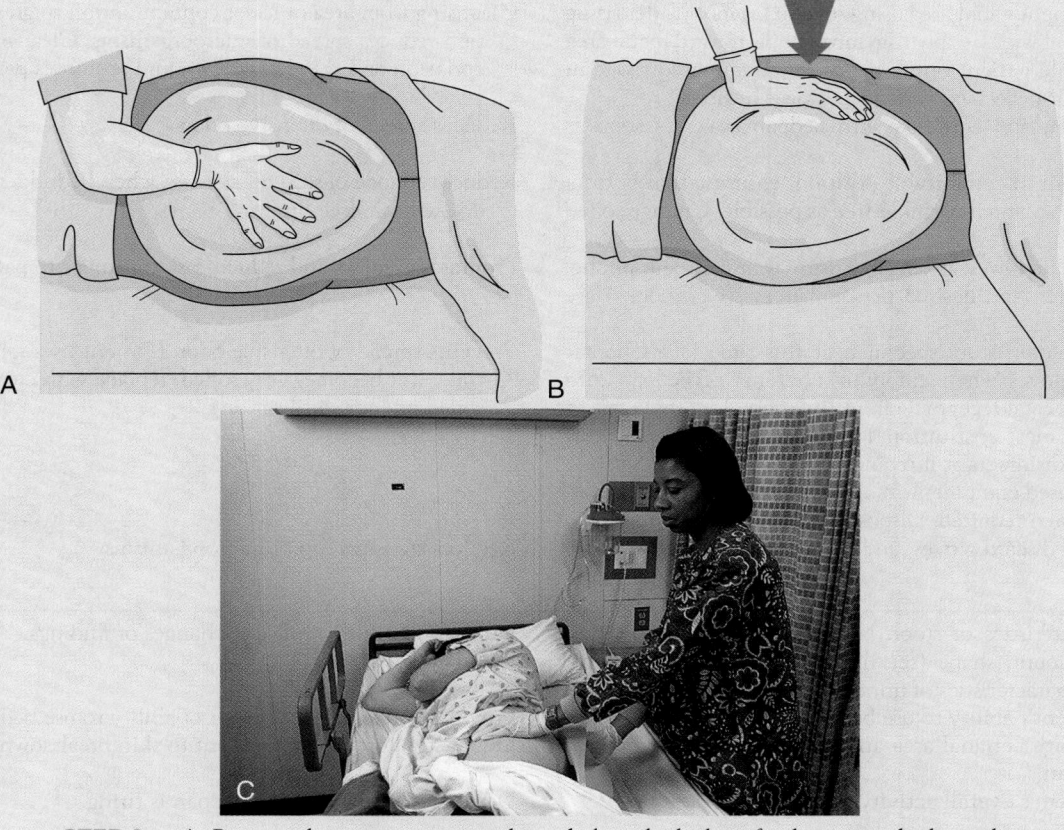

STEP 8c   **A,** Position the patient on one side, and place the bedpan firmly against the buttocks. **B,** Push down on the bedpan and toward the patient. **C,** Nurse places bedpan in position. (**A** *and* **B** *from Sorrentino SA:* Mosby's textbook for nursing assistants, *ed 6, St. Louis, 2006, Mosby.*)

STEP	RATIONALE
16 Collect basin of warm water.	Allows patient to perform hand hygiene after wiping perineal area (if appropriate); also allows nurse, wearing gloves, to use water to wash patient's perineal area if patient is unable to wipe thoroughly.
17 Raise bed to working height. Lower side rail and move aside upper linens; keep patient covered.	Maintains privacy.
18 Determine if patient is able to wipe own perineal area.	
19 Remove bedpan of mobile patient.	
a Ask patient to flex knees, placing body weight on lower legs, feet, and upper torso; lift buttocks up from bedpan. At same time, place hand farthest from patient on side of bedpan to support it (prevent spillage) and place other hand (closest to patient) under sacrum to assist in lifting. Have patient lift, remove bedpan, then place it on bedside chair.	Avoids pulling or forcing pan from under hips because this action pulls skin and causes tissue injury.
b Offer patient opportunity to perform perineal hygiene and then hand hygiene after having wiped perineal area (if appropriate).	Reduces spread of microorganisms.
20 Remove bedpan of immobile patient.	
a Lower head of bed.	Facilitates turning of patient.
b Assist patient with rolling onto side away from you and off bedpan. Hold bedpan flat while patient is rolling off it; otherwise, spillage will occur. Place bedpan and contents on bedside chair.	

STEP	RATIONALE
c Wipe patient's anal area using several layers of toilet tissue or perineal wipes, wipe from mons pubis toward rectal area (for female patient only); deposit contaminated tissue in bedpan. If necessary, perform perineal hygiene.	Cleansing from area of lesser contamination to greater contamination reduces spread of microorganisms. Cleansing prevents excoriation and skin breakdown and promotes personal hygiene.
21 Cover bedpan and contents with bedpan cover as soon as possible.	Reduces spread of offensive odors.
22 Return patient to comfortable position, ensuring that bottom linens are clean and as wrinkle-free as possible. Change soiled linens.	Reduces chance of skin breakdown when bedridden patient lies on dry, wrinkle-free linens.
23 Place bed in its lowest position. Ensure that call bell, phone, drinking water, and desired personal items (e.g., books) are within easy access.	Promotes comfort and reduces risk for injury to patient.
24 If ordered, obtain stool specimen at this time (see Chapter 43). Wear gloves when emptying contents of bedpan into toilet or in special receptacle in utility room. Use spray faucet attached to most institution toilets to rinse bedpan thoroughly. Use disinfectant if required by institution.	Prevents spread of offensive odor. (Patient uses same bedpan each time. If it becomes very soiled, replace with clean one and send soiled one for sterilization).
25 Replace all used equipment in appropriate location for subsequent use when required. Dispose of soiled linens correctly.	
26 Remove and discard gloves, and perform hand hygiene.	Reduces transmission of microorganisms.

EVALUATION

1 Assess characteristics of stool. Note color, odor, consistency, frequency, amount, shape (see illustration), and constituents. Also, assess characteristics of urine, if patient voided in bedpan.	Helps to identify significant changes or findings.
2 Evaluate patient's ability to use bedpan.	Provides continual assessment of ability to use bedpan.
3 Inspect patient's perianal area and surrounding skin while removing bedpan.	Liquid stool predisposes patient to skin breakdown.
4 Evaluate patient's overall activity tolerance and comfort.	Defecation and use of the bedpan is tiring.

The Bristol Stool Form Scale

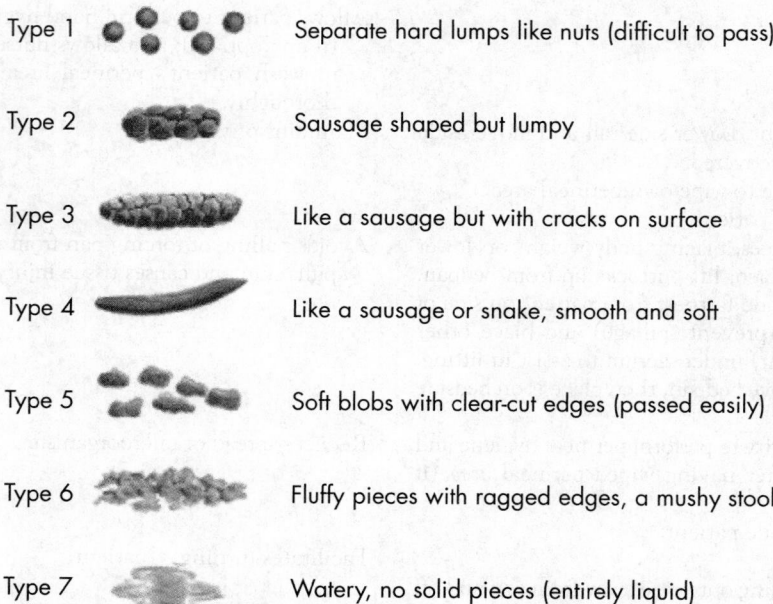

Type 1   Separate hard lumps like nuts (difficult to pass)

Type 2   Sausage shaped but lumpy

Type 3   Like a sausage but with cracks on surface

Type 4   Like a sausage or snake, smooth and soft

Type 5   Soft blobs with clear-cut edges (passed easily)

Type 6   Fluffy pieces with ragged edges, a mushy stool

Type 7   Watery, no solid pieces (entirely liquid)

Step 1   Bristol Stool Form Scale. (*From O'Donnell LJ, Virjee J, Heaton KW. Detection of pseudodiarrhoea by simple clinical assessment of intestinal transit rate, Br Med J, 300:439. ©1990. Reprinted with permission of the BMJ Publishing Group.*)

Unexpected Outcomes

1 Patient is unable to use bedpan.
2 Patient is incontinent of stool, resulting from patient's embarrassment in using bedpan or nursing staff's delay in offering bedpan.

3 Patient is constipated, resulting from pain of defecation, immobility, or unnatural position for defecation.

4 Patient develops irritation and breakdown of skin around perianal area.
5 Blood in stool or black stool.

Related Interventions

- If patient's mobility allows, obtain order for use of a bedside commode.
- Establish a regular schedule of offering bedpan, or improve responsiveness when patient calls for assistance.
- Discuss with staff the need to answer patient's request for toileting assistance promptly.
- Consult with health care provider regarding administration of a stool softener.
- Try offering dietary foods high in fiber.
- Increase fluid intake if appropriate for patient's medical condition.
- Administer perianal skin care using moisture barrier.
- Perform fecal occult blood testing (FOBT) (see Chapter 43).

Recording and Reporting

- Record type of assistance needed and if tolerates getting on/off bedpan, character and amount of stool, and urine output if patient also voids.
- Complete laboratory requisition if you collected stool or urine specimen, and send to laboratory.

Teaching Considerations

- Some patients on complete bed rest have overhead trapeze frame connected to bed to help lift them on and off bedpan. Teaching this activity helps to maintain strength of patient's arms.

Pediatric Considerations

- Constipation in early childhood results from environmental changes, such as being hospitalized and reluctance to use a bedpan.
- Repeated withholding of stool leads to stretching or dilating of the rectum and decreases the sensation or "urge" to defecate (Hockenberry and Wilson, 2007).

Gerontological Considerations

- Older adults have some loss of sphincter control and often will require a quick response when requesting a bedpan.
- Incidence of constipation is greater because there is impaired rectal sensation to defecate. As a result, the older adult does not perceive the need to defecate (Ebersole and others, 2008).
- Reinforce with older adult patients that as long as the consistency of the stool remains normal and the bowel movements occur with regularity there is no need to have a bowel movement daily. Therefore patients should not place themselves on laxatives to avoid constipation (Ebersole and others, 2008; Meiner and Lueckenotte, 2005).
- With increased age, transit time through the bowel increases, causing a normal lengthening of the time between bowel movements (Meiner and Lueckenotte, 2005).

SKILL 34-2 Removing Fecal Impaction Digitally

Constipation is a relatively common health problem for many adults who believe that a regular bowel habit requires having a daily bowel movement or a bowel movement at the same time each day (or both) (Bosshard and others, 2004). Medically, constipation is defined as infrequent stools. However, functional constipation includes two or more of the following factors. Each factor occurs for at least 3 months: (1) straining with defecation at least one quarter of the time, (2) lumpy or hard stools (or both) one quarter of the time, (3) sensation of incomplete evacuation one quarter of the time, or (4) two or fewer bowel movements in a week (Bosshard and others, 2004). There are varieties of interventions that successfully relieve constipation. However, there are patients who develop obstipation, which is the absolute inability to pass stool.

Fecal impaction, the inability to pass a hard collection of stool, occurs in all age-groups. Physically and mentally incapacitated persons and institutionalized older adult patients are at greatest risk (Kyle and Prynn, 2004). Symptoms of fecal impaction include constipation, rectal discomfort, anorexia, nausea, vomiting, abdominal pain, diarrhea (around the impacted stool), and urinary frequency. Prevention is the key to fecal impaction. However, once it occurs, digital removal of stool is the only alternative (Kyle and Prynn, 2004). This procedure is very uncomfortable and embarrassing for the patient. Excessive rectal manipulation causes irrita-

tion to the mucosa, bleeding, and stimulation of the vagus nerve, which causes a reflex slowing of the heart rate.

Delegation Considerations

The skill of removing a fecal impaction digitally cannot be delegated to NAP. When delegating care of a patient who has undergone digital removal of stool, the nurse directs the NAP to:
- Provide perineal care following each bowel movement.
- Observe any evacuated stool for color and consistency.
- Immediately report any signs of blood or bloody mucous discharge to the nurse for further assessment.

Equipment

- ❑ Clean gloves
- ❑ Water-soluble local anesthetic lubricant (NOTE: Some institutions require use of water-soluble lubricant without anesthetic when nurse performs procedure.)
- ❑ Waterproof, absorbent pads
- ❑ Bedpan
- ❑ Bedpan cover
- ❑ Bath blanket
- ❑ Basin, washcloths, towels, and soap
- ❑ Vital signs equipment

STEP	RATIONALE

ASSESSMENT

1 Assess patient:

  a Note medical history of fecal impaction.

    Disabled or institutionalized patients often have recurrent constipation (Wilson, 2005b).

  b Determine last bowel movement.

    Infrequent defecation increases chances of hard stool forming in rectum (Bosshard and others, 2004).

  c Observe consistency of stool or seepage of liquid stool. This situation occurs particularly in immobilized patients. Patient is continually or frequently incontinent of liquid stool.

    This is symptomatic of an impaction high in colon. Some patients are able to pass small pieces of hard stool or have episodes of passing small amounts of liquid stool (Wilson, 2005b).

  d Patient expresses desire to defecate but is unable to do so.

    Large fecal mass causes rectal distention and increases perception of urge to evacuate the rectum (Bosshard and others, 2004).

  e Patient complains of pain when trying to defecate.

    Pain often suppresses urge to defecate and compounds problem.

  f Note normal bowel patterns; eating habits; exercise pattern or level of mobility; medications, especially narcotic analgesics.

    Determines if these are contributing factors. Attempt to include nursing actions in care plan that help to prevent situation from recurring.

  g Obtain baseline vital signs.

    Provides baseline measurement. The sacral branch of the vagus nerve is stimulated during digital stimulation; this stimulation results in reflex slowing of heart rate (Seidel and others, 2007).

Critical Decision Point *Because of the potential to stimulate the sacral branch of the vagus nerve, patients with a history of dysrhythmias or heart disease have a greater risk for changes in heart rhythm. Be sure to monitor patient's pulse before and during procedure. This procedure is often contraindicated in cardiac patients; if in doubt, verify with the health care provider.*

  h Assess bowel sounds and abdominal distention.

    Indicates presence of peristalsis but does not conclusively confirm GI patency. Distention contributes to constipation.

2 Check patient's record to determine if health care provider's order exists to remove stool manually. Using two identifiers check patient's identification.

  Obtain written order before performing procedure, because this procedure involves excessive stimulation of the vagus nerve. Ensures right patient.

NURSING DIAGNOSES

- Acute pain
- Constipation
- Diarrhea

Individualize related factors based on patient's condition or needs.

PLANNING

1 Expected outcomes following completion of procedure:

- Impacted stool is successfully removed.

  Indicates rectum is clear of stool.

- Patient is free of abdominal or rectal discomfort.

  Fecal impaction causes direct pain to rectum and indirect abdominal discomfort through abdominal distention.

- Vital signs remain within patient's baseline.

  Indicates absence of vagal stimulation.

2 Explain procedure to patient.

  Information reduces anxiety and encourages patient participation in a therapeutic elimination protocol.

IMPLEMENTATION

1 Perform hand hygiene, and apply gloves.

  Prevents transmission of microorganisms.

2 Obtain assistance to help change patient's position, if necessary. Raise bed horizontally to comfortable working height.

  Promote patient safety and use of good body mechanics by nurse.

3 Pull curtains around bed or close door to room.

  Maintains patient's sense of privacy and prevents unnecessary exposure of body parts.

4 Lower side rail on patient's right side. Keeping the far side rail raised, assist patient to left side-lying position with knees flexed and back toward nurse.

  Promotes patient safety. Provides access to rectum.

5 Drape patient's trunk and lower extremities with bath blanket, and place waterproof pad under patient's buttocks.

  Maintains patient's sense of privacy and prevents unnecessary exposure of body parts.

6 Place bedpan next to patient.

7 Apply clean gloves. Lubricate gloved index finger and middle finger of dominant hand with anesthetic lubricant.

  Permits smooth insertion of finger into anus and rectum.

STEP	RATIONALE

Critical Decision Point   *Observe for the presence of perianal skin irritation, which indicates the need for additional postprocedure skin care to the perianal region to reduce pain during subsequent bowel elimination.*

STEP	RATIONALE
8 Instruct patient to take slow deep breaths. Gradually and gently insert gloved index finger, and feel anus relax around the finger. Then insert middle finger.	Slow deep breaths help to relax patient. Gradual insertion of index finger helps to dilate anal sphincter (Kyle and Prynn, 2004).
9 Gradually advance fingers slowly along rectal wall toward umbilicus.	Allows nurse to reach impacted stool high in rectum.
10 Gently loosen fecal mass by moving fingers in a scissors motion to fragment the fecal mass. Work fingers into hardened mass.	Loosening and penetrating mass allows nurse to remove it in small pieces, resulting in less discomfort to patient (Kyle and Prynn, 2004).
11 Work stool downward toward end of rectum. Remove small sections of feces and discard into the bedpan.	Prevents need to force finger up into rectum and minimizes trauma to mucosa.
12 Periodically assess heart rate, and look for signs of fatigue.	Vagal stimulation slows heart rate and causes dysrhythmias. Procedure often exhausts patient.

Critical Decision Point   *Stop procedure if heart rate drops or rhythm changes from the patient's baseline.*

STEP	RATIONALE
13 Continue to clear rectum of feces, and allow patient to rest at intervals.	Rest improves patient's tolerance of procedure, allowing heart rate to return to normal.
14 After removal of impaction, perform perineal hygiene.	Promotes patient's sense of comfort and cleanliness.
15 Remove bedpan, and inspect feces for color and consistency. Dispose of feces. Remove gloves by turning inside out and discarding in proper receptacle.	Reduces transmission of microorganisms.
16 Assist patient to toilet or clean bedpan. (Nurse may follow procedure with enema or cathartic.)	Removal of impaction stimulates defecation reflex.
17 Perform hand hygiene.	Reduces transmission of microorganisms.

EVALUATION

1 Perform rectal examination for stool, and observe anal and perianal area for irritation or skin breakdown	Determines if rectum is clear.
2 Reassess vital signs, and compare to baseline values. Continue to monitor patient for 1 hour for bradycardia.	Determines extent of vagal stimulation.
3 Assess bowel sounds.	Determines presence of peristaltic activity.
4 Palpate abdomen to determine if it is soft and nontender.	Discomfort is relieved.

Unexpected Outcomes	Related Interventions
1 Patient experiences bleeding from rectum.	• Assess anal and perianal region for source of bleeding. • Stop if bleeding is excessive.
2 Changes from baseline vital signs occur.	• Stop procedure, and retake vital signs. • Notify prescriber if vital signs remain altered.
3 Patient experiences autonomic dysreflexia, unique to patients with spinal cord injury. Symptoms include palpitations, sweating, headache, flushing, and severe hypertension.	• Remove impacted stool. • Prevent by instituting an appropriate bowel regimen (Kyle and Prynn, 2004).
4 Diarrhea is present.	• Assess patient for continuing impaction. • Administer suppositories or enemas as ordered. • Increase patient's fluid intake and dietary fiber.

Recording and Reporting

- Record patient's tolerance to procedure, amount and consistency of stool removed, vital signs, and adverse effects.
- Report any changes in vital signs and adverse effects to health care provider.

Teaching Considerations

- If constipation and subsequent impaction are diet related, teach patient about high-fiber nutritional products to increase bulk and the need for adequate fluid intake.
- If necessary, teach family caregivers about the effects of immobility, hydration, and nutrition on normal bowel elimination.

Pediatric Considerations

- Do not digitally remove stool in a pediatric patient because of the risk for anal fissures and pain that trigger stool withholding (Hockenberry and Wilson, 2007).

Gerontological Considerations

- Many older adult patients are especially prone to dysrhythmias and other problems related to vagal stimulation; monitor heart rate and rhythm closely.
- For older adults, instituting a diet adequate in dietary fiber (6 to 10 g per day) adds bulk, weight, and form to stool and improves defecation (Ebersole and others, 2008).
- Consider development of a regular toileting routine that includes responding to the urge to defecate (Meiner and Lueckenotte, 2005).

SKILL 34-3 Administering an Enema

Basic / Elimination Assistance / Administering a Cleansing Enema

An enema is the instillation of a solution into the rectum and sigmoid colon. Enemas promote defecation by stimulating peristalsis. The volume or type of fluid breaks up the fecal mass, stretches the rectal wall, and initiates the defecation reflex.

Typically an enema treats constipation or empties the bowel before diagnostic procedures or certain types of abdominal surgery. Preoperative enemas are common for some surgeries (Schmelzer and others, 2004).

Cleansing enemas promote complete evacuation of feces from the colon. They act by stimulating peristalsis through infusion of large volumes of solution. Oil-retention enemas act by lubricating the rectum and colon. Feces absorb oil and become softer and easier to pass. Medicated enemas contain pharmacological therapeutic agents. Some are prescribed to reduce dangerously high serum potassium levels, as with use of a sodium polystyrene sulfonate (Kayexalate) enema, or to reduce bacteria in the colon before bowel surgery, as with use of a neomycin enema. Types of enemas include the following:

Tap water (hypotonic) enema should not be repeated after first installation because water toxicity or circulatory overload can develop.

Physiological normal saline is safest. Infants and children can tolerate only this type because of their predisposition to fluid imbalance. Mix 500 mL (1 pint) tap water with 1 teaspoon table salt, if preparing solution at home.

Hypertonic solution is useful for patients who cannot tolerate large volumes of fluid. Only 120 to 180 mL (4 to 6 oz) is usually effective (e.g., commercially prepared Fleet enema).

Harris Flush enema is a return flow enema that helps to expel intestinal gas. Fluid alternately flows into and out of the large intestine. This stimulates peristalsis in the large intestine and assists in expelling gas.

Soapsuds enema (SSE) is pure castile soap added to either tap water or normal saline, depending on patient's condition and frequency of administration. Use *only* castile pure soap. Recommended ratio of pure soap to solution is 5 mL (1 teaspoon) to 1000 mL (1 quart) warm water or saline. Add soap to enema bag **after** water is in place to reduce excessive suds.

Oil-retention enema uses an oil-based solution. The colon absorbs a small volume, which allows the oil to soften stool for easier evacuation.

Carminative solution provides relief from gaseous distention. An example is MGW solution, which contains 30 mL of magnesium, 60 mL of glycerin, and 90 mL of water.

Delegation Considerations

The skill of administering an enema can be delegated to NAP unless medication is instilled via an enema. The nurse directs the NAP about:

- The proper way to position patients who have mobility restrictions or therapeutic equipment present.
- Informing the nurse about patient's abdominal pain (*exception:* a patient reports cramping) or rectal bleeding.
- Informing the nurse immediately about the presence of blood in the stool or around the rectal area, any change in patient vital signs, or new symptoms so the nurse can further evaluate the patient.

Equipment

- ❑ Clean gloves
- ❑ Water-soluble lubricant
- ❑ Waterproof, absorbent pads
- ❑ Toilet tissue
- ❑ Bedpan, bedside commode, or access to toilet
- ❑ Basin, washcloths, towel, and soap
- ❑ Intravenous (IV) pole

Enema Bag Administration

- ❑ Clean gloves
- ❑ Enema container (Fig. 34-3)
- ❑ Tubing and clamp (if not already attached to container)
- ❑ Appropriate-size rectal tube (adult: 22 to 30 Fr; child: 12 to 18 Fr)
- ❑ Correct volume of warmed solution (adult: 750 to 1000 mL; adolescent: 500 to 700 mL; school-age child: 300 to 500 mL; toddler: 250 to 350 mL; infant: 150 to 250 mL)

Prepackaged Enema

- ❑ Prepackaged enema container with rectal tip (Fig. 34-4)

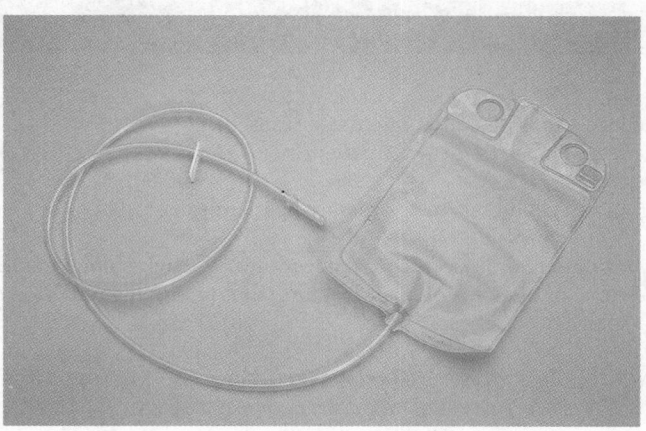

FIG 34-3   High-volume enema bag with tubing.

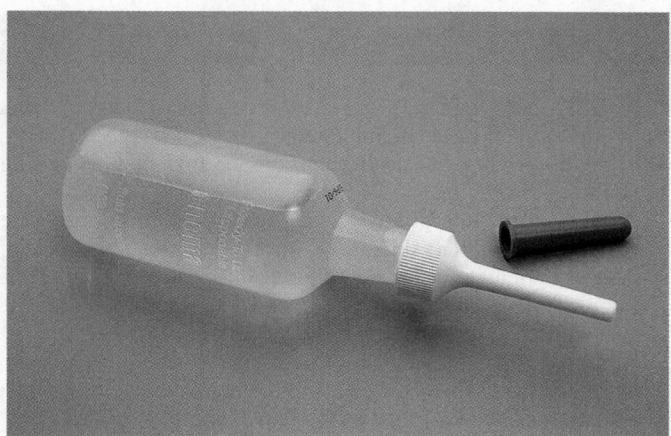

FIG 34-4   Prepackaged enema container with rectal tip.

STEP	RATIONALE

ASSESSMENT

1 Assess status of patient: last bowel movement, normal versus most recent bowel pattern, presence of hemorrhoids, mobility, and presence of abdominal pain.

Determines need for enema and the type of enema used. Also establishes baseline for bowel function.

2 Assess medical record for presence of increased intracranial pressure, cardiac disease, glaucoma, or recent abdominal, rectal, or prostate surgery.

Conditions contraindicate use of enemas.

3 Inspect abdomen for presence of distention and auscultate for bowel sounds.

Establishes baseline for determining effectiveness of enema.

4 Determine patient's level of understanding of purpose of enema.

Allows nurse to plan for appropriate teaching measures.

5 Check patient's medical record to clarify rationale for enema.

Determines purpose of enema administration: preparation for special procedure or relief of constipation.

6 Review order in the medical record for type and how many enemas required.

Order by health care provider is usually required for hospitalized patient.

Critical Decision Point   *"Enemas until clear" order means that you repeat enemas until patient passes fluid that is clear of fecal matter. Check agency policy, but usually patient should receive only three consecutive enemas to avoid disruption of fluid and electrolyte balance.*

NURSING DIAGNOSES

• Acute pain   • Constipation   • Risk for constipation

Individualize related factors based on patient's condition or needs.

PLANNING

1 Expected outcomes following completion of procedure:
   • Stool is evacuated.
   • Enema return is clear.
   • Abdomen is flat, nontender, with no distention.
2 Collect appropriate equipment, and arrange at bedside.
3 Using two identifiers correctly identify patient, and explain procedure.
4 Place prepackaged enema bottle in basin of warm water for patient comfort.

Solution clears rectum and lower colon of stool.
Indicates that all solid fecal material in colon has passed.
Gas and feces are expelled.
Ensures smooth procedure.
Ensures right patient undergoes right treatment. Information promotes patient cooperation and reduces anxiety.
Brings solution to body temperature.

STEP	RATIONALE

IMPLEMENTATION

1 Perform hand hygiene, and apply gloves.	Reduces transmission of microorganisms.
2 Provide privacy by closing curtains around bed or closing door.	Reduces embarrassment for patient.
3 Raise bed to appropriate working height for nurse; raise side rail on patient's left side.	Promotes good body mechanics and patient safety.
4 Assist patient into left side-lying (Sims') position with right knee flexed. You can place a child in dorsal recumbent position.	Allows enema solution to flow downward by gravity along natural curve of sigmoid colon and rectum, thus improving retention of solution.

Critical Decision Point   *If patient has poor sphincter control, position the patient on the bedpan in comfortable dorsal recumbent position. Patients with poor sphincter control cannot retain all of enema solution. Administering enema with patient sitting on toilet is unsafe because curved rectal tubing can abrade rectal wall.*

5 Place waterproof pad under hips and buttocks.	Prevents soiling of linen.
6 Cover patient with bath blanket, exposing only rectal area, clearly visualizing anus.	Provides warmth, reduces exposure of body parts, and allows patient to feel more relaxed and comfortable.
7 Separate buttocks, and examine perianal region for abnormalities, including hemorrhoids, anal fissure, and rectal prolapse.	Findings will influence nurse's approach to insertion of enema tip. Prolapse contraindicates enema.
8 Place bedpan or bedside commode in easily accessible position. If patient will be expelling contents in toilet, ensure that toilet is free. (Place patient's slippers and bathrobe in easily accessible position, if able to ambulate to bathroom.)	In case patient is unable to retain enema solution.
9 Administer enema.	
a Administer prepackaged disposable commercial Fleet enema:	
(1) Remove plastic cap from tip of container. Tip of nozzle is already lubricated, but you can apply more water-soluble jelly as needed.	Lubrication provides for smooth insertion of rectal tube without causing rectal irritation or trauma. With presence of hemorrhoids, extra lubricant is an added comfort.
(2) Gently separate buttocks, and locate rectum. Instruct patient to relax by breathing out slowly through mouth.	Breathing out promotes relaxation of external rectal sphincter.
(3) Expel any air from the enema container.	Introducing air into colon causes further distention and discomfort.
(4) Insert nozzle of container gently into anal canal, and angle nozzle toward the umbilicus (Rushing, 2005) (see illustration). *Adult:* 7.5 to 10 cm (3 to 4 inches) (see illustration) *Adolescent:* 7.5 cm to 10 cm (3 to 4 inches) *Child:* 5 to 7.5 cm (2 to 3 inches) *Infant:* 2.5 to 3.75 cm (1 to 1½ inches)	Gentle insertion prevents trauma to rectal mucosa.

STEP	RATIONALE

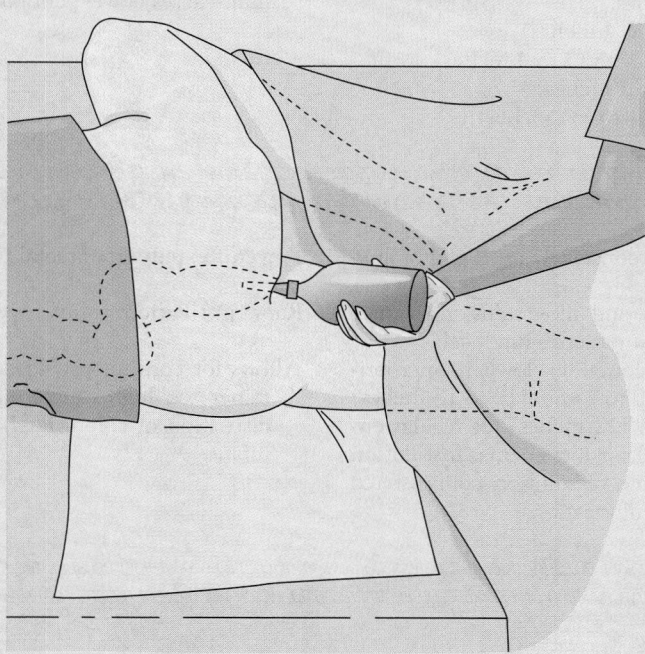

STEP 9a(4)   The tip of the commercial enema is inserted into the rectum. *(From Sorrentino SA:* Mosby's textbook for nursing assistants, *ed 6, St. Louis, 2006, Mosby.)*

Critical Decision Point   *If pain occurs or you feel resistance at any time during procedure, stop and discuss with prescriber.*

(5)   Roll plastic bottle from bottom to tip until all of solution has entered rectum and colon. Instruct patient to retain solution until urge to defecate occurs, usually 2 to 5 minutes.

Prevents instillation of air into colon and ensures all content enters rectum. Hypertonic solutions require only small volumes to stimulate defecation.

b   Administer enema using enema bag:

(1)   Add 750 to 1000 mL of warmed solution to enema bag: warm tap water as it flows from faucet, place saline container in basin of warm water before adding saline to enema bag, and check temperature of solution by pouring small amount of solution over inner wrist.

Hot water will burn intestinal mucosa. Cold water will cause abdominal cramping and is difficult to retain.

(2)   If SSE ordered, add castile soap after water.

Prevents bubbles in bag.

(3)   Raise container, release clamp, and allow solution to flow long enough to fill tubing.

Removes air from tubing.

(4)   Reclamp tubing.

Prevents further loss of solution.

(5)   Lubricate 6 to 8 cm (2½ to 3 inches) of tip of rectal tube with lubricating jelly.

Allows smooth insertion of rectal tube without risk for irritation or trauma to mucosa.

(6)   Gently separate buttocks, and locate anus. Instruct patient to relax by breathing out slowly through mouth. Then, touch patient's skin next to anus with tip of rectal tube.

Breathing out and touching skin with the tube promotes relaxation of external anal sphincter.

STEP	RATIONALE

(7) Insert tip of rectal tube slowly by pointing tip in direction of patient's umbilicus (see illustration). Length of insertion varies:
Adult: 7.5 to 10 cm (3 to 4 inches)
Adolescent: 7.5 cm to 10 cm (3 to 4 inches)
Child: 5 to 7.5 cm (2 to 3 inches)
Infant: 2.5 to 3.75 cm (1 to 1½ inches)

Careful insertion prevents trauma to rectal mucosa from accidental lodging of tube against rectal wall. Insertion beyond proper limit causes bowel perforation.

Critical Decision Point   *If tube does not pass easily, do not force. Consider allowing a small amount of fluid to infuse, and then try to reinsert the tube slowly. The instillation of fluid relaxes the sphincter and provides additional lubrication. Also, remove an impaction (see Skill 34-2) before administering the enema.*

(8) Hold tubing in rectum constantly until end of fluid instillation.

Prevents expulsion of rectal tube during bowel contractions.

(9) Open regulating clamp, and allow solution to enter slowly with container at patient's hip level.

Rapid instillation stimulates evacuation of rectal tube.

(10) Raise height of enema container slowly to appropriate level above anus: 30 to 45 cm (12 to 18 inches) for high enema, 30 cm (12 inches) for regular enema, 7.5 cm (3 inches) for low enema. Instillation time varies with volume of solution administered (e.g., 1 L/10 min) (see illustration).

Allows for continuous, slow instillation of solution; raising container too high causes rapid instillation and possible painful distention of colon. High pressure causes rupture of bowel in infant.

Critical Decision Point   *Lower container or clamp tubing if patient complains of cramping or if fluid escapes around rectal tube. Have patient breathe slowly in through nose and out through mouth. Temporary cessation of instillation prevents cramping, which will prevent patient from retaining all fluid, altering effectiveness of enema. Aids in relaxing and stops abdominal cramps.*

10 Instill all solution, then clamp tubing.

Prevents entrance of air into rectum.

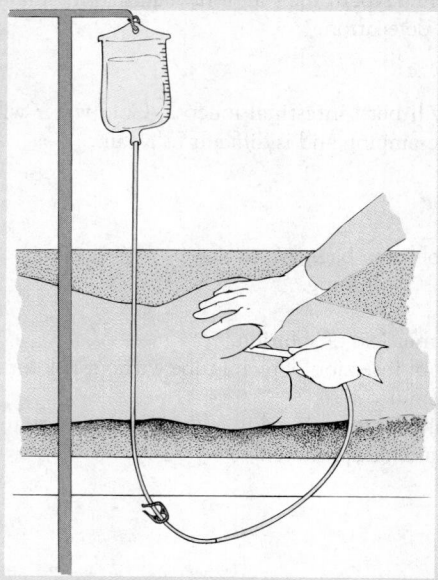

STEP 9b(7)   Insertion of rectal tube into rectum.

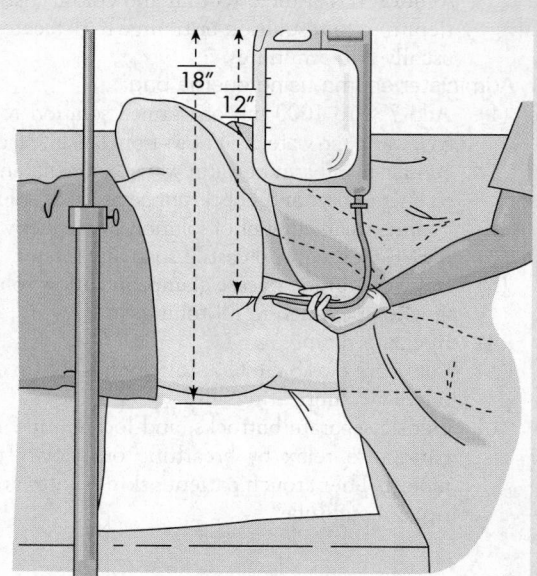

STEP 9b(10)   An enema is given in the Sims' position. The IV pole is positioned so that the enema bag is 12 inches above the anus and approximately 18 inches above the mattress (depending on the patient's size). (*From Sorrentino SA:* Mosby's textbook for nursing assistants, *ed 6, St. Louis, 2006, Mosby.*)

STEP	RATIONALE
11 Place layers of toilet tissue around tube at anus, and gently withdraw rectal tube and tip.	Provides for patient's comfort and cleanliness.
12 Explain to patient that some distention and abdominal cramping is normal. Ask patient to retain solution as long as possible while lying quietly in bed (Schmelzer and others, 2004). (For infant or young child, gently hold buttocks together for few minutes.)	Solution distends bowel. Length of retention varies with type of enema and patient's ability to contract rectal sphincter. Promotion of stimulation of peristalsis and defecation is more effective if retained longer.
13 Discard enema container and tubing in proper receptacle.	Reduces transmission and growth of microorganisms.
14 Assist patient to bathroom, or help to position patient on bedpan.	Normal squatting position promotes defecation.
15 Observe character of feces and solution (caution patient against flushing toilet before inspection).	

Critical Decision Point *When enemas are ordered "until clear," it is essential to observe contents of solution passed. The enema return is "clear" when no solid fecal material exists, but the solution may be yellowish in color.*

STEP	RATIONALE
16 Assist patient as needed with washing anal area with warm soap and water (if nurse administers perineal care, use gloves). If patient is using toilet, caution against flushing before inspection of enema return.	Fecal contents irritate skin. Hygiene promotes patient's comfort.
17 Remove and discard gloves, and perform hand hygiene.	Reduces transmission of microorganisms.

EVALUATION

1 Inspect color, consistency, and amount of stool, odor, and fluid passed.	Determines if stool is evacuated or fluid is retained. Note abnormalities such as presence of blood or mucus.
2 Assess condition of abdomen.	Determines if distention is relieved.

Unexpected Outcomes	Related Interventions
1 Abdomen becomes rigid and distended.	• Stop enema. • Obtain vital signs. • Notify prescriber.
2 Abdominal cramping or pain develops.	• Decrease height of enema bag. Slow rate of instillation. Have patient take slow, deep breaths in through nose and out through mouth.
3 Bleeding occurs.	• Stop the enema. • Notify prescriber. • Obtain vital signs, and assess abdomen and rectum.
4 Retention of enema solution is difficult for patient.	• Give enema slowly to aid in absorption. If patient is full of stool, retention is difficult. As stool is evacuated, there is more room in colon for additional fluid.
5 Patient evacuates fecal material after three large-volume enemas.	• Contact health care professional if order reads "enemas until clear."

Recording and Reporting

• Record type, volume of enema given, time of administration, characteristics of results, and patient's tolerance of the procedure.
• Report failure of patient to defecate and any adverse effects.

Teaching Considerations

• Instruct patient that enemas are not to treat cause of constipation. Instruct in lifestyle changes to encourage peristalsis.
• Instruct the patient in self-administration. Patient needs to lie in dorsal recumbent position with knees and hips flexed toward chest.

Pediatric Considerations

• The use of oral stool softeners is the initial recommended treatment of constipation in children.
• Children and infants usually do not receive prepackaged hypertonic enemas because hypertonic solutions cause rapid fluid shift (Hockenberry and Wilson, 2007).

Gerontological Considerations

• Caution is necessary when enemas are ordered "until clear" in the older adult population. Some older adults become fatigued, are at risk for fluid and electrolyte imbalances, and experience changes in vital signs.
• Instruct older adults and their caregivers in how to modify diet to avoid constipation.
• Some older adults may have difficulty retaining fluid. The nurse may gently hold buttocks together to assist.

Home Care Considerations

• Assess patient's and primary caregiver's ability and motivation to administer enema, and provide instruction as needed.
• Assess patient's ability to manipulate equipment and self-administer enema.
• Assess patient's environment to identify location for administering enema with privacy.

SKILL 34-4   Inserting and Maintaining a Nasogastric Tube for Gastric Decompression

Intermediate / Enteral Nutrition / Inserting a Nasogastric Tube

There are times following major surgery or with conditions affecting the GI tract when normal peristalsis is temporarily altered. Because peristalsis is slowed or absent, a patient cannot eat or drink fluids without causing abdominal distention. The temporary insertion of a nasogastric tube into the stomach serves to decompress the stomach, keeping it empty until normal peristalsis returns (Phillips, 2006).

An NG tube is a pliable tube inserted through the patient's nasopharynx into the stomach. The tube has a hollow lumen that allows the removal of gastric secretions and the introduction of solutions into the stomach. There are times when a nasogastric tube is used for enteral feedings, but a softer small-bore feeding tube is preferred for feeding purposes (see Chapter 31). The Levin and Salem sump tubes are the most common for stomach decompression. The Levin tube is a single lumen tube with holes near the tip (Fig. 34-5). You connect the tube to a drainage bag or an intermittent suction device to drain stomach secretions. The Salem sump tube is preferable for stomach decompression (Phillips, 2006). The tube has two lumina: one for removal of gastric contents and one to provide an air vent, which prevents suctioning of gastric mucosa into eyelets at the distal tip of a tube. A blue "pigtail" is the air vent that connects with the second lumen (Fig. 34-6). When the sump tube's main lumen is connected to suction, the air vent permits free, continuous drainage of secretions. **Never clamp off the air vent, connect to suction, or use for irrigation.** The heath care provider will order the suction setting, which is usually low intermittent.

Nasogastric tube insertion does not require sterile technique. Clean technique is adequate. The procedure is uncomfortable, with patients experiencing a burning sensation as the tube passes through the sensitive nasal mucosa. One of the greatest nursing care challenges is keeping the patient comfortable because the tube is a constant irritation to mucosa. Routinely assess the condition of the nares and mucosa for inflammation and excoriation. Supportive care includes changing soiled tape or fixation devices when they become soiled, keeping the nares lubricated and clean, and providing frequent mouth care to minimize the dehydration from mouth breathing.

Delegation Considerations

The skill of inserting and maintaining an NG tube cannot be delegated to NAP. Instead, the nurse directs the NAP to:
- Measure and record the drainage from an NG tube.
- Provide oral and nasal hygiene measures.
- Perform selected comfort measures, such as positioning, offering ice chips if allowed.
- Anchor the tube to the patient's gown during routine care to prevent accidental displacement.

Equipment
- ❑ 14 or 16 Fr NG tube (smaller-lumen catheters are not used for decompression in adults because they must be able to remove thick secretions)
- ❑ Water-soluble lubricating jelly
- ❑ pH test strips (measure gastric aspirate acidity)
- ❑ Tongue blade
- ❑ Flashlight
- ❑ Emesis basin
- ❑ Asepto bulb or catheter-tipped syringe
- ❑ 1-inch (2.5-cm) wide hypoallergenic tape or commercial fixation device
- ❑ Safety pin and rubber band
- ❑ Clamp, drainage bag, or suction machine with pressure gauge if wall suction is to be used
- ❑ Towel
- ❑ Glass of water with straw
- ❑ Facial tissues
- ❑ Normal saline
- ❑ Tincture of benzoin (*optional*)
- ❑ Suction equipment
- ❑ Clean gloves

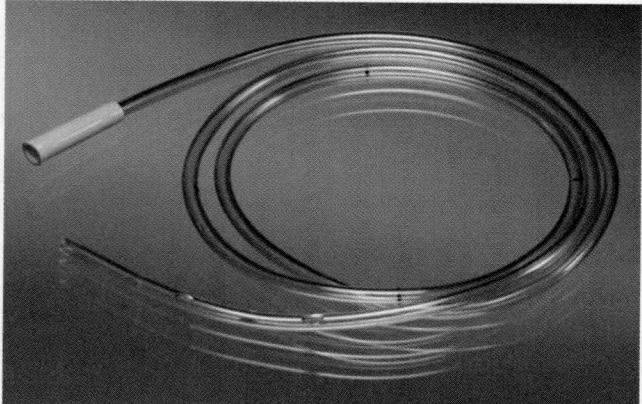

FIG 34-5   Levin tube. (*Courtesy Bard Medical, Covington, Ga.*)

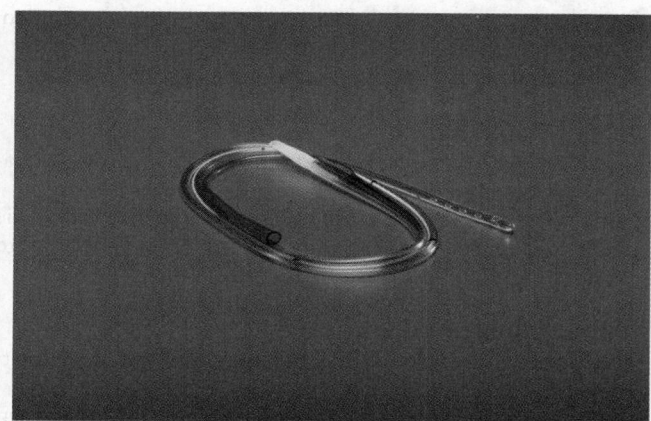

FIG 34-6   Salem sump tube. (*Courtesy Covidien, Mansfield, Mass.*)

STEP	RATIONALE

ASSESSMENT

1. Perform hand hygiene. Inspect condition of patient's nasal and oral cavity.

   Prevents transmission of infection. Determines need for special nursing hygiene measures after tube placement.

2. Ask if patient has had history of nasal surgery or congestion and allergies, and note if deviated nasal septum is present.

   *Alerts nurse to potential obstruction. Insert tube into **uninvolved** nasal passage. Procedure may be contraindicated if surgery is recent.*

3. Auscultate for bowel sounds. Palpate patient's abdomen for distention, pain, and rigidity.

   Decreased bowel sounds occur with peritonitis and paralytic ileus. In presence of diminished or absent bowel sounds, auscultate abdomen at least 1 minute in each quadrant, making sure that no sounds are missed (Seidel and others, 2006). Documents baseline for any abdominal distention and GI function, which later serves as comparison once tube is inserted.

4. Assess patient's level of consciousness and ability to follow instructions.

   Determines patient's ability to assist in procedure.

Critical Decision Point   *If patient is confused, disoriented, or unable to follow commands, obtain assistance from another staff member to insert the tube.*

5. Determine if patient had previous NG tube and which naris was used.

   Patient's previous experience will complement any explanations and prepares patient for NG tube placement.

6. Verify order for type of NG tube to be placed and whether tube is to be attached to suction or drainage bag.

   Requires an order from health care provider. Adequate decompression depends on NG suction.

NURSING DIAGNOSES

- Acute pain
- Deficient knowledge regarding purpose of gastric decompression
- Impaired oral mucous membrane
- Risk for impaired skin integrity

Individualize related factors based on patient's condition or needs.

PLANNING

1. Expected outcomes following completion of procedure:
   - Stomach will remain soft, nontender, and without distention.

     Correctly positioned NG tube remains patent, drains gastric secretions, and relieves gastric distention.
   - Patient's nares and surface of nose remain clear, without abrasions or excoriation.

     Ensures absence of irritation from NG tube.
   - Patient's nasal mucosa will remain moist and intact.

     Reduces risk for erosion developing.

2. Prepare equipment at the bedside. Have a 4-inch (10-cm) piece of tape ready with one end split in half or have NG tube fixation device available.

   Ensures well-organized procedure. Apply tape to hold tube in place after insertion.

3. Identify patient using two identifiers, and explain procedure. Inform patient there will be a burning sensation in nasopharynx as tube is passed. Develop hand signal with patient.

   Increases patient's cooperation and ability to anticipate nurse's action. If patient is unable to tolerate procedure, use of hand signal will alert nurse.

IMPLEMENTATION

1. Perform hand hygiene, and apply clean gloves.

   Reduces transmission of microorganisms.

2. Place patient in high-Fowler's position. Place pillows behind head and shoulders. Raise bed to horizontal level comfortable for nurse.

   Promotes patient's ability to swallow during procedure. Good body mechanics prevents injury to nurse or patient.

3. Place bath towel over patient's chest; give facial tissues to patient. Allow to blow nose if necessary. Place emesis basin within reach.

   Prevents soiling of patient's gown. Tube insertion through nasal passages may cause tearing and coughing with increased salivation.

4. Pull curtain around the bed, or close room door.

   Provides privacy.

5. Wash bridge of nose with soap and water or alcohol swab.

   Removes oils from nose to allow tape to adhere.

6. Stand on patient's right side if right-handed, left side if left-handed.

   Allows easiest manipulation of tubing.

7. Instruct patient to relax and breathe normally while occluding one naris. Then repeat this action for other naris. Select nostril with greater airflow.

   Tube passes more easily through naris that is more patent.

STEP	RATIONALE

8 Measure distance to insert tube:
  a *Traditional method:* Measure distance from tip of nose, to earlobe, then to xiphoid process (see illustration).
  b *Hanson method:* First mark 50-cm point on tube, and then do traditional measurement. Tube insertion should be to midway point between 50 cm (20 inches) and traditional mark.
	Approximates distance from naris to stomach; distance varies with each patient. Tube tip should enter stomach.

9 With a small piece of tape placed around tube, mark length you will insert.	Indicates length of tube you will insert.
10 Curve 10 to 15 cm (4 to 6 inches) of end of tube tightly around index finger, then release.	Aids insertion and decreases stiffness of tube.
11 Lubricate 7.5 to 10 cm (3 to 4 inches) of end of tube with water-soluble lubricating gel.	Minimizes friction against nasal mucosa and aids insertion of tube. Water-soluble lubricant is less toxic than oil-soluble lubricant if aspirated.
12 Alert patient when procedure will begin.	Decreases patient anxiety and increases patient cooperation.
13 Initially instruct patient to extend neck back against pillow; insert tube gently and slowly through naris with curved end pointing downward.	Facilitates initial passage of tube through naris and maintains clear airway for open naris.
14 Continue to pass tube along floor of nasal passage, aiming down toward patient's ear. If you feel resistance, apply gentle downward pressure to advance tube (do not force past resistance).	Minimizes discomfort of tube rubbing against upper nasal turbinates. Resistance caused by posterior nasopharynx. Downward pressure helps tube curl around corner of nasopharynx.
15 If you meet continued resistance, try to rotate the tube, and see if it advances. If still resistant, withdraw tube, allow patient to rest, lubricate tube again, and insert into other naris.	Forcing against resistance causes trauma to mucosa. Allowing patient to rest helps relieve anxiety.

Critical Decision Point   *If unable to insert tube in either naris, stop procedure and notify prescriber.*

STEP	RATIONALE

16 Continue insertion of tube until just past nasopharynx by gently rotating tube toward opposite naris.
  a Once past nasopharynx, stop tube advancement, allow patient to relax, and provide tissues.
 	
  b Explain to patient that next step requires that patient swallow. Give patient glass of water unless contraindicated.
	
	Relieves patient's anxiety; tearing is natural response to mucosal irritation, and excessive salivation may occur because of oral stimulation.
	Sipping water aids passage of NG tube into esophagus.

17 With tube just above oropharynx, instruct patient to flex head forward, take a small sip of water, and swallow. Advance tube 2.5 to 5 cm (1 to 2 inches) with each swallow of water. If patient is not allowed fluids, instruct to dry swallow or suck air through straw. Advance tube with each swallow.	Flexed position closes off upper airway to trachea and opens esophagus. Swallowing closes epiglottis over trachea and helps move tube into esophagus. Swallowing water reduces gagging or choking. Remove water from stomach by suction after insertion.

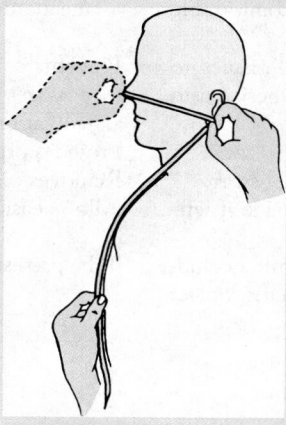

STEP 8a Technique for measuring distance to insert NG tube.

STEP	RATIONALE
18 If patient begins to cough, gag, or choke, withdraw tube slightly and stop advancement. Instruct patient to breathe easily and take sips of water.	Cough reflex is initiated when tube accidentally enters larynx. Withdrawal of the tube reduces risk for laryngeal entry. Small sips of water frequently reduce gagging. Give water cautiously to reduce the risk for aspiration.

Critical Decision Point   *If vomiting occurs, assist patient in clearing airway. Perform oral suctioning as needed.*

STEP	RATIONALE
19 If patient continues to cough during insertion, pull tube back slightly.	Tube may enter larynx and obstruct airway.
20 If patient continues to gag and cough or complains tube feels as though it is coiling behind throat, check back of oropharynx using flashlight and tongue blade. Withdraw the tube until tip is back in oropharynx, if coiled. Then reinsert with patient swallowing.	Tube may coil around itself in the back of the throat and stimulate gag reflex.
21 After patient relaxes, continue to advance tube with swallowing until you reach tape or mark on tube that signifies the tube is in the desired distance. Temporarily anchor tube to patient's cheek with piece of tape until tube placement is verified.	Tip of tube needs to be within stomach to decompress properly. Anchoring of tube prevents accidental displacement while tube placement is verified.
22 Verify tube placement (check agency policy for preferred methods for checking tube placement):	
a Ask patient to talk.	Patient is unable to talk if NG tube has passed through vocal cords.
b Inspect posterior pharynx for presence of coiled tube.	Tube is pliable and will coil up behind the pharynx instead of advancing into esophagus.
c Attach Asepto or catheter-tipped syringe to end of tube. Aspirate gently back on syringe to obtain gastric contents, observing color (see illustration).	Gastric contents are usually cloudy and green, but are sometimes off-white, tan, bloody, or brown. Aspiration of contents provides means to measure fluid pH and thus determine tube tip placement in GI tract.
	If the tube is improperly placed or migrates to other regions, the aspirate colors change. For example, yellow or bile-stained aspirates often indicate duodenal placement, or if the tube is in the esophagus, saliva-appearing aspirate may or may not be present.
d Measure aspirate for pH with color-coded pH paper. This ranges from 1 to 11 (see illustration).	Gastric aspirates have decidedly acidic pH values, typically 4 or less, compared with intestinal aspirates, which are usually greater than 4, or respiratory secretions, which are usually greater than 5.5 (Metheny and others, 2005).

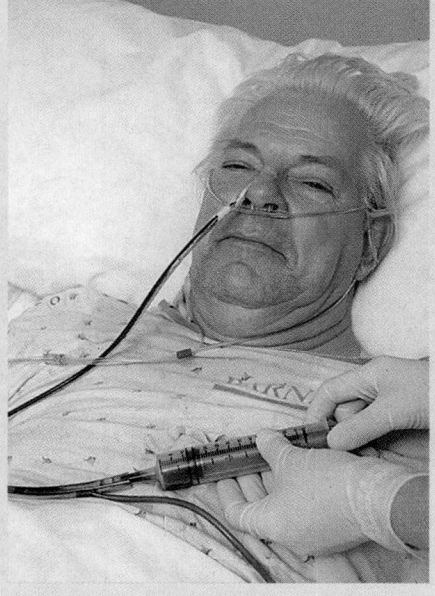

STEP 22c   Aspiration of gastric contents.

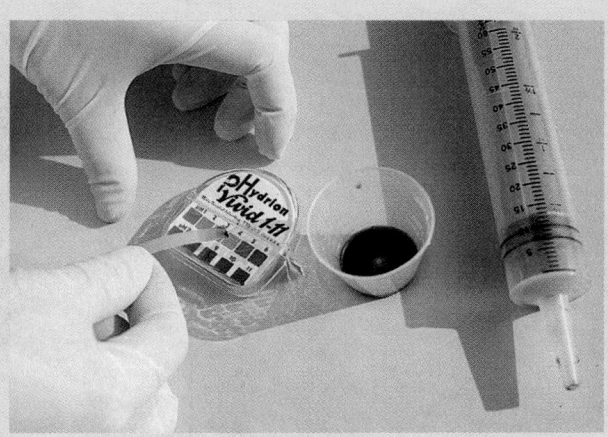

STEP 22d   Checking pH of gastric aspirate.

STEP	RATIONALE

e Have ordered x-ray examination performed of chest/ abdomen.

f If tube is not in stomach, advance another 2.5 to 5 cm (1 to 2 inches), and repeat Steps 22a to 22d to check tube position.

23 Anchor tube:

a Clamp end of tube, or connect tube to drainage bag or suction machine, after properly inserted.

b Tape tube to nose; avoid putting pressure on nares.
(1) Apply small amount of tincture of benzoin to lower end of nose, and allow drying before taping tube to nose *(optional)*. Apply prepared tape to nose, leaving split end free. Be sure top end of tape over nose is secure.
(2) Carefully wrap two split ends of tape around tube.
(3) *Alternative:* Apply tube fixation device using shaped adhesive patch (see illustration).

c Fasten end of NG tube to patient's gown by looping rubber band around tube in slipknot. Pin rubber band to gown.

d When using a Salem sump tube, keep pigtail above level of stomach.

e Unless prescriber orders otherwise, elevate head of bed 30 degrees.

f Explain to patient that sensation of tube decreases somewhat with time.

g Remove and discard gloves, and perform hand hygiene.

24 Once placement has been confirmed:

a Keep either red mark or tape on tube to indicate where tube exits nose.

b *Alternative:* Measure length of tube from nares to connector.

c Document length of tube in patient's record.

X-ray film is best verification of initial placement of the tube (Metheny and Titler, 2001).

Tube must be in stomach to provide decompression.

Use gravity for drainage bag. Intermittent suction is most effective for decompression. Patient going to operating room often has tube clamped.

Prevents tissue necrosis. Tape anchors tube securely.

Benzoin prevents loosening of tape if patient perspires or has oily skin.

Reduces pressure on nares if tube moves. Provides slack for movement without dislodging the NG tube.

Prevents siphoning action that clogs the tube.

Helps prevent esophageal reflux and minimizes irritation of tube against posterior pharynx.

Helps patient to adapt to continued sensory stimulus.

Reduces transmission of microorganisms.

The mark on tube or tape is guide to indicate continuous correct tube placement (Sanko, 2004).

Information assists in determining tube placement.

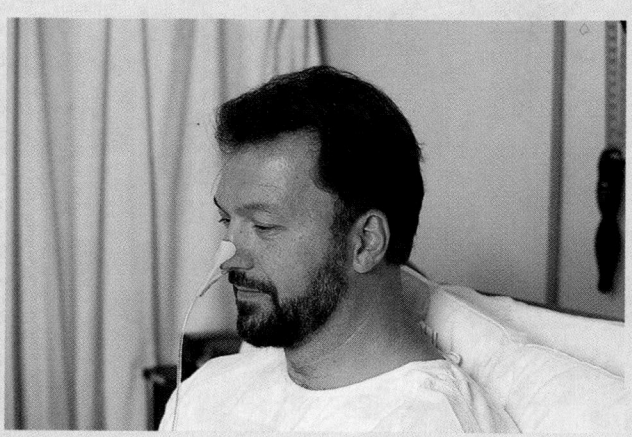

STEP 23b(3)   Patient with tube fixation device.

STEP	RATIONALE
25 Attach NG tube to suction as ordered.	Suction setting is usually ordered low intermittent, which decreases gastric irritation from NG tube.

Critical Decision Point *If lumen of tube is narrow and secretions are thick, NG tube will not drain as desired. Irrigate tube (Step 26). Consult with prescriber for higher suction setting if unable to irrigate tube due to thick secretions.*

STEP	RATIONALE
26 Irrigate tube:	
a Perform hand hygiene, and apply gloves.	Reduces transmission of microorganisms.
b Check for tube placement in stomach (see Step 22). Reconnect NG tube to connecting tube.	Prevents accidental entrance of irrigating solution into lungs.
c Draw up 30 mL of normal saline into Asepto or catheter-tip syringe.	Use of saline minimizes loss of electrolytes from stomach fluids.
d Clamp NG tube. Disconnect from connecting tubing, and lay end of connection tubing on towel.	Reduces soiling of patient's gown and bed linen.
e Insert tip of irrigating syringe into end of NG tube. Remove clamp. Hold syringe with tip pointed at floor, and inject saline slowly and evenly. Do not force solution.	Position of syringe prevents introduction of air into vent tubing, which causes gastric distention. Solution introduced under pressure causes gastric trauma.

Critical Decision Point *Do not introduce saline through blue pigtail air vent of Salem sump tube; it will clog the tube.*

STEP	RATIONALE
f If resistance occurs, check for kinks in tubing. Turn patient onto left side. Repeated resistance should be reported to health care provider.	Tip of tube may lie against stomach lining. Repositioning on left side may dislodge tube away from the stomach lining. Buildup of secretions will cause distention.
g After instilling saline, immediately aspirate, or pull back slowly on syringe to withdraw fluid. If amount aspirated is greater than amount instilled, record difference as output. If amount aspirated is less than amount instilled, record difference as intake.	Irrigation clears tubing, so stomach should remain empty. Measure and document irrigation inserted in tube as intake.
h Use an Asepto syringe to place 10 mL air into blue pigtail.	Ensures patency of air vent.
i Reconnect NG tube to drainage or suction. (Repeat irrigation if solution does not return.)	Reestablishes drainage collection; may repeat irrigation or repositioning of tube until NG tube drains properly.
j Remove and discard gloves, and perform hand hygiene.	Reduces transmission of microorganisms.
27 Discontinue NG tube:	
a Verify order to discontinue NG tube.	An order is required for procedure.
b Explain procedure to patient, and reassure that removal is less distressing than insertion.	Minimizes anxiety and increases cooperation. Tube passes out smoothly.
c Perform hand hygiene, and apply clean gloves.	Reduces transmission of microorganisms.
d Turn off suction, and disconnect NG tube from drainage bag or suction. Insert 20 mL of air into lumen of NG tube. Remove tape or fixation device from bridge of nose, and unpin tube from gown.	Have tube free of connections before removal. Clears gastric fluids from tube to prevent aspiration of contents or soiling of clothing and bedding.
e Stand on patient's right side if right-handed, left side if left-handed.	Allows easiest manipulation of tube.
f Hand patient facial tissue; place clean towel across chest. Instruct patient to take and hold breath.	Some patients wish to blow nose after tube is removed. Towel keeps gown from soiling. Temporary airway obstruction occurs during tube removal.
g Clamp or kink tubing securely, and then pull tube out steadily and smoothly into towel held in other hand while patient holds breath.	Clamping prevents tube contents from draining into oropharynx. Reduces trauma to mucosa and minimizes patient's discomfort. Towel covers tube, which is an unpleasant sight. Holding breath helps to prevent aspiration.
h Inspect intactness of tube.	
i Measure amount of drainage, and note character of content. Dispose of tube and drainage equipment into proper container.	Provide accurate measure of fluid output. Reduces transfer of microorganisms.
j Clean nares, and provide mouth care.	Promotes comfort.

STEP	RATIONALE
k Position patient comfortably, and explain procedure for drinking fluids, if not contraindicated. Instruct patient to notify you if nausea occurs.	Depends on the health care provider's order. Sometimes patients are not allowed anything by mouth (NPO) for up to 24 hours. When fluids are allowed, orders usually begin with small amount of ice chips each hour and increases as patient is able to tolerate more.
28 Clean equipment, and return to proper place. Place soiled linen in utility room or proper receptacle.	Proper disposal of equipment prevents spread of microorganisms and ensures proper exchange procedures.
29 Remove and discard gloves, and perform hand hygiene.	Reduces transmission of microorganisms.

EVALUATION

1 Observe amount and character of contents draining from NG tube. Ask if patient feels nauseated.	Determines if tube is decompressing stomach of contents.
2 Auscultate for presence of bowel sounds. Turn off suction while auscultating.	The sound of the suction apparatus is sometimes misinterpreted as bowel sounds.
3 Palpate patient's abdomen periodically. Note any distention, pain, and rigidity.	Determines success of abdominal decompression and the return of peristalsis.
4 Inspect condition of nares and nose.	Evaluates onset of skin and tissue irritation.
5 Observe position of tubing.	Prevents tension applied to nasal structures.
6 Ask if patient feels sore throat or irritation in pharynx.	Evaluates level of patient's discomfort.

Unexpected Outcomes	Related Interventions
1 Patient's abdomen is distended and painful.	• Assess patency of tube. NG tube may not be in stomach. • Irrigate tube. • Verify that suction is on as ordered.
2 Patient complains of sore throat from dry, irritated mucous membranes.	• Perform oral hygiene more frequently. • Ask prescriber whether patient can suck on ice chips, throat lozenges, or numbing medication.
3 Patient develops irritation or erosion of skin around naris.	• Provide frequent skin care to area. • Tape tube on naris to avoid pressure. • Consider switching tube to other naris.
4 Patient develops signs and symptoms of pulmonary aspiration: fever, shortness of breath, or pulmonary congestion.	• Perform complete respiratory assessment. • Notify prescriber. • Obtain chest x-ray examination as ordered.

Recording and Reporting

- Record length, size, and type of gastric tube inserted and through which nostril you inserted it. Also, record patient's tolerance of procedure, confirmation of tube placement, character of gastric contents, pH value, whether the tube is clamped or connected to drainage bag or to suction, and the amount of suction supplied.
- Record difference between amount of normal saline instilled and amount of gastric aspirate removed on I&O sheet. Record the amount and character of contents draining from NG tube every shift in nurses' notes or flow sheet.

- Record removal of tube "intact," the patient's tolerance of procedure, and final amount and character of drainage.

Gerontological Considerations

- Check for ill-fitting dentures, and remove them for the patient's safety and comfort during the insertion.
- Oral and nasal mucosal drying is sometimes present. Adequately lubricate the tube for insertion.

CRITICAL THINKING EXERCISES

Mr. Simon is a 66-year-old man with a history of severe osteoarthritis who is hospitalized following a total right knee replacement performed 2 days ago. At present he is allowed touch-down weight bearing on his right leg. Mr. Simon's last bowel movement was the day before surgery, so he has gone 3 days without a bowel movement. Since surgery, he received pain medication through his IV and began taking oral pain medication last night.

His abdomen is nontender, slightly distended, with active bowel sounds in all four quadrants. He attempted a bowel movement with a great deal of straining and expelled small, hard, brown stool. You have talked to the primary care provider and obtained orders for a Fleet enema.

1 You have explained the enema procedure to Mr. Simon and have prepared your supplies. You need to provide a bedpan or commode for Mr. Simon to expel the fecal material following the enema. Please make your selection of the type of bedpan or use of commode, and provide the rationale.
2 Mr. Simon is ordered to receive a Fleet enema. What is the expected outcome of Mr. Simon's enema? What, if any, instructions will you give to the NAP?
3 The NAP just reported to you that Mr. Simon is complaining of stomach pain. From the following, select and prioritize the correct actions:
  A Notify the health care provider.
  B Instruct the NAP to palpate Mr. Simon's abdomen.
  C Give postoperative pain medication as ordered.
  D Perform an abdominal assessment.
  E Obtain vital signs, and instruct the NAP to obtain vital signs every 15 to 30 minutes thereafter.
4. Two days later Mr. Simon had the same symptoms as before receiving the enema. This time he has liquid stool seeping from the rectum. You obtain an order to check for an impaction. You explain the procedure to Mr. Simon and begin the skill as required. As you are removing stool, the NAP who is helping you by monitoring Mr. Simon's vital signs reports that his pulse is 48 beats per minute. How do you proceed?

 REVIEW QUESTIONS

1 One risk associated with digital removal of impacted stool is stimulation of the vagus nerve. For what adverse effect should the nurse monitor the patient?
  1 Urinary incontinence
  2 An elevated pulse rate
  3 Abdominal cramping
  4 A drop in the heart rate
2 During insertion of a nasogastric tube, the nurse has the patient flex head forward at a specific time. What is the rationale for having the patient assume this position?
  1 It closes off the epiglottis so tube enters esophagus.
  2 It facilitates the tube passing through the nasal passages.
  3 It prevents stimulation of the gag reflex.
  4 It gives the patient something to do during the procedure.
3 The nurse is placing a bedpan under a frail, underweight female patient. The nurse's actions are appropriate if what method is followed?

  1 Slide the bedpan under the patient.
  2 Roll the patient onto a fracture bedpan.
  3 Shove the bedpan under the patient.
  4 Keep the patient flat after rolling her on the bedpan.
4 A patient has an order for enemas "until clear" in preparation for bowel surgery. What information in the patient's medical record would cause the nurse to question the physician's order?
  1 Hemorrhoid surgery 5 years ago
  2 Periodic fecal incontinence
  3 Taking medication for an enlarged prostate
  4 A history of glaucoma
5 A patient has a nasogastric tube for gastric decompression after intestinal surgery yesterday. The patient is nauseated, and his abdomen is distended. The nurse irrigated the tube without any resistance. What action should the nurse now take?
  1 Irrigate the tube again with more normal saline.
  2 Place the patient in high-Fowler's.
  3 Advance the nasogastric tube several inches.
  4 Turn the suction on continuous instead of intermittent.

REFERENCES

Centers for Disease Control and Prevention: Severe *Clostridium difficile*-associated disease in populations previously at low risk—four states, *MMWR Morb Mortal Wkly Rep* 54(47):1201, 2005.
Ebersole P and others: *Toward healthy aging: human needs and nursing response*, ed 7, St. Louis, 2008, Mosby.
Fletcher K: Elimination: geriatric self-learning module, *Medsurg Nurs* 14(2):127, 2005.
Hockenberry MJ, Wilson D: *Wong's nursing care of infants and children*, ed 8, St. Louis, 2007, Mosby.
Lawrence P, Rozmus C: Culturally sensitive care of the Muslim patient, *J Transcult Nurs* 12(3):228, 2001.
Lehne RA: *Pharmacology for nursing care*, ed 6, St. Louis, 2007, Mosby.
McKinney L and others: *Mosby's pharmacology in nursing*, ed 22, St. Louis, 2006, Mosby.
Meiner S, Lueckenotte AG: *Gerontologic nursing*, ed 3, St. Louis, 2005, Mosby.
Rushing J: Administering an enema to an adult, *Nursing* 33(11):28, 2005.
Seidel HM and others: *Mosby's guide to physical examination*, ed 6, St. Louis, 2006, Mosby.
Sorrentino SA: *Mosby's textbook for nursing assistants*, ed 6, St. Louis, 2006, Mosby.
Stanley M and others: *Gerontological nursing: promoting successful aging with older adults*, ed 7, Philadelphia, 2005, FA Davis.
Todd B: *Clostridium difficile*: familiar pathogen, changing epidemiology, *Am J Nurs* 106(5):33, 2006.
Wilson L: Understanding bowel problems in older people, part I, *Nurs Older People* 17(8):19, 2005, Part I.
Wilson L: Understanding bowel problems in older people, part II, *Nurs Older People* 17(9):15, 2005, Part II.

RESEARCH REFERENCES

Benoit R, Watts C: The effect of a pressure ulcer prevention program and the bowel management system in reducing pressure ulcer prevalence in an ICU setting, *J Wound Ostomy Continence Nurs* 34(2):163, 2007.
Bosshard W and others: The treatment of chronic constipation in elderly people—an update, *Drugs Aging* 21(14):911, 2004.
Kyle G, Prynn P: An evidence-based procedure for the digital removal of faeces, *Nurs Times* 100(48):71, 2004.
Metheny NA, Titler MG: Assessing placement of feeding tubes, *Am J Nurs* 101(5):36, 2001.
Metheny N and others: Effect of feeding tube properties on residual volume measurements in tube-fed patients, *J Parenter Enteral Nutr* 29(3):192, 2005.
Phillips N: Nasogastric tubes: an historical context, *Medsurg Nurs* 15(2):84, 2005.
Sanko J: Aspiration assessment and prevention in critically ill enterally fed patients: evidence-based recommendations for practice, *Gastroenterol Nurs* 27(6):279, 2004.
Schmelzer M and others: Safety and effectiveness of large-volume enema solutions, *Appl Nurs Res* 17(4):265, 2004.

Ostomy Care

MEDIA RESOURCES

- **evolve** http://evolve.elsevier.com/Perry/skills
  learning system
  - Review Questions
  - Video Clips

- [View Video!] Mosby's Nursing Video Skills, 3.0

- [NSO] Nursing Skills Online

OBJECTIVES

Mastery of content in this chapter will enable the nurse to:
- Identify types of fecal and urinary diversions.
- Explain differences in color and consistency of effluent based on the type of ostomy.
- Pouch a fecal or urinary diversion.
- Describe methods used to maintain integrity of the peristomal skin.
- Catheterize a urinary diversion.

Certain diseases or conditions require surgical intervention to create an opening into the abdominal wall for fecal or urinary elimination. Examples of these conditions include cancer, inflammatory bowel disease, infections such as diverticulitis that lead to perforation in the colon, neurological disease, or trauma. The opening is called a stoma and is constructed from a section of colon or small intestine. The output from the stoma is called the effluent. An opening in the large intestine or colon is a colostomy (Fig. 35-1), and the fecal effluent will vary in consistency depending on where the opening in the colon is surgically created. A colostomy in the descending or sigmoid colon generally results in a stool similar to that normally passed through the rectum. If the opening is in the transverse or ascending colon, the effluent will vary from thick liquid to semiformed stool. An opening in the ileal portion of the small intestine is an ileostomy (Fig. 35-2), and the fecal effluent will be watery to thick liquid and contain some digestive enzymes.

Fecal ostomies are either temporary or permanent, depending on the underlying condition and the surgical procedure performed. A urostomy or ileal conduit (Fig. 35-3) is created from a 6- to 8-inch portion of the intestine that is resected from the ileum. One end of the conduit is sutured closed, and the ureters are implanted through the mucosa. The other end is brought out on the abdominal wall, and a stoma is formed for urine to exit the body. This ostomy is permanent. The patient with a colostomy, ileostomy, or ileal conduit has no sensation or control over the time or frequency of the output and must wear a pouch to collect the effluent.

Surgical procedures to create continent internal fecal or urinary pouches have evolved over the last 25 years. These procedures eliminate the need for an external pouch. The continent ileostomy is a pouch made from a segment of the ileum and placed under the abdominal wall. The surgeon brings a narrow section of the ileum out on the abdominal wall to form a small flat stoma. At the open-

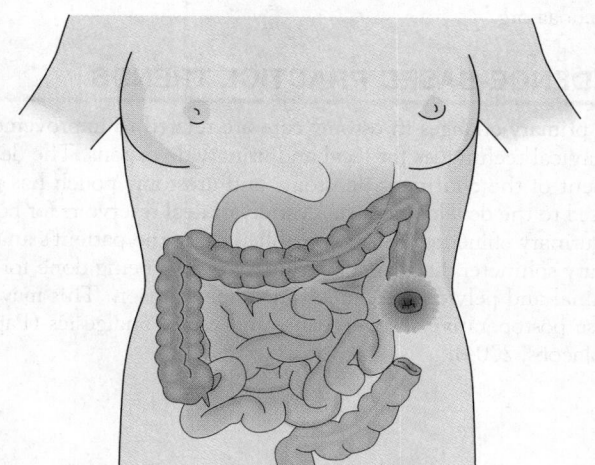

FIG 35-1   Sigmoid colostomy.

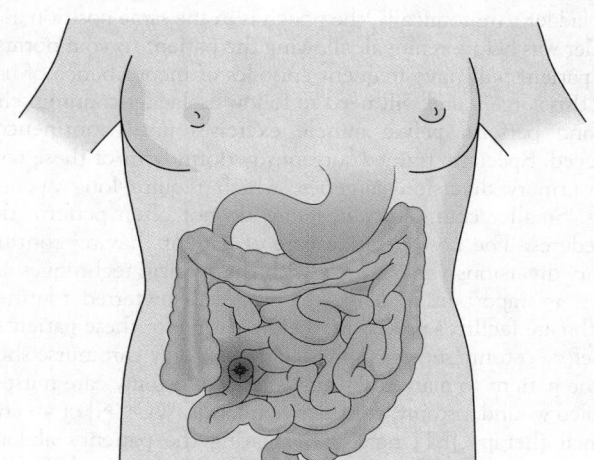

FIG 35-2   Ileostomy.

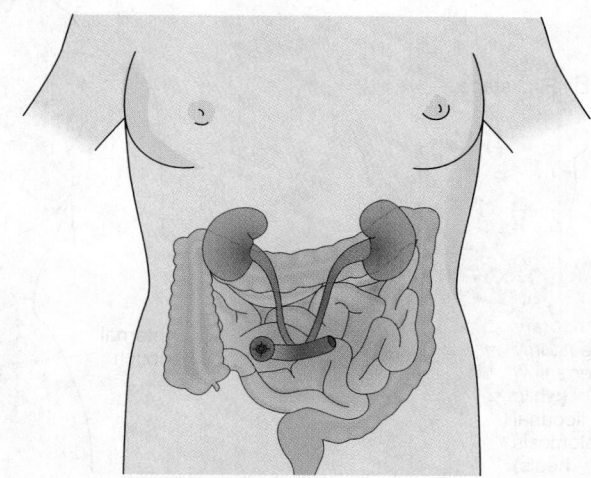

FIG 35-3   Urostomy (ileal conduit).

ing of the pouch, a one-way valve is surgically created. The patient inserts a large catheter through the stoma, and this catheter slips through the one-way valve and into the internal pouch. This allows for emptying of the pouch at regular intervals during the day. Only a few centers in the United States and Canada are still doing this procedure, because there are other surgical options available with higher long-term success rates. In the ileal pouch anal anastomosis the surgeon creates a **J**- or **S**-shaped internal reservoir from a segment of the ileum that is then connected to the anal canal just above the anal sphincter (Fig. 35-4). The patient will have four to six bowel movements per day. Most frequently the surgeon will perform a temporary ileostomy that will allow the fecal effluent to be diverted from the reservoir until it completely heals in about 3 months.

There are two types of continent urinary diversions. One is a continent urinary reservoir (Fig. 35-5) created from a distal portion of the ileum and proximal portion of the colon. The ureters are imbedded in the reservoir. This reservoir is situated under the abdominal wall and has a narrow ileal segment brought out through the abdominal wall to form a small stoma. The ileocecal valve creates a one-way valve in the pouch through which a catheter is inserted to empty the urine from the pouch. Patients must be able and willing to catheterize the pouch 4 to 6 times a day for the rest of their lives. The other type of continent urinary diversion is an orthotopic neobladder, which also uses an ileal pouch to replace the bladder. Anatomically, the pouch is in the same position as the bladder was before removal, allowing the patient to void normally. The patient will have frequent episodes of incontinence of urine after this surgery and will need to follow a bladder-training schedule and perform pelvic muscle exercises until continence is achieved. Specially trained surgeons perform both of these continent urinary diversion surgeries, which require long operating times. Smaller community hospitals do not often perform these procedures. The postoperative care of patients having continent urinary diversions varies widely with the surgical techniques used, and it is important to learn the surgeon's preferred routine or health care facility's procedures before caring for these patients.

Before ostomy surgery a physician or ostomy care nurse should see the patient to mark the stoma site. (An ostomy care nurse is a certified wound, ostomy, continence nurse [CWOCN] or an enterostomal therapy [ET] nurse.) Evaluating the patient's abdomen while the patient is lying, sitting, and standing allows the nurse and the patient to find an optimal location so that the new stoma is easy to pouch and maintain (ASCRS and WOCN, 2007).

With any ostomy requiring a pouching system, a secure seal to prevent leakage of the effluent and protect the skin around the stoma (peristomal skin) is vital to assisting the patient in resuming normal activities and accepting the changes in their bodies as a result of the surgery. In addition to the stress of illness and surgical recovery, patients with ostomies face body image changes, fear of social rejection, concern about sexual function and intimacy, and the need for help with personal care. It is very important to provide an effective pouching system to facilitate the emotional adjustment to the ostomy (Colwell and others, 2004). Do not act offended by the odor or appearance of the effluent in the pouch. A negative reaction from caregivers only reinforces the patient's feelings that this alteration in bodily function makes them personally and socially unacceptable. A supportive nurse makes the initial period of adjustment easier (Hyland, 2002). When a patient comes to the hospital with an ostomy, encourage the patient to resume self-care as soon as possible. Respect a patient's routine of care even if it differs from usual care in the facility.

Use a variety of teaching strategies for each patient based on the patient's physical ability, learning style, and emotional readiness to learn. Whenever possible, make a referral to an ostomy care nurse (Marquis and others, 2003). Ostomy groups throughout the country also are available to provide support for the patient. Information about these groups is available from the ostomy care nurse or on the United Ostomy Association of America website, http://www.uoaa.org.

EVIDENCE-BASED PRACTICE TRENDS

The primary changes in ostomy care are related to improvements in surgical techniques for fecal and urinary diversions. The development of the continent ileostomy and urostomy pouch has progressed to the development of a variety of ileal reservoirs for bowel and urinary effluent that are controlled using the patient's anal or urinary sphincter. Laparoscopic surgery is now being done for abdominal and pelvic procedures and stoma creation. This may decrease postoperative recovery time and use of analgesics (Pappas and Jacobs, 2004).

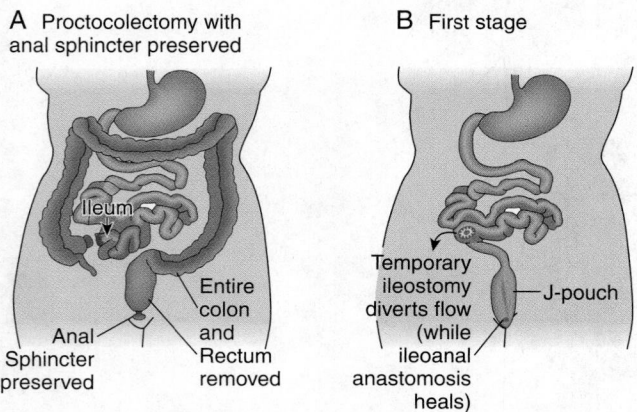

A Proctocolectomy with anal sphincter preserved

Ileum
Anal Sphincter preserved
Entire colon and Rectum removed

B First stage

Temporary ileostomy diverts flow (while ileoanal anastomosis heals)
J-pouch

FIG 35-4   Ileal pouch anal anastomosis.

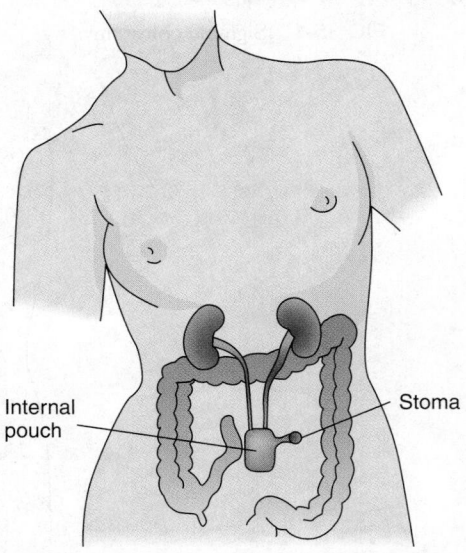

Internal pouch
Stoma

FIG 35-5   Continent urinary diversion.

Stoma care has improved, because pouching systems are more effective and adhesive technology more advanced. These improvements include a wider variety of sizes and shapes of skin barriers, depths of convexity from shallow to deep, and degrees of flexibility. The current trend is to apply the pouch directly to clean dry skin without using skin preparations, paste, or added adhesives unless the patient has a specific problem in keeping the pouch intact (WOCN, 2007). The adhesives on the skin barriers are pressure and heat sensitive, so have the patient apply gentle pressure with the hand over the skin barrier for several minutes to facilitate the adherence of the barrier to the skin. There are new and improved accessory products such as rings or seals for managing abdominal contours that are uneven or peristomal skin that is not intact. Some pouches have effective gas filters that allow flatus to escape slowly from the pouch through a charcoal filter. This filter absorbs odor and does not allow leakage of liquid effluent through the filter. All of the ostomy companies now have pouches with integrated closures. A Velcro-like closure eliminates the need for a clip to close the bottom of the pouch. It also requires less manual dexterity in emptying the pouch (Colwell and others, 2004). A wider selection of products for neonatal and pediatric use has improved the care of that population (Rogers, 2003).

CULTURAL CONSIDERATIONS

In any culture the presence and care of an ostomy presents unique challenges. New ostomies require monitoring and observation, and patients from other cultures often find this more invasive and embarrassing. Most cultures consider bowel and urinary secretions unfit for public display. Exposure of the lower torso, which is needed for ostomy care, is generally avoided among Asians, Africans, Hispanics, Hindus, Muslims, Arabs, Orthodox Jews, and Amish groups. When caring for patients with ostomies from these cultures, it helps to assign gender-congruent caregivers if possible and to allow presence of a family member if requested by the patient.

As you communicate with a patient during an ostomy procedure, be sensitive and avoid communicating anything that the patient may interpret as disrespect or disgust. As always, prepare adequately for the procedure, seek necessary assistance, and maintain a calm, professional demeanor.

Skill Performance Guidelines

1 Know how to assess your patient's stoma.
   - *Color/Moisture:* Stoma should be red or pink and moist. If it is gray, purple, or black, report this to the charge nurse or physician.
   - *Size:* In the 4 to 6 weeks after surgery, the stoma will likely decrease in size. Measure with each pouch change.
   - *Type:* Recognize the difference between a contour-budded stoma (Fig. 35-6) and a flush or retracted stoma (Fig. 35-7).
2 Know how to assess differences in the peristomal skin: intact, reddened but intact, raw, presence of blisters or a rash.
3 Know what type of effluent is expected from the ostomy.
   - *Colostomy:* Soft or formed stool.
   - *Ileostomy:* Liquid drainage.
   - *Ileal conduit:* Urine will have mucus in it because of flow through intestinal segment.
4 Know the pouching options available.

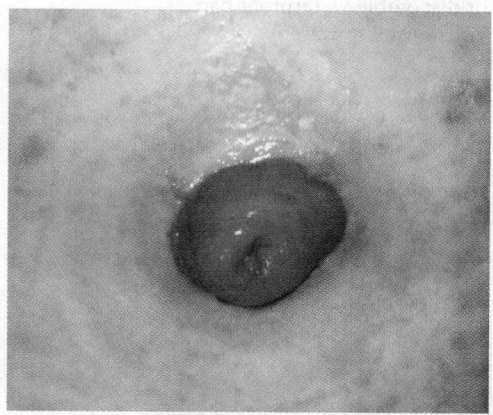

FIG 35-6   Budded stoma. (*Courtesy Jane Fellows.*)

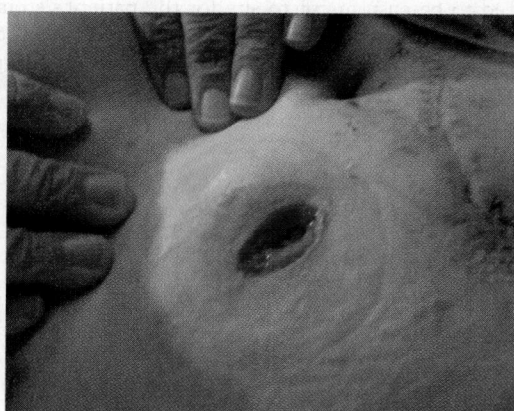

FIG 35-7   Retracted stoma. (*Courtesy Jane Fellows.*)

SKILL 35-1 Pouching a Colostomy or an Ileostomy

 Intermediate / Ostomy Care / Pouching a Colostomy

NSO *Ostomy Module / Lessons 1, 3, and 4*

Immediately after a fecal surgical diversion, it is necessary to place a pouch over the newly created stoma to contain effluent when the stoma begins to function. The pouch will keep the patient clean and dry, protect the skin from drainage, and provide a barrier against odor. Use a cut-to-fit, transparent pouching system that will cover the peristomal skin without constricting the stoma and allow for visibility of the stoma.

In the immediate postoperative period the stoma may be edematous and the abdomen distended. These symptoms will resolve over a 4- to 6-week period after surgery, but during this time it will be necessary to revise the pouching system to meet the changing size of the stoma and the changes in body contours (Erwin-Toth and Thomas-Hess, 2003).

There are many types of pouching systems, but all will have a protective layer that adheres to the skin called a skin barrier and a pouch. A one-piece pouching system (Fig. 35-8) has the two parts integrated together. A two-piece system (Fig. 35-9) has a separate skin barrier and pouch. The flush or retracted stoma may require a convex wafer (Fig. 35-10) for successful pouching. This type of skin barrier will provide gentle pressure on the peristomal skin to push the stoma through the opening in the wafer. You apply the pouch to the skin barrier by attaching it to a flange (a plastic ring) on the barrier. You must use the skin barrier with a flange that fits the corresponding size pouch from the same manufacturer to avoid leakage between the skin barrier and the pouch. Some pouching systems have precut openings in the barrier for the stoma, whereas others need to be custom cut to size for the patient's stoma measurement. It is important to understand how to use each of these different pouching systems before applying them on the patient.

The websites for the companies that make ostomy supplies have both patient and health care provider instructions that are helpful in understanding how to use the pouching systems. Three of these are http://www.convatec.com, http://www.us.coloplast.com, and http://www.hollister.com.

Delegation Considerations
The skill of pouching a new ostomy/ileostomy cannot be delegated to nursing assistive personnel (NAP). In some agencies care of an established ostomy (4 weeks postoperative or more) can be delegated to NAP. The nurse directs the NAP about:
- The expected amount, color, and consistency of drainage from the ostomy.
- The expected appearance of the stoma.
- Special equipment needed to complete procedure.
- Change in the patient's stoma and surrounding skin integrity that should be reported.

Equipment
- ❏ Skin barrier/pouch—clear drainable one-piece or two-piece, cut-to-fit or precut size
- ❏ Pouch closure device, such as a clip, if needed
- ❏ Ostomy measuring guide
- ❏ Adhesive remover (*optional*)
- ❏ Clean gloves
- ❏ Washcloth
- ❏ Towel or disposable waterproof barrier
- ❏ Basin with warm tap water
- ❏ Scissors

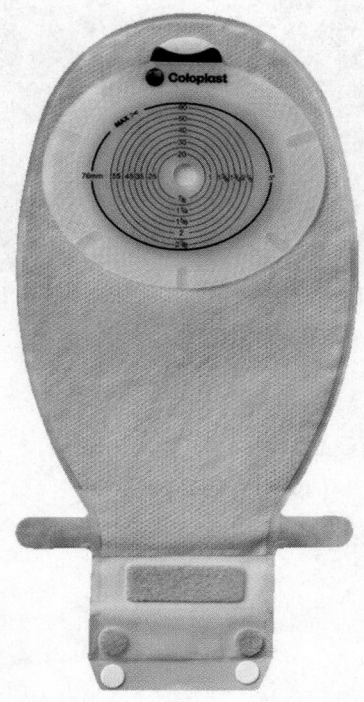

FIG 35-8 One-piece pouch with Velcro closure. (*Courtesy Coloplast, Minneapolis, Minn.*)

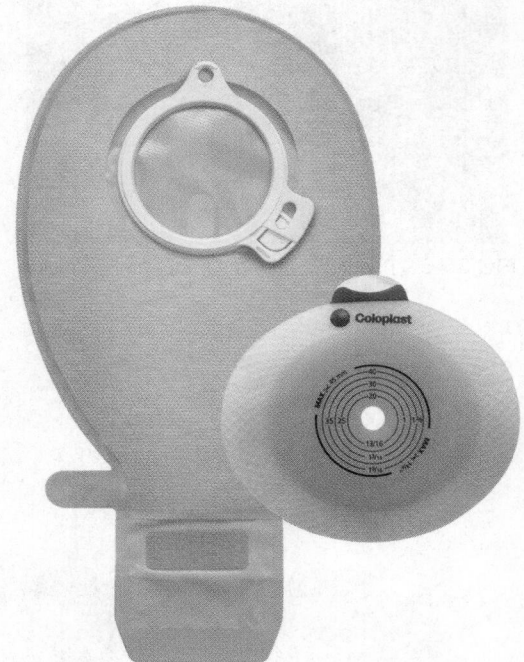

FIG 35-9 Two-piece pouching system with separate skin barrier and attachable pouch. (*Courtesy Coloplast, Minneapolis, Minn.*)

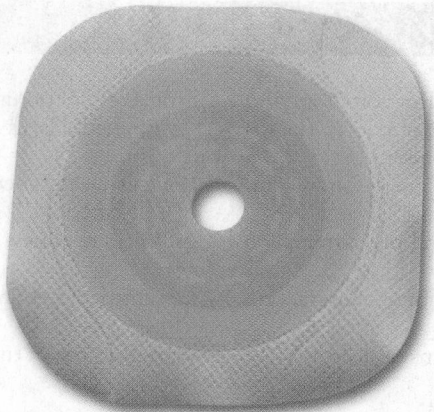

FIG 35-10 Convex skin barrier wafer. (*Courtesy Hollister Incorporated, Libertyville, Ill.*)

STEP	RATIONALE

ASSESSMENT

1 Perform hand hygiene and if necessary apply gloves (e.g., if there is drainage). Observe existing skin barrier and pouch for leakage and length of time in place. The pouch should be changed every 3 to 7 days, not daily (Colwell and others, 2004). Depending upon type of pouching system used (such as opaque pouch), you may have to remove pouch to fully observe stoma. Clear pouches permit viewing of stoma without their removal.

Assesses effectiveness of pouching system and allows for early detection of potential problems To minimize skin irritation, avoid unnecessary changing of entire pouching system, but if the effluent is leaking under the wafer, change it because skin damage from the effluent will cause more skin trauma than early removal of the wafer. Repeated leaking may indicate the need for a different type of pouch.

Critical Decision Point   *If the ostomy pouch is leaking, change it. Taping or patching it to contain effluent leaves the skin exposed to chemical or enzymatic irritation.*

2 Observe amount of effluent in the pouch, and empty the pouch if it is more than one-third to one-half full by opening the clip and draining it into a container for measurement of the output. Note consistency of the effluent, and record intake and output.

Pouches must be emptied when they are one-third to one-half full because the weight of the pouch may disrupt the seal of the adhesive on the skin.
Monitors fluid balance, return of bowel function after surgery.

3 Observe stoma for location, color, swelling, trauma, and healing or irritation of the peristomal skin. Assess type of stoma. Remove gloves.

Stoma characteristics are one of the factors to consider in selecting an appropriate pouching system. Convexity in the skin barrier is often necessary with a flush or retracted stoma.

4 Observe abdomen for best type of pouching system. Consider:
   a Abdominal contour
   b Presence of scars or incisions

Determines pouching system selection. Abdominal contours, scars, or incisions affect type of system and adhesion to skin surface.

5 Explore patient's attitude toward learning self-care, and identify others who will be assisting patient after leaving the hospital.

Facilitates teaching plan and timing of care to coincide with availability of caregivers.

NURSING DIAGNOSES

- Readiness for enhanced knowledge
- Risk for impaired skin integrity

Individualize related factors based on patient's condition or needs.

PLANNING

1 Expected outcomes following completion of procedure:
   - Stoma is moist and reddish pink. Skin is intact and free of irritation; sutures are intact.

Normal findings in a patient with postoperative ostomy that is healing. Stoma initially is edematous and shrinks over next 4 to 6 weeks.

STEP	RATIONALE

- Stoma drains moderate amount of liquid or soft stool and flatus in pouch. Flatus is noted by bulging of pouch. (Flatus may not be observable if pouch has a gas filter.)

Stoma is functioning normally. Snug seal around stoma has been attained. Flatus indicates return of peristalsis after surgery.

- Patient, family, and/or significant others observe stoma and steps of procedure.

Reveals acceptance of alteration in body image and interest in self-care.

- Patient asks questions about procedure and may attempt to assist with pouch change.

Indicates readiness to learn and to begin self-care.

2   Explain procedure to patient; encourage patient's interaction and questions.

Lessens patient's anxiety and promotes patient's participation.

3   Assemble equipment, and close room curtains or door.

Optimizes use of time; provides privacy.

IMPLEMENTATION

1   Position patient in semireclining position. If possible, provide patient a mirror for observation.

When patient is semireclining, there are fewer skin wrinkles, which allows for ease of application of pouching system.

2   Perform hand hygiene, and apply clean gloves.

Reduces transmission of microorganisms.

3   Place towel or disposable waterproof barrier across patient's lower abdomen

Protects bed linen; maintains patient's dignity.

4   If not done during assessment, remove used pouch and skin barrier gently by pushing skin away from barrier. An adhesive remover may be used to facilitate removal of skin barrier.

Reduces skin trauma. Improper removal of pouch and barrier can cause peristomal skin irritation or breakdown.

5   Cleanse peristomal skin gently with warm tap water using a washcloth; do not scrub skin. Pat the skin dry.

Avoid soap. It leaves residue on skin, which interferes with pouch adhesion (WOCN, 2007). Pouch does not adhere to wet skin.

6   Measure stoma (see illustration).

Allows for proper fit of pouch that will protect peristomal skin.

7   Trace pattern on pouch/skin barrier (see illustration).

Prepares for cutting opening in the pouch.

8   Cut opening on skin barrier wafer (see illustration).

Customizes pouch to provide appropriate fit over stoma.

9   Remove protective backing from adhesive (see illustration).

Prepares skin barrier for placement.

10   Apply pouch over stoma (see illustration). Press firmly into place around stoma and outside edges. Have patient hold hand over pouch to apply heat to secure seal.

Pouch adhesives are heat activated and will hold more securely at body temperature.

11   Close end of pouch.

Contains effluent.

12   Properly dispose of used pouch, and remove drape from patient.

Avoids odor in room.

13   Remove gloves. Perform hand hygiene.

Reduces transmission of microorganisms.

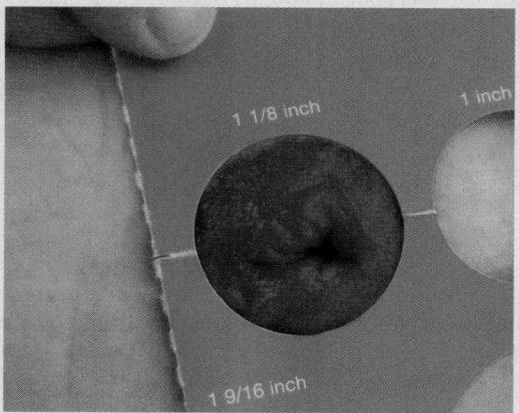

STEP 6   Measure stoma. (*Courtesy Coloplast, Minneapolis, Minn.*)

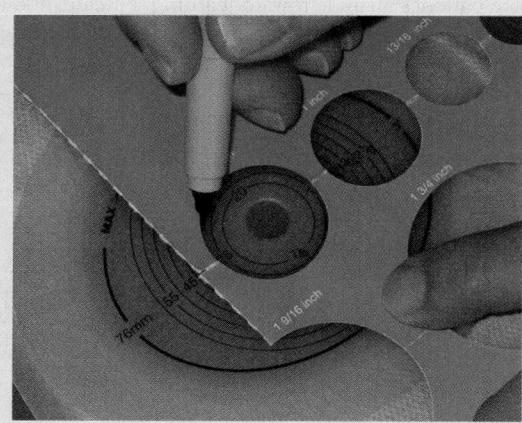

STEP 7   Trace measurement. (*Courtesy Coloplast, Minneapolis, Minn.*)

STEP	RATIONALE

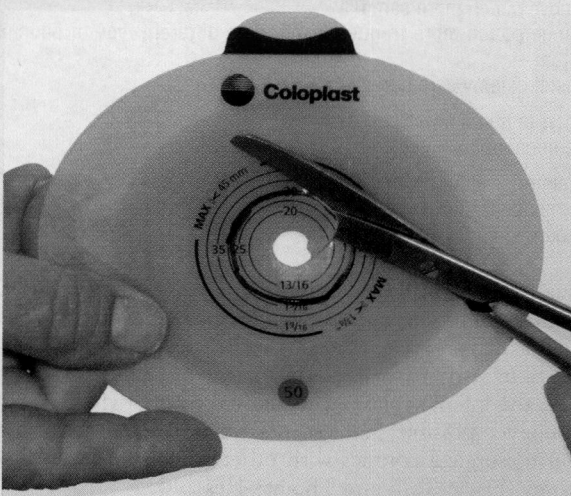

STEP 8   Cut opening in wafer. (*Courtesy Coloplast, Minneapolis, Minn.*)

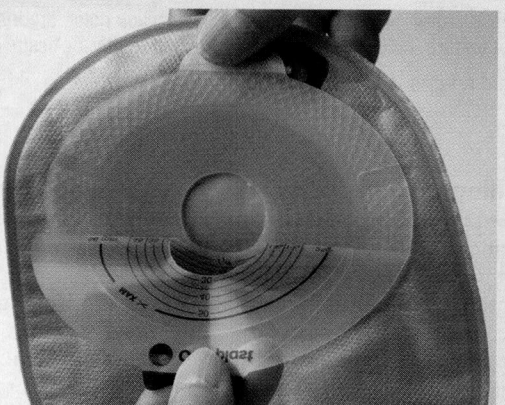

STEP 9   Remove protective backing. (*Courtesy Coloplast, Minneapolis, Minn.*)

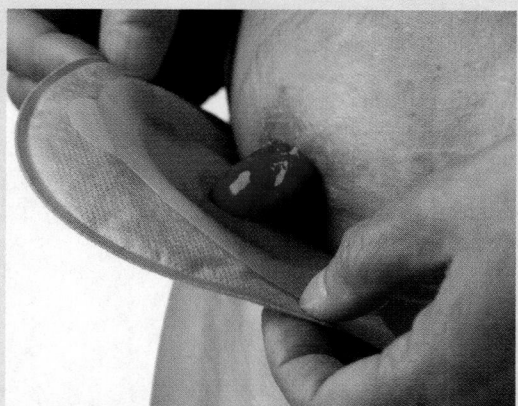

STEP 10   Apply pouch over stoma. (*Courtesy Coloplast, Minneapolis, Minn.*)

EVALUATION

1 Observe condition of skin barrier and adherence to abdominal surface.	Determines presence of leaks.
2 Observe appearance of stoma, peristomal skin, abdominal contours, and suture line during pouch change.	Provides information if another type of pouching system or additional skin care products are needed.

Critical Decision Point   *If peristomal skin is raw, blistered, or weeping, the skin surface will be moist and the pouch will not adhere, making the patient vulnerable to more severe skin breakdown. Consult the ostomy care nurse before proceeding with placing a pouch over moist, damaged skin.*

3 Observe patient's, family member's, or significant other's willingness to view stoma and ask questions about procedure.	Determines level of adjustment and understanding of stoma care and pouch application. Allows planning for future education needs and progress toward acceptance of altered body image.

Unexpected Outcomes	Related Interventions
1 Skin around stoma is irritated, blistered, or bleeding, or a rash is noted. May be caused by undermining of pouch seal by fecal contents, allergic reaction, or fungal skin eruption.	• Remove pouch more carefully. • Change pouch more frequently, or use a different type of pouching system. • Consult ostomy care nurse.
2 Necrotic stoma is manifested by purple or black color, dry instead of moist texture, failure to bleed when washed gently, or tissue sloughing.	• Report to nurse/physician. • Document appearance.
3 Patient refuses to view stoma or participate in care.	• Obtain referral for ostomy care nurse. • Allow patient to express feelings. • Encourage family support.

Recording and Reporting

- Record type of pouch and skin barrier applied, amount and appearance of effluent in pouch, size and appearance of stoma, condition of peristomal skin.
- Record patient/family level of participation, teaching that was done, and response to teaching.
- Report any of the following to nurse and/or physician: abnormal appearance of stoma, suture line, peristomal skin, or character of output.

Teaching Considerations

- Include family members or significant other(s) in teaching to facilitate patient's readiness to learn (Colwell and others, 2004).
- Some patients acknowledge stoma with minimal emotional difficulty; some may never completely adjust to it. Individualize care according to patient's situation and circumstances (Hyland, 2003).
- Give patient teaching materials that clearly state each step for a pouch change. Audiotaped or videotaped instructions are also available. For patients with learning disabilities, consider using materials that have illustrations for each step.
- Give patients a list of equipment and name, address, and phone number of a supplier.

Pediatric Considerations

- Select pediatric pouches designed especially for neonates, infants, and children; these pouches are smaller and have a more skin-sensitive adhesive on the barrier (Fig. 35-11).
- Because most ostomy surgery done on neonates is for emergencies, often no time is available for preoperative selection of stoma site. The surgery is usually done because the baby has necrotizing enterocolitis (NEC), Hirschsprung's disease, imperforate anus, or other congenital disorders (Rogers, 2003). The stomas are frequently temporary with closure of the ostomy when the surgical repair has healed and the baby is medically ready for surgery. Children and adolescents may have ostomy surgery for conditions such as cancer, inflammatory bowel disease, and trauma.
- Neonates may have multiple stomas on their tiny abdomens that are the result of corrective bowel surgeries. Select a cut-to-fit pouch that allows multiple stoma openings in skin barrier, yet still fits on neonate's abdomen (Colwell and others, 2003).
- Because babies swallow large amounts of air while sucking, it is normal to expect flatus. Make sure pouch can accommodate increased amount of flatus after feeding, or be prepared to release flatus frequently (Rogers, 2003).
- The skin of a preterm infant is not fully developed and is more absorbent than the skin of a full-term infant. Do not use skin sealants and adhesive removers unless they are approved for preterm infant use (Rogers, 2003).

- Usually a baby triples its birth weight in the first year. As a baby grows in size, so does the stoma. Measure the stoma frequently, and make appropriate adjustments in pouching and skin barrier size. Skin barriers for preterm infants must have flexibility to cover the infant's rounded abdominal contour (Rogers, 2003).
- Whenever possible, adolescents requiring an ostomy benefit from presurgical contact with other adolescents who have an ostomy (Erwin-Toth and Thomas-Hess, 2003).

Gerontological Considerations

- Evaluate the older adult's cognitive status for understanding of ostomy self-care instructions.

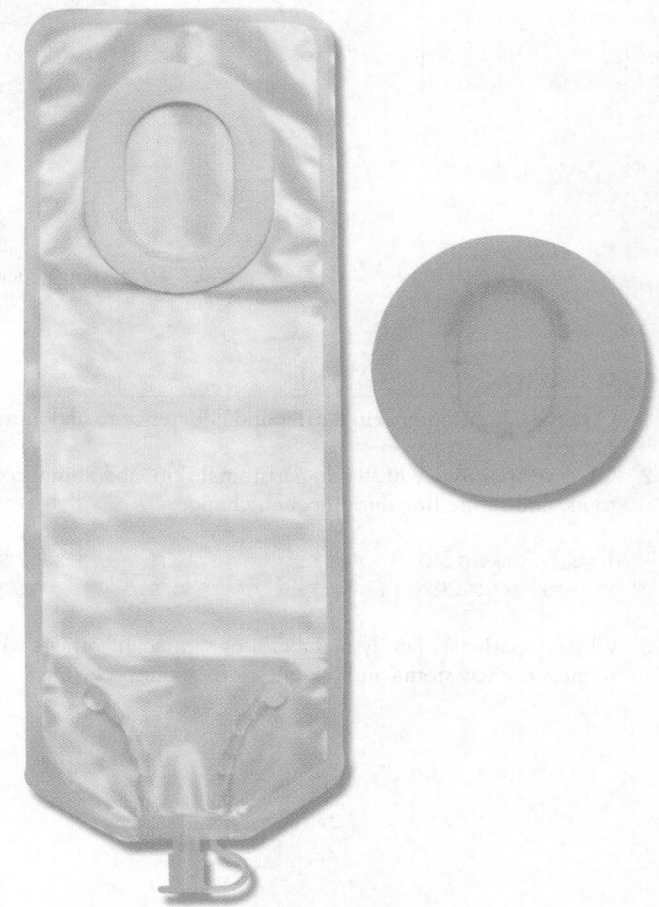

FIG 35-11 Newborn ostomy pouch. (*Courtesy Hollister, Incorporated, Libertyville, Ill.*)

- Some older patients have impaired manual dexterity or limited vision, so make adaptations for this while teaching. For patients who are unable to custom cut the size of their skin barriers, consider having barriers precut by an ostomy equipment supplier or using a precut pouching system.
- Financial concerns about cost of ostomy supplies and reimbursement are an important issue for patients on fixed income.

Home Care Considerations
- Evaluate patient's home toileting facilities and patient's ability to position self to empty pouch directly into the toilet.
- Patient may shower without covering pouch.
- Patients should avoid storing pouches in extremely hot or cold locations because temperature will affect barrier and adhesive materials.

SKILL 35-2 Pouching a Urostomy

 Intermediate / Ostomy Care / Pouching a Ureterostomy

Because urine flows continuously from an incontinent urinary diversion, placement of the pouch is more challenging than with the fecal diversion. In the immediate postoperative period, urinary stents extend out from the stoma (Fig. 35-12). A surgeon places the stents to prevent stenosis of the ureters at the site where the ureters are attached to the conduit. The stents will be removed during the hospital stay or at the first postoperative visit with the surgeon. The stoma is normally red and moist. It is made from a portion of the intestinal tract, usually the ileum. The stoma should protrude above the skin. An ileal conduit is usually located in the right lower quadrant. While the patient is in bed, the pouch may be connected to a bedside drainage bag to decrease the need for frequent emptying. When the patient goes home, the bedside drainage bag may be used at night to avoid having to get up to empty the pouch. Each type of urostomy pouch comes with a connector for the bedside drainage bag.

Delegation Considerations
The skill of pouching a new incontinent urinary diversion cannot be delegated to NAP. You can delegate care of an established incontinent urinary diversion (see agency policy). This will vary. The nurse directs the NAP about:

- Expected appearance of the stoma.
- Expected amount and character of the output, and when to report changes.
- Change in the patient's stoma and surrounding skin integrity that should be reported.
- Special equipment needed to complete procedure.

Equipment
❑ Skin barrier/urinary pouch (with antireflux flap)—clear, drainable one-piece or two-piece, cut-to-fit or precut size (Fig. 35-13)
❑ Appropriate adapter for connection to bedside drainage bag
❑ Measuring guide
❑ Bedside urinary drainage bag
❑ Clean gloves
❑ Washcloth
❑ Towel or disposable waterproof barrier
❑ Basin with warm tap water
❑ Scissors
❑ Adhesive remover
❑ Absorbent wick made from gauze rolled tightly in the shape of a tampon.

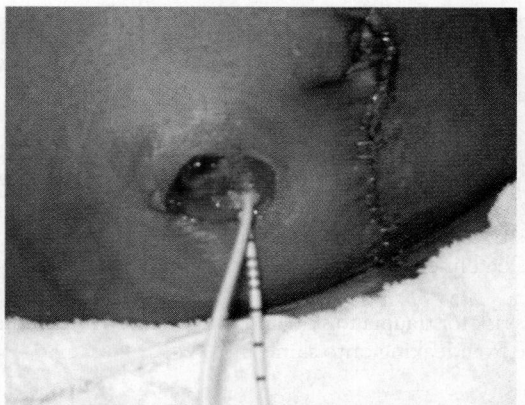

FIG 35-12 Urostomy stoma with stents in place. (*Courtesy Jane Fellows.*)

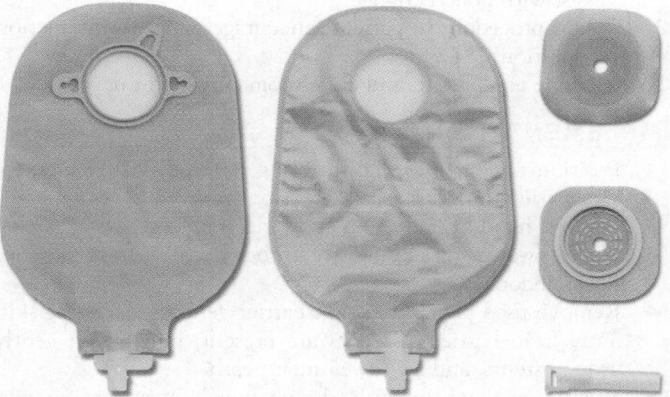

FIG 35-13 Urostomy pouching system with adapter to connect pouch to bedside drainage bag. (*Courtesy Hollister Incorporated, Libertyville, Ill.*)

STEP	RATIONALE

ASSESSMENT

1. Perform hand hygiene and apply gloves. Observe existing skin barrier and pouch for leakage and length of time in place. The pouch should be changed every 3 to 7 days, not daily (Colwell and others, 2004).

    Assesses effectiveness of pouching system and allows for early detection of potential problems To minimize skin irritation, avoid unnecessary changing of entire pouching system. If urine is leaking under the wafer, it should be changed because the patient's clothing and bed will be wet. Repeated leakage may indicate need for different type of pouch to provide a reliable seal.

2. Observe urine in the pouch or bedside drainage bag. Empty the pouch if it is more than one-third to one-half full by opening the valve and draining it into a container for measurement.

    Urine output provides information about renal status and whether volume is within acceptable limits (minimum of 30 mL/hr). Empty pouches when they are one-third to one-half full so that the weight of the pouch does not disrupt the seal.

3. Observe stoma for color, swelling, trauma, and healing of the peristomal skin. Assess type of stoma. Remove gloves.

    Stoma characteristics are one of the factors to consider in selecting an appropriate pouching system. Convexity in the skin barrier is often necessary with a flush or retracted stoma.

4. Explore patient's attitude toward learning self-care, and identify others who will be assisting patient after leaving the hospital.

    Facilitates teaching plan and timing of care to coincide with availability of caregivers.

NURSING DIAGNOSES

- Readiness for enhanced knowledge
- Risk for impaired skin integrity

Individualize related factors based on patient's condition or needs.

PLANNING

1. Expected outcomes following completion of procedure:
    - Stoma is moist, reddish-pink with stents protruding from it. Peristomal skin is free of irritation and is intact. Sutures are intact.

        Normal findings for postoperative urinary diversion.

    - Urine drains freely from stents or stoma. Urine is yellow with mucus shreds and is without foul odor. The urine may be pink or contain small blood clots after surgery. Volume of output is within acceptable limits (30 mL/hr).

        These are normal findings postoperatively. Mucous shreds are normal when urine flows through an intestinal segment.

    - Patient, family member, and/or significant others observe stoma and procedural steps.

        Shows adjustment to body image change and willingness to learn self-care.

    - Patient asks questions about procedure and may attempt to assist with pouch change.

        Indicates readiness to learn and to begin self-care.

2. Explain procedure to patient; encourage patient's interaction and questions.

    Lessens patient's anxiety and promotes patient's participation.

3. Assemble equipment, and close room curtains or door.

    Optimizes use of time; provides privacy.

IMPLEMENTATION

1. Position patient in a semireclining position. If possible provide patient a mirror for observation.

    When patient is semireclining, there are fewer skin wrinkles, which allows for ease of pouch application.

2. Perform hand hygiene, and apply clean gloves.

    Reduces transmission of microorganisms.

3. Place towel or disposable waterproof barrier across patient's lower abdomen.

    Protects bed linen; maintains patient's dignity.

4. Remove used pouch and skin barrier gently by pushing skin away from barrier. If stents are present, pull pouch gently around stents, and lay towel underneath.

    Reduces risk for trauma to skin and risk for dislodging stents. Keeps urine from leaking onto skin.

5. Wick stoma continuously during pouch measurement and change. Place rolled gauze wick at stomal opening.

    Using a wick at stoma opening prevents peristomal skin from becoming wet with urine during pouching-change procedure.

6. Cleanse peristomal skin gently with warm tap water using washcloth; do not scrub skin. Pat the skin dry.

    Avoid soap. It leaves residue on skin, which interferes with pouch adhesion (WOCN, 2007). Pouch does not adhere to wet skin.

7. Measure stoma (see Skill 35-1).

    Allows for proper fit of pouch that will protect peristomal skin.

8. Trace pattern on pouch/skin barrier (see Skill 35-1).

    Prepares for cutting opening in the pouch.

9. Cut opening in pouch (see Skill 35-1).

    Customizes pouch to provide appropriate fit over stoma.

10. Remove protective backing from adhesive surface (see Skill 35-1). Remove wick.

    Prepares pouch for application to skin.

STEP	RATIONALE
11 Apply pouch. Press firmly into place around stoma and outside edges. Have patient hold hand over pouch to apply heat to secure seal.	Pouch adhesives are heat activated and will hold more securely at body temperature.
12 Use adapter provided with pouches to connect pouch to bedside urinary bag.	Provides for collection and measurement of urine. Allows patient to rest without frequent emptying of the pouch.
13 Properly dispose of used pouch and soiled equipment.	Avoids odor in room.
14 Remove gloves; perform hand hygiene.	Reduces transmission of microorganisms.

EVALUATION

1 Observe appearance of stoma, peristomal skin, and suture line during pouch change.	Determines condition of stoma and peristomal skin and progress of wound healing.
2 Evaluate character and volume of urinary drainage.	Determines if stoma and/or stents are patent. Character of urine reveals degree of concentration and alterations in renal function.
3 Observe patient's, family member's, or significant other's willingness to view stoma and ask questions about procedure.	Determines level of adjustment and understanding of stoma care and pouch application.

Unexpected Outcomes	Related Interventions
1 Skin around stoma is irritated, blistered, or bleeding, or a rash is noted, possibly due to chronic exposure to urine.	• Check stoma size and opening in skin barrier. Resize skin barrier opening if necessary. • Remove pouch more carefully. • Consult ostomy care nurse.
2 No urine output for several hours, or output is less than 30 mL/hr. Urine has foul odor.	• Increase fluid intake. • Notify physician. • Obtain urine specimen for culture and sensitivity if ordered by the physician.
3 Patient, family member, or significant other is unable to observe stoma, ask questions, or participate in care.	• Consult ostomy care nurse. • Allow patient to express feelings. • Encourage family support.

Recording and Reporting

- Record type of pouch, time of change, condition and appearance of stoma and peristomal skin, and character of urine.
- Record urinary output on intake and output form.
- Document patient's, family's, or significant other's reaction to stoma and level of participation.
- Report abnormalities in stoma or peristomal skin and absence of urinary output to nurse in charge or physician.

Teaching Considerations

- Use opportunity to teach whenever doing pouch change even if patient does not appear interested. Do not insist that patient look at stoma; allow time for adjustment.
- Teach patients significance and importance of drinking 1½ to 2 quarts of fluid daily to prevent urinary tract infections (UTIs). Teach patients that some mucus in urine is expected, but they should report any blood in their urine, excessively cloudy urine, chills, fever (101° F or higher), and back (flank) pain to their physician.
- Give patient teaching materials that state each step clearly. Audiotaped or videotaped instructions are also available. For patients with learning disabilities, consider using material that has illustrations for each step.
- Give patients a list of equipment and name, address, and phone number of a supplier.

Pediatric Considerations

- In neonates, urinary diversions are less common than fecal ostomies. Surgical repair of congenital urinary abnormalities usu-

ally occurs in stages and focuses initially on drainage of the upper urinary tract to preserve renal function.
- Select pediatric pouches designed especially for neonates, infants, and children; these pouches are smaller and have a more skin-sensitive adhesive on the barrier.

Gerontological Considerations

- Older patients have decreased thirst and may not normally consume adequate fluids. Instruct patient in importance of fluid intake to promote healthy renal function and decrease risk for urinary tract infection.
- Evaluate older adult's cognitive status for understanding of ostomy self-care instructions.
- Some older patients have impaired manual dexterity or limited vision, so make adaptations for this while teaching. For patients who are unable to custom cut the size of their skin barriers, consider having barriers precut by ostomy equipment supplier or using a precut two-piece system.
- Financial concerns about cost of ostomy supplies and reimbursement are an important issue for patients on fixed income.

Home Care Considerations

- Instruct patient that pouch can be connected to straight drainage at night. Make sure patient understands that adapter will be needed to connect pouch to the bedside drainage bag.
- Patient may shower without covering pouch.
- Patients should avoid storing pouches in extremely hot or cold locations because temperature will affect barrier and adhesive materials.

SKILL 35-3   Catheterizing a Urinary Diversion

Catheterization of a urinary diversion is the only way to obtain an accurate culture and sensitivity specimen for screening for infection. When necessary to obtain a urine specimen from a urinary diversion, the best method is to insert a sterile catheter into the stoma. Obtaining a specimen of urine in a pouch does not provide an accurate finding because of the likely risk for contamination by microorganisms. With the use of strict aseptic technique, catheterization is relatively safe and easy. If a patient uses a two-piece system, you can remove the pouch from the skin barrier and replace it after the procedure without disturbing the skin barrier. If a patient uses a one-piece system, you have to remove the pouch to obtain the specimen and then replace it after the procedure.

Delegation Considerations

The skill of catheterizing a urinary diversion cannot be delegated to NAP. The nurse directs the NAP to:
- Inform nurse if patient complains of peristomal pain or back pain.

- Inform nurse if there is a change in color, odor, or amount of urine or if there is blood in the urine.

Equipment

☐ Urinary catheterization supplies (may be contained in pre-packaged sterile catheter kit or may need to be gathered separately)
  - 14 to 16 Fr sterile catheter
  - Water-soluble lubricant
  - Antiseptic swabs (e.g., povidone-iodine or chlorhexidine)
  - Sterile gloves
  - Sterile specimen container
☐ Absorbent wick
☐ Bed protection barrier
☐ Towels
☐ Urinary pouch if needed
☐ Clean gloves

STEP	RATIONALE
ASSESSMENT	
1 Observe for signs and symptoms of UTI such as elevated temperature, chills, foul-smelling urine, elevated white blood cell (WBC) count.	Determines need to perform catheterization to obtain a sterile specimen from urinary diversion. Urinary diversion poses risk for reflux of urine back to kidneys, resulting in infection.
2 Obtain physician's order for catheterization.	Invasive procedure requires physician's order.
3 Assess patient's understanding of need for procedure and how procedure is done.	Determines willingness to cooperate and reduces patient's anxiety.
NURSING DIAGNOSES	
• Deficient knowledge regarding catheterization procedure	• Risk for infection
Individualize related factors based on patient's condition or needs.	
PLANNING	
1 Expected outcomes following completion of procedure:	
• Urine specimen will not be contaminated with bacteria during the procedure.	Urine obtained correctly. Laboratory results will be accurate.
• Patient describes risks for infection and techniques to prevent infection.	Demonstrates patient's learning.
2 Assemble equipment.	Optimizes use of time.
3 Close room curtains or door.	Provides privacy.
4 Explain procedure to patient; if possible; attempt to obtain specimen when patient is due to change pouch if using one-piece system.	Lessens anxiety and promotes patient's cooperation. Changing pouch too frequently could result in skin trauma.
IMPLEMENTATION	
1 Check patient's identity using two identifiers (neither can be patient's room number). Position patient sitting, if possible, and drape towel across lower abdomen.	Ensures right patient undergoes right procedure. Gravity facilitates flow of urine. Maintains patient's dignity. Towel absorbs urine.
2 Perform hand hygiene, and put on clean gloves.	Reduces transmission of microorganisms.
3 Remove pouch. If patient uses two-piece system, remove pouch but leave barrier attached to skin.	Allows access to stoma.
4 Remove gloves, and perform hand hygiene. Open sterile catheterization set according to instructions, or open needed equipment and place on sterile barrier using aseptic technique (see Chapter 7). If not using catheterization kit, place gauze pad on sterile field, and squeeze small amount of lubricant onto gauze. Apply sterile gloves.	Avoids contamination.

STEP	RATIONALE
5 If needed, have patient hold absorbent wick on stoma.	Prevents leakage of urine on peristomal skin, linens, and clothing.
6 Cleanse surface of stoma with antiseptic swabs using circular motion from center outward. Using new swab each time, repeat twice. Wipe off excess antiseptic with dry sterile gauze or cotton ball.	Removes surface bacteria.

Critical Decision Point   *If patient has stents in place, use antiseptic swab to cleanse the ends of the stents and place the stents in the sterile cup. Allow urine to drip into the cup until an adequate amount for a specimen has been obtained.*

STEP	RATIONALE
7 Lubricate tip of catheter with water-soluble lubricant.	Lubricant facilitates passage of catheter through stoma.
8 Remove lid from specimen container. Place distal end of catheter into specimen container. Hold catheter in container with nondominant hand.	Because the conduit is for passage of urine rather than storage, only a small volume of urine will be obtained; take care to direct urine into container.
9 With dominant hand, gently insert catheter into stoma. Do not force catheter, redirect course as needed. Use gentle but firm pressure similar to regular catheterization of urethra. Have patient cough or turn slightly to facilitate flow of urine.	Use care to avoid trauma to conduit. Movement and coughing may facilitate flow of urine.
10 Maintain container below level of stoma. If needed, wait several minutes to get adequate amount of urine.	Culture and sensitivity studies only require 3 to 5 mL of urine (check agency policy).
11 After withdrawing catheter, place absorbent pad over stoma.	Keeps skin dry.
12 Put lid on specimen container.	Prevents accidental spillage.
13 Reapply new pouch, or reattach pouch if patient uses a two-piece system (see Skill 35-2).	Pouch is necessary to contain urine.
14 Dispose of used pouch and equipment properly.	Avoids unpleasant odor in room.
15 Remove gloves; perform hand hygiene. Label specimen, place in biohazard bag, and send to laboratory at once.	Labeling ensures acceptance of specimen by laboratory and processing. Allowing urine to sit for long periods at room temperature will adversely affect laboratory results.

EVALUATION

1 Await laboratory report, and compare results of culture and sensitivity with expected findings. Mucus is a normal finding in the urine of a patient with an ileal conduit.	Determines presence of infection. If contamination appears likely, second specimen will be necessary.
2 Instruct patient about signs and symptoms of UTI.	An informed patient will seek attention for a problem earlier if aware of signs and symptoms (Colwell and others, 2004).

Unexpected Outcomes	Related Interventions
1 Unable to obtain urine specimen.	• Reposition patient. • If there is still no urine, push fluids and try again later.
2 Skin or stoma reveals complications.	• Notify nurse and/or physician. • Consult with ostomy care nurse.

Recording and Reporting
- Record time specimen collected, patient's tolerance of procedure, and appearance of urine, skin, and stoma.
- Report results of laboratory test to nurse in charge or physician.

Teaching Considerations
- Explain common symptoms of UTI: flank pain, dark or bloody urine, foul-smelling urine, fever (101° F or higher), confusion.
- Encourage patient to notify physician if symptoms of infection develop.
- Reinforce importance of fluid intake (2 L/day).

CRITICAL THINKING EXERCISES

1 You are assigned to care for Janeé Bell, a 28-year-old engineer. She has been admitted for elective colon removal secondary to a 10-year history of ulcerative colitis. She is scheduled for an ileal pouch anal anastomosis with J-pouch construction and will have a temporary ileostomy. As part of her preoperative preparation, she should have:
   A A chance to empty a pouch
   B A nutrition consultation
   C Stoma site marking with a qualified ostomy care nurse
   D A barium enema
   Explain your choice.

2 When Janeé returns from surgery, you assess the stoma. You should expect the stoma to:
   A Be red and moist
   B Be just below the skin level
   C Have stents protruding from it
   D Be pink and dry
   Explain your choices.

3 When teaching Janeé about care at home, you explain that her ostomy pouch should be:
   A Changed daily
   B Emptied when it is one-third to one-half full
   C Emptied every 4 to 6 hours
   D Changed weekly
   Explain your choice.

4 Janeé notes that her bowel movement is always liquid and asks when it will be formed as it was before she got sick. You tell her:
   A It will be formed after she completely recovers from the surgery
   B To eat foods that are constipating until her bowel movement is a normal consistency
   C This is a normal output for an ileostomy
   D To reduce her fluid intake and it will become more formed
   Explain your choice.

 REVIEW QUESTIONS

1 The nurse has inserted a catheter into a patient's urinary diversion, but only a small amount of urine has drained. What action should the nurse perform first to try to obtain an adequate sample?
   1 Remove the catheter, and obtain urine from the pouch.
   2 Gently insert the catheter a little more.
   3 Massage the patient's abdomen.
   4 Have the patient turn to side.

2 A patient has a new urostomy secondary to bladder cancer. Which patient behavior suggests the most acceptance of his body image?
   1 He watches you change his pouch.
   2 He asks questions about how the ostomy works.
   3 He empties his pouch.
   4 He looks at his stoma.

3 The nurse is caring for a patient with a new permanent sigmoid colostomy and explaining information about care once the patient returns home. Which statement by the patient indicates that the patient requires further instruction on the topic?
   1 "I know that when I wash the stoma, a little bleeding is perfectly normal."
   2 "If I eat the right foods, the stool will be soft and formed."
   3 "I will need to regularly look at the skin around the stoma; it should not become excessively red."
   4 "The stoma will stay the shape it is so it will be easy to buy bags that fit."

4 A patient anticipating an ileostomy because of severe ulcerative colitis asks, "Will I really be able to have a normal life after having this procedure?" What is the most appropriate reply?
   1 "Let's talk about this when you are recovering from the surgery."
   2 "I'm going to have a person with an ostomy visit you before the surgery."
   3 "Why don't you talk with your surgeon about your concerns?"
   4 "Tell me the specific questions you have about life after the surgery."

5 A patient notes a raw, weeping area of the skin in an area under the skin barrier. Patient teaching would be effective if the patient takes which action?
   1 The patient cleans the area with alcohol to help dry it.
   2 The ostomy care nurse is consulted.
   3 The patient schedules an appointment next week with the physician.
   4 The patient continues his usual skin care regimen.

REFERENCES

ASCRS and WOCN joint position statement on the value of preoperative stoma marking for patients undergoing fecal ostomy surgery, 2007, Mount Laurel, NJ, 2007, The Association, http://www.wocn.org/pdf/wocn_Library/Position_statements/stomamarkingpositionstatement0807.pdf, accessed October 17, 2008.

Colwell J and others: *Fecal and urinary diversions: management principles*, St. Louis, 2004, Mosby.

Erwin-Toth P, Thomas-Hess C: Ostomy pearls: a concise guide to stoma siting, pouching systems, patient education, and more, *Adv Skin Wound Care* 16(3):146, 2003.

Hyland J: The basics of ostomies, *Gastroenterol Nurs* 25(6):241, 2002.

Pappas T, Jacobs D: Laparoscopic resection for colon cancer—the end or the beginning? *N Engl J Med* 350(20):2091, 2004.

Rogers VE: Ostomy care: managing preemie stomas—more than just the pouch, *J Wound Ostomy Continence Nurs* 30(2):100, 2003.

WOCN guidelines: basic ostomy care for healthcare providers and patients, Mount Laurel, NJ, 2007, The Association.

RESEARCH REFERENCE

Marquis P and others: Quality of life in patients with stomas: the Montreux study, *Ostomy Wound Manage* 49(2):48, 2003.

Preoperative and Postoperative Care

SKILLS AND PROCEDURES

MEDIA RESOURCES

-  http://evolve.elsevier.com/Perry/skills
  learning system
  - Review Questions
  - Video Clips

- Mosby's Nursing Video Skills, 3.0

KEY TERMS

Analgesia
Anesthesia
Aspiration
Atelectasis
Coagulopathies
Decompression
Dehiscence
Ecchymosis
Evisceration
Hemostasis
Hemovac drain
Homans' sign
Hypovolemic
  shock
Incentive
  spirometer
Informed consent
Jackson-Pratt
  drain
Malignant
  hyperthermia

Nasogastric (NG)
  tube
Paralytic ileus
Penrose drain
Phlebothrombosis
Positive expiratory
  pressure
Postanesthesia
  care unit (PACU)
Postoperative
Postural
  hypotension
Preoperative
Preoperative
  checklist
Procedural
  sedation
Thrombophlebitis
Urinary retention
Venous thrombo-
  embolism (VTE)

OBJECTIVES

Mastery of content in this chapter will enable the nurse to:

- Describe the activities needed to prepare a patient for surgery.
- Explain the rationale for preoperative procedures.
- Discuss cultural differences that might affect the implementation of preoperative and postoperative procedures.
- Adequately prepare a patient for surgery.
- Describe the benefits of structured preoperative teaching.
- Explain the rationale for each of the four postoperative exercises.
- Successfully instruct a patient in performing postoperative exercises.
- Discuss the differences in nursing assessment during the immediate postoperative period and the convalescent phase of recovery.
- Conduct an assessment of a postoperative patient.

The health care industry is in a continuous state of technological advancement. These constant changes are responsible for the development of new diagnostic and interventional devices (e.g., endoscopic examination and laser surgery) that have contributed to a shortened surgical length of stay and changes in roles for care providers. A majority of patients now undergo surgery in an ambulatory care setting. Most surgical patients who must be hospitalized are not admitted until the day of surgery.

Any form of surgery is a stressful event, whether it is a major surgical procedure occurring in a large medical center or a minor procedure occurring in an outpatient center. A patient must frequently make decisions to undergo procedures that are associated with pain, possible disfigurement, dependence, or even the threat of death. Psychologically, the experience of surgery can cause considerable fear and anxiety. Physiologically, the more complex the surgery, the more likely it is a patient will undergo changes in most major body systems.

Nurses use a variety of skills to help a surgical patient adequately prepare for the physiological and psychological stressors of surgery. During the preoperative phase, you will perform a thorough assessment of the patient's physical and emotional status. A variety of diagnostic tests are coordinated to ensure the surgeon and anesthesia care provider have the information needed to determine the patient's risks during surgery and postoperative period. In preparation for surgery, you will instruct the patient and family concerning postoperative care in compliance with The Joint Commission's patient and family education standards (Box 36-1). The instructional topics enable patients and their families to actively participate in the recovery process. Occasionally you will have to perform certain procedures, such as surgical skin preparation, the insertion of an indwelling catheter (see Chapter 33) or nasogastric (NG) tube (see Chapter 34) to protect the patient from risks associated with surgery.

It is imperative that you inquire about cultural practices and religious beliefs that will alter a patient's and/or family's acceptance of perioperative teaching and procedures. Remain nonjudgmental, and adapt the patient's care to encompass these practices and beliefs whenever possible. Individualize the patient's plan of care to provide an improved state of wellness and to maximize the patient's ultimate level of independence. Pertinent information is to be communicated to all members of the health care team so that the patient receives comprehensive and holistic care.

Although preoperative education improves patient outcomes postoperatively, the shift in the provision of surgical services poses special challenges to meet patients' educational needs in a reduced time frame. It is essential that ambulatory care patients receive adequate information to ensure that they or family members can manage postoperative care activities in the home setting. If a patient is to be admitted for same-day surgery, you can perform the preoperative assessment and teaching of postoperative care instructions several days before surgery. The surgeon's office nurse or, more typically, the preoperative nurse in the outpatient department does this. The nurse ensures the completion of operative permits, blood work, testing (e.g., electrocardiogram [ECG]), and any other ordered procedures before the start of the procedure.

During the postoperative phase, when a patient returns from the operating room (OR), you are initially responsible for assessing the patient's physical status to monitor any changes during the recovery process. Once the patient's condition stabilizes, you will focus your efforts on returning the patient to a functional level of wellness as soon as possible within the limitations created by surgery. The speed of a patient's recovery depends on how effectively you anticipate potential complications, initiate necessary supportive and preventive therapies, and actively involve the patient and family in the recovery process.

EVIDENCE-BASED PRACTICE TRENDS

Several evidence-based initiatives target the improvement of surgical care. These initiatives focus on decreasing surgical site infections (SSIs), adverse cardiac events, and postoperative venous thromboembolism (VTE). The Centers for Disease Control and Prevention (CDC), the Institute for Healthcare Improvement (IHI), The Joint Commission, Centers for Medicare and Medicaid Services (CMS), Association of periOperative Registered Nurses

---

| BOX 36-1 | The Joint Commission Patient and Family Education Standards |

Education provided is appropriate to the patient's needs. The assessment of learning needs addresses cultural and religious beliefs, emotional barriers, desire to learn, physical or cognitive limitations, and barriers to communication as appropriate. When called for by the age of the patient and the length of stay, the hospital assesses and provides for patient's education needs. Patients are educated about:

- The plan for care, treatment, and services (i.e., postoperative monitoring)
- Basic health practices and safety (i.e., out of bed [OOB] only with assistance)
- The safe and effective use of medication (i.e., the patient is only one allowed to self-administer patient-controlled analgesia [PCA])
- Nutrition interventions, modified diets, or oral health (i.e., progression of diet postoperatively)
- Safe and effective use of medical equipment or supplies when provided by the hospital (i.e., incentive spirometer)
- Pain—understanding pain, the risk for pain, the importance of effective pain management, the pain assessment process, and methods for pain management (i.e., reporting of pain, frequency of medications, nonmedication pain-relief techniques)
- Habilitation or rehabilitation techniques to help them reach the maximum independence possible (i.e., early ambulation)

Modified from The Joint Commission: *Accreditation manual for hospitals,* Chicago, 2008, The Commission.

(AORN), and others have implemented evidence-based initiatives that promote a culture of safety and protect patients from surgical complications.

The CDC's National Nosocomial Infections Surveillance (NNIS) system (2007a) reports that SSIs account for 22% of hospital-acquired infections. Current research indicates 40% of hospital-acquired infections are SSIs (Odom-Forren, 2006). Four evidence-based guidelines are identified to reduce SSIs:

- Do not remove hair unless it will interfere with the operation, and remove it using only electric clippers if possible.
- Give the correct antibiotic preoperatively and at the appropriate time.
- Maintain blood glucose level postoperatively, especially for patient undergoing cardiac surgery.
- Maintain normothermia.

There are also strict guidelines for use of antibiotics. The goal of prophylactic antibiotic therapy is to protect the patient from infection with as little risk as possible. To achieve this goal, antibiotics must be administered when they will be most beneficial. In addition, providers must select the most effective antibiotic to provide maximum coverage. Overall, it is recommended that prophylactic antibiotics be given as close to the time of incision as possible (within 30 to 60 minutes) and not be given for longer than 24 hours postoperatively. However, vancomycin and fluoroquinolones may be given up to 2 hours before incision because of their longer infusion times. Antibiotic use after incision closure does not reduce infection rate, and when the antibiotics are continued, infections are more likely to be caused by a resistant organism (CDC, 2007a; Odom-Forren, 2006).

Hyperglycemia inhibits the body's ability to fight infection. Immediate postoperative glucose control is also correlated with a reduction in surgical infection. The presence of hyperglycemia in the immediate postoperative period increases the risk for infection in both diabetic and nondiabetic patients. The higher the serum glucose level, the higher the potential for infection in both patient groups (QualityNet, 2007).

In addition to the above initiatives, maintaining normal body temperature also decreases risk for SSI in some patient populations (Dellinger and others, 2005). Hypothermia is associated with both impaired wound healing and infection.

Another category of recommendations for preventing surgical complications focuses on the prevention of adverse cardiac events. This initiative calls for the continued use of beta-blocker therapy before and after surgery. Often this medication may be missed because the surgeon is not the patient's primary care provider or the patient continues to be allowed nothing by mouth (NPO) for a period after surgery. This is one of many reasons why The Joint Commission now requires medication reconciliation on admission (or patient encounter with ambulatory care patients), with each transfer, and discharge.

It is reported that approximately 10% of all hospital deaths can be attributed to pulmonary embolus (PE). In addition, it is reported that 15% to 40% of routine surgical patients develop deep vein thrombosis (DVT). This rate is higher for some patients, such as those following orthopedic procedures or in critical care units (Geerts and others, 2004). In response to this, the American College of Chest Physicians recommends the use of prophylactic pharmacological and mechanical therapies to prevent VTE. The term *VTE* is now used because it incorporates both DVT and PE. Each patient's risk for VTE should be assessed, and patients treated appropriately. Mechanical therapies include the use of graduated compression stockings (see Chapter 10) along with intermittent

pneumatic compression (IPC) or venous foot pump. The venous foot pump is primarily limited to when IPC cannot be used, such as when surgery or injury occurs to the affected lower extremity. Pharmacological regimens include the administration of low-dose unfractionated heparin, low-molecular-weight heparin, factor Xa inhibitor (fondaparinux), or warfarin.

Another trend seen in the United States is the increased prevalence of obesity. Researchers estimate that 66% of adults aged 20 years and older are overweight or obese with 32.9% of the adult population considered obese (CDC, 2007b). Being overweight or obese increases the risk for many diseases and health conditions, including hypertension, dyslipidemia, type 2 diabetes, coronary heart disease, stroke, sleep apnea, and respiratory problems. These conditions increase risks of postoperative complications. Patients presenting with obstructive sleep apnea (OSA) have a higher incidence of failed endotracheal intubation than the general population (Marley and others, 2005). In addition, postoperatively patients with OSA have a greater incidence of airway management problems in the postanesthesia care unit (PACU) and postoperative pulmonary complications. Longer lengths of stay, as well as unanticipated postoperative admission to the intensive care unit, are common (Marley and others, 2005).

CULTURAL CONSIDERATIONS

To provide culturally competent care to a surgical patient, begin by assessing the family hierarchy to determine who needs to be involved in the patient's decisions regarding surgery. Collectivist groups such as African Americans, Asians, and Hispanics make decisions as a group. When providing preoperative teaching, include family members. Use of professional interpreters will prove beneficial.

Preoperatively it is important to accommodate a patient's religious and cultural needs. The preoperative and postoperative time is valued as a family time to support a patient by many cultures such as African Americans. For example, allow religious articles (e.g., medals, under clothing) to be worn until just before surgery. It is important to request information from the patient, family, or religious leader about how to remove these articles if absolutely necessary. Similarly, return these same articles promptly after surgery. Some Mormons who have received full sacraments request to wear an undergarment. A male Sikh may request to wear a turban, wear a metal bracelet, and keep his long hair and beard. An East Indian woman may wish to wear her wedding necklace.

Preoperatively and postoperatively it will be helpful to assess patient preferences for pain medication. Certain groups such as Filipinos believe that pain medication leads to addiction. Buddhists and Hindus prefer to endure the pain without medication (Andrews and others, 2007). Cultures (Latinos and Muslims) that value men being in control of their emotions may prevent members from verbalizing pain.

Skill Performance Guidelines

1. Know the type and nature of any previous surgery. Anatomical and physiological alterations affect a patient's health care needs.
2. Identify the factors and conditions that increase a patient's risks during surgery. Preoperative preparation and postoperative care depend upon the knowledge of these risk factors.
3. Know the rationale for and extent of impending surgery. Each type of surgical procedure requires a different type of nursing care.

4 Administer pain-relief therapies according to a patient's needs perioperatively. Pain can slow a surgical patient's recovery.

5 Encourage a patient's independence as soon as possible during the postoperative period. This minimizes the occurrence of postoperative complications.

6 Anticipate how surgery will affect a patient's ability to return home to a functional lifestyle. Early discharge planning, patient education, referral to community resources, and rehabilitation measures are needed to prepare a patient to return home.

7 Identify cultural and religious beliefs and practices that affect patients' and/or family members' reactions to the surgical experience, such as who can give consent, blood transfusions, and disposal of body parts, including hair.

SKILL 36-1 Preparing a Patient for Surgery

 Intermediate / Preoperative Nursing Care / Performing a Preoperative Assessment Preparing a Patient for Surgery

Preparing a patient for surgery involves activities and procedures that help to decrease anxiety, ensure patient safety, and decrease the risk for complications. A thorough nursing assessment is necessary to document baseline data for future comparisons to determine the effect of instruction and to monitor patients at risk for complications during the perioperative experience.

Anxiety interferes with the effectiveness of anesthesia and the ability of patients to actively participate in their care. Provide information to patients about what will occur during the periopera-

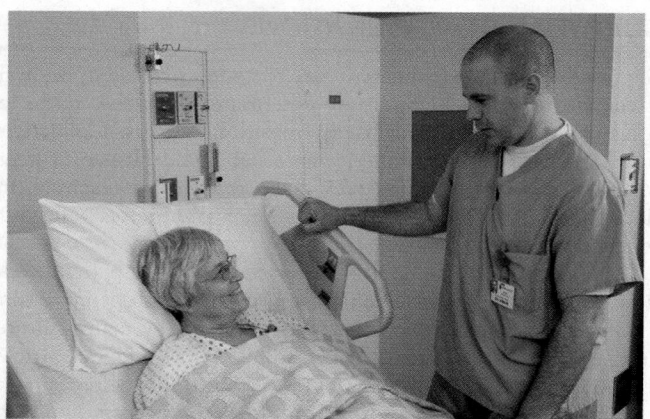

FIG 36-1 Nurse establishes a trusting relationship with patient.

tive experience, as well as what sensations a patient can expect to feel. Demonstration of a caring attitude toward the patient, family members, and significant others will increase feelings of trust and reduce anxiety (Fig. 36-1). Provide assurance that comfort measures will be implemented to manage pain (see Chapter 15).

You ensure patient safety through a number of interventions and activities. Informed consent is required by law to help protect patients' rights, their autonomy, and their privacy. The surgeon should give the patient information about the extent and type of surgery, alternative therapies, usual risks and benefits, and consequences of not having surgery in a nonthreatening manner as outlined in *The Patient Care Partnership*, developed by the American Hospital Association (2003) (Table 36-1). The patient or the patient's legal guardian must sign a surgical consent form that includes this information. If the patient's cultural practices include male dominance, the husband, father, or oldest brother of a female patient may also need to sign the consent form. The consent must also be signed by a witness to verify that the person who signed the consent is the patient so named or the patient's legal guardian. It is your ethical (not legal) responsibility, acting as the patient's advocate, to ensure that the patient understands the information and that the form has been signed and witnessed before the patient receives preoperative medication. See institutional policy regarding consent.

Some patients with "do not resuscitate" (DNR) orders require surgery for palliative care. DNR orders should not routinely be

TABLE 36-1	Information Needed for Informed Consent
Parameters	**Examples**
Name of procedure/surgery	Abdominal hysterectomy under general anesthesia.
Description of procedure/surgery	Removal of uterus only through an incision in the abdominal wall at the top of the pubic hairline, done while unconscious.
Person performing the procedure/surgery	Dr. Richard Jones assisted by Dr. William Smith.
Benefits of procedure/surgery	To remove uterus with fibroids and stop excessive bleeding. Abdominal route is necessary due to anticipated adhesions from prior abdominal surgery.
Potential risks and adverse effects of procedure/surgery	Risks of hemorrhage and infection from surgery, risks of excessive sedation and allergic reaction to drugs used with general anesthesia, accidental damage to bladder, intestines, and/or nerves controlling these organs.
Approximate length of time for procedure/surgery	About 1 hour; 1 to 2 hours in recovery room.
Approximate length of time needed for recovery	3 to 4 days on surgical unit; 4 to 6 weeks before resuming physically stressful work.
Alternative treatments	Removal of uterus vaginally, radiation to shrink fibroids.
Consequences of refusing treatment	Continuation of pain and vaginal bleeding, risk for developing anemia. After menopause, fibroids should regress.

upheld nor should they be routinely suspended during anesthesia and surgery. A patient's physicians are responsible for discussing and documenting issues with the patient and/or family to determine whether to maintain the DNR order or whether it should be partially or completely suspended during surgery. This discussion should describe potential resuscitation efforts that may be required during surgery and whether withholding resuscitation initiatives would alter the patient's goals for having the surgery. Considerations that should be included in the discussion are the goals of the surgical treatment, the possibility of resuscitative measures, a description of what these measures include, and possible outcomes with and without resuscitation. If the patient has opted to alter the DNR order during the intraoperative period, clear documentation should be in the medical record indicating when the DNR order is to be reinstated (AORN, 2007d).

Another aspect of maintaining safety is to minimize risk for patient injury due to falls. Patient activity is typically restricted after administration of preoperative sedatives. You must complete the preoperative checklist (Fig. 36-2) to ensure that all procedures have been carried out and all necessary information and documentation for safe delivery of care is in the patient's chart.

The risks for postoperative complications are decreased in a number of ways, some of which are specific to the type of procedure. For example, any patient with a surgical incision of the thorax or abdomen will have pain postoperatively, and this reduces lung expansion. The patient will be encouraged to learn how to use an incentive spirometer to reduce the incidence of atelectasis postoperatively. Deep breathing and coughing exercises are examples of other procedures used to reduce complications.

Food and fluids are routinely withheld for a period of time preoperatively. Practice guidelines for preoperative fasting in healthy patients undergoing elective procedures allow for the consumption of clear liquids up to 2 hours before surgery, a light breakfast (e.g., tea and toast) 6 hours before the procedure, and a heavier meal 8 hours beforehand (Baril and others, 2007; Stuart, 2006). Each patient should have orders written by anesthesia personnel outlining preoperative fasting requirements. In general, food and fluids are withheld for 4 to 8 hours before surgery requiring general anesthesia to minimize the risk for aspiration. The patient may need to be NPO even when spinal or epidural anesthesia is administered. Hypotension due to autonomic nervous system blockade can induce nausea and vomiting (Lewis and others, 2007). Patients who are dehydrated or are at risk for hypovolemia will have intravenous (IV) fluids ordered. Medications may be given to decrease respiratory and gastrointestinal (GI) secretions, as an adjunct to anesthesia, and to decrease the risk for infection and development of stress ulcers.

The type of surgery determines the preparation required preoperatively; for example, low-residue and clear liquid diets, enemas, cathartics, and oral antibiotics are for patients who undergo bowel surgery. Povidone-iodine douches are used for many gynecological procedures.

Encourage patients who smoke to stop the use of all tobacco products for at least 30 days before surgery. Nicotine delays wound healing and increases the risk for wound infection by constricting blood flow (Moller and others, 2006). Patients whose blood work indicates a low hemoglobin level and/or abnormal electrolyte levels or coagulopathies often require inpatient therapy before surgery.

Because many patients are admitted on the day of surgery, much of the preoperative preparation is often the responsibility of the patient or the primary caregiver. Therefore it is important that there is a preadmission nurse or nurse in the surgeon's practice to provide adequate instructions. Patient teaching should include any food and fluid restrictions, which medications, if any, are permitted on the morning of surgery, and the need for surgical site preparation the evening before surgery. It is also important to include action a patient will need to take if any of these instructions are mistakenly omitted. Written instructions are a useful adjunct to teaching because a patient and/or family can refer to them for any points that are unclear or forgotten. Videos and pamphlets are also useful adjuncts in preparing patients and their families.

In 2003 The Joint Commission (2003ab) implemented the Universal Protocol for Preventing Wrong Site, Wrong Procedure, Wrong Person Surgery. This protocol was implemented as an added safety measure to ensure the correct person, procedure, and surgical site are verified at the time of scheduling the procedure, upon admission or entry into the facility, and each time the responsibility for care of the patient is transferred to another caregiver. A final verification check occurs immediately before the start of the procedure involving the entire surgical team. If the case involves laterality (right versus left), multiple structures (e.g., fingers, toes, lesions) or multiple levels (e.g., spine), then the final verification should include a site marking by the person performing the procedure. The site markings need to be visible after the patient has been prepared and draped. Involve patients in this process when they are awake and aware if possible. Immediately before starting the procedure a "time out" is called. The entire operative team, using active communication, verifies the correct patient identity, correct side and site, agreement on the procedure to be done, correct patient position, and availability of correct implants and any special equipment or special requirements. This final verification process should be documented.

Delegation Considerations

The skills of assessment and teaching cannot be delegated to nursing assistive personnel (NAP). The nurse directs the NAP to:
- Maintain unique precautions needed for the assigned patient.
- Administer an enema or a douche (as necessary).
- Apply antiembolism stockings.
- Assist patients in removing clothing, jewelry, and prostheses.

Equipment

- ❑ Stethoscope
- ❑ Informed consent form
- ❑ Preoperative checklist
- ❑ Enema set and prescribed solution (if ordered—see Chapter 34)
- ❑ Douche set and prescribed solution (if ordered)
- ❑ Intravenous (IV) solutions and equipment (if ordered—see Chapter 31)
- ❑ Indwelling catheter set (if ordered—see Chapter 33)
- ❑ Antiembolism stockings and/or Intermittent pneumatic compression device (if ordered—see Chapter 10)
- ❑ Medications (if ordered—see Chapter 20)

A-1c4 NURSE'S DETAILED PERIOPERATIVE NOTE

DATE

HOSP. #

NAME

BIRTH DATE

ADDRESS

SS#

IF NOT IMPRINTED, PLEASE PRINT DATE, HOSP. #, NAME AND LOCATION

1. Place initials in the space preceding the appropriate response (YES/NO, MET/NOT MET, NOT APPLICABLE)
2. Explain any "NO" or "NOT MET" in the space provided adjacent to the item or in the comment section provided, except for * items.
3. Record additional information in the comment section.
4. Record initials immediately following narrative entry.

PERIOPERATIVE TRANSPORT BY:	METHOD:	PREOPERATIVE UNIT/AREA:
TIME RECEIVED IN PRESURGICAL CARE UNIT:	TIME RECEIVED IN OR:	

PATIENT ASSESSMENT/PREPARATION	YES	NO	COMMENT
PATIENT IDENTIFIED			ID Band Location
BLOOD BAND PRESENT*			#/Location
ALLERGIES* (If yes, please list)			
LATEX PRECAUTIONS INDICATED*			
CONSENT			
NPO			
HEALTH CHANGED SINCE LAST APPT			If Yes, Specify: Physician Notified:
INFECTIONS, PROBLEMS WITH HEART OR LUNGS			If Yes, Specify: Physician Notified:
TAKING ANY NEW MEDICATIONS			If Yes, Specify: Physician Notified:
PREOPERATIVE ORDERS COMPLETED			
SKIN ASSESSMENT COMPLETED			
VITALS OBTAINED DAY OF SURGERY			
HISTORY AND PHYSICAL PRESENT			
LAB VALUES REVIEWED			
LEVEL OF CONSCIOUSNESS—Answers questions/responds appropriately for age			
IMPLANTS/PROSTHESIS* (If yes, please list)			

Preoperative pain score (0–10)
Surgical site verified and marked with patient □
Patient voided @ _____ Belongings:
Nursing comments

NURSING DIAGNOSIS	NURSING ORDERS/INTERVENTIONS	EXPECTED PATIENT OUTCOMES
ANXIETY—Risk of, Related to Surgical Intervention and Outcomes	1. Psychologic & physiologic comfort measures are provided. ___ Yes ___ No	The patient reports and/or demonstrates a reduction in anxiety. ___ MET ___ NOT MET
KNOWLEDGE DEFICIT—Risk of, Related to Surgical Intervention	1. The patient's understanding is assessed and questions/concerns are addressed by the appropriate individuals. ___ Yes ___No	The patient's (guardian's) description of surgery corresponds with the Operative Consent (G-2d). ___ MET ___ NOT MET
INJURY—Risk for, Related to Tubes, Catheters, Lines ___ Not Applicable	1. Integrity of tubes, catheters, and lines is maintained. ___Yes ___ No Catheters/Tubes/Drains/Lines:	The patient's risk for injury related to care and management of tubes, catheters, and lines is minimized. ___ MET ___ NOT MET

Initials	Standards Implemented By:	Initials	Standards Implemented By:

26304/9-01/MH05859   **UNIVERSITY OF IOWA HOSPITALS AND CLINICS**

Side tab labels: A -1c4 / B CLIN. NOTES / C LABORATORY / D X-RAY EXAM / E CONSULTATION / F SPEC. EXAM / G THERAPY / H PATHOLOGY / I PT. QUES.

FIG 36-2   Preoperative assessment form. (*Courtesy University of Iowa Hospitals and Clinics.*)

STEP	RATIONALE

ASSESSMENT

1 Correctly identify patient by having patient state (if able) name and a second patient identifier (verify agency policy regarding identifiers to use, such as date of birth or patient registration number). Verify correct information on identification band.

Ensures correct patient. You need to use two distinct identifiers to verify correct patient identification (The Joint Commission [TJC], 2008).

2 Determine ability of patient to answer questions regarding health history and pending surgery.

Identifies reliability of patient and need to supplement with information from family members or significant others. Indicates need for further information for informed consent.

3 Collect nursing history, and identify risk factors (Table 36-2, p. 946) (see Chapter 6).

Allows for anticipation of possible complications and planning for interventions to reduce risks. Allergies, particularly to latex, can be life threatening.

Critical Decision Point   *If patient is having emergency surgery, focus on assessment of primary body system affected.*

4 Perform physical examination (Table 36-2 and Chapter 6). Focus on body systems surgery will affect.

Provides baseline data for future assessments and interventions. Also confirms or disputes information from history and may uncover new information.

5 Apply allergy/sensitivity band, and other safety bands if applicable.

Alerts health care providers to potential safety issues such as patient's allergies and sensitivities, risk for falls, presence of obstructive sleep apnea or other conditions.

6 Ask about patient's and family members' expectations of surgery and care. Include questions concerning fears, cultural practices, and religious beliefs if applicable.

Allows you to anticipate patient's/family's priorities and to adapt plan so that you can give appropriate instruction and support.

7 Review patient's preoperative orders.

Identifies specific procedures and diagnostic tests and medications patient will receive.

8 If patient is same-day admit or ambulatory patient, validate that preoperative preparations were completed as ordered. Specific preparations to review include NPO status, administration of medications, skin preparation, and bowel preparation if applicable.

Failure to complete preparation could lead to perioperative or postoperative complications and may necessitate the postponement or cancellation of surgery.

9 Ask if patient has an advance directive. If so, place it in patient's record.

Document conveys patient's wishes if life support measures are necessary.

NURSING DIAGNOSES

- Acute pain
- Anxiety
- Deficient knowledge regarding the surgical experience
- Fear
- Impaired gas exchange

- Impaired oral mucous membrane
- Impaired physical mobility
- Ineffective airway clearance
- Ineffective breathing pattern
- Ineffective tissue perfusion
- Risk for aspiration

- Risk for disturbed body image
- Risk for impaired skin integrity
- Risk for infection
- Risk for perioperative-positioning injury

Individualize related factors based on patient's condition or needs.

PLANNING

1 Expected outcomes following completion of procedure:
   - Patient can state what surgical procedure is being performed and risks and benefits of surgery.

   Identifies readiness to sign informed consent.

   - Patient participates in preoperative and postoperative care.

   Preoperative preparations are effective.

   - Patient states anxiety is decreased.

   Anxiety interferes with effectiveness of teaching and anesthesia.

2 Prepare patient's chart using preoperative checklist, and assemble equipment as needed.

Ensures that all preoperative procedures will be completed.

3 Explain procedures, and allow patient, family members, and significant others to ask questions and express concerns.

Decreases anxiety and increases cooperation.

STEP	RATIONALE

IMPLEMENTATION

1 Orient patient to room or presurgical (holding) area.

Decreases anxiety and promotes feelings of control.

2 Physician obtains informed consent. Act as patient advocate as needed; include considering any culturally sensitive issues. Witness form if allowed by agency.

Surgery cannot be legally performed without informed consent. Patient must receive information about need and extent of the surgery, alternatives, risks, and benefits. Patient and/or family may be afraid to ask questions or express concerns regarding diverse practices.

Critical Decision Point   *Patients who are illiterate can sign with a mark if properly witnessed. Minors, unless married or declared emancipated, and individuals considered incompetent cannot legally sign a consent form. Parent or legal guardian must provide consent. Some cultures do not allow female members to give consent. Refer to institutional protocol for implementing informed consent.*

3 Check medical record, and review or complete preoperative checklist (see Fig. 36-2).

Ensures that pertinent laboratory and diagnostic test results are available and that all preoperative preparations are completed.

4 Provide preoperative teaching, including explanation of postoperative exercises (see Skill 36-2), skin preparation, pain-control measures (see Chapter 15), and postoperative care in recovery room and nursing division (see Skill 36-3).

Decreases anxiety and promotes cooperation in care.

Critical Decision Point   *Patient may brush teeth but should not swallow water. Patient may take oral medications with sips of water (30 mL) if they are specially ordered to be taken preoperatively (e.g., antiarrhythmic or seizure medications). Withhold all other oral medications. You must later check postoperative orders to ensure that scheduled medications unrelated to surgery are not forgotten.*

5 Assess that any preoperative orders for enemas, douches, and skin preparations have been followed. Insert IV and/or indwelling catheter if ordered.

May delay or postpone surgery if not completed. IV and/or indwelling catheter may be inserted in holding or preanesthesia area.

6 Provide for hygiene measures, ensuring patient privacy. Instruct patient to remove all clothing, including undergarments, and to apply disposable cap and hospital gown with opening in back.

Prevents patient's hair from contaminating sterile surfaces and provides easy access to patient's body in OR.

7 Instruct patient to remove hairpins, clips, wigs, hairpieces, jewelry, including rings used in body piercing, and makeup (including nail polish and acrylic nails). Religious medals may be pinned to gown if agency policy permits. Some institutions allow you to remove acrylic nails or nail polish from only one finger if using a pulse oximeter. Check institution's policy.

Hair appliances and jewelry anywhere on the body may become dislodged and cause injury during positioning and intubation. Rings decrease circulation in fingers. Makeup, nail polish, and false nails impede assessment of skin and oxygenation. In addition, acrylic nails harbor pathogenic organisms (AORN, 2007a).

Critical Decision Point   *Tape wedding rings that cannot be removed. Be careful not to create tourniquet effect with tape around finger.*

8 Assist patient in removing prostheses, including dentures and oral appliances, glasses and contact lenses, artificial limbs and eyes, artificial eyelashes, and hearing aids. Inventory items, and give to family members or have security put them in a locked area. Document list of items and their location in preoperative checklist and/or nurses' notes per agency policy.

Prostheses can be lost or damaged during surgery and could cause injury. Oral appliances may occlude airway.

Critical Decision Point   *If patient needs to follow instructions in the OR, leave hearing aid in place. Decision may be made to leave wig or dentures in place until entering OR suite if removal will cause embarrassment. Check agency policy.*

9 Secure all valuables, or give to family member or significant other. Have release form signed if required by agency.

Valuables left in patient's room may be lost or stolen.

10 Apply antiembolism stockings as ordered (see Chapter 10).

Promotes venous return and reduces risk for thrombus formation.

11 Assess vital signs immediately before going to OR.

Abnormal vital signs indicate conditions that increase risk for surgery.

Critical Decision Point   *Report vital signs not within normal range or patient's baseline to physician. These results may require surgery to be postponed. Document abnormal vital signs and any action taken in nurses' notes and/or preoperative checklist according to agency policy.*

STEP	RATIONALE
12 If patient does not have an indwelling catheter, assist him or her in voiding before receiving preoperative medication.	Prevents incontinence and bladder distention during surgery and urinary retention with overflow postoperatively. Preoperative medication causes drowsiness and decreased voiding sensation.
13 Administer preoperative medications as ordered. (These medications may be given in preoperative or holding area. Check preoperative orders.)	Reduces pain, anxiety, respiratory secretions, and amount of anesthesia required. Promotes relaxation. Antibiotics may be ordered prophylactically but are given within 30 to 60 minutes of incision.

Critical Decision Point *Check that informed consent is signed before giving preoperative medications. Times on consent form and on medication administration record (MAR) must attest to this. Preoperative medications may alter level of consciousness and make the consent invalid.*

STEP	RATIONALE
14 Patient is placed on bed rest with call light within reach and is told not to get out of bed without assistance. Allow family members to remain at bedside until patient is transferred to surgical area. Maintain quiet and relaxing environment.	There is an increased chance of injury in attempting to ambulate to void when patient is sedated and unattended.

EVALUATION

1 Have patient describe surgical procedure and its benefits and risks.	Confirms level of knowledge needed to sign informed consent.
2 Compare all assessment data with patient's baseline and expected normal levels.	Evaluates patient's risk for complications and possible need to postpone surgery.
3 Have patient repeat preoperative instructions and demonstrate postoperative exercises.	Provides evidence that patient understands preoperative instructions and can perform exercises.
4 Monitor patient for signs and symptoms of anxiety, and ask how patient and family are feeling.	Increased heart rate and blood pressure, dilated pupils, dry mouth, increased sweating, and muscle rigidity or shaking are responses to stress and anxiety. Asking patient about feelings gives permission to express concerns, which can be further explored.

Unexpected Outcomes	Related Interventions
1 Patient is unable to give consent, and family member is unavailable.	• In emergency situations, obtain telephone consent from next of kin. Two persons must witness oral consent. • Documentation must include explanation of situation and fact that oral consent was obtained and witnessed. • At the earliest opportunity, person giving oral consent must sign a written consent. Signed telegram or signed fax may also be considered oral consent. Follow agency policy.
2 Vital signs are above or below patient's baseline or expected range.	• This indicates possible infection, anxiety, pain, or cardiovascular dysfunction, which increases surgical risk. • Patients who are dehydrated or malnourished may require hydration with IV solutions (see Chapter 28), parenteral nutrition (see Chapter 32), or antibiotic therapy before surgery.
3 Informed consent has not been signed and witnessed. Physician did not provide information and/or ensure that consent form was signed.	• Patient is not ready for surgery. Patient must sign consent before administration of preoperative medications or any medication that alters central nervous system. Notify physician/surgeon.
4 Patient did not remain NPO, which may indicate that the patient did not understand instructions or forgot.	• Notify surgeon and anesthesiologist. Surgery may be postponed or cancelled.
5 Patient is unable to state instructions or demonstrate postoperative exercises.	• Assessment of patient's level of understanding or method of instruction was insufficient. Revision of instruction and reteaching is necessary.
6 Patient did not void before receiving preoperative medication.	• Patient did not need to void or was unable to void. Assess for bladder distention. If distended, have patient use urinal or bedpan, or you may need order for catheterization (see Chapter 33).

Recording and Reporting

- Document all preoperative preparations in nurses' notes and/or checklist.
- Document patient's condition on transfer to OR in nurses' notes and/or on flow sheet.
- Document presence of any allergies/sensitivities on armband, in medical record, and in medication administration record.
- Record disposition of patient valuables/belongings (i.e., whether locked up according to agency policy or sent with family).
- Report and record any abnormal assessment findings, lack of signed and witnessed consent form, or failure of patient to maintain NPO status and action taken.
- Report and record patient's cultural practices and/or religious beliefs that affect perioperative care and any modification of care planned.

Teaching Considerations

- The Joint Commission patient and family education standards are guidelines to ensure that patient, family member, and/or primary caregiver know about surgical procedure, healing process, sutures, dressing, drains, feeding tubes, pain control, and diet with rationale for each. Adults learn best when they understand the purpose or meaning of what is being taught (TJC, 2008).

Pediatric Considerations

- Involve parents in preoperative preparation to decrease children's anxiety. Preadmission programs to prepare parents and children for same-day surgery have been shown to decrease anxiety in both parents and children. Part of preoperative teaching needs to include giving children the opportunity to handle equipment they will see, such as an anesthesia mask or drainage tube.
- Take the developmental level of child into consideration during preoperative preparation. Use toys and games to demonstrate preoperative procedures (Hockenberry and Wilson, 2007).
- Allow parents to accompany their child to the holding area.

Gerontological Considerations

- Physiological changes that occur with aging may require admission to hospital before surgery for additional diagnostic tests and stabilization of condition (Table 36-3).
- Focus on wellness and the person's strength.
- Teach when patient is alert and rested. Keep teaching sessions short.
- Age-related changes such as decreased vision, hearing, and short-term memory may require presence of family members or primary caregiver during preoperative preparation.

Home Care Considerations

- Instruct patients admitted on day of surgery about NPO status, skin preparation, and procedures such as enemas and douches before admission. Patients often use enemas or douches at home.
- Patients having surgery performed in ambulatory surgery centers must be accompanied by a family member or friend to allow for discharge after the procedure (Box 36-2).

TABLE 36-2	Assessment of the Surgical Patient
Assessment Category	**Key Criteria**
Nursing history	Previous personal/family experience with surgery (e.g., complications) and anesthesia (e.g., malignant hyperthermia)
Physical examination	General system review: • Head and neck • Integument • Thorax and lungs • Heart and vascular • Abdomen • Neurological status • Age • Nutrition • Radiotherapy, chemotherapy, medications that depress immune system • Fluid and electrolyte balance • Preexisting infection • Chronic respiratory disease (emphysema, bronchitis, asthma) • Immunological disorders (leukemia, acquired immunodeficiency syndrome) • Allergies/sensitivities (including medications, food, latex, and environmental)
Risk factors	Medication history (prescription, over-the counter [OTC], and herbal remedies) Physical or mental impairments Mobility limitations Prostheses (including hearing aids) Smoking habits Alcohol ingestion Family support and coping mechanisms Occupation Emotional health Temperature, blood pressure, pulse and respiratory rates Height and weight Oxygen saturations Electrocardiogram Laboratory values (e.g., Hgb, K^+, glucose, coagulation studies) Radiology and diagnostic test findings

TABLE 36-3 | Physiological Factors That Place Older Adult Patients at Risk for Surgery

Alterations	Surgery Risks	Nursing Implications
Cardiovascular		
Degenerative change in myocardium and valves Rigidity of arterial walls and reduction in sympathetic and parasympathetic innervation to heart Increase in calcium and cholesterol deposits within small arteries; arterial walls thickened	Reduced cardiac reserve. Predisposes patient to postoperative hemorrhage and rise in systolic and diastolic blood pressure. Predisposes patient to clot formation in lower extremities.	Assess baseline vital signs. Maintain adequate fluid balance to minimize stress to the heart. Ensure blood pressure is adequate to meet circulatory demands. Instruct patient in techniques for performing leg exercises and proper turning. Apply antiembolism stockings, sequential compression devices (SCDs) (see Chapter 10).
Integumentary System		
Decreased subcutaneous tissue and increased fragility of skin	Prone to pressure ulcers and skin tears.	Assess skin every 4 hours; pad all bony prominences during surgery. Turn or reposition (see Chapter 9).
Pulmonary		
Rib cage stiffens and enlarges Reduced diaphragm excursion Lung tissue less distensible; alveoli enlarged	Reduced vital capacity. Greater residual capacity or volume of air left in lung after normal breath increases, reducing amount of new air brought into lungs with each inspiration. Reduced blood oxygenation.	Instruct patient in proper technique for coughing and deep breathing exercises and use of spirometer. Encourage deep breathing. Use incentive spirometer to enhance exhalation. Assess oxygen saturation via oximetry (SpO_2).
Renal		
Reduced blood flow to kidneys Reduced glomerular filtration rate and excretory times Reduced bladder capacity	Blood loss causes a decrease in circulation to the kidney. Limits ability to remove drugs or toxic substances. Voiding frequency increases, and larger amount of urine stays in the bladder after voiding. Sensation of need to void may not occur until bladder is filled.	Monitor urinary output and laboratory data (i.e., blood urea nitrogen [BUN], creatinine). Assess for adverse effects of medications. Instruct patient to notify nurse immediately when sensation of bladder fullness develops. Keep call light or bedpan within easy reach.
Neurological		
Sensory losses, including reduced tactile sense, increased pain tolerance Decreased reaction time	Patient less able to respond to early warning signs of surgical complications. Patient becomes confused easily after anesthesia.	Inspect bony prominences for signs of pressure. Orient patient to surrounding environment. Observe for nonverbal signs of pain. Maintain safe environment. Institute fall precautions.
Metabolic		
Lower basal metabolic rate Reduced number of red blood cells and hemoglobin levels Change in total amounts of body potassium and water volume	Reduced total oxygen consumption and nutritional needs. Reduces ability to carry adequate oxygen to tissues. Greater risk for fluid or electrolyte imbalance.	Ensure adequate nutritional intake once diet is resumed. Administer necessary blood products. Assess for adequacy of oxygenation, fatigue, and infection. Monitor electrolyte levels.

BOX 36-2 | Postanesthesia and Ambulatory Surgery Discharge Criteria

Postanesthesia Discharge Criteria
- Patient awake (or returns to baseline)
- Vital signs stable
- No excess bleeding or drainage
- No respiratory depression
- SaO_2 greater than 90%
- Pain controlled
- Report given

Ambulatory Surgery Discharge Criteria
- All postanesthesia care unit (PACU) discharge criteria met
- No intravenous (IV) narcotics for last 30 minutes
- Minimal nausea and vomiting
- Pain controlled
- Voided (if appropriate to surgical procedure/orders)
- Able to ambulate if age-appropriate and not contraindicated
- Responsible adult present to accompany patient
- Discharge instructions given and understood

SKILL 36-2 Demonstrating Postoperative Exercises

Intermediate / Preoperative Nursing Care / Teaching About Postoperative Exercises and Pain Management Promoting Family Support and Participation

Structured preoperative teaching has a positive influence on a surgical patient's recovery (Lewis and others, 2007). You will provide information and teach skills to help patients understand the surgical experience and participate actively in the recovery process. The skills of coughing, deep breathing, turning, and use of an incentive spirometer are important in preventing circulatory and respiratory postoperative complications.

In the past, teaching occurred the evening before surgery when patients were most anxious. As a result of cost reduction efforts, many patients are admitted to the hospital or ambulatory surgery center the day of surgery. Preoperative teaching is not highly effective at this time because of the patient's high anxiety level. Many health care institutions have developed comprehensive outpatient patient education programs to better enable patients to receive the knowledge and skills needed to participate in their own care before coming to the hospital or ambulatory care center. Teaching booklets and videotapes are often available to supplement any instruction a nurse provides.

Postoperative exercises include diaphragmatic breathing and effective coughing, turning, and leg exercises. You can also use an incentive spirometer, a device that provides visual feedback for incentive spirometry, to encourage voluntary deep breathing (see Chapter 23, Skill 23-3). The physician may order incentive spirometry for patients especially at risk for atelectasis or pneumonia (e.g., chronic smokers or patients on prolonged bed rest). During the discussion of these exercises, you will explain the relationship between the exercises and the physiological principles that make them important. Through specific explanations and guided practice you will help develop patient commitment to the recovery process. Demonstrate the exercises, and then continue to coach the patient through several return practice sessions.

Whenever possible, include family members or other significant persons in the practice sessions. Frequently these individuals are with the patient during the postoperative period and can thus serve as coaches. You will also provide patients with information about the sensations typically experienced after surgery, such as incisional pain, nausea, tightness of dressings, and what interventions will alleviate them. The information helps patients interpret realistically the events that occur in the postoperative period. As a result, patients are able to decrease anxiety, conserve their energy, and attend to performing the exercises that assist in their recovery.

A potential postoperative complication is venous thromboembolism, including deep vein thrombosis and pulmonary embolism. Approximately 10% of hospital deaths are attributed to PE (MacDougall and others, 2006). One of the simplest ways to prevent the formation of DVT is to encourage and assist the patient in early ambulation and leg exercises. When this is not possible or the patient's age, past history, or surgical procedure place him or her at an increased risk, use additional devices to help prevent the formation of DVT. Compression stockings are frequently applied before surgery and remain on patients until they are able to fully ambulate. Intermittent pneumatic compression devices are also frequently used on surgical patients (see Chapter 10). These devices compress the leg and increase venous

flow, thereby decreasing venous pooling and stasis. Another device used in the prevention of DVT is the venous plexus foot pump (Fig. 36-3). This pump mimics the natural action of walking by intermittently compressing the sole of the foot and then relaxing it, so the venous plexus can fill with blood. Neither the intermittent pneumatic compression device nor the venous plexus foot pump should be used on patients with an acute DVT, significant peripheral vascular ischemia, large open wounds or skin grafts, or cancer of the extremity. None of these devices should replace the need for early and frequent ambulation.

Delegation Considerations

The skill of teaching postoperative exercises cannot be delegated to NAP. The NAP can reinforce and assist patients in performing postoperative exercises. The nurse directs the NAP about:
- Maintaining precautions unique to a particular patient.
- When to report if the patient is unable or unwilling to perform the exercises correctly.

Equipment

- ❑ Pillow (*optional;* used to splint the incision when coughing to reduce discomfort)
- ❑ Incentive spirometer
- ❑ Positive expiratory pressure (PEP) device
- ❑ Stethoscope

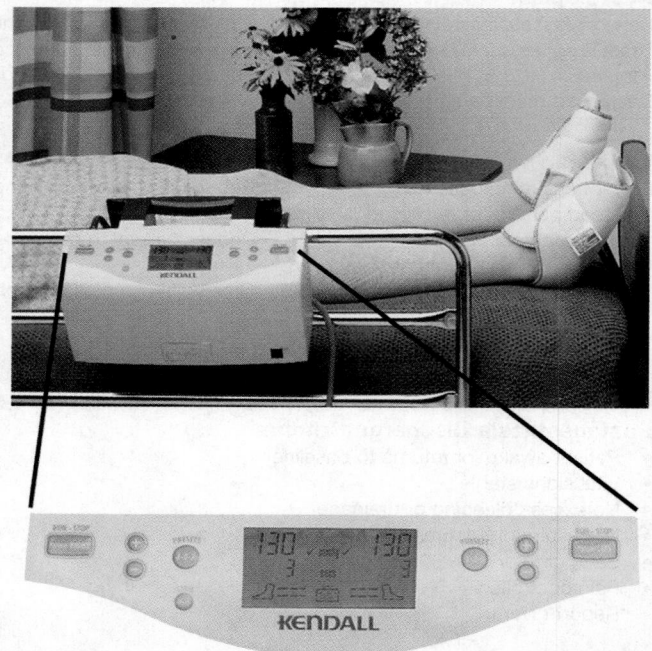

FIG 36-3 Venous plexus foot pump with bedside controls. (*Courtesy Tyco Healthcare Group LP.*)

STEP	RATIONALE

ASSESSMENT

1 Assess patient's risk for postoperative respiratory complications: identify presence of chronic pulmonary condition (e.g., emphysema, chronic bronchitis, asthma); any condition that affects chest wall movement, such as obesity, advanced pregnancy, thoracic or abdominal surgery; history of smoking; and presence of reduced hemoglobin level.

General anesthesia predisposes patient to respiratory problems because lungs are not fully inflated during surgery, cough reflex is suppressed, and mucus collects within airway passages. Postoperatively, inadequate lung expansion can lead to atelectasis and pneumonia. Chronic lung conditions create greater risk for developing respiratory complications. Smoking damages ciliary clearance and increases mucus secretion. A reduced hemoglobin level can lead to reduced oxygen delivery.

Critical Decision Point   *Assess and report to physician and/or anesthesiologist if patient has had a cold or upper respiratory infection within past week.*

2 Auscultate lungs.

Establishes baseline for postoperative comparison.

3 Assess patient's ability to deep breathe and cough by placing hand on patient's abdomen, having patient take a deep breath, and observing movement of shoulders, chest wall, and abdomen. Measure chest excursion during a deep breath (see Chapter 6). Ask patient to cough into tissue after taking a deep breath.

Reveals maximum potential for chest expansion and ability to cough forcefully; serves as baseline to measure patient's ability to perform exercises postoperatively. Diaphragmatic breathing allows for complete lung expansion and improved ventilation and increases blood oxygenation. Deep breathing also allows air to pass by partially obstructing mucous plugs, thus increasing force with which to expel mucous plug. Coughing loosens secretions and helps to remove them from pulmonary alveoli and bronchi.

4 Assess patient's risk for postoperative thrombus formation. (Older adults, immobilized patients, patients with personal or family history of clots, and women over 35 who smoke and are taking birth control pills are most at risk.) Observe the calves for redness, swelling, warmth, and tenderness. Palpate pedal pulses. Check for a Homans' sign, calf pain on dorsiflexion of the foot (which may or may not be present) (see Chapter 6, Skill 6-6). Calf pain is usually unilateral. Compare legs for bilateral equality.

Following general anesthesia, circulation slows, causing a greater tendency for clot formation. Immobilization results in decreased muscular contraction in lower extremities, which promotes venous stasis. The physical stress of surgery creates a hypercoagulable state in most individuals. Manipulation and positioning during surgery may inadvertently cause trauma to leg veins.

Critical Decision Point   *Homans' sign is not always present when a deep vein thrombosis exists (Kneale, 2005). Checking for Homans' sign is contraindicated in a suspected DVT because some researchers think that vigorous dorsiflexion may dislodge a thrombus. If you suspect a thrombus, notify physician and refrain from manipulating extremity any further. Surgery will usually be postponed. Antiembolism stockings or pneumatic compression cuffs may be ordered for patients at risk for thrombus formation (see Chapter 10).*

5 Assess patient's ability to move independently while in bed.

Patients confined to bed rest, even for limited periods, will need to turn regularly. Determines existence of any mobility restrictions.

6 Assess patient's willingness and capability to learn exercises; note factors such as attention span, anxiety level, level of consciousness, language skills, and level of pain, if any.

Capacity to learn depends on readiness, ability, and learning environment.

Critical Decision Point   *Highly anxious patients or those in severe pain have difficulty learning and performing postoperative exercises.*

7 Assess family member's or significant other's willingness to learn and to support patient postoperatively.

Family's or significant other's presence postoperatively can be a potential motivating factor for patient's recovery; a family member or significant other can coach patient on exercise performance.

8 Assess patient's medical orders preoperatively and postoperatively.

Requires adaptations in way patient performs exercises.

NURSING DIAGNOSES

- Acute pain
- Impaired gas exchange
- Impaired memory

- Impaired physical mobility
- Ineffective airway clearance
- Ineffective breathing pattern

- Ineffective tissue perfusion
- Risk for impaired skin integrity
- Risk for infection

Individualize related factors based on patient's condition or needs.

STEP	RATIONALE

PLANNING

1 Expected outcomes following completion of procedure:
- Patient is able to correctly deep breathe, use incentive spirometer, cough, turn, and perform leg exercises throughout postoperative period.

Patient's ability to perform exercises reduces risk for postoperative complications.

- Postoperatively, chest excursion meets or exceeds preoperative level.

Turning, deep breathing, and coughing exercises help patient maintain full lung expansion and clear airways postoperatively.

- Lungs are clear upon auscultation both preoperatively and postoperatively.

Absence of secretions reduces risk for postoperative pneumonia.

- No redness, warmth, or tenderness in lower extremities; pedal pulses palpable.

Leg exercises prevent the occurrence of circulatory and mobility problems postoperatively.

- Patient initiates exercises spontaneously.

Patient values importance of exercises to recovery.

2 Prepare equipment as needed.

3 Prepare room for teaching.

Quiet, private area free from distractions enhances patient's ability to learn.

IMPLEMENTATION

1 Teach diaphragmatic breathing:

  a Assist patient to comfortable sitting or standing position. If patient chooses to sit, raise head of bed to semi-Fowler's or Fowler's position, assist to side of bed or to upright position in chair. If patient is sitting in a chair, knees should be at or higher than hips. Use stool if necessary.

Upright position facilitates diaphragmatic excursion by using gravity to keep abdominal contents away from diaphragm. Prevents tension on abdominal muscles, which allows for greater diaphragmatic excursion.

Critical Decision Point *Postoperatively patient can usually be positioned upright with head of bed elevated. If patient must remain flat in bed, stress that exercises can still be performed.*

  b Stand or sit facing patient.

Patient will be able to observe breathing exercises performed by nurse.

  c Instruct patient to place palms of hands across from each other along lower borders of anterior rib cage; place tips of third finger lightly together. Demonstrate for patient.

Position of hands allows patient to feel movement of chest and abdomen as diaphragm descends and lungs expand inside chest wall.

  d Have patient take slow, deep breaths, inhaling through nose, and pushing abdomen against hands (see illustration). Explain that patient will feel normal downward movement of diaphragm during inspiration. Demonstrate for patient.

Slow, deep breath allows for more complete lung expansion and prevent panting or hyperventilation. Inhaling through nose warms, humidifies, and filters air. Explanation and demonstration focus on normal ventilatory movement of chest. Patient learns to understand how diaphragmatic breathing feels.

  e Avoid using chest and shoulder muscles while inhaling, and instruct patient in same manner.

Using auxiliary chest and shoulder muscles during breathing increases unnecessary energy expenditures and does not promote full lung expansion.

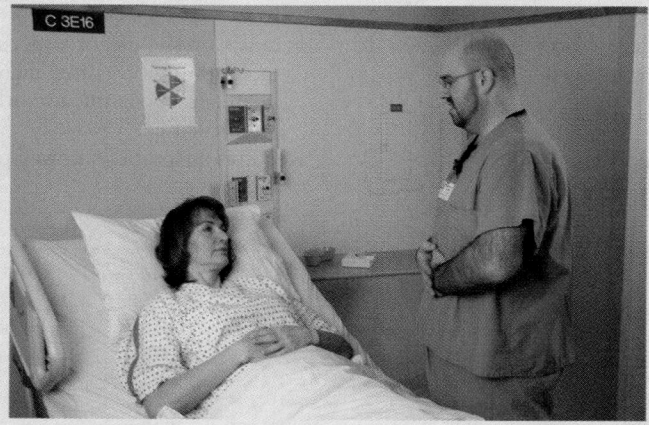

STEP 1d Patient and nurse practice deep breathing.

STEP	RATIONALE
f Take a slow, deep breath and hold for count of three, and then slowly exhale through mouth as if blowing out a candle (pursed lips).	Allows for gradual, controlled expulsion of air.
g Repeat breathing exercise three to five times.	Allows patient to observe slow, rhythmic breathing pattern.
h Have patient practice exercise. Patient is instructed to take 10 slow, deep breaths every 1 hour while awake during postoperative period until mobile. Another option is to have patient use incentive spirometry (see illustration).	Repetition of exercise reinforces learning. Regular deep breathing will prevent or minimize postoperative respiratory complications. Incentive spirometer gives a visual incentive to breathe as deeply as possible.
2 Teach positive expiratory pressure therapy and "huff" coughing:	
a Set positive expiratory pressure device for setting ordered.	Higher settings require more effort.
b Instruct patient to assume semi-Fowler's or high-Fowler's position, and place nose clip on patient's nose (see illustration).	Promotes optimum lung expansion and expectoration of mucus.
c Have patient place lips around mouthpiece. Instruct patient to take a full breath and then exhale 2 or 3 times longer than inhalation. Repeat pattern for 10 to 20 breaths.	Ensures that patient does all breathing through mouth. Ensures that patient uses the device properly.
d Remove device from mouth, and have patient take a slow, deep breath and hold for 3 seconds.	Promotes lung expansion before coughing.
e Instruct patient to exhale in quick, short, forced "huffs."	"Huff" coughing, or forced expiratory technique, promotes bronchial hygiene by increasing expectoration of secretions.
3 Teach controlled coughing:	
a Explain importance of maintaining an upright position.	Position facilitates diaphragm excursion and enhances thorax and abdominal expansion.
b Demonstrate coughing. Take two slow, deep breaths, inhaling through nose and exhaling through (pursed lips) mouth.	Deep breaths expand lungs fully so that air moves behind mucus and facilitates effective coughing.
c Inhale deeply a third time, and hold breath to count of three. Cough fully for two to three consecutive coughs without inhaling between coughs (see illustration, p. 952). (Tell patient to push all air out of lungs.)	Consecutive coughs help remove mucus more effectively and completely than one forceful cough.

Critical Decision Point   *Coughing may be contraindicated after brain, spinal, or eye surgery due to an increase in intracranial pressure.*

STEP	RATIONALE
d Caution patient against just clearing throat instead of coughing deeply.	Clearing throat does not remove mucus from deeper airways.
e If surgical incision is to be either thoracic or abdominal, teach patient to place either hands or a pillow over incisional area and place hands over pillow to splint incision (see illustration, p. 952). During breathing and coughing exercises, press gently against incisional area for splinting and support.	Surgical incision cuts through muscles, tissues, and nerve endings. Deep breathing and coughing exercises place additional stress on suture line and cause discomfort. Splinting incision with hands or pillow provides firm support and reduces incisional pulling and pain.

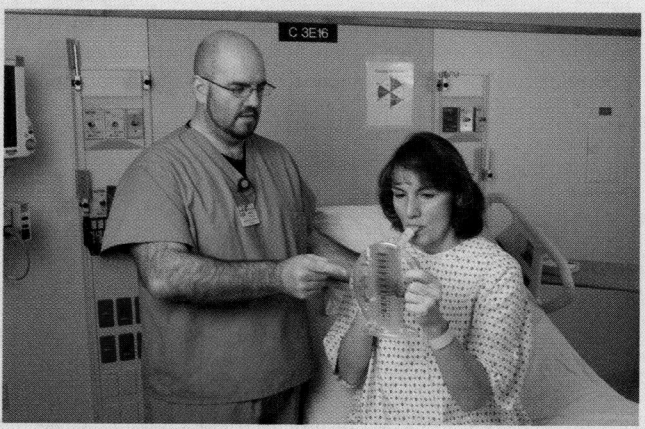

STEP 1h   Patient demonstrates incentive spirometry.

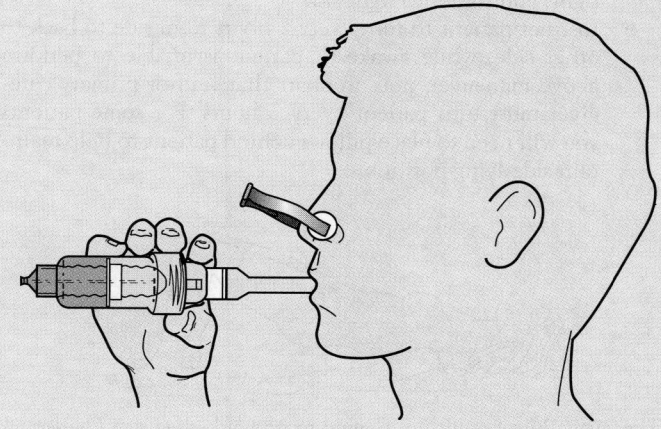

STEP 2b   Diagram of use of positive expiratory pressure device.

STEP	RATIONALE

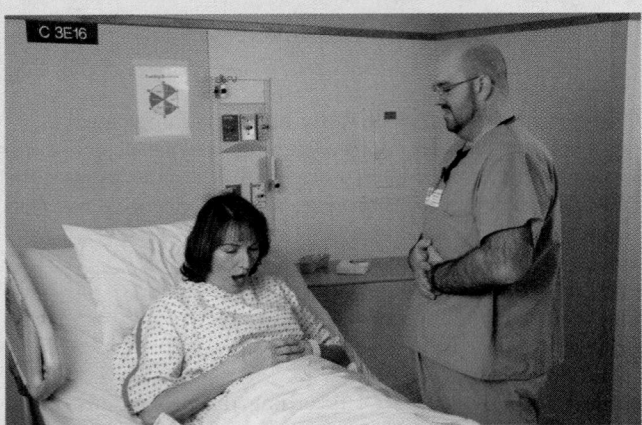

STEP 3c   Deep breathing exercise—placement of hands on upper abdomen during inhalation.

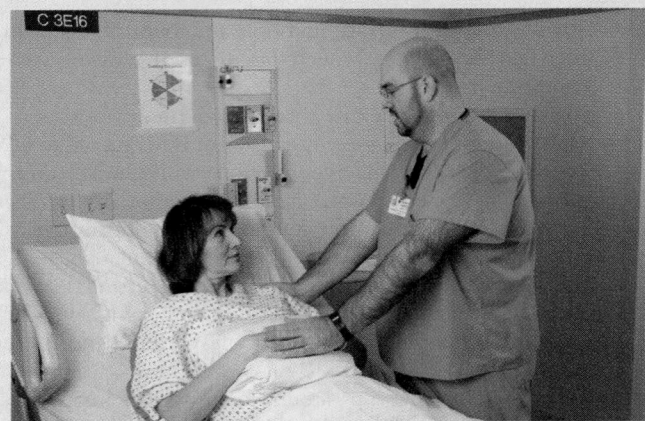

STEP 3e   Patient splinting abdomen with pillow.

f Patient continues to practice coughing exercises, splinting imaginary incision. Instruct the patient to cough two to three times every hour while awake.	Deep coughing with splinting effectively expectorates mucus with minimal discomfort.
g Instruct patient to examine sputum for consistency, odor, amount, and color changes and to notify nurse if any changes are noted.	Sputum consistency, odor, amount, and color changes indicate the presence of a pulmonary complication such as pneumonia.

Critical Decision Point   *For patients with preexisting pulmonary disease, know usual character of mucus to determine if change has occurred.*

4 Teach turning: (*Example:* Turning on right side)	
a Instruct patient to assume supine position and move toward left side of the bed. Patient can do this by bending knees and pressing heels against mattress to raise and move buttocks (see illustration).	Positioning begins in this example on left side of bed so that turning to right side will not cause patient to roll off bed's edge. Buttocks lift prevents shearing force from body moving against sheets.
b Instruct patient to place the right hand or a pillow over incisional area to splint it.	Splinting incision supports and minimizes pulling on suture line during turning.
c Instruct patient to keep right leg straight and flex left knee up (see illustration).	Straight leg stabilizes the patient's position. Flexed left leg shifts weight for easier turning.

Critical Decision Point   *Some patients, such as those who have had back surgery or vascular repair, are restricted from flexing their legs postoperatively. Some patients are restricted from turning or may need assistance for positioning (see Chapter 9).*

d Have patient grab right side rail with left hand, pull toward right, and roll onto right side.	Pulling toward side rail reduces effort needed for turning.
e Instruct patient to turn every 2 hours from side to back to other side, while awake. If patient is unable to perform above maneuver, note in chart that staff or primary caregiver must turn patient every 2 hours. For some patients you will need to place pillows behind patient to help maintain side-lying position.	Reduces risk for vascular complications by contraction of leg muscles around veins to improve venous return. Also reduces pulmonary complications by shifting mucus to prevent consolidation.

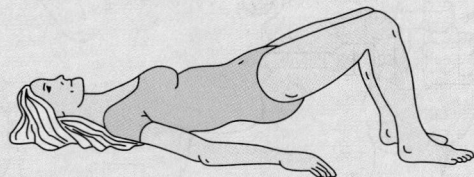

STEP 4a   Buttocks lift for moving to side of bed. (*From Lowdermilk D, Perry S: Maternity nursing, ed 7, St. Louis, 2006, Mosby.*)

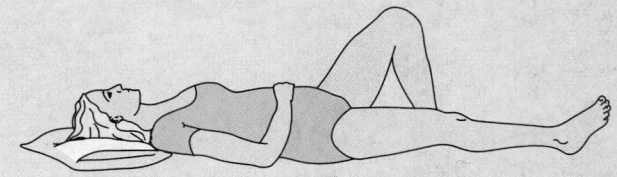

STEP 4c   Leg position when turning to the right. (*From Lowdermilk D, Perry S: Maternity nursing, ed 7, St. Louis, 2006, Mosby.*)

STEP	RATIONALE

5   Teach leg exercises:

   a   Have patient assume supine position in bed. Demonstrate leg exercises by performing passive range-of-motion exercises and simultaneously explaining exercise.

Provides for normal anatomical position of lower extremities and normal joint motion of each joint of lower extremities.

Critical Decision Point   *If patient's surgery involves one or both lower extremities, surgeon must order leg exercises in postoperative period. You can safely exercise leg unaffected by surgery unless patient has preexisting phlebothrombosis (blood clot formation) or thrombophlebitis (inflammation of vein wall).*

   b   Rotate each ankle in one direction and then in the other direction. Instruct patient to draw imaginary circles with big toe (see illustration). Repeat five times.

Ankle circle exercises maintain joint mobility and promote venous return.

   c   Alternate dorsiflexion and plantar flexion by moving both feet, pointing toes up toward head and then down toward end of mattress. Direct patient to feel calf muscles contract and relax alternately (see illustration). Repeat five times.

Calf pumping stretches and contracts gastrocnemius muscles, which enhances venous return.

   d   Perform quadriceps setting by tightening thigh and bringing knee down toward mattress, then relaxing (see illustration). Repeat five times.

Quadriceps-setting exercises contract muscles of upper legs, maintain knee mobility, and improve venous return to the heart.

   e   Patient alternately raises each leg from bed surface; patient begins by keeping leg straight and then bends leg at hip and knee (see illustration). Repeat five times.

Leg raise promotes contraction and relaxation of quadriceps muscles and promotes hip and knee movements by keeping leg straight and bending hip and knee joints.

Critical Decision Point   *If patient is unable to perform exercises, note on Kardex or in electronic medical record (EMR) that staff or primary caregiver must do passive range of motion to lower extremities every 2 hours while awake. Alternatively, notify surgeon, and request an order for pneumatic compression cuffs (see Chapter 10).*

   f   Have patient continue to practice exercises at least every 2 hours while awake. Patient is instructed to coordinate turning and leg exercises with diaphragmatic breathing, incentive spirometry, and coughing exercises.

Repetition of exercise sequence reinforces learning. Establishes routine for exercises that develops habit for performance. Sequence of exercises is leg exercises, turning, deep breathing, and coughing. Exercises before coughing enhance ability to move secretions so that they may be expectorated.

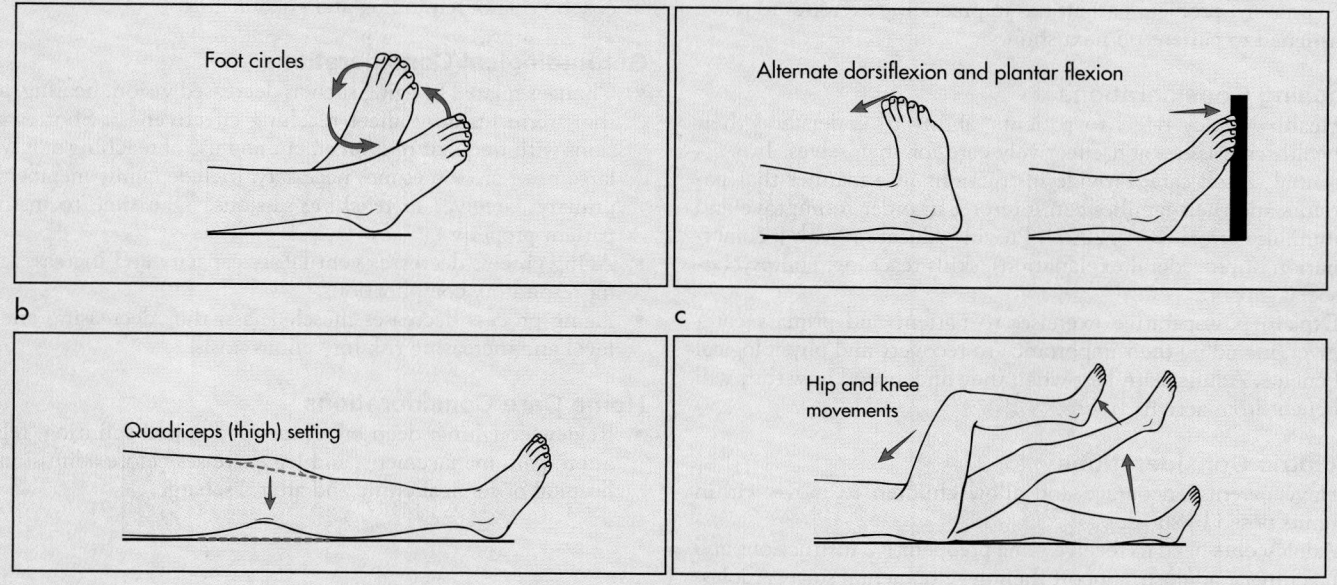

STEP 5b-e   **b**, Foot circles. **c**, Alternate dorsiflexion and plantar flexion. **d**, Quadriceps (thigh) setting. **e**, Hip and knee movements. (*From Lewis S and others:* Medical-surgical nursing: assessment and management of clinical problems, *ed 7, St. Louis, 2007, Mosby.*)

STEP	RATIONALE
EVALUATION	
1 Observe patient performing all four exercises independently.	Provides opportunity for practice and return demonstration of exercises. Ensures patient has learned correct technique.
2 Observe family member's or significant other's ability to coach patient.	Family member or significant other can assist positively or interfere with correct technique.
3 Evaluate patient's chest excursion.	Determines extent of lung expansion.
4 Auscultate patient's lungs.	Breath sounds reveal if airways are clear.
5 Palpate calves for redness, warmth, swelling, and tenderness. Assess pedal pulses.	Absent signs and normal pulses usually indicate that no venous thrombosis is present.

Unexpected Outcomes	Related Interventions
1 Patient is unwilling to perform exercises due to incisional pain of thorax or abdomen (deep breathing and coughing, turning) or due to surgery in lower abdomen, groin, buttocks, or legs (leg exercises).	• Instruct patient to ask for pain medication 30 minutes before performing postoperative exercises or use patient-controlled analgesia (PCA) immediately before exercising.
2 Patient is unable to perform exercises correctly. Anxiety and fatigue alter patient's performance.	• Repeat teaching using more demonstrations. • Patient may benefit from stress reduction techniques. • Assess for presence of anxiety, pain, and fatigue.
3 Patient develops pulmonary complications such as atelectasis postoperatively. Breaths are shallow; cough is ineffective.	• Notify physician or health care provider of findings. • Start oxygen as ordered, and increase frequency of coughing exercises. • Assess breath sounds in all lobes. • Place patient in upright position.
4 Patient develops circulatory complications such as venous stasis or thrombophlebitis postoperatively.	• Notify physician or health care provider of findings. • Place patient on bed rest with affected leg elevated as ordered. • Continue to have patient do exercises with unaffected leg.

Recording and Reporting

• Record physical assessment findings in nurses' notes or flow sheet.
• Report and record any assessed complications and action taken.
• Record in nurses' notes which exercises you have demonstrated to patient and whether or not patient can perform exercises independently.
• Report any problem patient has in practicing exercises to nurse assigned to patient on next shift.

Teaching Considerations

• Health literacy refers to patients' ability to understand their health care issues and effectively care for themselves. It is essential to self-care. Provide instructions in a manner that patients and their families can interpret in order to improve and minimize errors (Ross, 2007). Provide education with a combination of procedural explanations, skills teaching, and psychosocial support.
• Explain postoperative exercises to patient and primary caregiver, including their importance to recovery and physiological benefits. Adults learn best when they understand how they will benefit from activity.

Pediatric Considerations

• Have parents encourage and allow children to move within limits posed by surgery.
• Adolescents need to receive same preoperative instructions and teaching as adults to support their developmental stage. Adoles-

cents are searching for identity, and treating them with respect will enhance their self-esteem and independence and will increase compliance.
• Young children's normal responses of crying and moving extremities will maintain lung expansion and peripheral circulation. Therefore teaching coughing, deep breathing, and leg exercises is not usually necessary for young children.
• Children need family members and/or nursing staff to assume coach's role of reminding and encouraging.

Gerontological Considerations

• Changes related to aging such as decreased vision, hearing, and short-term memory affect teaching effectiveness. Shorter sessions with frequent reinforcement and use of teaching aids with large print are sometimes necessary. Include family members or primary caregiver in teaching sessions. Take time to instruct patient properly.
• Aging process decreases ventilatory capacity and increases risk for respiratory complications.
• Aging process decreases muscle mass, thus decreasing energy level and increasing risk for venous stasis.

Home Care Considerations

• Review coughing, deep breathing, abdominal splinting, relaxation, pain management, and leg exercises before admission to hospital or surgical clinic and after discharge.

SKILL 36-3 Performing Postoperative Care of a Surgical Patient

Intermediate / Postoperative Nursing Care / Providing Postoperative Care Managing Pain

Nursing care of a postoperative surgical patient is divided into two phases: immediate recovery and postoperative convalescence. During both phases you will make comprehensive and detailed assessments of a patient's condition. The effects of anesthesia and the physiological stressors imposed by surgery can place a patient at risk for a variety of physiological alterations. It is also important for you to facilitate communication among all members of the health care team, the patient, and the patient's family or significant other.

The first phase of postoperative care takes place during the immediate recovery period. For hospitalized patients this extends from the time a patient leaves the OR to the time the patient has stabilized in the recovery room (RR), postanesthesia room (PAR), or PACU, meets the discharge criteria, and has been transferred to the nursing unit. For an ambulatory surgical patient, the first phase of recovery normally lasts 1 to 2 hours before discharge home. The first phase is the most critical postoperative phase for assessing after effects of anesthesia, including airway clearance, cardiovascular complications, temperature control, and neurological function. A patient's condition can change rapidly. The nurse in the recovery area must make timely, intelligent, and accurate assessments to select the most appropriate measures of care for a patient.

Each hospital has its own policies for directing the process for recovering patients during the immediate postoperative period. Frequently, for example, patients undergoing cardiac or central vascular repair transfer from the OR to an intensive care unit (ICU). In this situation the patient is not sent to the RR/PACU area. The condition of these patients is potentially so unstable as to require the monitoring available only in an ICU.

The second phase of recovery is the postoperative convalescent period. This period extends from the time a patient is discharged from the RR or PACU to the time the patient is discharged from the hospital for inpatient patients. Outpatient surgical patients undergo convalescence at home. All patients who have undergone surgical procedures have similar postoperative needs. However, nursing care becomes very individualized and depends on the nature of a patient's surgery, preexisting medical conditions, the onset of complications, and the speed of recovery. Not all surgical patients recover at the same rate. During the convalescent period, you begin preparation for discharge and actively include the patient, family, and significant others in the process. You promote the patient's independence, educate the patient and/or family about any limitations imposed by surgery, and provide resources needed for the patient to assume an improved state of wellness.

Delegation Considerations

The skill of initiating and managing postoperative care of a patient cannot be delegated to NAP. The nurse directs NAP to:

- Report specific changes in patient's vital signs, behavior, or level of consciousness to the nurse.
- Obtain vital signs at specific intervals.
- Provide comfort and hygiene measures.

Equipment

Phase 1: Immediate Recovery Period

- ❏ Stethoscope, sphygmomanometer, or automatic blood pressure machine
- ❏ Thermometer
- ❏ Pulse oximeter and monitor
- ❏ IV fluid poles/infusion pump(s) and IV fluids ordered
- ❏ Emesis basin
- ❏ Oxygen equipment such as mask, nasal cannula, tubing, and oxygen regulator
- ❏ Continuous suction equipment (to suction airway)
- ❏ Intermittent suction (for NG tube suction if ordered) and irrigation supplies (irrigation setup, normal saline, pH paper)
- ❏ Dressing supplies
- ❏ Warmed blankets or active rewarming device
- ❏ Graduated container for measuring output
- ❏ Emergency equipment and medications
- ❏ Additional equipment for physical assessment as ordered

Phase 2: Postoperative Convalescent Period

- ❏ Stethoscope, sphygmomanometer, thermometer
- ❏ IV fluid poles and IV fluids ordered
- ❏ Intermittent external pneumatic compression equipment (if ordered)
- ❏ Emesis basin
- ❏ Washcloth and towel
- ❏ Waterproof pads
- ❏ Equipment for oral hygiene
- ❏ Pillows
- ❏ Facial tissue
- ❏ Oxygen equipment (if ordered)
- ❏ Continuous suction equipment (for airway suction and wound drainage systems if ordered)
- ❏ Intermittent suction (for NG suction if ordered) and irrigation supplies (irrigation setup, normal saline, pH paper)
- ❏ Dressing supplies
- ❏ Orthopedic appliances (if skeletal traction ordered)
- ❏ Graduated containers for measuring output
- ❏ Clean gloves

STEP	RATIONALE

ASSESSMENT

1 Phase 1: Immediate recovery period

   a Receive report from circulating nurse and/or anesthesia provider, including procedure performed, range of vital signs, any complications, estimated blood loss (EBL), other fluid loss, fluid replacement, type of anesthesia, medications given, type of airway and size, extent of surgical wound, restrictions to movement of position during surgery, and any preoperative medical and/or nursing diagnoses.   Determines patient's general status and allows nurse to anticipate need for special equipment, nursing care, and activities in RR/PACU.

> **Critical Decision Point**   *Patient's usual first complaint is of pain. Know how much sedative and/or analgesic have already been given and how long ago.*

   b Upon patient's arrival in RR/PACU, obtain report from surgeon and anesthesia provider.   Review provides detailed analysis of patient's physiological status, allowing nurse to make appropriate observations and interventions. Provides baseline data to determine any change in condition.

   c Consider type of surgical procedure, restrictions to movement, and type of anesthesia used.   Influences type of assessments nurse initiates, type of complications to observe for, and specific nursing interventions needed.

   d After receiving report, perform a thorough patient assessment, including vital signs, pulse oximetry, and respiratory, cardiac, neurological, GI, genitourinary (GU), and fluid status. Monitor patient's temperature, surgical site and drains, skin integrity, comfort, safety, and anxiety level.   Provides baseline for ongoing postoperative evaluations. Identifies priority nursing interventions.

> **Critical Decision Point**   *Be sure to turn patient on side (when possible) to observe underlying skin and accumulation of blood or serous drainage not visible otherwise.*

2 Phase 2: Convalescent period

   a Obtain phone report from nurse in RR/PACU.   Allows you to prepare hospital room with necessary supplies and equipment for patient's special needs.

   b Upon patient's arrival at division, collect more detailed report from nurse accompanying patient.   Detailed report helps you plan appropriate assessment and nursing care measures. Data provide baseline to detect any change in patient's condition.

   c Review patient's chart for information pertaining to type of surgery, complications, medications administered, preoperative medical risks, baseline vital signs, and patient's usual medications given/not given preoperatively.   Nature of surgery, intraoperative complications, and presence of medical risks dictate complications for which to observe. Vital signs provide means to measure postoperative changes. List of patient's usual medications may necessitate a call to physician for orders concerning timing and dose of drugs not given preoperatively.

   d Review postoperative orders.   Offers additional guidelines for type of care to provide.

   e Assess patient's knowledge and expectations of surgical recovery.   Patient will be better prepared to participate in care.

NURSING DIAGNOSES

- Acute confusion
- Acute pain
- Deficient fluid volume
- Deficient knowledge regarding postoperative care
- Disturbed sensory perception: visual, auditory

- Excess fluid volume
- Impaired gas exchange
- Impaired physical mobility
- Impaired skin integrity
- Impaired spontaneous ventilation
- Impaired swallowing
- Impaired verbal communication

- Ineffective airway clearance
- Ineffective breathing pattern
- Ineffective protection
- Ineffective thermoregulation
- Ineffective tissue perfusion
- Risk for aspiration
- Urinary retention

Individualize related factors based on patient's condition or needs.

STEP	RATIONALE

PLANNING

1 Expected outcomes following completion of procedure:

- Patient's vital signs, including oxygen saturation, remain within previous baseline or normal expected range.

  No occurrence of cardiovascular, pulmonary, or thermoregulatory changes except those expected from effects of anesthetic or analgesic.

- Patient reports relief of discomfort after analgesic or other pain-relief measures.

  Pain-relief measures effectively alter patient's reception or perception of pain.

- Surgical wound remains intact without redness, edema, ecchymosis, or discharge. If opaque dressing covers incision, dressing remains dry and intact. Drains, if present, remain patent.

  Indicates wound healing without signs of bleeding or infection.

- Breath sounds remain clear to auscultation; mucus is clear.

  Postoperative exercises and activity promote lung expansion and alveolar stability.

- Normal bowel sounds and/or return of flatus present within 48 to 72 hours after bowel or abdominal surgery and/or general anesthetic. Normal bowel sounds present within 24 hours in cases of minor surgery.

  Indicates return of intestinal peristalsis.

- Intake and output (I&O) remain relatively in balance with urinary output greater than 30 mL/hr.

  Adequate urinary elimination maintained. Fluid intake (IV and/or by mouth [PO]) adequately maintained.

- Legs remain without signs and symptoms of thrombophlebitis.

  Postoperative leg exercises and early ambulation minimize venous stasis and clot formation.

- Patient is able to discuss recovery and discharge plans. Verbalizes no specific physical complaints.

  Patient coping with physical and psychological stress of surgery.

2 Prepare the equipment as necessary at bedside, and test equipment for function.

Prepared for use if needed.

3 Explain to patient all procedures you are to perform and rationale for each. On nursing division include family members and/or significant other in explanations. In ambulatory surgery centers, families are allowed at the bedside during recovery period.

Involves patient in plan of care and minimizes anxiety. As recovery progresses, patient is able to make more choices regarding how procedures should be performed. Family can serve as coach and can help patient remember explanations given.

IMPLEMENTATION

1 Phase 1: Immediate recovery period:

- **a** Perform hand hygiene.

  Reduces transmission of microorganisms.

- **b** Check equipment setup in cubicle of RR/PACU.

  All equipment must be operational and ready to use on patient's arrival.

- **c** As patient enters RR/PACU on stretcher, immediately attach oxygen tubing to regulator, hang IV fluids, check IV flow rates, and attach pulse oximeter (see Chapter 5; Skill 5-6). Connect any drainage tubes to gravity drainage, continuous or intermittent suction as ordered. Attach cardiac monitor. Ensure indwelling catheter and bag are in drainage position and patent.

  Maintaining oxygenation and circulation are two priorities. Inhaled oxygen improves percentage delivered to alveoli. Pulse oximeter provides information on arterial oxygen saturation. IV fluids maintain circulatory volume and provide route for emergency drugs. Drainage tubes must remain patent and in proper position to allow fluid to drain.

- **d** Conduct complete assessment of all vital signs. Compare findings with patient's normal baseline. Continue assessing vital signs at least every 15 minutes until patient stabilizes. Provide warm blankets as needed for patient comfort.

  Vital signs reveal onset of postoperative complications, for example, respiratory depression, hypothermia or hyperthermia, pulse irregularity, or hypotension. Respiratory depression can result from anesthetics. Hypotension can result from anesthetics or acute blood loss. Acute blood loss may lead to hypovolemic shock with signs of reduced blood pressure, elevated heart and respiratory rates, pale skin, and restlessness. General anesthetic may affect temperature-regulating center, and lower metabolic rate causes hypothermia. Malignant hyperthermia is a rare inherited condition that develops after receiving an anesthetic and is a medical emergency (AORN, 2007b).

Critical Decision Point *If patient underwent a short procedure under procedural sedation, check agency policy for sedation recovery guidelines. The registered nurse (RN) monitoring a patient who receives procedural sedation/analgesia should have no other responsibilities that compromise continuous patient monitoring (AORN, 2007c). Monitor oxygenation periodically until patients are no longer at risk for hypoxemia. Monitor ventilation and circulation at regular intervals until patients are suitable for discharge. Design discharge criteria to minimize the risk for central nervous system or cardiorespiratory depression following discharge from observation by trained personnel (American Society of Anesthesiologists, 2004).*

STEP	RATIONALE
e Maintain patent airway:	
(1) Position patient on side with head facing down and neck slightly extended (see illustration). Never position patient with hands over chest (reduces chest expansion).	Extension prevents occlusion of airway at pharynx. Downward position of head moves tongue forward, and mucus or vomitus can drain out of mouth, preventing aspiration.
(2) Place small folded towel or small pillow under patient's head. If patient is restricted to supine position, elevate head of bed approximately 10 to 15 degrees, extend neck, and turn head to side. Have emesis basin available if patient becomes nauseated.	Supports head in extended position. Prevents aspiration if patient should vomit.
(3) Position patients with spinal anesthetic supine, without elevation of head, for up to 24 hours. Encourage fluid intake.	To prevent spinal headache from loss of cerebrospinal fluid. Increased IV or PO fluids aid body in replacing cerebrospinal fluid.

Critical Decision Point   *If patient is not able to hyperextend neck, turn head to side if possible; suction oropharynx (see Chapter 25) frequently.*

(4) Encourage patient to cough and deep breathe on awakening and every 15 minutes.	Promotes lung expansion and expectoration of mucous secretions.
(5) Suction artificial airway and oral cavity as secretions accumulate.	Clears airway of secretions.
(6) Once gag reflex returns, patient spits out oral airway (see illustration). Do not tape oral airway.	Indicates patient can clear airway independently. If airway is taped, patient will gag and may obstruct airway.

Critical Decision Point   *Because of shorter half-life of drugs used today, many patients have oral airway removed before leaving the OR. PACU nurse must assess that respiratory effort is adequate; otherwise airway may need to be replaced, and patient may need a ventilator.*

f Call patient by name in moderate tone of voice. If there is no response, attempt to arouse patient by touching or gently moving a body part. Explain that patient is in RR/PACU.	Determines patient's level of consciousness and ability to follow commands.
g Assess circulatory perfusion by inspecting color of nail beds, mucous membranes, and skin. Palpate for skin temperature. Test for capillary refill.	Pink or normal color of skin, nail beds, and mucous membranes and brisk (3 seconds or less) capillary refill indicate adequate perfusion. Warm extremities reveal adequate circulation.
h Monitor drainage:	
(1) Observe condition of dressing and drains for any evidence of bright red blood. Also look underneath patient for any pooling of bloody drainage.	Hemorrhage from surgical wound usually occurs within first few hours, indicating that a blood vessel was incompletely tied or cauterized during surgery. When dressing becomes saturated, blood oozes down patient's side and collects underneath patient.
(2) Inspect surgical area for swelling or discoloration. Note condition of surgical dressing, including amount, color, odor, and consistency of drainage. Mark dressing with circle around drainage using a black pen. Place time of marking, and check area every 10 to 15 minutes, marking any changes and noting vital signs.	A progressive increase in or changes in characteristics of drainage warrants call to surgeon because it could indicate hemorrhage (Academy of Medical-Surgical Nurses, 2004). Determines extent of fluid loss and condition of underlying wound. Size, location, and depth of wound influence amount of drainage.

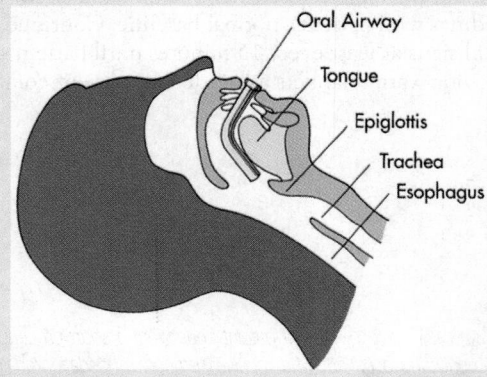

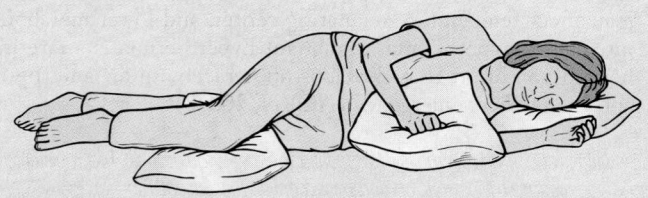

STEP 1e(1)   Position of patient during recovery from general anesthesia. *(From Lewis S and others:* Medical-surgical nursing: assessment and management of clinical problems, *ed 7, St. Louis, 2007, Mosby.)*

STEP 1e(6)   Oral airway position before removal.

STEP	RATIONALE
(3) Reinforce pressure dressing, or change simple dressing as ordered and needed (see Chapter 39). Make observations of condition of incision, surrounding tissue, and amount and color of any drainage if incision is exposed or covered with transparent dressing.	Pressure dressing should not be removed because it helps to maintain hemostasis (termination of bleeding) and to absorb drainage. Changing dressings immediately postoperatively can disrupt wound edges and aggravate drainage. First dressing changes most often occur 24 hours postoperatively and are usually done by physician. Minor surgical wounds may not have dressings but simply skin closure, or wounds may be covered with transparent dressing, which allows for observation of incision and surrounding tissue (Academy of Medical-Surgical Nurses, 2004).
(4) Inspect condition and contents of any drainage tubes and collecting devices. Note character and volume of drainage (see illustration). See Chapter 38 for other types of drains and collection devices.	Determines drainage tube patency and extent and character of wound drainage.
(5) Observe patency and intactness of urinary catheter system (if present). Note volume and character of urine.	Patent drainage system prevents bladder distention. Urine volume monitors renal function and perfusion. Decreased output (less than 30 mL/hour in an adult) is an early sign of hypovolemic shock.
(6) If NG tube is present, validate correct placement, and irrigate per protocol (see Chapter 34) with normal saline, if ordered.	Maintains patency of tube to ensure gastric decompression (removal of pressure caused by gas or liquid). Normal saline is isotonic and will not increase loss of fluid and electrolytes from stomach.
(7) Continue monitoring of IV fluid rates. Observe IV site for signs of infiltration, such as swelling, edema, redness, warmth, discomfort, and leakage of IV fluid (see Chapter 28).	Continuous regular infusion of IV fluids maintains patient's fluid intake to maintain adequate hydration and circulatory function.
i As patient awakens, provide mouth care by placing moistened washcloth to lips, swabbing oral mucosa with dampened toothette, or applying petrolatum to lips. Sips of tap water and ice chips may also be ordered.	Patient remains at risk for aspiration and should not receive fluids to rinse mouth. Moist cloth, toothette, or sips of water and/or ice chips can be soothing to dry mucosa.
j Assess level of pain as patient awakens. Provide pain medication as ordered and when vital signs have stabilized (TJC, 2007).	Pain increases the stress response and interferes with postoperative exercises. Pain medication can affect vital signs if effect of anesthetic is still present. Patient with spinal anesthesia is unable to feel sensation below level of spinal cord. Patient will need pain medication as regional anesthetic wears off.

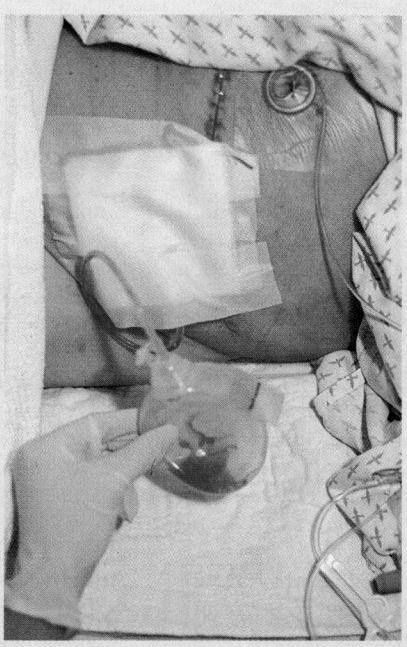

STEP 1h(4) Jackson-Pratt drain charged (collapsed) and patient's wound.

STEP	RATIONALE
k Encourage patient to begin deep breathing and coughing exercises.	Deep breathing allows for greater lung expansion, improved ventilation, and increased blood oxygenation. Coughing aids in loosening and removing secretions from pulmonary alveoli. This will decrease risk for pulmonary atelectasis, which could lead to pneumonia.
l Encourage patient to practice ankle circles and calf-pumping exercises.	These leg exercises encourage venous return. If spinal or epidural anesthetic was used, leg exercises help effects of regional anesthetic to wear off once drug has been substantially metabolized by liver.
m Explain to patient how he or she is progressing and that plans for transfer to a nursing division are being made.	Helps patient remain oriented to surroundings and recovery activities.
n Once all physiological signs have stabilized, contact physician for order to release patient to nursing unit. Measure all I&O before transferring patient to nursing division.	Physician is responsible for dictating level of observation and care required by patient. I&O while in PACU is important baseline information to include in report to nurse in nursing division.

Critical Decision Point   *If patient is to be discharged to home, ensure that patient has someone to drive him or her home and to observe patient for signs and symptoms of complications. Review with patient and driver reportable signs and symptoms and emergency care needed.*

STEP	RATIONALE
2 Phase 2: Convalescent period:	
a Make final check of equipment setup in patient's room, including emesis basin and waterproof pads. Be sure bed is in high position (level with stretcher) and wheels are locked.	During transfer, patient's status may change, necessitating quick interventions upon arrival. Availability of equipment ensures smooth transfer process. Locked wheels prevent bed from moving during transfer.
b Upon arrival at patient's room assist RR/PACU staff, and use three-person carry or slide board to transfer patient to bed (see Chapter 9).	Technique avoids strain on nurses' back muscles and maintains patient's safety.
c Once patient is transferred to bed, immediately attach any existing oxygen tubing, hang IV fluids, check IV flow rate, attach NG tube to suction, and place indwelling catheter in drainage position.	Maintains patient's oxygenation, circulation, and elimination functions. Allows for frequent monitoring of I&O. Provides for patient's comfort. Prevents potentially contaminated urine backflow into sterile bladder, thus decreasing incidence of bladder infections.
d Conduct complete assessment of all vital signs. Compare findings with vital signs in recovery area and patient's baseline values. Continue monitoring as ordered and as condition warrants (e.g., a typical order might read: VS q 15 min × 4, q 30 min × 2, q 1 hr × 4). Do not assume that further monitoring is unnecessary if the patient appears normal during the initial assessment.	Patient should be stabilized once transferred to nursing division. Change in vital signs reveal onset of postoperative complications.

Critical Decision Point   *Report to the anesthesiologist and/or physician any findings that differ from previous assessment.*

STEP	RATIONALE
e Maintain patient's airway:	
(1) Position patient on side (if allowed); if patient remains sleepy or lethargic, keep head extended.	Positioning minimizes chances of aspiration.
(2) Encourage deep breathing and coughing using pillow as an incisional splint every 1 to 2 hours.	Promotes lung expansion and expectoration of mucus.
f Be sure any drainage tubes are connected to proper suction or drainage device. If NG tube is present, validate correct placement, and irrigate as ordered and connect to proper drainage device (see Chapter 34).	Maintains drainage tube patency so that wound beds remain dry for healing. Occlusion of NG tube can lead to abdominal distention, vomiting, and aspiration.
g Assess patient's surgical dressing for intactness and presence and character of drainage. Reinforce as ordered. If no dressing present, inspect condition of wound (see Chapter 38).	Wound can hemorrhage quickly during early postoperative period. Observations of wound and dressings provide data to measure progress of wound healing.

Critical Decision Point   *If unable to change dressing, mark area of drainage, and label with time, date, and initials. Record frequency of reinforcement. Never use felt tip marker to mark dressing because ink can bleed into gauze, contaminating incision site.*

STEP	RATIONALE
h Assess for bladder distention if patient does not have indwelling catheter. Offer bedpan (see Chapter 34) or urinal (see Chapter 33) if patient senses urge to void.	Anesthetics and analgesics depress sensation of bladder fullness. Patient may still have no sensations below level of spinal or epidural anesthetic.

STEP	RATIONALE

Critical Decision Point *Initiate measures to stimulate voiding within 4 hours of surgery or removal of indwelling catheter to prevent urinary retention with overflow.*

i Measure and record all sources of fluid I&O (IV, irrigation fluids, ice chips, PO fluids; Foley/voided urine, NG drainage, wound drainage, and excessive perspiration) (see Chapter 6).	Assists in monitoring fluid and electrolyte balance.
j Position patient for comfort, maintaining airway and correct body alignment. Avoid positioning on surgical wound site or with pressure on popliteal space.	Good positioning reduces stress on suture line and decreases risks of aspiration and impaired circulation. Comfortable position helps patient relax.
k Encourage patient to continue with leg exercises every 1 to 2 hours. If patient is unable or unwilling to do them, do passive range of motion (see Chapter 10).	Leg exercises increase venous return, which decreases risk for thrombophlebitis. Range-of-motion exercises maintain joint mobility.
l If ordered, apply elastic stockings or pneumatic compression cuffs to lower extremities, and attach to compressor (see Chapter 10). Explain to patient that compression cuffs will inflate and deflate intermittently.	Increases venous return. Explanation decreases anxiety and fosters cooperation.
m Explain to patient that you have completed all observations and that you will ask family members or significant other to enter room. Place bed in lowest position and call light within reach, and raise side rails as appropriate.	Promotes patient's orientation and sense of well-being. Lowest position minimizes injury if patient becomes confused and tries to get out of bed. Call light and side rail positioning ensure patient's safety as effects of anesthetic continue to diminish.
n Explain patient's general status to family and/or significant other, describe purpose of any equipment in room, and explain reason for frequent observations and procedures.	Family and significant others are normally anxious to learn about patient's status. Unfamiliar sights (equipment and patient's appearance) also cause anxiety. Family's and significant other's understanding can promote their participation in patient's care.

Critical Decision Point *It is often helpful to give family simple tasks to perform, such as wiping patient's face with washcloth and coaching postoperative exercises.*

o Refer to recovery record to determine if pain medication was administered. Always ask patient to rate the severity of pain on an analog scale and to indicate the amount of analgesic he or she wants (TJC, 2008). Administer analgesic if vital signs remain stable, or initiate PCA if ordered (see Chapter 15).	Pain relief is essential for patient to be able to begin postoperative exercises. Patient is best judge of his or her pain. Pain scale provides an objective measure for nurse to interpret patient's progress.
p Provide oral hygiene, and repeat as needed.	Maintenance of moist mucous membranes facilitates expectoration of secretions and promotes comfort.
q As patient stabilizes over the next hours or days, perform the following measures:	
(1) Have patient participate in postoperative exercises.	Promotes pulmonary and circulatory function to minimize onset of postoperative complications.
(2) Encourage use of incentive spirometer if ordered. Watch patient use spirometer first few times to judge efficacy of breathing pattern. Chart level that patient can achieve.	Promotes lung expansion. Helps monitor progress and demonstrates if you need to encourage patient to inhale more deeply.
(3) Begin activity orders. Assess vital signs first time patient sits or stands to judge tolerance.	Early ambulation promotes circulation, lung expansion, and peristalsis. Sudden positional changes cause postural hypotension.
(4) Monitor bowel sounds per protocol. There is evidence that the return of flatus is more accurate than bowel sounds in detecting return of peristalsis after abdominal surgery (Madsen and others, 2005). Begin dietary orders slowly according to patient's tolerance. Medicate with antiemetic if patient is nauseated. Give analgesic with antiemetic until patient is eating well.	Promotes normal fluid and electrolyte balance, restores nutritional intake, and promotes normal GI function and wound healing. Analgesics often cause nausea on an empty stomach.
(5) Assist patient in assuming normal urinary voiding pattern (see Chapter 33). Male patients often need assistance to stand to void. Female patients need to sit on bedpan in bed or chair so legs can be bent and dangling or helped to bathroom.	Promotes normal urinary elimination and prevents bladder distention and urinary retention with overflow. A more natural position will help patient to void.

Critical Decision Point *If patient does not void within 8 hours after surgery or bladder becomes distended, notify physician. You may have to insert urinary catheter.*

STEP	RATIONALE
(6) Closely monitor progress of wound healing, and change dressings as ordered.	Wound infection occurs most often within 3 to 6 days postoperatively. Wound dehiscence occurs most often 3 to 11 days postoperatively.

Critical Decision Point   *Delayed wound healing may result in wound dehiscence or evisceration. This occurs most frequently after coughing, sneezing, vomiting, or getting up from a sitting position. Remind patient to use caution during these activities and to use pillow to splint incision. Evisceration is a medical emergency (see Chapter 39).*

STEP	RATIONALE
(7) Monitor and maintain wound drainage devices, such as Jackson-Pratt, Hemovac, or Penrose drains. Jackson-Pratt and Hemovac drainage systems must be emptied whenever they are half full of drainage or air and be recharged (compressed to discharge air) (see illustration).	Wound drainage devices promote healing from inside to outside and relieve pressure on suture line. Compressing a flexible closed container and then plugging drainage hole creates negative suction pressure.
(8) Monitor drainage for color, consistency, and amount every 4 to 8 hours. Compare to previous assessment.	Drainage should progress from sanguineous to serosanguineous to serous in color, become more watery, and decrease in amount as wound heals.
r Gradually increase patient's involvement in decision making and in any explanations about surgery and related implications.	Promotes patient's sense of control and independence. Encourages feeling of self-esteem.
s Teach patient and family signs and symptoms of complications such as infection, dehiscence, excessive bleeding, and need for nutrition for wound healing and techniques of wound care if needed.	Early discharge necessitates patient and family involvement because complications often occur after patient goes home.
t Discuss with patient and family or significant other plans for discharge.	Allows nurse to anticipate patient's needs in home setting and discuss any problems that might arise.
u Prepare to make referral for home care or convalescent care as patient's condition dictates. Get order from physician.	If patient continues to need nursing care or rehabilitation after discharge, physician's order is necessary. Referral provides continuity of care.

EVALUATION

1 Compare all vital sign assessment measurements with patient's baseline and expected normal levels.	Allows you to evaluate patient's respiratory, cardiovascular, and thermoregulatory status throughout recovery.
2 Measure patient's perception of pain after pain-relief measures, such as positioning, and use of analgesics.	Determines level of comfort achieved and effectiveness of pain-relief measures.
3 Monitor changes in surgical wound at least every shift.	Provides data for nurse to measure progress of wound healing.
4 Monitor lung sounds following postoperative exercises.	Determines status of airways.
5 Auscultate bowel sounds at least each shift.	Allows you to evaluate return of peristalsis and diet tolerance.
6 Monitor I&O balance for each shift.	Indicates onset of fluid imbalances.
7 Discuss with patient general level of comfort and progress toward recovery.	Gives patient sense of participation in care. Patient's perceptions are helpful in noting onset of complications. Reveals readiness to learn about discharge.
8 Conduct physical assessments appropriate for patient's unique type of surgery.	Allows nurse to monitor course of recovery.

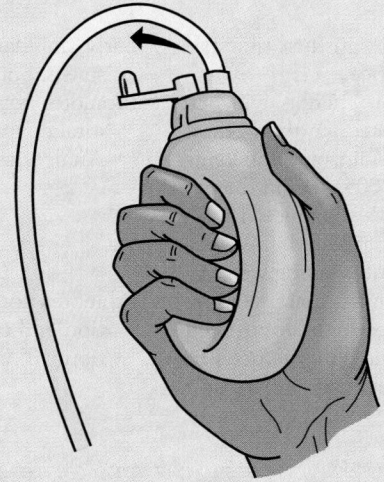

STEP 2q(7)   Charging a Jackson-Pratt drainage system.

Unexpected Outcomes	Related Interventions
1 Vital signs are above or below patient's baseline or expected range.	• Alterations may result from anesthetic effects. Ensure patient is fully awake from anesthesia before giving large doses of opioids. Ensure patient's family does not medicate patient with PCA. Monitor geriatric patient closely for opiate sensitivity—patient may require use of opiate antagonist such as Narcan in presence of bradypnea. • Medicate for pain as indicated; titrate analgesics to maximize pain relief; assess patient's use of and understanding of PCA device. • Notify physician or health care provider for symptoms of internal bleeding or shock such as hypotension or tachypnea.
2 Patient continues to experience incisional pain. Analgesic dosage may be insufficient.	• Initiate different nonpharmacological relief measures. Call physician or health care provider for additional analgesic orders. • Perform pain assessment.
3 Abnormal or diminished breath sounds are auscultated. This is sometimes due to bronchial constriction, mucous secretions in large airways, or atelectasis.	• Notify physician or health care provider, and request order for incentive spirometer, if not already ordered. • Change position to promote chest expansion. • Encourage patient to turn, deep breathe, and cough more often. • Investigate history of asthma or allergic response to medication when wheezing or stridor is auscultated.
4 Patient exhibits signs of hypovolemia related to hemorrhage.	• Elevate legs, but do not lower head past flat position. • Administer oxygen as ordered. • Increase rate of IV fluid, or administer blood products as ordered. • Monitor pulse and blood pressure every 5 to 15 minutes. • Apply pressure dressing to external wound if not contraindicated.
5 Patient complains of calf tenderness and warmth; may exhibit redness and edema in lower extremity.	• These are signs and symptoms of venous thrombosis or thrombophlebitis. Notify physician or health care provider, and anticipate orders for bed rest, leg elevation, and initiation of anticoagulation (e.g., heparin intravenous drip). • Do not massage affected leg. • Continue to have patient do leg exercises with unaffected leg.
6 Bowel sounds are absent or decreased.	• Paralytic ileus can develop as a common complication after bowel surgery. Intestinal motility may return slowly depending on anesthetic effects. • Keep IV in place. • Encourage turning and ambulation. • Assess for bowel sounds and flatus every 4 hours. • Report findings to physician or health care provider.
7 Patient develops fever, tenderness, and pain at wound site; increased white blood cell count or purulent drainage is present.	• These are signs and symptoms of wound infection. Notify physician or health care provider, and anticipate orders for culture of wound drainage and IV antibiotics.
8 Patient reports feeling something in wound "give way." Increased serosanguineous drainage occurs.	• Possibly indicates wound dehiscence or evisceration. Report wound dehiscence and/or evisceration to surgeon immediately because it could be life threatening. • If evisceration has occurred, cover abdominal contents with sterile gauze saturated with sterile normal saline, and prepare patient for emergency surgery.
9 I&O measurements reflect imbalance.	• Indicates possible fluid volume excess or deficit. Continue to monitor strict I&O, and contact physician or health care provider if 24-hour totals continue to reflect imbalance.
10 Patient is unable to discuss discharge plans or has negative view of recovery.	• Possibly indicates patient is coping poorly with stress of surgery. Discuss discharge plans and instructions with significant family member or friend. • Encourage patient to express fears and concerns. • Refer patient to support group if appropriate. • Notify physician or health care provider, and request referral for counseling if necessary.

Recording and Reporting
- Document patient's arrival in RR/PACU or nursing division; record vital signs, level of consciousness, assessment findings, and all nursing measures initiated in nurses' notes. Continue documentation every 15 minutes until stable, then every 30 minutes times 2, every hour times 4, then every 4 to 8 hours as condition warrants.
- Record vital signs and I&O on appropriate flow sheets.
- Report any abnormal assessment findings and signs of complications to nurse in charge and/or physician or health care provider.

Teaching Considerations
- If patient had spinal or epidural anesthetic, remind family or significant other that loss of extremity movement is normal for several hours.
- Reinforce preoperative teaching regarding coughing, deep breathing, leg exercises, and information concerning ambulation and pain control.
- Instruct patient and primary caregiver to identify signs and symptoms and appropriate actions to take for infection, respiratory, circulatory, or GI difficulties and wound disruptions.
- Provide important phone numbers to patient and primary caregiver for use in event of emergency and for follow-up care on discharge.
- Teach patient about appropriate wound care, diet recommendations, and activity restrictions.

Patient Teaching for Ambulatory Surgical Patients
- Physician's office telephone number (24-hour answer)
- Surgery center's telephone number
- Follow-up appointment, date, time
- Review of prescribed medications
- Guidelines related to specific surgery
- Dressing and wound care
- Pain control
- Activity restrictions
- Guidelines related to anesthesia
- Dietary restrictions
- Activity restrictions
- Signs and symptoms of complications

Pediatric Considerations
- Keep parent-child separation to minimum time possible. When a parent cannot be present, it is important to leave a favorite possession with child.
- Be alert for allergic responses and signs and symptoms of malignant hyperthermia in children who have not been exposed to drugs or anesthetic agents. Family history of allergies makes child at high risk for experiencing similar reactions.
- Vomiting is a major concern in young children because of increased risk for fluid and electrolyte imbalances and risk for aspiration. Vomiting is also more likely because surgery in children is often necessitated by accidental injuries without benefit of NPO status.
- Mandatory fluid intake guidelines are not usually necessary because of aggressive fluid replacement in children.
- Voiding before discharge from ambulatory surgery is not usually required for young children.
- Undermedicating young children may be based on myth that opiates are more dangerous for infants. The fact is that "by 3 to 6 months of age, healthy infants can metabolize opioids similarly to older children" (Hockenberry and Wilson, 2007). Observing the normalizing of vital signs and behavior after administration of analgesics is a valuable clue that pain really existed before treatment (Hockenberry and Wilson, 2007).

Gerontological Considerations
- The ability of older adults to tolerate surgery depends on extent of physiological changes that have occurred with aging, presence of any chronic diseases, and duration of surgical procedure.
- Undermedicating older adults is common. Asking patients to rate their pain before and after administration of analgesics and asking what numerical rating is acceptable to them are better methods of individualizing care.

Home Care Considerations
- Teach primary caregiver about any postoperative exercises, pain management, home modifications, or activity limitations.
- If patient is discharged with dressing changes, bedroom or bathroom is usually an ideal location for procedure. Have primary caregiver perform return demonstration of dressing change.

CRITICAL THINKING EXERCISES

You are assigned to care for Mrs. Edmonds, an obese 52-year-old African American. She is married with three adult children and is employed as an attorney. You just received her from the postanesthesia care unit following an abdominal hysterectomy for fibroid tumors and a bladder neck suspension. Her previous medical history includes 30-year 2-pack-per-day cigarette smoking and type 2 diabetes, and she has been on birth control pills for 20 years. She has an abdominal dressing that has a small amount of shadowing on it, is on oxygen at 2 L via nasal cannula, and has both a Foley catheter and a suprapubic catheter draining pink-tinged urine. She has an IV of $D_5\frac{1}{2}NS$ infusing at 125 mL/hr and a morphine PCA device. She received Ancef IV piggyback approximately 45 minutes before her incision was made and is to receive her second dose 8 hours later.

1 What risk factors does Mrs. Edmonds have for developing an SSI, and what is your role in prevention at this point in her care?
2 What topics should be included in Mrs. Edmonds' postoperative teaching, and who should be included?

3 What other postoperative complications is Mrs. Edmonds at risk for developing? Provide the rationale.
4 Before performing postoperative exercises, what should the patient be instructed to do?

REVIEW QUESTIONS

1 Prevention of surgical site infections requires numerous actions by both the surgical team and the patient. Select the measures that are used to reduce surgical site infections. Select all that apply.
   1 Discharge the patient from the hospital as soon as possible.
   2 Hair should be shampooed before neck or back surgery.
   3 Prophylactic antibiotic therapy should be given as close to the time of incision as possible.
   4 Excess hair should be shaved with a razor just before the surgery begins.

5 Control hyperglycemia in diabetic patients as well as nondiabetic patients.

6 Give a shower or bath after the preoperative enema is evacuated.

2 There are numerous measures to prevent venous thromboembolism during the postoperative period. Which intervention would be most appropriate before the surgery begins?

1 Performing an assessment for Homans' sign

2 Applying compression devices of some type

3 Teaching the patient coughing and breathing techniques

4 Instructing the patient how to ambulate after surgery

3 A female patient's culture requires that a male member of the family give consent for the scheduled surgery. Which approach by the nurse is the most appropriate?

1 Find out how much the patient understands about the scheduled procedure.

2 Have the patient sign the consent first with the male family member observing and then signing afterward.

3 Have the male member sign the consent form first, and then have the patient sign.

4 Refer to the institution's protocol for implementing this type of informed consent,

4 The risk manager is explaining the use of DNR orders in the surgical environment during an in-service that is being held for the new surgical team. Which statement is true regarding DNR orders?

1 DNR orders should remain in effect throughout all stages of surgical procedures.

2 DNR orders should automatically be suspended during and immediately following surgical procedures.

3 The physicians should discuss and document issues with the patient and/or family to determine whether DNR orders are to be maintained or modified during surgical procedures.

4 Patients with DNR orders typically are not generally candidates for surgical procedures.

5 A patient was admitted from the PACU to the medical-surgical unit following colectomy. Upon initial examination a dime-size amount of shadowing is noted on the abdominal dressing. Which intervention should be implemented next?

1 Do nothing because this is an expected outcome for the postoperative patient.

2 Mark the dressing with a circle around the drainage.

3 Remove the dressing to assess the exact amount of bleeding.

4 Immediately notify the physician.

REFERENCES

Academy of Medical-Surgical Nurses: *Core curriculum for medical-surgical nursing*, ed 3, Pitman, NJ, 2004, The Academy.

American Hospital Association: *The patient care partnership*, Chicago, 2003, The Association.

American Society of Anesthesiologists: *Standards for postanesthesia care*, approved by House of Delegates on October 12, 1988, and last amended on October 27, 2004.

Andrews M and others: *Transcultural concepts in nursing care*, ed 5, Philadelphia, 2007, Lippincott.

Association of periOperative Registered Nurses: *Standards, recommended practices and guidelines*, Denver, 2007a, The Association.

Association of periOperative Registered Nurses: *Standards and recommended practices for perioperative nursing: malignant hyperthermia guideline*, Denver, 2007b, The Association.

Associate of periOperative Registered Nurses: *Standards and recommended practices for perioperative nursing: managing the patient receiving moderate sedation/analgesia*, Denver, 2007c, The Association.

Association of periOperative Registered Nurses: *Standards and recommended practices for perioperative nursing: perioperative care of patients with do-not-resuscitate (DNR) orders*, Denver, 2007d, The Association.

Centers for Disease Control and Prevention: *Estimates of healthcare-associated infections*, www.cdc.gov/ncidod/dhqp/hai.html, accessed November 1, 2007a.

Centers for Disease Control and Prevention, National Center for Health Statistics: *Prevalence of overweight and obesity among adults: United States, 2003-2004*, last modified May 30, 2007, www.cdc.gov/nchs/products/pubs/pubd/hestats/overweight/overwght_adult_03.htm, accessed November 1, 2007b.

Dellinger EP and others: Hospitals collaborate to decrease surgical site infections, *Am J Surg* 190(1):9, 2005.

Hockenberry M, Wilson D: *Nursing care of infants and children*, ed 7, St. Louis, 2007.

Kneale J: *Orthopaedic nursing*, ed 2, Philadelphia, 2005, Elsevier.

Lewis S and others: *Medical-surgical nursing, assessment and management of clinical problems*, ed 7, St. Louis, 2007, Mosby.

Lowdermilk D, Perry S: *Maternity nursing*, ed 7, St. Louis, 2006, Mosby.

Madsen D and others: Listening to bowel sounds: an evidence-based practice project, *Am J Nurs* 105(12):40-49, 2005.

Marley R and others: Perianesthesia respiratory care of the bariatric patient, *J Perianesth Nurs* 20(6):404, 2005.

Mosby's dictionary of medicine, nursing, and health professions, ed 7, St. Louis, 2006, Mosby.

QualityNet: *Specifications manual for national hospital quality measures*, version 2.1d, 2007, www.qualitynet.org, accessed October 31, 2007.

Ross J: Health literacy and its influence on patient safety, *J Perianesth Nurs* 22(3)220, 2007.

The Joint Commission: *Implementation expectations for the universal protocol for preventing wrong site, wrong procedure and wrong person surgery*, Chicago, 2003a, The Commission.

The Joint Commission: *Universal protocol for preventing wrong site, wrong procedure, wrong person surgery*, Chicago, 2003b, The Commission.

The Joint Commission: *Accreditation manual for hospitals*, Chicago, 2008, The Commission.

RESEARCH REFERENCES

Baril P and others: Preoperative fasting: knowledge and perceptions, *AORN J* 86(4):609, 2007.

Geerts W and others: Prevention of venous thromboembolism: the Seventh ACCP Conference on Antithrombic and Thrombolytic Therapy, *Chest* 126:338S, 2004.

MacDougall D and others: Economic burden of deep-vein thrombosis, pulmonary embolism and post-thrombotic syndrome, *Am J Health Syst Pharm* 63(20):S5, 2006.

Moller A and others: Risk reduction: perioperative smoking intervention, *Best Pract Res Clin Anesthesiol* 20(2):237, 2006.

Odom-Forren J: Preventing surgical site infections, *Nursing* 36(6):59, 2006.

Stuart P: The evidence base behind modern fasting guidelines, *Best Pract Res Clin Anesthesiol* 20(3):457, 2006.

37

Intraoperative Care

MEDIA RESOURCES

• **evolve** *learning system* http://evolve.elsevier.com/Perry/skills

  • Review Questions
  • Video Clips

OBJECTIVES

Mastery of content in this chapter will enable the nurse to:
- Describe the meaning of a sterile conscience.
- Describe the roles of a registered nurse in the operating room.
- Identify guidelines for use of sterile technique in the operating room.

- Correctly perform surgical hand antisepsis.
- Correctly don a sterile surgical gown.
- Correctly apply sterile gloves using the closed technique.

Perioperatively a nurse practicing in the operating room supports a patient's surgical experience from the preoperative throughout the intraoperative period and into the postoperative phase (see Chapter 36). The standards of clinical practice that registered nurses (RNs) follow within the operating room provide an optimal level of care that ensures a patient's safety and comfort (Association of periOperative Registered Nurses [AORN], 2007b). In addition, you exercise judgment, critical thinking, and interpersonal communication skills in applying the nursing process to ensure patients receive appropriate nursing care during the perioperative experience.

Members of the surgical team include the surgeon (doctor of medicine [MD] or doctor of osteopathy [DO]), physician's assistant (PA), registered nurse first assistant (RNFA), certified registered nurse anesthetist (CRNA) and/or physician anesthesiologist (MD or DO), circulating nurse (RN), and scrub nurse/technician (RN, licensed practical nurse [LPN], or certified surgical technologist [CST]). The intraoperative phase begins when a patient enters the OR suite and ends with admission to the postanesthesia care unit (PACU). During the intraoperative phase, the RN assumes the role of first assistant to the surgeon, scrub nurse, or circulating nurse. The RNFA is a nurse with advanced education who assists the surgeon with the surgical procedure, performing a combination of nursing and delegated medical functions and/or skills (Box 37-1). The scrub nurse/technician (Box 37-2) is a "sterile" team member who provides the surgeon with instruments and supplies, disposes of soiled sponges, and accounts for sponges, sharps, and instruments on the surgical field. RNs, LPNs, or CSTs may assume the scrub nurse role. The circulating nurse (Box 37-3) is always an RN who is the charge nurse in the room (AORN, 2007b). The circu-

lating nurse is a "nonsterile" member of the surgical team who assumes responsibility and accountability for maintaining patient safety and continuity of quality care. This includes supervising the conduct of the scrub technician and delegating tasks to licensed and unlicensed nursing assistive personnel (NAP) as appropriate. The circulating nurse is also an assistant to the first assistant, scrub nurse/technician, and surgeon.

It is essential that perioperative nurses fully understand and follow the principles of aseptic technique and develop a sterile conscience. A sterile conscience requires knowledge of the principles of aseptic technique; self-discipline; good communication skills to identify, address, and correct any breaks in sterile technique; and the maturity to overcome personal preferences. If any question exists about sterility of an item, the item is unsterile. For example, if a sterile gown touches the floor while you are putting it on, you discard it and exchange it for a new one; the scrub nurse/technician who accidentally touches the faucet with one hand while rinsing will rescrub. These are examples of following your sterile conscience and being committed to safe, quality patient care.

EVIDENCE-BASED PRACTICE TRENDS

The practice of surgical scrubbing in perioperative settings is changing. In recent years manufacturers have introduced new hand scrub products that are replacing traditional lengthy scrub routines that use water, brushes, and nonalcohol antiseptic solu-

---

BOX 37-1 | Role and Responsibilities of a Registered Nurse First Assistant

The RNFA role is an expansion of the traditional perioperative nursing role, and areas of responsibility will overlap. Responsibilities specific to the practice of first assisting include:

- Participating in "time out" procedure with other surgical team members (safety measure taken to ensure correct patient, correct procedure, correct site and side, correct patient position, and correct implants/equipment present) (The Joint Commission, 2008)
- Providing surgical exposure (assisting in retraction of tissues and suctioning of surgical field)
- Providing hemostasis (control of bleeding)
- Handling and/or cutting tissue
- Using surgical instruments/medical devices and suturing
- Performing wound closure
- Applying human anatomical and physiological considerations in practice; recognizing structure, function and location of tissues and organs; manipulating tissues accordingly to avoid injury
- Ensuring preoperative and postoperative patient management in collaboration with other health care providers

From Association of periOperative Registered Nurses: Position statement: AORN official statement on RN first assistants. In *AORN standards and recommended practices for perioperative nursing*, Denver, 2007a, The Association. *RNFA*, Registered nurse first assistant.

BOX 37-2 | Role of the Scrub Nurse

- Assists circulating nurse in preparing OR, opening supplies
- Performs surgical hand antisepsis and dons sterile gown and gloves
- Prepares sterile field with procedure-appropriate supplies and instruments, verifying all are in working order
- Participates in "time out" procedure with other surgical team members (safety measure taken to ensure correct patient, correct procedure, correct site and side, correct patient position, and correct implants/equipment present) (The Joint Commission, 2003)
- Performs sponge, sharps, and instrument counts with circulating nurse before incision is made, at the beginning of wound closure, and at the end of the surgical procedure
- Labels all liquids and/or medications on sterile field with sterile marking pen when liquid or medication is out of the original container or package
- Gowns and gloves surgeons and assistants as they enter the OR
- Assists surgeons with sterile draping of patient
- Keeps sterile field orderly and monitors progress of procedure and any breaks in aseptic technique
- Passes sterile instruments and supplies to surgeons and assistants
- Handles surgical specimens per institutional policy
- Constantly monitors location of all sponges and sharps in the sterile field

OR, Operating room.

tions. Recent research demonstrates that hand scrub preparations containing 50% to 90% alcohol combined with chlorhexidine gluconate are just as effective as the traditional scrubbing method

- Organizes and prepares OR before start of surgical procedure; checks to see that equipment works properly
- Gathers supplies for surgical procedure and opens sterile supplies for scrub nurse/technician
- Counts sponges, sharps, and instruments with scrub nurse/technician before incision is made, at the beginning of wound closure, and at the end of the surgical procedure
- Ensures all liquids and/or medications on the sterile field are labeled with sterile marking pen when liquid or medication is out of the original container or package
- Sends for patient at appropriate time
- Conducts preoperative patient assessment, including the following:
  - Explains role and identifies patient
  - Reviews medical record and verifies procedure and consents
  - Confirms dentures and prostheses removed
  - Confirms patient's allergies, nothing by mouth (NPO) status, laboratory values, electrocardiogram (ECG), x-ray studies, skin condition, circulatory and pulmonary status
- Safely assists patient to operating table and positions patient according to surgeon preference and procedure type, using safety precautions (e.g., safety belt, securing arms, padding bony prominences)
- Participates in "time out" procedure with other surgical team members (safety measure taken to ensure correct patient, correct procedure, correct site and side, correct patient position, and correct implants/equipment present) (The Joint Commission, 2003)
- Applies conductive pad to patient if electrocautery used; may prepare patient's skin; may apply ECG electrodes
- Applies antiembolism stockings and sequential compression device per physician order
- Explains briefly to patient what the circulating nurse and the scrub nurse/technician are doing
- Assists surgical team by tying gowns and arranging equipment
- Assists anesthesia personnel during induction and extubation
- Continuously monitors procedure for any breaks in aseptic technique and anticipates needs of the team; opens additional sterile supplies for scrub nurse/technician
- Handles surgical specimens per institutional policy
- Documents on perioperative nurses' notes
- Communicates to family and PACU personnel during the surgical procedure

OR, Operating room; *PACU,* postanesthesia care unit.

in preventing surgical site infections (Parienti and others, 2002). The benefits of using a brushless, alcohol-based surgical hand product (with added emollients) include fast and easy application, limited or decreased damage to the user's skin, improved compliance with hand antisepsis protocols, simplified application technique, and reduced material waste (i.e., water, brushes, and packaging) (Conner, 2003).

Another evidence-based practice initiative found in many ORs is double gloving (wearing two pairs of sterile surgical gloves). Much of the research on surgical gloves focuses on holes created by contact with sharps during surgery. The 2002 Cochrane review, which summarizes findings from 18 studies, indicates that double gloving significantly reduces perforations to the innermost glove (Tanner and Parkinson, 2002). In addition, double gloving better protects the patient from surgical wound contamination. Therefore benefits of double gloving during surgery include decreasing the risk for exposure to blood-borne pathogens for the surgical team members and decreasing the risk for surgical wound infection for the patient (Twomey, 2000).

Skill Performance Guidelines

1 All items used within a sterile field must be sterile.
2 Gowns used by scrub persons must be sterile before donning. Once in place, gowns are sterile from the front chest and shoulders to table level and on the sleeves to 5 cm (2 inches) above the elbow.
3 Sterile persons must keep their hands in view, above waist level and below neckline, to avoid contamination.
4 When wearing a sterile gown, do not fold arms with hands tucked in the axillary region. This area is not considered sterile once you have donned the gown. Perspiration can lead to strike through, or contamination that occurs when moisture permeates a sterile barrier.
5 Sterile draped tables are sterile only at table level. Sides of the drape extending below table level are unsterile.
6 All personnel moving around or within a sterile field must do so in a manner consistent with maintaining the sterility of that field. Scrubbed persons move from sterile areas to other sterile areas, contacting a sterile field only with sterile gowns and gloves. Unscrubbed persons always stay at least 1 foot away from the sterile field while keeping it in constant view; they touch only unsterile areas.
7 Group all sterile supplies and equipment around the sterile-draped patient.
8 Unsterile persons must avoid reaching over the sterile field.
9 Scrubbed persons remain close to the sterile field. When changing position, turn face to face or back to back.

SKILL 37-1 Surgical Hand Antisepsis

In the operating room setting it is imperative that you achieve surgical hand antisepsis through effective surgical scrub or antiseptic hand rub (Boyce and Pittet, 2002). To reduce the risk for patients' acquiring postoperative infections, use of an antimicrobial preparation for hand antisepsis is an integral part of the presurgical scrubbing procedure for operating room personnel. Although the skin cannot be sterilized, you can greatly reduce the number of microorganisms by chemical, physical, and mechanical means.

The surgical hand scrub has been the traditional method for surgical asepsis. Through the use of an antimicrobial agent and sterile brushes or sponges, the surgical hand scrub removes debris and transient microorganisms from the nails, hands, and forearms; reduces the resident microbial count to a minimum; and inhibits rapid/rebound growth of microorganisms (AORN, 2007d). New evidence suggests that a brushless technique, with or without water, containing at least 60% alcohol, is an alternative to the traditional hand scrub with a brush with the same microbial efficacy (Gruendemann and Bjerke, 2001). Both hand antiseptic methods are currently used in operating room settings. This skill will address both techniques.

You wear surgical attire (i.e., scrubs) in the operating room to reduce the chance for contamination from surgical personnel to patients, and vice versa. Keep your fingernails short (¼ inch long), clean, and healthy. If you wear polish, make sure it is not chipped or older than 4 days. Never wear artificial nails or extenders (AORN, 2007d). Remove all rings, watches, and bracelets before the surgical scrub.

The Association of periOperative Registered Nurses (AORN) recommends a 3- to 4-minute hand and arm scrub with an approved antimicrobial agent for all surgical procedures. The institution should standardize the surgical hand scrub procedure for all staff using either the anatomical timed scrub or the counted stroke method (AORN, 2007d) (see agency policy). Some procedures, described as clean procedures (e.g., laryngoscopy and proctoscopy),

require performing hand hygiene but not necessarily surgical hand antisepsis.

Delegation Considerations

The skill of surgical hand antisepsis can be delegated to a surgical technologist or licensed practical nurse.

- The registered nurse routinely observes surgical hand antisepsis for staff compliance.

Equipment

- ❑ Deep sink with foot or knee controls for dispensing water and soap
- ❑ Antimicrobial agent approved by agency (dispenser with foot controls)
- ❑ Surgical scrub brush with plastic nail file
- ❑ Paper face mask, cap or hood, surgical shoe covers
- ❑ Sterile towel
- ❑ Sterile pack containing sterile gown
- ❑ Protective eyewear/face shield

STEP	RATIONALE
ASSESSMENT	
1 Determine type and length of time for hand hygiene per agency policy.	Guidelines vary regarding ideal time needed for surgical scrub.
2 Remove bracelets, rings, and watches.	Jewelry harbors and protects microorganisms from removal. Allergic skin reactions may occur as a result of scrub agent or glove powder accumulating under jewelry.
3 Inspect fingernails, which must be short (¼ inch), clean, and healthy. Nail polish that is chipped should be removed before entering surgical area. Never wear artificial nails or extenders.	Long nails and chipped or old polish harbor greater numbers of bacteria (AORN, 2009). Long fingernails can puncture gloves, causing contamination. Artificial nails harbor gram-negative microorganisms and fungus (AORN, 2007d).
4 Inspect condition of cuticles, hands, and forearms for presence of abrasions, cuts, or open lesions.	Personnel cuts, abrasions, exudative lesions, fresh tattoos, or hangnails tend to ooze serum, which may contain pathogens. These individuals should not have patient contact until conditions are healed (AORN, 2009).

NURSING DIAGNOSIS

- Risk for infection

Individualize related factors based on patient's condition or needs

PLANNING

1 Expected outcomes following completion of procedure: • Patient will not develop signs of surgical wound infection.	Indicates microorganisms are not transferred to the patient and sterile field.

IMPLEMENTATION

1 Don surgical shoe covers, cap or hood, face mask, and protective eyewear.	Protective eyewear prevents exposure to blood or body fluids splashing from the sterile field, causing the risk for infection (e.g., human immunodeficiency virus [HIV], hepatitis B virus [HBV]).

Critical Decision Point *Laser surgery requires special protective eyewear to prevent eye damage from stray laser energy.*

2 Perform a prescrub wash at beginning of work shift.
  a Turn water on using foot or knee control, and adjust to comfortable temperature.
  b Wet hands thoroughly with water. Follow manufacturer's directions for application of soap.
  c Rub hands, covering all surfaces, including the backs of hands, fingertips, inner webs, and palms, washing for at least 15 seconds.
  d Rinse well to remove all soap. Dry hands thoroughly with a disposable towel and discard towel.
	Prevents contamination of hands after scrub.
	
	A short prescrub wash/rinse at least 15 seconds at the beginning of the work shift removes gross debris and superficial microorganisms (AORN, 2009).

STEP	RATIONALE

3 Surgical hand scrub (with sponge)

a Turn on water using foot or knee control. Clean under nails of both hands using a disposable nail pick or cleaner. Rinse hands and forearms under running water (see illustration).

Removes dirt and organic materials that harbor microorganisms.

b Dispense the antimicrobial scrub agent according to manufacturer's instructions. Apply agent to wet hands and forearms using a soft, nonabrasive sponge.

Ensures removal of resident microorganisms on all surfaces of hands and arms (AORN, 2009).

c Time a 3 to 5 minute scrub (follow manufacturer's instructions). Visualize each finger, hand, and arm as having four sides (see illustration A). Wash all four sides effectively, keeping the hand elevated, elbow down. Repeat for other hand, fingers, and arm (see illustration B).

Times will vary by product.
Scrubbing all surfaces ensures removal of resident microorganisms on hands and arms (AORN, 2009).

d Avoid splashing surgical attire. Discard sponges in appropriate container.

e Rinse hands and arms, running water from fingertips to elbows in one continuous motion (see illustration).

Hands remain cleanest part of upper extremities.

f Turn off water using foot or knee controls, and back into operating room holding hands higher than elbows and away from surgical attire.

g Approach sterile setup, and grasp sterile towel, taking care not to drip water on the sterile field (see illustration).

Water contaminates the field.

h Keeping hands and arms above the waist and outstretched, carefully grasp one end of the sterile towel to dry one hand thoroughly, moving from fingers to elbow in a rotating motion (see illustration).

Avoids sterile towel's contacting unsterile scrub attire and transferring contamination to hands. Dry skin from cleanest (hands) to least clean (elbows).

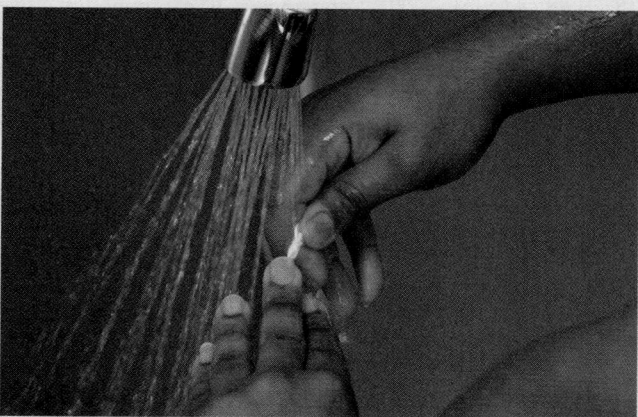

STEP 3a   Cleaning under fingernails.

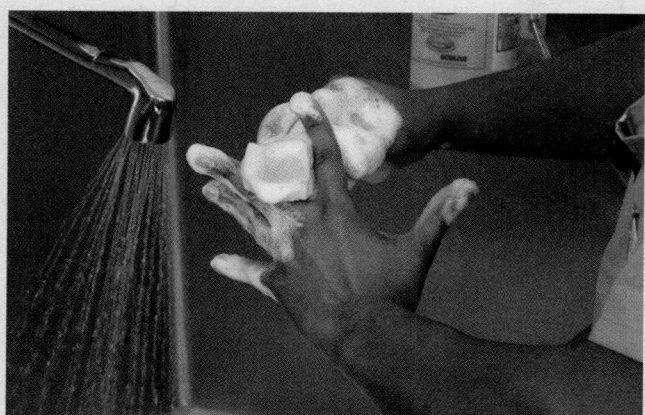

STEP 3c, *A*   Scrubbing sides of fingers.

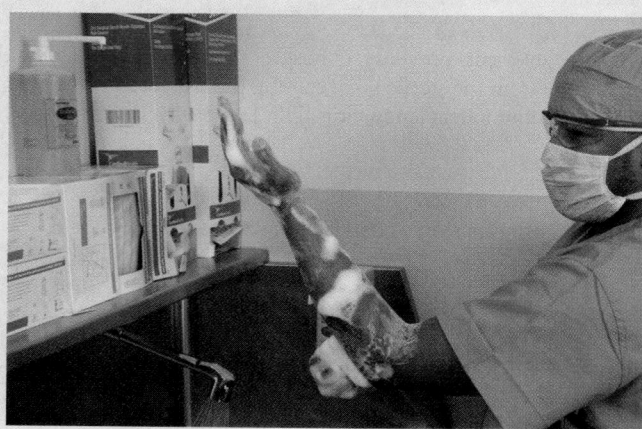

STEP 3c, *B*   Scrubbing forearms.

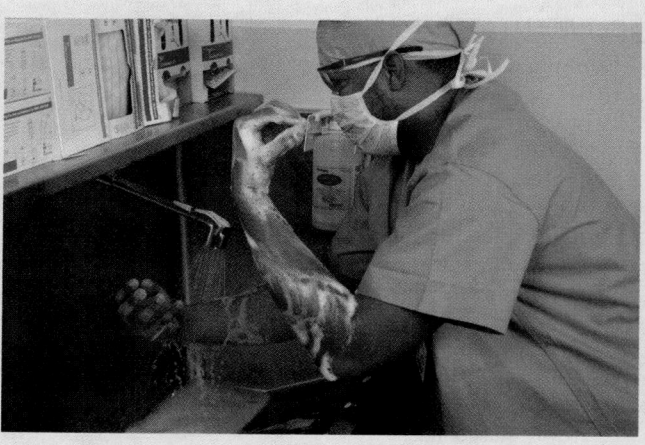

STEP 3e   Rinsing arms.

STEP	RATIONALE
i Use the opposite end of the towel to dry the other hand.	Avoids transfer of microorganisms from elbow to opposite hand.
j Drop towel into linen hamper or into circulating nurse's hand.	
4 Perform spongeless surgical hand scrub with an alcohol-based hand-rub product.	
a After prescrub wash (Step 2) Turn on water using foot or knee control. Clean under nails of both hands using a disposable nail pick or cleaner, rinse hands and forearms under running water. Dry hands thoroughly with a paper towel. Turn off water.	
b Dispense the manufacturer's recommended amount of the antimicrobial agent hand preparation (see illustration). Apply the agent to the hands and forearms according to manufacturer's instructions for application, recommended volume, and specified time.	Promotes reduction in microorganisms on all surfaces of hands and arms (AORN, 2009).
c Repeat the antimicrobial product application if indicated in manufacturer's instructions.	
d Rub thoroughly until completely dry (see illustration). Then proceed to OR to don gloves.	

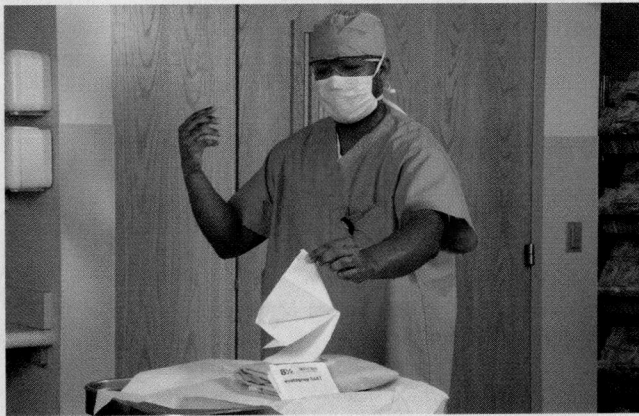

STEP 3g   Grasping sterile towel.

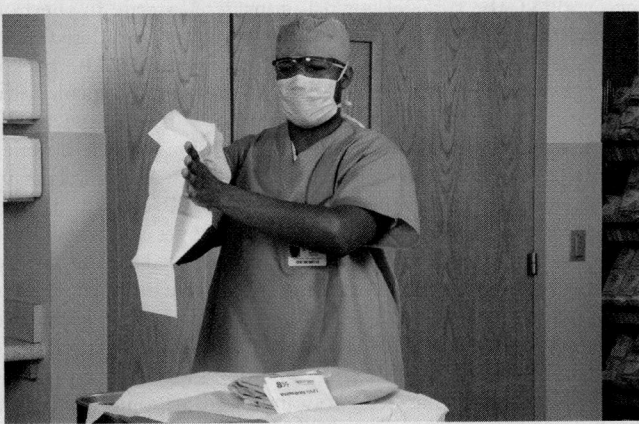

STEP 3h   Drying hands thoroughly.

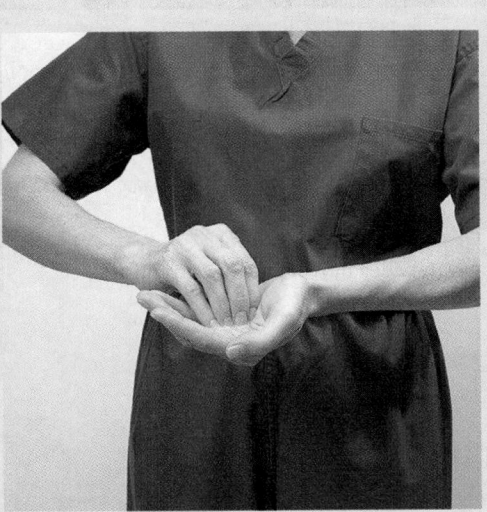

STEP 4b   Application of antimicrobial agent for brushless hand scrub. (*Photos Courtesy 3M Health Care.*)

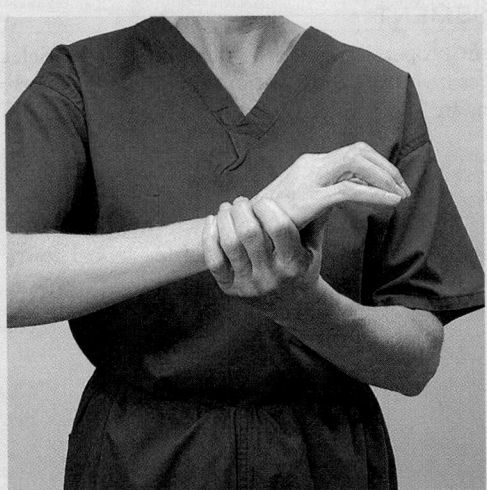

STEP 4d   Rub thoroughly until completely dry. (*Photos Courtesy 3M Health Care.*)

STEP	RATIONALE

EVALUATION

1   Monitor patient postoperatively for signs of surgical wound infection (usually occurs 2 to 3 days postoperatively).

Signs of infection include redness, heat, swelling, pain, and purulent drainage.

Unexpected Outcomes
1   Redness, heat, swelling, pain, or purulent drainage may develop at surgical site, which often indicates a wound infection.

Related Interventions
• Individualize interventions based on patient's situation (e.g., wound care, antibiotic therapy).

Recording and Reporting
• No recording is required for surgical hand antisepsis. Record area and description of surgical site postoperatively to provide baseline for monitoring wound.

Teaching Considerations
• Instruct patient and family or significant other to observe surgical site for signs of infection.

SKILL 37-2   Donning a Sterile Gown and Closed Gloving

Immediately following surgical hand antisepsis, apply a sterile gown and then apply sterile gloves. All members of the surgical team must prepare in this manner before entering the sterile field. Once applied, the surgical gown is considered sterile in the front from chest to waist or table level. The sleeves are considered sterile from 5 cm (2 inches) above the elbow to fingertips. The back of the gown is not considered sterile when worn. Surgical gowns should cover all garments worn underneath. All sterile gowns that are free of tears, punctures, strain, and abrasion provide an effective barrier against microorganisms, particulates, and fluids passing between unsterile and sterile areas (AORN, 2007c).

Use the closed-glove method to apply gloves when you enter the sterile field. If a glove becomes contaminated during the surgery, the circulating nurse, wearing protective unsterile gloves, grasps the outside of the glove and pulls off the glove inside out, leaving the stockinette cuff of the gown in place. Another sterile team member assists in regloving. The open method can be used when only one glove has been contaminated. In some settings the scrub nurse will wear two pairs of sterile gloves. If both the scrub nurse/technician's gloves become contaminated, the nurse regowns and regloves using the closed-glove method.

Delegation Considerations
The skill of donning a sterile gown and closed gloving can be delegated to a surgical technologist or licensed practical nurse.
• The RN routinely observes sterile gown application and closed gloving for staff compliance.

Equipment
❑ Package of proper-size sterile gloves (latex-free if nurse or patient has sensitivity or allergy)
❑ Sterile pack containing sterile gown
❑ Clean, flat, dry surface (table or Mayo stand) on which to open gown and gloves
❑ Paper face masks, cap or hood, surgical shoe covers
❑ Protective eyewear/face shield

STEP	RATIONALE

ASSESSMENT

1   Select proper size and type of sterile gloves. Select latex-free gloves if you know the patient or any surgical personnel in the room are latex sensitive.

Proper fit ensures ease of handling instruments and supplies. Prevents latex allergic response.

Critical Decision Point   *Know your institutional policy, because double gloving may be recommended to reduce the risk for glove perforation during a surgical procedure.*

2   Select proper size and type of sterile surgical gown.

Ill-fitting gown impedes movement of extremities.

STEP	RATIONALE

NURSING DIAGNOSIS

- Risk for infection

Individualize related factors based on patient's condition or needs.

PLANNING

1 Expected outcomes following completion of procedure: • Patient will not develop signs of surgical wound infection.	Nurse maintains aseptic technique and does not contaminate gown or gloves.

IMPLEMENTATION

1 Donning a sterile gown:

a Open sterile gown and glove package on a clean, dry, flat surface. Scrub nurse (before scrubbing hands) or circulating nurse can do this, preferably on a small table separate from the sterile field containing the sterile instruments and supplies.	Provides sterile area for gloving.
b Perform surgical hand antisepsis (see Skill 37-1). Dry hands thoroughly.	
c Pick up gown (folded inside out) from sterile package, grasping the inside surface of gown at the collar.	The hands are not completely sterile. The inside surface of the gown will contact the skin's surface and is thus considered contaminated.
d Lift folded gown directly upward, and step back, away from the table.	Prevents gown from touching unsterile object.
e Locate neckband; with both hands, grasp the inside front of gown just below neckband.	Clean hands may touch inside of gown without contaminating outer surface.
f Keeping gown at arm's length away from body, allow gown to unfold with the inside of gown toward body. Do not touch outside of gown or allow it to touch the floor.	Outside of gown remains sterile.
g With hands at shoulder level, slip both arms into armholes simultaneously (see illustration). Do not allow hands to move through cuff opening. Have circulating nurse pull gown over shoulders by reaching inside arm seams. Gown is pulled on, leaving sleeves covering hands.	Careful application prevents contamination. Gown covers hands to prepare for closed gloving.
h Have circulating nurse tie gown at neck and waist (see illustration). If gown is wraparound style, sterile front flap is not touched until the scrub nurse/technician has gloved (see Step 3b).	Secures gown without contaminating it.

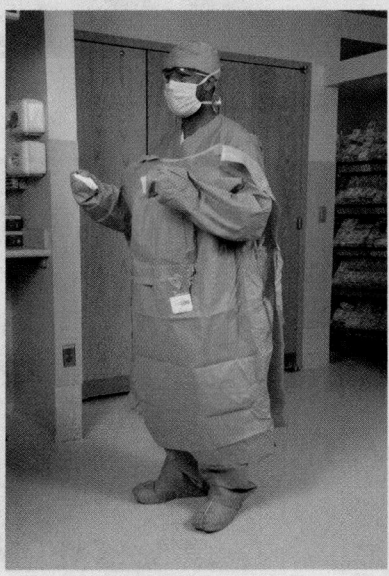

STEP 1g Placing arms in sleeves.

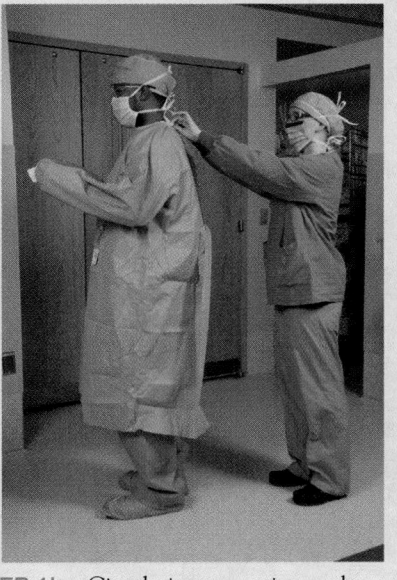

STEP 1h Circulating nurse ties scrub gown.

STEP	RATIONALE
2 Applying gloves using the closed-glove method:	
a With hands covered by gown cuffs and sleeves, open inner sterile glove package (see illustration).	Sterile gown cuff will touch sterile glove surface.
b Grasp folded cuff of glove for dominant hand with the nondominant hand.	Sterile gown touches sterile glove.
c Extend dominant forearm forward with palm up, and place palm of glove against palm of dominant hand. Gloved fingers point toward elbow.	Positions glove for application over cuffed hand, keeping glove sterile.
d While holding glove cuff through gown with dominant hand on which it was placed, grasp back of glove cuff with nondominant hand and turn glove cuff over end of dominant hand and gown cuff (see illustration).	Positions glove over gown for hand insertion.
e Grasp top of glove and underlying gown sleeve with covered nondominant hand. Carefully extend fingers into glove, being sure glove's cuff covers gown's cuff.	
f Glove nondominant hand in same manner with gloved, dominant hand (see illustration A). Keep hand inside sleeve. Be sure fingers are fully extended into both gloves (see illustration B).	Gloves remain sterile.

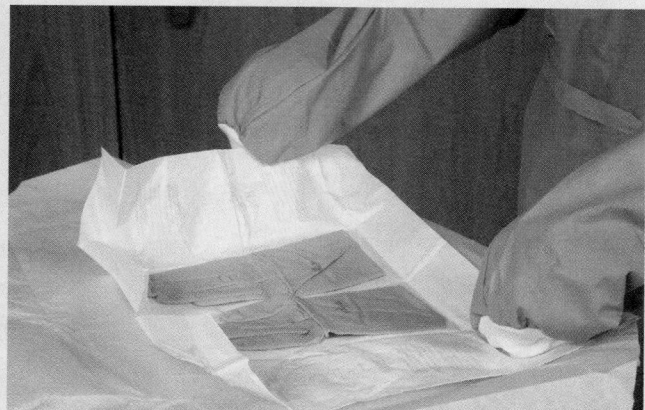

STEP 2a   Scrub nurse opens glove package.

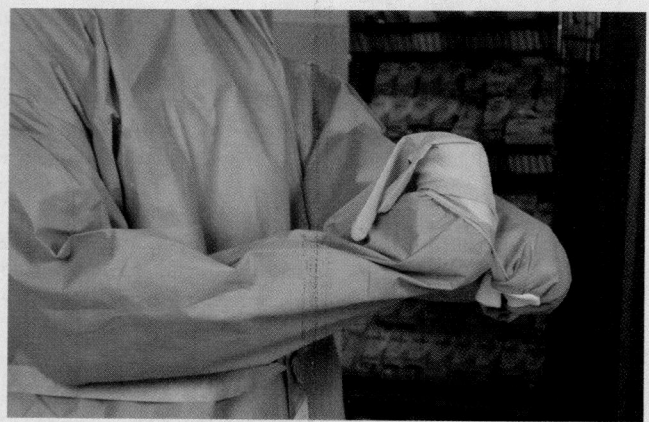

STEP 2d   Glove applied as hands remain inside cuffs.

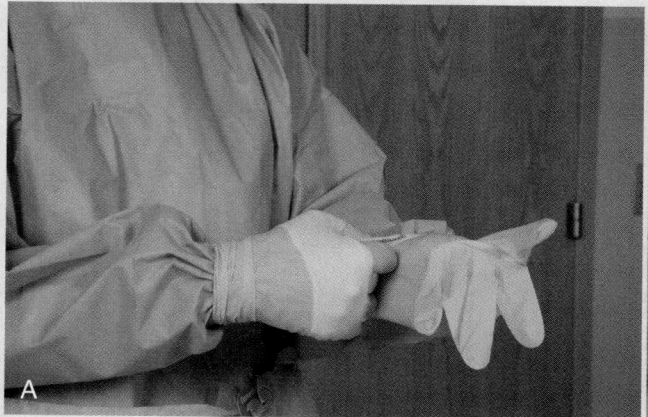

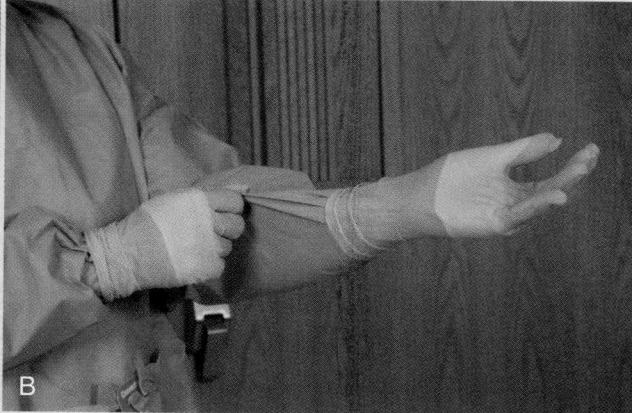

STEP 2f   **A,** Second glove applied. **B,** Gloved fingers extended.

STEP	RATIONALE
3 Donning a wraparound gown:	
a Grasp sterile front flap/paper tab with gloved hands, and untie.	Front of gown is sterile.
b Pass the sterile paper tab to a member of the sterile surgical team, or to a nonsterile team member (such as the circulating nurse) (see illustration). Keep gown tie in right hand. The circulating nurse stands still as the scrub nurse/technician turns.	Nonsterile team member uses caution not to touch the sterile tie when taking the sterile paper tab while the scrub nurse/technician turns.
c Allowing margin of safety, turn to the left one-half turn, covering back with extended gown flap. Retrieve sterile tie only from team member, and secure both ties in place.	Maneuver covers entire body with gown. Nonsterile team member pulls off paper tab and discards.

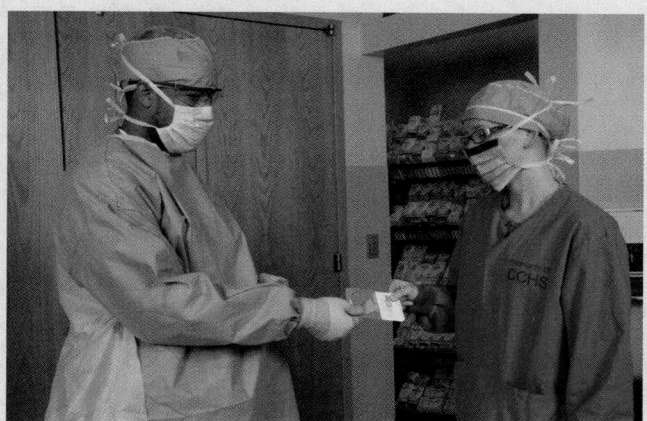

STEP 3b Paper tab on disposable gown is passed to circulating nurse.

EVALUATION

1 Monitor patient postoperatively for signs of surgical wound infection (usually occurs 2 to 3 days postoperatively).	Signs of infection include redness, heat, swelling, pain, and purulent drainage.

Unexpected Outcomes

1 Redness, heat, swelling, pain, or purulent drainage develops at surgical site, which often indicates a wound infection.

Related Interventions

• Individualize interventions based on patient's situation (e.g., wound care, antibiotic therapy).

Recording and Reporting

• No recording is required for sterile gowning and gloving. Record area and description of surgical site postoperatively to provide baseline for monitoring wound.

Teaching Considerations

• Instruct patient and family or significant other to observe surgical site for signs of infection.

CRITICAL THINKING EXERCISES

You are assigned to be the circulating nurse for Mrs. Alvarez, who is having an umbilical hernia repair. She is a 38-year-old Hispanic bookkeeper and mother of five children with no significant medical history except for postpartum hypothyroidism. The surgical team includes Dr. M. Klein; L. Relling, RNFA; Sarah Scott, CST (certified surgical technologist); and Dr. L. Bates, anesthesiologist. Sarah has recently completed an extended orientation, but still needs much supervision.

1 Sarah is running late because of the staff meeting this morning. You notice that she omits the prescrub hand wash before performing a brushless antiseptic hand rub. What should you do? Explain your choice.
   A Tell Sarah to apply extra hand antiseptic to both hands.
   B Tell Sarah she must start over and perform the prescrub hand wash first.
   C Tell Sarah she must now perform a surgical hand scrub with a brush.
   D Do nothing, because she is going to apply sterile gloves anyway.

2 Sarah just had artificial nails applied last night because she is in a wedding tonight. They are polished with no signs of chipping. Is it okay for Sarah to scrub for Mrs. James' hernia repair today? Explain your choice.
   A Yes, because the polish was applied just last night
   B Yes, because the polish is not chipped
   C No, because artificial nails may not be worn

3 While Sarah prepares the sterile field with the appropriate instruments and supplies for the umbilical hernia surgery, you notice that she reaches down to scratch the top of her leg. She continues to set up the sterile field without taking any action. What should she have done?

 REVIEW QUESTIONS

1 Many individuals play a vital role as part of the surgical team. What is included in the responsibilities of the circulating nurse?
   1 Performing the surgical hand scrub and donning a sterile gown and gloves
   2 Assisting in the retraction of tissues and suction of surgical field
   3 Conducting perioperative assessment and reviewing medical records for accuracy and completeness
   4 Helping the surgeons and assistants gown and glove as they enter the operating room

2 Many newer methods for the surgical scrub have been researched. Which method, however, is the traditional method for surgical asepsis?
   1 The surgical hand scrub
   2 Alcohol foam rub
   3 Brushless scrub
   4 Waterless scrub

3 The scrub nurse is getting ready to do her surgical scrub. What should be done before beginning the scrub?

1 Remove nail polish even if it is not chipped.
2 Inspect areas from fingertips to elbows for abrasions or open areas.
3 Move rings higher on the knuckles before beginning the scrub.
4 Remove bracelets and artificial nails.

4 The closed-glove method is standard in the operating room for many of the participants. The scrub nurse is performing it correctly if which procedure is observed?
   1 Both hands are covered with the cuffs of the gown.
   2 Both hands are exposed through the cuffs of the gown.
   3 The dominant hand is covered with the cuff of the gown.
   4 The nondominant hand is covered with the cuff of the gown.

5 Surgical personnel must have a sterile conscience to provide optimum patient safety. Which situation denotes a breach of sterile conscience?
   1 The scrub nurse accidentally touches the faucet with one hand while scrubbing, then rescrubs his hands.
   2 The circulating nurse accidentally touches a sterile item, then removes it from the sterile field.
   3 The surgeon thinks he contaminated a sterile glove and has the suspect glove changed.
   4 Before the scrub nurse dries her hands, she drips water on the sterile gown she is about to put on but does not replace the gown.

REFERENCES

Association of periOperative Registered Nurses: Position statement: AORN official statement on RN first assistants. In AORN standards and recommended practices for perioperative nursing, Denver, 2007a, The Association.

Association of periOperative Registered Nurses: Position statement—statement on one perioperative registered nurse circulator dedicated to every patient undergoing a surgical or other invasive procedure. In AORN standards, recommended practices, and guidelines, Denver, 2007b, The Association.

Association of periOperative Registered Nurses: Recommended practices for selection and use of surgical gowns and drapes. In AORN perioperative standards and recommended practices, Denver, 2007c, The Association.

Association of periOperative Registered Nurses: Recommended practices for surgical hand antisepsis/hand scrubs. In AORN perioperative standards and recommended practices, Denver, 2007d, The Association.

Association of periOperative Registered Nurses: Recommended practices for surgical hand hygiene, http://www.rpauthor.aorn.org. Accessed January 17, 2009.

Conner R: Clinical issues: fire blankets, alcohol-based hand scrubs, peel pouch indicators, aseptic technique definitions, shaving, AORN J 78(3):484, 2003.

The Joint Commission: Universal protocol for preventing wrong site, wrong procedure, wrong person surgery, Oakbrook Terrace, Ill, 2008, The Commission.

RESEARCH REFERENCES

Boyce JM, Pittet D: Guidelines for hand hygiene in health care settings, Am J Infect Control 30(8):S1, 2002.

Gruendemann BJ, Bjerke NB: Is it time for brushless scrubbing with an alcohol-based agent? AORN J 74(6):859, 2001.

Parienti JJ and others: Hand-rubbing with an aqueous alcoholic solution vs. traditional surgical hand-scrubbing and 30-day surgical site infection rates: a randomized equivalence study, JAMA 288(6):722, 2002.

Tanner J, Parkinson H: Double gloving to reduce surgical cross-infection, Cochrane Database Syst Rev 2002(3):CD003087.

Twomey CL: Double gloving: a risk reduction strategy, Jt Comm J Qual Saf 29(7):369, 2003.

Wound Care and Irrigations

38

MEDIA RESOURCES

- **evolve** *learning system* http://evolve.elsevier.com/Perry/skills
  - Review Questions
  - Video Clips

- [View Video!] Mosby's Nursing Video Skills, 3.0

- [NSO] Nursing Skills Online

KEY TERMS

Dehiscence
Eschar
Evisceration
Granulation tissue
Healing ridge
Hemostasis
Hemovac drain
Irrigation
Jackson-Pratt (JP) drain
Keloid
Penrose drain
Primary intention
Secondary intention
Tertiary intention
Staples

OBJECTIVES

Mastery of content in this chapter will enable the nurse to:

- Discuss the body's response during each stage of the wound-healing process.
- Differentiate between primary and secondary intention.

- Explain factors that impair or promote normal wound healing.
- Perform a wound assessment.
- Perform wound irrigation.
- Remove sutures or staples.
- Demonstrate care of a wound-drainage system.

Proper wound care is necessary to promote healing that results in an intact skin layer. Intact skin is the body's first line of defense against invasion by infectious microorganisms. The skin defends the body in other ways by serving as a sensory organ for pain, touch, and temperature, and it has an acid pH, which is often called the "acid mantle."

The skin or integument is the largest external organ. It has two layers: the epidermis and the dermis (Fig. 38-1). The outer layer, the epidermis, has five layers. The outermost layer, the stratum corneum, consists of flattened dead keratinized cells. The thin layer of the

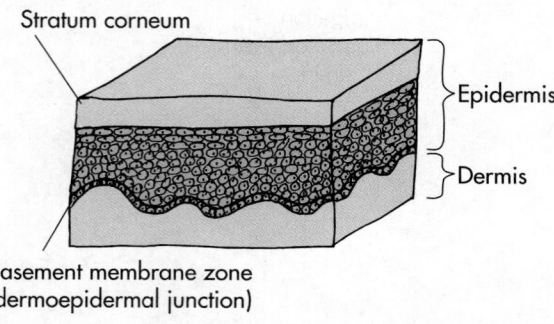

FIG 38-1   Layers of the integument.

| BOX 38-1 | Phases of Wound Healing (Full-Thickness Wounds) |

Hemostasis Phase
- Blood vessels constrict; clotting factors activate coagulation pathways to stop bleeding. Clot formation seals the disrupted vessels so blood loss is controlled and acts as a temporary bacterial barrier. Growth factors are released, which attract cells needed to begin the repair process.

Inflammatory Phase
- Vasodilatation occurs, allowing plasma and blood cells to leak into the wound, noted as edema, erythema, and exudate. Leukocytes (white blood cells) arrive in the wound to begin wound cleanup. Macrophages, a type of white blood cell, appear and begin to regulate the wound repair. The result of the inflammatory phase is a clean wound bed in the patient with a noncomplicated wound.

Proliferative Phase
- Epithelialization (the construction of new epidermis) begins. At the same time new granulation tissue is formed. New capillaries (angiogenesis) are created, restoring the delivery of oxygen and nutrients to the wound bed. Collagen is synthesized and begins to provide strength and structural integrity to the wound. Contraction, which occurs in open wounds, reduces the size of the wound.

Remodeling Phase
- Collagen is remodeled to become stronger and provide tensile strength to the wound. Outer appearance in an uncomplicated wound will be that of a well-healed scar.

Data from: Doughty DB, Sparks-Defriese B: Wound healing physiology. In Bryant RA, Nix DP, editors: *Acute and chronic wounds: current management concepts,* ed 3, St. Louis, 2007, Mosby.

stratum corneum prevents dehydration of underlying cells and is a physical barrier to the entry of certain chemicals. The barrier is selective; it does allow absorption of topical medications in paste, ointment, and dermal patch forms. The next layers of the epidermis are the stratum lucidum, stratum granulosum, and stratum spinosum. The innermost layer of the epidermis, the stratum germinativum, is sometimes called the basal layer. It is from this single layer of keratinocytes that cells migrate up toward the stratum corneum. Important features of the stratum germinativum are the epidermal protrusions, or "peaks and valleys" that point downward into the dermis. These provide resiliency and integrity to the skin structure. Melanocytes, the cells that give the skin its color, are also in this layer. The area that separates the epidermis from the dermis is called the dermoepidermal junction or the basement membrane zone.

Beneath the epidermis is the dermis. Collagen (a tough fibrous protein layer), blood vessels, and nerves compose the dermal layer. Collagen composes about 70% of the dermis and is extremely important in wound healing. The dermis restores the physical properties of the skin and its structural integrity. Restoration of both the epidermal and dermal layers is necessary to promote healing. Risk for local or systemic infection, impaired circulation, and breakdown of tissue directly impair the wound-healing ability of the skin layers (Doughty and Sparks-Defriese, 2007).

Physiologically, wound healing occurs in the same way for all patients, with skin cells and some tissues (including the vascular tissues) regenerating quickly and others regenerating slowly or not at all. The latter group includes cells of the liver, renal tubules, and central nervous system neurons.

Wound healing is complex and involves a series of physiological processes among cells and tissues. The location, severity, and extent of the injury and the tissue layer or layers involved all affect the wound-healing process (Doughty and Sparks-Defriese, 2007). A partial-thickness wound (loss of tissue limited to epidermis and partial dermis) heals by the process of regeneration. However, a full-thickness wound (total loss of skin layers as well as some deeper tissues) heals by scar formation (Box 38-1). In addition, there are underlying factors that prevent the ability of cells and tissues to regenerate, return to normal structure, or resume normal functioning (Box 38-2).

| BOX 38-2 | Systemic Factors Affecting Wound Healing |

- Tissue perfusion and oxygenation
- Nutritional status
- Infection
- Diabetes mellitus
- Corticosteroid therapy or hypercortisolemia
- Chemotherapy and radiation
- Age
- Stress—both psychological and physiological
- Immunosuppression
- Systemic conditions that affect health status such as renal or hepatic disease, sepsis, cancer
- Hematopoietic disorders

From Doughty DB, Sparks-Defriese B: Wound healing physiology. In Bryant RA, Nix DP, editors: *Acute and chronic wounds: current management concepts,* ed 3, St. Louis, 2007, Mosby.

The healing process proceeds in a series of events, generally described as phases. In a full-thickness wound the phases are hemostasis, inflammatory, proliferative, and maturation. Collagen deposition begins in the inflammatory phase and peaks during the proliferative phase. It is important for nurses to assess for the accumulation of this new tissue. This "healing ridge" is composed of newly formed collagen, and you can usually feel it along a healing wound (Doughty and Sparks-Defriese, 2007) (Fig. 38-2). It is usually present directly under the suture line between days 5 and 9 (Whitney, 2007). Lack of a ridge is cause for concern (Fig. 38-3), and you will need to begin interventions to reduce mechanical strain on the wound promptly (Whitney, 2007).

Types of healing are primary intention, secondary intention, and tertiary intention (Fig. 38-4). Healing by primary intention occurs when the edges of a clean surgical incision remain close together. The wound heals quickly, and tissue loss is minimal or absent (Doughty and Sparks-Defriese, 2007). The skin cells quickly regenerate, and capillary walls stretch across under the suture line to form a smooth surface as they join.

Wounds that are left open and allowed to heal by scar formation are classified as healing by secondary intention (Doughty and Sparks-Defriese, 2007). There is tissue loss and open wound edges. Granulation tissue gradually fills in the area of the defect with scar tissue (Fig. 38-5). This process is typical of severe laceration or massive surgical intervention with skin loss. In secondary intention there is some gap between the edges. Connective tissue develops, which supports new capillaries. This form of healing results in the formation of scar tissue to close the wound. The slowness of this process places a patient at greater risk for infection.

Healing by tertiary intention is sometimes called delayed primary intention or closure. It occurs when surgical wounds are not closed immediately but left open for 3 to 5 days to allow edema or infection to diminish. Then the wound edges are sutured or stapled closed. Scarring is usually minimal (Doughty and Sparks-Defriese, 2007). During the healing process a wound may have some type of dressing covering it.

The percentage and type of tissue in the wound base healing by secondary intention indicates the extent to which the wound is progressing toward healing (Nix, 2007). Viable tissue is normally red to pink in color and moist in appearance (Table 38-1). This type of tissue is called granulation tissue and indicates a wound moving toward healing. Black, brown, or tan tissue in the wound is eschar and should be removed before the wound healing can begin.

Do not remove an initial surgical dressing for direct wound inspection until a physician writes a medical order for removal. Certain situations and some institutional policies govern who changes the dressing the first time. Pay special attention to maintaining the position of drains during dressing changes (Doughty

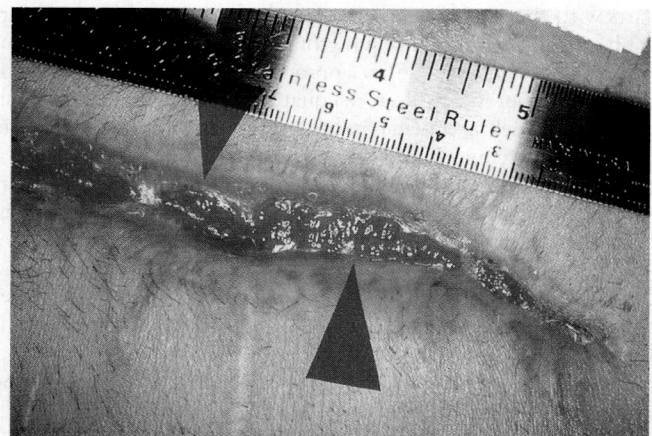

FIG 38-2 Surgical wound with epithelialization occurring: epithelial healing ridge apparent. *(From Bryant RA, Nix DP, editors: Acute and chronic wounds: current management concepts, ed 3, St. Louis, 2007, Mosby.)*

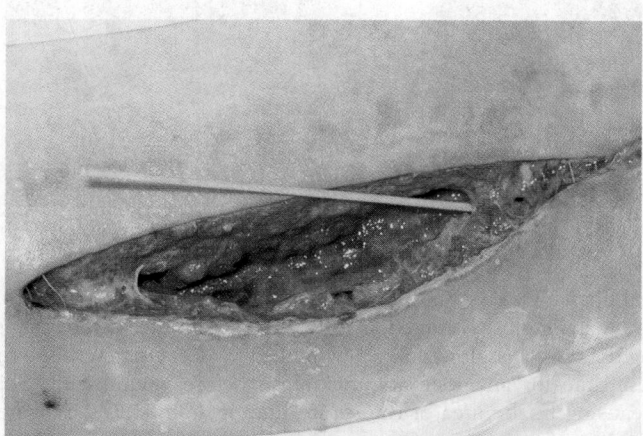

FIG 38-3 Surgical wound lacking evidence of healing epithelial ridge. *(From Bryant RA, editor: Acute and chronic wounds, ed 2, St. Louis, 2000, Mosby.)*

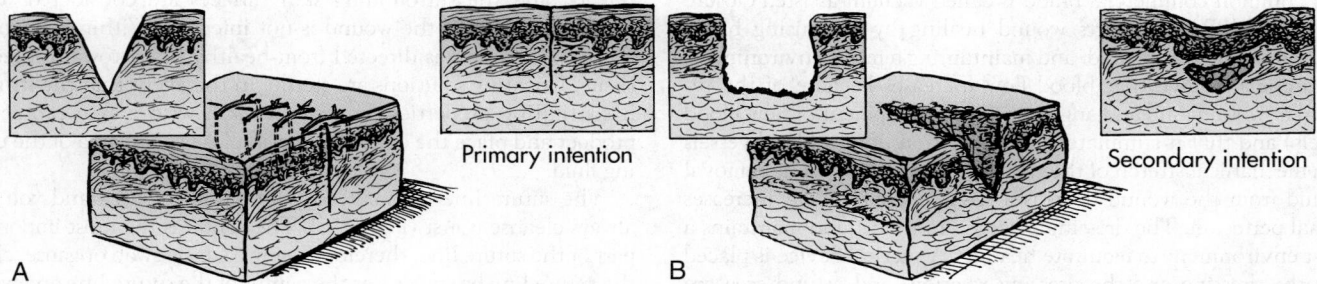

Primary intention

Secondary intention

A

B

FIG 38-4 **A,** Wound healing by primary intention, such as with a surgical incision. Wound healing edges are pulled together and approximated with sutures, staples, or adhesive tapes, and healing occurs by connective tissue deposition. **B,** Wound healing by secondary intention. Wound edges are not approximated, and healing occurs by granulation tissue formation and contraction of the wound edges. *(Used with permission: Bryant RA, editor: Acute and chronic wounds: nursing management, ed 2, St. Louis, 2000 Mosby.)*

TABLE 38-1	**Wound Color/Tissue**
Black/brown wounds/eschar	Black or brown tissue is eschar, which represents full-thickness tissue destruction. Black is used to describe necrotic tissue or desiccated tissue such as tendon. It is also noted as related to gangrenous lesions secondary to peripheral vascular disease. If the goal for a wound covered with eschar is debridement, sharp debridement is used to quickly remove the tissue, chemical debridement is used to soften the tissue for removal or a moist dressing is also considered to loosen the tissue. The method of debridement will depend upon the overall goal of the patient.
Yellow wounds/slough	Yellow tissue represents nonviable tissue and in some cases the presence of an infection. It is often yellow, cream-colored, or gray slough, which is usually accompanied by purulent drainage. For patients with a low infection risk, the use of moisture-retentive dressings enhances debridement. These moisture-retentive dressings may include moist dressings, as well as hydrocolloids, hydrogels, or alginates. If the wound is infected, topical antimicrobials are used.
Red wounds/granulation	Red tissue represents the presence of granulation tissue. The red color is the result of an increasing amount of new blood vessels in the wound and is considered healthy. The goal in management of a red granulated wound is to select a dressing that maintains a clean and moist wound environment and minimizes damage to healing tissue.

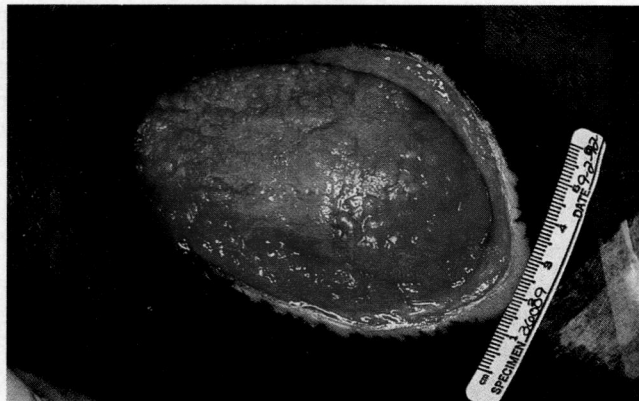

FIG 38-5   Open wound with granulation tissue.

and Sparks-Defriese, 2007). To promote patient comfort, administer an analgesic, as ordered, usually 30 to 45 minutes before changing the dressing. However, you will need to assess to determine the best time for analgesic administration before wound care. Skin cleansing in the area of the suture line or drain site is indicated when an excessive amount of drainage occurs. The presence of wound exudate is an expected stage of epithelial cell growth.

Negative pressure wound therapy (NPWT) is a mechanical wound care treatment that uses controlled negative pressure to assist and accelerate wound healing (Frantz and others, 2007). The most common commercial brand is called vacuum-assisted closure (V.A.C.). NPWT supports wound healing by optimizing blood flow, removing wound fluid, and maintaining a moist environment. Researchers believe that blood flow increases because of the removal of wound fluid and angiogenesis (development of new blood vessels) and that it stimulates the production of new blood vessels via a mechanical stretch of the tissue (Frantz, 20007). The removal of fluid from the wound decreases tissue edema, which increases dermal perfusion. The dressing placed into the wound maintains a moist environment to facilitate healing. A suction device is placed over the dressing and the dressing, suction, and wound area are covered with a transparent dressing, which provides the airtight seal necessary for NPWT. The dressing is changed on a scheduled basis, usually no earlier than 48 hours. Chronic wounds such as pressure ulcers, diabetic ulcers, traumatic wounds, and venous stasis ulcers are approved for NPWT (see Chapter 39).

While cleansing a wound, use meticulous hand hygiene and proper infection control procedures before and after removing soiled dressings to limit the risk for health care–acquired infection. Use clean gloves while cleansing a wound, to prevent exposure to body fluids, exudate, or bloody drainage from a wound. During wound cleansing, you deliver fluid or cleansing solution to the wound surface by means of a specific mechanical force. This force assists with the separation and removal of necrotic debris and surface bacteria (Rolstad and Ovington, 2007). To accomplish effective wound cleansing, use an appropriate solution that does not harm the tissue and uses an adequate force to agitate and wash away surface debris and devitalized tissue that contain bacteria (Rolstad and Ovington, 2007).

Irrigation is the most common method of wound cleansing. Irrigation uses the mechanical force (either high or low) of a stream of solution to remove debris, bacteria, and necrotic tissue from a wound. The pressure needed to irrigate wounds is between 4 and 15 psi. In addition to cleansing via irrigation (Table 38-2), prescribed medications are often added to the wound irrigant. Principles of basic wound irrigation include the following:

1 Cleanse in a direction from the least contaminated area to the most contaminated.
2 When irrigating, all the solution flows from the least contaminated to the most contaminated area.

When irrigating a wound, be sure that the flow of irrigation moves from the area being cleansed to an area that is both distal and lower. In wound care, the area you are cleansing is considered "clean" and the surrounding skin surfaces are considered "contaminated" even if the wound is not infected. Within the wound the irrigation flow is directed from healthy tissue toward infected tissue. Irrigating solutions are sterile. In the event that the irrigant has irritating properties, protect the skin with a skin protectant product and place the collection basin close to the area of the exiting fluid.

The suture line is the "least contaminated" area and you will always cleanse it first (Fig. 38-6). The center is the most important part of the suture line; therefore, using a sterile swab or gauze, clean the suture line by starting at the center of the suture line and working toward one end. With another sterile swab or gauze, start at the center of the incision and work toward the other end. All other cleansing involves moving from one end to the other on each side of the incision. Work in straight lines, moving away from the suture line with each successive stroke.

TABLE 38-2 | Wound Cleansing Protocol

Phase of Healing	Mechanical Force	
	High-Pressure Inflammatory	**Low-Pressure Proliferative**
Wound base characteristics	Presence of necrotic tissue (eschar, fibrin slough), debris, or other particulate matter Significant bacterial burden Moderate/large amount of exudate Residue from wound care products	Presence of granulation tissue or new epithelial cells Non/minimum serous or serosanguineous exudate Residue from wound care products
Clinical outcome(s)	Loosen, soften, and remove devitalized tissue from wound Separate eschar from fibrotic tissue/fibrotic tissue from granulating base Remove wound care product residue	Prevent trauma to viable wound tissue Remove wound care product residue
Solutions: Wound cleansers	Normal saline Volume of solution depends on size of wound	Normal saline Volume of solution depends on size of wound
Delivery systems*	35-mL syringe/19-gauge angiocatheter Irrijet DS	Pouring saline directly from bottle Bulb syringe Piston syringe

From Barr JE: Principles of wound cleansing, *Ostomy Wound Manage* 7A(suppl 41):15S, 1995.
*This is not an all-inclusive list of delivery systems available. Inclusion does not imply endorsement.

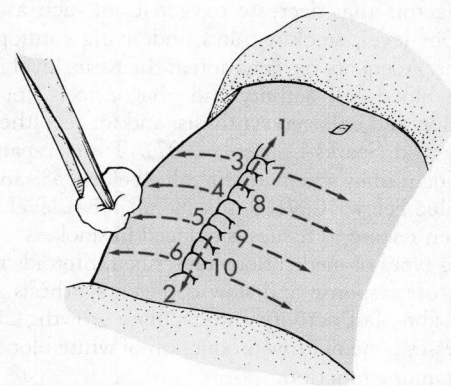

FIG 38-6 Method of cleansing the suture line area.

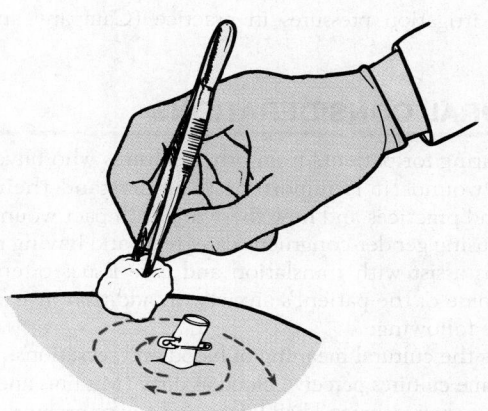

FIG 38-7 Cleansing a drain site.

If a drain is present, cleanse the drain site using a circular stroke starting with the area immediately next to the drain (Fig. 38-7). Using a new swab, cleanse immediately next to drain and attempt to cleanse a little further out from the drain. Continue this process with subsequent swabs until the skin surrounding the drain is cleansed.

Infection is present in a wound when microorganisms invade tissues and there is a systemic response. An infected acute wound usually demonstrates signs of local inflammation; redness and warmth in the area; presence of drainage, pain, or tenderness; and an unusual odor. Surgical wound infection is defined as a surgical site infection (SSI). It involves the site of surgery and presents within 1 year of the procedure. Superficial incision infection involves only skin and subcutaneous tissue at the incision. Deep incision infection involves organs or body cavities in the area of surgery (Stotts, 2007).

Dehiscence, a failure of wound healing in which the surgical wound breaks, separates, and opens to the fascial level, occurs 4 to 14 days after surgery with a mean of 8 days (Doughty, 2005). The wound edges open, and serosanguineous drainage is present. If the wound is allowed to heal by secondary intention, lightly pack wound with a moist dressing covered with a dry dressing, and change as needed. Factors contributing to surgical wound dehiscence include anemia, malnutrition, obesity, and use of steroids.

Evisceration is also a failure of wound healing, with total separation of the layers of the wound and protrusion of the internal organs through the wound. This is a surgical emergency, and you need to cover the wound with a moist saline dressing, notify the surgeon immediately, and prepare the patient for emergent surgery.

EVIDENCE-BASED PRACTICE TRENDS

Guidelines for the nursing care of wounds are developed to support clinical practice by providing consistent, research-based clinical decisions. The Wound, Ostomy and Continence Nurses Society (WOCN) developed four guidelines: *Guideline for Prevention and Management of Pressure Ulcers* (2003), *Guidelines for Management of*

Wounds in Patients With Lower Extremity Arterial Disease (2003), *Management of Patients With Lower Extremity Neuropathic Disease* (2004), *and Management of Patients With Lower Extremity Venous Disease* (2005). A panel of experts performed extensive searches on available literature on wounds and then established a level of evidence rating that provides the best available evidence on management. All of the guidelines are posted on the National Guidelines Clearing House website. A wound care team is an effective strategy to improve patient outcomes for chronic wounds and to decrease costs of supplies and nursing visits related to wound care (Sylvia and Perla, 2004). The wound care team provides early identification of patient needs, facilitates continuity of patient care, and acts as a resource for evidence-based practice related to wound care.

Research shows that wound cleansing and debridement are effective methods to prevent wound infection (Moscati and others, 2007). Irrigation of wounds by nurses is a technique used for wound cleansing. You achieve effective wound irrigation best through the use of a 35-mL syringe with a 19-gauge needle or angiocatheter with irrigation pressures delivered between 4 and 15 psi (Granick and others, 2007). When irrigation pressures exceed 15 psi, additional harm occurs to the tissues (WOCN, 2003). There is an increased risk for wound infection because the high pressures drive bacteria into the wound. Professional nurses need to be knowledgeable about correct wound irrigation techniques and able to achieve effective irrigation pressures in practice (Campany and others, 2000).

CULTURAL CONSIDERATIONS

When caring for patients from other cultures who have acute or chronic wounds it is important to understand their cultural beliefs and practices and how these might impact wound care. In general, using gender-congruent caregivers and having the family or friends assist with translation and care issues often helps to relieve some of the patient's anxiety. In addition, it is important to do the following:

- Assess the cultural meaning of blood and secretions.
  - Some cultures perceive blood as dirty (Muslims and Hindus); thus change stained bed linens and gowns promptly.
  - Some Asians believe that blood is the life force; hence explain the presence of blood-stained secretions and drainage thoroughly.
  - Some Africans perceive showing negative reactions toward a patient's bloody secretions as disrespectful.
- Recognize family members when giving explanations about the nursing care regimen.

- In collectivist cultures, presence of family members at the bedside is customary.
  - Among Arabic families, at least one family member, usually a female, stays at the bedside all the time (Miller and Petro-Nustas, 2002).
- Remind patients that traditional home remedies and practices need to be avoided because they may increase the risk for infection in open wounds.

Skill Performance Guidelines

1 Know the patient's age. With age, vascular changes occur, collagen tissue is less pliable, and scar tissue is tighter. Because the dermoepidermal junction becomes flatter in older adults, their skin tears more easily from mechanical trauma such as tape removal.

2 Know the patient's nutritional status. Tissue repair and infection resistance are directly related to adequate nutrition, including proteins, carbohydrates, lipids, vitamins, and minerals. Patients who are malnourished are at increased risk for wound infections and wound infection–related sepsis (Stotts, 2007).

3 Understand the risks of obesity. Inadequate vascularization decreases delivery of nutrients and cellular elements required for healing. The patient is at greater risk for wound infection and dehiscence or evisceration (Gallagher-Camden, 2007).

4 Identify factors that decrease oxygenation, such as decreased hemoglobin level, smoking, and underlying cardiopulmonary conditions. Adequate oxygenation at the tissue level is essential for white blood cell activity and phagocytosis, for fibroblast proliferation and collagen synthesis, and for reepithelialization (Doughty and Sparks-Defriese, 2007). Tissue repair is negatively influenced by a hematocrit value below 33% and a hemoglobin value below 10 g/100 mL. Hemoglobin level is reduced and oxygen release to tissues is reduced in smokers.

5 Know the types of medications prescribed. Steroids reduce the inflammatory response and slow collagen synthesis. Cortisone depresses fibroblast activity and capillary growth. Chemotherapy depresses bone marrow production of white blood cells and impairs immune function.

6 Identify the presence of chronic diseases or chronic trauma, such as diabetes or radiation. Decreased tissue perfusion and failure to release oxygen to tissues result from diabetes. In radiation therapy, wound healing is most effective when surgery is performed within 4 to 6 weeks of irradiation before the anticipated vascular scarring and fibrosis.

7 Unwounded skin is always stronger than healed skin.

PROCEDURAL GUIDELINE 38-1 Performing a Wound Assessment

Intermediate / Wound and Pressure Ulcer Care / Assessing Wounds

[NSO] *Wound Care Module / Lesson 1*

Wound assessment provides the baseline for planning and evaluating the wound care plan. Normal wound healing occurs in an organized fashion, and evaluating the wound status provides an ongoing assessment of wound healing and aids in determining wound treatments. The frequency of the wound assessment depends on the patient's overall condition, the policy of the health care setting, type of dressings used, and the overall patient goals (Nix, 2007). There are a variety of wound assessment tools; use will depend upon the facility's policy.

Routine wound assessments provides valuable information regarding the status of the wound. For example, is wound healing progressing as expected, or is it delayed; is there new drainage? Sometimes a wound increases in size. This often occurs in a wound with necrotic tissue. Removal of the necrotic tissue may result in a larger wound. This is not a negative finding. Obtain physician's order, (when needed) for consultations, such as a wound, ostomy and continence nurse or clinical nurse specialist (CNS) to discuss findings. If there is an increase in the amount

PROCEDURAL GUIDELINE 38-1   Performing a Wound Assessment—cont'd

and consistency of the drainage and if there is new presence of odor, these factors may indicate a wound infection, and a wound culture is often necessary to support appropriate antibiotics.

The following parameters are included in a wound assessment:

- *Location:* Note the anatomical position of the wound on the body.
- *Type of wound:* If possible, note the etiology of the wound—surgical, pressure, trauma.
- *Extent of tissue involvement:* Full-thickness wound involves both the dermis and epidermis. Partial-thickness wound involves only the epidermal layer. If it is a pressure ulcer, use the staging system of the National Pressure Ulcer Advisory Panel (NPUAP) (see Chapter 18).
- *Type and percentage of tissue in wound base:* Describe the type of tissue—granulation, slough, eschar—and the approximate amount.
- *Wound size:* Determine facility policy on how to measure dimensions, which will include width and length and, in some cases, depth.
- *Wound exudate:* Describe the amount, color, and consistency.
- *Presence of odor:* Note the presence or absence of odor.
- *Periwound area:* Assess the color, temperature, and integrity of the skin.

Delegation Considerations

The skill of wound assessment cannot be delegated to nursing assistive personnel (NAP). It is the nurse's responsibility to assess and document wound characteristics. The nurse directs the NAP by:

- Instructing the NAP to report drainage from the wound that is present on sheets or as strike through from the dressing.
- Discussing the importance of reporting the presence of odor in the area of the wound.

Equipment

- ❑ Protective equipment: clean gloves, gown, and goggles if splash/spray risk exists
- ❑ Agency tool to document assessment: measuring guide
- ❑ Cotton-tipped applicator
- ❑ Dressing supplies
- ❑ Disposable garbage bag

Procedural Steps

1 Determine the facility's approved assessment tool, and review the frequency of wound assessment. Examine the last wound assessment to use as comparison for this wound assessment.
2 Assess comfort level or pain on a scale of 0 to 10, and identify symptoms of anxiety.
3 Explain procedure of wound assessment to patient.
4 Close room door or bed curtains, and position patient.
   a Position comfortably to permit observation of wound in a well-lighted room.
   b Expose wound only.
5 Perform hand hygiene, and form a cuff on waterproof biohazard bag and place near bed.
6 Apply clean gloves, and remove soiled dressings.
7 Examine dressings for quality of drainage (color, consistency), presence or absence of odor, and quantity of drainage (note if dressings were saturated, slightly moist, or had no drainage). Discard dressings in waterproof bag. Discard gloves.

8 Perform hand hygiene, and apply clean gloves
9 Use the agency-approved assessment tool, and assess the following features:
   a The anatomical location of the wound on the body.
   b Extent of tissue loss: Determine if the wound is full or partial thickness. A partial-thickness wound heals by reepithelialization, whereas a full-thickness wound heals by the creation of scar tissue and will take longer to heal (Doughty and Sparks-Defriese, 2007).
   c The type and the percentage of tissue, noting granulation tissue, slough tissue, and/or eschar.
   d Size of wound in centimeters: Measure length, width, and depth (Nix, 2007) (see illustration).
      (1) Insert a cotton-tipped applicator into the deepest section of the wound to measure depth. Discard applicator in biohazard bag.
   e Presence of exudate from wound (amount, color, and consistency). Indicate amount of exudate by using part of dressing saturated or in terms of quantity (e.g., scant, moderate, copious). Expect amount to decrease as healing takes place. Serous drainage is clear like plasma; sanguineous or bright-red drainage indicates fresh bleeding; serosanguineous drainage is pink; purulent drainage is thick and yellow, pale green, or white.
   f Odor: State whether or not there is odor. A change in wound odor may indicate the presence of a wound infection (Stotts, 2007).
   g Periwound skin integrity: Include color, texture, temperature, and a description of any areas that are open, stripped, or have a rash. Periwound assessment gives clues on the effectiveness of the wound treatment, as well as possible wound extension (Nix, 2007).
10 Reassess patient's pain and level of comfort.
11 Reapply dressings as per order.
12 Discard biohazard bag, soiled supplies, and gloves as per agency policy; perform hand hygiene.
13 Record wound assessment findings, and compare assessment with previous wound assessments to monitor wound healing.

Critical Decision Point   *Once you compare the wound assessment to previous assessment, determine progress toward healing. If there is no movement toward healing, or if you notice deterioration, consider a wound care consultation. Lack of wound healing is often related to infection. Notify physician and wound care nurse or team.*

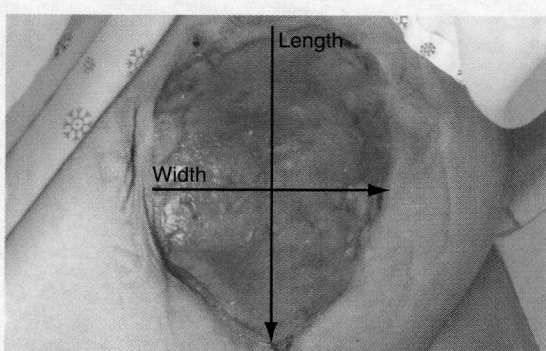

STEP 9d   Measuring wound length and width.

SKILL 38-1 Performing Wound Irrigation

Intermediate / Wound and Pressure Ulcer Care / Irrigating Wounds

Use sterile technique for cleaning and irrigating surgical wounds or clean technique for some chronic wounds, such as pressure ulcers. Introduce the cleansing solution directly into the wound with a syringe, syringe and catheter, shower, or whirlpool. When using a syringe, the tip remains 2.5 cm (1 inch) above the wound. If the patient has a deep wound with a narrow opening, attach a soft catheter to the syringe to permit the fluid to enter the wound. Irrigation should not cause tissue injury or discomfort. Avoid fluid retention in the wound by positioning the patient on the side to encourage the flow of the irrigant away from the wound. It is often helpful to use a 35-mL syringe with a 19-gauge needle to facilitate optimal pressure for cleansing with minimal risk for tissue injury (Rolstad and Ovington, 2007). Ambulatory patients often benefit from the use of a handheld shower for wound cleansing, holding the shower spray approximately 30 cm (12 inches) from the wound. For patients who require mechanical debridement and cleansing but cannot tolerate the above methods, whirlpool is a useful method. In most facilities the physical therapy department performs whirlpool treatments.

There are two types of wound irrigation: high-pressure and pulsatile high-pressure lavage. High-pressure irrigation is the cleansing of a necrotic wound with irrigating fluid delivered at 4 to 15 psi, with a 35-mL syringe and a 19-gauge angiocatheter. This procedure provides force to remove wound debris without damaging healthy tissue. Pulsatile high-pressure lavage is an alternative to high-pressure irrigation. It is the use of a machine to deliver intermittent high-pressure irrigation combined with suction to remove the irrigant and wound debris (Ramundo, 2007). Use a whirlpool to remove bacteria and debris from the surface of large wounds. Additional benefits include softening and loosening of adherent necrotic tissue and cleansing and removal of wound exudate (Ramundo, 2007).

Wound irrigations promote wound healing through removing debris from a wound surface, decreasing bacterial counts, and loosening and removing eschar. Eschar is black or brown necrotic tissue and may be loose or firmly adherent, hard, soft, or soggy (WOCN, 2003). Solutions used for irrigations include normal saline, warm water, and commercially available wound cleansers such as CarraKlenz or SAF Clens. Skin cleansers are not the same as wound cleansers, and you never substitute a skin cleanser for a wound cleanser.

Delegation Considerations
The skill of sterile wound irrigation cannot be delegated to NAP. However, you can delegate the cleansing of chronic wounds using clean technique. It is the nurse's responsibility to assess and document wound characteristics. The nurse directs the NAP by:
- Discussing modifications of the skill, such as increased frequency of wound cleansing other than once a shift.
- Instructing what to report when a wound is cleansed (e.g., wound color, presence of bleeding, drainage).
- Instructing to report patient pain.

Equipment
- ❑ Irrigant/cleansing solution (volume 1.2 to 2 times the estimated wound volume)
- ❑ Irrigation delivery system, depending on amount of pressure desired: sterile irrigation 35-mL syringe with sterile soft angiocatheter or 19-gauge needle (WOCN, 2003) or handheld shower or whirlpool
- ❑ Protective equipment: clean gloves, gown, and goggles if splash/spray risk exists
- ❑ Waterproof underpad, if needed
- ❑ Dressing supplies (Table 38-3)
- ❑ Disposable waterproof biohazard bag
- ❑ Extra towels and padding (to use to protect bed)
- ❑ Wound assessment supplies (see Procedural Guideline 38-1)

TABLE 38-3	Common Wound Dressing Categories			
Category	**Description/Function**	**Indications**	**Side Effects**	**Examples**
Hydrogel	Composed of water or glycerin Provides moisture to wound bed Available in sheets or in amorphous gel (usually in a tube) Autolytic debridement	Partial- and full-thickness wounds Dry to minimal exudate Necrotic wounds	Not indicated for heavily exudating wounds	Curasol Intrasite Gel Vigilon
Alginate	Calcium-sodium alginate fibers that form moisture-retentive gel on contact with wound fluid Absorption Available in pads and ropes for packing Autolytic debridement	Moderate to heavy wound exudate Infected wounds Hemostasis	May contribute to wound desiccation if wound exudate is minimal and gel dries	Restore Sorbsan Algisite M
Foams	Absorption Available in adhesive and non-adhesive forms	Absorption of moderate to heavy exudate Infected wounds	May promote wound dehydration and desiccation if minimal exudate	Allevyn Lyofoam PolyMem
Gauze	Absorption Woven gauze is 100% meshed cotton fabric woven into squares, rolls, and packing strips Available in sterile and nonsterile packing	Protection of surgical wounds Autolytic debridement (saline-moistened) Absorption of minimal to heavy exudate Deliver solution to wound	May adhere to healthy tissue and cause injury on removal Some products may shed, leaving lint in wound	Curity Gauze Sponges KERLIX Super Sponge KLING gauze rolls NU GAUZE packing strips
Hydrocolloids	Absorption Made of gelatin, pectin and carboxymethylcellulose particles suspended in adhesive base Maintain moist environment	Autolytic debridement Absorption of minimal to moderate exudate	May promote hypertrophic granulation tissue Some products leave residue in wound on removal	DuoDERM Restore Tegasorb

Data from Rolstad BS, Ovington LG: Principles of wound management. In Bryant RA, Nix DP, editors: *Acute and chronic wounds: current management concepts,* ed 3, St. Louis, 2007, Mosby.

STEP	RATIONALE

ASSESSMENT

1 Review order for irrigation of open wound and type of solution to be used.

> Open wound irrigation requires medical order including type of solution(s) to use.

2 Perform wound assessment, and examine recent charted assessment of patient's open wound (see Procedural Guideline 38-1).

3 Assess patient for history of allergies to antiseptics, medications, tapes, or dressing material.

> Known allergies suggest application of a sample of prescribed wound treatment as skin test before flushing wound with large volume of solution or selection of different tape or dressing material.

NURSING DIAGNOSES

- Acute pain
- Chronic pain
- Impaired skin integrity
- Impaired tissue integrity
- Risk for injury

Individualize related factors based on patient's condition or needs.

PLANNING

1 Expected outcomes following completion of procedure:
- Patient states acceptable level of comfort on 0 to 10 pain scale after wound irrigation.

> Premedication, gently administered irrigation, application of clean dressing, and repositioning patient ensure comfort.

- Wound begins to heal; dressing is clean and dry; wound is free of drainage and inflammation, or drainage decreases in amount or type (e.g., less bloody or serous as opposed to serosanguineous).

> Healing progresses in absence of debris and presence of protective covering.

- Skin integrity is maintained; no redness, edema, or inflammation noted in surrounding tissue.

> No further skin and tissue damage has resulted from wound irrigation.

STEP	RATIONALE
2 Identify patient using two identifiers. Explain procedure of wound irrigation and cleansing.	Ensures right patient receives right treatment. Information will reduce patient's anxiety.
3 Administer prescribed analgesic 30 to 45 minutes before starting wound irrigation procedure.	Promotes pain control and permits patient to move more easily and be positioned to facilitate wound irrigation (Krasner and others, 2007).
4 Obtain appropriate supplies for wound irrigation and wound dressing.	
5 Close room door or bed curtains, perform hand hygiene, and position patient.	Maintains privacy; frequent hand hygiene reduces microorganisms.
a Position comfortably to permit gravitational flow of irrigating solution over wound and into collection receptacle (see illustration).	Directing solution from top to bottom of wound and from clean to contaminated area prevents further infection. Position patient during planning stage, keeping in mind the bed surfaces needed for later preparation of equipment.
b Position patient so that wound is vertical to collection basin. Place container of irrigant/cleansing solution in basin of hot water to warm solution to body temperature.	Warmed solution increases comfort and reduces vascular constriction response in tissues.
6 Place padding or extra towel in the bed.	Protects bedding.
7 Expose wound only.	Prevents chilling of patient.

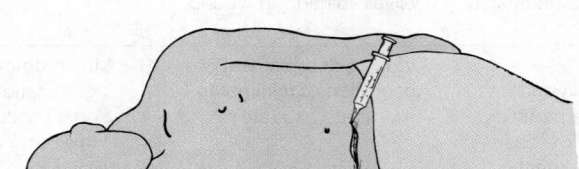

STEP 5a   Patient position for wound irrigation.

IMPLEMENTATION

1 Form cuff on waterproof biohazard bag, and place near bed.	Cuffing helps to maintain large opening, thereby permitting placement of contaminated dressing without touching waste bag itself.
2 Apply gown and goggles.	Protects nurse from splashes or sprays of blood and body fluids (Centers for Disease Control and Prevention [CDC], 1997).
3 Perform hand hygiene, and prepare equipment; open sterile supplies (see Chapter 8).	Reduces transmission of microorganisms.
4 Apply sterile gloves.	Prevents transfer of microorganisms to wound surface.
5 Irrigate wound with wide opening:	
a Fill 35-mL syringe with irrigation solution.	Flushing wound helps remove debris and facilitates healing by secondary intention.
b Attach 19-gauge angiocatheter or 19-gauge needle.	Catheter lumen delivers ideal pressure for cleansing and removal of debris (Ramundo, 2007).
c Hold syringe tip 2.5 cm (1 inch) above upper end of wound and over area being cleansed.	Prevents syringe contamination. Careful placement of the syringe prevents unsafe pressure of the flowing solution.
d Using continuous pressure, flush wound; repeat Steps a, b, and c until solution draining into basin is clear.	Clear solution indicates removal of all debris.
6 Irrigate deep wound with very small opening:	
a Attach soft catheter to filled irrigating syringe.	Catheter permits direct flow of irrigant into wound. Expect wound to take longer to empty when opening is small.
b Gently insert tip of catheter into opening about 1.3 cm (½ inch).	Prevents tip from touching fragile inner wall of wound.

Critical Decision Point   *Do not force catheter into the wound because this will cause tissue damage.*

STEP	RATIONALE
c Using slow, continuous pressure, flush wound.	Use of slow mechanical force of a stream of solution loosens particulate matter on the wound surface and promotes healing (Ramundo, 2007).
d Pinch off catheter just below syringe while keeping catheter in place.	Prevents aspiration of solution into syringe and contamination of sterile solution (Dochterman and Bulechek, 2004).
e Remove and refill syringe. Reconnect to catheter, and repeat until solution draining into basin is clear.	

Critical Decision Point *Pulsatile high-pressure lavage is often the irrigation of choice for necrotic wounds. The amount of irrigant is wound-size dependent. Pressure settings on the device need to remain between 4 and 15 psi. Do not use pulsatile high-pressure lavage on exposed blood vessels, muscle, tendon, and bone. Do not use this type of irrigation with graft sites. Use this irrigation with caution in patients receiving anticoagulant therapy (Ramundo, 2007).*

7 Cleanse wound with handheld shower:	
a With patient seated comfortably in shower chair, adjust spray to gentle flow; make sure water is warm.	Useful for patients able to shower with assistance or independently. May be accomplished at home.
b Shower for 5 to 10 minutes with shower head 30 cm (12 inches) from wound.	Ensures wound is thoroughly cleansed.
8 When indicated, obtain cultures (see Chapter 43) after cleansing with nonbacteriostatic saline.	The WOCN (2003) recommends using quantitative bacterial cultures (tissue biopsy or needle aspiration) rather than swab cultures, which often detect only surface bacterial contaminants.

Critical Decision Point *Consider culturing a wound if it has a foul, purulent odor; inflammation surrounds the wound; a nondraining wound begins to drain; or patient is febrile.*

9 Dry wound edges with gauze; dry patient after shower.	Prevents maceration of surrounding tissue from excess moisture.
10 Apply appropriate dressing (see Chapter 39).	Maintains protective barrier and healing environment for wound.
11 Remove gloves, mask, goggles, and gown.	Prevents transfer of microorganisms.
12 Assist patient to comfortable position.	
13 Dispose of equipment and soiled supplies, and perform hand hygiene.	Reduces transmission of microorganisms.

EVALUATION

1 Have patient rate level of comfort on scale of 0 to 10.	Patient's pain should not increase as a result of wound irrigation.
2 Monitor type of tissue in wound bed.	Identifies wound healing progress and determines type of wound cleansing and dressing needed.
3 Inspect dressing periodically.	Determines patient's response to wound irrigation and need to modify plan of care.
4 Evaluate periwound skin integrity.	Determines if extension of wound has occurred or if signs of infection are present (warm red periwound skin).
5 Observe for presence of retained irrigant.	Retained irrigant is a medium for bacterial growth and subsequent infection.

Unexpected Outcomes	**Related Interventions**
1 Bleeding or serosanguineous drainage appears.	• Flush wound during next irrigation using less pressure. • Notify physician of bleeding.
2 Increased pain or discomfort occurs.	• Decrease force of pressure during wound irrigation. • Assess patient for need for additional analgesia before wound care.
3 Suture line opening extends.	• Notify physician. • Reevaluate amount of pressure to use for next wound irrigation.

Recording and Reporting

- Record wound assessment before and after irrigation; amount, color, and odor of drainage on dressing removed; amount and type of solution used; irrigation device used; patient's tolerance of the procedure; type of dressing applied after irrigation.
- Immediately report to attending physician any evidence of fresh bleeding, sharp increase in pain, retention of irrigant, or signs of shock.

Teaching Considerations

- Instruct patient and primary caregiver regarding wound care technique, observe them doing a return demonstration, and provide written instructions.
- Explain the need for specialized supplies such as irrigating solutions and dressings and the need to maintain asepsis when performing care.

- Instruct patient and primary caregiver in signs of improper wound healing and wound infection.
- Teach patient and caregiver how to make normal saline, especially if cost is an issue. You make normal saline by using 8 teaspoons of salt in 1 gallon of distilled water and keeping it refrigerated for 1 month. The saline solution should be allowed to reach room temperature before use (Fellows and Crestodina, 2006).

Pediatric Considerations

- Some pediatric patients are very frightened. They might verbally and physically try to prevent nurse from cleaning wound. Having child active in parts of procedure or working out child's feelings about wound irrigation using play therapy on a doll with a wound will help child to be more cooperative with procedure.
- Neonatal skin is immature and is easily damaged from pressure and wound care products. Check that products are approved for use with this population. Remember that in neonates the skin readily absorbs products.
- Common topical anesthetic solutions include 2% and 4% lidocaine jelly that inactivate exposed wound pain receptors.

Gerontological Considerations

- Wound irrigations are traumatic, frightening, and painful to some older patients. Assess patient's cooperation before doing wound irrigation. Be aware of patient's cognitive level of understanding when performing wound irrigation.
- With aging comes a 20% loss in dermal thickness, making the skin of older adults almost transparent in appearance. The skin thus is less resilient, and wound irrigation can easily result in skin tears and other trauma (Ratliff and Fletcher, 2007).

Home Care Considerations

- Assess patient's home environment to determine adequacy of facilities for performing wound care; check especially for adequate lighting, running water, and storage of supplies.
- Plan wound care in conjunction with patient's total rehabilitation goals. The objective of wound care management in a subacute care setting is to return the patient to his or her home environment (Beshara and others, 2000).
- Provide support for the patient and caregiver during the wound-healing process. Chronic wounds do not heal properly and do not close in a timely manner (Doughty and Sparks-Defriese, 2007).
- Some patients need to receive wound care management in an outpatient wound care clinic. Be sure patient has directions to clinic and knows where to park and where to obtain dressing supplies.

SKILL 38-2   Performing Suture and Staple Removal

Institutional policy determines whether *only* the physician or the physician *and* nurse may remove sutures and staples. Always obtain the physician's written order before implementing either skill. The time of removal is based on the stage of incision healing and the extent of surgery.

Sutures and staples are generally removed within 7 to 10 days after surgery if healing is adequate. Retention sutures usually remain in place 14 to 21 days. Timing the removal of sutures and staples is important. They must remain in place long enough to ensure initial wound closure with enough strength to support internal tissues and organs. Leaving the sutures in too long increases the risk for infection at the puncture sites. Sutures left in longer than 14 days generally leave scar marks (Autio and Olson, 2002). The physician determines and orders removal of all sutures or staples at one time or removal of every other suture or staple as the first phase, with the remainder removed in the second phase.

Sutures are threads of wire or other materials used to sew body tissues together. Sutures come in different sizes and are absorbent or nonabsorbent. Sutures are placed within tissue layers in deep wounds and superficially as the final means for wound closure. The deeper sutures are usually an absorbable material that disappears in several days. Superficial sutures repair the skin using nonabsorbent sutures (Autio and Olson, 2002).

Staples are stainless steel wire. The location of the incision sometimes restricts their use, because there must be adequate distance between the skin and structures that lie below the skin, including bone and vascular structures. The cosmetic result is not always as desirable as that obtained with finer suture material. Staples do provide ample strength. Removal requires a sterile staple extractor and aseptic technique.

The patient's history of wound healing, site of wound, tissues involved, and the purpose of the sutures determine the suture material selected. For example, a patient with repeated abdominal surgeries might require wire sutures for greater strength to promote wound closure.

The physician and/or nurse judge whether to remove all sutures if any sign of suture line separation is evident during the process of suture or staple removal. It is not uncommon to remove every other suture initially, removing the balance several days to a week later.

Delegation Considerations

The skill of staple and/or suture removal cannot be delegated to NAP. The nurse directs the NAP by:

- Instructing the NAP to report drainage, bleeding, swelling at the site or an elevation in the patient's temperature to the nurse.
- Instructing the NAP to report patient's complaints of pain to the nurse.
- Providing information about any special hygiene practices following suture removal.

Equipment

- ❑ Disposable waterproof bag
- ❑ Sterile suture removal set (forceps and scissors) or sterile staple extractor
- ❑ Sterile applicators or antiseptic swabs
- ❑ Steri-Strips or butterfly adhesive strips
- ❑ Clean gloves
- ❑ Sterile gloves

STEP	RATIONALE

ASSESSMENT

1   Identify patient with need for suture or staple removal:
   a   Check physician's order.

   b   Review specific directions related to suture or staple removal.

   c   Determine history of conditions that may pose risk for impaired wound healing: advanced age, cardiovascular disease, diabetes, immunosuppression, radiation, obesity, smoking, poor cellular nutrition, very deep wounds, and infection.

2   Assess patient for history of allergies.

3   Assess patient's comfort level or pain on a scale of 0 to 10.

4   Assess healing ridge and skin integrity of suture line for uniform closure of wound edges, normal color, and absence of drainage and inflammation.

Rationale:

Physician's order is required for removal of sutures.
Indicates specifically which sutures are to be removed (e.g., every other suture).
Preexisting health disorders affect speed of healing and sometimes result in dehiscence.

Determines if patient is sensitive to antiseptic.
Provides baseline of patient's comfort level to determine response to therapy.
Indicates adequate wound healing for support of internal structures without continued need for sutures or staples.

Critical Decision Point   *If wound edges are separated or signs of infection are present, wound has not healed properly. Notify physician because sutures or staples may need to remain in place and/or other wound care initiated.*

NURSING DIAGNOSES

• Impaired skin integrity   • Risk for impaired skin integrity   • Risk for infection

Individualize related factors based on patient's condition or needs.

PLANNING

1   Expected outcomes following completion of procedure:
   • All suture material or staples are removed.
   • Suture line is intact.
   • Patient states acceptable level of comfort on 0 to 10 scale following removal of sutures or staples.

2   Explain to patient that suture removal is usually not a painful procedure, but patient may feel pulling or tugging of the skin.

Rationale:

Removes source of infection or irritation from retained sutures.
Wound is healing and does not require protective dressings.
Some patients require pain medicine before suture or staple removal.

Gains patient cooperation and reduces anxiety.

IMPLEMENTATION

1   Close curtains or room door.

2   Identify patient using two identifiers. Position patient comfortably, while exposing suture line.

Rationale:

Provides privacy.
Ensures right patient undergoes right treatment. Prepares area for staple or suture removal.

Critical Decision Point   *For patient who is highly anxious or who has an extensive wound, consider need to administer analgesic 30 minutes before suture removal.*

3   Ensure direct lighting is on suture line.

4   Perform hand hygiene.

5   Place cuffed waterproof disposal bag within easy reach.

6   Prepare materials needed for suture/staple removal:
   a   Open sterile suture removal kit or staple extractor kit.
   b   Open sterile antiseptic swabs, and place on inside surface of kit.
   c   Obtain gloves, sterile gloves if policy indicates.

Rationale:

Aids visibility and correct placement of forceps or extractor during removal process, ultimately reducing soft tissue injury.
Reduces risk for infection.
Provides for easy disposal of contaminated dressings and prevents passing items over sterile work area.

STEP	RATIONALE
7 Apply clean gloves. Carefully remove dressing, and discard dressing and clean gloves in prepared refuse disposal bag.	Reduces transmission of infection.
8 Inspect wound and suture line (see illustration).	Determines adequacy of wound healing.
9 Apply sterile gloves, if required by policy, or clean gloves.	
10 Cleanse sutures or staples and healed incision with antiseptic swabs.	Removes surface bacteria from incision and sutures or staples.
11 Remove staples:	
a Place lower tips of staple extractor under first staple. As you close handles, upper tip of extractor depresses center of staple, causing both ends of staple to be bent upward and simultaneously exit their insertion sites in the dermal layer (see illustration).	Avoids excess pressure to suture line and secures smooth removal of each staple.
b Carefully control staple extractor.	Avoids suture-line pressure and pain.
c As soon as both ends of staple are visible, move it away from skin surface, and continue on until staple is over refuse bag (see illustration).	Prevents scratching tender skin surface with sharp pointed ends of staple for comfort and infection control.
d Release handles of staple extractor, allowing staple to drop into refuse bag.	Avoids contaminating sterile field with used staples.
e Repeat Steps a to d until all staples are removed.	
12 Remove sutures (see illustration). Steps below demonstrate removal of intermittent sutures:	
a Place gauze a few inches from suture line. Grasp scissors in dominant hand and forceps in nondominant hand.	Gauze serves as receptacle for removed sutures. Placement of scissors and forceps allows for efficient suture removal.

Critical Decision Point   *Placement of scissors and forceps is very important. Avoid pinching the skin around the wound when lifting up the suture. Likewise, avoid cutting the skin around the wound by accident when snipping the suture.*

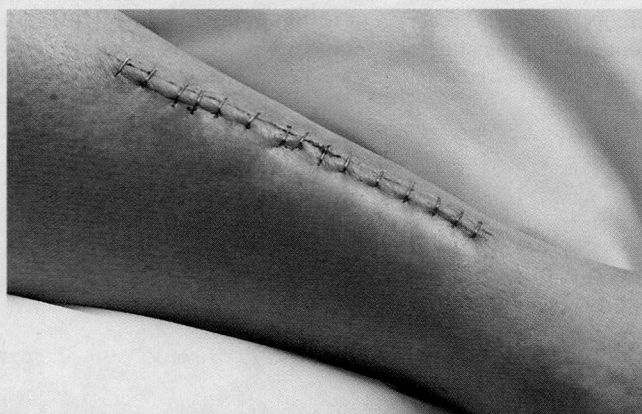

STEP 8   Suture line secured with staples.

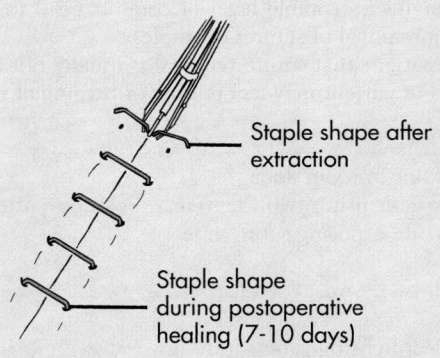

Staple shape after extraction

Staple shape during postoperative healing (7-10 days)

STEP 11a   Staple extractor placed under staple.

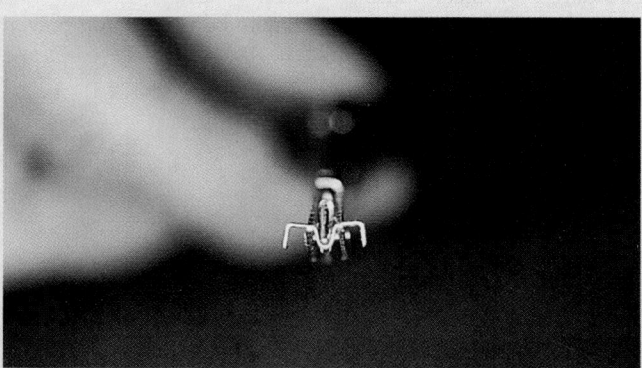

STEP 11c   Metal staple removed by extractor.

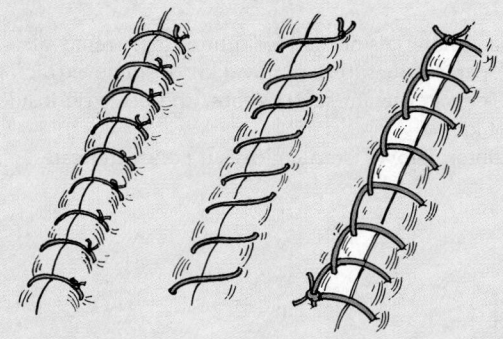

STEP 12   Types of sutures: *Left,* Intermittent; *middle,* continuous; *right,* blanket.

STEP	RATIONALE

b   Grasp knot of suture with forceps, and gently pull up knot while slipping tip of scissors under suture near skin (see illustration).

Releases suture.

c   Snip suture as close to the skin as possible at end distal to the knot.

Critical Decision Point   *Never snip both ends of suture; there will be no way to remove the part of the suture situated below the surface.*

d   Grasp knotted end with forceps, and in one continuous smooth action pull the suture through from the other side (see illustration). Place removed suture on gauze.

Smoothly removes suture without additional tension to suture line.

Critical Decision Point   *Never pull exposed surface of any suture into tissue below epidermis. The exposed surface of any suture is considered contaminated.*

e   Repeat Steps a to d until you have removed every other suture.

f   Observe healing level. Based on observations of wound response to suture removal and physician's original order, determine whether remaining sutures will be removed at this time. If so, repeat Steps a to d until you have removed all sutures.

Determines status of wound healing and if suture line will remain closed after all sutures are removed.

g   If any doubt, stop and notify physician.

13 Remove continuous sutures, including blanket stitch sutures:

a   Place sterile gauze a few inches from suture line. Grasp scissors in dominant hand and forceps in nondominant hand.

Gauze serves as receptacle for removed sutures. Placement of scissors and forceps allows for efficient suture removal.

b   Snip first suture close to skin surface at end distal to knot.

Releases suture.

c   Snip second suture on same side.

Releases interrupted sutures from knot.

d   Grasp knotted end, and gently pull with continuous smooth action, removing suture from beneath the skin. Place suture on gauze compress.

Smoothly removes sutures without additional tension to suture line. Prevents pulling of contaminated portion of suture through the skin.

e   Repeat Steps a to d in consecutive order until the entire line is removed.

14 Inspect incision site to make sure all sutures are removed and to identify any trouble areas. Gently wipe suture line with antiseptic swab to remove debris and cleanse wound.

Reduces risk for further incision line separation.

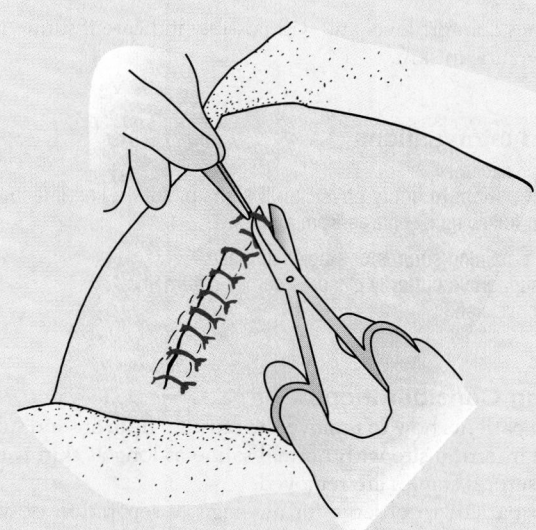

STEP 12b   Removal of intermittent suture. Nurse cuts suture as close to skin as possible, away from the knot.

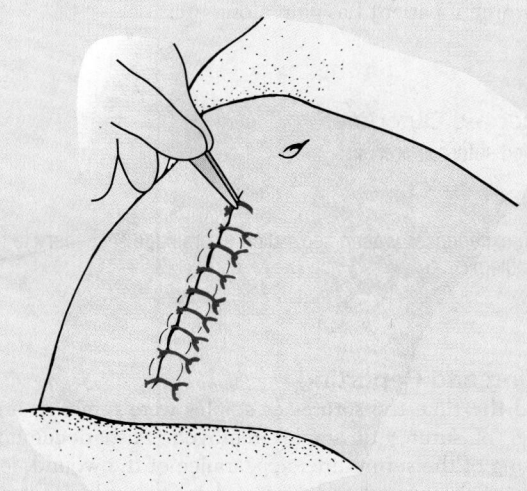

STEP 12d   Nurse removes suture and never pulls the contaminated stitch through tissues.

STEP	RATIONALE

Critical Decision Point *Make sure that you remove the entire suture and that no part is retained in the patient's wound.*

15 Apply Steri-Strips if *any* separation greater than two stitches or two staples in width is apparent to maintain contact between wound edges.	Supports the wound by distributing tension across the wound and eliminates closure technique scarring (Autio and Olson, 2002).
a Cut Steri-Strips to allow strips to extend 4 to 5 cm (1½ to 2 inches) on each side of the incision.	
b Remove backing, and apply across incision (see illustration).	
c Instruct patient to take showers rather than soak in bathtub according to physician's preference.	Steri-Strips are not removed and are allowed to fall off gradually.
16 Apply light dressing, or expose to air if no clothing will come in contact with suture line. Instruct patient about applying own dressing if it will be needed at home.	Healing by primary intention eliminates need for dressing.
17 Discard all contaminated materials, and remove and dispose of gloves.	Reduces transmission of infection.
18 Route reusable items such as staple extractor for resterilization, and perform hand hygiene.	Reduces transmission of infection.

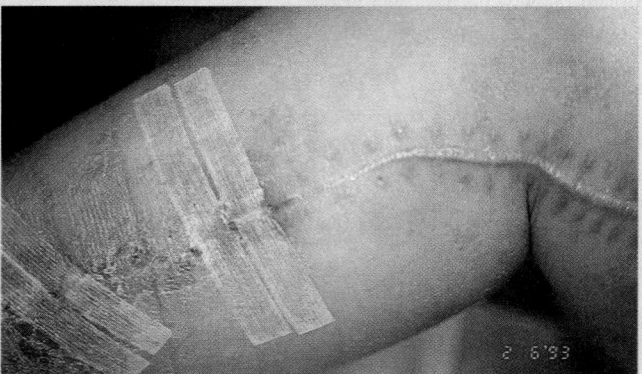

STEP 15b   Steri-Strips over incision.

EVALUATION

1 Assess site where sutures or staples were removed; inspect condition of soft tissues, including skin. Look for any pieces of removed suture that were left behind.	Ensures that sources of infection have been removed.
2 Determine if patient has pain along incision.	Determines comfort level and will possibly indicate if suture material remains in skin.

Unexpected Outcomes

1 Retained suture is present.

2 Patient experiences wound separation or drainage secondary to healing problems.

Related Interventions

- Notify physician.
- Instruct patient to notify physician if signs of suture line infection develop following discharge from agency.

- Leave remaining sutures or staples in place.
- Place supportive butterfly closures across suture line.
- Notify physician.

Recording and Reporting

- Record the time the sutures or staples were removed and the number of sutures or staples removed. Also document the cleansing of the suture line, appearance of the wound, level of healing of the wound and type of dressing applied. Document the patient's response to suture or staple removal.
- Immediately report to physician if suture line separation, dehiscence, evisceration, bleeding, or purulent drainage occurs.

Teaching Considerations

- Teach patients how to remove the crusting from around sutures/staple insertion site with normal saline as long as skin is intact once sutures/staples are removed.
- Teach patient to observe for any sign of separation of wound edges before removing remaining sutures/staples and to inspect incision for continued healing.

- Continue instruction in resumption of bathing and showering activities, prevention of abdominal strain during defecation, and provision of adequate nutrition and ambulation.
- Teach patient not to put additional stress on suture line from such activities as lifting or bending (Dochterman and Bulechek, 2004). Patients with abdominal surgery or injury need to avoid lifting heavy packages or equipment for several weeks.
- Instruct patient that sometimes there is a small amount of drainage from wound immediately after suture removal.
- Instruct patient to avoid exposing wounds to the sun because this increases scarring (Autio and Olson, 2002).

Pediatric Considerations

- Assistance is sometimes necessary to keep babies from moving during the suture removal procedure.
- Topical anesthetic solutions (e.g., lidocaine, EMLA) applied to intact skin may provide short-term (20 minutes) anesthesia (Krasner and others, 2007).

Gerontological Considerations

- Some older adults need reassurance about suture/staple removal procedure. Depending on their mental status, they may not understand procedure.
- Older skin is often at higher risk for dehiscence after sutures/staples are removed.

SKILL 38-3 Managing Drainage Evacuation

 Intermediate / Wound and Pressure Ulcer Care / Using a Wound Drainage System

NSO *Wound Care Module / Lesson 2*

If drainage accumulates in the wound bed, wound healing is delayed. Drainage is removed by using either a closed or open drain system, even if the amount of drainage is small. The drain is inserted directly through the suture line into the wound or through a small stab wound near the suture line into the area of the wound.

An open drain system (e.g., a Penrose drain [Fig. 38-8]) removes drainage from the wound and deposits it onto the skin surface. Insert a sterile safety pin through this drain, outside the skin, to prevent the tubing from moving into the wound.

To remove the Penrose drain the physician advances the tubing in stages as the wound heals from the bottom up. Nursing interventions include caution to prevent accidental removal of the drain during dressing changes and to protect skin surfaces in direct contact with the irritating drainage. Because of the danger of accidental dislodgment and the need to assess the drain placement accurately, do not delegate the care of Penrose drains that are covered with gauze pads to nursing assistive personnel. Some Penrose drains are contained within wound pouches because of the high volume of drainage from the wound.

A closed drain system, such as the Jackson-Pratt (JP) drain (Fig. 38-9) or Hemovac drain (Fig. 38-10), relies upon the presence of a vacuum to withdraw accumulated drainage from around the wound bed into the collection device. A JP drain collects fluid that is in the range of 100 to 200 mL/24 hr, whereas the Hemovac drain accommodates more drainage, usually up to 500 mL/24 hr. The collection device is connected to a clear plastic drain with multiple

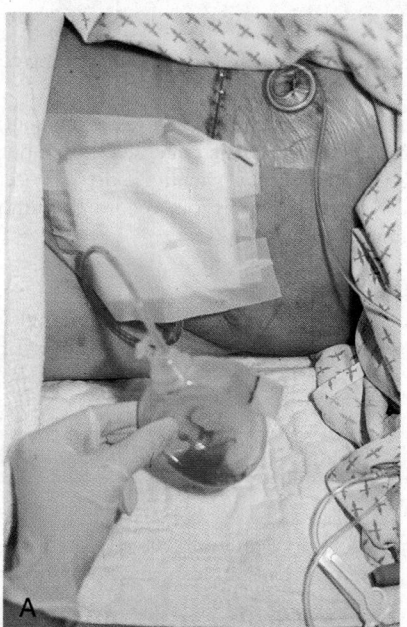

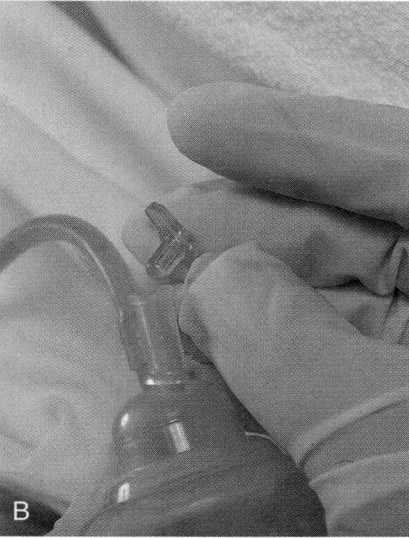

FIG 38-9 A, Jackson-Pratt wound drainage system. **B,** Emptying Jackson-Pratt device.

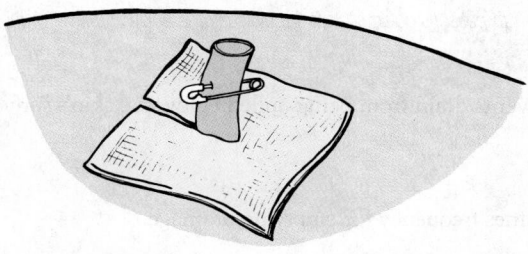

FIG 38-8 Penrose drain with a drain-split gauze.

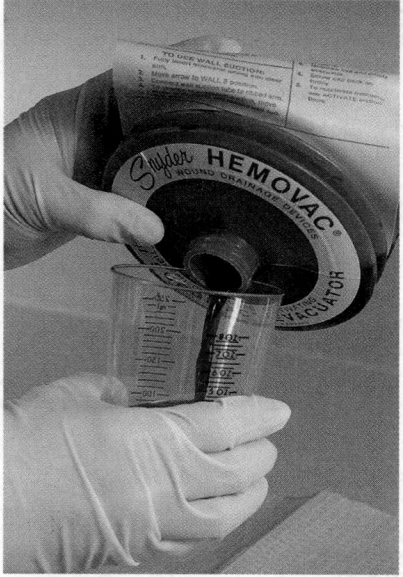

FIG 38-10   Hemovac contents drained into measuring container.

Hemovac
- Connect graduated adapter to emptying port and then to wall suction tubing.
- Set suction level as prescribed or on low if suction level not specified.

Jackson-Pratt
- Attach tubing to evacuator.
- Squeeze evacuator flat to allow all air to be evacuated, and close port.

you may delegate emptying a closed drainage container or pouch, measuring the amount of drainage, and reporting the amount on the patient's intake and output (I&O) record to NAP. The nurse directs the NAP by:

- Discussing any modification of the skill such as increased frequency of emptying the drain other than once a shift.
- Instructing to report any change in amount, color, or odor of drainage.
- Reviewing the I&O procedure.

Equipment
- Graduated measuring cylinder
- Alcohol sponge
- Gauze sponges
- Goggles if needed
- Sterile specimen container, if culture is needed
- Sterile dressings or pouch, if drain is needed
- Clean gloves
- Safety pin(s)

perforations. Drainage collects in a closed reservoir, suction bladder, or bag (Box 38-3). The closed system collects fluid but operates only if the tubing is patent and a vacuum exists. You empty the drainage periodically from the reservoir, record the amount, and reestablish the vacuum.

Delegation Considerations
The assessment of wound drainage and maintenance of drains and the drainage system cannot be delegated to NAP. However,

STEP	RATIONALE

ASSESSMENT

1 Identify presence, location, and purpose of closed wound drain and drainage system as patient returns from surgery. Assess drainage present on patient's dressing.

2 Identify number of wound drain tubes and what each one will be draining. Label each drain tube with a number or label.

3 Assess if drain tube needs self-suction, wall suction, or no suction by checking physician's orders.

4 Inspect system to determine presence of one straight tube or Y-tube arrangement with two tube insertion sites.

5 Inspect system to ensure proper functioning. A complete systematic inspection includes the insertion site, drainage moving through tubing in direction of reservoir, patency of drainage tubing, airtight connection sites, and presence of any leaks or kinks in the system.

Drainage tubing is usually placed within wound or through small surgical incision near major wound.

Assigning a labeling system to each drain helps with consistent documentation when patient has multiple drainage tubes.

Some drain tubes, such as Hemovacs, are used with self-suction or wall suction.

Allows nurse to plan skin care and identifies quantity of sterile dressing supplies needed.

Properly functioning system maintains suction until reservoir is filled. Tension on drainage tubing increases injury to skin and underlying muscle.

Critical Decision Point   *Attach tape and a safety pin to drainage tubing with tape and pin to patient's gown so that the evacuator is below the level of the wound and does not pull on insertion site.*

6 Be sure Penrose drain has a sterile safety pin in place. Penrose drains are sometimes covered with a gauze dressing or a wound pouch. Use caution, and do not accidentally pull on drain while positioning gauze.

7 Identify type of drainage containers patient has.

Pin prevents drain from being pulled below the skin's surface.

Determines frequency for emptying drainage.

STEP	RATIONALE

NURSING DIAGNOSES

- Impaired skin integrity
- Risk for infection
- Risk for injury

Individualize related factors based on patient's condition or needs.

PLANNING

1 Expected outcomes following completion of procedure:	
• Wound healing continues.	Patient will be comfortable, and wound drainage will be collected.
• Vacuum is reestablished.	Suction system is intact.
• Tubing is patent.	Fluid is draining away from wound area.
2 Explain procedure to patient.	Promotes patient's cooperation and reduces anxiety.

IMPLEMENTATION

1 Close room door or bedside curtains.	Provides privacy.
2 Perform hand hygiene, and apply gloves.	Reduces transmission of microorganisms.
3 Place open specimen container or measuring graduate on bed between you and patient.	Permits measuring and discarding of wound drainage.
4 When emptying evacuator, maintain asepsis while opening port:	Avoids entry of pathogens.
a Hemovac (see Fig. 38-10):	
(1) Open plug on port indicated for emptying drainage reservoir.	Vacuum will be broken, and reservoir will pull air in until chamber is fully expanded.
(2) Tilt evacuator in direction of plug.	Drains fluid toward plug.
(3) Slowly squeeze two flat surfaces together while draining into sterile laboratory specimen container if culture is ordered, then drain remainder into graduated cylinder. Cover specimen container.	Prevents splashing of contaminated drainage.
(4) Hold uncovered alcohol sponge in dominant hand; place evacuator on flat surface with open outlet facing upward; continue pressing downward until bottom and top are in contact; hold surfaces together with one hand, quickly cleanse opening and plug with other hand, and immediately replace plug; secure evacuator on patient's bed.	Compression of surface of Hemovac creates vacuum. Cleansing of plug reduces transmission of microorganisms into drainage evacuation.
(5) Check evacuator for reestablishment of vacuum, patency of drainage tubing, and absence of stress on tubing.	Facilitates wound drainage and prevents tension on drainage tubing.
b Jackson-Pratt evacuator (see Fig. 38-9, *A*):	
(1) Open emptying cap on side of bulb-shaped reservoir (see Fig. 38-9, *B*).	Breaks vacuum for drain.
(2) Tilt evacuator in direction of plug, and drain toward opening. Empty drainage from evacuator.	
(3) Compress bulb over drainage container. Cleanse ends of emptying port with alcohol sponge while continuing to compress container. Replace cap immediately. Secure evacuator below wound site with safety pin through indicated perforation to patient's gown.	Reestablishes vacuum. Reduces transmission of microorganisms into drainage evacuator and prevents tension on drainage tubing.
5 Place and secure drainage reservoirs to prevent any pull on tubing insertion sites. Be sure there is slack in tubing from reservoir to wound.	Pinning drainage tubing to patient's gown will prevent tension or pulling on tubing and insertion site (Dochterman and Bulechek, 2004).
6 Send labeled specimen to laboratory (if ordered by physician).	Allows for culture testing to determine infection.
7 Discard soiled supplies, remove gloves, and perform hand hygiene.	Reduces transmission of microorganisms.

STEP	RATIONALE
8 Apply new clean gloves, and proceed with dressing change (see Chapter 39) around drain site and inspection of skin if indicated or ordered. Split-drain sponge dressings are often used around drain tubes (see illustrations) and then taped in place.	Prevents entrance of bacteria into surgical wound.
9 Discard contaminated materials, and perform hand hygiene.	Reduces transmission of microorganisms.

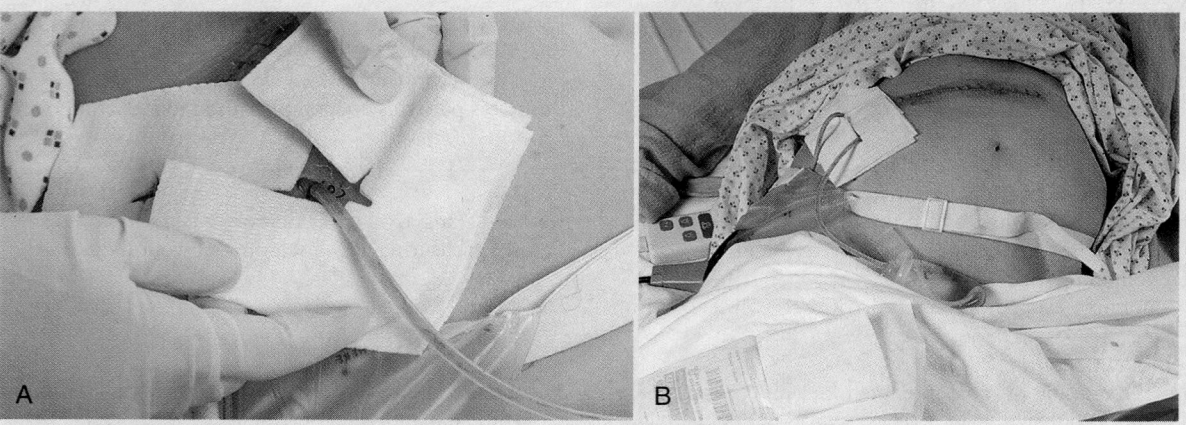

STEP 8   **A,** Applying Jackson-Pratt (JP) split gauze dressing around a JP drain tube. **B,** Split dressing in place around a JP drain tube.

EVALUATION

1 Observe for drainage in drainage evacuator.	Indicates presence of vacuum, patency of tubing, and functioning of drainage evacuator.

Critical Decision Point   *Clots or large collections of debris may block drainage flow. The Y site in the drainage tubing is especially prone to clogging.*

2 Inspect wound for drainage or collection of drainage fluid under the skin, causing a seroma.	Drainage should not be significant under suture line. May indicate inadequate functioning of drainage evacuator.
3 Measure drainage, empty drainage system, record on I&O form.	Empty drainage collection reservoir every 8 to 12 hours and as needed for large drainage volume. Collect diagnostic specimen in the presence of unexpected purulence or pungent odor, reports findings to physician, and record in progress note.
4 Assess patient's level of comfort using the 0 to 10 scale.	Ensures that procedure does not increase patient's pain.

Unexpected Outcomes	Related Interventions
1 Wound becomes infected.	• Notify physician about the presence of signs of infection: purulent drainage, odor, reddened site, increased white blood cell count, and temperature elevation. • Use aseptic technique when changing dressings.
2 Bleeding appears.	• Determine amount of bleeding, and notify physician if excessive. • Assess for tension on patient's drainage tubing. • Secure tubing to prevent pulling and pain.
3 Patient experiences pain.	• Assess patient's level of pain. • Medicate patient. • Stabilize drainage tubing to reduce tension and pulling against incision. • Notify physician if signs of wound infection are present.
4 Drainage evacuator system is not accumulating drainage.	• Assess drainage tubing for clots. • Assess drainage system for air leaks or kinks. • Notify physician.

Recording and Reporting

- Record emptying of the drainage evacuator; reestablishment of vacuum in evacuator; amount, color, odor of drainage; dressing change to drain site; and appearance of drain insertion site.
- Record amount of drainage on I&O record.
- Immediately report a sudden change in amount of drainage, either output or absence of drainage flow, to the physician. Also report pungent odor of drainage or new evidence of purulence, severe pain, or dislodgment of the drainage tube to the physician.

Teaching Considerations

- Instruct patient about anticipated postoperative drainage, expected progress of wound healing and drainage volume, and estimated date of removal of drain as volume diminishes.
- Instruct patient or caregiver in how to empty and record amount of drainage. If patient is going home with drainage device, ask patient or caregiver to record amount emptied and bring the recording to the next outpatient visit.

Pediatric Considerations

- Have parents help to prevent pediatric patients from dislodging drainage tubes.

Gerontological Considerations

- Be aware that older adult patients with large amounts of drainage will need additional fluid intake because they are more likely to become dehydrated.
- Take measures to prevent a confused patient from pulling out drain collector.

Home Care Considerations

- Provide written instructions in drain care.
- Arrange for home care nurse if needed.

? CRITICAL THINKING EXERCISES

You are assigned to care for Mrs. Pereira, who was readmitted to the hospital with wound dehiscence and infection following a colon resection. Her past medical history includes chronic obstructive lung disease as well as diverticulitis.

1 Which factors listed below from Mrs. Pereira's history contributed to her poor wound healing? Select all that apply. Explain your choices.
  A Takes prednisone daily for respiratory disease
  B Has type 2 diabetes mellitus
  C Takes aspirin daily because of myocardial infarction (MI) 6 years earlier
  D Eats six small high-protein meals a day
  E Is 74 years old
  F Drinks 2 L of water daily

2 When performing the wound assessment you note that the wound base is covered with red, moist granulation tissue. Is the presence of granulation tissue a good finding? Explain your answer.

3 Wound irrigation daily was ordered for Mrs. Pereira. How should you position Mrs. Pereira for the wound irrigation? Explain your choice.
  A Supine with irrigation basin vertical to wound
  B High-Fowler's with basin at base of wound
  C Lying on her side with basin vertical to wound
  D Low-Fowler's with basin at base of wound

4 Which intervention will help to reduce the risk for infection during wound irrigation? Select all that apply.
  A Use sterile technique.
  B Direct the flow of solution from healthy tissue to infected tissue.
  C Warm irrigation solution to body temperature.
  D Clean suture line after doing wound irrigation.
  E Irrigate with a continuous pressure of 3 psi.

5 Mrs. Pereira has a Jackson-Pratt (JP) drain near the wound. The order is to empty the JP drain collection device every 8 hours. After draining the fluid from the container, how will you reestablish the closed suction system?
  A There is no need to reestablish the suction; closing the port achieves the closed suction setup.
  B Compress the bulb portion of the container, and close the port.
  C Pump the container several times before closing.
  D Leave 10 mL of wound fluid in the container to keep the level of suction constant.

✓ REVIEW QUESTIONS

1 A patient has a large abdominal wound, which will require irrigation and packing after discharge from the hospital. Which statement made by the patient indicates a need for further teaching related to her wound irrigation?
  1 "I'll lie so the wound is vertical to the basin during the irrigation."
  2 "I'll use slow continuous pressure while irrigating my wound."
  3 "I'll warm the irrigation solution to body temperature before I use it."
  4 "I'll irrigate the wound starting at the bottom and move to the top."

2 The patient tells the nurse that the physician said his sutures are coming out today. Which nursing action is most important before removing the sutures?
  1 Assemble the required equipment.
  2 Check that there is a physician's order for the suture removal.
  3 Perform hand hygiene in view of the patient.
  4 Explain to the patient what will be happening during the suture removal.

3 A patient has an extensive abdominal wound and is to have half of the staples removed and the incision line cleaned. Which actions should the nurse take during the preparation and actual interaction with the patient? Select all that apply.
  1 Position the patient in a semi-Fowler's position.
  2 Place upper tip of staple remover under staple to ease removal.
  3 Administer an analgesic 30 minutes before the staple removal.
  4 Lift up on the staple when depressing the extractor handles.
  5 Clean the incision before removing the staples, starting at the sides next to the incision.
  6 Remove all of the staples at the top of the incision, and leave the rest, beginning at the middle of the incision.

4 The patient is to have sutures removed from his back after surgery. The nurse is performing the procedure correctly by taking which step?
  1 Snip the suture at the end proximal to the knot.
  2 Wipe the area with a disinfectant swab to prevent wound infection.
  3 Remove the suture in a smooth continuous manner.
  4 Hold the scissors in your nondominant hand and the pickups in your dominant hand.

5 The nurse notes approximately 60 mL of very red drainage in the Jackson-Pratt drain 6 hours after surgery. Which nursing interventions should be included in the care for this patient? Select all that apply.

   1 Empty the drain 24 hours from now.

   2 Pin the drainage tubing to the patient's gown.

   3 Place Vaseline gauze around the tube insertion site.

   4 Secure the drain above the level of the wound.

   5 Empty the drain now.

   6 Squeeze the drain flat before putting in the drainage plug.

REFERENCES

Autio L, Olson KK: The four S's of wound management: staples, sutures, Steri-Strips, and sticky stuff, *Holist Nurs Pract* 16(2):80, 2002.

Barr JE: Principles of wound cleansing, *Ostomy Wound Manage* 7A(suppl 41):15S, 1995.

Beshara M and others: Practice development in acute and long-term care settings. In Bryant RA, editor: *Acute and chronic wounds: nursing management,* ed 2, St. Louis, 2000, Mosby.

Bryant RA, editor: *Acute and chronic wounds,* ed 2, St. Louis, 2000, Mosby.

Bryant RA, Nix DP, editors: *Acute and chronic wounds: current management concepts,* ed 3, St. Louis, 2007, Mosby.

Centers for Disease Control and Prevention: *Part II: recommendations for isolation precautions in hospitals,* 1997, http://wonder.cdc.gov/wonder/prevguid/p000049/p0000419.asp.

Dochterman JC, Bulechek GM: *Nursing interventions classification (NIC),* ed 4, St. Louis, 2004, Mosby.

Doughty DB: Preventing and managing surgical wound dehiscence, *Adv Skin Wound Care* 18(6):319, 2005.

Doughty DB, Sparks-Defriese B: Wound-healing physiology. In Bryant RA, Nix DP, editors: *Acute and chronic wounds: current management concepts,* ed 3, St. Louis, 2007, Mosby.

Fellows J, Crestodina L: Home-prepared saline: a safe, cost-effective alternative for wound cleansing in home care, *J Wound Ostomy Continence Nurs* 33(6):606, 2006.

Frantz RA and others. In Bryant RA, Nix DP, editors: *Acute and chronic wounds: current management concepts,* ed 3, St. Louis, 2007, Mosby.

Gallagher-Camden S: Skin care needs of the obese patient. In Bryant RA, Nix DP, editors: *Acute and chronic wounds: current management concepts,* ed 3, St. Louis, 2007, Mosby.

Krasner DL and others: Managing wound pain. In Bryant RA, Nix DP, editors: *Acute and chronic wounds: current management concepts,* ed 3, St. Louis, 2007, Mosby.

Nix DP: Patient assessment and evaluation of healing. In Bryant RA, Nix DP, editors: *Acute and chronic wounds: current management concepts,* ed 3, St. Louis, 2007, Mosby.

Ramundo J: Wound debridement. In Bryant RA, Nix DP, editors: *Acute and chronic wounds: current management concepts,* ed 3, St. Louis, 2007, Mosby.

Ratliff CR, Fletcher KR: Skin tears: a review of the evidence to support prevention and treatment, *Ostomy Wound Manage* 53(3):32, 2007.

Rolstad BS, Ovington LG: Principles of wound management. In Bryant RA, Nix DP, editors: *Acute and chronic wounds: current management concepts,* ed 3, St. Louis, 2007, Mosby.

Stotts NA: Nutritional assessment and support. In Bryant RA, Nix DP, editors: *Acute and chronic wounds: current management concepts,* ed 3, St. Louis, 2007, Mosby.

Sylvia C, Perla J: The team approach to total education and management, *J Wound Ostomy Continence Nurs* 31(3S):S21, 2004.

Whitney JD: Acute surgical and traumatic wounds. In Bryant RA, Nix DP, editors: *Acute and chronic wounds: current management concepts,* ed 3, St. Louis, 2007, Mosby.

Wound, Ostomy and Continence Nurses Society: *Guideline for prevention and management of pressure ulcers,* WOCN clinical practice guidelines series, Glenview, Ill, 2003.

RESEARCH REFERENCES

Campany E and others: Nurses' knowledge of wound irrigation and pressures generated during simulated wound irrigation, *J Wound Ostomy Continence Nurs* 27:296, 2000.

Granick MS and others: Comparison of wound irrigation and tangential hydro dissection in bacterial clearance of contaminated wounds: results of a randomized, controlled clinical study, *Ostomy Wound Manage* 53:46, 2007.

Miller J, Petro-Nustas W: Context for care of Jordanian women, *J Transcult Nurs* 13(3):228, 2002.

Moscati RM and others. A multicenter comparison of tap water versus sterile saline for wound irrigation, *Acad Emerg Med* 14:404, 2007.

Dressings, Bandages, and Binders

SKILLS AND PROCEDURES

KEY TERMS

Dead space
Debridement
Dehiscence
Epithelialization
Erythema
Evisceration
Excoriation
Exudate
Granulation
Hydrocolloid
Hydrogel

Macerated
Negative pressure wound therapy
Neovascularization
Occlusive dressing
Pressure dressing
Primary dressing
Secondary dressing
Wound vacuum-assisted closure

MEDIA RESOURCES

- **evolve** learning system http://evolve.elsevier.com/Perry/skills
  - Review Questions
  - Video Clips

-  Mosby's Nursing Video Skills, 3.0

- **NSO** Nursing Skills Online

Mastery of content in this chapter will enable the nurse to:
- Properly assess a wound.
- Discuss the purposes of dressings, bandages, and an abdominal binder.
- Choose the correct dressing for a wound.
- Understand the technique of a dressing, bandage, or binder application.

- State advantages and disadvantages of the types of dressings used.
- Correctly apply dry, moist-to-dry, pressure, transparent, and synthetic dressings.
- Correctly change a negative pressure wound therapy dressing.
- Correctly demonstrate the technique for applying turned bandages.
- Correctly apply an abdominal binder.

Wound healing is complex. Wounds heal best in a moist environment because it facilitates healing and prevents wound tissue from drying or incorporating gauze fibers into healing tissue (Bolton, 2007). The concept of moist wound healing revolutionized wound management, causing the development of many moisture-retentive dressings. As a result, wound dressings act like the skin and maintain a physiological environment promoting adequate moisture, temperature, pH, blood supply, and pathogen control (Rolstad and Ovington, 2007).

There are two types of dressings, primary and secondary. A primary dressing comes in direct contact with the wound bed. Secondary dressings cover or hold primary dressings in place. Dressings serve several functions: maintaining a moist environment, protecting from outside contaminants, protecting from further injury, preventing the spread of microorganisms, increasing patient comfort, and controlling bleeding. The ideal dressing is based on the purpose of the dressing (Box 39-1). For example, apply a pressure dressing to control bleeding. Use a highly absorbent dressing to manage wound drainage. Use an alginate, foam, or hydrocolloid dressing in a noninfected wound that is draining a moderate to large amount of exudate.

Another factor to consider when choosing a dressing is ease of application. The dressing should conform to body contours, be durable yet flexible, and be able to absorb or contain exudate. It should also be cost-effective, easily removed without damage to the healing surface, and acceptable in appearance (Rolstad and Ovington, 2007).

When changing a dressing you need to know about wound healing and how to differentiate a normal or expected appearance from abnormal change in a wound. Assessment of the exudates absorbed by the dressing provides valuable diagnostic information (see Chapter 38, Procedural Guideline 38-1).

Primary healing takes place when tissue is cleanly cut and the margins are reapproximated. Repair frequently occurs without complication. New capillary circulation bridges the wound quickly in 3 to 4 days, and once normal tissue oxygenation is achieved, the wound is healed. A wound closed for primary healing is most susceptible to infection during the first 4 days.

Healing by secondary intention occurs when a wound is left open. Healing results in the formation of granulation tissue from the bottom of the wound and eventual epithelialization from the sides of the wound to close the defect. During the process of epithelialization, epithelial cells migrate and proliferate from the wound edges to cover the wound surface. Burns, infected wounds, and deep pressure ulcers heal in this manner (Doughty and Sparks-DeFriese, 2007).

The type of dressing depends on the wound characteristics and the goal of wound management, which can be wound debridement or wound healing. Various types of dressings are applied to wounds. Given the many types of available dressings, it may be difficult to decide which dressing is best to use on a particular wound. Fig. 39-1 is helpful for selection of an appropriate dressing for a particular wound.

Dry woven gauze dressings do not interact with the wound tissues and cause little wound irritation. These are most often used in wounds with minimal damage (Table 39-1). Telfa gauze dressings contain a shiny, nonadherent surface on one side that does not stick to the wound. Drainage passes through the nonadherent surface to the outer gauze dressing. A dry dressing is not used for debriding wounds. When a dry dressing inadvertently adheres to the wound, moisten the dressing with sterile normal saline or sterile water before removing gauze to minimize wound trauma. *Moistening the gauze only applies to dry dressings and is not applicable for moist-to-dry dressings.*

Moist dressings are used with full-thickness wounds that resemble craters. Granulation tissue and new capillary networks must form to fill in the defect (Fig. 39-2, p. 1003). Moist-to-dry dressings are for wounds requiring debridement (see Skill 39-1). A moist-to-dry dressing has a moist contact dressing layer that touches the wound surface. The moistened gauze increases the absorptive ability of the dressing to collect exudate and wound debris. This layer dries and adheres to dead cells, thus debriding the wound when removed. Isotonic solutions, such as normal saline or lactated Ringer's solution are used to moisten dressings because they aid mechanical debridement and create an environment conducive to tissue growth. The outer absorbent layer is a dry dressing that protects the wound from invasive organisms.

A moist-to-dry dressing is a method of debridement that can cause trauma to new healthy granulation tissue (Milne and Houle, 2002). Recent advances in wound care therapies have created a number of new debriding products for use along with moist gauze for debriding necrotic wounds. Autolytic debriding products are applied to wounds to allow the enzymes to self-digest dead tissue.

BOX 39-1   Dressing Recommendations

- Is nontraumatic and reduces volume of exudate, but does not allow the wound to dry
- Maintains a stable physiological wound environment
- Keeps the wound bed continuously moist, but also keeps the surrounding (periwound) intact skin dry
- Resolves the amount of periwound erythema by 1 week
- Reduces by 50% wound dimensions or depth of sinus tract within 2 weeks
- Reduces volume of exudate
- Reduces by 25% the amount of necrotic tissue (eschar) by 1 week
- Reduces pain intensity during dressing changes
- Easy to apply and remove with easy-to-follow patient/family instructions
- Cost-effective: reimbursable and/or affordable
- Appropriate for infected wounds

Data from Rolstad BS, Ovington LG: Principles of wound management. In Bryant RA, Nix DP: *Acute and chronic wounds: nursing management,* ed 3, St. Louis, 2007, Mosby; Hall P, Schumann L: Wound care: meeting the challenge, *J Am Acad Nurse Pract* 13(6):258, 2001.

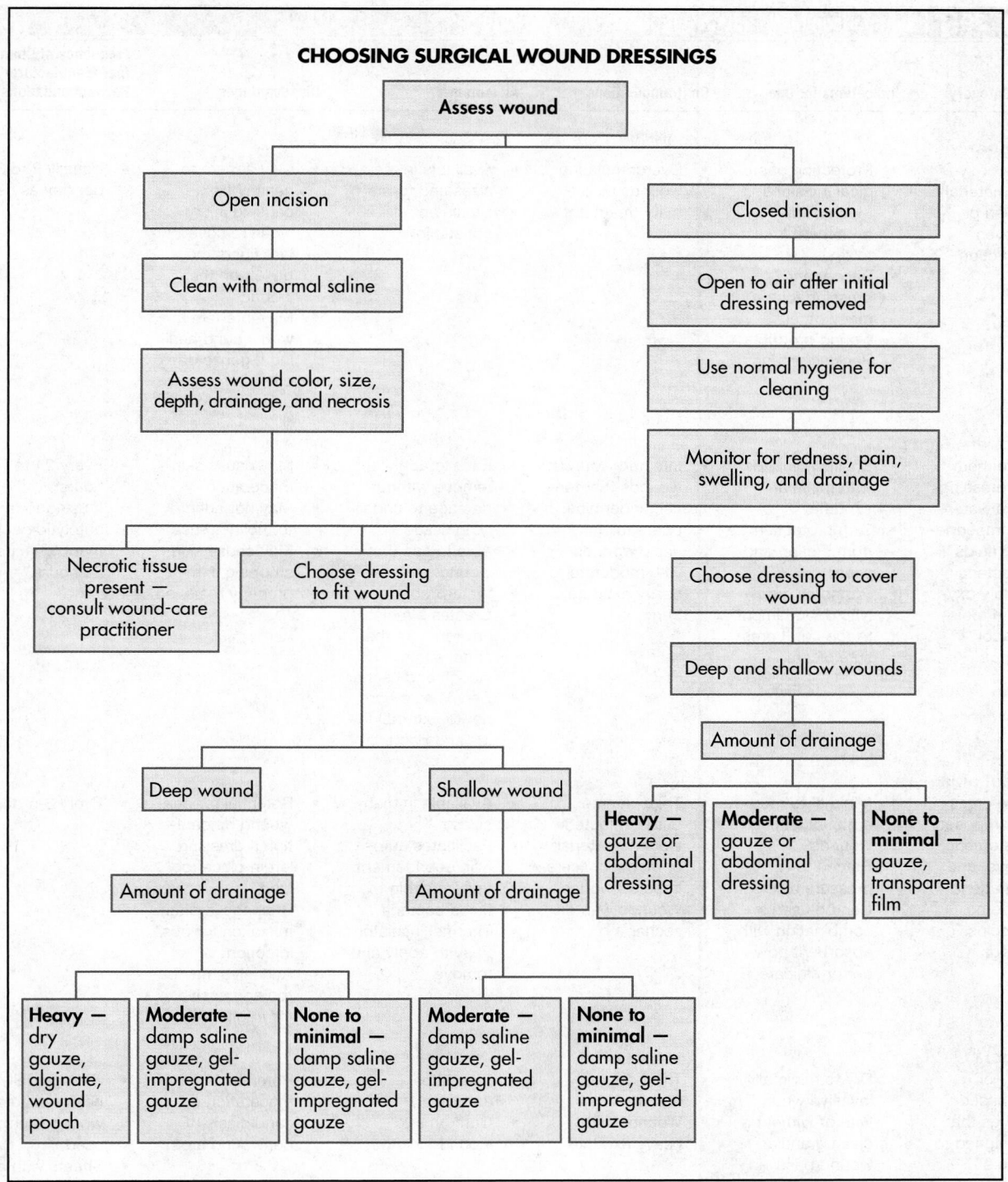

FIG 39-1 Flow chart for dressing selection.

TABLE 39-1	Comparison of Wound Care Products				
Product Category	**Indications for Use**	**Contraindications**	**Advantages**	**Disadvantages**	**Frequency of Change (per Manufacturer's Recommendations)**
Gauze Dressings A cotton or synthetic material of woven or nonwoven construction.	• Protection of surgical incisions • Mechanical debridement (moist to dry) • Secondary dressing for many other wound products • Packing wounds	• Overgranulating wounds as primary treatment	• Available in many sizes and forms • Sterile and nonsterile	• May adhere to healthy tissue, causing injury when removed • Lint fibers may be left on the wound • May interfere with wound healing if gauze dries out in a moist-to-dry dressing	• Usually 2 to 3 times per day as needed.
Transparent Films Adhesive membrane dressings that are waterproof, impermeable to fluids and bacteria and allow oxygen and moisture vapor exchange.	• Shallow wounds with minimal exudate • Skin protection from friction and shear • Promotes autolytic debridement • Stage I or II pressure ulcers	• Infected wounds, wounds that tunnel, undermine, or are full thickness; wounds with moderate to heavy exudate; burns	• Easy to apply and remove without damage to underlying tissue • Able to see the wound • Waterproof • Creates a moist environment that softens thin slough and eschar • Serves as a barrier to external fluids and bacteria	• May cause skin maceration • May not adhere to moist areas • May cause skin stripping if improperly removed	• Every 24 to 72 hours. • If using to facilitate autolytic debridement, change every 24 hours.
Hydrocolloids Adhesive dressings composed of elastomeric, adhesive, and gelling agents. Considered semiocclusive dressings.	• Minimal to moderate exudating wounds • Stage I to IV pressure ulcers • Can be used in combination with absorbent powder or alginate	• Third-degree burns, infected wounds; arterial or diabetic ulcers • Infected wound • Wounds with dry eschar	• Available in many sizes • Facilitates autolytic debridement • Impermeable to fluids/bacteria • Thermal insulator • Easy to apply and remove	• Potential for periwound maceration if dressing left in place too long • Drainage is often mistaken for pus/infection • Adhesive may be too aggressive for fragile skin	• Every 3-5 days.
Hydrogel Glycerin- or water-based dressings that are designed to hydrate a wound. They may also absorb a small amount of exudate.	• Dry to minimally invasive wound with or without a clean granular wound base • Shallow or deep wounds • Wounds with undermining • Necrotic wounds	• Third-degree burns • Wounds with heavy exudate	• Facilitates autolysis • Conforms to wound	• Potential for maceration or candidiasis of periwound area	• Change daily if adhesive sheets or wound fillers are not used. • Sheets with adhesive covers are changed up to 3 times per week.

TABLE 39-1	Comparison of Wound Care Products—cont'd				
Product Category	**Indications for Use**	**Contraindications**	**Advantages**	**Disadvantages**	**Frequency of Change (per Manufacturer's Recommendations)**
Alginates Highly absorbent, nonwoven material that forms a gel when exposed to wound drainage; fibrous product derived from brown seaweed.	• Moderate to heavily exudating wounds with or without depth • Full-thickness, tunneling wounds • Partial- and full-thickness wounds • Leg ulcers, donor sites, traumatic wounds	• Third-degree burns • Nondraining wounds • Dry necrotic wounds	• Nonadhering • Nonocclusive • May be packed into tunneled areas • Promotes autolytic debridement in exudating wounds • Highly absorbent	• More expensive than gauze or gauze packing strips • May not be practical for large wounds • Gelled material may be mistaken for purulence	• Loosely pack wound. • Layer dressings in a deep wound. • Change every 24 hours.
Foam Dressings An absorbent, nonadherent polyurethane pad used to protect wounds and maintain a moist healing environment.	• Moderate or heavily exudating wounds • Partial- and full-thickness wounds • Stages II, II, and IV pressure ulcers	• Third-degree burns, wounds that tunnel, wounds with sinus tracts, nondraining wounds, caution with infected wounds	• Provides high absorbency while maintaining moist wound environment • May be used with other dressings (films, absorbers) • Nonadherent to wound bed	• Nonadhesive foams require a secondary dressing • Maceration of periwound may occur if dressing is left on too long	• Change up to 3 times per week. • When using foam wound fillers, change once per day.

Modified from Rolstad BS, Ovington LG: Principles of wound management. In Bryant RA, Nix DP: *Acute and chronic wounds: nursing management,* ed 3, St. Louis, 2007, Mosby; Nelson D, Dilloway MA: Principles, products, and practical aspects of wound care, *Crit Care Nurs Q* 25(1):33, 2002.

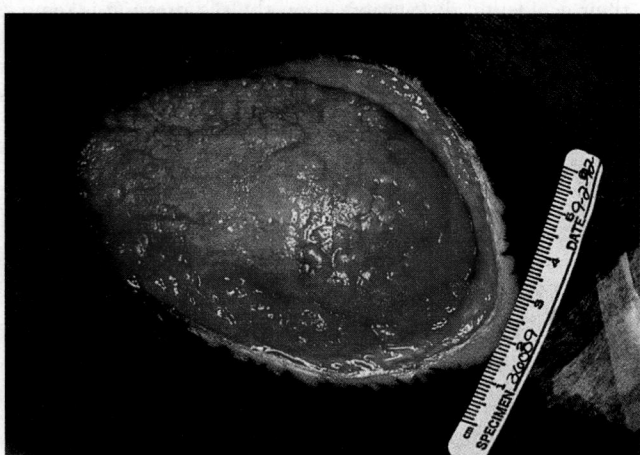

FIG 39-2   Granulation tissue in an open wound.

Enzymatic debriding agents are applied directly to the wound bed and act by breaking down dead tissue (Harvey, 2005). Both autolytic and enzymatic products are used in combination with moist-to-dry gauze, but may also come as prepackaged dressings that do not require any additional gauze.

Dressings are also available as thin, self-adhesive transparent films (e.g., OpSite and Tegaderm) (see Skill 39-3). These dressings are a synthetic permeable membrane that acts as a temporary second skin (see Table 39-1). The film is ideal for small, superficial wounds. This type of dressing uses autolysis to debride a necrotic wound. It is also useful as a dressing over an intravenous (IV) catheter site. The transparent film allows you to assess the wound without removing the dressing.

The hydrocolloid dressings (DuoDERM, Restore, and Tegasorb) represent a category of hydroactive dressings (see Skill 39-4). These dressings provide a moist environment for wound healing while facilitating the softening and subsequent removal of wound debris. The dressing promotes wound healing by providing a semi-occlusive protective barrier that absorbs drainage from the wound into the dressing (see Table 39-1).

Hydrogel dressings (e.g., Curisol, IntraSite Gel, and Vigilon) have a high moisture content (95%), causing them to swell and retain fluid (see Skill 39-4). They are useful over clean, moist, or macerated tissues (see Table 39-1). These nonadherent dressings are very soothing and cooling, thus making them especially useful for painful burn wounds.

Alginate dressings (e.g., Algisite M, Restore, and Sorbsan) are highly absorbent and absorb serous fluid or exudate to form a hydrophilic gel that conforms to the shape of the wound (Rolstad and

Ovington, 2007). Because these dressings absorb and hold exudate, they create a moist environment and promote granulation, epithelialization, and autolysis (see Skill 39-4). A secondary dressing is often used over the alginate.

Foam dressings (e.g., Allevyn, PolyMem, and Lyofoam) absorb light-to-heavy amounts of exudate, are conformable, and can easily be made to fit a wound (see Skill 39-4). These properties make them especially useful for treating draining ulcers (see Table 39-1).

EVIDENCE-BASED PRACTICE TRENDS

Moist wound healing (MWH) changed the way wounds are managed. An evidence-based report card supports the impact of a moist wound environment on the speed and quality of wound healing (Bolton, 2007). Water vapor transmission rate (WVTR) through a wound dressing is a reliable measure of the moisture retention capacity of the dressings. Low rates indicate a small amount of water vapor transmission, whereas the higher rates indicate increased water vapor transmission. Low WVTR occurs with hydrocolloid or film dressings, medium WVTR occurs with foam dressings, and high WVTR occurs with gauze or impregnated gauze dressings. Understanding the need for MWH and how dressing types affect water transmission is important in selecting proper wound dressings for specific wounds (Bolton, 2007).

The type of wound care and dressing change required also determines whether to use clean or sterile technique. The Wound, Ostomy and Continence Nurses Society (WOCN) supports the use of clean technique for the management of chronic wounds, except when sharp debridement is used at the bedside (Wooten and others, 2005). Current practice recommends using sterile gloves for postoperative dressing changes in the first 24 to 48 hours after surgery.

Different types of dressings demonstrate comparable healing outcomes for wounds but vary in cost. Hydrocolloid and collagen dressings are equally effective in healing pressure ulcers. However, the collagen dressings are more expensive. Dressing selection needs to be individualized to the goals of wound healing (Gray and Weir, 2007).

CULTURAL CONSIDERATIONS

Different cultures and religious practices attribute different meanings to wounds and trauma. It is important to assess and try to understand the different meaning of blood and wounds and how it affects patients and their families. Some East Asian cultures interpret loss of blood and secretions as loss of one's spiritual and vital life energy. Some Muslims and Hindus perceive blood as dirty; hence you need to dispose of soiled dressings and linens (Galanti, 2004). When possible and appropriate, be sure to accommodate cultural care modalities such as heat and cold when performing wound irrigations. If permitted, use warm or room temperature solutions when the condition is categorized as cold to achieve balance and healing.

Dressing changes always require a respect for a patient's privacy. However, sometimes patients from other cultures have additional privacy needs such as the need for gender-congruent caregivers, especially if dressings are located in areas considered private.

Dressing changes are at times painful. Take time to understand cultural differences in expressions of pain and beliefs toward pain medications.

- Patients from northern European and Asian backgrounds are often more stoic about pain expression, and you will need to offer the pain medication even if the patient does not complain of pain (Galanti, 2004).
- Some patients, for example those from Korea, may express somatic symptoms such as improved sleep and appetite.

Skill Performance Guidelines

1 Determine the goals of wound management. For example, certain dressings are used to debride wounds, whereas others are used to maintain a moist wound environment necessary for granulation tissue to fill wound defects in a clean wound.

2 Know the cause or type of wound. Wounds caused by vascular insufficiency, diabetes mellitus, pressure, trauma, and surgery are all very different and must have an individualized treatment plan. Not knowing the cause of the wound can have serious negative effects if you use treatments that are contraindicated for certain types of wounds.

3 Know the expected amount and type of wound exudate or drainage (Box 39-2). Wounds with large amounts of drainage require more frequent dressing changes or need absorptive dressing.

4 Know the type of dressing ordered. Moist-to-dry dressings require more equipment than do dry dressings. Pressure dressings require elastic bandages to maintain the pressure.

5 Determine if wound drainage tubes are present. This prevents their accidental dislocation when the old dressing is removed (see Chapter 38, Skill 38-3).

6 Determine the presence of any further break in skin integrity adjacent to the wound. Breaks in skin integrity further increase the patient's risk for infection.

BOX 39-2	Types of Wound Exudate

- *Serous,* which is a clear, watery plasma
- *Sanguineous,* which indicates fresh bleeding, bright red
- *Serosanguineous,* which is a pale, red, more watery drainage than sanguineous drainage
- *Purulent,* which is a thick, yellow, green, or brown drainage

SKILL 39-1   Applying a Dressing (Dry and Moist-to-Dry)

 Intermediate / Wound and Pressure Ulcer Care / Changing a Dressing

NSO *Wound Care Module, Lesson 3*

Dry dressings are for wound healing by primary intention with little drainage. The dressing protects the wound from injury, prevents introduction of bacteria, reduces discomfort, and speeds healing.

Dry dressings are commonly used for abrasions and nondraining postoperative (primary intention healing) incisions. The dry dressing does not debride the wound; hence it is not for wounds requiring debridement. In addition, a dry dressing is not appropriate for an open wound that is healing by secondary intention. If a dry dressing adheres to a wound, moisten the dressing with sterile normal saline or water before removing the woven gauze. Moistening the dressing in this manner decreases the adherence of the dressing to the wound and reduces the risk for further trauma to the wound.

Moist-to-dry dressings are gauze moistened with an appropriate solution. For this reason, moist-to-dry dressings are sometimes called wet-to-dry or damp-to-dry dressings. The primary purpose of moist-to-dry dressings is to mechanically debride a wound. The moistened contact layer of the dressing (primary dressing) increases the absorptive ability of the dressing to collect exudate and wound debris (Ovington, 2001a). As the dressing dries, it adheres to the wound and debrides the wound of the tissue when the dressing is removed (Table 39-1). A dressing that is too wet causes tissue maceration and bacterial growth (Table 39-2). It also does not dry out and therefore does not remove the necrotic tissue when being removed from the wound (Gray and Weir, 2007). The moistened gauze must be covered with a secondary dressing layer that is dry. Disadvantages of moist-to-dry dressings are that the dressing needs to be changed every 4 to 6 hours and the removal of the dry dressing is likely to cause pain to the patient.

Use woven gauze to pack wounds. Principles for correctly packing a wound are provided in Box 39-3. Commonly used wetting agents include normal saline and lactated Ringer's solution, which are isotonic solutions that aid in mechanical debridement. Acetic acid is effective against *Pseudomonas aeruginosa* but is toxic to fibroblasts in standard dilutions.

Povidone-iodine, usually one-quarter to one-half strength, is a rapid-acting antimicrobial agent for cleansing *intact* skin and is never used on a healthy granulating wound bed. This agent is used only in select situations for short-term use (e.g., preventing surgical site infection). Research has not proven that bacteria levels decrease in chronic open wounds when povidone-iodine is applied (Joanna Briggs Institute, 2008). Other antibiotic solutions may be ordered, although their use is controversial. See Chapter 38 for a more detailed discussion of appropriate solutions to use to clean wounds. Because they can harbor microorganism growth, solutions should be discarded 24 to 48 hours after opening and replaced with fresh solutions. Clearly label all solution bottles with date and time of opening.

TABLE 39-2	Problems Associated With Wounds Requiring Debridement
Problem	**Nursing Activities**
Solutions used may be irritating to healthy skin around wound.	Protect healthy skin with protective barrier, such as Stomahesive, or apply topical ointments, such as zinc oxide. If zinc oxide is used, it should be removed with mineral oil. Avoid scrubbing of the skin because the scrubbing can cause harm to the epithelial layer.
Wound becomes excessively dry.	Continually moist dressing (with a health care provider's order) might be tried. Eliminate fine mesh gauze, and lightly pack wound with fluffy gauze dampened with prescribed solution.
Wound is deep, and retention of dressing in cavity is suspected.	Irrigate wound copiously with prescribed solution to loosen dressing for removal. Use continuous "ribbon" or strip of gauze to dress deep wounds.
Wound drainage is damaging healthy tissue.	Protect healthy tissue with skin barrier, such as a hydrocolloid. Wounds with large amounts of drainage may benefit from occlusive drainage collection device.
Patient's skin is irritated by tape.	Use hydrocolloid under tape, use Montgomery ties as needed, use fabric tape that has multidirectional stretch, secure dressing with binder, or wrap with roll gauze if on extremity.

BOX 39-3	Principles for Packing a Wound

- Use the wound characteristics to decide what type of packing is appropriate.
- Make sure the packing material can be safely used to pack a wound.
- Moisten the packing material with a noncytotoxic solution such as normal saline. Never use cytotoxic solutions (e.g., povidone-iodine) to pack a wound.
- If using woven gauze, fluff it before packing it into the wound.
- Loosely pack the wound.
- Do not let the packing material drag or touch the surrounding wound tissue before you put it into the wound.
- Fill all the wound dead space with the packing material.
- Pack the wound until you reach the wound surface; never pack the wound higher than the wound surface.

Delegation Considerations

The skill of applying dry and moist dressings to the new acute wound cannot be delegated to nursing assistive personnel (NAP). In some settings the skill of applying a dry dressing or changing the top dressing can be delegated to NAP (refer to agency policy). The nurse is responsible for assessment of the wound. The nurse directs the NAP about:

- Any unique modifications of the skill, such as the need for use of special tape or taping techniques to secure the dressing.
- Reporting pain, fever, bleeding, or wound drainage to the nurse immediately.

Equipment

- ❑ Clean gloves
- ❑ Sterile gloves
- ❑ Sterile dressing set (scissors, forceps) (may be *optional*, check institution policy)
- ❑ Sterile drape (*optional*)
- ❑ Sterile dressings: fine mesh gauze, 4 × 4 inch gauze, abdominal (ABD) pads
- ❑ Sterile basin (*optional*)
- ❑ Antiseptic ointment (as prescribed)
- ❑ Cleansing solution as prescribed
- ❑ Sterile normal saline or prescribed solution
- ❑ Tape, ties, or bandage as needed (include nonallergenic tape if necessary)
- ❑ Protective waterproof underpad
- ❑ Waterproof bag
- ❑ Adhesive remover (*optional*)
- ❑ Measurement device (*optional*): tape measure, camera (*optional*)
- ❑ Protective gown, goggles, mask used when splashing from wound is a risk
- ❑ Additional lighting if needed (e.g., flashlight, treatment light)

STEP	RATIONALE

ASSESSMENT

1 Assess size of wound (see Chapters 18 and 38).	Assists nurse in planning for proper type and amount of supplies needed.
2 Assess location of wound.	Determines dressing type needed and if assistance is needed to hold dressings in place.
3 Determine patient's level of comfort using a scale of 0 to 10. Administer prescribed analgesic as needed 30 minutes before dressing change.	Comfortable patient will be less likely to move suddenly, causing wound or supply contamination. Serves as baseline to measure response to dressing therapy.
4 Assess patient's knowledge of purpose of dressing change.	Determines level of support and explanation required by patient.
5 Assess need and readiness for patient or family member to participate in dressing wound.	Prepares patient or family member if dressing must be changed at home.
6 Review medical orders for dressing change procedure.	Indicates type of dressing or applications to use.
7 Identify patients with risk factors for wound-healing problems, including:	Physiological changes resulting from aging, chronic illness, poor nutrition, medications, and cancer treatments have the potential to affect wound healing (Rolstad and Ovington, 2007).
a Aging	Physiological changes of aging alter the immune system, resulting in decreased resistance to pathogens (Ebersole and others, 2008).
b Prematurity	The skin of premature babies is not mature and does not have the immune functions of normal skin (Hockenberry and Wilson, 2007).
c Obesity	Subcutaneous tissue has diminished vascularity.
d Diabetes	Vascular changes associated with diabetes reduce blood flow to peripheral tissues; also leukocyte malfunction occurs secondary to hyperglycemia.
e Compromised circulation	Results in inadequate supply of nutrients, blood cells, and oxygen to wound.
f Poor nutritional state	Impairs stages of inflammation and collagen formation states.
g Immunosuppressive drugs	Decreases inflammatory response and decreases collagen synthesis.
h Irradiation in area of wound	Decreases blood supply to tissues.
i High levels of stress	Increased cortisol levels reduce number of lymphocytes and decrease inflammatory response.
j Steroids	Slows rate of epithelialization and neovascularization and inhibits contraction.

NURSING DIAGNOSES

• Acute pain	• Deficient knowledge regarding dressing application	• Impaired skin integrity • Risk for infection

Individualize related factors based on patient's condition or needs.

STEP	RATIONALE

PLANNING

1 Expected outcomes following completion of procedure:
  • Patient's wound is free of infection; drainage decreases, and wound closure is progressing.
  • Patient reports improved comfort.
  • Patient or family explains method of dressing application.
2 Explain procedure to patient.

Indicates wound is healing appropriately.

Indicates dressing procedure and choice are appropriate.
Indicates learning has occurred.
Decreases patient's anxiety. Relieves anxiety.

IMPLEMENTATION

1 Close room or cubicle curtains. Perform hand hygiene. Apply gown, goggles, and mask if risk for splashing exists.

Provides for privacy and reduces transmission of microorganisms.

2 Check patient's identification using two identifiers; one cannot be the patient's room number.

Ensures correct patient receives correct therapy.

3 Position patient comfortably, and drape to expose only wound site. Instruct patient not to touch wound or sterile supplies.

Draping provides access to wound while minimizing exposure. Dressing supplies become contaminated when touched by patient's hand.

4 Place disposable waterproof bag within reach of work area. Fold top of bag to make cuff. Put on clean disposable gloves (see illustration).

Ensures easy disposal of soiled dressings. Prevents contamination of bag's outer surface.

5 Apply clean gloves. Remove tape, bandages, or ties: Pull parallel to skin, toward dressing, and hold down uninjured skin. If over hairy areas, remove in the direction of hair growth. Secure patient permission to clip or shave area (check agency policy). Remove any adhesive from skin.

Pulling tape toward dressing reduces stress on suture line or wound edges and reduces irritation and discomfort.

6 With gloved hand or forceps remove dressing one layer at a time. Carefully remove outer secondary dressing first, and then remove inner primary dressing that is in contact with the wound bed. If drains are present, slowly and carefully remove dressings and avoid tension on any drainage devices. Keep soiled undersurface from patient's sight.

The purpose of the primary dressing is to remove necrotic tissue and exudate. Appearance of drainage may be upsetting to patient. Avoids accidental removal of drain.

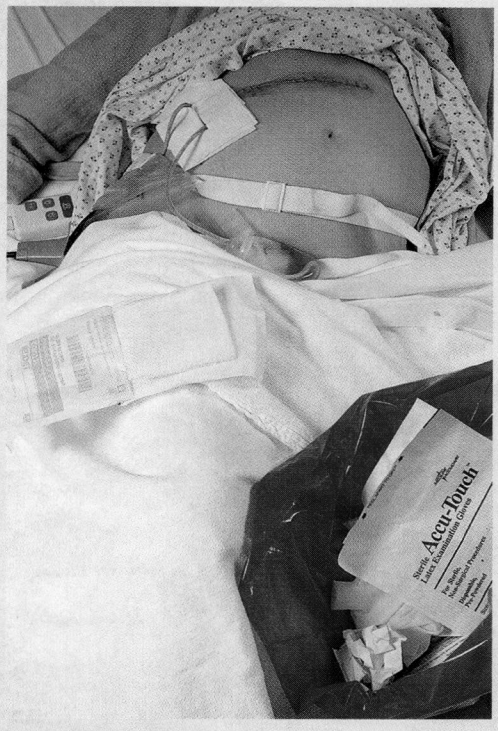

STEP 4 Disposable waterproof bag placed near work area.

STEP	RATIONALE

a If dressing sticks on a wet-to-dry dressing, gently free dressing and alert patient of discomfort.

Wet-to-dry dressing should debride wound (Ramundo, 2007). Do not wet the dressing, it should be dry.

b If dressing sticks on dry dressing, moisten with saline and remove.

Prevents tearing of wound edges.

7 Fold dressing with drainage contained inside, and remove gloves inside out. With small dressings, remove gloves inside out over the dressing (see illustration). Dispose of gloves and soiled dressing according to agency policy.

Provides containment of soiled dressings, prevents contact of nurse's hands with drainage, and reduces cross contamination.

8 Inspect wound for color, drains, exudate, integrity, and presence of drains (see illustration). Observe appearance of drainage on dressing. Assess for odor. Gently palpate the wound edges for drainage, bogginess, or patient report of increased pain. Measure wound size (length, width, and depth [if indicated]) (see Chapters 18 and 38).

Provides assessment of drainage and of wound's condition. Indicates status of healing.

9 Describe the appearance of the wound and any indicators of wound healing to the patient.

Wounds may appear unsettling and frightening to patients; it is helpful for the patient to know that the wound appearance is as expected and that healing is taking place.

10 Create sterile field with a sterile dressing tray or individually wrapped sterile supplies on over-bed table (see illustration). Pour any prescribed solution into sterile filed.

Sterile dressings remain sterile while on or within sterile surface. Preparation of all supplies prevents break in technique during dressing change.

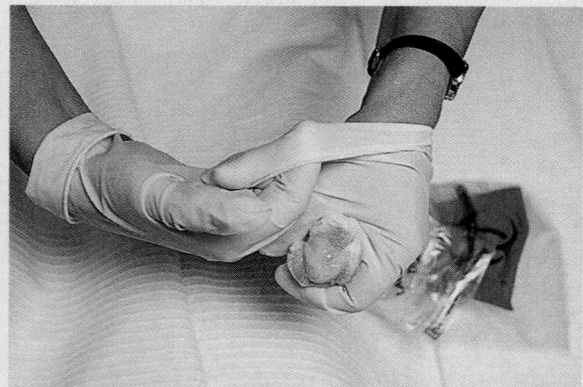

STEP 7   Removal of disposable glove over contaminated dressing.

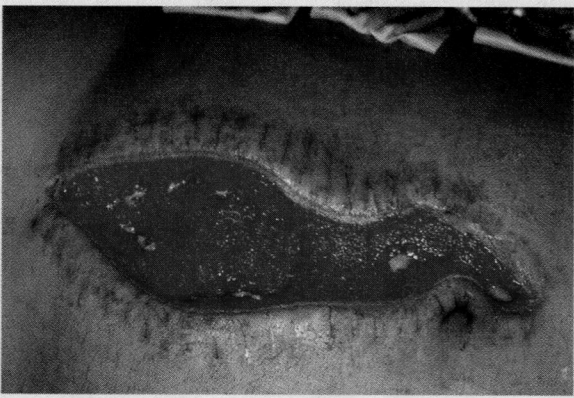

STEP 8   Abdominal wound with beefy red granulation tissue present and attached wound edges. (*From Bryant RA, Nix DP: Acute and chronic wounds: nursing management, ed 3, St. Louis, 2007, Mosby.*)

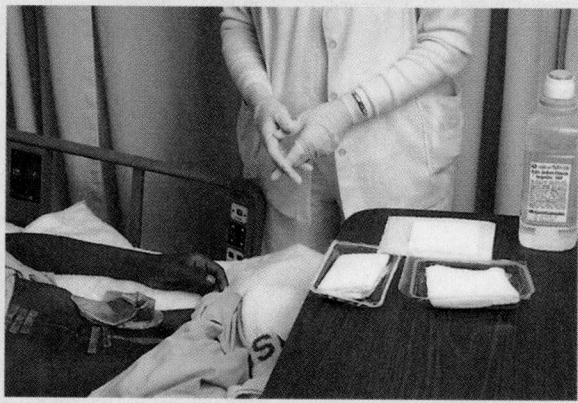

STEP 10   Sterile dressing field.

STEP	**RATIONALE**
11 Cleanse wound (see Chapter 38):	
a Apply clean gloves. Use an aseptic swab for each cleansing stroke, or spray wound surface.	Prevents transfer of organisms from previously cleaned area (Harvey, 2005).
b Clean from least contaminated area to most contaminated (see Chapter 38) (see illustration).	Cleansing in this direction prevents introduction of organisms into wound.
c Cleanse around the drain (if present), using circular stroke starting near drain and moving outward and away from the insertion site (see Chapter 38).	Correct aseptic technique in cleansing prevents contamination.
12 Use dry gauze to blot in same manner as in Step 11 to dry wound.	Drying reduces excess moisture, which could eventually harbor microorganisms.
13 Apply antiseptic ointment if ordered, using same technique to apply as for cleansing.	Helps reduce growth of microorganisms.
14 Apply dressing:	A dressing over a wound helps patients gradually adjust to changes in body image (Whitney, 2007).
a Dry dressing	
(1) Apply sterile gloves.	
(2) Apply loose woven gauze as contact layer.	Promotes proper absorption of drainage.
(3) If drain is present, apply a precut 4 × 4 inch gauze flat around drain.	Secures drain and promotes drainage absorption at site.
(4) Apply additional layers of gauze as needed.	Ensures proper coverage and optimal absorption.
(5) Apply thicker woven pad (e.g., Surgipad, abdominal dressing).	This type of dressing is often used on postoperative wounds where there is excessive drainage (Harvey, 2005).
b Moist-to-dry dressing	
(1) Apply sterile gloves.	
(2) Place fine mesh gauze in container of prescribed sterile solution. Wring out excess solution.	Moist gauze absorbs drainage and, when allowed to dry, traps debris.

Critical Decision Point *If a "packing strip" is used to pack the wound, use sterile scissors to cut the amount of dressing that you will use to pack the wound. Do not let the packing strip touch the side of the bottle. Pour prescribed solution over the packing gauze or strip to moisten it.*

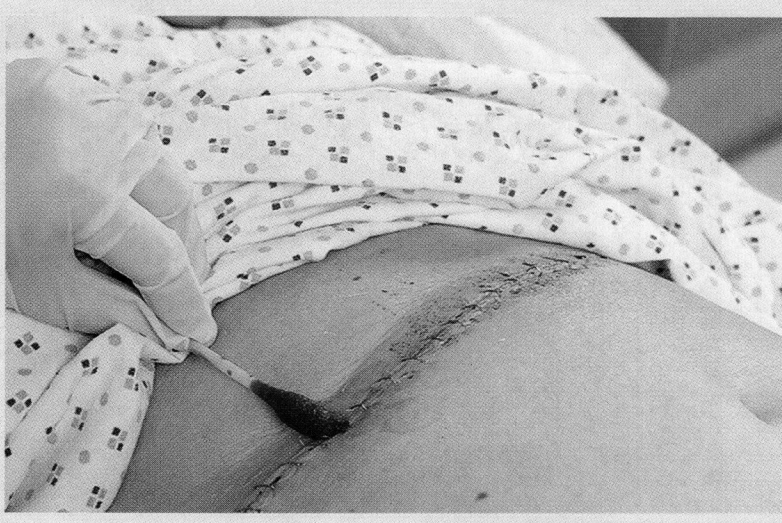

STEP 11b Cleansing wound.

STEP	RATIONALE

(3) Apply moist fine-mesh, open-weave gauze as a single layer directly onto wound surface. If wound is deep, gently pack gauze into wound with sterile gloved hand or forceps until all wound surfaces are in contact with moist gauze (see illustration A). Be sure gauze does not touch periwound skin (see illustration B).

Inner gauze should be moist, not dripping wet, to absorb drainage and adhere to debris. Wound is loosely packed to facilitate wicking of drainage into absorbent outer layer of dressing. Moisture that escapes the dressing often macerates the periwound area (Gray and Weir, 2007).

Critical Decision Point *If wound is deep, gently lay moistened woven gauze over wound surface with forceps until all surfaces are in contact with moist gauze and the wound is loosely filled. Fill the wound, but avoid packing the wound too tightly or having the gauze extend beyond the top of the wound.*

(4) Observe packing to ensure that any dead space from sinus tracts, undermining, or tunneling is loosely packed with gauze.

Do not overpack the wound too tightly; it can cause wound trauma when the dressing is removed (Nelson and Dilloway, 2002).

(5) Apply dry sterile gauze over moistened gauze 4 × 4.

Dry layer pulls moisture from wound.

(6) Cover with an ABD pad, Surgipad, or gauze (see illustration).

Protects wound from entrance of microorganisms.

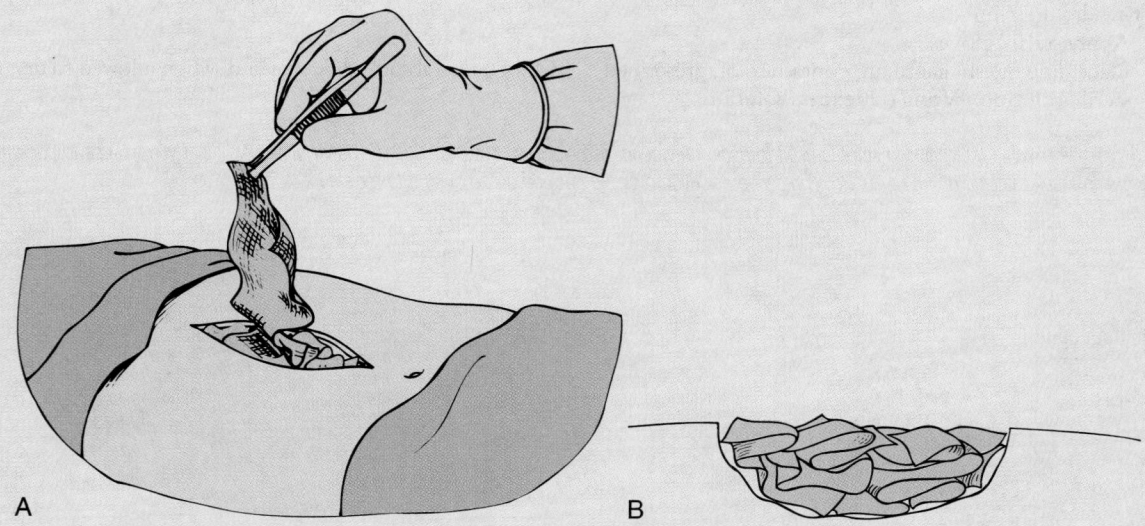

STEP 14b(3)   **A,** Packing wound. **B,** Wound packed loosely.

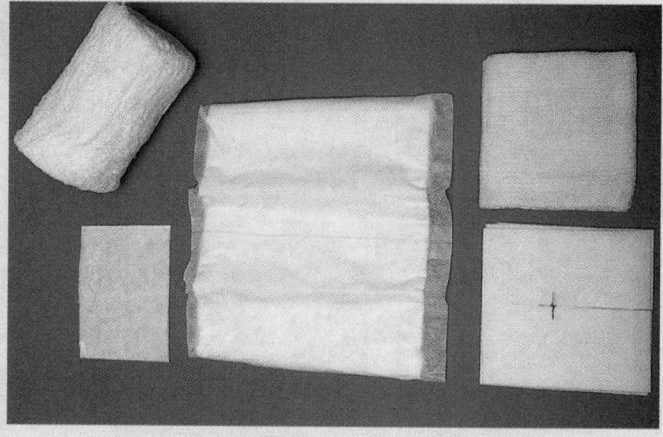

STEP 14b(6)   Secondary wound dressings.

STEP	RATIONALE
15 Secure dressing with roll gauze (for circumferential dressings) (see illustration A), tape, Montgomery ties or straps (which are applied perpendicular to the wound) (see illustration B), or binder.	Supports wound and ensures placement and stability of dressing.
16 Dispose of all dressing supplies. Remove cover gown and goggles, and remove gloves inside out; dispose of them according to agency policy.	Reduces transmission of microorganisms. Clean environment enhances patient comfort.
17 Write date and time dressing applied, on tape in ink (not marker).	
18 Assist patient to comfortable position.	Promotes patient's sense of well-being.
19 Perform hand hygiene.	Reduces transmission of microorganisms.

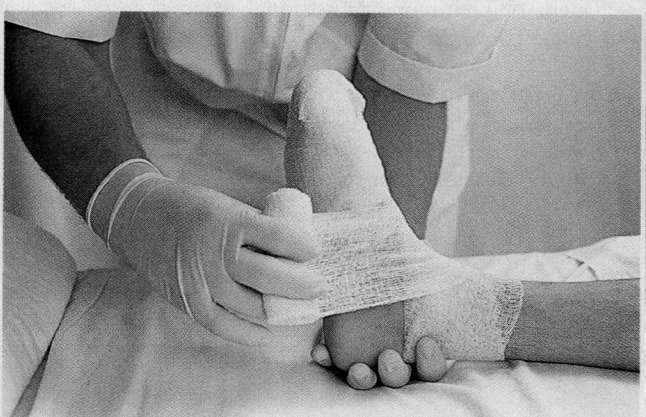 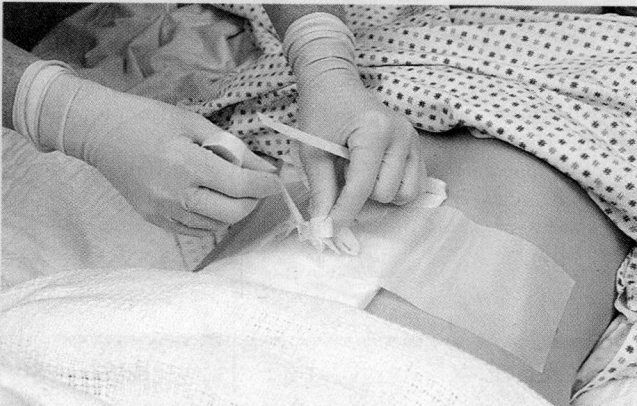

STEP 15   **A,** Application of roll gauze. **B,** Securing Montgomery ties.

EVALUATION

1 Observe appearance of wound for healing, including size of wound, amount, color, and type of drainage, and periwound erythema or swelling.	Determines rate of healing.
2 Ask patient to rate pain using a scale of 0 to 10.	Increased pain is often an indication of wound complications, such as infection, or a result of dressing pulling tissue.
3 Inspect condition of dressing at least every shift.	Determines status of wound drainage.
4 Ask patient to describe steps and techniques of dressing change.	Evaluates patient's learning.

Unexpected Outcomes	Related Interventions
1 Wound appears inflamed and tender, drainage is evident, and/or an odor is present.	• Monitor patient for signs of infection. • Notify health care provider. • Obtain wound culture.
2 Wound bleeds during dressing change.	• Observe color and amount of drainage. If excessive, apply pressure dressing. • Inspect area along dressing and directly underneath patient to determine the amount of bleeding. • Obtain vital signs as needed. • Notify health care provider.
3 Patient reports sensation that "something has given way under the dressing."	• Observe wound for increased drainage or dehiscence (partial or total separation of wound layers) or evisceration (total separation of wound layers and protrusion of viscera through wound opening). • Protect wound. Cover with sterile moist dressing. • Instruct patient to lie still. • Remain with patient to monitor vital signs. • Notify health care provider.

Recording and Reporting

- Record appearance of wound, color, presence and characteristics of exudate, change in wound characteristics, especially drainage amount, type and amount of dressings applied, and tolerance of patient to dressing change.
- Report any unexpected appearance of wound drainage, accidental removal of drain, bright red bleeding, or evidence of wound dehiscence or evisceration.

Teaching Considerations

- Explain expected wound appearance and risks of improper wound care. Provide patient with a written list of signs to report to the health care provider.
- After demonstrating wound care, allow patient or caregiver to perform dressing change with and without supervision.

Pediatric Considerations

- Some pediatric patients are fearful of dressing changes. Obtain patient's cooperation, and/or have another person available to keep child from moving during dressing change procedure (Hockenberry and Wilson, 2007).
- Older child may need something to do during dressing changes. Listening to music or watching video helps to relieve some of the boredom or stress during procedure (Hockenberry and Wilson, 2007).

Gerontological Considerations

- Adhesive tape is often too irritating to older adults' skin and causes skin tears. Use paper tape, nonallergenic tape, or wraps or mesh without tape contacting the patient's skin.
- Normal aging changes of skin tissue may also delay wound-healing process (Meiner and Lueckenotte, 2006).

Home Care Considerations

- Consider the ability of caregiver and amount of time needed to change a particular dressing when selecting a dressing procedure in the home care setting. More expensive dressings may be used to decrease frequency of dressing changes.
- For adequate reimbursement, payers require a signed health care provider's order and treatment plan. Documentation of need for services and status of wound healing is needed for reimbursement or continuing professional wound care services in the home (Bryant and others, 2007).

Long-Term Care Considerations

- Centers with subacute care units often provide specialized wound care. Patients are admitted to center for continued wound care management.

SKILL 39-2 Applying a Pressure Bandage

A pressure bandage is a temporary treatment to control excessive bleeding. The bleeding is a sudden and unanticipated event. It follows surgical intervention, or it may be a life-threatening occurrence related to accidental trauma, stabbing, suicide attempt, or other injury. Following application of the pressure dressing itself, immobilizing devices are placed adjacent to the dressing to augment pressure.

An adult weighing 154 lb (70 kg) has a total volume of 5 L of circulating blood. Quickly and effectively implement nursing interventions when excessive blood loss occurs. Once pressure is applied, it must continue until the health care team completes definitive actions. Surgical repair is most often the option of choice.

Delegation Considerations

The skill of applying a pressure dressing cannot be delegated to NAP. The nurse directs the NAP to:

- Observe the pressure dressing during care activities to make sure that it remains in place and that there is no visible bleeding from the site.
- Observe under the patient for bleeding.

EQUIPMENT

- ❑ Sterile gauze
- ❑ Gauze roll bandage
- ❑ Adhesive tape
- ❑ Clean gloves
- ❑ Sandbags
- ❑ Protective gown, goggles, mask (used when spray from wound is a risk)
- ❑ Equipment for vital signs

STEP	RATIONALE
ASSESSMENT	

1 Identify patients at risk for unexpected bleeding:
    a Traumatic injury
    b Donor graft site
    c Arterial puncture sites
    d Postoperative wounds
    e Wounds after surgical debridement
    f History of bleeding disorder
	Be familiar with conditions associated with unexpected bleeding to rapidly respond to bleeding.

Phase I: Immediate Action—First Nurse	
1 Identify patient with sudden hemorrhage:	Factors contributing to bleeding could still be present.

STEP	RATIONALE
a Locate external bleeding site.	Maintaining asepsis and privacy are considered only if time and severity of blood loss permit inclusion of these activities. NOTE: Wounds to the groin area can result in large amounts of blood loss, which is not always visible.
b Apply direct pressure immediately.	Hemostasis maintained as supplies are prepared.
2 Seek assistance.	Bandage must be quickly secured.

Phase II: Applying Pressure Bandage—Second Nurse

STEP	RATIONALE
1 Quickly observe location of bleeding.	
• *Arterial bleeding* is bright red and gushes forth in waves, related to heart rhythm; if vessel is very deep, flow will be steady.	
• *Venous bleeding* is dark red and flows smoothly.	
• *Capillary bleeding* is oozing of dark red blood; self-sealing controls this bleeding.	
• *Hemorrhage* is loss of a large amount of blood either externally or internally in short period of time.	Bleeding source determines method and supplies needed for applying pressure bandage.
2 Quickly observe area underneath patient for blood.	Blood will flow with gravity to the lowest point. Frequently a large volume of blood may be underneath patient and not initially visible.
3 Quickly assess patient's pulse, blood pressure, skin color, anxiety/restlessness, and changes in level of consciousness. Reassess every 5 to 15 minutes until patient is stabilized.	Findings of tachycardia, hypotension, diaphoresis, restlessness, and diminished urinary output indicate impending hypovolemic shock.

NURSING DIAGNOSES

- Decreased cardiac output
- Deficient fluid volume
- Impaired skin integrity
- Ineffective peripheral tissue perfusion

Individualize related factors based on patient's condition or needs.

PLANNING

STEP	RATIONALE
1 Expected outcomes following completion of procedure:	
• Bleeding is temporarily controlled.	Source of bleeding is controlled with pressure.
• Circulation to distal parts is adequate.	Blood flow to periphery is maintained.
• Fluid loss is minimal.	Loss of blood is controlled.
• Patient's blood pressure and pulse remain within normal range.	

IMPLEMENTATION

STEP	RATIONALE
1 Apply clean gloves. *If patient's condition permits*, perform hand hygiene, apply clean gloves, and provide privacy.	Maintaining asepsis and privacy are considered only if time and severity of blood loss permit inclusion of these activities.
2 First person presses on site of bleeding. Second person unwraps roller bandage and places within easy access.	Hemostasis maintained as supplies are prepared. Pressure dressing provides interim control of bleeding.
3 Second person quickly cuts three to five lengths of adhesive tape and places them within easy reach.	Bandage must be quickly secured.
4 In *simultaneous coordinated actions*:	
a Rapidly cover bleeding area with multiple thicknesses of gauze compresses. First person slips fingers out as other nurse exerts adequate pressure to continue controlling bleeding.	Gauze is absorbent. Layers provide bulk against which local pressure can be applied to bleeding site.

Critical Decision Point   *As soon as possible, elevate extremity or area of bleeding. Elevation assists in decreasing the rate of blood loss.*

STEP	RATIONALE
b Place adhesive strips 7 to 10 cm (3 to 4 inches) beyond width of dressing with even pressure on both sides of the fingers as close as possible to central bleeding source. Secure tape on distal end, pull tape across dressing, and maintain firm pressure as proximate end of tape is secured.	Tape exerts downward pressure, promoting hemostasis. To ensure blood flow to distal tissues and prevent tourniquet effect, adhesive tape must not be continued around entire extremity.
c Remove fingers temporarily, and quickly cover center of area with third strip of tape.	Provides pressure to source of bleeding.

STEP	RATIONALE
d Continue reinforcing area with tape as each successive strip is overlapped on alternating sides of center strip. Also continue applying pressure.	Prevents tape from loosening.
e When pressure bandage is on extremity, apply roller gauze: apply two circular turns tautly on both sides of fingers that are pressing gauze. Compress over bleeding site. Simultaneously remove finger pressure and apply roller gauze pressure over center. Continue with figure-eight turns. Secure end with two circular turns and strip of adhesive (see Skill 39-6).	Roller gauze acts as pressure bandage, exerting more even pressure over extremity.

Critical Decision Point   *Start pressure bandage from distal to proximal, working toward the heart.*

STEP	RATIONALE
5 Remove gloves, and perform hand hygiene.	Reduces the spread of microorganisms.

EVALUATION

STEP	RATIONALE
1 Immediately evaluate patient to determine response to pressure dressing.	
a Observe for control of bleeding	Effective pressure bandage controls bleeding without blocking distal circulation.
b Evaluate adequacy of circulation (distal pulse, skin characteristics)	Determines level of perfusion to distal body parts.
c Estimate volume of blood loss (e.g., count number of dressings used, weigh saturated dressing)	Determines blood and fluid replacement needs.
d Measure vital signs	Identifies patient's adaptation to blood loss and early stages of hypovolemic shock.

Unexpected Outcomes

1 Uncontrolled hemorrhaging progresses to fluid and electrolyte imbalance, tissue hypoxia, confusion, hypovolemic shock, cardiac arrest, and death.

Related Interventions

- Initiate IV therapy (health care provider's order is required) for fluid replacement.
- Initiate nothing-by-mouth (NPO) order because surgical intervention may be needed.
- Apply pressure to pressure point as needed; place patient in Trendelenburg's position; provide warmth.
- Monitor vital signs every 5 to 15 minutes (apical, distal rate, blood pressure).
- Monitor dressing for signs of bleeding.
- Reinforce dressing with tape as needed to prevent seepage. If dressing is saturated, replace only top layers so as not to disturb any clot formation at the wound site.

Recording and Reporting

- Report immediately to health care provider present status of patient's bleeding control, time bleeding was discovered, estimated blood loss, nursing interventions (including effectiveness of applied pressure bandage), apical and distal pulses, blood pressure, mental status, signs of restlessness, and need for health care provider to administer to patient without delay.
- Record and implement health care provider's verbal orders in response to above reporting. (NOTE: Institutional policy on telephone/verbal orders varies.)

Teaching Considerations

- Explain need to monitor vital signs.
- Explain need for patient to remain quiet and stay in position to reduce bleeding.

Pediatric Considerations

- Child will calm down if care providers and family remain calm.

Gerontological Considerations

- Due to the normal changes of aging, the older adult has an increased risk for vascular and tissue changes distal to the pressure dressing. Therefore assess skin and pulse distal to the pressure bandage frequently.

Home Care Considerations

- At home patient may apply pressure with clean towels or linen.
- Emergency system (9-1-1) should be activated.
- Position patient to promote elevation of affected body part (if extremity) and promote relaxation.
- If a puncture wound occurs from a penetrating object (e.g., knife, toy, building materials), do not remove the object. Removal of object will cause more rapid blood loss and may damage underlying structures.

SKILL 39-3   Applying a Transparent Dressing

NSO   *Wound Care Module / Lesson 3*

A transparent dressing is a clear, adherent, nonabsorptive, polyurethane moisture and vapor-permeable dressing (Fig. 39-3). These dressings manage superficial, minimally draining wounds and are often used following laparoscopic surgery, for protection over high-friction areas, and as a dressing over an IV catheter. This synthetic permeable membrane acts as a temporary second skin, adheres to undamaged skin to contain exudate, minimizes wound contamination, and allows the wound to "breathe."

With the use of a transparent dressing, a moist exudate forms over the wound surface, which prevents tissue dehydration and allows for rapid, effective healing by speeding epithelial cell growth (Rolstad and Ovington, 2007). Because these dressings are clear, you can observe the wound without removing the dressing. For best results these dressings are applied over clean, debrided wounds that are not actively bleeding. The accumulation of fluid with a white, opaque appearance and erythema of the surrounding tissue usually indicate an infectious process, and the dressing should be removed and a wound culture obtained.

Delegation Considerations

The skill of applying a transparent dressing for select wounds can be delegated to NAP (refer to agency policy). The assessment of the wound and care of sterile or new acute wounds cannot be delegated to NAP. The nurse directs the NAP about:

- Explaining how to adapt the skill for a specific patient.
- Reporting any signs of bleeding, drainage, infection, or poor wound healing immediately to the nurse.

Equipment

- ❑ Sterile gloves (*optional*)
- ❑ Dressing set (*optional*)
- ❑ Sterile saline or other agent (as ordered)
- ❑ Clean gloves
- ❑ Cotton swabs
- ❑ Waterproof bag for disposal
- ❑ Transparent dressing (size as needed)
- ❑ Sterile 4 × 4 inch gauze pads
- ❑ Skin preparation materials (*optional*)
- ❑ Moisture-proof gown, goggles, and mask (used when splashing from wound is a risk)

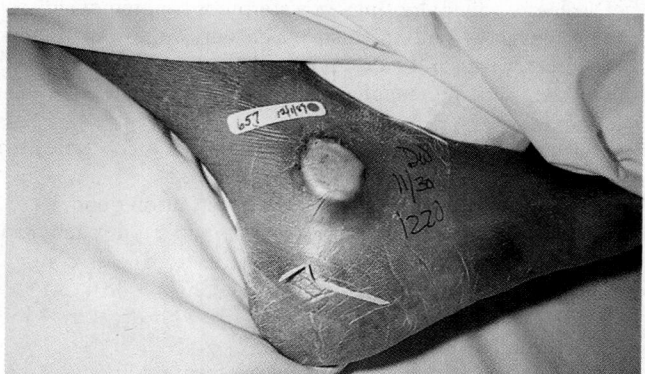

FIG 39-3   Transparent dressing.

STEP	RATIONALE

ASSESSMENT

1 Assess location and size of wound (see Chapter 38).	Determines supplies and assistance needed.
2 Review health care provider's orders for frequency and type of dressing change.	Health care provider orders frequency of dressing changes and special instructions.
3 Determine patient's level of comfort using a scale of 0 to 10. Administer prescribed analgesic as needed 30 minutes before dressing change.	Comfortable patient will be less likely to move suddenly, causing wound or supply contamination. Serves as baseline to measure response to dressing therapy.
4 Assess patient's knowledge of purpose of dressing.	Identifies patient's learning needs.
5 Assess risk for impaired wound healing.	Physiological changes due to aging, chronic illness, poor nutrition, medications, and cancer treatments have the potential to affect wound healing (Doughty and Sparks-DeFriese, 2007).

NURSING DIAGNOSES

• Acute pain	• Impaired skin integrity	• Risk for infection

Individualize related factors based on patient's condition or needs.

PLANNING

1 Expected outcome following completion of procedure: • Wound heals rapidly with little pain and mobility restriction for patient.	Dressing effective in preventing infection and promoting healing.
2 Explain procedure to patient.	Relieves anxiety and promotes understanding of healing process.
3 Position patient comfortably and to allow access to dressing site.	Facilitates application of dressing.

STEP	RATIONALE

IMPLEMENTATION

1   Close door or cubicle curtains; keep sheet or gown draped over body parts not requiring exposure.

Provides privacy and decreases transfer of microorganisms.

2   Check patient's identification using two identifiers; one cannot be the patient's room number. Expose wound site, minimizing exposure. Instruct patient not to touch wound or sterile supplies.

Ensures correct patient receives correct therapy. Dressing supplies become contaminated when touched by patient's hand.

3   Cuff top of disposable waterproof bag, and place within reach of work area.

Cuff prevents accidental contamination of tip of outer bag.

4   Perform hand hygiene, and apply clean gloves. Apply moisture-proof gown, mask, and eye goggles if there is risk for splashing.

Reduces transmission of infectious organisms from soiled dressings to nurse's hands.

5   Remove old dressing by pulling back slowly in a direction parallel to the wound rather than upward.

Reduces excoriation or irritation of skin following dressing removal.

6   Dispose of soiled dressings in waterproof bag, remove disposable gloves by pulling them inside out, dispose of them in waterproof bag, and perform hand hygiene.

Reduces transmission of microorganisms.

7   Prepare dressing supplies. Use sterile supplies for new wounds.

Reduces risk for break in sterile technique.

8   Pour saline or prescribed solution over 4 × 4 inch sterile gauze pads.

Maintains sterility of dressing.

9   Apply clean or sterile gloves (check institution policy).

Allows nurse to handle dressings.

10 Cleanse area gently with moist 4 × 4 inch sterile gauze pads, or spray with wound cleanser. Cleanse from least contaminated to most contaminated area (see Chapter 38).

Reduces introduction of organisms into wound.

11 Pat dry skin around wound thoroughly with dry 4 × 4 inch sterile gauze pads.

Transparent dressing with adhesive backing does not adhere to damp surface (Rolstad and Ovington, 2007).

12 Inspect wound for tissue type, color, odor, and drainage; measure if indicated.

Provides a baseline for monitoring wound healing.

Critical Decision Point   *If wound has a large amount of drainage, choose another dressing that can absorb this amount of wound drainage rather than transparent film dressing, which can absorb only light to moderate amounts of drainage.*

13 Apply transparent dressing according to manufacturer's directions. *Do not stretch film during application.* Avoid wrinkles in film.

Wrinkles provide tunnel for exudate drainage.

   a   Remove paper backing, taking care not to allow adhesive areas to touch each other.

   b   Place film smoothly over wound without stretching (see illustration).

The stretching action breaks the seal to increase ease of removal (Rolstad and Ovington, 2007).

   c   Label dressing with date, your initials, and time of dressing change on outer label of dressing (see Fig. 39-3).

Provides record for determining when to next change dressing.

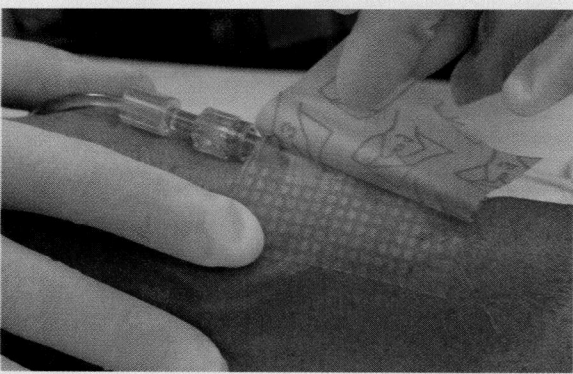

STEP 13b   Transparent dressing placed smoothly over an IV site.

STEP	RATIONALE
14 Discard soiled dressing materials properly. Remove protective equipment and gloves by pulling them inside out, and discard in prepared bag. Perform hand hygiene.	Reduces transfer of microorganisms.
15 Assist patient to comfortable position.	Enhances patient comfort and relaxation.

EVALUATION

1 Inspect appearance of wound and amount of drainage.	Determines status of wound healing. Wound is easy to view.
2 Inspect periwound areas.	Identifies any injury to surrounding skin.
3 Ask patient to rate pain using a scale of 0 to 10.	Determines any change in pain during procedure.

Unexpected Outcomes	Related Interventions
1 Wound is inflamed, tender; drainage and/or an odor is present.	• Remove dressing, and obtain wound culture according to agency policy. • Different type of dressing may be required.
2 Dressing does not stay in place.	• Evaluate size of dressing used for adequate wound margin (2.5 to 3.75 cm [1 to 1½ inches]). • Dry patient's skin thoroughly before reapplication.
3 Outer layer of patient's skin tears on removal of dressing.	• Adhesive backing may be too strong for fragile skin. • Consider other non–adhesive-backed transparent dressing.

Recording and Reporting
- Record appearance of wound, color, any odor, characteristics, and patient response to dressing change.
- Report signs of infection to health care provider.

Teaching Considerations
- Explain need to change dressing should edges loosen.
- Explain to patient and family that collection of wound fluid under dressing is not "pus," but normal interaction of body fluids with dressing.

Pediatric Considerations
- Adhesive backing may cause skin tears on premature babies' immature skin (Hockenberry and Wilson, 2007).
- Children may find this procedure more tolerable if they know that the longer the dressing is left on, the easier it is to remove (Hockenberry and Wilson, 2007).

Gerontological Considerations
- Adhesive backing may be too strong for the skin of older adults. Do not use a film dressing that has an adhesive backing that has a stronger bond to the epidermis than the epidermis has to the dermis (Meiner and Lueckenotte, 2006).

Home Care Considerations
- Wound may be cleansed in shower, if approved by physician.
- Many types of transparent dressings exist. Explore types with patient, and recommend type patient has easy access to and finds easy to apply.

SKILL 39-4 Applying Hydrocolloid, Hydrogel, Foam, or Absorption Dressings

 Intermediate / Wound and Pressure Ulcer Care / Changing a Dressing

Hydrocolloid dressings are composed of elastometric, adhesive, and gelling agents. There are a variety of reasons to use these dressings: (1) maintaining a moist wound environment for healing of clean, shallow to moderately deep wounds; (2) autolytic debriding of necrotic wounds; (3) protecting high-friction areas on intact skin; (4) protecting from contamination; and (5) providing absorption of minimal amount of exudates in superficial and shallow wounds (Rolstad and Ovington, 2007). A hydrocolloid dressing is usually applied beneath Montgomery ties or on bony prominences to reduce injury to the subcutaneous tissues. Hydrocolloid dressings help diminish pain and discomfort because the "cushioning" effect provides protection to the wound and skin beneath bony prominences. These adhesive-backed dressings conform well to different body contours. Hydrocolloids come in the form of granules, paste, or wafer dressings. Wound exudate is absorbed into the dressing, forming a jellylike substance next to the wound surface. The dress-

ing maintains a moist, insulated environment that promotes rapid, effective healing.

Hydrogel dressings are glycerin- or water-based dressings designed to hydrate the wound (Rolstad and Ovington, 2007.) They are nonadherent and have some absorptive properties. Hydrogel dressings serve the same functions as a hydrocolloid dressing. These dressings are available in several forms, including a "sheet," amorphous gels, and impregnated gauze that can be placed in the wound. These dressings facilitate wound debridement by rehydration. They absorb exudate and encourage healing by maintaining a moist wound-healing environment (Fig. 39-4). The gel dressings are nonadherent and must be covered with a secondary dressing to hold them in place.

The hydrocolloid or hydrogel dressings are used frequently over venous stasis ulcers, arterial ulcers, and pressure ulcers. Hydrocolloid dressings are one of the most frequently used dressings for

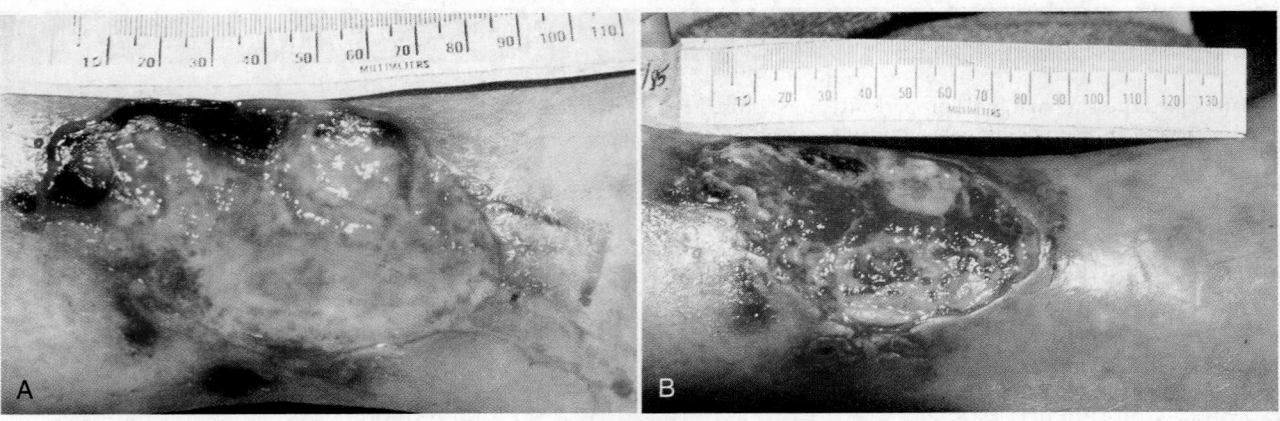

FIG 39-4 **A,** Highly exudative venous ulcer with slough present in wound bed and eschar present along superior aspect. **B,** One week after treatment with hydrocolloids and compression therapy, venous ulcer has granulation tissue present. The amount of slough and eschar is reduced. *(From Bryant RA, Nix DP: Acute and chronic wounds: nursing management, ed 3, St. Louis, 2007, Mosby.)*

pressure ulcers in home and long-term care settings (Rolstad and Ovington, 2007). Because of their "cooling" and soothing properties, hydrogel dressings are also used with burns and to protect the skin from radiation.

Foam dressings absorb moderate to heavy exudates in superficial or deep wounds, protect friable periwound skin, provide autolytic debridement, pad and protect high-trauma areas (e.g., pretibial area and forearms), and are often used with infected wounds following appropriate intervention and close monitoring of wound healing. The foam dressings protect the wound surface while maintaining a moist, insulated environment. The result is a well-hydrated wound bed that can heal rapidly with little discomfort to the patient. Application directions for the different brands of foam dressings vary. Read and follow the specific manufacturer's directions for the particular brand of foam dressings used.

Alginate dressings include calcium alginate materials, which are manufactured from natural material (seaweed) and are known for their absorptive properties, forming a gel over the wound surface as exudate is contained. The exudate absorbers are nonadhesive, nonocclusive dressings that conform to the shape of the wound. These dressings are appropriate for full-thickness wounds with moderate to high amounts of drainage. You can safely pack deep tracking wounds with calcium-sodium alginate preparation, which allows easy removal with little risk for retained dressing deep in the wound cavity. Generally alginate dressings require a secondary dressing, and that dressing can be changed as needed. Alginate dressings are changed as often as needed; in some cases these are changed daily depending on the volume of exudate (Rolstad and Ovington, 2007).

Delegation Considerations
The skill of applying a hydrocolloid, hydrogel, foam, or absorption dressing cannot be delegated to NAP. The nurse directs the NAP about:

- Approach to assist in positioning patient during dressing application.

Equipment
- ❑ Sterile gloves *(optional)*
- ❑ Dressing set *(optional)* (Fig. 39-5)
- ❑ Sterile saline or other cleansing solution (as ordered)
- ❑ Clean gloves
- ❑ Waterproof bag for disposal
- ❑ Wound measurement devices, tape measure, tracing paper, camera *(optional)*
- ❑ Dressing (size as needed) as prescribed (hydrocolloid, hydrogel, foam, absorption)
- ❑ Sterile 4 × 4 inch gauze pads
- ❑ Secondary dressing of choice (if needed)
- ❑ Protective gown, goggles, and mask (used when splashing from wound is a risk)

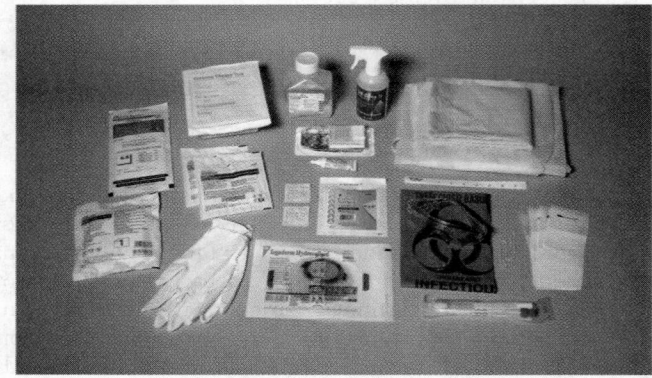

FIG 39-5 Dressing set

STEP	**RATIONALE**

ASSESSMENT

1 Assess wound location and size of wound (see Chapter 38, Procedural Guideline 38-1).

Allows nurse to determine supplies and assistance needed. Provides baseline of wound condition.

2 Determine the type of dressing. ***Do not use alginate or absorptive dressings on nonexudative wounds.***

Most of these dressings are designed to absorb moderate to large amounts of wound drainage and therefore should not be used in wounds with minimal or no drainage (Rolstad and Ovington, 2007).

> **Critical Decision Point** *Some brands of hydrocolloid dressings are available in custom shapes and sizes to better fit certain difficult body parts such as the sacrum, heels, or elbows. The variety of shapes aids in flexibility of dressing selection and better dressing adherence.*

3 Review health care provider's orders for frequency and type of dressing change.

Health care provider orders mode of therapy.

4 Determine patient's level of comfort using a scale of 0 to 10. Administer prescribed analgesic as needed 30 minutes before dressing change.

Comfortable patient will be less likely to move suddenly, causing wound or supply contamination. Serves as baseline to measure response to dressing therapy.

5 Assess patient's knowledge of purpose of dressing.

Identifies patient's learning needs.

NURSING DIAGNOSES

- Acute pain
- Deficient knowledge regarding wound care
- Impaired skin integrity
- Risk for infection

Individualize related factors based on patient's condition or needs.

PLANNING

1 Expected outcomes following completion of procedure:
   - Wound heals rapidly with little pain and mobility restriction for patient.

   Dressing effective in preventing infection and promoting healing.

   - Wound exudate is adequately absorbed.

   Dressing effective in exudate management for draining wounds.

   - Wound drainage is contained, and skin surrounding wound remains intact.

   Dressing effective in controlling wound exudate.

   - Patient explains procedure correctly.

   Indicates learning has occurred.

2 Explain procedure to patient.

Relieves anxiety and promotes understanding of healing process.

3 Position patient to allow access to dressing site.

Facilitates application of dressing.

IMPLEMENTATION

1 Close room door or cubicle curtains.

Provides for patient privacy and reduces transfer of microorganisms.

2 Check patient's identification using two identifiers; one cannot be the patient's room number. Position patient comfortably, expose wound site, and drape patient. Instruct patient not to touch wound or sterile supplies.

Ensures correct patient receives correct therapy. Draping provides access to wound while minimizing exposure. Dressing supplies become contaminated when touched by patient's hand.

3 Cuff top of disposable waterproof bag, and place within reach of work area.

Cuff prevents accidental contamination of top of outer bag. Nurse should not reach across sterile field.

4 Perform hand hygiene, and put on clean gloves. Moisture-proof gown, mask, and goggles are worn when risk for splashing exists.

Reduces transmission of infectious organisms.

5 Remove old dressing. For easier removal, pull back slowly across dressing in direction of hair growth.

Reduces irritation and possible injury to skin.

> **Critical Decision Point** *Check removal directions for specific brand of dressing used. Some brands need to have old dressing soaked or moistened for removal. With some types of dressings, use adhesive remover to ease off dressing. Use caution to avoid contact of adhesive remover with the wound.*

6 Dispose of soiled dressings in waterproof bag. Remove disposable gloves by pulling them inside out, and dispose of them in waterproof bag.

Reduces transmission of microorganisms.

STEP	RATIONALE

Critical Decision Point   *Hydrocolloid dressings interact with wound fluids and form a soft whitish-yellowish gel, which is hard to remove and may have a faint odor. Normal discoloration often occurs with some brands of foam dressings. A residual gel substance occurs in wound beds with some brands of absorption dressings. These are normal occurrences; do not confuse these findings with pus or purulent exudate, wound infection, or deterioration of the wound.*

STEP	RATIONALE
7 Prepare sterile dressing supplies.	Reduces risk for break in sterile technique.
8 Pour saline or prescribed solution over 4 × 4 inch sterile gauze pads, or open spray wound cleanser.	Maintains sterility of dressing.
9 Apply sterile or clean gloves (check agency policy).	Allows nurse to handle dressings.
10 Cleanse area gently with moist 4 × 4 inch sterile gauze pads, swabbing exudate away from wound, or spray with wound cleanser (see Chapter 38).	Reduces introduction of organisms into wound. Cleansing effectively removes any residual dressing gel without injuring newly formed delicate granulation tissue in the healing wound bed.
11 Thoroughly pat wound surface dry with dry 4 × 4 inch sterile gauze pads. Dry intact skin around the wound.	Dressing will not adhere to damp surface. Periwound skin should be kept dry to prevent breakdown.
12 Inspect wound for tissue type, color, odor, and drainage. Measure wound size and depth.	Appearance and measurement indicate state of wound healing.
13 Apply dressing according to manufacturer's directions.	Ensures proper application of dressing. Different brands of dressings require different application techniques.
a Hydrocolloid dressings:	

Critical Decision Point   *For some brands of hydrocolloid wafers, the size of the dressing needs to extend onto intact periwound skin at least 2.5 cm (1 inch) (Rolstad and Ovington, 2007).*

STEP	RATIONALE
(1) Apply hydrocolloid wafer over wound. In the case of a deep wound, hydrocolloid granules or paste are applied before the wafer. Dressing should not be stretched during application. Avoid wrinkles that would provide tunnel for exudate drainage.	Hydrocolloid granules/paste assist in absorbing drainage to increase wearing time of dressing (Rolstad and Ovington, 2007).

Critical Decision Point   *Edges may be notched to help mold around wound. Consider using custom shapes to better conform to certain parts of the body such as heels, elbows, and sacrum.*

STEP	RATIONALE
(2) Hold the dressing in place for 30 to 60 seconds following application.	Hydrocolloid dressings are most effective at body temperature. Holding the dressing in place for a short period of time facilitates dressing action (Rolstad and Ovington, 2007).
(3) Apply a secondary addressing (e.g., ABD pad) if needed.	Fluid gels take form of cavity type of wounds. A secondary dressing is used with a hydrogel to hold it in place because it has no adhesive.
(4) When a secondary dressing is not used, apply nonallergenic paper tape around the edges of the hydrocolloid dressing.	Prevents edges of dressing from rolling or adhering to sheets and clothing.
b Foam dressings:	
(1) Know removal and application characteristics of specific brand of foam dressing you are using. Most foam dressings should be applied smoothly; avoid wrinkles.	May be used with absorptive dressings to accommodate more highly draining wounds.
(2) Cut the foam to extend 2.5 cm (1 inch) onto intact periwound skin. (Make sure you know which side of foam dressing should be placed toward wound bed and which side should be facing away from wound bed; check manufacturer's instructions).	Ensures proper absorption and keeps wound exudate away from wound bed (Rolstad and Ovington, 2007).
(3) Some brands of foam dressings need slight tension on the dressing while being applied. Some brands of foam dressings need to be covered with a secondary dressing (Rolstad and Ovington, 2007).	
c Absorption or alginate dressings:	
(1) Fill wound cavity, but fill one-half to two-thirds full.	Allows for expansion with absorption.
(2) Cut dressing to fit wound size or loosely pack into the wound bed.	Loose packing allows space for alginate dressing to expand to fill wound bed.

STEP	RATIONALE
(3) Apply secondary dressing, such as a transparent film (see Skill 39-3), hydrogen, foam, or hydrocolloid.	Alginates are primary dressings and absorb and hold exudate and create a moist environment to promote granulation, epithelization, and autolysis (Rolstad and Ovington, 2007). The secondary dressing prohibits drainage on bed linens and clothing.
14 Discard soiled dressing materials properly. Remove gloves by pulling them inside out, and discard in prepared bag. Perform hand hygiene.	Reduces transfer of microorganisms.
15 Assist patient to comfortable position.	Enhances patient comfort and relaxation.

EVALUATION

1 Inspect condition of wound on ongoing basis. Note drainage and odor.	Determines status of wound healing.
2 Evaluate patient's level of comfort.	Determines if pain resulted from procedure.
3 Ask patient to explain wound care method.	Evaluates patient's level of learning.

Unexpected Outcomes	Related Interventions
1 Wound develops more necrotic tissue and increases in size.	• In rare instances, some wounds will not tolerate hypoxia induced by hydrocolloid dressings. In these patients, discontinue use. • Evaluate appropriateness of wound care protocol. • Evaluate patient for other impediments to wound healing.
2 Dressing does not stay in place.	• Evaluate size of dressing used for adequate margin (2.5 to 3.75 cm [1 to 1½ inches]), or dry skin more thoroughly before reapplication. • Consider custom shapes for difficult body parts. "Picture frame" the edges of the hydrocolloid dressing using tape. • Dressing may be secured with roll gauze, tape, transparent dressing, or dressing sheet.
3 Wound drainage is more than dressing can absorb.	• Change type of dressing to one that can absorb amount of wound drainage. • Foam dressings may be used over wound exudate absorbers.

Recording and Reporting

• Record characteristics of wound tissue type: color, odor, viscosity, and amount of drainage; application of dressing; and patient's tolerance to dressing change. Graph wound surface area or volume if wound is chronic wound. Write date, time, and nurse's initials in ink (not marker) on the dressing.

• Report unusual observations immediately; then chart what was reported and when.

Teaching Considerations

• Explain expected wound appearance, fluid or gel accumulation in wound bed, and possible odor with use of specific dressing.

• Because application technique can vary with different brands, tell patient and caregiver not to purchase a brand different from the one for which nurse gave them instructions. If a different brand must be used, patient and caregiver should check with nurse for any additional instructions or modifications in application and removal techniques.

Pediatric Considerations

• See Pediatric Considerations for Skills 39-1, 39-2, and 39-3.

Gerontological Considerations

• See also Gerontological Considerations for Skills 39-1, 39-2, and 39-3.

• Avoid early and frequent removal of a hydrocolloid dressing to reduce injury to surrounding intact skin.

SKILL 39-5 Negative Pressure Wound Therapy

Negative pressure wound therapy (NPWT) is a type of therapy that speeds wound healing by applying localized negative pressure to draw the edges of a wound together. It is commonly used for acute, chronic, traumatic, and dehisced wounds (Figs. 39-6 and 39-7); pressure ulcers; partial-thickness burns; and as a bolster for skin grafts (Aguinaga and others, 2007; Reisler, 2007). NPWT accelerates wound healing through faster granulation tissue formation and faster surface area reduction (Braakenburg and others, 2006; Hunter and others, 2007) and through reducing excess moisture in a wound and increasing perfusion (Jerome, 2007). The system generates a negative pressure at a wound surface through a foam pad, which increases oxygen tension, decreases bacterial counts, and increases granulation formation (Reisler, 2007). NWPT applies suction to the wound, which assists in removing exudate, promoting contraction of the wound bed, preparing the wound for closure, and promoting formation of granulation tissue (Aguinaga and others, 2007). Added benefits of NPWT include improved patient comfort and a reduction in the frequency of dressing changes (Braakenburg, 2006) (Fig. 39-8). In addition, Braakenburg (2006) found the therapy highly effective with patients with diabetes.

Contraindications for NPWT include malignancy in the wound bed, osteomyelitis, certain fistulas, necrotic tissue with eschar, and treatment with hyperbaric oxygen therapy (Aguinaga and others, 2007).

A physician or wound care specialist orders the cycle and amount of negative pressure to a wound (Mendez-Eastman, 2005). The negative pressure is continuous or intermittent, depending on the stage of wound healing. The target negative pressures for wound healing ranges from −50 mm Hg to −175 mm Hg, but a setting of −125 mm Hg is most common. However, there is now a V.A.C. Instill system that allows clinicians to add solutions to a wound, as well as apply negative pressure. The V.A.C. Instill involves continuous or intermittent pressure between −50 and −200 mm Hg (Jerome, 2007). An example of a cycle for a V.A.C. Instill is instillation of a solution for 1 to 2 minutes (saturates foam pad), hold time of 1 second to 1 hour, and continuous negative pressure for 1 minute to 12 hours (Jerome, 2007). To optimize wound healing, the negative pressure of a traditional NPWT unit is maintained 22 out of 24 hours per day (Kinetic Concepts, Inc. [KCI], 2004). As the wound heals, the settings may change.

Once NPWT is initiated, it must remain intact from 24 hours to 5 days (Franz and others, 2007). The schedule for changing NPWT dressings varies. An infected wound may need a dressing change every 24 hours, whereas a clean wound can be changed 3 times a week. As the wound heals, the wound base becomes redder and granulation tissue lines the surface of the wound. The wound has a stippled or granulated appearance. Paler areas develop as the wound heals. This indicates an increase in fibrous tissue (Mendez-Eastman, 2005).

Delegation Considerations

The skill of NPWT cannot be delegated to NAP. The nurse directs the NAP to:

- Use caution in positioning or turning patient to avoid tubing displacement.
- Report any change in integrity of the dressing.
- Report any change in patient's temperature or comfort level.

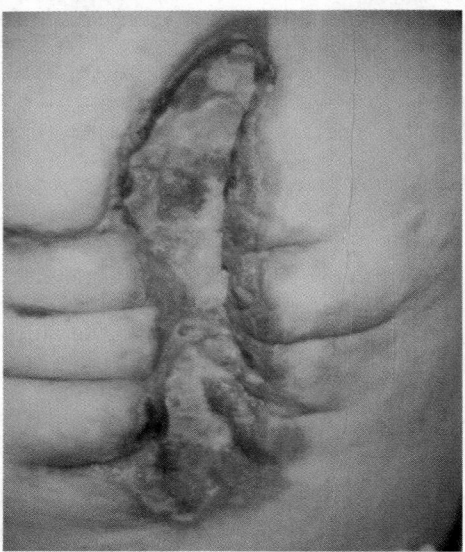

FIG 39-6 Dehisced wound before V.A.C. therapy. (*Courtesy Kinetic Concepts, Inc. [KCI], San Antonio, Tex.*)

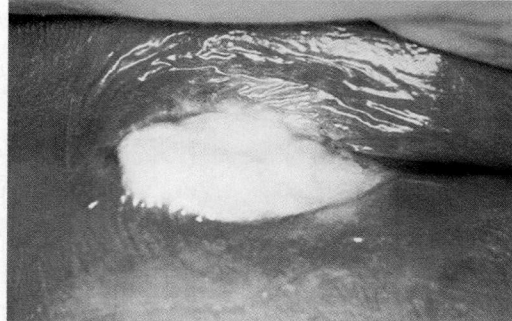

FIG 39-7 Dehisced wound after V.A.C. therapy. (*Courtesy Kinetic Concepts, Inc. [KCI], San Antonio, Tex.*)

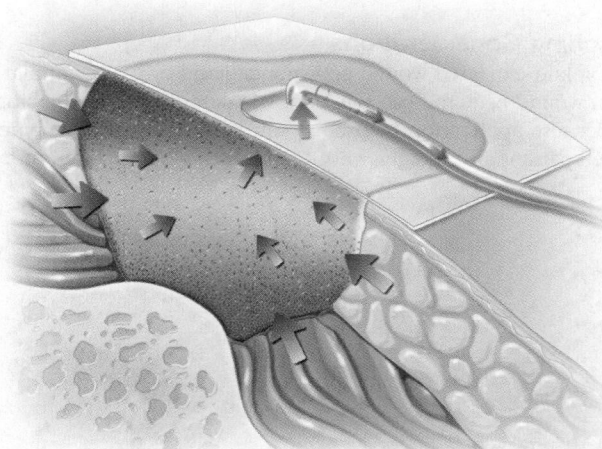

FIG 39-8 V.A.C. system using negative pressure to remove fluid from area surrounding the wound, reducing edema, and improving circulation to area. (*Courtesy Kinetic Concepts, Inc. [KCI], San Antonio, Tex.*)

Equipment

- ❑ 3 Pairs gloves, clean and sterile
- ❑ Scissors, sterile
- ❑ Stethoscope
- ❑ Waterproof bag for disposal
- ❑ Skin protectant/Stomahesive/hydrocolloid dressing/skin barrier
- ❑ Linen bag
- ❑ Protective gown, mask, goggles (used when splashing from wound is a risk)

Negative Pressure Wound Therapy

- ❑ NPWT, such as a V.A.C. unit, requires health care provider's order (Fig. 39-9)
- ❑ NPWT foam dressing
- ❑ NPWT transparent dressing
- ❑ Tubing for connection between NPWT unit and NPWT dressing
- ❑ *Optional:* 0.25% bupivacaine solution, syringe and 19-gauge needle, alcohol swab

V.A.C. Instill

- ❑ V.A.C. Instill unit (requires health care provider's order)
- ❑ V.A.C. foam dressing
- ❑ V.A.C. transparent dressing
- ❑ Instillation solution in clearly marked 250- to 500-mL bags intended for wound instillation
- ❑ V.A.C. Instill infusion tubing—labeled and with Luer-Lok connectors that do not fit standard IV tubing

- ❑ V.A.C. Instill pad
- ❑ V.A.C. Instill vacuum pad

FIG 39-9 V.A.C. unit. *Top to bottom:* V.A.C. unit, connective tubing to go between V.A.C. unit and V.A.C. dressing, absorbent foam. (*Courtesy Kinetic Concepts, Inc. [KCI], San Antonio, Tex.*)

STEP	RATIONALE

ASSESSMENT

1. Assess location, appearance, and size of wound (see Chapter 38).

   Provides information about status of wound, presence of complications, and type of supplies and assistance needed to apply V.A.C. dressing. NPWT is effective with some types of chronic wounds, such as burns and pressure ulcers, but not effective in osteomyelitis, and further study is needed (Gregor and others, 2008).

2. Review health care provider's orders for frequency of dressing change, type of negative pressure (traditional NPWT or V.A.C. Instill), type of foam to use, amount of negative pressure, and cycle (intermittent or continuous).

   Physician orders frequency of dressing changes and any special instructions.

3. Determine patient's level of comfort using a scale of 0 to 10. Administer prescribed analgesic as needed 30 minutes before dressing change.

   Comfortable patient will be less likely to move suddenly, causing wound or supply contamination. Serves as baseline to measure response to dressing therapy.

4. Assess patient's and family member's knowledge of purpose of dressing and whether they will participate in dressing wound.

   Identifies patient's learning needs. Prepares patient and family if dressing will need to be changed at home.

5. If patient is to receive irrigation via V.A.C. Instill system, assess for allergies to irrigation solution.

   Reactions range from a rash and burning sensation or increased pain to anaphylaxis (Jerome, 2007).

NURSING DIAGNOSES

- Acute pain
- Deficient knowledge regarding wound care
- Impaired skin integrity
- Risk for infection

Individualize related factors based on patient's condition or needs.

PLANNING

1. Expected outcomes following completion of procedure:
   - Patient's wound shows evidence of healing by smaller size and less drainage, redness, or swelling.

     Dressing effective in promoting healing and preventing infection.

   - Patient reports less pain during and after dressing changes.

     Analgesic and comfort measures effective in controlling patient pain.

   - Dressing remains intact with airtight seal and prescribed negative pressure.

     Dressing effective in maintaining negative pressure and promoting healing.

   - Patient or family member demonstrates correct method of dressing changes.

     Indicates patient and family learning has occurred.

STEP	RATIONALE
2 Explain procedure to patient.	Relieves anxiety and promotes understanding of healing process.
3 Before removal of old dressings, put system into "de-Vac" mode (see steps below) over a period of 45 minutes.	Found to loosen foam dressing for easier, less painful removal (Price and others, 2006).
4 Offer to administer ordered analgesic 30 minutes before dressing change.	Reduces patient discomfort during manipulation of wound tissues.

IMPLEMENTATION

STEP	RATIONALE
1 Close room door or cubicle curtains.	Provides for patient privacy and reduces transmission of organisms.
2 Check patient's identification using two identifiers; one cannot be patient's room number. Position patient comfortably, expose wound site, and drape patient. Instruct patient not to touch wound or sterile supplies.	Ensures correct patient receives correct therapy. Draping provides access to wound while minimizing exposure. Dressing supplies become contaminated when touched by patient's hand
3 Cuff top of disposable waterproof bag, and place within reach of work area.	Cuff prevents accidental contamination of top of outer bag.
4 Perform hand hygiene, and put on clean disposable gloves. If risk for spray exists, apply protective gown, goggles, and mask.	Reduces transmission of infectious organisms from soiled dressings to nurse's hands.
5 When an NPWT unit is in place, begin by pushing therapy on/off button.	Deactivates therapy and allows for proper drainage of fluid in drainage tubing.
a Keeping tube connectors with NPWT unit, disconnect tubes from each other and raise tubing connectors above level of unit to drain fluids into canister.	Allows for proper drainage of fluid in drainage tubing (KCI, 2004). Change NPWT canister unit when full or at least once a week to control odor.
b Before lowering, tighten clamp on canister tube.	

Critical Decision Point *In the past, practice involved introduction of normal saline into tubing to soak underneath foam for easier removal. Research has shown presence of microorganisms in the tubing, which could recontaminate wound if saline is instilled. An effective alternative is to clamp the dressing tube, clean the external surface of the transparent dressing with alcohol, and, using sterile technique, inject 0.25% bupivacaine through the dressing into the sponge. After 15 to 20 minutes the dressing can be removed less painfully for patient (Price and others, 2006).*

STEP	RATIONALE
6 Gently stretch transparent film horizontally, and slowly pull up from the skin.	Reduces stress on suture line or wound edges and reduces irritation and discomfort.
7 Remove old dressing, observe surface area, tissue type, color, odor, and drainage within wound. Use caution to avoid tension on any drains that are present. Discard dressing, and remove and discard gloves in waterproof bag. Avoid having patient see old dressing because the sight of wound drainage may be upsetting to the patient. Perform hand hygiene.	Determines condition of wound and need for replacement of dressing. Avoids accidental removal of drains. Reduces transmission of microorganisms.
8 Apply sterile or clean gloves (see agency policy). Irrigate the wound with normal saline or other solution ordered by the health care provider. Gently blot to dry (see Chapter 38).	Irrigation removes wound debris and cleanses wound bed.

Critical Decision Point *If this is a new surgical wound, sterile technique may be required. Use clean technique with chronic wounds.*

STEP	RATIONALE
9 Measure wound as ordered: at baseline, first dressing change, weekly, and discharge from therapy.	Objectively documents wound measurement, staging, color, and odor of drainage (Bryant and Nix, 2007).

Critical Decision Point *Physician may order wound cultures on a routine basis. However, when drainage looks purulent or has a foul odor, or if there is a change in amount or color, obtain wound culture even when not ordered for that particular dressing change (Jerome, 2007).*

STEP	RATIONALE
10 Apply skin protectant, barrier film, Stomahesive wafer, or hydrocolloid dressing to skin around the wound.	Maintains airtight seal needed for negative pressure wound therapy and protects the periwound skin from moisture-associated skin damage (Jerome, 2007).
11 Remove and discard gloves. Perform hand hygiene.	Prevents transmission of microorganisms.
12 Depending on the type of wound, apply sterile or new clean gloves.	Fresh sterile wounds require sterile gloves. Chronic wounds require clean technique. Do not use the same gloves worn to clean wound, because cross contamination may occur.

STEP	RATIONALE
13 Prepare NPWT foam (see illustration).	
a If needed, measure wound and then select appropriate foam dressing.	Establishes baseline for wound size.
	Black polyurethane (PU) foam has larger pores and is most effective in stimulating granulation tissue and wound contraction. It is hydrophobic and does not absorb fluid but stays moist and promotes exudate removal (Jerome, 2007).
	White polyvinyl alcohol (PVA) soft foam is denser with smaller pores and is used when the growth of granulation tissue needs to be restricted. It is hydrophilic (Franz and others, 2007).
b Using sterile scissors, cut foam to exact wound size, making sure to fit the size and shape of the wound, including tunnels and undermined areas.	Proper size of foam dressing maintains negative pressure to entire wound.

Critical Decision Point   *Use of black foam may cause patients to experience more pain because of excessive wound contraction. You will need to switch patient to the PVA soft foam.*

14 Gently place foam in wound, being sure that the foam is in contact with entire wound base, margins, and tunneled and undermined areas.	Maintains negative pressure to entire wound. Edges of the foam dressing must be in direct contact with the patient's skin .

Critical Decision Point   *For deep wounds, regularly reposition tubing to minimize pressure on wound edges. Reposition patients with restricted mobility or sensation frequently so that they do not lie on the tubing and cause skin damage (KCI, 2004).*

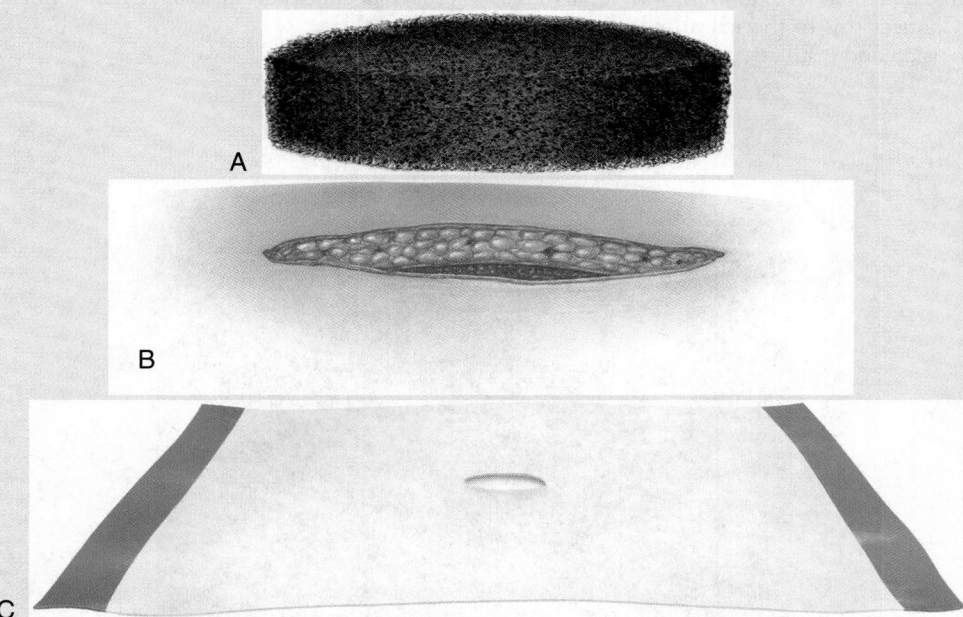

STEP 13   Dressing application. **A,** Properly sized foam to cover wound. **B,** Wrinkle-free transparent dressing applied over foam. **C,** Secure tubing to the foam and transparent dressing unit (Step 15). *(Courtesy Kinetic Concepts, Inc. [KCI], San Antonio, Tex.)*

STEP	RATIONALE
15 Apply NPWT transparent dressing.	
a Cover the NPWT foam and 3 to 5 cm (1.2 to 2 inches) of surrounding healthy tissue.	Ensure that the wound is properly covered and a negative pressure seal can be achieved (Box 39-4, p. 1028).
b Apply transparent dressing, keeping it wrinkle-free.	
c Secure tubing of NPWT unit to transparent film, aligning drainage hole to ensure an occlusive seal. Do not apply tension to drape and tubing.	Excessive tension may compress foam dressing and impede wound healing. Excessive tension also produces a shear force on peri-wound area (KCI, 2004).
16 Secure tubing several centimeters away from the dressing.	Prevents pull on the primary dressing, which can cause leaks in the negative pressure system (KCI, 2004).
17 After the wound is completely covered, follow the steps to connect the tubing from the dressing to the tubing from the canister and NPWT unit (see illustration).	Intermittent or continuous negative pressure can be administered at −50 mm Hg to −175 mm Hg, according to physician orders and patient comfort. The average is −125 mm Hg (Franz and others, 2007).
a Remove canister from sterile packaging, and push into NPWT unit until a click is heard. **An alarm will sound if the canister is not properly engaged.**	Canister collects drainage.
b Connect the dressing tubing to the canister tubing. Make sure both clamps are open.	
c Place NPWT unit on a level surface, or hang from the foot of the bed. **The unit will alarm and deactivate therapy if the unit is tilted beyond 45 degrees.**	
d Press in green-lit power button, and set negative pressure as ordered. Wound will be completely encased.	Activates negative pressure and seals wound.
18 **V.A.C. Instill option:**	V.A.C. Instill is useful for wounds that are not responding to conventional negative pressure wound therapy and for initial management of high-risk wounds (Jerome, 2007).
a Check the name and strength of irrigation solution against physician's orders.	Ensures patient is receiving correct medication.
b Follow Steps 1 to 15b.	
c Place the V.A.C. Instill instillation pad at the highest (nondependent) aspect of the wound and the vacuum pad at its most dependent aspect (Jerome, 2007). Connect the tubing from the vacuum pad to the V.A.C. Instill unit.	Instillation pad instills irrigation solution as vacuum pad delivers negative pressure.
d The V.A.C. Instill pad has an extension, with a Luer-Lok connection. Connect this to the irrigation solution bag. Label the extension and instillation tubing.	Proper labeling prevents inadvertent connection to an intravenous line.

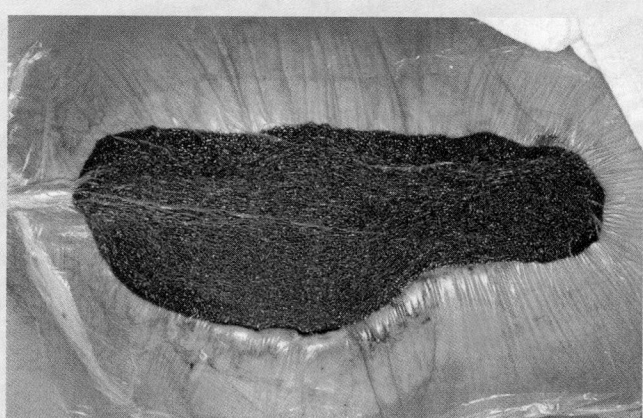

STEP 17 Foam dressing, transparent dressing, and V.A.C. tubing secured over existing wound. (*Courtesy Kinetic Concepts, Inc. [KCI], San Antonio, Tex.*)

STEP	RATIONALE
e Initiate the touch screen on the V.A.C. Instill system. Three functions are available: utilities, therapy, and on-off. Using the **therapy function,** select continuous or intermittent negative pressure and the ordered negative pressure. Select instillation of solution as ordered and a holding time (Jerome, 2007).	V.A.C. Instill allows for continuous or intermittent negative pressure with infusion of a sterile solution to irrigate the wound.
f Be sure all tubing is connected and settings entered. Then select the on switch to begin therapy.	
g Measure and document the volume of fluids instilled and drained during treatment. Canister requires more frequent changing than traditional NPWT.	Monitors fluid balance and amount of wound drainage.
19 Discard soiled dressing materials properly. Perform hand hygiene.	Reduces transmission of microorganisms.
20 Inspect system to verify that negative pressure is achieved.	Negative pressure is achieved when an airtight seal is achieved (see Box 39-4).
a Verify that display screen reads THERAPY ON.	
b Be sure clamps are open and tubing is patent.	
c Identify air leaks by listening with stethoscope over wound edges or by moving hand around edges of wound while applying light pressure.	Determines presence of air leaks.
d If a leak is present, use strips of transparent film to patch areas around the edges of the wound.	
21 Assist patient to a comfortable position. Patients may ambulate with an NPWT.	Enhances patient comfort and relaxation.
22 Discard gloves, and perform hand hygiene	Prevents transmission of microorganisms.

EVALUATION

1 Inspect condition of wound on ongoing basis; note drainage and odor.	Determines status of wound healing.
2 Ask patient to rate pain using a scale of 0 to 10.	Determines patient's level of comfort following the procedure.
3 Verify airtight dressing seal and correct negative pressure setting.	Determines effective negative pressure being applied.
4 Measure wound drainage output in canister on a regular basis. More frequent emptying will be necessary with V.A.C. Instill.	Monitors fluid balance and wound drainage.
5 Observe patient's or family member's ability to perform dressing change.	Indicates that learning has occurred.

Unexpected Outcomes	Related Interventions
1 Wound appears inflamed and tender, drainage has increased, and an odor is present.	• Notify the health care provider. • Obtain wound culture. • Increase frequency of dressing changes.
2 Patient reports increase in pain.	• Patient may need more analgesia when NPWT is initiated or changed. • If using black foam, switch to the PVA foam. • Negative pressure may need to be reduced and gradually titrated upward.
3 Negative pressure seal has broken.	• Take preventive measures (see Box 39-4). • Clip or shave surrounding skin (check agency policy).
4 Patient or caregiver is unable to perform dressing change.	• Provide additional teaching and support. • Obtain services of home care agency.

Recording and Reporting

- Chart in the nurses' notes the appearance of wound, color, characteristics of any drainage, presence of wound healing augmentation, such as NPWT pressure setting, dressing change, and patient response to dressing change.
- Record date and time of dressing change on new dressing.
- Report brisk, bright red bleeding, evidence of poor wound healing, evisceration or dehiscence, and possible wound infection to physician.

Teaching Considerations

- Instruct patient and caregiver in the type of signs and symptoms that indicate development of an infection and to report to health care provider immediately.
- Explain expected wound appearance with use of dressing. Instruct patient and caregiver in appearance of foam dressings.
- Instruct patient and family in points to follow to maintain negative pressure seal.
- Explain frequency of dressing changes required. Often the dressing is not changed daily.
- Explain need to change NPWT canister when full or at least once a week to help to control odor (KCI, 2004).

Pediatric Considerations

- V.A.C. therapy is not appropriate for fragile neonatal skin.
- Parents need to actively participate in NPWT treatment.

Gerontological Considerations

- Use skin care practices to protect periwound tissue. Transparent film may be irritating to fragile skin. Skin protectant is one method to reduce the risk for tissue injury.

- Therapy may need to start with lower negative pressures such as −75 mm Hg and slowly down to −125 mm Hg (KCI, 2004).
- Visual impairment may prevent self-care and require home care services.

Home Care Considerations

- Patient and family may benefit from visits with home care agency to monitor initial treatments.
- Provide information to family and caregiver regarding proper disposal of contaminated product.

BOX 39-4   Maintaining an Airtight Seal

Once Wound V.A.C. therapy is initiated, the wound must stay sealed to avoid wound desiccation. Wounds around joints and near the sacrum are problem areas to seal. The following points may assist in maintaining an airtight seal:

- Choose a wound suitable for therapy.
- Clip or shave hair around wound (check agency policy).
- Cut transparent film to extend 3 to 5 cm beyond wound perimeter.
- Avoid wrinkles in transparent film.
- Dressing should be cut or molded to fit wound.
- Use multiple small strips of transparent film to hold dressing in place before covering dressing with large piece of transparent film.
- Avoid adhesive remover because it leaves a residue that hinders film adherence.

From Thompson G: An overview of negative pressure wound therapy (NPWT), *Wound Care* 6:523, 2008.

SKILL 39-6   Applying Gauze and Elastic Bandages

 Intermediate / Wound and Pressure Ulcer Care / Changing a Dressing

NSO *Wound Care Module / Lesson 3*

Gauze and elastic bandages secure or wrap hard-to-cover areas of the body. The bandages secure dressings on extremities, amputation stumps, and the hand (Table 39-3). For example, a dressing covering the length of a patient's lower leg is held in place more firmly when a well-secured gauze bandage surrounds the dressing. An elastic bandage applies compression to a body part. Elastic compression to a lower extremity prevents edema by promoting the return of blood from the peripheral circulation to the central circulation. Compression also supports varicosities. Many patients use elastic bandages in the form of stockings to reduce dependent edema in the extremities.

Other uses of elastic bandages include support of the knee, ankle, elbow, and wrist in conditions such as strains and sprains (Phipps and others, 2006). When fully stretched, an elastic bandage extends to 270 cm (3 yards). Shorter lengths of 135 cm (1½ yards) are available for bandaging the wrist or a child's foot or knee. Gauze bandages likewise come in a variety of lengths. Gauze and elastic bandages are available in widths ranging from 1.5 to 7.5 cm (½ to 3 inches).

Elasticized bandages are available in rolls of various widths and materials, including gauze, elasticized knit, elastic webbing, and muslin. Gauze bandages are lightweight and inexpensive, mold easily around contours of the body, and permit air circulation to prevent skin maceration, the softening and breakdown of the skin due to fluid. Elastic bandages conform well to body parts but also exert pressure over a body part. Elastic compression bandages are either long-stretch or short-stretch. Long-stretch bandages provide sustained compression regardless of a patient's activities. Short-stretch bandages provide compression only when a patient activates his or her calf muscle pump, as in walking. Continuous compression therapy, the treatment of choice for chronic venous insufficiency, has multiple therapeutic benefits, including reducing venous hypertension, stimulation of fibrinolysis, and increased local oxygenation. Nurses require advanced training to apply continuous compression bandages, which is beyond the scope of this text.

When applying a gauze or elastic bandage, you select a type of bandage turn and bandage width depending on the size and shape of the body part to be bandaged. For example, 3-inch bandages are most commonly used for the adult leg. A smaller 2-inch bandage is normally used for the wrist. Gauze and elastic bandages come supplied in a roll with an inner and outer surface for easy application. In preparation for bandaging, place the outer surface next to the skin and then roll it around the surface to be covered. Apply even tension during application. When applying an elastic bandage to an extremity, start the bandage at the site farthest from the heart (distal) and proceed toward the heart (proximal).

TABLE 39-3 | Types of Bandage Turns

Type	Description	Purpose or Use
Circular Circular turns.	Bandage turn overlapping previous turn completely	Anchors bandage at the first and final turn; covers small part (finger, toe)
Spiral Spiral turns.	Bandage ascending body part with each turn overlapping previous one by one-half or two-thirds width of bandage	Covers cylindrical body parts such as wrist or upper arm
Spiral-reverse Spiral-reverse turns.	Turn requiring twist (reversal) of bandage halfway through each turn	Covers cone-shaped body parts such as the forearm, thigh, or calf; useful with nonstretching bandages such as gauze or flannel
Figure eight Figure-eight turns.	Oblique overlapping turns alternately ascending and descending over bandaged part; each turn crossing previous one to form figure eight	Covers joints, applies low-grade pressure for venous return; snug fit provides excellent immobilization
Recurrent Recurrent turns.	Bandage first secured with two circular turns around proximal end of body part; half turn made perpendicular up from bandage edge; body of bandage brought over distal end of body part to be covered with each turn folded back over on itself	Covers uneven body parts such as head or stump

Delegation Considerations

The skill of applying an elastic bandage for compression cannot be delegated to NAP. A nurse assesses the condition of any wound or dressing before applying a bandage. The skill of applying bandages to secure nonsterile dressings can be delegated to NAP (refer to agency policy). The nurse directs the NAP to:

• Modify the bandage application, such as special taping.

• Report a patient's complaint of pain, numbness, or tingling after a bandage has been applied or any changes in patient's skin color or temperature.

Equipment

❑ Correct width and number of gauze or elastic bandages
❑ Clips or adhesive tape
❑ Clean gloves, if wound drainage is present

STEP	RATIONALE

ASSESSMENT

1   Review patient's medical record and Kardex for specific orders related to application of gauze or elastic bandage. Note area to be covered, type of bandage required, frequency of change, and previous response to treatment.

Specific prescription may direct procedure, including such factors as extent of application (e.g., toe to knee, toe to groin) or duration of treatment.

2   Apply clean gloves if drainage or break in skin is present. Inspect skin of area to be bandaged for alterations in integrity as indicated by presence of abrasion, discoloration, or chafing. Palpate for swelling. Pay close attention to areas over bony prominences.

Altered skin integrity may contraindicate use of elastic bandage to be applied directly to the skin because of applied pressure. May require a dressing before bandage is applied.

3   Inspect the condition of any wound for size, integrity of tissues, and presence and character of drainage, and be sure it is covered with a proper dressing.

Inspection provides baseline for wound condition. Surgical dressing replacement or reinforcement precedes application of any bandage. Prevents soiling of bandage.

4   Observe adequacy of circulation by noting surface temperature, skin color, pulses (distal to area to be bandaged), presence of edema, and sensation and movement of body parts to be wrapped.

Comparison of area before and after application of bandage is necessary to ensure continued adequate circulation. Impairment of circulation may result in pain, coolness to touch when compared with opposite side of body, cyanosis or pallor of skin, diminished or absent pulses, edema or localized pooling, and numbness and/or tingling of body part.

5   Determine patient's level of comfort using a scale of 0 to 10. Administer prescribed analgesic as needed before dressing change.

Comfortable patient will be less likely to move suddenly, causing wound or supply contamination. Serves as baseline to measure response to dressing therapy.

6   Assess for size of bandage.

a   *Gauze or basic elastic bandage to secure a dressing:* Assess size of area to be covered. Each successive roll of gauze/elastic should overlap previous layer. Use smaller widths for upper extremities, larger widths for lower extremities.

Proper size bandage avoids bulkiness and ensures adequate coverage.

b   *Elastic bandage to provide simple compression:* Assess circumference of lower extremity before or shortly after patient gets out of bed in the morning or after patient has been in bed for at least 15 minutes. Select width that will cover and overlap without bulkiness.

Assures clinician that dependent edema is at a minimum, so true leg circumference can be estimated. Compression bandages not applied correctly may produce pressures that are either too low or too high to promote venous return.

7   Identify patient's and primary caregiver's present knowledge level and ability to manipulate bandage if bandaging will be continued at home.

Ensures that planning and teaching are individualized.

NURSING DIAGNOSES

- Acute pain
- Chronic pain
- Deficient knowledge regarding bandage application
- Impaired physical mobility
- Impaired tissue integrity

Individualize related factors based on patient's condition or needs.

PLANNING

1   Expected outcomes following completion of procedure:
- Patient states pain or discomfort is decreased or absent on a scale of 0 to 10.

Indicates proper application of bandage without excess pressure or compression that could impair local blood flow.

- Patient denies tingling or numbness.

Bandage is not causing pressure on peripheral nerves or arterial circulation.

- Distal parts (toes, fingers) feel warm (symmetrically) to touch, pulse is present, no cyanosis or blanching is present, and motion is not unnecessarily impaired.

Indicates adequate circulation to distal regions.

- Dressing remains in place with gauze bandage smooth and intact.

Gauze bandage applied correctly.

- Localized edema is reduced.

Elastic bandage promotes venous return.

- Patient applies bandage correctly.

Demonstrates learning and ensures continuity of care after discharge.

STEP	**RATIONALE**
2 Explain procedure to patient.	Promotes cooperation, reduces anxiety, and ensures technique for self-application.
3 Teach skill to patient or significant other when bandage will be applied in the home.	Reduces anxiety and ensures continuity of care.

IMPLEMENTATION

1 Close room door or curtains.	Maintains patient's comfort and dignity.
2 Assist patient with assuming comfortable, anatomically correct position lying in bed.	Maintains alignment. Facilitates application of bandage in anatomical position.
3 Perform hand hygiene, and apply gloves if drainage is present.	Reduces transmission of microorganisms.

Critical Decision Point   *With patient in bed, elevation of dependent extremities for 15 minutes before elastic bandage application enhances venous return.*

4 Apply gauze or elastic bandage to secure dressing	
a Hold roll of bandage in dominant hand, and use other hand to lightly hold beginning layer of bandage at distal body part. While rolling bandage around body part, in two circular turns, continue transferring roll to dominant hand as bandage is wrapped.	Maintains appropriate and consistent bandage tension.
b Apply bandage from distal point toward proximal boundary (see illustration 4b, 1) using variety of turns to cover various shapes of body parts (see Table 39-3). (For bandaging of amputation stump, see illustration 4b, 2).	Apply bandage in manner that conforms evenly to body part and promotes venous return.

Critical Decision Point   *Except in cases in which toes or fingers are treated because of wounds, toes or fingertips should remain uncovered and visible for follow-up circulatory assessment.*

c While unrolling elastic bandage, stretch bandage slightly. Explain to patient that smooth, even pressure will be applied to improve venous circulation, prevent clot formation, reduce or prevent swelling, immobilize body part, secure surgical dressings, and provide pressure.	Maintains uniform bandage tension.

Critical Decision Point   *Avoid wrapping bandage too tightly because this may cause numbness and tingling from impaired circulation and/or pressure on peripheral nerves.*

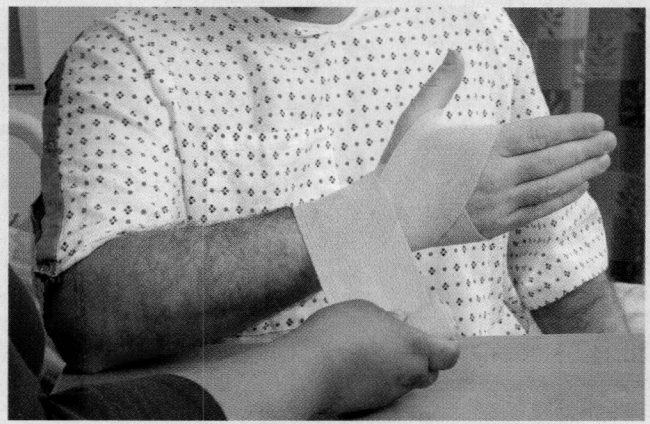

STEP 4b(1)   Hold bandage in dominant hand. Use other hand to lightly hold beginning layer while applying two circular turns.

STEP	RATIONALE

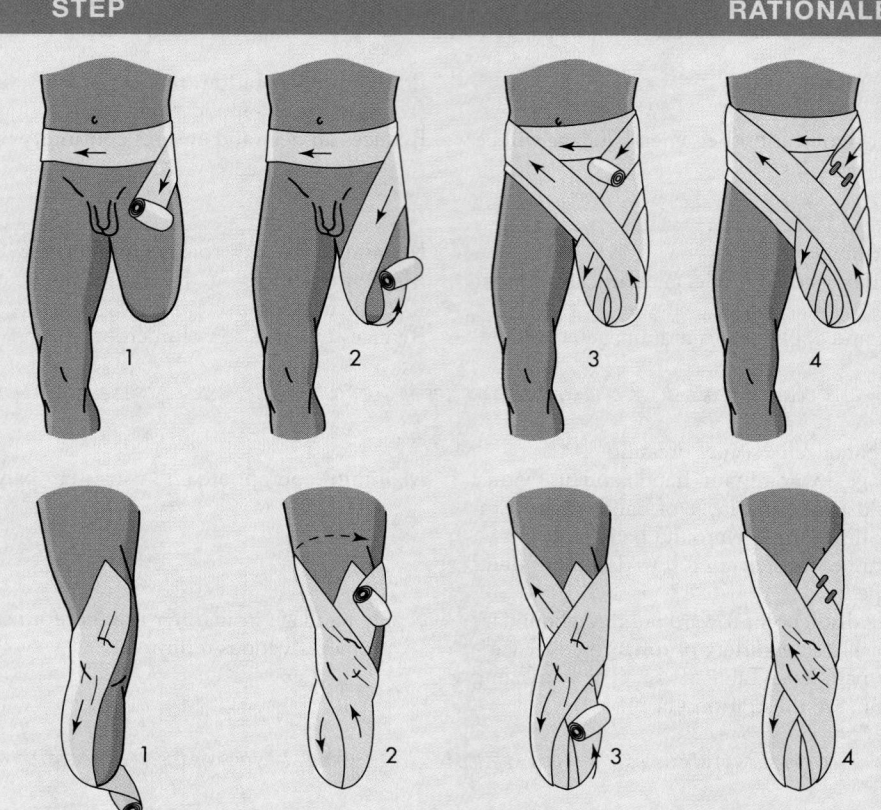

STEP 4b(2)   *Top,* Correct method for bandaging midthigh amputation stump. Note that bandage must be anchored around patient's waist. *Bottom,* Correct method for bandaging midcalf amputation stump. Note that bandage need not be anchored around the waist. (*From Monahan F, Phipps J and others: Phipp's Medical-surgical nursing: health and illness perspectives, ed 8, St. Louis, 2006, Mosby.*)

STEP	RATIONALE
d Overlap turns by one-half to two-thirds width of bandage roll (see illustration).	Prevents uneven bandage tension and circulatory impairment.
e Secure first bandage with clip or tape before applying additional rolls (see illustration).	Maintains a smooth bandage surface.
f Apply additional rolls without leaving any uncovered skin surface. Secure last bandage applied.	Prevents wrinkling or loose ends.
5 Apply elastic bandage for simple intermittent compression:	
a Have patient lie in bed with leg slightly elevated.	Promotes venous return during application.
b Hold roll of bandage in dominant hand, and use other hand to lightly hold beginning layer of bandage at distal body part. While rolling bandage around body part, continue transferring roll to dominant hand as you apply bandage.	Maintains appropriate and consistent bandage tension.
c Apply the highly elastic conformable bandage using a figure-eight turn. Apply from distal (just above toes) to most proximal boundary.	Applies higher compression pressure at the ankle while reducing pressure at the thigh to promote venous return.
d Stretch bandage slightly while applying.	Maintains uniform tension.
e After applying only one layer of bandage, secure with tape or clips.	Prevents excess pressure over limb.

Critical Decision Point   *Do not apply multiple layers of elastic bandage without special training.*

STEP	RATIONALE
6 Remove gloves if worn, and perform hand hygiene.	Reduces transmission of microorganisms.
7 Remove and reapply elastic bandage once every 8 hours unless otherwise directed by physician.	Single-layer bandage can slip easily, causing excess pressure where bandage rests.

STEP	RATIONALE

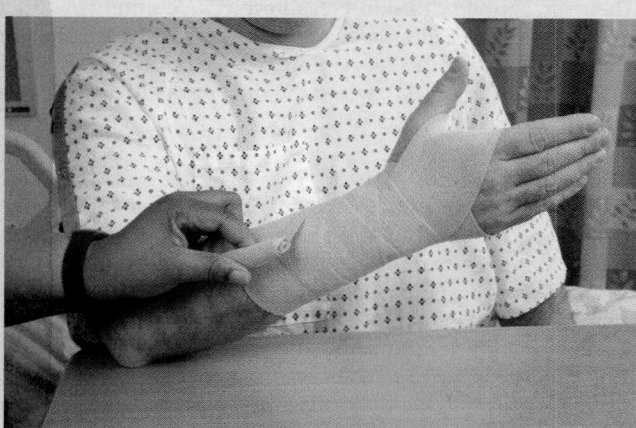

STEP 4d   Apply bandage from distal to proximal.

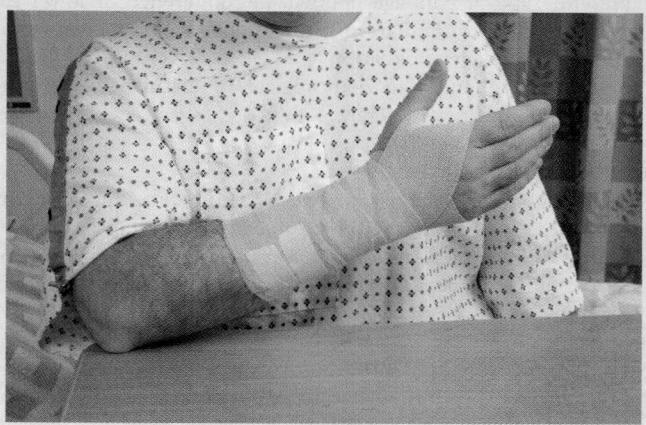

STEP 4e   With bandage overlapped, tape before applying an additional, continuous roll.

EVALUATION

1 Evaluate distal circulation when bandage application is complete and at least twice during 8-hour period.

Measurements determine if bandage is too tight, compromising circulation or movement.

   a Observe skin color for pallor or cyanosis.

Determines if circulation is compromised.

   b Palpate skin for warmth.

   c Palpate pulses, and compare bilaterally.

Early detection and management of circulatory impairment ensures healthy neurovascular status.

   d Ask patient to rate any pain on scale of 0 to 10 and to describe any numbness, tingling, or other discomfort.

Neurovascular changes indicate impaired venous return.

   e Observe mobility of extremity.

Determines if bandage is too tight, which restricts movement, or if intended therapeutic joint immobility is attained.

2 Evaluate bandage for wrinkles, looseness, or tightness; patient discomfort or itchiness; and changes, including drainage.

Slippage of bandage can cause pressure on underlying tissue, leading to impaired circulation or pressure on nerves.

3 Have patient demonstrate bandage application.

Return demonstration validates patient's learning.

Unexpected Outcomes	Related Interventions
1 Circumferential ridging develops with deep indentations into skin; patient may note tingling, numbness, or pain.	• Bandage is too tight, causing impaired circulation. • Remove, and wait 30 minutes before reapplying.
2 Extremity distal to wrap is cool, cyanotic, or blanched.	• Remove bandage. • Notify health care provider.
3 Dressing is loose, slipping, or improperly wrapped, providing improper support.	• Remove dressing. • Reapply using correct technique.
4 Extremity has decreased range of joint motion.	• Notify health care provider. • Check dressing for correct application.

Recording and Reporting

- Document condition of wound or skin, integrity of dressing if present, type of bandage applied, circumference of lower extremity, status of circulation, and patient's comfort level before and after bandage application.
- Report any changes in neurological or circulatory status to nurse in charge or physician.

Teaching Considerations

- Applying elastic bandage to oneself is difficult. Teach significant other if treatment will continue after hospitalization.
- Unless total immobilization is prescribed for patient, instruct on proper range-of-motion exercises. Encourage patient to practice regularly.

Pediatric Considerations

- Use adhesive tape rather than loose clips or safety pins to fasten bandage on small child or infant.

Gerontological Considerations

- As patients age, skin becomes more fragile, which increases their susceptibility to skin breakdown. Once skin/tissue injury occurs, wound healing is delayed. Assess these patients more frequently for evidence of skin breakdown or decrease in circulation over the areas covered by and distal to the bandage (Ebersole and others, 2008).

Home Care Considerations

- Advise patient on best resources for obtaining bandage supplies. Consult with home care nurse as needed.
- Assess patient's and primary caregiver's ability, motivation, willingness to leave bandage in place and availability to participate in bandaging procedure.
- Assess patient's environment to determine potential for permitting bandaged area to remain free from contaminants.
- Have patient wash elastic bandage and place in large folds over a line to dry. Do not use an electric dryer because bandage can shrink.

SKILL 39-7 Applying an Abdominal and Breast Binder

Binders are bandages made of large pieces of material specially designed to fit a specific body part. Most binders are made of elastic or cotton. The most common type of binders are the abdominal binder and breast binder. An abdominal binder supports large abdominal incisions (e.g., following hernia repair) that are vulnerable to tension or stress as a patient moves or coughs (Fig. 39-10). A breast binder looks like a tight-fitting sleeveless vest. It conforms to the shape of the chest wall and is available in various sizes. Breast binders provide support after breast surgery. You secure a binder with Velcro strips or metal fasteners.

Binders are indicated for the support of underlying muscles and large incisions. The muscles and viscera surrounding an operative site may require support during the postoperative period to reduce trauma and edema. This promotes healing and permits a patient to move more freely without additional discomfort. The basic shape of an abdominal binder is a rectangle that is wide enough to extend from the groin to the waistline and long enough to encircle the abdomen with an overlap for closure.

Delegation Considerations

The skill of applying a binder can be delegated to NAP. A nurse assesses the condition of any incision, the skin, and patient's ability to breathe before binder application. The nurse directs the NAP about:

- How to modify the skill, such as special wrapping or manner of securing the binder.
- Reporting patient's complaint of pain, numbness, tingling, or difficulty breathing after applying abdominal binder, or any changes in patient's skin color or temperature.

Equipment

- ☐ Clean gloves, if wound drainage present
- ☐ Gauze bandage as needed
- ☐ Correct size cloth/elastic straight binder
- ☐ Safety pins (6 to 8) unless Velcro closure or metal fasteners are attached

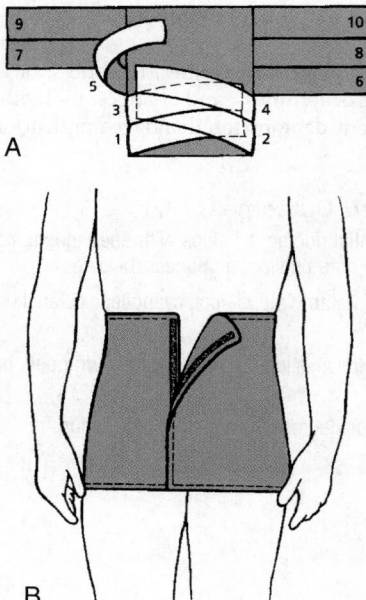

FIG 39-10 Straight abdominal binder with Velcro closure.

STEP	RATIONALE

ASSESSMENT

1 Observe patient who needs support of thorax or abdomen; observe ability to breathe deeply, cough effectively, and turn or move independently.	Baseline assessment determines patient's ability to breathe and cough. Impaired ventilation of lung can lead to alveolar atelectasis and reduced oxygenation.

STEP	RATIONALE
2 Review medical record for order for binder.	Application of a binder can be based on nursing judgment, but in some institutions a health care provider's order is required (check agency policy).
3 Inspect skin for actual or potential alterations in integrity. Observe for irritation, abrasion, and skin surfaces that rub against each other.	Actual impairments in skin integrity can be worsened with application of a binder. Binder can cause pressure and excoriation.
4 Inspect any surgical dressing for intactness, presence of drainage, and coverage of incision. Change any soiled dressing before applying binder.	Dressing replacement or reinforcement precedes application of any binder. If left uncovered, a wound can be damaged from rubbing of binder.
5 Determine patient's level of comfort using a scale of 0 to 10. Administer prescribed analgesic 30 minutes before dressing change.	Comfortable patient will be less likely to move suddenly, causing wound or supply contamination. Serves as baseline to measure response to dressing therapy.
6 Gather necessary data regarding size of patient and appropriate binder to use (see manufacturer's guidelines).	Ensures proper fit of binder.
7 Determine patient's knowledge of purpose of binder.	Improves patient's ability to cooperate with application and adhere to its placement.

NURSING DIAGNOSES

- Acute pain
- Deficient knowledge regarding binder application
- Impaired physical mobility
- Impaired skin integrity
- Impaired tissue integrity
- Ineffective breathing pattern

Individualize related factors based on patient's condition or needs.

PLANNING

1 Expected outcomes following completion of procedure:	
• Patient's respirations are unrestricted. Coughing is effective, and secretions are expectorated.	Ability to fully expand lungs and cough must continue after application of binder to enhance oxygenation and avoid pulmonary complications.
• Patient is able to move within prescribed limits and states pain is absent or reduced.	Support to incision from binder promotes comfort during turning, ambulation, or deep breathing.
• Patient's suture line is intact, with no drainage or separation.	Binder decreases tension on suture line to promote healing. Snug support helps maintain intact suture line.
2 Explain procedure to patient.	Promotes patient's understanding and cooperation.
3 Teach skill to patient or significant other.	Reduces anxiety and ensures continuity of care after discharge.

IMPLEMENTATION

1 Close curtains or room door.	Maintains patient's comfort and dignity.
2 Perform hand hygiene, and apply clean gloves (if likely to contact wound drainage).	Reduces transmission of microorganisms.
3 Apply abdominal binder:	
a Position patient in supine position with head slightly elevated and knees slightly flexed.	Minimizes muscular tension on abdominal organs.
b Assist patient in rolling on side away from you toward raised side rail while firmly supporting abdominal incision and dressing with hands. Fanfold far side of binder toward midline of binder.	Reduces pain and discomfort. Positions patient for binder application.
c Place binder flat on bed, right side up. Fanfold far side of binder toward midline of binder.	Gathers binder together so patient can roll over with minimal effort.
d Place fanfolded ends of binder under patient.	Permits placement and centering of binder with minimal discomfort.
e Instruct or assist patient in rolling over folded binder. For overweight patients consider asking nurse colleague to assist (see Chapter 9).	Positions patient over binder.
f Unfold and stretch ends out smoothly on far side of bed. Then stretch out ends on near side of bed.	Smooth, even binder maintains skin integrity and comfort.
g Instruct patient to roll back into supine position.	Facilitates an even application of binder over abdomen.
h Adjust binder so that supine patient is centered over binder, using symphysis pubis and costal margins as lower and upper landmarks.	Centers support from binder over abdominal structures, which reduces incidence of decreased lung expansion while ensuring adequate wound support.

STEP	RATIONALE
i If patient is very thin, pad iliac prominences with gauze bandage.	Reduces pressure on prominences.
j Close binder. Pull one end of binder over center of patient's abdomen. While maintaining tension on that end of binder, pull opposite end of binder over center (see illustration) and secure with Velcro closure tabs, metal fasteners, or horizontally placed safety pins.	Provides continuous wound support and comfort.

Critical Decision Point   *Recheck patient's ability to breathe deeply and cough effectively. Shallow respirations, continuing after a tight binder has been loosened, may indicate beginning of serious respiratory problems, including alveolar atelectasis and pulmonary embolus, among others.*

STEP	RATIONALE
k Assess patient's comfort level, and adjust binder as necessary.	Helps determine effectiveness of binder placement. Promotes comfort and chest expansion
4 Apply breast binder:	
a Assist patient to sit up and place arms through binder's armholes.	Eases binder placement.
b Assist patient to supine position if needed.	Facilitates position of breasts for binder placement.
c Pad area under breasts if needed.	Prevents skin contact with undersurface.
d Using Velcro closures tabs, secure binder at nipple in the front. Continue closure process above and then below nipple line until binder is closed.	Horizontal placement of closures may reduce risk for uneven pressure.
e Adjust shoulder straps and waistline darts to reduce binder size if needed.	
f Assess patient's comfort level and adjust binder as necessary.	Promotes comfort and chest expansion.
5 Remove gloves, and perform hand hygiene.	Prevents cross infections.

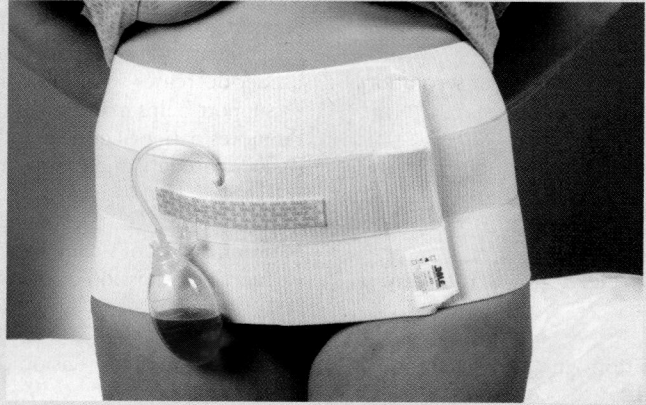

STEP 3j   Abdominal binder with Velcro closures. (*Courtesy Dale Medical Products, Inc., Plainsville, Mass.*)

EVALUATION

1 Ask patient to rate pain on a scale of 0 to 10.	Binder should not increase discomfort.
2 Remove binder and surgical dressing to assess skin and wound characteristics at least every 8 hours.	Determines that binder has not resulted in complications (e.g., rubbing or abrasion of skin, disruption of wound).
3 Evaluate patient's ability to ventilate properly, including deep breathing and coughing, every 4 hours.	Identifies any impaired ventilation and potential pulmonary complications.
4 Identify patient's need for assistance with activities such as hair combing, dressing, and ambulating.	Mobility of upper extremities may be limited, depending on severity and location of incision.

Unexpected Outcomes

1 Impaired breathing as evidenced by shallow, rapid respirations leads to ineffective oxygenation.

2 Tight binder impairs circulation to tissues.

3 Skin integrity is impaired, resulting from uneven pressure and irritation.

4 Pain and discomfort are increased.

Related Interventions

• Remove binder.
• Reapply binder using correct technique.

• Remove binder.
• Consult with health care provider, and reapply if appropriate.

• Remove binder.
• Administer skin care according to agency policy .
• Consult with health care provider, and reapply if appropriate.

• Remove binder and reapply using correct technique.

Recording and Reporting

• Record type and application of binder, condition of skin, circulation, integrity of underlying dressing, and patient's comfort level.
• Report any complications (e.g., pain, skin irritation, impaired ventilation) to nurse in charge.
• Report reduced lung expansion to health care provider immediately.

Teaching Considerations

• Consider patient's dexterity in reapplying binder to self, opportunities to practice skill, and need to teach family caregiver.

Pediatric Considerations

• Use adhesive tape rather than loose clips or pins to fasten binder on small child or infant. Be sure child is not allergic to adhesive.

Gerontological Considerations

• As patients age, skin becomes more fragile, which increases their susceptibility to skin breakdown. Once skin/tissue injury occurs, healing is delayed. Assess these patients more frequently for evidence of skin breakdown over area covered by binder (Ebersole and others, 2008).

Home Care Considerations

• Assess primary caregiver's understanding, ability, and motivation to participate in application of binder.
• Assess patient's understanding of purpose of binder and willingness to permit binder to remain in place.
• Instruct family to wash breast or abdominal binders and hang to dry.

[?] CRITICAL THINKING EXERCISES

Mr. Williams is a 62-year-old patient who has a chronic diabetic leg ulcer. The ulcer has reoccurred several times over the last 5 years. He cares for it at home by applying a hydrogel dressing.

1 The patient tells you he has trouble applying the dressing. What step is he likely having difficulty performing?

2 What assessment findings suggest the wound is not healing?
Mr. Williams' response to the dressing remains poor. While he is in the clinic, you observe that the ulcer is now 6.0 cm in diameter and draining a dark yellow, foul-smelling drainage. The skin around the ulcer is inflamed. The physician has decided to try NPWT therapy.

3 Mr. Williams asks you, "What is the advantage of using NPWT?" What would be your response?

4 You prepare to apply the NPWT system. Because Mr. Williams already has presence of inflammation around the wound site, what action do you take to reduce periwound irritation and inflammation?

5 After applying the NPWT dressing, you temporarily leave Mr. Williams' room. When you return, he tells you he thought he heard a swishing sound around the dressing. You hear nothing. What might Mr. Williams be describing, and how would you assess for it?

[✓] REVIEW QUESTIONS

1 The nurse is removing a moist-to-dry dressing from a packed wound 6 hours after it was placed in the wound. What observation indicates that the packing technique was incorrectly done?
   1 The patient experiences some pain when the dressing is removed.
   2 The gauze removed is still wet.
   3 Necrotic tissue is seen in the removed packed gauze.
   4 The wound bed looks pink with some granulation tissue.

2 A patient is having a wound debrided. Which measure used in this type of wound treatment is most appropriate?
   1 A dry Telfa pad is used between the wound and the outer layer of the dressing.
   2 A moist dressing against the wound increases the ability of the dressing to collect exudate.
   3 Dry sterile gauze pads are most effective in protecting granulation tissue.
   4 Self-adhesive transparent film, such as Tegaderm, is preferred for debriding large draining wounds.

3 The nurse is caring for a patient with a painful burn wound. The wound care would be appropriate if the nurse applied which type of dressing?
   1 Hydrocolloid
   2 Hydrogel
   3 Alginate
   4 Foam

4 The wound care nurse is reviewing the charts of the group of patients he will be seeing in the clinic. Which patients are at risk for wound-healing problems? Select all that apply.
   1 A 58-year-old woman who is on immunosuppressive drugs for arthritis
   2 A 34-year-old man who has had diabetes mellitus since the age of 12
   3 A 42-year-old woman who has been using steroids for asthma
   4 A 65-year-old African American man who is 10 pounds overweight
   5 An 80-year-old woman with a history of osteoporosis
   6 A 20-year-old man who is receiving radiation near the wound

5 After the nurse applies an abdominal binder to a patient, the patient begins to experience shallow, rapid respirations. What is the appropriate nursing action?
   1 Notify the physician.
   2 Elevate the head of the bed.
   3 Check the patient's vital signs.
   4 Remove, then reapply the abdominal binder.

REFERENCES

Aguinaga A and others: Positive steps towards negative pressure wound therapy, *Medsurg Nurs* 16(3):181, 2007.

Bryant RA, Nix DP: *Acute and chronic wounds: nursing management,* ed 3, St. Louis, 2007, Mosby.

Bryant RA and others: Billing, coding, and reimbursement. In Bryant RA, Nix DP: *Acute and chronic wounds: nursing management,* ed 3, St. Louis, 2007, Mosby.

Doughty D, Sparks-DeFriese B: Wound-healing physiology. In Bryant RA, Nix DP: *Acute and chronic wounds: nursing management,* ed 3, St. Louis, 2007, Mosby.

Ebersole P and others: *Toward healthy aging: human needs and nursing response,* ed 7, St. Louis, 2008, Mosby.

Franz RA and others: Device and technology in wound care. In Bryant R, Nix D: Acute and chronic wounds: current management and concepts, ed 3, St. Louis, 2007, Mosby.

Galanti GA: *Caring for patients from different cultures,* ed 3, Philadelphia, 2004, University of Pennsylvania Press.

Harvey C: Wound healing, *Orthop Nurs* 23(2):143, 2005.

Hockenberry MJ, Wilson D: *Wong's nursing care of infants and children,* ed 8, St. Louis, 2007, Mosby.

Jerome D: Advances in negative pressure wound therapy: the VAC Instill, *J Wound Ostomy Continence Nurs* 34(2):191, 2007.

Kinetic Concepts, Inc: *The V.A.C. vacuum assisted closure: V.A.C. therapy clinical guidelines: a reference source for clinicians,* product information, San Antonio, Tex, 2004, Kinetic Concepts, Inc.

Mendez-Eastman S: Using negative-pressure wound therapy for positive results, *Nursing* 35(5):48, 2005.

Phipps J and others: *Medical-surgical nursing: health and illness perspectives,* ed 7, St. Louis, 2003, Mosby.

Ramundo J: Wound debridement. In Bryant R, Nix, D: *Acute and chronic wounds: current management and concepts,* ed 3, St. Louis, 2007, Mosby.

Reisler T: A simple method of securing an interface dressing and vacuum-assisted closure foam pad to difficult wounds, *Ann Plast Surg* 59(2):230, 2007.

Rolstad BS, Ovington LG: Principles of wound management. In Bryant RA, Nix DP: *Acute and chronic wounds: nursing management,* ed 3, St. Louis, 2007, Mosby.

Whitney JD: Acute surgical and traumatic wounds. In Bryant RA, Nix DP: *Acute and chronic wounds: nursing management,* ed 3, St. Louis, 2007, Mosby.

Wooten M and others: *WOCN position statement: clean versus sterile: management of chronic wounds,* Glenview, Ill, 2005, Wound, Ostomy and Continence Nurses Society.

RESEARCH REFERENCES

Bolton L: Operational definition of moist wound healing, *J Wound Ostomy Continence Nurs* 34(1):23, 2007.

Braakenburg A and others: The clinical efficacy and cost effectiveness of the vacuum-assisted closure technique in the management of acute and chronic wounds: a randomized controlled trial, *Plast Reconstr Surg* 118(2):390, 2006.

Gray N, Weir D: Prevention and treatment of moisture-associated skin damage (maceration) in the periwound skin, *JWOCN* 34(2):153, 2007.

Gregor S and others: Negative pressure wound therapy: a vacuum of evidence? *Arch Surg* 143(2):189, 2008.

Hunter JE and others: Evidence-based medicine: vacuum-assisted closure in wound care management, *Int J Wound J* 4:256, 2007.

Joanna Briggs Institute: Solutions, techniques, and pressure in wound cleansing, *Nursing Standard* 22(27):35, 2008.

Price RD and others: Local anesthetic for change of vacuum-assisted closure dressings, *Plast Reconstr Surg* 117(7):2537, 2006.

Thompson G: An overview of negative pressure wound therapy (NPWT), *Wound Care* 6:523, 2008.

Warm and Cold Therapy

KEY TERMS

Compress
Conduction
Cryotherapy
Evaporation
Insulator
Neuropathy

Piloerection
Sitz bath
Vasoconstriction
Vasodilation

MEDIA RESOURCES

- evolve http://evolve.elsevier.com/Perry/skills
  learning system
  - Review Questions

Mastery of content in this chapter will enable the nurse to:
- Identify the effects of heat and cold on the patient.
- Differentiate the types of injuries or conditions that benefit from heat and cold applications.
- Identify the risks to patients related to heat and cold applications.
- Explain common guidelines used to protect patients who receive heat and cold applications.
- Correctly apply heat and cold applications.

The local application of moderate heat and cold to body parts has beneficial effects. To use heat and cold therapies safely, you need to understand how the body normally responds to temperature variations and the risks connected with these applications.

Exposure to heat or cold causes both systemic and local responses (Table 40-1). The hypothalamus is the body's thermostat, and it regulates heat production and heat loss. Systemically, when the skin is exposed to warm or hot temperatures, vasodilation and perspiration occur to promote heat loss. As perspiration evaporates from the skin, cooling occurs. In cryotherapy, when the skin is exposed to cool or cold temperatures, the systemic response includes vasoconstriction and piloerection to conserve heat. Shivering occurs in response to cooler temperatures, producing heat through skeletal muscle contraction.

The local response to heat and cold results from changes in blood vessel size, which affects blood flow to the exposed area. This physiological response explains the effectiveness of heat and cold therapies.

The stimulation of heat or cold receptors sends sensory impulses that travel via somatic afferent fibers to the hypothalamus and cerebral cortex. The cerebral cortex makes a person aware of temperature sensations. The body also has a protective reflex response for exposure to temperature extremes. Exposure to an extremely hot or cold stimulus sends impulses traveling to the spinal cord, synapsing at the spinal cord, and returning by way of motor nerves to cause withdrawal from the stimulus. The person becomes aware of the discomfort as withdrawal occurs.

Sensory adaptation to local temperature extremes can occur quickly within the body. Although a person may initially feel a temperature extreme, once the sensory receptors adapt, the person may become unaware of any temperature variation. Eventually excessive heat causes a burning sensation; excessive cold causes a numbing sensation before pain is sensed. Because of this physiological phenomenon, the risk for tissue injury from heat and cold applications is high. Certain patients are more at risk than others for injury from warm and cold applications (Table 40-2). You play an important role in maintaining patients' safety in the application of heat and cold. An order for a heat or cold application is always necessary, and it should include the duration of the treatment and the desired temperature to be used when settings can be controlled (Table 40-3). In health care agencies, materials distribution departments typically set temperature settings on heat and cold devices. Because many of these therapies can be used at home, instruct patients and their families in the proper use of these therapies.

When using heat or cold therapies, you can use either dry or moist applications. The selection of dry or moist application depends on the nature of temperature conduction and the result desired from therapy. Temperature travels from an external source such as a compress or water pad to the skin's surface. A substance that conducts temperatures poorly is a good insulator and thus a protector for skin and tissues. For example, cloth placed over a heating pad insulates the skin from hot temperature extremes. Plastic, which is the external covering for most commercial heating pads, and the fluid in moist compresses both conduct heat well,

TABLE 40-1	Pathophysiologic Effects of Hot and Cold Modalities	
	Cold	**Hot**
Pain	↓	↓
Spasm	↓	↓
Metabolism	↓	↑
Blood flow	↓	↑
Inflammation	↓	↑
Edema	↓	↑
Extensibility	↓	↑

Data from Nadler S and others: The physiologic basis and clinical applications of cryotherapy and thermotherapy for the pain practitioner, *Pain Physician* 7(3):395, 2004.

TABLE 40-2	Characteristics of Hot and Cold Application		
	Examples of Conditions Treated	**Precautions**	**Adverse Treatment Effects**
Cold applications	Immediately after direct trauma such as sprain, strains, fractures, muscle spasms; after superficial lacerations or puncture wounds; after minor burns; chronic pain of arthritis, joint trauma; delayed-onset muscle soreness; inflammation	Circulatory insufficiency Cold allergy Advanced diabetes	Cardiovascular effects (bradycardia) Raynaud's phenomenon Cold urticaria Nerve and tissue damage Slowed wound healing Frostbite
Hot applications	Inflamed or edematous body part; new surgical wound; infected wound; arthritis; degenerative joint disease; localized joint pain, muscle strains; low back pain; menstrual cramping; hemorrhoidal, perianal, and vaginal inflammation; local abscess	Pregnancy Laminectomy sites Spinal cord Malignancy Vascular insufficiency Eyes, testes, heart	Burns Infections Increased pain Increased inflammation

Data from Nadler S and others: The physiologic basis and clinical applications of cryotherapy and thermotherapy for the pain practitioner, *Pain Physician* 7(3):395, 2004.

thus placing the patient at risk for injury during heat applications. However, there are distinct advantages to using both dry and moist applications (Table 40-4). Be familiar with the effects of each application type.

EVIDENCE-BASED PRACTICE TRENDS

The application of ice, or cryotherapy, is one of the most widely used therapeutic modalities in the management of acute musculoskeletal injuries (McGuire and Hendricks 2006). The use of cryotherapy for various injuries has a positive effect on pain relief and is effective in the postoperative period after reconstructive surgery of the knee (Kullenberg and others, 2006; McGuire and Hendricks, 2006). Cryotherapy reduces analgesic medication use after shoulder and foot surgery, knee arthroscopy, and knee arthroplasties (McGuire and Hendricks, 2006). Cold also reduces recovery time as part of the rehabilitation program for the treatment of both acute and chronic injuries (Janwantanakul, 2004). The reduction of temperature creates positive physiological and biological effects, such as pain relief, reduction of muscle spasm, decrease of nerve conduction velocity, and decrease in inflammation edema by constriction of blood vessels (Janwantanakul, 2004). According to Kullenberg and others (2006), simultaneous application of cold and compression is a better treatment. Compression acts with cold to reduce the blood flow and edema formation, while compression provides support to the soft tissues.

There is very little information comparing the effects of heat to the effects of cold. Use of heat and cold create different physiological responses. Treatment choice of heat or cold therapy depends on local responses desired. The early application of cold initially diminishes swelling and pain. The application of ice—but not heat—also reduces edema. Heat may increase swelling and subsequently slow recovery. According to Nadler and others (2004), contrast therapy, which alternates between hot and cold treatment modalities, provides no additional therapeutic benefits when compared with hot or cold therapy alone.

After traumatic brain injury, temperature elevations resulting from damage to the hypothalamus are often harmful, and interventions to prevent an increase in temperature are necessary (Johnston and others, 2006; Thompson and others, 2007). Research shows that inducing mild hypothermia at 32° to 34° C (89.6° to 93.2° F) for 12 to 24 hours can prevent brain damage after cardiac arrest (Calver and others, 2005; Lasater, 2005).

The hypothermia-hyperthermia blanket raises, lowers, or maintains body temperature through conductive heat or cold transfer between the blanket and a patient. The significance of maintaining normal body temperature or normothermia in colorectal surgery patients led the Centers for Disease Control and Prevention (CDC) and Centers for Medicare and Medicaid Services (CMS) Surgical Care Improvement Project (SCIP) (2007) to include this measure in its set of quality measures.

Scott and Buckland (2006) performed a systematic review of 26 randomized control studies examining whether preventing hypothermia during surgery prevents postoperative complications and improves outcomes for patients. They concluded that prevention of intraoperative hypothermia should be considered standard practice in all perioperative departments. This is especially important for patients undergoing major surgery. The studies examined several warming methods: passive external/surface rewarming (i.e., placing warm blankets on top of the patient or controlling the room temperature), active external/skin surface rewarming (i.e., forced-air warming or circulating-fluid warming), and active internal/core rewarming (i.e., infusing warmed IV fluids or use of warmed ventilator gases). No single method was judged to be superior in preventing hypothermia, and one (i.e., warming of ventilator gases) was identified as lacking efficacy (Scott and Buckland, 2006). Hypothermia may result in longer patient stays in postanesthesia care units (PACUs), as well as increased risk for intraoperative blood loss, postoperative wound infections, pressure ulcers, and myocardial ischemia (Good and others, 2006; Wicks, 2006). Planned hypothermia is sometimes part of the care plan for patients undergoing neurological or cardiovascular surgery (Bitner and others, 2007). Studies based on these specialized modes of temperature control were not included in the Scott and Buckland systematic review.

Recent research documents the therapeutic effects of warming preoperative patients (Cooper, 2006; Wagner and others, 2006). Active warming using a forced-air blanket before the induction of anesthesia reduces the incidence and degree of hypothermia in patients undergoing off-pump coronary artery bypass surgery (Kim and others, 2006; Wicks, 2006). Prevention appears to be the best approach, but hypothermia remains an ongoing problem. Patient temperatures should always be monitored, and it is recommended that normothermia should be part of the discharge criteria from the PACU (Scott and Buckland, 2006).

TABLE 40-3	Temperature Ranges for Warm and Cold Applications	
Temperature	**Celsius Range (Degrees)**	**Fahrenheit Range (Degrees)**
Hot	37-41	99-106
Warm	34-37	93-99
Tepid	26-34	79-93
Cool	18-26	64-79
Cold	10-18	50-64

TABLE 40-4	Choice of Dry or Moist Warm Application	
Type	**Advantages**	**Disadvantages**
Moist application	Reduces drying of skin and softens wound exudate Conforms well to body area being treated Penetrates deeply into tissue layers Lessens sweating and insensible fluid loss	Can cause maceration of the skin with prolonged exposure Cools rapidly because of moisture evaporation Creates greater risk for burns to skin because moisture conducts heat
Dry application	Less likely to burn skin Does not cause skin maceration Retains temperature longer because not influenced by evaporation	Increases body fluid loss through sweating Does not penetrate deep into tissue Causes increased drying of skin

CULTURAL CONSIDERATIONS

When explaining the use of warm and cold therapy to patients, the meaning and significance of the therapy can take on very different interpretations based on a patient's culture. It is therefore important to assess the culture-specific applications of warm and cold principles for the patient and family members.

- Assess how warm and cold are used normally in the care of the patient in the home.
- Many cultures, such as Hispanic, Arab, Asian, African, Caribbean, and Eastern European, adhere to the hot and cold theory. It is believed that too much exposure to something "hot" or "cold" causes an illness (Giger and Davidhizar, 2004).
  - In Asian therapy, hot and cold concepts are part of the yin and yang concept that integrates balance and holistic health.
  - The goal of hot and cold principles is restoring balance by giving the opposite of the cause or problem. Pneumonia, cramps, and colic are considered "cold" diseases. For example, wrapping extremities and layering of blankets are common treatments for colds.
  - In general, patients treat cold conditions with "hot" therapies and hot conditions with "cold" therapies. A patient with a cold condition might avoid bathing, air-conditioning, and ice or cold beverages.
- Accommodate generic beliefs and practices of the patient.
- Use cultural brokers such as family members, physicians, and religious leaders to increase acceptance of critical therapies such as hypothermia or ice packs that contradict the patient's/family's beliefs and practices.
- Some patients refuse being exposed to reduce body temperature.

 Skill Performance Guidelines

1. Protect damaged skin. Exposed layers of skin are more sensitive to temperature variations than intact skin.
2. Know the temperature of the application being used. Many devices, such as heating pads or water flow pads (e.g., Aqua-K pads), have thermostats to regulate temperature. Always check the temperature of a device, and check the temperature of a moist compress applied directly to the skin.
3. Certain body parts, such as the extremities or perineum, are more sensitive than others to temperature extremes. Modify the intensity of heat and cold when treating sensitive skin areas.
4. Check the patient frequently during a heat or cold application. The condition of the skin indicates whether tissue injury is occurring. Be observant for signs of excessive redness, maceration, or blistering.
5. Know the patient's risk for injury from heat or cold. Certain patients are more predisposed to injury than others (see Table 40-2).
6. Do not allow the patient to adjust temperature settings. It is common for the patient to adapt to a temperature extreme and then want to adjust the temperature.
7. Never position patients so that they cannot move away from the temperature source. This avoids the risk for injuries from temperature exposure. The hospitalized patient should always have a call light within reach.
8. Do not leave a patient unattended if the person is unable to sense temperature changes or move away from the temperature source. You are responsible for the patient's safety.
9. Discourage the patient from moving an application. This may cause injury to an unprotected area of the body and decrease the effectiveness of therapy.

SKILL 40-1   Application of Moist Heat (Compress and Sitz Bath)

Heat is primarily for acute muscular strain injuries and can selectively affect either superficial or deep tissue (Nadler and others, 2004). If deep muscle penetration is desired, moist heat is the preferred application method. When areas are prone to muscle spasm in response to an acute injury, you apply heat for 20 to 30 minutes every 2 hours. Due to the analgesic effects of moist heat, patients will usually be more compliant with treatment. Warm compresses and commercial heat packs (Fig. 40-1) are examples of moist heat applications. A warm compress is a section of sterile or clean gauze moistened with a prescribed heated solution (i.e., normal saline or sterile water). You apply it directly to an open wound or the skin's surface. A sterile compress is necessary only when there is a break in skin integrity. Commercially packaged sterile, premoistened compresses are available in some agencies. They require the use of a special infrared lamp to heat. You heat plain sterile or clean gauze by adding the gauze to a container of warmed solution. You can apply an aquathermia heating pad over a compress to deliver a continuous, controlled source of heat to improve the application's therapeutic effects (see Skill 40-2). Moist warm compresses improve circulation, relieve edema, promote consolidation of exudate in a wound, and promote comfort.

Moist heat application also includes the use of warm baths, soaks, and sitz baths. A warm bath or soak involves immersion of a body part into a warmed solution. Warm soaks and sitz baths promote circulation, reduce edema and inflammation, promote muscle relaxation, debride wounds, and apply medicated solutions. If a body part is too large to immerse, you can soak it by wrapping the affected body part in a dressing saturated with the prepared, warmed solution.

You give a sitz bath with a special tub or chair basin that allows a patient to sit in water without immersing the legs, feet, and upper trunk (Fig. 40-2). Sitz basins are disposable and especially easy to use in the home. Portable baths fit easily on top of toilets. Patients who have undergone perineal or rectal surgery, who have had an

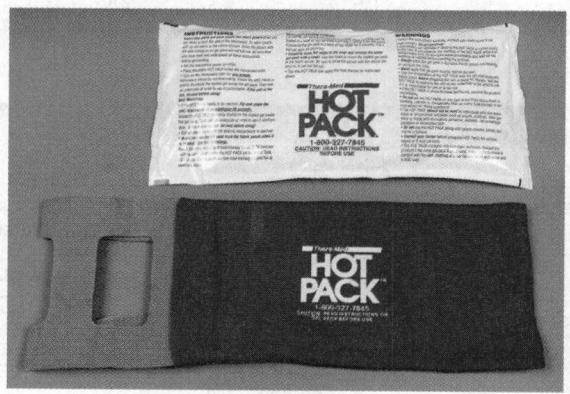

FIG 40-1   Commercial heat pack.

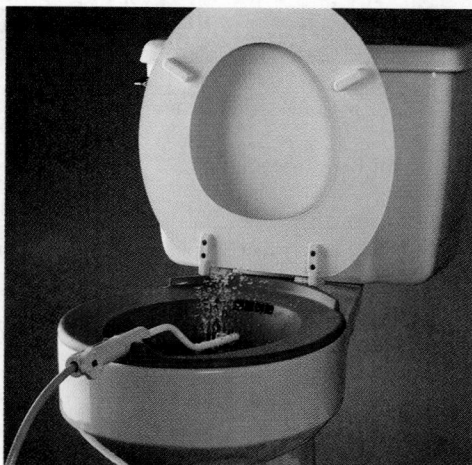

FIG 40-2   Disposable sitz bath.

- Maintain proper temperature of the application throughout the treatment and keep the application in place for only the required length of time.
- Inform the nurse if any discomfort develops, requiring termination of the treatment.
- Inform the nurse if the patient complains of dizziness or lightheadedness.
- Report when treatment is complete so that an evaluation of the patient's response can be made.

Equipment
Moist Compress
- ❏ Absorbent gauze dressing, cloth rolls, or commercially prepared compresses
- ❏ Dry bath towel, bath blanket
- ❏ Clean gloves
- ❏ Sterile gloves (see agency policy)
- ❏ Waterproof pad
- ❏ Ties or tape
- ❏ Commercial heat pack (*optional*)
- ❏ Aquathermia or electric heating pad (*optional*)
- ❏ Prescribed medication (if ordered)
Sitz Bath
- ❏ Clean basin, tub, or sitz bath (basin may need to be sterile if body part to be soaked has an open wound)
- ❏ Prescribed solution warmed to appropriate temperature (tap water is commonly used for sitz baths)
- ❏ Prescribed medication (if ordered)
- ❏ Dry bath towel
- ❏ Clean gloves
- ❏ Sterile gloves (see agency policy)
- ❏ Waterproof pad
- ❏ Bath blanket

episiotomy during childbirth, or who have painful hemorrhoids or perineal inflammation benefit from a sitz bath.

When preparing a soak or bath, remember that the heated solution is in direct contact with the patient's skin. Be sure to check water temperature frequently and carefully to prevent burns. It is desirable to keep the solution temperature constant to enhance the moist heat's therapeutic effects. Whenever you add heated solution to a soak basin or bath, remove the patient's body part and then reimmerse once the solution has mixed.

Delegation Considerations
When the patient is stable and there are no risks or complications, the skill of applying moist heat can be delegated to nursing assistive personnel (NAP). The nurse directs the NAP to:

STEP	RATIONALE
ASSESSMENT	
1 Refer to physician's order for type of moist heat application, location and duration of application, desired temperature, and institutional policies regarding temperature.	Ensures safe and correct application.
2 Assess skin around area you are treating for sensitivity to temperature and pain by measuring light touch or pinprick as appropriate for the body part involved and temperature sensation (see Chapter 18). Monitor those patients insensitive to heat or cold sensations closely during treatment.	Certain conditions alter conduction of sensory impulses that transmit temperature and pain, predisposing patients to injury from heat applications.

Critical Decision Point   *Patients with diabetes mellitus, victims of stroke or spinal cord injury, and patients with peripheral neuropathy and rheumatoid arthritis are particularly at risk for thermal injury (Nadler and others, 2004).*

3 Refer to patient's medical record to identify any systemic contraindications to moist heat application: history of myocardial infarction, angina pectoris, or hypotension, and use of nitroglycerin transdermal patch or ointment and smoking cessation patches.	Certain cardiovascular conditions and side effects of certain medications place patient at risk for sudden changes in blood pressure and blood flow caused by vasodilation. Heat causes vasodilation, which aggravates active bleeding (Nadler and others, 2004).

Critical Decision Point   *Use caution when there is an area of active bleeding or inflammation.*

4 Assess patient's blood pressure and pulse.	Establishes a baseline to determine response to therapy.
5 Assess patient's mobility: ability to position self for soak application, position self in bath, sit up from bath.	Determines level of assistance needed to position patient for treatment.

STEP	RATIONALE
6 Assess patient's level of comfort using an appropriate pain scale (0 to 10).	Provides baseline for patient's comfort level.
7 Assess patient's understanding of application and its purpose.	Determines need for health teaching.

NURSING DIAGNOSES

- Acute pain
- Chronic pain
- Deficient knowledge regarding moist heat applications

- Disturbed sensory perception (tactile)
- Impaired physical mobility
- Impaired skin integrity

- Ineffective peripheral tissue perfusion
- Risk for injury

Individualize related factors based on patient's condition or needs.

PLANNING

1 Expected outcomes following completion of procedure:	
• Affected area is pink and warm to touch immediately after heat application.	Vasodilation increases blood flow to site.
• After multiple applications, wound shows signs of healing (e.g., granulation; reduced edema, inflammation, drainage).	Moist heat increases blood flow, enhances white blood cell infiltration, and removes waste products from cells (Nadler and others, 2004).
• Patient denies burning sensation.	Indicates appropriate temperature applied.
• Patient will report a measurable decrease in pain.	Heat reduces edema/inflammation and relaxes stiff and strained muscles. Heat applications cause pain signals to be overridden as they enter dorsal horn of spinal column and decrease pain perception in cerebral cortex (Nadler and others, 2004).
• Blood pressure and pulse are within patient's normal range.	No systemic vascular changes occur. The goal of therapy is to achieve a localized vascular response.
• Patient able to safely apply therapy.	Measures level of learning.
2 Assemble and prepare equipment and supplies.	Organization of supplies prevents unnecessary delays in procedure.
3 Explain steps of procedure and purpose to patient. Describe the sensation the patient will feel, such as decreasing warmth and wetness. Explain precautions to prevent burning.	Minimizes patient's anxiety and promotes cooperation during procedure.

IMPLEMENTATION

1 Close door if in private room, and/or close bedside curtains. Check patient's identity using two identifiers; one cannot be patient's room number.	Decreases drafts, thus decreasing the transmission of microorganisms. Provides for privacy. Ensures right patient receives right treatment.
2 Perform hand hygiene.	Reduces transmission of microorganisms.
3 Moist sterile compress:	
a Assist patient in assuming comfortable position in proper body alignment, and place waterproof pad under area to be treated.	Compress remains in place for several minutes. Limited mobility in uncomfortable position causes muscular stress. Pad prevents soiling of bed linen.
b Expose body part to be covered with compress, and drape patient with bath blanket.	Prevents unnecessary cooling and exposure of body part.
c Apply clean gloves. Remove any existing dressing covering wound. Dispose of gloves and dressings in proper receptacle.	Reduces transmission of microorganisms.
d Assess condition of wound and surrounding skin. Inflamed wound appears reddened, but surrounding skin is less red in color.	Provides baseline to determine response to moist heat.

Critical Decision Point *If skin surrounding wound is reddened, application may be contraindicated.*

e Perform hand hygiene.	Reduces transmission of microorganisms.
f Prepare compress.	
(1) Open sterile supplies (see Chapter 8). Pour solution into sterile container.	Sterile compress is needed when applied to open wound.
(2) Use sterile technique to drop gauze compress into container to become immersed in solution.	

STEP	RATIONALE
(3) If using portable heating source, warm solution. Commercially prepared compresses may remain under infrared lamp until just before use.	

Critical Decision Point   *To avoid injury to patient, test temperature of sterile solution by applying drop to your forearm (without contaminating solution). It should feel warm to the skin without burning.*

STEP	RATIONALE
g Prepare aquathermia pad (see Skill 40-2) or commercial heat pack (if needed).	
h Apply sterile gloves if dressing change is sterile, otherwise you may use clean gloves.	Allows you to manipulate sterile dressing and touch open wound.
i Pick up one layer of immersed gauze, wring out any excess solution, and apply it lightly to open wound and avoid surrounding skin.	Excess moisture macerates skin and increases risk for burns and infection. Skin is sensitive to sudden change in temperature.
j In few seconds, lift edge of gauze to assess for redness.	Increased redness indicates burn.
k If patient tolerates compress, pack gauze snugly against wound. Be sure to cover all wound surfaces by warm compress.	Packing of compress prevents rapid cooling from underlying air currents.
l Cover moist compress with dry sterile dressing and bath towel. If necessary, pin or tie in place. Remove sterile gloves.	Dry sterile dressing will prevent transfer of microorganisms to wound via capillary action caused by moist compress. Towel insulates compress to prevent heat loss.
m Apply aquathermia or waterproof heating pad over the towel (*optional*) (see Skill 40-2) or commercial heat pack. Keep it in place for desired duration of application.	Provides constant temperature to compress.
n If an aquathermia pad or heat pack is *not* used to maintain temperature of application, change warm compress using sterile technique every 5 to 10 minutes or as ordered during duration of therapy.	Prevents cooling and maintains therapeutic benefit of compress.
o After prescribed time, apply disposable gloves, and remove pad, towel, and compress. Reassess wound and condition of skin, and replace dry sterile dressing as ordered.	Continued exposure to moisture will macerate skin. Prevents entrance of microorganisms into wound site.
p Assist patient to preferred comfortable position.	Maintains patient's comfort.
q Dispose of equipment and soiled compress. Perform hand hygiene.	Reduces transmission of microorganisms.
4 Sitz bath or soak to intact open skin:	
a Apply clean gloves. Remove any existing dressing covering wound. Dispose of gloves and dressings in proper receptacle.	Reduces transmission of microorganisms.
b Assess condition of wound and surrounding skin. Pay particular attention to suture line.	Provides baseline to determine response to warm soak.
c Fill basin or tub in bathroom with warmed solution. Check temperature.	Checking for correct temperature reduces risk for burns.

Critical Decision Point   *Test temperature of solution by applying small amount to your forearm. It should feel warm to touch without burning.*

STEP	RATIONALE
d Assist patient to bathroom to immerse body part in tub or basin.	Prevents falls.
e Assess heart rate. Make sure patient does not feel lightheaded and that call light is within reach.	Provides baseline to determine if vascular response to vasodilation occurs during treatment.
f Cover patient with bath blanket or towel as desired.	Prevents chilling and enhances patient's ability to relax.
g Maintain constant temperature throughout 15- to 20-minute soak:	Ensures proper therapeutic effect.
(1) Keep large sheet or blanket over container or basin.	Prevents heat loss through evaporation. Therapeutic effects of soak can be obtained only from constant temperature.
(2) After 10 minutes, remove body part from soak, check to see that skin is not burned, empty cooled solution, add newly heated solution, and reimmerse body part.	Presence of burn contraindicates completing the soak. Adding warmed solution to basin with body part immersed can cause burn.
h After 15 to 20 minutes, remove patient from soak or bath; dry body parts thoroughly. (Wear clean gloves if drainage is present.)	Avoids chilling. Enhances patient's comfort.

STEP	RATIONALE
i Drain solution from basin or tub. Clean and place in proper storage area. Dispose of soiled linen and gloves (if used); perform hand hygiene.	Reduces transmission of microorganisms.

EVALUATION

STEP	RATIONALE
1 Inspect condition of body part or wound treated for redness, burns, and pain.	Evaluates effectiveness of treatment and risk for potential injury.
2 Question patient regarding presence of burning sensation, severity of pain, and general response to therapy.	Determines if patient was exposed to temperature extreme, resulting in burn. Evaluates patient's subjective response to therapy.
3 Assess vital signs if patient complains of dizziness or light-headedness.	Determines if systemic vascular response to vasodilation has occurred.
4 Have patient demonstrate application of therapy and explain its purpose.	Measures level of learning and ability to perform application.

Unexpected Outcomes	Related Interventions
1 Patient's skin is reddened and sensitive to touch. Extreme warmth caused burning of skin layer.	• Discontinue moist application immediately. • Notify physician.
2 Patient complains of burning and discomfort. Individuals vary in their tolerance to heat and pain.	• Reduce temperature. • Assess for skin breakdown. • Notify physician.
3 Patient is unable to explain purpose of application or performs it incorrectly.	• Provide reinstruction or clarification.

Recording and Reporting

- In nurses' notes, record procedure and who performed it (if delegated), noting type, location, and duration of application, as well as solution and temperature.
- Record condition of body part, wound, and skin before and after treatment and patient's response to therapy.
- Record preprocedure and postprocedure vital signs (as indicated).
- Record any instructions given and patient's ability to explain and perform procedure.
- Report all patient complaints and any unusual findings to nurse in charge or physician.

Teaching Considerations

- If a patient needs to continue heat applications after discharge, have the patient or family member give a return demonstration before discharge.
- Teach the patient to gently pack wound to avoid discomfort.
- Caregivers and patients need to learn that careful assessment is needed for patients with reduced sensation to determine if temperature of compress is too hot.

Pediatric Considerations

- The skin of infants and children is thin and fragile and therefore easily damaged. Use special caution in this population (Hockenberry and Wilson, 2007). Remain with children during procedure for safety and effectiveness.
- It is often helpful to incorporate play into the time a child is required to soak. Placing items in the basin for the child to interact with is helpful. Place boats or other similar water toys in the bath with a child who requires a bath soak. Adult supervision is necessary.

Gerontological Considerations

- An older adult patient who is receiving long-term steroid therapy or is malnourished can develop thin, fragile skin, which is more easily damaged. Skin becomes less elastic and more prone to tears with aging.
- An older adult may have impaired circulation to a given skin region or impaired sensation for pain or temperature (Meiner and Lueckenotte, 2006).
- Older adult patients, whose aging process has resulted in loss of subcutaneous tissue and fat and consequently the insulating effect of these tissues, may experience alterations in thermoregulation (Lien, 2007).
- In some frail, older patients with cardiac conditions, it is necessary to monitor vital signs throughout procedure.

Home Care Considerations

- When necessary, assess availability of primary caregiver to assist patient in application of moist heat, family caregiver's understanding of purpose of procedure, and willingness of caregiver to comply with procedure and not leave patient.
- Assess physical environment to determine adequacy of facilities for use by patient. Patient may need assistive devices to get in/out of a tub or a commode chair to set up a sitz bath.

SKILL 40-2 Applying Aquathermia and Heating Pads

Aquathermia and heating pads are common forms of dry heat therapy (Fig. 40-3). Both are covered and applied directly to the skin's surface, and for this reason you need to take extra precautions to prevent burns. The aquathermia pad (water flow pad) used in health care settings, consists of a waterproof rubber or plastic pad connected by two hoses to an electrical control unit that has a heating element and motor. Distilled water circulates through hollowed channels in the pad to the control unit where water is heated (or cooled). You adjust the temperature setting by inserting a plastic key into the control unit. In most health care institutions, the central supply department sets the temperature regulators to the recommended temperature, approximately 40.5° to 43° C (105° to 109.4° F). Always check the temperature on a unit. Because of the constant temperature control, aquathermia pads tend to be safer than heating pads but still need to be checked because they can malfunction. If distilled water in the unit runs low, simply add more distilled water to the reservoir at the top of the control unit. Rubber and plastic conduct heat, so wrap the pad in a towel or pillowcase to avoid direct exposure to the skin.

The conventional heating pad, used in the home care setting, consists of an electric coil enclosed in a waterproof cover. A cotton or flannel cloth covers the outer pad. The pad connects to an electrical cord that has a temperature-regulating unit for high, medium, or low settings. Because it is so easy to readjust temperature settings on heating pads, instruct patients not to turn the setting higher once they have adapted to the temperature. It is wise to avoid using the highest setting.

Delegation Considerations
The skill of applying an aquathermia or heating pad can be delegated to NAP (see agency policy). Assess the condition of the area you will treat, and explain the purpose of the treatment. If there are risks or complications, this skill cannot be delegated. The nurse directs the NAP to:
- Maintain proper temperature of the application throughout the treatment and keep the application in place for only the length of time specified based on physician order or hospital policy.
- Check patient's skin for excessive redness and pain during application and report any changes to the nurse.
- Report when treatment is complete so that an evaluation of the patient's response can be made.

Equipment
Aquathermia (Acute Care)
- ❑ Electrical control unit
- ❑ Distilled water (for aquathermia pad)
- ❑ Bath towel or pillowcase
- ❑ Tape ties or gauze roll

Heating Pad (Home Care)
- ❑ Electrical control unit
- ❑ Bath towel or pillowcase

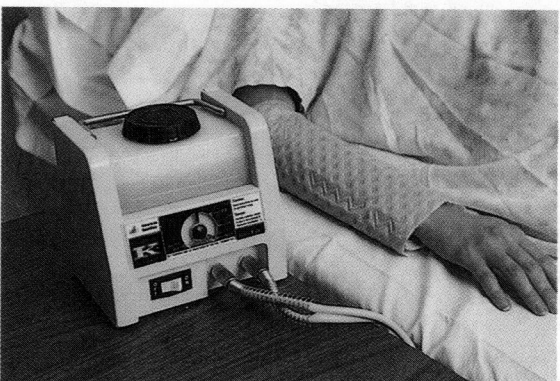

FIG 40-3 Aquathermia pad.

STEP	RATIONALE

ASSESSMENT

1 Refer to physician's order for location of application and duration of therapy. Institutional policy usually sets recommended temperature for aquathermia pad.

Order required to help ensure patient's safety.

2 Assess condition of skin in area where you will apply the pad.

Provides baseline to determine change in skin condition after heat application.

3 Assess level of discomfort (using a pain scale of 0 to 10) and range of motion if patient is being treated for muscle sprain.

Provides baseline to determine if pain relief is achieved.

4 Assess area you will treat for sensitivity to temperature, light touch, and pain (see Chapter 18).

Determines if patient is insensitive to heat extremes.

5 Check electrical plugs and cords for obvious fraying or cracking.

Prevents injury from accidental electrical shock.

6 Determine patient's or family member's knowledge of procedure, including steps for application and safety precautions.

Heating pads are frequently used in the home. Assessment determines extent of health teaching required.

NURSING DIAGNOSES

- Acute pain
- Chronic pain
- Deficient knowledge regarding dry heat applications

- Disturbed sensory perception (tactile)
- Impaired physical mobility
- Impaired skin integrity

- Ineffective peripheral tissue perfusion
- Risk for injury

Individualize related factors based on patient's condition or needs.

STEP	RATIONALE

PLANNING

1 Expected outcomes following completion of procedure:
  - Skin is pink and warm to touch after application.

    Vasodilation from heat exposure increases blood flow to affected part.
  - Patient reports less discomfort of inflamed tissues or strained muscles.

    Thermoreceptors, special temperature-sensitive nerve endings, are activated by changes in skin temperature. These receptors initiate nerve signals that block the pain signal (Nadler and others, 2004).
  - Patient may be able to move strained muscles more freely.

    Heat reduces stiffness and improves range of motion (Nadler and others, 2004).
  - Patient correctly applies pad.

    Documents learning.

2 Prepare equipment and supplies.

  Organization of supplies prevents unnecessary delays in procedure.

3 Explain procedure and precautions.

  Improves likelihood of patient's compliance with therapy.

IMPLEMENTATION

1 Close door if in private room, and/or close bedside curtains.

  Provides for patient's privacy.

2 Check patient's identity using two identifiers; one cannot be patient's room number.

  Ensures right patient receives right treatment.

3 Perform hand hygiene, and position patient comfortably so area you will treat is exposed.

  Reduces transfer of microorganisms. Patient must be able to assume position for several minutes during application.

4 For aquathermia or uncovered heating pad, cover or wrap area to be treated with bath towel, or enclose the pad with pillowcase.

  Prevents heated surface from touching patient's skin directly and increasing risk for injury to patient's skin.

Critical Decision Point *Do not pin the wrap to pad because this may cause a leak in device.*

5 Place pad over affected area (see Fig. 40-3), and secure with tape, tie, or gauze as needed.

  Pad delivers dry warm heat to injured tissues. Pad should not slip onto different body part.

Critical Decision Point *Never position patient so that patient is lying directly on pad. This position prevents dissipation of heat and increases risk for burns.*

6 Turn heating pad on to low or medium setting. Check temperature setting.

  Prevents exposure of patient to temperature extremes.

7 Turn on aquathermia pad and monitor condition of skin every 5 minutes during application, and question patient regarding sensation of burning.

  Determines if heat exposure is resulting in burn.

8 After 20 to 30 minutes (or time ordered by physician), remove pad and store.

  Continued exposure results in burns. Some patients should not have access to pad without supervision.

9 Assist patient in returning to preferred comfortable position, dispose of soiled linen, and perform hand hygiene.

  Promotes relaxing environment. Reduces transmission of microorganisms.

EVALUATION

1 Inspect condition of skin exposed to heat.

  Evaluates response of skin to heat exposure.

2 Ask patient if strained muscle or inflamed area continues to be painful. Evaluate pain severity.

  Heat reduces edema and relieves pain from muscle stiffness and spasm (Nadler and others, 2004).

3 Note if patient is able to move strained muscle with less discomfort.

  Heat relaxes strained muscle.

Critical Decision Point *Do not have patient actively exercise muscle to evaluate results of therapy. Active exercise can aggravate muscle strain.*

4 Observe patient apply pad to be used in the home.

  Measures level of learning.

Unexpected Outcomes	Related Interventions
1 Skin is reddened and sensitive to touch. Symptoms indicate first-degree burn.	• Remove the pad, and reassess in 5 to 10 minutes. • If symptoms continue, notify nurse in charge, or contact physician.
2 Edema and inflammation are increased. Applying heat too soon after an injury can increase edema through vasodilation.	• Notify nurse in charge, or contact physician.
3 Body part is painful to move. Movement stretches burn-sensitive nerve fibers in skin.	• Discontinue aquathermia or heating pad use. Wait for swelling to resolve before attempting to reapply. • Notify nurse in charge, or contact physician.
4 Patient applies heat incorrectly or is unable to relate precautions.	• Reinstruct patient or family caregiver as necessary.

Recording and Reporting

- Record site of application, duration of therapy, and patient's response.
- Describe any instruction given and patient's success in demonstrating procedure.
- Report changes in skin integrity such as burns.

Teaching Considerations

- Highlight safety precautions as they are followed during application.

Pediatric Considerations

- Because of the risk for injury from heating pads, providers rarely use this treatment for children.
- The skin of infants and children is thin and fragile and therefore easily damaged. Use special caution in this population. Remain with children during procedure for safety and effectiveness.

- Assess body temperature gain and loss, which occurs more readily in pediatric patients.

Gerontological Considerations

- Older adults are more at risk for burns because of loss of heat sensation. Check site frequently during all treatments.
- Older patients have thin, more fragile skin that is susceptible to burns.

Home Care Considerations

- Assess patient and primary caregiver as to their understanding, ability, and motivation to comply with procedure.
- Assess home environment for facilities (e.g., condition of electrical outlets and condition of equipment) to comply with implementation of procedure.

SKILL 40-3 Applying Cold Applications

There are a variety of cold (cryotherapy) modalities, such as moist cold compresses, chemical or cold packs, electromechanical or compression devices, or cold soak immersion of a body part. Cold therapy treats localized inflammatory responses that lead to edema, hemorrhage, muscle spasm, or pain (see Table 40-1). Cold exerts a profound physiological effect on the body, reducing inflammation caused by injuries to the musculoskeletal system (Janwantanakul, 2004; Kullenberg and others, 2006; McGuire and Hendricks, 2006). Because reduction of inflammation is the primary goal, cryotherapy is the treatment of choice for the first 24 to 48 hours after an injury.

Vasoconstriction resulting from cold application reduces blood flow to the injured part and thus reduces fluid accumulation and slows bleeding and hematoma formation associated with trauma. The lower temperature also suppresses muscle spasm and produces a local anesthetic response, resulting frequently in the reduction of the use of analgesic medications (McGuire and Hendricks, 2006). When used appropriately, cold applications significantly lessen pain and immobility by reducing swelling of injured tissues (Janwantanakul, 2004; Kullenberg and others, 2006; McGuire and Hendricks, 2006). This is an important point for nurses to know when deciding on the choice of heat or cold for the treatment of acute injuries. Cold is also indicated as an adjunct analgesic for chronic pain and spasticity control.

A cold compress usually consists of a commercial cold pack or a gauze dressing or a washcloth that has been immersed in iced or chilled solution to achieve the desired temperature. The compress may be sterile or clean; however, a clean compress is most common. Any open wounds require sterile applications. There are many sizes or thicknesses of gauze to use, depending on the site of injury. For example, a cold compress to the eye requires thicker gauze that fits a small area to maintain a cold temperature. Thin gauze works more effectively for larger areas such as the face.

Ice bags and cold packs come in a variety of sizes to fit different body parts (Fig. 40-4). When a commercial ice bag or cold pack is unavailable, use a plastic bag or glove filled halfway with crushed ice. Squeeze the bag or glove to expel air, which hampers cold conduction. In the home, a patient can substitute a bag of frozen vegetables for an ice bag. Wrap all of these items in a towel or cloth before application.

There are electrically controlled cooling devices that simultaneously provide cold and compression (Fig. 40-5). Compression acts synergistically with cold to reduce the blood flow and edema formation while providing support to the soft tissues. The cooling pad has the advantage of delivering a constant cool temperature. This type of machine can be recommended as an alternative aid to

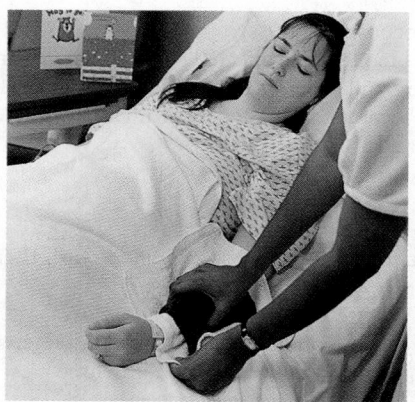

FIG 40-4 Placement of ice pack (or bag) on extremity.

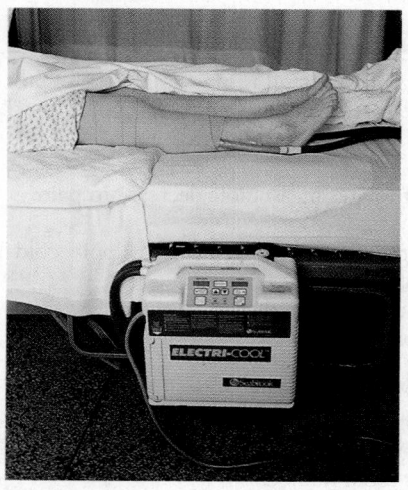

FIG 40-5 Compression cooling device.

postoperative pain management in patients undergoing total knee arthroplasty (Kullenberg and others, 2006). Elevating the extremity during treatment further augments venous return. A person who undergoes treatment with one of these devices is simultaneously receiving all five components of the protection, rest, ice, compression, and elevation (PRICE) method for managing this type of injury (Ivins, 2006).

Delegation Considerations

The skill of applying cold applications can be delegated to NAP in special situations (see agency policy). Assess the patient, and explain the purpose of the treatment. If there are risks or complications, this skill is not delegated. The nurse directs the NAP to:

- Maintain proper temperature of the application throughout the treatment and keep the application in place for only the length of time specified in the physician's order.
- Check patient's skin for excessive redness or pain and report immediately to the nurse if any adverse reactions occur.

- Report when treatment is complete so that a nurse can evaluate the patient's response.

Equipment

- ❑ Sterile gloves (*option:* see agency policy)
- ❑ Clean gloves (if blood or body fluids are present)
- ❑ Tapes, ties or gauze roll, or elastic wrap bandage
- ❑ Towel or pillowcase
- ❑ Cold compress
  - Absorbent gauze (clean or sterile) folded to desired size
  - Clean or sterile basin with ice and water at desired temperature
  - Bath towel or absorbent pad
- ❑ Ice bag or collar with water
  - Ice pack
- ❑ Cool water flow pad
  - Cooling pad and electrical pump
- ❑ Compression device with appropriate extremity attachments

STEP	RATIONALE
ASSESSMENT	
1 Refer to physician's order for type, location, and duration of application. Temperature of an electronic device will be ordered.	Physician's order is required for all cold applications.
2 Inspect condition of injured or affected part. Gently palpate area for edema.	Provides baseline for determining change in condition of injured tissues.

> **Critical Decision Point**   *Keep injured part in alignment and immobilized. Movement can cause further injury to strains, sprains, or fractures.*

STEP	RATIONALE
3 Consider time in which injury occurred.	Apply cold as soon as possible after an injury to prevent edema. (Ivins, 2006).
4 Ask patient to describe severity and character of pain on a scale of 0 to 10, if able (or other pain scale when applicable).	Provides baseline for determining pain relief with therapy.
5 Assess area you will treat for sensitivity to temperature, light touch, and pain and for adequate circulation (see Chapter 18).	Determines if patient is insensitive to cold extremes.
6 Assess patient's understanding of procedure.	Determines need for health teaching.

NURSING DIAGNOSES

• Acute pain	• Deficient knowledge regarding cold applications	• Impaired skin integrity
• Chronic pain		• Ineffective peripheral tissue perfusion
	• Impaired physical mobility	• Risk for injury

Individualize related factors based on patient's condition or needs.

STEP	RATIONALE
PLANNING	
1 Expected outcomes following completion of procedure:	
• Affected area is slightly pale and cool to touch.	Result of vasoconstriction.
• Extent of edema is decreased.	Cold reduces blood flow to affected part, reducing edema formation (Kullenberg and others, 2006; McGuire and Hendricks, 2006).
• Patient relates measurable decrease in pain.	Cold creates local anesthetic effect (Kullenberg and others, 2006; McGuire and Hendricks, 2006).
• Patient correctly states how to apply cold and provides demonstration.	Documents learning.
2 Prepare equipment and supplies.	Organization prevents unnecessary delays.
3 Explain procedure and precautions.	Improves likelihood of patient's compliance with therapy.
IMPLEMENTATION	
1 Close room door and bedside curtain. Perform hand hygiene.	Provides privacy for patient. Reduces spread of microorganisms.
2 Check patient's identity using two identifiers; one cannot be patient's room number.	Ensures right patient receives right treatment.

STEP	RATIONALE
3 Position patient carefully, keeping body part in proper alignment and only exposing area you will treat.	Prevents further injury to body part. Avoids unnecessary exposure of body parts, maintaining patient's comfort and privacy.

Critical Decision Point   *Keep body part affected by strains, sprains, or fractures aligned to prevent further injury.*

STEP	RATIONALE
4 Place towel or absorbent pad under area you will treat.	Prevents soiling of bed linen.
5 Apply clean gloves.	Reduces spread of infection.
6 Apply cold compress:	
a Check temperature of solution, and submerge gauze into basin filled with cold solution; wring out excess moisture.	Extreme temperature can cause tissue damage. Dripping gauze is uncomfortable to patient.
b Apply compress to affected area, molding it gently over site.	Ensures that cold is directed over site of injury.
7 Apply electrically controlled cooling device:	
a Wrap flow pad in towel or pillowcase.	Prevents adverse reactions from cold such as burn or frostbite.
b Wrap cool water flow pad around body part	Ensures even application of cold temperature.
c Turn pad on, and be sure correct temperature is set.	Ensures effective therapy.
d Secure with elastic wrap bandage, gauze roll, or ties (see Fig. 40-5).	
8 Apply ice bag or collar:	
a Fill bag with water, secure cap, and invert.	Ensures that there are no leaks.
b Empty water, and then fill bag two-thirds full with small ice chips.	Bag is easier to mold over body part when it is not full.
c Release excess air from bag by squeezing its sides before securing cap.	Excess air interferes with cold conduction.
d Wipe bag dry.	Prevents skin maceration.
e Wrap prepared bag with towel or pillowcase, if desired. Apply over injury. Secure with tape as needed.	Protects patient's tissue and absorbs condensation. Prevents direct exposure of cold against patient's skin.
9 Apply ice pack:	
a Squeeze or knead a commercial cold pack.	Releases alcohol-based solution to create cold temperature.

Critical Decision Point   *Moisture may form on outside of bag if room temperature is warm. This does not indicate a leak.*

STEP	RATIONALE
b Wrap prepared bag or pack with towel or pillowcase. Apply pack directly over injury.	Protects patient's tissue and absorbs condensation. Prevents direct exposure of cold against patient's skin.

Critical Decision Point   *Do not reapply ice pack to red or bluish areas; continual use of ice pack makes ischemia worse.*

STEP	RATIONALE
10 Remove gloves, and dispose of in proper container.	Reduces transmission of microorganisms.
11 Check condition of skin every 5 minutes for duration of application.	Determines if there are adverse reactions to cold (e.g., mottling, redness, burning, blistering, numbness) (Nadler and others, 2004).
a Edema reduces sensation, so use extra caution during cold therapy.	
b Numbness and tingling are common sensations with cold applications and indicate adverse reactions only when severe and coupled with other symptoms. Stop when patient complains of burning sensation or skin begins to feel numb.	When applying cold, skin will initially feel cold, followed by relief of pain. As cryotherapy continues, patient will feel a burning sensation, then pain in the skin, and finally numbness (Nadler and others, 2004).
12 After 15 to 20 minutes (or as ordered by the physician), apply clean gloves, remove compress or pad, and gently dry off any moisture.	Drying prevents maceration of skin.

Critical Decision Point   *Areas with little body fat (such as knee, ankle, and elbow) do not tolerate cold as well as fatty areas (such as thigh and buttocks). For bony areas, decrease time of cold application to lower range.*

STEP	RATIONALE
13 Assist patient to comfortable position.	Maintains relaxing environment.

STEP	RATIONALE
14 Remove and dispose of supplies. Empty basin, if used, and dry. Dispose of soiled linen and gloves. Perform hand hygiene.	Reduces transmission of microorganisms.

EVALUATION

1 Inspect affected area for changes in condition of skin.	Determines reaction to cold application.
2 Palpate affected area gently.	Determines level of edema.
3 Assess level of severity of pain.	Determines if pain has been relieved.
4 Ask patient to apply cold application and explain risks of treatment.	Measures level of learning.

Unexpected Outcomes	Related Interventions
1 Skin takes on mottled, reddened, or bluish-purple appearance as a result of prolonged exposure.	• Stop the treatment. • Notify nurse in charge or physician. • Injury from prolonged exposure requires different therapy.
2 Patient complains of burning type of pain and numbness.	• Stop the treatment because these are signs of ischemia. • Notify nurse in charge or physician.
3 Patient is unable to describe application or use compress correctly.	• Provide reinstruction and clarification.

Recording and Reporting

- In nurses' notes, record procedure, including type, location, duration of application, and patient's response.
- Describe any instruction given and patient's success in demonstrating procedure.
- Report undesirable changes in condition of skin to nurse in charge or physician.

Teaching Considerations

- Injuries requiring this type of therapy usually occur away from acute care settings. Patients active in sports should know steps to take to minimize extent of injury.

Pediatric Considerations

- A greater metabolic rate and larger trunk in relation to the rest of the body make children more prone to hypothermia (Hockenberry and Wilson, 2007). Exercise caution with young patients.
- Infants have an unstable temperature control mechanism, so mottling of extremities is common and does not always indicate an adverse reaction (Hockenberry and Wilson, 2007).

- Cool soaks also decrease itching with some skin lesions. Use the same precautions and use of play as with warm soaks.

Gerontological Considerations

- Older adults are more at risk for tissue damage due to altered responses to change in body temperature (Lien, 2007). Check site frequently during all treatments.

Home Care Considerations

- Assess patient and primary caregiver as to understanding, ability, and motivation to comply with procedure.
- Assess patient's home environment for adequacy of facilities and equipment with which to implement procedure.
- Patients can make an ice pack by placing ice cubes in a zippered plastic bag or by using a bag of frozen peas or corn. Place a thin towel between bag and skin.

SKILL 40-4 Caring for Patients Requiring Hypothermia or Hyperthermia Blankets

The hypothermia-hyperthermia blanket raises, lowers, or maintains body temperature through conductive heat or cold transfer between the blanket and the patient. When placed on top of the patient, the cooling blanket helps to reduce the patient's body temperature (Fig. 40-6). When operated manually, the unit maintains a set temperature regardless of the patient's temperature. Because you assess the patient's temperature using conventional thermometers, the unit's temperature is manually adjusted to reach a different temperature setting. When operating in the automatic setting, the unit continually monitors the patient's temperature using a thermistor probe (rectal, skin, or esophageal). The system increases or decreases the temperature of the circulating water in response to the preset target temperature and actual measured patient temperature.

Patients can have high, prolonged fevers from infectious and neurological diseases and as side effects from anesthesia. Recent research shows that induced hypothermia improves neurological outcomes in traumatic brain injury (Johnston and others, 2006) and acute stroke (Guluma, 2004) and is a management option when patients are resuscitated after cardiac arrest (Haugk and others, 2007; Howes and Green, 2007).

Delegation Considerations

This skill can be delegated to NAP (see agency policy). The patient is assessed, and the purpose of the treatment is explained. If there are risks or complications, this skill is not delegated. The nurse directs the NAP to:

- Maintain proper temperature of the application throughout the treatment and discontinue the application as specified in the physician's order.
- Inform the nurse of any unexpected outcomes such as shivering or redness to the skin.
- Report when treatment is complete so that an evaluation of the patient's response can be made.

Equipment

- ❑ Hypothermia or hyperthermia blanket with control panel and rectal probe
- ❑ Sheet or thin bath blanket
- ❑ Distilled water to fill the units if necessary
- ❑ Clean gloves
- ❑ Rectal thermometer

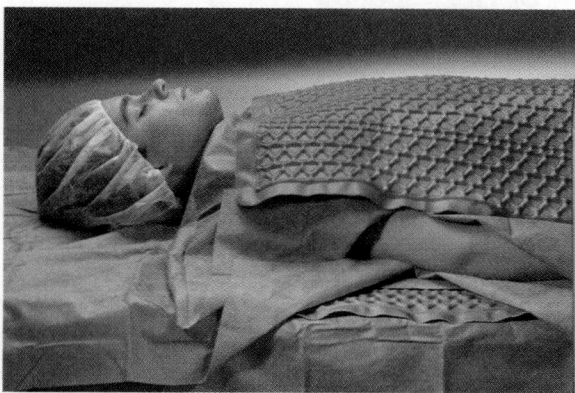

FIG 40-6 Hypothermia cooling blanket is applied over paper sheet before additional top sheet is applied to bed. (*Courtesy Cincinnati Sub-Zero Maxi-Therm Hyper-Hypothermia Blanket.*)

STEP	RATIONALE
ASSESSMENT	
1 Refer to physician's order, and double-check that patient's current body temperature requires use of hypothermia or hyperthermia blanket.	Institution of therapy requires physician's order.
2 Assess vital signs, neurological status, mental status, and peripheral circulation.	Establishes baseline data to use for comparison during therapy.
3 Verify that other, less intensive measures cannot return patient's body temperature to normal.	Use of hypothermia and hyperthermia blanket is not without risk and should be instituted only when other measures are not effective.

Critical Decision Point *Antipyretic therapy may be attempted for fever. Physiological manifestations of fever include increased oxygen consumption, increased heart rate, increased cardiac output, and elevated levels of catecholamines, which are harmful to seriously or critically ill patients (Lasater, 2005).*

4 Assess patient's skin on chest and extremities, paying close attention to bony prominences such as hands and feet.	These areas are more exposed to blanket and consequently are at greater risk for injury. Baseline data enable you to quickly determine if injury to skin is result of therapy.

NURSING DIAGNOSES

- Deficient knowledge regarding implications of hypothermia or hyperthermia blanket
- Disturbed sensory perception (tactile)
- Hyperthermia
- Impaired skin integrity
- Ineffective peripheral tissue perfusion
- Risk for injury

Individualize related factors based on patient's condition or needs.

STEP	RATIONALE

PLANNING

1   Expected outcomes following completion of procedure:
   - Temperature is within normal range. Indicates that therapy is effective.
   - Absence of shivering with hypothermia blanket. Shivering increases metabolic rate and heat production but also increases oxygen consumption. This mechanism contributes to body temperature elevation and can cause patient's body temperature to rise. In addition, shivering causes vasoconstriction, which can injure skin of distal body regions.
   - Skin clear without signs of injury or burns. Distal regions of patient's skin are at greatest risk for injury from blanket. Indicates that treatment is causing no adverse effects.

2   Explain procedure to patient. Increases cooperation and reduces anxiety.
3   Position patient comfortably.
4   Prepare blanket according to agency policy and manufacturer's instructions. Manufacturer's instructions are usually located on machine. Agencies have specific policies on maintaining equipment in functional order. Each type of blanket varies from one manufacturer to another.

IMPLEMENTATION

1   Perform hand hygiene, and apply clean gloves. Reduces transmission of microorganisms.
2   Check patient's identity using two identifiers; one cannot be patient's room number. Ensures right patient receives right treatment.
3   Measure temperature, pulse, respirations, and blood pressure. Provides baseline for determining response to therapy.
4   Apply lanolin or mixture of lanolin and cold cream to patient's skin where it will touch blanket. Helps protect skin from heat and cold sensations.
5   Turn on blanket, and observe that cool or warm light is on. Precool or prewarm blanket, setting pad temperature to desired level. Verifies that blanket is correctly set to assist in reducing (cool) or increasing (warm) patient's body temperature. Prepares blanket for prescribed therapy.
6   Verify that pad temperature limits are set at desired safety ranges. Safety ranges prevent excessive cooling or warming. The blanket automatically shuts off when preset body temperature is achieved.
7   Cover the hypothermia or hyperthermia blanket with a thin paper or cloth sheet or bath blanket. Protects patient's skin from direct contact with blanket, thus reducing risk for injury to skin. Sheet or blanket covers plastic and provides insulation between patient and appliance.
8   Position hypothermia or hyperthermia blanket on top of patient. Provides wide distribution of blanket against patient's skin.

Critical Decision Point   *When using a blanket for hypothermia, the patient has the potential to develop pressure ulcers because of decreased blood flow in the skin.*

   a   Wrap patient's hands and feet in gauze. Reduces risk for thermal injury to body's distal areas.
   b   Wrap scrotum with towels. Protects sensitive tissue from direct contact with cold.
9   Lubricate rectal probe and insert into patient's rectum. When using hypothermia or hyperthermia blanket, it is imperative that you continuously monitor patient's core interior (rectal) temperature.
10 Turn and position patient regularly to protect from pressure ulcer development and impaired body alignment (see Chapter 10). Keep linens free of perspiration and condensation. Patient has an increased risk for pressure ulcer development because of skin moisture created by blanket and patient's body temperature.
11 Double-check fluid thermometer on control panel of blanket before leaving room. Verifies that pad temperature is maintained at desired level.
12 Remove gloves, and perform hand hygiene. Reduces transmission of microorganisms.

EVALUATION

1   Monitor patient's temperature and vital signs every 15 minutes during first hour, and every 30 minutes of therapy thereafter. Provides continuous evaluation of response of patient's body temperature to therapy during initial and continual therapy.
2   Evaluate automatic temperature control every 30 minutes visually and every 4 hours by taking patient's rectal temperature. Ensures removal of hypothermia or hyperthermia blanket when patient's temperature returns to desired level. Decreases risk for subnormal body temperature. Verifies accuracy of rectal probe and automatic temperature control device.

Critical Decision Point   *It is generally accepted to discontinue hypothermia treatment when the patient's core temperature is 1° F above desired temperature.*

STEP	RATIONALE
3 Observe skin for indications of burns, change in color, and other signs of injury.	Hypothermia and hyperthermia blankets have the potential to cause skin injuries.
4 Observe patient for signs of shivering.	Early signs of shivering, which may harm patient, include electrocardiographic changes, facial muscle twitching, or hyperventilation.
5 Determine patient's level of comfort.	Therapy has the potential to cause discomfort. Prompt assessment reduces risk for severe injuries.

Unexpected Outcomes

1 Patient's core body temperature decreases or rises rapidly. This indicates that temperature is too extreme and might produce injury to patient.

2 Patient's core temperature remains unchanged.

3 Patient begins to shiver. Shivering increases metabolic rate and heat production, causing patient's core body temperature to rise, and increases oxygen consumption.

4 Skin breaks down, indicating that patient's skin may have received thermal injury (frostbite or burn) from blanket.

Related Interventions

• Adjust blanket temperature no more than 1° F every 15 minutes to avoid complications.

• Patient may need hypothermic or hyperthermic treatment of additional sites, such as axilla, groin, and neck, in addition to those covered by blanket.
• Discuss use of an antipyretic with physician.

• Adjust the temperature to a more comfortable range, and assess if shivering decreases.
• If shivering continues, stop treatment and notify physician.

• Stop treatment.
• Notify physician.

Recording and Reporting

• Record baseline data: vital signs, neurological and mental status, status of peripheral circulation, and skin integrity when therapy was initiated.
• Note type of hyperthermia-hypothermia unit used; control settings (manual or automatic, and temperature settings); date, time, duration, and patient's tolerance of treatment.
• Chart on temperature graphic repeated measurements of vital signs to document response to therapy.
• Report any unexpected outcome to physician. Further treatment may be needed.

Teaching Considerations

• Instruct patients and their families not to move patient off blanket.

Pediatric Considerations

• A greater metabolic rate and larger trunk in relation to the rest of the body make children more prone to hypothermia. Exercise caution with young patients.
• Infants have an unstable temperature control mechanism, so mottling of extremities is common and does not always indicate an adverse reaction.

Gerontological Considerations

• Some older adults are more at risk for tissue damage because of loss of cold sensation. Check patient frequently during all treatments.

[?] CRITICAL THINKING EXERCISES

You are assigned to care for Adam Montgomery, an 82-year-old male diabetic patient who is postoperative day 1 for total knee arthroplasty. The surgeon has ordered a cold compression cuff device to be applied for 2 to 3 hours followed by a 1- to 2-hour break with compression loosened. Your patient has been confused off and on since returning to the patient care unit and is receiving hydrocodone 5/500 1 to 2 tablets every 4 hours for pain.

1 What do you need to do to begin Mr. Montgomery's cold application? Select all that apply. Explain your choice(s).
   A Refer to physician's order for location and duration of the application.
   B Assess current pain level.
   C Assess condition of injured or affected body part.
   D Explain the procedure and precautions to avoid injury to the skin.

2 Risks for cold applications include which of the following? Select all that apply.
   A A chronic pain condition
   B A condition causing circulatory insufficiency to extremities
   C An acute injury less than 2 days old
   D An inability to provide feedback about tissue temperature

3 What conditions put Mr. Montgomery at risk? Can you delegate this treatment to NAP? Why or why not?

4 Localized cold therapy is used primarily after orthopedic surgery or injury to reduce swelling and as a pain management tool. Depending on the application method and duration, the physiological effects of cold therapy may include which of the following? Select all that apply.
   A Reducing localized pain
   B Vasodilation
   C Muscle relaxation
   D Vasoconstriction

☑ REVIEW QUESTIONS

1 A patient has been diagnosed with severe muscle strain of the lower back, and the physician has ordered heat applications to the lower back for 48 hours. Which nursing intervention has the greatest priority in this situation?
   1 Frequent assessment of the setting on the heat delivery system
   2 Placement of a plastic wrap over the compress for better penetration
   3 Frequent assessment of the area where the heat is being applied
   4 Encouragement of the patient to increase his oral fluid intake

2 There are many conditions that can increase the risk for injury from heat applications. Which of the following patients would be at risk? Select all that apply.
   1 A patient with a lot of body fat
   2 A patient being treated for anxiety
   3 A patient with peripheral vascular disease
   4 A patient with type 1 diabetes
   5 A patient with dehydration
   6 A malnourished patient
   7 A patient who has been on long-term steroid therapy

3 The nurse has just completed a cold application to a patient's knee. Which observation would be expected as a result of the treatment?
   1 The affected area is slightly pale and cool to touch.
   2 The amount of edema has increased.
   3 The patient relates a measurable increase in pain.
   4 The affected area is mottled or bluish purple.

4 The nurse is preparing to apply a cold application to a patient's elbow. What nursing intervention would be indicated?
   1 Decrease the length of time the cold application would normally be applied.
   2 Increase the time the cold application would normally be applied.
   3 Keep the time length of the cold application the same as when the application is over a fatty area.
   4 Leave the cold application in place until it naturally cools to allow for deeper penetration.

5 A patient placed on a hypothermia blanket begins to shiver. Why should the nurse be concerned about the patient's response to this therapy?
   1 Shivering decreases the patient's metabolic rate and amount of heat loss.
   2 The shivering decreases the amount of oxygen consumption by the patient.
   3 The shivering increases the patient's metabolic rate and heat production.
   4 Shivering causes general vasoconstriction, which is contraindicated for this patient.

REFERENCES

Calver P and others: The big chill: improving the odds after cardiac arrest, *RN* 68:58, 2005.

Centers for Medicare and Medicaid Services: *Surgical Care Improvement Project*, http://www.medqic.org/SCIP, accessed September 17, 2007.

Cooper S: The effect of preoperative warming on patients' postoperative temperatures, *AORN J* 83(5):1074, 2006.

Giger J, Davidhizar R: *Transcultural nursing: assessment and interventions*, ed 4, St. Louis, 2004, Mosby.

Good KK and others: Postoperative hypothermia—the chilling consequences, *AORN J* 83(5):1055, 2006.

Guluma K: Therapeutic hypothermia in threatening acute stroke, *Endovasc Today*, May, 2004, p 72.

Hockenberry MJ, Wilson D: *Wong's nursing care of infants and children*, ed 8, St. Louis, 2007, Mosby.

Howes D, Green RS: Stock your emergency departments with ice packs: a practical guide to therapeutic hypothermia for survivors of cardiac arrest, *Can Med Assoc J* 176(6):759, 2007.

Ivins D: Acute ankle sprains: an update, *Am Fam Physician* 74(10):1714, 2006.

Lasater M: The role of thermoregulation in cardiac resuscitation, *Crit Care Nurs Clin North Am* 17:97, 2005.

Lien CA: *Thermoregulation in the elderly*, http://www.asahq.org/clinical/geriatrics/thermo.htm, accessed September 17, 2007.

McGuire DA, Hendricks SD: Incidences of frostbite in arthroscopic knee surgery postoperative cryotherapy rehabilitation, *Arthroscopy* 22(10):1141, 2006.

Meiner SE, Lueckenotte AG: *Gerontologic nursing*, ed 3, St. Louis, 2006, Mosby.

Wicks TC: Take our patient warming quiz and get all the answers to the most burning questions about unplanned hypothermia, *Outpatient Surg Mag* 7(4):36, 2006.

RESEARCH REFERENCES

Bitner J and others: A team approach to the prevention of unplanned postoperative hypothermia, *AORN J* 85(5):921, 2007.

Haugk M and others: Feasibility and efficacy of a new non-invasive surface cooling device in post-resuscitation intensive care medicine, *Resuscitation* 75:76, 2007.

Janwantanakul P: Different rate of cooling time and magnitude of cooling temperature during ice bag treatment with and without damp towel wrap, *Phys Ther Sport* 5:156, 2004.

Johnston NJ and others: Body temperature management after severe traumatic brain injury: methods and protocols used in the United Kingdom and Ireland, *Resuscitation* 70:254, 2006.

Kim JY and others: The effect of skin surface warming during anesthesia preparation on preventing redistribution hypothermia in the early operative period of off-pump coronary artery bypass surgery, *Eur J Cardiothorac Surg* 29:343, 2006.

Kullenberg B and others: Postoperative cryotherapy after total knee surgery: a prospective study of 86 patients, *J Arthroplasty* 21(8):1175, 2006.

Nadler S and others: The physiologic basis and clinical applications of cryotherapy and thermotherapy for the pain practitioner, *Pain Physician* 7(3):395, 2004.

Scott EW, Buckland R: A systematic review of intraoperative warming to prevent postoperative complications, *AORN J* 83(5):1090, 2006.

Thompson HJ and others: Intensive care unit management of fever following traumatic brain injury, *Intensive Crit Care Nurs* 23:91, 2007.

Wagner D and others: Effects of comfort warming on preoperative patients, *AORN J* 84(3):426, 2006.

Home Care Safety

MEDIA RESOURCES

- **evolve** http://evolve.elsevier.com/Perry/skills
  learning system
  - Review Questions

KEY TERMS

Alzheimer's disease

Dementia

Polypharmacy

Reminiscing

Respite care

Wandering

OBJECTIVES

Mastery of content in this chapter will enable the nurse to:
- Identify patients at risk for safety problems and possible accidents.
- Promote self-care of patients in the home.
- Describe factors within a home environment that create risks for injury for patients.
- Perform a home safety risk assessment.
- Identify interventions that modify the home environment for physical safety.
- Identify interventions to reduce safety risks for patients with sensory, cognitive, and mental status alterations.
- Recommend strategies to ensure safe drug administration within the home.
- Perform a geriatric fall risk assessment.

Safety is being in an environment and feeling secure in your surroundings. In Maslow's hierarchy of needs (1954), safety includes security, stability, protection, and freedom from fear and anxiety. Safety has both a physical and an emotional component. For example, if a wheelchair-bound patient removes door frames to allow for better bathroom access, the physical improvements will enhance the patient's confidence to maneuver within the home. When a patient's environment is safe, the potential to provide self-care is maximized. In addition, the patient will emotionally feel less anxious about trying to move about and to interact within the environment.

Healthy People 2010 identifies injury and violence prevention as a focus area, with the reduction of death from falls as an objective (U.S. Department of Health and Human Services [USDHHS], 2007). The two main goals of *Healthy People 2010* are to increase quality and years of life and eliminate health disparities. In accordance with *Healthy People 2010,* home care nurses must assess the patient and home environment for risk. Patients with chronic conditions such as diabetes mellitus, for example, may be at risk for falls due to neuropathies. Patients living in socioeconomically disadvantaged areas by contrast may be at risk for injury due to violence or poor living conditions.

Accident prevention begins with making timely and adequate home repairs. However, many patients do not have the resources for maintaining a safe home environment. The nurse plays an important role in improving and maintaining a patient's safety by collaborating with patients, family members, caregivers, and other health care providers in the community in finding the best approaches for meeting a patient's safety needs. The ultimate goal is to create an environment in which the patient and family can provide self-care safely and effectively.

Family caregiving is on the rise as more people are providing ongoing support to family members and friends in the home. Many older adults are opting to age in place and remain in their homes rather than enter a long-term care facility. Home care nurses become very adept at partnering closely with patients and family caregivers so that the patient's nursing care needs are met within the home without disrupting normal lifestyles unnecessarily. Nurses in any setting need to assess for patterns of health care problems (e.g., falls, burns, or medication errors) that point to safety problems in the home.

Home care patients include the chronically ill, disabled children with physical and mental impairment, victims of acute medical illness and traumatic accidents, and the terminally ill. Older adults are significantly at risk for threats to safety within the home because of the physiological changes that accompany aging. Despite older adults' risks, they learn how to negotiate their environments relatively well and are usually more aware of potential dangers. Thus older adults may often be more cautious than younger persons about changes in their environment, even if those changes will bring a sense of security and safety. The onset of an acute illness requires special effort to restore the older adult's sense of security.

A common misconception about aging is that cognitive impairments are widespread among older adults. However, when an older adult does begin to experience disorientation, loss of language skills, loss of the ability to calculate, and poor judgment, you need to investigate the underlying cause. Dementia is a generalized impairment of intellectual functioning, with the most common form being Alzheimer's disease. As Alzheimer's disease progresses, safety becomes a key concern. Patients with dementia often experience cognitive, behavioral, and social challenges. These patients are at risk for falls, as well as burns or lacerations (Poulin de Courval and others, 2006). Alzheimer's disease accounts for 50% of all dementia diagnoses (Wallace, 2006).

Fall prevention is a critical aspect of care for older adults. You can address fall prevention by taking a patient history to assess for reasons for recent falls and plan appropriate interventions. After a fall an older adult will experience greater functional decline in activities of daily living; therefore prevention is key (Akyol, 2007). Serious injury and even death can result from a fall, so constantly reassess the home environment and communicate effectively with the patient and caregivers.

EVIDENCE-BASED PRACTICE TRENDS

Preschool children are at great risk for injury in the home. Environmental hazards, as well as electric shock, falls, accidental poisonings, and kitchen burns, are risks for preschoolers. A recent study of mothers' awareness of risks identifies major areas of concern, including a lack of knowledge of safety locks, unstable furniture, and antislip materials (Al-Khameesa, 2007). Perform a needs assessment for childproofing the home, and use the opportunity to teach parents about a variety of safety issues that will assist the family in remaining injury free.

An important source of evidence-based practice guidelines for patient safety is in the area of fall prevention, and the older adult is of special concern. Environmental hazards, gait disturbances, muscle weakness, and visual impairments are some of the causes of falls in older patients (Rao, 2005). Polypharmacy adds to the risk. The risk for falls substantially increases for individuals with a number of risk factors. Health care providers should perform a fall assessment, with routine physical examinations and diagnostic tests as indicated (Rao, 2005). The home care nurse also performs the assessment at the initial visit, as well as follow-up visits to reassess the patient and environment as indicated. Multifactorial interventions are the most successful types of interventions, including exercise programs with gait and balance training, proper use of assistive devices, strength training, Tai Chi, and removal or modification of environmental hazards (Rao, 2005; USDHHS, 2007). Addressing the individual patient needs and providing appropriate intervention(s) assist patients in remaining safe in their home.

CULTURAL CONSIDERATIONS

A patient's culture influences lifestyle and the manner in which the patient structures and maintains the home environment. Consider the following to promote safety within the patient's home:

- At the first visit, perform a cultural assessment to understand the patient's beliefs, values, and practices to determine appropriate nursing interventions within a cultural context (Andrews, 2007).
- Collaborate with the patient in assessing the home environment. Assess cultural practices that pose risks, such as burning incense (Asian cultures) and lighting candles (Jewish and Asian cultures) when a patient is on oxygen therapy.
- Assess for culture-specific health-related practices that pose a risk to the patient's safety, such as coining. Coining is a practice in which a coin is rubbed over the body to expel "bad winds" believed to cause illness. Coining can leave abrasions on the skin (Andrews, 2007).
- The Amish are sometimes reluctant to discuss alternative, complementary, or nontraditional therapy practices. Question these patients in a gentle, respectful, and nonjudgmental manner (Graham and Cates, 2006).
- Perform a nutritional assessment. Discuss diet and food preparation concerns of the patient. Provide assistance in meeting a culturally relevant diet within the patient's ability and resources.
- When assessing the availability of family caregivers in the home, recognize that many collectivist cultures (e.g., Jewish, Hispanic, Arabic, Asian) value an active presence and caring for ill family members. With the patient's permission, include these family members when performing the safety assessment.
- Facilitate patient access to necessary support services. Family obligation is a burden for many Asian families whose support system is decreased markedly by immigration. Occasionally, other family members will not accept seeking outside help in caring for elder parents. Some patients with limited English language proficiency are not able to access support services on their own.
- Time orientation is different for each culture. For example, Asians and Native Americans focus on the past and value long-standing traditions. These patients may look to ancestors for guidance in issues of illness and protection. You must recognize this, and talk with the patient to address safety issues in a culturally congruent manner that respects this time orientation (Andrews, 2007).
- Establish a mutually respectful atmosphere of communication with the patient and family caregivers before attempting to discuss home safety issues and concerns. Address the patient in a manner that is appropriate. For example, some Asian and European cultures write their last name first; avoid confusion and the risk for offending the patient (Andrews, 2007).
- Regarding medication safety, be sure that medication labels are not confusing for a patient. For example, the Spanish word for "eleven" is written as "once." A Spanish patient could confuse a medication direction that requires them to take a medication 1 time a day, as 11 times a day.

Skill Performance Guidelines

1. When assisting the patient with changing the home environment, retain as much of the patient's independence and ability to provide self-care as possible. Be respectful of the patient/family autonomy and self-determination.
2. Reinforce with family or friends who assume the role of caregiver the importance of preserving patient autonomy as much as possible.
3. Make modifications to the home environment only after consulting with and considering patients' physical strengths, remaining functional abilities, and resources for making change.

SKILL 41-1   Modifying Safety Risks in the Home Environment

The home environment should be a place where individuals feel healthy, comfortable, and safe. People want to be able to move about freely within their homes, regardless of the home's size, and to have a sense of control over daily living routines. This requires maintenance of personal space and a sense of privacy. All persons seek to create a personal space in their homes with which they can identify and maneuver about without having to think about every action or movement. As the home care nurse, you can help a patient maintain independence and reduce risk in the home environment by conducting a safety assessment.

Patients requiring home care often experience physical alterations that require changes in their home environment. In the case of older adults, the progressive physical changes of aging create the same type of need. The changes need to complement the patient's remaining strengths. For example, if a patient has poor balance but good upper arm strength, make modifications so that the patient can safely walk or move throughout the house, ascend and descend stairs, and enter and exit a bathtub or shower. Teaching a patient to safely use a walker helps the patient increase mobility and maintain independence (Fig. 41-1).

Respect the concept of personal space. Making changes too rapidly without the patient's consent will cause more problems than benefits. Appreciate the arrangement of the patient's space within the home, and do not move things or suggest modifications

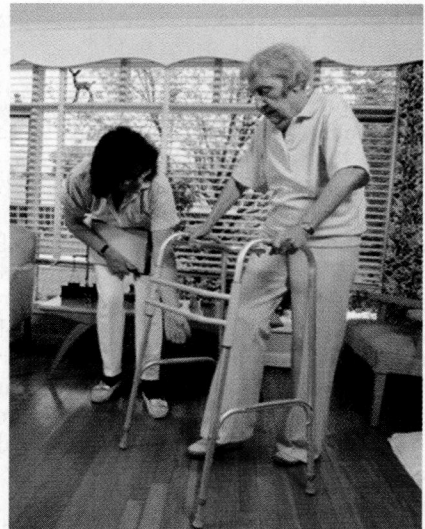

FIG 41-1   Use of a walker may help a patient remain mobile.

without permission. Knowing the rooms the patient most frequently uses helps in making the adjustments to create a safe environment.

Delegation Considerations

The skill of conducting an initial home safety assessment cannot be delegated to nursing assistive personnel (NAP). However, principles involved in changing the home environment are both practical and commonsense in approach. The nurse directs the NAP by:

- Having NAP inform the nurse when they make suggestions for ways to make the home safer.

Equipment

☐ Home safety checklist

STEP	RATIONALE
ASSESSMENT	
1 Review previous physical findings, or assess the patient's vision, hearing, musculoskeletal, and neurological function.	Reveals sensory alterations or problems with strength, coordination, or balance that predispose patient to injury.
2 Determine if patient has had a history of falls or other injuries within the home. Be specific in your assessment. Use the mnemonic SPLATT (Meiner and Lueckenotte, 2006): **S**ymptoms at time of fall **P**revious fall **L**ocation of fall **A**ctivity at time of fall **T**ime of fall **T**rauma postfall	Key symptoms are helpful in identifying cause of fall. Onset, location, and activity associated with fall provide further details on causative factors and how to prevent future falls.
3 Have patient who has had a near fall or actual fall maintain a fall diary (Box 41-1, p. 1067).	Information in a fall diary is very helpful in determining antecedents and consequences of falling (Meiner and Lueckenotte, 2006).
4 Conduct a timed Get Up and Go test for basic mobility. Instruct the patient to rise from a standard chair, walk approximately 3 m (10 feet), turn around, walk back to the chair, and sit in the chair again. Time the patient while he or she performs the activity. Have patient perform the test three times, and then calculate the mean score.	Simple screening examination is very useful in detecting difficulties with balance or gait (Pettersson and others, 2005). The normal required time to finish the test is less than 20 seconds, with no staggering when turning or need to hold on to something (Ebersole, 2008). Individuals who cannot complete the test probably have mobility problems, especially if the time is greater than 20 seconds (Shumway-Cook, 2000).
5 Review risk factors that predispose patients to accidents within the home:	
a Known visual impairment	Reduced visual function alters patient's balance, depth perception, or adaptation to the dark or glaring light.
b Hearing impairment	Prevents patient from hearing normal environmental sounds clearly as a source of orientation. Also prevents clear perception of any home-installed alarms (e.g., smoke alarm).
c Neuromuscular dysfunction (e.g., lower extremity weakness, unsteady gait, impaired balance, poor ankle dorsiflexion)	Factors predispose patients to fall. Recurrent falls are associated with difficulty standing up from a chair.
d Reduced energy or fatigue	Predisposes to falls.
e Incontinence or nocturia	Frequent trips to bathroom often cause patient with other deficits to accidentally trip or fall over barriers. It is difficult for patient to get up and move quickly (Aykol, 2007).
f History of stroke, parkinsonism, delirium, seizures, dementia, arrhythmias, gait disturbances, muscle weakness, and syncope	These factors are predominant causes of falls in older adults (Aykol, 2007; Rao, 2005).
g Postural hypotension, palpitations, difficulty breathing, or shortness of breath	Dizziness or light-headedness predisposes to falls (Aykol, 2007).
h Medication usage and history, including polypharmacy and use of sedatives, antihypertensives, antidepressants, and diuretics	Multiple use of medications has been associated with falls. Medications that alter sensorium affect balance and judgment. Diuretics cause increased trips to bathroom (Rao, 2005).
6 Determine if patient has a fear of falling. Possible indicators include apprehension during ambulation (observed in facial expressions), sweating or trembling while ambulating, clutching persons or objects while ambulating, reluctance to change position or ambulate, and new onset of wobbly, reduced mobility after a fall.	Fear of falling occurs variably in older adult population. This fear is related to an increase in incidence of falls, restriction of activities, gait deficits, and decreased functional mobility (Brewer and others, 2007).

Critical Decision Point   *Use family members or caregiver as a resource in assessments because they may witness accident trends or patterns.*

STEP	RATIONALE
7 Partner with patient, family, and caregivers to conduct a home safety assessment:	Provides comprehensive review of all areas within home that pose hazardous situations.
a Front and back entrances	
(1) Are walkways to the front/back door even and free from holes or cracks?	Entrances pose barriers in surfaces over which patient must walk.
(2) Are home entrances well lit, including walkways?	Poorly lit areas prevent individuals from seeing variations in walking surface.
(3) Does patient have nonskid strips/safety treads or bright-colored paint on outdoor steps? What colors are most easily seen by patient? Are these colors used?	Nonskid surfaces cause fewer slips on stairs. Color on steps permits individual to see edges, accommodating for any reduced depth perception.
(4) Are doormats in good repair with nonskid backing and tapered edge?	Raised edges pose risk for tripping.
(5) Are doors in good repair, and do they open and close easily? Can patient open and close all doors easily?	Act of opening and closing door can cause a fall.
(6) Is there a sturdy handrail on both sides of stairs leading to entrance?	Handrails provide greater support while ascending and descending stairs.
(7) Are steps in good condition with even, flat surfaces?	Uneven surfaces predispose to tripping.
b Kitchen	Kitchen is one of the most hazard-oriented rooms in a home and poses serious hazards for fire.
(1) Does patient wear clothing with short or close-fitting sleeves when cooking?	Short or close-fitting sleeves are less likely to accidentally catch on fire when a person works at a stove.
(2) Does patient always stay in kitchen when cooking?	Lack of attention when using fire is a risk.
(3) Does patient have a loud timer to signal when food is cooked?	Prevents burning of food and risk for fire.
(4) Does patient keep stove top and oven clean and grease free?	Grease is highly flammable.
(5) Are stove control dials easy to see and use?	Patient may accidentally use higher flame than is necessary for cooking safely.
(6) Is a charged, easy-to-use fire extinguisher close at hand?	Extinguisher should be ready for use at all times.

Critical Decision Point   *Have patient demonstrate steps of how to use extinguisher.*

STEP	RATIONALE
(7) Are there emergency numbers for police, fire, and poison control posted on or near telephone?	Emergency phone numbers and extinguisher ensure quick response if fire occurs.
(8) Can items in kitchen cabinets and shelves be reached without climbing on a stool or chair? Is step stool sturdy and in good repair?	Climbing on step stools or chairs creates risks for falls.
(9) Is there adequate lighting over sink, stove, and work areas?	Poor lighting makes it difficult to see control knobs or dials or provides inadequate illumination when using sharp knives or utensils.
(10) Are kitchen throw rugs and mats slip resistant?	Rugs or mats not slip resistant can easily slide on tile or wood floors.
c Bathrooms	
(1) Can patient unlock bathroom door from both sides of door?	Functional locks prevent person from being trapped in bathroom.
(2) Is tub or shower equipped with nonskid mats, abrasive strips, or surfaces that are not slippery?	Bathrooms are hazardous. Wet floors and tub or shower bottoms can be very slippery, creating risk for falls.
(3) Does bathroom floor have nonslip surface or rug with nonskid backing?	Slippery tile predisposes to falls.
(4) Does patient avoid using slippery bath oils when bathing?	Use of bath oils makes tub surface slippery and increases risk for falls.
(5) Do bathtub and shower have at least one grab bar that is a different color than that of the wall?	Grab bars provide extra support while maneuvering into and out of tubs or showers.
(6) Is patient careful not to place towels on grab bars?	Some patients accidentally grab towel instead of bar when needing support. Towel can slip off bar.
(7) Does shower have stable stool or chair and handheld sprayer?	Shower stool allows patient to sit while showering.

STEP	RATIONALE
(8) Are cold and hot water faucets clearly marked, and is temperature on water heater 120° F or lower?	Accidental burns can occur from exposure to hot water.
d Bedroom	
(1) Is a night-light placed in bedroom and/or bath?	Older adults have poor night vision.
(2) Is a working smoke detector just outside bedroom door?	Alarm situated just outside bedroom can awaken person early enough to escape fire.
(3) Can patient turn on light without having to get out of bed in the dark?	Getting out of bed, without proper lighting or ability to adjust to light changes, and reaching for necessary objects puts patient at risk for falls.
(4) Is furniture arranged to provide clear path from bed to bathroom?	Obstructed path creates barrier that causes tripping and falls.
(5) Is phone with emergency numbers within easy reach of bed?	Some patients develop physical symptoms while in bed, requiring easy access to phone.
(6) Are other alarm systems available? Push buttons that call for help? Nursery listening devices for invalid patients?	Alarm systems placed in readily accessible location can alert family/caregivers when person requires immediate assistance.
e Living room/family room	
(1) Are electrical or extension cords removed from under furniture and carpeting? Kept out of the way of traffic?	Patients can easily trip or fall over electrical cords.
(2) Can patient turn on light without having to walk into dark room?	Darkened room can disorient and prevent patient from seeing uneven surfaces.
(3) Are hallways and walkways free from objects and clutter?	Objects and clutter in the common walkway can cause falls.
(4) Are loose area rugs securely attached to floor and not placed over carpeting? (For best safety, consider removing throw rugs.)	Loose edges of rugs are easy for persons to trip over.
(5) Is furniture arranged in each room so that patient can walk around easily?	Furniture creates obstacles to walking in a room.
(6) Is all furniture steady and without sharp edges?	Patients often use edge of furniture for support when standing.
f Around the house	
(1) Are all living areas and stairways well lit?	Adequate lighting helps persons to see any barriers or uneven walking surfaces.
(2) Is flooring or carpeting throughout house in good repair?	Frayed carpet or irregular surfaces can cause tripping and result in a fall.
(3) Are all thresholds level with floor or no more than ½ inch in height?	Uneven thresholds can cause tripping.
(4) Is there a light switch at both top and bottom of stairs?	Prevents individual from having to walk a portion of stairs in dark.
(5) Does lighting produce glare or shadows on stairs?	Older adults are sensitive to glare.
(6) Do handrails run continuously from top to bottom of flights of stairs?	Handrails provide a source of physical support when ascending and descending stairs.
(7) Are handrails securely attached to wall?	
(8) Are step coverings in good condition? Stairs free of clutter?	
(9) Are guns kept in the house? Are trigger locks installed on all guns? Are guns stored unloaded? Is ammunition in a secure location?	Following gun safety standards decreases the risk for injury and death related to gun use (Hockenberry and Wilson, 2007).
g General fire safety	
(1) Does patient have properly working smoke detectors with good batteries?	Smoke alarms properly located, well functioning, and with batteries replaced twice a year can provide timely alert for fire.
(2) Are there fire or electrical hazards?	Elders are at a risk for fires because many are on fixed incomes and cannot afford home repairs (Ebersole, 2008).

Critical Decision Point   *Check to see when battery was last changed; battery should be changed every 6 months. Instruct patients to change battery each time they change their house clocks for daylight savings.*

STEP	RATIONALE
(3) Does patient have several emergency exit plans in case of fire?	Exit plan helps persons to anticipate route of escape when fire does occur. Exit should not have locks that are difficult to open or any physical barriers.

STEP	RATIONALE
(4) Has family determined a meeting place in event of emergency, such as at mailbox in front of home?	Use of a common emergency meeting location is an efficient method for determining that all family members are safely out of the house.
(5) Does patient use portable space heaters? Are they kept 3 feet away from flammable items?	Heaters, furnaces, and chimneys pose risks for fire.
(6) Is furnace area free of things that can catch on fire?	
(7) Does a qualified professional check furnace and chimney annually?	
(8) Does patient who smokes report smoking in bed?	Approximately one of every four fire deaths in 2003 was attributed to smoking materials. Older adults have the highest risk for death or injury due to smoking-material fires (National Fire Protection Association [NFPA], 2007).
h General electrical safety	
(1) Are electrical cords in good condition, not frayed, spliced, or cracked?	Damaged cords can short-circuit and lead to fire.
(2) Are electrical cords kept away from water?	Use of any appliance or device that is exposed to water creates risk for electrical shock.
(3) Does patient use extension cord/outlet extenders with built-in circuit breaker or fuse?	Prevents overloading of circuit that can lead to fire.
(4) Do all wall outlets and switches have cover plates?	Prevents physical contact with wiring.
(5) Does patient use lightbulbs of correct wattage for each fixture?	Use of excessive wattage can lead to fire.
(6) Is main electrical fuse box for home easily accessible and clearly labeled?	In event of emergency, fuse box should be easy to access so that proper circuit can be cut off.
i Carbon monoxide prevention	
(1) Are furnace flues checked regularly for patency?	Common cause of carbon monoxide toxicity.
(2) Is there a carbon monoxide detector in home?	
8 Assess patient's financial resources; determine monthly income used for ongoing expenses.	Determines potential for making repairs to home. Reveals need for low-cost community service support.
9 Assess patient's and family member's willingness to make changes. Has patient accepted limitations that pose risk for injury? Determine how important functional independence is for patient.	Some patients perceive attempts to improve safety within home as intrusive. If you show that necessary revisions to home environment will preserve independence, patient will participate more willingly.

NURSING DIAGNOSES

- Anxiety
- Deficient knowledge regarding home safety risks
- Disturbed sensory perception (visual, auditory, and/or tactile)

- Health-seeking behaviors regarding home safety
- Impaired home maintenance
- Impaired memory

- Impaired physical mobility
- Ineffective health maintenance
- Risk for injury

Individualize related factors based on patient's condition or needs.

PLANNING

1 Expected outcomes following completion of procedure:	
• Patient and/or family will describe potential environmental risks within home that predispose to accidents.	During home safety assessment nurse instructs patient in those risks that are of greatest concern.
• Patient and/or family will initiate actions to correct environmental risks, making home safer.	Patient sees value in altering living environment.
• Patient will remain free of injury.	Environmental barriers are reduced or removed to minimize injuries.
2 Prioritize with patient and family environmental barriers that pose greatest risk.	Patient's own physical and/or cognitive deficits will make certain environmental risks more hazardous. Prioritization helps patient make best choices.
3 Recommend calling in reliable contractor if major home repairs are necessary.	Ensures repairs are made safely and correctly.

STEP	RATIONALE

IMPLEMENTATION

1   Recommend steps to take to reduce physical hazards that predispose patient to falls:

a   Paint edges of concrete stairs bright yellow, orange, or white.

Patient can see edge of stairs more clearly.

b   Install treads with uniform depth of 22.5 cm (9 inches) and 9-inch risers (vertical face of steps)

If stairs are of uniform size, patient does not have to continually adjust vision or stride.

c   Rearrange furniture to open up space through hallways and major rooms.

Creates unobstructed pathway for ambulation.

d   Reduce clutter within living areas (e.g., footstools, flower pots, extension cords, children's toys, stacked newspapers or magazines).

Mobility hazards resulting from clutter are especially a risk at night (Ebersole and others, 2008).

e   Secure all carpeting, mats, and tile; place nonskid backing under small rugs and doormats.

Reduces chance of patient slipping when stepping on rug surface.

f   Pad floor, and use specialized tile that absorbs impact of falls.

Cushions person's fall.

g   Use low-rise beds, or use futon beds or a mattress on the floor.

Lowers distance to floor surface.

h   Have enough electrical outlets installed to be able to plug light or electronic device (e.g., TV, video) into nearby outlet. Secure electrical cords against baseboards.

Prevents need to run extension cords across walkways.

i   Install nonskid strips on surface of bathtub and/or shower stall.

Reduces chances of slipping on tub/shower stall surface.

j   Have grab bar installed in studs at tub, toilet, and/or shower (see illustration). Have patient select vertical or horizontal placement if choice available. Be sure bar is different color than wall

Bar provides stability for maneuvering in bathroom. Should be easy to see.

k   Have handrails installed along the side of any stairway (see illustration). Be sure stairways are well lighted, with switches at top and bottom of steps.

Older adults have difficulty seeing edges of stairs.

l   Install appropriate broad-beam lighting for outside walkways.

Provides full illumination.

m   Keep a lighted phone easily accessible, next to the patient's bed.

Prevents patient from having to get up out of bed, often in the dark.

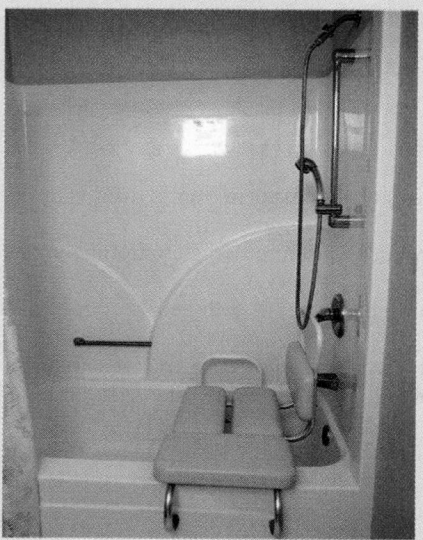

STEP 1j   Grab bars and safety seat installed in a shower.

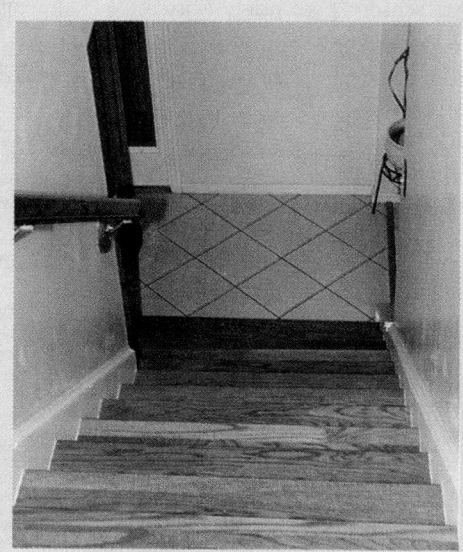

STEP 1k   Handrails installed along stairways provide security for patients with visual, balance, and coordination problems.

STEP	RATIONALE

n   Install motion sensor exterior lighting for walkways/driveway.

Reduces risk for patient falls due to dark surroundings.

o   Have patient use padding or types of clothing that will cushion bony prominences, especially high-risk bony prominences (e.g., hips). Specially designed hip protectors are available.

Helps to absorb impact of falling body.

2   Make modifications to promote safe practice of activities of daily living (ADLs):

a   Provide direct light source in areas where patient reads, cooks, uses tools, or conducts hobby work. High-intensity light on object or surface that is involved works best.

Visual changes in the older adult include sensitivity to glare, increased lens opacities, decreased visual acuity and decreased visual accommodations (Ross and Summerlin, 2007).

Critical Decision Point   *Avoid fluorescent lighting because it creates excessive glare.*

b   Consider satin and nongloss finishes for walls, cabinets, and countertops in kitchen. Have sheer curtains or adjustable shades in other living areas.

Reduces glare for older adults.

c   Apply colored tape or paint to color code controls of stove, oven, dryer, toaster, and other appliances.

Patients with reduced visual acuity may adjust appliance to wrong setting, creating potential risk for fire or burning.

d   Consider installing lazy Susans or pull-out drawers with glide mechanisms in kitchen cabinets. Install C-ring handles in lower cabinets.

Makes access to food and kitchen supplies easier.

3   Take steps to prevent spread of infection in shared kitchens and bathrooms:

a   Instruct patient in cleaning practices to prevent spread of infection.

Families often provide home care, and they need instruction in infection control practices.

b   Instruct patient not to share eating and drinking utensils.

Some infections are spread by saliva.

c   Instruct patient to clean appliances and surfaces daily.

Regular cleaning will prevent the risk for contamination and spread of infection.

4   Take steps to eliminate fire hazards:

a   Have smoke detectors installed near each bedroom, in kitchen, and in basement of home. Be sure detector is on each floor of home.

Fires most frequently start in basement near furnace, dryer, or electrical wiring; kitchen; or in living areas where there is extensive wiring. Alarm should be close by to alert patient and family when sleeping.

b   Have patient select fire extinguisher that is easy to handle and manipulate (see illustration). Ask patient to read instructions and demonstrate its proper use.

Some older adults or patients with disabilities have difficulty gripping mechanisms on certain extinguishers.

c   Have area around furnace cleared of any flammable items.

Reduces risk for fire.

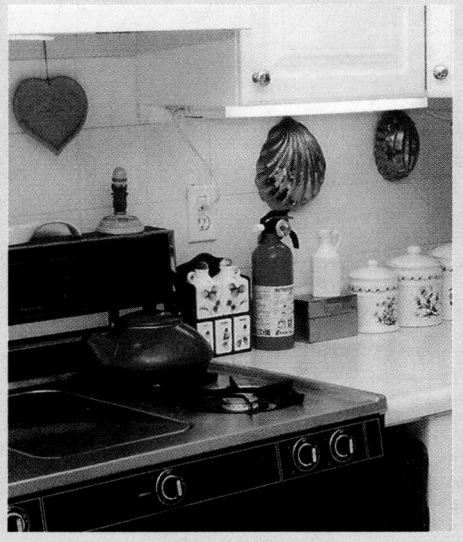

STEP 4b   Fire extinguisher accessible in kitchen.

STEP	RATIONALE
d Instruct patient to never place portable space heater within 3 feet of flammable items (Meiner and Lueckenotte, 2006).	Intense heat will ignite flammable items easily.
e Have patient make appointments for maintenance of furnace and chimney cleaning in appropriate season.	Furnace maintenance prevents short circuits and fires. Accumulation of creosote on chimney walls can lead to fire.
f Have patient check lightbulb wattage in all fixtures.	Ensures proper wattage being used.
g Have patient establish routine during cooking that keeps patient in kitchen. Be sure cooking range is clean and items such as potholders and towels are away from burners.	Food cooking on stove can easily boil over or begin to burn when unattended.
h If patient is a smoker, review need to keep ashtrays clean and emptied. Placing a small amount of water or sand in bottom of ashtray is useful if patient is visually impaired.	Patient with reduced vision may be unable to tell if cigarette, cigar, or match has extinguished.
i Strongly discourage smoking in bed, smoking in a chair when there is a possibility of falling asleep, and smoking after taking a medication that diminishes alertness.	Risks factors for burns, as well as fire.
j Recommend patient install power strips or surge protectors for plugging in multiple appliances/devices.	Prevents risk for electrical short, which can cause a fire.
5 Take steps to reduce chances of injury from burns:	
a Have setting on hot water heater adjusted to 49° C (120° F) or lower.	Prevents scalding burns (Meiner and Lueckenotte, 2006).
b Instruct patient to always turn cold water on first.	Prevents direct exposure to hot water.
c Install touch pads on lamps.	Light is easy to turn on without risk for touching hot lightbulb.
d Use color codes of red for hot and blue for cold on water faucets. (If patient cannot distinguish colors, choose two that are easily distinguished.)	Prevents accidental burning from turning on wrong faucet.
6 Take steps to prevent carbon monoxide exposure in the home:	
a Have condition of furnace venting checked annually just before time of season when furnace is turned on.	Improper venting prevents escape of carbon monoxide, a poisonous gas that alters hemoglobin to prevent formation of oxyhemoglobin and reduces oxygen supply to tissues.
b Caution patients against using a gas stove or barbecue grill for heating inside of home.	Both are sources of carbon monoxide.
c Have carbon monoxide detector installed in home (see illustration).	Detector alarms when carbon monoxide reaches unsafe levels.

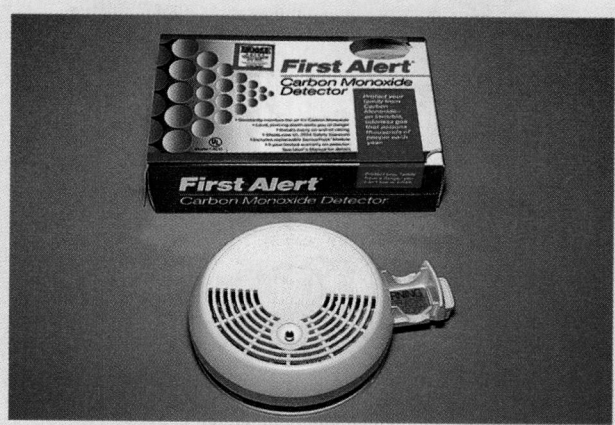

STEP 6c   Carbon monoxide detector.

STEP	RATIONALE

EVALUATION

1 Have patient and family member(s) identify safety risks revealed in home safety assessment.

2 During follow-up visit or call to home ask patient to discuss plans for making any modifications, and observe what changes patient has implemented.

3 During follow-up visits or calls ask if patient has experienced any falls or other injuries within home.

4 Reassess for progression of dementia.

Demonstrates what patient recognizes as a risk and its relative importance for changing.

Evaluates extent to which patient sees risks as potentially harmful and complies with suggested changes.

Reveals if risks have been eliminated, depending on patient's previous history of injury.

Assesses for potential risk to patient and caregiver.

Unexpected Outcomes

1 Patient and family do not acknowledge risks identified from home safety assessment.

2 Patient fails to make changes agreed on in previous plan.

3 Patient suffers fall or burn within home.

Related Interventions

- Determine if reluctance to make changes is due to limited resources, disbelief concerning need to make changes, fear of loss of autonomy, or other reasons.
- Review implications of risks to patient's safety and welfare.
- Determine reason for failure to make changes.
- Help prioritize greatest risks.
- Conduct an assessment of contributing factors and conditions in environment at time of injury.
- Make revisions based upon assessment findings.

Recording and Reporting

- Retain copy of home safety assessment in patient's home care record.
- Record any instruction provided, patient's response, and changes made within environment in progress notes.

Teaching Considerations

- Family and caregivers will benefit from learning how to safely assist patient in ambulating or transferring from bed to chair or wheelchair to chair, depending on patient's mobility limitations (see Chapter 9).
- Instruct patient and caregiver in what to do in case patient falls, including access to emergency assistance and how to prevent further injury. Many communities have a service available for persons who live alone. The service company provides a small device that a patient wears around the neck and a special monitor connected to patient's telephone. Patients summon help by pressing button on device if phone is inaccessible. When company receives an alarm, it calls the patient to determine the problem. If there is no answer, the company will contact family members, friends, or a rescue squad to check on patient. This service is a valuable option to frail older adults who live alone or are left at home alone for periods of time.

Pediatric Considerations

- Caution parents when working in the kitchen to never pour hot liquids when an infant or young child is near.
- Remove all crib toys that are strung across crib or playpen when child begins to push up on hands or knees (4 to 7 months).
- Keep faucets out of reach of children.
- Keep guns and ammunition in separate, secured places.
- Install safety measures appropriate to developmental level (i.e., cabinet locks and gates).

Gerontological Considerations

- If patient is wheelchair-bound, lower light switches and other control devices within easy reach. Similarly, redesign kitchen cabinets and other storage closets for better access. Install a raised toilet seat or high-rise toilet to make it easier for the patient to get on and off the toilet. A handheld showerhead or lift system will also assist the older adult and caregiver in regular hygiene practices (USDHHS Administration on Aging, 2007). Another option is placing a bedside commode (with bedpan removed) over a conventional toilet seat. Commode level is usually higher than toilet and can also be moved near the bed for nighttime use.

Long-Term Care Considerations

- Maintain close supervision of confused patients.

BOX 41-1   Fall/Near Fall Diary

- Keep a notebook and across the longest edge of the paper, write the headings: "Date," "Time of Fall," "Activity at Time of Fall," "Symptoms," and "Injury."
- As soon as possible after the fall, patient completes information under each heading.
- If a family member witnesses the fall, the family member records what happened on a separate piece of paper.
- List emergency contact numbers in the diary for patient to call in case a fall results in serious injury.
- Instruct patient to bring diary to the health care provider's office at the next scheduled visit or share information with home care nurse on next home visit.

Modified from Meiner SE, Lueckenotte AG: *Gerontologic nursing,* ed 3, St. Louis, 2006, Mosby.

SKILL 41-2 Adapting the Home Setting for Patients With Cognitive Deficits

An important aspect of safety is a person's ability to perform routine ADLs and instrumental activities of daily living (IADLs) to make correct decisions about home management activities. ADLs include the patient's ability to bathe, dress, go to the toilet, transfer, maintain continence, and feed oneself, whereas IADLs include the ability to use a telephone, prepare meals, travel, do housework, take medication, and shop. Some patients who are unable to perform these activities or who require assistance from another have physical disabilities and/or cognitive limitations. Cognitive limitations threaten the person's autonomy. Family members often misunderstand certain behaviors associated with cognitive changes and become concerned as to whether the individual can function safely within the home. You may face situations where you have to make decisions as to whether a patient is competent to perform self-care.

Two of the most common cognitive conditions affecting patients in the home are dementia and depression. Dementia is a chronic generalized impairment of intellectual functioning that leads to a decline in the ability to perform basic and instrumental activities of daily living. Dementia is characterized by a gradual, progressive, irreversible cerebral dysfunction. Alzheimer's disease is the most common form of dementia. It has the characteristic progressive symptoms of loss of memory (amnesia), loss of the ability to recognize objects and persons (agnosia), loss of the ability to perform familiar tasks (apraxia), and loss of language skills (aphasia). As Alzheimer's disease progresses, older adults become more dependent on caregivers for assistance.

Individuals who are in the early to middle stage of dementia are at risk for wandering. A wandering patient may walk around the house trying repeatedly, but ineffectively, to carry out a task independently. Another example of wandering is when the patient tries to leave his or her place of residence but is stopped by family caregivers. If wandering is a problem, instruct the family or caregiver to provide current photographs of the patient to local police and install locks and bells on doors (Ross and Summerlin, 2007).

Depression is a chronic, insidious emotional disorder characterized by feelings of sadness, melancholy, dejection, and worthlessness that are inappropriate and out of proportion to reality. It occurs alone or in combination with cognitive disorders such as dementia. Depression occurs secondary to isolation when the older adult is homebound and has few social visitors.

Delegation Considerations
Aspects of the skill of adapting the home environment for patients with cognitive deficits can be delegated. However, the nurse is responsible for the assessment of cognitive function. The nurse directs the NAP by:
- Reviewing their suggestions for helping patients adapt approaches to performing daily activities.
- Having NAP inform nurse when there is a change in patient's mood, memory, and ability to maintain home.

Equipment
- ❏ Mini-Mental State Examination (MMSE)
- ❏ Short Geriatric Depression Scale (SGDS)
- ❏ Calendar
- ❏ Paper for making lists
- ❏ Medication organizer (*optional*)
- ❏ Bulletin board or poster board (*optional*)
- ❏ Motion detector (*optional*)

STEP	RATIONALE

ASSESSMENT

1	Assess patient over a short period of time, and be sensitive to patient's sensory needs or disabilities.	Respects the human dignity of the patient.
2	Be sure the room in which you meet with patient and family is well lit with minimal outside noises or interruptions. Speak clearly and in normal tone of voice.	An optimal environment for the assessment of the patient's cognitive and mental status will provide a more valid assessment.
3	Ask patient to describe own level of health, and have him or her describe how it affects the ability to perform self-care skills (e.g., bathing, dressing, eating, toileting).	Question will require patient to attend to one topic. Allows nurse to assess attention and concentration. Also determines if patient is fully perceptive of physical capabilities.

Critical Decision Point *Do not create situation in which patient feels you are not listening to his or her views. The additional person supplements answers with the patient's consent, but the patient remains the focus of the interview.*

4	Ask how the patient is doing with home management responsibilities: "Tell me what bills you pay each month. Can you tell what each one is for? Can you tell me about your normal day—when do you get up, eat meals, dress? Do you have problems dressing or bathing?"	Provides good comparison of patient and family perceptions. Interaction will help to measure short-term memory, judgment, and problem solving.
5	Assess patient's medications. Review number and type of medications, purpose as prescribed, time of day taken, and dosages. Assess where patient stores medications. Give special attention to pain medications, anticonvulsants, antihypertensives (especially beta-adrenergic blockers), diuretics, digoxin, aspirin, and anticoagulants. Have patient or caregiver keep updated list of medications that can be brought to emergency room if needed.	Older adults frequently suffer drug interactions from polypharmacy, the concurrent prescribing of multiple medications. Some drugs and/or combinations of drugs place patient at risk for side effects that increase chances of injury as a result of physical or cognitive changes. Keeping a list of medications will allow health care provider easy access to medication history.

STEP	RATIONALE
6 Determine if patient has family member or friend who assists with self-care or home management responsibilities. What level of support is provided by caregiver? How frequent is the caregiver available? Does patient perceive satisfaction in caregiver's support? What level of satisfaction does caregiver perceive? Does caregiver have access to and/or take advantage of respite care?	The relationship between a family caregiver and a patient helps define how difficult it is to provide caregiving support. The role of family caregiver is often stressful, particularly if the individual has other responsibilities such as parenting, work, or school. Determines availability of resource to patient and quality of that support.
7 During discussion, observe patient's dress, nonverbal expressions, appearance, and cleanliness.	Conditions such as depression and dementia can result in patient's inability to attend to personal appearance.

Critical Decision Point *Do not confuse behavioral changes with lack of available resources to maintain hygiene. Also be aware of signs and symptoms of abuse or neglect. Report suspected abuse to appropriate social service agency.*

STEP	RATIONALE
8 Observe immediate home environment. Is it well kept and orderly (see Skill 41-1)?	Behavioral changes associated with cognitive dysfunction are evident in disorderly home and inappropriate placement of objects (e.g., carton of orange juice placed inside kitchen cabinet instead of in refrigerator).
9 If you suspect a cognitive or mental status change: a Complete a Mini-Mental State Examination (e.g., Folstein's examination) for dementia. b Complete Short Geriatric Depression Scale for depression.	Test screens orientation, attention and calculation, recall, language, and intelligence. SGDS is a valid 15-item screening tool for depression in older adults (Yesavage, 1988).
10 If you suspect a patient is wandering, observe for the following behaviors (family caregivers might provide information as well): • Repeated shadowing or seeking whereabouts of caregiver • Revisiting one destination many times • Inability to locate landmarks or getting lost in a familiar setting • Going into unauthorized or private places • Searching for "missing" people or places • Walking with no apparent destination or purpose • Haphazard or continuous moving, walking, or pacing • Walking that cannot easily be redirected	Alerts family and caregivers of potential safety risks. When wandering extends outside the safe environment, the patient is at increased risk for injury or death (Aud, 2004).
11 Assess what current environmental strategies family caregivers are using in dealing with wandering (e.g., latches and alarms on doors, visual cues such as STOP signs, constant supervision).	Assists in determining level of intervention necessary.
12 Assess caregiver for signs and symptoms of stress.	Assists in determining if caregiver is feeling burdened or overwhelmed and is in need of assistance.

NURSING DIAGNOSES

- Acute confusion
- Caregiver role strain
- Disturbed thought processes
- Impaired home maintenance
- Impaired memory
- Ineffective health maintenance
- Ineffective role performance
- Risk for injury
- Self-care deficit (feeding, toileting, bathing/hygiene, dressing/grooming)
- Wandering

Individualize related factors based on patient's condition or needs.

PLANNING

1 Expected outcomes following completion of procedure: • Patient is able to complete home management responsibilities within existing limitations. • Patient receives appropriate combination of medications for diagnosed conditions. • Patient is able to perform self-care activities. • Family caregivers will describe steps to take to minimizing wandering. • Patient experience fewer episodes of wandering. • Caregiver identifies community resources for support.	Modifications are made that help patient apply remaining cognitive functions. Assistive devices enable patient to follow prescribed medication regimen. Interventions preserve patient's autonomy and maximize patient's functionality. Instruction will prepare caregivers with wandering management strategies. Wandering management strategies will be effective. Services available can include respite care, adult day care programs, and support groups.

STEP	RATIONALE
2 If patient has difficulty with self-care skills, or fine motor skills refer family to occupational therapy, homemaker services, or respite care as appropriate.	Occupational therapists provide assistive devices and recommend self-care adaptations. Homemaker services provide added resource for meal preparation and home cleaning. Respite care provides family caregiver temporary rest away from continuous responsibilities.
3 Offer assistive devices to make bathing, dressing, writing, and feeding easier (see illustrations).	Assistive eating devices have larger handles and cup handles or plate edges to assist with meals. Assistive clothing uses Velcro, large zippers, and elastic to facilitate independence when dressing.
4 Consider patient's level of cognitive impairment when making changes in patient's living environment. Some patients may require only minor adaptations, and others will depend more on assistance of caregivers.	Retention of patient's independence and autonomy is ultimate goal.
5 Determine best time of day for approaches that result in desired response.	Some patients are more alert and responsive in morning versus afternoon or vice versa.

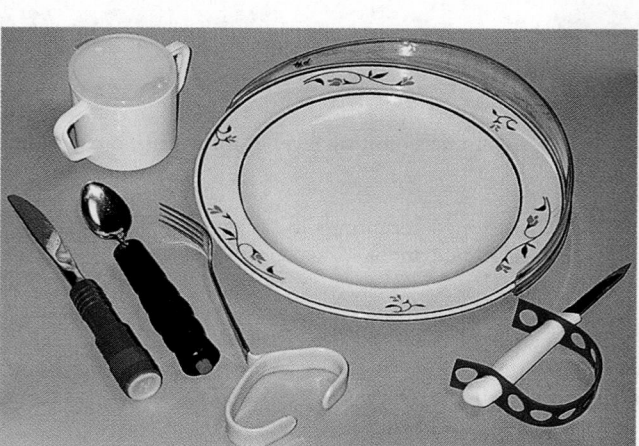 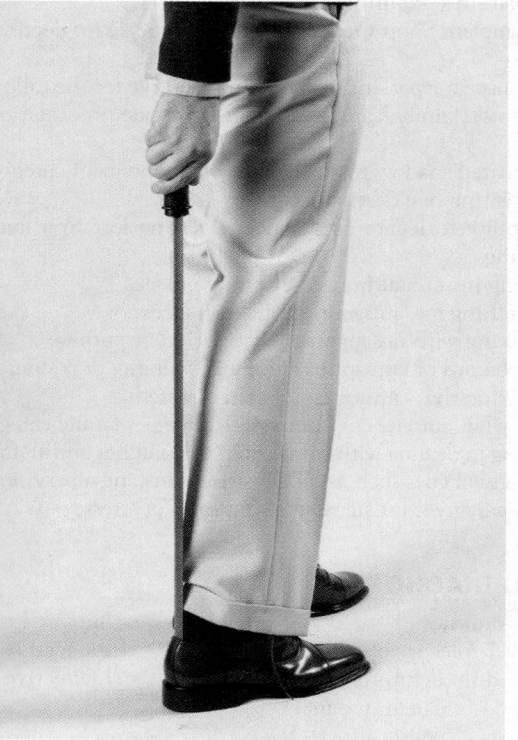

STEP 3   A, Assistive feeding devices. **B,** Assistive device to aid in putting on shoes. (*Courtesy Gold Violin, all rights reserved*)

IMPLEMENTATION

1 If patient has difficulty remembering when to perform tasks (e.g., paying bills, taking medicines), help to create a list, or post reminder notes in a conspicuous location (e.g., bulletin board, front of refrigerator), provide a medication container organized by days of week, recommend a wristwatch with alarm to signal medication administration times.	Memory function in older adults tends to be preserved for relevant, well-learned material (Meiner and Lueckenotte, 2006). Lists and organizers will help patient cope with memory loss and still safely perform activities.
2 When patient has difficulty completing tasks such as writing checks for bills or bringing groceries into home from store, reduce steps it takes to complete task. Consolidate steps or simplify task.	Prevents frustration in completing task and/or forgetting step that leads to task being unfinished.

STEP	RATIONALE
3 Help patient and caregiver determine routine schedule for daily activities such as eating, bathing, daily exercise, home cleaning, and napping. Have large calendar posted in conspicuous area to write in appointments or special planned events.	Consistency creates sense of security and keeps patient oriented to daily activities. Routines are important in providing security, but patient also needs to have the option of making changes as necessary.
4 Instruct caregiver to focus on patient's abilities rather than disabilities. Use abilities in modifying approaches to perform daily activities. For example, if patient has limited use of right hand, try approaches that maximize use of left hand.	Retains patient's autonomy and sense of self-worth.
5 Have caregiver assist with setting-up activities so that patient can complete task (e.g., chopping up vegetables before actual cooking, placing wash basin on table in bedroom for sponge bath, placing clothes to wear for the day on bed, unpacking groceries on countertop for eventual storage, arranging food on plate with items in clockwise orientation—vegetables at 9, salad at 3, meat at 6).	Helps patient master task even though unable either physically or cognitively to perform all steps.
6 Discuss with patient, caregiver, and primary care provider options for scheduling multiple medications:	Drugs sometimes cause physiological changes that create risk for injury.
a Administer medications that are likely to cause confusion at bedtime.	Reduces risk for confusion during waking hours contributing to disorientation and risk for falling.

Critical Decision Point *Do not recommend this if patient has nocturia.*

STEP	RATIONALE
b Space antihypertensives and antiarrhythmics at different times to minimize side effects.	These drugs cause blood pressure changes and dizziness, thus increasing risk for falls.
c Reduce number of pain medications used when possible.	Drugs create sedative effects, increasing risk for falls.
d Have diuretics taken early in day and not at night.	Diuretic effect occurs during the day while patient is awake.
e Discuss possibility of taking medications at the same time with health care provider.	If safe and appropriate, taking medications at the same time will alleviate problem of patient remembering multiple administration times.
7 Instruct caregiver in how to use simple and direct communication:	Relays care and support through therapeutic communication techniques.
a Sit or stand in front of patient in full view.	Promotes reception of verbal and nonverbal messages.
b Face the patient with a hearing impairment while speaking; do not cover the mouth.	Patient can see speaker's lips. Prevents voice distortion.
c Use a calm and relaxed approach.	
d Use eye contact and touch.	Helps to reinforce messages.
e Speak slowly, in simple words and short sentences.	Enhances understanding of messages.
f Use nonverbal gestures that complement verbal messages.	
8 Place clocks, calendars, and personal mementos (e.g., pictures, scrapbooks) throughout rooms within the home. Enhance the environment with addition of tactile boards or three-dimensional art.	Maintaining familiar surroundings will maximize cognitive function (Small, 2007).
9 Have caregiver routinely orient patient to who caregiver is and what activities they are going to complete.	This strategy is useful in patients with progressive dementia. Behavioral symptoms in later stages include delusions, agitation, and hallucinations (Alzheimer's Association, 2005).
10 Be sure patient has regular naps or rest periods during the day.	Fatigue adds to any mental status changes. Provides patient energy to perform planned activities.
11 Have caregiver encourage and support frequent visits by family and friends. Instruct caregiver in how to use humor and reminiscing of favorite stories to promote social interaction.	Participation in social activities prevents boredom and restlessness.
12 Provide a safe place for a person to wander (e.g., large family room or fenced yard).	Reduces risk for injury and leaving residence.
13 Use labels to cue or remind the person (Alzheimer's Association, 2005).	Assists in reorienting the patient.
14 Recommend family of wandering patient install door locks or electronic guards.	Reduces chance of wandering (Small, 2007).
15 Create a calm, safe setting that is appropriate for the patient's abilities (Alzheimer's Association, 2005).	Prevents falls and minimizes behavioral symptoms.

STEP	RATIONALE
16 Monitor patient for personal comfort (e.g., hunger, thirst, constipation, full bladder, and comfortable temperature) (Alzheimer's Association, 2005).	Reduces stimuli that prompt wandering.
17 Install a motion detector near an exit site, with a portable alarm that can accompany caregiver.	Alerts caregiver to patient's attempt to exit residence.

EVALUATION

1 During follow-up visits ask patient to review the home management activities completed the morning of that day, as well as the previous day.	Determines patient's ability to recall events and evaluates if patient completed planned activities.
2 Review with patient and caregiver revised schedule for medication administration.	Evaluates understanding of regimen.
3 Have caregiver keep track of doses patient takes over a 1-week period.	Tracking doses will confirm if patient is adherent to regimen.
4 Ask caregiver to describe ways that will increase patient's success in completing home management and self-care activities.	Measures learning.
5 Have caregiver show schedules of daily routines and review specific approaches used. Observe environment for presence of reality orientation cues.	Determines caregiver's success in applying information and making environmental changes.
6 Have family caregivers describe options for minimizing wandering.	Measures learning.
7 Have family caregivers report number of occurrences of wandering.	Determines if reduction in wandering has occurred.

Unexpected Outcomes	Related Interventions
1 Patient is unable to complete daily activities as planned.	• Further modifications are sometimes necessary. • Reassess what occurred when a task was not completed.
2 Patient experiences drug interaction from multiple medications.	• Have physician evaluate patient's medication regimen. • Recommend feasibility of pharmacy consultation.
3 Caregiver is unable to describe/implement techniques that will improve patient's orientation and ability to complete activities.	• Reinstruction and discussion are necessary. • Support for caregiver is sometimes necessary before caregiver can learn how to support someone else. • Consider that caregiver is not able to provide necessary support; need to analyze other options.
4 Caregiver is unable to describe/implement strategies to decrease wandering.	• Reinstruction and discussion are necessary. • Caregiver may not have resources available to adapt environment.
5 Patient's wandering increases.	• Reconsider strategies used. • Reassess factors prompting wandering.

Recording and Reporting

- Record assessment of patient's cognitive and mental status, recommended interventions, and patient's and caregiver's response in progress notes.
- Report to health care provider any change in patient's behavior that reflects a decline in cognitive or mental status.

Teaching Considerations

- Instruct caregiver in signs and symptoms of dementia and depression. If patient's functionality continues to decline, caregiver may choose to learn more ADL support skills (e.g., how to assist with hygiene, dressing, transfer and turning, toileting).

Pediatric Considerations

- Children with cognitive impairment are often not aware of inherent dangers during play and other activities. Parental supervision is critical.

Gerontological Considerations

- Early diagnosis of the cause of dementia is best for the patient and caregiver so that prompt treatment can begin, the patient can be included in treatment decisions as much as possible, and the caregiver has an understanding of the behavior (Alzheimer's Association, 2005).

SKILL 41-3 Medication and Medical Device Safety

Patients frequently must manage the administration of medications and the use of medical devices such as syringes, blood glucose monitoring equipment, dressing supplies, and even intravenous (IV) devices. This includes administration, storage, and disposal of medications and medical devices. Safety is critical in ensuring that the patient administers medications correctly, uses devices properly, and cleans and removes waste from equipment. Infection control is just one principle the patient and/or caregiver must learn for the home setting. The Environmental Protection Agency recommends placing soiled dressings in securely fastened plastic bags before adding to regular trash. Make sure patients know local regulations regarding waste disposal and follow the procedures consistent with local laws.

One of the nurse's responsibilities within the home environment is to assist the patient with sensory, mobility, or cognitive deficits. Patients who require special consideration include those with acute sensory or neurological impairment, those with chronic illness such as diabetes or arthritis, and older adults, who frequently have physical limitations that make manipulation of medical devices and dispensing of medications difficult.

For example, patients with arthritic hands are sometimes unable to open medication containers because of weakness in the hands and the pain created by pressure on the joints. This skill reviews steps to take to ensure safe use of medications and medical devices.

Delegation Considerations
The skill of assessing for and monitoring medication and medical device safety cannot be delegated to NAP. However, the NAP can make suggestions that further ensure patient safety regarding the use of basic infection control practices and how to dispose of sharps, needles, and contaminated supplies.

Equipment
- ❏ Colored marking pens
- ❏ Labels
- ❏ Puncture-resistant sharps container or 2-L soda bottle with cap
- ❏ Duct, masking, or adhesive tape
- ❏ Assistive devices (e.g., syringe magnifier)
- ❏ Medication organizers

STEP	RATIONALE
ASSESSMENT	
1 Assess patient's sensory, musculoskeletal, and neurological function.	Reveals any deficits that will affect preparation and use of medications or medical devices.
2 If family or caregiver provides routine assistance, assess his or her function as above.	Determines level of assistance caregivers can provide.
3 Assess patient's medication regimen and length of time patient has been receiving each drug.	Determines complexity of medication regimen and how familiar patient is with regimen.
4 Ask patient to show you where medications are stored in home. Look at each container.	Determines condition and labeling of containers.
5 Assess the temperature of storage area.	Medication should not be stored in extreme heat. Insulin should be kept in a cool place.
6 Have patient describe daily schedule for drug administration and whether there are any problems in following that schedule.	Helps to reveal patient's adherence to or misunderstanding of instructions.
7 If patient self-administers injections, ask to see where patient stores those supplies and what patient uses to dispose of used syringes and needles.	Determines sterility of equipment and whether method of disposal creates risk to patient or family for needle-stick injuries.
8 If patient uses a glucose-monitoring device, ask to see where monitor, lancets, and glucose strips are stored. Also ask about how patient disposes of lancets.	Allows nurse to examine cleanliness of equipment, sterility of lancets, and condition of glucose strips. Sharps should be disposed of in puncture-proof container.
9 If patient applies dressings to a wound, ask to see where patient stores dressings and determine how patient disposes of soiled dressings.	Determines if patient stores and discards dressing supplies properly.

NURSING DIAGNOSES

- Deficient knowledge regarding medication and medical device safety
- Health-seeking behaviors regarding medication safety
- Ineffective health maintenance
- Noncompliance (sharps disposal)
- Risk for infection
- Risk for injury

Individualize related factors based on patient's condition or needs.

STEP	RATIONALE

PLANNING

1 Expected outcomes following completion of procedure:

- Patient and caregiver will discuss principles of medication safety.

Nurse provides knowledge base for safe medication administration.

- Patient and caregiver will prepare medications independently.

Adaptations successfully accommodate patient's and/or caregiver's deficits in handling and manipulating equipment.

- Patient and caregiver will identify correct conditions for storing medications, medical devices, and supplies.

Instruction focuses on infection control measures.

- Patient and caregiver will dispose of used medical equipment and supplies correctly.

Appropriate receptacles and methods for disposal are made available.

IMPLEMENTATION

1 Instruct patient and caregiver in principles to ensure medications are safe to use:

a Never take a medicine prescribed for another member of household.

Medications must be of full strength and used for the appropriate pharmacological reason to have therapeutic benefit.

b Do not take any medicine more than a year old or past expiration date on container.

Expired medication is sometimes toxic or no longer effective.

c Do not place different medicines in same container.

Prevents accidental "mix-up" of medications and medication error.

d Do not place medications in different containers than their original ones.

Prevents accidental "mix-up" of medications and confusion as to expiration dates.

e Always finish a prescribed medication; do not save for a future illness.

Prevents underdosing or inappropriate dosing.

f Wash hands before and after administering/taking medication.

Contaminated hands are a source of infection transmission.

2 Recommend approaches for preparation of medications:

a For patients with weakened grasp or pain of hands and fingers, have local pharmacist place medications in a screw-top container.

Tops of childproof containers are difficult to remove, especially if hand and finger grasp are weakened.

Critical Decision Point   *If patient has children or grandchildren who have easy access to medication storage area or patient's purse, be sure medications are stored in secure place.*

b For patients with visual alterations, have pharmacy type larger labels on all medication containers.

Ensures patient is able to read drug name and dosage schedule clearly.

c For patients who are legally blind, have braille labels placed on medication containers.

Labels embossed with drug name, strength, and prescription numbers are easy to read for patient trained in use of Braille.

d For patients taking multiple medications, introduce a color-coding system. Use the same color for drugs that patient needs to take at the same time. Mark tops of bottle caps with a colored marking pen.

Technique helps ensure patient takes correct drugs and doses at correct times of day.

e Provide specially designed syringes with large numerals or syringe magnifier for patients with visual alterations (see illustration).

Ensures accurate dose of drug is prepared in syringe.

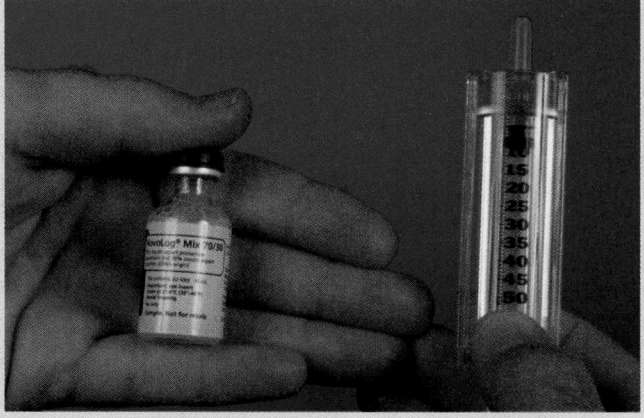

STEP 2e   Syringe with magnifier.

STEP	RATIONALE
f For patients who have difficulty manipulating syringes, offer a spring-loaded needle insertion aid.	Delivers injection safely without manipulation of plunger.

Critical Decision Point   *Instruct family caregivers in knowing what to do following a needle-stick injury: wash the affected area thoroughly with soap and water, then dry. If patient has acquired immunodeficiency syndrome (AIDS), hepatitis, or other communicable disease, caregivers should pursue appropriate laboratory testing.*

STEP	RATIONALE
g Instruct caregivers in how to properly draw up prescribed volume of medication into syringe. When necessary, have caregiver prepare extra prefilled syringes for patient's use when caregiver is absent.	Ensures caregiver knows proper preparation techniques. Ensures patient has access to injections.
3 Recommend approaches for medication and supply storage:	
a Store medications in a safe place, preferably in the kitchen.	Moisture in bathroom may cause medications to decompose.
b Keep liquid medications and parenteral drugs, especially insulin, in a cool place.	Prevents decomposition of drug.

Critical Decision Point   *Insulin may be stored in refrigerator, but it is not necessary. Patients can store insulin at room temperature for up to 30 days without losing potency as per manufacturer's guidelines (Cohen and others, 2007). If insulin is stored in refrigerator, be sure drug is in a bin or container, away from food.*

STEP	RATIONALE
c Keep medical supplies such as syringes, dressing supplies, and glucose meter in airtight container (e.g., plastic storage bin), and store in cool place, such as bedroom closet.	Ensures supplies are not exposed to moisture or other contaminants.
d Instruct patient and caregiver to use new needle with each medication administration.	Multiple use of same needle puts patient at risk for infection.
4 Review for patient and caregiver the proper techniques for disposal of medications, "sharps," and disposable medical supplies:	
a Discard unused portions of drugs or outdated drugs in sink or toilet.	Ensures that no one in household uses drug not prescribed for their use or drugs that will be ineffective pharmacologically.
b Obtain sharps container from medical supply store or IV equipment supplier. (If finances are limited, have patient use a small-neck plastic bottle, such as a soda bottle.) Dispose of all needles and lancets in container (see illustration).	Puncture-proof container prevents exposure to contaminated needle stick. Small-neck container makes it difficult for anyone to easily retrieve a used needle or sharp.
c Caution against filling container to a point where needles protrude out opening. Discard when three-fourths full, securing top with duct tape or adhesive tape.	Prevents needle sticks.
d Store sharps container in an area inaccessible to children.	Prevents injury to child.

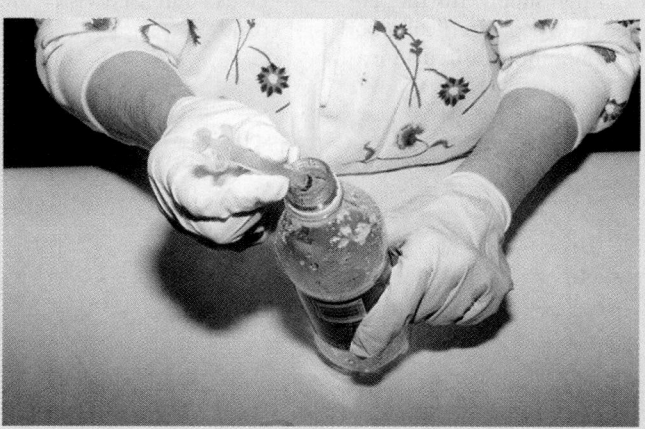

STEP 4b   Disposing of syringe in plastic soda bottle.

STEP	RATIONALE
e Dispose of soiled dressings, used glucose testing reagent strips, and IV tubing in a separate, sealed, plastic garbage bag. Then place in second plastic bag (double bagged), and discard appropriately as trash.	Prevents contamination with other items in home. Minimizes chances of caregiver being exposed to infectious waste.
f Consult local public health department or community authorities regarding proper way to dispose of waste.	Most communities have strict guidelines for waste disposal.

EVALUATION

1 Have patient and/or caregiver describe steps to take to ensure medications are safe to use.	Demonstrates learning.
2 Observe patient and/or caregiver prepare and administer a medication dose.	Evaluates ability to physically manipulate medications and necessary equipment.
3 Observe home setting for location of medications and supplies.	Evaluates patient's and/or caregiver's adherence to recommendations.
4 Have patient describe how sharps or medical equipment is discarded.	Demonstrates learning.
5 Do pill counts (pills remaining in containers) at successive intervals, such as twice a week for 2 weeks.	Verifies patient takes correct number of medications over a period of time.

Unexpected Outcomes	Related Interventions
1 Patient and/or caregiver is unable to recall principles for safe use of drugs.	• Reinstruction necessary, or patient and caregiver need chance to ask more questions regarding benefit of precautions. • Offer written, simple, and clear instructions.
2 Patient and/or caregiver has difficulty or is unable to prepare and self-administer a medication.	• Offer further assistance in setting up equipment. • Offer assistive aids. • Reinstruct in steps used to prepare medication.
3 Medications and medical devices are not stored in a secure or appropriate location.	• Assess whether patient chooses to store items conveniently rather than safely or has limited resources. • Reinstruction and discussion are necessary.
4 Sharps and disposable medical equipment are not disposed of properly.	• Provide reinstruction. • Arrange to provide appropriate containers.
5 Excess or insufficient number of pills found during pill count.	• Review with patient daily drug prescribed. Reevaluate use of dosage reminders.

Recording and Reporting
• Record instructions and recommendations to patient and caregiver and results of return demonstrations in progress notes.

Teaching Considerations
• Instruct patients in care of linen. Use of lancets or application of dressings causes soiling of patient's linen supply. Instruct patient to keep infected or soiled linen in a separate, leakproof plastic bag. Instruct patient to wash contaminated items separately from household laundry in hot water with 1 cup of bleach and detergent for *two* regular wash cycles.

Pediatric Considerations
• It is vital to keep medications and other equipment out of the reach of small children. If teaching self-management skills, include adult supervision and input. Never refer to medications as candy.

CRITICAL THINKING EXERCISES

Mrs. James is a 79-year-old woman who lives with her 84-year-old sister in a split-level four-bedroom home. Mrs. James has a history of metastatic bone cancer and was recently diagnosed with heart failure. In addition to taking multiple oral medications, she undergoes weekly intravenous chemotherapy for progression of her cancer. Mrs. James has no other family closer than a 2-hour drive, and her older sister has advanced glaucoma and diminished hearing. Both women refuse to move from their home, even at the urging of Mrs. James' three children to move closer to one of them. Mrs. James can no longer drive, nor does her sister, and she is unable to climb the few steps needed to move beyond the lower living level of the home. Because of this immobility, Mrs. James cannot reach the upstairs bathrooms, which contain showers, and she relies on her older sister to help care for her and maintain the house on a daily basis.

1 Based upon her medical history, offer two reasons why Mrs. James is at risk for falls.
2 Mrs. James' children expressed concern that their mother is getting confused as to her medication regimen. To assess the patient's adherence to her medication regimen:
 A Ask patient to show you where medications are stored in home
 B Have patient describe daily schedule for drug administration
 C Determine caregiver's knowledge of medication schedule
 D Examine the condition of storage area for medications
3 Mrs. James' children tell you they are concerned about their mother's and aunt's safety, "We worry that they will get injured. We have tried to convince them to move to a one-level apartment near us, but they refuse." What advice might you give the family?
4 The family is also concerned that their aunt is being overburdened with taking care of their mother. What questions might you ask the aunt to determine if she is feeling overburdened? What suggestions would you give to the family to assist the aunt in the care of their mother?

 ## REVIEW QUESTIONS

1 A woman found wandering in her nightclothes is also dirty but does not appear to have any injuries. What topics would an emergency department nurse include in his discussion with the patient and her family? Select all that apply.
 1 The medications she is taking and who supervises them
 2 Any decrease in cognitive function seen within the past few months
 3 Whether she pays her bills or who does
 4 Any history of wandering
 5 When she was last visited by family
 6 When she was last seen by a physician
2 A 50-year-old teacher with severe rheumatoid arthritis is noting some changes in her mobility. What simple screening examination could be used to detect difficulties with balance or gait?
 1 The Mini-Mental State Examination
 2 The timed Get Up and Go test
 3 The SPLATT screening tool
 4 A fall diary
3 A patient at home is changing a dressing daily on a foot ulcer. In what type of container should the nurse teach the patient to place the old dressing for disposal?
 1 In a wide-mouth plastic bottle
 2 In a small plastic container
 3 In the standard garbage can
 4 In a plastic garbage bag placed into a second plastic bag

4 A patient has recently noticed that she almost falls more often. Her physician recommended that she begin an exercise program. When teaching this patient, the nurse would explain that a program with which focus would be most effective for her?
 1 Endurance exercises
 2 Maintaining range of motion
 3 Incorporating the patient's activity patterns
 4 Strength, gait, and balance
5 An older adult patient with diabetes mellitus asks the home care nurse how to make things easier because she is insulin dependent. Which suggestion by the nurse would be most helpful in assisting the patient in maintaining a stable blood glucose level?
 1 Discard the used syringes in a small-neck bottle such as a screw-top soda bottle.
 2 Keep the insulin vials in the refrigerator until shortly before they are needed.
 3 Keep the insulin vials on the kitchen counter until all the insulin has been used.
 4 Keep the glucose meter strips in an airtight bag in the closet until they have been used.

REFERENCES

Alzheimer's Association: *Basics of Alzheimer's disease: what it is and what you can do,* 2005, http://www.alz.org/documents/national/basics_of_alz_low.pdf.
Andrews MM: Cultural diversity and community health nursing. In Nies MA, McEwen M, editors: *Community/public health nursing: promoting the health of populations,* ed 4, St. Louis, 2007, Elsevier.
Ebersole P and others: *Toward health aging: human need & nursing response,* ed 7, St. Louis, 2008, Mosby.
Hockenberry M, Wilson D: *Wong's nursing care of infants and children,* ed 8, St. Louis, 2007, Mosby.
Maslow A: *Motivation and personality,* ed 2, New York, 1954, Harper and Row.
Meiner SE, Lueckenotte AG: *Gerontologic nursing,* ed 3, St. Louis, 2006, Mosby.
National Fire Protection Association: *Smoking materials–related fires,* 2007, http://www.nfpa.org/itemDetail.asp?categoryID=294&itemID=19303&URL=Research%20&%20Reports/Fact%20sheets/Safety%20in%20the%20home/Smoking%20material-related%20fires.
Ross MET, Summerlin E: Senior health. In Nies MA, McEwen M, editors: *Community/public health nursing: promoting the health of populations,* ed 4, St. Louis, 2007, Elsevier.
Small GW: *Dementia,* http://www.americangeriatrics.org/products/finalGRS4Demo/chapter/text.html, accessed September 25, 2007.
U.S. Department of Health and Human Services: *Healthy People 2010,* 2007, http://www.healthypeople.gov/default.htm.
U.S. Department of Health and Human Services Administration on Aging: *Home modifications and assistive devices,* http://www.aoa.gov/press/nfc_month/2004/fact_sheets/Fact%20Sheet%20-%20Home%20Modification%20and%20Assistive%20Devices.pdf.
Wallace M: Older adult. In Edelman CL, Mandle CM, editors: *Health promotion throughout the lifespan,* ed 6, St. Louis, 2006, Mosby.

RESEARCH REFERENCES

Al-Khamees NA: Prevention of home-related injuries of preschoolers: safety measures taken by mothers, *Health Educ J* 65(3):24 2006.
Aud MA: Dangerous wandering: elopements of older adults with dementia from long-term care facilities, *Am J Alzheimers Dis Other Demen* 19(6):361, 2004.
Aykol AD: Falls in the elderly: What can be done? *Int Nurs Rev* 54(2):191, 2007.
Brewer K and others: Falls in community dwelling older adults: introduction to the problem, *PT—Magazine of Physical Therapy* 15(7):8 2007.
Cohen VC and others: Room-temperature storage of medications labeled for refrigeration, *Am J Health Syst Pharm* 64(16):1711, 2007.
Graham LL, Cates JA: Health care and sequestered cultures: a perspective from the Old Order Amish, *J Multicult Nurs Health* 12(3):60, 2006.
Pettersson AF and others: Motor function in subjects with mild cognitive impairment and early Alzheimer's disease, *Dement Geriatr Cogn Disord* 19(5-6):299, 2005.
Poulin de Courval LP and others: Reliability and validity of the Safety Assessment Scale for people with dementia living at home, *Can J Occup Ther* 73(2): 2006.
Rao SS: Prevention of falls in older patients, *Am Fam Physician* 72(1):81, 2005.

Home Care Teaching

MEDIA RESOURCES

- evolve *learning system* http://evolve.elsevier.com/Perry/skills
  - Review Questions
  - Video Clips

OBJECTIVES

Mastery of content in this chapter will enable the nurse to:
- Identify factors that influence patients' abilities to learn and care for themselves at home.
- Discuss the collaborative nature of home care teaching.
- Assess safety factors that often impair or prohibit a patient's ability to perform skills in the home setting.
- Discuss situations and conditions that require a patient and/or family to learn skills that support and achieve health maintenance.
- Choose appropriate teaching strategies to use in the home setting.
- Implement and evaluate appropriate learning strategies that support patients' ability to care for selves in the home.

Changes in the health care delivery system have shifted where patients receive care. Although acute and long-term care settings continue to provide inpatient services, many patients recover from or are treated for illnesses in their homes. Patients assume greater responsibility for managing their own care, resulting in a greater demand for home care nurses. In addition to attending to the physical, emotional, and financial needs of patients, the home care nurse also provides patient education on a variety of complex topics (Falvo, 2004).

Patient teaching is an essential part of nursing practice. Evidence-based practice guidelines, which include patient education, are widely used in health care settings to improve the quality of care (Redman, 2007). For example, intensive patient education about self-management principles is integral to successful diabetes management. Interdisciplinary teams that include nurses, physicians, advanced practice nurses, dietitians, pharmacists, and mental health professionals provide diabetes self-management education on topics such as control of blood glucose level, dietary choices, and prevention of long-term and short-term complications of diabetes (American Diabetes Association, 2007).

All nurses, including home care nurses, have an ethical responsibility to teach their patients. Information needs to be relevant, current, and clearly presented. When describing the rights of patients, the American Hospital Association (2003) includes the patient's right to make informed decisions about health care. The Joint Commission (2007b) launched the "Speak Up" initiative, encouraging patients to ask questions about their health care, their medications, and their rights. Therefore the home care nurse clarifies information provided to the patient by other health care professionals and often becomes the patient's primary source of information.

An additional challenge facing home care nurses today is illiteracy. Patients who are illiterate often have difficulty reading, writing, and speaking English. They also have difficulty completing mathematical computations and solving problems related to self-care (Falvo, 2004). To overcome challenges presented by illiteracy, assess the patient's ability to learn and understand information in different ways before, during, and after patient education is provided (Jones, 2007). For example, assess patients' reading abilities and understanding by asking patients to review printed information and answer open-ended questions, such as, "After looking over this medication teaching sheet, tell me how this medication will help you" (Osborne, 2004). To assess math skills, ask patients to calculate dosages of prescribed medications. To assess the ability to problem solve, describe real-life problems and ask patients to solve them. For example, when helping an obese male patient with a weight management program, ask him to identify healthy food choices from a restaurant's menu.

Patient education is an essential component of home care and a major factor in patients' compliance with therapies (Bastable, 2006). Home care nurses thoroughly assess factors that affect a patient's abilities and willingness to manage self-care. If a person does not want to learn, it is unlikely that learning will occur. However, you can motivate many patients, even those with a history of not complying with treatment recommendations, to learn and make significant behavior changes (Levensky and others, 2007).

When teaching patients, present information in an organized manner and include only essential information, allowing adequate time for the patient to learn. Assess a patient's learning preferences carefully (Mayer and others, 2007; Risica and Phipps, 2006). For example, does the patient prefer information verbally, in print, or over the Internet? Reinforce verbal instructions with printed culturally appropriate patient education information, and use other audiovisual materials when possible. Make sure patient education material is at a level that matches the patient's ability to read and understand information. Break complex skills into smaller parts, and ensure that the patient understands each part before progressing to the next step. For example, to teach a woman how to feed her husband though a feeding tube, first teach how to measure the tube feeding and how to use the equipment. Once she understands this part of the process, describe how to administer the feeding. Provide illustrated written materials that outline the steps for administering the tube feeding. Assess learning by observing her perform a return demonstration of the tube feeding.

Home care nurses are creative and adapt teaching to meet each patient's unique physical, psychosocial, and cultural needs. It is very important for the patient to become an active partner in the plan of care. Refer the patient to community resources to help overcome barriers (e.g., lack of transportation or inadequate funds for medications), and collaborate with the patient, family, or other caregivers, as well as interdisciplinary teams (e.g., pharmacists, physical therapists, and occupational therapists). Many times a variety of other social services and health-related organizations are involved in making the patient's home care plan successful. For collaboration to be successful, identify who is involved in the patient's care and establish mutual trust and respect for each person's abilities and contributions through open and honest communication. When home care nurses successfully implement individualized teaching plans, patients and families improve their quality of life, make fewer physician visits, reduce their health care expenses, and regain health or gain more control over illness.

EVIDENCE-BASED PRACTICE TRENDS

Patients need to understand how to manage their diseases and related care at home. However, knowledge alone does not necessarily predict a change in health-related behaviors (Bastable, 2006; Falvo, 2004). As a result, researchers investigate factors leading to improved health behaviors in a variety of populations. Analysis of current research indicates that patients perceived teaching provided by nurses as important, and patient education provided by nurses enhanced patient outcomes (Suhonen and Leino-Kilpi, 2006). For example, in one study, women who were more knowledgeable about coronary heart disease were more likely to practice health promotion behaviors to reduce their risk for heart disease (Thanavaro and others, 2006). Intentional patient education provided by nurses in another study markedly reduced the occurrence of falls on a medical telemetry unit (Jeske and others, 2006). If a patient has a lack of understanding, nurses need to be available and accessible to provide, clarify, and reinforce meaningful and relevant patient education.

Patients who are informed are more likely to manage their health problems better than those who are not informed (Behar-Horenstein and others, 2005; Kutzleb and Reiner, 2006). However, many times people who are members of vulnerable populations do not pursue or have access to necessary health care. Two vulnerable populations in the community are people of lower socioeconomic status and people living with chronic illnesses.

There are different educational strategies that enhance the outcomes of patient education in these populations. For example, a sample of English- and Spanish-speaking women who were patients at a low-income prenatal clinic indicated that they preferred to receive education from multiple sources. Overall, they preferred information provided verbally by their health care providers, but many also used printed material and videos (Risica and Phipps, 2006). In another study, men who had a radical prostatectomy and survived prostate cancer received care from advanced practice nurses that included patient education. The men reported that they were better able to communicate with their spouses and understand their illness after discharge from the hospital (McCorkle and others, 2007).

Tailored education also is effective in helping patients who have diabetes achieve control of their blood glucose levels. One study randomized patients who were on insulin pumps or who took multiple insulin injections into two groups. One group received frequent, individualized teaching, whereas the other group received standard care. The group that received the intensive teaching intervention achieved significantly better control of their blood glucose levels (Skeie and others, 2007). Another study also assigned patients with diabetes to two different groups. One group was asked to visit a website daily. They received intense educational interventions in text messages from their cellular phones and from the website. The other group received standard care. The patients who received the computerized educational intervention had significantly better blood glucose control (Kim, 2007). The results of these studies indicate that individualized educational interventions provided by nurses to meet the needs of vulnerable populations were successful in helping these patients attain positive outcomes.

Regardless of the population or the skill or information you present, the results of research indicate that individualized, interdisciplinary teaching efforts that are theoretically based are the most effective in promoting behavior change (Bastable, 2006; Levensky and others, 2007; Scharf Donovan, 2007). Therefore nurses need to lead and participate in interdisciplinary teams to provide individualized teaching and facilitate self-directed learning and problem solving in their patients.

CULTURAL CONSIDERATIONS IN HOME CARE TEACHING

When caring for patients from different cultures, you need to have knowledge of a patient's cultural background and beliefs, as well as the patient's ability to understand instructions developed outside of his or her native language. When educating patients of different ethnic groups, be aware of the distinctive aspects of each culture, being careful not to stereotype patients. Collaborate with other nurses and educators to assist in dealing with cultural diversity and ask for help from the people in the cultural group to share values and beliefs. Ethnic nurses are excellent resources who are able to provide input through their experiences to improve the care provided to members of their own community (Bastable, 2003). When patients cannot understand English, use certified health care interpreters to provide health care information (Cutilli, 2006; The Joint Commission [TJC], 2007a).

In addition, be aware of intergenerational conflict of values. This occurs when immigrant parents uphold their traditional values and their children, who are exposed to American values in social encounters, develop beliefs similar to those of their American peers. Consider this conflict in values when providing information to families or groups that have members from different generations. To enhance patient education in culturally diverse populations, know when and how to provide education while respecting cultural values. Modify teaching regarding interventions or desired behaviors to accommodate for cultural differences. Effective educational strategies often require you to use different patterns of communication (Cutilli, 2006; TJC, 2007a).

Skill Performance Guidelines

1 Assess the patient's and caregiver's physical, cognitive, emotional, cultural, environmental, and social resources to enhance successful learning and skill performance.

2 Present information in an understandable and orderly manner directed toward the patient's and caregiver's learning style and abilities.

3 Individualize the teaching care plan based on assessed physical, psychosocial, cultural, educational, and cognitive abilities of the patient and caregiver.

4 Assess if the patient in the home setting is able to safely perform a skill. If the patient is unable to execute the skill independently, identify a caregiver who will help provide the skill safely in the home setting.

5 Assess and determine if the patient has home medical equipment and is able to meet health care needs in the home environment to promote successful self-care management.

6 Include teaching interventions for other persons in the household who positively or negatively influence the patient's self-care management.

SKILL 42-1   Teaching Body Temperature Measurement

An elevation in body temperature sometimes is an early warning sign of serious health problems. Patients susceptible to temperature alterations (e.g., patients who are immunosuppressed) or their caregivers need to know how to measure temperature correctly so that they can seek medical attention early when alterations occur. Parents need to know how to measure their children's temperature because children can develop seriously high fevers very quickly,

and older adults or their caregivers need to know the techniques for temperature measurement because older adults have impaired temperature control mechanisms. Teach patients the skills of measuring body temperature and lowering temperature when a fever occurs at home.

A variety of body temperature thermometers are currently available, including mercury, disposable single-use, electronic digital, and tympanic thermometers. Mercury thermometers pose a significant risk to the environment and are not recommended. If a mercury thermometer breaks, and it is not disposed of properly, the mercury gets into the air, posing a major health risk in the home (Environmental Protection Agency [EPA], 2007). Educate patients about the environmental hazards associated with mercury in the home, and encourage patients to purchase mercury-free thermometers.

Help a patient choose the most appropriate thermometer to use in the home based on the patient's dexterity, vision, and financial resources. For example, a patient with visual changes from glaucoma or retinopathy is able to read a thermometer with a large digital display more easily. The need for an oral, rectal, or axillary temperature depends on the patient's age and health status. (See Chapter 5 for guidelines on use of all types of thermometers.)

Delegation Considerations
The skill of teaching patients to measure body temperature cannot be delegated to nursing assistive personnel (NAP).

Equipment
- ❑ Thermometer
- ❑ Disposable probe cover if thermometer requires it
- ❑ Water-soluble lubricant (for rectal measurements only)
- ❑ Paper or logbook and pencil or pen if frequent measurements are to be taken
- ❑ Disposable gloves (for rectal temperature taken by a caregiver)

STEP	RATIONALE
ASSESSMENT	
1 Assess patient's/caregiver's ability to manipulate and read thermometer. Have patient put on eyeglasses if necessary.	Physical restrictions in handling or reading thermometer prevent patient from being able to read thermometer and often require instruction of family member or significant other instead of patient.
2 Assess patient's knowledge of normal temperature range, symptoms of fever and hypothermia, and patient's risk for body temperature alterations.	Identifies patient's ability to initiate preventive health measures and recognize alterations in body temperature.
3 Assess patient's ability to determine appropriate type of thermometer to be used in varying situations (see Chapter 5).	Determines knowledge of age-related or medical conditions that determine selection of oral, rectal, or axillary temperature.
4 Assess patient's/caregiver's previous knowledge and experience in measuring temperature. Have patient/caregiver perform return demonstration if they indicate ability to measure temperature.	Allows assessment of patient's knowledge and use of safety precautions, aseptic technique, and time period for insertion.

NURSING DIAGNOSES

- Deficient knowledge regarding temperature measurement
- Health-seeking behaviors (temperature measurement)
- Readiness for enhanced therapeutic regimen management
- Risk for imbalanced body temperature
- Risk for infection

Individualize related factors based on patient's condition or needs.

PLANNING

1 Expected outcomes following completion of procedure:	
• Patient/caregiver is able to correctly measure temperature.	Indicates skills are effectively learned.
• Patient/caregiver demonstrates proper cleaning and storage of equipment.	Prevents transfer of microorganisms and maintains integrity of thermometer.
• Patient states normal temperature range and factors that affect temperature, signs and symptoms of fever and hypothermia, and measures to take with abnormal temperatures.	Cognitive learning is achieved.
2 Select setting in home where patient is most likely to measure temperature.	Practicing in same environment where skill is routinely performed facilitates comprehension and learning (Redman, 2007).
3 Discuss and demonstrate with patient or family member normal temperature ranges and proper way to position patient before thermometer insertion; instruct family member to remain with patient if age or physical status requires.	Discussion and demonstration promotes patient's understanding of comfort and safety principles, as well as technique to ensure accurate measurement (Bastable, 2006).

IMPLEMENTATION

1 Demonstrate steps of thermometer preparation, insertion, and reading. Provide rationale for steps to patient or caregiver.	Demonstration is best technique for teaching psychomotor skills (Falvo, 2004). Adults learn best when they understand purpose of procedure.

STEP	RATIONALE
2 Perform hand hygiene. If taking rectal temperature, instruct patient to lubricate tip with water-soluble lubricant, wear clean, disposable gloves, and use only rectal thermometer for rectal temperatures.	Lubrication prevents trauma to rectal tissue. Implementing body substance isolation prevents transmission of microorganisms.
3 Have patient perform each step with guidance from nurse. Do not rush patient.	Allows for correction of errors in technique as they occur and for discussion of potential consequences of errors.
4 Instruct patient to take temperature at least 30 minutes after smoking or ingesting hot or cold liquids or foods.	Waiting at least 30 minutes after drinking hot or cold liquids or foods improves accuracy of temperature reading (Quatrara and others, 2007).
5 Discuss common symptoms of fever: warm, dry, flushed skin; feeling warm; chills; piloerection; malaise; and restlessness.	Patient needs to recognize onset of fever in self or family member for early detection and intervention.
6 Discuss common signs and symptoms of hypothermia: cool skin, uncontrolled shivering, loss of memory, and signs of poor judgment. Explain that persons with inadequate home heating, older adults, or those unaware of potential dangers of cold conditions are at risk.	Patient needs to recognize onset of hypothermia in self or family member.

Critical Decision Point *Teach patient to take temperature after chills/shivering subsides to obtain an accurate temperature.*

STEP	RATIONALE
7 Discuss importance of notifying health care provider when temperature elevations occur, and review common therapies for temperature reduction that are safe to perform at home, including use of antipyretics, exposing the skin to air, reducing room temperature, increasing air circulation, applying cool moist compresses to the skin (e.g., forehead), and drinking fluids (Hockenberry and Wilson, 2007).	Treating fever enhances patient comfort (Hockenberry and Wilson, 2007).
8 Instruct patient in proper method for storing thermometer (when applicable), and select suitable storage location.	Thermometer is stored properly so it does not break or become inaccurate when not in use.
9 Provide set of written guidelines for patient's reference, and offer guidance regarding when additional action (such as notifying health care provider) needs to be taken.	Clear, concise written instructions that include pictures minimize anxiety and reinforce verbal instructions, enhancing learning and promoting patient confidence (Wingard, 2005).
10 Give patient a logbook or piece of paper to record temperature and the time temperature was taken if patient needs to measure temperatures frequently. Instruct patient to use written record to report temperatures to health care provider.	Keeping organized record of temperatures helps patient validate and report temperature fluctuations to health care provider.

EVALUATION

1 Have patient independently demonstrate technique for temperature measurement, including ability to read thermometer three separate times.	Feedback through return demonstration of psychomotor skill is best means of evaluating mastery of skill (Bastable, 2006).
2 Watch patient clean and store equipment.	Proper cleaning prevents bacterial growth, and proper storage preserves accuracy of thermometer.
3 Ask patient to identify normal temperature range and influence of smoking and hot and cold liquids or foods on oral readings; discuss safety implications for temperature measurement.	Measures cognitive learning and confirms understanding of information.
4 Have patient describe common signs and symptoms of fever and hypothermia and methods for control.	Measures cognitive learning.
5 *Optional:* Watch patient record temperature values and times in logbook. Review patient's logbook periodically to ensure that temperatures are being recorded correctly.	Health care providers make changes in patient care based on information provided by the patient. To ensure changes are made appropriately, patient needs to record accurate information.

Unexpected Outcomes	Related Interventions
1 Patient/caregiver is unable to measure temperature, clean thermometer correctly, or verbalize information about temperature that was taught.	• Ask patient/caregiver to describe difficulties experienced while performing temperature measurement. • Use a different teaching strategy. • Plan for patient to perform return demonstration during next scheduled home care visit, or plan to teach family caregiver.
2 Patient reports mercury glass thermometer has broken.	• Instruct patient in the steps to safely dispose of the thermometer (Box 42-1).

Recording and Reporting

- Record information taught and patient's response in home care record.
- Record temperature in home care record and home documentation system (e.g., logbook).

Teaching Considerations

- Instruct patient or family never to force thermometer into rectum and never to use rectal thermometer after rectal surgery, when the patient has a rectal disorder such as tumor or severe hemorrhoids, when the patient has a low platelet count, or when it is difficult to position patient for proper thermometer placement.
- Use caution in recommending aspirin or any other over-the-counter drug or antipyretic medicine in patients whose conditions contraindicate their use (e.g., gastric ulcer, bleeding tendencies, risk for Reye's syndrome in children, allergic reactions, drug interactions, liver or kidney dysfunction). Encourage patient to contact health care provider before using over-the-counter antipyretics.
- Instruct patient to never use sponging with isopropyl alcohol to lower fever because of neurotoxic effects (Hockenberry and Wilson, 2007).

Pediatric Considerations

- Stage of growth and development of child will determine site of measurement and type of equipment used (see Chapter 5).
- Different types of thermometers are available for use with children (e.g., temporal artery, tympanic, pacifier). Reliability of these different thermometers varies; ensure that parents know how to use the equipment correctly and how to detect the signs and symptoms of a fever (Braun, 2006; Robinson and others, 2005; Schuh and others, 2004).
- Teach the family to take a child's temperature whenever a child feels warm to the touch, even if the temperature was recently normal. Accurate assessment of a child's temperature positively affects the child's outcomes to a medical condition (Hockenberry and Wilson, 2007).

Gerontological Considerations

- Mean oral temperature for older adults often ranges from 35° to 36.1° C (95° to 97° F); therefore temperature considered within normal range sometimes reflects a fever in the older adult (Ebersole and others, 2008).
- Older adults are more sensitive to temperature changes and tend to demonstrate symptoms of delirium or dementia with variations of body temperature.
- Altered internal temperature regulation or dehydration occurs frequently in frail, debilitated patients. Temperature measurement becomes very important to prevent severe states of hypothermia or hyperthermia.
- Teaching sessions need to involve active learner participation. Patients learn best when they are rested and alert. Sessions need to be shorter in duration depending on factors such as fatigue.
- Consider common age-related sensory changes in the older adult, and direct teaching strategies to compensate for any alterations, such as a magnifying glass to read thermometer.

BOX 42-1 | **Steps to Take in the Event of a Mercury Spill**

- If possible, close the room off from the rest of the house, and increase ventilation in the affected room by opening windows or turning on a fan.
- Put on rubber or latex gloves. Do not touch mercury.
- Pick up glass pieces, place them in a folded paper towel, and place glass and towel into plastic zip lock bag.
- Use an eyedropper or a piece of heavy paper (e.g., playing card) to pick up visible mercury beads. Then put shaving cream on a small brush and "dot" the area or press duct tape in area to pick up smaller beads.
- Place mercury, material used to pick up mercury, and broken glass in a plastic zip lock bag. Triple bag the contaminated objects (place in a total of three sealed bags).
- Place gloves, mercury, and all other wastes into a trash bag. Secure and label the bag.
- Call local health department to determine where to dispose of mercury safely.
- If possible, keep windows open and room well ventilated for 2 days.
- Instruct patient not to use a vacuum cleaner, a broom, or household cleaners when cleaning up mercury spill. Also instruct patient not to put mercury down the drain or place contaminated clothing into the washing machine.

Data from Environmental Protection Agency: *Mercury,* 2007, http://www.epa.gov/mercury/index.htm.

SKILL 42-2 Teaching Blood Pressure and Pulse Measurement

Patients with a variety of illnesses such as cardiac, kidney, or vascular diseases are susceptible to wide variations in their blood pressure (BP) and pulse. They benefit from knowing how to assess their own BP and pulse because they are able to seek medical attention early when readings outside their acceptable ranges occur. Examples of patients who need to know these skills include those with heart disease and those involved in cardiac rehabilitation programs. In addition, healthy people who exercise learn how their body responds to exercise and are able to determine appropriate exercise plans based on knowing what their pulse and BP are before, during, and after exercise.

Research demonstrates that patients who frequently monitor their BP at home experience better BP control and have decreased health care costs (Canzanello and others, 2005; Cappuccio and others, 2004; Funahashi and others, 2006). Furthermore, measurements of BP and pulse help health care providers establish baseline data about their patients and analyze trends as a result of medications, exercise, or rehabilitation programs (Karavatas, 2005). In order to have this essential information about patients who are living at home, teach patients to measure their BP and pulse regularly and to interpret readings that are outside of individualized normal values. For example, teach patients about factors that affect the accuracy of BP readings such as cuff placement, movement of the tubing, and position of the patient.

Aneroid sphygmomanometers are available to measure BP in the home (see Chapter 5). Mercury manometers have a potential environmental risk associated with mercury and therefore have become less available. Aneroid manometers are safe, lightweight, compact, and portable. In the home, many patients choose to use electronic BP devices that are commercially available. These devices, which often also measure pulse rate, produce a BP measurement without needing to use a stethoscope. A cuff around the arm, the wrist, or a fingertip is used, and a reading is displayed electronically for the patient. Although electronic monitors are easier to use, they often provide systolic readings that are a little lower than the reading obtained by a health care professional, and the diastolic readings are often a little higher (Canzanello and others, 2005). Therefore it is essential to compare BP obtained by a health care provider with BP obtained by the electronic monitor to assess the accuracy of the home monitor.

One factor that affects the accuracy of BP monitoring is cuff size (Pickering and others, 2005). BP cuffs that are too small tend to overestimate BP, whereas cuffs that are too large tend to underestimate BP (Jones and others, 2003). Not all electronic home BP monitors come with interchangeable cuff sizes, further complicating the monitoring of BP at home. Help patients/caregivers investigate issues surrounding cuff size and calibration and accuracy of electronic equipment before they determine which type of BP monitor to purchase (Jones and others, 2003).

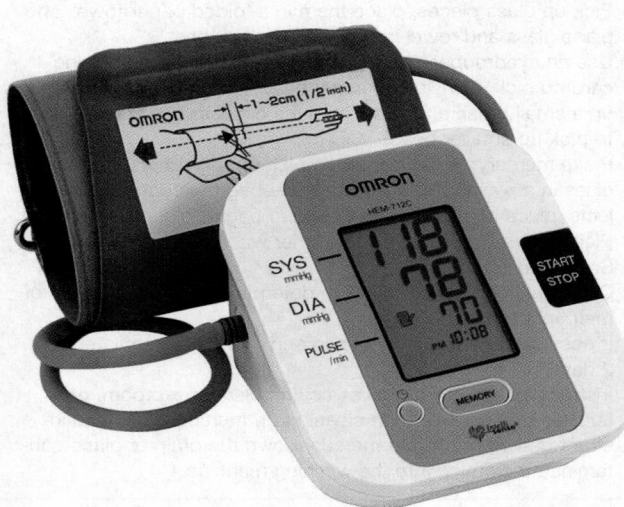

FIG 42-1   Home blood pressure monitoring device. (*Courtesy Omron Healthcare, Bannockburn, Illinois.*)

Delegation Considerations
The skill of teaching patients to measure BP and pulse cannot be delegated to NAP.

Equipment
For Blood Pressure
❑ Sphygmomanometer or electronic BP reading device (Fig. 42-1) with bladder and cuff: bladder should completely encircle arm without overlapping; cuff should be secure and fit snugly (Box 42-2)
❑ Stethoscope (two-headed teaching stethoscope is ideal) if using sphygmomanometer
For Pulse
❑ Wristwatch or clock with a second hand
For Both
❑ Pen or pencil and logbook or paper for recording

BOX 42-2	**Guidelines for Blood Pressure Cuff Size**

Adult Sizes
- For arm circumference of 22 to 26 cm, use "small adult" size: 12 × 22 cm
- For arm circumference of 27 to 34 cm, use "adult" size: 16 × 30 cm
- For arm circumference of 35 to 44 cm, use "large adult" size: 16 × 36 cm
- For arm circumference of 45 to 52 cm, use "adult thigh" size: 16 × 42 cm

Pediatric Sizes
- For newborn or premature infants, use "newborn" size: 4 × 8 cm
- For infants, use "infant" size: 6 × 12 cm
- For older children, use "child" size: 9 × 18 cm
- A standard adult cuff, a large adult cuff, and a thigh cuff for use in children with very large arms may be needed

Data from Pickering TG and others: Recommendations for blood pressure measurement in humans: an AHA scientific statement from the Council on High Blood Pressure Research Professional anad Public Education Subcommittee, *J Clin Hypertens* 7(2):102, 2005.

STEP	**RATIONALE**

ASSESSMENT

1 Assess patient's/caregiver's visual and auditory acuity, as well as ability to properly use BP monitoring equipment, see clock or watch with second hand, and/or feel pulse.

Physical restrictions affecting use of equipment requires adaptation of equipment or instruction of family member instead of patient.

2 Assess patient's knowledge of normal BP and pulse ranges and symptoms and common causes of high or low readings.

Identifies patient's ability to know when to initiate preventive health measures and recognize alterations in BP and pulse.

3 Assess patient's knowledge of what BP and pulse measure, specific medical issues that affect them, and why an awareness of variations is important to patient's well-being.

Identifies patient's understanding of potential cause-and-effect relationships between variations in BP and pulse and health status.

4 Assess patient's previous knowledge and experience in measuring BP. Have patient/caregiver perform return demonstration if they indicate ability to measure BP.

Allows nurse to assess patient's knowledge and skill performance.

STEP	RATIONALE
5 Assess home environment for a favorable place to measure BP and pulse (e.g., quiet room with a comfortable place to sit).	Ensures more accurate measurement.

NURSING DIAGNOSES

- Deficient knowledge regarding blood pressure/pulse monitoring
- Health-seeking behaviors (BP and pulse measurement)
- Ineffective health maintenance

Individualize related factors based on patient's condition or needs.

PLANNING

1 Expected outcomes following completion of procedure:	
• Patient/caregiver accurately monitors BP and pulse.	Learning has occurred.
• BP and pulse are within range expected for patient's age and condition (see Chapter 5).	Cardiovascular status is stable at level that is acceptable for patient.
• Patient explains importance of measuring BP and pulse, best time for measurement, and when to communicate with health care provider to evaluate changes in treatment regimen.	Measures cognitive learning.
2 Encourage patient to perform measurements on routine schedule for a long-term monitoring plan.	Daily activities and many extrinsic and intrinsic factors affect measurement fluctuations. A routine schedule allows for daily comparisons.
3 Encourage patient to avoid exercise, caffeine, and smoking for 30 minutes before assessment to avoid inaccurate reading.	These factors cause elevations in BP and pulse.
4 Have patient perform measurement in a comfortable position, with arm supported and feet flat on floor, and in warm and quiet environment.	Maintains patient's comfort during measurement. Systolic and diastolic BP increases with crossed-leg position.
5 In teaching phase, explain procedure to patient, and have patient rest at least 5 minutes before measurement.	Reduces anxiety that can falsely elevate readings.
6 Describe symptoms that indicate the need to perform BP and/or pulse measurement.	Promotes understanding of health status alterations that need medical intervention.

IMPLEMENTATION

1 Blood pressure measurement:	
a Discuss with patient the best sites for assessing BP. For self-measurement, brachial artery is almost always used. Explain to avoid applying cuff to arm with: • Intravenous (IV) catheter with or without fluids infusing • Arteriovenous shunt • Breast or axillary surgery • Trauma, inflammation, or disease • Cast or bulky bandage	Most accessible sites are easiest to measure for accuracy of assessment. Appropriate site selection promotes accuracy in reading and minimizes potential for trauma. Application of pressure from inflated bladder temporarily impairs blood flow and compromises circulation in extremity that already has impaired circulation.
b Demonstrate steps for measuring BP (see Chapter 5):	Demonstration is best technique for teaching psychomotor skill (Falvo, 2004).
(1) Use of sphygmomanometer and stethoscope:	
(a) Teach palpation of artery, positioning of cuff, wrapping of cuff, placement of stethoscope, inflation and release of cuff, listening for Korotkoff sounds.	Prepares patient/caregiver for measurement of BP.
(b) Describe sounds of measurement and relationship to observation of gauge during BP reading. Caution patient about level and length of time appropriate for cuff inflation.	Ensures accurate reading. Prolonged inflation of cuff impairs circulation of limb.
(c) Teach patient to routinely clean diaphragm of stethoscope with rubbing alcohol or damp cloth.	Stethoscopes are frequently contaminated with microorganisms. Cleaning stethoscope routinely prevents transmission of microorganisms.

Critical Decision Point *If patient/caregiver needs to use stethoscope to take BP, use double-headed teaching stethoscope to verify accuracy of reading, or perform BP 1 to 2 minutes after patient's attempt to verify accuracy. If patient is having difficulty hearing BP, ensure that patient is applying cuff appropriately and using the correct size cuff. Also determine correct use of equipment (e.g., cuff may have been deflated too quickly or too slowly; cuff may not have been pumped high enough for systolic readings).*

STEP	RATIONALE

(2) Use of electronic BP monitor:

    (a) Teach correct placement of cuff, use of electronic equipment for proper cuff inflation, and procedure for changing batteries.

Using electronic equipment correctly helps ensure accurate BP readings.

2 For pulse measurement:

  a Discuss with patient the best sites for assessing pulse: radial and carotid.

Radial and carotid sites are accessible and usually the easiest to palpate.

Critical Decision Point   *If carotid site is chosen, caution patient against vigorously massaging neck while attempting to locate pulse or attempting to locate both arteries at the same time. Stimulation of carotid sinus leads to reflex slowing of heart rate from vagal stimulation. In addition, simultaneous occlusion of both carotid arteries decreases blood to brain, resulting in fainting.*

  b Demonstrate steps for palpating pulse (see Chapter 5): position of artery on wrist or neck, how to locate artery, use of fingertips for palpation, compression of artery, palpation of pulse before counting, counting pulse, and calculating pulse rate.

Demonstration is best technique for teaching psychomotor skills.

    (1) Instruct use of gentle pressure; reinforce not to press hard over pulse site.

Pressing too hard may occlude the artery.

    (2) Instruct in use of watch or clock with a second hand to count pulse.

Ensures correct timing of pulse.

    (3) Instruct to count for a full 60 seconds, starting with second hand at 12:00 position.

Consistent timing of procedure will reduce confusion, forgetfulness about time period, or starting point used for pulse measurement. A full 60-second count increases accuracy of measure.

3 Educate patient about normal desired BP and pulse ranges, purposes for monitoring, and when to take measurements (e.g., before and after taking heart or antihypertensive medications; before, during, and after exercise).

Patient needs to be able to determine when values are not in desired ranges and when measurements need to be taken.

Critical Decision Point   *Discuss importance of notifying health care provider and withholding medications when abnormal values in BP or pulse occur (e.g., hypotension or bradycardia). Patient needs to understand preventive measures to take and to follow prescriber's directions if alterations develop.*

4 Have patient attempt each step of skill on nurse or family member.

Nurse can correct any errors in technique as they occur.

5 Observe patient demonstrate techniques on self (see illustration). When measuring BP, do not allow multiple repetitive BP attempts on any one limb.

After developing confidence in measuring values in others, patient is ready to measure own values. Making repeated BP attempts restricts circulation.

6 Teach patient to monitor BP and pulse even if they remain in normal range.

Continuous monitoring provides important information that evaluates effectiveness of medications or other treatments.

7 Provide patient with printed instructions with written or pictorial guide, or provide patient with a videotape demonstrating procedure if possible.

Printed and audiovisual references for patient promote confidence for independent performance (Bastable, 2006).

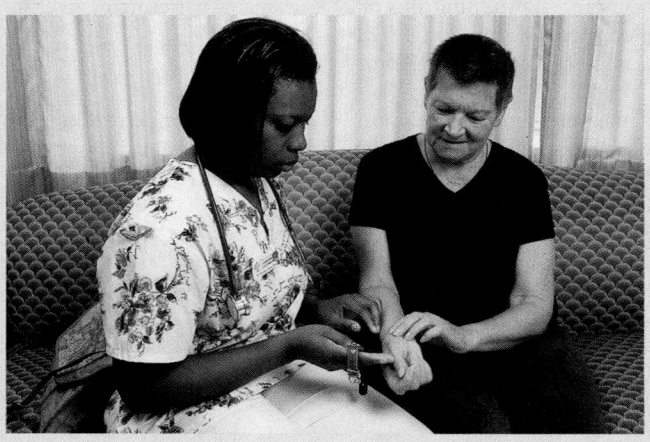

STEP 5   Nurse observing patient checking pulse.

STEP	RATIONALE
8 Give patient a logbook or piece of paper to record BP and pulse and the time they were taken. In addition, patient records whether or not medications that affect BP or pulse were taken. Instruct patient to use written record to report readings to health care provider.	Keeping organized record of BP and pulse readings and medications empowers patient and provides accurate information to health care providers (Rassin and others, 2007).
9 Instruct patient in proper care of equipment (e.g., storage, cleaning, and battery care).	Improper care and storage of equipment affects accuracy of measurement.

EVALUATION

1 Observe patient demonstrate technique for BP and/or pulse measurement on at least three different occasions, and verify patient adds information to logbook correctly.	Feedback through return demonstration of psychomotor learning is best means to evaluate learning (Bastable, 2006).
2 Ask patient if readings are within desired range and when to report abnormal readings to health care provider.	Determines patient's ability to know when readings are within proper range and what to do when abnormal readings are obtained.
3 Ask patient to describe reason for BP and pulse monitoring and any related medications (e.g., antihypertensives, antidysrhythmics) or treatment (e.g., diet and exercise).	Determines if patient understands monitoring and related therapies.
4 Have patient demonstrate proper care of equipment.	Demonstrates learning.

Unexpected Outcomes	Related Interventions
1 Patient or caregiver is unable to measure BP or pulse due to cognitive or sensory problems (e.g., inability to manipulate equipment, visualize numbers on equipment or clock).	• Alter teaching plan to accommodate patient's problems (e.g., use other types of equipment that are easier to manipulate, see, or hear). • Reinforce information taught, and continue to plan return demonstrations until patient is able to perform skill. • Teach skill to family, friend, or other caregiver.
2 Patient has difficulty in explaining purposes of measurement or implications of therapy.	• Review and reinforce information that patient does not understand.

Recording and Reporting

• Record teaching and patient responses in home care record.
• Record BP and pulse in home care record and home documentation system (e.g., logbook).

Teaching Considerations

• Educate patient about risks for hypertension (see Chapter 5).
• Ensure patient understands prescriber's recommendations for treatment regimen, including potential side effects and interactions of any medication therapies. For example, educate patient about when to withhold medications in event of alterations in BP or pulse alteration. Instruct patients taking thyroid medications to withhold medications when BP is above normal range or pulse is above 100 beats per minute. Beta-adrenergic blockers (e.g., propranolol), calcium channel blockers (e.g., verapamil hydrochloride), or cardiac glycosides (e.g., digoxin) often are withheld if BP is below normal range and/or pulse is below 60 beats per minute. Confirm specific guidelines for BP and pulse with prescriber, document information in home care record, and provide clear, written instructions for the patient.

Pediatric Considerations

• Readings (BP or pulse) are often inaccurate if the infant or child is anxious and uncooperative. BP is also inaccurate when the cuff size is inappropriate. Having others divert the child's attention or taking the child's BP or pulse while the child is seated on the parent's lap usually helps calm the child (Hockenberry and Wilson, 2007).

• Young children will be more likely to cooperate if allowed to touch and/or play with equipment before procedure. Consider performing the procedure first on the parent or another person significant to child. This allows the child to observe that the procedure is safe.
• Use the radial pulse in children over 2 years of age. Femoral or brachial pulse is best site for palpation of pulse for children under 2 (Hockenberry and Wilson, 2007; White and others, 2004). The older the child, the easier it will be for the parent to assess heart rate (White and others, 2004).
• In infants, teach parents to observe and count the pulse on anterior fontanel. Remind parents **not** to palpate the pulse.

Gerontological Considerations

• Musculoskeletal changes such as arthritis or other joint conditions may impair abilities to position limb comfortably and/or perform fine motor skills required for patient to measure BP and pulse (Meiner and Lueckenotte, 2006).
• Older adults, especially those who are frail or who have lost upper arm mass, require a smaller BP cuff.
• Current national guidelines support that normal BP limits are the same regardless of age. Therefore older adults need to maintain a BP less than 120/80 mm Hg. Patients with hypertension and diabetes or renal disease need to have blood pressures less than 130/80 (National Institutes of Health [NIH], 2003).
• Home BP monitoring is not a replacement for BP monitoring by health care professionals in older adults, but it reduces the number of required office visits if the older adult patient is able

to accurately use the equipment and if the equipment is accurate (Cappuccio and others, 2004).

- Teach older adult patients how to exercise safely. Cardiac output is lower in older adults. Therefore the heart cannot adapt as well to sudden demands for increased oxygen (Ebersole and others, 2008). Use the following calculation to determine a safe maximum heart rate during exercise in the older adult population: (220 − age) × 0.70. For example, if the patient is 77 years old, using this formula yields a safe maximum heart rate of 100 beats per minute.

SKILL 42-3 Teaching Intermittent Self-Catheterization

Most patients urinate and empty their bladder four or five times a day. However, some patients are not able to empty their bladders. Infections in the bladder or kidneys and damage to the kidneys sometimes result from incomplete emptying of the bladder. Clean intermittent self-catheterization (CIC) is a safe and effective way to empty the bladder. Patients who use CIC have a variety of health problems that affect the neuromuscular control of the bladder (e.g., spinal cord injury, multiple sclerosis, spina bifida, bladder outlet obstruction, or continent urinary diversion). In the past, nurses used strict aseptic technique when inserting intermittent or indwelling urinary catheters in hospital or home settings. However, current research shows that CIC does not increase the risk for urinary tract infections (UTIs) (Society of Urologic Nurses and Associates [SUNA], 2006). Today, some hospital policies recommend sterile technique, whereas others recommend clean technique (Lemke and others, 2005). In the home setting, clean technique is recommended because when patients are in their home, they are not exposed to bacterial organisms that will cause urinary tract infections (SUNA, 2006).

Using CIC has several benefits. For example, some patients feel that they are more in control of their care, which enhances their quality of life. CIC also helps some patients become continent again, maintain a positive body image, and experience less anxiety and embarrassment. In addition, CIC allows patients to express their sexuality and sustain satisfying relationships with significant others. However, the skill requires physical and manual dexterity, and patients sometimes experience urinary tract infections, inflammation of the urethra (urethritis), and urethral bleeding (Roberts and Naik, 2006; Robinson, 2007). When the patient is unable to perform CIC independently, teach the patient's significant other or caregiver how to perform the skill.

Delegation Considerations
The skill of teaching intermittent self-catheterization cannot be delegated to NAP.

Equipment
- ❑ Soap, water, and clean washcloth
- ❑ Mirror *(optional)*
- ❑ Urethral catheter (smallest size that is able to pass easily into the bladder and completely drain the patient's urine)
- ❑ Lubricant (e.g., water-soluble jelly)
- ❑ Container for collection of urine (e.g., urinal)—not needed for patients emptying urine directly into toilet
- ❑ Mild soap (e.g., Ivory)
- ❑ Catheter storage item or container (e.g., brown paper bag, clean towel)
- ❑ Paper or logbook and pencil or pen *(optional)*

STEP	RATIONALE

ASSESSMENT

1. Review patient's medical record, including order for CIC, and nurses' notes. Gather information about voiding history, existing medical and surgical history, patient's usual daily fluid intake, postvoid residual amounts, and daily voiding routine.

Determines reason for CIC, frequency of catheterization, and previous responses to patient education (Robinson, 2006a).

2. Assess patient's ability to perform CIC, including developmental level, level of consciousness, motor function, and psychosocial status.

Physical or cognitive impairment indicates need to teach family member or other caregiver. Psychological aspects of CIC (e.g., embarrassment, fear, poor self-image) interfere with successful teaching (Robinson, 2006a).

3. Assess patient's and/or caregiver's knowledge about CIC, and observe performance of CIC.

Effective patient education builds on previous knowledge; observation is effective way to evaluate performance of psychomotor skills (Bastable, 2006).

NURSING DIAGNOSES

- Impaired urinary elimination
- Overflow urinary incontinence
- Readiness for enhanced therapeutic regimen management
- Readiness for enhanced urinary elimination
- Reflex urinary incontinence
- Urinary retention

Individualize related factors based on patient's condition or needs.

PLANNING

1. Expected outcomes following completion of procedure:
   - Patient or family caregiver states signs and symptoms that indicate need for CIC.

Indicates patient or family member is able to identify appropriate times to use CIC.

STEP	RATIONALE
• Patient or family correctly demonstrates how to perform CIC and clean and store equipment.	Return demonstration of skill indicates learning (Bastable, 2006).
• Patient or family verbalizes signs and symptoms of complications of CIC (e.g., UTI, urethral bleeding) and when to contact health care provider.	Urinary complications are common in patients who use CIC (Kovindha and others, 2004). Verbalization of signs and symptoms of complications helps patients identify potential problems early and seek appropriate care.
2 Select setting in home that patient or family will most likely use when performing CIC.	Practicing skill in home setting where it is routinely performed decreases anxiety and enhances patient learning (Robinson, 2007).
3 Help patient select catheter that is the easiest to use, causes the least amount of trauma, and is the most comfortable. Some patients use different catheters depending on whether they are at home or are out (Robinson, 2007).	A variety of single-use and reusable catheters are currently available.

IMPLEMENTATION

STEP	RATIONALE
1 Teach patient how to perform appropriate hand hygiene using soap and water.	Prevents risk for urinary infection and trauma, which can lead to urethral strictures (Robinson, 2006a).
2 Help patient get into a comfortable position in a place that has adequate lighting.	Patient needs adequate lighting to perform skill. Some men prefer to stand, whereas others prefer to sit. Female patients often need to try different positions to decide which position is the most comfortable (Robinson, 2007; SUNA, 2006).
3 Teach patient how to clean urethral meatus:	
a *For women:* Teach patient to spread labia with one hand and cleanse urethral opening with warm soapy water and a clean washcloth with the other hand.	Retraction of labia allows for female urethral meatus to be cleaned, reducing risk for infection.
b *For men:* If patient has not been circumcised, teach patient to retract foreskin to expose urethral meatus. Teach patient to hold penis perpendicular to the body with one hand and cleanse urethral opening with warm soapy water and a clean washcloth with the other hand.	Ensures cleaning of meatus and reduces risk for infection.
4 Teach female patient how to insert catheter:	
a Using mirror, help patient locate meatus. Explain it is just below the clitoris and just above the vaginal opening.	Mirror helps female patient visualize anatomy.

Critical Decision Point *If female patient is unable to visualize anatomy or wants to learn how to find meatus while in a sitting position, teach touch technique by helping patient use fingers to find her clitoris and her vaginal opening. Teach patient to put one finger over the clitoris and another finger over the vaginal opening. Then, help her use these two fingers to find the urethral opening. Another method is the tunnel technique. When women sit with their hips flexed forward, the labia create a "tunnel" that leads to the urethral opening. Teach the woman to slightly separate labia near the clitoris and angle the catheter backward into the urethral opening while placing a finger over the vaginal opening (Williams, 2005).*

STEP	RATIONALE
b Lubricate tip of catheter with water-soluble jelly. Rotate tip to spread lubricant around bottom 2.5 to 5 cm (1 to 2 inches) of catheter.	Lubrication reduces urethral trauma.
c Place outflow end of catheter into urine collection container or let hang over toilet bowl. Slowly and gently insert the tip of the catheter 5 to 10 cm (2 to 4 inches) into the meatus until urine begins to flow.	Appearance of urine indicates catheter tip is in bladder.

Critical Decision Point *If patient feels resistance at the internal sphincter, teach patient to apply firm, gentle, steady pressure until muscles relax and allow catheter to pass (SUNA, 2006).*

STEP	RATIONALE
5 Teach male patient how to insert catheter:	
a Lubricate the tip of catheter with water-soluble jelly. Rotate tip to spread lubricant around bottom 13 to 18 cm (5 to 7 inches) of catheter.	Lubrication reduces urethral trauma.
b Place outflow end of catheter into urine collection container or let hang over toilet bowl. Slowly and gently insert the tip of the catheter 15 to 20 cm (6 to 8 inches) into the meatus until urine begins to flow. Tell patient catheter often needs to be inserted to the end of the catheter for urine to begin to flow.	Male urethra is longer than female urethra. Flow of urine indicates catheter tip is in bladder.

STEP	RATIONALE

Critical Decision Point *Some men experience some resistance when the catheter reaches the prostatic urethra or the neck of the bladder. If patient feels resistance, teach him to apply firm, gentle, steady pressure to fatigue the external sphincter and cause muscle relaxation (SUNA, 2006).*

STEP	RATIONALE
6 Instruct patient to hold catheter in place while urine flows into container or toilet.	Release of catheter during procedure often causes catheter to accidentally come out before bladder is completely emptied.
7 When the urine flow stops, teach patient to slowly and gently remove the catheter and perform hand hygiene.	Removing catheter slowly allows the pockets of urine that can accumulate at base of bladder to drain (SUNA, 2006).
8 Give patient logbook or piece of paper to record amount of urine if needed.	Some patients need to keep track of their urinary output.
9 Instruct patient to clean catheter with mild soap (e.g., Ivory) and water immediately after use. Rinse catheter completely and allow to air dry then store in a clean dry towel or in a brown paper bag.	Prevents urinary tract infections.
10 Teach patient to replace catheter every month or when it becomes cracked or brittle, has any build up of sediment, or loses its form.	Appropriate disposal and replacement of equipment prevents complications of CIC (Oh and others, 2006; SUNA, 2006).

EVALUATION

1 Observe patient independently demonstrate technique for CIC.	Feedback through return demonstration of psychomotor skill is best means of evaluating learning of skill.
2 Ask patient to identify plan for timing of CIC and steps to take when problems arise.	Measures patient's cognitive learning and ability to problem solve.
3 Review patient's logbook, and observe patient enter information about urine output if indicated.	Confirms patient understands record keeping and importance of tracking urine output.

Unexpected Outcomes	Related Interventions
1 Patient is unable to easily pass catheter into bladder.	• Teach patient not to force catheter into bladder. • Tell patient to go to nearest urgent care center or emergency department if bladder is full and patient is unable to insert catheter. • Consider initiating consultation with urologist.
2 Patient states he or she is having symptoms of UTI (e.g., flank or abdominal pain, malaise, fever, chills).	• Inform patient's health care provider of symptoms, and anticipate treatment with antibiotic.

Recording and Reporting

- Record information taught and patient's response in home care record.
- Record urine output in home care record and home documentation system (e.g., logbook).

Teaching Considerations

- Patients who perform CIC routinely will usually have abnormal findings (e.g., blood or small amounts of bacteria in urine). Teach them that this is to be expected and that taking antibiotics routinely is not recommended (SUNA, 2006).

Pediatric Considerations

- Children who are motivated and are physiologically and developmentally ready need to learn how to catheterize themselves (SUNA, 2006).
- When teaching children CIC, use developmentally appropriate teaching strategies, such as role play, games, computers, and written materials with pictures (Bray and Sanders, 2007; Merenda, 2005).

- Concerns of children and adolescents who use CIC include leakage and being wet. They also are often concerned about what their peers know. Allow children to voice their concerns, and help them problem solve what they will do in a variety of situations (Edwards and others, 2004).

Gerontological Considerations

- Current evidence shows CIC is very effective in older adults. For example, it helps restore continence, decreases urinary urge and nocturia, and improves quality of life (Pilloni and others, 2005).
- Musculoskeletal and/or neurological changes such as arthritis or cerebral vascular accident (stroke) often impair a patient's ability to manipulate catheter or get into a comfortable position for CIC. Try different adaptive devices to enable patient to be independent if possible. If adaptive device does not work, instruct a caregiver to perform the procedure (Robinson, 2006b; Robinson, 2007).

SKILL 42-4   Using Home Oxygen Equipment

Home oxygen therapy is usually administered via nasal cannula or different types of masks (e.g., simple mask, reservoir mask, or non-rebreather mask) (Duck, 2006; Edwards, 2006). When a patient has a permanent tracheostomy, however, a T tube or tracheostomy collar is used. Oxygen-conserving devices (OCDs) reduce the amount of oxygen the patient uses, resulting in an overall cost reduction to the patient (Lewarski, 2006). There are three types of OCDs:

1 *Reservoir nasal cannula:* Stores oxygen in a chamber during the expiratory phase of respirations
2 *Demand oxygen delivery systems:* Deliver a burst of oxygen only during inspiration
3 *Transtracheal oxygen catheter:* Delivers oxygen through a catheter permanently inserted into the trachea, thus allowing the patient to speak and bypassing anatomical dead space (Petty and others, 2005) (Table 42-1)

In the home, three types of oxygen delivery systems are available: compressed oxygen, oxygen concentrators (Fig. 42-2, A), and liquid oxygen. Some oxygen tanks are large and stationary.

Portable tanks are easy to move, weigh more than 10 lb, are not designed to be carried (Fig. 42-2, B), and deliver oxygen for about 5 hours at 2 L/min. Ambulatory tanks weigh less than 10 lb, are designed to be carried, and deliver oxygen for at least 4 hours at 2 L/min. Table 42-2 compares the different types of home oxygen delivery systems.

Compressed oxygen requires a regulator and flowmeter. The patient receives delivery of several large oxygen tanks to the home. The size of the tank and flow rate determine how long compressed oxygen tanks will last (Table 42-3). Liquid systems take up less space because oxygen is stored in a liquid state. Liquid oxygen is stored at or below −297° F and requires the use of a small ambulatory tank that is filled from a reservoir in the home (Fig. 42-3). Table 42-4 shows how long a liquid oxygen system will last depending on the prescribed flow rate. The oxygen concentrator method extracts oxygen from the room air and supplies oxygen to the patient at prescribed flow rates. Oxygen concentrators deliver a lower percentage of oxygen to the flowmeter. Therefore, if a patient is switched to a concentrator, the flow rate usually needs to be

TABLE 42-1	Oxygen Flow and Appropriate Uses for Oxygen Delivery Devices		
Device	**Flow (L/min)**	**FiO₂ Range (%)**	**Uses**
Nasal cannula	¼-8	22-45	Patients receiving long-term oxygen therapy
Transtracheal catheter	¼-4	22-45	Patients who require high oxygen flow through a tracheostomy tube
Simple oxygen mask	6-12	35-50	Patients who require short-term oxygen therapy with moderate FiO₂ needs
Reservoir mask	6-10	35-60	Patients in acute respiratory distress with moderate FiO₂ needs
Nonrebreather mask	10-15	80-100	Patients in acute respiratory failure or in emergency situations

Data from Petty TL: *Guide to prescribing home oxygen: home oxygen options,* National Lung Health Education Program, http://www.nlhep.org/resources/Prescrb-Hm-Oxygen/home-oxygen-options-4.html, accessed November 17, 2007.

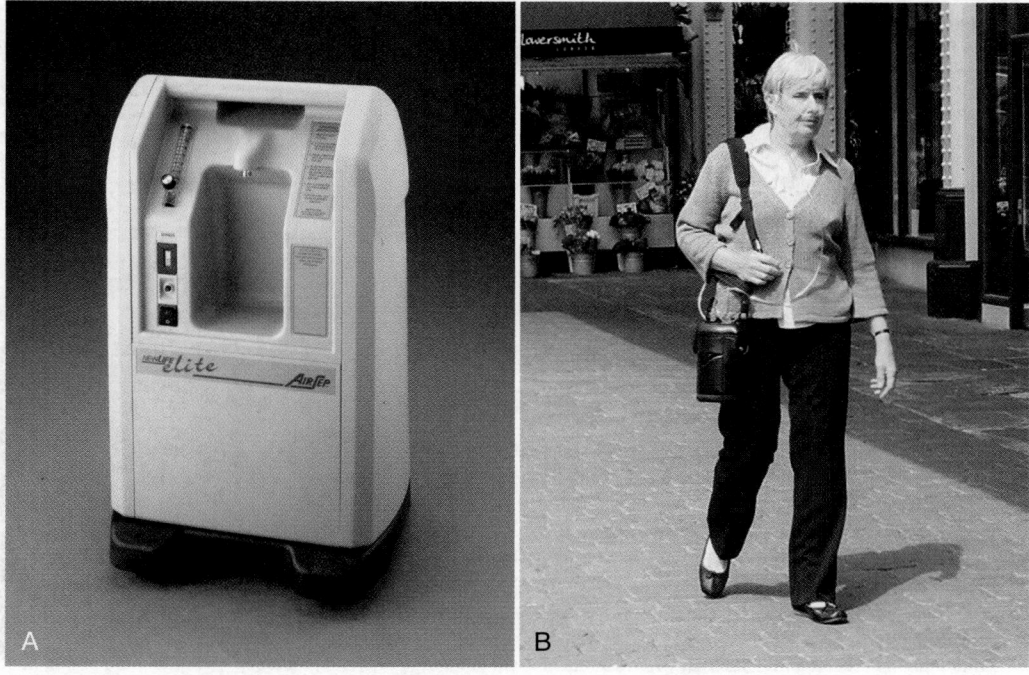

FIG 42-2   **A,** Portable oxygen concentrator for home use. **B,** Ambulatory tank is small enough to be easily carried. (*Courtesy AirSep Corporation.*)

TABLE 42-2 | Home Oxygen Systems

Primary Use	Advantages	Disadvantages
Compressed Oxygen Intermittent therapy, such as for exercise or sleep only	100% oxygen stored in steel or aluminum cylinders; relatively inexpensive; no loss of gas during storage; relatively portable; delivery of up to 15 L/min; does not require electrical source; smaller tanks available	Bulky and heavy; frequent refilling necessary with continuous use; patient must know how to read regulator and must understand when to call medical supplier for replacement cylinder; portable cylinders weigh 15 lb and empty quickly when in use; may require weekly deliveries
Liquid Oxygen Systems System of choice for high-volume users and active patients	100% oxygen; more oxygen can occupy a smaller space; convenient ambulatory units refilled at home can be carried as a shoulder bag, backpack, or wheeled luggage cart; delivery of up to 6 L/min; patient can be taught how to safely fill ambulatory units from larger reservoir; quiet and easy operation; does not require electricity for operation; requires relatively fewer deliveries of oxygen (as few as 8 times per year)	Evaporates, especially in warmer temperatures and when not in use; potential for connections to freeze together or form frost at connections if tight connection not maintained during filling; can be costly in setup and delivery fees
Concentrators Cost-effective for patients requiring low-flow continuous oxygen and patients with limited mobility inside or outside home	Inexpensive, fixed monthly costs; most units with delivery of up to 4 or 5 L/min; good choice for people who do not leave their homes frequently; no cylinders or tanks to refill	Oxygen concentration decreases as liter flow increases (usually 85% to 90%); power supply necessary; increased electrical costs (around $30 or more a month); is not an ambulatory unit, therefore requires second system for portability (usually gas cylinders); requires regular maintenance and a backup system

Data from Petty TL: *Guide to prescribing home oxygen: home oxygen options,* National Lung Health Education Program, http://www.nlhep.org/resources/Prescrb-Hm-Oxygen/home-oxygen-options-4.html, accessed November 17, 2007.

TABLE 42-3 | Oxygen Cylinder Timetable*

	Large (H-K) Tank		Small (E) Tank	
L/min	**2200 lb** **Full**	**1000 lb** **½ Full**	**625 L** **Full**	**284 L** **½ Full**
1	115 hr	52 hr	10 hr	5 hr
2	56 hr	26 hr	5 hr	2 hr
3	37 hr	17 hr	3 hr	1 hr
4	28 hr	13 hr	3 hr	1 hr
5	22 hr	10 hr	2 hr	54 min
6	18 hr	8 hr	<2 hr	47 min

The following formulas can also be used to determine the length of time a tank will last:

For E Cylinders
Pressure on cylinder gauge (psi) − 500 psi (safety factor) × 0.3 (E cylinder factor) ÷ L/min = minutes

For H Cylinders
Pressure on cylinder gauge (psi) − 500 psi (safety factor) × 3.1 (H cylinder factor) ÷ L/min = minutes

EXAMPLE: If E cylinder reads 1500 psi and liter flow rate is 4 L/min
Time left: 1500 − 500 × 0.3 ÷ 4 = 1000 × 0.3 ÷ 4 = 300 ÷ 4 = 75 minutes (1 hr 15 min)
NOTE: Do not allow oxygen cylinder pressure to fall below 500 psi, or the patient may run out of oxygen.

*All times are approximate.

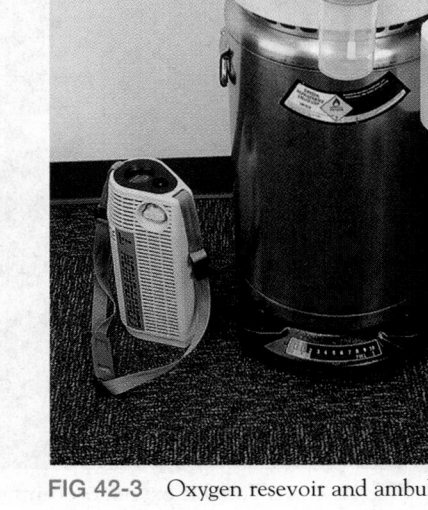

FIG 42-3   Oxygen resevoir and ambulatory tank.

adjusted. The patient who uses a concentrator needs to have a backup system, such as a portable oxygen tank, in case of power failure.

Home oxygen equipment is designated as durable medical equipment (DME) in the home care setting. Governmental or private insurance often pays for home oxygen therapy if there are written orders prescribed by the physician or advanced practice nurse. A certificate of medical necessity (CMN) is required for patients who receive Medicare (Centers for Medicare and Medicaid Services, 2006). Specific guidelines need to be met before Medicare coverage begins (Box 42-3).

Patients requiring home oxygen need extensive teaching to use their oxygen therapy efficiently and safely. To enhance home safety, The Joint Commission's 2008 Home Care National Patient Safety Goals (2007c) require completion of a home risk appraisal that includes presence of working smoke detectors, fire extinguishers, and a home safety plan. In addition, provide patient education about the safe use of oxygen in the home (Box 42-4). When initiating and managing ongoing oxygen therapy, collaborate with the patient, prescriber, caregivers, DME provider, and payer.

Delegation Considerations

The skill of teaching patients how to use home oxygen equipment cannot be delegated to NAP.

Equipment
- Nasal cannula, oxygen mask (see Skill 23-1), OCD, or other prescribed delivery device
- Oxygen tubing
- Home oxygen delivery system (compressed oxygen, oxygen concentrator, or liquid oxygen) with all required equipment (varies with supplier and system used)
- "No Smoking/Oxygen in Use" sign for each entrance to the home

TABLE 42-4 Liquid Oxygen Timetable

	Stationary Reservoirs		Portable Units	
L/min	41 L	31 L	½ L	1 L
0.25	1400 hr	1060 hr	28 hr	44 hr
0.50	1125 hr	850 hr	18 hr	27 hr
1	560 hr	425 hr	9 hr	15½ hr
1.5	375 hr	283½ hr	6 hr	11½ hr
2	281 hr	213 hr	4½ hr	8½ hr
3	187½ hr	142 hr	3 hr	6 hr

BOX 42-3 Medicare Qualifications for Home Oxygen Therapy

Oxygen Therapy at Rest
- PaO_2 ≤55 mm Hg or SaO_2 ≤88% at room air
- PaO_2 = 56-59 mm Hg or SaO_2 ≤89% *and one of the following:*
  - Dependent edema suggesting congestive heart failure
  - Cor pulmonale or pulmonary hypertension as evidenced on ECG, echocardiogram, gated blood pool scan, or pulmonary artery pressure measurement
  - Erythrocythemia as evidenced by hematocrit >56%

Nocturnal Oxygen Therapy
- PaO_2 ≥56 mm Hg or SaO_2 ≥89% at room air while awake *and one of the following:*

- PaO_2 ≤55 mm Hg or SaO_2 ≤88% during sleep
- PaO_2 falls more than 10 mm Hg during sleep
- SaO_2 falls more than 5% with signs and symptoms of hypoxemia during sleep

Exercise Oxygen Therapy
- PaO_2 ≥56 mm Hg or SaO_2 ≥89% at room air while at rest *and one of the following:*
  - PaO_2 ≤55 mm Hg during exercise
  - SaO_2 ≤88% during exercise

Data from Positive Air, Inc: *Medicare requirements for the home use of oxygen,* http://positiveair.com/medicare_home_use_of_oxygen.htm, accessed November 17, 2007. *PaO₂,* Arterial oxygen tension (partial pressure); *SaO₂,* oxygen saturation in blood; *ECG,* electrocardiogram.

BOX 42-4 Safe Home Oxygen Therapy Principles

Fire Safety
- Although oxygen is not flammable, it will support combustion, therefore:
  - Use and store oxygen in a well-ventilated area.
  - Do not use petroleum-based ointments (e.g., Vaseline) around the nose—use of these ointments could cause burns.
  - Keep all oxygen equipment at least 8 feet from open flames (e.g., matches, fireplaces, stoves, space heaters, candles).
  - Do not allow smoking in the house.
  - Avoid using electrical appliances that produce sparks (e.g., electric razors).
  - Install smoke detectors, and have a fire extinguisher available in the home.
  - Help patient and family plan a fire evacuation route.

Oxygen Storage and Handling
- Store oxygen tanks upright in carts or stands to prevent tipping or falling, or place tanks flat on the floor when not in use.

- Do not store oxygen tanks in the trunk of a car.
- When transporting oxygen in a vehicle, ensure tanks are secured properly in the passenger area with the windows opened 2 to 3 inches to allow adequate ventilation.

Concentrator Safety
- Plug concentrators into properly grounded outlets.
- Do not use extension cords, power strips, or multioutlet adapters with concentrators.
- Ensure power supply or circuit meets or exceeds the amperage requirements of the concentrator.

Liquid Oxygen Safety
- Avoid direct contact with liquid oxygen because it can cause frostbite.
- Do not touch connectors that are frosted or icy.
- Keep ambulatory tanks upright; do not lay them down or place on their side.

Data from City of Tyler, Texas: *Home oxygen safety,* 2007, http://www.cityoftyler.org/Default.aspx?tabid5707.

STEP	RATIONALE

ASSESSMENT

1 While patient is still in the hospital, determine patient's or family's ability to use oxygen equipment correctly (if appropriate and possible). In the home setting reassess for appropriate use of equipment.

Physical or cognitive impairments indicate need to instruct family member or significant other in how to operate home oxygen equipment. Determines specific components of skill that patient and family are able to easily complete.

2 Assess home environment for adequate electrical service if oxygen concentrator is used.

Oxygen concentrators require electricity to work (Petty, 2007). Continuous oxygen therapy must not be interrupted.

3 Assess patient's and/or family's knowledge of purpose of oxygen and ability to observe for signs and symptoms of hypoxia: apprehension, anxiety, decreased ability to concentrate, decreased levels of consciousness, increased fatigue, dizziness, behavioral changes, increased pulse, increased respiratory rate, pallor, and cyanosis.

Hypoxia sometimes occurs at home when patient uses oxygen. Possible causes of hypoxia include poor tubing connections, use of long oxygen tubing, or worsening of patient's physical problem with a change in respiratory status.

4 Determine appropriate resources in community for equipment and assistance, including maintenance and repair services and medical equipment supplier.

Ensures readily available assistance for patients with home oxygen systems.

5 Determine appropriate backup systems for compressor in event of power failure (e.g., notify local emergency medical services [EMS]). Have a spare oxygen tank available for emergency use.

Many municipalities require that patients who have home oxygen equipment notify EMS before putting the equipment in the home. When there is a power outage, EMS will call the home, and in some cases the home is on priority list for having power restored.

NURSING DIAGNOSES

- Anxiety
- Deficient knowledge regarding home oxygen therapy
- Ineffective health maintenance

Individualize related factors based on patient's condition or needs.

PLANNING

1 Expected outcomes following completion of procedure:
- Patient receives oxygen at the prescribed rate.
- Patient and family will verbalize purpose and correct use of home oxygen.
- Patient and family will demonstrate how to maintain oxygen system.
- Patient and family will state indications for calling DME provider to replenish oxygen supply and reorder oxygen delivery supplies.
- Patient and family will verbalize safety guidelines for oxygen use (e.g., place "No Smoking/Oxygen in Use" signs at entrances to home).
- Patient and family will verbalize emergency plan of care.

Oxygen system set up correctly.
Provides measurable criteria to determine level of understanding.

Provides return demonstration of skills needed to use home oxygen system.
Patient needs constant supply of oxygen at home.

Provides measure of understanding of oxygen use.

Ensures safe, continuous delivery of home oxygen.

2 Select setting in home where patient is most likely to use oxygen equipment.

Practicing in same environment where skill is routinely performed facilitates comprehension and learning.

IMPLEMENTATION

1 Perform hand hygiene.

Reduces transmission of microorganisms.

2 Place oxygen delivery system in a clutter-free environment that is well ventilated, away from walls, drapes, curtains, bedding, combustible materials, and at least 8 feet from heat sources (City of Tyler, Texas, 2007).

Keeps system balanced and prevents injury.

Critical Decision Point   *Do not place oxygen delivery system in a closet.*

3 Demonstrate steps for preparation and completion of oxygen therapy:
  a Compressed oxygen system:
    (1) Turn cylinder valve counterclockwise two to three turns with wrench.

Demonstration is reliable technique for teaching psychomotor skill (Falvo, 2004) and enables patient to ask questions.

Turns on oxygen.

STEP	RATIONALE
(2) Check cylinders by reading amount on pressure gauge.	Verifies adequate oxygen supply for patient use.
(3) Store wrench with oxygen tank or in other safe place.	Storing wrench in a safe place ensures it is available whenever needed.
b Oxygen concentrator system:	
(1) Plug concentrator into appropriate outlet.	Provides power safely to concentrator.
(2) Turn on power switch.	Starts concentrator motor.
(3) Alarm will sound for a few seconds.	Alarm turns off when desired pressure inside concentrator is reached.
c Liquid oxygen system:	
(1) Check liquid system by depressing button at lower right corner and reading the dial on the stationary oxygen reservoir or the ambulatory tank.	Verifies adequate oxygen supply for patient use.
(2) Collaborate with DME provider to provide instruction in refilling ambulatory tank.	Ambulatory tanks of liquid oxygen need to be filled when empty.

Critical Decision Point   *Only fill ambulatory tanks when they are empty. Liquid oxygen is stored at or below −297° F inside reservoir, and the temperature inside the ambulatory tank is warmer. If cold oxygen from the reservoir mixes with warmer oxygen left in the ambulatory tank, the ambulatory tank malfunctions.*

STEP	RATIONALE
(3) To refill liquid oxygen tank:	
(a) Wipe both filling connectors with a clean, dry, lint-free cloth.	Removes dust and moisture from system.
(b) Turn off flow selector of ambulatory unit.	
(c) Attach ambulatory unit to stationary reservoir by inserting female adapter from ambulatory tank into male adapter of stationary reservoir (see illustration).	Secures connection between oxygen reservoir and ambulatory tank.
(d) Open fill valve on ambulatory tank (e.g., lever, button, key), and apply firm pressure to top of stationary reservoir (see illustration). Stay with unit while it is filling. You will hear a loud hissing noise. Tank should be filled in about 2 minutes.	Prevents leakage of oxygen during filling process. If oxygen leaks during filling process, connection between ambulatory tank and reservoir potentially ices up and ambulatory and reservoir tanks stick together.

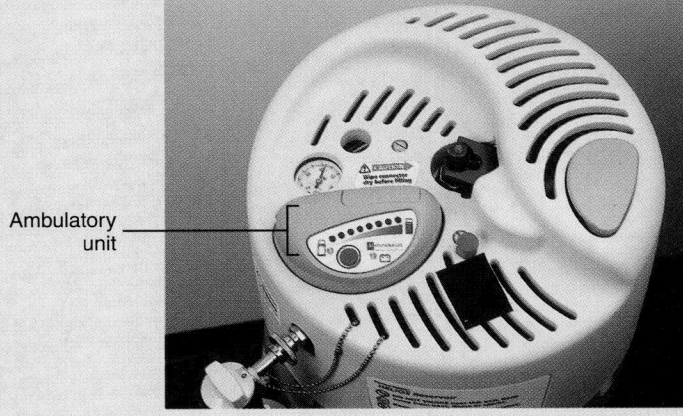

Ambulatory unit

STEP 3c(3)(c)   Top view of stationary reservoir.

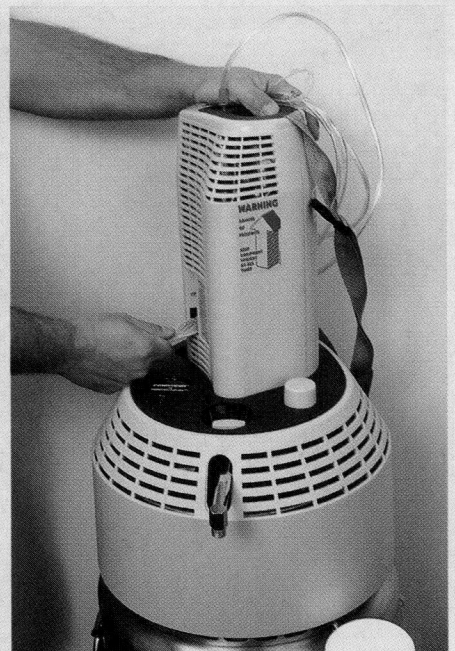

STEP 3c(3)(d)   Fill valve on ambulatory tank is opened while applying firm pressure to top of ambulatory tank.

STEP	RATIONALE
(e) Disconnect ambulatory unit from stationary reservoir when hissing noise changes and vapor cloud begins to form from stationary unit.	Overfilling causes ambulatory unit to malfunction due to high pressure in tank.

Critical Decision Point   *If ambulatory unit does not separate easily, valves from reservoir and ambulatory unit are frozen together. Wait until valves warm to disengage (about 5 to 10 minutes). Do not touch any frosted areas because contact with skin causes skin damage from frostbite.*

STEP	RATIONALE
(f) Wipe both filling connectors with clean, dry, lint-free cloth.	Ice often forms during filling process. Removes moisture from oxygen system.
4 Connect oxygen delivery device (e.g., nasal cannula) to oxygen delivery system (see Chapter 23) (see illustration).	Connects oxygen source to delivery method.
5 Adjust oxygen flow rate (L/min).	Ensures appropriate oxygen delivery.
6 Place oxygen delivery device (e.g., nasal cannula) on patient (see Chapter 23). Ensure patient has two sets of oxygen delivery devices (e.g., nasal cannula) and tubing.	Delivers oxygen to patient. Extra set of equipment is used when equipment is cleaned or in case of equipment malfunction.
7 Perform hand hygiene.	Reduces transmission of microorganisms.
8 Instruct patient not to change oxygen flow rate.	Provides prescribed amount of oxygen. Exceeding prescribed amount of oxygen is sometimes harmful (e.g., patient with chronic obstructive pulmonary disease [COPD]).
9 Have patient or family member perform each step with guidance. Provide written material for reinforcement and review.	Allows for correction in any errors in technique and discussion of their implications.
10 Instruct patient or family to notify health care provider if signs or symptoms of hypoxia or respiratory tract infection occur (e.g., fever, increased sputum, change in color of sputum, foul sputum odor).	Respiratory tract infections increase oxygen demand and often affect oxygen transfer from lungs to blood, creating exacerbation of patient's pulmonary disease.
11 Discuss emergency plans for power loss, natural disaster, and acute respiratory distress. Have family caregiver or patient call 9-1-1 and notify health care provider and home care agency.	Ensures appropriate response and can prevent worsening of patient's condition.
12 Instruct patient in safe home oxygen practices, including placing "No Smoking/Oxygen in Use" signs at each entrance to home, not allowing smoking in the house, keeping oxygen tanks 8 feet away from open flames, and storing oxygen tanks upright.	Ensures safe use of oxygen in the home and prevents injury to patient and family (City of Tyler, Texas, 2007).

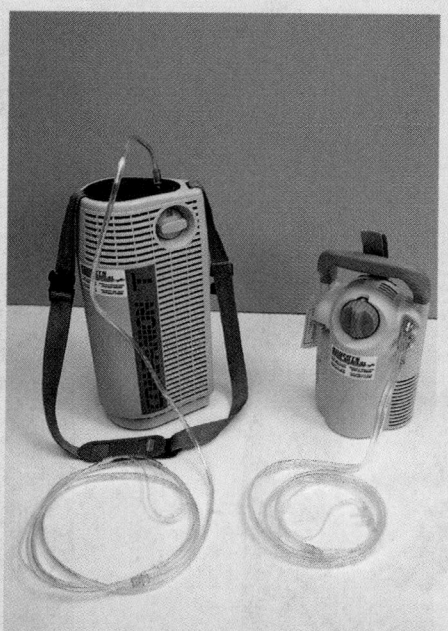

STEP 4   Oxygen delivery device (nasal cannulas) and tubing attached to ambulatory oxygen tanks.

STEP	RATIONALE
13 Record teaching plan, information given to patient, and validation of learning.	Provides written documentation of teaching plan for patient and family. Documents patient learning.

EVALUATION

1 Monitor rate at which oxygen is delivered.	Determines if patient is regulating oxygen at prescribed rate.
2 Ask patient/family caregiver about ease or problems associated with home oxygen.	Determines ability of patient or family to deal with stressors associated with home oxygen use. Also indicates patient's risk for inappropriate oxygen use.
3 Ask patient and family to state safety guidelines, emergency precautions, and emergency plan.	Determines patient's knowledge of what to do if power fails, there is a failure in equipment, or patient's status worsens.

Unexpected Outcomes	Related Interventions
1 Patient has signs and symptoms associated with hypoxia (see Assessment, Step 3).	• Determine if oxygen delivery device and oxygen source are delivering oxygen properly. • Determine if prescribed oxygen flow rate is set properly. • Assess patient for change in respiratory status, such as airway plugging, respiratory tract infection, or bronchospasm. • Instruct patient and family when to notify health care provider or activate EMS because of signs of hypoxia.
2 Patient uses unsafe practices with oxygen therapy, uses oxygen around fire or cigarette smoking, or sets incorrect flow rate.	• Reinforce patient education, and perform follow-up reassessment (see Box 42-4). • Include family caregiver in instruction, and set up problem-solving exercises with patient.
3 Patient is unable to fill ambulatory system.	• Identify and instruct family caregiver who can help patient fill tank.

Recording and Reporting

- Record teaching plan and information provided to patient in home care record.
- Record validation of patient or family learning.
- Communicate patient's or family's learning progress to other health care providers involved in patient's care.
- Record oxygen delivery system, related supplies, and prescribed oxygen flow rate.

Teaching Considerations

- Potential for oxygen desaturation and decreased oxygen delivery to brain impairs patient's ability to remember previous learning. Provide frequent teaching sessions and written or pictorial instructions to reinforce previous learning of teaching plan.
- Instruct patient and caregiver in appropriate cleaning, disinfecting, and maintenance of all oxygen delivery systems and supplies. Verify instructions with manufacturer's guidelines and DME provider's instructions.
- Instruct patient and caregiver to check mask and tubing by placing hands or face over mask or cannula to feel airflow and to check to be sure mask is not too tight; tight mask often leaves

marks on skin. Apply cotton or gauze sponge at pressure points.

Pediatric Considerations

- Keep equipment and matches out of reach of any children in home. Playing with fire and manipulating dials or flowmeters have disastrous effects on oxygen safety.
- Home oxygen therapy in children often creates a lot of stress in the family, especially when the child is a premature infant, because of the complex demands placed on the parents. Home visits by a nurse and other health care professionals and referral to support groups help parents better cope with the demands of caring for a child requiring oxygen at home (Kelly, 2006).

Gerontological Considerations

- Older adults have less efficient respiratory systems and less surface area for gas exchange, so they are at greater risk for cerebral anoxia and confusion when they experience decreased oxygen levels. They sometimes are unable to recognize respiratory problems or problems with their oxygen delivery system; therefore they need frequent contact with a designated caregiver.

SKILL 42-5   Teaching Home Tracheostomy Care and Suctioning

Performing tracheostomy care and suctioning in the home are similar to tracheostomy care and suctioning in the hospital except for one key variable: the use of *medical asepsis* or *clean technique*. Aseptic technique is used in the hospital because the patient is more susceptible to infection and because more virulent or pathogenic microorganisms are usually present. In the home setting, the majority of patients use clean technique, whereas some need to use aseptic technique. Use judgment in choosing the correct technique for each patient. For example, use aseptic technique with patients who are immunocompromised, who are infected (not colonized), or who have caregivers infected with viral, bacterial, or fungal microorganisms. Patients living in unclean conditions also need to be suctioned using aseptic technique whenever possible to try to prevent infection. All caregivers need to use standard precautions when suctioning with either clean or aseptic technique.

Caring for a tracheostomy (also called a trach) at home begins in the hospital (see Chapter 25) with teaching and return demonstration. The patient or caregiver usually learns better when instruction in less invasive techniques such as tracheal stoma care precedes more invasive techniques such as inner cannula care and suctioning. Continually develop, implement, and evaluate the teaching plan based on patient performance. Some patients and their families learn quickly, whereas others do not. Therefore begin teaching as soon as it is feasible. It is imperative that patients and their families have the ability to suction many times before discharge to develop confidence with skill performance; otherwise, arrangements to provide 24-hour care are necessary before discharge.

Delegation Considerations

The skill of teaching home tracheostomy (or trach) care and suctioning cannot be delegated to NAP.

Equipment

- ❑ Suction machine with connecting tube
- ❑ Clean or sterile gloves
- ❑ Three small basins
- ❑ Mild soapy water or solution of 3% hydrogen peroxide
- ❑ Normal saline
- ❑ Clean 4 × 4 inch gauze pads (nonshredding)
- ❑ Appropriate size of sterile or clean and disinfected suction catheter (diameter no greater than half the diameter of the tracheostomy tube; e.g., if the tracheostomy tube is 8 mm, then use 16 Fr or smaller suction catheter)
- ❑ Tracheostomy care kit or clean 4 × 4 inch gauze pads (nonshredding)
- ❑ Small nylon bottle brush or pipe cleaners or disposable inner cannula
- ❑ Cotton-tipped applicators
- ❑ Tracheostomy ties (twill ⅜-inch preferably)
- ❑ Mirror
- ❑ Wet washcloth or paper towel *(optional)*
- ❑ Dry cloth, towel, or paper towel *(optional)*
- ❑ Protective eyewear *(optional)*
- ❑ Trash bag (plastic, leakproof preferred)
- ❑ Disposable apron *(optional)*
- ❑ Bag-valve-mask (BVM) with oxygen supply *(optional)*

STEP	RATIONALE

ASSESSMENT

1 Assess patient's ability to perform tracheostomy care and suctioning properly, including level of consciousness, ability to attend and problem solve, and fine motor function.

Instructing family member or significant other is essential if patient's physical and cognitive impairment prevents ability to perform tracheostomy care and suctioning. Emergency situations usually require family member or significant other to suction.

2 Assess patient's and family member's knowledge of need to perform:
  a Tracheostomy care, including presence of excess peristomal secretions, excess intratracheal secretions, soiled or damp tracheostomy dressing/ties, and diminished airway through tracheostomy tube.

Allows patient to accurately evaluate need to provide tracheostomy care. Signs and symptoms are related to presence of secretions at stoma site or within tracheostomy tube.

  b Suctioning, including the presence of gurgling, tactile fremitus, wheezes or crackles on inspiration or expiration, restlessness, ineffective coughing, absent or diminished breath sounds, tachypnea, cyanosis, acutely decreased level of consciousness, hypertension or hypotension, tachycardia or bradycardia, acutely shallow respirations, or acute dyspnea.

Allows patient to accurately evaluate need to perform tracheostomy tube suctioning. Physical signs and symptoms result from lower airway obstruction and tissue hypoxia.

3 Observe patient or family member performing complete tracheostomy tube care and suctioning.

Determines which specific components of skill patient or family member can easily complete and which are more difficult and require reinforcement.

STEP	RATIONALE

NURSING DIAGNOSES

- Deficient knowledge regarding tracheostomy care
- Ineffective health maintenance
- Risk for caregiver role strain
- Risk for infection

Individualize related factors based on patient's condition or needs.

PLANNING

1. Expected outcomes following completion of procedure:

   - Patient or family member identifies signs and symptoms indicating need for tracheostomy care and suctioning.

     Patient or family member is able to institute preventative means to maintain airway.

   - Patient or family member states factors that influence tracheostomy airway functioning.

     Tracheostomy often impairs normal airway clearance, humidification, and gas exchange.

   - Patient or family member correctly demonstrates complete tracheostomy tube care and suctioning in controlled setting.

     Provides validation of ability to perform procedure.

   - Patient or family member identifies signs of stoma inflammation or respiratory tract infection and when to notify physician.

     Measures cognitive learning.

   - Lower and upper airways are cleared of secretions, as evidenced by absent or diminished crackles, wheezes, tactile fremitus, and gurgles in large airways; return of breath sounds that were absent or diminished; normalization of vital signs; increased depth of respirations; absence of cyanosis; improved color; and decreased dyspnea.

     Suctioning is successful.

   - Stoma site is clean and free of infection and transesophageal fistula; inner cannula is free of secretions.

     Tracheostomy care is successful.

2. Select setting in home that patient or family member is most likely to use when completing tracheostomy tube care.

   Practicing skill in same setting where skill will be routinely performed facilitates comprehension and learning (Bastable, 2006).

3. Discuss and demonstrate with patient or family member proper position for procedure (high-Fowler's position in front of a mirror).

   Promotes understanding of comfort and safety principles and facilitates visibility.

IMPLEMENTATION

1. Suctioning:

   a. Verify health care provider's orders for suctioning.

      Invasive procedure requires an order.

   b. Perform hand hygiene.

      Reduces transmission of microorganisms.

   c. Teach and demonstrate step-by-step preparation and completion of tracheostomy tube suctioning using either open suctioning or closed suctioning (see Chapter 25) (see illustration).

      Demonstration is reliable technique for teaching psychomotor skill and enables patient or family member to ask questions throughout procedure (Falvo, 2004). Steps used to suction patients in the hospital are also used in the home.

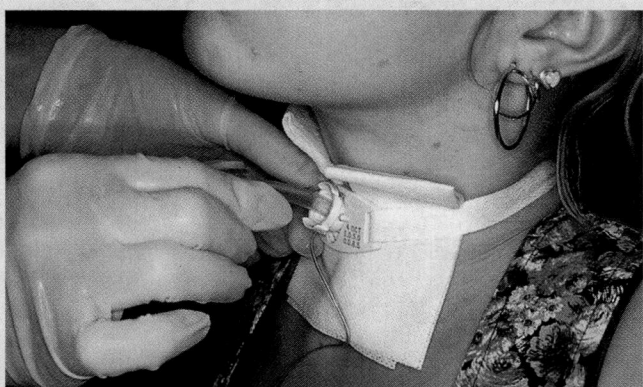

STEP 1c Insertion of suction catheter into tracheostomy tube.

STEP	RATIONALE

Critical Decision Point   *Instillation of normal saline before suctioning, once a common practice, is no longer recommended because it can cause a fall in PaO₂, an increased risk for infections, and tachycardia (Celik and Kanan, 2006).*

d After suctioning patient, teach to suction nasal and oral pharynx, and give mouth care. Encourage patient or family member to brush teeth with small soft toothbrush 2 times a day, and use mouth moisturizer and moisturize lips every 2 to 4 hours.

Dental plaque harbors microorganisms. Suctioning removes secretions from upper airway and prevents risk for infection, especially in patients who are mechanically ventilated (Cason and others, 2007; Seckel, 2007).

e At conclusion of procedure have patient take two to three deep breaths and determine if symptoms that necessitated suctioning are no longer present.

Deep breathing reduces oxygen loss and prevents hypoxia. Expect patient's respiratory status to improve following suctioning.

f Disconnect suction catheter; coil and discard catheter in appropriate receptacle. If catheter is to be cleaned and disinfected, set aside. Remove soiled gloves, and perform hand hygiene.

Prevents transmission of microorganisms.

2 Trach care:

a Teach skills of tracheostomy care, including cleaning stoma and tracheostomy tube, and changing tracheostomy ties (see illustrations and Chapter 25).

Steps used to provide tracheostomy care in the hospital are also used in the home. *Exception:* Mild soap and water can be used to cleanse a tracheostomy tube. Use hydrogen peroxide solution only to remove heavy secretions.

Critical Decision Point   *During tracheostomy care the patient is at risk for tracheostomy tube coming out. Never remove the old tracheostomy tube ties until the new ties are properly secured. Keep two tracheostomy tubes, one the same size as the patient's and one a size smaller, at the patient's bedside so you can insert a new tube if the tube comes out.*

b Clean reusable supplies in warm soapy water. Rinse thoroughly, and dry between two layers of clean paper towels. Store supplies in loosely closed clear plastic bag.

Prevents transmission of microorganisms. Air must circulate, or humidity in bag can promote microorganism growth.

c Remove and discard gloves. Perform hand hygiene.

Reduces transmission of microorganisms.

d Reusable supplies need to be disinfected at least weekly. To disinfect supplies use one of the methods described below:

Removes organisms and reduces risk for infection.

(1) *Method 1:* Boil reusable (boilable) supplies for 15 minutes. Allow to cool and dry.

(2) *Method 2:* Soak reusable supplies in equal parts of vinegar and water for 30 minutes. Remove, rinse thoroughly, and dry.

(3) *Method 3:* Soak reusable supplies in prepared solutions of quaternary ammonium chloride compounds according to manufacturer's instructions. Rinse and dry.

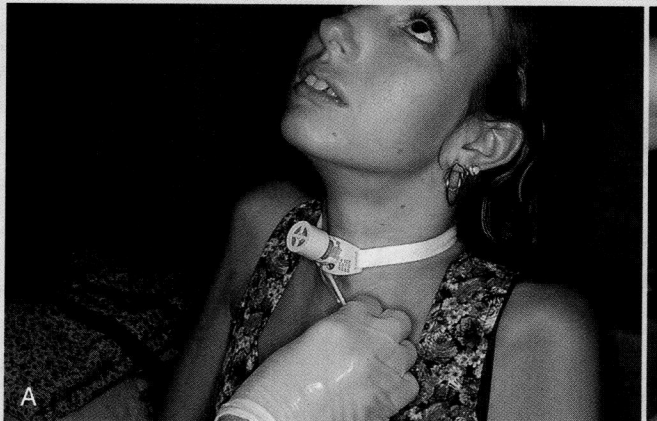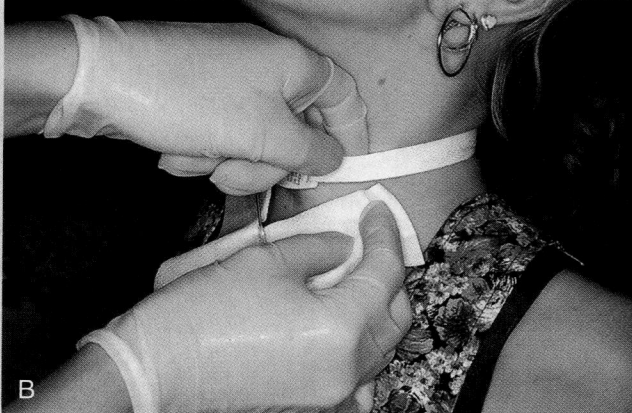

STEP 2a   **A,** Cleaning area around tracheal stoma. **B,** Applying clean tracheostomy dressing.

STEP	RATIONALE
3 Have patient or family member perform each step with guidance from you.	Adults learn psychomotor skills best by active participation, and you can correct any errors in technique as they occur and discuss their implications (Falvo, 2004).

4 Discuss signs and symptoms of the following:
  a Stoma infection (redness, tenderness, drainage)
  b Respiratory tract infection (fever, increased sputum, change in color of sputum, foul sputum odor, increased cough, chills, night sweats)
  c Transesophageal fistula (air leaking through stoma, nose, or mouth with cuff properly inflated; more air needed to inflate cuff; aspiration of food or liquid during suctioning; excessive belching; coughing when swallowing)
	Patient and caregiver must be able to recognize onset of complications associated with long-term tracheostomy use early so that medical treatment can begin, reducing risk for more serious negative outcomes. Emphasize importance of notifying physician when signs and symptoms of complications occur.

EVALUATION

1 Ask patient to state signs of stoma or respiratory tract complications.	Prompt identification of symptoms results in early treatment and decreases risk for complications that may lead to hospital readmission.
2 Observe patient or family member demonstrating technique for tracheostomy tube care and suctioning.	Feedback through independent demonstration of psychomotor skill is reliable method to evaluate learning.

Unexpected Outcomes	Related Interventions
1 Stoma site is reddened or hard, with or without drainage.	• Evaluate patient's or caregiver's technique. • Increase frequency of tracheostomy care.
2 Copious colored secretions are present around stoma or when patient is suctioned.	• Use sterile technique for suctioning and tracheostomy care. • Evaluate for adequate humidity (use room humidifier or tracheostomy collar humidity, if needed) (see Chapter 23). • Notify health care provider.
3 Bloody secretions are suctioned.	• Evaluate suctioning technique, suctioning frequency, and size of catheter used. • Alter suction depth by going no more than 1 to 2 cm past the end of the tracheostomy tube in adults (take length of tube and add 1 cm) to avoid making contact with the carina (Brosche and others, 2005). • Assess for signs of infection.
4 No secretions are suctioned.	• Evaluate fluid status, need for increased humidity. • Determine if appropriate size of suction catheter is used. • Reassess suction frequency.
5 Tracheostomy tube comes out.	• Replace tracheostomy tube to maintain an airway. • Activate emergency medical system if needed.
6 Skin breakdown is present at stoma site.	• Assess site for pressure areas or site infection. • Remove pressure source.

Recording and Reporting

• Record patient instruction and accuracy of care delivered by patient or family member.
• Develop a system of recording home care for patient or caregiver to document and keep track of tracheostomy care provided.

Teaching Considerations

• Some patients benefit by using a mirror to visualize stoma area.

Pediatric Considerations

• Encourage parents to give trach care as soon as child is stable in the hospital. The more time they have to practice these skills, the more comfortable they become in caring for the child at home.

• Children with tracheostomies need to socialize and play with other children who are close to their own age. Encourage parents to take children out of the home. However, an additional adult needs to travel in the car with the child to assist if problems arise while in the car (Hockenberry and Wilson, 2007).

• To prevent hypoxia, teach parents that suctioning needs to last no more than 5 seconds. Allow the child to rest for at least 30 to 60 seconds between suctioning passes, and do not suction more than three times (Hockenberry and Wilson, 2007).

• Teach families and significant others infant or child cardiopulmonary resuscitation, including use of bag-valve-mask or mouth-to-trach technique. They also need to notify the local EMS of the child's condition and the presence of a tracheostomy and provide EMS with a list of equipment in the home (Hockenberry and Wilson, 2007).

- Encourage parents to have a cool mist humidifier in same room as child; humidity helps keep secretions thin and decreases the likelihood of mucous plugging (Hockenberry and Wilson, 2007).
- Caring for a child with a tracheostomy often disrupts parents' ability to socialize. Develop a plan that includes respite care to allow parents time to meet their own needs (Montagnino and Mauricio, 2004).
- Tracheostomy tubes are changed every 3 to 4 weeks in adults and every 1 to 2 weeks in children (Hockenberry and Wilson, 2007). Two people are required to change the tracheostomy tube. Procedural Guideline 42-1 provides guidelines for changing a tracheostomy tube at home.

Gerontological Considerations

- Older adults lose some properties of elastic recoil and often have greater difficulty in clearing airway secretions through cough. As a result, they require more suctioning and airway care and have increased risk for infection (Ebersole and others, 2008).
- Assess for cognitive, mobility, or sensory impairments that impair ability to manage artificial airway at home and teach caregiver if patient is unable to manage airway independently.
- Anxiety accompanies decreased ability to breathe and may cause the older adult to become too nervous to perform suctioning independently.

PROCEDURAL GUIDELINE 42-1   Changing a Tracheostomy Tube at Home

Delegation Considerations

The skill of changing a tracheostomy tube cannot be delegated to NAP.

Equipment

- ❏ Clean gloves
- ❏ Suction catheter
- ❏ Suction machine
- ❏ Bag-valve-mask
- ❏ Face mask
- ❏ New sterile tracheostomy tube

Procedural Steps

1 Do not allow patient to have anything by mouth (NPO), or hold tube feedings for at least 1 hour before procedure.
2 Explain procedure to patient before tracheostomy is changed to alleviate anxiety. Have family member assist.
3 Perform hand hygiene, and put on clean gloves.

4 Remove new tube from sterile container. Remove the inner cannula and insert obturator into outer cannula. Attach clean tracheostomy ties to neck plate, checking integrity of cuff.
5 Suction tracheostomy tube, and have bag-valve-mask and face mask available.
6 Have family member stabilize tracheostomy face plate. Loosen tracheostomy ties, and deflate tracheostomy tube cuff (if tracheostomy has one).
7 Family member pulls the old tracheostomy tube out with gentle, steady pressure in the same direction as an inner cannula would be removed.
8 Apply sterile gloves. Push new tracheostomy into tracheostomy site using gentle force, while pushing back and then down. Remove the obturator. Allow air to flow in, then insert inner cannula.
9 Secure new tracheostomy ties, inflate cuff, and place dressing around stoma if necessary.

SKILL 42-6   Teaching Medication Self-Administration

Researchers estimate that many patients who are prescribed drug regimens at home fail to take medications correctly (Haynes and others, 2007). A recent literature review indicates that 20% to 40% of patients with acute illnesses fail to follow their medication schedule. This percentage increases to 30% to 60% in patients with chronic illnesses and 80% for patients who take preventive medications (Christensen, 2004). Consequently, many admissions to hospitals and nursing homes, medical malpractice suits, therapeutic failures, and medical emergencies result from inaccurate medication use. Patients have difficulty in taking prescribed medications regularly for several reasons: patients stop taking medications once symptoms subside, regimens involving multiple drugs at a variety of times are confusing, the consequences of not taking medications are poorly understood, prescriptions are costly, and many patients fear addiction. A large portion of patients who do not comply are older adults, who frequently suffer psychomotor, cognitive, sensory, and mobility problems. Some older adults also have poor social support, interfering with the ability to prepare and take medications correctly (Metlay and others, 2005). Medication education is associated with enhanced patient outcomes (Muir-

Cochrane and others, 2006). Educating patients about their medications could save 120,000 lives and $45.6 billion per year in the United States alone (Schommer and others, 2002). The following skill is an outline to help prepare patients for following drug regimens in the home.

Delegation Considerations

The skill of teaching patients medication self-administration cannot be delegated to NAP. The nurse directs the NAP to:

- Communicate to the nurse problems patients are having with medication administration.

Equipment

- ❏ Medication
- ❏ Liquid to take with medication
- ❏ Medication administration record, computer printout, or other up-to-date list of current medications from prescriber
- ❏ Container for daily or weekly preparation
- ❏ Measuring devices as needed (e.g., medicine cup, teaspoon)
- ❏ Teaching tools (e.g., charts, written instructions, color codes)

STEP	RATIONALE

ASSESSMENT

1   Assess patient's cognitive, sensory, and motor function; level of consciousness, sight, hearing, touch, literacy, swallowing ability, mobility, activity tolerance, social support, and willingness to cooperate (see Chapter 20).

Cognitive, sensory, and motor deficits frequently influence patient's ability to take or prepare prescribed medication correctly and to participate in instruction (Metlay and others, 2005).

2   Assess resources patient has to obtain medications when needed: finances, social support, and transportation.

Lack of resources is a major factor that will negatively affect compliance with medication self-administration regimen (Muir-Cochrane and others, 2006).

3   Assess patient's learning readiness and ability to attend; consider presence of pain, fatigue, patient interest in instruction.

Presence of significant illness, frailty, or confusion will affect teaching plan. Indicates need to rely on caregiver for learning and implementation (if available) on a short- or long-term basis (Curry and others, 2005).

4   Assess patient's and/or family member's knowledge regarding medication therapy: names of drugs, how to administer, purpose or action, daily doses and times to be taken, side effects to expect, and what to do if problems occur.

Reveals patient's level of understanding and need for instruction. Family member or support person is important resource to help patient comply with or adhere to medication therapy.

5   Assess patient's belief in need for drug therapy. Consider cultural values, religious beliefs, personal experiences with medications, and significant others' values about drugs.

Many factors influence patient's willingness to follow drug regimen.

6   Check patient's prescribed and over-the-counter (OTC) medications, including use of herbal supplements: Has more than one health care provider prescribed medications? Are medications obviously inappropriate? Are labels clearly marked? Are time schedules confusing? Do different drugs look alike? Does patient store medications together or out of original containers? Are expiration dates on bottles still current?

Determines sources of confusion affecting patient's compliance. Noncompliance with medication therapy (especially in older adults) is often aggravated by multiple chronic conditions, which are often treated with multiple medications sometimes prescribed by more than one health care provider. Compliance is more difficult when medication regimens are complex (Metlay and others, 2005).

7   Assess patient's understanding of effects and interactions between prescribed medications and ingestion of certain foods, OTC drugs, and herbal supplements.

Medication interactions, including those with OTC drugs, herbals, and certain foods, can seriously affect medication effectiveness and/or create negative side effects (Curry and others, 2005).

NURSING DIAGNOSES

- Anxiety
- Deficient knowledge regarding medication administration
- Health-seeking behaviors (medication self-administration)
- Ineffective health maintenance
- Ineffective individual or family therapeutic regimen management
- Readiness for enhanced knowledge

Individualize related factors based on patient's condition or needs.

PLANNING

1   Expected outcomes following completion of procedure:
- Patient/family member is able to state purpose of each medication and why it is beneficial.

Demonstrates cognitive learning.

- Patient identifies common adverse effects and relief measures.

Enhances compliance with medication therapy.

- Patient is able to state when to notify physician about medication problems.

Empowers patient to participate in care.

- Patient reads each label and explains when each drug should be taken.

Prevents medication administration errors.

- Patient/family member demonstrates self-administration of medication by prescribed route (see illustrations).

Demonstrates skill achieved.

2   Prepare environment for teaching session:
   a   Select room that is well lit.
   b   Provide comfortable seating.
   c   Be sure patient is close and can see nurse clearly.
   d   Control sources of noise and distractions.

Room environment needs to minimize existing sensory alterations. Comfortable environment free of distractions promotes patient's attention (Bastable, 2006).

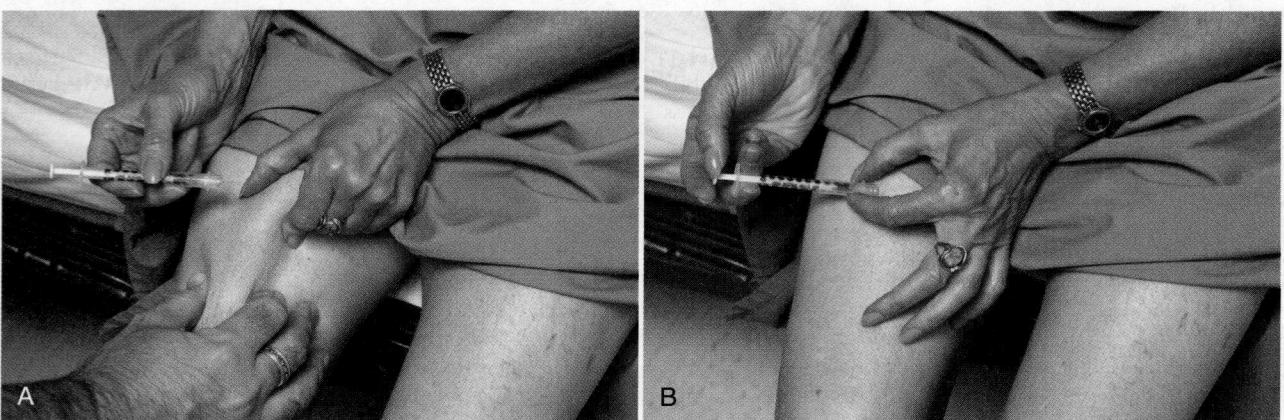

STEP 1   Patient demonstrating self-injection technique.

STEP	RATIONALE

3 Prepare teaching materials:
  a Use materials printed in large bold letters (set in 14 point or larger type).
  b Provide illustrations of safety guidelines.
  c Give written schedules or individualized instruction sheets.
	Provide teaching materials designed to meet patient's learning needs and patient's capacity to learn.

4 Ensure patient is wearing glasses or hearing aids if needed during teaching session.	Use of glasses or hearing aids increases patient's sensory perception and increases likelihood of attending to teaching session and understanding content (Redman, 2007).
5 Consult with prescriber to review medications patient is receiving and to simplify regimen if possible.	Review of medications helps minimize risk for drug interactions from multiple medications and ensures accuracy of medication regimen. Simplification of regimen improves compliance, particularly related to daily frequency of prescribed doses (Haynes and others, 2007).
6 Arrange teaching time to allow participation of family members (see illustration).	Family can serve as positive resource to patient and often reinforce information provided.

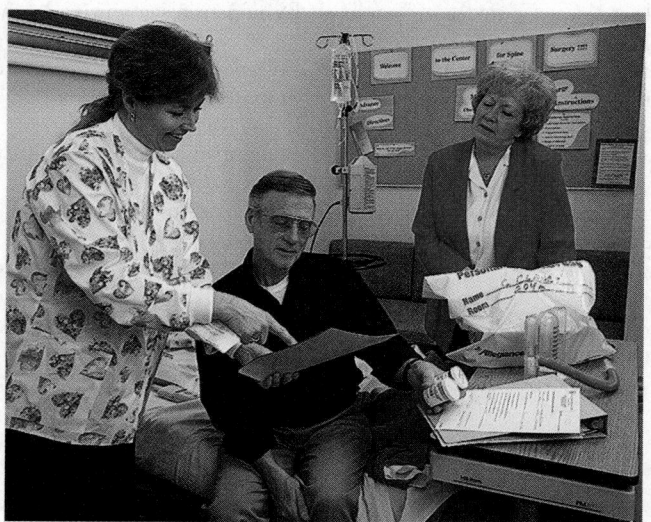

STEP 6   Patient and family participating in medication self-administration teaching program.

STEP	RATIONALE

IMPLEMENTATION

1 Present information clearly and concisely:
   a Face learner in well-lit room.

   b Use short sentences, and speak in slow, low-pitched voice.
   c Provide descriptions in understandable terms.

2 Provide frequent pauses so that patient can ask questions and express understanding of content.
3 Instruct patient/family member on the following content: purpose of regularly scheduled and prn drugs and their desired effects, how drug works and why it helps, dosage schedules and rationale, common side effects, what to do to relieve side effects, what to do if dose is missed, when to call with problems, who to call with problems, drug safety guidelines, and implications when medications are not taken.
4 Instruct patient in appropriate route of medication delivery, including oral, subcutaneous, intramuscular, topical, etc.

5 Provide frequent, short teaching sessions. Plan to have several teaching sessions, especially if patient needs to take multiple medications. Leave instruction aids in the home for patient to review if possible.
6 Provide teaching about OTC medications and herbal supplements.
7 Provide patient with special charts, diagrams, learning aids, written information, and Internet/intranet resources (see illustration).

Rationale column:

Improves patient's ability to attend and understand.
Allows visualization of patient's nonverbal responses to education. Patient with hearing loss or visual problem is able to see your expressions, read written information, and hear your voice more clearly.
Enhances understanding of information.
Prevents confusion of terminology. Patients learn more quickly when you present information at the level of the learner (Redman, 2007).
Increases patient's participation in learning process. Ongoing feedback ensures that patient is acquiring information.
Provides patient with sufficient information to understand and take medications safely at home.

Patient needs to be proficient in all routes of medication administration. Adverse effects often occur if medications are administered incorrectly.
Frequent sessions improve patient's attention and retention of information discussed. Reference to charts, written information, and other teaching tools as a resource enhances learning (Haynes and others, 2007).
Many patients do not understand effects of OTC and herbal supplements (Curry and others, 2005).
Clear written information, charts, and other resources, such as the Internet/intranet enhance patient learning and allow for reinforcement of information (Institute of Safe Medical Practice [ISMP], 2003).

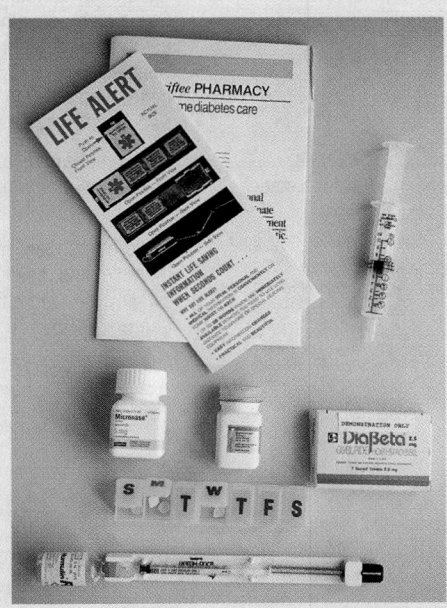

STEP 7   Examples of aids for patient medication self-administration.

STEP	RATIONALE
8 Offer assistance as patient practices preparing medication (e.g., "Let's prepare the medications you will take with your meals or prepare the medicines you take first in the morning").	Allows for observation of patient's ability to read labels correctly and prepare all medications for prescribed times.
9 Have pharmacy provide clear, large-print labels for medication bottles and medication teaching handouts if appropriate.	Improves patient's ability to read and follow directions.
10 Have pharmacy provide containers that patient can open independently if manual dexterity is limited.	Most pharmacies dispense pills in "childproof" containers, which the patient with limited mobility of fingers/hands often finds difficult to manipulate or open.

Critical Decision Point   If there are pets or small children in home or children who frequently visit home, help patient establish a "safe place" for medication, to reduce risk for accidental ingestion by pets or children.

STEP	RATIONALE
11 Facilitate arrangements for pharmacy to receive written prescriptions in a timely fashion if required for dispensing. Arrange for pharmacy to deliver medications to home if patient is unable to arrange for transportation to pharmacy.	Availability of drugs influences compliance.

EVALUATION

1 Ask patient and family member to explain information about each drug: purpose; actions; routes; timing of medications and maximum frequency of use of either prescribed or OTC medications; side effects and interactions; and foods, herbals, or OTC medications to avoid.	Feedback measures patient's cognitive learning and helps to ensure compliance with medication therapy.
2 Identify patient's problem-solving abilities (e.g., when to call health care provider or refer to printed information for resources).	Developing techniques to gain information and solve problems will assist in patient compliance and reduce potential problems from medication regimen (Curry and others, 2005).
3 Have patient or family member prepare doses for all prescribed medications.	Indicates understanding of medication dosages and schedules.
4 Ask patient to verbalize any remaining questions regarding medication management.	Offers opportunity for clarification and minimizes any remaining confusion or misunderstanding.

Unexpected Outcomes

1 Patient makes errors in preparing medications or is unable to recall and/or explain information discussed in teaching sessions.

2 Medication self-administration plan is not possible due to patient's self-care deficits. This is very common when the patient develops cognitive changes.

3 Patient refuses to take medications as prescribed.

Related Interventions

- Provide additional instruction and/or teaching materials for consultation when information is forgotten or unclear.
- Ensure written instructions are at patient's level of understanding. Some commercially prepared booklets contain instructions that are too complex or contain medical jargon that is difficult to understand.
- Consider use of pictures, color coding, diagrams, and tape-recorded instructions for the reading or sight impaired.
- Periodically observe patient prepare and administer medications.
- Develop alternative plan, which often relies on family/caregivers to provide safe administration of home medication regimen.
- Explore and identify reasons for noncompliance, which often include the following: cost, side effects, complexity of regimen, problems with swallowing, and cultural preferences.
- See Box 42-5.

Recording and Reporting

- Document instruction provided and learning outcomes achieved by patient in home care record.
- Develop system of recording for patient or family member to use to document compliance.
- Develop a patient recording mechanism of dosage schedules and self-monitoring of regimen.

Teaching Considerations

- See Chapter 41 for guidelines for medication safety.
- If it is difficult to plan a separate teaching session, instruct patient while administering medications.
- Examples of learning aids include homemade calendars for each week that contain plastic bags containing medications to take at specific times, egg cartons divided into color-coded sections with medications for the day, clock faces for patients who cannot read or see clearly, color coding for drug types (e.g., blue for sedative, red for pain pill), and pillboxes that identify days of the week and times of day.

Pediatric Considerations

- Instruct adults to keep all medications safely and securely out of reach of children.
- Encourage caregivers not to tell children that medications are treats, because this increases the risk for child overdosing by mistaking medicine for candy.
- Successful medication teaching involves the child's parents or other caregivers and the child and siblings whenever possible. To provide effective medication teaching to children, take the child's developmental and cognitive abilities into consideration when planning teaching sessions (Hockenberry and Wilson, 2007).
- Parents need to supervise older children as they begin taking responsibility for their own treatment.

Gerontological Considerations

- Capacity for learning new information remains as people age (in the absence of dementia); however, older patients often need additional time to accomplish learning. Allow adequate time and number of teaching sessions to support successful learning. Effective teaching strategies for older adults include memory aids, information written in large letters (14 point is recommended), involvement of family member or caregiver, follow-up teaching sessions either over the telephone or in person, and computer-assisted teaching guides (Ebersole and others, 2008).
- Cognition problems coupled with complexity of medication regimens have a negative effect on safe medication self-administration in older adults. Attempt to decrease the complexity of medication regimens in patients with cognitive deficits whenever possible to promote safe medication self-administration practices (Curry and others, 2005).
- Older adults often have to take medications in multiple routes (e.g., oral, inhaled, injections). Many times, problems with physical dexterity, eyesight, cognitive skills, and memory negatively affect adherence to medication schedules. Establish a therapeutic nurse-patient relationship in helping patients overcome these barriers to adherence.

BOX 42-5 | Evidence-Based Nursing Interventions to Enhance Compliance With Medication Therapy

- Be available for the patient, and make frequent meaningful contacts, especially when a new therapy is initiated or changes are made (Lucas and others, 2007).
- Make home visits to patients when needed, and collaborate with other disciplines when providing information; home visits by home care nurses enhance compliance with medication therapy (McCoy and others, 2007).
- Help patients develop a variety of strategies to remind them to take their medications (e.g., pillboxes, text messages on cellular phones) (Sidat and others, 2007).
- Schedule medication dosages at times that fit into the patient's daily routine (Sidat and others, 2007).
- Instruct patients about benefits of medications and the complications that may happen if medications are not taken correctly or if they are not taken at all (Sidat and others, 2007).
- Provide interdisciplinary medication education in settings that are private and convenient for the patient and enhance learning (Lucas and others, 2007).
- Identify patients who are at risk for noncompliance, and intervene early and frequently (Hudson and others, 2004).

- Use theory-based interventions (e.g., Prochaska and DiClemente's Transtheoretical Model of Change) to enhance motivation to comply with medication schedules (Levensky and others, 2007).
- Use motivational interviewing to enhance understanding of current behaviors and patient's readiness to change (Levensky and others, 2007). Motivational interviewing consists of the following principles:
  - *Express empathy:* Communicate acceptance of the patient's experience and feelings about taking (or not taking) medications as prescribed.
  - *Develop a discrepancy:* Use reflective listening, ask open questions, support the patient during interactions, and use summary statements to become aware of inconsistencies between the patient's unhealthy choices and personal goals or values.
  - *Roll with resistance:* Do not impose new perspectives on the patient; instead, allow patient to answer questions and develop potential solutions.
  - *Support self-efficacy:* Express your belief in the patient's ability to take medications as prescribed; ask patient to identify successful behaviors and to identify successful behaviors in other people.

SKILL 42-7 Managing Feeding Tubes in the Home

Enteral nutrition therapy in the home setting is usually effective when the patient tolerates at least 70% of feeding intake without complications, the patient is medically stable, the patient or caregiver is able to administer feedings, and the patient or caregiver has sufficient time in a controlled environment to learn the skill. The majority of patients requiring home enteral nutrition are older adults, people with disorders of the central nervous system, and people with dysphagia (Silver and others, 2004). Patients benefit when they are able to see tube feeding equipment and devices when learning how to administer home enteral nutrition. Provide hands-on experience and patient involvement with decision making about home enteral nutrition whenever possible.

This procedure in the home setting follows the guidelines and skills described in Chapter 31. This skill focuses on the teaching of the patient or caregiver in the home. Frequently in this setting the nurse is responsible for reinsertion of nasogastric and gastrostomy feeding tubes, and the physician or advanced practice nurse is responsible for reinsertion of jejunostomy tubes. See Skills 31-1 through 31-5 for insertion, feeding, and replacement procedures.

Delegation Considerations

The skill of management of feeding tubes in the home cannot be delegated to NAP. The nurse inserts feeding tubes, verifies tube placement, assesses for residual volume, and administers medications through feeding tubes. However, administration of enteral tube feeding via syringe is sometimes delegated to NAP (verify agency policy). The nurse directs the NAP to:
- Report when patient has difficulty with feeding, coughing, gagging, respiratory distress, discomfort, or vomiting.

Equipment

See Skill 31-1 for equipment for insertion, Skill 31-2 for placement, and Skills 31-3 through 31-5 for irrigating and administering feedings.
- ❑ Documentation records (daily weights, intake and output [I&O], temperature, feeding residuals)

STEP	RATIONALE

ASSESSMENT

1	Assess patient's health status, including presence of discomfort and fatigue and ability to successfully manage enteral feedings in the home.	Increases successful home management with fewer complications.
2	Assess patient's or caregiver's physical, emotional, financial, and community resources.	Increases ability for self-care and home management.
3	Assess environmental conditions of home (sanitation, storage of equipment, work area, supplies, and power source).	Ensures safe environment and decreases risks of infection and complications.
4	Assess patient's and caregiver's understanding of purpose of enteral feedings and positive expected outcomes.	Understanding rationale of treatment is critical to enhancing participation and cooperation in care (Bastable, 2006).
5	Assess patient's and caregiver's understanding of storage and management of equipment and supplies and where and how to obtain supplies.	Ensures safe home management and decreases risk for complications.
6	Assess patient's and caregiver's ability to manipulate feeding equipment.	Sometimes caregiver needs to administer enteral feedings.

NURSING DIAGNOSES

- Anxiety
- Deficient knowledge regarding administration of enteral feedings
- Feeding self-care deficit
- Imbalanced nutrition: less than body requirements
- Ineffective health maintenance
- Readiness for enhanced therapeutic regimen management
- Risk for aspiration

Individualize related factors based on patient's condition or needs.

PLANNING

1	Expected outcomes following completion of procedure:	
	• Patient and caregiver will verbalize the purpose of enteral feedings and enhanced nutritional health.	Provides measurable criteria to determine level of cognitive understanding.
	• Patient and caregiver will demonstrate proper use of equipment and handling of formulas.	Provides demonstration of skills needed to manage home enteral nutrition.
	• Patient and caregiver will demonstrate accurate administration of enteral feedings and medications.	Provides demonstration of skills needed to administer home enteral nutrition.
	• Patient and caregiver will verbalize understanding of signs and symptoms and management of complications of feeding.	Confirms patient and caregiver are able to administer feeding safely.

STEP	RATIONALE

IMPLEMENTATION

1 Perform hand hygiene.
   Reduces transmission of microorganisms.

2 Discuss with patient and caregiver purpose of enteral feeding and enhanced nutritional health.
   Reinforces importance of regular feedings.

3 Assist patient or caregiver in determining a feeding schedule that will maintain nutritional requirements and that will fit within the patient's or family's schedule.
   Promotes compliance with enteral nutrition therapy.

Critical Decision Point *Explain that caregiver needs to communicate changes in feeding schedules made to fit daily routine.*

4 Demonstrate how to identify placement of feeding tube: aspiration of gastric fluid, checking pH of gastric fluid, and acceptable pH range (see Skill 31-2).
   Some nasally placed tubes are inadvertently placed in respiratory system and migrate to esophagus or into respiratory tract. Check pH periodically. Aspirated secretions with low pH are strong indicator of gastric placement. However, high pH cannot differentiate between aspirated secretions obtained from respiratory and intestinal tube placements (Metheny, 2006).

Critical Decision Point *Instruct patient to avoid administration of all feedings, flushes, or medications if there is any doubt as to placement of enteral feeding tube.*

5 Observe patient and caregiver in determining placement of nasally placed tube.
   Identifies if there are areas for further teaching.

6 Observe patient or caregiver aspirate gastric contents. Instruct to return gastric contents after aspiration.
   Aspirates more than 200 mL indicate need to initiate interventions such as changing from intermittent to continuous feedings, evaluating possibility of decreasing opioid analgesics, and starting a medication that enhances gastric motility (e.g., metoclopramide) to reduce aspiration risk (Metheny, 2006).

Critical Decision Point *If gastric aspirates are more than 200 mL, instruct patient or caregiver to return gastric contents and delay tube feeding for 1 hour. If aspirates remain more than 200 mL after an hour, instruct patient or caregiver to contact home care nurse or health care provider.*

7 Discuss use of medical asepsis in setting up and changing administration sets, mixing formulas (do not add formula to hanging bag), refrigeration of unused formula, limiting amount of formula "hung" at one time to amount that can be infused in a 4- to 6-hour period (less time in warmer weather), and maintenance and care of bag.
   Medical aseptic technique minimizes risk for microorganism contamination. Refrigeration and limiting "hang" time reduces microorganisms. Changing administration sets every 24 hours reduces microorganism growth.

8 Instruct patient or caregiver that the patient needs to sit up in a chair or have the head of the bed elevated at least 30 to 45 degrees while receiving feedings or medications or when tube is flushed. If this is not possible, place the patient in reverse Trendelenburg's position.
   Decreases risk for aspiration (Metheny, 2006). Aspiration is indicated by increased coughing, difficulty in breathing, or vomiting.

9 Observe patient or caregiver mixing, administering, and storing formulas; changing administration sets; and cleaning bags. Discuss flushing of tube after administration of feedings or medications.
   Identifies competence and need for further teaching. Regular flushing of tube prevents clogging.

10 Observe patient or caregiver administering medications and flushing tube (see Skill 21-2).
   Ensures medications are given correctly.

Critical Decision Point *Verify that medications do not include any sublingual, enteric-coated, or sustained-release medications.*

11 Discuss and observe use of infusion pump if patient is receiving continuous feeding (see Chapter 31).
   Use of tube-feeding infusion pumps is complex and requires reinforcement.

12 Discuss measures to stabilize feeding tube in patients with abdominal tubes and to protect skin integrity.
   Prevents tube from dislodging and prevents skin breakdown.

13 Provide contact information for ordering equipment and supplies or whom to call in case of equipment failure.
   Ensures family is able to respond in an emergency.

14 Discuss emergency plan and actions to take for signs and symptoms of aspiration, such as elevating the head of the bed and calling health care provider.
   Ensures understanding of management of equipment, supplies, emergency plan, and collaboration.

STEP	RATIONALE
15 Discuss whom to contact and when for signs of diarrhea, constipation, or weight loss.	Provides support to patient and family.
16 Perform hand hygiene.	Reduces transmission of microorganisms.

EVALUATION

1 Ask patient and caregiver to state purpose of home enteral nutrition therapy.	Demonstrates cognitive learning.
2 Observe patient and caregiver performing medical asepsis techniques, checking tube placement, aspirating residuals, administering medications and solutions, and using equipment.	Demonstrates psychomotor learning.
3 Ask patient and caregiver to state measures used to prevent complications (e.g., verification of tube position before each feeding, elevation of patient during feeding, stabilization and flushing of tubing).	Ensures safe home management and identification of areas for teaching.
4 Ask patient and caregiver how to care for open formula cans.	Ensures safe home management and identification of areas of teaching.
5 Ask patient and caregiver about management of complications (e.g., signs of intolerance: nausea, abdominal distention, diarrhea, skin problems, and fluid deficit).	Ensures safe home management and identification of areas of teaching.

Unexpected Outcomes	Related Interventions
1 Displacement of feeding tube occurs.	• Instruct family to notify home care nurse whenever this happens and stop feeding. • Nurse will reposition feeding tube, and verify placement before initiating any enteral feeding.
2 Signs and symptoms of aspiration are present.	• Stop feeding. Raise head of bed. • Verify tube position. • Notify health care provider.
3 Patient develops diarrhea.	• Notify health care provider. • Consider change in strength, type, or rate of enteral feeding or administration of antidiarrheal agents.
4 Skin surrounding stoma or tube insertion site (nares) breaks down, or drainage around insertion site develops.	• Reposition feeding tube at nares to avoid pressure. • Cleanse stoma area more frequently. • Apply antibiotic ointment around stoma as ordered. • Contact health care provider.

Recording and Reporting

- Record instructions given to patient and caregivers and their response in home care record.
- Record specifics of enteral feeding plan, including type and size of tube in home, formula, and amounts to be administered in specific time frames.
- Patient and caregivers need to document I&O, daily weights, amount of gastric fluid aspirated before each feeding (or every 4 hours if receiving continuous feeding), date and time of feedings, amount and type of formula, any additives, and date and time administration sets are changed.

Teaching Considerations

- Performing skill without nurse in attendance provokes anxiety. Always leave a phone number and instructions about how to reach home care nurse if needed.

Pediatric Considerations

- Children are at risk for aspiration and fluid and electrolyte imbalance, so teach parent to monitor child carefully.
- Children who receive long-term home enteral feedings often experience developmental and growth delays. Other common problems include sleep disturbance, tube blockages, problems with delivery of equipment and equipment malfunction. Therefore these children require close follow-up and frequent nutritional monitoring (Evans and others, 2006).
- Teach parents to position children who cannot sit up during or after a tube feeding on their right side during the tube feeding and for at least 1 hour after the feeding (Hockenberry and Wilson, 2007).
- Children with special health needs are living longer and are becoming adults. Many services for these children decrease dramatically as they become young adults. Nurses need to carefully collaborate with interdisciplinary teams to ensure these individuals become as independent as possible.

Gerontological Considerations

- Assess for changes and limitations in sensory function, mobility, or dexterity that indicate a need to teach a significant other how to administer feedings.
- Home enteral therapy in older adults requires frequent monitoring, assessment, and intervention from interdisciplinary teams that include nurses and dietitians (Silver and others, 2004).

SKILL 42-8   Managing Parenteral Nutrition in the Home

Patients who cannot take in enough nutrition by mouth and who cannot receive enteral feedings because they do not have a functioning gastrointestinal tract receive parenteral nutrition (PN) in the home. Patients who receive PN at home have a variety of health problems, such as pancreatitis, liver failure, or Crohn's disease. Patients who have organ failure, uncontrolled diabetes mellitus, or electrolyte imbalances that cannot be corrected are poor candidates for home PN (Newton and Delegge, 2007). Nurses who manage PN in the home collaborate frequently with registered dietitians and other health care providers to ensure the patient receives appropriate calories, protein, and fluid. PN is administered through a long-term central venous catheter (CVC), such as a tunneled CVC (e.g., Groshong or Hickman catheter), an implantable port, or a peripherally inserted central catheter (PICC). PICCs are used when PN administration will last for a few weeks (Brogden, 2004; Mirtallo and others, 2004). The administration of PN in the home is very similar to administration of PN in the acute care setting. Because it is more expensive than enteral feedings and has greater risks for complications (e.g., hyperglycemia, infection, fatty liver, or pneumothorax), PN is used only when other types of nutritional support cannot be used (Sudakin, 2006).

PN is individually formulated to meet each patient's nutritional needs. This nutritionally complete supplement often includes a mixture of amino acids, dextrose, fat emulsions, vitamins, electrolytes, minerals, and trace elements. In the home care setting, PN is often called total nutrient admixture (TNA). TNA is a three-in-one mixture of amino acids, lipids, and dextrose. Usually administration of PN in the home takes about 12 hours. Therefore many patients choose to receive their PN while they sleep. Because of the risks involved with PN and because managing PN in the home is very complex, patients receive at least their first infusion of PN in an acute care setting, and they receive frequent visits from the home care nurse once they are home. Carefully assess the reaction of the patient and family to the use of the technology needed to administer PN at home, and provide emotional support. Although administering PN in the home increases patients' autonomy, it often interferes with their ability to maintain their normal routines. Consult with other health care professionals (e.g., clinical psychologists) when needed (Lehoux and others, 2004). These safeguards ensure patient safety and promote optimal nutritional outcomes.

Nurses who help patients manage PN in the home often face a variety of ethical issues, especially if the patient has a terminal illness or is in a progressive vegetative state. It is usually more difficult to withdraw supplemental nutrition once it is started. Therefore ensure that patients and their families are aware of the benefits and burdens associated with the long-term administration of PN, and provide psychosocial support as they go through the decision-making process (Sudakin, 2006).

Delegation Considerations
The skill of managing parenteral nutrition in the home cannot be delegated to NAP.

Equipment
- ❑ IV solution of PN or TNA
- ❑ IV tubing with optional filter (0.2 μm for dextrose/amino acids, 1.2 μm for TNA)
- ❑ Electronic IV infusion pump with alarms and protection from free flow
- ❑ Home blood glucose monitoring equipment
- ❑ Alcohol swabs
- ❑ Clean gloves
- ❑ Paper or logbook and pencil or pen

STEP	RATIONALE

ASSESSMENT

1 Assess patient's nutritional status and risk for malnutrition using a nutrition screening tool (see Chapter 30). Identify signs and symptoms of malnutrition (e.g., weight loss or weight below ideal level; muscle atrophy, wasting, or weakness; lethargy; unable to eat for more than 6 days). Include measurement of vital signs.

Use of screening tool provides consistent way to identify patient's risk factors and signs or symptoms of malnutrition that indicate long-term need for PN (Sudakin, 2006).

2 Assess patient's fluid and electrolyte levels, as well as serum albumin, total protein, transferrin, prealbumin, triglycerides, and glucose levels.

Provides baseline assessment data. Patients who have severe nutritional deficits are at risk for refeeding syndrome and need close monitoring (Btaiche and Khalidi, 2004).

3 Assess patient's venous access device for edema, drainage, tenderness, and signs of inflammation (see Chapter 28). Measure circumference of upper arm if patient has PICC; mark place on arm where measurement was taken.

Infection is a common complication when patient has a venous access device. Measurement of arm helps detect infiltration of PICC. Mark on arm ensures consistent measurements over time.

4 Verify prescriber's order for nutrients, vitamins, minerals, trace elements, electrolytes, and flow rate.

Ensures safe and accurate PN administration.

5 Assess patient's or caregiver's anxiety level and readiness to learn.

Anxiety prevents learning. Skill is highly complex, and patient needs to be ready to learn.

6 Assess patient's or caregiver's previous knowledge and experience in managing PN in the home. Have patient or caregiver perform return demonstration if able to perform skill.

Determines level of understanding before beginning teaching session.

STEP	RATIONALE

NURSING DIAGNOSES

- Adult failure to thrive
- Anxiety
- Caregiver role strain
- Fatigue
- Imbalanced nutrition: less than body requirements
- Readiness for enhanced nutrition
- Risk for infection
- Social isolation

Related factors are individualized based on patient's condition or needs.

PLANNING

STEP	RATIONALE
1　Expected outcomes following completion of procedure:	
• Patient or caregiver is able to correctly administer PN.	Indicates skills are effectively learned.
• Patient or caregiver demonstrates proper care of CVC.	Prevents infection and ensures patency of venous access device.
• Patient or caregiver states signs and symptoms that need to be reported to health care provider.	Ensures safe administration of PN in home.
2　Select setting in home where patient is most likely to administer PN.	Practicing in same environment where skill is routinely performed facilitates comprehension and learning (Redman, 2007).

IMPLEMENTATION

STEP	RATIONALE
1　Provide name and phone number of persons or resources that are available 24 hours a day, 7 days a week in case problems arise.	Provides assurance and allows patient or caregiver to troubleshoot problems and answer questions (American Society for Parenteral and Enteral Nutrition [ASPEN], 2005).
2　Explain the type/name of infusion, dosage, expected outcomes, and components of PN. Explain that PN needs to be stored in the refrigerator.	Allows patient or caregiver to verify that correct PN is infused and patient or caregiver understands expected outcomes of care. Refrigeration maintains integrity of PN.
3　Have patient or caregiver perform each step with guidance from nurse. Do not rush patient.	Allows you to correct errors in technique as they occur and discuss implications.
4　Instruct patient or caregiver to inspect the label of the bag, ensure the patient's name is on the label, ensure that the bag has not expired, and check the bag for leaks.	Ensures right patient receives right PN. Bag needs to be intact to maintain closed system and ensure patient receives all prescribed nutrients (ASPEN, 2005).
5　Suggest taking PN solution out of the refrigerator for 30 to 60 minutes before scheduled infusion time.	Chilled solution often causes discomfort; allowing solution to warm enhances comfort during infusion (Mirtallo and others, 2004).
6　Perform hand hygiene.	Reduces risk for infection.
7　Explain need to inspect fluid in bag for color and precipitates.	Changes in color or precipitates in bag indicate disruption in the PN.

Critical Decision Point　*If precipitate appears, components of mixture are separated, or color changes, explain that solution needs to be discarded (ASPEN, 2005).*

STEP	RATIONALE
8　Demonstrate how to attach IV tubing to bag, how to attach filter to IV tubing (*optional*), how to prime IV tubing, and how to load IV tubing into electronic infusion pump (see Chapter 28).	Prepares PN solution for IV administration.
9　Put on clean gloves. Wipe CVC port with alcohol, and show how to flush CVC and connect IV tubing to port (see Chapter 28). Use needleless system whenever possible.	CVC needs to be patent, and IV tubing needs to connect to CVC to allow PN to be administered. Needleless systems prevent needle-stick injuries.
10　Explain how to determine appropriate rate of infusion and how to program infusion pump (see Skill 28-2).	Ensures PN is administered at appropriate rate (ASPEN, 2005).
11　Remove and dispose of gloves; perform hand hygiene.	Prevents spread of microorganisms.
12　When infusion is completed, explain how to disconnect IV tubing and flush CVC (see Chapter 28). Ensure patient or caregiver performs hand hygiene before and after disconnecting line.	Flushing CVC following infusion maintains patency of vascular access device. Meticulous hand hygiene prevents infection.
13　Describe appropriate use and storage of infusion pump and supplies. Explain appropriate tubing replacement schedules (e.g., every 24 hours for TNA, 72 hours for three-in-one solutions) (Mirtallo and others, 2004).	Maintains integrity of equipment; appropriate timing of tubing changes prevents infection.
14　Assist in developing plan for appropriate disposal of supplies, including needles, syringes, and unused medications or solutions, using principles of standard precautions.	Implementation of standard precautions is necessary to prevent transmission of communicable diseases and prevents needle-stick injuries.

STEP	RATIONALE
15 Demonstrate appropriate care of CVC site; discuss how to change dressings, frequency of dressing changes, and signs of infection (see Skill 28-6).	Prevents infection at CVC insertion site (Brogden, 2004).
16 Teach patient and/or caregiver about signs and symptoms that indicate potential complications from PN therapy (e.g., infection at CVC site, refeeding syndrome, hyperglycemia, hypernatremia, hypophosphatemia, hypokalemia, hypomagnesemia) and when to call for help (Btaiche and Khalidi, 2004).	Knowledge of complications of PN therapy allows for early detection and appropriate action (ASPEN, 2005).
17 Demonstrate use of self–blood glucose monitor. Explain frequency of testing, normal glucose values, and what to do if values fall outside of expected range (ASPEN, 2005) (see Chapter 43).	PN increases blood glucose levels, which negatively affects patient outcomes (Debaveye and Van den Bergh, 2006). Frequent monitoring of glucose level helps detect problems early. Expect testing frequency to decrease as patient's condition and response to PN stabilizes.
18 Provide patient with a logbook to record administration of PN, weights, I&O, and blood glucose levels.	Allows health care providers and patients to evaluate outcomes and detect adverse effects of nutritional therapy.
19 Help patient develop a plan to reorder supplies, PN fluid, and prescribed additives; also help develop an emergency plan (e.g., what to do if the electricity goes out), and a home safety plan (e.g., fire prevention, how to get to bathroom without tripping).	Plans allow for continuous, safe, and effective administration of PN (ASPEN, 2005).

EVALUATION

1 Have patient or caregiver independently demonstrate initiation, infusion, and discontinuation of PN infusion as well as CVC site care.	Feedback through return demonstration of psychomotor skill is best means of evaluating mastery of skill (Bastable, 2006).
2 Watch patient clean and store PN, equipment, and supplies.	Proper cleaning and storage prevents bacterial growth.
3 Ask patient to identify expected outcomes of nutritional therapy.	Measures patient cognitive learning and confirms understanding of information.
4 Have patient describe common signs and symptoms of infection and other complications of PN.	Measures cognitive learning.
5 Watch patient record information in logbook. Review patient's logbook periodically to ensure information is being recorded correctly.	Health care providers make changes in patient care based on information provided by the patient. To ensure changes are made appropriately, patient needs to record accurate information.

Unexpected Outcomes

1 Patient is unable to manage home PN therapy or verbalize information that was taught.

2 Patient reports signs and symptoms of complications from PN or CVC.

Related Interventions

- Ask patient to describe difficulties experienced while performing skill.
- Use a different teaching strategy.
- Teach family caregiver, and evaluate need to increase frequency of home visits to ensure safe administration of PN at home.
- Inform health care provider.
- Tell patient to call EMS if signs and symptoms are severe.

Recording and Reporting

- Record information taught and patient's response in home care record.
- Record information that evaluates outcomes of PN therapy (e.g., weight, electrolyte and glucose levels, physical assessment findings) in home care record and home documentation system (e.g., logbook).

Teaching Considerations

- Assess patient's psychosocial status while providing information. Many patients experience a decrease in the quality of life when PN feedings are started in the home, which often increases anxiety and decreases comprehension of information (Joque and Jatoi, 2005).
- Eating is often a social event. When patients do not eat, they tend to feel socially isolated. Teach patients and caregivers the importance of maintaining social relationships and enhancing social support during PN therapy. Refer patient to support groups and other resources, such as the Oley Foundation (http://oley.org/index.html) (Sudakin, 2006).

Pediatric Considerations

- The risk for displacement of the CVC increases as the child grows. Ensure that the placement of the venous access device is confirmed with x-ray examination as the child grows (Mirtallo and others, 2004).
- Teach the family to socialize child with other children to enhance development (Hockenberry and Wilson, 2007).

Gerontological Considerations

- Frail older adults are at high risk for electrolyte disturbances. Frequently assess and monitor their response to PN and their laboratory values.
- Carefully assess patient's ability to perform skill. Management of PN at home is complex and requires manual dexterity and visual acuity, as well as high-level critical thinking and decision-making skills. Include caregiver or other family members in teaching plan to help with management of home PN.

 Critical Thinking Exercises

You are scheduled to visit Mr. Anderson, a 75-year-old retired banker who is widowed. Mr. Anderson was recently hospitalized for atrial fibrillation, an abnormal heart rhythm, and was sent home on digoxin, a cardiac glycoside, to control his arrhythmia. Mr. Anderson has impaired visual acuity and is hard of hearing. In addition to his recent arrhythmia, he also has benign prostatic hypertrophy that has worsened and now requires him to catheterize himself. Despite his new health problems, Mr. Anderson is very active and is very interested in learning about his new medical condition and medication. This is your first home visit.

1. What information would you like to have about Mr. Anderson before you go to his home to assist him with safely managing his new medication and learning how to catheterize himself?
2. You teach Mr. Anderson how to take his pulse before he takes his digoxin. How long do you tell him to take his pulse? Explain your choice.
   A. For 15 seconds and then multiply by 4
   B. For 30 seconds and then multiply by 2
   C. For a full minute
   D. For 2 minutes
3. Mr. Anderson tells you he cannot feel his radial pulse after repeated attempts. What is your next step?
4. Describe three teaching strategies you could use to enhance Mr. Anderson's learning.
5. You are preparing to teach Mr. Anderson how to perform CIC. Put the following steps in the order in which you need to teach them:
   A. Slowly and gently remove catheter from bladder, and perform hand hygiene.
   B. Hold penis perpendicular to the body, and cleanse urethral meatus with soapy water and clean washcloth.
   C. Get into a comfortable position.
   D. Lubricate tip of catheter, and spread lubricant around bottom 13 to 18 cm (5 to 7 inches) of catheter.
   E. Teach how to clean and store catheter.
   F. Perform hand hygiene.
   G. Insert catheter 15 to 20 cm (6 to 8 inches) into the meatus until urine begins to flow.
   H. Hold catheter in place while urine flows into toilet or urine collection container.

REVIEW QUESTIONS

1. A patient has purchased a new electronic blood pressure monitoring device. Which nursing action will verify the accuracy of the patient's blood pressure monitor?
   1. Call the patient after 2 weeks of monitoring, and ask for the readings obtained.
   2. Have the patient check her neighbor's blood pressure with the new monitor.
   3. Check the patient's blood pressure with a manual aneroid sphygmomanometer 1 to 2 minutes after the patient checks her blood pressure with her monitor.
   4. Ask the patient to describe when and how she should take her blood pressure using her new monitor.
2. A patient is being discharged from the hospital with home oxygen therapy. What should be included in the nurse's teaching session with him and his family? Select all that apply.
   1. The patient should not allow people in the home to smoke.
   2. The patient should be able to attend his son's Boy Scout campfire.
   3. The patient should use an electric razor when shaving.
   4. The patient should have two complete sets of oxygen delivery devices.
   5. The oxygenation delivery systems can be placed behind the bedroom curtains so the room looks neat and uncluttered.
   6. When filling an ambulatory liquid tank from the stationary reservoir, the first thing to do is to wipe the connectors of both tanks with a lint-free cloth.
3. A patient's family is being taught how to suction the patient's tracheostomy in preparation for her discharge home. What information should be included in the teaching session? Select all that apply.
   1. Instill normal saline to help prevent hypoxia during suctioning.
   2. Set the suction pressure on the suction machine between 160 and 180 mm Hg.
   3. Determine if the patient needs several breaths of 100% oxygen before suctioning.
   4. Place the patient in a supine position.
   5. Grasp the suction catheter with the nondominant hand.
   6. Apply intermittent suction for no more than 15 seconds.

4 An 83-year-old patient cares for himself at home. Which nursing intervention will enhance compliance with his medication regimen?
  1 Teach him everything he needs to know in 1 day, and then check back in 2 weeks.
  2 Include him in deciding the system used to help him remember to take his medications.
  3 Provide printed, large-print instructions that are written in dark blue ink.
  4 Provide medication information when his daughter and infant grandchild are visiting him.

5 An older adult patient had a recent stroke and is receiving home enteral nutrition. What action should the nurse have instructed the family to take if the patient begins to have difficulty breathing and coughing? Select all that apply.
  1 Call the physician.
  2 Put the head of the bed higher.
  3 Verify tube placement.
  4 Stop the feeding.

REFERENCES

American Diabetes Association: Standards of medical care in diabetes, *Diabetes Care* 30(suppl 1):S4, 2007.

American Hospital Association: *Patient care partnership: understanding expectations, rights, and responsibilities,* Chicago, 2003, The Association.

American Society for Parenteral and Enteral Nutrition: Standards for specialized nutrition support: home care patient, *Nutr Clin Pract* 20(5):579, 2005.

Bastable SB: *Nurse as educator: principles of teaching and learning for nursing practice,* Sudbury, Mass, Jones & Bartlett, 2003.

Bastable SB: *Essentials of patient education,* Sudbury, Mass, Jones & Bartlett, 2006.

Bray L, Sanders C: Teaching children and young people intermittent self-catheterization, *Urol Nurs* 27(3):203, 2007.

Brogden B: Current practice in administration of parenteral nutrition: venous access, *Br J Nurs* 13(18):1068, 2004.

Brosche TA and others: Consult stat: how to dodge the dangers of deep suctioning, *RN* 68(9):60, 2005.

Btaiche I, Khalidi N: Metabolic complications of parenteral nutrition in adults, part I, *Am J Health Syst Pharm* 61(15):1938, 2004.

Centers for Medicare and Medicaid Services: *Your Medicare benefits,* 2006, http://www.medicare.gov/Publications/Pubs/pdf/10116.pdf.

Christensen AJ: Patient adherence to medical treatment regimens: bridging the gap between behavioral science and biomedicine, New Haven, 2004, Yale University Press.

City of Tyler, Texas: *Home oxygen safety,* 2007, http://www.cityoftyler.org/Default.aspx?tabid=707.

Curry LC and others: Teaching older adults to self-manage medications, *J Gerontol Nurs* 31(4):32, 2005.

Cutilli CC: Do your patients understand? Providing culturally congruent patient education, *Orthop Nurs* 25(3):218, 2006.

Debaveye Y, Van den Bergh G: Risk and benefits of nutritional support during critical illness, *Annu Rev Nutr* 26:513, 2006.

Duck A: Respiratory care: cost-effectiveness and efficacy in long-term oxygen therapy, *Nurs Times* 102(7):46, 2006.

Ebersole P and others: *Toward healthy aging: human needs and nursing response,* ed 7, St. Louis, 2008, Mosby.

Edwards M: Caring for patients with COPD on long-term oxygen therapy, *Br J Community Nurs* 10(9):404, 2006.

Environmental Protection Agency: *Mercury,* 2007, http://www.epa.gov/mercury/index.htm.

Evans S and others: Home enteral feeding audit 1 year post-initiation, *J Hum Nutr Diet* 19(1):27, 2006.

Falvo DR: *Effective patient education: a guide to increased compliance,* ed 3, Boston, 2004, Jones & Bartlett.

Hockenberry MJ, Wilson D: *Wong's nursing care of infants and children,* ed 8, St. Louis, 2007, Mosby.

Institute of Safe Medical Practice: Helping to remove the barriers to patient education, *ISMP Medication Safety Alert* 8(20):1, 2003, http://www.ismp.org/Newsletters/acutecare/articles/20031002.asp.

Jones DW and others: Measuring blood pressure accurately: new and persistent challenges, *JAMA* 289(8):1027, 2003.

Jones JH: Patient illiteracy, *AORN J* 85(5):951, 2007.

Joque L, Jatoi A: Total parenteral nutrition in cancer patients: why and when? *Nutr Clin Care* 8(2):89, 2005.

Kelly MM: The medically complex premature infant in primary care, *Journal of Pediatric health Care* 20(6):367, 2006.

Levensky ER and others: Motivational interviewing: an evidence-based approach to counseling helps patients follow treatment recommendations, *Am J Nurs* 107(10):50, 2007.

Lewarski JS: Oxygen conserving devices: optimizing the benefits, *AARC Times* 30(9):38, 2006.

Meiner SE, Lueckenotte AG: *Gerontologic nursing,* ed 3, St. Louis, 2006, Mosby.

Merenda LA: Key elements of bladder and bowel management for children with spinal cord injuries, *SCI Nurs* 22(1):8, 2005.

Metheny NA: Preventing respiratory complications of tube feedings: evidence-based practice, *Am J Crit Care* 15(4):360, 2006.

National Institutes of Health: *The seventh report of the Joint National Committee on Prevention, Detection, Evaluation, and Treatment of High Blood Pressure,* http://www.nhlbi.nih.gov/guidelines/hypertension/express.pdf , 2003.

Newton AF, Delegge MH: Home initiation of parenteral nutrition, *Nutr Clin Pract* 22(1):57, 2007.

Osborne H.: *Health literacy from A to Z: practical ways to communicate your health message,* Sudbury, Mass, 2004, Jones & Bartlett.

Petty TL: *Guide to prescribing home oxygen: home oxygen options,* National Lung Health Education Program, http://www.nlhep.org/resources/Prescrb-Hm-Oxygen/home-oxygen-options-4.html, accessed November 17, 2007.

Petty TL and others: *Long-term oxygen therapy (LTOT): history, scientific foundations, and emerging technologies,* http://www.nlhep.org/pdfs/lt_oxygen.pdf, 2005.

Pickering TG and others: Recommendations for blood pressure measurement in humans: an AHA scientific statement from the Council on High Blood Pressure Research Professional and Public Education Subcommittee, *J Clin Hypertens* 7(2):102, 2005.

Pilloni S and others: Intermittent catheterization in older people: a valuable alternative to an indwelling catheter? *Age Ageing* 34(1):57, 2005.

Positive Air, Inc: *Medicare requirements for the home use of oxygen,* http://www.positiveair.com/medicare_home_use_of_oxygen.htm, accessed November 17, 2007.

Redman B: *The practice of patient education,* ed 10, St. Louis, 2007, Mosby.

Robinson J: Intermittent self-catheterization: principles and practice, *Br J Community Nurs* 11(4):144, 2006a.

Robinson J: Intermittent self-catheterization appliances for disabled patients, *Br J Community Nurs* 11(12):520, 2006b.

Robinson J: Intermittent self-catheterization: teaching the skill to patients, *Nurs Stand* 21(29):48, 2007.

Sudakin T: TEN or TPN, *Nursing* 36(12):52, 2006.

The Joint Commission: *National strategies needed to better serve increasingly diverse patient population in American hospitals,* 2007a, http://www.jointcommission.org/NewsRoom/NewsReleases/jc_report_032907.htm.

The Joint Commission: *Speak up,* http://www.jointcommission.org/GeneralPublic/Speak+Up, 2007b.

The Joint Commission: 2009 *Patient safety goals: home care program,* 2007c, http://www.jointcommission.org/PatientSafety/NationalPatientSafetyGoals/08_ome_npsgs.htm.

Williams ME: Clinical consultation: how do we teach clean intermittent self-catheterization using touch technique? *Rehabil Nurs* 30(5):171, 2005.

Wingard R: Patient education and the nursing process: meeting the patient's needs, *Nephrol Nurs J* 32(2):211, 2005.

RESEARCH REFERENCES

Behar-Horenstein LS and others: Improving patient care through patient-family education programs, *Hosp Top* 83(1):21, 2005.

Braun CA: Accuracy of pacifier thermometers in young children, *Pediatr Nurs* 32(5):413, 2006.

Canzanello VJ and others: Improved blood pressure control with a physician-nurse team and home blood pressure measurement, *Mayo Clin Proc* 80(1):31, 2005.

Cappuccio FP and others: Blood pressure control by home monitoring: meta analysis of randomized trials, *BMJ* 329(7458):145, 2004.

Cason CL and others: Nurses' implementation of guidelines for ventilator-associated pneumonia from the Centers for Disease Control and Prevention, *Am J Crit Care* 16(1):28, 2007.

Celik SA, Kanan N: Current conflict: use of isotonic sodium chloride solution on endotracheal suctioning in critically ill patients, *Dimens Crit Care Nurs* 25(1):11, 2006.

Edwards M and others: Neuropathic bladder and intermittent catheterization: social and psychological impact on children and adolescents, *Dev Med Child Neurol* 46(3):168, 2004.

Funahashi J and others: The economic impact of the introduction of home blood pressure measurement for the diagnosis and treatment of hypertension, *Blood Press Monit* 11(5):257, 2006.

Haynes RB and others: Interventions for enhancing medication adherence, *Cochrane Database Syst Rev,* 2008(1):CD000011, DOI:10.1002/14651858.CD000011.pub3, http://www.cochrane.org/reviews/en/ab000011.html.

Hudson TJ and others: A pilot study of barriers to medication adherence in schizophrenia, *J Clin Psychiatry* 65(2):211, 2004.

Jeske L and others: Partnering with patients and families in designing visual cues to prevent falls in hospitalized elders, *J Nurs Care Qual* 21(3):236, 2006.

Karavatas SG: Status of research on selected cardiopulmonary tests and measures utilized in the rehabilitation of geriatric patients, *Top Geriatr Rehabil* 21(3):221, 2005.

Kim H: A randomized controlled trial of a nurse short-message service by cellular phone for people with diabetes, *Int J Nurs Stud* 44(5):687, 2007.

Kovindha A and others: Reused silicone catheter for clean intermittent catheterization (CIC): is it safe for spinal cord–injured men? *Spinal Cord* 42(11):638, 2004.

Kutzleb J, Reiner D: The impact of nurse-directed patient education on quality of life and functional capacity in people with heart failure, *J Am Acad Nurse Pract* 18(3):116, 2006.

Lehoux P and others: The use of technology at home: what patient manuals say and sell vs. what patients face and fear, *Sociol Health Illn* 26(5):617, 2004.

Lemke JR and others: Intermittent catheterization for patients with a neurogenic bladder: sterile versus clean—using evidence-based practice at the staff nurse level, *J Nurs Care Qual* 20:302, 2005.

Lucas GM and others: Adherence, drug use, and treatment failure in a methadone-clinic-based program of directly administered antiretroviral therapy, *AIDS Patient Care STDS* 21(8):564, 2007.

McCorkle R and others: Effects of advanced practice nursing on patient and spouse depressive symptoms, sexual function, and marital interaction after radical prostatectomy, *Urol Nurs* 27(1):65, 2007.

McCoy ML and others: A correlational pilot study of home health nurse management of heart failure patients and hospital readmissions, *Home Health Care Manage Pract* 19(5):392, 2007.

Mayer DK and others: Cancer survivors information seeking behaviors: a comparison of survivors who do and do not seek information about cancer, *Patient Educ Couns* 65(3):342, 2007.

Metlay JP and others: Medication safety in older adults: home-based practice patterns, *J Am Geriatr Soc* 53(6):976, 2005.

Mirtallo J and others: Safe practices for parenteral nutrition, *JPEN J Parenter Enteral Nutr* 28(6):S38, 2004.

Montagnino BA, Mauricio RV: The child with a tracheotomy and gastrostomy: parental stress and coping in the home—a pilot study, *Pediatr Nurs* 30(5):373, 2004.

Muir-Cochrane E and others: Self-management of medication for mental health problems by homeless young people, *Int J Ment Health Nurs* 15(3):163, 2006.

Oh SJ and others: Effect of a "centralized intensive education system" for clean intermittent self-catheterization in patients with voiding dysfunction who start catheterization for the first time, *Int J Urol* 13(7):905, 2006.

Quatrara B and others: The effect of respiratory rate and ingestion of hot and cold beverages on the accuracy of oral temperatures measured by electronic thermometers, *Medsurg Nurs* 16(2):105, 2007.

Rassin M and others: Personal medical documents management—how patients perceive, keep and manage their medical documents: a qualitative study, *Int J Nurs Stud* 44(6):862, 2007.

Risica PM, Phipps MG: Educational preferences in a prenatal clinic population, *Int J Childbirth Educ* 21(4):4, 2006.

Roberts K, Naik R: Urinary catheters: catheterization options following radical surgery for cervical cancer, *Br J Nurs* 15(19):1038, 2006.

Robinson JL and others: Accuracy of parents in measuring body temperature with a tympanic thermometer, *BMC Family Practice* 6(1):3, 2005.

Scharf Donovan H and others: An update on the representational approach to patient education, *J Nurs Scholarsh* 39(3):259, 2007.

Schommer JC and others: Interdisciplinary medication education in a church environment, *Am J Health Syst Pharm* 59(5):423, 2002.

Schuh S and others: Comparison of the temporal artery and rectal thermometry in children in the emergency department, *Pediatr Emerg Care* 20(11):736, 2004.

Seckel M: Implementing evidence based practice guidelines to minimize ventilator-associated pneumonia, *AACN News* 24(1):8, 2007.

Sidat M and others: Experiences and perceptions of patients with 100% adherence to highly active antiretroviral therapy: a qualitative study, *AIDS Patient Care STDS* 21(7):509, 2007.

Silver HJ and others: Older adults receiving home enteral nutrition: enteral regimen, provider involvement, and health care outcomes, *JPEN J Parenter Enteral Nutr* 28(2):92, 2004.

Skeie S and others: Accurate self-monitoring of blood glucose (SMBG) and tailored education improves metabolic control in type 1 diabetes (the MEASURE study), *Diabetes* 56(suppl 1): pA115, 2007.

Society of Urologic Nurses and Associates: Clinical practice guidelines: adult clean intermittent catheterization, 2006, http://www.suna.org/cgi-bin/WebObjects/SUNAMain.woa/wa/viewSection?s_id=1073743840&ss_id=536873467.

Suhonen R, Leino-Kilpi H: Adult surgical patients and the information provided to them by nurses: a literature review, *Patient Educ Couns* 61(1):5, 2006.

Thanavaro JL and others: Predictors of health promotion behavior in women without prior history of coronary heart disease, *Appl Nurs Res* 19(3):149, 2006.

White J and others: Parents measuring pulses: an observational study, *Arch Dis Child* 89(3):274, 2004.

Specimen Collection

KEY TERMS

Aseptic technique
Aspirate
Blood culture
Clean-voided specimen
Culture
Double-voided specimen
Dysuria
Expectorate
Glucose monitoring
Guaiac test
Hematuria

Ketones
Melena
Midstream collection
Occult blood
Point-of-care test
Reagent
Sensitivity
Timed urine collection
Urgency
Vacutainer tube
Venipuncture
Void

MEDIA RESOURCES

- **evolve** *learning system* http://evolve.elsevier.com/Perry/skills
    - Review Questions
    - Video Clips

-  Mosby's Nursing Video Skills, 3.0

- **NSO** Nursing Skills Online

Mastery of content in this chapter will enable the nurse to:

- Explain the rationale for the collection of each specimen.
- Identify special conditions necessary for collection of each specimen.
- Explain instructions to encourage patient cooperation for successful collection of the specimen.
- Recognize the impact of sociocultural issues that affect patient's cooperation with collection of specimen.
- Identify measures to minimize anxiety and promote safety during specimen collection.
- Discuss nursing responsibilities for processing a specimen after collection.
- Chart appropriate information in a patient's record after collection of the specimen.
- Properly collect clean-voided, timed, and catheterized urine specimens.

- Correctly measure glucose, ketones, protein, blood, and pH in urine.
- Correctly check for the presence of occult blood in a stool specimen.
- Correctly perform measures to detect occult blood in gastric secretions.
- Properly collect specimens for culture from the nose and throat, urethra and vagina, sputum, and wound.
- Properly perform venipuncture.
- Properly collect blood specimen from peripheral and central venous access.
- Properly collect specimens for blood cultures.
- Correctly perform blood glucose monitoring.
- Use infection control practices to prevent transmission of pathogens.
- Properly perform arterial puncture for blood gas measurement.

Proficiency in performing point-of-care (POC) tests and assisting with diagnostic testing and specimen collection and analysis are nursing responsibilities. Skill and judgment in obtaining specimens affect patient comfort and ensure accuracy and quality of diagnostic procedures. Accountability, attention to monitoring patient outcomes, and current health care economics increase the demand for accurate and timely laboratory tests.

Laboratory examination of urine, stool, sputum, blood, and wound drainage specimens provides important information about body functioning and contributes to the assessment of a patient's health status. Laboratory test results aid in the diagnosis of health care problems, provide information about the stage and activity of a disease process, and measure a patient's response to therapy.

Normal values for laboratory tests are found in reference books. In addition, a laboratory may establish its own values for each test. These values are usually readily available on the agency's laboratory slips. Discuss any major deviations with the health care provider or physician immediately.

Patients are often embarrassed or uncomfortable when giving a sample of body excretions or secretions. Excretion is the process by which the body eliminates or sheds substances by organs or tissues. Secretion is the release of chemical substances manufactured by cells of glandular organs. When collecting specimens, wear gloves and perform hand hygiene. Also, handle excretions discretely. Invasive collection procedures and fear of unknown test results often cause patients anxiety. Patients who receive clear explanation about the purpose of the specimen and how you will obtain it are more cooperative. Give patients proper instruction in collecting their own specimens of urine, stool, and sputum, thus avoiding embarrassment.

Laboratory tests are expensive. You can minimize unnecessary costs by using the correct procedure for obtaining and processing specimens. Consult the institution's procedure manual, or call the laboratory with questions about laboratory tests.

The assurance of confidentiality is an important issue associated with laboratory testing. Disclosure of confidential information can result in discrimination in a variety of circumstances. Agencies must have clearly written and enforced policies regarding disclosure of test results and maintenance of confidentiality throughout the health care system (U.S. Department of Health and Human Services, 2006).

EVIDENCE-BASED PRACTICE TRENDS

Positive patient identification is a term that means the patient is positively identified before the procedure. Before obtaining a laboratory specimen, use at least two identifiers, such as the identification number on the admission armband and asking the patient's name. Be aware of agency policies that govern obtaining laboratory specimens. Correct identification of patients for laboratory tests, as well as the delivery of care, are in the National Patient Safety Goals of The Joint Commission (TJC) (2008).

The U.S. Food and Drug Administration (FDA) approved at least 18 self-testing home kits, including serum cholesterol, human immunodeficiency virus (HIV), prothrombin time (PT), and glucose. Nurses usually perform these tests as point-of-care testing at the bedside. Patients who self-test with point-of-care tests need education about issues related to these tests. The testing kits are self-testing, not self-diagnosing (Corbett, 2008).

The role of the nurse is extremely important in specimen collection. Proper specimen collection technique minimizes need for additional specimen collection, unnecessary treatments, and higher cost of medical care (Barclay and Murata, 2007; Beall and others, 2007; Dock, 2005). Needleless and needle safety devices enable health care providers to collect blood specimens more safely with a lowered risk for needle-stick injuries (see Chapter 22).

CULTURAL CONSIDERATIONS

Assess cultural beliefs associated with specimen collection. For example, Southeast Asians consider blood as irreplaceable. They may become anxious about a needle penetrating the skin, allowing blood to seep out. The insertion of a foreign object into the mouth to collect specimens may be threatening to the Southeast Asian patient who believes that diseases can be introduced through the mouth and that the head is the seat of one's life force (D'Avanzo, 2008).

Consider both cultural and language barriers when delegating specimen collection to the patient and family members. For example, Muslims and Hindus designate which hand is to be used for clean and dirty tasks. Collecting their own stool and urine specimens may be difficult because only the left hand can be used for "dirty" activities. Provide for hygienic needs of patients after the procedure, including hand hygiene and cleansing of the anus and urinary meatus. Language barriers make it difficult to explain the purpose of tests and collection techniques. Be sure to provide repeated return demonstrations to ensure the patient or family member understands how to perform a procedure.

Whenever possible, use gender-congruent caregivers when collecting specimens (vaginal, rectal, and urinary) from patients whose cultural values uphold distinct separation of gender roles and modesty. Provide privacy when giving instructions and during specimen collection.

 Skill Performance Guidelines

1 Adapt to the patient's need and ability to perform and/or participate in specimen collection procedures.
2 Recognize that specimen collection may cause anxiety, embarrassment, and/or discomfort.
3 Provide support for patients who are fearful of the results of a specimen examination.
4 Adapt to age-related factors that affect patient's compliance with specimen collection.
5 Recognize that children require simple explanations and demonstration of procedures and benefit from support of parents/ family members.
6 Adapt sociocultural variations that affect patient's compliance with specimen collection.
7 Verify patient's identity by using at least two forms of identifiers. Verify the type of procedure scheduled and the procedure site with the patient. Ensures accurate patient identification

and improves patient safety. Use of patient's room number is not an acceptable identifier (TJC, 2008).
8 Obtain specimens in accordance with specific prerequisite conditions (e.g., fasting, nothing by mouth [NPO]) as required.
9 Follow standard precautions (see Chapter 7) when collecting specimens of blood or other body fluids.
10 Collect specimens in appropriate containers, at the correct time, and in the appropriate amount.
11 Properly label all specimens with the patient's identification; complete laboratory requisition as necessary.
12 Deliver specimens to the laboratory within the recommended time, or ensure that they are stored properly for later transport.
13 Follow procedures for special conditions (e.g., iced specimens, special containers with preservatives) required for transport of specimens.
14 Know institutional policy regarding infection control practices for transportation of all specimen containers of body substances.
15 Follow procedure for medications or dietary intake that may result in some deviations from normal values.
16 Follow precautions for collecting specimens from patients who are in protective isolation.

SKILL 43-1   Urine Specimen: Midstream (Clean-Voided) Urine; Sterile Urinary Catheter Specimen

Intermediate / Specimen Collection / Collecting a Midstream Urine Specimen
Urinary Catheter Management / Obtaining a Sterile Urine Specimen

[NSO] *Specimen Collection Module / Lessons 1 and 2*

A common test performed on urine is a culture and sensitivity measurement. In the laboratory a few drops of urine are placed on a special medium to determine whether or not bacteria are present. Readings are made at 24- and 48-hour intervals, and the final reading is made after 72 hours. If bacteria are present, sensitivity testing reveals which antibiotics will be effective against the microorganism.

When patients can void voluntarily, collect a midstream urine specimen for culture and sensitivity testing. You may need to assist some patients who are unable to collect a specimen independently. A patient begins to urinate and during the middle portion of voiding collects a specimen. The initial stream flushes the urethral orifice and meatus of possible bacteria. It is easiest for a patient to obtain a clean-voided specimen while using toilet facilities rather than a bedpan or urinal.

A patient who has an indwelling catheter may require the collection of a urine specimen. Use strict aseptic technique to ensure sterility and to avoid introducing bacteria into the urinary tract. Do not collect a urine specimen for culture tests from a urine drainage bag unless it is the first urine to drain into a new sterile bag. Bacteria grow rapidly in drainage bags and can give a false measurement of bacteria in the urine.

Delegation Considerations

The skill of collecting a midstream (clean-voided) or sterile urine from an indwelling catheter can be delegated to NAP. The nurse directs the NAP by:

- Informing about any mobility restrictions patient has that will affect collection technique.
- Informing when to obtain specimens.
- Instructing about reporting when blood, mucus, or foul odors are present in the specimen.

Equipment

❏ Completed identification labels with proper patient identifiers.
❏ Completed laboratory requisition with date, time, name of test, patient identification, and source of culture
❏ Clean gloves
❏ Small biohazard plastic bag for delivery of specimen to laboratory (or container specified by agency)

Clean-Voided Specimen

❏ Commercial kit (Fig. 43-1) for clean-voided urine containing:
  - Sterile cotton balls and/or 2 × 2 inch gauze pads, cleansing towelette, or two 4 × 4 inch gauze pads
  - Antiseptic solution (chlorhexidine or povidone-iodine solution)
  - Sterile water or normal saline
  - Sterile specimen container
❏ Sterile and clean gloves
❏ Soap, water, washcloth, and towel
❏ Bedpan (for nonambulatory patient), specimen hat (Fig. 43-2) (if all urine needs to be measured), potty-chair (for young child)

Sterile Urine Specimen From an Indwelling Catheter

❏ 3-mL safety syringe with 1-inch needle (21 gauge) (for culture) or 3-mL Luer-Lok syringe (for needleless port)
❏ 20-mL safety syringe with 1-inch needle (21 gauge) (for routine urinalysis) or 20-mL Luer-Lok syringe (for needleless port)
❏ Alcohol, chlorhexidine, or other disinfectant swab
❏ Clamp or rubber band
❏ Specimen container (nonsterile for routine urinalysis, sterile for culture)
❏ Clean gloves

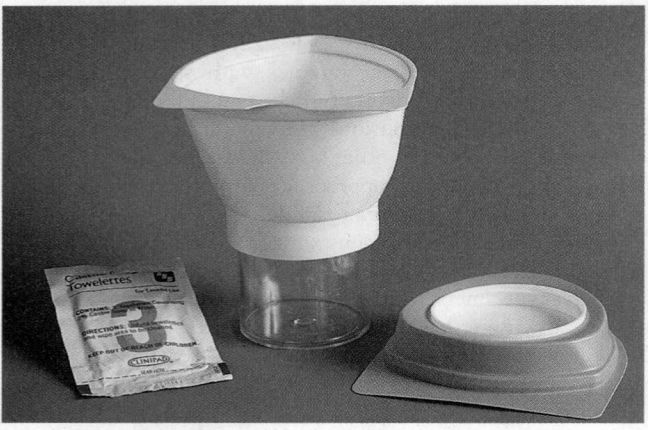

FIG 43-1   Clean-voided specimen collection kit.

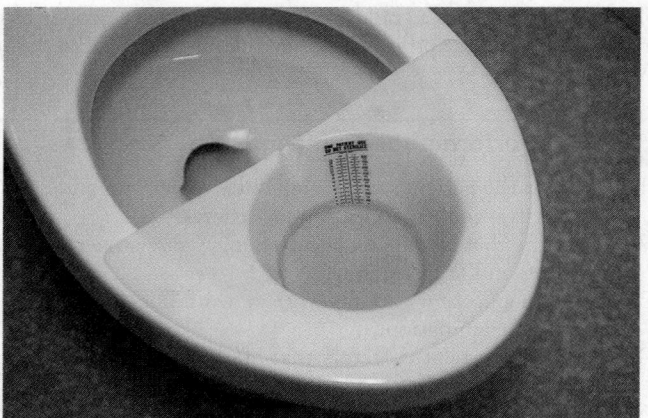

FIG 43-2   Specimen hat.

STEP	RATIONALE

ASSESSMENT

1   Assess patient's or family members' understanding of purpose of test and method of collection.

2   Assess for signs and symptoms of urinary tract infections: frequency; urgency; dysuria; hematuria; flank pain; fever; cloudy, malodorous urine; burning pain on urination; voiding in small amounts; an inability to void; and incomplete emptying of the bladder.

3   Refer to medical record for indications of urinary infection.
   a   Assess risks for urinary tract infection (e.g., poor perineal hygiene, improperly handled diagnostic instruments, previous urinary catheterization).

4   Refer to agency procedures for specimen collection methods.

5   Complete procedure-related assessment
   a   Clean-voided specimen
      (1)   Assess patient's mobility, balance, and coordination in being able to cleanse own perineum and use toilet facilities independently.
   b   Sterile specimen from urinary catheter
      (1)   Assess indwelling catheter for type of built-in sampling port and type of material from which it is made (Dock, 2005).

Rationale:

Information allows nurse to clarify misunderstanding; promotes patient compliance.
Indicates bacteria in urine.

Allows nurse to anticipate need to test patient's urine for bacteria.
Helps nurse explain purpose of specimen procedure for patient.

Agency policies may vary regarding collection and/or handling of specimens.

Determines level of assistance required by patient.

Provides appropriate place for removal of urine from catheter and selection of correct equipment. Port prevents leakage of urine from catheter. For needle port it is safe to insert needle directly into self-sealing rubber catheter. For needleless Luer-Lok port the one-way valve prevents leakage. Do not puncture Silastic, silicone, or plastic catheters with a needle. These are not self-sealing.

NURSING DIAGNOSES

- Acute pain
- Anxiety
- Deficient knowledge regarding specimen collection
- Risk for infection

Individualize related factors based on patient's condition or needs.

PLANNING

1   Expected outcomes following completion of procedure:
   - Patient produces midstream urine specimen that is not contaminated with feces or toilet tissue.
   - Urine has normal characteristics.

Proper collection technique prevents substances from changing normal characteristics of urine.
Specimen collected correctly provides evidence of absence of infection.

STEP	RATIONALE
• Patient will discuss purpose and benefits of midstream urine collection.	Evaluate patient's learning.
• Urine specimen is obtained from the catheter without contamination.	Procedure is safely performed.
• Urinary catheter and drainage system remain intact.	There is no indication (e.g. leaking of urine) that catheter or drainage system was punctured by needle or valve dislodged during specimen collection.

2 Offer patient appropriate fluids to drink (if permitted) before attempting to collect specimen.

Enhances patient's ability to void.

3 Explain procedure to patient and/or family member.
   a Explain reason midstream specimen is needed.
   b Inform how to obtain specimen free of feces and tissue.
   c Explain why catheter will need to be clamped for 30 minutes before obtaining urine specimen and why it is not obtained from drainage bag.
   d Emphasize that although some types of indwelling catheter need a syringe with needle to remove urine from the catheter, the patient will not experience any discomfort.

.

Promotes cooperation and participation.

Feces and tissue alter chemical composition of specimen.

Prevents development of anxiety over catheter clamping and promotes understanding of need to collect urine coming from bladder.

Prevents anxiety when nurse manipulates catheter and aspirates urine with syringe and/or needle. Promotes patient cooperation.

IMPLEMENTATION

1 Verify patient's identity by using at least two forms of identifiers, neither of which is the patient's room number. Verify the type of procedure scheduled and the procedure site with the patient.

Ensures accurate patient identification and improves patient safety. Use of patient's room number is not an acceptable identifier (TJC, 2008).

2 Perform hand hygiene, and label specimen container.

Reduces transfer of microorganisms. Labeling before collection decreases mislabeling or not labeling after collection (Ernst, 2007).

3 Provide privacy for patient; close curtains around bed, or close room door. Allow mobile patients to collect specimen in bathroom.

Privacy allows patient to relax and produce a specimen more easily.

4 Collect clean-voided specimen.
   a Give patient cleansing towelette or towel, washcloth, and soap to cleanse perineum. If patient is dependent, don clean gloves and assist patient with cleansing perineum.
   b Assist bedridden patient onto bedpan (see illustration). Raise head of bed.
   c Using surgical asepsis, open sterile kit or prepare sterile tray.
   d Apply sterile gloves (when assisting dependent patient).

   e Pour antiseptic solution over cotton balls (unless kit contains prepared gauze pads in antiseptic solution).
   f Open specimen container, and place cap with sterile inside surface up, and do not touch inside of container.

Patients prefer to wash their own perineal areas when possible. Cleansing prevents contamination of specimen after urine passes from urethra.

Provides easy access to perineal areas to collect specimen. Semisitting position eases voiding.

Maintains sterility of equipment.

Prevents introduction of microorganisms on nurse's hands into specimen.

Cotton ball or gauze is used to cleanse perineum.

Contaminated specimen is a frequent reason for inaccurate reporting on urine cultures and sensitivities.

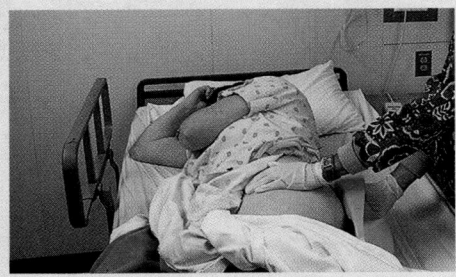

STEP 4b   Nurse assisting patient on a bedpan.

STEP	RATIONALE
g Assist or allow patient to independently cleanse perineum and collect specimen. The amount of assistance needed varies with each patient.	Maintains patient's dignity and comfort.
(1) Male patient	
(a) Nurse or patient will hold patient's penis with one hand. Using circular motion and antiseptic swab, cleanse meatus, moving from center to outside (see illustration). In uncircumcised men, retract the foreskin before cleansing.	Reduces number of microorganisms at urethral meatus and moves from areas of least to most contamination.
(b) If agency procedure indicates, rinse area with sterile water and dry with cotton balls or gauze pad.	Prevents contamination of specimen with antiseptic solution.
(c) After patient has initiated urine stream into toilet or bedpan, pass urine specimen container into stream and collect 30 to 60 mL of urine (see illustration).	Initial urine flushes out microorganisms that normally accumulate at urinary meatus and prevents collection in specimen.
(2) Female patient	

Critical Decision Point   *If patient is menstruating, record this information on laboratory slip.*

STEP	RATIONALE
(a) Either nurse or patient will spread patient's labia minora with thumb and forefinger or forefinger and middle finger of nondominant hand.	Provides access to urethral meatus.
(b) Use dominant hand to cleanse urethral area with swab (cotton ball or gauze), moving from front (above urethral orifice) to back (toward anus). Using a fresh swab each time, repeat front-to-back motion three times (begin with left side, then right side, then down center) (see illustration).	Prevents contamination of urinary meatus with fecal material. Cleansing down center last decreases contamination from labia.

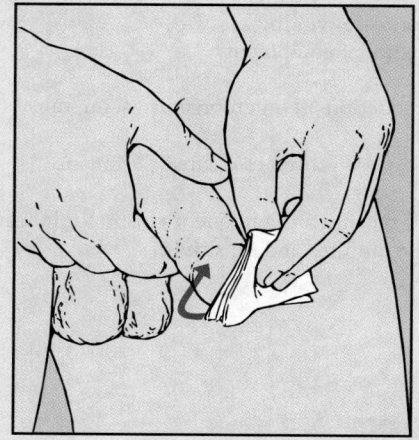

STEP 4g(1)(a)   Cleansing technique (male).

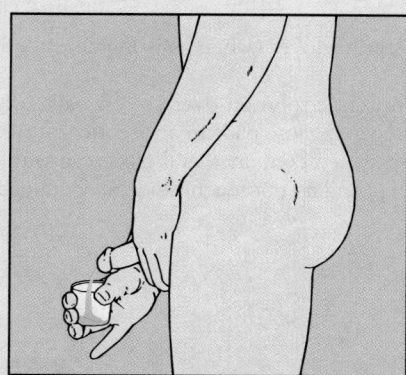

STEP 4g(1)(c)   Collecting midstream urine specimen (male).

STEP	RATIONALE

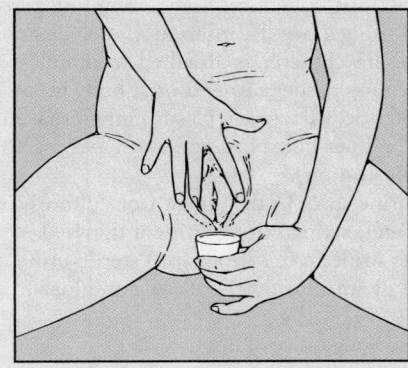

STEP 4g(2)(b)   Cleansing technique (female).

STEP 4g(2)(d)   Collection of midstream urine specimen (female).

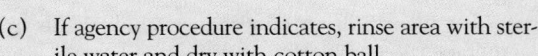

(c) If agency procedure indicates, rinse area with sterile water and dry with cotton ball.

Prevents contamination of specimen with antiseptic solution.

(d) While continuing to hold labia apart, patient should initiate urine stream into toilet or bedpan; after stream is achieved, pass specimen container into stream and collect 30 to 60 mL of urine (see illustration).

Initial stream flushes out resident microorganisms that accumulate at urethral meatus.

h Remove specimen container before flow of urine stops and before releasing labia or penis. Patient finishes voiding into bedpan or toilet. Offer or assist with personal hygiene as appropriate.

Prevents contamination of specimen with skin flora.

i Replace cap securely on specimen container (touch only outside).

Retains sterility of inside of container and prevents spillage of urine.

j Cleanse urine from exterior surface of container.

Prevents transfer of microorganisms to others.

k Empty bedpan (if applicable), remove and discard gloves, and perform hand hygiene.

Reduces transmission of microorganisms.

5 Sterile urinary catheter specimen

a Clamp drainage tubing with clamp or rubber band for 30 minutes.

Permits collection of fresh sterile urine in catheter tubing rather than draining into bag.

b Return to room, and inform patient that procedure to collect specimen from catheter will begin.

Allows patient to anticipate manipulation of urinary catheter and cope more effectively with discomfort that may occur when catheter is moved.

c Perform hand hygiene, label specimen container, and put on clean gloves.

Reduces transfer of microorganisms.

d Position patient so that catheter is easily accessible.

Allows for easy collection of specimen.

e Cleanse entry port for needle or port to attach Luer-Lok syringe with disinfectant swab. Wait until disinfectant is dry.

Prevents entry of microorganisms into catheter.

STEP	RATIONALE

f Perform urine collection from a sampling port.

    (1) If using a needle, insert at 45-degree angle just above where catheter is attached to drainage tube in self-sealing rubber catheter or at built-in sampling port in Silastic, silicone, or plastic catheter (see illustration).

    Ensures entrance of needle into catheter lumen. Prevents accidental puncture of lumen that leads to balloon that holds catheter in place in bladder. Aspiration of water from lumen can result in catheter slipping out of bladder.

    (2) For Luer-Lok port, screw on syringe to attach (see illustration).

g Draw urine into 3-mL syringe (for culture), or draw urine into 20-mL syringe (for routine urinalysis).

    Allows collection of urine without contamination. Proper volume is needed to perform test.

h Transfer urine from syringe into sterile urine container for culture or into nonsterile urine container for routine urinalysis.

    Prevents contamination of urine during transfer procedure.

i Place lid snug on container.

    Prevents contamination of specimen by air and spillage.

j Unclamp catheter, and allow urine to flow into drainage bag.

    Allows urine to drain by gravity and prevents stasis of urine in bladder, which can cause discomfort and potential damage to kidneys.

6 Dispose of soiled supplies, remove and discard gloves, and perform hand hygiene.

    Reduces transmission of microorganisms.

7 Attach laboratory requisition to specimen.

    Incorrect identification of specimen could result in diagnostic or therapeutic errors.

8 Take specimen to laboratory within 15 to 20 minutes. Refrigerate specimen if it not taken to the laboratory within 2 hours.

    Transport specimen to laboratory immediately. If this is not possible, specimen may be refrigerated (Pagana and Pagana, 2007).

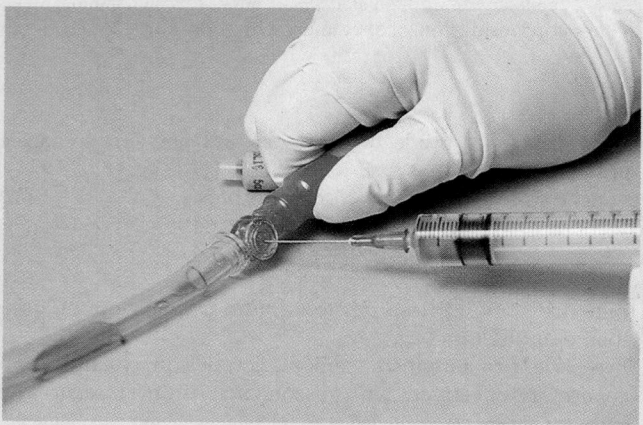

STEP 5f(1) Insertion of needle through self-sealing port.

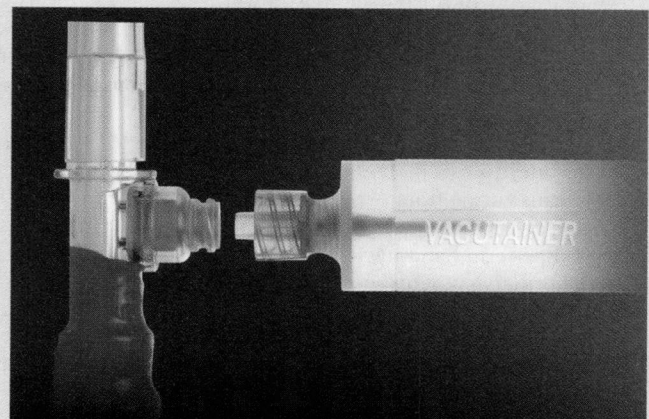

STEP 5f(2) Needle-free sampling port. (*Courtesy Becton Dickinson and Co.*)

EVALUATION

1 Observe characteristics of urine and contaminants such as toilet paper or feces.

    Contaminants prevent specimen from being used.

2 Assess patient's urine culture and sensitivity report for bacterial growth.

    Routine cultures identify organism(s), and sensitivity study identifies antimicrobial medications that may be effective against pathogen.

3 Observe urinary drainage system to ensure that it is intact and patent.

    System must remain closed to remain sterile.

4 Ask patient to describe midstream urine collection procedure.

    Validates patient's understanding.

Unexpected Outcomes	Related Interventions
1 Urine specimen is contaminated with feces or toilet paper.	• Repeat patient instruction and specimen collection. If unable to obtain specimen through clean voiding, patient may need catheterization (see Skill 33-1).
2 Urine specimen is accidentally discarded.	• Repeat specimen collection.
3 Patient is unable to urinate on demand.	• Offer fluids if permitted. Allow more time for urine to accumulate in bladder. Try obtaining specimen after 30 minutes.
4 Urine culture reveals bacterial growth (determined by colony count of more than 10,000 organisms per milliliter).	• Report findings to health care provider. • Administer medications as ordered. • Monitor patient for fever and dysuria.
5 Lumen leading to balloon that holds catheter in bladder is punctured.	• Notify health care provider. • Prepare for removal and insertion of new catheter. • Collect specimen.
6 Patient has pain during procedure.	• Stop and continue to monitor patient. • Notify health care provider. • Administer pain medication if ordered.

Recording and Reporting

- Record collection of specimen in nurses' notes or per agency policy; note time and date, appearance, odor and color of urine, and disposition to laboratory.
- Report any abnormal findings.

Teaching Considerations

- Discuss signs and symptoms of urinary tract infection.
- Explain significance of cleansing genital area before collecting specimen.
- Explain to female patient importance of cleansing labia from front to back.

Pediatric Considerations

- Use a sterile plastic urine collecting bag that adheres to the perineum of a non–toilet-trained child. Special considerations for boys: place penis and scrotum inside the bag (Fig. 43-3). Researchers have found cleansing procedure before the urine collection is not beneficial for non–toilet-trained children (Behrman and others, 2004). Cleansing is effective with toilet-trained children. To cleanse the perineum use soap and water to decrease contamination of a midstream urine collection (Vaillancourt and others, 2007).
- Give instructions and/or explanations regarding cleansing and collecting the specimen to children in an age-appropriate manner such as use of a doll to help with explanation. This will encourage cooperation and decrease anxiety during the collection process.
- It may be easier to collect a midstream urine specimen in a young girl by having the child sit facing the back of the toilet. In this position the labia are naturally separated, decreasing the chance of contamination (Hockenberry and Wilson, 2007).
- The greatest number and variety of real and imagined fears present during the preschool years. The best method to help preschool children with procedures is to actively involve them in practical methods to deal with frightening experiences (Hockenberry and Wilson, 2007).

Gerontological Considerations

- Assistance for older adults depends on ability and independence. Clear and concise explanation about procedure and reason for sample will increase cooperation. Make sure all equipment is available at bedside within easy reach to allow proceeding with obtaining specimen by the patient or when ready for assistance by the nurse or designated person.

Home Care Consideration

- Ideally, specimens for culture should not be collected at home because time delay before laboratory culture would greatly enhance bacterial growth. If patient collects the urine specimen, the patient should keep it on ice until it reaches the laboratory for testing.

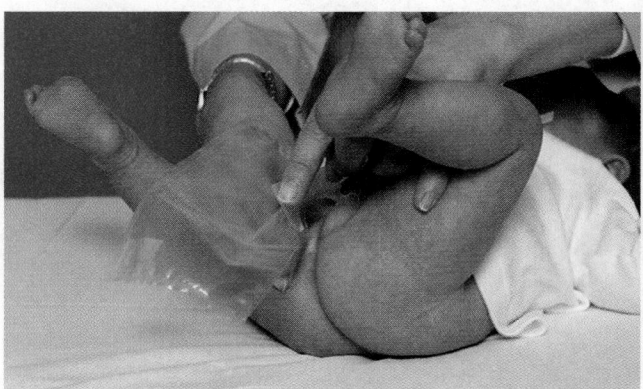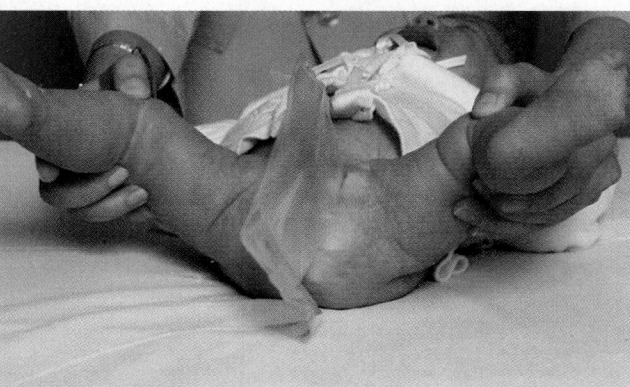

FIG 43-3   Application of urine collection bag. (*From Hockenberry MJ, Wilson D: Wong's nursing care of infants and children, ed 8, St. Louis, 2007, Mosby.*)

PROCEDURAL GUIDELINE 43-1   Collecting a Timed Urine Specimen

Some tests of renal function and urine composition require urine to be collected over 2 to 72 hours. The 24-hour timed collection is most common. The tests measure for elements such as amino acids, creatinine, hormones, glucose, and adrenocorticosteroids, the levels of which fluctuate throughout the day. A timed urine collection can also provide a means to measure the concentration or dilution of urine.

Timed urine collections begin after a patient urinates. The nurse discards the first specimen and then collects every successive specimen until the time period has ended. Each specimen is transferred immediately to a large collection bottle kept in the patient's bathroom. Any missed specimens make test results inaccurate. The patient should always provide the last specimen as close as possible to the end of the collection period.

Delegation Considerations

The skill of collecting a timed urine specimen can be delegated to NAP. However, you are responsible for determining purpose of timed urine specimen collection, timed period collection, if fluid or dietary requirements or medications are administered in conjunction with test, patient's ability to correctly collect specimen, if specimen needs to be on ice, and if preservatives are used in the collection bottle. The nurse directs the NAP about:

- When timed collection begins and the proper way to store the specimen during the collection period.
- Placing signs in patient's toileting area indicting a timed urine collection is taking place and to collect all urine for the specified time.
- Reporting when blood, mucus, or foul odors are present in the urine specimen.

Equipment

- ❑ Large collection bottle with cap that usually contain a chemical for urine preservation
- ❑ Bedpan, urinal, specimen hat, bedside commode, or pediatric potty-chair
- ❑ Graduated measuring container, if intake and output (I&O) are to be recorded
- ❑ Basin large enough to hold collection bottle surrounded by ice if immediate refrigeration is required
- ❑ Specimen identification label
- ❑ Laboratory requisition
- ❑ Signs to save urine for timed specimen collection
- ❑ Clean gloves
- ❑ Small biohazard plastic bag for delivery of specimen to laboratory (or container specified by agency)
- ❑ Instructional signs that remind patient and staff of timed urine collection

Procedural Steps

1. Explain the reasons for specimen collection, how patient can assist, and that urine must be free of feces and toilet tissue.
2. Place specimen collection container in the bathroom and, if indicated, in a pan of ice. Post signs to remind staff and patient of timed urine collection. If patient leaves unit, be sure that personnel in receiving area collect and save all urine.
3. Apply clean gloves, and collect first specimen and discard. Indicate time on laboratory requisition. Begin collecting all urine for designated time.
4. Measure volume of each voiding if output is to be recorded.
5. Place all voided urine in labeled specimen bottle with appropriate additives. Remind patient not to place toilet tissue in the bottle and to empty urine into bottle before defecating.
6. Encourage patient to empty bladder during last 15 minutes of urine collection period.
7. At end of period, send labeled specimen to laboratory with appropriate requisition.
8. Remove signs and inform patient that specimen collection period is completed.

PROCEDURAL GUIDELINE 43-2 Measuring Chemical Properties of Urine: Glucose, Ketones, Protein, Blood, and pH

Intermediate / Specimen Collection / Screening Urine for Chemical Properties

Tests for chemical properties of urine are part of the routine urinalysis completed in the laboratory or as a point-of-care test performed quickly at the bedside or in the home. Urine testing for glucose and acetone monitors glucose and ketone bodies. The test is easy to perform and causes no pain; however, it is being replaced by testing capillary blood, which is obtained by skin puncture (see Skill 43-8). Capillary blood monitoring is an accurate assessment of current serum glucose levels (Pagana and Pagana 2007).

You assess the chemical properties of urine by immersing a special chemically prepared strip of paper into a clean urine specimen or by combining drops of urine with chemically prepared tablets. The change in color of the strip or tablet indicates the presence of any of these substances.

Delegation Considerations
The skill of obtaining a specimen, performing the test, and reporting the results of the test can be delegated to NAP. However, you are responsible for the assessment of the patient's ability to obtain a specimen, to follow any specific health care provider orders, and to understand the procedure. The nurse directs the NAP to:
- Report any odor, blood, or mucus in the urine specimen.

Equipment
☐ Bedpan, urinal, specimen hat, bedside commode, or pediatric potty-chair

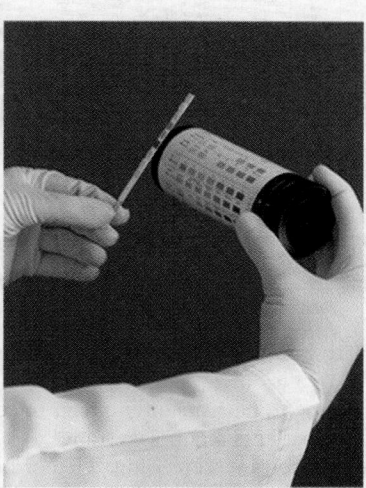

FIG 43-4   Testing urine using a reagent strip.

☐ Watch with second hand
☐ Reagent strip or tablets (check expiration date)
☐ Container with color strip code
☐ Paper towel
☐ Clean gloves
☐ Small biohazard plastic bag for delivery of specimen to laboratory (or container specified by agency)

Procedural Steps
1 Determine if double-voided specimen is needed for testing. If required:
  a Ask patient to collect random urine specimen and discard.
  b Have patient drink a glass of water.
  c Have patient collect another specimen 30 to 45 minutes later.
2 Perform hand hygiene, and apply clean gloves.
3 Use Multistix reagent test strip. It may simultaneously assess for up to 10 chemical properties: specific gravity, pH, protein, glucose, ketones, blood, bilirubin, urobilinogen, leukocytes, and nitrites (Hamill, 2007).
  a Immerse end of chemically impregnated test strip into urine.
  b Remove strip from container immediately, and tap it gently against side of container.
  c Time for number of seconds specified on container, and compare color of strip with color chart (Fig. 43-4, Table 43-1).
4 Remove and discard gloves; perform hand hygiene.
5 Record results immediately on appropriate testing flow sheet. Report reading to nurse or health care provider.

TABLE 43-1	Color Chart for Reagent Strip	
Test	**When to Read**	**Range of Results**
pH	Anytime	4.6-8.0
Protein	Anytime	None or up to 8 mg/100 mL
Glucose	10 seconds (qualitative)	(−) to +4
	30 seconds (quantitative)	(−) to +4 (270)
Ketones	15 seconds	(−) to +3 (large)
Blood	25 seconds	(−) to +3 (large)

SKILL 43-2 Measuring Occult Blood in Stool

Intermediate / Specimen Collection / Performing Fecal Occult Blood Testing

NSO *Specimen Collection Module / Lesson 4*

A common test performed on fecal material is the guaiac test for fecal occult blood. Fecal occult blood testing detects blood in the stool and is useful as a colorectal cancer screening test because cancers and adenomatous polyps bleed more than normal mucosa. The test measures microscopic amounts of blood in the feces. Normally a person loses small amounts of blood daily in the feces as a result of minor abrasions of the nasopharyngeal or oral mucosa. If greater than 50 mL of blood enters the feces from the upper gastrointestinal tract, the blood causes melena (darkening of feces). The guaiac test helps to reveal blood that is visually undetectable.

The test is a useful diagnostic tool for conditions such as colon cancer, upper gastrointestinal (GI) ulcers, and localized gastric parasitic infections or intestinal irritation. The amount of bleeding increases with the size of the polyp and stage of cancer. People with small polyps (less than 1 cm in diameter) bleed scarcely more than those without polyps.

The test is easy to perform. Patients are often instructed in how to collect fecal specimens for the test in the home. Only a small amount of stool is needed to perform the test successfully. The most common guaiac tests are the Hemoccult slides and the Hematest tablets.

Delegation Considerations

The skill of testing stool for occult blood can be delegated to NAP. The nurse directs the NAP to:

- Report immediately if blood is detected and not to discard stool from a positive test, so that the nurse may repeat the testing.

Equipment

- ❑ Soap, water, washcloth, and towel
- ❑ Paper towel
- ❑ Clean gloves
- ❑ Wooden applicators

Hemoccult Test (Fig. 43-5)
- ❑ Cardboard Hemoccult slide
- ❑ Hemoccult developing solution

Hematest
- ❑ Hematest tablets (tablets must be protected from moisture, heat, and light)
- ❑ Guaiac paper (reagent tablet produces blue reaction on guaiac paper if fecal smear contains blood)
- ❑ Sink with running water

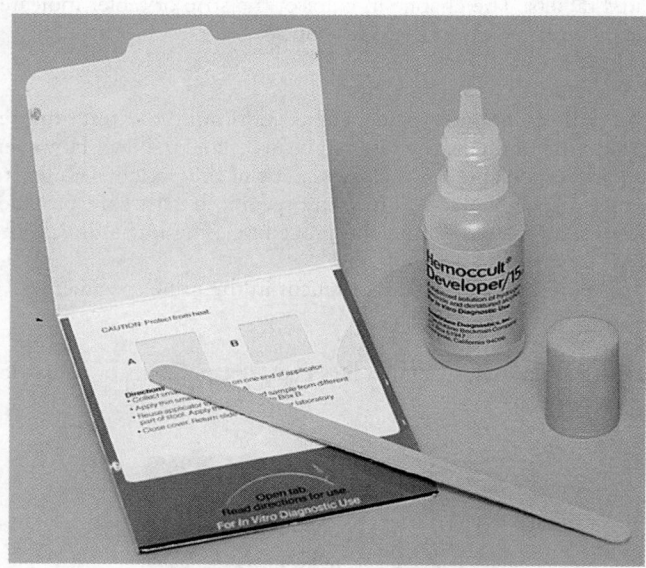

FIG 43-5 Hemoccult testing kit for measuring occult blood.

STEP	RATIONALE

ASSESSMENT

STEP	RATIONALE
1 Assess patient's or family members' understanding of need for stool test.	Provides nurse with information on which to base necessary health teaching.
2 Assess patient's ability to cooperate with procedure and collect specimen.	To avoid embarrassment, patients often prefer to collect own stool specimen. Some patients require assistance.
3 Assess patient's medical history for bleeding, GI disorder, or hemorrhoids.	Nurse can institute routine screening. Hemorrhoids can cause bleeding that may be misinterpreted as upper GI bleeding.
4 Obtain patient's medication history. Note drugs that can cause GI mucosal bleeding.	Anticoagulants increase risk for bleeding in GI tract, even from minor trauma to mucosa. Long-term use of steroids, nonsteroidal antiinflammatory drugs (NSAIDs), and acetylsalicylic acid (aspirin) can irritate mucosa and result in bleeding.
5 Refer to health care provider's orders for medication or dietary modifications or restrictions before test.	Specimens will be positive if contaminated by menstrual blood, hemorrhoid blood, or povidone-iodine. Diets rich in meats, green leafy vegetables, poultry, and fish may produce false-positive results. Drugs that affect results include alcohol, antiinflammatory agents, ascorbic acid (vitamin C), and nonsteroidal agents (Pagana and Pagana, 2007).

STEP	RATIONALE

NURSING DIAGNOSES

- Anxiety
- Bowel incontinence
- Constipation
- Deficient knowledge regarding collection and testing of stool specimen
- Diarrhea

Individualize related factors based on patient's condition or needs.

PLANNING

1   Expected outcomes following completion of procedure:
- Test for occult blood is negative.

   Patient has only small amount of blood in feces because of normal nasopharyngeal and oral mucosa abrasions.

- Patient will discuss purpose and benefits of testing stool for blood.

   Validates learning.

2   Explain procedure to patient and/or family member. Discuss reason for specimen collection and how patient can assist. Explain that feces must be free of urine and toilet tissue.

   Patient who understands procedure is more likely to cooperate and may be able to obtain specimen independently. Also prevents accidental disposal of specimen.

3   Arrange for any needed dietary or medication restrictions.

   Ensures accuracy of test results.

IMPLEMENTATION

1   Perform hand hygiene, and apply clean gloves.

   Reduces transmission of microorganisms.

2   Obtain uncontaminated stool specimen.

   Specimen is placed in clean, dry container and not contaminated with urine, water, or toilet tissue. If frank red blood is observed within stool, report these findings immediately to the health care provider.

3   Use tip of wooden applicator to obtain small portion of feces.

   Small specimen is sufficient for measuring blood content.

4   Measure for occult blood.

   a   Perform Hemoccult slide test:

   (1)   Open flap of slide, and apply thin smear of stool on paper in first box.

   Guaiac paper inside box is sensitive to fecal blood content.

   (2)   Obtain second fecal specimen from different portion of stool, and apply thinly to slide's second box (see illustration).

   Occult blood from upper GI tract is not always equally dispersed throughout stool. Findings of occult blood are more conclusive for GI bleeding when entire specimen is found to contain blood.

   (3)   Close slide cover, and turn slide over to reverse side. Open cardboard flap, and apply two drops of Hemoccult developing solution on each box of guaiac paper (see illustration).

   Developing solution penetrates underlying fecal specimen. Change in color of guaiac paper indicates blood.

   (4)   Read results of test after 30 to 60 seconds. Note color changes.

   Ensures correct results. Bluish discoloration indicates occult blood (guaiac positive). No change in color of guaiac paper indicates negative results.

   (5)   Dispose of gloves and test slide in proper receptacle. Perform hand hygiene.

   Reduces transfer of microorganisms.

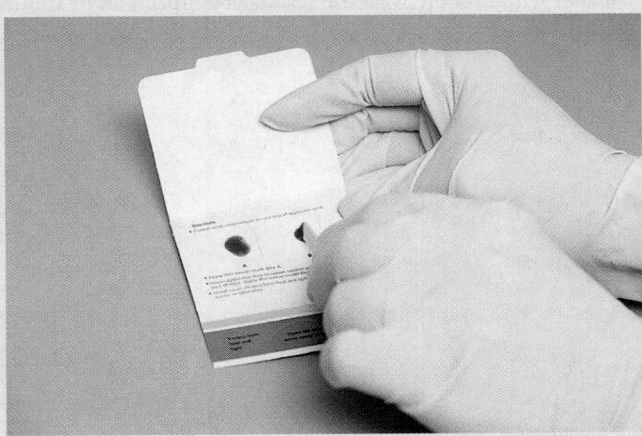

STEP 4a(2)   Application of stool specimen.

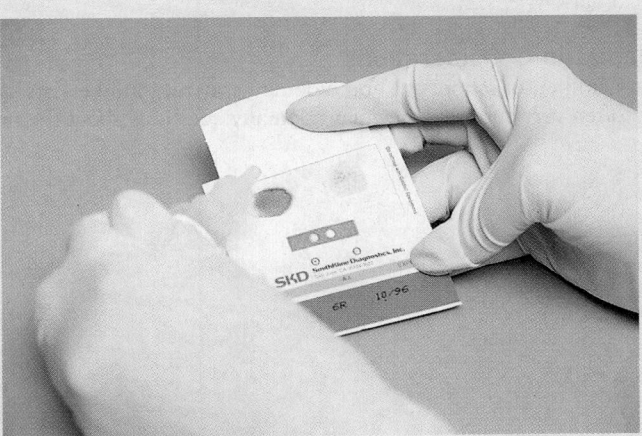

STEP 4a(3)   Application of developing solution.

STEP	RATIONALE
b Perform test using Hematest tablets:	Tablet contains solid form of developing solution.
(1) Place stool on guaiac paper and Hematest tablet on top of stool specimen. Apply 2 to 3 drops of tap water to tablet, allowing water to flow onto guaiac paper	Tap water dissolves Hematest tablet and thus dispenses developing solution over specimen and guaiac paper.
(2) Observe color of guaiac paper within 2 minutes.	Bluish discoloration is guaiac positive. Do not read color after 2 minutes. False findings may occur.
(3) Dispose of tablet and paper in proper receptacle.	Reduces spread of infection.
(4) Wrap wooden applicator in paper towel, grasp in nondominant hand, and remove gloves over to contain; then dispose in proper receptacle. Perform hand hygiene.	Reduces spread of infection.

EVALUATION

1 Ask patient to explain collection procedure.	Documents level of learning.
2 Note color changes in guaiac paper.	Reveals blood in feces.

Critical Decision Point   *Single positive test result does not confirm bleeding or indicate colorectal cancer. For confirmed positive results, test must be repeated at least three times while patient is on meat-free, high-residue diet. More in-depth diagnosis is needed with positive result (Fischbach and Dunning, 2008).*

3 Note character of stool specimen.	Certain abnormal constituents of stool may be visible.

Unexpected Outcomes	**Related Interventions**
1 Test for occult blood is positive.	• Continue to monitor patient.
	• Notify health care provider.

Recording and Reporting

- Record results of test in nurses' notes.
- Record any unusual characteristics of stool in nurses' notes
- Report positive test results to health care provider.

Teaching Considerations

- Explain rationale regarding why patient needs to obtain specimens from two different areas of stool specimen.
- If patient has been on long-term steroid or anticoagulant drug therapy, explain how these drugs may result in occult blood in stools.
- If health care provider orders meat-free diet before test, explain its significance to test results (red meats can cause false-positive results).
- Discuss reason for multiple testing of stool for occult blood. Patients are usually requested to obtain specimen every day for 3 days.

Pediatric Considerations

- Children of school age and older are concrete thinkers and are often very curious. They may ask many questions about the test.

- Answer questions honestly and at child's level of understanding. Allow child to watch, if desired, while performing test.
- Testing reagent is often poisonous, so keep it out of reach of the small child.

Gerontological Considerations

- Serial fecal specimens collected in the home for an older adult require assistance from a family member or friend.

Home Care Considerations

- Many patients are instructed to collect specimens at home and return them to clinic or health care provider's office.
- Patients who collect specimens at home are asked to prepare slides with feces, close cardboard slide, and return it to office or clinic.
- Alert patient that presence of home products such as toilet bowl cleaner will interfere with the results (Fischbach and Dunning, 2008).

SKILL 43-3 Measuring Occult Blood in Gastric Secretions (Gastroccult)

Intermediate / Specimen Collection / Performing Gastric Occult Blood and pH Testing

NSO *Specimen Collection Module / Lesson 3*

Analysis of gastric secretions or emesis can detect blood that is not always visible. Gastroccult testing helps to reveal bleeding in the esophagus or stomach. The test can verify the presence of blood when red or black coloration of the gastric contents is noted or when the gastric contents or emesis has the appearance of coffee grounds. The test measures microscopic amounts of blood in the gastric secretions. The guaiac test identifies blood that is visually undetectable. The test is a useful diagnostic tool for conditions such as upper ulcers or bleeding. Because the test is easy to perform, patients are often instructed in how to test emesis in the home.

Delegation Considerations
The skill of Gastroccult testing can be delegated to NAP for test on emesis. You cannot delegate the skill of Gastroccult testing to NAP if the specimen is collected from a nasogastric (NG) or nasoenteral tube. The nurse directs the NAP to:
- Report immediately if blood or coffee ground emesis is visible in NG or nasoenteral tube secretions.
- Save specimen for repeat testing.

Equipment
- ❑ Facial tissues
- ❑ Emesis basin
- ❑ Wooden applicator or 3-mL syringe
- ❑ 60-mL bulb or catheter tip syringe
- ❑ Gastroccult test cardboard slide
- ❑ Gastroccult developing solution
- ❑ Clean gloves

STEP	RATIONALE
ASSESSMENT	
1 Assess patient's or family members' understanding of need for test.	Provides nurse with information on which to base necessary health teaching.
2 Assess patient's medical history for bleeding or GI disorders.	Nurse can institute routine screening.
3 Obtain patient's medication history. Note drugs that can cause GI mucosal bleeding.	Anticoagulants increase risk for bleeding in GI tract, even from minor trauma to mucosa. Long-term use of steroids, NSAIDs, and acetylsalicylic acid (aspirin) can irritate mucosa.

NURSING DIAGNOSES
- Anxiety
- Deficient knowledge regarding occult blood testing
- Fear

Individualize related factors based on patient's condition or needs.

STEP	RATIONALE
PLANNING	
1 Expected outcomes following completion of procedure:	
• Test for occult blood is negative.	Patient has only small or no amount of blood in gastric secretions.
• Patient will discuss purpose and benefits of testing gastric contents for blood.	Validates learning.
2 Explain procedure to patient and/or family member. Discuss reason for specimen collection.	Patient who understands procedure is more likely to be less anxious and more cooperative.
IMPLEMENTATION	
1 Perform hand hygiene, and apply clean gloves.	Reduces transmission of microorganisms.
2 Verify NG tube placement (see Chapter 34).	Ensures aspiration of gastric contents.
3 Obtain specimen by disconnecting tube from suction or gravity drainage from nasogastric or nasoenteral tube. Using a bulb or catheter tip syringe, aspirate 5 to 10 mL.	Aim is to test gastric contents.

Critical Decision Point *Observe specimen. If you notice red blood or coffee-ground material, report these findings immediately.*

STEP	RATIONALE
4 To obtain sample of emesis, use a 3-mL syringe or wooden applicator to get sample from emesis basin.	Small specimen is sufficient for measuring blood content.
5 Perform Gastroccult slide blood test:	
a Using wooden applicator or syringe, apply one drop of gastric sample to Gastroccult blood test slide.	Sample must cover test paper for test reaction to occur.

STEP	RATIONALE
b Apply two drops of commercial developer solution over sample and one drop between positive and negative performance monitors (see illustration).	
c Verify that performance monitor turns blue in 30 seconds.	Indicates slide is working properly.
d After 60 seconds compare color of gastric sample with that of performance monitor.	If sample turns blue, test is positive for occult blood. If sample turns green, it is negative for occult blood.
e Dispose of test slide, wooden applicator, and syringe in proper receptacle. If needed, reconnect NG tube to drainage system. Remove gloves. Perform hand hygiene.	Reduces spread of infection.

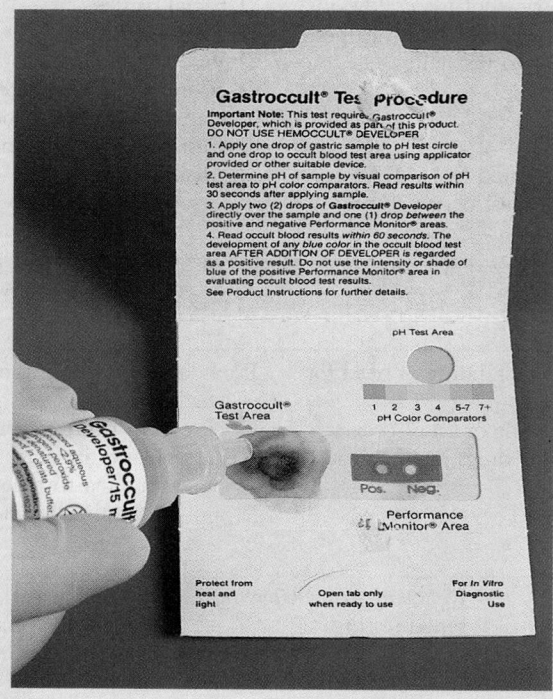

STEP 5b   Applying developing solution to Gastroccult test area.

EVALUATION

1 Ask patient to explain reason for procedure.	Validates level of understanding.
2 Note color changes in guaiac paper.	Reveals blood in gastric secretions.
3 Note character of gastric secretions.	Blood may be visible, or coffee-ground material denoting blood may be observed.

Unexpected Outcomes	Related Interventions
1 Test for occult blood is positive.	• Continue to monitor patient. • Notify health care provider.

Recording and Reporting
- Record results of test in nurses' notes.
- Record any unusual characteristics of gastric contents in nurses' notes.
- Report positive test results to health care provider.

Teaching Considerations
- Explain to patient why specimen is necessary.
- If patient has been on long-term steroid or anticoagulant drug therapy, explain how these drugs may result in occult blood.

Pediatric Considerations
- Children of school age and older are concrete thinkers, often very curious, and may ask many questions about test. Answer questions honestly and at child's level of understanding. Allow child to watch, if desired, while test is performed.

Gerontological Considerations
- Reassure patient that the specimen collection procedure is not uncomfortable if being obtained from an NG or nasoenteral tube.

Home Care Considerations
- Many patients can perform the Gastroccult test on emesis.

SKILL 43-4 Collecting Nose and Throat Specimens for Culture

A nose or throat culture specimen is a diagnostic tool for determining the nature of the patient's nose and/or throat problem. Laboratory personnel place the specimen on a culture medium to determine if pathogenic organisms will grow.

This specimen collection can cause discomfort to sensitive mucosal membranes. Collection of a throat culture sometimes causes gagging. Patient's clear understanding of the specimen collection technique minimizes anxiety or discomfort.

Delegation Considerations

The skill of collecting nose and throat specimens for culture cannot be delegated to NAP. The nurse directs the NAP to:

- Report any complaint of shortness of breath, difficulty breathing, and other signs of respiratory distress.

Equipment

- ❑ Two sterile swabs in sterile culture tubes (flexible wire swab with cotton tip may be used for nose cultures)
- ❑ Nasal speculum (*optional*)
- ❑ Emesis basin or clean container (*optional*)
- ❑ Tongue blades
- ❑ Penlight
- ❑ Facial tissues/gauze
- ❑ Clean gloves
- ❑ Completed identification labels with proper patient identifiers
- ❑ Completed laboratory requisition (date, time, name of test, patient identification, source of culture)
- ❑ Small biohazard plastic bag for delivery of specimen to laboratory (or container specified by agency)

STEP	RATIONALE
ASSESSMENT	
1 Assess patient's understanding of purpose for procedure and ability to cooperate. Nurse may need assistance to obtain throat cultures from confused, combative, or unconscious patients.	Provides basis to determine need for health teaching and need for assistance.
2 Assess condition of and drainage from nasal mucosa and sinuses.	Reveals physical signs that indicate infection or allergic irritation. Clear drainage usually indicates allergy. Yellow, green, or brown drainage usually indicates infection.
3 Determine if patient experiences postnasal drip, sinus headache or tenderness, nasal congestion, sore throat, or exposure to others with similar symptoms.	Symptoms help reveal nature of problem.
4 Assess condition of posterior pharynx.	Will reveal local inflammation or lesions of pharynx.

Critical Decision Point *Pay particular attention to areas of inflammation or purulent drainage. Identification of inflamed or purulent areas allows nurse to swab those sites quickly.*

STEP	RATIONALE
5 Assess patient for systemic signs of infection: fever, chills, and/or fatigue.	Infection originating within nasopharynx can become systemic, requiring antibiotic therapy.
6 Review health care provider's orders to determine if nose, throat, or both cultures are needed.	Prevents exposing patient to unnecessary discomfort of repeated cultures.

NURSING DIAGNOSES

- Acute pain
- Chronic pain
- Deficient knowledge regarding specimen collection
- Risk for infection

Individualize related factors based on patient's condition or needs.

PLANNING

STEP	RATIONALE
1 Expected outcomes following completion of procedure:	
• There is no bacterial growth in specimens.	Absence of infection.
• Patient does not experience bleeding of nasal mucosa.	Procedure is atraumatic.
• Specimen is not contaminated.	Evidenced by results of laboratory analysis.
• Patient will discuss purpose of nose and throat cultures.	Validates learning.
2 Plan to do culture before mealtime or at least 1 hour after eating.	Procedure often induces gagging; timing will decrease patient's chances of vomiting.
3 Explain procedure to patient and/or family member. Discuss reason for specimen collection and how patient can assist.	Understanding of procedure usually decreases anxiety and promotes cooperation.
4 Explain that patient may have tickling sensation or gagging during swabbing of throat. Nasal swab may create urge to sneeze. Both procedures require only a few seconds.	Helps patient to relax.

STEP	RATIONALE

IMPLEMENTATION

1. Verify patient's identity by using at least two forms of identifiers, neither of which is the patient's room number. Verify the type of procedure scheduled and the procedure site with the patient.

   Ensures accurate patient identification and improves patient safety. Use of patient's room number is not an acceptable identifier (TJC, 2008).

2. Ask patient to sit erect in bed or chair facing you. Acutely ill patient or young child may lie back against bed with head of bed raised to 45-degree angle.

   Provides easy access to nasal or oral structures.

3. Have swab in tube ready for use. Loosen top so that swab can be removed easily.

   Allows nurse to grasp swab easily without danger of contamination. Most commercially prepared tubes have tops that fit securely over end of swab, which allows nurse to touch outer tops without contaminating swab stick.

4. Collect throat culture:
   a. Perform hand hygiene, and apply clean gloves.

      Reduces transmission of microorganisms.

   b. If possible, schedule procedure when patient's stomach is empty.

      Throat swabbing can cause the patient to gag. Obtaining specimen on an empty stomach reduces the risk for vomiting.

   c. Instruct patient to tilt head backward. For patients in bed, place pillow behind shoulders.

      Facilitates visualization of pharynx.

   d. Ask patient to open mouth and say "ah." To visualize the pharynx, depress tongue with tongue blade and note inflamed areas of pharynx or tonsils. Depress anterior third of tongue only. (Illuminate with penlight as needed.)

      Permits exposure of pharynx, relaxes throat muscles, and minimizes gag reflex.
      Area to be swabbed should be clearly visualized.

Critical Decision Point *Placement of tongue blade along back of tongue more likely initiates gag reflex. If patient gags, remove tongue blade and allow patient to relax before reinserting.*

   e. Insert swab without touching lips, teeth, tongue, cheeks, or uvula.

      Prevents contamination with organisms from the oral cavity (Garza and Becan-McBride, 2005).

   f. Gently but quickly swab tonsillar area side to side, making contact with inflamed or purulent sites (see illustration).

      These areas contain most microorganisms.

   g. Carefully withdraw swab without touching oral structures. Immediately place swab in culture tube. Place gauze around ampule, and crush ampule at bottom of tube. Push tip of swab into liquid medium (see illustrations).

      Retains microorganisms within culture tube. Mixing swab tip with culture medium ensures life of bacteria for testing.

   h. Place top on culture tube securely.

      Prevents contamination from microorganisms.

   i. Discard tongue depressor into trash; remove gloves and discard. Perform hand hygiene.

      Reduces transmission of microorganisms.

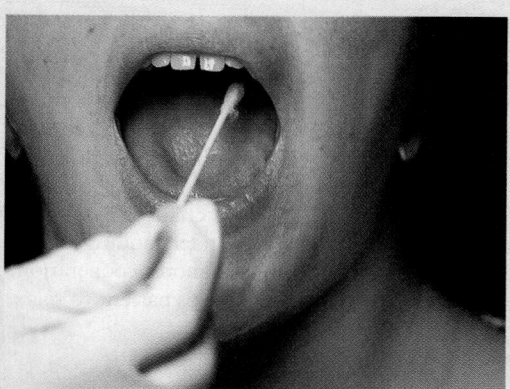

STEP 4f Obtaining tonsillar swab.

STEP	**RATIONALE**

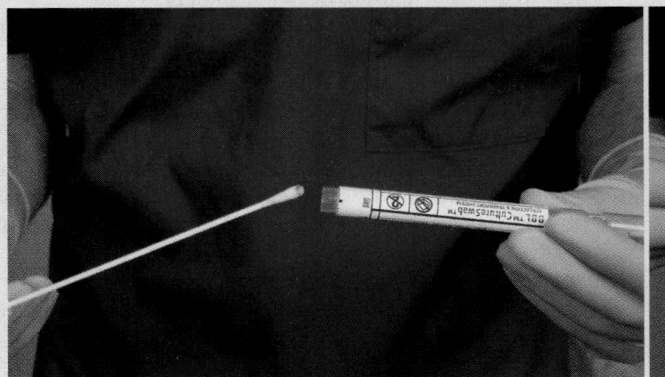 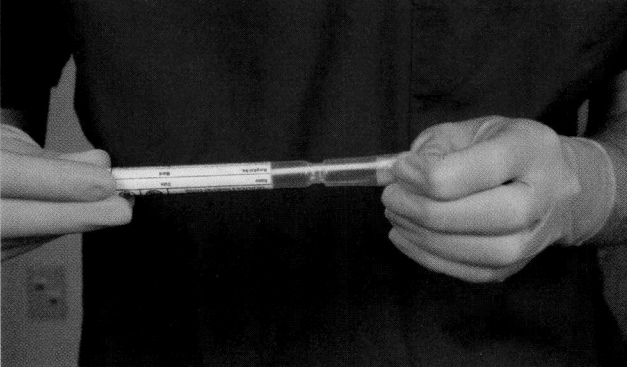

STEP 4g   Activating culture tube. **A,** Place swab into tube. **B,** Crush end of tube to release liquid medium.

5 Collect nasal culture:	
a Perform hand hygiene, and apply clean gloves.	Reduces transmission of microorganisms.
b Encourage patient to blow nose.	Clears nasal passages of mucus containing resident bacteria.
c Ask patient to alternatively occlude each nostril and exhale.	Determines nostril with greater patency.
d Ask patient to tilt head back. Patients in bed should have small pillow behind shoulders.	Provides access to nasal passages and facilitates visualization of nasal septum and sinuses.
e Gently insert nasal speculum in one nostril (*optional*).	Allows retraction of mucosa for easier swab insertion.
f Carefully pass swab through center of speculum (if used) into nostril until it reaches that portion of mucosa that is inflamed or containing exudate. Rotate swab quickly.	Swab should remain sterile until it reaches area to be cultured. Rotating swab covers all surfaces where exudate is present.
g Remove swab without touching sides of speculum or nose.	Prevents contamination of swab by resident bacteria.
h Carefully remove nasal speculum (if used), and place in basin. Offer patient facial tissue.	Minimizes period of time patient will experience discomfort.
i Insert swab into culture tube. Crush ampule at bottom of tube, and push tip of swab into liquid medium.	Retains microorganisms within culture tube. Mixing swab tip with culture medium ensures life of bacteria for testing.
j Place top on tube securely.	Prevents contamination from microorganisms.
k Remove gloves, discard, and perform hand hygiene.	Reduces transmission of microorganisms.
6 Collect nasopharyngeal culture:	
a Follow Step 5, a through k, except for Step 5f use a special swab on a flexible wire that can be flexed downward to reach nasopharynx via nose. Need to advance swab to nasopharynx.	Only this specially designed swab allows access to difficult-to-reach nasopharyngeal area.
7 Securely attach properly completed identification label and laboratory requisition to culture tube. Agency policy dictates type of information to place on label. Note on laboratory requisition if patient is taking antibiotic or if specific organism is suspected (e.g., *Bordetella pertussis*).	Incorrect identification of specimen could result in diagnostic or therapeutic errors.
8 Send specimen to laboratory immediately, or refrigerate.	Fresh specimen provides most accurate test results.

EVALUATION

1 Check laboratory record for results of culture test.	Results reveal type of organisms in nose or pharynx and antibiotics most likely to be effective.
2 Ask patient to explain purpose of culture.	Demonstrates learning.

Unexpected Outcomes	Related Interventions
1 Nose and throat cultures reveal bacterial growth.	• Notify health care provider of findings. • Administer medications as ordered.
2 Patient experiences nasal bleeding.	• Apply pressure and ice pack over bridge of nose. • Notify health care provider of patient's condition.
3 Specimen is contaminated.	• Repeat specimen collection.

Recording and Reporting
- Record specimen collection, date, time, and disposition in nurses' notes.
- Describe appearance of nasal and oral mucosal structures in nurses' notes.
- Report unusual test results to health care provider.

Teaching Considerations
- Instruct patient that procedure is painless but gagging is common.
- Discuss patient's role in collecting specimen.
- Explain how and why you are collecting specimen.
- Discuss relationship between culture results and medication.
- Discuss reason for time delay in receiving culture results.

Pediatric Considerations
- Allowing young children to visualize and examine speculum decreases their fear of it.
- Immobilization of child's head and arms is important when obtaining nose or throat culture. You should do this in firm, gentle, kind manner. Ask another nurse to assist, if necessary.

- Ask parents to act as coach with their child.
- Showing tongue blade and penlight to child and demonstrating how to say "ah" helps to decrease anxiety.
- School-age child will be more cooperative if given opportunity to ask questions about procedure and results.
- Respiratory syncytial virus (RSV) is in respiratory secretions, usually obtained by nasopharyngeal aspiration (Hockenberry and Wilson, 2007).
- Do not attempt throat culture if you suspect acute epiglottitis because trauma from swab might cause increase in edema and resulting occlusion of airway (Hockenberry and Wilson, 2007).

Gerontological Considerations
- Some older adults need assistance in keeping mouth open to obtain specimen.
- Some older adults have poor dentition. Take care not to break a tooth, and consider removal of dentures.
- In confused patients, you may need someone to hold patient's hands while collecting a sample.

SKILL 43-5   Obtaining Vaginal or Urethral Discharge Specimens

Normally, there is minimal discharge from the vagina or urethra. Factors such as poor hygiene practices cause an accumulation of discharge. If a patient develops an increased amount of discharge or if there is a change in the character of discharge from the vagina or urethra, medical follow-up is necessary.

Drainage from the vagina or urethra is normally thin, nonpurulent, whitish or clear, and small in amount. A woman will have bloody discharge during menstruation. A newborn infant may have bloody discharge from the vagina for 2 to 4 weeks after birth because of the abrupt decrease in maternal hormones at birth.

The patients most commonly requiring cultures of vaginal or urethral discharge have signs and symptoms of sexually transmitted disease or urinary tract infection. Patients suspected of having a sexually transmitted disease may be embarrassed by their condition. Show respect and understanding toward the patient. If the patient undergoes a complete diagnostic workup, the list of questions you will ask is often exhausting and causes anxiety. When collecting vaginal or urethral specimens, work quickly and calmly, maintaining the patient's privacy at all times.

Delegation Considerations
The skill of obtaining vaginal or urethral discharge culture samples cannot be delegated to NAP.

Equipment
- ❑ Sterile swab in sterile culture tube (commercially available culture tubes have swab and tube with ampule containing special transport medium)
- ❑ Sheet, blanket, or paper drape
- ❑ Clean gloves
- ❑ Penlight or gooseneck lamp
- ❑ Completed identification labels with proper patient identifiers
- ❑ Completed laboratory requisition (date, time, name of test, patient identification, source of culture)
- ❑ Small biohazard plastic bag for delivery of specimen to laboratory (or container specified by agency)

STEP	RATIONALE
ASSESSMENT	
1 Assess understanding of need for culture and ability to cooperate with procedure.	Provides nurse with information on which to base necessary health teaching.
2 Assess condition of external genitalia. Observe urethra, meatus, and vaginal orifice for redness, swelling, complaint of tenderness, and discharge that is whitish, mucoid, or purulent, or a woman may have whitish discharge like cottage cheese.	Assessment findings and specimen test results reveal nature of problem.
3 Ask patient if dysuria, localized pruritus of genitalia, or lower abdominal pain have been experienced.	Symptoms of urinary tract or vaginal infection.
4 If symptoms suggest sexually transmitted disease, gather and record sexual history of patient.	Determine sexual activity and if there has been sexual contact with a person known to have a sexually transmitted disease. If culture results are positive, tell patient to receive treatment and to have sexual partners evaluated (Pagana and Pagana, 2007).
5 Refer to health care provider's order to determine if culture is to be vaginal or urethral.	Patient may require one or both types of cultures.

STEP	RATIONALE

NURSING DIAGNOSES

- Acute pain
- Anxiety
- Deficient knowledge regarding specimen collection
- Risk for infection

Individualize related factors based on patient's condition or needs.

PLANNING

STEP	RATIONALE
1 Expected outcomes following completion of procedure.	
• Specimen is not contaminated.	Results on laboratory test will reveal whether skin cells or mucosal cells have contaminated specimen.
• Vaginal or urethral cultures do not reveal growth of microorganisms.	Evidence of absence of infection.
2 Explain procedure to patient and/or family member. Discuss reason for specimen collection and how patient can assist. Instruct female patient not to douche 24 hours before culture is obtained. Male is not to urinate 1 hour before urethral culture.	Patient who understands procedure is less anxious and more likely to cooperate. Douching of vaginal canal would remove discharge containing pathogens. Urinating by male washes secretions out of urethra (Pagana and Pagana, 2007).
3 Maintain nonjudgmental attitude while obtaining data.	Demonstrates respect for patient.

IMPLEMENTATION

STEP	RATIONALE
1 Verify patient's identity by using at least two forms of identifiers, neither of which is the patient's room number. Verify the type of procedure scheduled and the procedure site with the patient.	Ensures accurate patient identification and improves patient safety. Use of patient's room number is not an acceptable identifier (TJC, 2008).
2 Perform hand hygiene.	Reduces transmission of microorganisms.
3 Draw bedside curtains, or close room door. Place "Do Not Enter" sign on door (if available).	Provides privacy for patient and demonstrates nurse's respect for patient's well-being.
4 Assist patient to proper position, raise gown, and drape body parts to be exposed:	Provides easy access to perineal area. Draping minimizes exposure of body parts, minimizing anxiety.
a *Female:* Dorsal recumbent position with sheet draped over each leg and genitalia.	
b *Male:* Sitting on chair or bed or lying supine with sheet draped across lower trunk and genitalia.	
5 Apply clean gloves.	Prevents contamination of nurse's hands from discharge.
6 Direct light source onto perineum (may not be needed for male patient).	Allows better visualization of external urethral or vaginal structures.
7 Open culture tube, and hold swab in dominant hand.	Provides for easier manipulation of swab during culture collection.
8 Instruct patient to deep breathe slowly.	Helps patient to relax. Tensing of muscles around pelvic floor may cause discomfort during swabbing.
9 Obtain specimens:	
a Female	
(1) With nondominant hand, fully separate labia to expose vaginal orifice.	Exposes perineum and ensures specimen is of vaginal discharge.
(2) Touch tip of swab into discharge pool, being careful not to touch skin or mucosa along perineum or vaginal canal. If no discharge is visible, gently insert swab 1 to 2.5 cm (½ to 1 inch) into vaginal orifice and rotate before removal.	Discharge contains the greatest concentration of microorganisms.
(3) To expose urethral meatus, use nondominant hand to pull gently on labia minora upward and back to separate.	Allows better visualization of urethral orifice.
(4) Use clean swab, gently apply to tip of meatus where discharge is visible. Avoid touching labia.	Discharge contains greatest concentration of microorganisms.

Critical Decision Point   *If discharge near vagina appears different from discharge along perineum, collect separate specimens from each area because if there are two organisms present, they could be cross contaminated on a single swab. Label specimen with area of patient's body you swabbed.*

STEP	RATIONALE
b Male	
(1) Grasp patient's penis proximal to glans with nondominant hand; if male is uncircumcised, gently retract foreskin.	Provides clear exposure of urethral meatus.

STEP	RATIONALE
(2) Use dominant hand to hold swab. Apply gently to area of discharge at urinary meatus.	Discharge contains greatest number of microorganisms.
(3) If no discharge is apparent, health care provider may order swab to be introduced into urinary meatus. Hold male genitalia firm but gently.	Excess manipulation can cause erection.
(4) Return foreskin to natural position.	Tightening of foreskin around shaft of penis can cause localized discomfort, edema, and potential necrosis.
10 Return each swab to culture tube, and secure top.	Retains microorganisms within tube.
11 Remove and discard gloves.	Reduces spread of microorganisms.
12 If using commercial culture tube, wrap ampule with gauze to prevent injury to nurse's fingers while crushing. Immediately squeeze end of tube to crush ampule (see Skill 43-4, Implementation, Step 4g). Push tip of swab into fluid medium.	Medium supports life of microorganisms until culture is analyzed.
13 Label each culture tube with identification label, and affix completed requisition.	Incorrect specimen identification could lead to diagnostic or therapeutic error.
14 Send specimen immediately to laboratory, or refrigerate.	Bacteria multiply quickly. Prompt analysis ensures accurate results.
15 Assist patient to comfortable position, offer or assist with personal hygiene, replace gown, and remove drape; discard into correct receptacle. Perform hand hygiene.	Reinforces patient's sense of self-esteem. Reduces transmission of microorganisms.

EVALUATION

1 Review laboratory results for evidence of pathogens.	Results will reveal type of organisms present. Certain organisms are common to vaginal tract. Urethra should be free of microorganisms.
2 Continue to monitor whether discharge is present, and if so, observe color and amount.	Characteristics of discharge indicate specific type of infection.
3 Observe specimen for presence of feces.	Need to obtain another specimen if it contains feces.

Unexpected Outcomes	Related Interventions
1 Vaginal or urethral cultures reveal growth of pathogenic microorganisms.	• Notify health care provider of findings, and follow new orders. • Continue to monitor patient.
2 Specimen is contaminated with epidermal cells.	• Repeat specimen collection.

Recording and Reporting

- In nurses' notes record types of cultures obtained and date and time sent to laboratory.
- Describe character of discharge and appearance of vaginal orifice or urethral meatus.
- Report laboratory results to nurse in charge or health care provider.

Teaching Considerations

- Discuss symptoms of vaginal or urethral infection with patient as appropriate.
- Explain relationship between genital discomfort and infection of vaginal or urinary tract.
- Explain time required to obtain results of culture.
- Discuss sexuality and safe sexual practices with patient if appropriate.
- Patients with urethral or vaginal discharge often require instruction about perineal hygiene measures.
- If topical treatments (e.g., suppositories) are ordered, instruct patient in proper administration of medication (see Chapter 21).

Pediatric Considerations

- Young child will probably desire parents' presence, whereas adolescent usually will not.
- In collection from infant or young child, another nurse can assist with specimen by gently holding child's legs apart in froglike position. Have parent present to encourage cooperation.
- Parents should understand that obtaining specimen would not affect virginity of child.
- Be sensitive to cultural variations and beliefs pertaining to genitalia (i.e., female circumcisions).
- In addition to collecting the specimen on adolescent patients, this may also open up the possibility of discussions related to sexuality in which they may have questions, but are not comfortable opening discussions on their own.

Gerontological Considerations

- When obtaining sample from older adult, assist patient to comfortable position and drape for privacy.
- Clear explanation regarding importance of obtaining sample is extremely helpful to alleviate or diminish anxiety and to gain cooperation.

Procedural Guideline 43-3   Collecting a Sputum Specimen by Expectoration

Delegation Considerations

The skill of collecting a sputum specimen by expectoration can be delegated to NAP. The nurse directs the NAP by:

- Instructing to immediately report the presence of blood in the sputum or changes in the patient's vital signs.

Equipment

- ❑ Completed identification labels (with appropriate patient identifiers)
- ❑ Completed laboratory requisition, including appropriate patient identification, date, time, name of test, and source of culture
- ❑ Small biohazard plastic bag for delivery of specimen to laboratory (or container as specified by agency)
- ❑ Sterile specimen container with cover
- ❑ Clean gloves
- ❑ Facial tissues
- ❑ Emesis basin (*optional*)
- ❑ Toothbrush (*optional*)

Procedural Steps

1   Explain importance that patient coughs and expectorates sputum. Patient cannot imply clear throat and expectorate saliva.

2   Provide opportunity to cleanse or rinse mouth with water. Patient should not use mouthwash or toothpaste because the products may alter culture results.

3   Apply clean gloves. Provide sputum cup and instruct patient not to touch the inside of the container.

4   Have the patient take three to four deep breaths. Emphasize to patient that breaths should include slow, full exhalation. Then after a full exhalation ask patient to cough forcefully, expectorating sputum directly into specimen container.

5   Repeat until 5 to 10 mL (½ to 2 teaspoons) of sputum (not saliva) has been collected.

6   Secure top on container tightly. If any sputum is present on outside of container, wipe it off with disinfectant.

7   Offer patient tissues after patient expectorates, dispose of tissues, and offer mouth care.

8   Remove and dispose of gloves.

9   Securely attach properly completed identification label and laboratory requisition to side of specimen container (not lid).

10 Enclose specimen in a plastic biohazard bag.

11 Send specimen immediately to laboratory.

SKILL 43-6   Collecting Sputum Specimen by Suction

 Intermediate / Specimen Collection / Collecting a Sputum Specimen

Sputum is produced by cells lining the respiratory tract. Although production is minimal in the healthy state, disease states can increase the amount or change the character of sputum. Examination of sputum aids in the diagnosis and treatment of several conditions ranging from simple bronchitis to lung cancer.

Suctioning is often indicated to collect sputum from patients unable to spontaneously produce a sample for laboratory analysis. Sometimes suctioning provokes violent coughing, causes vomiting and aspiration of stomach contents, and induces constriction of pharyngeal, laryngeal, and bronchial muscles. In addition, suctioning may cause hypoxemia or vagal overload, causing cardiopulmonary compromise and increases in intracranial pressure.

Three major types of sputum specimens are sputum for cytology, culture and sensitivity, and acid-fast bacilli (AFB). Cytological or cellular examination of sputum may identify aberrant cells or cancer. You can use sputum collected for culture and sensitivity testing to identify specific microorganisms and determine antibiotics that are most sensitive. The AFB smear is used to support the diagnosis of tuberculosis (TB). A definitive diagnosis of TB also requires a sputum culture and sensitivity.

Delegation Considerations

The skill of collecting sputum specimens by suction cannot be delegated to NAP. The nurse directs the NAP to:

- Notify the nurse when the patient expectorates bloody sputum.

Equipment

Suctioned Specimen

- ❑ Completed identification labels with proper patient identifiers
- ❑ Completed laboratory requisition, including patient identification, date, time, name of test, and source of culture
- ❑ Suction device (wall or portable)
- ❑ Sterile suction catheter (size 14, 16, or 18 Fr—not large enough to cause trauma to nasal mucosa)
- ❑ Sterile gloves and clean gloves
- ❑ Sterile saline in container
- ❑ In-line specimen container or sputum trap
- ❑ Small plastic bag for delivery of specimen to laboratory (or a container as specified by agency)
- ❑ Oxygen therapy equipment if indicated
- ❑ Protective eyewear
- ❑ Disinfectant wipe

STEP	RATIONALE

ASSESSMENT

1   Check health care provider's orders for type of sputum analysis and specifications (e.g., amount of sputum, number of specimens, time of collection, method to obtain). Specimens for AFB require three consecutive morning samples, and cultures can take up to 8 weeks.

Specific test to dictate when or how frequently specimens are collected. Ideal time to collect sputum is early morning because bronchial secretions tend to accumulate during the night. Bacteria also accumulate as secretions pool.

STEP	RATIONALE
2 Assess patient's level of understanding of procedure and its purpose.	Provides baseline for nurse to establish teaching plan.
3 Assess when patient last ate a meal (or had a tube feeding). Wait 1 to 2 hours after eating.	Patient may gag, vomit, and aspirate stomach contents during procedure.
4 Determine type of assistance needed by patient to obtain specimen.	Positioning, postural drainage, deep breathing, and coughing exercises may improve ability to cough productively. Suctioning is often indicated when a patient is unable to cough and expectorate.
5 Assess patient's respiratory status, including respiratory rate, depth, pattern, and color of mucous membranes.	Active coughing may alter respiratory status. Respiratory status can depend on amount of sputum in tracheo-bronchial tree.

NURSING DIAGNOSES

- Deficient knowledge regarding specimen collection procedures
- Ineffective airway clearance
- Ineffective breathing pattern
- Risk for aspiration
- Risk for infection

Individualize related factors based on patient's condition or needs.

PLANNING

1 Expected outcomes following completion of procedure:	
• Patient's respirations are same rate and character as before procedure.	Specimen collection did not alter respiratory status.
• Patient is relaxed, able to answer questions (if no artificial airway present).	Suctioning tends to cause anxiety.
• Sputum is not contaminated by saliva or oropharyngeal flora.	Sputum must originate from tracheobronchial tree for accurate results.
• Laboratory tests do not reveal abnormal cells or micro-organisms.	Absence of infection or abnormal cells.
• Patient will discuss purpose and benefit of sputum collection.	Validates learning.
2 Explain steps of procedure and purpose. Instruct patient to breathe normally during suctioning to prevent hyperventilation.	Promotes understanding and cooperation.

Critical Decision Point *When you will suction patient, stress importance of relaxing and breathing at normal rate.*

IMPLEMENTATION

1 Verify patient's identity by using at least two forms of identi-fiers, neither of which is the patient's room number. Verify the type of procedure scheduled and the procedure site with the patient.	Ensures accurate patient identification and improves patient safety. Use of patient's room number is not an acceptable identifier (TJC, 2008).
2 Perform hand hygiene.	Reduces transmission of microorganisms.
3 Close curtains or room door.	Provides privacy.
4 Position patient in high- or semi-Fowler's position for suction-ing.	Promotes full lung expansion and facilitates ability to cough.

Critical Decision Point *If patient has surgical incision or localized area of discomfort, have patient place hands firmly over affected area or place pillow over area. Splinting of painful area minimizes muscular stretching and discomfort during coughing and thus makes cough more productive.*

5 Apply clean glove to nondominant hand. Prepare suction machine or device, and determine if it functions properly.	Adequate amount of suction is necessary to aspirate sputum.
6 Connect suction tube to adapter on sputum trap.	Establishes suction that passes through sputum trap to aspirate specimen.

STEP	RATIONALE
7 Using sterile technique, apply sterile glove (required only for dominant hand if use sleeved catheter).	Tracheobronchial tree is sterile body cavity. Allows nurse to manipulate suction catheter without contamination.
8 With gloved hand, connect sterile suction catheter to rubber tubing on sputum trap.	Aspirated sputum will go directly to trap instead of to suction tubing.
9 Other hand should have clean glove on for application of suction. Thumb should be on trap prepared to provide suction, and trap should be covered.	
10 Gently insert tip of suction catheter through nasopharynx, endotracheal tube, or tracheostomy tube without applying suction (see Chapter 25).	Minimizes trauma to airway as catheter is inserted.
11 Advance catheter into trachea gently and quickly.	Entrance of catheter into larynx and trachea triggers cough reflex.
12 As patient coughs, apply suction for 5 to 10 seconds, collecting 2 to 10 mL of sputum.	Ensures collection of sputum from deep within tracheobronchial tree. Suctioning longer than 10 seconds can cause hypoxia and mucosal damage.
13 Release suction and remove catheter; then turn off suction.	Suction can damage mucosa if applied during withdrawal.
14 Detach catheter from specimen trap, and dispose of catheter in appropriate receptacle.	Decreases risk for spreading microorganisms.
15 Secure top on specimen container tightly. For sputum trap, detach suction tubing and connect rubber tubing on sputum trap to plastic adapter (see illustration).	Contains microorganisms within container, preventing exposure to personnel handling specimen.
16 If any sputum is present on outside of container, wash it off with disinfectant.	Prevents spread of infection to persons handling specimen.
17 Offer patient tissues after expectorating. Dispose of tissues in emesis basin or trash container.	Maintains cleanliness and comfort.
18 Remove and dispose of gloves.	Reduces transmission of microorganisms.
19 Offer patient mouth care, if desired.	Promotes comfort.
20 Perform hand hygiene.	Reduces spread of microorganisms.
21 Label specimen with identification label to side of specimen container (not lid).	Incorrect identification could lead to diagnostic or therapeutic error.
22 Place specimen in small plastic bag (or container specified by agency), and attach requisition.	Plastic bag or container reduces risk for health care worker's exposure to sputum.
23 Send specimen immediately to laboratory, or refrigerate.	Bacteria multiply quickly. Prompt analysis ensures accurate results.

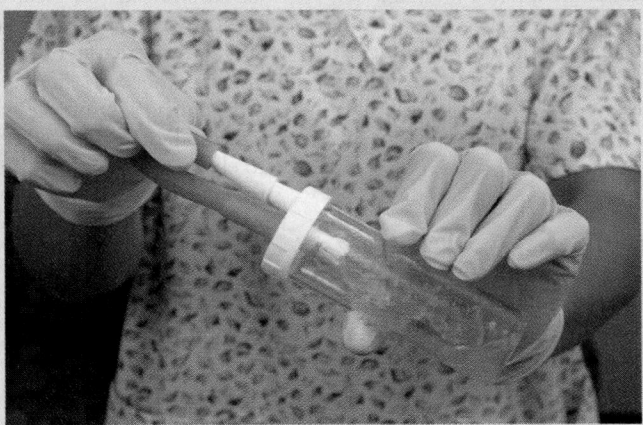

STEP 15   Securing top on sputum specimen container.

STEP	RATIONALE

EVALUATION

1 Observe patient's respiratory status throughout procedure, especially during suctioning.

Excessive coughing or prolonged suctioning can alter respiratory pattern and cause hypoxia.

2 Note anxiety or discomfort in patient.

Procedure can be uncomfortable. If patient becomes short of breath, anxiety will develop.

3 Observe character of sputum: color, consistency, odor, volume, viscosity, and/or presence of blood.

Characteristics may indicate disease entities.

4 Refer to laboratory reports for test results.

Indicates if abnormal cells or microorganisms in sputum.

5 Evaluate patient's ability to describe/demonstrate sputum collection process.

Reinforces patient's ability to collect future expectorated specimens.

Unexpected Outcomes	Related Interventions
1 Patient becomes hypoxic; increased respiratory rate and effort are necessary; patient feels short of breath.	• Discontinue procedure until stable. • Provide oxygen therapy as needed (if ordered). • Notify health care provider of patient's condition. • Continue to monitor patient's vital signs and pulse oximetry.
2 Patient remains anxious or complains of discomfort from suction catheter.	• Discontinue procedure until stable. • Provide oxygen therapy as needed (if ordered). • Notify health care provider of patient's change in condition. • Continue to monitor patient's vital signs and pulse oximetry.
3 Inadequate amount of sputum collected.	• Repeat specimen collection after patient takes several deep breaths.
4 Specimen contains blood, pathogenic organisms, or abnormal cells.	• Stop suctioning further. • Report findings to health care provider.
5 Patient complains of pain when coughing to produce sputum.	• Encourage patient who is recovering from a surgical procedure to splint incision before coughing. • Obtain order for pain medication as needed (prn). • Inform health care provider of changes in patient's condition.

Recording and Reporting

• Record method used to obtain specimen, date and time collected, type of test ordered, and laboratory receiving specimen in nurses' notes. Describe characteristics of sputum specimen. Describe patient's tolerance of procedure.

• Report unusual sputum characteristics to nurse in charge or health care provider.

• When laboratory reports are available, report abnormal findings to health care provider. If AFB sputum culture is positive, initiate appropriate isolation techniques.

• Many agencies require nurse to note on specimen requisition if patient is receiving antibiotics.

Teaching Considerations

• Nurse can demonstrate proper splinting technique for postoperative patients.

• If aerosol treatment is indicated, teach patient purpose of procedure, explaining that it will stimulate coughing and sputum expectoration.

Pediatric Considerations

• Children need very clear instructions or demonstration for deep breathing. Infants and young children will be unable to cooperate; aerosol treatment may be indicated.

• You may need assistance restraining a young child's head and arms during suctioning; parent may assist by providing support.

• Use smaller catheter size for young children. It may be possible to elicit a cough by tickling the back of the throat with the suction catheter.

SKILL 43-7 Obtaining Wound Drainage Specimens

Intermediate / Specimen Collection / Collecting a Specimen for Wound Culture

NSO *Specimen Collection Module / Lesson 5*

When caring for a patient with a wound, assess the wound's condition and observe for the development of infection. Localized inflammation, tenderness, and warmth at the wound site and purulent drainage usually signify wound infection. Identification of the causative organism confirms an infection and provides accurate treatment. A specimen of wound drainage is analyzed to determine the type and number of pathogenic microorganisms.

Never collect a wound culture sample from old drainage. Empty drainage devices and collect fresh drainage for the specimen. Resident colonies of bacteria on the skin grow in wound exudate and may not be the true causative organisms of infection. You will use separate techniques to collect specimens for measuring aerobic versus anaerobic microorganisms. Aerobic organisms grow in superficial wounds exposed to the air. Anaerobic organisms grow deep within body cavities, where oxygen is not normally present.

Delegation Considerations

The skill of obtaining wound drainage specimens cannot be delegated to NAP. The nurse directs the NAP to:
- Report foul odor, increase in drainage, and increase in temperature or patient complaint of discomfort.

Equipment

- ❑ Culture tube with swab and transport medium for aerobic culture
- ❑ Anaerobic culture tube with swab (tubes contain carbon dioxide or nitrogen gas)
- ❑ 5- to 10-mL syringe and 19-gauge needle
- ❑ Clean gloves
- ❑ Sterile gloves
- ❑ Protective eyewear
- ❑ Antiseptic swab
- ❑ Sterile dressing materials (determined by type of dressing)
- ❑ Paper or plastic disposable bag
- ❑ Completed specimen identification label with proper patient identifiers
- ❑ Completed laboratory requisition (date, time, name of test, patient identification, and source of culture)
- ❑ Small plastic biohazard bag for delivery of specimen to laboratory (or container specified by agency)

STEP	RATIONALE

ASSESSMENT

1 Assess patient's understanding of need for wound culture and ability to cooperate with procedure.

Use data to develop teaching plan. Wound is painful site. Collection of specimen may cause anxiety or fear.

2 Assess patient for signs of fever, chills, or excessive thirst. Note in laboratory results if white blood cell count is elevated.

Signs and symptoms indicate systemic infection.

3 Ask patient about extent and type of pain at wound site. If patient requires analgesic before dressing changes, give medication 30 minutes before to reach peak effect.

Pain at wound site often increases with infection.

4 Determine when dressing change is scheduled (see Chapter 39). You may perform wound assessment as part of the actual procedure.

5 Review health care provider's orders for aerobic or anaerobic culture.

Specimens are taken from different sites and placed in different containers, depending on type of culture.

6 Wear clean gloves to remove any soiled dressings covering wound. Apply sterile gloves, and assess condition of wound carefully. Observe for swelling, opening of wound edges, inflammation, and drainage. Palpate gently along wound edges and note tenderness or drainage. While you are changing dressing, patient may prefer not to see wound or soiled dressing.

Gloves minimize exposure to microorganisms

Surface of open wound is considered sterile. Sterile gloves allow nurse to palpate area without wound contamination. Signs indicate wound infection.

NURSING DIAGNOSES

- Acute pain
- Anxiety
- Chronic pain

- Deficient knowledge regarding wound drainage culture procedure
- Impaired tissue integrity

- Risk for infection
- Risk for injury

Individualize related factors based on patient's condition or needs.

PLANNING

1 Expected outcomes following completion of procedure:
- Wound culture does not reveal bacterial growth.
- Culture swab is not contaminated by bacteria from skin.
- Patient will discuss purpose and procedure for specimen collection.

Wound remains free of pathogenic microorganisms.
Test results indicate type of cells present.
Validates learning.

STEP	RATIONALE
2 Determine if patient may receive analgesic before dressing change and/or specimen collection. Administer as ordered.	Minimizes discomfort during procedure.
3 Explain reason for wound culture and how it will be collected.	Promotes understanding and cooperation and eases anxiety.
4 Explain that patient may feel tickling sensation when wound is swabbed.	Anticipation of expected sensations minimizes anxiety.

IMPLEMENTATION

STEP	RATIONALE
1 Verify patient's identity by using at least two forms of identifiers, neither of which is the patient's room number. Verify the type of test scheduled with the patient.	Ensures accurate patient identification and improves patient safety. Use of patient's room number is not an acceptable identifier (TJC, 2008).
2 Perform hand hygiene.	Reduces transfer of microorganisms.
3 Close bedside curtains or door to room.	Provides privacy.
4 Apply clean gloves. Remove old dressing, and assess each dressing removed for exudate and drainage. Fold soiled sides of dressing together, and dispose of in appropriate receptacle.	Protects hands from contact with drainage.
5 Cleanse area around wound edges with antiseptic swab. Remove old exudate.	Removes skin flora, preventing possible contamination of specimen.
6 Discard swab, and dispose of soiled gloves in appropriate receptacle. Perform hand hygiene.	Reduces spread of infection.
7 Open packages containing sterile culture tube and dressing supplies.	Provides sterile field for picking up and handling sterile supplies.
8 Apply sterile gloves.	Allows nurse to maintain sterility of items while collecting specimen.
9 Collect cultures:	
a Aerobic culture	
(1) Take swab from culture tube, insert tip into wound in area of drainage, and rotate swab gently. Remove swab, and return to culture tube. (Wrap ampule with gauze to prevent injury to your fingers.) Crush ampule of medium, and push swab into fluid.	Swab should be coated with fresh secretions from within wound. Medium keeps bacteria alive until analysis is complete.
b Anaerobic culture	
(1) Take swab from special anaerobic culture tube, swab deeply into draining body cavity, and rotate gently. Remove swab, and return to culture tube.	Specimen is taken from deep cavity where oxygen is not present. Carbon dioxide or nitrogen gas keeps organisms alive until analysis is complete. Air injected into tube would cause organisms to die.
(2) Another method is to insert tip of syringe (without needle) into wound and aspirate 5 to 10 mL of exudate. Attach 19-gauge needle, expel all air, and inject drainage into special culture tube.	

Critical Decision Point   *Never collect exudate from skin unless it is separate culture and labeled as such.*

STEP	RATIONALE
10 Place correct specimen label on each culture tube.	Ensures correct results for correct patient.
11 Ask another nurse to attach labels and proper requisitions to each tube. Note on specimen requisition if patient is receiving antibiotics. Send specimens to laboratory immediately.	Bacteria multiple rapidly. Prompt analysis ensures accurate results.
12 Clean wound as ordered, and apply new sterile dressing.	Protects wound from further contamination, aids in absorbing drainage and debridement of the wound.
13 Remove gloves. Dispose of gloves and soiled supplies in appropriate receptacle according to agency policy.	Reduces spread of infection.
14 Secure dressings with tape or ties.	Keeps dressing securely in place over wound.
15 Assist patient to comfortable position.	Promotes patient's ability to relax.
16 Perform hand hygiene.	Reduces transmission of microorganisms.

EVALUATION

STEP	RATIONALE
1 Obtain laboratory report for results of cultures.	Report indicates if pathogenic organisms are identified.
2 Observe character of wound drainage.	Characteristics can reveal abnormal status.
3 Observe edges of wound for redness and bleeding.	Indicates trauma to healing tissue.
4 Ask patient about purpose of wound culture.	Validates learning.

Unexpected Outcomes

1 Wound cultures reveal heavy bacterial growth.

2 Wound culture is contaminated from superficial skin cells.

3 Patient describes increased pain.

Related Interventions

- Monitor patient for fever, chills, or excessive thirst, which indicate systemic infection.
- Inform health care provider of findings.

- Monitor patient for fever and pain.
- Inform health care provider of findings.
- Repeat collection of specimen as ordered.

- Provide analgesia.
- Repeat culture.

Recording and Reporting

- Record types of specimens obtained, source, and time and date sent to laboratory in nurses' notes.
- Describe appearance of wound and characteristics of drainage in nurses' notes.
- Report any evidence of infection to charge nurse and health care provider.
- Record patient's tolerance of procedure and response to analgesics.

Teaching Considerations

- Notify patient before beginning of possible discomfort during procedure.
- Instruct patient to inform nurse if procedure causes pain or need to stop because unable to tolerate pain.
- Teach patient to assess status of wound for changes.
- Discuss signs and symptoms of infection.

Pediatric Considerations

- If procedure is to be performed on a child and is anticipated to be painful, some agencies prefer performing procedure in area other than child's room, thus maintaining feeling that child's room is safe place (Hockenberry and Wilson, 2007).
- It is often helpful to have an additional nurse or other adult available to assist with a specimen collection in a young child or infant.

Home Care Considerations

- When applicable, discuss ways to prevent infection.
- Teach patient antiseptic practices (e.g., hand washing, disposal of dressings, and clean technique for applying dressing).

Long-Term Care Considerations

- Carefully monitor wound drainage to prevent spread of infection to other residents (e.g., in a nursing home).

SKILL 43-8   Collecting Blood Specimens and Culture by Venipuncture (Syringe Method and Vacutainer Method)

Advanced / Intravenous Fluid Therapy Administration / Performing Venipuncture

NSO *Vascular Access / Drawing Blood and Administering Fluid Module*

Blood tests are one of the most commonly used diagnostic aids in the care and evaluation of patients. In any health care setting blood tests can yield valuable information about a patient's nutritional, hematological, metabolic, immune, and biochemical status. Tests allow health care providers to screen patients for early signs of physical alterations, plot the course of existing disease, and monitor responses to therapies.

The nurse is often responsible for collecting blood specimens; however, many institutions have specially trained phlebotomists who are responsible for drawing venous blood, and some may allow respiratory therapist to draw blood for arterial blood gas analysis. Be familiar with your institution's policies and procedures and your state's Nurse Practice Act regarding guidelines for drawing blood samples.

The three methods of obtaining blood specimens are (1) skin puncture, (2) venipuncture, and (3) arterial puncture. All procedures require sterile technique. Anticipate the patient's anxiety. The procedures are painful, and often just the appearance of a needle is frightening, especially to children. A calm approach and skilled technique help to limit anxiety.

Venipuncture, the most common method, involves inserting a hollow-bore needle into the lumen of a large vein to obtain a specimen. You may use a needle and syringe, a Vacutainer and test tubes, or draw from an existing peripheral intravenous (IV) line or central venous catheter (CVC) that allows the drawing of multiple blood samples. Because veins are major sources of blood for labora-

tory testing and routes for IV fluid or blood replacement, maintaining their integrity is essential. You need to be skilled in venipuncture to avoid unnecessary injury to veins.

Skin puncture, also called capillary puncture, is the least traumatic method of obtaining a blood specimen. A sterile lancet or needle is used to puncture a vascular area on a finger, earlobe, toe, or heel. Recent studies indicate the option of obtaining blood from other sites but the sites have limitations. Manufacturer's instructions will indicate ability to use alternative sites. You place a drop of blood on a test slide or collect it within a thin glass capillary tube for laboratory analysis. POC clinical laboratory tests at the bedside most frequently use skin puncture (Pagana and Pagana, 2007).

Blood cultures aid in detection of bacteria in the blood. It is important that at least two culture specimens be drawn from two different sites. Because bacteremia may be accompanied by fever and chills, blood cultures should be drawn when the patient is experiencing these clinical signs (Pagana and Pagana, 2007). Bacteremia exists when both cultures grow the infectious agent. Only one culture growing bacteria is considered contamination.

Because blood culture specimens obtained from an IV catheter are frequently contaminated, tests using them should not be performed unless catheter sepsis is suspected. Draw cultures before antibiotic therapy begins because the antibiotic may interrupt the organism's growth in the laboratory. If the patient is receiving antibiotics, notify the laboratory and inform them of specific antibiotics the patient is receiving (Pagana and Pagana, 2007).

Delegation Considerations
The skill of collecting blood specimens by venipuncture can be delegated to specially trained NAP. In some institutions, phlebotomists are the persons responsible for obtaining venipuncture samples. Agency and government regulations and policies differ regarding personnel who may draw blood specimens. However, you are responsible for assessing the patient before, during, and after the procedure.

Equipment
All Procedures
- ❏ Alcohol 70% or antiseptic swab (check agency policy for specific antiseptic solution)
- ❏ Clean gloves
- ❏ Small pillow or folded towel
- ❏ Sterile 2 × 2 inch gauze pads
- ❏ Tourniquet
- ❏ Adhesive bandage or adhesive tape
- ❏ Appropriate blood tubes
- ❏ Completed identification labels with proper patient identifiers
- ❏ Completed laboratory requisition (appropriate patient identification, date, time, name of test, and source of culture)
- ❏ Small plastic biohazard bag for delivery of specimen to laboratory (or container specified by agency)
- ❏ Sharps container

Venipuncture With Syringe
- ❏ Sterile needles (20 to 21 gauge for adults; 23 to 25 gauge for children)
- ❏ Sterile syringe of appropriate size
- ❏ Sterile syringe attached to butterfly IV catheter with extension tubing

Venipuncture With Vacutainer
- ❏ Vacutainer and safety access device

- ❏ Vacutainer blood tubes with Luer-Lok adapter (for Luer-Lok syringe) (Fig. 43-6)
- ❏ Sterile double-ended needles (20 to 21 gauge for adults; 23 to 25 gauge for children)

CVC Collection
- ❏ Two empty 10-mL sterile syringes
- ❏ Sterile 10-mL normal saline flushes
- ❏ Vacutainer and safety device to transfer blood to tube

Blood Cultures
- ❏ Sterile needles (20 to 21 gauge for adult; 23 to 25 gauge for children)
- ❏ Two 20-mL sterile syringes
- ❏ Anaerobic and aerobic culture bottles (check agency policy)

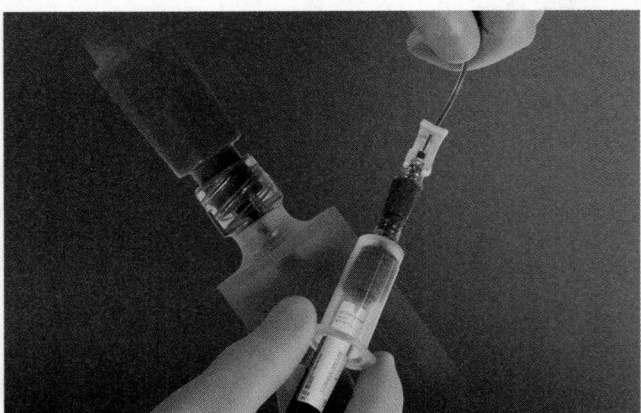

FIG 43-6 Vacutainer tube with Luer-Lok adapter. (*Courtesy and copyright Becton Dickinson.*)

STEP	RATIONALE

ASSESSMENT

1 Determine patient's understanding of purpose of procedure and method you will use.

Provides data for nurse to establish teaching plan and provide emotional support. Some patients' past experiences increase anxiety.

2 Determine if special conditions need to be met before specimen collection.

Some tests require meeting specific conditions to obtain accurate measurement of blood elements (e.g., fasting blood sugar, drug peak and trough level, timed endocrine hormone levels).

3 Assess patient for possible risks associated with venipuncture: anticoagulant therapy, low platelet count, bleeding disorders (history of hemophilia). Review medication history.

Patient history may include abnormal clotting abilities caused by low platelet count, hemophilia, or medications that increase risk for bleeding and hematoma formation.

4 Determine patient's ability to cooperate with procedure.

Some patients may need assistance. Procedure may appear threatening to patient. Reassure child that body continuously makes more blood as blood is collecting in tube or syringe (Hockenberry and Wilson, 2007).

5 Assess patient for contraindicated sites for venipuncture: presence of IV fluids, hematoma at potential site, arm on side of mastectomy, or hemodialysis shunt.

Drawing specimens from such sites can result in false test results or may injure patient. Samples taken from vein near IV infusion may be diluted or may contain concentrations of IV fluids. Postmastectomy patient may have reduced lymphatic drainage in arm on operative side, increasing risk for infection from needle sticks. Never use arteriovenous shunt to obtain specimens because of risks for clotting and bleeding. Hematoma indicates existing injury to vessel wall.

6 Review health care provider's orders for type of tests.

Multiple samples are often needed. Health care provider's order is required.

STEP	RATIONALE

Critical Decision Point *Some specimens have special collection requirements before or following specimen collection, for example:*
- *Cryoglobulin levels: Use prewarmed test tubes.*
- *Ammonia and ionized calcium levels: Place tube in ice for delivery to laboratory.*
- *Lactic acid levels: Do not use tourniquet.*
- *Vitamin levels: Avoid exposure of test tube to light.*

NURSING DIAGNOSES

- Anxiety
- Deficient knowledge regarding blood specimen collection process
- Fear
- Risk for infection
- Risk for injury

Individualize related factors based on patient's condition or needs.

PLANNING

1 Expected outcomes following completion of procedure: • Venipuncture site shows no evidence of continued bleeding or hematoma after specimen collection. • Patient denies anxiety or discomfort. • Laboratory tests show normal findings. • Patient will discuss purpose, procedure, and benefits of venipuncture. 2 Explain procedure to patient: describe purpose of tests; explain how sensation of tourniquet, alcohol swab, and needle stick will feel.	Indicates hemostasis achieved. Removal of painful stimulus lessens anxiety. Some patients are not anxious about procedure. No abnormalities are found in blood. Validates learning. Anticipatory guidance helps to reduce anxiety.

IMPLEMENTATION

1 Verify patient's identity by using at least two forms of identifiers, neither of which is the patient's room number. Verify the type of procedure with the patient.	Ensures accurate patient identification and improves patient safety. Use of patient's room number is not an acceptable identifier (TJC, 2008).
2 Perform hand hygiene.	Reduces transfer of microorganisms.
3 Bring equipment to bedside and organize.	Facilitates procedure.
4 Close bedside curtain or room door.	Provides for privacy.
5 Raise or lower bed to comfortable working height.	Reduces strain on nurse's back muscles and improves access to venipuncture site.
6 Assist patient to supine or semi-Fowler's position with arms extended to form straight line from shoulders to wrists. Place small pillow or towel under upper arm. If in clinic or health care provider's office, use chair with special arm extension.	Helps to stabilize extremity because arms are most common sites of venipuncture. Supported position in bed reduces chance of injury to patient if fainting occurs.
7 Apply tourniquet 5 to 10 cm (2 to 4 inches) above venipuncture site selected (antecubital fossa site is most often used). Encircle extremity, and pull one end of tourniquet tightly over other, looping one end under other. Apply tourniquet so you can remove it by pulling an end with a single motion.	Tourniquet blocks venous return to heart from extremity, causing veins to dilate for easier visibility.

Critical Decision Point *Palpate distal pulse (e.g., brachial) below tourniquet. If pulse is not palpable, reapply tourniquet more loosely. If tourniquet is too tight, pressure will impede arterial blood flow.*

8 Do not keep tourniquet on patient longer than 1 minute.	Prolonged tourniquet application causes stasis, localized acidemia, and hemoconcentration (Pagana and Pagana, 2007).
9 Ask patient to open and close fist several times, finally leaving fist clenched. Instruct patient to avoid vigorous opening and closing of fist.	Facilitates distention of veins by forcing blood up from distal veins. Vigorous open and close may cause erroneous laboratory results from hemoconcentration (Pagana and Pagana, 2007).
10 Quickly inspect extremity for best venipuncture site, looking for straight, prominent vein without swelling or hematoma.	Straight and intact veins are easiest to puncture.

STEP	RATIONALE
11 Palpate selected vein with fingers. Palpate for firm vein that rebounds. Do not use vein that feels rigid, cordlike, and rolls when palpated (see illustration).	Patent, healthy vein is elastic and rebounds on palpation. Thrombosed vein is rigid, rolls easily, and is difficult to puncture.
12 Select venipuncture site. In case of blood cultures, two different sites are selected. Release tourniquet. (If vein cannot be palpated or viewed easily, remove tourniquet and apply warm, wet compress over extremity for 10 minutes.)	Prevents discomfort to patient and inaccurate test results (Garza and Becan-McBride, 2005). Warming increases arterial blood flow, making veins more prominent (Garza and Becan-McBride, 2005).
13 Perform hand hygiene, and apply clean gloves.	Standard for venipuncture is to apply gloves just before site preparation (Baer, 2005).

14 Obtain blood sample:
  a **Syringe method**
    (1) Reapply tourniquet and relocate vein. Have syringe with appropriate needle securely attached.
	Needle must not dislodge from syringe during venipuncture.

(2) Cleanse venipuncture site with antiseptic swabs, moving in circular motion from selected site, approximately 5 cm (2 inches) (see illustration). Allow to dry.	Antimicrobial agent cleans skin surface of resident bacteria so organisms do not enter puncture site. Allowing antiseptic to dry completes its antimicrobial task and reduces "sting" of venipuncture. Alcohol left on skin can cause hemolysis of sample and retraction of tissue away from puncture site.
(a) If drawing sample for blood alcohol level or blood cultures, use only antiseptic swab, not alcohol swab.	Ensures accurate test results.
(3) Remove needle cover, and inform patient that "stick" lasts only a few seconds.	Patient has better control over anxiety when prepared about what to expect.

Critical Decision Point   *Observe needle for defects, such as burrs, which can cause increased discomfort and damage to the patient's vein.*

STEP	RATIONALE
(4) Place thumb or forefinger of nondominant hand 2.5 cm (1 inch) below site, and gently pull and stretch skin distal to patient until skin is taut and vein stabilized.	Stabilizes vein and prevents rolling during needle insertion.
(5) Hold syringe and needle at 15- to 30-degree angle from patient's arm with bevel up.	Reduces chance of penetrating both sides of vein during insertion. Bevel up decreases chance of contamination by not dragging bevel opening over the skin and allows point of needle to first puncture skin, reducing trauma.
(6) Slowly insert needle into vein (see illustration). (a) With experience nurse will feel "pop" as needle enters vein.	Prevents puncture through vein to opposite side.

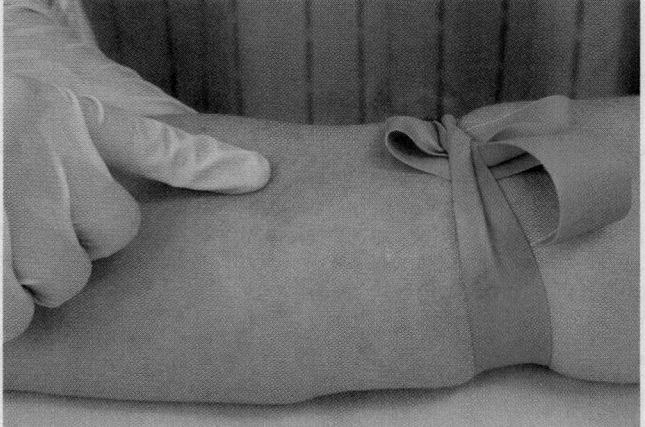

STEP 11   Palpation of vein.

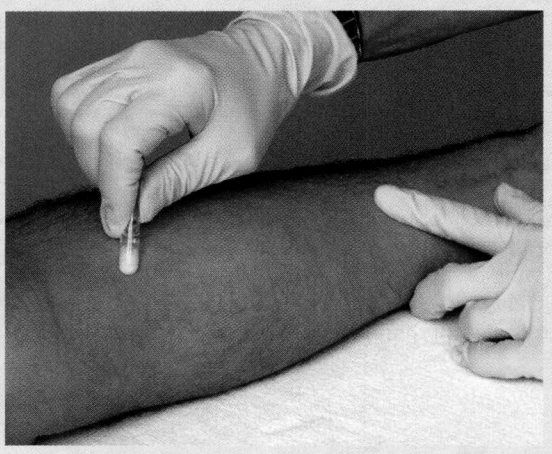

STEP 14a(2)   Cleansing site.

STEP	RATIONALE
(7) Hold syringe securely, and pull back gently on plunger.	Syringe held securely prevents needle from advancing. Pulling on plunger creates vacuum needed to draw blood into syringe. If plunger is pulled back too quickly, pressure may collapse vein.
(8) Observe for blood return (see illustration).	If blood flow fails to appear, needle may not be in vein.
(9) Obtain desired amount of blood, keeping needle stabilized.	Test results are more accurate when required amount of blood is obtained. You cannot perform some tests without minimal blood requirement. Movement of needle increases discomfort.
(10) After obtaining specimen, release tourniquet.	Reduces bleeding at site when needle is withdrawn.
(11) Apply 2 × 2 inch gauze pad without applying pressure. Quickly but carefully withdraw needle from vein, and apply pressure following removal of needle (see illustration). Check for hematoma.	Pressure over needle can cause discomfort. Careful removal of needle minimizes discomfort and vein trauma. Hematoma may cause compression injury (Baer, 2005).
(12) Clinical and Laboratory Standards Institute (CLSI) and Occupational Safety and Health Administration (OSHA) recommend activating safety feature of the needle used to access a vein, removing and discarding it, and replacing it with a safety-transfer device to fill the tubes (Baer, 2005).	Prevents needle-stick injury. Vacuum in tube will draw in blood and fill to correct amount.
(13) Fill blood tubes using safety transfer device. If tubes contain additives, invert back and forth 8 to 10 times.	Additives prevent clothing. Shaking can cause hemolysis of RBCs.
b Vacutainer method (vacuum tube system method)	
(1) Reapply tourniquet and relocate vein. Attach double-ended needle to Vacutainer tube (see illustration).	Long end of needle is used to puncture vein. Short end fits into blood tubes.

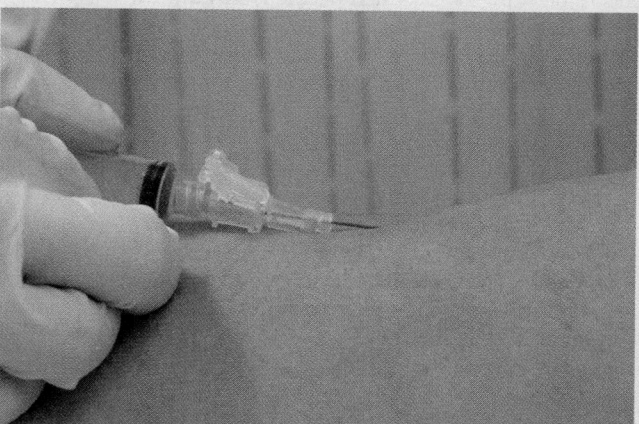

STEP 14a(6)   Inserting needle into vein.

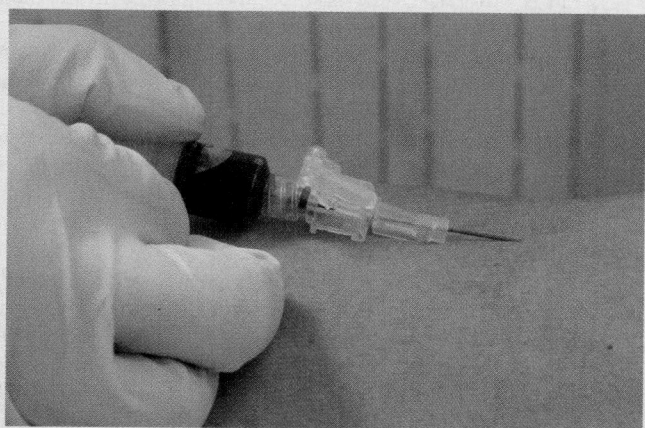

STEP 14a(8)   Blood return as nurse pulls back on plunger.

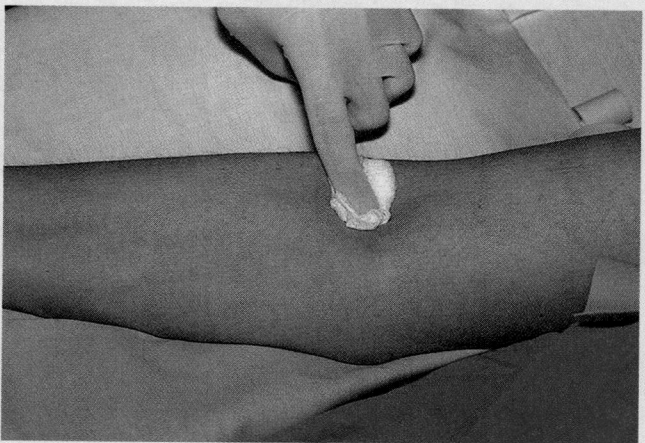

STEP 14a(11)   Application of gauze to puncture site.

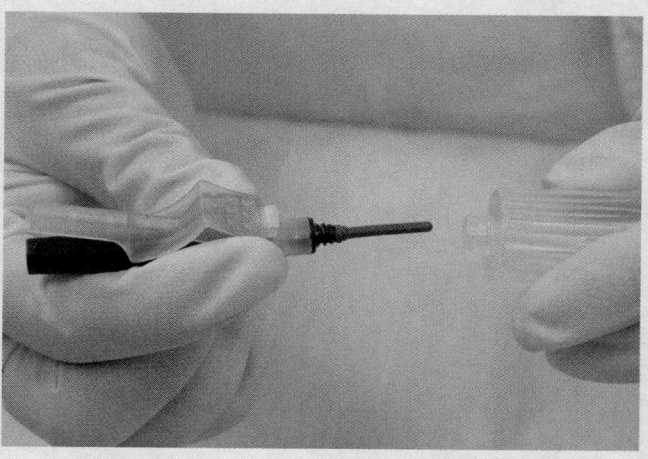

STEP 14b(1)   Attaching needle to Vacutainer tube.

STEP	RATIONALE
(2) Have proper blood specimen tube resting inside Vacutainer, but do not puncture rubber stopper.	Puncturing causes loss of tube's vacuum.
(3) Cleanse venipuncture site with antiseptic swab, moving in circular motion out from site for approximately 5 cm (2 inches). Allow to dry.	Cleans skin surface of resident bacteria so that organisms do not enter puncture site.
(4) Remove needle cover, and inform patient that "stick" will occur.	Patient has better control over anxiety when prepared about what to expect.
(5) Place thumb or forefinger of nondominant hand 2.5 cm (1 inch) below site, and gently pull and stretch skin distal to patient until skin is taut and vein stabilized.	Helps to stabilize vein and prevent rolling during needle insertion.
(6) Hold Vacutainer needle at 15- to 30-degree angle from arm with bevel up.	Smallest and sharpest point of needle will puncture skin first. Reduces chance of penetrating sides of vein during insertion. Keeping bevel up causes less trauma to vein.
(7) Slowly insert needle into vein (see illustration).	Prevents puncture on opposite side.
(8) Grasp Vacutainer securely, and advance specimen tube into needle of holder (do not advance needle in vein).	Pushing needle through stopper breaks the vacuum and causes flow of blood into tube. If needle in vein advances, vein may become punctured on other side.
(9) Note flow of blood into tube (should be fairly rapid) (see illustration).	Failure of blood to appear indicates that vacuum in tube is lost or needle is not in vein.
(10) After specimen tube is filled to correct level, grasp Vacutainer firmly, and remove tube. Insert additional specimen tubes as needed. If tubes contain additives, invert back and forth immediately 8 to 10 times.	Vacuum in tube stops flow at amount to be collected. Grasping prevents needle from advancing or dislodging. Tube should fill completely because additives in certain tubes are measured in proportion to filled tube. Ensures proper mixing with additive to prevent clotting.
(11) After last tube is filled and removed from Vacutainer, release tourniquet.	Reduces bleeding at site when needle is withdrawn.
(12) Apply 2 × 2 inch gauze pad over puncture site without applying pressure, and quickly but carefully withdraw needle with Vacutainer from vein.	Pressure over needle can cause discomfort. Careful removal of needle minimizes discomfort and vein trauma.
(13) Immediately apply pressure over venipuncture site with gauze or antiseptic pad for 2 to 3 minutes or until bleeding stops. Observe for hematoma. Tape gauze dressing securely.	Direct pressure minimizes bleeding and prevents hematoma formation. A hematoma may cause compression and nerve injury. Pressure dressing controls bleeding.

c Blood Cultures

STEP	RATIONALE
(1) Reapply tourniquet and relocate vein. Carefully prepare proposed venipuncture site with antiseptic swab (check agency policy). Allow antiseptic to dry.	Antimicrobial agent cleans skin surface so organisms do not enter puncture site or contaminate culture. Drying ensures complete antimicrobial action.
(2) Clean bottle tops of vacuum tubes or culture bottles. Check agency policy regarding cleaning with 70% alcohol after cleaning with antiseptic solution and air-drying.	Ensures specimen is sterile.

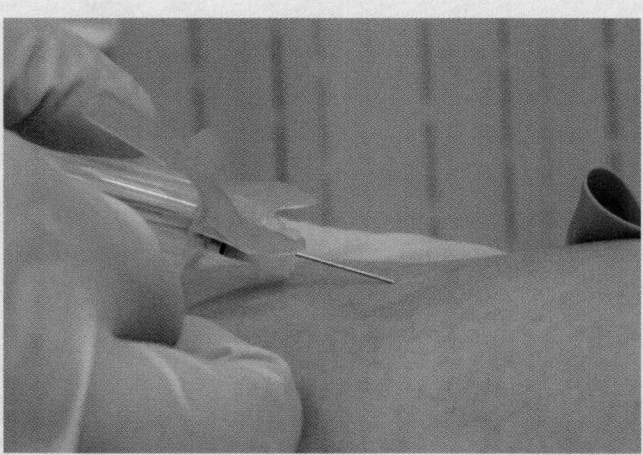

STEP 14b(7)   Inserting Vacutainer needle into vein.

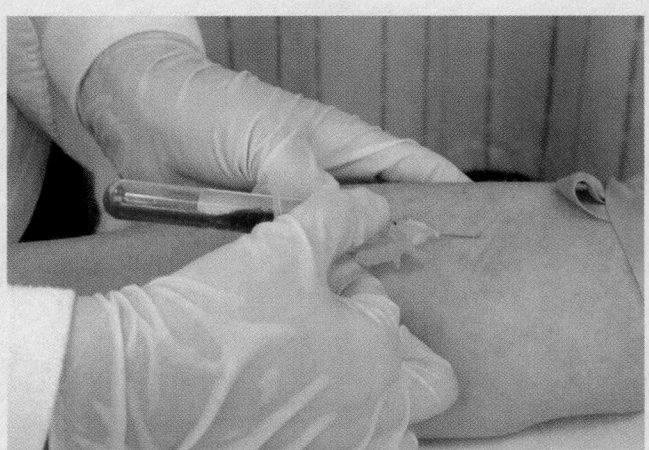

STEP 14b(9)   Blood flowing into tube.

STEP	RATIONALE
(3) Collect 10 to 15 mL of venous blood by venipuncture (see steps 14a[1-12]) in 20-mL syringe from each venipuncture site.	Culture specimens must be obtained from two sites. If one site produces bacteria, but not the other, assumption is that bacteria in first culture may be a contaminant and not the infecting agent. When infecting agent grows in both cultures, bacteremia exists and is due to organism in culture (Pagana and Pagana, 2007).
(4) Activate safety guard, and discard needle. Replace with new sterile needle before injecting blood sample into culture bottle.	Maintains sterile technique and prevents contamination of specimen.
(5) If both aerobic and anaerobic cultures are needed, inoculate anaerobic first.	Anaerobic organisms may take longer to grow (Pagana and Pagana, 2007).
(6) Mix gently after inoculation.	Mixes medium and blood.
d CVC Blood Collection	
(1) Select appropriate port. Turn off all IV pumps and clamp lumens (see illustration).	If more than one lumen, select a lumen not in use if possible. Prevents dilution of sample with medication or total parenteral nutrition (TPN).
(2) Wipe cap (all caps are Luer-Lok) with alcohol wipe or antiseptic solution. Attach 10-mL flush to selected port. Aspirate gently for blood return. Flush with 5 to 10 mL normal saline (NS) (check agency policy). Do not use syringe smaller than 5 mL.	To ensure patency of selected lumen. To ensure line is clear. Pressure from small syringe may damage the catheter.
(3) Wipe cap with alcohol wipe. Attach syringe to selected lumen, aspirate 5 mL of blood, and discard in appropriate receptacle.	To ensure is blood sample not contaminated with IV fluids, medication, or other products.
(4) Wipe cap with alcohol wipe. Attach empty 10-mL syringe and aspirate blood. Use Vacutainer holder with Luer-Lok attachment; fill desired tubes.	Tubes have vacuum and automatically fill to necessary amount.
(5) When necessary tubes are filled, discard syringes into appropriate receptacles.	Reduces risk for contamination by blood-borne pathogens.
(6) Attach 10-mL NS flush. Flush with 5 to 10 mL NS using push, pause method. Ensure positive pressure for lumen. Cap with spring automatically has positive pressure so syringe can be removed then lumen locked (see illustration). For caps without positive pressure, hold syringe plunger steady at completion of flush, lock off lumen with slide clamp, then remove syringe.	Push, pause creates turbulence that assists in clearing lumen. Positive pressure prevents blood from flowing into the tip of the catheter and forming a clot.

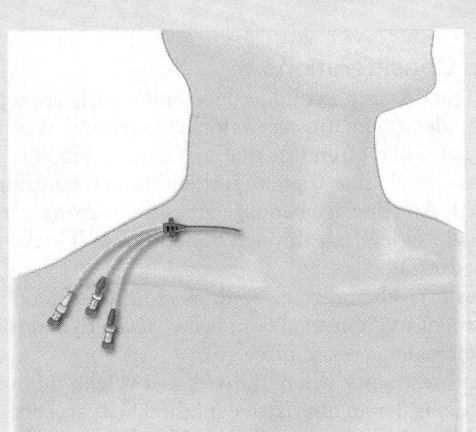

STEP 14d(1) Triple lumen central venous catheter; select appropriate port.

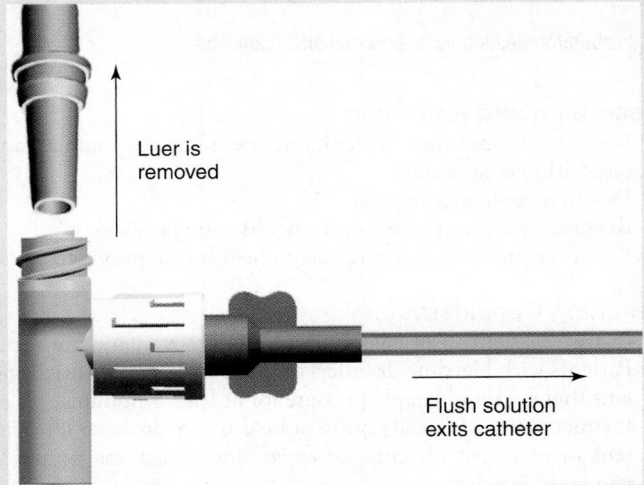

Luer is removed

Flush solution exits catheter

STEP 14d(6) Positive pressure cap helps maintain the patency of vascular access device. (*With permission, courtesy ICU Medical, Inc., San Clemente, Calif.*)

STEP	RATIONALE
(7) Take blood tubes containing additives; gently rotate back and forth 8 to 10 times.	Additives mix with blood to prevent clotting. Shaking can cause hemolysis of red blood cells, producing inaccurate test results.
15 Inspect puncture site for bleeding, and apply adhesive tape with gauze.	Keeps puncture site clean and controls any final oozing.
16 Check tubes for any sign of external contamination with blood. Decontaminate with 70% alcohol if necessary.	Prevents cross contamination. Reduces risk for exposure to pathogens present in blood.
17 Assist patient to comfortable position.	.
18 Securely attach properly completed identification label to each tube, and affix proper requisition.	Incorrect identification of specimen could result in diagnostic or therapeutic errors.
19 Dispose of needles, syringe, Vacutainer, and soiled equipment in proper container. Do not recap needles.	Prevents cross contamination through needle sticks and contact with blood.
20 Place specimens in bag to be sent to laboratory.	
21 Remove clean gloves after specimen is obtained and any spillage is cleaned.	Reduces risk for exposure to blood-borne pathogens.
22 Perform hand hygiene after procedure.	Reduces transfer of microorganisms.
23 Send specimens immediately to laboratory. Blood cultures must be sent to laboratory within 30 minutes (Pagana and Pagana, 2007).	Fresh specimen ensures accurate results. Bacteria multiply quickly.

EVALUATION

1 Reinspect venipuncture site.	Determines if bleeding has stopped or hematoma has formed.
2 Determine if patient remains anxious or fearful.	Some patients require more blood tests in the future. Address concerns, and let patient express anxiety.
3 Check laboratory report for test results.	Reveals constituents of blood specimen.
4 Ask patient to explain purposes of tests.	Validates learning.

Unexpected Outcomes	Related Interventions
1 Hematoma forms at venipuncture site.	• Apply pressure. • Continue to monitor patient for pain and discomfort.
2 Bleeding at site continues.	• Apply pressure to site. • Instruct patient to apply pressure. • Monitor patient. • Notify health care provider.
3 Signs and symptoms of infection at venipuncture site occur.	• Notify health care provider. • Apply moist heat to site (see Chapter 40).
4 Patient becomes dizzy or faints during venipuncture.	• Assist patient into chair. • Lower patient's head between knees. • Remain with patient.
5 Laboratory tests reveal abnormal blood constituents.	• Notify health care provider.

Recording and Reporting

- Record date and time of venipuncture, samples obtained, and disposition of specimen.
- Describe venipuncture site.
- Report any STAT test results to health care provider.
- Report any abnormal test results to health care provider.

Teaching Considerations

- Instruct patient to briefly apply pressure to venipuncture site. Patients with bleeding disorders or those undergoing anticoagulant therapy should apply pressure for at least 5 minutes.
- Instruct patient to notify nurse or health care provider if persistent or recurrent bleeding or expanding hematoma occurs at venipuncture site.

Pediatric Considerations

- Explain procedure to child at developmentally appropriate age, and provide atraumatic care (Hockenberry and Wilson, 2007).
- Because children often fear that loss of their blood is a threat to their lives, explain to them that their blood is continually being produced. An adhesive bandage gives them assurance that their blood will not leak out through puncture site (Hockenberry and Wilson, 2007).
- At times it is advantageous to draw children's blood specimens in treatment room instead of in bed or room to maintain feeling that their room is a safe place.
- Only use restraints when the risk outweighs not using a restraint. Consider an alternative method first, and document the method (Hockenberry and Wilson, 2007).

- When performing venipuncture on children, you need to explore a variety of sources for vein access: scalp, antecubital fossa, saphenous, and hand veins.
- Application of EMLA cream may be ordered to reduce pain in infants and young children (Hockenberry and Wilson, 2007).
- Vacutainers are not recommended in children under 2 years of age due to possible vein collapse with their use.

Gerontological Considerations
- Older adults have fragile veins that are easily traumatized during venipuncture. Sometimes application of warm compresses may help in obtaining samples. Using small-bore catheter may be beneficial.

Home Care Considerations
- In home care setting a blood pressure cuff, rather than a tourniquet, can be used for venipuncture.

SKILL 43-9 Blood Glucose Monitoring

Intermediate / Specimen Collection / Performing Blood Glucose Testing

Obtaining capillary blood by skin puncture is an alternative when you cannot perform venipuncture, to reduce the frequency of needle sticks, and for self-management of diabetes mellitus. The procedure is less painful than venipuncture, and the ease of the skin puncture method makes it possible for patients to perform this procedure. The development of reagent strips, home glucose monitors, and the skin puncture method has revolutionized home management care of patients with diabetes mellitus.

There are two methods for self-testing of blood glucose level. Both methods require obtaining a large drop of blood by skin puncture. You can use a handheld single-use lancet or automatic lancet-holder device. You then apply a drop of blood to a specially prepared chemical reagent strip.

The first self-testing method involves visually reading the reagent strip by comparing it to the color chart on the container. Examples of such strips include Chemstrip bG, Glucostix, and Trendstrips. If the color on the strip falls between two reference blocks on the chart, you may need to estimate the results. Thus results of blood glucose measurement may not always be accurate.

The second type of blood glucose monitoring uses reflectance meters (Fig. 43-7). A variety of meters are on the market, including the Glucometer II (Ames), Accu-Chek III (Boehringer Mannheim), Glucoscan 3000 (LifeScan), and OneTouch (LifeScan). After a drop of blood from the skin puncture is dropped onto the reagent strip, the meter provides an accurate measurement of blood glucose level in less than 60 seconds.

The meters use a wet-wash or dry-wipe method of testing. To perform a wet wash, the user flushes the blood-coated reagent strip with water before inserting the strip into the glucose meter. The dry-wipe method requires the user to wipe off the blood-coated reagent strip with a dry cotton ball before making a reading. Some products do not require blood to be flushed or wiped before a reading. The various methods allow measurement of blood glucose between 20 and 800 mg/dL, thus providing a sensitive measurement of blood glucose level.

These meters differ in several ways, including amount of blood needed for each test, testing speed, overall size, ability to store test results in memory, cost of the meter, and cost of test strips (FDA, 2005). Some larger meters are voice activated, which is a nice support for the older adult patient with visual impairments. Glucose readings may be from 0 to 800 mg/dL. The amount of time to complete the glucose testing with the current glucose meters varies from 5 seconds to 50 seconds. You can program some meters to monitor the glucose levels for a continuous 72 hours.

Most meters allow for an alternative site, including the forearm, palm, and thigh. Two new methods of obtaining glucose measurement are available on the market. A minimally invasive glucose meter uses a very small fine plastic sensor inserted through the abdomen and provides continuous readings of blood glucose levels. A biosensor is taped on the external abdomen (Fig. 43-8). The patient using a handheld wireless meter activates the biosensor to transmit the blood glucose level at any time without puncturing the skin. Another model, the noninvasive glucose meter, does not puncture the skin with a needle but uses laser technology to puncture the skin. For the patient with diabetes mellitus who requires assessment of trends and patterns these systems are ideal (FDA, 2005).

Delegation Considerations
The skill of measuring blood glucose level after skin puncture (capillary puncture) can be delegated to NAP who are specifically instructed in performing the skill. You must first assess the patient to

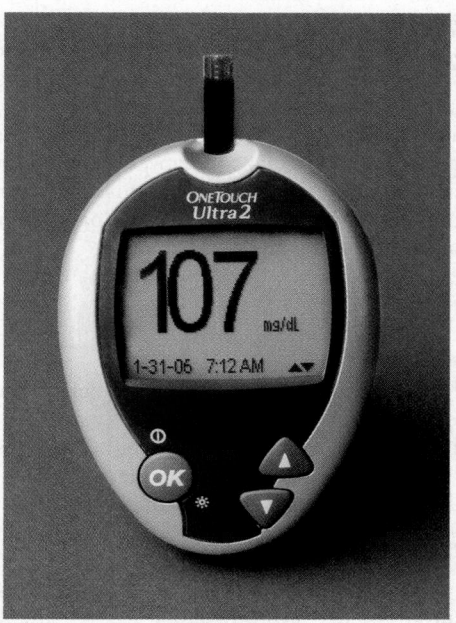

FIG 43-7 Blood glucose monitor. (*Courtesy LifeScan, Inc., Milpitas, Calif.*)

determine that serum glucose monitoring is appropriate for delegation. When the patient's condition changes frequently, you should not delegate this skill to NAP. The nurse directs the NAP by:

- Explaining appropriate sites to use for puncture and when to obtain glucose levels.
- Reviewing expected levels and when to report to the nurse unexpected glucose levels.

Equipment

- ❑ Antiseptic swab
- ❑ Cotton ball
- ❑ Sterile lancet or blood-letting device
- ❑ Heel-warming device *(optional)*
- ❑ Paper towel
- ❑ Blood glucose meter (e.g., OneTouch)
- ❑ Blood glucose reagent strips (brand determined by meter used)
- ❑ Clean gloves

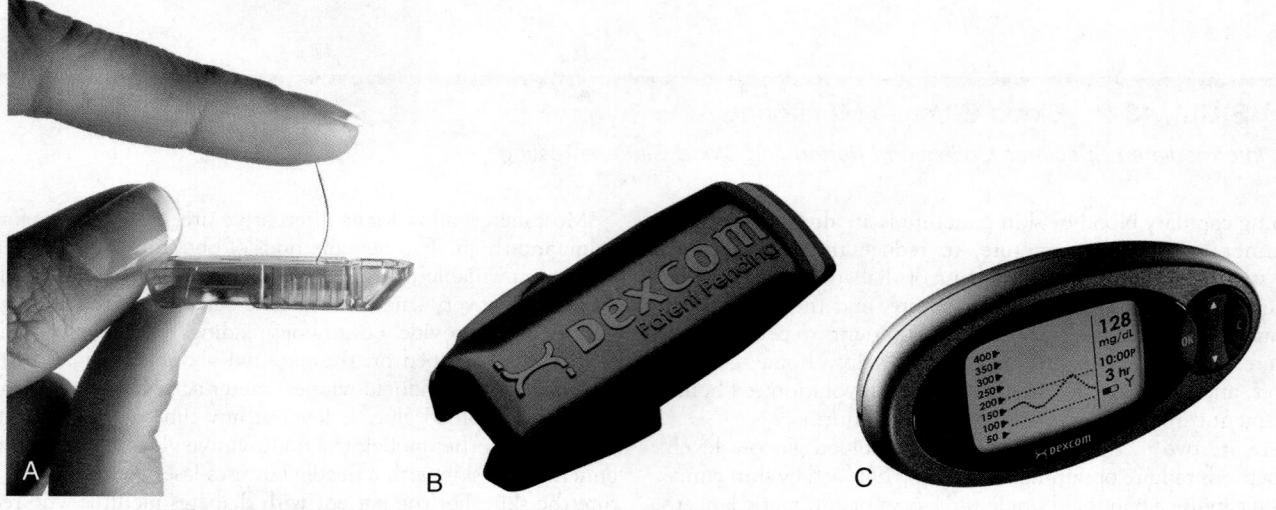

FIG 43-8   A, Tiny sensor implanted under skin transmits continuous reading to receiver **B,** to alert wearer of any deviation from desired glucose target range. **C,** Monitor displays and stores readings. *(Courtesy DexCom, Inc.)*

STEP	RATIONALE

ASSESSMENT

1 Assess understanding of procedure and purpose. Determine if patient with diabetes mellitus understands how to perform test and realizes importance of glucose monitoring.

Data set guidelines for nurse to develop teaching plan.

2 Determine if specific conditions need to be met before or after sample collection (e.g., with fasting, after meals, after certain medications, before insulin doses).

Dietary intake of carbohydrates and ingestion of concentrated glucose preparations alter blood glucose levels.

3 Determine if risks exist for performing skin puncture (e.g., low platelet count, anticoagulant therapy, bleeding disorders).

Abnormal clotting mechanisms increase risk for local ecchymosis and bleeding.

4 Assess area of skin you will use as puncture site. Inspect fingers, toes, and heel. Alternative sites are the palm, arm, or thigh. Avoid areas of bruising and open lesions.

Sides of fingers, toes, and heels are commonly selected because they have fewer nerve endings.

Measurements from alternative sites are meter specific and may be different than those from traditional sites (Corbett, 2008). The puncture site should not be edematous, inflamed, or recently punctured because these factors cause increased interstitial fluid and blood to mix and also increase the risk for infection.

5 Review health care provider's order for time of frequency of measurement.

Health care provider determines test schedule on basis of patient's physiological status and risk for glucose imbalance.

6 For diabetic patient who performs test at home, assess ability to handle skin-puncturing device. If patient chooses, he or she may wish to continue self-testing while in hospital.

Patient's physical health may change (e.g., vision disturbance, fatigue, pain, disease process), preventing patient from performing test.

NURSING DIAGNOSES

- Anxiety
- Deficient knowledge regarding blood glucose monitoring
- Disturbed sensory perception (tactile)
- Ineffective health maintenance
- Ineffective therapeutic regimen management

Individualize related factors based on patient's condition or needs.

STEP	RATIONALE

PLANNING

1 Expected outcomes following completion of procedure:	
• Puncture site shows no evidence of bleeding or tissue damage.	Hemostasis achieved. Lancet or needle did not puncture skin too deeply.
• Blood glucose level is normal.	Normal fasting glucose is 70 to 110 mg/dL, indicating good metabolic control.
• Patient demonstrates procedure.	Demonstrates psychomotor learning.
• Patient explains test results.	Validates knowledge.
2 Explain procedure and purpose to patient and/or family. Offer patient and family opportunity to practice testing procedures. Provide resources/teaching aids for patient.	Promotes understanding and cooperation.

IMPLEMENTATION

1 Perform hand hygiene before procedure.	Reduces transfer of microorganisms.
2 Instruct adult to perform hand hygiene with soap and warm water, if able.	Promotes skin cleansing and vasodilatation at selected puncture site. Hand washing establishes practice for patient when test is performed at home.
3 Position patient comfortably in chair or in semi-Fowler's position in bed.	Ensures easy accessibility to puncture site. Patient will assume position when self-testing.
4 Remove reagent strip from container; then tightly seal cap. Check the code on the test strip vial.	Protects strips from accidental discoloration due to exposure to air or light. Code on test strip vial must match code entered into the glucose meter.
5 Turn on glucose meter, if necessary.	Activates meter.

Critical Decision Point   *Some monitors are activated when the reagent strip is inserted and therefore do not have a specific on/off switch.*

6 Insert strip into glucose meter (refer to manufacturer's directions), and make necessary adjustments (see illustration).	Some machines must be calibrated; others require zeroing of timer. Each meter is adjusted differently.
7 Remove unused reagent strip from meter, and place on paper towel or clean, dry surface with test pad facing up (see manufacturer's directions).	Moisture on strip can alter accuracy of final test results.
8 Apply clean gloves.	Reduces risk for contamination by blood.
9 Choose puncture site. Puncture site should be vascular. In adult, select lateral side of finger; be sure to avoid central tip of finger, which has more dense nerve supply.	Ensures free flow of blood following puncture.

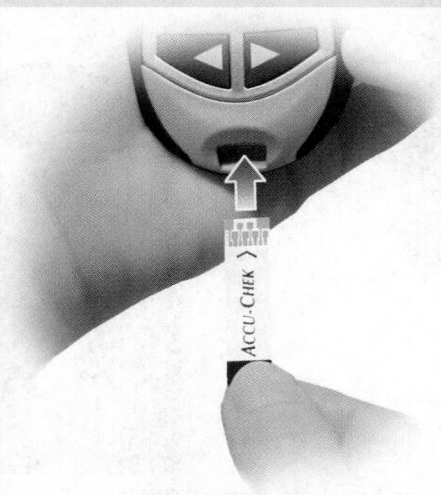

STEP 6   Load test strip into meter. *(Courtesy Accucheck Glucometer.)*

STEP	RATIONALE
10 Hold finger you will puncture in dependent position while gently massaging finger toward puncture site.	Increases blood flow to area before puncture.
11 Clean site with antiseptic swab, and *allow it to dry completely*.	Alcohol can cause blood to hemolyze.
12 Remove cover of lancet or blood-letting device. Hold lancet perpendicular to puncture site, and pierce finger or heel quickly in one continuous motion (do not force lancet).	Cover keeps tip of lancet/needle sterile.
13 Some agencies use lancet devices with an automatic blade retraction system. This reduces the possibility of self-sticks, preventing exposure to blood-borne pathogens. Place blood-letting device firmly against side of finger and push release button, causing needle to pierce skin (see illustration).	Blood-letting devices are designed to pierce skin for specific depth, ensuring adequate blood flow. Perpendicular position ensures proper skin penetration.
14 Wipe away first droplet of blood with cotton ball. (See manufacturer's directions for meter used.)	First drop of blood may contain more serous fluid than blood cells.
15 Lightly squeeze puncture site (without touching) until large droplet of blood has formed (see illustration). Repuncturing is necessary if large enough drop does not form to ensure accurate test results. (See manufacturer's direction regarding how blood is applied.)	Adequate-size droplet is needed to activate monitor and obtain accurate results. Excessive squeezing of tissues during blood sample collection may contribute to pain, bruising, scarring, and hematoma formation (Pagana and Pagana, 2007).

Critical Decision Point   *Diabetic patients frequently have peripheral vascular disease, making it difficult to produce a large drop of blood after a finger stick. Be sure to hold finger in dependent position before puncturing to improve blood flow.*

16 Obtain test results.	Exposure of blood to test strip for prescribed time ensures proper results.

Critical Decision Point   *Some meters (such as OneTouch [LifeScan]) require blood sample to be applied to test strip already in the meter. Once the drop of blood is applied, the meter automatically calculates the reading.*

a Be sure meter is still on. Bring test strip in the meter (in this example, an *ACCU-CHEK*) to the drop of blood (see illustrations). The blood will be wicked onto the test strip (see manufacturer's instructions).	Blood enters strip, and glucose device will show message on screen to signal enough blood is obtained.

Critical Decision Point   *Do not scrape blood onto the test strips or apply blood to wrong side of test strip. This prevents accurate glucose measurement.*

b The blood glucose test result will appear on the screen (see illustration). Some devices will "beep" when completed.

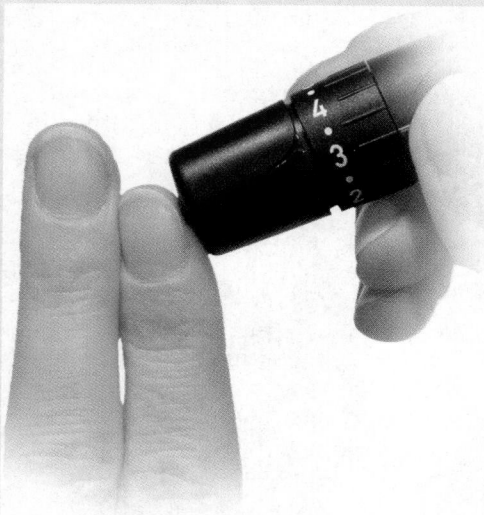

STEP 13   Prick side of finger with lancet. (*Courtesy Accucheck Glucometer.*)

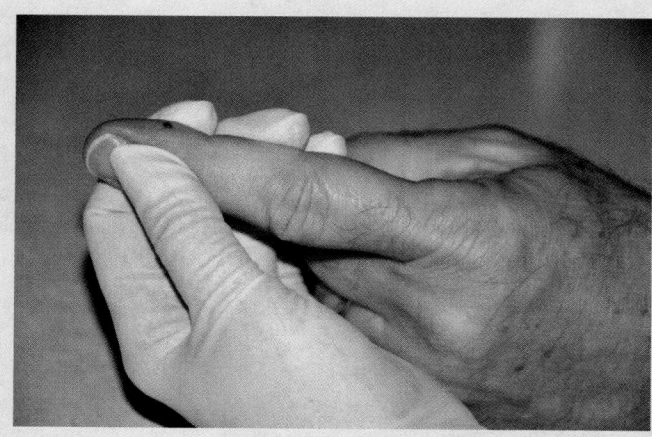

STEP 15   Squeeze puncture site until a large droplet of blood is formed.

STEP	RATIONALE

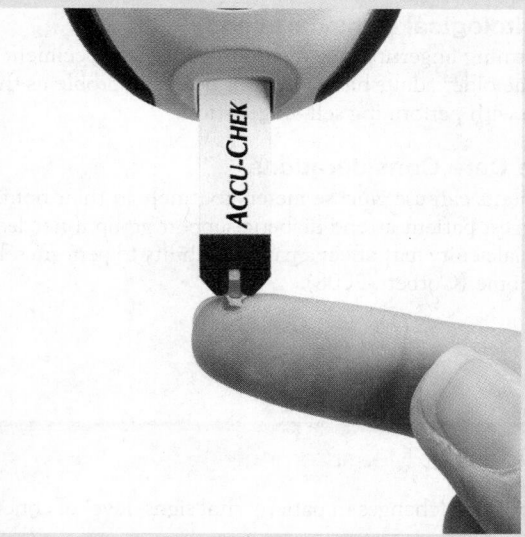

STEP 16a   Touch the test strip to the blood drop. Blood is absorbed into the test strip. (*Courtesy Accucheck Glucometer.*)

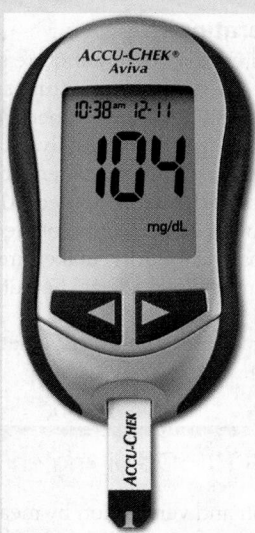

STEP 16b   Results appear on meter screen. (*Courtesy Accucheck Glucometer.*)

17   Turn meter off. Dispose of test strip, lancet, and gloves in proper receptacle.

Meter is battery powered. Proper disposal reduces risk for needle-stick injury and spread of infection.

18   Discuss test results with patient.

Promotes participation and compliance with therapy.

EVALUATION

1   Reinspect puncture site for bleeding or tissue injury.

Site is possibly a source of discomfort and infection.

2   Compare glucose meter reading with normal blood glucose levels and previous test results.

Determines if glucose level is normal.

3   Ask patient to discuss procedure.

Validates level of learning.

4   Ask patient to explain test and results.

Results of test may cause anxiety. Patient may misunderstand specific step of procedure.

Unexpected Outcomes	Related Interventions
1 Puncture site is bruised or continues to bleed.	• Apply pressure. • Notify health care provider.
2 Blood glucose level is above or below target range.	• Continue to monitor patient. • Check if there are medication orders for deviations in glucose level. • Administer insulin or carbohydrate source as ordered depending on glucose level. • Notify health care provider.
3 Glucose meter malfunctions.	• Review instructions for troubleshooting glucose meter. • Repeat test.
4 Patient expresses misunderstanding of procedure and results.	• Repeat instructions to patient. • Have patient demonstrate procedure.

Recording and Reporting

• Record procedure and glucose level in nurses' notes or special flow sheet and action taken for abnormal range.
• Describe response, including appearance of puncture site, in nurses' notes.
• Describe explanations or teaching provided in nurses' notes.
• Record and report abnormal blood glucose levels.

Teaching Considerations

• Provide information on where patient with diabetes mellitus can obtain testing supplies if applicable. When possible, teach with the same meter the patient will use at home.
• Provide patient with information on where to obtain assistance if glucose meter has malfunctioned.
• Instruct patient in what to do and whom to contact if glucose meter malfunctions.

- Stress importance of the timing of blood glucose levels, particularly in patients with diabetes mellitus.

Pediatric Considerations
- Allow young children to choose puncture site.
- Heel and great toe are common puncture sites in infants.
- Assess for localized complications in heels of premature infants who must have blood drawn repeatedly.
- Heel warming helps to obtain specimen from a neonate.
- Infection or abscess of the heel and necrotizing osteochondritis are the most serious complications of heel-stick puncture in infants. To avoid osteochondritis make sure the puncture is not deeper than 2.4 mm and is made at the outer aspect of the heel (Hockenberry and Wilson, 2007).
- Use earlobe to obtain blood in older pediatric patients (Pagana and Pagana, 2007).

- Allow young child with parent to demonstrate technique; incorporate a play activity for further understanding.

Gerontological Considerations
- Warming fingertips may facilitate obtaining specimen.
- Some older adults have vision or dexterity problems that interfere with performing self–finger sticks.

Home Care Considerations
- Patients can use glucose meters routinely in their homes.
- Suggest patient attend diabetic support group if needed.
- Visual acuity may affect a patient's ability to perform self-testing at home (Corbett, 2008).

SKILL 43-10 Obtaining an Arterial Specimen for Blood Gas Measurement

You assess oxygenation and ventilation by measuring arterial blood gases (ABGs). Measurement of ABGs provides valuable information in assessing and managing a patient's respiratory and metabolic disturbances (Pagana and Pagana, 2007). The parameters measured include arterial blood pH, partial pressure of oxygen (PaO_2), partial pressure of carbon dioxide ($PaCO_2$), and arterial oxygen saturation (SaO_2). The ABG sample is easy to obtain and analyze to provide a clear picture of acid-base balance, oxygenation, and ventilation. Alterations from normal show the nurse how the patient is adapting to the disease process.

Measuring ABGs aids the nurse in assessment of acid-base balance. Nurses should check agency policy regarding who is allowed to obtain ABG samples. Many institutions allow only nurses in critical care areas to obtain ABG samples, others specify a certified respiratory therapist, and some require institutional certification of this skill. A decision to draw ABG samples frequently may be a direct result of the nurse's physical assessment (see Chapter 6).

Delegation Considerations
The skill of obtaining an arterial blood sample cannot be delegated to NAP. The nurse directs the NAP to:
- Report any bleeding from puncture site of the specimen obtained.

- Report any changes in patient vital signs, level of conciousness, restlessness.

Equipment
- ☐ Commercial blood gas kit or individual supplies, including:
  - ☐ 3-mL heparinized syringe
  - ☐ 23- or 25-gauge needle with safety guard
  - ☐ Filter cap (allows expelling of air and retains blood)
  - ☐ Alcohol swabs (2)
  - ☐ 2 × 2 inch gauze pad
  - ☐ Tape
  - ☐ Heparin (1:1000 solution)
- ☐ Cup or plastic bag with crushed ice
- ☐ Completed identification labels with proper patient identifiers
- ☐ Completed laboratory requisition with date, time, name of test, patient identification and source of specimen
- ☐ Clean gloves
- ☐ Protective eyewear
- ☐ Commercial blood gas kits are available
- ☐ Small plastic biohazard bag for delivery of specimen to laboratory (or container specified by agency)

STEP	RATIONALE

ASSESSMENT

1 Determine need to obtain ABG sample and presence of health care provider's order. Signs and symptoms of alteration in respiratory status requiring sampling include dyspnea, sudden change in respiratory rate or pattern, unequal breath sounds, unequal chest expansion, cyanosis, change in level of consciousness, self-extubation without need for immediate reintubation, and increased work of breathing.

Some situations and medical conditions place patients at risk for alteration in acid-base balance and ventilation status. Health care provider's order is required for ABG sample.

2 Assess for factors that influence ABG measurements:
  a Patient who has just awakened
  b Immediately after suctioning
  c Less than 20 to 30 minutes after oxygen therapy or ventilator setting change

Allows nurse to eliminate factors that cause inaccurate results.

STEP	RATIONALE

   d Patient whose oxygen has not been in place continually for at least 20 to 30 minutes

   e Body temperature.

3 Perform physical assessment of thorax and lungs.

Physical signs and symptoms will indicate need for ABG sample.

4 Identify medications that may influence ABG measurement (e.g., anticoagulants, diuretics).

Certain medications increase risk for bleeding at puncture site.

5 Review criteria for choosing site for ABG sample.

Prevents causing compromised circulation from puncture.

Critical Decision Point   *Factors that contraindicate use of arterial site include amputation, contractures, localized infection, dressing or cast, mastectomy, or arteriovenous shunts.*

   a Assess collateral blood flow. Perform Allen's test:

Allen's test assesses collateral circulation before performing arterial puncture on radial artery. Positive Allen's test ensures there is collateral circulation to hand in case thrombosis of radial artery occurs following puncture (Pagana and Pagana, 2007).

     (1) Have patient make tight fist and raise hand above heart.

Removes as much blood from hand as possible.

     (2) Apply direct pressure to both radial and ulnar arteries (see illustration).

Obstructs arterial blood flow to hand.

     (3) Have patient lower hand and open hand (see illustration).

Fingers and hand should be pale and blanched, indicating lack of arterial blood flow.

     (4) Release pressure over ulnar artery; observe color of fingers, thumbs, and hand (see illustration).

Flushing identifies that circulation through ulnar artery is good and the ulnar artery alone is capable of providing blood supply to entire hand. Therefore you can use the radial artery for puncture.

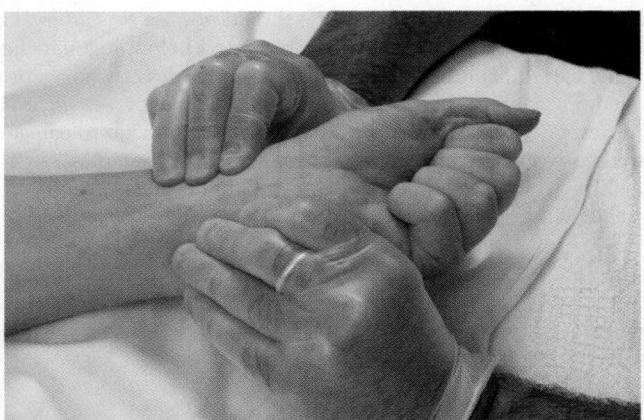

STEP 5a(2)   Applying pressure to radial and ulnar arteries.

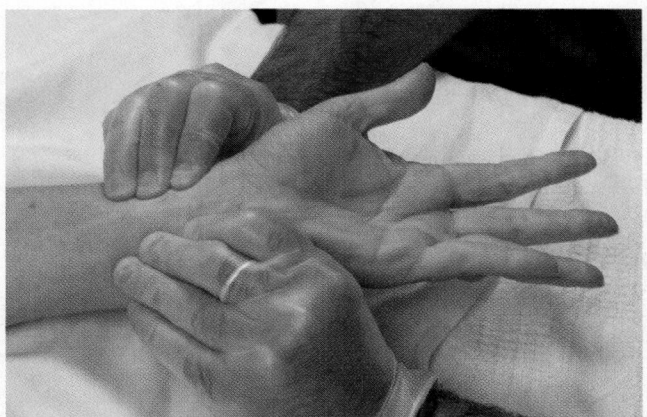

STEP 5a(3)   Patient opening hand; note color.

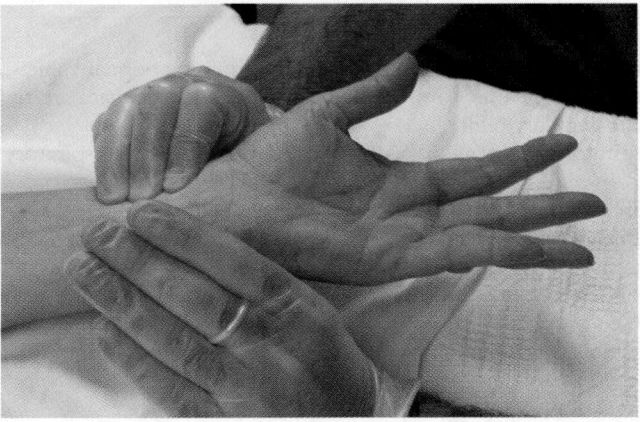

STEP 5a(4)   Releasing pressure over ulnar artery, and noting color of hand.

STEP	RATIONALE
b Accessibility of vessel.	Palpating, stabilizing, and performing venipuncture of a superficial artery is easier. Superficial arteries are located at distal ends of extremities.

Critical Decision Point *If there is no flushing in 15 seconds, Allen's test is negative and you should repeat this test on the other arm or choose another artery for puncture (Pagana and Pagana, 2007).*

c Tissue surrounding artery.	Muscle, tendon, and fat have decreased sensation to pain. Bony periosteum and nerves are highly sensitive to pain.
d Arteries not directly adjacent to veins.	Helps reduce chance of venous puncture and possibility of inaccurate samples.
6 Assess best arterial sites for use in obtaining specimen.	Arterial blood may be obtained from areas where strong pulses are palpable (i.e., radial, brachial, or femoral artery) (Pagana and Pagana, 2007).

Critical Decision Point *Previous puncture sites or preexisting conditions may eliminate potential sites. Artery should be easily accessible.*

a Radial artery	Safest, most accessible site for puncture; is superficial, is not adjacent to large veins, usually has adequate collateral circulation by ulnar artery, and is relatively painless if periosteum is avoided. Used when Allen's test is positive.
b Brachial artery	Has reasonable collateral blood flow, is less superficial, is more difficult to palpate and stabilize, carries increased risk for venous puncture, and results in increased discomfort for patient if brachial nerve is punctured. Used when radial artery is inaccessible or Allen's test is negative.
c Femoral artery	Nurses without specialized training should not use this artery. Has no adequate collateral flow if obstructed below inguinal ligament, is difficult to stabilize, is deep, and is directly adjacent to femoral vein. Is best artery to use in emergency (e.g., cardiac arrest or hypovolemic shock when pulses are difficult to palpate).
7 Determine baseline ABG values for patient.	Provides basis for comparison and evaluation of therapies.
8 Determine patient's knowledge about ABG procedure.	Obtaining blood specimen is painful. Patient who is knowledgeable will be more cooperative.

NURSING DIAGNOSES

- Anxiety
- Deficient knowledge regarding arterial blood gases
- Impaired gas exchange
- Ineffective airway clearance
- Ineffective breathing pattern
- Ineffective peripheral tissue perfusion
- Risk for injury

Individualize related factors based on patient's condition or needs.

PLANNING

1 Expected outcomes following completion of procedure:	
• Patient's ABG values are within normal ranges.	Determining normal values is essential for accurate interpretation.
• Patient's extremity distal to puncture remains warm, pink, and free of pain and has adequate capillary refill.	Documents adequate arterial circulation to extremity.
• Patient denies anxiety, and respiratory rate remains within baseline.	Anxiety increase respiratory rate, which can alter ABG results.
• Patient discusses ABG procedure.	Documents learning.
2 Prepare heparinized syringe (if heparinized syringes are unavailable, kits have heparinized syringe).	Heparin mixes with specimen to prevent clotting.
3 Aspirate 0.5 mL sodium heparin (1000 units/mL) into syringe from vial or ampule.	Prevents blood sample from clotting before reaching laboratory. Excessive heparin can affect pH of arterial sample.
4 Withdraw plunger entire length of syringe, and maintain asepsis.	Coats barrel of syringe with heparin.

STEP	RATIONALE
5 Eject all heparin in barrel out of syringe.	In hub of syringe 0.15 to 0.25 mL of sodium heparin remains; 0.05 mL of sodium heparin adequately anticoagulates 1 mL of blood; 0.15 mL adequately anticoagulates 3 mL without affecting pH level.
6 Explain steps and purpose of procedure to patient.	Reduces anxiety and promotes understanding and cooperation.

IMPLEMENTATION

1 Verify patient's identity by using at least two forms of identifiers, neither of which is the patient's room number. Verify the type of procedure scheduled and the procedure site with the patient.	Ensures accurate patient identification and improves patient safety. Use of patient's room number is not an acceptable identifier (TJC, 2008).
2 Perform hand hygiene.	Reduces transmission of infection.
3 Palpate selected radial, femoral, or brachial site with fingertips.	Determines area of maximal impulse for puncture site.
4 Using radial artery, elevate the patient's wrist with a small pillow, and ask the patient to extend the fingers downward. Stabilize artery by slight hyperextension of wrist.	This flexes the wrist and positions the radial artery closer to the surface (Fischbach and others, 2008). Reduces mobility of artery and makes insertion of needle easier.
5 Put on clean gloves. Clean area of maximal impulse with alcohol swab or antiseptic swab per agency procedure, wiping in circular motion away from site. Allow to dry.	Reduces number of resident bacteria on skin's surface. Drying maximizes antibacterial effects.
6 Hold 2 × 2 inch gauze pad with same fingers used to palpate artery.	Keeps gauze pad accessible for covering of puncture site when necessary.
7 Use corner of sterile gauze pad or alcohol wipe to point to chosen site.	Maintaining location of artery improves likelihood of successful puncture.
8 Hold needle bevel up and insert at 45-degree angle into artery, with bevel directed proximally. Prepare patient for needle stick because radial sticks are painful.	Angle allows for better arterial flow into needle. Oblique hole in artery seals more easily. Prepared patient will be less likely to withdraw arm.
9 Stop advancing needle when blood is noted returning into hub of needle or syringe.	Quick return of blood indicates that arterial flow is obtained. Prevents puncturing through both sides of artery.
10 Allow arterial pulsations to pump 2 to 3 mL of blood into heparinized syringe slowly (see illustration).	Allowing pulsations to assist in filling syringe reduces presence of air bubbles in sample. Bubbles alter ABG results.
11 When sampling is complete, hold 2 × 2 inch gauze pad over puncture site, withdraw syringe and needle, and activate safety guard over needle.	Pad minimizes pulling of skin as needle is withdrawn. Decreases contamination from blood and accidental needle stick.
12 Apply pressure over and just proximal to puncture site with pad (see illustration).	Insertion of needle into artery is just proximal to insertion site through skin. Gauze absorbs any blood that might ooze from site.
13 Maintain continuous pressure on and proximal to site for 3 to 5 minutes (approximately 15 minutes if patient is undergoing anticoagulant therapy or has bleeding disorder) (Pagana and Pagana, 2007).	To avoid hematoma formation, apply and hold pressure, or apply a pressure dressing to the arterial puncture site for 3 to 5 minutes (Pagana and Pagana, 2007).

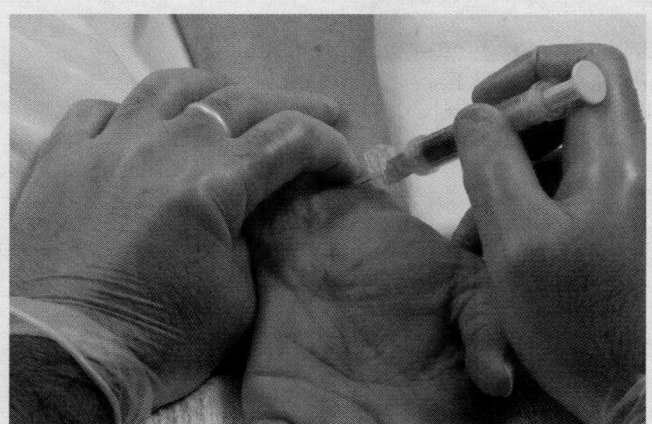

STEP 10 Blood flowing into syringe.

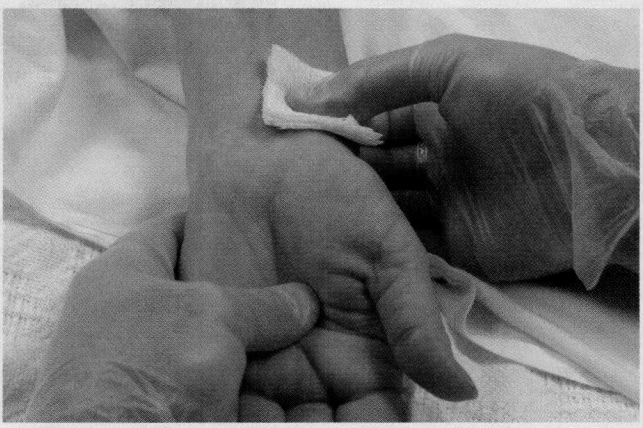

STEP 12 Applying firm pressure to arterial puncture site.

STEP	RATIONALE

14 Visually inspect site for signs of bleeding or hematoma formation.

Determines if continued need exists to exert pressure. Because an artery rather than a vein has been accessed, monitor puncture site for bleeding.

15 Palpate artery below or distal to puncture site.

Determines if pulse quality has changed, indicating alteration in arterial flow.

16 Remove gloves, and perform hand hygiene.

Reduces transmission of microorganisms.

17 Take syringe, remove safety needle, and attach a filter cap (available in kit) to expel air, or cover tip of syringe with 2 × 2 inch sterile gauze to expel air (see agency procedure). Some kits may have all supplies, including syringe with heparin, needle with safety needle cap, and a filter cap that allows air to vent and not blood (see illustration).

Decreases chance of contamination from room air. Air bubbles in the specimen can falsely elevate or decrease the results, depending on the patient's blood gas status (Leeuwen and others, 2006).

18 Prepare syringe for laboratory analysis according to agency policy. Common principles include:
  • Place patient identification label on syringe.
  • Place syringe in cup of crushed ice.

  • Attach properly labeled requisition to blood gas sample.

  • Indicate amount of any supplemental oxygen (e.g., 2 L O_2, 70% by mask, room air) on requisition.

  • Indicate patient's temperature.

Permits proper identification of sample for laboratory.
Failure to place the ABG sample in an ice bath may affect results of the pH, PaO_2, and $PaCO_2$ (Leeuwen and others, 2006).
Prevents mislabeled specimens in laboratory. Ensures correct results received for correct patient.
Information for laboratory should include the fraction of inspired oxygen (FiO_2) which is 21% for room air (Fischbach and others, 2004).
Temperature affects the amount of gas in solution. Fever will increase actual PaO_2 and $PaCO_2$ (Leeuwen and others, 2006).

19 Send sample to laboratory immediately.

Prevents alteration in gas tensions resulting from metabolic processes that continue after blood is drawn (Fischbach and others, 2008).

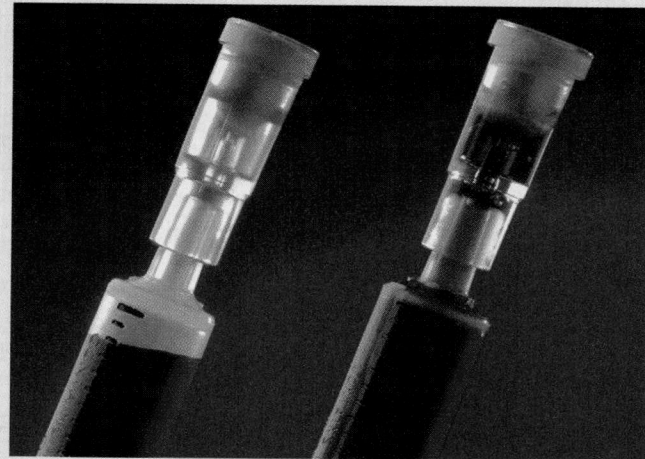

STEP 17 Filter-Pro Air Bubble Removal Device expels air safely from syringe without accidentally expelling blood and aerosolizing the sample. (*With permission from Smiths Medical, Carlsbad, Calif.*)

EVALUATION

1 Inspect puncture site and area distal to puncture site for complications.

Obstruction of artery can develop or penetration of important structures anatomically juxtaposed to an artery (Pagana and Pagana, 2007).

2 Review results of sample as soon as possible.

Identifies any abnormality and expedites initiation of treatment.

Unexpected Outcomes

1 Patient has abnormal ABG values.

2 Patient has hematoma formation at puncture site.

3 Puncture site is bruised or continues to bleed.

Related Interventions

- Continue to monitor patient.
- Notify health care provider of findings, and obtain further orders.

- Apply warm compresses to enhance absorption of blood (see Chapter 40).
- Continue to monitor patient.
- Notify health care provider.

- Apply pressure.
- Notify health care provider.

Recording and Reporting

- Record results of Allen test.
- Record puncture site and disposition of specimen to laboratory in nurses' notes.
- Report ABG results to health care provider as soon as available.
- Report patient's FiO_2 and any ventilator settings (e.g., tidal volume [V_T], respiratory frequency [RF] mode of ventilation).
- Record results of test and condition of puncture site in nurses' notes.
- Record patient's tolerance of the procedure.

Teaching Considerations

- Teach patient to report numbness, burning, and/or tingling during and after in hand that had radial artery puncture.

Pediatric Considerations

- In neonatal and pediatric patients, you can use capillary blood gas. Procedures are similar to those for obtaining heel sticks.
- When dealing with neonatal patients, especially premature infants, normal values for ABGs often differ from those of adults.
- Arterial blood samples from punctures are painful and cause crying and breath holding that affect the accuracy of blood gas values (decreases PaO_2) (Hockenberry and Wilson, 2007).

Gerontological Considerations

- Pay special attention during interpretation of ABGs for patients with chronic pulmonary conditions. In these patients compensatory mechanisms may allow normal pH in face of markedly elevated $PaCO_2$.

[?] CRITICAL THINKING EXERCISES

Mrs. Yamamoto is a 76-year-old who was admitted with pneumonia today. She has a productive cough. She also has diabetes mellitus. Her blood glucose level on admission is 208 mg/dL. She speaks minimal English. Her daughter translates for her and states her blood glucose level is normally well controlled with oral hypoglycemic medication.

1 Which test(s) would you expect to be ordered? Select all that apply.
  A Sputum specimen today
  B Throat culture in morning
  C Midstream urine culture at noon
  D Finger stick for blood glucose levels before meals and at bedtime
2 Immediate results will be available for which of the tests?
3 Briefly describe how you would teach Mrs. Yamamoto about providing a sputum specimen.
4 What do you need to assess to determine Mrs. Yamamoto's ability to test her own blood glucose levels at home?

[✓] REVIEW QUESTIONS

1 A urine specimen for culture and sensitivity is being collected from a male patient. Which steps would be used to obtain an accurate specimen? Select all that apply.
  1 Two patient identifiers are checked.
  2 Help the patient to perform pericare before the sterile part of the procedure.
  3 Wipe the head of the penis back and forth three times with each swab.
  4 Collect 10 to 20 mL for the sample.
  5 Have the patient initially void into a bedpan or clean container.
  6 Have patient hold penis above the sterile specimen cup and complete voiding to obtain the specimen.
2 A 24-hour urine (timed urine collection) is being started. Which step is essential in order to have an accurate collection?
  1 Discard the first urine specimen.
  2 Include the first specimen for the test.
  3 Discard both the first and last specimen.
  4 Discard the last specimen.
3 A patient is scheduled to obtain a stool for occult blood several days from now. Which food should be avoided before the stool sample is obtained because it can alter the results of the test?
  1 Potatoes
  2 Tomatoes
  3 Bananas
  4 Apples
4 The nurse is preparing to obtain a throat culture. Which steps would facilitate obtaining an accurate specimen? Select all that apply.
  1 Place the patient in a sitting position or at a 45-degree angle.
  2 Have the patient lean her head forward.
  3 Have the patient swallow a small amount of water to rinse away food from the culture site before swabbing the area.
  4 Swab the tonsillar area.
  5 Swab the uvula.
  6 Have the patient blow her nose.
5 The nurse is preparing to obtain a culture from a male patient with a urethral discharge. Before obtaining the culture, what objective data should the nurse observe the genital area for?
  1 Redness
  2 Lower abdominal discomfort
  3 Urethral stinging
  4 Itching

REFERENCES

Baer D: Tips from the clinical experts: standards for transporting specimens, *Med Lab Obs* 37(11):36, 2005.

Barclay L, Murata P: *Perineal cleaning during urine collection may minimize contamination,* http://www.medscape.com/viewarticle/556640, May 17, 2007.

Beall A and others: Blackboard basics for lab 101: microbiology, garbage in garbage out, *MLO Med Lab Obs* 39(3):12, 2007, http://www.mlo-online.com.

Behrman RE and others: *Nelson textbook of pediatrics,* ed 17, Philadelphia, 2004, Elsevier.

Corbett JV: *Laboratory tests and diagnostic procedures with nursing diagnoses,* ed 7, Upper Saddle River, NJ, 2008, Prentice-Hall.

D'Avanzo CE: *Cultural health assessment,* ed 4, St. Louis, 2008, Mosby.

Dock B: Improving the accuracy of specimen labeling, *Clin Lab Sci* 18(4):210, 2005.

Fischbach F, Dunning MB.: *A manual of laboratory and diagnostic tests,* ed 8, Philadelphia, 2008, Lippincott Williams & Wilkins.

Garza D, Becan-McBride: *Phlebotomy handbook: blood collection essentials,* ed 7, Upper Saddle River, NJ, 2005, Prentice-Hall.

Hamill T: *Point of care testing: Multistix and Uristix urinalysis,* San Francisco, March 8, 2007, UCSF Clinical Laboratory.

Hockenberry MJ, Wilson D: *Wong's nursing care of infants and children,* ed 8, St. Louis, 2007, Mosby.

Leeuwen A and others: *Davis's comprehensive handbook of laboratory and diagnostic tests with nursing implications,* ed 2, Philadelphia, 2006.

Pagana K, Pagana T. *Mosby's diagnostic and laboratory test reference,* ed 8, St. Louis, 2007, Elsevier/Mosby.

The Joint Commission: *2009 National patient safety goals,* Oakbrook, Ill, 2008, The Commission, accessed December 14, 2008, http://www.jointcommission.org.

U.S. Department of Health and Human Services, Office of the Secretary: HIPAA administration simplification: enforcement; final rule, part III, 45 CFR, parts 160 and 164 (*Fed Regist* vol 71, No. 32, February 16, 2006, http://www.hhs.gov/ocr/hipaa/FinalEnforcementRules06.pdf.

U.S. Food and Drug Administration: *Diabetic information: glucose meters and diabetes management,* June 14, 2005, http://www.fda.gov/diabetes/glucose.html.

Vaillancourt S and others: To clean or not to clean: effect on contamination rates in midstream urine collections in toilet-trained children, *Pediatrics* 11(6):21288, 2007.

Diagnostic Procedures

MEDIA RESOURCES

- **evolve** http://evolve.elsevier.com/Perry/skills
  learning system
  - Review Questions
  - Audio Glossary

KEY TERMS

Abdominal girth	Lumens
Aldrete score	Manometer
Aspiration	Medullary
Biopsy	Minimal sedation
Bone marrow	Moderate sedation
Cerebrospinal fluid (CSF)	Modified Ramsay sedation scale
Cytology	Percutaneous coronary intervention (PCI)
Deep sedation	
Epidural blood patch	Peritoneal fluid
Fiberoptic	Precordial
Herniation	Radiopaque
Intestinal obstruction	Stopcock
	Subarachnoid space
Intravenous conscious sedation (IV sedation)	Thrombocytopenia
	Tracheobronchial tree
Lavage	Trocar

OBJECTIVES

Mastery of content in this chapter will enable the nurse to:
- Identify physiological indications for diagnostic procedures.
- Demonstrate organizational skills in planning diagnostic procedures.
- Describe the procedural responsibilities for all health care providers or physicians and nursing assistive personnel.
- Perform appropriate physical and psychological assessments before, during, and after diagnostic procedures.

- Effectively assist the physician or other health care professionals with angiogram, cardiac catheterization, intravenous pyelogram, bone marrow aspiration/biopsy, lumbar puncture, paracentesis, thoracentesis, bronchoscopy, and endoscopy.
- Demonstrate understanding of nursing responsibilities related to the use of intravenous sedation during the diagnostic/surgical procedure.

You will perform diagnostic tests at the patient's bedside or in specially equipped rooms within a hospital or outpatient care setting. Your responsibilities include assessing the patient's knowledge of the procedure, preparing the patient, providing a safe environment and emotional support throughout the procedure, and providing preprocedural and postprocedural assessment, care, and documentation. Supervise any nursing care delegated to nursing assistive personnel (NAP). When testing is completed in an outpatient setting, provide detailed printed home care instructions and teach postprocedure care to the patient or caregiver. The physician is responsible for providing the patient with an explanation of the test, risks, benefits, treatment options, and outcomes.

EVIDENCE-BASED PRACTICE TRENDS

Intravenous (IV)sedation is often used for diagnostic or surgical procedures that do not require complete anesthesia in acute care, surgical care, and outpatient care settings. The current terminology used for procedural sedation is now classified as "minimal," "moderate," or "deep" sedation/analgesia. Moderate sedation was previously known as *conscious* sedation (American Academy of Pediatrics, 2006; American Society of Anesthesiologists, 2004a). In procedures that require sedation, agencies maintain standards for preassessment, preparation, and monitoring of patients. Objective scales for preassessment determine if a patient is at risk for undesirable outcomes. Use of an objective scale, such as the American Society of Anesthesiologists (ASA) classification, helps reduce the risk for complications by determining when it is prudent to involve an anesthesiologist to help manage the care of a complicated patient condition (ASA, 2004a). These objective scales provide evidence-based criteria that, when followed, help reduce the risk for complications.

The use of a vascular closure device is now common after procedures involving an arteriotomy or opening in an artery. The devices apply manual compression to prevent bleeding at the arterial site. Vascular closure devices are available in varieties that mechanically "plug" the arteriotomy or that percutaneously apply pressure over the site. Research on these devices show that vascular closure devices decrease the time needed for hemostasis (cessation of bleeding) and return to ambulation, and as a result, increase patient comfort and mobility. However, because each device leaves behind foreign material (e.g., clip, sealant, or suture), infection is an increased concern (Kim, 2006).

Causes of postpuncture headache after lumbar puncture (LP) continue to affect patients. The symptoms can last for several days and are incapacitating. Current literature includes practice guidelines for managing postpuncture headaches; these guidelines include prevention of headaches. Interventions to prevent headaches include adequate hydration and fever control before the lumbar puncture (Oedit and others, 2005). Another effective intervention includes postprocedure application of an epidural blood patch for pain management (Ahmed and others, 2006).

Skill Performance Guidelines

Before the procedure:

1. Perform the essential patient safety steps of proper identification of the patient and procedure (and site, where applicable). Check agency policy for required steps. This includes verbal verification and documentation of the above upon patient arrival, again in the procedure room, and just before starting the procedure (The Joint Commission [TJC], 2008a).

2. Obtain a medication history, identify any medications for which uninterrupted dosing is required (e.g., anticonvulsants, antibiotics, certain cardiac medications). If the procedure requires a status of nothing by mouth (NPO), discuss medications with the physician or health care provider. When insulin or oral hypoglycemic medications are administered to patients before procedures, arrange to have either the patient's meal or other nutritional support available on completion of the test.

3. Determine patient factors that can affect the procedure or the patient's responses:

FACTOR	POSSIBLE EFFECT(S)
Level of anxiety, educational level, previous experience, language barrier, sensory deficits	Impaired ability to understand and give informed consent. Impaired ability to understand and cooperate with instructions during the procedure. Impaired ability to understand postprocedure instructions.
Previous positive or negative experience with diagnostic testing	Influences the amount of teaching and support needed. IV or oral sedation is often needed.
Physical limitations	Impaired ability to maintain needed position during the procedure.
Cultural factors	Affect the patient's acceptance and response to the procedure. Some cultures are less expressive about communicating discomfort.

4. When patients have chronic illness, fatigue, or decreased functional status, plan diagnostic testing schedules to provide rest periods between multiple tests performed on the same date.

5. Verify that informed consent was obtained. The physician or health care provider performing the procedure is responsible for obtaining informed consent from the patient. In some agencies after the physician or health care provider discusses the procedure and obtains verbal consent, the nurse obtains the patient's signature on the consent form. (Check agency policy to deter-

mine if a consent form is required and the expectations of the registered nurse [RN] in this process). When there is no evidence of informed consent in the patient medical record, hold any preprocedure medications that alter the patient's level of consciousness, and notify the physician or health care provider performing the procedure, as well as staff in any receiving area.

During the procedure:

1 *Procedures involving the use of radiation:* Minimize the amount of radiation exposure by using protective shielding devices such as a lead apron and goggles, radioprotective gloves, and thyroid shield. Remain positioned as far away from the radiographic equipment as possible, while still performing required patient care (Lombardi, 2006).

2 Provide reassurance to the patient throughout the procedure. Most of these procedures cause moderate discomfort, and the patient tolerates the procedure better if you remain at the patient's side and explain each step.

3 Monitor physiological parameters indicated by the procedure.

4 Assist the physician or health care provider with the procedure, repositioning the patient as needed, providing equipment and supplies, and obtaining and preparing specimens for testing.

After the procedure:

1 Monitor physiological parameters indicated by the procedure.

2 Provide the patient and any caregivers with discharge instructions that include:
   • Complications that may occur
   • How to handle complications
   • Physical signs and symptoms to report to the physician or health care provider

3 Follow agency policy for disposal of waste materials from the procedure.

SKILL 44-1 Intravenous Moderate Sedation During a Diagnostic Procedure

Certain diagnostic or therapeutic procedures require the patient to receive IV moderate sedation. Moderate sedation helps improve the patient's cooperation with the procedure, allows a rapid return to the preprocedure status, and minimizes the risk for injury. In addition, it often raises the patient's pain threshold and provides amnesia concerning the actual procedural events. Moderate sedation is a drug-induced depression of consciousness during which patients respond purposefully to verbal commands, either alone or accompanied by light tactile stimulation. In addition, no interventions are required to maintain a patent airway, and spontaneous ventilation is adequate (ASA, 2004a).

Deep sedation is one risk associated with moderate sedation when the patient's level of consciousness depresses past the point at which a patent airway can be maintained. Because of this risk, the use of IV moderate sedation is closely controlled and normally restricted to physicians and nurses who receive specialized training or credentialing (American Association of Nurse Anesthetists [AANA], 2004; Association of periOperative Registered Nurses [AORN], 2006). Know the agency policy for recommended and maximum doses of medications, as well as monitoring and documentation requirements when using IV sedation.

The most common types of medications used to achieve moderate sedation include benzodiazepines and opiates. Benzodiazepines reduce anxiety and promote muscle relaxation. Midazolam (Versed) also produces an amnesic effect. Opiates, such as meperidine, help control pain while achieving sedation. Propofol, a rapid-acting hypnotic, is also commonly used.

Patient risks during IV sedation include hypoventilation, airway compromise, hemodynamic instability, and/or altered levels of consciousness that include an overly depressed level of consciousness or agitation and combativeness. Emergency equipment appropriate for the patient's age and size (see Chapter 27) and staff with skill in airway management, oxygen delivery, and use of resuscitation equipment is essential. During and after the procedure, patients need continuous monitoring of vital signs, oxygen saturation, heart rhythm, lung sounds, and level of consciousness.

Delegation Considerations

The skill of assisting with intravenous sedation cannot be delegated to NAP. In most agencies a registered nurse or health care provider or physician assesses and monitors the patient's level of sedation, airway patency, and level of consciousness. Roles in monitoring depend on scope-of-practice guidelines as determined by state regulations and by agency policy and practitioner credentialing. Check agency procedures regarding specific monitoring parameters and frequency required before, during, and after the procedure.

Equipment

❏ Protective equipment: gloves, mask, gown
❏ Sedation agent as prescribed: diazepam (Valium), midazolam (Versed), fentanyl (Sublimaze)
❏ Emergency equipment: crash cart, defibrillator, and endotracheal equipment in various sizes
❏ Equipment for insertion of a peripheral intravenous catheter (see Chapter 28)
❏ Oxygen and airway supplies: bag and mask device, oral/nasopharyngeal airways, suction equipment
❏ Sphygmomanometer or noninvasive blood pressure monitor
❏ Pulse oximeter
❏ Electrocardiogram (ECG) machine
❏ Appropriate reversal drugs (e.g., flumazenil for reversal of benzodiazepines, naloxone for reversal of opiates)
❏ Pain medication for procedures anticipated to cause discomfort

---

STEP	RATIONALE

ASSESSMENT

1 Verify patient's identity by using at least two forms of identifiers, neither of which is the patient's room number. Verify the type of procedure scheduled and the procedure site with the patient.

Ensures accurate patient identification and improves patient safety. Use of patient's room number is not an acceptable identifier (TJC, 2008).

STEP	RATIONALE
2 Verify that a preprocedure history and physical examination was completed.	Accrediting agencies, such as The Joint Commission, require a documented preprocedure history and physical before the administration of procedural IV sedation.
3 Verify that informed consent was obtained.	Federal regulations, many state laws, and accreditation agencies require informed consent for procedure.
4 Assess the patient's past history of adverse reaction to IV sedation (e.g., hemodynamic instability, nausea and vomiting, airway compromise, altered level of consciousness).	Patients with a history of these reactions are at higher risk for procedural complications if IV sedation is used.
5 Verify the patient's ASA Physical Status Classification (Box 44-1, p. 1170).	The ASA recommends that patients receiving a classification of 3 or higher have an anesthesia consultation before receiving IV sedation (ASA, 2004a).

Critical Decision Point   *If the patient has an ASA classification of 3 to 6 or history of or evidence for difficult intubation, sleep apnea, or complications related to sedation/anesthesia, then consultation with an anesthesiologist is often required by the agency.*

STEP	RATIONALE
6 Assess the patient's current or past history for substance abuse.	A history of substance abuse usually requires dose adjustment of the sedative.
7 Verify that the patient has not ingested food or fluids, except for oral medications, for at least 4 hours. Verify specific agency requirements.	Because a risk of moderate sedation is loss of airway protection, an empty stomach reduces the risk for aspiration.
8 Determine if patient is allergic to latex, antiseptic, or anesthetic solutions.	Allergic reactions to latex range from mild skin reaction to anaphylaxis. Common allergic reactions to local anesthetic agents include central nervous system (CNS) depression, respiratory difficulty, and hypotension.
9 Assess patient's level of understanding of procedure, including any concerns.	Determines extent of instruction or level of support required and decreases anxiety.
10 Assess baseline heart rate, breath sounds, respiratory rate, blood pressure, level of consciousness, pain level, and oxygen saturation.	Establishes a baseline for comparison during the procedure.
11 Determine patient's height and weight.	Needed to calculate drug dosages.
12 Assess and document the patient's baseline status via the agency's designated scoring system. Many agencies use an "Aldrete score" (Table 44-1, p. 1170).	Establishes a baseline for comparison after the procedure.

NURSING DIAGNOSES

- Acute pain
- Anxiety
- Deficient knowledge regarding purpose and steps of procedure
- Risk for aspiration
- Risk for injury

Individualize related factors based on patient's condition or needs.

PLANNING

1 Expected outcomes following completion of procedures: • Patient's airway remains patent.	Moderate sedation is monitored successfully without progression to deep sedation.
• Patient's level of comfort is equivalent to a score of 4 or less on a pain scale of 0 to 10.	Use of a standardized pain scale provides reliable detection of increasing pain and pain relief.
2 Explain to patient that the IV sedation will cause relaxation, but that he or she will be awake during the procedure. If the patient will not be able to verbalize because of the nature of the procedure, teach patient agreed-upon nonverbal signals for things such as "yes," "no," and "pain."	Encourages cooperation and minimizes risks and anxiety about the procedure.
3 Explain to patient that close monitoring of vital signs and frequent checks to determine that the patient is awake are normal and do not mean that there are problems.	Reduces patient anxiety during the procedure.
4 Explain to patient the major steps of the procedure.	Reduces patient anxiety during the procedure.
5 Position the patient as needed for the procedure.	
6 Take "time out" to verify patient's name, type of procedure scheduled, and procedure site with patient.	"Time out" verification just before starting the procedure includes the physician and all personnel and is a safety precaution to prevent wrong patient, wrong site, and wrong procedure errors (TJC, 2008).

STEP	RATIONALE
IMPLEMENTATION	
1 Establish a peripheral IV access (see Chapter 28).	Provides access for administration of sedation and any emergency changes (as needed).
2 During the diagnostic procedure, monitor heart rate and oxygen saturation (SpO$_2$) continuously via pulse oximetry equipment. Monitor airway patency, respiratory rate, blood pressure, and appropriate level of consciousness and responsiveness every 5 to 15 minutes.	Vital signs provide a comparison with patient's baseline status.
3 Observe for verbal or nonverbal evidence of pain, facial grimacing, and eye opening.	Physical responses indicate level of sedation.
4 Monitor level of consciousness/responsiveness to physical and/or verbal stimulation. Assess level of sedation using the Modified Ramsay Sedation Scale (Table 44-2, p. 1170) or other criteria adopted by the agency.	Determines the patient's level of sedation. Use of a numeric rating scale ensures consistency in assessments and an accurate judgment of the patient's changing status, verbal/physical stimulation.

Critical Decision Point *Report a Ramsay sedation score higher than 3 to the physician.*

EVALUATION	
1 Monitor the patient throughout the procedure using the Ramsay Sedation Scale.	Provides data to verify patient's expected return to baseline status.
2 After procedure: Use Aldrete score and monitor airway patency, oxygen saturation, and pain score every 5 minutes for at least 30 minutes, then every 15 minutes for an hour, and then every 30 minutes until the patient meets the discharge criteria on the agency's designated scoring system.	Enables prompt detection of any suppression of airway and protective reflexes due to delayed action of medication.
3 Ask patient to repeat back what he or she understands regarding the procedure or any postprocedure patient instructions.	Verifies patient understanding of procedure or discharge education.
4 Have patient's "designated driver" explain any postprocedure education and sign appropriate documents.	Patients who receive conscious sedation are restricted from driving for 24 to 48 hours depending on the procedure, type of sedation, and postprocedure restrictions.

Unexpected Outcomes

1 Oversedation, evidenced by:
  - Decreasing oxygen saturation; cyanosis; slow, shallow respirations with periods of apnea
  - Tachycardia
  - Sedation score of 4 or higher on the Modified Ramsay Sedation Scale, score less than 8 on Aldrete Scale.

2 Patient develops cardiac instability evidenced by irregular heart rate, change in pulse rate, or change in blood pressure.

Related Interventions

- Support patient's breathing via positioning and manual bagging.
- Immediately notify physician or health care provider.
- Be prepared to administer reversal agents. Naloxone is for reversal of opioids and flumazenil is for reversal of benzodiazepines.

- Obtain electrocardiogram as ordered.
- Immediately notify physician or health care provider.

Recording and Reporting

- Document vital signs, oxygen saturation, and sedation level at baseline, then every 5 minutes during the procedure, and every 15 minutes for at least 30 minutes after the procedure according to agency policy.
- Record dosage, route, time of drugs administered during and after the procedure, including the use of reversal agents and significant patient reactions during the procedure. Include IV fluids and blood products, if administered.
- Immediately report to patient's physician or health care provider any respiratory distress, cardiac compromise, or altered mental status.

Teaching Considerations

- Explain that it is unlikely for patients to remember the procedure, because of the amnesic effect of the sedative.

Pediatric Considerations

- Sedation is used in pediatric patients to attain their cooperation with procedures. For this reason, deep sedation is used more often than conscious sedation in children under age 6 or those who did not progress as expected through their developmental stages (American Academy of Pediatrics, 2006).

- Children are more likely than adults to sustain a serious complication resulting from anesthesia. Such complications are often linked to either the cardiovascular or respiratory system. For this reason the American Academy of Pediatrics recommends that personnel who are able to manage a child's airway be present for the procedure (American Academy of Pediatrics, 2006).
- A preprocedure medical evaluation is required. To safely administer sedation to the pediatric patient consider anatomical and physiological variations, preprocedure assessments, and pharmacological techniques (American Academy of Pediatrics, 2006).
- During the preprocedure assessment, answer the parent's questions in a relaxed and confident manner. When communicating with children, take into account the child's developmental stage.

Gerontological Considerations

- Closely monitor the effects of medications on patient's respiratory status and pulse. These drugs interfere with breathing or increase or decrease heart rate due to the reduced drug clearance through the kidneys or the liver (Lewis and others, 2007).

- Physical limitations of the patient, including hearing and vision loss, contribute to frustration and confusion, compounding the sense of loss of control.

Home Care Considerations

- Instruct the patient to avoid making any legally binding decisions until at least 24 hours after the procedure.

BOX 44-1	Physical Status Classification

1 =	Healthy patient; no organic, physiological, or psychiatric disturbances.
2 =	Presence of mild systemic disease without functional limitations.
3 =	Presence of severe systemic disease with significant systemic effects and significant functional limitation.
4 =	Presence of medical condition that is poorly controlled, associated with significant dysfunction, and is a potential threat to life.
5 =	Presence of critical medical condition associated with little chance of survival.
6 =	Presence of brain death.

From American Society of Anesthesiologists: *Relative value guide,* 2004, The Society.

TABLE 44-1	Aldrete Scoring System	
		Score
Activity (Moving voluntarily on command)	4 extremities	2
	2 extremities	1
	0 extremities	0
Respiration	Able to deep breathe and cough freely	2
	Dyspnea, shallow or limited breathing	1
	Apneic	0
Circulation	BP ± 20 mm Hg of presedation level	2
	BP ± 20-50 mm Hg of presedation level	1
	BP ± 50 mm Hg of presedation level	0
Consciousness	Fully awake	2
	Arousable on having name called	1
	Not responding	0
Color	Normal	2
	Pale, dusky, blotchy, jaundiced or other change	1
	Cyanotic	0

From Aldrete JA: The post-anesthesia recovery score revisited, *J Clin Anesth* 7:89, 1995; Aldrete JA: Post-anesthetic recovery score, *J Am Coll Surg* 205(5):3, 2007.
BP, Blood pressure.

TABLE 44-2	Modified Ramsay Sedation Scale	
Minimal sedation (anxiolysis)	1	Anxious and agitated or restless or both
	2	Cooperative, oriented, and tranquil
Moderate sedation/analgesia (conscious sedation)	3	Responds to commands spoken in a normal voice
Deep sedation/analgesia	4	Brisk response to a light forehead tap or loud auditory stimulus
	5	Sluggish response to a light forehead tap or loud auditory stimulus
	6	No response to a light forehead tap or loud auditory stimulus

Data from Ramsay MA and others: Controlled sedation with alphaxalone-alphadolone, *Br Med J* 2(920):656, 1974; American Society of Anesthesiologists: *Continuum of depth of sedation definition of general anesthesia and levels of sedation/analgesia,* Oct 31, 1999, http://www.asahq.org/publicationsAndServices/standards/20.htm, accessed Jan 18, 2004.

SKILL 44-2   Contrast Media Studies: Angiogram, Cardiac Catheterization, and Intravenous Pyelogram

Contrast media studies involve visualization of blood vessels and internal organs by intravascular injection of a radiopaque medium. An arteriogram (angiogram) permits visualization of the vasculature of an organ and the organ's arterial system (Fig. 44-1). Arteriography is most frequently performed by a radiologist to diagnose occlusions, stenosis, emboli, thromboses, aneurysms, tumors, congenital malformations, or trauma of the arteries of the brain, heart, lung, kidneys, or lower extremities.

Cardiac catheterization is a specialized form of angiography in which a catheter is inserted into the left or right side of the heart via a major peripheral vessel. The test studies pressures within the heart, cardiac volumes, valvular function, and patency of coronary arteries. Cardiac catheterizations are performed in specially equipped laboratories (Fig. 44-2). A contrast medium is injected, and the structures and functions of the heart are assessed.

Cardiac catheterizations are contraindicated in patients who would refuse needed surgery, are allergic to iodine contrast media, are uncooperative or cannot lie still during the entire procedure, or are susceptible to dye-induced renal failure. Precautions to help prevent dye-induced renal failure include making sure the patient is well-hydrated, premedicating with acetylcysteine (Mucomyst) before, during, and after the procedure, and using nonionic (instead of ionic) contrast media (Murray and others, 2006).

Intravenous pyelography (IVP) is a venographic examination of the flow of radiopaque contrast medium through the kidneys, ureters, and bladder to identify obstruction, hematuria, stones, bladder injury, or renal artery occlusion. Dye is injected into a peripheral vein, and serial radiographs are taken over the subsequent 30 minutes.

Delegation Considerations

The skill of assisting with angiography and intravenous pyelography can be delegated to NAP if the patient is stable and if no IV sedation is used. The nurse directs the NAP about:

- When to obtain and report vital signs.
- What signs and symptoms to report to the nurse.
- Accompanying the patient to the procedure room and assisting specially trained and licensed radiology personnel with the specific angiography procedure.

You can delegate the skill of assisting with cardiac catheterization to specially trained NAP with an RN continuously present. The RN presence is needed because of the required continuous assessment and monitoring for serious complications. The NAP helps with patient transport, positioning, and obtaining needed supplies.

Equipment

- ❑ Protective supplies: mask, goggles, sterile gown, and gloves
- ❑ Sterile packs containing catheters/equipment for performing procedures
- ❑ Equipment for IV access
- ❑ Medications, such as diazepam (Valium), midazolam (Versed), proprfol, or other sedative for IV sedation as indicated
- ❑ Emergency equipment: oxygen, emergency cart, defibrillator, cardiac monitor, pulse oximeter, and sedative reversal agents

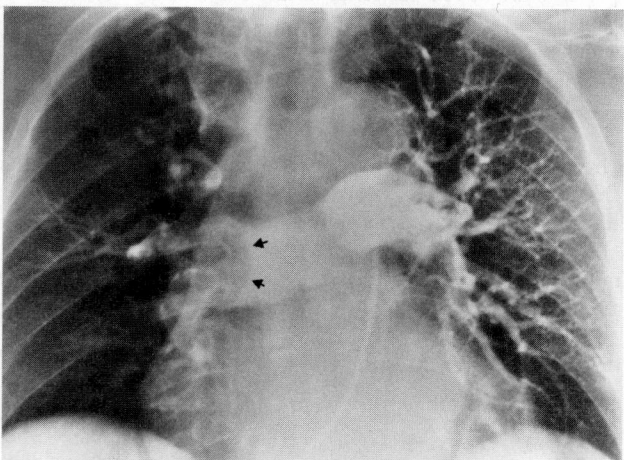

FIG 44-1   Pulmonary arteriogram shows obstruction (*arrows*) of right pulmonary artery. (*From Eisenberg R, Johnson N: Comprehensive radiographic pathology, ed 4, St. Louis, 2007, Mosby.*)

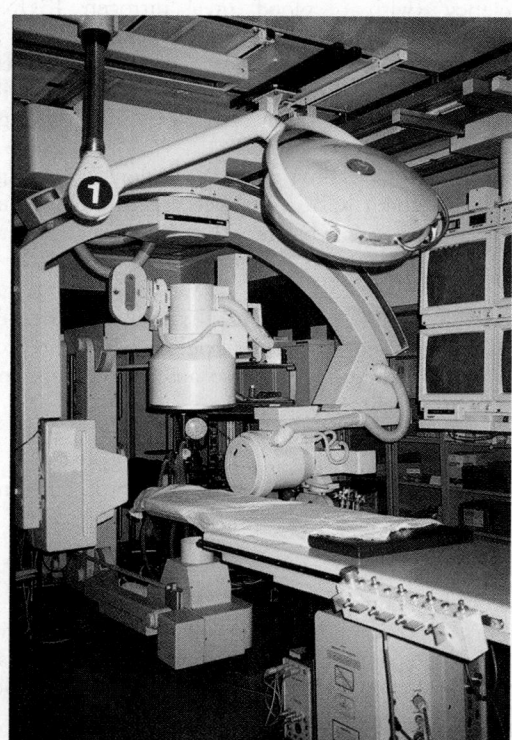

FIG 44-2   Cardiac catheterization laboratory. (*From Hockenberry MJ, Wilson D: Wong's nursing care of infants and children, ed 8, St. Louis, 2007, Mosby.*)

STEP	RATIONALE

ASSESSMENT

1 Verify patient's identity by using at least two forms of identifiers, neither of which is the patient's room number. Verify the type of procedure scheduled and the procedure site with the patient.

Ensures accurate patient identification and improves patient safety. Use of patient's room number is not an acceptable identifier (TJC, 2008).

2 Verify that informed consent was obtained.

Federal regulations, many state laws, and accreditation agencies require informed consent for procedure.

3 Determine if patient is taking anticoagulants.

Medication increases risk for bleeding and is often stopped before the procedure.

4 Assess patient for allergies to iodine dye, latex, shellfish; if so, notify cardiologist or radiologist.

Patients with allergies to iodine, shellfish, or other contrast media are at risk for anaphylactic reactions. A hypoallergenic contrast medium is sometimes used.

5 Examine medical record for contraindications:
   a *All contrast media:* Pregnancy unless the benefits of the test outweigh the risks to the fetus.

Radioactive iodinated contrast media crosses the blood-placental barrier.

   b *Angiography contraindications:* Anticoagulant therapy, bleeding disorders, thrombocytopenia, dehydration, uncontrolled hypertension, renal insufficiency, and pregnancy.

Anticoagulants and bleeding disorders are contraindications for arterial procedures because they interfere with the patient's blood clotting abilities and may cause blood loss.

Dehydration and renal insufficiency are contraindications to the use of ionic radiographic contrast media because the patient has an impaired ability to excrete the contrast media via the kidneys.

   c *Cardiac catheterization contraindications:* Severe cardiomyopathy, severe dysrhythmias, uncontrolled congestive heart failure (CHF)

Introduction of a catheter into the myocardium increases the risk for dysrhythmias (Pagana and Pagana, 2007).

   d *IVP contraindications:* Dehydration, known renal insufficiency (with a blood urea nitrogen [BUN] level >40 mg/100 mL) (Pagana and Pagana, 2007).

Iodinated dye is sometimes nephrotoxic and worsens existing kidney disease.

   e Determine whether patient took the drug metformin hydrochloride (Glucophage) within the previous 48 hours. If so, notify the physician or health care provider immediately.

Taking metformin hydrochloride (Glucophage) 48 hours before receiving iodinated contrast media can lead to acute renal failure and lactic acidosis (Ott, 2008).

6 Assess patient's bleeding and coagulation status (e.g., complete blood count [CBC], platelets, prothrombin time [PT]) and assess patient's renal function (e.g., electrolytes, BUN, creatinine levels) before the procedure.

Abnormal laboratory findings may contraindicate the procedure because of potential complications of hemorrhage and/or renal failure. Report elevated BUN or creatinine levels because such patients are at risk for renal failure induced by contrast media (Pagana and Pagana, 2007).

7 Obtain vital signs and peripheral pulses. For arterial procedures, mark patient's peripheral pulses before the procedure. For cardiac catheterization, also auscultate heart and lungs and obtain weight.

Provides baseline data and locations for comparison with findings during and after procedure.

8 Determine patient's hydration status.

Severe dehydration can cause renal failure (Pagana and Pagana, 2007).

9 Assess patient's level of understanding of procedure, including any concerns.

Determines extent of instruction or level of support required.

10 Remove all of patient's jewelry and metal objects.

Eliminates objects that interfere with radiography visualization of the vessels.

11 Preprocedure preparation:
   a *For IVP:* Verify that patient has completed the necessary bowel preparation of an orally administered evacuation preparation 24 hours before the test and evacuation enema 8 hours before test (check agency policy).

An evacuated lower intestine and bowel improves visualization of urinary structures.

   b *For cardiac catheterization:* Determine whether the hair at site of catheter insertion needs clipping or preparation with antiseptic just before the procedure. Allow antiseptic to dry.

Reduces risk for site-related infection. Drying promotes maximal antibacterial activity.

12 Determine type of arteriogram scheduled (e.g. carotid, femoral, brachial). If cardiac catheterization, verify if test is for right or left heart. For IVP, ask if the study is for one or both kidneys.

Enables you to anticipate patient teaching needs and postprocedure interventions.

STEP	RATIONALE
13 Determine and document last time of ingested food. NOTE: Exceptions occur for patients at risk for contrast media–induced renal impairment who are specifically instructed to drink increased fluids in the hours before the procedure.	Prevents possible aspiration because patient is sedated. Excessive hydration causes dilution of the contrast medium, making structures more difficult to visualize. Patients should be NPO for 6 to 8 hours before procedure. Good preprocedure hydration reduces the risk for renal impairment caused by contrast media (Pagana and Pagana, 2007).
14 Review physician's or health care provider's orders for preprocedure medications for IV sedation:	Increased sedation is necessary in anxious or confused patients.
a Atropine	Decreases salivary secretions and increases heart rate when bradycardia is present.
b Diphenhydramine (Benadryl)	Used prophylactically to block histamine and decrease allergic response.
c Preprocedural sedative	Decreases anxiety and promotes relaxation.
15 Review order for IV sedation during procedure.	See Skill 44-1.

NURSING DIAGNOSES

- Acute pain
- Anxiety
- Decreased cardiac output
- Deficient knowledge regarding purpose and steps of procedure
- Fear
- Risk for infection
- Risk for injury

Individualize related factors based on patient's condition or needs.

PLANNING

1 Expected outcomes following completion of procedure: • Patient does not have any complications or significant changes in vital signs or peripheral pulses. No allergic response.	Procedure performed without complication.
• Patient's level of comfort is equivalent to a score of 4 or less on a pain scale of 0 to 10. Expected discomfort includes soreness at catheter insertion site and possible backache.	Patient tolerates procedure. Use of a standardized pain scale provides reliable detection of increasing pain and pain relief.
• Patient is able to tolerate increased fluid intake and urinate sufficient output (at least 30 mL/hr) to excrete the radiographic dye.	Adequate renal function.
• Patient recovers from IV sedation without respiratory complications or change in level of consciousness.	Appropriate level of sedation.
2 Explain to patient purpose of the procedure and what will happen during the procedure.	Helps to minimize patient's anxiety.
3 For cardiac catheterization, it is common to verify the availability of emergent cardiac surgery due to the risk for complete coronary artery occlusion from dislodged plaque or inadvertent perforation of the vasculature (check agency policy).	Prepares backup plan for possible procedural outcomes that would require emergency surgery.

IMPLEMENTATION

1 Perform hand hygiene, and apply appropriate protective equipment.	Reduces transmission of microorganisms.
2 Have patient empty bladder before procedure.	Ensures that patient will not need to void during procedure.
3 Prepare monitoring equipment, including cardiac monitor, pulse oximetry, blood pressure cuff.	Provides easy access to equipment for monitoring patient status during and after procedure.
4 Provide IV access using large-bore cannula, and remove gloves.	Provides access for delivery of intravenous fluids and/or drugs.
5 Monitor vital signs, obtain weight, and (for arterial procedures) palpate peripheral pulses.	Provides baseline data for comparison during and after procedure.
6 Assist patient in assuming a comfortable supine position on x-ray table or in a slight Trendelenburg's position. Immobilize the extremity that will be injected with contrast media.	For arterial procedures, patient needs to maintain position for 1 to 3 hours.
7 Take "time out" to verify patient's name, type of procedure scheduled, and procedure site with the patient.	"Time out" verification just before starting the procedure includes the physician and all personnel and is a safety precaution to prevent wrong patient, wrong site, and wrong procedure errors (TJC, 2008).

STEP	RATIONALE
8 Tell patient that during the injection of the dye, he or she may experience some chest pain and a severe hot flash that is quite uncomfortable but lasts only a few seconds.	Dye causes a feeling of warmth, flushing, or a metallic taste shortly after injection.
9 Physician cleanses site for catheter insertion (femoral, carotid, or brachial) with antiseptic.	Reduces transmission of microorganisms.
10 All team members apply mask and goggles, sterile gown, cap, and gloves. (All technologists and assistants do the same.) Drape patient with sterile drapes, leaving puncture site exposed.	Maintains surgical asepsis.
11 Anesthetize the skin overlying the arterial puncture site.	Provides local anesthetic to area of incision or puncture.
12 For arterial procedures:	
a Physician performs needle puncture of artery; inserts guidewire through needle and angiographic (or cardiographic) catheter threaded over wire.	Permits access to artery and prevents coiling of catheter in artery.
b Advance catheter to desired artery or cardiac chamber, and inject contrast medium.	Permits radiographic visualization of structures, aneurysms, occlusions, or anomalies.
13 During dye injection, specialized machinery takes rapid sequence of x-ray films.	Permits radiographic records of visualization of dye through artery and any abnormalities present.
14 If indicated iodinated dye is used, observe patient for signs of anaphylaxis, including respiratory distress, palpitation, itching, and diaphoresis.	Allergic reactions can be life threatening.
15 For cardiac catheterization, the nurse assists with measuring cardiac volumes and pressure.	Provides data related to cardiac output, central venous pressure (CVP), ventricular pressures, and pulmonary artery pressure. Pressure on puncture site promotes clotting and prevents bleeding.

Critical Decision Point   *Be prepared to end the cardiac catheterization procedure early in the event of severe unrelieved chest pain, neurological symptoms of a cerebrovascular accident, cardiac dysrhythmias, or hemodynamic changes (Pagana and Pagana, 2007).*

16 Nurse administering IV sedation monitors level of sedation and level of consciousness (see Skill 44-1).	Proper IV sedation does not cause loss of consciousness.
17 Physician withdraws catheter and applies pressure to puncture site for 5 to 15 minutes.	Five to fifteen minutes of manual pressure is often enough to stop active site bleeding. However, a certain amount of bed rest is needed to achieve reliable hemostasis. Check agency policy for postprocedure bed rest requirements. This is often up to 6 hours when no vascular closure device is used.

Critical Decision Point   *Before removing sheaths, check for physician's or health care provider's orders for instructions for treating a vasovagal reaction. Manual pressure applied to the groin can stimulate the baroreceptors and cause a vasovagal reaction in which the patient becomes bradycardic and hypotensive. Vasovagal reactions are usually brief and self-limiting. When applying pressure to the groin after sheath removal, be alert for a vasovagal reaction and be prepared to treat it by lowering the head of the bed to the flat position and giving a bolus of intravenous fluids.*

18 An alternative to applying manual pressure is a vascular closure device.	Vascular closure devices include Angio-Seal, VasoSeal, Duett, and Perclose. Each has a unique method for providing closure of the arterial site. They provide a pretied suture knot that closes the arterial access site after the procedure. This knot provides rapid hemostasis (Kim, 2006).
19 If a percutaneous coronary intervention (PCI), such as a percutaneous transluminal coronary angioplasty (PTCA) or directional coronary atherectomy (DCA), was performed during the cardiac catheterization, a femoral sheath is often left in place and removed in several hours.	Postinterventional sheaths provide emergency access to the vasculature in the event that the coronary artery becomes occluded, allowing time for anticoagulants to wear off.
20 Remove and discard gloves.	
21 After the procedure:	
a For arterial procedures:	
(1) Keep affected extremity immobilized for 6 to 8 hours after removal of sheath, according to agency protocol. Use orthopedic bedpan for female patient as needed while on bed rest.	Allows time for the body's natural hemostatic mechanisms to form stable initial repair at the insertion site.
(2) Emphasize the need to lay flat for 6 to 12 hours (and possibly overnight if the sheath is left in the groin).	Helps to prevent disruption of hemostasis.

STEP	RATIONALE
b Encourage patient to drink 1 to 2 L of fluid after procedure.	Facilitates elimination of contrast material and prevents renal damage (Pagana and Pagana, 2007).

EVALUATION

1 Assess patient's body position and comfort during procedure.	
2 Monitor vital signs and oxygen saturation and assess for signs of cardiac complications every 15 minutes for 1 hour, every 30 minutes for 2 hours, or until vital signs are stable.	Verifies patient's physiological status and evaluates effect of procedure. Signs of cardiac complications include chest pain or pressure, new dysrhythmias, and/or shortness of breath.
3 Monitor for complications:	
a Perform neurovascular checks by palpating peripheral pulses on affected extremity and by comparing right and left extremities for skin color, temperature, and sensation. Use a Doppler ultrasonic stethoscope to locate pulses that are not palpable (see Chapter 6).	Enables prompt detection of circulatory impairment caused by intravascular clotting or bleeding at the procedure site. Signs of reduced circulation include diminishing distal pulses and/or coolness, mottling, pallor, pain, numbness, and tingling in affected extremity.
b Assess vascular access site for bleeding and hematoma.	Verifies expected sealing of puncture.
c Auscultate heart and lungs, and compare with preprocedure findings.	Evaluates patient response to procedure.
d Observe patient for possible delayed reaction to iodine dye (if used)—dyspnea, hives, tachycardia, and rash (Pagana and Pagana, 2007).	Reaction occurs up to 6 hours after injection of dye.
4 Assess for level of sedation, level of consciousness, and oxygen saturation. Use the Aldrete Scale (see Skill 44-1).	Determines patient's response to IV sedation.
5 Assess postprocedure laboratory values—CBC, prothrombin time.	Detects changes in laboratory values that indicate the onset of complications, such as bleeding.
6 Observe patient for signs of discomfort.	Early sign of complication.

Critical Decision Point *Patient's report of any feelings of pain, dyspnea, numbness or tingling, or other untoward symptoms usually indicates cardiac complications or procedure site complications. Immediately report these to the physician or health care provider.*

Unexpected Outcomes	Related Interventions
1 Vasovagal response occurs (at time of femoral puncture or after procedure with femoral pressure). Symptoms include feeling faint, dizzy, light-headed, and possible momentary loss of consciousness. Bradycardic pulse is caused by stimulation of the vagus nerve via baroreceptors.	• Support airway. • Lower table or head of bed to flat position or to Trendelenburg's position. • Be prepared to administer bolus of IV fluid.
2 Evidence of oversedation: • Prolonged reduced level of consciousness	• See Skill 44-1.
3 Pedal pulses are nonpalpable bilaterally 2 hours after an arteriogram.	• Assess pulse with Doppler. • Immediately notify physician or health care provider.
4 Hematoma or hemorrhage is present at catheter insertion site.	• Apply pressure over insertion site. • Monitor catheter site every 30 minutes for 2 to 3 hours, then as needed. • Notify physician or health care provider if interventions do not stop the bleeding of if patient demonstrates symptoms of acute blood loss (hypotension, tachycardia).
5 Patient has allergic reaction to contrast medium: • Symptoms of flushing, itching, and urticari	• Continue monitoring. • Assess patient for anaphylaxis. • Monitor vital signs. • Notify physician or health care provider. • Follow specific postprocedural orders related to findings. • Administer antihistamine or epinephrine if ordered.
6 Renal toxicity from contrast medium occurs: • Urine output less than 30 mL/hr	• Place on strict intake and output monitoring. • Monitor closely for signs of fluid overload. • Review electrolyte, urea nitrogen, and creatinine levels.
7 Patient experiences retroperitoneal bleeding (when femoral access site is used): • Low back pain radiating to both sides of the body (hallmark sign)	• Prepare patient for emergency surgery. • Monitor vital signs every 5 to 15 minutes. • Monitor distal pulses hourly.

Recording and Reporting

- Record patient's status: vital signs, oxygen saturation, status of peripheral pulses for equality and symmetry, blood pressure for hypotension, temperature and color of catheterized extremity, condition of IV site, and level of patient responsiveness. Record any drainage from puncture site, appearance of dressing, and condition of puncture site.
- Report to physician or health care provider changes in vital signs, excessive bleeding or increasing hematoma at puncture site, decreased or absent peripheral pulses, persistent pain, altered neurological status, dysrhythmias, decreased oxygen saturation, or decreased responsiveness after sedation.

Teaching Considerations

- Before the procedure, confirm that patient made arrangements for transportation home. In addition, prepare patient to stay in the hospital if complications occur or if an intervention necessitates prolonged postprocedure vascular checks.
- Because the dye can transfer to breast milk, teach women who are breast-feeding to substitute formula for breast milk for 24 hours after the procedure (Pagana and Pagana, 2007).

Pediatric Considerations

- Cardiac catheterizations in infants have the highest risk for complications and death in infants weighing less than 5 kg (Cheatham, 2001; McMahon and others, 2003).
- Infants and children are particularly susceptible to the diuretic effects of radiocontrast dyes, due to their small body size. In addition, those with congenital cardiac anomalies develop compensatory erythrocytosis and thus will experience complications from dehydration very quickly. Emphasize the importance of fluid intake with the child and parent(s) (Hockenberry and Wilson, 2007).

Gerontological Considerations

- Physical exposure and room temperature contribute to hypothermia in frail older adults who are unable to communicate that they are cold. Use heated blankets or forced-air heat to maintain core temperature at comfortable, safe levels (Negishi and others, 2003).
- In the older adult, slight alterations in vital signs or behavior are signs for impending problems; therefore close monitoring is very important.

Home Care Considerations

- On discharge, provide patient with written instructions to contact the physician or health care provider (or affiliated emergency department) if the following occur after arteriogram or cardiac catheterization:
  - Bleeding from the catheterization puncture site; apply gentle pressure with a clean gauze or cloth
  - Formation of a knot or lump under the skin that increases in size
  - Worsening of a bruise or its movement down the extremity rather than disappearing
  - Pain at puncture site or in the extremity used for the catheterization
  - Extremity is pale and cool to the touch where arterial puncture is made
  - Appearance of redness, swelling, or warmth of the affected extremity
- After arteriogram or cardiac catheterization, instruct patient not to drive or climb stairs for 24 hours; to avoid sports, strenuous housework, and lifting for 3 days; and to avoid taking baths until wound is healed.
- On discharge after an IVP, instruct patient to:
  - Drink at least three 8-ounce glasses of water to help flush the contrast media through the kidneys
  - Watch for signs of a delayed reaction to the contrast medium for 24 hours after the procedure and call his or her physician or health care provider or go to the nearest emergency department

---

SKILL 44-3   Assisting With Aspirations: Bone Marrow Aspiration/Biopsy, Lumbar Puncture, Paracentesis, and Thoracentesis

Aspirations are sterile invasive procedures involving the removal of body fluids or tissue for diagnostic procedures (Table 44-3). Informed consent is required for these invasive procedures.

Bone marrow aspiration is the removal of a small amount of the liquid organic material in the medullary canals of selected bones, in particular the sternum and the posterior superior iliac crests in adults. In children the anterior or posterior iliac crests are used, and in infants the proximal tibia is used (Hockenberry and Wilson, 2007; Pagana and Pagana, 2007). A biopsy is the removal of a core of marrow cells for laboratory analysis. Both aspiration and biopsy diagnose and differentiate leukemia, certain malignancies, anemia, and thrombocytopenia. The marrow is examined in a laboratory to reveal the number, size, shape, and development of red blood cells (RBCs) and megakaryocytes (platelet precursors). Bone marrow cultures help differentiate infectious diseases such as tuberculosis (TB) or histoplasmosis. This procedure takes about 20 minutes.

Potential complications of bone marrow aspiration or biopsy include bleeding, especially if a coagulopathy is present, infection, and less commonly organ puncture. The nurse assists with aspiration procedures and must know normal hematological laboratory values.

A lumbar puncture (LP), called a spinal puncture or spinal tap, involves the introduction of a needle into the subarachnoid space of the spinal column. The purpose of the test is to measure pressure in the subarachnoid space; obtain cerebrospinal fluid (CSF) for visualization and laboratory examination; and to inject anesthetic, diagnostic, or therapeutic agents. CSF is examined in a laboratory to help diagnose spinal cord tumors, CNS infections, hemorrhage, and degenerative brain disease. The procedure takes about 30 minutes.

The major contraindication for LP is evidence of greatly increased intracranial pressure (ICP). The LP causes a sudden release of pressure and possible herniation of the brain structures through the foramen magnum. This herniation compresses the brain stem, which contains the vital cardiac, respiratory, and vasomotor centers, and sudden death results. In elective LP, preprocedure computed tomography results are reviewed for evidence of brain shift to rule out ICP.

Abdominal paracentesis involves aspiration of peritoneal fluid from the abdomen. The aspirate undergoes cytologic studies and is analyzed for bacteria, blood, glucose, and protein to help diagnose the causes of an abdominal effusion. Paracentesis is also a palliative measure to provide temporary relief of abdominal and respiratory

TABLE 44-3 | Summary of Aspiration Procedures

Aspiration Procedure	Preparation/Assessment Specific to Test	Position and Site	Special Considerations
Bone marrow aspiration	Assess complete blood count for abnormalities.	 Sternum Superior illiac crest Proximal tibia "X" marks site of aspiration. (*From Ignatavicius DD, Workman ML: Medical-surgical nursing: critical thinking for collaborative care, ed 5, 2006, Saunders.*)	Patients with arthritis or orthopnea may have difficulty assuming this position. Pressure is applied to the site following procedure.
Lumbar puncture	Assess neurological status, including movement, sensation, and muscle strength of legs to provide a baseline for comparison.	 Lateral decubitus position L1 L3 L5 L2 L4 Subarachnoid space (*From Ignatavicius DD, Workman ML: Medical-surgical nursing: critical thinking for collaborative care, ed 5, 2006, Saunders.*)	*Risk for spinal headache:* Instruct patient to remain flat and logroll according to physician orders. Observe for excessive drainage at the site. Fluid loss at the site can predispose patient to headache and infection.
Paracentesis	Assess bladder for distention, and determine last voiding. Weigh patient, assess abdomen, and measure abdominal girth at largest point. Mark location.	 (*From Pagana KD, Pagana TJ: Mosby's manual of diagnostic and laboratory tests, ed 3, St. Louis, 2006, Mosby.*)	After fluid is removed, pressure on diaphragm is released and breathing becomes much easier. *Risk for trauma:* Have patient empty urinary bladder before procedure.

Continued

TABLE 44-3 | Summary of Aspiration Procedures—cont'd

Aspiration Procedure	Preparation/Assessment Specific to Test	Position and Site	Special Considerations
Thoracentesis	Assess respiratory rate and depth, symmetry of chest on inspiration and expiration, cough and sputum. Assist patient with remaining still during the procedure to prevent trauma to the visceral pleura. Patient will need to hold breath and avoid coughing during the procedure.	Area for needle insertion Ribs Parietal pleura Visceral pleura Lung tissue (parenchyma) Pleural effusion Syringe Diaphragm	Monitor blood pressure for hypotension if large quantity of fluid is removed. *Risk for pneumothorax:* Observe for sudden shortness of breath, tracheal deviation, anxiety, and altered vital signs and decreased oxygen saturation.

discomfort causes by severe ascites. Lavage paracentesis, in which a lavage of solution is instilled then withdrawn, is done to detect the presence of bleeding, as in cases of blunt abdominal trauma, or tumor cells, when cancer is suspected. Although not contraindicated, paracentesis is performed with caution in patients with coagulopathies, with portal hypertension with abdominal collateral circulation, and in those who are pregnant. The procedure takes about 30 minutes.

Thoracentesis is performed to analyze or remove pleural fluid or to instill medications intrapleurally. Cytology studies are performed, and specimens are examined for blood, glucose, amylase, lactate dehydrogenase (LD), and cellular composition. Cytological specimens are examined for malignancy, differentiated between transudative and exudative characteristics, and cultured for pathogens. The following cause transudate in the pleural space: ascites, cirrhosis (hepatic), congestive heart failure, hypertension (pulmonary, systemic), nephritis, and nephrosis. Blocked lymphatic drainage, empyema, esophageal rupture, infarction (pulmonary), infection, neoplasm, pancreatitis, rheumatoid arthritis, systemic lupus erythematosus, thoracic duct disruption, accidental injury, and tuberculosis cause exudates in the pleural space. Therapeutic thoracentesis relieves pain, dyspnea, and signs of pleural pressure. The test takes about 30 minutes.

Delegation Considerations

The skill of assisting with aspirations can be delegated to NAP if the patient is stable (refer to agency policy). Assessment of the patient's condition cannot be delegated. The nurse directs the NAP about:

- How to properly position the patient during the procedure.
- When to take and report vital signs.
- What signs and symptoms experienced by the patient to immediately report to the nurse.

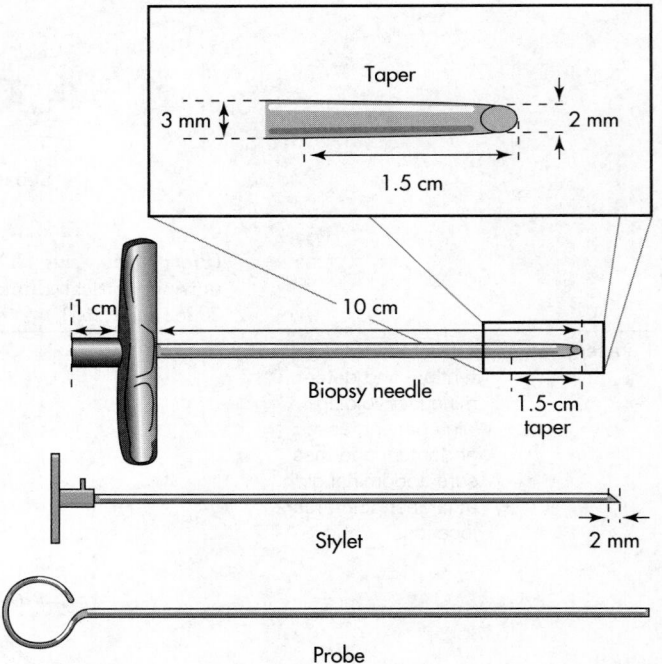

FIG 44-3 Bone marrow biopsy needle showing shape and size. (*From Monahan F and others:* Phipps' medical-surgical nursing: health and illness perspectives, *ed 8, St. Louis, 2007, Mosby.*)

Equipment

- ❑ Protective equipment: masks, goggles, gowns, gloves for all health care personnel
- ❑ Test tubes, sterile specimen containers, laboratory requisitions, and labels

❑ Analgesia if ordered, given 30 minutes before procedure
❑ Antiseptic solution
❑ 4 × 4 inch gauze pads, tape, Band-Aid
❑ Aspiration tray: Most institutions provide trays specific to the aspiration procedure. Standard equipment includes antiseptic solution (e.g., povidone-iodine; chlorhexidine); gauze sponges (4 × 4 inch); sterile towels; local anesthetic solution (e.g., lidocaine 1%); two 3-mL sterile syringes with 16- to 27-gauge needles. Additional equipment for specific aspirations includes:

- Bone marrow aspiration: additional two bone marrow needles with inner stylet (Fig. 44-3)
- Lumbar puncture: manometer to measure spinal pressure and at least four test tubes
- Paracentesis: IV fluids as ordered, vacuum bottles, stopcock with extension tubing, sterile collection containers, measuring tape
- Thoracentesis: vacuum bottles, stopcock with extension tubing
- Sphygmomanometer, pulse oximeter

STEP	RATIONALE

ASSESSMENT

1 Verify patient's identity by using at least two forms of identifiers, neither of which is the patient's room number. Verify the type of procedure scheduled, purpose, and the procedure site with the patient and medical record.

Ensures accurate patient identification and improves patient safety. Use of patient's room number is not an acceptable identifier (TJC, 2008a).

2 Verify that informed consent was obtained.
3 Review medical record for contraindications.
  a *Lumbar puncture:* Increased intracranial pressure (IICP), spinal deformities, and clotting disorders.

Factors can cause hemorrhage, and ICP can cause brain stem herniation.

  b *Paracentesis:* Caution is needed with patients with clotting disorders, intestinal obstructions, and pregnancy.

Paracentesis in pregnant woman can injure fetus.

4 Determine patient's ability to assume position required for procedure and ability to remain still. Discuss with the physician or health care provider the need for premedication for very anxious patients.

Movement during the procedure can cause complications, such as bleeding and injury to nerves or tissue. The required position depends on site used for aspiration.

5 Before procedure: Obtain vital signs, oxygen saturation value, and weight. For paracentesis obtain an abdominal girth measurement. (Use ink pen to mark location of position of abdominal girth measurement). For lumbar puncture obtain baseline assessment of lower extremity movement, sensation, and muscle strength.

Provides baseline for comparison with postprocedure vital signs. Patients will have decreased abdominal girth and lose weight after paracentesis.

6 Instruct patient to empty bladder.

Reduces risk for bladder trauma during paracentesis. Promotes patient comfort.

7 Assess patient's coagulation status: use of anticoagulants, platelet count, and prothrombin time.

Invasive procedures are contraindicated in patients with coagulation disorders due to risk for bleeding (Pagana and Pagana, 2007).

8 Determine whether patient is allergic to antiseptic, latex, or anesthetic solutions.

Decreases chance of allergic reactions.

9 Assess patient's level of understanding of procedure, including any concerns.

Determines extent of instruction and level of support required.

10 Obtain baseline pain level.

Determines need for preprocedure analgesia. Pain control helps patients maintain proper position and tolerate aspiration procedure.

NURSING DIAGNOSES

- Acute pain
- Anxiety
- Deficient knowledge regarding purpose and steps of procedure
- Fear
- Impaired gas exchange
- Impaired mobility
- Ineffective breathing pattern
- Risk for infection
- Risk for injury

Individualize related factors based on patient's condition or needs.

PLANNING

1 Expected outcomes following completion of procedure:
  - Patient describes the purpose of the procedure.

Demonstrates patient understanding and improves the likelihood of cooperation.

  - Patients assume and maintains the required position and remains still throughout the procedure.

Correct position facilitates safe and timely completion of the procedure.

STEP	RATIONALE

• There is no bleeding at needle insertion site.

• Amount of aspirate is sufficient to perform laboratory testing.

• Patient's level of comfort is equivalent to a score of 4 or less on a pain scale of 0 to 10.

• Respiratory rate, heart rate, and blood pressure remain within normal limits during and after aspiration procedure.

2 Explain steps of skin preparation, anesthetic injection, needle insertion, position required.

3 Before thoracentesis verify recent chest x-ray examination.

Precautions during procedure prevent bleeding.

Use of a standardized pain scale provides reliable detection of increasing pain and pain relief.

Removal of abdominal (ascites) or pleural fluid increases lung expansion and improves gas exchange.

Anticipation of expected sensations and procedural activities reduces anxiety.

Provides a preprocedure baseline to determine the location of pleural fluid.

IMPLEMENTATION

1 Perform hand hygiene.

2 Premedicate for pain, if ordered.

3 Set up sterile tray, or open supplies to make accessible for physician or health care provider.

4 Take "time out" to verify patient's name, type of procedure scheduled, and procedure site with patient.

5 Assist patient in maintaining correct position. Reassure patient while explaining procedure.

  a *Bone marrow:*

    • *Adults:* For sternal biopsy place patient in supine position. For iliac crest biopsy place patient in prone or lateral recumbent position.

    • *Children:* For iliac crest biopsy place patient in prone or lateral recumbent position.

  b *Lumbar puncture:* Position patient in lateral recumbent (fetal) position with head and neck flexed (see Table 44-3).

  c *Paracentesis:* Position in bed in semi-Fowler's position or sitting upright on side of bed or in chair with feet supported (see Table 44-3).

  d *Thoracentesis:* Place patient in the orthopneic position (upright position with arms and shoulders raised and supported on a padded over-bed table) (see Table 44-3). If patient is unable to tolerate this position, assist patient to side-lying position with the affected lung positioned upward.

Reduces transmission of microorganisms.

Reduces the discomfort of the procedure.

Maintains integrity of sterile field and promotes prompt completion of procedure.

"Time out" verification just before starting the procedure includes the physician and all personnel and is a safety precaution to prevent wrong patient, wrong site, and wrong procedure errors (TJC, 2008).

Decreases chance of complications occurring during procedure. Explanations increase patient comfort and relaxation.

Provides spinal column full curvature. Spinal column is flexed as much as possible to allow maximal space between vertebrae.

Position uses gravity to cause fluid to accumulate in the lower abdominal cavity, where it is drained more easily.

Expands intercostal space for needle insertions.

Critical Decision Point   *Emphasize the importance of remaining immobile during procedure to prevent trauma, especially with the lumbar puncture, because sudden movement is a risk for spinal cord nerve root damage; sudden movement during paracentesis or thoracentesis risks damage of the abdominal or pulmonary structures. Also, instruct patient not to cough, sneeze, or breathe deeply during the procedures, because these actions increase the risk for needle displacement and damage of other structures.*

6 Explain to patient that pain can occur when lidocaine is injected into the tissues. Pressure may also occur when the tissue or fluid is aspirated.

7 Physician applies sterile gloves, mask, and goggles; cleanses skin with antiseptic solution; and drapes site with sterile drape.

8 Physician injects local anesthetic. Allow time for anesthesia to occur.

9 Physician inserts needle or trocar into the spinal space or body cavity involved (see Table 44-3). To aspirate tissue or body fluids for specimen analysis, a syringe is attached to the trocar or needle and aspirate is placed into a specimen container.

Aspiration is painful, but lasts for only a few moments. Preprocedure analgesia decreases discomfort. If the patient is having a bone marrow aspirate, a deep pressure feeling is frequently experienced as the bone marrow is withdrawn (Pagana and Pagana, 2007).

Removes surface bacteria from skin at area of puncture site. Creates a sterile field.

Provides optimal effect of local anesthesia.

STEP	RATIONALE

10 Assess patient's condition during procedure, including respiratory status, vital signs if indicated, and complaints of pain.

Identifies any changes that indicate complication.

Critical Decision Point   *For patients who have a paracentesis or thoracentesis, increased or worsening abdominal or thoracic pain is significant. Severe abdominal pain indicates a possible bowel perforation following a paracentesis. Following a thoracentesis abdominal pain results from diaphragmatic, liver, or spleen perforation. Inspiratory chest pain results from perforation of the lung.*

11 Note characteristics of aspirate:
   a *Bone marrow aspirate:* Marrow may appear red or yellow.
   b *Lumbar puncture:* Record opening pressure; observe fluid for color, cloudiness, or blood.
   c *Paracentesis:* Fluid may appear yellow, cloudy, bile-stained green, or blood tinged. Gastric lavage fluid may appear bright red.

   d *Thoracentesis:* Pleural fluid may appear clear yellow, pus-like, or cloudy.

Normal marrow.
Normal CSF is clear and colorless. Cloudiness is the result of protein, which indicates an infection.
Blood-tinged fluid is caused by a traumatic tap. In a trauma patient a paracentesis tap is used to lavage the peritoneum to identify active bleeding.
Transudate and exudates are typically yellow, straw color. Blood-stained fluid indicates a malignancy, pulmonary infarction, or severe inflammation. Puslike fluid is indicative of an infection (empyema); milky fluid indicates a chylothorax, a leak from the thoracic duct resulting in lymphatic drainage in the pleural cavity (Allibone, 2006).

12 Properly label specimens, and transport to laboratory.

Nurse is responsible for labeling tubes correctly. Specimens are labeled in order of collection.

13 Physician removes needle/trocar and applies pressure over insertion site until drainage ceases. If necessary, assist with direct pressure and gauze dressing.

Assists in homeostasis and secures insertion site.

EVALUATION

1 Monitor level of consciousness, vital signs, and oxygen saturation. Check agency policy; sometimes you will measure as often as every 15 minutes for 2 hours.

Verifies patient's physiological status in response to procedure or any potential complications.

2 Inspect dressing over puncture site for bleeding, swelling, tenderness, and erythema. Inspect area under patient for bleeding. Avoid disrupting a healing clot at the site if a pressure dressing is present.

Determines further blood loss from puncture site. Infection is a potential complication, especially if the patient is leukopenic (Pagana and Pagana, 2007).

3 Assess pain score to determine if patient's level of comfort is equivalent to a score of 4 or less on a pain scale of 0 to 10.

Use of a standardized pain scale provides reliable detection of increasing pain so that postprocedure analgesia is given.

4 Following a paracentesis, measure abdominal girth.

Determines the amount of change in size following procedure.

Unexpected Outcomes	Related Interventions
1 Oversedation occurs	• See Skill 44-1.
2 Site complications occur:	• Notify physician or health care provider, and obtain further orders.
a *Bone marrow:* Tenderness or erythema at site	• Administer analgesic as ordered. • Continue to monitor site.
b *Lumbar puncture:*	
(1) Postprocedural headache (PPH) is evidenced by headache, blurred vision, and tinnitus.	• Monitor fluid loss. • Notify physician, who may inject a blood patch into the epidural space. • Medicate for pain as ordered.
(2) Excess loss of CSF is indicated by decreased level of conciousness, dilated pupils, and increased intracranial pressure.	• Maintain airway. • Notify physician. • Transfer to intensive care unit (ICU).
c *Paracentesis:* Leakage of fluid from site and acute abdominal pain occur.	• Reinforce dressing, may also be instructed to place a sterile collection bag over site. • Monitor vital signs and oxygen saturation. • Assess abdomen for bowel sounds.
d *Thoracentesis:* Pneumothorax is evidenced by sudden dyspnea, tachypnea, and asymmetrical chest excursion.	• Administer oxygen. • Monitor vital signs and oxygen saturation. • Notify physician. • Anticipate chest x-ray examination and possible chest tube insertion.

Recording and Reporting

- Record in patient's chart name of procedure; preprocedure preparation; location of puncture site; amount, consistency, and color of fluid drained or specimen obtained; duration of procedure; patient's tolerance of the procedure (e.g., vital signs, oxygen saturation); and comfort level; laboratory tests ordered; specimen sent; type of dressing; postprocedure activities (e.g., chest x-ray examination); and other procedure-specific assessments (e.g., extremity assessment, abdominal girth, level of conciousness).
- Immediately report to physician or health care provider any change in vital signs, oxygen saturation, unexpected pain/discomfort, and any excessive drainage from dressing over puncture site.

Teaching Considerations

- Instruct patient that some persons experience tenderness at the puncture site for several days after the study and that mild analgesia often helps to relieve some of the discomfort.

Pediatric Considerations

- Conscious or unconscious sedation is commonly used. If using unconscious sedation, an anesthesiologist or nurse anesthetist will be needed for the procedure.

- Prepare preschool children before the procedure; make a game out of having child recall the next procedural step, which can serve as distraction mechanism (Hockenberry and Wilson, 2007).

Gerontological Considerations

- Older adults with arthritis need help to sustain the required position.
- Older adults have reduced elastic lung recoil, weaker cough efficiency, and decreased chest expansion. Restlessness may indicate hypoxia following thoracentesis.
- Be aware that older adults may have specific fears and anxiety related to postprocedure falling and fatigue.

Home Care Considerations

- Teach patients and caregivers about specific postprocedure complications and when to report them to the physician or health care provider.
- If patient is transferred to long-term care facility, ensure thorough communication between facilities regarding results of procedure and patient condition.

SKILL 44-4 Assisting With Bronchoscopy

Bronchoscopy is the examination of the tracheobronchial tree through a lighted tube containing mirrors. A flexible fiberoptic bronchoscope has lumens that allow both visualization and simultaneous administration of oxygen (Fig. 44-4). The fiberoptic bronchoscope is used for obtaining sputum, foreign bodies, and biopsy specimens. Laser ablation of endotracheal lesions is also performed through the bronchoscope.

Bronchoscopy may be an emergency or elective procedure and is performed for diagnostic and therapeutic reasons. The main purposes of this procedure are to aspirate excessive sputum or mucous plugs that airway suctioning cannot remove; to visualize the tracheobronchial tree for assessment of abnormalities of the mucosa, abscesses, aspiration pneumonia, strictures, and tumors; to obtain deep tissue biopsy and sputum specimens; and to remove foreign bodies. This procedure is contraindicated in patients who cannot tolerate interruption of high-flow oxygen unless intubated. Potential complications of bronchoscopy include fever, infection, hypoxemia, bronchospasm and laryngospasm, pneumothorax, aspiration, dysrhythmias and hypotension, hemorrhage (after biopsy), and cardiac arrest. When needed, perform airway suctioning before assisting with the procedure.

The procedure is performed at the bedside or in a specially equipped endoscopy room. Usually a pulmonary specialist or surgeon performs this procedure in about 30 to 45 minutes.

Delegation Considerations

The skill of assisting with bronchoscopy cannot be delegated to NAP because this skill requires repeated performance of nursing assessments for patient tolerance of the procedure and for life-threatening complications requiring emergency intervention. The NAP takes baseline and postprocedure vital signs and assists with patient positioning, as long as a nurse is continuously present during the procedure. In addition, this procedure involves the use of IV moderate sedation, which requires the continuous presence of a nurse. The nurse directs the NAP about:

- Immediately reporting to the nurse if the patient has possible respiratory distress or is coughing up blood.
- How to assist with patient positioning.

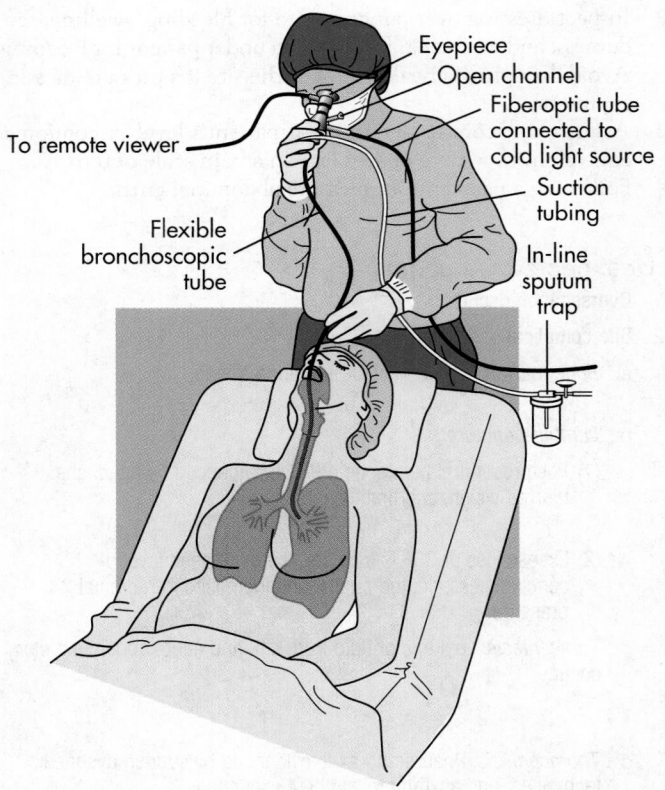

FIG 44-4 Flexible fiberoptic bronchoscopy.

Equipment

❑ Bronchoscopy tray, if available from central supply, which may include flexible fiberoptic bronchoscope (see Fig. 44-4); 4 × 4 inch gauze sponges; local anesthetic spray (lidocaine); sterile tracheal suction catheters; diazepam (Valium), midazolam (Versed), or other sedative for IV sedation

❑ Oxygen, resuscitative equipment, pulse oximeter, cardiac monitor

❑ Sterile gloves

❑ Sterile water-soluble lubricating jelly (NOTE: Petroleum-based lubricants are not used because of the hazard of aspiration and subsequent pneumonia.)

❑ Protective equipment: mask, gown, gloves, and goggles for all physicians or health care providers

❑ Emesis basin

❑ Tracheal suction equipment

❑ Stethoscope, sphygmomanometer

STEP	RATIONALE
ASSESSMENT	
1 Verify patient's identity by using at least two forms of identifiers, neither of which is the patient's room number. Verify the type of procedure scheduled and the procedure site with the patient.	Ensures accurate patient identification and improves patient safety. Use of patient's room number is not an acceptable identifier (TJC, 2008a).
2 Verify that informed consent was obtained.	Federal regulations, many state laws, and accreditation agencies, such as The Joint Commission, require informed consent for procedure.
3 Assess patient's history for inability to tolerate interruption of high-flow oxygen, unless intubated.	Determines need for oxygen administration during procedure.
4 Obtain vital signs and oxygen saturation value.	Baseline data provide for comparison with findings during and after procedure.
5 Assess respiratory status: type of cough, sputum produced, and lung sounds.	Provides for comparison with respiratory status during and after procedure.
6 Determine purpose of procedure: for sputum aspiration, assessment, tissue biopsy, or for removal of foreign body.	Anticipates needs of patient and physician.
7 Determine whether patient is allergic to local anesthetic used for spraying throat (usually lidocaine).	Allergy causes laryngeal edema or laryngospasm.
8 Assess need for preprocedure medication (usually atropine and opioid or sedative).	Atropine decreases secretions and inhibits vagally stimulated bradycardia; opioids or sedatives relieve anxiety and decrease discomfort.
9 Assess time patient last ingested food. Patient must be NPO for at least 8 hours before a bronchoscopy.	Reduces risk for aspiration.
10 Assess patient's level of understanding of procedure, including any concerns.	Determines extent of instruction and level of support required.

NURSING DIAGNOSES

- Anxiety
- Deficient knowledge regarding purpose and steps of procedure
- Fear

- Impaired gas exchange
- Ineffective airway clearance
- Ineffective breathing pattern

- Risk for aspiration
- Risk for infection
- Risk for injury

Individualize related factors based on patient's condition or needs.

STEP	RATIONALE
PLANNING	
1 Expected outcomes following completion of procedure:	
• Patient recovers from sedation without respiratory complications or change in level of consciousness.	Sedation adequate and patient tolerates procedure.
• Patient's level of comfort is equivalent to a score of 4 or less on a pain scale of 0 to 10.	Minimal trauma caused by bronchoscope. Use of a standardized pain scale provides reliable detection of increasing pain so that postprocedure analgesia is given.
• Physician is able to observe, suction, and obtain specimens from tracheobronchial tree.	Indicates that purpose of procedure was achieved.
• Patient explains procedure and assumes the appropriate position.	Demonstrates patient's understanding.
2 Explain procedure to patient.	Reduces anxiety and increases cooperation.
3 Assist patient in maintaining position desired by physician: semi-Fowler's, side-lying, or supine.	Provides maximal visualization of lower airway and adequate lung expansion.
4 Remove and safely store patient's dentures.	Minimizes chance of airway obstruction.

STEP	RATIONALE

IMPLEMENTATION

1. Perform hand hygiene, and apply protective equipment.

Reduces transmission of microorganisms.

2. Assess current IV access, or establish new IV access with large-bore cannula (see Chapter 28).

Provides immediate access for IV fluids or medications if an emergency occurs.

3. Assist patient in maintaining position, usually semi-Fowler's position.

Best position to provide visualization of the lower airway and maintain optimal lung expansion.

4. Take "time out" to verify patient's name, type of procedure scheduled, and procedure site with patient.

"Time out" verification just before starting the procedure includes the physician and all personnel and is a safety precaution to prevent wrong patient, wrong site, and wrong procedure errors (TJC, 2008a).

5. Position tip of suction catheter for easy access to patient's mouth.

Drains secretions to reduce risk for aspiration.

6. Physician sprays nasopharynx and oropharynx with topical anesthetic. Lidocaine is commonly used 10 to 15 minutes before procedure. When a patient is intubated or has a tracheostomy, anesthetic spray is usually not needed.

Provides swift anesthesia of oropharynx.

7. Instruct patient not to swallow local anesthetic; provide emesis basin for expectoration of local anesthetic.

Reduces unintended anesthesia of esophagus.

8. Attach bronchoscope to machine for light source.

Another physician or surgery personnel attaches machine cable to bronchoscope.

9. Physician applies goggles, mask, and sterile gloves; then introduces bronchoscope into mouth to pharynx; and passes through glottis and into trachea and bronchi (see Fig. 44-4). More anesthetic spray may be used at glottis to prevent cough reflex. For intubated patients, the flexible bronchoscope is introduced through the endotracheal tube.

Bronchoscope must be passed through upper airway structures to promote visualization of lower airways. Trachea and bronchi are observed for lesions and obstructions. Adaptor accompanies bronchoscope and is used for bag-valve-mask or ventilator use.

10. Mucus is suctioned and bronchial washing performed with cytological specimens taken with a wire brush or curette. Biopsy specimens may also be obtained.

Cytologic specimens are obtained to diagnose carcinoma.

11. Assist patient through procedure with explanations.

Although premedicated and drowsy, remind patient not to change position and to cooperate. Reinforce that patient will be able to breathe during procedure.

12. Assess patient's respiratory status during procedure: observe degree of restlessness and respiratory rate; observe capillary refill, color of nail beds, and pulse oximetry.

Bronchoscope can cause feelings of suffocation and vasovagal response, as well as laryngospasm. In addition, because airway is partially occluded, patient can develop hypoxia during the procedure.

13. Note the characteristics of suctioned material. Expect a small amount of blood mixed with the aspirate because of tissue trauma.

Information used to record and report and to make further patient observations.

14. Using gloved hand, wipe patient's mouth and nose to remove lubricant after bronchoscope is removed.

Promotes hygiene and comfort.

15. Instruct patient not to eat or drink until the tracheobronchial anesthesia has worn off and gag reflex has returned, usually 2 hours. Use tongue depressor to touch pharynx to test for presence of gag reflex.

Prevents aspiration.

16. Remove protective equipment, and perform hand hygiene.

Reduces transmission of microorganisms.

EVALUATION

1. Monitor vital signs and oxygen saturation.

Verifies physiological response.

2. Observe character and amount of sputum. Physician may order serial sputum collection for 24 hours for cytological examination.

Assesses for complication of bronchial perforation, indicated by severe hemoptysis. Slight blood-tinged sputum is normal after this procedure.

3. Observe respiratory status closely, palpate for facial or neck crepitus.

Detects an early sign of bronchial perforation (Chernecky and Berger, 2008).

4. Instruct patient not to try to swallow sputum until gag reflex returns. Provide emesis basis for expectoration of sputum. Assess for return of gag reflex. Gag reflex usually returns in approximately 2 hours.

Helps prevent aspiration pneumonia, which is a risk until gag reflex returns.

5. Ask patient to describe postprocedure normal and abnormal symptoms.

Evaluates patient's understanding.

Unexpected Outcomes	Related Interventions
1 Vasovagal response caused by stimulation of the baroreceptors during bronchoscope insertion, causing bradycardia. Symptoms include: • Feeling faint, dizzy, and light-headed • Diaphoresis with a slow, steady pulse • Unconsciousness for a few seconds	• Lower head of table. • Support airway.

2 Laryngospasm and bronchospasm as evidenced by:
• Sudden, severe shortness of breath
	• Call physician immediately.
	    • Prepare emergency resuscitation equipment.
	    • Anticipate possible cricothyrotomy.

3 Hypoxemia as evidenced by: • Gradual shortness of breath • Decreasing level of consciousness	• Maintain airway and breathing. • Notify physician immediately. • Monitor oxygen saturation.
4 Hemorrhage: • Acute blood loss • Hypotension and tachycardia • Decreasing level of consciousness	• Notify physician immediately. • Follow specific postprocedural orders related to findings.
5 Oversedation (see Skill 44-1)	

Recording and Reporting

• Record name of procedure (include biopsy if performed), duration of procedure, patient's tolerance of procedure, and complications, and collection and disposition of specimen. Document return of gag reflex.

• Report excessive bleeding or respiratory difficulty after procedure or changes in vital signs beyond patient's normal limits to physician immediately. Report results of procedure to appropriate health care personnel.

Teaching Considerations

• Before the procedure, instruct patient to perform good mouth care to decrease risk for introducing bacteria into lungs during procedure.

• Instruct patient to arrange for transportation home after an ambulatory procedure because (at most agencies) patient will not be permitted to drive for 24 hours after receiving sedation.

• Instruct patient in how to perform controlled coughing techniques for obtaining serial sputum samples, if ordered (see Chapter 43).

Pediatric Considerations

• In children the procedure is most frequently performed under general anesthesia to remove foreign bodies from larynx or trachea. Follow-up care after the foreign body is removed includes chest physiotherapy as needed, monitoring for respiratory distress, and education of parents.

• Children are at higher risk for hypoxemia than adults because their bronchus is smaller and the bronchoscope decreases the available breathing space (Pagana and Pagana, 2007).

Gerontological Considerations

• Physical exposure and room temperature contribute to hypothermia in frail older adults who are unable to communicate that they are cold. Use heated blankets or forced-air heat to maintain core temperature at comfortable, safe levels (Negishi and others, 2003).

• Postprocedure restlessness often indicates hypoxemia or pain. Thoroughly assess pulmonary capacity before administering opioids, which could depress the respiratory centers.

Home Care Considerations

• Instruct ambulatory care patients to notify the physician if the following symptoms develop: fever, chest pain or discomfort, dyspnea, wheezing, or hemoptysis.

• Throat discomfort is managed with throat lozenges or warm saline gargles.

SKILL 44-5 Assisting With Gastrointestinal Endoscopy

Endoscopy allows direct visualization of an internal organ or structure by means of a long, flexible fiberoptic scope with a light source attached (Fig. 44-5). For visualization of the upper gastrointestinal (GI) tract, esophagoscopy, gastroscopy, gastroduodenojejunoscopy (GJD) or duodenoscopy is performed; or more frequently, esophagogastroduodenoscopy (EGD), which permits visualization of esophagus, stomach, and duodenum in one examination. Besides direct observation, endoscopy enables biopsy of suspicious tissue, polyp removal, and performance of many other procedures, such as direct visual guidance for fine-needle aspiration biopsies and dilation and stenting of strictures. For visualization of the hepatobiliary tree and pancreatic ducts, an endoscopic retrograde cholangiopancreatography (ERCP) is performed. For visual examination of the lower GI tract, proctoscopy, sigmoidoscopy, or colonoscopy is performed. Typically, these patients receive IV moderate sedation.

Risks of endoscopic procedures include intestinal perforation, hemorrhage, peritonitis, aspiration, respiratory depression, and myocardial infarction secondary to vasovagal response. Both upper and lower GI endoscopic examinations are performed in a specially equipped endoscopic unit.

Delegation Considerations

The skill of assisting with endoscopy cannot be delegated to NAP because this skill requires repeated performance of nursing assessments for patient tolerance of the procedure and for life-threatening complications requiring emergency intervention. This procedure often involves the use of IV moderate sedation, which requires the continuous presence of a nurse. The nurse directs the NAP about:

- How to assist with patient positioning.

Equipment

- ❏ Protective equipment: mask, gown, gloves, goggles for all health care personnel
- ❏ Endoscopy tray
- ❏ Fiberoptic endoscope and camera (see Fig. 44-5)
- ❏ Solutions for biopsy specimens
- ❏ Local anesthetic spray
- ❏ Tracheal suction equipment (see Chapter 25)
- ❏ Blood pressure equipment

- ❏ Sterile water-soluble jelly
- ❏ Sterile gloves for health care provider or physician
- ❏ Emesis basin
- ❏ IV fluid and equipment for IV start (*optional*)
- ❏ Diazepam (Valium), midazolam (Versed), or other sedative for IV sedation (*optional*)
- ❏ Carbon dioxide source (for lower GI procedures)
- ❏ Oxygen, resuscitative equipment, pulse oximeter, sphygmomanometer

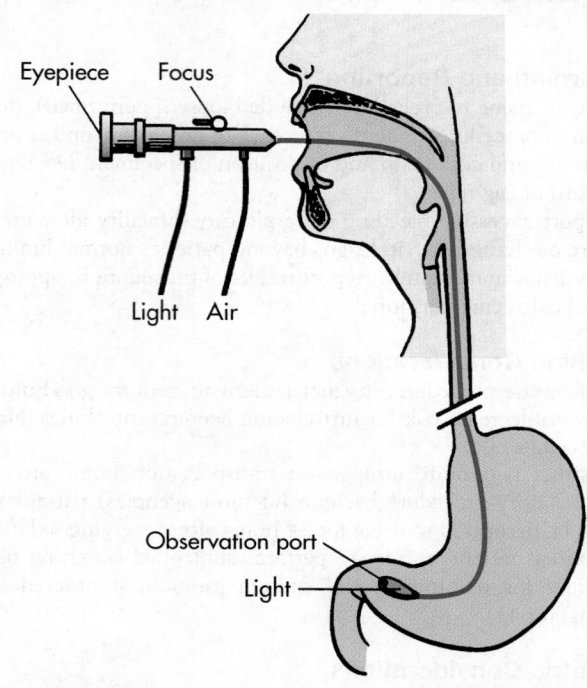

FIG 44-5 Stomach may be visualized by means of a fiberscope.

STEP	RATIONALE

ASSESSMENT

1 Verify patient's identity by using at least two forms of identifiers, neither of which is the patient's room number. Verify the type of procedure scheduled and the procedure site with the patient.

Ensures accurate patient identification and improves patient safety. Use of patient's room number is not an acceptable identifier (TJC, 2008a).

2 Verify that informed consent was obtained.

Federal regulations, many state laws, and accreditation agencies, such as The Joint Commission, require informed consent for procedure.

3 Determine if GI bleeding is present. Observe character of emesis, stool, and nasogastric (NG) tube drainage for frank blood or material that looks like coffee grounds.

Test is contraindicated in patients with severe upper GI bleeding because viewing lens becomes covered with blood clots, preventing visualization (Pagana and Pagana, 2007).

Critical Decision Point *If patient is actively bleeding, physician may order lavage of the stomach and aspiration to clear clots before procedure is attempted.*

STEP	RATIONALE
4 Determine purpose of procedure: biopsy, examination, or co-agulation of bleeding sites.	Anticipates appropriate equipment needs.
5 Verify that patient has been NPO for at least 8 hours for endos-copy of upper GI tract.	Introduction of endoscope increases risk for vomiting resulting from stimulation of the gag reflex. Empty stomach reduces risk for aspiration of stomach contents.
6 For lower GI studies (proctoscopy, sigmoidoscopy, or colonos-copy), verify that the patient followed a clear liquid diet for 2 days and has completed any ordered bowel-cleansing regimen.	An empty intestinal tract promotes endoscopic insertion and good visualization of the interior walls.
7 Assess patient's level of understanding of procedure, including any concerns.	Determines extent of instruction and level of support required.

NURSING DIAGNOSES

- Acute pain
- Anxiety
- Deficient knowledge regarding purpose and steps of procedure

- Fear
- Impaired gas exchange
- Ineffective breathing pattern
- Risk for aspiration

- Risk for infection
- Risk for injury

Individualize related factors based on patient's condition or needs.

PLANNING

1 Expected outcomes following completion of procedure:	
• Patient does not aspirate and has no postprocedure bleeding.	Indicates absence of complications and tolerance of procedure.
• Patient's level of comfort is equivalent to a score of 4 or less on a pain scale of 0 to 10.	Use of a standardized pain scale provides reliable detection of in-creasing pain so that postprocedure analgesia is given.
• Patient is without respiratory complications or change in level of consciousness.	Recovers from sedation.
• Patient describes purposes and steps of procedure.	Documents patient understanding.
2 Prepare patient:	
a Explain steps of procedure, including sensations to expect.	Relieves anxiety and answers patient's questions.
b Administer pain medication or preprocedure medication.	Promotes relaxation and reduces anxiety.

IMPLEMENTATION

1 Perform hand hygiene, and apply protective equipment.	Reduces transmission of microorganisms.
2 Remove patient's dentures or other dental appliances.	Prevents dislodgment of dental structures during intubation phase.
3 Take "time out" to verify patient's name, type of procedure scheduled, and procedure site with patient.	"Time out" verification just before starting the procedure includes the physician and all personnel and is a safety precaution to prevent wrong patient, wrong site, and wrong procedure errors (TJC, 2008a).
4 Ensure IV line is patent, and administer IV sedation as or-dered (see Skill 44-1).	Provides route for emergency medications.
5 Assist patient through procedure:	
a Anticipate needs, and promote comfort.	Patient is unable to speak after tube is passed into throat.
b Tell patient what is happening as each portion of the procedure is carried out.	Reassures patient about procedure and how long it will last.
c Place tissue specimens in proper laboratory containers.	Ensures proper labeling and preparation of specimens for micro-scopic examination.
d Assist patient to comfortable position.	Promotes rest and relaxation.
6 Physician performs hand hygiene and applies protective equipment.	Reduces transmission of microorganisms.
7 Assist physician to spray nasopharynx and oropharynx with local anesthetic.	Topical anesthetic decreases the gag reflex caused by passage of the endoscope, thus improving safety and comfort.
8 For upper GI procedures, assist patient in maintaining left lateral Sims' position. For lower GI procedures, assist patient in maintaining left lateral decubitus position. Drape patient for privacy and comfort.	Position allows easy passage of upper or lower endoscope.
9 Administer atropine, if ordered (upper GI studies).	Atropine reduces the quantity of secretions, therefore reducing risk for aspiration for upper GI endoscopic procedures.

STEP	RATIONALE
10 Position tip of suction cannula for easy access in the patient's mouth (upper GI studies).	Drains oral secretions to reduce risk for aspiration.
11 *Upper GI studies:* Physician slowly passes endoscope into mouth, esophagus, stomach, or duodenum, and advances to desired depth while visualizing the walls. *Lower GI studies:* A lubricant-coated flexible fiberoptic endoscope is inserted through the anus and slowly advanced through the rectum and colon, while visualizing the walls.	Provides visualization of structures.
12 Physician insufflates air through endoscope into upper GI tract. For colonoscopy, carbon dioxide is used.	Distends GI structures for better visualization. Carbon dioxide insufflation produces less postprocedure abdominal cramping than air insufflation (Chernecky and Berger, 2008).
13 Physician examines, photographs, or performs biopsy of structures and then slowly removes the endoscope.	
14 Place tissue specimens in laboratory containers. Provide slides and containers for specimens, and seal as needed.	Provides specimen preservation for accurate histopathological examination.
15 Assist patient to comfortable position.	Promotes relaxation.
16 Suction if there are excessive oral secretions or vomitus.	Prevents aspiration of oral secretions or gastric contents.
17 Inform patient not to eat or drink until gag reflex returns.	Reduces risk for aspiration.

EVALUATION

1 Monitor vital signs and oxygen saturation according to agency policy, which can be every 15 minutes for 2 hours.	Change in vital signs may indicate new bleeding in GI tract or oversedation.
2 Assess for level of sedation and level of consciousness (see Skill 44-1).	Determines patient's response to IV sedation.
3 Ask patient to describe level of comfort using a 0 to 10 pain scale. Observe for pain.	Monitors for sudden abdominal pain, which can indicate rupture of abdominal organs.
4 Evaluate emesis or aspirate for frank or occult blood (see Chapter 43).	Monitors for gastrointestinal bleeding.
5 Assess for return of gag reflex, usually in 2 to 4 hours. Provide oral hygiene when gag reflex returns.	Determines when effects of anesthetic have disappeared. Gag reflex prevents aspiration.
6 Ask patient to state postprocedure dietary and activity limitations.	Evaluates patient understanding.

Unexpected Outcomes	Related Interventions
1 Vasovagal response caused by stimulation of the baroreceptors during endoscope insertion as evidenced by: • Feeling faint, dizzy, and light-headed • Diaphoresis with a slow, steady pulse • A few seconds of unconsciousness	• Lower head of table. • Support airway.
2 Damage to the intestinal wall as evidenced by: • Abdominal pain, fever, or bleeding	• Continue to monitor vital signs. • Notify physician of findings.
3 Aspiration pneumonia as evidenced by: • Dyspnea, tachypnea • Decreasing trend in oxygen saturation • Fever	• Support airway. • Follow specific postprocedural orders related to findings. • Monitor oxygen saturation. • Notify physician.
4 Oversedation occurs: • Decreasing level of consciousness	• See Skill 44-1.

Recording and Reporting

- Record the procedure, duration, patient's tolerance, complications and interventions, and collection and disposition of specimen.
- Report onset of bleeding, abdominal pain, dyspnea, and vital sign changes to physician. Report the duration of procedure, patient's tolerance, and changes in vital signs or condition.

Teaching Considerations

- Upper GI endoscopy:
  - Explain method for endoscope insertion. Prepare the patient for a slight feeling of not being able to breathe. Assure patient that this feeling is common, but that air is delivered through the endoscope and suffocation will not occur.
  - Teach the patient simple hand signals for pain or discomfort, because he or she will not be able to speak after the endoscope is positioned in the esophagus.
- Lower GI procedures (colonoscopy, sigmoidoscopy, proctoscopy):
  - Explain that it is normal to experience increased flatus and abdominal cramping.
  - Small amounts of blood in the stool are common if a biopsy was taken.

Pediatric Considerations

- Child requires deep sedation or general anesthesia (American Academy of Pediatrics, 2006).
- Introduction of the endoscope in infants and small children who have a narrow and collapsible airway may result in respiratory distress.

Gerontological Considerations

- Older adult patients frequently have reduced drug clearance from decreased glomerular filtration rate (GFR) and nephron activity or decreased hepatic function. Therefore it is important to monitor the effects of medications given to the older adult patient (Meiner and Lueckenotte, 2006).
- Because of age-related changes in the older adult, the gastric mucosa is thinner, which increases the incidence of irritation and ulceration (Meiner and Lueckenotte, 2006).
- Physical exposure and room temperature contribute to hypothermia in frail older adults who are unable to communicate that they are cold. Use heated blankets or forced-air heat to maintain core temperature at comfortable, safe levels (Negishi and others, 2003).
- Some older adults experience dehydration, electrolyte imbalance, and exhaustion from test preparation. If the procedure is done on an ambulatory care basis, it is helpful to have someone stay with the patient.

Home Care Considerations

- Explain that patient might have hoarseness or a sore throat after procedure. Patient can have ice chips or anesthetic lozenges after gag reflex returns.
- Instruct patient or family to notify physician if patient has a fever, chest pain or discomfort, dysphasia, dyspnea, wheezing, or hemoptysis.

SKILL 44-6   Obtaining an Electrocardiogram

An electrocardiogram (ECG) is a graphic representation of the heart's electrical activities, or conduction system. The electrical impulse for each heartbeat originates within the sinoatrial (SA) node, the "pacemaker" of the heart. The SA node is in the right atrium. The rate of impulses initiated at the SA node for an adult at rest is about 60 to 100 beats per minute. The electrical impulses are then transmitted through the atria to the atrioventricular (AV) node. The AV node assists with atrial emptying by delaying the impulse before transmitting it through the bundle of His and the ventricular Purkinje network.

The electrical activity of the conduction system is recorded on an ECG. An ECG is completed to determine baseline cardiac function (e.g., preoperative, prediagnostic testing), to help evaluate response to cardiac medications, to help monitor recovery after an MI, or when a patient experiences chest discomfort. An ECG monitors the regularity and path of the electrical impulse through the conduction system; however, it does not reflect muscular work of the heart.

The normal sequence on the ECG is called normal sinus rhythm (NSR), which contains PQRST waves (Fig. 44-6). The PR interval represents atrial depolarization during which the atria empty their blood supply into the ventricles. The QRS interval represents ventricular depolarization, during which ventricular contraction occurs. The remainder of the waveform through the end of the T wave signifies ventricular repolarization.

Disturbances in conduction result when impulses cannot travel through the normal pathways. These rhythm disturbances are called dysrhythmias, meaning a deviation from the normal sinus heart rhythm (Table 44-4). Dysrhythmias occur as a response to ischemia, valvular abnormality, anxiety, drug toxicity, or acid-base or electrolyte imbalance. Some common dysrhythmias include tachycardia (greater than 100 beats per minute), bradycardia (less than 60 beats per minute), premature ventricular contractions (PVCs), or heart block (delayed or absent beat).

The electrical impulses are conducted to the body's surface and are detected by electrodes placed on the limbs and torso. The electrodes carry these impulses to a continuously running graph that plots the ECG wave pattern. The appearance of the ECG pattern helps diagnose whether there are any abnormalities in the electrical conduction through the heart. The 12-lead ECG equipment is composed of 10 electrodes that are connected to the 10 lead wires

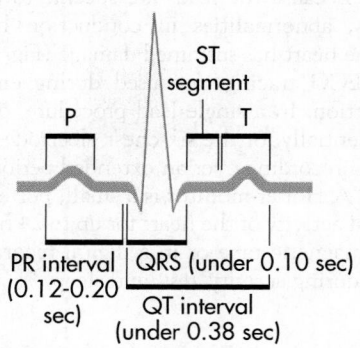

FIG 44-6   Normal ECG waveform. (*From Pagana KD, Pagana TJ: Mosby's manual of diagnostic and laboratory tests, ed 3, St. Louis, 2006, Mosby.*)

TABLE 44-4	Common Basic Cardiac Dysrhythmias	
Rhythm Characteristics	**Appearance**	**Clinical Significance**
Sinus tachycardia: Regular rhythm, rate 100-180 beats per minute, normal PQRS complex	 *(From Wellens HJJ, Conover MB: The ECG in emergency decision making, ed 2, Philadelphia, 2006, Saunders.)*	Normal response to exercise, emotion, pain, fever, hyperthyroidism, and certain drugs
Sinus bradycardia: Regular rhythm, rate less than 60 beats per minute, normal P, PR interval, and QRS complex	 *(From Potter PA, Perry AG: Fundamentals of nursing: ed 6, St. Louis, 2007, Mosby.)*	Associated with decreased cardiac output, dizziness, syncope, and chest pain
Premature ventricular contractions (PVCs): Irregular rhythm followed by compensatory pause	 *(From Potter PA, Perry AG: Basic nursing: a critical thinking approach, ed 6, St. Louis, 2007, Mosby.)*	Caused by irritable focus; if more than 6 per minute or in pairs, indicates increased ventricular irritability
Ventricular tachycardia: Rhythm slightly irregular, rate 100-200 beats per minute, P wave absent, PR interval absent, QRS complex wide and bizarre	 *(From Wellens HJJ, Conover MB: The ECG in emergency decision making, ed 2, Philadelphia, 2006, Saunders.)*	Often a forerunner of ventricular fibrillation; may cause decreased cardiac output because of decreased ventricular filling time

of an ECG machine. One electrode is placed on each of the four extremities, and six electrodes are placed at specific sites on the chest for a total of 10 electrodes. The 12 "leads" that are produced are 12 different graphical pictures, based on how the electricity flows between specific electrodes. They are the bipolar limb leads I, II, III; augmented limb leads aV_R, aV_L, aV_F; and precordial chest leads V_1 to V_6. Because the leads are specific to portions of the heart's anatomy, abnormalities in conduction help determine which part of the heart has sustained damage (Fig. 44-7).

Single-lead ECG tracings are used during emergencies and pacemaker insertion. In a single-lead procedure, one electrode is substituted sequentially for the six chest electrodes. If you need a continuous ECG recording over an extended period of time, use a Holter monitor. A Holter monitor is a small, portable device that records electrical activity of the heart for up to 24 hours. The ECG is recorded on magnetic tape or in a digital record and monitors cardiac rhythm during activity, rest, and sleep.

Delegation Considerations

Because an electrocardiogram is noninvasive and poses no risk to the patient, the skill of assisting with the electrocardiogram is routinely delegated to NAP who are specifically trained in obtaining the measurement. The nurse directs the NAP to:

- Immediately summon the nurse if the patient states that he or she is having chest pain or if the patient appears anxious.

Equipment

- ☐ 12-lead ECG machine
- ☐ ECG leads or electrodes (self-stick adhesive)
- ☐ Electrode gel *(optional)*
- ☐ Alcohol wipes
- ☐ Scissors

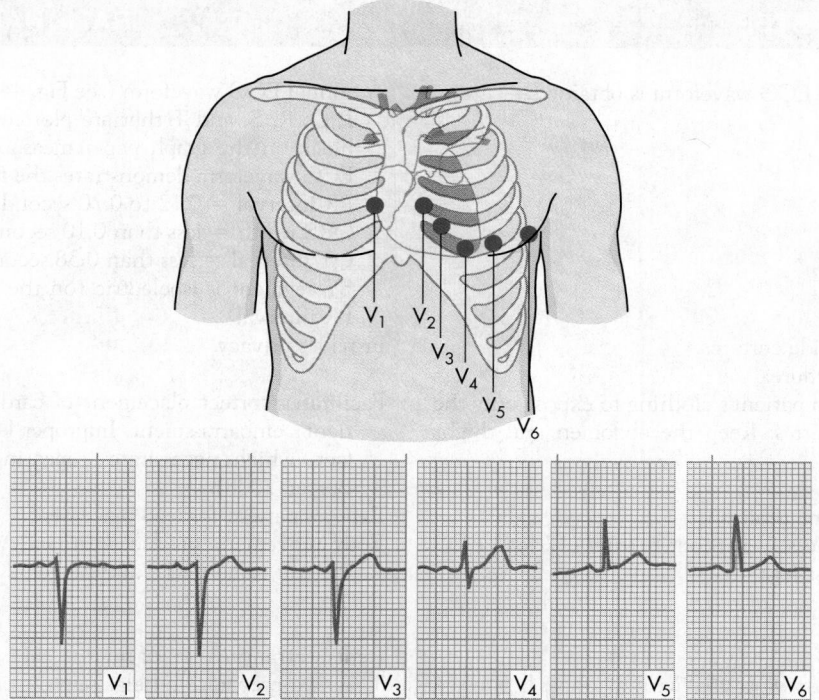

FIG 44-7 Anatomical placement of precordial leads. (*From Monahan F and others:* Phipps' medical-surgical nursing: health and illness perspectives, *ed 8, St. Louis, 2006, Mosby.*)

STEP	RATIONALE

ASSESSMENT

1 Verify patient's identity by using at least two forms of identifiers, neither of which is the patient's room number. Verify the type of procedure scheduled and the procedure site with the patient.

Ensures accurate patient identification and improves patient safety. Use of patient's room number is not an acceptable identifier (TJC, 2008a).

2 Determine rationale for obtaining ECG.

ECG determines baseline cardiac function (e.g., preoperative, prediagnostic testing), to help evaluate response to cardiac medications, to help monitor recovery after a myocardial infarction, or when patient experiences chest discomfort (Chernecky and Berger, 2008). If the ECG is ordered for active chest pain, perform it right away.

3 Assess patient's level of understanding of procedure, including any concerns.

Determines extent of instruction and level of support required.

4 Assess patient's ability to follow directions and remain still in a supine position.

Provides clear, accurate recording without artifacts.

NURSING DIAGNOSES

- Acute pain
- Anxiety
- Deficient knowledge regarding purpose and steps of procedure
- Fear

Individualize related factors based on patient's condition or needs.

PLANNING

1 Expected outcomes following completion of procedure:
- Patient tolerates procedure without anxiety or discomfort.

Appropriate preparation decreases anxiety.

STEP	RATIONALE
• Clear recording of the ECG waveform is obtained.	A normal ECG waveform (see Fig. 44-6) consists of specific waves P, Q, R, S, and T that are plotted on graph paper. Each small block on the graph paper measures 0.04 second. A "normal" ECG waveform demonstrates the following characteristics: PR interval = 0.12 to 0.20 second QRS width = less than 0.10 second QT interval = less than 0.38 second ST segment is isoelectric (on the same horizontal level as the PR interval)
2 Close room door or bedside curtains.	Provides privacy.
3 Prepare patient for procedure:	
a Remove or reposition patient's clothing to expose only the patient's chest and arms. Keep the abdomen and thighs covered.	Facilitates correct placement of cardiac leads and minimizes patient's embarrassment. Improper lead placement produces artifact, which necessitates repeating the test (Chernecky and Berger, 2008).
b Place patient in supine position.	Exposes patient for lead placement.
c Instruct patient to lie still without talking (12-lead ECG only) and to not cross legs.	Body movement produces artifact, which necessitates repeating the test (Chernecky and Berger, 2008).

IMPLEMENTATION

1 Perform hand hygiene.	Reduces transmission of microorganisms.
2 Cleanse and prepare skin; wipe sites with alcohol. It is often necessary to clip hair from the chest if large amounts of hair are present. In patients who are very thin and emaciated, it is difficult to secure electrodes because of bony structure and decreased amount of subcutaneous tissue.	This skin preparation helps remove oils that prevent adherence of the electrodes.
3 Apply self-sticking electrode, being careful to use pressure on the perimeter only, and attach leads. (If self-sticking leads are not available, apply electrode paste to skin before attaching leads.) For 12-lead ECG:	Position of leads promotes proper display of ECG on paper. Pressure on the center of the lead displaces the electroconductive gel and results in a poor tracing.
a Chest (precordial leads) (see Fig. 44-7):	Proper position of leads promotes accurate display of ECG on paper.
(1) V_1—Fourth intercostal space (ICS) at right sternal border	
(2) V_2—Fourth ICS at left sternal border	
(3) V_3—Midway between V_2 and V_4	
(4) V_4—Fifth ICS at midclavicular line	
(5) V_5—Left anterior axillary line at level of V_4 horizontally	
(6) V_6—Left midaxillary line at level of V_4 horizontally	
b Extremities: one lead on each extremity. Place on lower portion of each extremity, avoiding any bone prominences.	Positioning of leads in this manner produces fewer artifacts.
(1) aV_r—Right wrist	
(2) aV_l—Left wrist	
(3) aV_f—Left ankle	
(4) aV_7—Right ankle	
4 Turn on machine, enter required demographic information, and obtain tracing.	Transfers electrocardiac conduction to ECG tracing paper for subsequent analysis by cardiologist. Chest pain experienced during the study is often correlated to an arrhythmia on the ECG (Pagana and Pagana, 2007).
a *Simultaneous 12-channel recording:* Enter patient's name and medical record number into the ECG machine menu. Obtain test tracing. Reposition leads as needed. Activate machine to obtain a simultaneous tracing of all 12 leads. If patient experiences chest pain during the procedure, document occurrence of chest pain on the resulting printout.	

STEP	RATIONALE
b *Single-channel recording:* After placing the limb electrodes, dispense electroconductive gel over the V_1 to V_6 locations (described above). Turn the lead selector to lead "1," turn on the machine, and begin the recording. If the tracing is clear, run sequential 6-second tracings for leads I, II, III, aV_R, aV_L, and aV_F by turning the lead selector to the corresponding settings. Then stop the machine, position the V electrode over the V_1 position and run a 6-second tracing. Repeat sequentially by moving the V electrode over V_2, V_3, V_4, V_5, and V_6 positions.	
5 Disconnect leads, and wipe off excess electrode paste from chest.	Promotes comfort and hygiene.
6 Deliver ECG tracing to appropriate laboratory, physician, or health care provider.	Provides for review of ECG by cardiologist.

EVALUATION

1 Although the procedure is painless, it is important to note and document if the patient is experiencing any chest discomfort during the procedure.	Helps correlate ECG changes to symptoms of chest pain.

Unexpected Outcomes

1 ECG is uninterpretable:
- Absence of tracing in one or more leads
- The presence of artifact in the ECG tracings

2 Patient has chest pain or anxiety.

Related Interventions

- Inspect electrodes for secure placement.
- Reposition any wires that move as a result of patient breathing or movement or vibrations in the environment.
- Remind patient who is moving that lying still is necessary to obtain a good tracing. Manually hold any extremities, if needed.
- If artifact looks like 60-cycle interference (looks like a very thick-lined waveform), unplug battery-operated equipment in the room one item at a time to see if the interference disappears. NOTE: 60-cycle interference is rare.
- Repeat the tracing.

- Continue to monitor.
- Reassess factors contributing to anxiety.
- Follow specific postprocedural orders related to findings.
- Notify physician or health care provider.

Recording and Reporting

- Record when ECG was obtained (date and time) and where tracing was sent, rationale for obtaining ECG (e.g., pain, discomfort, preoperatively, postoperatively), and baseline vital signs. Include rhythm strip in the patient's chart (check agency policy).
- Report any unexpected outcomes immediately.

Teaching Considerations

- If you select Holter monitoring, instruct patient to maintain an accurate diary of activities (detailed documentation of activities and occurrence of chest pain assist in diagnoses of condition). Also, inform patient that the Holter monitoring interpretation will be available in a few days.

Gerontological Considerations

- Be aware that medications, such as digitalis and antiarrhythmics, can affect results.

CRITICAL THINKING EXERCISES

Mr. Hall, a 67-year-old African American, is a retired executive. He is scheduled for a cardiac catheterization under moderate sedation. The prescription for the procedure faxed from the health care provider's or physician's office lists "new-onset chest pain" as the clinical indication for the procedure.

1 What other information would you assess about this patient?
2 What laboratory data would you review as part of your preparation of Mr. Hall for his procedure?
   A CBC, levels of prealbumin and blood gases
   B CBC, platelet prothrombin time, and levels of BUN and creatinine
   C Lipid panel, blood glucose level, and electrolyte levels
3 Describe the steps you would take to perform patient verification safety procedures for Mr. Hall.
4 Cardiac catheterization often involves the use of intravenous moderate sedation. The health care provider or physician has not requested the presence of an anesthesiologist during the procedure. You are responsible for verifying Mr. Hall's ASA classification before the procedure. What ASA classification would you consider appropriate for Mr. Hall?
   A 1
   B 2
   C 3
   D 4
   E 5
   F 6
5 When you review Mr. Hall's chart, you see that the consent form for the procedure is unsigned. When you inquire of him whether the health care provider or physician explained the procedure and the risks and ask if he has any questions, he replies, "My doctor told me that I needed this to find out why my chest pain is happening. But I don't know how risky it is." What would you do?
   A Ask Mr. Hall to sign the consent form, and tell him to ask about the risks when the doctor arrives.
   B Hold the consent form until health care provider or physician arrives to speak with Mr. Hall. Proceed with preparation by administering the preprocedure Valium to Mr. Hall.
   C Hold the consent form until the health care provider or physician arrives to discuss the information needed for informed consent. Hold the preprocedure Valium until after informed consent is obtained.
6 Mr. Hall's cardiac catheterization procedure is finished. The right femoral site was used for catheter insertion. Which items take priority in your postprocedure assessments of Mr. Hall?
   A Heart rate and rhythm, respiratory effort, oxygen saturation, procedure site for bleeding control, pedal pulses
   B Blood pressure, pain level, neurological checks, complete blood count, electrolytes
   C Pupil checks, level of consciousness, breath sounds, bowel sounds

REVIEW QUESTIONS

1 A patient scheduled for a diagnostic procedure requiring intravenous moderate sedation has an ASA physical status classification of 4. Which action should the nurse take before the beginning of the procedure?
   1 Assess breath sounds and the current pulse oximetry value.
   2 Check the patient's comfort level and peripheral pulses.
   3 Determine that the patient has had nothing to eat or drink for 4 hours.
   4 Notify the physician scheduled to perform the procedure of the ASA score.
2 The nurse is reassessing a patient who is recovering after a cardiac catheterization. Which set of postprocedure assessment data should be reported immediately to the physician?
   1 Increase in heart rate from 92 to 116 beats per minute, and low back pain radiating to the sides
   2 Occasional PVCs, and mild tenderness at catheter insertion site
   3 Urine output of 40 mL in the first hour postcatheterization, and decrease in oxygen saturation from 99% to 96%
   4 Bloody drainage visible at the edge of the dressing
3 On the urological unit, each of the nurse's patients is scheduled for an intravenous pyelogram. For which patient is this procedure contraindicated?
   1 The patient with renal failure
   2 The patient with a urinary tract infection
   3 The patient with possible kidney stones
   4 The patient with only one kidney
4 The nurse is assisting a patient who has just had a paracentesis performed. Which assessment data indicate that the desired results from the procedure have occurred?
   1 Increased abdominal girth, decreased respiratory effort, increased respiratory rate
   2 Increased abdominal girth, increased respiratory effort, decreased respiratory rate
   3 Decreased abdominal girth, decreased respiratory effort, decreased respiratory rate
   4 Decreased abdominal girth, increased respiratory effort, increased respiratory rate
5 The nurse is giving a 77-year-old man instructions about how to prepare for his colonoscopy next week. What information should be included in his instructions?
   1 Eat only soft foods for 3 days before the day of the procedure. Administer a cleansing enema in the morning before the test. Consume no food or fluids for 4 hours before the procedure.
   2 Have a full-liquid diet the day before the procedure. Drink a bowel-cleansing preparation the night before the procedure. Take the prescribed antibiotic the morning of the procedure.
   3 No diet modifications are needed in the days before the procedure. Fast from food and fluids, except for medications, the night before the procedure. Have a bowel movement the morning before the procedure.
   4 Consume clear liquids only for 2 days before the procedure. Complete the bowel preparation the night before the procedure. Fast from food and fluids for 8 hours before the procedure.

REFERENCES

Allibone C: Assessment and management of patients with pleural effusion, *Nurs Stand* 20(22):55, 2006.

American Academy of Pediatrics: Guidelines and management of pediatric patients during and after sedation for diagnostic and therapeutic procedures: an update, *Pediatrics* 118:2387, 2006.

American Association of Nurse Anesthetists: *AANA-ASA joint statement regarding propofol administration*, 2004, accessed September 29, 2007.

American Society of Anesthesiologists: *Continuum of depth of sedation definition of general anesthesia and levels of sedation/analgesia*, 2004a, http://www.asahq.org/publicationsandservices/standards/29thm.

American Society of Anesthesiologists: *Relative value guide*, Park Ridge, Ill, 2004b, The Society.

Association of periOperative Registered Nurses: *Standards, recommended practices, and guidelines*, Denver, 2006, The Association.

Chernecky CC, Berger BJ: *Laboratory tests and diagnostic procedures*, ed 5, Philadelphia, 2008, Elsevier.

Eisenberg R, Johnson N: *Comprehensive radiographic pathology*, ed 4, St. Louis, 2007, Mosby.

Hockenberry MJ, Wilson D: *Wong's nursing care of infants and children*, ed 8, St. Louis, 2007, Mosby.

Ignatavicius DD, Workman ML: *Medical-surgical nursing: critical thinking for collaborative care*, ed 5, 2006, Saunders.)

Lewis S and others: *Medical-surgical nursing*, ed 7, St. Louis, 2007, Mosby.

Lombardi M: *Radiation safety in nuclear medicine*, ed 2, San Diego, 2006, CRC Press.

Meiner SE, Lueckenotte AG: *Gerontologic nursing*, St. Louis, 2006, Mosby.

Monahan F and others: *Phipps' medical-surgical nursing: health and illness perspectives*, ed 8, St. Louis, 2007, Mosby.

Murray P and others: Prevention of acute renal failure in the intensive care unit. In *Intensive care in nephrology*, London, 2006, Taylor & Francis.

Ott L: Assessing blood flow with CT angiography, *Nursing* 28(1):26, 2008.

Pagana KD, Pagana TJ: *Mosby's diagnostic and laboratory tests*, ed 8, St. Louis, 2007, Mosby.

From Potter PA, Perry AG: *Basic nursing: a critical thinking approach*, ed 4, St. Louis, 1999, Mosby.

The Joint Commission, *2009 National patient safety goals*, Oakbrook Terrace, Ill, 2008, The Commission, accessed November 26, 2008.

RESEARCH REFERENCES

Ahmed SV and others: Post lumbar puncture headache, *Postgrad Med J* 82(973):713, 2006.

Aldrete JA: The post-anesthesia recovery score revisited, *J Clin Anesth* 7:89, 1995.

Aldrete JA: Post-anesthetic recovery score, *J Am Coll Surg* 205(5):3, 2007.

Cheatham JP: Intervention in the critically ill neonate and infant with hypoplastic left heart syndrome and intact atrial septum, *J Interv Cardiol* 14(3):357, 2001.

Kim MC: Vascular closure devices, *Cardiology Clin* 24:277, 2006.

McMahon CJ and others: Cardiac catheterization in infants weighing less than 2500 grams, *Cardiol Young* 13(2):117, 2003.

Negishi C and others: Resistive-heating and forced-air warming are comparably effective, *Anesth Analg* 96(6):1683, 2003.

Oedit R and others: Efficacy of the epidural blood patch for the treatment of post lumbar puncture headache BLOPP: a randomized, observer-blind, controlled clinical trial, *BMC Neurol* 5(1):12, 2005.

Ramsay MA and others: Controlled sedation with alphaxalone-alphadolone, *Br Med J* 2(920):656, 1974.

Wellens HJJ, Conover MB: *The ECG in emergency decision making*, ed 2, Philadelphia, 2006, Saunders.

Answer Key

CHAPTER 1

Answers to Critical Thinking Exercises

1   A PICO question with an intervention focus would be "Does a low-carbohydrate diet compared with a high-carbohydrate diet reduce the frequency of diarrhea in adult patients with ulcerative colitis?" If the literature search were to be broader with respect to diet options, the PICO question might be "Does diet therapy reduce the frequency of diarrhea in adult patients with ulcerative colitis?"

2   A systematic review summarizes all research studies (usually randomized controlled trials [RCTs]) that have been conducted on the same research question to determine the strength of the evidence in answering the question.

3   A case control study

4   Because Maria is Hispanic, her cultural orientation may have a strong influence on her food choices. Jeanne must partner with Maria to determine if there are foods that Maria is willing to try and that meet diet guidelines.

Answers to Review Questions

1   3 Rationale: Evidence-based practice is founded upon data obtained by using established methods of research.

2   1, 3, 4, 6 Rationale: The health care provider's permission would be needed only if the nursing measures would potentially interfere adversely with a patient's outcome, but that patient would have been eliminated from the study population. The focus is also on nursing, not medical orders. Publication of the findings is not a required step, but communication of results is required. It is hoped that new findings would be shared.

3   2 Rationale: A knowledge-focused trigger is a question regarding new information about a topic.

4   4 Rationale: A PICO question should have the following components: an identified patient population, the intervention thought to be worthwhile, a comparison of interest, and the desired outcome.

5   1 Rationale: Determining whether data are relevant for the situation requires value determination, feasibility, and use of the data for making a change.

CHAPTER 2

Answers to Critical Thinking Exercises

1   Additional information that would be helpful as the nurse assumes care for Mrs. Hampton includes:
  • Level of consciousness and findings from neurological assessment
  • Patient's medical history, including medications; information regarding any recent changes in medication or treatment plan
  • Blood glucose level, home insulin schedule and dosages, whether home insulin was administered before presenting to hospital
  • Results of any testing completed, such as computed tomography (CT) scan of head or magnetic resonance imaging (MRI)
  • Patient's plans or expectations for discharge (e.g., plans to return home with assistance of husband)
  • Referrals that have been made for physical therapy and speech therapy
  • Discharge planning that has been started by the discharge planner or case manager

2   You introduce yourself to Mr. and Mrs. Hampton, explain that you are the nurse that will be caring for Mrs. Hampton during the day shift, and accompany them to the assigned room. Orient them to the room and help put Mrs. Hampton's belongings away after making sure all her personal belongings were brought with her. Show the Hamptons the call light system and how to get help if needed. Provide Mr. Hampton with a comfortable chair, and support his interactions with his wife.

Allow Mr. Hampton to participate in the care of Mrs. Hampton to the extent that he is comfortable. Reinforce the reasons for the transfer, and answer any questions that the Hamptons have about the transfer. Allow them the opportunity to express their anxiety about the move from the intensive care unit.

3   Ask Mr. Hampton to bring a copy of the advance directive to the hospital. Notify the physician that Mrs. Hampton has an advance directive. Document in the medical record the presence of an advance directive and the request made for Mr. Hampton to bring the document to the hospital. Ask Mrs. Hampton to explain the substance of the advance directive to determine her understanding of the advance directive. Place a copy of the advance directive in the medical record.

4   Recognize that Mr. Hampton's anxiety is normal, and allow him to express his concerns related to taking his wife home. Ask Mr. Hampton about family or other help that is available. Have Mr. Hampton describe the home and identify what problems there may be related to Mrs. Hampton's mobility and risk for falls. Discuss with Mr. Hampton changes that can be made in the home to improve safety (e.g., removal of throw rugs, having grab bars installed in the bathroom at the toilet and tub). Have the discharge planner or case manager work with Mr. Hampton to get the home equipment that is needed to help Mrs. Hampton bathe and navigate through her home.

Answers to Review Questions

1   1, 2, 4, and 6 Rationale: The nurse is responsible for identifying allergies, and if present, places an allergy band on the patient. It is also the nurse's role to clarify the specific details pertaining to the patient's advance directive. All the other activities may be done by the admission clerk.

2   4 Rationale: The discharge planning process is comprehensive and multidisciplinary, including representatives from all the services who provided care.

3   2 Rationale: The patient's current status must be accurate to anticipate the needs that may occur during the transfer or discharge.

4   2 Rationale: Toddlers do better in unfamiliar settings when they have items that they are used to having to comfort them. They also think in the present, so having something they can hold onto is most important. The other information from the parents regarding the child's rituals and preferences is important but might not be used, depending on the medical needs of the child.

5   4 Rationale: It is important to first assess the situation with information from the patient that focuses on his needs. There may be an underlying patient concern that when discovered may cause a reversal of this behavior. Restraints, whether physical or chemical, cannot be used unless the patient's well-being or the safety of others is in jeopardy.

CHAPTER 3

Answers to Critical Thinking Exercises

1   Contact a linguistic service, show empathy and respect, obtain an accurate health history.

2   Pause and consider your own feelings and thoughts about Mrs. Garcia and the anger she has expressed. Have the linguistic translator tell you what Mrs. Garcia is saying. Try a calm, firm approach using a comfortable voice.

3   Have any other nurses or the person who picks up the food tray leave the room. This encourages the patient to express herself rather than provoke anger. Keep an adequate distance from the patient. This prevents pressuring Mrs. Garcia.

4   Answer questions appropriately. If patient asks a power struggle type of question (e.g., challenging why she needs to be restricted moving about), redirect the discussion and set limits by giving clear explanation. Inform patient of consequences.

Answers to Review Questions

1 4 Rationale: A therapeutic nurse-patient relationship is goal directed, which can also include the need to assist a patient in discussing any pertinent topics, whether comfortable or uncomfortable.

2 1 Rationale: Therapeutic communication is goal directed, which in this situation is better pain management for the patient.

3 3 Rationale: The use of "why" questions may cause defensiveness in the patient and may hinder communication. The other options promote communication by encouraging the patient to communicate.

4 3 Rationale: The nurse needs to first assess the level of anxiety so appropriate communication techniques and strategies can be used. The patient may not have the insight to understand what is currently causing his or her behavior.

5 2 Rationale: Speaking louder and bringing in other team members may be perceived as threatening and may cause the patient's behavior to become out of control faster. The patient may not be aware of his or her behavior, and therefore asking about comfort measures to relieve the patient's threatening behavior may also cause him or her to escalate. The nurse may need to leave the room quickly and by positioning himself or herself near the door, the nurse should not be trapped by the patient.

CHAPTER 4

Answers to Critical Thinking Exercises

1 Vital signs and glucose testing can be recorded by nursing assistive personnel (NAP) on flow sheets. It is appropriate for the NAP to document repetitive care aspects. As a nurse, you must give the NAP specific information as to when you want to be notified about vital sign data (e.g., temperature above 99° F orally, heart rate greater than 100 beats per minute, blood pressure less than 100/70 mm Hg or greater than 130/85 mm Hg, and glucose measurement less than 60 mg/dL or greater than 120 mg/dL). Pain assessment and preoperative teaching must be done and recorded by the nurse.

2 You specify in your report to the NAP that the NAP is to notify you if there is any change in the pain; if there are any symptoms of dizziness, pallor, or confusion; and if the patient expresses any lack of understanding about the preoperative teaching.

3 Include the following elements: location of pain, description of type of pain, duration, information obtained from palpation of area, pain intensity on a scale of 0 to 10, patient comments, results of pain relief measures.

4 The following are your actions in order of priority:
   a Fully assess the patient.
     (1) *History:* Determine what is meant by "feels dizzy and sweaty." She could be weak and feel faint, she could feel increased pain, or because of her type 2 diabetes she could be hypoglycemic or hyperglycemic.
     (2) *Laboratory data:* Obtain a glucose measurement.
     (3) *Physical assessment:* Obtain vital signs; auscultate chest, heart, and abdomen; assess skin color and temperature.
     (4) *Actions:* Administer a simple sugar such as orange juice followed by a complex carbohydrate and protein, such as an apple and peanut butter.
   b Notify the health care provider. Rationale: Notification of the health care provider after your assessment of the patient provides some objective data for the health care provider to evaluate. Merely calling the health care provider and reporting that the NAP reported that the patient "feels dizzy and sweaty" provides little objective information. Remember, it is the nurse's responsibility to assess the patient and to report and document the findings.
   c Perhaps you may want to increase the frequency of the patient's vital sign measurements until the health care provider sees her. Provide the NAP with specific instructions about what information you want reported and when you want the information reported to you.

5 The following are your actions in order of priority:
   a Fully assess the patient's current understanding of the preoperative teaching.
     (1) History:
       (a) If possible, gather data about what the patient correctly understands.
       (b) Clarify the teaching that the patient understands, and repeat any areas that the patient found unclear or confusing.
   b Have the patient repeat or return demonstrate teaching to validate learning has taken place.

Answers to Review Questions

1 2 Rationale: Documentation is to be entered by the nurse who rendered the care or made the observation.

2 3 Rationale: Military time is one 24-hour time cycle, so for this example you would begin with 1200 (noon) and add 4 (four) hours, which adds up to 1600 hours in military time.

3 1 Rationale: Focus charting begins with the concern or problem being experienced (data), what was done about the problem (action) and the patient's outcome (response).

4 3 Rationale: The fourth purpose is identification of trends in clinical care.

5 3 Rationale: The patient's health care providers understand what is happening with the patient and how best to meet the identified needs using a unified approach.

CHAPTER 5

Answers to Critical Thinking Exercises

1 All of the routine vital signs can be delegated. Temperature should be tympanic or temporal, because patient is confused and may not be able to hold an oral thermometer.

2 Possible explanations for differences are technique, equipment, and patient-related findings. Technique includes site of blood pressure measurement and whether the nursing assistive personnel (NAP) used the proper method. The nurse may want to observe the NAP's technique in blood pressure measurement. Equipment differences include using a cuff that is too small. An example of a patient-related finding is that the patient may be normotensive but was anxious in the emergency department, thus raising blood pressure. The intervention indicated is for the nurse to repeat the blood pressure.

3 The NAP should be told to report any temperature over 98.6° F. A temperature of 99.4° F may reflect a significant fever in an older adult.

4 The NAP should be told to wake the patient if needed to obtain the temperature and pulse rate.

Answers to Review Questions

1 3 Rationale: The nurse needs to assess more than just the vital signs when a patient is experiencing a variety of abnormal signs and symptoms.

2 3 Rationale: The patient needs a brief period of rest before an accurate blood pressure measurement can be obtained.

3 3 Rationale: The nurse needs to recheck the blood pressure and make sure the equipment is working properly. The nurse can make additional assessments as needed.

4 1 Rationale: The sensor needs repositioned because of a low reading and irregular waveform pattern even though the patient says that his breathing is better.

5 4 Rationale: It will be accurate even with a decreased blood flow. The ear can be used effectively even if the patient has a history of peripheral vascular disease.

CHAPTER 6

Answers to Critical Thinking Exercises

1 Focused systems assessments would include cardiovascular and peripheral neurovascular, respiratory, abdominal and perineal, intake and output.

a Key elements of each system:
(1) *Cardiovascular:* Blood pressure (BP); heart rate (HR); inspection, palpation, and auscultation of the heart
(2) *Peripheral neurovascular:* Inspection and palpation of extremities; checking peripheral pulses, edema, skin color and temperature, capillary refill of nail beds; sensation, movement
(3) *Respiratory:* Checking rate and depth of respirations, chest excursion, lung sounds
(4) *Abdominal:* Checking size and shape of abdomen, palpating bladder, assessing bowel sounds
(5) *Intake and output:* Intake, output (Foley, Jackson-Pratt drain), intravenous site patency

2 A crackling noise upon inspiration indicates crackles. Crackles indicate fluid in the alveoli and small airways. Priority nursing diagnosis is ineffective airway clearance.

3 This indicates a normal heart rate, which is between 60 and 100 beats per minute, regular rate and rhythm.

4 The nurse must listen for 5 minutes over each quadrant before deciding bowel sounds are absent. It is common for bowel sounds to be hypoactive postoperatively for 24 hours or more following abdominal surgery.

5 See Skill 6-4 for specifics. Unilateral leg edema is one of the most reliable findings of deep vein thrombosis. Other symptoms include pain or tenderness, erythema, increased warmth, and firmness of affected area.

6 For risk factors, see Skill 6-6, Assessment Step 1. For teaching musculoskeletal health, see Skill 6-6, Teaching Considerations and Gerontological Considerations.

Answers to Review Questions

1 4 Rationale: Palpation or percussion of the abdomen can cause bowel sounds to be heard, although peristalsis can be absent. All the other responses are correct.

2 3 Rationale: Comparison of areas side to side is extremely important in evaluating a patient's neurological system. This prevents omissions between the affected and unaffected areas.

3 2 Rationale: Diarrhea would cause the bowel sounds to be hyperactive, and because so much fluid had already been lost, the urine would be darker, therefore concentrated.

4 3 Rationale: Having the patient breathe deeper enables the nurse to fully assess lung sounds in the bases of patients' lungs.

5 780 mL Rationale: 3 ounces = 90 mL (orange juice) + 120 mL (milk) + 90 mL (popsicle) + 360 mL (cola) + 120 mL ice (ice is calculated as half its volume).

CHAPTER 7

Answers to Critical Thinking Exercises

1 Joe should wash his hands with soap and water and then put on gloves to continue his assessment, explaining the rationale for this to Mr. Nesbitt. He should put Mr. Nesbitt on contact precautions because the drainage from his sacral wound may contain pathogens. His gloves should be changed if they become soiled

2 After assessing the wound, if his gloved hand contacted the wound, it would be necessary to remove the gloves, perform hand hygiene, and reglove before checking the Foley catheter, especially if he touches the catheter. However, gloves would not be necessary to visually inspect the position and condition of the tubing. Hand hygiene should be performed when Joe leaves the patient's room.

3 Contact precautions do not require use of a mask. However, if the nurse has a respiratory infection, he or she might choose to wear a mask to protect the patient from exposure.

Answers to Review Questions

1 4 Rationale: Soap and water is essential for visibly dirty hands according to the Centers for Disease Control and Protection.

2 2 Rationale: Lathering the hands with the cleansing agent using friction is the best method to remove dirt and transient bacteria.

3 1-5 Rationale: All of the first five factors apply.

4 2 Rationale: A mask provides a barrier when the patient has droplet precautions.

5 3 and 4 Rationale: Gowns are used once and discarded because of the chance of being contaminated. Hand hygiene should always be performed before and after going into a room.

CHAPTER 8

Answers to Critical Thinking Exercises

1 Insertion of an indwelling urinary catheter requires wearing sterile gloves. Clean gloves are used for nasogastric (NG) tube and intravenous catheter insertion. No gloves are necessary to measure blood pressure.

2 Discard the used catheter, reprepare the skin at a new site, and open a new catheter for insertion into the vein.

3 Ask Mrs. Lorenzo if she has ever had a previous reaction to the following items within hours of exposure: adhesive tape, dental or face mask, golf club grip, ostomy bag, rubber band, balloon, bandage, elastic underwear, IV tubing, rubber gloves, condom. Use latex-free products when caring for Mrs. Smith.

4 Nothing. Only 1 inch from the border of the drape to the edge is considered contaminated.

Answers to Review Questions

1 1 Rationale: Gloves, then mask, eyewear, and cap

2 2 Rationale: Holding or moving the object below the waist

3 1 Rationale: Grab only the inside of the glove with the ungloved hand.

4 4 Rationale: Individuals with spina bifida are at risk for latex allergy, and so a nonlatex catheter should be used, as well as nonlatex gloves by the nurse. Individuals with spina bifida who have a latex sensitivity may also be allergic to bananas, avocados, kiwi fruit, and tomatoes, but not eggs.

5 3 Rationale: The label of the bottle should be facing the student's palm, so the label will not become distorted or ruined if fluid runs down the bottle.

CHAPTER 9

Answers to Critical Thinking Exercises

1 Additional information may include the following:
• Physiological capacity to transfer, including ability to move hands and arms. Presence of paralysis and level of orientation and alertness (cognitive status). Patient's level of comfort.

2 A, B, and C are correct answers. Mr. Clark is in pain most likely related to his lacerations and fractures. Pain management is a priority at this time. In addition to pain management, explaining to Mr. Clark the purpose of the computed tomography (CT) scan will help elicit his cooperation. Mr. Clark is most likely fearful of movement because of his pain and uncertainty of his condition. Describing the method of transfer and showing him that there will be additional personnel to help transfer him to the stretcher will increase his trust and cooperation. D is incorrect. You may inform Mr. Clark that it is a physician's order, but the patient has the right to refuse treatment. You are more likely to elicit Mr. Clark's cooperation by determining the underlying reasons for Mr. Clark's refusal to transfer.

3 Logrolling Mr. Clark will maintain proper alignment by moving all body parts at the same time, preventing tension or twisting of the spinal column.

4 A nurse must supervise and aid nursing assistive personnel when moving a patient who has suffered a spinal cord injury to keep the spinal column in straight alignment to prevent further injury.

Answers to Review Questions

1 2 Rationale: Patient should be transferred using this ability to partially bear weight on one leg and use his upper body strength. The bariatric transfer device is recommended.

2 3 Rationale: Keeping the knees bent allows for better balance and leverage; keeping the trunk erect helps prevent muscle fatigue because the muscles are working together.

3   3 Rationale: A transfer belt is contraindicated around the patient's waist after abdominal surgery. It is far better to have the patient sit on the side of the bed dangling for a few minutes with the nurse there to allow for a smoother transition from supine to upright position for the first time.

4   2 Rationale: The patient's pain may be at a level at which he does not want to move. There are no data to support any of the other options.

5   2 Rationale: The patient's skeleton must be kept in alignment, which requires the patient to be turned as a total unit, using enough staff for the turning and positioning. The patient should not participate in the activity because of the instability of the spinal cord.

CHAPTER 10

Answers to Critical Thinking Exercises

1   Mr. Timber reports a pain level of 8 on a scale of 0 to 10. A nursing priority is to provide pain management strategies and lower his level to an agreed-upon range. In addition, Mr. Timber may have concerns about his ability to safely ambulate without falling or injuring himself. Spending time with Mr. Timber explaining about and demonstrating the use of crutches will assist in minimizing his anxiety and concerns.

2   Mr. Timber has at least two major risk factors associated with orthostatic hypotension: his history of diabetes mellitus and his age. To minimize the complications, allow Mr. Timber to sit with the head of the bed elevated for several minutes before dangling him on the side of the bed. During dangling, instruct Mr. Timber to take several deep breaths and move his feet up and down and in a circular motion to promote venous return via intermittent contraction and relaxation of the skeletal leg muscles.

3   Assess the safety of the continuous passive motion (CPM) machine by inspecting the electrical cord for fraying and damage. In addition, put the CPM machine through one full cycle before applying to patient to ensure the machine is functioning properly. Assess the setup of the machine before placing on the patient's bed: check the stability of the frame, the flexion/extension controls, padding to exposed metal parts or hard surfaces, and the on/off switch.

4   The appropriate crutch gait for Mr. Timber is the three-point alternating, or three-point gait that requires the patient to bear all of his weight on one foot. Several teaching considerations are needed for Mr. Timber. It is important that these considerations are individualized to meet the learning needs of the patient. Some examples of teaching considerations for Mr. Timber are the following:
- Instruct patient with axillary crutches about the dangers of pressure on the axillae that occurs when leaning on the crutches to support body weight.
- Explain why patient must use crutches measured for him or her.
- Demonstrate how to routinely inspect crutch tips. Rubber tips should be securely attached to the crutches. When tips are worn, they should be replaced. Rubber crutch tips increase surface friction and help prevent slipping.

Answers to Review Questions

1   2 Rationale: Range-of-motion exercises are done only until resistance is met, not pain.

2   4 Rationale: Risk for activity intolerance is common for patients who have been immobile for a period of time and are beginning to exert more energy.

3   3 Rationale: If a blood clot is suspected in a leg, the patient should be kept calm and quiet in bed. There should be no rubbing or movement of the leg. The elastic stockings and sequential compression devices are for prevention and should not be applied if a clot is suspected.

4   3 Rationale: Nursing assistive personnel can make sure the patient's environment is free from potential threats to patient safety such as spills or clutter.

5   4 Rationale: A caregiver of the same gender should walk with the patient because the patient will need to be touched during the activity. The caregiver will stand on the patient's right side for support.

CHAPTER 11

Answers to Critical Thinking Exercises

1   The correct answer is C. A fiberglass cast sets up and is dry in 15 to 20 minutes, so it is not necessary to prevent indentation nor does the cast remain damp after that time period. A plaster of Paris cast will take much longer and is susceptible to indentation and dampness and the need to assist in the drying process.

2   The correct answer is B. The patient is receiving pain medication, and the assessment data indicate muscles spasms. You do not release the traction because she has a fracture.

3   The correct answer is D. A heating pad would increase the swelling at this point. The key data are increased swelling and pain that is out of proportion to what is expected, given that she is being medicated and the extremity is elevated. The concern is compartment syndrome and altered neurovascular status. To bivalve the cast, cut it in two lengthwise along each side. In addition, the wadding underneath is cut to relieve the pressure. Although a window may be cut in a cast to visualize a wound underneath, it does not relieve pressure.

4   The correct answer is B. Traction is not removed when a patient has a fracture. Skin maceration and breakdown can occur if the linens are not changed. The patient in Buck's extension traction can be rolled briefly to the unaffected side while maintaining the traction in order to change the linens or to administer back care.

Answers to Review Questions

1   3 Rationale: The patient needs to learn the proper use of the trapeze, so alignment can be maintained and the activities can be done as easily as possible for both patient and staff. The patient needs to cough, deep breathe, and change position as able to prevent pneumonia.

2   1 Rationale: Elevation and ice decrease the blood flow to the area and thereby decrease swelling, but the ice would be more effective than the use of only one pillow.

3   1 and 6 Rationale: The skin under a cast undergoes a change from soft and uniform to many layers being in place, because the normal sloughing that occurs cannot occur under the cast. Lotion is used after the cleaning with the enzyme wash to help remove dead skin, not to soften the skin. Activity resumption occurs with a physician's order and after possible evaluation by a physical therapist. Friction and hot water are contraindicated because the skin is fragile for at least a month.

4   4 Rationale: Pain on passive motion may signify compartment syndrome.

5   3 Rationale: The other patients must be kept either flat (for Bryant's and Dunlop's) or not higher than 30 degrees (for Buck's).

CHAPTER 12

Answers to Critical Thinking Exercises

1   Complete assessment with emphasis on pressure ulcer risk, current mobility status, and skin integrity.

2   Determine patient's level of pressure ulcer risk, and then determine whether pressure reduction or relief is needed. Mr. Hoji is at high risk for pressure ulcers. He has decreased mobility and sensation. Mr. Hoji needs pressure relief. The rationale is that he has no ability to independently change position. In addition, because of impaired sensation, he cannot perceive pressure on his skin and tissues.

3   Anxiety and nausea are common with air-suspension beds; a patient's comfort can be improved with pharmacological agents to reduce anxiety and nausea. In addition, when lateral rotation is also used, a patient's nausea increases. When patients are prescribed an antiemetic, such as Compazine, be sure that this medication is given routinely as opposed to an "as needed" (prn) order. Explaining to the patient that these sensations are temporary and will gradually improve is important. However, the patient cannot really process this information unless he or she is comfortable. For these reasons pharmacological agents to control anxiety, nausea, and any pain are beneficial to patients on support surfaces.

Answers to Review Questions

1 3 Rationale: Patients tend to perspire on this bed. The surface of the bed quickly removes fluids from contact with the patient's skin, so the evidence of perspiration may be minimized. The perspiration and/or diaphoresis can go undetected, and the increase in insensible fluid loss may not be noticed until the patient develops dehydration or electrolyte changes.

2 2 Rationale: Stop the rotation of the bed, and assess the patient further. The patient may experience orthostatic hypotension when the bed rotates. Stopping rotation while remaining with the patient and conducting further blood pressure assessments will indicate if the problem diminishes. The rotation can begin again, perhaps at a decreased angle and at a slower cycle.

3 4 Rationale: Consider changing to a pressure-relief device because this patient is not responding to pressure reduction. The patient needs to move to a pressure-relief system because of the development of pressure ulcers on more than one position area (e.g., supine and left lateral positions).

4 1 Rationale: The patient's ability to assist with transfer to the bed is the least factor to be considered. A severely overweight patient has problems with mobility and therefore needs a bed that will enable the caregiving staff to reposition and provide care while relieving pressure on the skin.

5 1 Rationale: A patient should never be placed in prone position on an air-fluidized bed because of the chance of suffocation. All of the other options are appropriate.

CHAPTER 13

Answers to Critical Thinking Exercises

1 Diarrheal stools may cause Mr. Werneck to have to get out of bed often to use toilet facilities. The diarrhea can cause electrolyte and fluid imbalances that increase risk for dizziness or orthostatic hypotension. The weakness in his leg and his sense of fatigue also add to his risk. Antihypertensive medications increase risk for orthostatic hypotension, which increases fall risk. Isolation after visiting hours might prompt him to walk more on his own. Finally, his age is a risk factor as well.

2 Provide a bedside commode to eliminate the need to walk to the bathroom. Inform his wife of her husband's risk for falls, and involve her in reminding the patient to sit up and dangle his feet before he attempts to get up to sit on the commode. Keep the call light close by, and respond promptly if the patient complains of discomfort or needs assistance to get up. Place a nonskid pad alongside the bed. Place Mr. Werneck in a room close to the nurses' station.

3 Call for help, assess the patient for injury, and stay with the patient until assistance arrives.

Answers to Review Questions

1 4 Rationale: A safe environment is important, but the patient's behaviors and risks must be matched with the interventions to be used. Restraints are always a last resort and are not considered a safe fall prevention strategy. A bed alarm can be useful in fall prevention but should be combined with appropriate behavioral therapies.

2 1, 3, 4, and 5 Rationale: Visitors should limit their visitation to approximately 30 minutes per day. Anyone entering the patient's room must be aware that radiation is present. This overrides the patient's privacy. All of the other strategies are correct.

3 4 Rationale: Because of his weight and limited mobility, the most appropriate method for evacuating this patient is by rolling him out of his room in his bed. The other methods would increase the risk for injury to the nurse(s) involved.

4 1, 2, and 4 Rationale: The facility would outline the alternative strategies to be used before initiating the use of restraints, as well as the documentation required when restraints are applied. It is not required to notify the patient's next of kin when restraints are applied. All of the other options are correct.

5 3 Rationale: The patient should not be involved in securing the fire. The patient should be evacuated as quickly and safely as possible.

CHAPTER 14

Answers to Critical Thinking Exercises

1 Rescue workers should wear respiratory and skin personal protective equipment (PPE) and locate selves upwind and uphill unless cyanide is suspected.

2 A 22-year-old with cyanosis, a respiratory rate of 35 breaths per minute, and confusion would be color coded immediate, red. A 14-year-old with a diffuse red rash on the extremities would be color coded minimal, green. A 56-year-old with controlled bleeding of deep lacerations received from falling debris would be color coded delayed, yellow. A 41-year-old with burns on 50% of the body would be color coded immediate, red. Those coded red would receive highest priority.

3 The primary objective for initial care is decontamination. Decontamination is the process used to remove harmful contaminants from the surface of the skin. It is achieved by removing clothing and scrubbing the skin and by hydrolysis, a process of chemical dilution using large volumes of water.

4 Clothing should be cut off rather than pulled over the head to prevent contamination of the head and hair. Clothing should then be placed in a biohazard bag, labeled, and sealed to reduce the likelihood of secondary chemical contamination.

5 Children may be frightened by separation from their parents, the appearance of rescue workers in PPE, and decontamination procedures. Do not immediately pick up a child to avoid secondary contamination. Offer verbal encouragement and praise to facilitate treatment. Observe children closely for symptoms of exposure because they are more prone to the effects of chemical toxins (being closer to the ground and having a higher respiratory rate than adults). Children are also more susceptible to hypothermia with decontamination procedures.

Answers to Review Questions

1 1 Rationale: Practice makes staff more familiar with disaster protocols in the event of a true disaster.

2 4 A nurse who must inform a mother that her three children did not survive would have the most difficult job.

3 2 Rationale: A disaster victim who arrives at the emergency department with labored respirations, cool skin, a pulse of 120 beats per minute, and a blood pressure of 90/60 mm Hg should receive the highest level of priority of care because of the presenting signs. This victim stands a good chance of survival with appropriate care.

4 2 Rationale: Contact isolation is needed because of the mechanism of transmission.

5 1 Rationale: The health care workers must be protected first because of the chance of spreading whatever contamination may be present. If the health care workers become infected, then no one will be available to care for the victims.

CHAPTER 15

Answers to Critical Thinking Exercises

1 The correct answer is B: When the pain is severe, a mild analgesic will relieve the pain only slightly, if at all. A strong opioid is necessary for this patient's severe level of pain. However, an assessment is needed to establish the extent of pain and to rule out developing other complications.

2 The correct answer is A. The standard pain-intensity tool used for adults is the 0 to 10 scale. The pain should be assessed frequently; every hour would be good initially, until the pain is controlled. Use your judgment to reassess as often as needed, but assessing with each set of vital signs would be appropriate when the pain is well controlled with a PCA. Choice B is fine after the pain is under control, but not at this point. There is no indication that Mrs. Koby would need an alternative scale, as in choice C. The FACES Scale has not been tested on the adult population; it is recommended primarily for children. Every 8 hours is not often enough for a patient in severe pain with uncontrolled pain. Although there is nothing wrong with observing her behavior, as in choice D, she is able to self-report pain, which is the "gold standard" for pain assessment. Assessing every 12 hours is not often enough for uncontrolled pain.

3 The correct answer is D. The PCA computer has a built-in program for locking out the delivery of a medication dose if it has not been the prescribed interval; this keeps a patient safe from overdose as long as the machine is correctly programmed and correctly functioning. You must make sure that this is happening. Choice A implies that it does not matter if she receives an overdose. Although it is important for her to receive as large a dose as needed and cancer patients often can tolerate large doses, the medication dosages must be increased gradually and are still very closely monitored for safety. Choice B implies that only the nurses' watching the PCA keeps it safe. The correct programming is most important. Although the machine is closely monitored by one nurse, it is only necessary to have two nurses check it when the PCA is initiated and whenever the programming needs to be changed. Choice C indicates the patient has to monitor the PCA visually herself around-the-clock, an impossibility for anyone, especially a very sick patient. The patient only needs to push the button when she needs a dose of medication. Everything else is monitored by the machine and the nurse.

4 If a PCA is discontinued, federal regulations dictate the process. The law governing this is the Controlled Substances Act. If any medication remains in the cassette, the amount must be recorded with two nurses witnessing the wastage. The date and time and type of medication and reason for wastage are also recorded. Both nurses must sign the record. The empty cassette is discarded or returned to the pharmacy per agency policy.

Answers to Review Questions

1 2 Rationale: Patients in chronic pain are very familiar with the medications and therapies they use for pain relief. These patients usually require higher doses of analgesics without suffering adverse reactions. Relaxation is often very beneficial for patients in chronic pain. Patients with chronic pain do not usually have autonomic signs or symptoms.

2 3 Rationale: The patient should be encouraged to use the PCA when feeling discomfort to achieve pain control. The device prevents delivery of an overdose. If the patient is sleeping, it likely means she has achieved pain relief. The family member should never push the button of the PCA for the patient. The PCA is designed so that there is minimal risk of overdose.

3 2 Rationale: Itching (pruritus) is a common side effect of intraspinal opioids and is not related to an allergic reaction and does not require change in the infusion rate or notification of health care provider.

4 2 Rationale: Nonpharmacological therapies are very effective in patients who express fear or anxiety. If the therapies seem unappealing, they are less likely to be effective. Patients who have complete pain relief from pharmacological measures likely will not gain added benefit. Massage is contraindicated in cases of bone injury.

5 3 Rationale: The use of anticoagulants sometimes contraindicates the placement of an epidural catheter due to the risk for epidural hematoma at the insertion site.

CHAPTER 16

Answers to Critical Thinking Exercises

1 Because you do not know what he has been told about his situation, begin by exploring his perceptions of his health status and validate his feelings. "Tell me what you were told about your illness. I would like to understand better." Discussion helps reveal misperceptions or the need for factual information to help Mr. Lange gain a sense of control. Mr. Lange has also opened the door for a conversation about his emotional state. Paraphrase by saying, "It sounds like you are feeling all alone and don't know where to go for help. Is that right?" Sit down while speaking, and ensure privacy by closing the door.

2 The correct answer is C. Patients do not experience grief exactly as the theorists describe. Perhaps Mr. Lange is denying that his cancer has spread, considers bargaining with other health care providers, and feels angry and sad at the same time, and in no particular order. Sometimes care providers take the patient's anger personally and withdraw, just when the patient needs support the most. Talk with Mr. Lange, validate that his anger is a normal response to loss, and find out how you can best support him.

3 The correct answer is B. The nurse should gather more assessment data before selecting an intervention (choices A and D). Perform a physical assessment of the patient's abdomen, and ask about normal bowel patterns, current pain medications, and recent diet and fluid intake. Assess the type, timing, location, precipitating and relieving factors, and intensity of Mr. Lange's abdominal pain. Allow Mr. Lange to describe his own symptoms instead of asking his wife (choice C). Ask him about other symptoms he may be experiencing.

4 Assess what Mr. Lange and his wife already know about hospice care and what it means to them. Realize that people face many changes when opting to receive home hospice care. Their familiar health care patterns and relationships will change, and caregivers will come into their home. To accept hospice care admits that death is presumed likely within the next few months or sooner. Symptom management becomes the primary focus of care. Assess the Lange family's degree of openness and awareness concerning death. The family must provide the care for all daily activities, necessitating some temporary changes in roles and schedules. Families do, however, have access to professional and volunteer hospice team members throughout their experience. Hospice professionals provide teaching, support, counseling, home visits as needed, and 24-hour contact for medical emergencies or questions. Family members need a support system to meet the challenges of helping their loved one die at home.

5 The correct answer is D. Both family members and health care providers want to offer solutions to problems that cause distress to patients (choices A, B, and C). Disease process, medications, social withdrawal, and a slowing of bodily functions, however, cause persons nearing the end of life to lose their interest in food. Encouraging or forcing Mr. Lange to eat when he does not feel hungry causes unnecessary stress for him and his wife. While difficult, Mr. Lange's family should support his decisions to eat when and what he wants, in the quantity he desires.

Answers to Review Questions

1 3 Rationale: It is essential to have the patient's input in the planning stages of palliative care to hear what the patient's priorities and values are. An open-ended question always elicits more information than a closed-ended one.

2 4 Rationale: Overwhelming grief does not allow the individual to feel in touch with everyday situations and responsibilities, including work. The individual may need counseling to be able to cope with the situation.

3 2 Rationale: Patients identify pain as their most common and severe symptom.

4 4 Rationale: Whenever a change occurs in a patient, assessment is indicated. Many conditions can cause restlessness, such as a decrease in oxygenation caused by a twisted nasal cannula, a clogged urinary catheter, or the need to be turned.

5 2 Rationale: Placing him supine with the head of the bed elevated approximately 30 degrees helps to decrease livor mortis (purple discoloration of the skin).

CHAPTER 17

Answers to Critical Thinking Exercises

1 The correct answers are A, B, and D. The description of the nail in choice C is what a healthy nail should look like. The other choices describe abnormal physical changes that if left untreated could result in the development of a pressure ulcer, which could lead to gangrene and potential amputation, especially in diabetic patients.

2 The correct answers are A, C, and D. Patients with diabetes should wear socks made of natural fibers to aid in absorption of perspiration. Cotton socks are most commonly recommended. A professional should trim nails to minimize chance of injury and infection. It is recommended that diabetic patients should not soak feet for two reasons. Decreased sensation in lower extremities makes it difficult to judge temperature. The second reason is that soaking feet can lead to dry skin, which can result in breaks in the skin. This puts patients at risk for infection.

3 The correct answer is B. Annual foot inspection by a professional is a must for diabetic patients. Also, if any change in the condition of the feet is identified, the patient should seek immediate help.

Answers to Review Questions

1 3 Rationale: The moving of a cloth on the skin during bathing not only cleans, but also removes dead skin cells.

2 4 Rationale: The patient with arthritis in her neck may have limited movement, as well as pain. This could cause a problem when her head is turned and repositioned while her hair is washed.

3 4 Rationale: A thermal bath in bed provides a more thorough bath in the safest environment for both the patient and the caregiver should the patient become aggressive or uncooperative.

4 3 Rationale: Only the left hand is used for cleaning the genital area by Muslims. The right hand is reserved for eating and praying. As long as the caregiver is a woman, it is not necessary to have another woman present. If the nurse is right-handed, she should switch and perform the pericare using her left hand to show respect for her patient's beliefs. Gloves should be used for all patients when doing pericare.

5 4 Rationale: Before administering oral care to an unconscious patient, check the gag reflex to determine risk for aspiration. A pupil check will indicate if intracranial pressure is developing. The Glasgow Coma Scale measures level of consciousness. It is important to inspect the oral cavity, but this will not reveal any risk for aspiration.

CHAPTER 18

Answers to Critical Thinking Exercises

1 Ms. Willett is unable to move well in bed or change position because of the immobilizer and the pain that she is experiencing. She is also on bed rest. She is a high risk under the activity subscale on the Braden Scale because of her bed rest.

2 The correct answer is B, eschar. Granulation tissue is red and moist and is found in wounds that are moving toward healing. Slough tissue can be tan, yellow, brown, or gray, is moist, and is found in wounds that require interventions to clean this tissue from the wound. Erythema is intact red skin that is warm to the touch. Eschar, the correct answer, is dead devitalized tissue that may need to be removed to allow the area to heal.

3 The correct answer is A. A sheet burn will open the top layer of skin, and the area will be slightly moist. Blistering is caused when the two layers of skin, dermis and epidermis, separate and allow fluid to accumulate. A blistered area is intact. Bruising results in breakage of the local capillaries and discoloration of the tissues. The correct answer is erythema.

4 It is likely that the erythema has occurred because of unrelieved pressure over Ms. Willet's sacrum. She is on bed rest and not moving well because of her pain and the immobilizer. This area is at risk for pressure ulcer development. The nurse should palpate the reddened area. If it does not blanch, the nurse can suspect tissue damage.

Answers to Review Questions

1 2 Rationale: This provides an early baseline assessment, as well as periodic reassessment throughout the confinement.

2 2 Rationale: The patient has numerous risk factors that necessitate the consultation with the wound clinical nurse specialist about the most appropriate bed surface to reduce pressure.

3 4 Rationale: This pressure ulcer cannot be staged because the wound base must be visible to assess the depth of tissue destruction.

4 2 Rationale: This type of dressing protects the wound base and provides a moist environment, which in this case is essential to support the growth of new tissue.

5 2 Rationale: The head is the most common site of pressure ulcers in neonates and very young children because the skin is thin, little hair is present to absorb pressure, and they are often unable to reposition themselves adequately to reduce pressure.

CHAPTER 19

Answers to Critical Thinking Exercises

1 First, determine if there was secondary injury to his eyes; for example, observe eyes for any redness or drainage, ask him about any eye discomfort, visual changes, or blurred vision. Then determine his contact lens care routine; for example, determine what he uses to clean his lenses and how he proceeds with cleaning. Last, identify who can help him with contact lens care if it is needed.

2 Mrs. Wong should report any drainage, excessive dryness, pain, or odor to her health care provider. This can indicate injury or infection in the socket and may require further treatment. How to clean the artificial eye; proper storage of the artificial eye; situations, such as pain or infection, when she must contact her health care provider; and the need to have her artificial eye carefully examined each year for any damage.

3 Dogs are particularly attracted to the smell of hearing aids and may play with the aid and damage it, or they may actually ingest the hearing aid. These are small aids, and if ingested by a child my cause severe breathing problems. Hearing aid batteries are toxic if ingested and must be kept away from children.

Answers to Review Questions

1 2 Rationale: The patient will be unable to care for her contact lenses immediately after surgery. No signs or symptoms have been presented to justify any of the other choices.

2 4 Rationale: Some disposable contact lenses are intended to be cleaned and reused. Furthermore, there is increased risk for infection with any contact lens use.

3 4 Rationale: The chemical should be removed as soon as possible to minimize the risk for permanent damage to the eye. Although a basin may be positioned to catch a dislodged contact lens, taking time to remove the lens delays removing the chemical from the eye and increases the risk for permanent damage. Testing the pH of secretions may be performed after an initial period of irrigation to determine the need to continue.

4 1 Rationale: The artificial eye should be cleaned only as often as necessary to prevent discomfort. The other statements are correct and indicate adequate teaching.

5 2 and 3 Rationale: Make sure the patient can see your face to facilitate comprehension. Speaking more slowly while using the same appropriate tone causes less frustration for the patient while allowing you to assess whether other approaches need to be used. Raising voice volume distorts the voice and may make understanding more difficult. If the patient appears not to understand, a different choice of words may help, but a rapid series of statements or questions deprives the patient of the longer processing time needed to compensate for a hearing impairment. Gestures may not be helpful in many circumstances.

CHAPTER 20

Answers to Critical Thinking Exercises

1 The antidepressant, hormone, cardiac drug (beta-blocker), and antihypertensive medications can all potentially create adverse effects in older adults.

2 The weakness and dizziness are likely side effects of the Lopressor and the antihypertensive. Because he takes multiple medications, there should be concern that there is possible drug interaction, with either summation or synergism occurring.

3 The physician has the option of lowering the dose in the older adult to determine if therapeutic effects can still be achieved.

4 $\dfrac{\text{Dose ordered}}{\text{Dose on hand}} \times \text{Amount on hand} = \text{Amount to administer}$

$$\frac{75 \text{ mg}}{50 \text{ mg}} \times 1 \text{ tablet} = 1.5 \text{ tablets}$$

5 You would need to evaluate if the patient has the motor dexterity or visual acuity to split tablets.

Answers to Review Questions

1 1 Rationale: Many medications bind to albumin (protein). If a patient is malnourished, the level of protein can be lowered and toxicity can be a problem, especially if the medication would normally bind to the protein. The patient should always be watched for the other problems.

2 1 Rationale: The trough is drawn when the level of the medication is the lowest, which occurs right before the next dose is due.

3 1 Rationale: The patient is nauseated; therefore it is important to judge which route is best for the patient, because of the chance of vomiting the medication.

4 4 Rationale: 0.5 g = 500 mg. If each tablet is 250 mg, then two tablets are needed.

5 4 Rationale: The nurse must know how the medication is metabolized and excreted, whether through the liver, kidneys, or intestines. Whichever system is affected can affect the manner and amount of drug absorbed or excreted.

CHAPTER 21

Answers to Critical Thinking Exercises

1 A spacer device would be helpful for Mrs. Martin. She would just need to breathe in and out of the spacer device to receive the medication after pressing the metered-dose inhaler (MDI) canister.

2 The order for the albuterol is for 2 puffs 4 times a day, or 8 puffs a day. Dividing 200 actuations by the 8 per day, the canister will last for about 25 days. Mrs. Martin should mark her calendar a few days before the 25 days will pass in order to get the medication refilled in time.

3 The nurse should explain to Mrs. Martin that the old medication should be removed before applying new medication. The layer of old medication will reduce the antibacterial action of the ointment. The nurse should demonstrate to Mrs. Martin how to do the wound care, then watch as Mrs. Martin performs it herself.

4 The nurse needs to review the correct technique for transdermal patch application and removal with Mrs. Martin. The old patches should be removed, folded with sticky sides together, wrapped in paper, and discarded. The new patch should be applied to a new area of skin, and the old site washed with soap and water to remove residue. Mrs. Martin may need to check to see if her physician would like her to have a nitrate-free period overnight. If so, then the patch would be removed at bedtime and a new patch applied in the morning.

5 The nurse needs to explain that sublingual nitroglycerin tablets are to be placed under the tongue and allowed to dissolve completely before swallowing the saliva. Chewing the medication during an episode of chest pain will reduce its effectiveness.

Answers to Review Questions

1 4 Rationale: An oral-dosing syringe has the appropriate markings for accuracy and usually has a protective colored tip to prevent its being lost in the infant's environment.

2 3 The nurse must explain that the tablet should not be crushed, broken, or chewed.

3 4, 5, 6 Rationale: The tube should be adequately flushed after the last dose of medication to decrease the chance of crusting inside the tube and to ensure that all the medication has left the tube. Gastric residual should be checked before giving the medications. If too much gastric content is still left in the stomach, there may be a problem with the patient's rate of absorption, which can affect the medication absorption, as well. The head of the bed should be left elevated to prevent aspiration.

4 2 Rationale: Because the patient is immunocompromised and has a large wound, sterile gloves should be used when applying medication because of the risk for infection.

5 1 Rationale: Applying the patch to a different area each time prevents skin irritation, which would affect the absorption rate.

CHAPTER 22

Answers to Critical Thinking Exercises

1 Before you give the medication, you need the following information:
- The drug classification, desired effect, and nursing implications associated with heparin therapy, such whether or not a filter needle is needed with medication preparation
- The safe dose for the medication and compare it with the ordered dose
- The amount of medication in milliliters to be administered
- If heparin comes in a vial or an ampule
- If any of the patient's current medications, diet, or herbal supplements have potential interactions with heparin or put the patient at increased risk for bleeding
- The anticipated adverse effects of heparin

2 You need to know:
- The patient's weight
- If anything is affecting the blood flow to subcutaneous tissues of the abdomen
- Nutritional and fluid status and skin turgor
- Partial thromboplastin time to evaluate the desired effect

3 If institutional policy or pharmacy allows the multiple-dose vial to be used again, evaluate the vial for:
- Desired dose, including the amount of medication in each milliliter of solution
- Expiration date before opening the vial
- Color of solution in vial and whether precipitate is present

4 You should always use the smallest syringe possible when preparing medication. Usually a 25-gauge ⅜- to ⅝-inch needle will deposit medication into the subcutaneous tissue of a normal-size patient; however, this patient is overweight and may need a different size needle. Use the abdomen, staying 2.5 cm (1 inch) away from the umbilicus.

5 You need to know:
- If a medication needs to be diluted before you administer it by intravenous (IV) push
- The rate per minute of administration
- The patient's allergies to medications
- The compatibility of IV medications with IV fluids before administering the medication

Answers to Review Questions

1 2 Rationale: The nurse should calculate and determine how much medication needs to be injected into the patient, while considering which route is being used. This needs to be done before the diluent and powder are mixed.

2 1 Rationale: The medication from the vial is withdrawn first to prevent any contamination of the vial with medication from the ampule.

3 2 Rationale: A 22-gauge, 1½-inch needle will penetrate the ventrogluteal area and disperse the aqueous-based medication easily. The other needle sizes are either too small or too large.

4 1 Rationale: The patient is experiencing infiltration of the IV infusion, and the site needs to be changed.

5 1 Rationale: Assessment of the condition of the IV insertion site is the priority. If there is a problem with the site, the medication cannot be given.

CHAPTER 23

Answers to Critical Thinking Exercises

1 Additional information may include the following:
a Pulmonary system
  (1) Pulse oximetry
  (2) Observe breathing pattern.
  (3) Observe for use of accessory muscles and nasal flaring.
  (4) Auscultate lungs for adventitious sounds.

(5) Auscultate lungs to determine if adventitious lung sounds clear with coughing.

(6) Observe sputum for color, thickness, amount, and patient ability to clear airway.

b Cardiac system

(1) Vital signs

(2) Heart rate and rhythm

c Neurological system

(1) Level of consciousness (LOC)

(2) Orientation

(3) Ability to follow instructions

Rationale: Mr. Landon is very fatigued and short of breath, which makes taking a history difficult. Obtaining cardiopulmonary data through a focused assessment enables the nurse to identify pertinent data about the patient's status before treatment. In addition, a brief neurological examination obtains baseline LOC and orientation and assists in determining the patient's ability to follow instructions. These baseline data help to determine the patient's present cardiopulmonary and oxygenation status without increasing patient's level of fatigue. Remember, in patients without underlying cardiac disease, the body adapts to decreased oxygenation or increased oxygen demands by increasing heart rate and blood pressure. In addition, the nurse has a sense of the patient's understanding of care and ability to participate in care through coughing and deep breathing, anticipated oxygen therapy, etc.

2 Administration of oxygen therapy

a The FIO_2 level is between 24% and 28%.

b Hypercarbia is a risk for patients with chronic obstructive pulmonary disease (COPD) because the oxygen therapy may override the adapted respiratory drive. As a result, CO_2 is retained, and there is an increased risk for respiratory failure in this patient.

3 Comfort measures to use with oxygen therapy

a The strap on the cannula may be too tight or placed incorrectly. Inspect the external ears where the cannula strap rested to observe for any skin irritation. Adjust the fit of the cannula, and place pressure-relieving devices (e.g., ear protectors or folded 4×4) under the elastic strap of the cannula.

b The oxygen may dry out the nasal mucosa, and the cannula itself can irritate the patient's nares. Inspect nares for skin irritation. Evaluate the humidification level of the oxygen therapy; perhaps more humidification is needed.

4 The correct answer is D. Partial rebreather mask mixes exhaled carbon dioxide with oxygen and causes an increase in carbon dioxide. Because Mr. Landon has underlying COPD and pneumonia, he is at risk for carbon dioxide retention, and this risk is further increased by the partial rebreather mask.

5 Worsening of patient's oxygenation status

a Mr. Landon is confused at times, and his level of consciousness is decreased. Bilevel positive airway pressure (BiPAP) requires a snug-fitting face mask. It is possible that the patient will feel claustrophobic or be so confused that he will continually attempt to remove the mask. It is important that someone (e.g., nursing assistive personnel, family) be with him to reinforce why the mask is in place and to help relieve anxiety. If BiPAP is effective in a patient, the LOC and oxygenation levels usually improve within 20 to 30 minutes of therapy.

b There is a risk for carbon dioxide retention. Monitoring of continuous pulse oximetry provides oxygen saturation trends. Serial arterial blood gas (ABG) levels (e.g., ABG levels taken every hour) provide data to monitor carbon dioxide and pH levels.

6 The correct answer is B. As patients' oxygenation declines, they work harder; therefore the respiratory rate is increased. But the results of this work are ineffective, and the oxygen saturation falls, and they retain more carbon dioxide. As a result of the carbon dioxide retention, patients develop a carbon dioxide narcosis in which they become very sleepy. As patients improve, answer D would reflect part of the clinical picture.

Answers to Review Questions

1 1 A respiratory rate of 24 breaths per minute could be seen in a dyspneic patient because it is an elevated rate. All of the other options

would be seen when hypoxia has been present for a long time, not from a sudden onset.

2 2 Rationale: If the reservoir is deflated, the patient breathes in large amounts of carbon dioxide.

3 3 Rationale: The fluid from the humidification unit may have started to pool in the lowest level of the corrugated oxygen tubing and needs to be emptied away from the patient.

4 3 Rationale: Patients with an underlying diagnosis of chronic obstructive pulmonary disease are at risk for retaining carbon dioxide.

5 1 Rationale: This is the only option listed associated with low-pressure alarms. The other options are a result of situations associated with high-pressure alarms.

CHAPTER 24

Answers to Critical Thinking Exercises

1 Place bed in Trendelenburg's, and use three positions: left side-lying to drain right lower lobe bronchus, right side-lying to drain left lower lobe bronchus, and left side-lying with one-quarter turn back onto pillow to drain right middle lobe.

2 Chest examination revealed decreased breath sounds at bases posteriorly and over right lateral chest wall. There was decreased chest wall excursion, which was more pronounced on the right side. Patient complained of increased cough and sputum production and dyspnea. Respiratory rate increased to 30 breaths per minute, and oxygen saturation decreased to 85% on room air.

3 Improvement of lobar collapse on chest x-ray film is a common clinical finding after the successful application of chest physiotherapy (CPT). In addition, oxygenation usually improves, and dyspnea, tachypnea, fever, and leukocytosis begin to resolve.

4 Documentation includes the following: (a) tolerated CPT to bilateral lower lobes and right middle lobe using Trendelenburg's position; (b) breath sounds increased at both bases and right middle lobe area after treatment with decreases in rhonchi and palpable fremitus; (c) coughed up 30 mL of thick yellow secretions and drank two 8-ounce glasses of water during therapy session; (d) instructed family in how to position patient at home and how to do percussion and vibration; they performed an excellent return demonstration; and (e) repeat chest x-ray film showed reexpansion of right middle lobe and increased aeration of bilateral lower lobes.

Answer to Review Questions

1 1 Rationale: Right side-lying Trendelenburg's aids in the drainage from the left lower lobe.

2 1 Rationale: Sitting up in a chair and leaning backward onto a pillow will promote drainage from the area. The upright position will especially help with the air-filled abscesses.

3 2 Rationale: Postural drainage should be avoided for 1 to 2 hours after meals. If he finished his lunch at 1 PM, the soonest that postural drainage can be done is at 2 PM.

4 2 Rationale: Forceful cough is the best option given for this type of patient to clear his secretions. Increasing fluids will help thin the secretions but not help him to cough. Postural drainage as well as vibration and shaking are contraindicated because of the chance of fracturing a rib or causing injury to this frail patient.

5 3 Rationale: A current assessment of the patient is needed before decisions regarding treatment can be made. There can be a number of causes for the dyspnea and the bleeding. The physician will be notified but will expect current patient information to be available.

CHAPTER 25

Answers to Critical Thinking Exercises

1 The correct answer is A. Rationale: Yankauer suctioning is the method of choice; this enables the patient to clear oral secretions as needed, and it is a clean, nonsterile procedure.

2 The correct answer is B. The patient's pulmonary secretions are deep within the lungs, and the suction catheter must enter the trachea. The

Yankauer suction device is not designed to clear secretions within the lungs. Orotracheal suction risks introducing oral bacteria into the lungs, thus worsening the patient's pulmonary infections.

3 The correct answers are A, B, and C. Hand hygiene has a direct benefit in reducing nosocomial infections and the transfer of microorganisms to health care professionals. Sterile suction technique reduces nosocomial infection in patients in acute care settings, those with new artificial airways or new tracheostomies, or those patients with acute illnesses/trauma. Clean suction technique can be used in patients who have permanent airways, usually a tracheostomy, and are free of any pulmonary infections. Frequently clean technique is used in the home environment.

4 The correct answers are A, C, and E. Answer A: It is important to notify the physician or the nurse in charge because new care orders may be necessary for this patient; these orders may include antibiotics, chest physiotherapy, or diagnostic tests such as bronchoscopy. Answer C: In some patients increasing fluids may assist in liquefying pulmonary secretions. Before increasing fluids be sure to determine that it is not contraindicated for this patient. For example, patients with cardiac or renal diseases may not be able to tolerate an increase in fluids. Answer E: A sputum specimen for culture and sensitivity is needed because a change in thickness and/or sputum color frequently indicates an infectious process. The type of infection needs to be determined before administering an antibiotic. Frequently patients will have a sputum specimen obtained and then be treated with a very broad-spectrum antibiotic. Following the results of the sputum specimen culture and sensitivity, the antibiotics may be changed if necessary.

Answers to Review Questions

1 1 Rationale: Oropharyngeal suction uses a Yankauer or tonsillar tip suction device to remove large amounts of thick mucus. This would be most appropriate for a patient who cannot clear her airway by herself.

2 1 and 3 Rationale: The tracheal area must always be suctioned first because of the ease with which organisms can be introduced into the area, resulting in sepsis.

3 1 Rationale: When secretions narrow the lumen of the airway, the body compensates by raising the respiratory rate to provide adequate oxygenation.

4 3 Rationale: Whenever there is a drop in the patient's oxygen saturation, the patient should be assessed for an open airway. This follows the ABCs of cardiopulmonary assessment.

5 1 Rationale: This is one of the times notifying the physician is indicated. The patient has already been repositioned and suctioned, and there are no data that support that the nurse is allowed to reposition the endotracheal tube. The physician may need to order an x-ray film to check the placement of the endotracheal tube.

CHAPTER 26

Answers to Critical Thinking Exercises

1 Vitals signs will document patient's cardiopulmonary status and identify any early changes. Prompt detection and correction of air leaks related to the chest tube decrease the risks for chest tube complications and duration of chest tube placement. The hourly monitoring of chest tube drainage is to provide timely observations on the amount and type of drainage. During the first 3 hours 100 mL/hr is expected, and patient coughing and position changes can result in a temporary increase in drainage.

2 Avoid dependent chest tube loops; change position of patient and drainage tubes to prevent drained blood from pooling in the chest or tube.

3 This drainage is dark red, not bright red; it is not a large volume; and it is probably due to the rapid discharge of accumulated drainage from the chest. This discharge of fluid was probably stimulated by the patient's activity from bed to chair. However, because this is a fresh postoperative patient, you would take his vital signs to determine his tolerance to activity and to monitor cardiopulmonary status. You would also monitor chest tube drainage to be sure that the volume did not increase excessively, and you would implement measures to assist in

maintaining chest tube patency (see answer 2).

4 This is an emergent situation. Your patient has a recurrence of a pneumothorax or hemothorax or another unrelated problem, such as a myocardial infarction. Your actions are as follows: Notify health care provider of your findings, remain with patient, and get assistance in getting Mr. Robert into bed. It would also be important to make sure that supplemental oxygen is available and on and to verify that there is an adequate IV line. If the patient has had his oxygen and IV fluids discontinued, have someone bring the necessary equipment to the patient's bedside.

Answers to Review Questions

1 2 Rationale: Explaining that by controlling pain he will be able to be active and cough well is a true statement. Option 1 is very close, but there is no guarantee that the medication will not make him too sleepy.

2 3 Rationale: The pneumothorax is getting worse. The signs and symptoms are indicative of respiratory distress.

3 1 Rationale: Monitoring chest tube drainage and maintaining chest tube patency are the key priorities when a patient has a chest tube.

4 1 Rationale: Because the patient has a pneumothorax, and air, not fluid needs to be removed, the tubes are placed high. If fluid solely needs to be removed, the tubes would be lower. If the patient had both a pneumothorax and a hemothorax, there would be one tube placed high and one placed low.

5 3 Rationale: Place an occlusive dressing over chest tube site helps prevent the air leak from getting worse as well as helping prevent bacteria from entering the site. It is essential to check vital signs to assess the status of the patient.

CHAPTER 27

Answers to Critical Thinking Exercises

1 The correct answer is B. Rationale: Upon finding an unconscious patient, you must call for help immediately to mobilize necessary equipment for defibrillation.

2 The correct answer is A. Rationale: In a hospital setting where protected methods of artificial ventilation are available, mouth-to-mouth without a barrier device is not recommended because of the risk for microbial contamination.

3 The correct answer is A. Rationale: Need to verify that after successful ventilation the patient is pulseless before initiation of chest compressions or automated external defibrillator (AED) in adults.

4 The correct answer is B. Cardiopulmonary resuscitation (CPR) interruptions should be minimized. Only very brief interruptions should be allowed for changing CPR personnel during pulse checks, defibrillation, and intubation.

5 Reassessment of the primary ABCDs will continue even after the code team has arrived. Assisting the code team with performance of the secondary ABCDs may include handing off the requested supplies from the crash cart, setting up suction, establishing peripheral or central intravenous (IV) access, chest auscultation upon intubation, connection to a monitor/defibrillator, relaying significant patient information to the code team, or administering or handing off medications. Delegation of other actions may include having someone assist the victim's roommate or visitors away from the code scene, assigning pastoral care or other nurses to communicate with family members, delegating someone to remove excess furniture or equipment from the room, having someone bring the patient's chart to the bedside, assigning a fresh person to perform chest compressions, or assigning another nurse to record/document the events of the code.

Answers to Review Questions

1 4 Rationale: It may stimulate vomiting or laryngospasm if inserted in the semiconscious patient.

2 3 Rationale: It is essential to continue compressions if no pulse is present until the AED prompt says not to touch the patient.

3 3 Rationale: The jaw-thrust technique prevents head extension and neck movement, which is crucial to prevention of paralysis or spinal cord injury.

4   4 Rationale: Rapid and thorough compressions are essential for maintaining some degree of circulation during this time.

5   4 Rationale: There needs to be a brief pause physiologically before another shock is delivered.

CHAPTER 28

Answers to Critical Thinking Exercise

1   The correct microdrip rate would be 100 gtt/min. The correct macrodrip rate would be 25 gtt/min.

2   The following steps are necessary before initiating the IV:
   - You should first check the health care provider's order to ensure that there is a written order for the initiation of the IV, solution, rate of administration, additives, and medications.
   - Check the IV solution for integrity, including, but not limited to, discoloration, cloudiness, leakage, expiration date.
   - Obtain IV history from the patient. Provide explanation of the procedure to the patient. Allay any anxieties, and answer any questions the patient may have.
   - Obtain all equipment necessary for the procedure.
   - Check laboratory data to evaluate any abnormalities, such as K^+, that should be considered before starting the IV solution.

3   The presence of discomfort at the site warrants closer inspection for signs of phlebitis or infiltration. The nurse should also check to be sure the slower rate is not positional or that the IV tubing is not kinked. If the patient has early signs of phlebitis or infiltration, stop the infusion. Check with the physician to determine if new IV in the right arm will be sufficient. For phlebitis, apply a warm, moist compress to the site. For infiltration, elevate arm on pillow.

4   Document the following:
   - All signs and symptoms of complications of the IV catheter, such as tenderness and pain at site, redness, swelling
   - Discontinuation of the IV: size and length of catheter, amount of fluid infused, medication administered
   - Interventions initiated, such as warm compresses
   - Patient response to procedure

5   The following are teaching considerations:
   - Instruct the patient in the signs and symptoms of complications of IV catheters, such as tenderness and pain at site, redness, and swelling.
   - Instruct the patient in the need to keep IV tubing unobstructed and free of kinks, to notify the nurse if tubing comes disconnected, and to place pressure on the site if bleeding occurs at the site.
   - Instruct the patient in how to ambulate with the IV using a rolling IV pole and keeping the IV solution container in a gravity-dependent position with the IV site.
   - Instruct the patient in any complications associated with the infusing of the IV solution, such as free flow, flow stoppage, blood noticed in tubing.
   - Instruct the patient not to alter the EID settings and to notify the nurse if the alarm sounds.

Answers to Review Questions

1   2 Rationale: The formula is $\dfrac{1000 \text{ mL} \times 15 \text{ gtt/mL}}{12 \text{ hours} \times 60 \text{ min/hr}} = 21$ gtt/min

2   3 Rationale: Phlebitis is evidenced by what the patient is experiencing. Coolness and swelling would be seen with infiltration. There are no data to support the other two options.

3   4 Rationale: The tip of the catheter should be in the superior vena cava above the right atrium of the heart.

4   2 Rationale: Although it is desirable to place an IV infusion in the patient's nondominant hand, this patient has a medical condition that dictates that the IV catheter be placed in her dominant hand or arm.

5   1 Rationale: The patient is susceptible to bleeding, so pressure should be applied whenever a device such as a needle is removed from his body while he still has prolonged bleeding times. You or the patient can apply the pressure for the required period of time.

CHAPTER 29

Answers to Critical Thinking Exercises

1   You should review the potential benefits and risks associated with blood transfusions. Describe and discuss options such as autologous transfusion and blood alternatives. Ms. Cooper needs to know that bleeding and blood loss may occur with long bone surgery and bone marrow insult. Blood transfusion may be a theraputic regimen in her recovery. Also explain that comprehensive testing and screening of blood products now reduces incidence of infection and disease transmission. The patient's blood sample is mixed with the donor's blood sample to determine the compatibility of the two. This will ensure she gets the correct blood type. Explain the process for verification of the patient identification and blood unit label information to prevent transfusion errors.

   As with any invasive procedure, the risk for infectious transmission may occur. Because transfusions are administered directly in the vascular system, nurses perform hand hygiene to prevent infection.

   If transfusions are not used when clinically indicated, recovery may be impaired. Ms. Cooper has the right to refuse blood transfusions. Because Ms. Cooper's surgery is elective, she has the option of providing autologous blood, which is her own blood donated in advance, to be used in the event she requires postoperative blood products.

2   Ms. Cooper needs to schedule an appointment with the blood bank to donate her own blood for personal use. Her blood cell counts, including hemoglobin and hematocrit, must be within the normal range. No donations may be made within 72 hours of surgery.

3   Mrs. Cooper can receive all blood types in a transfusion. Her blood cells carry A and B antigens.

4   You should verify the health care provider's orders for the transfusion of the blood product. A signed consent form should be in the medical record. A vascular access device that is patent without complications must be assessed before initiation. You should have a 0.9% NaCl infusion setup with either a stopcock or Y-tubing for the blood product. Obtaining baseline vital signs is necessary.

   The patient's name and identification number on an arm identification bracelet should match the transfusion form information. The unit number, component, ABO and Rh on blood product and transfusion record should match. You must verify this information with another staff member as required by the facility's policy. Most facilities have a transfusion form that should be completed to record the name of the blood product, identification number and expiration date, the patient's and donor's blood type, and patient identification, including name and date of birth.

   The blood product should not be at room temperature for more than 30 minutes before the initiation of transfusion. When there is a delay in initiating the blood transfusion, the blood product should be returned to the blood bank. Once the product is initiated, the product should be infused within 4 hours to decrease the risk for pathogen growth.

   You should remain with the patient for the first 15 minutes of transfusion, and monitor the patient throughout the transfusion. You may direct the nursing assistive personnel to take frequent vital signs and inquire about the patient's comfort. However, you maintain responsibility for assessing and monitoring the patient. If any adverse signs and symptoms are present, you should implement appropriate actions and notify the physician. You are responsible for documenting the time and date transfusion was initiated; the size, location, and type of vascular access device; any additional measures taken, such as pressure bag or blood warmer; reporting and documenting any adverse signs and symptoms; recording any premedications given or therapeutic medications given for adverse signs and symptoms such as fever, itching, rash; recording any instructions or teaching provided to the patient; recording the time and date transfusion ended; and evaluating the patient's response.

5   You should slow the transfusion and assess the patient for rash or hives and respiratory symptoms such as coughing, wheezing, or throat or oral mucous membrane itching. You should ask the patient to describe when and where the signs and symptoms occurred. The assessment should include the back and trunk because this is a common area of occurrence. A set of vital signs should be taken. You should reassure the patient that sometimes sensitivities occur during blood transfusions.

You should notify the physician for orders, which usually include administration of antihistamine and continuing the transfusion. You should continue monitoring the signs and symptoms, noting whether they dissipate or get worse. If they continue to worsen, the physician should again be notified. You should record the response on the medical record.

Answers to Review Questions

1 3 Rationale: Normal saline is the only IV solution that should be used with blood because of its isotonic quality. Dextrose solutions cause hemolysis of the red blood cells.

2 3 Rationale: Only negative blood types can be given to a patient with a negative blood type.

3 4 Rationale: When blood is stored, there is continual destruction of red blood cells, which release potassium from the cells into the plasma. If blood is transfused rapidly, there may be transient hyperkalemia before the potassium is reabsorbed. The hematocrit and hemoglobin values would indicate whether a patient needs a blood transfusion. The sodium level is not relevant to this situation.

4 2 Rationale: Comparing the patient's identification bracelet with the blood bag label number is the most important step to take.

5 4 Rationale: It is essential to maintain an IV access, but you do not want the patient to receive any more of the current blood. Another blood administration set should be primed with a new bag of normal saline in case more blood needs to be given. Remember to keep the old blood bag and saline, as well as the administration set, and send them to the appropriate department per protocol for analysis.

CHAPTER 30

Answers to Critical Thinking Exercises

1 Mr. Jasper's body mass index is 18.9; he is at the lower limit of "normal weight." With his condition he is at risk for being underweight unless his nutritional status improves.

2 With the left-sided weakness from his stroke he may have difficulty chewing or swallowing, and he will likely have difficulty handling food utensils or cutting his own food.

3 The patient could be given additional snacks or be offered small meals 5 times a day. In addition, butter, margarine, and honey can be added to his pureed food to increase kcaloric density. Finally, you could arrange to have Mr. Jasper also receive oral nutritional supplements.

4 If Mr. Jasper is having swallowing difficulty, the daughter might encourage her father to position his head with the chin down while swallowing. The daughter should help her father eat slowly, taking smaller amounts of food in his mouth. It would be helpful for the daughter to know the signs and symptoms of aspiration so she can alert a staff member if her father develops problems.

Answers to Review Questions

1 2 Rationale: A score of 19 indicates that the patient is at risk for being malnourished. All of the measures are important, but the dietitian's expert knowledge of nutrition would be most appropriate initially and to find the most appropriate foods for the patient to eat now.

2 1 Rationale: It is a federally funded program aimed at identifying older adults at nutrition risk.

3 1 Rationale: The patient has glossitis and a possible B_{12} deficiency.

4 4 Rationale: Both the pain and the nausea must be addressed, and option 4 is the only one that does that. All of the other options could be used after the pain and nausea are addressed. This is an example of a situation in which the nurse identifies that physician intervention is crucial.

5 1 Rationale: The nurse has obtained a lot of information about the patient's condition, and if the patient is given something by mouth and aspirates, the patient could be injured. This is an example of "Do no harm." It is better to wait for further assessment, such as the results of swallow studies that might be ordered, than to risk patient injury.

CHAPTER 31

Answers to Critical Thinking Exercises

1 Assess Mr. Meeks' mental status, presence of a gag reflex, and ability to swallow. If he is unable to remain alert and chew or swallow food successfully, he is at risk for aspirating any regurgitated contents from a tube feeding.

2 Mr. Meeks may have difficulty understanding your explanation of the procedure. Use simple phrases, and take time to explain the procedure. Show him what the feeding tube looks like. He will possibly have trouble communicating, depending on his level of alertness. If he can communicate, have him use his right hand to make signals. You may need assistance to position him for the insertion. If he has a reduced gag reflex, you might not offer him water or ice chips for swallowing. Plan on having to coach him to successfully swallow during tube insertion.

3 Frequent aspiration of contents often leads to clogging of the tube.

4 For patients receiving continuous feeding, the aspirate will look like curdled enteral formula. The pH will likely be basic with a value of 5 or higher.

Answers to Review Questions

1 1 Rationale: Radiographic confirmation of nonrespiratory placement

2 2 Rationale: The tip of the tube is in the stomach. Because of the H_2 blocker, the volume of gastric acid secretion and the acid content of secretions are reduced, causing the pH value to be higher.

3 3 Rationale: The jejunostomy tube would be the safest route because it bypasses the face and is farthest from the lungs, decreasing the chance of aspiration the most, which is essential when facial injuries are present.

4 2 Rationale: Performing frequent hand hygiene has been found to be the most effective method of controlling nosocomial infections, regardless of the procedures. Bacteria from another patient can still be transmitted after the old gloves are removed if hand hygiene is not performed.

CHAPTER 32

Answers to Critical Thinking Exercises

1 Vital signs, electrolyte levels, weight, and fluid status (auscultating lung sounds, checking for edema)

2 Provides baseline for measuring tolerance to high concentration of glucose infusion

3 The fever is a likely indication of an infection, which could be the result of a catheter site or bloodstream infection. You should notify the physician immediately.

4 You would caution Mr. Giles about his enthusiasm and explain that it is unlikely he has gained all of the weight from a restoration in nutritional status. It is likely that some of the weight gain is from fluid retention. Your assessment would include auscultating lung sounds, checking for edema in the extremities, and comparing heart rate with baseline.

Answers to Review Questions

1 1 and 3 Rationale: The fluid for the total parenteral nutrition is hyperosmolar. However, you should avoid complex terms in the explanation. Explaining that the smaller veins cannot tolerate the concentration of the nutrients very well and become irritated easily is more easily understood by the patient.

2 1 Rationale: Elevated temperature, chills, nausea and vomiting, and chest pain are indicative of lipid infusion intolerance. Choice 2 could indicate a problem with the catheter placement. Choice 3 could indicate infection, and choice 4 is nonspecific.

3 2 Rationale: The Infusion Nurses Society recommends changing IV administration sets for 3:1 parenteral nutrition every 24 hours and immediately upon suspected contamination.

CHAPTER 33

Answers to Critical Thinking Exercises

1 The following assessments would be pertinent for this patient:
- Determine cultural considerations that would be appropriate as you care for this patient.
- Assess understanding and knowledge of her condition and treatment plan.
- Assess intake for the shift; check for trends in intake and output (I&O).
- Assess level of functional ability, including cognitive and physical ability.
- Determine if the patient has a distended bladder, if she feels as though she has to urinate, or is uncomfortable.
- Ask when the patient last voided.
- Assess patient's knowledge of condition.

2 Explain the term *postvoid residual* (PVR). Include when this assessment is important.
- Postvoid residual is an assessment to determine the amount of urine remaining in the bladder immediately after voiding.
- It is a procedure used when the patient is unable to empty the bladder completely or unable to urinate.
- Residual urine in the bladder predisposes the patient to bladder overdistention and urinary tract infection (UTI).

3 Before catheterizing this patient, it would be appropriate to question the order because a bladder scan is possible. The scanner is an accurate, noninvasive method used to determine the volume of urine in the bladder. It does not increase the risk for UTI development, whereas catheterization is an invasive procedure. Use of the bladder scanner will possibly eliminate the need for catheterization.

4 The following teaching would be appropriate before assessing PVR:
- The reason the patient needs to void before the procedure
- The need to measure her urine after voiding
- That she needs to notify you immediately after urinating so the procedure can be initiated within 10 to 15 minutes

Answers to Review Questions

1 4 Rationale: The elastic adhesive must be applied correctly to hold the condom catheter on, but should not be tight.

2 3 Rationale: Inserting the catheter close to the bifurcation ensures the inflation balloon will be in the bladder and not the urethra of a male patient.

3 4 Rationale: Turning the patient to a side-lying position may move the tip of the catheter in the bladder and increase irrigation fluid flow from the bladder.

4 2 Rationale: Having a fluid intake of at least 2000 mL daily promotes urinary flow and helps prevent blockage of the catheter.

5 1 Rationale: The cloudy effluent indicates possible peritonitis and must be treated immediately.

CHAPTER 34

Answers to Critical Thinking Exercises

1 A fracture bedpan is best; it is easier to place in patients with restricted mobility. Mr. Simon can assist with placement by using a side rail or a trapeze bar. A commode is contraindicated because Mr. Simon is only able to use touch-down weight bearing and therefore may not transfer from bed to commode easily or timely.

2 It is expected that the Fleet enema would stimulate a bowel movement, and the fecal material expelled may be hard or range from hard to soft stool. In addition, Mr. Simon may have subsequent bowel movements throughout the day. You must instruct the nursing assistive personnel (NAP) about the expected outcome of the enema. In addition, you must instruct the NAP to immediately report to you any complaints of abdominal pain or discomfort, rectal bleeding, blood in the stool, enlarged abdomen, or changes in vital signs.

3 The following three actions will occur rapidly:
 1 Choice D. Perform an abdominal assessment. Mr. Simon's pain could be due to many factors ranging from benign gas to perfora-

tion. You need to collect data as baseline to monitor progression of pain and other abdominal signs and symptoms. In addition, you need data when you call his health care provider.

 2 Choice E. Obtain vital signs, and instruct the NAP to obtain vital signs (VS) every 15 to 30 minutes thereafter. You need to obtain the first set of VS as a baseline and compare with the patient's range of VS. The NAP then monitors these VS at your direction for frequency. This obtains valuable information while you are contacting the health care provider.

 3 Choice A. Notify the health care provider. You should now have abdominal assessment and your VS measurement data to report. You do not do the following:
 Choice B. Instruct the NAP to palpate Mr. Simon's abdomen. Assessment is a nursing responsibility. You may, however, instruct the NAP to notify you if it appears that Mr. Simon's abdomen is getting bigger or his level of pain changes.
 Choice C. Give postoperative pain medication as ordered. Although Mr. Simon indeed has pain medication, that medication is to control postoperative knee pain. It will take away or diminish his abdominal pain. Until the cause of Mr. Simon's abdominal pain is identified, the presence of pain and changes in quality and intensity are important clinical assessment findings that should not be masked by analgesia.

4 Stop the procedure and assess vital signs. Call the prescriber if the pulse remains low.

Answers to Review Questions

1 4 Rationale: Stimulation of the vagus nerve can cause a reflex bradycardia. It is essential to check the patient's vital signs before the procedure to establish a baseline.

2 1 Rationale: Having the patient place his chin to his chest after the tube passes the back of the throat closes the epiglottis, which reduces the chance of the tube going into the trachea.

3 2 The frail, underweight patient should be rolled onto the bedpan. The choice of using a fracture bedpan is an individual decision, but it often works better for patients with these characteristics. The bedpan should never be shoved under the patient because of the chance of shearing the tissue and causing injury.

4 4 A history of glaucoma would alert you that enemas should be avoided because they can increase the intraocular pressure. You should contact the physician and not perform the procedure.

5 3 The nasogastric tube is most likely just above the level of the fluid in the stomach and was not positioned far enough during surgery. The patient would experience nausea, and the abdomen would be distended because of the accumulation of gastric fluids and nasogastric irrigation fluid. You may advance the tube because the surgery was performed on the intestines and not the stomach. Remember, never to touch the nasogastric tube or irrigate it if the surgery has been done on the stomach because of the chance of perforation unless specifically allowed by an order from the surgeon.

CHAPTER 35

Answers to Critical Thinking Exercises

1 The correct answer is C. Stoma site marking should be done preoperatively to avoid having a stoma in a location that would make pouching difficult, such as in a fold or crease or a location that the patient cannot see. Choice A: It is not feasible for her to empty a pouch until after surgery. Choice B: A nutrition consultation may be needed after surgery, but often there are few dietary restrictions with an ileostomy. Choice D: The diagnosis of ulcerative colitis has already been made, so this diagnostic test for colon disease would be unnecessary preoperatively.

2 The correct answer is A. The stoma should be red and moist. Choice B: Retraction of the stoma below skin level is usually secondary to necrosis and does not occur until about 2 weeks after surgery. Choice C: Stents protruding from a stoma are seen with a urostomy, not an ileostomy. Choice D: The stoma may be pink after surgery, but it would be moist and producing mucus.

3 The correct answer is B. To avoid having the pouch get too heavy and loosen from the skin, it should be emptied when it is one-third to one-half full. Choice A: The pouch should not be changed daily because this could cause skin breakdown. Choice C: Pouch emptying cannot be done on a prescribed schedule. The frequency will vary with food and fluid intake. Choice D: An expected wear time for an ileostomy pouch is 3 to 5 days.

4 The correct answer is C. The effluent from an ileostomy is always liquid, though it may be thick or thin liquid. This is a normal finding with an ileostomy. Choice A: A colostomy produces a formed bowel movement. With an ileostomy, she will not have a formed bowel movement. Choice B: Although foods eaten may affect the consistency of the output, they will not cause constipation or a more solid bowel movement. Choice D: Reducing fluid intake may cause electrolyte imbalance but will not cause the effluent from the ileostomy to be formed.

Answers for Review Questions

1 4 Rationale: The repositioning of the patient might facilitate additional drainage through the catheter.
2 3 Rationale: Active participation in his care shows the most acceptance of his body image.
3 4 Rationale: The stoma will initially be edematous. The swelling will decrease normally over 4 to 6 weeks.
4 4 Rationale: Assessment is the first step of the nursing process, and by using an open-ended question, you can determine the specific concerns the patient has. Shifting responsibility to the physician is inappropriate, and waiting until after the surgery to address the issue only increases the patient's anxiety. Having a person with an ostomy will be very helpful, but assessment needs to be done first.
5 2 Rationale: The patient needs assistance immediately before the enzymes from the drainage can continue to break down the skin. The ostomy care nurse is the best resource person to contact.

CHAPTER 36

Answers to Critical Thinking Exercises

1 Obesity, diabetes, and smoking place Mrs. Edmonds at increased risk for a surgical site infection (SSI). Antibiotics should not be given beyond 24 hours unless there is a clinical indication. You will need to instruct Mrs. Edmonds that she will not be allowed to smoke in the hospital and follow up to ensure she has an order for a substitute nicotine product if needed and offer smoking cessation instruction/consultation. Glycemic control must be maintained during the recovery period to promote incision healing.
2 You will need to reinforce with Mrs. Edmonds how to turn, cough, deep breathe, and use the incentive spirometer. Instruction in pain-control measures, including how to use the patient-controlled analgesia (PCA) device as well as how to splint her incision with a small pillow before coughing, turning, or ambulating, must also be reinforced. Early ambulation and the need to wear intermittent pneumatic compression (IPC) while in bed or up in chair must also be included. Include family in teaching, and reinforce that for safety reasons Mrs. Edmonds is the only person to activate the PCA device.
3 Given her history of smoking, following general anesthesia, she is at an increased risk for pulmonary complications. Include lung auscultation as part of routine assessment, and closely monitor respiratory rate, temperature, and presence of productive cough. A history of obesity, taking birth control pills, and undergoing pelvic surgery place her at an increased risk for deep vein thrombosis (DVT)/venous thromboembolism (VTE). Mrs. Edmonds will need anticoagulant therapy and must wear IPC while she is in bed or sitting up in the chair.
4 Patient should be instructed to use PCA device before ambulating/performing exercises and to splint incision with small pillow to decrease incisional discomfort.

Answers to Review Questions

1 1, 2, 3, 4, 5, and 6 Rationale: Hair is removed using an electric shaver so the skin is intact, thus reducing the chance of surgical site infection. All of the other statements are true.

2 2 Rationale: Compression devices are applied preoperatively and are generally some type of either knee-high or thigh-high compression hosiery. They prevent pooling of blood in the lower extremities. The pneumatic compression devices may or may not be used during surgery. The patient may not be able to ambulate after surgery due to the nature of the surgery, or physical therapy may be needed before ambulating.
3 4 Rationale: The institution's protocol needs to be followed, and possibly a representative of the institution who is familiar with these situations, such as a risk manager, may be helpful in this situation.
4 3 Rationale: The physicians should discuss and document issues with the patient and/or family to determine whether "do not resuscitate" (DNR) orders are to be maintained or modified during surgical procedures.
5 2 Rationale: Mark the dressing with a circle around the drainage and the time noted. This will give an objective assessment of the extent of the drainage and can be continually reassessed.

CHAPTER 37

Answers to Critical Thinking Exercises

1 The correct answer is B. Rationale: A short prescrub wash/rinse removes gross debris and superficial microorganisms and must be completed before performing surgical antisepsis.
2 The correct answer is C. Rationale: Artificial nails may not be worn because they may harbor gram-negative microorganisms and fungus, thereby increasing the risk for the patient's developing a surgical wound infection.
3 After scratching her leg, Sarah should have stopped and immediately changed the affected glove because the area of the gown below the waistline is considered contaminated, thereby increasing the risk for the patient's developing a surgical wound infection.

Answers to Review Questions

1 3 Rationale: The circulating nurse assumes responsibility and accountability for maintaining patient safety and continuity of quality care. This includes patient assessment, review of consents and the medical record, supervision of the scrub technician, and delegating tasks to licensed and unlicensed nursing assistive personnel as appropriate.
2 1 Rationale: The surgical hand scrub has been traditionally used for many years.
3 2 Rationale: All surfaces on both hands, extending from the fingertips just past the forearms, should be checked for the presence of abrasions, cuts, or open lesions. Rings should be removed totally, and artificial nails need to be removed weeks before being in a surgical environment in order for the nails and skin to heal after the artificial nails are removed.
4 1 Rationale: Both hands should be covered with the cuffs of the gown to provide sterility.
5 4 Rationale: Anything sterile touched by something or someone unsterile becomes unsterile.

CHAPTER 38

Answers to Critical Thinking Exercises

1 The correct answers are A, B, and E. Rationale:
   - Prednisone is a steroid. Steroids decrease the inflammatory response and slow collagen synthesis, impairing wound healing.
   - Diabetes mellitus impairs wound healing by decreasing tissue perfusion and hindering the release of oxygen at the tissue level.
   - Age impairs wound healing. Vascular changes, diminished pliability in collagen tissue, and scar tissue tightness contribute to impaired wound healing.
2 Granulation tissue is composed of new blood vessels that will bring nutrients and oxygen to the tissue. This type of tissue must be present in order for the wound to heal. Once a wound is filled with granulation tissue, healing will progress; thus a wound filled with granulation tissue is a good finding.

3 The correct answer is C. Rationale: This is the position of choice for abdominal wound irrigation. This position allows the flow of irrigation solution to go from the area being cleansed to an area that is distal and lower. The solution flows from a clean to a contaminated area. The collection basin helps to keep the patient's bed dry.

4 The correct answers are A and B. Use sterile technique, and direct the flow of solution from healthy tissue to infected tissue.

5 The correct answer is B. Rationale: A Jackson-Pratt drain is a closed suction setup. Once the collector is drained, push out the air by compressing the drain and closing it. When the collector is drained, all exudate should be removed and no pumping of the collector should be done.

Answers to Review Questions

1 4 Rationale: The fluid needs to drain from top to bottom, allowing gravity to help.

2 2 Rationale: If there is no order for the suture removal, then none of the other steps need to be taken. Nurses cannot remove staples or sutures merely because the patient said the physician said they could be.

3 3 Rationale: The patient should be premedicated because of the wound size. The patient should be positioned as flat as possible. The lower tip of the staple remover is placed under the staple, and there is no lifting up on the staple when depressing the extractor handles. The incision cleaning is started at the top of the incision and not the sides. When half the staples are removed, it means that every other staple is removed. This allows observation of how the wound is healing. In some instances, small strips of tape, called Steri-Strips, will be used where the staples were removed to help stabilize the tissue.

4 3 Rationale: The suture should be removed in a smooth continuous manner. The knot should have been snipped at the end distal to the knot. The scissors should have been held in your dominant hand and the pickups in your nondominant hand. Disinfectants are never used on living tissue because of their harsh chemical action. Antiseptics may be used on skin to remove organisms.

5 2, 5, 6 Rationale: The drainage needs to be emptied, measured, and recorded. After you have emptied the drainage, you need to depress or squeeze the drain flat before putting in the plug. This helps the suction mechanism to work. Attaching the drain to the patient's gown below the level of the wound helps to prevent the drain from pulling and also keeps it in a dependent position to allow for maximum drainage.

CHAPTER 39

Answers to Critical Thinking Exercises

1 He is likely not holding the dressing in place for 30 to 60 seconds, which helps dressing to conform. He also needs to apply a secondary dressing over the hydrogel.

2 The wound develops more necrotic tissue and increases in size. Drainage also increases.

3 NPWT applies negative pressure to a wound to improve granulation of tissue and reduction in the size of the wound. It has been very effective with diabetic patients. NPWT improves circulation to tissues. In addition, it eliminates the need for frequent dressing changes and is less painful.

4 You will apply a skin protectant or Stomahesive barrier to protect the skin.

5 Mr. Williams may be hearing an air leak through the edges of the dressing. You can use a stethoscope to auscultate around the edges of the dressing.

Answers to Review Questions

1 2 Rationale: To adequately debride a wound, the packing needs to be dry upon removal. The dressing was too wet when it was initially placed in the wound.

2 2 Rationale: The dampness of the gauze helps to attract drainage. It is essential that the gauze not be packed too tightly, which would decrease the open areas of the gauze that the exudate could fill.

3 2 Rationale: A hydrogel dressing is soothing and is the most appropriate one listed for a patient with burns.

4 1, 2, 3, and 6 Rationale: The following conditions, medications, or treatments interfere with wound healing: immunosuppressive drugs, diabetes, steroids, and irradiation.

5 4 Rationale: If the binder is placed either too high or too tight, the patient can experience shortness of breath, which would require you to release the binder and reapply it.

CHAPTER 40

Answers to Critical Thinking Exercises

1 You would need to do all of the choices. Hot and cold therapies require a physician order, validating location, duration, and temperature as prescribed in the order. Assessing current pain level and condition of the extremity provides a baseline assessment for care. Patient education regarding procedure, precautions, and signs and symptoms of frostbite should be explained to prepare the patient.

2 The correct answers are B and D. There is greater risk for tissue injury when there is diminished circulation. A confused patient may be unable to provide feedback about how the application is feeling and will need to be monitored more closely for signs and symptoms of adverse effects.

3 Mr. Montgomery's diabetes and confusion place him at risk. Diabetic patients frequently have peripheral vascular disease or neuropathy of the extremities. Confusion may decrease his ability to provide feedback about tissue temperature. The task can be delegated to the nursing assistive personnel (NAP), but you would need to increase monitoring to maintain patient safety.

4 The correct answers are A, C, and D. Localized cold therapy reduces blood flow to the injured body part, prevents edema formation, and reduces inflammation. Local analgesia is produced by slowing or blocking peripheral nerve conduction and preventing muscle spasm by decreasing spasticity.

Answers to Review Questions

1 3 Rationale: It is essential to assess the area being treated. It is important to monitor the machine, but the patient response is always the priority, especially because moist heat penetrates deeper into tissue layers.

2 3, 4, 5, 6, and 7 Rationale: Patients with decreased circulation, conditions that cause decreased fluid or nutrients to their systems, and the use of steroids for a long time are at risk for tissue injury.

3 1 Rationale: The area being treated would be slightly pale and cool to touch because of the decrease in circulation.

4 1 Rationale: Because the area being treated has little fat or tissue around it, the amount of time the cold is applied should be decreased.

5 3 Rationale: Shivering increases muscle activity, which in turn increases the patient's metabolic rate and therefore heat production, which is counterproductive.

CHAPTER 41

Answers to Critical Thinking Exercises

1 The multiple medications Mrs. James takes may cause dizziness and lead to falls. Her immobility is also a risk factor for falling because of muscle weakness due to lack of exercise and the risk for attempting to perform an activity she no longer can do safely.

2 The correct answer is B.

3 Despite older adults' risks, they learn how to negotiate their environments relatively well and are usually more aware of potential dangers. Thus older adults may often be more cautious than younger persons. Encourage the family to discuss with their mother what might provide a greater sense of security for both of them, such as installing an alarm system and a medical emergency alert system. Offer a home safety assessment.

4 Perform a caregiver burden assessment on the older sister, being careful to do so without offending either patient. Offer resources for respite care and home assistance as indicated. Discuss ways that the family can help the aunt even though they do not live nearby.

Answers to Review Questions

1. 1-6 Rationale: All of these topics would be covered to determine the physical and mental status of the patient and to check that the patient is not a victim of abuse or neglect.
2. 2 Rationale: The timed Get Up and Go test looks at how the person changes position and become mobile. The Mini-Mental State Examination (MMSE) is used to screen for cognitive changes. SPLATT is a mnemonic used to assess actual falls. A fall diary is used to record the events surrounding an actual fall. Safety is a priority for individuals of any age.
3. 4 Rationale: Soiled dressings should be double bagged in impervious plastic.
4. 4 Rationale: These are the physical abilities that the patient must have to help prevent falls.
5. 2 Rationale: The method of discarding the syringes has nothing to do with maintaining the blood glucose at a stable level. The kitchen temperature varies, and the insulin should be discarded by the expiration date just as the glucose meter strips should be discarded by the expiration date.

CHAPTER 42

Answers to Critical Thinking Exercises

1. Additional information needed:
   - List of current medications
   - Cognitive status
   - Problems with sensation or mobility
   - Recent vital signs, especially heart rate and rhythm—expect rate to be irregular if he is in atrial fibrillation
   - Motivation and willingness to learn
   - Insurance status and preferred or required durable medical equipment (DME) provider for purchase of catheterization supplies
   - Family or friends who are willing to help
2. The correct answer is C. The pulse of a patient with an arrhythmia should be taken for a full minute in case the pulse is irregular.
3. Mr. Anderson may be pressing too hard over the artery or is unable to locate it. Coach him in his technique, and reinstruct about artery location. You might also consider teaching him how to feel his carotid artery instead. If a cognitive deficit exists, teach a family member or friend how to check the pulse.
4. There are many teaching strategies you can employ to facilitate successful medication education in older adults (see Box 42-5). Some strategies to enhance Mr. Anderson's learning include the following:
   - Provide typewritten information in large print.
   - Provide information to the patient that he feels is important.
   - Repeat information that is important in the beginning and at the end of teaching sessions.
   - Develop a trusting relationship with Mr. Anderson.
   - Use a memory aid, such as a daily checklist, to help him remember to take his medications.
5. The correct order is F, C, B, D, G, H, A, E.

Answers to Review Questions

1. 3 Rationale: The best method of verifying accuracy is obtaining two readings within 1 to 2 minutes of each other using two different monitoring devices.
2. 1, 4, and 6 Rationale: He needs to stay away from anything that can cause a shock, such as short circuiting from an electric shaver. He also needs to stay away from an open flame, such as a campfire, unless very far away from it, but there still can be stray sparks, which can create a problem. A patient with home oxygen therapy needs an extra set of oxygen delivery devices in case one should fail. Using lint-free cloths for cleaning equipment reduces friction.
3. 3 and 6 Rationale: Instilling normal saline does not decrease hypoxia. The suction pressure stated is too high. The patient should not be flat. She should be elevated at least 30 to 45 degrees. The suction catheter would be in the sterile gloved dominant hand, which would allow for less chance of contamination.

4. 2 Rationale: He needs time and input to learn and participate in this important part of his care. There should not be anything or anyone that could distract his attention. There is no data to support that he needs enlarged written directions.
5. 1, 2, 3, and 4, Rationale: The patient is showing signs of aspiration. Raise the head of the bed and stop feeding. Then have the family caregiver notify the physician and verify tube placement. If difficult breathing continues, call 9-1-1.

CHAPTER 43

Answers to Critical Thinking Exercises

1. The correct answers are A and D. Testing sputum would be important to determine if Mrs. Yamamoto has pneumonia, identify the organism, and guide the health care provider in selecting the best treatment. Elevated blood glucose levels occur when a person with diabetes becomes ill. Mrs. Yamamoto's blood glucose level is elevated because of her pneumonia.
2. As a point-of-care laboratory test, finger sticks for blood glucose level would give immediate results. Sputum specimens need to be cultured and take 72 hours for results.
3. There are several issues to consider when deciding to teach Mrs. Yamamoto to provide a sputum specimen. Her limited use of English is a major barrier. The daughter translated previously. You could schedule a time convenient for the daughter to assist with translation. Pictures can be of assistance, as well as demonstration of what is desired. Determine if the hospital has translators, or use the free telephone service available in many areas.
4. You need to assess Mrs. Yamamoto's ability to perform a finger stick. The ideal is to demonstrate to Mrs. Yamamoto and then have her perform a demonstration when the next finger stick is needed.

Answers to Review Questions

1. 1, 2, 5, 6 Rationale: Answer 3 is incorrect; the head of the penis is wiped in a circular motion, not back and forth. Answer 4 is incorrect; the amount of urine needed is between 30 and 60 mL.
2. 1 Rationale: The first urine specimen is discarded. This signifies the beginning of the collection time, which ends 24 hours later. The patient is encouraged to void right before the collection time ends.
3. 2 Rationale: Tomatoes can change the result because of their high vitamin C content. Numerous other foods can alter the results.
4. 1, 4 Rationale: These are the only correct steps for this procedure.
5. 1 Rationale: Redness is the only objective data. All of the other choices are subjective, that is, what the patient says he is experiencing.

CHAPTER 44

Answers to Critical Thinking Exercises

1. Additional information may include the following:
   - Medical history
   - Relevant recent diagnostic testing
   - Home medications
   - Lifestyle assessment
   - Focused physical examination
2. The correct answer is B. Rationale: Cardiac catheterization poses a risk for blood loss and a risk for complications that would require emergency coronary artery bypass graft surgery. Hematocrit and hemoglobin values are needed to obtain a baseline hematological status that will be compared with possible repeat testing. Prothrombin time/international normalized ratio (PT/INR) is affected by warfarin, which Mr. Hall is taking for chronic atrial fibrillation. The physician needed to instruct Mr. Hall to stop his warfarin 1 to 2 nights before this procedure. A current PT/INR is needed to determine whether Mr. Hall is at risk for uncontrolled bleeding. Values for blood urea nitrogen and creatinine are needed to evaluate Mr. Hall's renal function and along with urine specific gravity to help determine whether Mr. Hall is dehydrated. Patients with baseline dehydration or impaired renal function are at risk for impaired excretion of the radiographic dye used during the cardiac catheterization procedure.

3 In the presence of another nurse, ask Mr. Hall the following upon arrival and just before starting the procedure: name; identifying number, such as birth date; purpose of visit. Also compare the information given verbally by Mr. Hall to his wrist identification band. Document both instances in Mr. Hall's medical record.

4 The correct answer is B. Mr. Hall falls into an American Society of Anesthesiologists (ASA) classification of "2—presence of mild systemic disease without functional limitations."

5 The correct answer is C. Patients who have not yet given informed consent need to wait until the health care provider provides explanation of the procedure. In addition, do not administer any medication that can reduce their level of consciousness, because it will impair their ability to give legal informed consent.

6 The correct answer is A. These assessments are in order of threat to life and tailored to the procedure that was done. Heart rate and rhythm are affected because of catheter irritation or injury to the heart. Respiratory effort and oxygen saturation are frequently insufficient if the intravenous sedation suppressed Mr. Hall past the level of "moderate" sedation. The procedure site can easily bleed if mechanically disrupted when Mr. Hall is transferred from the procedure table to a cart and then to his bed. A visual check is essential to make sure that the dressing, sandbag, or closure device is secure to prevent arterial bleeding. Fre-

quent pedal pulse checks help promptly detect any intravascular clotting that might occur at the procedure site and cause reduced circulation to the legs.

Answers to Review Questions

1 4 Rationale: The ASA score of 4 indicates that a consultation from an anesthesiologist may be indicated. This will vary among institutions, but the physician should be notified before the commencement of the procedure.

2 1 Rationale: The changes and assessment data indicate there is bleeding occurring internally.

3 1 Rationale: The patient with renal failure may not be able to filter out the chemicals in the intravenous pyelogram dye. The patient with one kidney may have total function of that kidney. It would not be contraindicated for the other patients.

4 3 Rationale: With the removal of fluid from the abdomen, the abdominal girth would be smaller, it would be easier to breathe, and the number of respirations per minute would be lower because of less fluid and pressure.

5 4 Rationale: Colonoscopy requires an empty bowel. Because sedation is used the patient needs to have nothing by mouth (NPO) for 8 hours before the procedure to decrease the need for aspiration.

Appendix

Terminology/Combining Forms: Prefixes and Suffixes

Medical terminology is similar to a foreign language. Many medical terms are derived from Latin and Greek sources. They often consist of two or more simple words or word elements. A word root or *combining form* may be put together with a *prefix* and a *suffix*.

Root—the basis of a word
    Example: *nephr/o/tic* (degenerative changes in the kidney)
    Root: nephr- (kidney)

Linking vowel—a vowel that joins the combining form to the suffix or another combining form
    Example: nephr/*o*/sis (disease of the kidneys)
    Linking vowel: o

Prefix—the beginning of a word
    Example: *hyper*/active (excessively active)
    Prefix: hyper- (excessive)

Suffix—the ending of a word
    Example: nephr/*itis* (inflammation of the kidney)
    Suffix: -itis (inflammation)

Combining form—the union of a word root with a linking vowel
    Example: *hepato*/megaly (enlargement of the liver)
    Combining form: hepato- (liver)

The following table provides some of the most commonly used terminology for your reference.

COMMON PREFIXES

PREFIX	DEFINITION
a-	without
ab-	away from
abd-	abdominal
acu-	sharp
ad-	toward
adip-	fat
ad lib-	freely, as wanted
aero-	air, gas
al-	toward
ambi-	both
an-	not
ana-	up
ante-	before, in front of
anti-	against
arteri-	artery
arthro-	joint
auto-	self
bi-	two
brady-	slow
cata-	down
chole-	bile
cili-	eyelid
circum-	around
co-	with, together
cogni-	know
colo-	colon
con-	with, together
contra-	against

PREFIX	DEFINITION
crani-	skull
cut-	skin
cyt-	cell
de-	from, lack of
demi-	half
dent-	tooth
derm-	skin
dia-	through, across
diplo-	double, twofold
dis-	to free or undo
dors-	back
dur-	hard
dy-	two
dys-	bad, painful, difficult, abnormal
ec-	out, out from
ecto-	outside
em-	in
embol-	to insert
encephalo-	brain
endo-	in, within
entero-	intestine
epi-	above, upon
erythro-	red
eso-	within, inward
et-	and
eu-	good, normal
ex-	out, away from
exo-	outside
extra-	outside
faci-	face
fiss-	split, cleft
fore-	before, in front of
gastro-	stomach
glosso-	relating to the tongue
glyco-	sugar
haplo-	simple, single
heme-	iron-based
hemi-	one half
hepat-	liver
hetero-	different
histo-	tissue
homo-	same
hydro-	wet, water
hyper-	excessive, above normal
hypo-	under, below
im-	not
in-	in, not
infra-	under, below
inter-	between
intra-	in, within
isch-	deficiency
iso-	equal, alike
lapis-	stone
lapra-	loin or flank, sometimes abdomen
latero-	side
macro-	large

PREFIX	DEFINITION
mal-	bad
meato-	opening
medi-	middle
melano-	black
mesa-	middle
meso-	middle
meta-	beyond, change
micro-	small
mono-	one
morpho-	form, structure
multi-	many, much
neo-	new
nephro-	kidney
oculo-	eye
onco-	tumor
oro-	mouth
osteo-	bone
pan-	all
para-	beside, beyond
per-	through, by
peri-	around
phago-	eating
poly-	many, much
post-	after, behind
pre-	before, in front of
primi-	first
pro-	before, in front of
pseudo-	false
quadri-	four
re-	again, backward
retro-	backward, behind
rhabdo-	rod-shaped, striated
rhodo-	red
scler-	hardening
semi-	one half
sub-	under, below
super-	above, excessive
supra-	above, excessive
stetho-	chest
sym-	together
syn-	union, together, joined
tachy-	rapid
tetra-	four
therm-	heat
trans-	through, across
tri-	three
ultra-	beyond, excess
uni-	one
vas-	vessel or duct
xantho-	yellow
xero-	dry

COMMON SUFFIXES

SUFFIX	DEFINITION
-ac	pertaining to
-agra	excessive pain
-al	pertaining to
-algia	painful condition, pain
-apheresis	removal
-ar	pertaining to

SUFFIX	DEFINITION
-ary	pertaining to
-ase	enzyme
-bi	two, double
-blast	developing cell
-cele	hernia, swelling, sac
-centesis	puncture of a cavity
-clasis	break, fracture
-clysis	irrigation, washing
-coccus	berry shaped
-crit	to separate
-cyte	cell
-desis	fusion, binding, fixation
-drome	to run
-dynia	pain
-ectasis	expansion, dilation
-ectomy	excision, removal of a body part
-emesis	vomiting
-emia	blood
-er	one who
-gen	forming, producing, origin
-genesis	forming, producing, origin
-genic	origin, formation
-grade	to go
-gram	the record made, mark
-graph	instrument for recording, machine
-graphy	the process, process of recording
-ia	condition
-iasis	morbid condition
-iatry	treatment, medicine
-ic/-ical	pertaining to
-icle	small, minute
-ism	condition
-ist	one who specializes in, specialist
-itis	inflammation
-lith	stone, calculus
-logist	specialist in the study of
-logy	process of study
-lysis	dissolution, setting free
-malacia	softening, soft
-megaly	enlargement
-meter	instrument for measuring
-metry	act of measuring
-odynia	pain
-oid	form, shape
-ole	small, minute
-ology	study or science of
-oma	tumor
-opsy	to view
-or	one who
-orrhea	flow, discharge
-osis	condition or state
-ous	pertaining to
-para	to bear (offspring)
-paresis	partial paralysis
-pathy	disease, suffering
-penia	deficiency, lack of, decrease
-pexy	fixation
-phagia	eating, swallowing
-phasia	speech
-philia	attraction for
-phobia	fear
-physis	to grow

SUFFIX	DEFINITION
-plasia	formation, growth
-plasm	growth, formation
-plasty	mold, shape, repair
-plegia	paralysis
-poiesis	formation, production
-ptosis	downward displacement, falling
-ptysis	spitting
-rrhage	bursting forth, rupture
-rrhaphy	suturing in place
-rrhea	flow, discharge
-rrhexis	rupture
-scope	instrument to visually examine
-scopy	process of examining, visual examination
-sepsis	infection
-sis	state of, condition
-spasm	involuntary spasm
-stalsis	constriction
-stasis	control, constant level, stop
-stenosis	narrowing, stricture
-stomy	creation of an opening
-therapy	treatment
-tic	pertaining to
-tome	instrument for cutting
-tomy	process of cutting, incision
-toxic	poison
-tresia	opening
-tripsy	surgical crushing
-trophy	nourishment
-ula	small, minute
-ule	small, minute
-y	process

Glossary

abdominal girth The measurement of the abdomen's circumference, taken at the same place with each measurement.

abduction Movement of an extremity away from the midline of the body.

accommodation reflex Adjustment of the eyes for near vision, composed of pupillary constriction, convergence of the visual axes, and increased convexity of the lens.

accurate empathy Communication technique used by a nurse to show understanding of a patient's feelings and experiences.

Acetest A test that measures the presence of ketone (acetone) bodies in the urine. A large quantity of acetone causes rapid change in the color of the Acetest tablet.

active listening An interpersonal process whereby a person hears a message, decodes the meaning, and conveys an understanding about the meaning to the sender.

active range-of-motion exercises Exercises of the joints performed by an individual without assistance.

active-assisted range-of-motion exercises Exercises of the joints performed by an individual with some assistance. A nurse, for example, helps support an extremity.

activity tolerance Kind and amount of exercise or work that a person is able to perform.

actual loss Any loss of a person or object that can no longer be felt, heard, known, or experienced.

acuity systems Systems to determine the right amount of staff according to weighted patient workload.

acute pain Severe pain with a rapid onset and of short duration.

addiction A compulsive physiological need for a habit-forming drug.

adduction Movement of an extremity toward the midline of the body.

adjuvant therapy The treatment of a disease with substances that enhance the action of drugs, especially drugs that promote the production of antibodies.

adrenergic drug A medication that mimics the effects of sympathetic nerve stimulation of the autonomic nervous system.

advance directive Document defining a patient's end-of-life care decisions.

adverse drug effect (ADE) Any noxious, unintended response to a drug that occurs at dosages normally used in humans for the prophylaxis, diagnosis, or therapy of disease.

adverse drug reactions (ADRs) Nontherapeutic effects of medications.

adverse reaction Unintended response to a drug.

aerobe A microorganism that lives and grows in the presence of free oxygen.

aerobic Pertaining to the presence of air or oxygen.

afebrile Without fever.

agglutinate A process by which cells that display antigens (red blood cells, bacteria) adhere to each other, or clump together.

air embolus A quantity of air that circulates in the bloodstream to eventually lodge in a blood vessel.

air fluidization The process of blowing warm air through a collection of microspheres to create a fluidlike environment; used in special mattresses designed to reduce pressure against a person's skin.

air leak Escaping air in closed chest drainage; may be patient centered or within the chest tube system.

air-fluidized bed A special bed designed to distribute weight evenly over its support surface. Fluidization is created by forcing a gentle flow of temperature-controlled air upward through a mass of fine ceramic microspheres.

air-suspension bed A device that supports a patient's weight on air-filled cushions, minimizing tissue damage from pressure and shear.

albumin An acute-phase protein involved in nutrient transport and the maintenance of oncotic pressure. Used as a measure of visceral protein status. Has a half-life of 14 to 20 days.

aldosterone A steroid hormone produced by the adrenal cortex that causes the kidney tubules to excrete potassium and reabsorb sodium and water.

Aldrete score Score based on the Aldrete Scoring System for determining a patient's postanesthesia recovery status.

allergen A substance that can produce a hypersensitive reaction in the body but that is not necessarily intrinsically harmful.

all-hazards event Multiple manmade or natural events with destructive capacity to cause multiple casualties.

all-hazards preparedness The comprehensive preparedness necessary to manage casualties resulting from a disaster regardless of etiology.

allogeneic Denoting a cell type that is from the same species but genetically distinct.

alopecia Partial or complete lack of hair.

Alzheimer's disease Dementia characterized by progressive confusion, memory failure, disorientation, restlessness, and speech disturbances. Cause is not fully understood.

amino acid An organic compound composed of one or more basic amino groups and one or more carboxyl groups. Amino acids are the building blocks that construct proteins and the end products of protein digestion.

amnesic syndrome Memory impairment in the absence of other cognitive impairments.

ampule Small sterile glass or plastic container that usually contains a single dose of solution to be administered parenterally.

anaerobic Pertaining to absence of air or oxygen.

analgesia A decreased or absent sensation of pain.

anaphylactic reaction Exaggerated hypersensitivity reaction to a previously encountered antigen. It is a severe and sometimes fatal systemic reaction characterized by itching, hyperemia, angioedema, and in severe cases vascular collapse, bronchospasm, and shock.

anaphylaxis An exaggerated hypersensitivity reaction to a previously encountered antigen. The reaction may be localized or generalized.

anastomosis A surgical joining of two ducts or blood vessels to allow flow from one to the other.

anemia A disorder characterized by a decrease in hemoglobin in the blood to levels below the normal range, decreased red cell production, or increased red cell destruction or blood loss.

anesthesia The absence of normal sensation, especially sensitivity to pain.

anesthetics Drugs or agents capable of producing a complete or partial loss of feeling.

anions Negatively charged ions.

anthropometry The science of measuring the human body as to height, weight, and size of component parts, including measurement of skinfolds.

antianginal A medication that dilates coronary arteries, improving blood flow to the myocardium to prevent angina.

antidysrhythmic A class of medications that possess properties for controlling abnormal cardiac rhythms (e.g., quinidine and propranolol [Inderal]).

antiemetic Of or pertaining to a substance or procedure that prevents or alleviates nausea and vomiting.

antipyretic Pertaining to a substance, such as a medication, that reduces fever.

apical pulse Measurement of the heartbeat as taken with the stethoscope placed over the apex of the heart.

apnea An absence of spontaneous respirations.

approximate To come together, as in the edges of a wound.

aqueous Watery or waterlike; referring to a medication prepared with water.

artificial airway Plastic or rubber device inserted into the upper or lower respiratory tract to facilitate ventilation or secretion removal.

ASA classification A classification system for ranking the level of a patient's physical health, established by the American Society of Anesthesiologists (ASA).

ascites Effusion and accumulation of serous fluid in the abdominal cavity.

asepsis The absence of disease-producing (pathogenic) organisms.

aseptic technique The methods used during patient care to prevent microbial contamination. They can be either clean (medical asepsis) techniques or sterile (surgical asepsis) techniques.

aspirant Fluid or particulate that is aspirated.

aspirate Withdrawal of fluid or air into the barrel of a syringe or suction device.

aspiration The entry of gastric contents into the tracheobronchial passages. This increases a patient's risk for aspiratory pneumonia.

astigmatism Abnormal condition of the eye in which the light rays cannot be focused clearly in a point on the retina because the spherical curve of the cornea is not equal in all meridians. Vision is blurred, and use of the eyes causes discomfort.

astringent A topical substance that causes constriction of tissues upon application; commonly used for cleansing the skin.

atelectasis An abnormal condition characterized by the collapse of lung tissue, preventing the respiratory exchange of carbon dioxide and oxygen.

atmospheric pressure Pressure exerted by the atmosphere. (Atmospheric pressure at sea level is 760 mm Hg.)

atrophy Wasting or diminution of size or physiological activity of a part of the body caused by disease or other influences.

audiologist A health professional with at least a master's degree who studies sense of hearing defects, diagnoses hearing loss, and works to provide rehabilitation of individuals with hearing loss.

auscultation The act of listening for sounds within the body to evaluate the condition of the heart, lungs, pleura, intestines, or other organs or to detect fetal heart sounds. Performed directly or most commonly through use of a stethoscope.

auscultatory gap The temporary disappearance of Korotkoff sounds when blood pressure is being auscultated. Occurs in hypertensive patients and may cause an underestimation of blood pressure.

autoclave An appliance used to sterilize medical instruments or other objects with steam under pressure.

Autolet A small instrument with a lancet used to obtain a capillary blood specimen.

autologous transfusion Transfusion of a patient's own blood through either predeposit, blood salvaged intraoperatively by a cell saver, or blood shed postoperatively.

automated external defibrillator (AED) Device used by basic cardiopulmonary resuscitation (CPR) providers to treat fast, irregular dysrhythmias with electrical shock to the heart using automated rhythm analysis and simplified functions.

autopsy Examination of the deceased's body performed to confirm or determine the cause of death.

autotransfusion The collection, anticoagulation, filtration, and reinfusion of blood from an active bleeding site. Used in cases of trauma and major surgery.

axillary Pertaining to the pyramid-shaped space that forms the underside of the shoulder between the upper part of the arm and the side of the chest.

bacteremia Presence of bacteria in the blood.

bacteriostatic Tending to inhibit development or reproduction of bacteria.

bag-valve-mask (BVM) or Ambu-bag Bag attached to a mask that provides artificial ventilations to a patient when squeezed.

balance Position in which a person's center of gravity is correct so that the risk for falling is reduced.

bariatric bed A specialized surface equipped with hand controls to allow for self-positioning, providing a stable, adaptable surface for managing the morbidly obese patient.

basal energy expenditure (BEE) The amount of energy required at rest for basic life processes such as breathing, maintaining body temperature, and cardiac function. Basal energy expenditure can be estimated or measured.

basal metabolism Energy needed to maintain the body's basic processes such as respiration, circulation, and temperature.

base of support Surface area on which an object rests.

bed rest Placement of a patient in bed for a prescribed period for therapeutic reasons.

belt restraints. Type of restraint used to secure a patient on a stretcher.

bias Influences that distort a research study's findings.

binder Bandage made of a large piece of material to fit and support a specific body part.

bioavailability The extent to which a dose of a drug reaches its site of action to produce an effect.

biohazard container Container used for medical waste that must be made of rigid material so as to be puncture-resistant and labeled with the words "Sharps Waste," and with a biohazard symbol and the word "Biohazard."

biological agent Bacteria or virus that, when released into the environment, has the potential to cause widespread and continuing infection and mass casualties.

biological disaster The unexpected release of a biological agent capable of causing widespread illness or contamination into the environment.

biopsy The removal and microscopic examination of tissue, performed to establish precise diagnosis.

bioterrorism/bioterrorist attack The release of a biological agent into a specified environment with the intent of causing mass casualties.

blood culture A laboratory test on serum to determine presence of infection in the blood.

blood group Classification of blood type based on the presence or absence of genetically determined antigens on the surface of the red cell.

blood plasma The liquid portion of the blood, free of its formed elements and particles.

blood transfusion Administration of whole blood or a blood component as cells to replace blood lost through trauma, surgery, or disease.

blood type Blood type identified by genetically determined antigens on the surface of red blood cells.

blunt-tip vial access cannula A needleless cannula designed to be inserted into vial adapter or for needleless access to fill a syringe.

body alignment Refers to the condition of joints, tendons, ligaments, and muscles in various body positions.

body mass index (BMI) A measurement of weight in comparison to height. Used to categorize an individual's degree of adiposity.

body mechanics Coordinated efforts of the musculoskeletal and nervous systems to maintain proper balance, posture, and body alignment.

bolus A large, round preparation of medicinal material for oral ingestion; a dose of a medication or a contrast material injected all at once intravenously.

bone marrow Specialized, soft tissue filling the spaces in cancellous bone of the epiphyses; responsible for red blood cell production.

borborygmus Audible abdominal sound produced by hyperactive intestinal peristalsis.

bradycardia An abnormality in heart rate in which the heart contracts steadily at a rate less than 60 contractions per minute.

bradypnea Breathing that is normal in rate but abnormally slow (less than 12 breaths per minute).

brain death The irreversible absence of all brain function, including brain stem function.

bronchophony An increase in intensity and clarity of vocal resonance that may result from an increase in lung tissue density, such as in the consolidation of pneumonia.

bronchospasm Abnormal contraction of the smooth muscles of the bronchi.

bronchus One of several large air passages in the lungs through which pass inspired air and exhaled gases.

bruit Abnormal sound or murmur created by turbulent blood flow heard while auscultating an organ, gland, or artery.

buccal Of or pertaining to the inside of the cheek; surface of a tooth or gum next to the cheek.

buccal medication Medication placed between the upper or lower molar teeth and cheek area and allowed to dissolve.

cadence Pace or rate of verbal communication.

calorie (Kcal) A calorie is the amount of heat required to raise the temperature of 1 g of water 1° C at atmospheric pressure.

cannula A small tube for insertion into a body cavity, duct, or vessel.

capillary closing pressure The amount of external pressure required to close off the blood flow to the capillaries.

carcinoma Malignant epithelial neoplasm that tends to invade surrounding tissue and spread to distant regions of the body.

cardiac Pertaining to the heart; pertaining to a person with heart disease.

cardiac arrest The cessation of circulating blood flow that eliminates oxygen transport or perfusion, usually precipitated by ventricular fibrillation or ventricular asystole.

cardiac output Volume of blood ejected by the ventricles of the heart in 1 minute; equal to stroke volume times heart rate.

cardiomegaly Enlargement of the heart; typical sign of heart failure.

cardiopulmonary arrest Sudden cessation of respirations, pulse, and circulation.

cardiopulmonary resuscitation (CPR) Basic emergency procedure for life support, consisting of artificial respiration and manual external cardiac massage.

caries Decay of a tooth; progressive decalcification of enamel and dentin of a tooth.

case management The assignment of a health care provider to assist a patient by assessing need for health care and social service systems and to ensure that required services are obtained.

cast Rigid plaster or fiberglass application molded over skin tissues to hold musculoskeletal tissues to permit healing of injuries.

cast brace Combination of a brace within a cast at a joint.

cast saw Saw used to cut through plaster to remove cast.

cast shoe Shoe worn over the foot encased in plaster.

cast syndrome A series of patient signs indicative of an untoward (claustrophobic) reaction to being in a cast.

casualty Any individual who is ill, injured, missing, or killed as a result of a mass casualty incident.

catheter A tubular device for insertion into vessels or body cavities for diagnostic or therapeutic purposes, to permit injection, or withdraw fluids.

cathartic Drug that acts to promote bowel evacuation.

catheterization Introduction of a tube through the urethra and into the bladder.

cations Positively charged ions.

cell cycle The sequence of events that occurs during the growth and division of tissue cells.

center of gravity Midpoint or center of body weight. In the adult it is the midpelvic cavity between the symphysis pubis and the umbilicus.

centigrade Temperature scale in which 0 degrees is the freezing point of water and 100 degrees is the boiling point of water at sea level; also called Celsius.

central venous access device (CVAD) A catheter placed in a large central vein to give medication, fluids, or blood product.

central venous pressure (CVP) Pressure in the great veins (superior and inferior vena cava) as blood returns to the heart.

cephalic vein One of the four superficial veins of the upper limb.

cerebrospinal fluid (CSF) Substance contained within the four ventricles of the brain, the subarachnoid space, and the central canal of the spinal cord.

cerumen Earwax; a waxy secretion produced by apocrine sweat glands in the external ear canal.

cervical halter Support for the head, made of cotton material, used for traction.

change-of-shift report Means through which nurses report information about their assigned patients to the nurses working the next shift for the purpose of providing continuity of care for patients. May be given orally in person, by audiotape recording, or during "walking-planning" rounds at each patient's bedside.

charting by exception (CBE) A charting methodology in which data are entered only when there is an exception from what is normal or expected. Reduces time spent documenting.

cheilosis Disorder of the lips and mouth characterized by scales and fissures.

chemical decontamination The process of removing or neutralizing contaminating chemical agents.

chemical warfare agent The use of the toxic properties of chemical substances to kill, injure, or incapacitate an enemy.

chemotherapy Use of drugs to prevent cancer cells from multiplying, invading adjacent tissue, and metastasizing.

chest physiotherapy Physical maneuvers, including postural drainage, chest percussion, vibration, rib shaking, and cough, to improve airway mucus clearance in patients with retained tracheobronchial secretions.

chest tube Catheter inserted through the chest wall into the intrapleural space by a physician.

chronic pain Pain that persists beyond the period of healing, ceases to serve a protective function, degrades patient function, and serves no adaptive purpose.

chronic venous insufficiency Abnormal circulatory condition characterized by decreased return of the venous blood from the legs to the trunk of the body.

circulating nurse A registered nurse (RN) considered to be the charge nurse in the operating room during a surgical procedure.

circumduction The circular movement of a limb; the motion of the head of a bone within an articulating cavity such as the hip joint.

clarifying An attempt to put into words vague ideas or unclear thoughts of a patient to enhance the nurse's understanding, or asking a patient to explain what he or she means.

clean technique (medical asepsis) The purposeful prevention of the transmission of microorganisms by using procedures such as hand hygiene and disinfection of equipment to reduce the number of microorganisms.

cleansing enema An enema, usually soapsuds, administered repeatedly until the colon is free of all formed fecal material.

clean-voided specimen A technique used to collect a urine specimen as free from bacterial contamination as possible without catheterizing the patient.

clinical guidelines Systematically developed statements about a plan of care for a specific set of clinical circumstances involving a specific patient population.

Clinitest A test that measures the amount of glucose and acetone in a urine specimen.

closed system suction catheter A suction catheter that is attached to the mechanical ventilator circuit encased within a sterile sheath. The catheter system permits sterile airway suctioning without interrupting mechanical ventilation or requiring the nurse to apply sterile gloves.

coagulopathies A disease or condition affecting the blood's ability to coagulate.

code event A declaration of or a state of medical emergency and call for medical personnel and equipment to attempt to resuscitate a patient, especially when in cardiac arrest or respiratory distress or failure.

colon Portion of large intestine from the cecum to the rectum.

colonization The reproduction of microorganisms at a specific site without the signs/symptoms of a disease or tissue invasion.

colonized The presence of bacteria on the surface or in the tissue of a wound without indications of infection such as purulent exudate, foul odor, or surrounding inflammation. All stage II, III, and IV pressure ulcers are colonized.

colostomy Surgical formation of an opening of the colon onto the surface of the abdomen through which fecal matter is emptied.

comforting Any nursing action taken to promote comfort of a patient, such as a back rub or change in position.

comminuted fracture A fracture in which the bone is broken into several fragments.

compartment syndrome Insufficient arterial perfusion to an extremity caused by trauma or stasis; leads to ischemia and tissue necrosis if not reversed.

compatibility The quality or state of existing together in harmony. The formation of a stable chemical or biochemical system, specifically in medication, so that two or more drugs can be administered at the same time without producing side effects.

compliance Fulfillment by a patient of the caregiver's prescribed course of treatment.

compound A substance composed of two or more different elements, chemically combined, that cannot be separated by physical means.

compress Soft pad of gauze or cloth used to apply heat, cold, or medications to the surface of a body part.

computer-based patient care record (CPCR) Record stored in a comprehensive computerized system that is used by all health care practitioners to permanently store information pertaining to a client's health status, clinical problems, and functional abilities. The CPCR can store numerous databases, including structured assessment data, clinical decision support systems, and diagnostic artificial intelligence. The CPCR will store information pertaining to a given client from any health care event and thereby provide access to information across a client's life span.

condition of participation A requirement that all patients be notified of their rights when entering a health care facility. Part of the Key Principles of Patient's Rights documentation.

conduction Mechanism of heat transfer involving flow of heat from one object to another with which it is in contact.

conjunctiva Mucous membrane lining the inner surfaces of the eyelids and anterior part of the sclera.

conjunctivitis A highly contagious eye infection. The crusty drainage that collects on eyelid margins can easily spread from one eye to the other.

constipation Condition characterized by difficulty in passing stool or an infrequent passage of hard stool.

contamination The introduction of infectious material on normally clean or sterile sites.

continent ostomy or diversion Results from a surgical procedure that leaves a patient with an internal pouch where either stool or urine is temporarily stored and the effluent is removed by intubation through the external stoma. It is continent because the effluent does not drain spontaneously from the stoma; instead, a catheter must be inserted through the stoma to drain the effluent from the internal pouch.

continent urinary diversion A surgical procedure that uses a distal portion of the ileum and proximal portion of the colon to create an ileal pouch. The ureters fromt the patient's kidneys are embedded in the pouch. A narrow ileal segment forms a stoma on the abdominal wall.

continuous subcutaneous infusion (CSQI or CSCI) A method of medication administration in which medication is administered continuously into the subcutaneous tissue using a medication infusion pump.

continuum of care Matching an individual's ongoing needs with the appropriate level and type of medical, psychological, health, or social care or services within an organization or across multiple organizations.

contractures Abnormal condition of a joint, characterized by flexion and fixation and caused by atrophy and shortening of muscle fibers or by loss of normal elasticity of the skin.

core temperature Temperature of deep body tissues and organs.

costovertebral angle (CVA) tenderness Palpation over this region can elicit tenderness. Tenderness is common with kidney infection or trauma to the region.

countertraction Use of patient's body weight or other weights, ropes, and pulleys to counter the pull of the traction weight.

crackles Fine bubbling sound heard on auscultation of the lung.

crepitation The sound and/or feeling produced when bone ends rub against each other. The patient describes the sound and feeling.

critical/collaborative pathway Tool used in managed care that incorporates the treatment interventions of caregivers from all disciplines who normally care for a client. Designed for a specific case type, a pathway is used to manage the care of a client throughout a projected length of stay.

crutch gait Gait assumed by a person on crutches by alternately bearing weight on one or both legs and on the crutches.

crutch palsy Temporary or permanent loss of sensation or movement resulting from pressure on axilla from crutch.

cryotherapy Therapy in which the skin is exposed to cool or cold temperatures; used to treat localized inflammatory responses.

cuff A plastic air- or foam-and-air-filled balloonlike attachment on the distal end of the endotracheal tube or tracheostomy tube that prevents loss of air from the lung and inhalation of foreign bodies around the tube.

culture Laboratory test involving the cultivation of microorganisms or cells in a special growth medium.

cutaneous stimulation Stimulation of the skin.

cuticle A thin edge of cornified epithelium at the base of a nail.

cyanosis Bluish discoloration of the skin and mucous membranes caused by an excess of deoxygenated hemoglobin in the blood or a structural defect in the hemoglobin molecule.

cycloplegic Pertaining to a drug that paralyzes ciliary muscles of the eye, causing pupillary dilation for ophthalmological examination or surgery.

cytology The study of cells, including their formation, origin, structure, function, biochemical activities, and pathologic characteristics.

dangling To sit on the side of a bed with legs dependent or feet on the floor.

DAR An acronym for a method of documentation that includes data (subjective and objective), action (nursing interventions), and response of the patient (evaluation of effectiveness).

dead space A cavity remaining in a wound.

debride To remove dead or damaged tissue from a wound; to remove dirt, foreign objects, damaged tissue, and cellular debris from a wound or burn to prevent infection and promote healing.

debridement Removal of dead tissue in a wound.

decompression Removal of pressure as from gas and fluid in the stomach and intestinal tract.

decontamination The process of removing foreign material such as blood, body fluids, or chemical, biological, or radioactive contaminants. It does not eliminate microorganisms but is a necessary step preceding disinfection or sterilization.

deep sedation An induced state of sedation characterized by depressed consciousness so that the patient is unable to continuously and independently maintain a patent airway and experiences a partial loss of protective reflexes.

deep tissue injury Purple or maroon localized area of discolored intact skin or blood-filled blister resulting from damage to underlying soft tissue from pressure and/or shear. The injured area may be preceded by tissue that is painful, firm, mushy, boggy, or warmer or cooler compared to adjacent tissue.

deep vein thrombosis A thrombus in one of the deep veins of the body, most often the iliac or femoral vein. Symptoms include tenderness, pain, swelling, warmth, and discoloration of the skin. It is potentially life-threatening.

de-escalation A communication strategy involving the reduction of anxious and/or agitated behaviors exhibited verbally or nonverbally by a patient; using a calm yet firm approach diffuses the patient's increasing anxiety and/or agitated state, thereby minimizing potentially violent outbursts.

defecation Passage of feces from the digestive tract through the rectum.

dehiscence The separation or opening of wound layers.

dementia A term used to describe a group of symptoms related to a loss or impairment of mental powers. These symptoms appear in a person who is awake and are demonstrated by symptoms of mental confusion, memory loss, disorientation, intellectual impairment, or similar problems.

dental caries Chalky white discoloration of teeth or presence of brown or black discoloration.

dentifrice A pharmaceutical compound used with a toothbrush for cleaning and polishing teeth.

Department of Homeland Security (DHS) The federal department that administers all matters relating to homeland security.

dermatitis An inflammatory condition of the skin characterized by erythema and pain or pruritus.

dermatological Pertaining to the skin.

detection and surveillance Awareness of the environment, recognizing what might be unusual or different, and knowing what these differences mean in terms of terrorism preparedness.

devitalized Tissues with reduced oxygen supply and blood flow.

dialysis A procedure that removes fluid and solid wastes from the blood or lymph.

diaphoresis Secretion of sweat typically associated with hyperthermia, physical exertion, and emotional stress.

diastolic pressure The lower blood pressure measurement, which reflects the pressure consistently exerted within the arterial system during the period of ventricular relaxation.

diffusion Movement of oxygen to the red blood cells at the alveolar level.

diluent Agent that makes a solution or mixture thinner or more liquid by admixture.

disaster A catastrophic and/or destructive event that disrupts normal functioning; it may include any anticipated or unexpected event whose effects lead to significant destruction and/or adverse consequences.

disaster management The discipline of dealing with and avoiding risks. It is a discipline that involves preparing for disaster before it occurs, providing disaster response, and supporting and rebuilding after disasters have occurred.

disaster response A phase of the disaster management cycle. Its preceding cycles aim to reduce the need for a disaster response or to avoid it.

disaster triage A model for sorting individuals by the seriousness of their condition and the likelihood of their survival.

discharge planning The process by which a nurse plans for a patient's eventual release from a health care agency; the process begins on a patient's admission to the agency.

distraction A pain-reduction technique that diverts an individual's attention away from the pain sensation.

do not resuscitate (DNR)

documentation Anything written or printed that is relied on as record or proof for authorized persons. It is a vital aspect of nursing practice and is a vital link between the provision and evaluation of health care.

documentation system Detailed information, in either written or computerized form, about a computer system, including its architecture, design, data flow, and programming logic.

dorsal Pertaining to the back or posterior.

dorsiflexion Flexion toward the back, as accomplished by a muscle (e.g., in the hand or foot).

dorsum The back of the hand.

double-void A procedure of discarding the first urine specimen and testing the second urine specimen that was obtained 30 to 45 minutes later; this procedure gives a more accurate amount of glucose being spilled into the urine at that particular time.

drawsheet A special sheet placed over the regular sheet on a bed and used to move a person in bed.

drop factor Refers to the calibration of intravenous (IV) tubing (IV infusion set) in drops per milliliter. For example, the drop factor of microdrip IV tubing is 60 gtt/mL.

drug tolerance (see Table 6-1) A decreased physiological response after repeated administration of a drug or a chemically related substance.

dry powder inhaler (DPI) Handheld device that disperses powdered medication for inhalation.

duration of action Length of time during which a drug is present in a concentration great enough to produce a therapeutic effect.

dysphagia Difficulty swallowing.

dyspnea Difficulty in breathing.

dysrhythmia An irregular, fast or slow heart rhythm.

dysuria Pain or burning on urination, may also be accompanied with difficulty in urination. Usually indicates an urinary tract infection.

ecchymosis Bluish discoloration of an area of skin or mucous membrane caused by the extravasation of blood into the subcutaneous tissues as a result of trauma to the underlying blood vessels or fragility of the vessel walls.

edema Abnormal accumulation of fluid in interstitial spaces of tissues.

effleurage A type of massage stroke that glides without manipulating deep muscles, smoothes and extends muscles, increases nutrient absorption, and improves lymphatic and venous circulation.

effluent The drainage that is expected from an ostomy.

egophony A change in the voice sound as heard on auscultation of a patient with pleural effusion. When patient is asked to make e-e-e sounds, the sound is heard over the peripheral chest wall as a-a-a.

elastic bandage Bandage of elasticized fabric that provides support and allows movement.

electrolyte An element or compound that, when melted or dissolved in water or another solvent, dissociates into ions and is able to carry an electric current.

electronic infusion device (EID) Used to infuse IV fluid at a prescribed rate. There are two types an infusion pump, which is designed to deliver a measured amount of fluid over a period of time, and an IV controller, which delivers fluid with the aid of gravity.

electronic medical record A medical record in digital format.

embolus (emboli) A foreign object, a quantity of air or gas, a bit of tissue or tumor, or a piece of thrombus that circulates in the bloodstream until it becomes lodged in a vessel.

emergency responders Those individuals whose job it is to respond to an emergency situation—typically police, fire, hazardous materials (HAZMAT), and emergency medical services (EMS) personnel.

empathy Ability to recognize and to some extent share the emotions and state of mind of another and to understand the meaning and significance of that person's behavior.

endemic The expected or normal incidence present in a geographical area or population.

end-of-life-care The human provision of physical, psychological, social, and spiritual support to a patient and patient's family at the end of life.

endotracheal intubation Placement of plastic tube into the trachea to provide artificial ventilations on a continuous basis.

endotracheal tube Artificial airway inserted through the mouth into the trachea.

enema Procedure involving introduction of a solution into the rectum for cleansing or therapeutic purposes.

enteral nutrition The administration of nutrition via the gastrointestinal tract (i.e., by mouth, tube feeding, or oral supplement).

enteral tube feeding The introduction of food or nutritive material directly into the digestive tract by nasogastric or gastric tube.

enteric coated Tablets coated with a substance that does not dissolve until reaching the intestine. Used when drug constituents are irritating to oral and gastric mucosa.

enucleation Removal of the eyeball, performed in cases of malignancy, severe infection, extensive trauma, or to control pain in glaucoma.

epidemic A disease that spreads rapidly through a demographic segment of the human population, with an incidence beyond what is expected.

epidemiology Study of the occurrence, distribution, and causes of disease.

epidural Administration of local anesthetic by way of a catheter into the epidural space of the spinal column. Designed to produce anesthesia of the pelvic, abdominal, or genital areas.

epidural analgesia Delivery of an analgesic into the epidural space in pain control.

epidural blood patch Procedure whereby a physician injects a small amount of autologous blood into the epidural space.

episiotomy A surgical procedure in which an incision is made in a woman's perineum to enlarge her vaginal opening for delivery of an infant; procedure prevents tearing of perineum.

epithelialization The process by which epidermal cells migrate (move) over the wound's surface to close the top or "resurface" the wound.

erythema Redness or inflammation of the skin or mucous membranes, result of dilation and congestion of superficial capillaries.

eschar Scab or dry crust that results from excoriation of the skin.

evaporation Mechanism of heat loss whereby moisture from the body's surface changes to vapor and transfers heat to the surrounding air.

eversion Turning outward or inside out, such as turning the foot outward at the ankle.

evidence-based practice (EBP) A problem-solving approach to clinical practice that combines the conscientious use of research-based evidence in combination with a clinician's expertise and patient preferences and values in making decisions about patient care.

evisceration The separation of wound layers with the protrusion of abdominal organs through the wound layers.

excoriation An injury to the surface of the skin or other part of the body caused by scratching or abrasion.

excretion The process of eliminating, shedding, or getting rid of substances by body organs or tissues.

exercise Performance of any physical activity for the purpose of conditioning the body, improving health, maintaining fitness, or as a therapeutic measure.

exit site Point at which a catheter leaves a body site.

exophthalmos Abnormal protrusion of one or both eyeballs caused by trauma, intracranial lesions, intraorbital disorders, or systemic disease, most commonly hyperthyroidism.

expectorant An agent that facilitates removal of bronchopulmonary secretions.

expectorate The act of coughing and spitting out mucus from the respiratory tract. Maneuver is useful in assisting a patient with clearing the airways of pulmonary secretions.

extension Movement increasing the angle between two adjoining bones.

external fixation Skeletal traction applied through the use of pins attached to a frame rather than weights.

external rotation Rotation of a joint outward.

external urethral sphincter Voluntary muscle that must relax in order for a patient to void or completely empty the bladder.

extravasation The inadvertent infiltration of intravenous fluids or medications into the subcutaneous tissues surrounding the infusion site.

extremity restraints Restraints used to immobilize one or all extremities.

exudate Any fluid that has been extruded from a tissue or its capillaries, more specifically because of injury or inflammation. It is characteristically high in protein and white blood cells.

Fahrenheit Temperature scale in which 32° is the freezing point of water and 212° is the boiling point of water at sea level.

fascia Fibrous connective tissue.

febrile Pertaining to or characterized by fever or an elevation in body temperature.

fenestrated drape A drape with a round or slitlike opening in the center.

fenestrated tracheostomy tube A tracheostomy tube containing a hole (fenestration) on the posterior aspect of the outer cannula that allows airflow over the vocal cords and speech in spontaneously breathing patients.

fenestration Surgical procedure in which an opening is created to gain access to the cavity within an organ or a bone.

fever An abnormal elevation of body temperature.

fiberoptic Pertaining to fiberoptics; referring to the transmission of an image along flexible bundles of coated glass or plastic fibers having special optical properties.

field triage tag Tags constructed of a high-density, water-resistant synthetic paper and printed using a special thermal printing process, allowing them to be used in field situations.

first responders Those public service providers required to be the first on the scene of a disaster, typically EMS, fire, or police personnel.

flexion Movement decreasing the angle between two adjoining bones; bending of a limb.

flora Microorganisms that reside on and within the body to compete with disease-producing microorganisms to provide a natural immunity against certain infections.

flossing Mechanical cleansing of tooth surfaces with the use of stringlike waxed or unwaxed dental floss.

flotation device A foam mattress with a gel-like pad located in its center, designed to protect bony prominences and distribute pressure more evenly against the skin's surface.

flotation pad A device constructed of foam or a silicone or polyvinyl chloride gel encased in a vinyl-covered square; protects bony prominences and distributes pressure more evenly against the skin's surface.

flow sheet A recording form used to document the same type of repeated measurements, procedures, or observations over time. Data on flow sheets allow the user to see trends over time.

fluid volume deficit (FVD) An alteration characterized by the loss of fluids and electrolytes in an isotonic fashion.

fluid volume excess (FVE) An alteration characterized by the abnormal retention of fluids and electrolytes in an isotonic fashion.

focus charting A charting methodology for structuring progress notes according to the focus of the note, for example, symptoms and nursing diagnosis. Each note includes data, action, and patient response.

fontanel A space covered by tough membranes between the bones of an infant's cranium.

footboard Board placed perpendicular to the mattress, parallel to and touching the plantar surface of a patient's feet and used to maintain dorsiflexion of the feet.

footdrop A falling or dragging of the foot from paralysis of the flexors of the ankle.

foramen magnum The large opening in the anterior and inferior part of the occipital bone, interconnecting the vertebral canal and cranial cavity.

four-poster cast Cast placed over the shoulders; contains four vertical posts or poles on the anterior and posterior lateral sides of the head to immobilize the cervical vertebrae.

Fowler's position Posture assumed by a patient when the head of the bed is raised approximately 45 to 90 degrees, as though the patient is sitting upright.

fracture pan A bedpan designed for patients with body or leg casts or patients restricted from raising their hips. It has a shallow upper end that slips easily under a patient.

friction Effect of rubbing, or the resistance that a moving body meets from the surface on which it moves; a force that occurs in a direction to oppose movement; in massage, technique in which deeper tissues are stroked or rubbed, usually through strong circular movements of the hand.

friction rub Dry grating sound heard during auscultation, caused by rubbing of tissue surfaces.

gag reflex A normal neural reflex elicited by touching the soft palate or posterior pharynx, the response being the elevation of the palate, retraction of the tongue, and contraction of the pharyngeal muscles. Tests for function of the vagus and glossopharyngeal nerves.

gait Manner or style of walking, including rhythm, cadence, and speed.

gait belt A leather or heavy canvas belt that encircles a patient's waist, it may or may not have handles. The purpose of the belt is for a nurse to hold when ambulating an unsteady patient to reduce risk for fall.

gastrostomy feeding tube Long, hollow, flexible tube inserted into the stomach through a stab wound in the upper left abdominal quadrant.

gingivae The gums of the mouth.

gingivitis Inflammatory condition in which the gums are red, swollen, and bleeding.

glucose monitoring A diagnostic test to determine the blood glucose level.

granulation The presence of red, granular, moist tissue that appears during the healing of open wounds; type of tissue containing new blood vessels that bleed readily.

granulation tissue Soft, pink, fleshy projection of tissue that forms during the healing process in a wound not healing by primary intention.

gravity The heaviness or weight of an object resulting from the effect of the attraction between any body of matter and any planetary body.

guaiac test Diagnostic test to detect blood in the stool.

guided imagery Technique in which patient focuses on an image, becoming less aware of pain.

gurgle Abnormal coarse sound heard during auscultation of the lung; produced by air entering large mucus-containing airways.

halitosis Offensive breath resulting from poor oral hygiene, dental or oral infections, ingestion of certain foods, or systemic diseases.

hand rolls Cylindrical rolls of cloth or gauze placed against the palmar surface of a patient's hand to maintain hand, thumb, and fingers in a functional position.

Harris splint Expandable splint that supports the thigh in skeletal traction.

hazard/hazard identification A condition or phenomenon that increases the probability of a loss that may result in injury or illness/recognition of conditions or agents creating risk.

healing ridge Induration of collagen deposits beneath the skin extending to about 1 cm on each side of the wound.

health care–acquired infection Infection that was not present or incubating at time of admission.

Health Insurance Portability and Accountability Act (HIPAA) A federal law designed to protect the privacy of patient health information.

heatstroke Condition characterized by core body temperature of 45° C (116° F).

heave A lift or thrust felt during palpation of the heart.

hematemesis Vomiting of blood.

hematology The study of blood cells.

hematoma Collection of extravasated blood trapped in the tissues of the skin or in an organ; results from trauma or incomplete coagulation.

hematopoiesis The formation and development of blood cells in bone marrow.

hematuria Abnormal presence of blood in the urine.

hemiparesis Muscular weakness of one half of the body.

hemiplegia Paralysis of one side of the body.

hemoconcentration The concentration of red blood cells in one area.

hemodialysis A procedure in which impurities or wastes are removed from the blood; used in treating renal insufficiency and various toxic conditions.

hemodynamics The study of movements of the blood and of the forces concerned therein.

hemolysis The destruction of red blood cells.

hemopneumothorax An accumulation of both air and blood in the intrapleural space. This condition is characterized by the signs and symptoms listed with pneumothorax and hemothorax.

hemoptysis Coughing up of blood from the respiratory tract.

hemorrhoids A varicosity in the lower rectum or anus caused by congestion in the hemorrhoidal veins.

hemostasis Termination of bleeding by mechanical or chemical means or by the coagulation process of the body.

hemothorax An accumulation of blood in the intrapleural space caused by a pulmonary infarction, tissue damage that occurs as a result of lung cancer or other chest trauma, or a complication of anticoagulant therapy after chest surgery.

Hemovac drain A type of closed drain system.

heparin lock An intravenous needle connected to a small "well" that allows for the intermittent injection of medication without the need for repeated venipuncture.

herniation The abnormal protrusion of an organ or other body structure through a defect or natural opening in a covering, membrane, muscle, or bone.

high-Fowler's position Placement of a patient in a semi-sitting position by raising the head of the bed more than 45 to 60 degrees.

hirsutism Excessive body hair in a masculine distribution, caused by heredity, hormonal dysfunction, or medication.

Homans' sign In the presence of phlebitis or when phlebitis is suspected, dorsiflexion of the foot elicits pain in the calf.

homeostasis The state of equilibrium (balance between opposing pressures) in the internal environment of the body, naturally maintained by adaptive responses that promote healthy survival.

hospice A system of family-centered care designed to assist the terminally ill person to be comfortable and to maintain a satisfactory lifestyle through the phase of dying.

Hoyer lift (mechanical/hydraulic lift) Mechanical device that uses a canvas sling to easily lift dependent patients for transferring.

Huber needle Special needle with a deflected point designed to prevent damage to the silicone septum of implanted infusion ports.

humectant A substance that promotes retention of moisture.

hydrocolloid An adhesive, moldable wafer made of a carbohydrate-based material, usually with a waterproof backing. This dressing usually is impermeable to oxygen, water, and water vapor and has some absorptive properties.

hydrogel A water-based, nonadherent, polymer-based dressing that has some absorptive properties.

hygiene The science of health. Self-care measures people use to maintain their health are called personal hygiene.

hypercalcemia Greater than normal amounts of calcium in the blood.

hypercapnia Elevated arterial $PaCO_2$ greater than 45 mm Hg; also called hypercarbia.

hyperemia Increased blood flow in part of the body, as in the inflammatory response, local relaxation of arterioles, or obstruction of the outflow of blood from an area.

hyperextension Movement of a body part beyond its normal resting extended position.

hyperkalemia Refers to solutions with potassium concentrations greater than 5.0 mEq/L.

hypermagnesemia Refers to solutions with magnesium concentrations greater than 2.5 mEq/L.

hypernatremia Refers to solutions with sodium concentrations greater than 147 mEq/L.

hyperopia A refractive error of the eye in which parallel rays of light focus behind the retina; causes difficulty seeing near objects.

hyperphosphatemia Refers to a higher than normal range of serum phosphorus. Normal range for serum phosphorus is 2.5 to 4.5 mg/100 mL (1.7 to 2.6 mEq/L).

hyperpigmentation Unusual darkening of the skin.

hypertension Condition characterized by an elevated blood pressure persistently exceeding 150/90 mm Hg.

hyperthermia Condition characterized by body temperature over 38° C (100.4° F).

hypertonic Having a greater concentration of solute than another solution, hence exerting more osmotic pressure a total electrolyte content of 375 mEq/L or greater.

hypodermoclysis The injection of an isotonic or hypotonic solution into subcutaneous tissue to supply a continuous and large amount of fluid, electrolytes, and nutrients.

hypokalemia Refers to solutions with potassium concentrations less than 3.5 mEq/L.

hypomagnesemia Refers to solutions with magnesium concentrations less than 1.5 mEq/L.

hyponatremia Refers to solutions with sodium concentrations less than 137 mEq/L.

hypoosmolar State in which there is an abnormal gain in water or loss of sodium-rich fluids with replacement by water only. As a result, there is a low concentration of solutes in the body fluids.

hypophosphatemia Refers to a lower than normal range of serum phosphorus. Normal range of serum phosphorus is 2.5 to 4.5 mg/100 mL (1.7 to 2.6 mEq/L).

hypotension Condition characterized by a low blood pressure that is inadequate to perfuse and oxygenate body tissue.

hypotheses Predictions about the relationships between or among a research study's variables.

hypothermia Condition characterized by body temperature below 36° C (96.8° F).

hypothermia therapy Techniques used to reduce elevated body temperature.

hypotonic Having a smaller concentration of solute than another solution, hence exerting less osmotic pressure.

hypovolemic shock State of physical collapse caused by massive blood loss, circulatory dysfunction, and inadequate tissue perfusion.

hypoxemia Abnormal deficiency of oxygen in arterial blood.

hypoxia Insufficient oxygen available to meet the metabolic needs of tissues and cells.

idiosyncratic reaction A response to a medication or therapy that is unique to an individual.

ileal conduit A method of urinary diversion through intestinal tissue. Ureters are implanted in a section of dissected ileum that is then sewed to an ostomy in the abdominal wall.

ileostomy Surgical formation of an opening of the ileum onto the surface of the abdomen, through which fecal matter is emptied.

immobility Pertaining to the inability of a body part or limb to be moved.

immunocompromised A state of defective or failed immune response that makes a person more likely to acquire an infection.

impaction Presence of large or hard fecal mass in the rectum or colon.

implanted subcutaneous port A central venous catheter with a reservoir surgically placed under the skin that may remain in place for a prolonged period to obtain blood samples and administer medications.

incentive spirometer Individual patient device used to encourage full lung expansion. Reduces the risk for atelectasis in the immobilized or postoperative patient.

incentive spirometry Method of deep breathing providing visual feedback to patients concerning their inspiratory volume.

Incident Command System (ICS) A "first-on-scene" structure in which the first responder to a scene has charge of the scene until the incident has been declared resolved; a superior-ranking responder arrives on scene and seizes command.

incident report Confidential document that describes any patient accident while the person is on the premises of a health care agency.

incompatibility Describes two medications of different chemical makeup that cannot be mixed together.

incontinence Inability to control urination or defecation.

incontinent diversion A urinary diversion that does not give a patient the ability to control when urine exits the stoma, requiring the use of an external ostomy pouch.

incubation period Period between exposure to a pathogenic organism and the appearance of symptoms. A patient is often contagious during this time and capable of spreading disease without realizing it.

induration Hardening of a tissue, particularly the skin.

infection The invasion and reproduction of microorganisms in a body tissue that can result in a local or systemic clinical response such as cellulitis or fever.

infiltration Presence of intravenous fluids within the subcutaneous space surrounding a venipuncture site.

informed consent Permission obtained from a patient to perform a specific test or procedure.

infusate Volume of parenteral fluid infused into a patient over an established period of time.

infusion Introduction of a fluid such as a drug, electrolyte, or nutrient directly into a vein by means of gravity flow.

infusion pump Device designed to deliver a measured amount of fluid over a period of time.

injection Act of forcing a liquid into the body by means of a syringe.

injection cap A rubber diaphragm covering a plastic cap. Permits needle insertion into a catheter or vial.

inspection A physical examination skill involving the examiner's looking at external and internal body parts for physical characteristics.

insulator A substance that conducts temperatures poorly used to protect skin and tissues from hot or cold therapies.

intake Measurement of the ingestion or infusion of liquids into the body, including all liquids and semiliquids, liquid medications, enteral tube feedings, intravenous therapy, blood components, and parenteral nutrition.

integument Skin and its appendages hair, nails, and sweat and sebaceous glands.

intercostal space (ICS) Space found between adjoining ribs.

internal rotation Rotation of a joint inward.

International Nursing Coalition for Mass Casualty Education (INCMCE) Now known as Nursing Emergency Preparedness Education Coalition (NEPEC); coordinated by Vanderbilt University School of Nursing. It was founded in response to recognition of the need for nurses to be more adequately prepared to respond to mass casualty events.

interviewing The process of conducting an organized, systematic conversation with a patient. Designed to gather information regarding a patient's level of health, response to care, or perception of symptoms or events.

intestinal obstruction Any obstruction that results in failure of the contents of the intestine to pass through the lumen of the bowel.

intraabdominal pressure Amount of tension within the abdominal cavity.

intracavitary Within a body cavity.

intracellular fluid Liquid within the cell membrane.

intraclavicular fossa Small pocket area or indentation just below the clavicle on both sides of the neck.

intradermal (ID) injection Form of injection in which a solution is introduced into the dermal skin layer.

intramuscular (IM) injection Form of injection in which a solution is introduced into the body of a muscle.

intrapleural Pertaining to, or affecting, the potential space between the parietal and visceral pleurae.

intrapulmonic Pertaining to, or affecting, the spaces within the lungs.

intraspinal Referring to both the epidural and intrathecal routes of medication administration.

intrathecal Of or pertaining to a structure, process, or substance within a sheath, as within the spinal canal.

intravenous conscious sedation (IVCS) The intravenous administration of pharmacological agents to provide a minimally depressed level of consciousness to provide comfort during diagnostic or treatment procedures.

intravenous (IV) injection Form of injection in which a solution is introduced into a vein.

introitus An entrance or orifice into a cavity.

intubation Passage of a tube into a body aperture.

invasive Referring to procedures that involve puncture, incision, or insertion of a foreign object into the body.

invasive procedure A procedure in which the normal protective barrier of the skin or mucous membrane is broken or compromised (e.g., an intravenous puncture or a bladder catheterization).

inversion Turning something upside down.

irrigate To flush with a fluid, usually with a slow, steady pressure on a syringe plunger. Done to cleanse a wound or clear tubing.

irrigation Gentle washing of an area with a stream of solution.

ischemia A decreased supply of oxygenated blood to a body organ or part.

isolation Infection control and prevention methods such as barrier technique that are used to decrease the transmission of microorganisms.

isometric contraction Increased muscle tension without muscle shortening.

isometric exercise The tightening or tensing of muscles without moving body parts.

isotonic A solution with a total electrolyte content of approximately 310 mEq/L.

isotonic solution Having the same concentration of solute as another solution, hence exerting the same amount of osmotic pressure as the solution.

IV plug A small rubber or plastic cap that connects to the open end of a patient's IV access catheter. Also referred to as injection cap because a needle can be inserted into the rubber cap for the administration or aspiration of fluids.

jacket restraints Vestlike restraints that usually cross on the back of a patient but may also cross on the front.

Jackson-Pratt drain A closed drain system.

jejunostomy feeding tube A hollow tube inserted into the jejunum through the abdominal wall for administration of liquefied foods.

joint Any one of the connections between bones.

karaya A natural gum product that softens with body heat and conforms to the contours around the stoma.

Kardex Trade name for card filing system that allows quick reference to the particular need of the patient for certain aspects of nursing care.

keloid An overgrowth of scar tissue at the site of skin injury, such as a wound or surgical incision.

ketone An organic chemical compound with two compounds attached to it.

kilogram The metric conversion for a pound; weight (pounds) ÷ 2.2 = kilograms.

kinesthetic Related to the ability to perceive the existence or direction of weight or movement.

laryngospasm Spasm of the muscles surrounding the larynx causing airway narrowing and stridorous breathing.

lateral flexion A range of joint motion exercise during which the head is tilted as far as possible toward each shoulder, maintains neck mobility.

latex allergy reaction Allergic response to products containing latex (e.g., gloves, medical devices). Can present as contact dermatitis, allergic rhinitis, or immediate life-threatening reactions leading to urticaria, bronchospasm, edema, etc.

lavage The irrigation or washing out of an organ or cavity.

let-down reflex A normal reflex in a lactating woman often elicited by tactile stimulation of the nipple, resulting in release of milk from the glands of the breast.

leukopenia A decrease in circulating white blood cells.

leverage Occurs when specific bones, such as the humerus, ulna, and radius, and the associated joints, such as the elbow joint, act together as a lever.

line of gravity An imaginary line that goes from the center of gravity to the base of support.

lipid emulsion A soybean oil.

lipodystrophy Any abnormality in metabolism and deposition of fat.

logrolling Maneuver used to turn a reclining patient from one side to the other or completely over without flexing the spinal column.

loss Absence of a significant other, object, or state of health to which the person must adapt through the grieving process.

lotion Liquid preparation applied externally to protect the skin or treat a dermatological disorder.

lumen The hollow channel within a tube.

lunula A semilunar structure, such as the crescent-shaped pale area at the base of the nail of a finger or toe.

macerate To soften, usually by soaking in water.

maceration Skin that becomes abnormally soft and breaks down because of prolonged exposure to moisture.

maculopapular Discolored elevated lesions on the skin.

malabsorption Impaired absorption of nutrients from the gastrointestinal tract.

malignant hyperthermia An autosomal dominant trait characterized by often fatal hyperthermia with rigidity of the muscles occurring in affected people exposed to certain anesthetic agents.

malnutrition Any disorder of nutrition.

manmade disaster A catastrophic event whose principal direct cause is attributable to human action.

manometer An instrument for measuring pressure or tension of liquids or gases.

manual defibrillator Device used by trained personnel to treat fast, irregular dysrhythmias with electrical shock to the heart.

mass casualty disaster/event/incident (MCI) Any event or situation that results in multiple casualties and/or deaths; an MCI exists when health care needs exceed health care resources.

mass casualty triage Move, Assess, Sort, and Send (MASS) approach to triage initially sorts victims into groups, which are then evaluated for transportation to treatment.

massage A form of cutaneous stimulation that involves the application of touch and movement to muscles, tendons, and ligaments.

mastication Chewing, tearing, or grinding food with the teeth while it mixes with saliva.

material safety data sheet (MSDS) A form containing data about the properties of the particular chemical and information for handling the substance in a safe manner (e.g., storage, disposal, protective equipment, and spill-handling procedures).

maturational loss A loss expressed as any change in a person's developmental process that is normally expected during a lifetime.

meatus Any opening or tunnel through any part of the body (e.g., the point at which the urethra opens to the skin).

mediastinal shift A condition in which the mediastinal contents move toward the unaffected side in the presence of a pneumothorax, hemothorax, or hemopneumothorax. The mediastinal shift causes compression of the organs and is a life-threatening situation.

medical asepsis The techniques used to reduce and prevent the spread of microorganisms (clean technique).

medical disaster A catastrophic event that results in human casualties that overwhelm the available health care resources.

medicated enema Administration of a medication via an enema. Usually used preoperatively with patients scheduled for bowel surgery.

medication administration record (MAR) The report that serves as a legal record of the medications administered to a patient at a facility by a nurse or other health care professional.

medication dependence Two types of medication dependence exist psychological (or addiction) and physical. In psychological dependence a patient desires the medication for some benefit other than the intended effect. The individual believes a desirable effect will result when taking the medication. Physical dependence involves a physiological adaptation to a medication that manifests itself by intense physical disturbance when the medication is withdrawn.

medication plateau Blood serum concentration reached and maintained after repeated, fixed doses.

medication tolerance Decreased physiological response after repeated administration of a medication or a chemically related substance.

medullary Of or pertaining to the medulla of the brain.

melanin Black or dark brown pigment that occurs naturally in the skin, hair, and iris.

melanocyte A body cell capable of producing melanin, the pigment of the skin.

melena Darkening of the feces by blood pigments.

metastasis Process by which tumor cells are spread to distant parts of the body.

metered-dose inhaler (MDI) A device designed to deliver a measured dose of an inhalation drug.

microorganisms Any microscopic entity capable of sustaining living processes, such as bacteria, virus, fungi, only some of which typically cause human disease.

microvasculature The portion of the circulatory system composed of the capillary network.

micturition Urination; act of passing or expelling urine voluntarily through the urethra.

midarm circumference (MAC) A measurement of the circumference of the upper arm used to estimate muscle mass.

midstream collection Procedure in which a patient initiates a stream of urine, inserts a sterile collection cup into the stream, and then withdraws the cup before the stream of urine stops.

milliequivalent per liter (mEq/L) Number of grams of a specific electrolyte dissolved in 1 L of plasma.

Minerva jacket Cast encasing the head (with face and ears exposed), continuing over the thorax and back to the iliac crests.

minimal sedation Lightest level of sedation; includes local and topical anesthetics and peripheral nerve blocks.

mitten restraints Thumbless mitten devices used to restrain a patient's hands.

mobility The amount and quality of physical activity.

moderate sedation A drug-induced depression of consciousness during which patients respond purposefully to verbal commands, either alone or accompanied by light tactile stimulation.

Modified Ramsay Sedation Scale A numeric rating scale used to evaluate patient's level of sedation.

moleskin Adhesive-backed tape used for some forms of skin traction.

morgue A unit of a hospital with facilities for the storage and autopsy of the dead.

mucociliary transport Process in which cilia lining the tracheobronchial tree sweep mucus upward toward the esophagus to keep airways clear of inhaled particulate.

mucopurulent Characteristic of a combination of mucus and pus.

mummy restraints Blanket or sheet folded in such a manner as to restrain a small child or infant.

mutual aid agreement Reciprocal agreement to provide help between two or more agencies.

mydriasis Dilation of the pupil of the eye caused by contraction of dilator muscles of the iris.

mydriatics Ophthalmic preparations that stimulate the sympathetic nerve fibers or block parasympathetic nerve fibers of the eye, temporarily paralyzing the iris sphincter muscle.

myelosuppression A decrease in the cellular components of the bone marrow.

nares The pairs of anterior and posterior openings in the nose that allow for passage of air to the pharynx and lungs.

nasal Of or pertaining to the nose and nasal cavity.

nasal cannula Device for delivering oxygen by way of two small tubes that are inserted into the nares.

nasogastric (NG) feeding tube A small tube that is passed via the nares into the stomach.

nasointestinal (NI) feeding tube Tungsten-weighted tube inserted through the naris to allow natural peristaltic movement of the tube through the pyloric sphincter into the duodenum or jejunum.

National Dysphagia Diet Released in October 2002, the National Dysphagia Diet provides recommendations for uniformity of dysphagia diets for all health care facilities. Solid and liquid diets are separated into four levels.

natural/environmental disaster A catastrophic event that results from an ecological event that exceeds the capacity of the community.

nebulization Vaporization or dispersion of a liquid in a fine spray.

nebulizer Device used to distribute medication throughout nasal passages and tracheobronchial airway by vaporizing the medication.

necrosis Localized tissue death.

necrotic Related to death of a portion of tissue.

negative pressure Pressure, measured in millimeters of Mercury (mm Hg), that is less than atmospheric pressure.

negative pressure ventilation Therapy used for patients with primary neuromuscular illnesses that interfere with normal respiratory muscle function. The patient is fitted with a poncho or shell that is connected to the ventilator. Air is removed from between the patient's chest wall and the interior wall of the poncho or shell, causing the patient to inhale.

negative pressure wound therapy The application of pressure less than the ambient atmospheric pressure (as in a vacuum) to a wound, to draw wound edges together, remove exudates and excess moisture, and promote healing.

negligence Omission of care.

neovascular assessment Series of eight observations required to measure neurological and circulatory status of a patient's peripheral tissue.

neovascularization The process by which the vascular network in a wound is generated. This can also be called angiogenesis.

neurological Pertaining to the study and treatment of the nervous system.

neuropathy An abnormal condition characterized by inflammation and degeneration of the peripheral nerves.

neurovascular assessment Series of eight observations (assessments) required to measure neurological and circulatory status of a patient's peripheral tissues.

neutropenia An abnormal decrease in the number of neutrophils in the blood.

neutropenic Having an abnormal decrease in the number of neutrophils, white blood cells, in the blood.

nitroglycerin Medication that causes dilation of coronary arteries.

noncontinent (incontinent) ostomy/diversion Results from a surgical procedure that leaves a patient with an external stoma through which either stool or urine drains. It is noncontinent/incontinent because the effluent drains spontaneously from the stoma and the patient must continuously wear an external ostomy pouch over the stoma.

noncoring Huber needle A specially designed needle (straight or a 90-degree needle) intended for use with a vascular access device. This needle permits penetration into the chamber of the vascular access device without causing damage and thus permits repeated administration of medication directly into a patient's bloodstream.

noninvasive ventilation (NIV) Noninvasive ventilation (NIV) maintains positive airway pressure and improves alveolar ventilation without the need for an artificial airway. In addition, this mechanical ventilator alternative reduces and reverses atelectasis, improves oxygenation, reduces pulmonary edema, and improves cardiac function.

nonopioids Analgesics that do not contain opioids.

nonpharmacological aids Interventions used to prevent illness and promote health without the use of or in addition to the use of medications.

nontunneled percutaneous central venous catheters

noxious Harmful, injurious, or detrimental to health.

NPO Nothing to be taken or given by mouth.

nuclear event The release of radiation by a device in an explosive manner as a result of a nuclear chain reaction.

nutritional risk The potential to become malnourished because of factors that are primary (e.g., inadequate intake) or secondary (e.g., disease).

nutritional screening The systematic process of identifying risk factors related to nutritional problems and malnutrition.

nutritional support nursing The care of individuals with potential or known nutrition alterations. The goal is to assist individuals in restoring and maintaining optimal nutritional health.

objective data Data obtained by an observer (nurse) through direct physical examination, including observation, palpation, and auscultation, and by laboratory analyses and radiological and other studies.

obstipation The absolute inability to pass stool.

obturator Small dull-pointed introducer inserted in outer cannula that facilitates insertion of tracheostomy tube by gradually widening or dilating stoma to width of tracheostomy tube.

occlusive dressing A dressing that prevents air from reaching a wound or lesion and retains moisture, heat, body fluids, and medication.

occult blood Blood that appears from a nonspecific source, with obscure signs and symptoms. May be detected by means of a chemical test or microscopic examination.

ocular Of or pertaining to the eye.

oil-retention enema An enema containing a small volume of an oil-based solution; used to soften fecal mass.

ointment A semisolid externally applied preparation, usually containing a drug.

olfaction The sense of smell.

oncology A branch of medicine regarding the study of tumors.

onset of medication action Period of time after a drug is administered for it to produce a response.

opening pressure The amount of tension measured in a manometer following insertion of a spinal needle into the subarachnoid space.

ophthalmic Of or pertaining to the eye.

opioids Pertaining to natural and synthetic chemicals that have opium-like effects although they are not derived from opium.

opposition The relation between the thumb and the other digits of the hand for the purpose of grasping objects between the thumb and fingers. This maneuver is used during range-of-joint-motion exercises to maintain grasping ability of a patient.

oral airway Minimally flexible curved piece of plastic extending from the exterior of the lips over the tongue to the pharynx.

Organ Procurement Agency (OPA) Community-based agency whose focus is to obtain donated organs for transplantation.

organ/tissue donation Families and significant others are offered the option of organ and/or tissue donation. This process includes, but is not limited to, the donation of heart, lung, kidneys, liver, corneal tissue, and bone.

orientation phase Period in the nurse-patient relationship when a nurse and patient first meet and set the tone for the rest of their relationship, assessing the patient's situation and setting goals.

orthopedics Branch of medicine devoted to the study and treatment of the skeletal system, its joints, muscles, and associated structures.

orthopnea An abnormal condition in which a person must sit or stand to breathe deeply or comfortably.

orthostatic hypotension A drop in blood pressure of 15 mm Hg or more when an individual rises from a sitting to a standing position.

orthotopic neobladder A type of continent urinary diversion that uses an ileal pouch to replace the bladder. The ileal pouch is the same anatomical position as the bladder. The patient uses pelvic muscle exercises and bladder training exercises to achieve urinary continence.

osteoblastic Physiological activity that leads to the formation of specific bone tissue, osteoblasts.

osteoblasts Osteoblasts synthesize the collagen and glycoproteins to form the matrix for bone formation.

osteoclastic Physiological activity producing osteoclast bone cells that function in the development and periods of bone growth and repair, such as the breakdown and resorption of osseous tissue.

ostomy A surgical procedure in which the elimination of stool or urine is re-routed from the usual exiting part of the patient. Instead, the stool or urine exits the body through a surgically created opening called a stoma.

otic Of or pertaining to the ear.

otitis media Inflammation or infection of the middle ear, a common childhood affliction.

ototoxic Having a harmful effect on the eighth cranial nerve or the organs of hearing and balance.

outer cannula Main portion of tracheostomy tube through which patient breathes that stays in place at all times. The pilot balloon and faceplate are connected to the outer cannula.

output Includes all liquids excreted, such as urine, vomitus, and diarrhea, and drainage from wounds, fistulas, and suction equipment.

overdose Oral or parenteral ingestion of an excessive quantity of a medication or drug.

over-the-counter (OTC) medication Drug available to a consumer without a prescription.

over-the-needle catheter (ONC) A type of angiocatheter. The needle used for peripheral IV access is encased in a catheter made of Teflon, plastic, or another flexible material. After the needle pierces the skin, the catheter is threaded into a vein and the needle is withdrawn. The catheter remains in the vein for the instillation of fluid.

oximetry Procedure used to measure amount of oxygenated hemoglobin.

oxygen mask A flexible mask that fits snugly and securely over a patient's nose and mouth for delivery of oxygen.

oxygen saturation Amount of hemoglobin that is fully saturated with oxygen expressed as percentage of total available hemoglobin.

oxygen therapy Administration of oxygen by any route to a patient to prevent or relieve hypoxia.

oxygen toxicity Administration of oxygen level greater than 50% for greater than 24 hours resulting in increased permeability of the alveolar wall, alveolar-capillary leakage, noncardiogenic pulmonary edema, decreased lung compliance, and respiratory failure.

pain Subjective, unpleasant sensation caused by noxious stimulation of sensory nerve endings.

pain intensity The degree or extent of pain perceived by an individual.

pain rating scales Graphic or numeric representations that allow patients to quantify their pain experience.

pain threshold The amount of pain stimulus required to produce a physical or psychological response.

pain tolerance Point at which a person is not willing to accept pain of greater severity or duration.

palliative care The prevention, relief, reduction, or soothing of symptoms of disease or disorders without effecting a cure.

pallor Unnatural paleness or absence of color in the skin.

palpation A technique used in physical examination in which the examiner feels the texture, size, consistency, and location of certain parts of the body with the hands.

palpebra Portion of the conjunctiva that lines the inner surface of the eyelids; it is thick, opaque, and highly vascular.

pandemic Occurring throughout the population of a country, a people, or the world.

paralysis An abnormal condition characterized by loss of muscle function or the loss of sensation.

paralytic ileus A decrease in or absence of intestinal peristalsis that may occur after abdominal surgery, illness, or trauma.

paraphrasing Transforming a patient's words into the nurse's words, keeping the meaning intact.

parenteral Not in or through the digestive system.

parenteral nutrition (PN) The administration of nutrition into the vascular system.

paresis Slight or partial paralysis related in some cases to local neuritis.

parietal pleura The pleural membrane that lines the thoracic cavity.

passive range-of-motion exercises Exercises of the joints performed for an individual by someone else.

patency Absence of obstruction such as clots within an intravenous needle or kinks within intravenous tubing; the state of being open and unblocked.

pathogen Microorganism capable of producing disease.

pathogenic microorganisms Those capable of producing an infection or disease.

Patient Care Partnership, The A list of patient's rights promulgated by the American Hospital Association; it offers some guidance and protection to patients by stating the responsibilities that a hospital and its staff have toward patients and families during hospitalization; it is not a legally binding document.

patient care profile (PCP) A report that is automatically updated each shift within a computerized medical record.

Patient Self-Determination Act Legislation that requires all Medicare and Medicaid recipient hospitals to provide patients with information on advance directives and their right to accept or reject medical treatment.

patient-controlled analgesia (PCA) Technique that allows patients to self-administer small, continuous doses of intravenous or subcutaneous opioids as they feel the need.

patient's rights The rights to which patients are entitled as recipients of medical care.

peak action Time it takes for a drug to reach its highest effective concentration.

peak airway pressure The highest amount of positive pressure needed to inflate the lung.

peak concentration The highest effective concentration of a drug in the serum.

Pearson attachment The support used under the leg in balanced-suspension skeletal traction.

pediculosis Infestation of the integument with blood-sucking lice.

peer reviewed Process by which experts in a field evaluate an article or report for the quality of its scholarship, relevance to its field, and appropriateness for publication in which it may appear. Only those articles judged to meet the highest standards will be published.

PEH Acronym for pseudoepitheliomatous hyperplasia; maceration of skin surrounding the stoma.

pelvic belt Girdle-shaped cotton belt or support that fits around the hips, lumbosacral area, and abdomen for attaching ropes and weights in pelvic belt traction.

pelvic sling A hammocklike sling that fits under a patient's lumbosacral area and hips and is then connected to ropes and weights; it suspends the pelvis off the bed as treatment for fractures of pelvic bones.

Penrose drain An open drain system.

perceived loss Any loss that is tangible and uniquely defined by the grieving patient. It may be less obvious to others.

percussion A technique in physical examination used to assess the size, borders, and consistency of some of the internal organs and to discover the presence and to evaluate the amount of fluid in a cavity of the body.

percutaneous Performed through the skin, such as a biopsy or the aspiration of fluid from a space below the skin using a needle, catheter, and syringe.

percutaneous coronary intervention (PCI) Procedures such as percutaneous transluminal coronary angioplasty (PTCA) or directional coronary atherectomy (DCA) performed during cardiac catheterization.

perfusion Effect of pulmonary circulation in moving blood to and from the blood-gas barrier so gas exchange can occur.

periodontal Referring to tissues surrounding the teeth, such as the gums and buccal mucosa.

periodontitis Receding gum lines, inflammation, gaps between teeth.

perioperative Related to the entire surgical experience.

peripherally inserted central catheter (PICC) A peripherally inserted catheter that extends to the superior vena cava or right atrium.

peristomal Referring to the area of skin surrounding a surgically created stoma.

peritoneal fluid Substance in the abdominal cavity for lubrication of peritoneal membrane and internal organs.

peritonitis Inflammation of peritoneum produced by bacteria or irritating substances introduced into the abdominal cavity by a penetrating wound or perforation of an organ in the gastrointestinal or reproductive tract.

PERRLA Acronym for pupils equal, round, reactive to light, and accommodation; the acronym is recorded in the physical examination if pupil assessment is normal.

petaling Finishing the raw or ragged edges of a plaster cast to prevent skin irritation or pressure.

pétrissage A massage technique in which the skin is gently lifted and squeezed.

pharmacokinetics The study of how medications enter the body, reach their site of action, are metabolized, and exit the body.

pharmacological agents Oral, parenteral, or topical substances used to alleviate symptoms and treat or control illness.

pharynx The throat.

phlebitis Inflammation of a vein.

phlebitis solution A hypertonic solution capable of causing inflammation of a vein.

phlebothrombosis Blood clot formation.

phlebotomy The incision of a vein for the letting of blood, as in collecting blood from a donor.

physical dependence A physiological state in which abrupt cessation of a drug results in a withdrawal syndrome.

physical restraint Any device, garment, material, or object that restricts a person's freedom of movement or access to one's body.

PICO A format approach for organizing a clinical question into four components; patient population, Intervention or area of interest, Comparison of interest, and Outcome.

PIE An acronym for problem, intervention, and evaluation, used as an organizing framework for narrative nurses' notes.

piggyback infusion Method for administering intravenous (IV) medications intermittently; a piggyback IV set is a supplementary set that connects with the primary IV tubing.

piloerection Erection of hair due to the action of the arrectores pilorum muscles, the smooth muscles attached to the hair follicles; commonly referred to as goose bumps.

plantar flexion Flexion of the foot and toes toward the sole.

plaque (dental) A thin film on teeth made up of mucin and colloidal material found in saliva and often secondarily invaded by bacteria.

plateau Blood serum concentration reached and maintained after repeated, fixed doses of a drug.

pleura Delicate serous membrane enclosing the lung.

pleural cavity Space between visceral and parietal pleurae; pressure within the cavity is negative when compared with atmospheric pressure.

pleural fluid Substance contained between visceral and parietal pleurae for lubrication of the membranes.

pneumonitis Inflammation of the lung; may be caused by a virus or may be a hypersensitivity reaction that occurs as a result of allergy to chemical or organic dusts.

pneumothorax An accumulation of air in the intrapleural space caused by a severe blow to the chest, extremely forceful cough, chest trauma, or open chest surgery.

podiatrist A health care professional trained to diagnose and treat diseases and disorders of the feet.

point of maximal impulse (PMI) Point at which the heartbeat can most easily be palpated through the chest wall, usually along the left midclavicular line at the fourth or fifth intercostal space.

point-of-care test Performing laboratory tests at the primary care setting, such as the bedside (e.g., glucose monitoring or assay of whole blood, plasma, or serum).

polypharmacy Concurrent prescription, administration, or use of multiple medications, some of which may not be indicated clinically.

POMR An acronym for problem-oriented medical record, used as an organizing framework for a patient's complete medical record.

positive end expiratory pressure (PEEP) The application of positive airway pressure at the end of exhalation through a ventilator or breathing device.

positive pressure Pressure, measured in millimeters of mercury (mm Hg), that is greater than atmospheric pressure.

positive-pressure ventilation Mechanical ventilation that delivers compressed gas to the airways at greater than ambient pressure.

postanesthesia care unit (PACU) Postsurgical recovery area where patients are closely monitored and stabilized before discharge to a specific nursing unit or in the case of same day surgery, to home.

postcast care Nursing interventions performed for and with patients in casts or after cast removal.

postmortem care Care provided to the body after death.

postoperative Period of time after completion of a surgical procedure wherein a nurse monitors a patient's recovery.

postural Position of body, usually refers to change of position from supine to sitting, sitting to standing.

postural drainage Gravitational clearance of airway secretions by assumption of one or more of 10 different body positions for 5 to 15 minutes each; each posture corresponds to specific segments of bronchi in the lung.

postural hypotension Condition in which a normotensive person becomes light-headed or dizzy and experiences low blood pressure when rising to an upright position.

posture Position of the body in relation to the surrounding space.

prealbumin A plasma protein with a half-life of only 2 days, used as a marker of nutritional status.

precordial Of or pertaining to the precordium, which forms the region over the heart and the lower part of the thorax.

preemptive analgesia A method of preventing pain while reducing opioid use.

premature ventricular contraction (PVC) A cardiac dysrhythmia characterized by a ventricular contraction preceding the expected contraction; it appears on an electrocardiogram as an early, wide QRS complex without a preceding P wave.

preoperative The period of time preceding induction of anesthesia and the beginning of a surgical procedure.

preoperative checklist Agency-specific list of guidelines for ensuring completion of nursing interventions. This list includes items to be assessed or verified, for example, verification that preoperative orders are written and completed, laboratory work is in the patient's medical record, the patient has voided, current vital signs are documented.

presbycusis Loss of hearing sensitivity and speech intelligibility, associated with aging.

presbyopia Farsightedness resulting from a loss of elasticity of the lens of the eye. The condition commonly develops with advancing age.

pressure dressing A temporary treatment for the control of excessive bleeding; pressure dressings require elastic bandages to maintain the pressure and may also require the application of sandbags adjacent to the dressing to augment pressure.

pressure ulcer A lesion that develops in the skin as a result of prolonged, unrelieved pressure.

primary dressing A dressing that comes in direct contact with the wound bed.

primary intention Primary union of the edges of a wound, progressing to complete scar formation with granulation.

prn "As needed." Administration times are determined by the patient's needs.

problem-oriented medical record (POMR) Method of recording data about the health status of a patient that fosters a collaborative problem-solving approach by all members of the health care team.

procedural sedation An anesthetic procedure in which analgesia and anesthesia are accomplished without loss of consciousness.

pronation Movement of a body part so the front or ventral surface faces downward.

proprioceptive function Sensation that is achieved through stimuli originating from within the body regarding spatial position and muscular activity.

prosthesis An artificial replacement for a missing part of the body.

pruritus The symptom of itching.

pseudoaddiction Exhibition of drug-seeking behaviors though the true driving factor is pain relief not physical addiction.

Pseudomonas A genus of gram-negative bacteria that includes several free-living species of soil and water and some opportunistic pathogens, isolated from wounds and sputum; may produce blue and yellow pigments.

pulleys Mechanical round, grooved disks over which ropes can move freely for traction pull.

pulmonary aspiration The entry of secretions or foreign material into the trachea and lungs.

pulmonary edema Accumulation of extracellular fluid in a patient's lung tissue and alveoli, commonly caused by left-sided heart failure, fluid overload.

pulse deficit Condition characterized by difference between apical pulse rate and peripheral pulse rate that results in a lack of peripheral perfusion.

pyrexia Fever. An elevation of the body temperature above the normal range.

pyrogen Any substance or agent that tends to cause a rise in body temperature, such as some bacterial toxins.

quality assurance In health care, any evaluation of services provided and of the results achieved as compared with accepted standards.

radial flexion A range-of-motion exercise during which there is a bending of the wrist medially toward the thumb; maintains wrist mobility.

radiopaque Not permitting the passage of x-rays or other radiant energy. Bones are relatively radiopaque and therefore show as white areas on an exposed x-ray film.

random voided specimen A urine specimen obtained at any point of a 24-hour period.

reactive hyperemia The return of blood to an area of tissue upon the release of externally applied pressure.

reagent Chemical used to indicate the presence of a particular substance.

reduction The alignment of fracture fragments through manipulation. Closed reduction is accomplished through manual manipulation and casting or traction.

reflecting A cognitive strategy that involves reappraisal of one's actions to evaluate outcomes. A communication strategy used to clarify what a patient is feeling and to affirm that the patient's feelings are acceptable.

refractive error Condition in which parallel rays of light are not brought to focus on the retina.

registered dietitian (RD) A health care professional who has successfully completed an examination and maintains continuing education requirements in nutritional care for individuals and groups.

registered nurse first assistant (RNFA) A nurse with advanced education who assists the surgeon with surgical procedures, performing a combination of nursing and medical functions.

reinfusion device An apparatus that is placed, usually intraoperatively during orthopedic or vascular procedures, into a space where significant blood loss is anticipated. This device collects the blood, filters it, and is then used to reinfuse that blood intravascularly.

relaxation A cognitive strategy that provides mental and physical pain relief or reduces pain.

reminiscing A form of therapy for older adults that provides a life review. Individual talks about remote memories, expression of related feelings, and recognition of positive experiences, as well as conflicts.

remission The partial or complete disappearance of the clinical and subjective characteristics of a chronic or malignant disease.

renal insufficiency Partial kidney failure characterized by less than normal urinary excretion and abnormal urinary laboratory results (e.g., creatinine, blood urea nitrogen level).

residual urine The volume of urine in the bladder after a normal voiding.

residual volume The amount of fluid that pools in the stomach or intestine that is able to be aspirated from a gastric or intestinal tube at any given time.

resistive isometric exercise Contracting of muscles while pushing against a stationary object or resisting the movement of an object.

respiratory arrest Cessation of respirations.

respiratory distress Difficulty breathing that may be associated with abnormal blood oxygen or carbon dioxide levels and may require supportive measures to preserve life.

respite care Provision of short-term relief or time off for people providing home care to an ill, disabled, or frail older adult.

restating A communication strategy involving the reiteration of a patient's verbal statements and/or questions using similar words; this affirms that the message was acknowledged by the nurse.

restating The process of verbally clarifying information provided by a patient or family.

restraint Device used to immobilize a patient or an extremity.

reverse Trendelenburg's position Position in which the lower extremities are low and the body and head are elevated on an inclined plane.

right atrial catheter An indwelling intravenous catheter inserted centrally or peripherally and threaded into the superior vena cava or right atrium.

rigidity Condition of hardness, stiffness, or inflexibility.

rigor mortis The rigid stiffening of skeletal and cardiac muscle shortly after death.

risk assessment tool for pressure ulcers Evaluation protocols for assessing the likelihood for the development of pressure ulcers; two such protocols are the Braden Scale and the Norton Scale, which assess the following five risk factors physical condition, mental state, activity, mobility, and incontinence.

rooting reflex A normal response in newborns when the cheek is touched or stroked along the side of the mouth to turn the head toward the stimulated side and begin to suck.

rotation A basic range of joint motion allowed by various joints the rotation of a bone around its central axis, such as shoulder rotation.

Rotokinetic bed A special bed equipped with an automatic turning device that completely immobilizes patients while rotating them from 90 to 270 degrees along a horizontal axis.

S₁ Symbol for the first heart sound in the cardiac cycle occurring with ventricular systole; it is associated with the closure of the mitral and tricuspid valves.

S₂ Symbol for the second heart sound in the cardiac cycle; it is associated with closure of the aortic and pulmonary valves just before ventricular diastole.

saline lock See heparin lock.

SBAR Stands for Situation-Background-Assessment-Recommendation technique that provides a framework for communication among a patient's health care team.

sclerosis Condition characterized by hardening of tissue resulting from any of several causes, including inflammation, the deposit of mineral salts, and infiltration of connective tissue cells.

scrub nurse Surgical nurse whose primary responsibility is to provide the surgeon with instruments and supplies during surgery, which requires strict surgical asepsis. In addition, this nurse along with the circulating nurse disposes of soiled sponges and accounts for sponges, needles, and instruments on the surgical field.

scrubbed team members Includes the surgeon and scrub nurse or technician and assisting physicians who are scrubbed.

sebaceous gland One of the small glands in the dermis that secretes an oily substance (sebum) on the skin's surface and in the hair.

seborrheic dermatitis A common and chronic inflammatory skin disease characterized by dry or moist greasy scales and yellow crusts.

sebum Oily secretion of the sebaceous glands of the skin. When combined with sweat, sebum forms a moist, oily, acidic film that is antibacterial and antifungal and protects the skin against drying.

secondary dressing A dressing used to cover or hold primary dressings in place.

secondary intention Wound closure in which the edges are separated, granulation tissue develops to fill the gap, and, finally, epithelium grows in over the granulation, producing a larger scar than results with primary intention.

secretion A product produced by a gland of the body.

seizure A hyperexcitation of neurons in the brain leading to a sudden, violent, involuntary series of muscle contractions that may be paroxysmal and episodic, as in a seizure disorder, or transient and acute, as after a head injury.

seizure precautions Measures that protect a patient from injury during a seizure.

self-catheterization The ability of individuals to insert a urinary catheter into their urinary meatus.

semi-Fowler's position Placement of patient in an inclined position, with the upper half of the body raised by elevating the head of the bed approximately 30 to 45 degrees.

sensitivity Laboratory test used in conjunction with culture; it measures the response of microorganisms to antibiotics that have been placed on a culture plate.

sentinel event An incident that involves serious physical or psychological injury or death or the risk thereof.

sepsis Infection, contamination.

serology Branch of medicine dealing with serum and blood products.

serum half-life The time it takes for the excretion process to lower the serum medication concentration by half.

shaking Physiotherapy technique in which a concurrent, compressive force is supplied to the chest wall.

sharps container A puncture-proof container that is used for the disposal of any used sharp items such as needles, disposable scissors, and scalpels.

shear An applied force or pressure exerted against the surface and layers of the skin as tissues slide in opposite but parallel planes.

shearing Pressure exerted against the surface and layers of the skin as tissues slide underneath the body as it moves against a surface.

shearing force An applied force or pressure exerted against the surface and layers of the skin as tissues slide in opposite but parallel planes.

sheet wadding Stretchable sheets of cotton padding used to cover skin before a cast is applied.

shelter-in-place To take refuge in a small interior room with no or few windows.

side effect An effect caused by a drug that is different from the therapeutic (desired) action; the effect may be harmless or injurious.

sigmoid colon The part of the large intestine that extends from the descending colon to the rectum.

sign Objective finding perceived by an examiner, such as a fever, rash, abnormal reflex, or abnormal breath sound.

silicone septum Silicone partition that covers the port chamber housed in the metal or plastic body of the implanted infusion port.

situational loss Loss due to any sudden, unpredictable external event.

sitz bath Special bath in which only the hips and buttocks are immersed in fluid.

skin barrier An artificial layer of skin, made of plastic or vinyl-like material, applied to skin before application of tape or ostomy drainage bags. Protects skin from chronic irritation.

sling Device used to support or limit movement, enhance circulation, and prevent edema of the arm, hand, or wrist.

slough Necrotic (dead) tissue in the process of separating from viable portions of the body.

smart pump Infusion devices, referred to as a "smart pump" by the Institute for Safe Medication Practices (ISMP), are commercially available infusion systems that perform a "test of reasonableness" to check that programming is within preestablished institutional limits before infusion can begin.

SOAP Acronym for *subjective, objective, assessment,* and *plan,* the four parts of the written account of a patient's health problem in a problem-oriented record.

SOAPIE See SOAP—Alternative acronym includes intervention and evaluation.

solute A substance dissolved in a solution.

solute solution Solutes are dissolved particles and are either electrolytes or nonelectrolytes. Solute solution refers to these particles when they are found in body fluids or plasma (i.e., solution).

solution A mixture of one or more substances dissolved in another substance.

spasm Involuntary muscle contraction.

speculum A retractor used to separate the walls of a cavity (e.g., the vaginal cavity).

sphygmomanometer Device used for noninvasive measurement of arterial blood pressure consisting of cuff, air bladder, inflation bulb, and gauge to indicate amount of air pressure being exerted.

spica cast An orthopedic cast applied to immobilize part or all of the trunk of the body and part or all of one or more extremities.

splinting Supporting the abdominal area to reduce pain caused by coughing or sneezing after surgery.

sponge Gauze dressing used to absorb blood in a surgical wound.

spore An inactive but viable state of microorganisms.

spreader bar A metal bar with curved hoop areas for attaching hooks or pins for traction.

sputum Lung mucus; normally thin, watery, and white or clear and watery.

standard precautions Techniques used to reduce the risk for the transmission of blood-borne pathogens or microorganisms present in moist body substances regardless of a patient's diagnosis or infection status.

standardized care plan Documentation that uses the nursing process format in specifying the plan of care for patient problems.

staples Stainless steel wire used to close a surgical wound.

stent A straw or tubelike device that is placed through the stoma into bowel to keep open the flow of effluent.

sterile Free from all life forms, including spores.

sterile conscience One's personal principles and morals that guide one to maintain strict asepsis and sterile techniques at all times.

sterile field A specified area, such as within a tray or a sterile drape, that is considered free from microorganisms.

sterilization Process by which microorganisms, including spores, are killed.

stockinette Stretchable cotton materials of various sizes and widths used immediately over the skin to protect tissues from the irritation of felt or plaster.

stoma Surgically created opening between a body cavity and the body's surface, such as a colostomy.

stomatitis Any inflammatory condition of the mouth.

stopcock A valve that controls the flow of fluid or air through a tube.

strategic national stockpile (SNS) A national repository of the Centers for Disease Control and Prevention for antibiotics, chemical antidotes, antitoxins, life-support medications, intravenous administration supplies, airway maintenance supplies, and medical/surgical items.

strike through Source of contamination by which moisture permeates a sterile field or barrier.

stroke volume (SV) The volume of blood ejected from the left ventricle with each ventricular contraction.

subarachnoid space Situated or occurring between the arachnoid and the pia mater membranes, which cover the brain and spinal cord.

subcutaneous emphysema The presence of free air or gas in the subcutaneous tissues.

subcutaneous injection Form of injection in which a solution is introduced into subcutaneous tissues.

subcutaneous tunnel A tunnel under the skin between the exit site of a catheter and the entrance into a body cavity (such as the epidural space) or vein.

subjective data Data collected from a patient.

sublingual Route for administering a drug beneath the tongue.

sublingual medication Medication placed under the tongue and allowed to dissolve.

suction The act of sucking up a substance by reducing air pressure over its surface.

suction catheter Thin plastic or rubber tubing used to remove secretions.

summarization Reworking a lengthy interaction or discussion into a few brief sentences.

summarizing A process in which an interviewer organizes and condenses information provided and verifies with the patient that the information is correctly interpreted.

summation Occurs when the combined effect of two drugs produces a result that equals the sum of the individual effects of each drug.

supination Movement of a body part so the front or ventral surface faces upward.

suppository A solid form of medication inserted into a body cavity (e.g., the rectum or vagina). The drug is absorbed after it dissolves in the cavity.

surgical asepsis Practices or techniques designed to render and maintain objects and areas free from pathogenic microorganisms. Also referred to as sterile techniques.

surgical scrub Process of removing as many microorganisms as possible from the hands and arms by mechanical washing and chemical antisepsis.

suspension A liquid in which small particles of a solid are dispersed, but not dissolved, and in which the dispersal is maintained by stirring or shaking the mixture.

sympathomimetic A pharmacological agent that mimics the effects of stimulation of organs and structures by the sympathetic nervous system.

synergistic reaction An undesired reaction that occurs when one drug potentiates the effect of another.

systemic Of or pertaining to the whole body rather than to a localized area.

systolic pressure The higher blood pressure measurement; reflects pressure within the arterial system during the period of ventricular contraction (systole).

T tube A T-shaped device that is attached to an endotracheal or tracheostomy tube for delivery of humidified air.

tachycardia An abnormality in heart rate in which the myocardium contracts regularly, but at a rate over 100 beats per minute.

tachypnea Condition characterized by respiratory rate greater than 20 breaths per minute.

tandem setup An infusion mini-bag and tubing inserted into an injection port farthest away from a patient; used for administration of a prepared intravenous admixture.

tartar A hard, gritty deposit that collects on the teeth.

technological disaster A catastrophic event in which people, property, community infrastructure, and economic welfare are adversely affected by the disruption of technology (e.g., industrial accidents and unplanned release of nuclear waste).

TENS (transcutaneous electrical nerve stimulation) A mild electrical stimulation that interferes with the transmission of painful stimuli.

tension pneumothorax A life-threatening situation caused by a rupture in the pleura, resulting in an increase in the amount of air in the pleural space and an increase in pressure, leading to the collapse of the lung.

tepid Moderately warm to the touch.

termination phase The period in the nurse-patient relationship when a nurse and patient examine and evaluate their relationship and its goals and results; the time when they deal with the emotional content involved in saying good-bye.

tertiary intention Wound healing that occurs when surgical wounds are not closed immediately, but left open for 3 to 5 days to allow edema or infection to diminish.

The Joint Commission A private, nongovernmental agency that establishes guidelines for the operation of health care facilities. The guidelines are the basis of accreditation, generally required for Medicare reimbursement. Formerly known as The Joint Commission on Accreditation of Healthcare Organizations.

therapeutic Treatments or interventions implemented to prevent illness and/or promote health.

therapeutic effect The intended or desired physiological response of a medication.

therapeutic silence The use of silence that encourages verbal description and reflection; avoidance of premature verbal communication that may be due to a nurse's anxiety.

thermoregulation Ability to control temperature within acceptable range.

third party payer An insurance plan, health maintenance organization (HMO), or preferred provider organization (PPO) that reimburses for health care services.

Thomas splint A long splint with a half or full ring at one end; covered with towels and lined with felt or other soft material, it is used to suspend the thigh in skeletal traction.

thrill A fine vibration felt by an examiner's hand on the body of a patient over the site of an aneurysm or on the precordium.

thrombocytopenia A decrease in circulating platelets.

thrombophlebitis Inflammation of a vein, often accompanied by formation of a clot.

thrombosis An abnormal vascular condition in which thrombus develops within a blood vessel of the body.

thrombus Accumulation of platelets, fibrin, clotting factors, and the cellular elements of the blood attached to the interior wall of a vein or artery, sometimes occluding the lumen of the vessel.

tidal volume Amount, in milliliters, of air inhaled with each breath. Spontaneous tidal volume is 5 to 10 mL/kg body weight.

tidaling A normal gentle rocking of fluid in a chest tube water-seal system or in the diagnostic indicator of waterless units. Indicates that the system is functioning properly.

timed collection The collection of a substance such as urine or stool for a specific period of time.

tinnitus Ringing heard in one or both ears.

tissue ischemia Decreased blood supply to body tissues.

TLC 1. Abbreviation for total lung capacity. 2. Informal abbreviation for tender loving care.

tolerance A phenomenon by which the body becomes increasingly resistant to a drug or other substance through continued exposure to the substance.

tongue-thrust reflex An immature form of swallowing in which the tongue is projected forward instead of retracted during swallowing.

topical Of or pertaining to a drug or treatment applied to the surface of a body part.

topical agents Pertaining to drugs or treatments applied to the surface part of the body.

toxic effects Severe and progressive negative effects of drugs.

tracheobronchial tree Anatomical divisions of the respiratory tract, including the combination of trachea, bifurcations into the right and left mainstem bronchi, and subsequent bifurcations into smaller bronchi and bronchioles.

tracheostomy Opening through the neck into the trachea with an indwelling tube inserted; created surgically to produce an airway.

tracheostomy collar Curved oxygen delivery device with an adjustable neck strap that fits around the tracheostomy.

traction Force or pull applied to limbs, bones, or other tissues to pull the tissues apart, often for realignment.

traction boot A foam rubber boot shaped to fit a forearm or leg, used for a type of skin traction.

transdermal Refers to a form of medication that is applied to the skin's surface and is absorbed across the dermal or outer skin layer.

transfusion reaction Systemic response by the body to the administration of blood incompatible with that of the recipient.

transfusion-related acute lung injury (TRALI) A serious blood transfusion complication characterized by the acute onset of noncardiogenic pulmonary edema after transfusion of blood product.

transmission-based precautions Techniques used to prevent the transmission of microorganisms from patients documented or suspected to be infected with highly transmissible pathogens for which additional precautions are needed beyond standard precautions. The three types are airborne, droplet, and contact precautions.

transtracheal oxygen therapy (TTOT) A method of administering oxygen to a patient by establishing a low-flow catheter route directly in the trachea.

Trendelenburg's position Position in which the head is low and the body and legs are elevated.

triage Establishing priorities of patient care for urgent treatment based on the seriousness of injuries and likelihood for survival; used in an emergency situation to maximize effectiveness of available resources.

trocar A sharp, pointed rod that fits inside a tube; used to pierce the skin and the wall of a cavity or canal in the body to aspirate fluids, to instill a medication or solution, or to guide the placement of a soft catheter.

trough concentration The point at which the lowest amount of drug is detected in the serum.

tuberculosis A chronic granulomatous infection caused by an acid-fast bacillus, *Mycobacterium tuberculosis*, generally transmitted by the inhalation or ingestion of infected droplets and usually affecting the lungs.

tunneled central venous catheters A catheter surgically inserted into a vein in the neck or chest and passed under the skin. Only the end of the catheter is brought through the skin; medications can be administered through this end of the catheter.

turning sheet Bed sheet folded in half, placed under a patient between shoulders and below the hips. Used by health care providers to lift, turn, and position a patient. Also called a lift sheet.

tympanic Pertaining to a structure that resonates when struck; drumlike.

ulnar flexion A range-of-motion exercise during which there is a lateral bending of the wrist toward the fifth finger; maintains wrist mobility.

undermining Condition of a wound in which the loss of underlying tissues is greater than the loss of the skin.

unit-dose system System of drug distribution in which a portable cart containing a drawer for each patient's medications is prepared by the pharmacy with a 24-hour supply of medications.

unscrubbed team members In surgical setting, includes the anesthesiologist or anesthetist and the circulating nurse, who wear surgical attire but are not gowned or gloved.

upper airway respiratory system All respiratory structures above the epiglottis, including nose, sinuses, mouth, and pharynx.

urethral meatus The opening to the canal for the discharge of urine.

urethral sphincter Voluntary muscle at the neck of the bladder that relaxes to allow micturition.

urgency The need to void immediately.

urinal Plastic or metal receptacle for urine.

urinary retention Inability to empty the bladder, resulting from a number of possible causes.

urinary stent A thin catheter threaded into segments of the ureter that carry urine, produced by the kidney, either down into the bladder internally or to an external collection system.

urinary tract infection Greater than normal level of pathogens in the urinary tract.

urine Fluid secreted by the kidneys, transported by the ureters, stored in the bladder, and voided through the urethra.

urine specific gravity Measurement of the degree of concentration of the urine.

urinometer Device used for determining specific gravity of urine.

urosepsis Systemic bacterial infection frequently resulting from a bacterial infection in the urine (bacteriuria). Bacteriuria leads to the spread of organisms into the kidney, which can lead to bacteremia or urosepsis.

urostomy The diversion of urine away from a diseased or defective bladder through a surgically created opening, or stoma, in the skin.

Vacutainer tube A glass tube with a rubber stopper; air has been removed to create a vacuum.

valgus An abnormal position in which a part of a limb is bent or twisted outward, away from the midline, such as the heel of the foot.

Valsalva maneuver Any forced expiratory effort against a closed airway, as when an individual holds the breath and tightens the muscles in a concerted, strenuous effort to move a heavy object or to change position in a bed.

variable A concept, characteristic, or trait that changes (e.g., takes on measurably different values) within an identified population in a research study.

variance Positive or negative changes in patient progress toward expected outcomes on a critical pathway. Deviations from the critical path plan most often used in the case management model of delivering health care.

varices Tortuous, dilated veins.

varus An abnormal position in which a part of a limb is turned inward toward the midline, such as the heel and foot.

vascular access device (VAD) An indwelling catheter, cannula, or other instrumentation used to obtain venous or arterial access.

vasoconstriction Narrowing of the lumen of any blood vessel, especially the arterioles and the veins in the blood reservoirs of the skin and abdominal viscera.

vasodilation An increase in the diameter of a blood vessel caused by inhibition of its vasoconstrictor nerves or stimulation of dilator nerves.

vein lumen Central opening through which blood flows in a vein.

vellus Soft, fine hair covering all parts of the body except the palms, soles, and areas where other types of hair are normally found.

venipuncture Technique in which a vein is punctured transcutaneously by a sharp rigid stylet (such as a butterfly needle), a cannula (such as an angiocatheter that contains a flexible plastic catheter), or a needle attached to a syringe.

venous thromboembolism (VTE) Terminology used to describe a condition that involves deep vein thrombosis and pulmonary embolus.

venous thrombosis A condition characterized by the presence of a clot in a vein in which the wall of the vessel is not inflamed.

ventilation Respiratory process by which gases are moved into and out of the lungs.

ventral Of or pertaining to an anterior position, toward the abdomen.

verbal order A physician's or nurse practitioner's order for a medication or other therapy that is spoken to the nurse to be entered into a patient's medical records.

vertigo A sensation of faintness or an inability to maintain normal balance in a standing or seated position, sometimes associated with giddiness, mental confusion, nausea, and weakness.

vesicant A drug capable of causing tissue necrosis when extravasated.

vial Glass container with a metal-enclosed rubber seal.

vibration Physiotherapy technique performed by contracting all the muscles in the caregiver's upper extremities to cause vibration while applying pressure to the chest wall.

viscera The internal organs enclosed within a body cavity, primarily the abdominal organs.

visceral pleura A serous membrane lining both lungs.

visceral protein status The amount of protein that pertains to the internal organs (e.g., abdominal).

vital signs Physiological parameters that reflect key body processes; refers to temperature, blood pressure, heart rate, respiratory rate, and oxygen saturation.

void The process of emptying the bladder of urine; urinate; micturate.

volume-control set (Volutrol) Used to administer hourly fluids and intermittent intravenous medications, usually to children. A fluid chamber holds 100 to 150 mL of fluid to be infused over a specific period.

walking heel Plastic or rubber heel placed in the sole of a leg cast to allow weight bearing.

wandering Meandering, aimless, or repetitive locomotion that exposes the individual to harm and is frequently incongruent with boundaries, limits, or obstacles.

weapons of mass destruction (WMD) Weapons that can kill large numbers of humans and/or cause great damage to structures (e.g., buildings), natural structures (e.g., mountains), or the biosphere.

weight Force exerted on a body by the gravity of the earth.

weight holder A metal, T-shaped bar that holds weights for traction.

weights Filled bags or metal disks of varying poundage used for traction.

whispered pectoriloquy The transmission of a whisper through the pulmonary structures so that it is heard as normal audible speech on auscultation.

windowing Cutting a small area of a cast to permit inspection of the tissues below.

working phase The period in the nurse-patient relationship when the focus is on communication strategies, interventions for problem resolution, and enhancement of self-concept.

wound vacuum-assisted closure (V.A.C.) A type of therapy that speeds wound healing by applying localized negative pressure to draw the edges of a wound together.

xerostomia Dryness of the mouth caused by the cessation of normal salivary secretions. It is a common symptom of a number of diseases such as diabetes, acute infections, and Sjögren's syndrome and is a common adverse reaction to drugs.

Yankauer suction A large filter-tipped rigid plastic suction catheter used mainly in the mouth or other large body cavity.

Zassi Bowel Management System An intrarectal catheter used to manage diarrhea. Catheter diverts feces while at the same time providing a means to administer medications.

Z-track method Method for injecting irritating medications into muscle without tracking residual medication through sensitive tissues.

Index

A

Abbreviations, medication errors and, 515, 516*t*

ABCD mnemonic
  for code management, 728
    primary survey, 732-735
    secondary survey, 735-737
  for melanoma, 114, 121*b*
  in nutritional assessment, 803

Abdomen
  abdominal muscle isometric exercises and, 238
  movement during inspiration and expiration, 85*f*
  quadrants of, 151
  washing of, 430

Abdominal aorta, 148*f*

Abdominal assessment, 151-155
  female patient and, 149-150, 155
  general survey in, 148-149
  indirect percussion in, 110*f*
  male patient and, 150, 155
  nursing diagnoses in, 150
  teaching considerations in, 156-157

Abdominal binder, 1034*t*, 1034-1037

Abdominal brace, 290

Abdominal distention, 152-153

Abdominal girth measurement, 152

Abdominal muscle isometric exercises, 238

Abdominal pain
  common causes of, 147*t*
  constipation and, 906

Abdominal paracentesis, 1176-1182, 1177-1178*t*, 1178*f*

Abdominal thrusts, 731*t*

Abducens nerve assessment, 162

Abduction in range-of-motion exercises, 231*t*
  fingers and, 234*t*
  hip and, 235*t*
  shoulder and, 232*t*
  thumb and, 234*t*
  toes and, 236*t*

Abduction pillow, 290, 290*f*

ABGs; *See* Arterial blood gases

ABO incompatibility, 786-787

ABO system, 786, 787*t*

Abrasion, 423*t*
  dry dressing for, 1005

Absorption dressing, 1017-1021, 1018*f*

Absorption of medication, 509*t*, 510
  older adult and, 523*t*

Abuse signs in general survey, 116

Acapella device, 656, 664, 664*f*

Accident prevention, 1058

Accidental decannulation, 694

Accu-Check III, 1153

Acetic acid for packing wound, 1005

Acetone, urine, 1127, 1127*f*

Achilles tendon pressure ulcer site, 465*f*

Acid-fast bacilli smear, sputum specimen for, 1139

Acidemia, 629

Acne, 423*t*

Acoustic stethoscope, 80*f*

Active-assisted range-of-motion exercises, 229-230, 232-236*t*

Active listening, 31*b*

Active range of motion, 161

Active range-of-motion exercises, 229-230, 231-236*t*

Active warming, 1041

Activities of daily living
  cognitive deficit and, 1068
  home care safety and, 1065
  incorporating range-of-motion exercises into, 231*t*

Activity apron, 332*f*

Actual body weight, 812, 814

Actual loss, 406

Acute care, pressure ulcer risk and, 474*t*

Acute eczematous rash, 423*t*

Acute hemolytic transfusion reaction, 788*t*, 797

Acute pain, 371, 372

Addiction, 371, 372*b*, 511

Addison's disease, 166

Additives to intravenous solutions, 742

Adduction in range-of-motion exercises, 231*t*
  fingers and, 234*t*
  hip and, 235*t*
  shoulder and, 232*t*
  thumb and, 234*t*
  toes and, 236*t*

Adhesive-backed medicated disk, 529

Adhesive membrane dressing, 1002*t*

Administration of medications, 515-520
  genetic and cultural factors in, 524
  isolation precautions and, 181-182
  nursing process in, 522-524
  preoperative, 945
  right documentation in, 520
  right dose in, 518*f*, 518-519
  right medication in, 515-518, 516*t*, 517*f*
  right patient in, 519, 519*f*
  right route in, 519
  right time in, 519-520
  routes in, 512, 512*t*, 513*t*

Admission of patient, 12*b*, 12-18
  admitting clerk or secretary role in, 12, 13*b*, 14*b*
  nurse role in, 14, 14*f*

Adolescent
  equipment for intubation and suctioning of, 675*t*
  health assessment of, 112-113
  heart rate and pulse of, 81
  insertion of indwelling urinary catheter and, 875

Adrenal gland, 148*f*

Adult cardiopulmonary resuscitation, 731*t*

Advance directive, 12, 14*b*, 404, 722

Advanced cardiovascular life support, 721

Adventitious breath sounds, 131, 133*t*

Adverse drug effects, 510-511, 511*f*, 511*t*
  medication errors and, 507
  patients at increased risk for, 510*b*

Aerobic culture of wound drainage, 1144

Aerosol medication, 508*t*

Aerosolized medication spray, 543-544

African-American version of Oucher Pain Scale, 376

Age
  fluid imbalances and, 745
  influence on apical pulse rate, 81
  influence on blood pressure, 92
  influence on body temperature, 69
  oral airway guidelines for size by, 723*t*
  pressure ulcer risk and, 471

Aging
  skin changes with, 120
  wound healing problems and, 1006

Agnosia, 1068

Air bubbles
  in infusion tubing, 747, 763
  in syringe, 583, 584, 585

Air embolism
  central parenteral nutrition-related, 850*t*
  central vascular access device-related, 782*t*

Air-fluidized bed, 298*t*, 305, 310*f*, 310-313

Air leak
  in chest tube, 713*t*
  in inflating cuff of endotracheal or tracheostomy tube, 697

Air mattress, 301, 305

Air mattress overlay, 302, 302*f*, 305

Air splint, 290

Air-suspension bed, 307*f*, 307-310

Airborne precautions, 179*b*, 184*t*

Airway management, 668-698
  airway suctioning and, 673-682
    after postural drainage, 656
    artificial airway and, 679-680
    assessment before, 675-676
    closed suction catheter and, 682
    endotracheal tube and, 674
    equipment for, 674, 674*f*, 675*t*
    home care considerations in, 681
    nasopharyngeal and nasotracheal, 673, 677-679

Index of Skills and Procedural Guidelines